SAUNDERS

COMPREHENSIVE REVIEW

for the NCLEX-PN® EXAMINATION

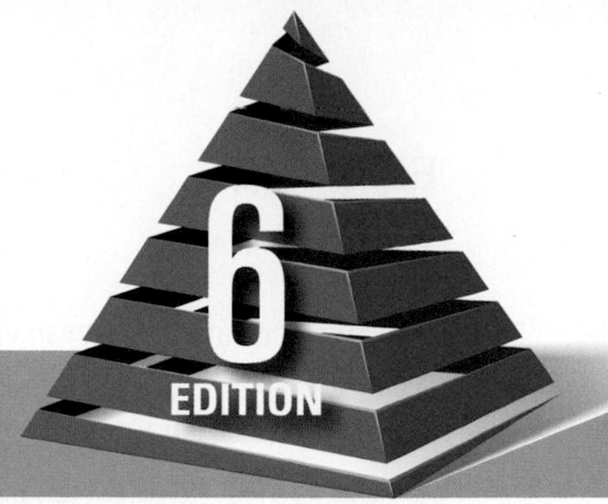

SAUNDERS

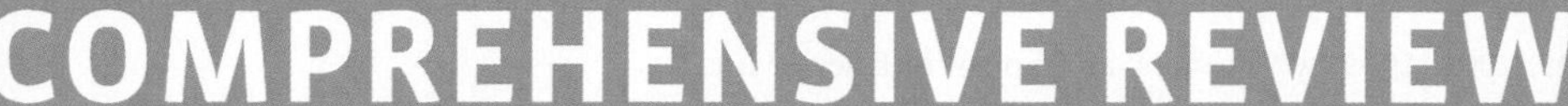

for the NCLEX-PN® EXAMINATION

LINDA ANNE SILVESTRI, PhD, RN

Instructor of Nursing
Salve Regina University
Newport, Rhode Island

President
Nursing Reviews, Inc.
Charlestown, Rhode Island
Professional Nursing Seminars, Inc.
Charlestown, Rhode Island
Nursing Reviews, Inc.
Las Vegas, Nevada

Elsevier Consultant
HESI NCLEX-RN® and NCLEX-PN® Live Review Courses

ELSEVIER

ELSEVIER

3251 Riverport Lane
St. Louis, Missouri 63043

SAUNDERS COMPREHENSIVE REVIEW FOR THE NCLEX-PN®
EXAMINATION, SIXTH EDITION ISBN: 978-0-323-28931-3

Notices

Knowledge and best practice in this field are constantly changing. As new research and experience broaden our understanding, changes in research methods, professional practices, or medical treatment may become necessary.

Practitioners and researchers must always rely on their own experience and knowledge in evaluating and using any information, methods, compounds, or experiments described herein. In using such information or methods they should be mindful of their own safety and the safety of others, including parties for whom they have a professional responsibility.

With respect to any drug or pharmaceutical products identified, readers are advised to check the most current information provided (i) on procedures featured or (ii) by the manufacturer of each product to be administered, to verify the recommended dose or formula, the method and duration of administration, and contraindications. It is the responsibility of practitioners, relying on their own experience and knowledge of their patients, to make diagnoses, to determine dosages and the best treatment for each individual patient, and to take all appropriate safety precautions.

To the fullest extent of the law, neither the Publisher nor the authors, contributors, or editors, assume any liability for any injury and/or damage to persons or property as a matter of products liability, negligence or otherwise, or from any use or operation of any methods, products, instructions, or ideas contained in the material herein.

Library of Congress Cataloging-in-Publication Data
Silvestri, Linda Anne, author.
Saunders comprehensive review for the NCLEX-PN examination/Linda Anne Silvestri. – 6 edition.
p. ; cm.
Comprehensive review for NCLEX-PN examination
Includes bibliographical references and index.
ISBN 978-0-323-28931-3 (pbk. : alk. paper)
I. Title. II. Title: Comprehensive review for NCLEX-PN examination.
[DNLM: 1. Nursing, Practical–Examination Questions. 2. Nursing Care–Examination Questions. WY 18.2]
RT62
610.73076–dc23 2014033430

Senior Content Strategist: Yvonne Alexopoulos
Content Development Manager: Laurie Gower
Content Development Specialist: Laura Goodrich
Marketing Manager: Danielle LeCompte
Publishing Services Manager: Jeff Patterson
Project Manager: Bill Drone
Designer: Margaret Reid

Printed in Canada
Last digit is the print number: 9 8 7 6 5 4 3 2 1

To my parents—
To my mother, **Frances Mary**,
and in loving memory of my father, **Arnold Lawrence**,
who taught me to always love, care, and be the best I could be.

To All Future Licensed Practical Nurses,

Congratulations to you!

You should be very proud and pleased with yourself on your most recent, well-deserved accomplishment of completing your nursing program to become a licensed practical nurse. I know that you have worked very hard to become successful and that you have proven to yourself that indeed you can achieve your goals.

In my opinion, you are about to enter the most wonderful and rewarding profession that exists. Your willingness, desire, and ability to assist those who need nursing care will bring great satisfaction to your life. In the profession of nursing, your learning will be a lifelong process. This aspect of the profession makes it stimulating and dynamic. Your learning process will continue to expand and grow as the profession continues to evolve. Your next very important endeavor will be the learning process involved to achieve success in your examination to become a licensed practical nurse.

I am excited and pleased to be able to provide you with the *Saunders Pyramid to Success* products, which will help you prepare for your next important professional goal: becoming a licensed practical nurse. I want to thank all of my former nursing students whom I have assisted in their studies for the NCLEX-PN exam for their willingness to offer ideas regarding their needs in preparing for licensure. Student ideas have certainly added a special uniqueness to all of the products available in the *Saunders Pyramid to Success*.

Saunders Pyramid to Success products provide you with everything you need to ready yourself for the NCLEX-PN exam. These products include material that is required for the NCLEX-PN exam for all nursing students regardless of educational background, specific strengths, areas in need of improvement, or clinical experience during the nursing program.

So let's get started and begin our journey through the *Saunders Pyramid to Success*, and welcome to the wonderful profession of nursing!

Sincerely,

Linda Anne Silvestri

Linda Anne Silvestri, PhD, RN

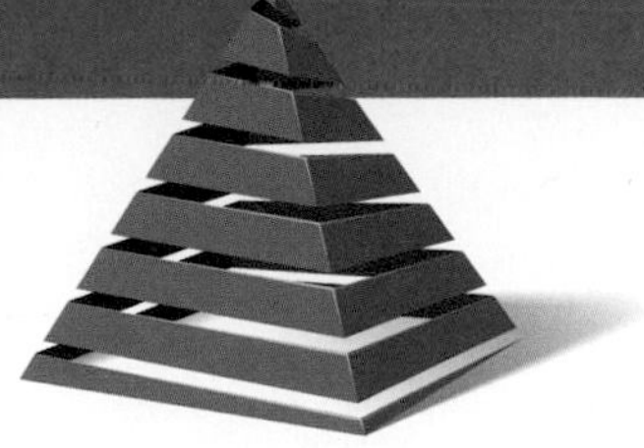

About the Author

Linda Anne Silvestri

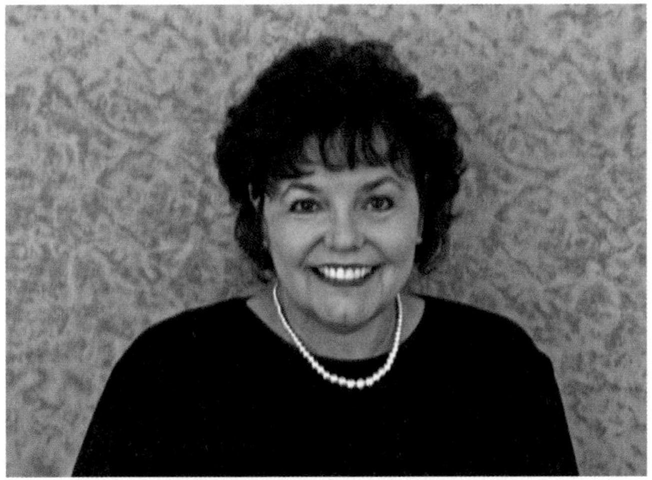

(Photo by Laurent W. Valliere.)

As a child, I always dreamed of becoming either a nurse or a teacher. Initially, I chose to become a nurse because I really wanted to help others, especially those who were ill. Then I realized that both of my dreams could come true: I could be both a nurse and a teacher. So I pursued my dreams.

I received my diploma in nursing at Cooley Dickinson Hospital School of Nursing in Northampton, Massachusetts. Afterward, I worked at Baystate Medical Center in Springfield, Massachusetts, where I cared for clients in acute medical-surgical units, the intensive care unit, the emergency department, pediatric units, and other acute care units. Later I received my associate degree from Holyoke Community College in Holyoke, Massachusetts; my BSN from American International College in Springfield, Massachusetts; and my MSN from Anna Maria College in Paxton, Massachusetts, with a dual major in nursing management and patient education. I received my PhD in nursing from the University of Nevada, Las Vegas (UNLV), and conducted research on self-efficacy and the predictors of NCLEX success. In 2012, I received the UNLV School of Nursing Alumna of the Year Award. I am also a member of the Honor Society of Nursing, Sigma Theta Tau International, Phi Kappa Phi, the Western Institute of Nursing, the Eastern Nursing Research Society, the Golden Key International Honour Society, the National League for Nursing, and the America Nurses Association.

As a native of Springfield, Massachusetts, I began my teaching career as an instructor of medical-surgical nursing and leadership-management nursing in 1981 at Baystate Medical Center School of Nursing. In 1989, I relocated to Rhode Island and began teaching advanced medical-surgical nursing and psychiatric nursing to RN and LPN students at the Community College of Rhode Island. While teaching there, a group of students approached me for assistance in preparing for the NCLEX examination. I have always had a very special interest in test success for nursing students because of my own personal experiences with testing. Taking tests was never easy for me, and as a student, I needed to find methods and strategies that would bring success. My own difficult experiences, desire, and dedication to assist nursing students to overcome the obstacles associated with testing inspired me to develop and write the many products that would foster success with testing. My experiences as a student, nursing educator, and item writer for the NCLEX exams aided me as I developed a comprehensive review course to prepare nursing graduates for the NCLEX examination.

In 1994, I began teaching medical-surgical nursing at Salve Regina University in Newport, Rhode Island, and I am currently there as an adjunct faculty member. I also prepare nursing students for the NCLEX examination at Salve Regina University.

I established Professional Nursing Seminars, Inc., in 1991 and Nursing Reviews, Inc., in 2000. These companies are located in Charlestown, Rhode Island. In 2012, I established an additional company, Nursing Reviews, Inc., in Las Vegas, Nevada. Both companies are dedicated to assisting students in their success with the NCLEX-RN and the NCLEX-PN examinations.

Today, I am the successful author of numerous review products. Also, I serve as an Elsevier consultant for HESI live reviews, the review courses for the NCLEX examination conducted throughout the country. I am so pleased that you have decided to join me on your journey to success in testing for nursing examinations and for the NCLEX examination!

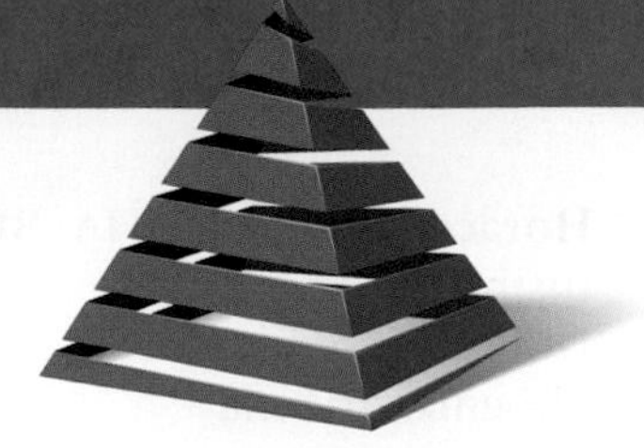

Contributors

Special Contributor

Mary Dowell, PhD, RN
Graduate Nursing Faculty
University of Phoenix
Phoenix, Arizona

Consultants

Dianne E. Fiorentino
Research Coordinator
Nursing Reviews, Inc.
Las Vegas, Nevada

James Guilbault, Jr., BS, PharmD
Clinical Pharmacist
Wilbraham, Massachusetts

Nicholas L. Silvestri, BA
Editorial and Communications Analyst
Nursing Reviews, Inc.
Las Vegas, Nevada

Angela Silvestri-Elmore, PhD, RN
Assistant Professor of Nursing
Touro University
Henderson, Nevada

Contributors

Kristen Bagby, RN, MSN
Staff Nurse
St. Louis Children's Hospital
St. Louis, Missouri

Keara Cobbs, LPN
Graduate
St. Charles Community College
St. Charles, Missouri

Marie du Toit, BSN, MSN
Assistant Professor
West Liberty University
West Liberty, West Virginia

Margie Francisco, EdD(c), MSN, RN
Nursing Professor
Illinois Valley Community College
Oglesby, Illinois

Marilyn L. Johnessee Greer, MS, RN
Associate Professor of Nursing
Rockford College
Rockford, Illinois

Joyce Hammer, RN, MSN
Adjunct Clinical Faculty
Monroe Country Community College
Monroe, Michigan

Terri Hood-Brown, MSN, RN
Assistant Professor, RN-to-BSN Coordinator
Ohio University
Athens, Ohio

Tiffany Jakubowski, BSN, RN
Adjunct Instructor
Front Range Community College
Longmont, Colorado

Tara McMillan-Queen, RN, MSN, ANP, GNP
Faculty II
Mercy School of Nursing
Charlotte, North Carolina

Heidi Monroe, MSN, RN-BC, CPAN, CAPA
Assistant Professor of Nursing
Bellin College
Green Bay, Wisconsin

Robin Moyers, PhD, RN-BC
Nursing Educator
Carl Vinson VA Medical Center
Dublin, Georgia

Terri Peterson, RN, BSN, MSNEd
Associate Professor
Program Coordinator, Practical Nursing/Nursing Assistant Programs
Bauder College
Atlanta, Georgia

Jennifer Ponto, RN, BSN
Faculty, Vocational Nursing Program
South Plains College
Levelland, Texas

Donna Russo, RN, MSN, CCRN
Nursing Instructor
Frankford Hospital School of Nursing
Philadelphia, Pennsylvania

Horace Smith, III MHA, BBA, LPN
Instructor
University of Phoenix
Phoenix, Arizona

Tiffany M. Smith, MSN/ED, BSN, RN
PhD Student
University of Nevada, Las Vegas
Las Vegas, Nevada

Russlyn A. St. John, RN, MSN
Professor, Practical Nursing
St. Charles Community College
Cottleville, Missouri

Claudia Stoffel, MSN, RN, CNE
Professor, Nursing
West Kentucky Community and Technical College
Paducah, Kentucky

Bethany Hawes Sykes, EdD RN, CEN, CCRN
Adjunct Faculty
Department of Nursing
Salve Regina University
Newport, Rhode Island

Laurent W. Valliere, BS, DD
Vice President of Nursing Reviews, Inc.
Professional Nursing Seminars, Inc.
Charlestown, Rhode Island

The author and publisher would also like to acknowledge the following individuals for contributions to the previous editions of this book:

Alicia M. Adams, MN, RN, CEN
Roosevelt, Utah

Katrina D. Allen, RN, MSN, CCRN
Chickasaw, Alabama

Sonya S. Beacham, MSN, RN
Wilmington, North Carolina

Carol Boswell, EdD, RN
Odessa, Texas

Sharen Brady, MSN, RN
Ogden, Utah

Joyce Campbell, RN, MSN, CCRN, FNP-C
Chattanooga, Tennessee

Brenda E. Caranicas, MS, RN
New Town, North Dakota

Brigitte L. Casteel, RN, BSN
Weber City, Virginia

Faith Chumchal Darilek, RN, MSN
Victoria, Texas

Jean DeCoffe, MSN, RN
Milton, Massachusetts

Stephanie A. Dupler
Lebanon, Pennsylvania

Mary Ann Hogan, MSN, RN, CS
Amherst, Massachusetts

Mary Joanne Hovey, MSN, RN
Wilmington, North Carolina

Lisa Ivers, BSN, RN
Hamilton, Ohio

Lula Johnson, MSN, RN
Detroit, Michigan

Misty D. Johnson, LPN
North Platte, Nebraska

Mary T. Kowalski, MSN, BA, RN
Ridgecrest, California

Nancy K. Maebius, PhD, RN
San Antonio, Texas

Barbara Magenheim, EdD, MSN, BSN, RN, CNE
Chandler, Arizona

Lois S. Marshall, PhD, RN
Miami, Florida

Beverly McNeese, RN
Baton Rouge, Louisiana

Jan H. Mearkle, MSN, RN, CSNP
Summit, Mississippi

Jo Ann Barnes Mullaney, PhD, RN, CS
Newport, Rhode Island

Victoria Oxendine, RN, MSN, FNPC
Wilmington, North Carolina

Joann E. Potts Peuterbaugh, MSN, RN
Alton, Illinois

Elizabeth Pratt, BSN, RNC
Magnolia, Arkansas

Bonnie L. Shipferling, PhD(c), MSN, BSBA, RN
Pasadena, Texas

Jennifer C. Spencer, RN, BSN
Wilmington, North Carolina

Louis M. Stackler, RN, BSN, MS
Tulsa, Oklahoma

Jacquelyn Stovall, RN, BSN
San Antonio, Texas

Ruth Chandley Threlkeld, MSN, BSN
Clark, Missouri

Julie Traynor, MS, RN
Devils Lake, North Dakota

Ann Leiphart Unholz, MS, RN
Highland Springs, Virginia

Paula A. Viau, PhD, RN
Kingston, Rhode Island

Margaret Wafstet, MN, RN
Missoula, Montana

Kim Webb, RN, MN
Tonkawa, Oklahoma

Mary Louise White, MSN, RN
University Center, Michigan

Patricia H. White, BSN, RNC
Wilmington, North Carolina

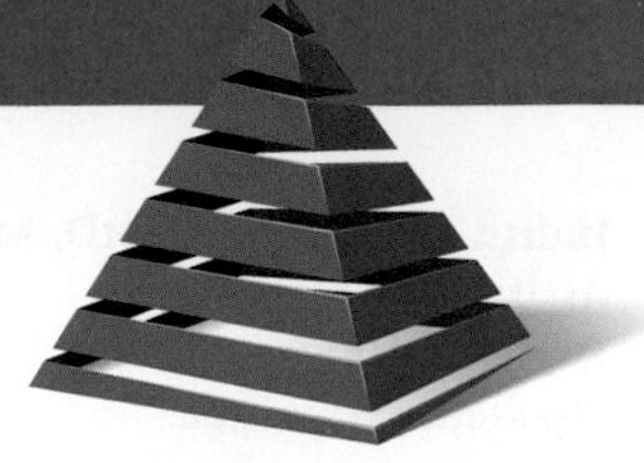

Reviewers

Carol Annesser, RN, MSN, BC, CNE
Assistant Professor, Nursing
Mercy College of Ohio
Toledo, Ohio

Dawn Baker, MSN, RN, WHNP-BC
Nursing Faculty
Oakland Community College
Bloomfield Hills, Michigan

Amanda Benz, RN, MSN
University of Saint Francis
Fort Wayne, Indiana

Sonya Blevins, DNP, RN, CMSRN, CNE
Assistant Professor of Nursing
University of South Carolina-Upstate
Greenville, South Carolina

Danese Boob, MSN/ED, RN-BC
Pennsylvania State University, Hershey and World Campus
Hershey, Pennsylvania

Collin Bowman-Woodall, MS, RN
Assistant Professor
Samuel Merritt University
San Mateo, California

Anna Brunch, RN, MSN
Nursing Professor
Illinois Valley Community College
Oglesby, Illinois

Jean Burt, MS, RN
Instructor, Nursing Program
Wilbur Wright College
Chicago, Illinois

Johnathan Carlos
Associate Professor
Southern California University of Health Sciences

Judy Carlyle, MNSC, RN
ARNEC
Nashville, Arkansas

Mary Carrico, MS Ed, RN
Professor of Nursing
West Kentucky Community and Technical College
Paducah, Kentucky

Judith Carrion, EdD, MSN/Ed, MSHS, BSN, RN-BC, CRRN, CNOR
Assistant Professor
Roseman University
Henderson, Nevada

Lori Catalano, JD, MSN, CCNS, PCCN
University of Cincinnati
Cincinnati, Ohio

Janie Corbitt, RN, MS
Retired, Instructor of Nursing

Michelle Cox, RN, MSN
Assistant Professor
Sinclair Nursing Department

Julie Darby, MSN, RN, CNE
Baptist College of Health Sciences
Memphis, Tennessee

Patricia Delmoe, RN, BSN, MN, MA
Boswell School of Nursing
Sun City, Arizona

Kathy Dillard, RN, BSN
Northwestern State University
Natchitoches, Louisiana

Sherry Donovan, MSN, RN-BC
Yakima, Washington

Christine Emch, MSN, RN
Mercy College of Ohio
Toledo, Ohio

Amber Essman, MSN, APRN, FNP-BC, CNE
Minute Clinic/Chamberlain College of Nursing
Grove City, Ohio/Columbus, Ohio

Mary Fabick, MSN, MEd, RN-BC, CEN
Associate Professor of Nursing
Milligan College
Milligan College, Tennessee

Donna Fabry, DNP
Clinical Assistant Professor
University at Buffalo, School of Nursing
Buffalo, New York

Abimbola Farinde, PharmD, MS
Clear Lake Regional Medical Center
Webster, Texas

Pamela B. Fouche, PhD
Senior Coordinator of Natural Science Online Course Delivery
Walters State Community College
Morristown, Tennessee

Margie Francisco, EdD, MSN, RN
Illinois Valley Community College
Oglesby, Illinois

Gwendolyn Gaston, MSN, RN
Dallas Nursing Institute
Dallas, Texas

Shari Gould, MSN, RN
Victoria College
Victoria, Texas

Mary Griffin, PhD, RN, CNE
Faculty, School of Nursing
Carolinas College of Health Sciences
Charlotte, North Carolina

Sheila Grossman, PhD, FNP-BC, APRN, FAAN
Fairfield University School of Nursing
Fairfield, Connecticut

Joyce Hammer, RN, MSN
Adjunct Clinical Faculty
Monroe Country Community College
Monroe, Michigan

Lilah Harper
Anderson Continuing Education

Jerry Harvey, MS, RN, BC
Assistant Professor of Nursing
Liberty University
Lynchburg, Virginia

Dorothy M. Hendrix, PhD, RHIT
East Los Angeles College
Monterey Park, California

Traci Hermann, RN, MSN, CNE
University of Cincinnati, Blue Ash College
Cincinnati, Ohio

Judith Hochberger, PhD, MS, RN
Assistant Professor
Roseman University of Health Sciences
Henderson, Nevada

Laura Hope, MSN, RN
Florence Darlington Technical College
Florence, South Carolina

Celeste Hughes, MSN, RN
Georgia Northwestern Technical College
Rome, Georgia

Renee Hyde, MSN, RN-BC
Faculty
Rowan Cabarrus Community College
Kannapolis, North Carolina

Katherine Kelly, RN, DNP, FNP-C
Assistant Professor, School of Nursing
California State University
Sacramento, California

Marci Langenkamp, MS, RN
Edison Community College
Piqua, Ohio

Cheryl Lehman, PhD, CNS-BC, RN-BC, CRRN
San Antonio, Texas

Sue McCann, MSN, RN, DNC
Advanced Practice Nurse, Clinical Research Coordinator
University of Pittsburgh Medical Center Presbyterian-Shadyside
Pittsburgh, Pennsylvania

Molly McClelland, PhD, RN, CMSRN, ACNS-BC
Associate Professor of Nursing
University of Detroit
Detroit, Michigan

Janie V. McCloskey, RN, MSN
Faculty
Carolinas College of Health Sciences
Charlotte, North Carolina

Nancy McManus, BSN, MEd, RN-BC, CGRS
Summa Health System Hospitals
Akron, Ohio

Tara McMillian Queen, RN, MSN, ANP, GNP
Faculty II
Mercy School of Nursing
Charlotte, North Carolina

Kathleen E. Meyer, DNP, CNE, APRN, ACHPN
Stafford Services, Inc.
Cleveland, Ohio

Helena Moissant, RN, MSN
Asante Rogue Regional Medical Center
Medford, Oregon

Ann Motycka, RN, MSN, CNE
Professor
Ivy Tech Community College
Evansville, Indiana

Robin Moyers, PhD, MSN, RN-BC
Nursing Educator
Carl Vinson VA Medical Center
Dublin, Georgia

Linda Nance, EdD, RN-BC, MSN, BSN, FNP
Professor of Nursing, Curriculum Development Facilitator
Scottsdale Community College
Scottsdale, Arizona

Lazette Nowicki, RN, MSN
Professor of Nursing
American River College
Sacramento, California

Becky Oglesby, DNP, RN

Terri Peterson, RN, BSN, MSNEd
Bauder College
Atlanta, Georgia

Heather Pollet, BSN, RN
Interim Nursing Director
Coffeyville Community College Nursing Program
Coffeyville, Kansas

Catherine Powers, MSN, FNP-BC
East Tennessee State University
Johnson City, Tennessee

Marty Richardson, RN, MS
Nursing Professor
Grayson College
Denison, Texas

Heather Roberts, RN, MSN
Faculty
Presbyterian School of Nursing
Queens University of Charlotte

Karen Robertson, MSN, MBA, PhD/ABD
Rock Valley College
Rockford, Illinois

Russlyn St. John, RN, BSN, MSNEd
Associate Professor, Program Coordinator
Practical Nursing/Nursing Assistant Programs
Bauder College
Atlanta, Georgia

Charlotte D. Strahm, DNSc, RN, CNS
Associate Professor
Colorado Mountain College
Glenwood Springs, Colorado

Serena Strain, RN, BSN, MSN
Nurse Faculty
Forsyth Technical Community College

Deema L. Tackett, MSN, RN, CNL
Assistant Professor of Nursing
Southern State Community College
Hillsboro, Ohio

Lisa Tardo-Green, MSN, RN
Faculty
Cabarrus College of Health Sciences
Concord, North Carolina

Lindsay Tucholski, MSN, RN
Assistant Professor
Cedarville University
Cedarville, Ohio

Tonya Turnage, MSN, RN
Nursing Faculty
Armstrong Atlantic State University
Savannah, Georgia

Amy Voris, DNP, AOCN, CNS
Assistant Professor of Nursing, Adjunct Clinical Faculty, and Clinical Site Coordinator
Cedarville University
Cedarville, Ohio

Donna Walker Hubbard, RN, MSN
Assistant Professor Retired
University of Mary Hardin Baylor
Belton, Texas

Donna Wilsker, MSN, RN
Dishman Department of Nursing
Lamar University
Beaumont, Texas

Karen Winsor, MSN, RN, ACNS-BC
Advanced Practice Nurse for Orthopedic Trauma
University Medical Center at Brackenridge
Austin, Texas

Tricia Winters, RRT, BBA
North Central State College
Mansfield, Ohio

Nancee Wozney, PhD, RN
Dean of Nursing and Allied Health
Southeast Technical Minnesota State College

Susan Yeager, MS, RN, CCRN, ACNP
Wexner Medical Center at The Ohio State University
Columbus, Ohio

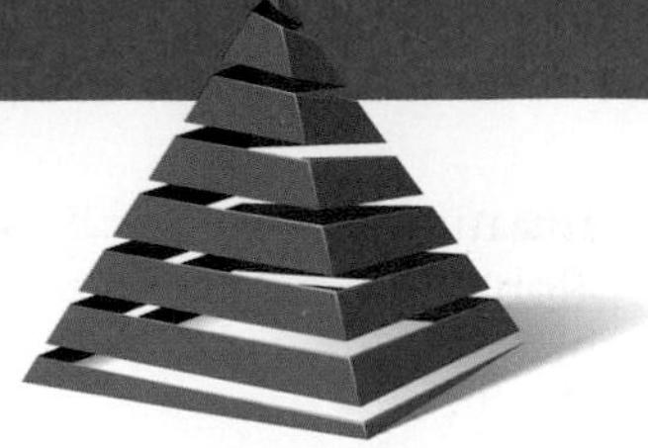

Preface

To laugh often and much, to appreciate beauty, to find the best in others, to leave the world a bit better, to know that even one life has breathed easier because you have lived, this is to have succeeded.

Ralph Waldo Emerson

Welcome to Saunders *Pyramid to Success!*

An Essential Resource for Test Success

Saunders Comprehensive Review for the NCLEX-PN® Examination is one in a series of products designed to assist you in achieving your goal of becoming a licensed practical nurse. This text provides you with a comprehensive review of all of the nursing content areas specifically related to the new 2014 test plan for the NCLEX-PN examination, which is implemented by the National Council of State Boards of Nursing. This resource will help you achieve success on your nursing examinations during nursing school and on the NCLEX-PN examination.

Organization

This book contains 20 units and 67 chapters. The chapters are designed to identify specific components of nursing content, and they contain practice questions, including a critical thinking question and both multiple-choice and alternate item formats that reflect the chapter content and the 2014 test plan for the NCLEX-PN exam. The final unit contains an 85-question Comprehensive Test.

The new test plan identifies a framework based on *Client Needs*. These Client Needs categories include Safe and Effective Care Environment, Health Promotion and Maintenance, Psychosocial Integrity, and Physiological Integrity. *Integrated Processes* are also identified as a component of the test plan. These include Caring, Communication and Documentation, Nursing Process, and Teaching and Learning. All the chapters address the components of the test plan framework.

Special Features of the Book

Pyramid Terms

Each unit begins with *Pyramid Terms* and their definitions. These *Pyramid Terms* are important to the discussion of the content in the chapters of the unit. Therefore, they are in bold blue type throughout the content section of each chapter.

Pyramid to Success

The *Pyramid to Success,* a feature part of the unit introduction, provides you with an overview, guidance, and direction regarding the focus of review in the particular content area, as well as the content areas of relative importance to the 2014 test plan for the NCLEX-PN exam. The *Pyramid to Success* reviews the Client Needs as they pertain to the content in that unit or chapter. These points identify the specific components to keep in mind as you review the chapter.

Pyramid Points

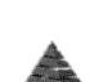

Pyramid Points are the little icons that are placed next to specific content throughout the chapters. The *Pyramid Points* highlight content that is important for preparing for the NCLEX-PN examination and identify content that typically appears on the NCLEX-PN examination.

Pyramid Alerts

Pyramid Alerts are the red text found throughout the chapters that alert you to important nursing information. These alerts identify content that typically appears on the NCLEX-PN examination.

Priority Nursing Actions

Numerous *Priority Nursing Actions* boxes have been placed throughout the chapters. These boxes present a clinical nursing situation and the priority actions to take in the event of its occurrence. A rationale is provided that explains the correct order of action, along with a reference for additional research.

Critical Thinking: What Should You Do? Questions

Each chapter contains a *Critical Thinking: What Should You Do?* question. These questions provide a brief clinical scenario related to the content of the chapter and ask you what you should do about the client situation presented. A narrative answer is provided along with a reference source for researching further information.

Special Features Found on Evolve

Pretest and Study Calendar

The accompanying Evolve site contains a 75-question pretest that provides you with feedback on your strengths and weaknesses. The results of your pretest will generate an individualized study calendar to guide you in your preparation for the NCLEX-PN examination.

Heart, Lung, and Bowel Sound Questions

The accompanying Evolve site contains *Audio Questions* representative of content addressed in the 2014 test plan for the NCLEX-PN exam. These questions are in NCLEX-style format, and each question presents an audio sound as a component of the question.

Video Questions

The accompanying Evolve site also contains new *Video Questions* representative of content addressed in the 2014 test plan for the NCLEX-PN exam. These questions are in NCLEX-style format, and each question presents a video clip as a component of the question.

Testlet Questions

The accompanying Evolve site contains testlet (case study) questions. These question types include a client scenario and several accompanying practice questions that relate to the content of the scenario.

Audio Review Summaries

The companion Evolve site includes three *Audio Review Summaries* that cover challenging subject areas under the 2014 NCLEX-PN test plan, including *Pharmacology, Acid-Base Balance,* and *Fluids and Electrolytes*.

Practice Questions

While preparing for the NCLEX-PN examination, it is crucial for students to practice taking test questions. This book contains 825 NCLEX-style multiple-choice and alternate item format questions. The accompanying software includes all the questions from the book, plus additional Evolve questions for a total of over 4500 questions.

Multiple-Choice and Alternate Item Format Questions

Starting with Unit II, each chapter is followed by a practice test. Each practice test contains several multiple-choice questions and an alternate item format question. The alternate item format questions at the end of the chapters and on the accompanying Evolve site may be presented as one of the following:

- Fill-in-the-blank question
- Multiple response question
- Prioritizing (ordered response) question, also known as a drag-and-drop question
- Figure/illustration question, also known as a hot spot question
- Graphic options question, in which each option contains a figure or illustration
- Chart/exhibit question
- Audio question that includes a heart, lung, or bowel sound
- Video question
- Testlet question

These questions provide you with practice in prioritizing, decision-making, and critical thinking skills.

Answer Section

The answer sections include the correct answer, rationale, test-taking strategy, question categories, and a reference. The structure for the answer section is unique and provides the following information:

- ***Rationale:*** The rationale provides you with the significant information regarding both correct and incorrect options.
- ***Test-Taking Strategy:*** The test-taking strategy provides a logical path for selecting the correct option and helps you to select an answer to a question on which you might have to guess. In each practice question, the specific strategy that will assist in answering the question correctly is highlighted in bold **blue** type. Specific suggestions for review are identified in the test-taking strategy and are highlighted in bold **magenta** type to provide you direction for locating the specific content in this book. The highlighting of the specific test-taking strategies and specific content areas in the practice questions will provide you with guidance on what topics to review for further remediation in *Saunders Strategies for Test Success: Passing Nursing School and the NCLEX® Exam* and in this book, the *Saunders Comprehensive Review for the NCLEX-PN® Exam.*
- ***Question Categories:*** Each question is tagged with categories based on the 2014 NCLEX-PN test plan. Additional content categories are provided with each question to assist you in identifying areas in need of review. The categories identified with each practice question include Level of Cognitive Ability, Client Needs, Integrated Process, and the specific nursing Content Area. New to this edition is a *Priority Concepts* code, which provides you with the specific concepts related to nursing practice. All categories are identified by their full names so you do not need to memorize codes or abbreviations. Additionally, every question on the accompanying Evolve site is

organized by these question codes, so you can customize your study session to be as specific or as generic as you need.

- *Reference:* A reference, including a page number, is provided so you can easily find the information that you need to review in your undergraduate nursing textbooks.

Pharmacology and Medication Calculations Review

Students consistently state that pharmacology is an area with which they need assistance. The 2014 NCLEX-PN test plan continues to incorporate pharmacology in the examination as it has in the past. Therefore, pharmacology chapters have been included for your review and practice. This book includes 13 pharmacology chapters, a medication and intravenous calculation chapter, and a pediatric medication calculation chapter. Each of these chapters is followed by a practice test that uses the same question format described earlier. This book contains numerous pharmacology questions. Additionally, more than 900 pharmacology questions can be found on the accompanying Evolve site.

How to Use This Book

Saunders Comprehensive Review for the NCLEX-PN® Examination is especially designed to help you with your successful journey to the peak of the Saunders *Pyramid to Success:* becoming a licensed practical nurse. As you begin your journey through this book, you will be introduced to all the important points regarding the 2014 NCLEX-PN examination, the process of testing, and unique and special tips regarding how to prepare yourself for this very important examination.

You should begin your process through the Saunders *Pyramid to Success* by reading all of Unit I in this book and becoming familiar with the central points regarding the NCLEX-PN examination. Read Chapter 4, which was written by a nursing graduate who recently passed the examination, and note what she has to say about the testing experience. Chapter 5, "Test-Taking Strategies," will provide you with the critical testing strategies that will guide you in selecting the correct option or assist you in selecting an answer to a question if you must guess. Keep these strategies in mind as you proceed through this book. Continue by studying the specific content areas addressed in Units II through XIX. Review the *Pyramid Terms* and *Pyramid to Success* notes, and identify the Client Needs specific to the test plan in each area. Read through the chapters, and focus on the *Pyramid Points* and *Pyramid Alerts* that identify the areas most likely to be tested on the NCLEX-PN examination. Pay particular attention to the Priority Nursing Actions boxes because they provide information about the steps that you will take in clinical situations requiring prioritization.

As you read each chapter, identify your areas of strength and those in need of further review. Highlight these areas, and test your abilities by answering the *Critical Thinking: What Should You Do?* question and taking all the practice tests provided at the end of the chapters. Be sure to review all the rationales and the test-taking strategies. The rationale provides you with information regarding both the correct and incorrect options. The test-taking strategy highlights the specific strategy in bold **blue** type and offers a logical path to selecting the correct option. The test-taking strategy also provides the content to review, highlighted in bold **magenta** type. Use the references to easily find any information you need to review.

After reviewing all the chapters in the book, turn to Unit XX, the Comprehensive Test. Take this examination, and then review each question, answer, and rationale. Identify any areas requiring further review; then take the time to review those areas again in both the book and the companion Evolve site.

Climbing the Pyramid to Success

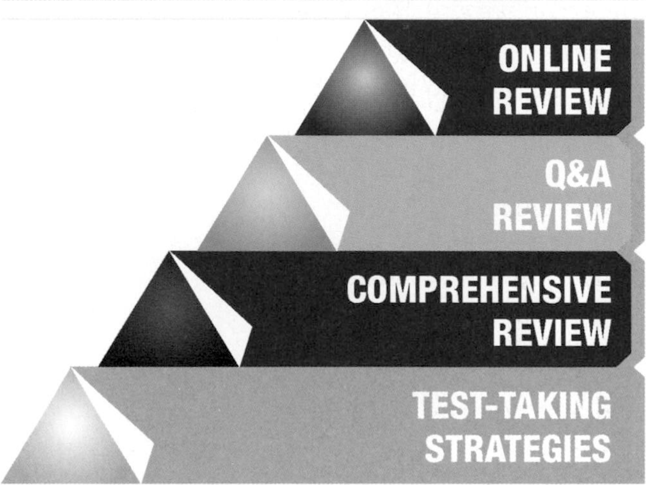

The purpose of this book is to provide a **comprehensive review** of the nursing content you will be tested on during the NCLEX-PN examination. However, *Saunders Comprehensive Review for the NCLEX-PN® Examination* is intended to do more than simply prepare you for the rigors of the NCLEX-PN. This book is also meant to serve as a valuable study tool that you can refer to throughout your nursing program, with customizable Evolve site selections to help identify and reinforce key content areas.

At the base of the *Pyramid to Success* are my **test-taking strategies**, which provide a foundation for understanding and unpacking the complexities of NCLEX-PN exam questions, including alternate item formats. *Saunders Strategies for Test Success: Passing Nursing School and the NCLEX® Exam* takes a detailed look at all the test-taking strategies you will need to know to pass any nursing examination, including the NCLEX-PN. Special tips are integrated for beginning nursing students, and there are over 1000 practice questions included so you can apply the testing strategies.

For on-the-go Q&A review, you can pick up *Saunders Q&A Review Cards for the NCLEX-PN® Examination*, which features 1200 practice NCLEX-type questions spanning all content areas.

Your final step on the *Pyramid to Success* is to master the online review. *Saunders Online Review for the NCLEX-PN® Examination* provides an interactive and individualized platform to get you ready for your final licensure exam. This online course provides 10 high-level content modules, supplemented with instructional videos, animations, audio, illustrations, testlets, and several subject matter exams. End-of-module practice tests are provided, along with several *Crossing the Finish Line* practice tests. In addition, you can assess your progress with a pretest and posttest comprehensive exam in a computerized environment that prepares you for the actual NCLEX-PN exam.

Using the Companion Evolve Site

The main website for Evolve is evolve.elsevier.com. There is a code located in the front cover of your book that you'll need to use to access the companion Evolve site for this book. The site contains more than 4500 questions and has three main functions:

- *Pretest and study calendar:* To assess your strengths and weaknesses, take the 75-question pretest. Your results will generate a customized study calendar.
- *Study:* Select questions by Client Needs, Integrated Process, Alternate Item Format Type, Priority Concepts, or specific Content Area. The answer, rationale, test-taking strategy, codes, and reference appear immediately after you answer each question.
- *Exam:* Select questions by Client Needs, Integrated Process, Alternate Item Format Type, Priority Concepts, or specific Content Area. Then select the number of questions you'd like to take in your exam: 10, 25, 50, or 100. When you have finished the exam, the percentage of questions you answered correctly will be shown in a table, and you can go back to review the questions and answers—as well as rationales, test-taking strategies, question codes, and reference(s)—for each question.

Good luck with your journey through the Saunders *Pyramid to Success*. I wish you continued success throughout your new career as a licensed practical nurse!

Linda Anne Silvestri, PhD, RN

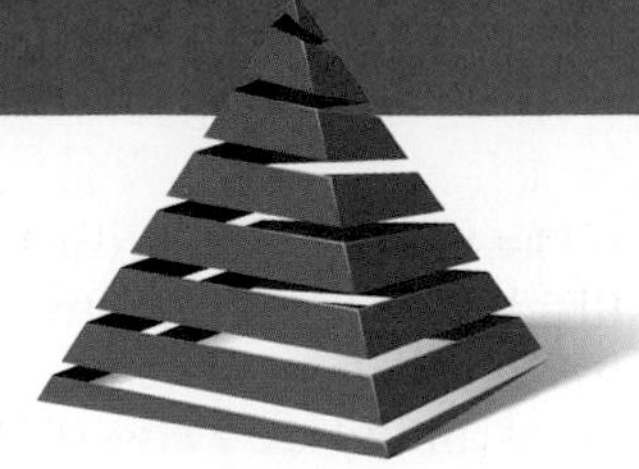

Acknowledgments

Sincere appreciation and warmest thanks are extended to the many individuals who in their own ways have contributed to the publication of this book.

First, I want to thank all my nursing students at the Community College of Rhode Island in Warwick who approached me in 1991 and persuaded me to help them prepare to take the NCLEX examination. Their enthusiasm and inspiration led to the commencement of my professional endeavors in conducting review courses for the NCLEX exam for nursing students. I also thank the numerous nursing students who have attended my review courses for their willingness to share their needs and ideas. Their input has certainly added a special uniqueness to this publication.

I wish to acknowledge all the nursing faculty who taught in my NCLEX review courses. Their commitment, dedication, and expertise have certainly helped nursing students achieve success with the NCLEX exam. Additionally, I want to acknowledge and sincerely thank my husband Laurent W. Valliere, or Larry, for his contribution to this publication, for teaching in my NCLEX review courses, and for his commitment and dedication in helping my nursing students prepare for the NCLEX from a nonacademic point of view. Larry has supported my many professional endeavors and was so loyal and loving to me each and every moment as I worked to achieve my professional goals. Larry, thank you so much! A special thank you also goes to Keara Cobbs, PN, for writing a chapter for this book about her experiences preparing for and taking the NCLEX-PN examination.

I sincerely acknowledge and thank two very important individuals from Elsevier who are so dedicated to my work in creating NCLEX products for nursing students. I thank Yvonne Alexopoulos, senior content strategist, for her continuous assistance, enthusiasm, support, and expert professional guidance as I prepared this publication. And I thank Laura Goodrich, content developmental specialist, for her tremendous amount of support and assistance, her weekly priority lists to keep me on track, her ideas for the product, and her professional and expert skills in organizing and maintaining an enormous amount of manuscript for production. I could not have completed this project without Laura! So a very special and sincere thank you extends to both Yvonne and Laura.

I also thank Angela E. Silvestri, PhD, RN, for reviewing content and practice questions and for her assistance with creating new practice questions; Mary Dowell for her expert assistance and contributions in the book and Evolve site; Elodia Dianne Fiorentino for researching content and preparing references for each practice question; Nicholas Silvestri for editing, formatting, and organizing manuscript files for me; and James Guilbault for researching and updating medications. A special thank you to all of you for providing continuous support and dedication to my work in preparing this publication and maintaining its excellent quality.

I want to acknowledge all of the staff at Elsevier for their tremendous assistance throughout the preparation and production of this publication and all of the Elsevier staff involved in the publication of previous editions of this outstanding NCLEX review product. A special thank you to all of them. I thank all the important people in the production department, including Bill Drone, senior project manager; Jeff Patterson, publishing services manager; Emily Ogle, multimedia producer; David Rushing, multimedia manager; and Maggie Reid, designer, who all played such significant roles in finalizing this publication. I sincerely thank those in the marketing department who helped with the promotion of this book, including Danielle LeCompte, marketing manager, and Julie Mark, marketing coordinator. And a special thank you to Laurie Gower, Content Development Manager, Kristin Geen, director, and Loren Wilson, SVP & GM, Content, for their years of expert guidance and continuous support for all the products in the *Pyramid to Success*.

I would also like to acknowledge Patricia Mieg, former educational sales representative, who encouraged me to submit my ideas and initial work for the first edition of this book to the W.B. Saunders Company.

I want to acknowledge my parents, who opened my door of opportunity in education. I thank my mother, Frances Mary, for all of her love, support, and assistance as I continuously worked to achieve my professional goals. I thank my father, Arnold Lawrence, who always provided insightful words of encouragement. My memories of his love and support will always remain in my heart. I am certain that he would be very proud of my professional accomplishments.

I also thank all my family for being continuously supportive, giving, and helpful during my research and preparation of this publication.

I want to especially acknowledge each and every individual who contributed to this publication: the contributors, item writers, and updaters for your expert input and ideas. I also thank the many faculty and student reviewers of the manuscript for their thoughts and ideas. A very special thank you to all of you!

I also need to thank Salve Regina University for the opportunity to educate nursing students in the baccalaureate nursing program and for its support during my research and writing of this publication. I would like to especially acknowledge my colleagues Dr. Eileen Gray, Dr. Ellen McCarty, and Dr. Bethany Sykes for all their encouragement and support.

I wish to acknowledge the Community College of Rhode Island, which provided me the opportunity to educate nursing students in the Associate Degree of Nursing Program, and a special thank you to Patricia Miller, MSN, RN, and Michelina McClellan, MS, RN, from Baystate Medical Center, School of Nursing, in Springfield, Massachusetts, who were my first mentors in nursing education.

Finally, I extend a very special thank you to all my nursing students, past, present, and future. All of you light up my life! Your love and dedication to the profession of nursing and your commitment to provide health care will bring never-ending rewards!

Linda Anne Silvestri, PhD, RN

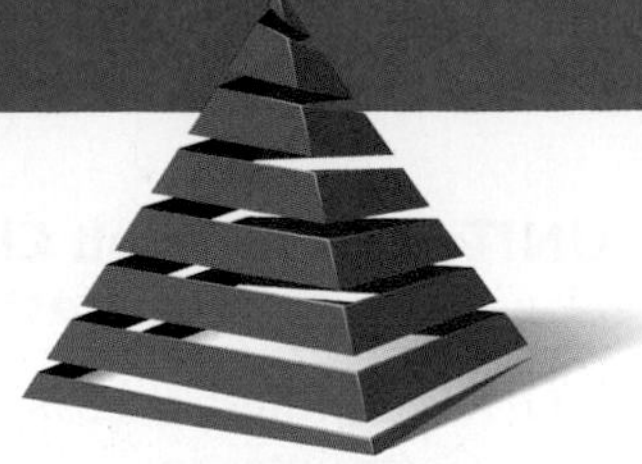

Contents

UNIT I

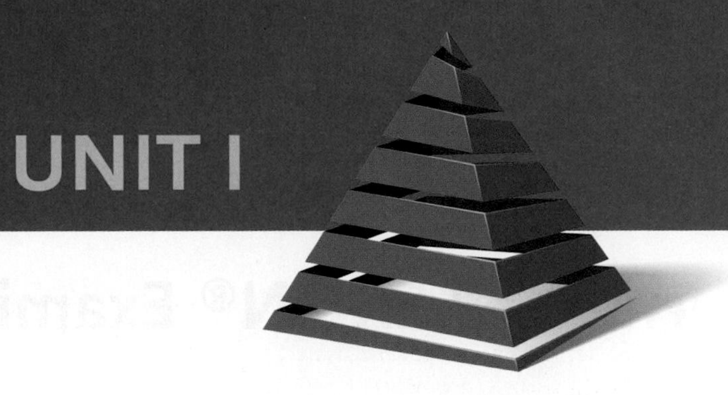

NCLEX-PN® Exam Preparation

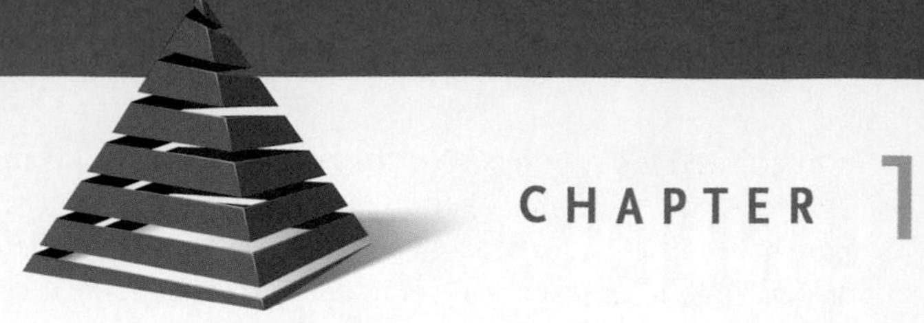

CHAPTER 1

The NCLEX-PN® Examination

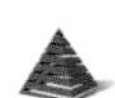

The Pyramid to Success

Welcome to the Pyramid to Success

Saunders Comprehensive Review for the NCLEX-PN® Examination is specially designed to help you begin your successful journey to the peak of the pyramid, becoming a licensed practical/vocational nurse. As you begin your journey, you will be introduced to all the important points regarding the NCLEX-PN examination and the process of testing, and to the unique and special tips regarding how to prepare yourself for this important examination. You will read what a nursing graduate who recently passed the NCLEX-PN examination has to say about the test. Important test-taking strategies are detailed. These details will guide you in selecting the correct option or assist you in selecting an answer to a question at which you must guess.

Each of the content areas in this book begins with the Pyramid to Success. The Pyramid to Success addresses specific points related to the NCLEX-PN examination, including the Pyramid Terms, and the Client Needs as identified in the test plan framework for the examination. Pyramid Terms are key words that are defined and are set in **bold purple** throughout each chapter to direct your attention to significant points for the examination. The Client Needs specific to the content of the chapter are identified.

Throughout each chapter, you will find Pyramid Point bullets that identify areas most likely to be tested on the NCLEX-PN examination. Read each chapter, and identify your strengths and areas that are in need of further review. Test your strengths and abilities by taking all the practice tests provided in this book and on the accompanying Evolve site. Be sure to read all the rationales and test-taking strategies. The rationale provides you with significant information regarding the correct and incorrect options. The test-taking strategy provides you with the logical path to selecting the correct option. The test-taking strategy also identifies the content area to review, if required. The reference source and page number are provided so that you can easily find the information that you need to review. Each question is coded with the Level of Cognitive Ability, the Client Needs category, the Integrated Process, and the nursing Content Area.

Following the completion of your comprehensive review in this book, continue on your journey through the Pyramid to Success with the companion book *Saunders Q&A Review for the NCLEX-PN® Examination*, which provides you with more than 4500 practice questions based on the NCLEX-PN examination test plan framework, with a specific focus on Client Needs and Integrated Processes. Then, you will be ready for *HESI/Saunders Online Review for the NCLEX-PN® Examination*. Additional products in Saunders Pyramid to Success include *Saunders Strategies for Test Success: Passing Nursing School and the NCLEX® Exam* and *Saunders Q&A Review Cards for the NCLEX-PN® Exam*. These products are described next.

HESI/Saunders Online Review for the NCLEX-PN® Examination

This product addresses all areas of the test plan identified by the National Council of State Boards of Nursing (NCSBN). The course contains a pretest that provides feedback regarding your strengths and weaknesses and generates an individualized study schedule in a calendar format. Content review is in an outline format and includes self-check practice questions and case studies, figures and illustrations, a glossary, and animations and videos. Numerous online exams are included. There are 2500 practice questions; the types of questions in this course include multiple-choice and alternate item formats.

Saunders Strategies for Test Success: Passing Nursing School and the NCLEX® Exam

This product focuses on the test-taking strategies that will help you pass your nursing examinations while in nursing school and will prepare you for the NCLEX examination. The chapters describe various test-taking strategies and include sample questions that illustrate how to use the strategies; over 1000 practice questions accompany this book, and each question provides a tip for the beginning nursing student. The practice questions reflect the framework and the content identified in the NCLEX-RN test plan and include multiple-choice and alternate item format questions. In addition to the focus on test-taking strategies, information about cultural characteristics and practices, pharmacology strategies, medication and intravenous calculations, laboratory values, positioning guidelines, and therapeutic diets is included.

Saunders Q&A Review Cards for the NCLEX-PN® Exam

This product is organized by content areas and the test plan framework of the NCLEX-PN test plan. It provides you with 1200 unique practice test questions on portable and easy-to-use cards. The cards have the question on the front, and the answer, rationale, and test-taking strategy are on the back. This product includes multiple-choice questions and alternate item format questions, including fill-in-the-blank, multiple-response, ordered-response, figure, graphic option, and chart/exhibit questions.

All the products in the Saunders Pyramid to Success can be obtained online by visiting elsevierhealth.com or by calling 800-545-2522.

Let's begin our journey through the Pyramid to Success.

The Examination Process

An important step in the Pyramid to Success is to become as familiar as possible with the examination process. Candidates facing the challenge of this examination can experience significant anxiety. Knowing what the examination is all about and knowing what you will encounter during the process of testing will assist in alleviating fear and anxiety. The information contained in this chapter addresses the procedures related to the development of the NCLEX-PN examination test plan, the components of the test plan, and the answers to the questions most commonly asked by nursing students and graduates preparing to take the NCLEX-PN examination. The information contained in this chapter related to the test plan was obtained from the NCSBN website (http://www.ncsbn.org) and from the NCSBN test plan for the NCLEX-PN examination (effective April 2014). You can obtain additional information regarding the test and its development by accessing the NCSBN website or by writing to the National Council of State Boards of Nursing, 111 East Wacker Drive, Suite 2900, Chicago, IL 60601. You are encouraged to access the NCSBN website because this site provides you with valuable information about the NCLEX and other resources available to an NCLEX candidate.

Computer Adaptive Testing

The acronym *CAT* stands for computer adaptive test, which means that the examination is created as the test-taker answers each question. All the test questions are categorized on the basis of the test plan structure and the level of difficulty of the question. As you answer a question, the computer determines your competency based on the answer you selected. If you selected a correct answer to a question, the computer scans the question bank and selects a more difficult question. If you selected an incorrect answer, the computer scans the question bank and selects an easier question. This process continues until the test plan requirements are met and a reliable pass-or-fail decision is made.

When a test question is presented on the computer screen, you must answer it or the test will not move on. This means that you will not be able to skip questions, go back and review questions, or go back and change answers. In a CAT examination, once an answer is recorded, all subsequent questions administered depend, to an extent, on the answer selected for that question. Skipping and returning to earlier questions are not compatible with the logical methodology of a CAT. The inability to skip questions or go back to change previous answers will not be a disadvantage to you; you will not fall into that "trap" of changing a correct answer to an incorrect one with the CAT system.

If you are faced with a question that contains unfamiliar content, you may need to guess at the answer. There is no penalty for guessing on this examination. With most of the questions, the answer will be right there in front of you. If you need to guess, use your nursing knowledge and clinical experiences to their fullest extent and all the test-taking strategies that you have practiced in this review program.

You do not need any computer experience to take this examination. A keyboard tutorial is provided and administered to all test-takers at the start of the examination. The tutorial will instruct you on the use of the on-screen optional calculator, the use of the mouse, and how to record an answer. In addition to the traditional four-option, multiple-choice question, the tutorial provides instructions on how to respond to alternate item format questions. This tutorial is provided on the NCSBN website, and you are encouraged to view the tutorial when you are preparing for the NCLEX examination. In addition, at the testing site, a test administrator is present to assist in explaining the use of the computer to ensure your full understanding of how to proceed.

Development of the Test Plan

The test plan for the NCLEX-PN examination is developed by the NCSBN. The NCLEX examination is a national examination; the NCSBN considers the legal scope of nursing practice as governed by state laws and regulations, including the Nurse Practice Act, and uses these laws to define the areas on the examination that will assess the competence of the test-taker for licensure.

The NCSBN also conducts an important study every 3 years, known as a practice analysis study, to determine the framework for the test plan for the examination. The participants in this study include newly licensed practical or vocational nurses. From a list provided, the participants select the nursing activities that they perform, the frequency of performing these specific activities, the impact of the activities on maintaining client safety, and the setting where the activities were performed. A panel of content experts at the NCSBN analyzes the results of the study and makes decisions regarding the test plan framework. The results of this recently conducted study provided the structure for the test plan implemented in April 2014.

Test Plan

The content of the NCLEX-PN examination reflects the activities identified in the practice analysis study conducted by the NCSBN. The questions are written to address Level of Cognitive Ability, Client Needs, and Integrated Processes as identified in the test plan developed by the NCSBN.

Level of Cognitive Ability

Most questions on the NCLEX examination are written at the application level or higher levels of cognitive ability. Box 1-1 presents an example of a question that requires you to apply data.

Client Needs

In the test plan implemented in April 2014, the NCSBN has identified a test plan framework based on Client Needs. The NCSBN identifies four major categories of Client Needs. Some of these categories are divided further into subcategories. The Client Needs categories include Safe and Effective Care Environment, Health Promotion and Maintenance, Psychosocial Integrity, and Physiological Integrity (Table 1-1).

BOX 1-1 Level of Cognitive Ability: Applying

The nurse notes blanching, coolness, and edema at the peripheral intravenous (IV) site. Based on these findings, the nurse should implement which **most appropriate** action?

1. Remove the IV
2. Apply a warm compress
3. Check for a blood return
4. Measure the area of infiltration

Answer: *1*

This question requires that you focus on the data identified in the question and determine that the client is experiencing an infiltration. Next you need to consider the harmful effects of infiltration and determine the action to implement. Because infiltration can be damaging to the surrounding tissue, the most appropriate action is to remove the IV to prevent any further damage.

TABLE 1-1 Client Needs Categories and Percentage of Questions on the NCLEX-PN® Examination

Client Needs Category	Percentage of Questions
Safe and Effective Care Environment	
Coordinated Care	16-22
Safety and Infection Control	10-16
Health Promotion and Maintenance	7-13
Psychosocial Integrity	8-14
Physiological Integrity	
Basic Care and Comfort	7-13
Pharmacological Therapies	11-17
Reduction of Risk Potential	10-16
Physiological Adaptation	7-13

Data from National Council of State Boards of Nursing (NCSBN). (2013). *2014 NCLEX-PN® Detailed Test Plan*. Chicago: NCSBN.

Safe and Effective Care Environment

The Safe and Effective Care Environment category includes two subcategories:

- Coordinated Care
- Safety and Infection Control

According to the NCSBN, Coordinated Care addresses content that tests the nurse's knowledge, skills, and ability required to collaborate with health care members to facilitate effective client care. The NCSBN indicates that Safety and Infection Control addresses content that tests the nurse's knowledge, skills, and ability required to protect clients, families, significant others, visitors, and health care personnel from health and environmental hazards. Box 1-2 presents examples of questions that address these two subcategories.

Health Promotion and Maintenance

The Health Promotion and Maintenance category addresses the principles related to expected stages of growth and development. According to the NCSBN, this Client Needs category also addresses content that tests the nurse's knowledge, skills, and ability required to assist others to prevent health problems; to recognize alterations in health; and to develop health practices that promote and support wellness. See Box 1-3 for an example of a question in this Client Needs category.

Psychosocial Integrity

The Psychosocial Integrity category addresses content that tests the nurse's knowledge, skills, and abilities required to promote and support the ability of the client, client's family, and client's significant other to cope, adapt, and problem solve during stressful events. The NCSBN also indicates that this Client Needs category addresses the emotional, mental, and social

BOX 1-2 Safe and Effective Care Environment

Coordinated Care

The nurse has received the client assignment for the day. Which client should the nurse attend to **first**?

1. The client who has a nasogastric tube attached to intermittent suction
2. The client who needs to receive subcutaneous insulin before breakfast
3. The client who is 2 days postoperative and is complaining of incisional pain
4. The client who has a blood glucose level of 50 mg/dL and complains of blurred vision

Answer: *4*

This question addresses the subcategory, Coordinated Care, in the Client Needs category, Safe and Effective Care Environment. It requires you to establish priorities by comparing the needs of each client and deciding which need is urgent. The client described in option 4 has a low blood glucose level and symptoms reflective of hypoglycemia. This client should be attended to first so that treatment can be implemented. Although the clients in options 1, 2, and 3 have needs that require attention, they are not the priority and can wait until the client in option 4 is stabilized.

Safety and Infection Control

The nurse prepares to care for a client on contact precautions who has a hospital-acquired infection caused by methicillin-resistant *Staphylococcus aureus* (MRSA). The client has an abdominal wound that requires irrigation and has a tracheostomy attached to a mechanical ventilator, which requires frequent suctioning. The nurse should assemble which necessary protective items before entering the client's room?

1. Gloves and a gown
2. Gloves, mask, and goggles
3. Gloves, mask, gown, and goggles
4. Gloves, gown, and shoe protectors

Answer: *3*

This question addresses the subcategory, Safety and Infection Control, in the Client Needs category, Safe and Effective Care Environment. It addresses content related to protecting oneself from contracting an infection and requires that you consider the methods of possible transmission of infection, based on the client's condition. Because splashes of infective material can occur during the wound irrigation or suctioning of the tracheostomy, option 3 is correct.

BOX 1-3 Health Promotion and Maintenance

The nurse is choosing age-appropriate toys for a toddler. Which toy is the **best** choice for this age?

1. Puzzle
2. Toy soldiers
3. Large stacking blocks
4. A card game with large pictures

Answer: *3*

This question addresses the Client Needs category, Health Promotion and Maintenance, and specifically relates to the principles of growth and development of a toddler. Toddlers like to master activities independently, such as stacking blocks. Because toddlers do not have the developmental ability to determine what could be harmful, toys that are safe need to be provided. A puzzle and toy soldiers provide objects that can be placed in the mouth and may be harmful for a toddler. A card game with large pictures may require cooperative play, which is more appropriate for a school-age child.

BOX 1-4 Psychosocial Integrity

A client with coronary artery disease has selected guided imagery to help cope with psychological stress. Which client statement indicates an understanding of this stress reduction measure?

1. "This will help only if I play music at the same time."
2. "This will work for me only if I am alone in a quiet area."
3. "I need to do this only when I lie down in case I fall asleep."
4. "The best thing about this is that I can use it anywhere, anytime."

Answer: *4*

This question addresses the Client Needs category, Psychosocial Integrity, and the content addresses coping mechanisms. Guided imagery involves the client's creation of an image in the mind, concentrating on the image, and gradually becoming less aware of the offending stimulus. It can be done anytime and anywhere; some clients may use other relaxation techniques or play music with it.

well-being of the client, family, or significant other. See Box 1-4 for an example of a question in this Client Needs category.

Physiological Integrity

The Physiological Integrity category includes four subcategories, described by the NCSBN as follows:

- Basic Care and Comfort: Addresses content that tests the nurse's knowledge, skills, and ability required to provide comfort and assistance to the client in the performance of activities of daily living.
- Pharmacological Therapies: Addresses content that tests the nurse's knowledge, skills, and ability required to administer medications and parenteral therapies, including dosage calculations and pharmacological pain management.
- Reduction of Risk Potential: Addresses content that tests the nurse's knowledge, skills, and ability required

to prevent complications or health problems related to the client's condition or any prescribed treatments or procedures.

- Physiological Adaptation: Addresses content that tests the nurse's knowledge, skills, and ability required to provide care to clients with acute, chronic, or life-threatening conditions.

See Box 1-5 for examples of questions in this Client Needs category.

Integrated Processes

The NCSBN identifies four processes that are fundamental to the practice of nursing. These processes are a component of the test plan and are incorporated throughout the major categories of Client Needs. The Integrated Process subcategories include:

- Caring
- Communication and Documentation
- Nursing Process (Clinical Problem-Solving Process)
  - Data Collection
  - Planning
  - Implementation
  - Evaluation
- Teaching and Learning

See Box 1-6 for an example of a question that incorporates the Integrated Process of caring.

BOX 1-5 Physiological Integrity

Basic Care and Comfort

A client with Parkinson's disease develops akinesia while ambulating, increasing the risk for falls. Which suggestion should the nurse provide to the client to alleviate this problem?

1. Use a wheelchair to move around.
2. Stand erect and use a cane to ambulate.
3. Keep the feet close together while ambulating and use a walker.
4. Consciously think about walking over imaginary lines on the floor.

Answer: 4

This question addresses the subcategory, Basic Care and Comfort, in the Client Needs category, Physiological Integrity, and addresses client mobility and promoting assistance in an activity of daily living to maintain safety. Clients with Parkinson's disease can develop bradykinesia (slow movement) or akinesia (freezing or no movement). Having these clients imagine lines on the floor to step over can keep them moving forward while remaining safe.

Pharmacological Therapies

The nurse monitors a client receiving digoxin (Lanoxin) for which **early** manifestation of digoxin toxicity?

1. Anorexia
2. Facial pain
3. Photophobia
4. Yellow color perception

Answer: 1

This question addresses the subcategory, Pharmacological and Parenteral Therapies, in the Client Needs category, Physiological Integrity. Digoxin is a cardiac glycoside that is used to manage and treat heart failure and to control ventricular rates in clients with atrial fibrillation. The most common early manifestations of toxicity include gastrointestinal disturbances such as anorexia, nausea, and vomiting. Facial pain, personality changes, and ocular disturbances (photophobia, light flashes, halos around bright objects, yellow or green color perception) are also signs of toxicity, but are not early signs.

Reduction of Risk Potential

A magnetic resonance imaging (MRI) study is prescribed for a client with a suspected liver tumor. The nurse should implement which action to prepare the client for this test?

1. Instruct the client about inhalation techniques.
2. Keep the client NPO for 6 hours before the test.
3. Shave the groin for insertion of a femoral catheter.
4. Remove all metal-containing objects from the client.

Answer: 4

This question addresses the subcategory, Reduction of Risk Potential, in the Client Needs category, Physiological Integrity, and the nurse's responsibilities in preparing the client for the diagnostic test. In an MRI study, radiofrequency pulses in a magnetic field are converted into pictures. All metal objects, such as rings, bracelets, hairpins, and watches, should be removed. In addition, a history should be taken to ascertain whether the client has any internal metallic devices, such as orthopedic hardware, pacemakers, or shrapnel. NPO status is not necessary for an MRI study of the liver. The groin may be shaved for an angiogram, and inhalation techniques may be necessary for a ventilation/perfusion lung scan.

Physiological Adaptation

A client with renal insufficiency has a magnesium level of 3.6 mg/dL. Based on this laboratory result, the nurse should recognize which finding as significant?

1. Hyperpnea
2. Drowsiness
3. Hypertension
4. Physical hyperactivity

Answer: 2

This question addresses the subcategory, Physiological Adaptation, in the Client Needs category, Physiological Integrity. It addresses an alteration in body systems. The normal magnesium level is 1.6 to 2.6 mg/dL. A magnesium level of 3.6 mg/dL indicates hypermagnesemia. Neurological manifestations begin to occur when magnesium levels are elevated and are noted as neurological depression, such as drowsiness, sedation, lethargy, respiratory depression, muscle weakness, and areflexia. Bradycardia and hypotension also occur.

BOX 1-6 Integrated Processes

A client is scheduled for angioplasty. The client says to the nurse, "I'm so afraid that it will hurt and will make me worse off than I am." Which response by the nurse is therapeutic?

1. "Can you tell me what you understand about the procedure?"
2. "Your fears are a sign that you really should have this procedure."
3. "Try not to worry. This is a well-known and easy procedure for the doctor."
4. "Those are very normal fears, but please be assured that everything will be okay."

Answer: 1

This question addresses the subcategory, Caring, in the category, Integrated Processes. Option 1 is a therapeutic communication technique that explores the client's feelings, determines the level of client understanding about the procedure, and displays caring. Option 2 demeans the client and does not encourage further sharing by the client. Option 3 diminishes the client's feelings by directing attention away from the client and to the health care provider's importance. Option 4 does not address the client's fears and puts the client's feelings on hold.

Types of Questions on the Examination

The types of questions that may be administered on the examination include:

- Multiple-choice
- Fill-in-the-blank
- Multiple-response
- Ordered response
- Figure
- Chart/exhibit
- Graphic option
- Audio
- Video

Some questions may require you to use the mouse and cursor on the computer. For example, you may be presented with a picture that displays the arterial vessels of an adult client. In this picture, you may be asked to "point and click" (using the mouse) on the area (hot spot) where the dorsalis pedis pulse could be felt. In all types of questions, the answer is scored as either right or wrong. Credit is not given for a partially correct answer. Additionally, all question types may include pictures, graphics, tables, charts, sound, or video. The NCSBN provides specific directions for you to follow with all question types to guide you in your process of testing. Be sure to read these directions as they appear on the computer screen. Examples of some of these types of questions are noted in this chapter. All question types are provided in this book and the accompanying Evolve site.

Multiple-Choice Questions

Most of the questions that you will be asked to answer will be in the multiple-choice format. These questions provide you with data about a client situation and four answers or options.

Fill-in-the-Blank Questions

Fill-in-the-blank questions may ask you to perform a medication calculation, determine an intravenous flow rate, or calculate an intake or output record on a client. You will need to type only a number (your answer) in the answer box. If the question requires rounding the answer, this needs to be performed at the end of the calculation. The rules for rounding an answer are provided in the tutorial provided by the NCSBN and are also provided in the specific question. Additionally, you must type in a decimal point if necessary; however, it is not necessary to type a "0" before the decimal point. See Box 1-7 for an example.

Multiple-Response Questions

For a multiple-response question, you will be asked to select or check all the options, such as nursing interventions, that relate to the information in the question. No partial credit is given for correct selections. You need to do exactly as the question asks, which will be to select all the options that apply. See Box 1-8 for an example.

BOX 1-7 Fill-in-the-Blank Question

A prescription reads: acetaminophen (Tylenol Extra Strength) liquid, 650 mg orally every 4 hours PRN for pain. The medication label reads: 500 mg/15 mL. The nurse prepares how many milliliters to administer one dose? **Fill in the blank.**

Answer: 19.5 *mL*

Formula:

$$\frac{Desired}{Available} \times Volume = mL$$

$$\frac{650\ mg}{500\ mg} \times 15\ mL = 19.5\ mL$$

In this question, you need to use the formula for calculating a medication dose. When the dose is determined, you will need to type your numeric answer in the answer box. Always follow the specific directions noted on the computer screen when answering the question. Also, remember that there will be an on-screen calculator on the computer for your use.

Ordered Response Questions

In this type of question, you will be asked to use the computer mouse to drag and drop your nursing actions in order of priority. Information will be presented in a question and based on the data you need to determine what you will do first, second, third, and so forth. The unordered options will be located in boxes on the left side of the screen, and you need to move all options in order of priority to ordered response boxes on the right side of the screen. Specific directions for moving the options are provided with the question. See Box 1-9 for an example.

Figure Questions

A question with a picture or graphic will ask you to answer the question based on the picture or graphic. The question could contain a chart, a table, or a figure or illustration. You also may be asked to use the computer mouse to point and click on a specific area in the visual. A figure or illustration may appear in any type of question, including a multiple-choice question. See Box 1-10 for an example.

Chart/Exhibit Questions

In this type of question, you will be presented with a problem and a chart or exhibit. You will be provided with tabs or buttons that you need to click to obtain the information needed to answer the question. A prompt or message may appear that may indicate the need to click on a tab or button. See Box 1-11 for an example.

BOX 1-8 Multiple-Response Question

The emergency department nurse is caring for a child suspected of acute epiglottitis. Which interventions apply in the care of the child? **Select all that apply.**

- ☐ 1. Obtain a throat culture.
- ☒ 2. Ensure a patent airway.
- ☒ 3. Prepare the child for a chest x-ray.
- ☐ 4. Maintain the child in a supine position.
- ☒ 5. Obtain a pediatric-size tracheostomy tray.
- ☒ 6. Place the child on an oxygen saturation monitor.

In a multiple-response question, you will be asked to select or check all the options, such as interventions, that relate to the information in the question. To answer this question, recall that acute epiglottitis is a serious obstructive inflammatory process that requires immediate intervention. Examination of the throat with a tongue depressor or attempting to obtain a throat culture is contraindicated because the examination can precipitate further obstruction. To reduce respiratory distress, the child should sit upright. The child is placed on an oxygen saturation monitor to monitor oxygenation status. A lateral neck and chest x-ray is obtained to determine the degree of obstruction, if present. Tracheostomy and intubation may be necessary if respiratory distress is severe. Remember to follow the specific directions given on the computer screen.

BOX 1-9 Ordered Response Question

The nurse is preparing to suction a client who has a tracheostomy tube and gathers the supplies needed for the procedure. What is the order of **priority** of the actions that the nurse takes to perform this procedure? **Arrange the actions in the order that they should be performed. All options must be used.**

Unordered Options

Hyperoxygenate the client.
Place the client in a semi-Fowler's position.
Turn on the suction device and set the regulator at 80 mm Hg.
Apply gloves and attach the suction tubing to the suction catheter.
Apply intermittent suction and slowly withdraw the catheter while rotating it back and forth.
Insert the catheter into the tracheostomy until resistance is met and then pull back 1 cm.

Ordered Response

Place the client in a semi-Fowler's position.
Turn on the suction device and set the regulator at 80 mm Hg.
Apply gloves and attach the suction tubing to the suction catheter.
Hyperoxygenate the client.
Insert the catheter into the tracheostomy until resistance is met and then pull back 1 cm.
Apply intermittent suction and slowly withdraw the catheter while rotating it back and forth.

This question requires you to arrange, in order of priority, the nursing actions that should be taken to suction a client who has a tracheostomy tube. The nurse positions the client first, and then turns the suction device on and sets the regulator. The nurse then dons gloves and attaches the suction tubing to the suction catheter. The nurse hyperoxygenates the client before and after suctioning. The nurse then inserts the catheter into the tracheostomy until resistance is met and pulls back 1 cm, applies intermittent suction, and slowly withdraws the catheter while rotating it back and forth. Remember that the client and equipment are prepared before performing the procedure. Also, remember that on the NCLEX examination, you will use the computer mouse to place the unordered options in an ordered response.

BOX 1-10 Figure Question

A client who experienced a myocardial infarction is being monitored via cardiac telemetry. The nurse notes the sudden onset of this cardiac rhythm on the monitor and should plan to take which **immediate** action? **Refer to figure.**

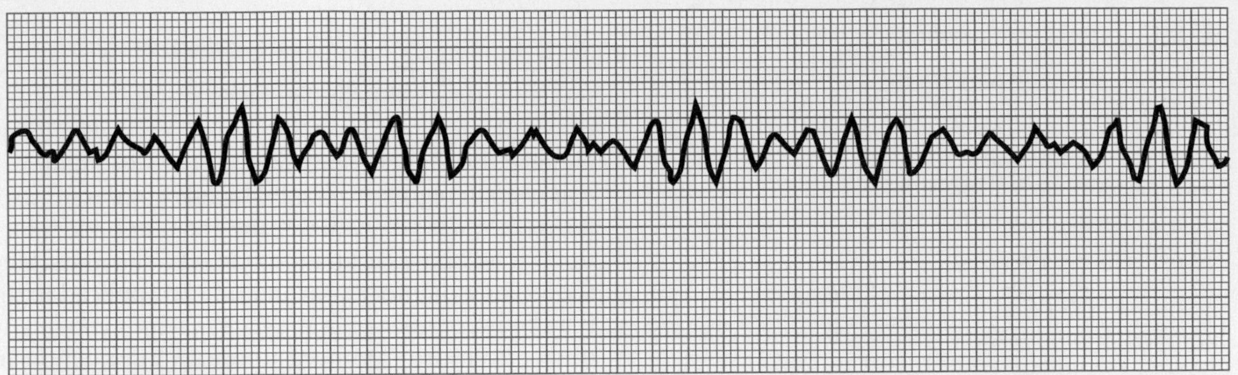

(Figure from Ignatavicius D, Workman M: *Medical-surgical nursing: Patient-centered collaborative care*, ed 7, Philadelphia, 2013, Saunders.)

1. Take the client's blood pressure.
2. Initiate cardiopulmonary resuscitation (CPR).
3. Place a nitroglycerin tablet under the client's tongue.
4. Continue to monitor the client for 5 minutes and then contact the registered nurse.

Answer: 2

This question requires you to identify the cardiac rhythm, and then determine the immediate nursing action. This cardiac rhythm identifies a coarse ventricular fibrillation (VF). The goals of treatment are to terminate VF promptly and convert it to an organized rhythm. The health care provider (HCP) or an advanced cardiac life support (ACLS)—qualified nurse or other HCP must immediately defibrillate the client. If a defibrillator is not readily available, CPR is initiated until the defibrillator arrives. Options 1, 3, and 4 are incorrect actions and delay life-saving treatment.

BOX 1-11 Chart/Exhibit Question

The nurse reviews the history and physical examination documented in the medical record of a client requesting a prescription for oral contraceptives. The nurse determines that oral contraceptives are contraindicated because of which documented item? **Refer to chart.**

CLIENT'S CHART		
History and Physical	**Medications**	**Diagnostic Results**
Item 1: Has renal calculi *Item 2:* Had thrombophlebitis 1 year ago	*Item 3:* Multivitamin orally daily	*Item 4:* Electrocardiogram: normal

Answer: 2

This chart/exhibit question provides you with data from the client's medical record and asks you to identify the item that is a contraindication to the use of oral contraceptives. Oral contraceptives are contraindicated in women with a history of any of the following: thrombophlebitis and thromboembolic disorders, cardiovascular or cerebrovascular diseases (including stroke), any estrogen-dependent cancer or breast cancer, benign or malignant liver tumors, impaired liver function, hypertension, and diabetes mellitus with vascular involvement. Adverse effects of oral contraceptives include increased risk of superficial and deep vein thrombosis, pulmonary embolism, thrombotic stroke (or other types of strokes), myocardial infarction, and accelerations of preexisting breast tumors.

Graphic Option Questions

In this type of question, the option selections will be pictures rather than text. Each option will be preceded by a circle, and you will need to use the computer mouse to click in the circle that represents your answer choice. See Box 1-12 for an example.

Audio Questions

Audio questions will require listening to a sound to answer the question. These questions will prompt you to use the headset provided and click on the sound icon. You will be able to click on the volume button to adjust the volume to your comfort level, and you will be able to listen to the sound as many times as necessary. Content examples include, but are not limited to, various lung sounds, heart sounds, or bowel sounds. Examples of these question types are located on the accompanying Evolve site. See Figure 1-1 for an example.

Video Questions

Video questions will require viewing an animation or video clip to answer the question. These questions will prompt you to click on the video icon. There may be sound associated with the animation and video, in which you will be prompted to use the headset. Content examples include, but are not limited to, data collec-

BOX 1-12 Graphic Option Question

The nurse should place the client in which position to administer a soapsuds enema? **Refer to figures 1–4.**

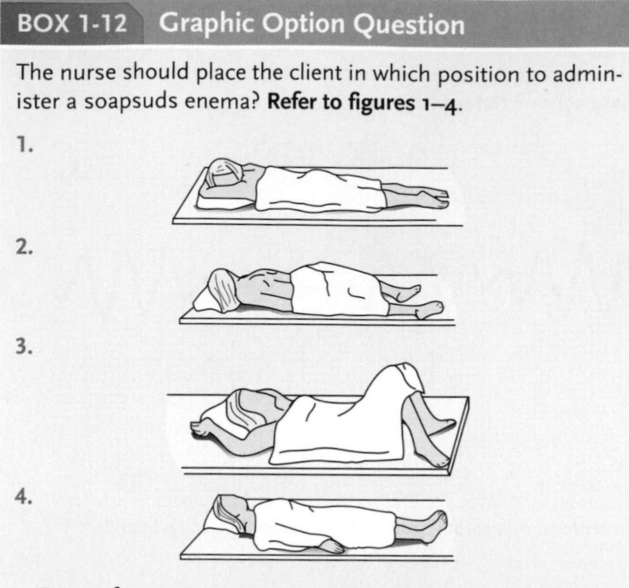

(Figures from Potter P, Perry A, Stockert P, Hall A: *Fundamentals of Nursing*, ed 8, St. Louis, 2013, Mosby.)

Answer: 2

This question requires you to select the picture that represents your answer choice. To administer an enema, the nurse assists the client into the left side-lying (Sims) position with the right knee flexed. This position allows the enema solution to flow downward by gravity along the natural curve of the sigmoid colon and rectum, improving the retention of solution. Option 1 is a prone position. Option 3 is a dorsal recumbent position. Option 4 is a supine position.

tion techniques, nursing procedures, or communication skills. Examples of these question types are located on the accompanying Evolve site. See Figure 1-2 for an example.

Registering to Take the Examination

It is important to obtain an NCLEX examination candidate bulletin from the NCSBN website at www.ncsbn.org because this bulletin provides all the information that you need to register for and schedule your examination. It also provides you with website and telephone information for NCLEX examination contacts. The initial step in the registration process is to submit an application to the state board of nursing in the state in which you intend to obtain licensure. You need to obtain information from the board of nursing regarding the specific registration process because the process may vary from state to state. When you receive confirmation from the board of nursing that you have met all of the state requirements, you can register to take the NCLEX examination with Pearson Vue. You may register for the examination through the Internet or by telephone. The NCLEX candidate website is http://www.pearsonvue.com/nclex.

Following the registration instructions and completing the registration forms precisely and accurately are important. Registration forms not properly completed or not accompanied by the proper fees in the required method of payment will be returned to you and will delay testing. You must pay a fee for taking

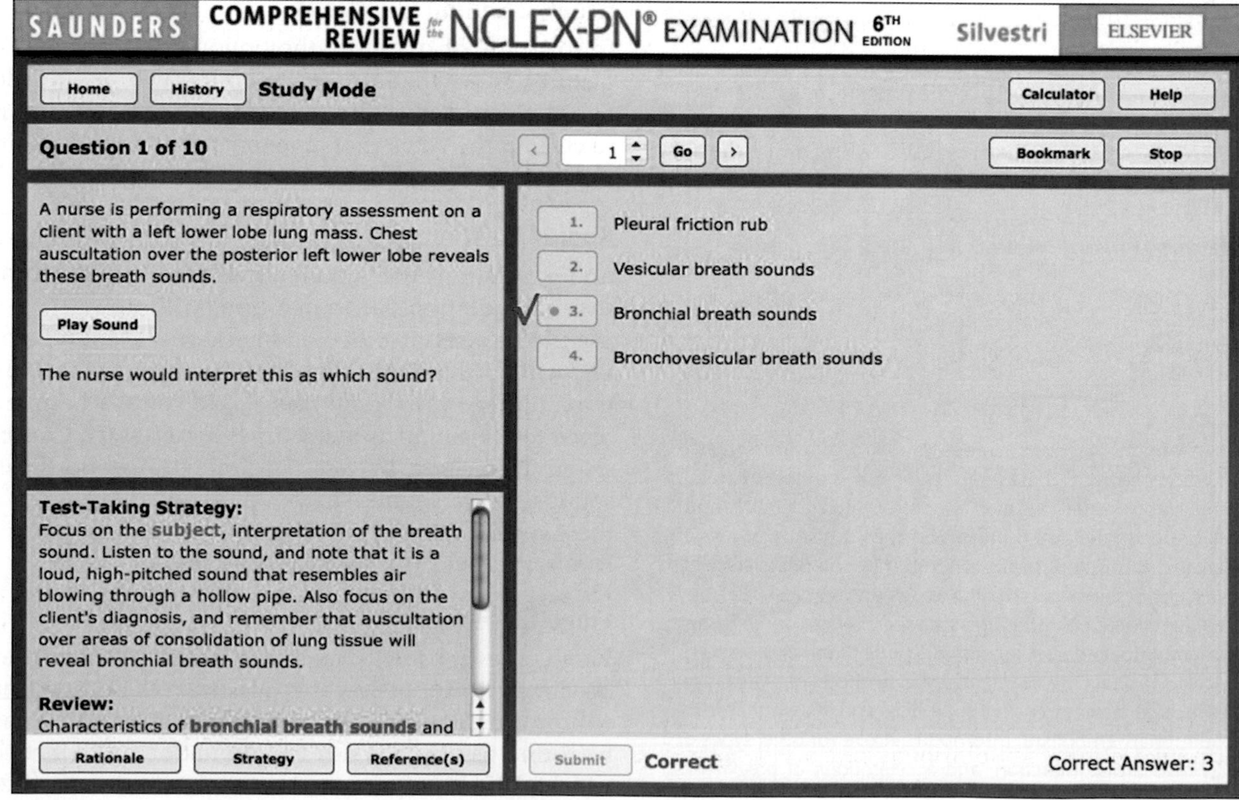

FIGURE 1-1 Audio Question

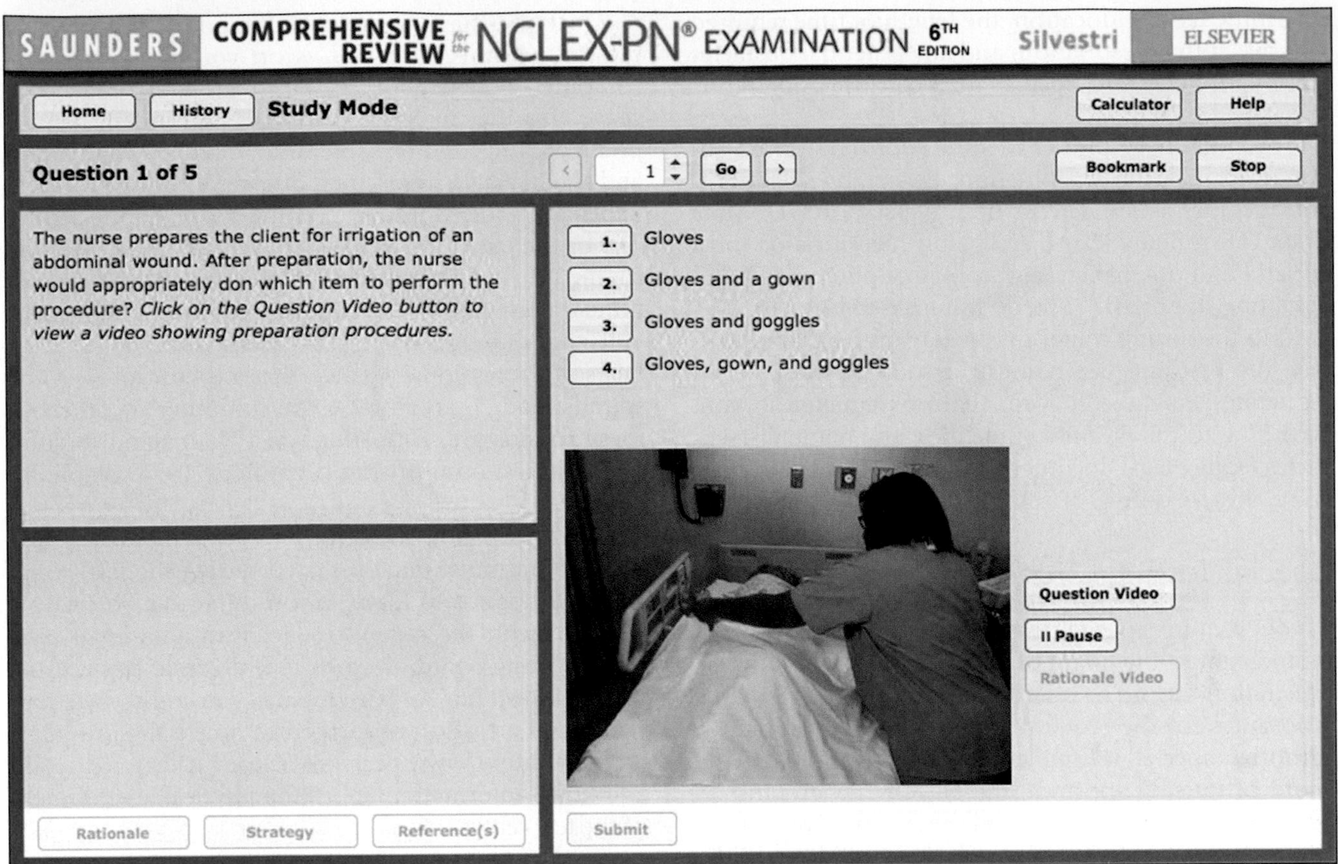

FIGURE 1-2 Video Question

the examination; you also may have to pay additional fees to the board of nursing in the state in which you are applying. You will then be made eligible by the licensure board and will receive an Authorization to Test (ATT) form via email. If you do not receive an ATT form within 2 weeks of registration, you should contact the candidate services at 866-496-2539 (U.S. candidates).

Authorization to Test Form and Scheduling an Appointment

You cannot make an appointment until the board of nursing declares eligibility and you receive an ATT form. Note the validity dates on the ATT form, and schedule a date and time when you receive the ATT. The examination will take place at a Pearson Professional Center. U.S. candidates can make an appointment through the Internet (http://www.pearsonvue.com/nclex) or by telephone (866-496-2539). You can schedule an appointment at any Pearson Professional Center. You do not have to take the examination in the same state in which you are seeking licensure. A confirmation of your appointment with the appointment date and time and the directions to the testing center will be sent to you via email.

Changing Your Appointment

If for any reason you need to cancel or reschedule your appointment to test, you can make the change on the candidate website (http://www.pearsonvue.com/nclex) or by calling candidate services. The change needs to be made 1 full business day (24 hours) before your scheduled appointment. If you fail to arrive for the examination or fail to cancel your appointment to test without providing appropriate notice, you will forfeit your examination fee and your ATT form will be invalidated. This information will be reported to the board of nursing in the state in which you have applied for licensure, and you will be required to register and pay the testing fees again.

Day of the Examination

It is important that you arrive at the testing center at least 30 minutes before the test is scheduled. If you arrive late for the scheduled testing appointment, you may be required to forfeit your examination appointment. If it is necessary to forfeit your appointment, you will need to re-register for the examination and pay an additional fee. The board of nursing will be notified that you did not take the test. A few days before your scheduled date of testing, take the time to drive to the testing center to determine its exact location, the length of time required to arrive at that destination, and any potential obstacles that might delay you, such as road construction, traffic, or parking sites.

You must have proper identification (ID) to be admitted to take the examination. Acceptable identification includes a U.S. driver's license, passport, U.S. state ID, or U.S. military ID. All acceptable identification must be valid and not expired and contain a photograph and signature (in English). You do not need to bring the ATT form to the testing center on the day of the exam; however, the first and last names on your ID must match the names on the ATT form that was emailed to you. According to the NCSBN guidelines, any name discrepancies require legal documentation, such as a marriage license, divorce decree, or court action legal name change.

Special Testing Circumstances

If you require special testing accommodations, you should contact the board of nursing before submitting a registration form. The board of nursing will provide the procedures for the request. The board of nursing must authorize special testing accommodations. Following board of nursing approval, the NCSBN reviews the requested accommodations and must approve the request. If the request is approved, the candidate will be notified and provided the procedure for registering for and scheduling the examination.

Testing Center

The test center is designed to ensure complete security of the testing process. Strict candidate identification requirements have been established. You must bring the required form of identification. You will be asked to read the rules related to testing. A digital fingerprint and palm vein print will be taken, and this procedure is usually done twice. A digital signature and photograph will also be taken at the test center. These identity confirmations will accompany the NCLEX exam results. In addition, if you leave the testing room for any reason, you may be required to perform these identity confirmation procedures again to be readmitted to the room.

Personal belongings are not allowed in the testing room. Secure storage, such as a locker and locker key, will be provided for you; however, storage space is limited, so you must plan accordingly. All electronic devices, including a cell phone, must be placed in a sealable bag provided by the test administrator and kept in the locker. Any evidence of tampering of the bag could result in an incident and a result cancellation. In addition, the testing center will not assume responsibility for your personal belongings. The testing waiting areas are generally small; friends or family members who accompany you are not permitted to wait in the testing center while you are taking the examination.

Once you have completed the admission process, the test administrator will escort you to the assigned computer. You will be seated at an individual work space area that includes computer equipment, appropriate lighting, and erasable note board or white board and a marker. No items, including unauthorized scratch paper, are allowed into the testing room. Eating, drinking, or the use of tobacco is not allowed in the testing room. You will be observed at all times by the test administrator while taking the examination. Additionally, video and audio recordings of all test sessions are made. Pearson Professional Centers has no control over the sounds made by typing on the computer by others. If these sounds are distracting, raise your hand to summon the test administrator. Earplugs are available on request.

You must follow the directions given by the test center staff and must remain seated during the test except when authorized to leave. If you think that you have a problem with the computer, need an additional erasable or white board, need to take a break, or need the test administrator for any reason, you must raise your hand. You are also encouraged to access the candidate website (http://www.pearsonvue.com/nclex) to obtain additional information about the physical environment of the test center.

Testing Time

The maximum testing time is 5 hours; this period includes the tutorial, the sample items, all breaks, and the examination. All breaks are optional and count against testing time. If you take a break, you must leave the testing room, and when you return, you may be required to perform identity confirmation procedures to be readmitted.

Length of the Examination

The minimum number of questions that you will need to answer is 85. Of these 85 questions, 25 will be pretest (unscored) questions. The maximum number of questions in the test is 205.

The pretest questions are questions that may be presented as scored questions on future examinations. These pretest questions are not identified as such. In other words, you do not know which questions are the pretest (unscored) questions.

Pass-or-Fail Decisions

All the examination questions are categorized by test plan area and level of difficulty. This is an important point to keep in mind when you consider how the computer makes a pass-or-fail decision because a pass-or-fail decision is not based on a percentage of correctly answered questions.

The NCSBN indicates that a pass-or-fail decision is governed by three different scenarios. The first scenario is the 95% Confidence Interval Rule, in which the computer stops administering test questions when it is 95% certain that the test-taker's ability is clearly above the passing standard or clearly below the passing standard. The second scenario is known as the Maximum-Length Exam, in which the final ability estimate of the test-taker is considered. If the final ability estimate is above the passing standard, the test-taker passes; if it is below the passing standard, the test-taker fails.

The third scenario is the Run-Out-Of-Time Rule (R.O.O.T). If the examination ends because the test-taker ran out of time, the computer may not have enough information with 95% certainty to make a clear pass-or-fail decision. If this is the case, the computer will review the test-taker's performance during testing. If the test-taker has not answered the minimum number of required questions, the test-taker fails. If the test-taker's ability estimate was consistently above the passing standard on the last 60 questions, the test-taker passes. If the test-taker's ability estimate falls to or below the passing standard, even once, the test-taker fails. Additional information about pass-or-fail decisions can be found in the 2014 NCLEX examination candidate bulletin located at www.ncsbn.org.

Completing the Examination

When the examination has ended, you will complete a brief computer-delivered questionnaire about your testing experience. After you complete this questionnaire, you need to raise your hand to summon the test administrator. The test administrator will collect and inventory all erasable or white boards and then permit you to leave.

Processing Results

Every computerized examination is scored twice, once by the computer at the testing center and again after the examination is transmitted to Pearson Professional Centers. No results are released at the test center. The board of nursing receives your result, and you will be notified 2 days to 2 weeks after you take the examination. In some states, an unofficial result can be obtained via the Quick Results Service 2 business days after taking the examination. This can be done through the Internet or telephone, and there is a fee for this service. Information about obtaining your NCLEX result by this method can be obtained on the NCSBN website under "candidate services."

Candidate Performance Report

A candidate performance report is provided to a test-taker who failed the examination. This report provides the test-taker with information about her or his strengths and weaknesses in relation to the test plan framework and provides a guide for studying and retaking the examination. If a retake is necessary, the candidate must wait 45 to 90 days between examination administration. Test-takers should refer to the state board of nursing in the state in which licensure is sought for procedures regarding when the examination can be taken again.

Interstate Endorsement

Because the NCLEX-PN examination is a national examination, you can apply to take the examination in any state. When licensure is received, you can apply for interstate endorsement, which is obtaining another license in another state to practice nursing in that state. The procedures and requirements for interstate endorsement may vary from state to state, and these procedures can be obtained from the state board of nursing in the state in which endorsement is sought. You may also be allowed to practice nursing in another state if the state has enacted a Nurse Licensure Compact. The state boards of nursing can be accessed via the NCSBN website at http://www.ncsbn.org. States that participate in the Nurse Licensure Compact can also be located on this website.

Nurse Licensure Compact

It may be possible to hold one license from the state of residency and practice nursing in another state under the mutual recognition model of nursing licensure if the state has enacted a Nurse Licensure Compact. To obtain information about the Nurse Licensure Compact and the states that are part of this interstate compact, access the NCSBN website at http://www.ncsbn.org.

Additional Information About the Examination

Additional information regarding the NCLEX-PN examination can be obtained through the NCLEX examination candidate bulletin located on the NCSBN website and from the NCSBN, 111 East Wacker Drive, Suite 2900, Chicago, IL 60601. The telephone number for the NCLEX examinations department is 866-293-9600. The website is http://www.ncsbn.org.

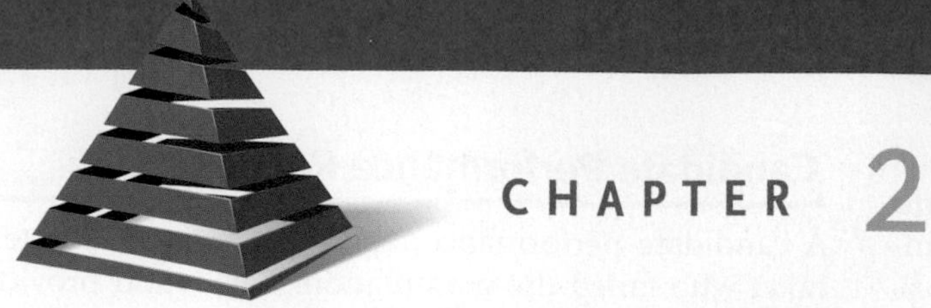

CHAPTER 2

NCLEX-PN® Preparation for Foreign-Educated Nurses

You have taken an important first step: seeking the information that you need to know to become a licensed practical nurse (LPN) in the United States. The challenge that is presented to you is one that requires great patience and endurance. The positive result of your endeavor will reward you professionally, however, and give you the personal satisfaction of knowing that you have become part of a family of highly skilled nurses.

National Council of State Boards of Nursing

The National Council of State Boards of Nursing (NCSBN) is the agency that develops and administers the NCLEX-PN® examination, the examination that you need to pass to become licensed as a nurse in the United States. Guidelines and procedures must be followed, and documents must be sought and submitted to become eligible to take this examination. This chapter provides general information regarding the process you need to pursue to become a licensed nurse in the United States. An important first step in the process of obtaining information about becoming a licensed nurse in the United States is to access the NCSBN website at http://www.ncsbn.org and obtain information provided for international nurses in the NCLEX website link. The NCSBN provides information about some of the documents you need to obtain as an international nurse seeking licensure in the United States and about credentialing agencies. The NCSBN also provides a resource manual for international nurses that contains all the necessary licensure information regarding the requirements for education, English proficiency, and immigration requirements such as visas and VisaScreens. You are encouraged to access the NCSBN website to obtain the most current information about seeking licensure as a nurse in the United States.

⚠ A first step is to access the NCSBN website at http://www.ncsbn.org and obtain the information provided for international nurses in the NCLEX website link. The resource manual can be located at www.ncsbn.org/Resource:manual_for_international_nurses.pdf.

State Requirements for Licensure

An important factor to consider as you pursue this process is that some requirements may vary from state to state. You need to contact the board of nursing in the state in which you are planning to obtain licensure to determine the specific requirements and documents that you need to submit. Boards of nursing can decide either to use a credentialing agency to evaluate your documents or to review your documents at the specific state board, known as in-house evaluation. When you contact the board of nursing in the state in which you intend to work as a nurse, inform them that you were educated outside of the United States and ask that they send you an application to apply for licensure by examination. Be sure to specify that you are applying for LPN licensure. You should also ask about the specific documents needed to become eligible to take the NCLEX exam. You can obtain contact information for each state board of nursing through the NCSBN website at http://www.ncsbn.org. When you have accessed the NCSBN website, select the link titled "Boards of Nursing." Additionally, you can write to the NCSBN regarding the NCLEX exam. The address is 111 East Wacker Drive, Suite 2900, Chicago, IL 60601. The telephone number for the NCSBN is (866) 293-9600; the fax number is (312) 279-1036.

⚠ Contact the board of nursing in the state in which you are planning to obtain licensure to determine the specific requirements and documents that you need to submit. Documents that you need to submit vary state by state.

Credentialing Agencies

The state board of nursing in the state in which you are seeking licensure may choose to use a credentialing agency to review your documents. If so, it is necessary that you use the credentialing agency that the state requires. The state board of nursing will provide you with the name and contact information of the credentialing agency. Seeking this information is important because you need to know where to send your required documents. Additionally, the NCSBN website (http://www.ncsbn.org) can provide information about credentialing agencies.

General Licensure Requirements

Required documents may vary, depending on the state requirements. These documents must be sent to either the state board of nursing or the credentialing agency specified by the state. Neither the credentialing agency nor the state board of nursing will accept these documents if they are sent directly from you. These documents must be official documents sent directly from the licensing authority or other agency in your home country to verify validity. Some of the general documents required are listed in Box 2-1; however, remember that the documents you need to submit vary state by state. Use the list provided in Box 2-1 as a checklist for yourself after you have found out about the documents you are required to submit.

When all of your documents have been submitted, they will be reviewed. If you have met the eligibility requirements to take the NCLEX examination, you will be notified that you are eligible. Then you need to obtain an application to take the NCLEX exam from the state in which you intend to seek licensure and submit the required fees. Your application will be reviewed and processed, and you will be notified that you can make an appointment to take the NCLEX exam. Additional information about the application process for the NCLEX exam can be obtained at the NCSBN website at www.ncsbn.org. Box 2-2 provides a brief guide of the general steps to take in the licensure process.

BOX 2-1 Some Documents Needed to Obtain Licensure

1. Proof of citizenship or lawful alien status
2. Work visa
3. VisaScreen certificate
4. Commission on Graduates of Foreign Nursing Schools (CGFNS) certificate
5. Criminal background check documents
6. Official transcripts of educational credentials sent directly to credentialing agency or board of nursing from home country school of nursing
7. Validation of a comparable nursing education as that provided in U.S. nursing programs; this may include theoretical instruction and clinical practice in a variety of nursing areas, including, but not limited to, medical nursing, surgical nursing, pediatric nursing, maternity and newborn nursing, community and public health nursing, and mental health nursing
8. Validation of safe professional nursing practice in home country
9. Copy of nursing license or diploma or both
10. Proof of proficiency in the English language
11. Photograph(s)
12. Social Security number
13. Application and fees

BOX 2-2 General Steps in the Licensure Process

1. Access the NCSBN website at http://www.ncsbn.org, and read the literature provided for international nurses.
2. Contact the board of nursing in the state in which you are planning to obtain licensure to determine the specific requirements and documents that you need to submit.
3. Have the required documents sent from the appropriate agency in your home country.
4. When you are notified about eligibility to take the NCLEX exam, obtain the application form from the state in which you intend to obtain licensure, complete the form, and submit it with required fees.
5. Schedule an appointment to take the NCLEX exam when you receive your Authorization to Test (ATT) form.
6. Take the NCLEX exam.
7. Become a licensed nurse in the United States.

⚠ Official documents must be sent directly from the licensing authority or other agency in your home country.

Work Visa

A foreign-educated nurse who wants to work in the United States needs to obtain the proper work visa or visas. Obtaining the work visa is a U.S. federal government requirement. To obtain information about the work visa and the application process, contact the Department of Homeland Security (DHS), Office of U.S. Citizenship and Immigration Services (USCIS). The website is http://www.immigrationdirect.com/index.html.

VisaScreen

U.S. immigration law requires certain health care professionals to complete a screening program successfully before receiving an occupational (work) visa (Section §343 of the Illegal Immigration Reform and Immigration Responsibility Act of 1996). To become a licensed nurse in the United States, you are required to obtain a VisaScreen certificate. You can ask about the VisaScreen certificate when you make your initial contact with the state board of nursing in which you are seeking licensure. The VisaScreen is a federal screening program, and the certificate needs to be obtained through an organization that offers this program.

⚠ Obtaining the work visa and the VisaScreen is a U.S. federal government requirement.

The Commission on Graduates of Foreign Nursing Schools (CGFNS) is an organization that offers this federal screening program. The VisaScreen components of this program include an educational analysis, license verification, assessment of proficiency in the English language, and an examination that tests nursing knowledge. When the applicant successfully achieves each component, the applicant is presented with a VisaScreen certificate. You can obtain information related to the VisaScreen through the CGFNS website at http://www.cgfns.org. The CGFNS website also provides you with specific information about the components of this program.

The Commission on Graduates of Foreign Nursing Schools (CGFNS) is also a credentialing agency and awards a CGFNS certificate to the applicant when all eligibility requirements are met. Some state boards of nursing use the CGFNS as a credentialing agency and require a CGFNS certificate, whereas others do not. Check with the state board of nursing regarding this certificate. The CGFNS certification program contains three parts, and you must complete all parts successfully to be awarded a CGFNS certificate. The three parts include a credentials review, a qualifying examination that tests nursing knowledge, and an English language proficiency examination. These components are similar to those needed to obtain the VisaScreen certificate. You can obtain information related to the CGFNS certificate through the CGFNS website at http://www.cgfns.org.

⚠ The NCLEX examination is administered in English only.

Registering to Take the NCLEX Exam

When you have completed all state and federal requirements and received documentation that you are eligible to take the NCLEX examination, you can register for the exam. You need to obtain information from the state board of nursing in the state in which you are seeking licensure regarding the specific registration process because the process may vary from state to state. The NCLEX candidate website is http://www.pearsonvue.com/nclex, and you are encouraged to access this site for additional information. Following the registration instructions and completing the registration forms precisely and accurately are important. You must pay a fee for taking the examination, and you may have to pay additional fees to the board of nursing in the state in which you are applying. When your eligibility is determined by the state licensure board, you will receive an Authorization to Test (ATT) form via email. You cannot make an appointment to test until the board of nursing declares eligibility and you receive an ATT form.

⚠ Registration forms for taking the NCLEX exam that are not properly completed or not accompanied by the proper fees in the required method of payment will be returned to you and will delay testing.

The examination takes place at a Pearson Professional Center, and you can make an appointment through the Internet or by telephone. You can schedule an appointment at any Pearson Professional Center. You do not have to take the exam in the state in which you are seeking licensure. NCLEX exam testing abroad is also available in some countries, and it is recommended that you visit the NCLEX website for current information about international testing sites. Chapter 1 contains additional information regarding the NCLEX exam and testing procedures. You can also obtain information about the registration process and testing procedures from the NCSBN website at http://www.ncsbn.org.

Preparing to Take the NCLEX Exam

When you have successfully completed the requirements to become eligible to take the NCLEX exam, you have one more important goal to achieve: to pass the NCLEX exam.

⚠ Begin preparing for the NCLEX exam as soon as possible; start preparing even before you begin the licensure process.

I highly recommend adequate preparation for the NCLEX exam because the examination is difficult. An important step that you have taken in preparing is that you are using this book, *Saunders Comprehensive Review for the NCLEX-PN® Examination*. After you have reviewed the content and answered the practice questions, the next step in your journey to success is to use the companion book, *Saunders Q&A Review for the NCLEX-PN® Examination*; this book provides you with more than 3200 practice questions based on the NCLEX-PN examination test plan framework, with a specific focus on Client Needs and Integrated Processes. Then you will be ready for *HESI/Saunders Online Review for the NCLEX-PN® Examination*. Additional products in Saunders Pyramid to Success include *Saunders Strategies for Test Success: Passing Nursing School and the NCLEX® Exam* and *Saunders Q&A Review Cards for the NCLEX-PN® Exam*. These additional products are described next.

HESI/Saunders Online Review for the NCLEX-PN® Examination addresses all areas of the test plan identified by the NCSBN. The course contains a pretest that provides feedback regarding your strengths and weaknesses and that generates an individualized study schedule in a calendar format. Content review is in an outline format and includes self-check practice questions and testlets (case studies), figures and illustrations, a glossary, and animations and videos. Numerous practice exams are included. There are more than 2500 practice questions, and the types of questions in this course include multiple-choice and alternate item formats.

Saunders Strategies for Test Success: Passing Nursing School and the NCLEX® Exam focuses on the test-taking strategies that will prepare you for the NCLEX-PN exam. The chapters describe all the test-taking strategies and include several sample questions that illustrate how to use the test-taking strategy. This book has 1000 practice questions. All the practice questions reflect the framework and the content identified in the NCLEX-PN test plan and include multiple-choice and alternate item format questions. In addition to the focus on test-taking strategies, information on cultural characteristics and practices, pharmacology strategies, medication and intravenous calculations, laboratory values, positioning guidelines, and therapeutic diets is included in the book.

Saunders Q&A Review Cards for the NCLEX-PN® Exam is organized by the test plan framework of the NCLEX-PN test plan. It provides you with 1200 unique practice test questions on portable and easy-to-use cards. The question is on the front of the card, and the answer, rationale, test-taking strategy, and content area code are on the back of the card. This product includes multiple-choice questions and alternate item format questions.

All the products in the Saunders Pyramid to Success can be obtained online by visiting http://elsevierhealth.com or by calling 800-545-2522.

Stay positive and confident, and believe that you can achieve your goal.

Finally, never lose sight of your goal. Patience and dedication contribute significantly to your achieving the status of a licensed nurse. Remember, success is climbing a mountain, facing the challenge of obstacles, and reaching the top of the mountain. I wish you the best success in your journey and beginning your career as a licensed nurse in the United States.

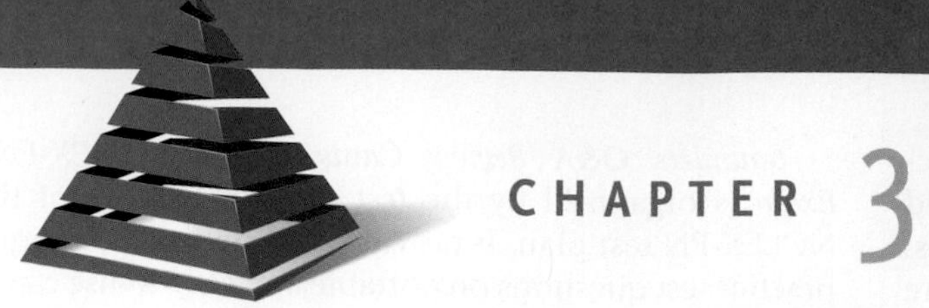

CHAPTER 3

Pathways to Success

Laurent W. Valliere, BS, DD

Pyramid to Success

Preparing to take the NCLEX-PN® exam can produce a great deal of anxiety. You may be thinking that the NCLEX-PN is the most important exam that you will ever have to take and that it reflects the culmination of everything for which you have worked so hard. The NCLEX-PN is an important exam because receiving that nursing license means that you can begin your career as a licensed practical/vocational nurse. Your success on the NCLEX-PN involves expelling all thoughts from your mind that allow this exam to appear overwhelming and intimidating; such thoughts will take complete control over your destiny. A positive attitude, a structured plan for preparation, and maintaining control of your pathway to success will ensure your achievement of reaching the peak of the Pyramid to Success (Fig. 3-1).

Pathways to Success (Box 3-1)

The Foundation

The foundation of the Pathways to Success begins with a positive attitude, the belief that you will achieve success, and the development of control. It also includes the creation of a list of your personal short- and long-term goals and a plan for preparation. A positive attitude, belief in yourself, control, and a list of personal goals will lead you to becoming a licensed practical/vocational nurse. Without these components, your Pathway to Success leads to nowhere and has no end point. You will expend energy and valuable time in your journey, but you will lack control over where you are heading, and you will experience exhaustion without any accomplishment. Therefore, it is imperative that you take the time to develop that positive attitude and to establish your short- and long-term goals.

Where do you start? To begin this process, find a location that offers solitude. Sit or lie in a comfortable position, close your eyes, relax, inhale deeply, hold your breath to a count of 4, exhale slowly, and, again, relax. Repeat this breathing exercise several times until you begin to feel relaxed, free from anxiety, and in control of your destiny. Allow your mind to become void of all of the mind chatter; you are now in control, and your mind can see for miles. Your highway of life has a multitude of destinations to which you may travel. Next, reflect on all that you have accomplished and the path that brought you to where you are today. Keep a journal of your reflections as you plan the order of your journey to the Pyramid to Success.

The List

It is time to create "The List." "The List" is your set of short- and long-term goals. Begin by developing the goals you wish to accomplish today, tomorrow, over the next month, and into the future. Allow yourself the opportunity to list all that is flowing from your mind. Write your goals in your personal journal. When "The List" is complete, put it away for 2 or 3 days. After that time, retrieve and review "The List," and begin the process of planning for preparing for the NCLEX-PN exam.

The Plan for Preparation

Now that you have "The List" in order, look at the goals that relate to studying for the licensing exam. The first task is to decide what study pattern works best for you. Think about what has worked most successfully for you in the past. There are questions that must be addressed to develop your plan for study. These questions are identified in Box 3-2.

The plan must include a schedule. Use a calendar to plan and document the times and nursing content areas for your study sessions. Establish a realistic schedule that includes your daily, weekly, and future goals, and adhere to it. This consistency will provide advantages to you and those supporting you. A daily schedule allows you to plan your content areas for study more carefully. Stick to your plan of study. Adherence to the plan helps you develop a rhythm that can only enhance your retention and positive momentum. The people who are supporting you will share this rhythm, and they will be able to schedule their activities and life better because you are consistent with your study schedule. You are moving forward, and you are in control!

The length of the study session will depend on you and your ability to focus and concentrate. What you need to think about is quality rather than quantity when you are determining a realistic amount of time for each

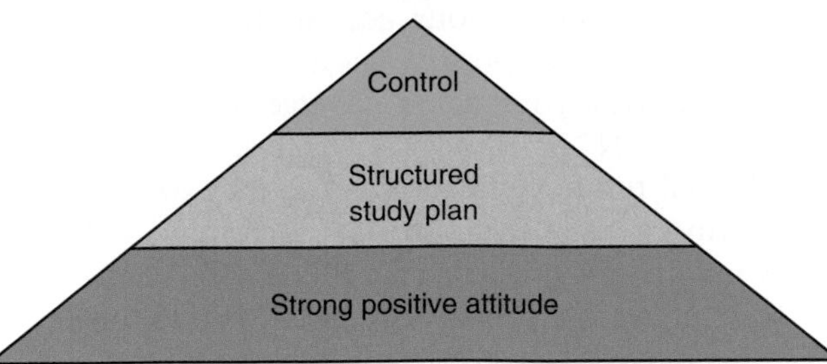

FIGURE 3-1 The Pyramid to Success.

BOX 3-1 Pathways to Success

The Foundation
- Maintaining a positive attitude
- Thinking about realistic short- and long-term goals
- Preparing a plan for preparation
- Maintaining control

The List
- Journaling realistic short- and long-term goals

The Plan for Preparation
- Developing a study plan and schedule
- Deciding on the place to study
- Balancing personal and work obligations with the study schedule
- Sharing the study schedule and personal needs with others
- Implementing the study plan

Positive Pampering
- Planning time for exercise and fun activities
- Establishing healthy eating habits
- Including activities in the schedule that provide positive mental stimulation

Final Preparation
- Reviewing and identifying goals that have been achieved
- Remaining focused to complete the plan of study
- Writing down the date and time of the exam and posting it next to your name with the letters "LPN" or "LVN" after it, along with the word "YES!"
- Taking a test drive to the testing center
- Enjoying relaxing activities on the day before the exam

The Day of the Exam
- Grooming yourself for success
- Eating a healthy and nutritious breakfast
- Maintaining a confident and positive attitude
- Maintaining control
- Meeting the challenges of the day
- Reaching the peak of the Pyramid to Success

session. Plan to schedule at least 2 hours of daily quality study time. If you can spend more than 2 hours studying, then by all means do so.

You may be asking yourself, "What do you mean by quality time?" Quality time means spending

BOX 3-2 Developing a Plan of Study

- Do I work better alone or in a group study environment?
- If I work best in a group, does the group consist of one, two, or more study partners?
- Who are these study partners?
- How long should my study sessions last?
- Does the time of day that I study make a difference for me?
- Do I retain more if I study in the morning?
- How does my work schedule affect my study pattern?
- How do I balance my family obligations with my need to study?
- Do I have a comfortable study area at home, or do I need to find another environment that is more conducive to my study needs?

uninterrupted quiet time focusing on your study session. This may mean that you will have to isolate yourself for these study sessions. Think again about what has worked for you during nursing school when you studied for exams, and select a study place that has also worked for you in the past. If you have a special study room at home that you have always used, then plan your study sessions in that special room. If you have always studied at a library, then plan your study sessions for the library. If you plan to study at home, make the time spent studying uninterrupted and quiet. Sometimes it is difficult to balance your study time with your family obligations and possibly a work schedule, but if you can, plan your study time for when you know that you will be at home alone. Try to eliminate anything that may be distracting during your study time. Shut off your cell phone so that you will not be disturbed. If you have small children, plan your study time during their nap time or school hours.

Your plan must include the ways in which you will manage your study needs and the demands of your work, family, and friends. Take time to think about how you will balance your everyday commitments with your plan for study. Your family and friends are key players in your life, and they are going to become a part of your Pyramid to Success. After you have established your study needs, communicate your needs and the importance of your study plan for achieving your goal of becoming a licensed practical/vocational nurse to your family and friends.

A difficult part of the plan may be how you will deal with those family and friends who choose not to participate in your Pathways to Success. What if an individual or individuals choose not to be part of your plan? For example, what do you do if a friend asks you to go to a movie during your scheduled study time? Your friend may say, "Come on. Take some time off. You have plenty of time to study. Study later when we get back!" Then you are faced with a decision. You must weigh all of the factors carefully. You must keep your goals in mind and remember that your need for positive momentum is critical. Your decision may not be an easy one, but it must be one that will help you ensure that your goal of becoming a licensed practical/vocational nurse is achieved. Remember, positive momentum and meeting your goals are most important.

Positive Pampering

Positive pampering means that you must continue to care for yourself holistically. Positive momentum can be maintained only if you are properly balanced. Proper exercise, diet, and positive mental stimulation are critical to achieving your goal of becoming a licensed practical/vocational nurse. Just as you have developed a schedule for study, you should have a schedule that includes some fun and some form of physical activity. It is your choice—aerobics, running, walking, weight lifting, bowling, or whatever makes you feel good about yourself. Time spent away from the hard study schedule and devoted to some form of fun and physical exercise pays its rewards 100-fold. You will feel alive and more energetic with a schedule that includes these activities.

Establish healthy eating habits. Stay away from fatty foods because they will slow you down. Eat lighter meals, and eat more frequently. Include complex carbohydrates in your diet for energy, and be careful not to include too much caffeine in your daily diet. Continue to feel good about yourself, because you are in control.

Take the time to pamper yourself with activities that make you feel even better about who you are. Make dinner reservations at your favorite restaurant with someone who is special and who is supporting your goal of becoming a licensed practical/vocational nurse. Take walks in a place that has a particular tranquility that enables you to reflect on the positive momentum that you have achieved and maintained. Whatever it is and wherever it takes you, allow yourself the time to do some positive pampering.

Final Preparation

You have established the foundation of your Pyramid to Success. You have developed your list of goals and your study plan, and you have maintained your positive momentum. You are moving forward, and you are in control. When you receive your date and time for the NCLEX-PN exam, you may immediately think, "I'm not ready!" Stop! Reflect on all that you have achieved. Think about your goal achievement and the organization of the positive life momentum with which you have surrounded yourself. Think about all those individuals who love and support your effort to become a licensed practical/vocational nurse. Believe that the challenge that awaits you is one that you have successfully prepared for and that will lead you to your goal of becoming a licensed practical/vocational nurse!

Take a deep breath, and organize the remaining days so that they support your educational and personal needs. Support your positive momentum with a visual technique. Write your name in large letters, and write the letters "LPN" or "LVN" after it. Post one or more of these visual reinforcements in areas that you frequent. This form of visual motivational technique works for many individuals preparing for this exam.

Through all that you have accomplished to this point, it is imperative that you not fall into the trap of expecting too much of yourself. The idea of perfection must not drive you to a point that causes your positive momentum to hesitate. You must believe in who you are as you are, and you need to stay focused on your goal. Allow yourself the opportunity to continue to carry out your plan in a manner that is the most conducive to who you are. The date and time are in hand. Write down the date and time, and underneath write the word "YES!" Post this next to your note with your name plus "LPN" or "LVN."

You must ensure that you know how to get to the testing center. A test run is a must. Time the drive, and allow for road construction or other problems that may slow down traffic. On the test run, when you arrive at the testing facility, you may want to walk into it. Walk in and become familiar with the lobby and the surroundings. This may help to alleviate some of the peripheral nervousness associated with entering an unknown building. Remember, you must do whatever it takes to keep yourself in control. If familiarizing yourself with the facility will help you to maintain positive momentum, then by all means be sure to do so. Who is in control? *You* are!

It is time to check your study plan and make the necessary adjustments now that a firm date and time are set. Adjust your review so that it flows to your needs and so that your study plan ends 2 days before the exam. Remember that the mind is like a muscle. If it is overworked, it has no strength or stamina. Your strategy is to rest the body and mind on the day before the examination. Your strategy is to stay in control and allow yourself the opportunity to be absolutely fresh and attentive on the day of the examination. This will help you to control the nervousness that is natural, achieve the clear thought processes required, and feel confident that you have done all that is necessary to prepare for and conquer this challenge. The day before the exam is to be one of pleasure. Treat yourself to what you enjoy the most.

Relax! Take a deep breath, hold it to a count of 4, and exhale slowly. You have prepared yourself well for the challenge of tomorrow. Allow yourself a good night's sleep, and wake up on the day of the exam knowing that you are absolutely ready to succeed. Look at your name with "LPN" or "LVN" after it and the word "YES!"

The Day of the Exam (Box 3-3)

Wake up believing in yourself and knowing that all you have accomplished is about to propel you to the

BOX 3-3 The Day of the Exam

Breathe—Inhale deeply, hold your breath to a count of 4, and exhale slowly.
Believe—Have positive thoughts today, and keep those thoughts focused on your achievements.
Control—You are in command!
Believe —This is your day!
Visualize—"LPN" or "LVN" with your name!

professional level of becoming a licensed practical/vocational nurse. Allow yourself plenty of time, eat a nutritious breakfast, and groom yourself for success. You are ready to meet the challenges of the day and overcome any obstacle that may face you. Your test day will soon be history, and then you will receive your test result, which will have your name with the letters "LPN" or "LVN" after it.

Be proud and confident of your achievements. You have worked hard to achieve your goal of becoming a licensed practical/vocational nurse. If you believe in yourself and your goals, no one person or obstacle can move you off the pathway that leads to success and to the peak of the Pyramid!

Congratulations! I wish you the very best in your career as a licensed practical/vocational nurse.

This Is Not a Test

1. What are the factors needed to ensure a productive study environment? **Select all that apply.**
   1. Secure a location that offers solitude
   2. Plan breaks during your study session
   3. Establish a realistic study schedule that includes your goals
   4. Continue with the study pattern that has worked best for you

Answer: *1, 2, 3, 4*

Rationale: A location of solitude helps to ensure concentration. Taking breaks during your study session helps to clear your mind and increase your ability to concentrate and focus. Establishing a realistic study pattern will keep you in control. Do not vary your study pattern. It has been successful for you until now, so why change it?

2. What are the key factors in your final preparation? **Select all that apply.**
   1. Remain focused on the study plan
   2. Visualize the "LPN/LVN" after your name
   3. Stop studying the day before the exam and relax
   4. Know where the testing facility is and how long it takes to get there

Answer: *1, 2, 3, 4*

Rationale: Focus on your plan of study, and success will follow. Positive reinforcement: Write your name in large letters on a piece of paper with LPN/LVN after your name and post it where you see it often. Allow yourself a day of pampering before the test. Wake up on the day of the test refreshed and ready to succeed. Ensure that you know where the testing facility is; map out your route and the average time it takes to arrive.

3. What key points do the Pathways to Success emphasize to help ensure your success? **Select all that apply.**
   1. A strong positive attitude
   2. Believing in your ability to succeed
   3. Being proud and confident in your achievements
   4. Maintaining control of your mind, surrounding environment, and physical being

Answer: *1, 2, 3, 4*

Rationale: A strong, positive attitude leads to success. Believe in who you are and the goals you have set for yourself. Be "proud and confident." If you believe in yourself, you will achieve success. Maintain control and all your goals will be attainable.

Final Result

Your Grade: A+

Continue to "Believe" and you will succeed.

LPN/LVN belongs to you!

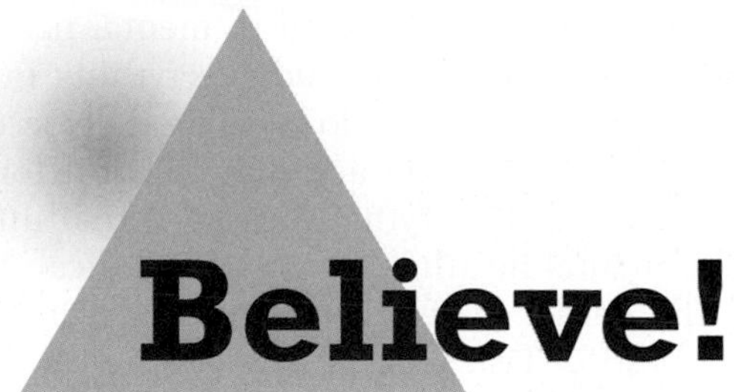

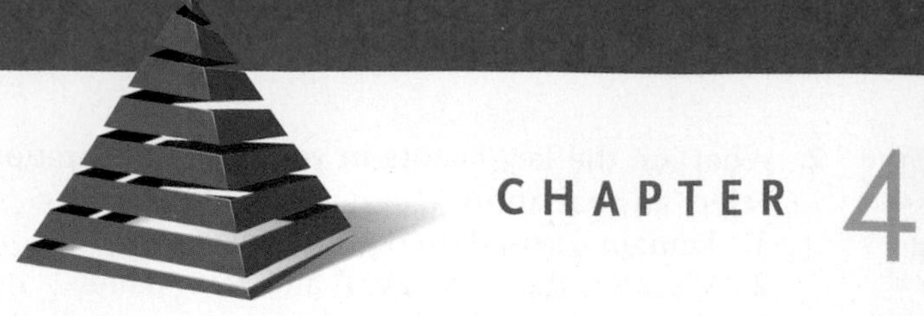

CHAPTER 4

The NCLEX-PN® Examination: From a Graduate's Perspective

Keara Cobbs, LPN

All nursing students know that passing the NCLEX® is the final test in becoming a nurse. All the hard work put in during nursing school is preparation for the biggest test of all: the NCLEX. Taking the NCLEX is more than just a test; it is a nursing graduate's nightmare. Your fate and future in becoming a nurse are based on passing the NCLEX. As everyone has heard, after taking the NCLEX, you may feel nauseated, lightheaded, and worried that you failed. I was the kind of person who would not believe it until it happened to me. Here is my story.

I bought several books to help me prepare for the NCLEX. I even purchased a book download on my phone. One negative thing immediately was that I had way too many books. I looked through each book, but with over 5000 questions combined, I felt like I was just flipping through the pages rather than studying. I recommend that you limit your study material purchases so you can focus on one resource at a time. I used the electronic software from *Saunders Strategies for Test Success: Passing Nursing School and the NCLEX® Exam,* which helped me to identify the areas I needed to work on.

Preparing for the NCLEX is different from preparing for a test in nursing school. In class, when we were going over a certain body system, we knew what might be on the test or what material to concentrate on. While studying for the NCLEX, you are likely to get questions ranging from medical–surgical to mental health. I felt there was no way I could study everything in time to take my test. So I decided to separate each section and focus my study time on a specific section for a week or two. I divided everything up: maternal/infant, pediatrics, mental health, and medical-surgical. I tried to study the harder material first and saved the material I knew best for last. I was always good with maternal/infant and pediatrics in nursing school but struggled in medical-surgical, so I spent more of my time on medical-surgical and just briefly reviewed the content areas I knew. My teacher at St. Charles Community College always told us to review the things you did not know more than the material you knew. Reviewing the topics you already feel comfortable with does not help you with topics you find more difficult. My goal was to strengthen my weaknesses.

I started studying at the end of March, after our NCLEX review class in nursing school. I scheduled my NCLEX test for May 7, so I had a month and a half to prepare. I took studying for the NCLEX very seriously. I studied five times a day for 1 or 2 hours, with breaks. I worked part-time on the weekends as a server, and while I was at work, I would review flash cards and exam questions during my breaks. The most important part of studying was going over the lab values and the drugs. There are so many drugs to remember. I used *Saunders Strategies for Test Success: Passing Nursing School and the NCLEX® Exam* to help me remember the different drug categories by the last letters in their names. Still, after all the studying I had done, I did not feel prepared enough but was told that this was a normal feeling. The day before the test, I relaxed and tried my best not to study. I was extremely nervous.

The night before my scheduled test, I woke up at least seven times from having nightmares about failing the exam. I can definitely say it was the worst night of my life. When I finally got up, I made breakfast, prayed, and got dressed. I felt so sick that praying was the only thing that kept me from passing out before even making it to the test center. I had driven to the center the day before to become familiar with the location, but the drive on testing day seemed longer than the previous day, even though I was an hour early. I sat in my car, prayed some more, and looked over some last-minute review materials. Sitting there, I became even more anxious waiting for my time to come that I just decided to go into the building. There was a man pacing back and forth in front of the building. I realized I wasn't the only person about to lose it.

The test day is like being searched at the airport, except this time you might look a little guilty just because you're so nervous. The receptionist took my picture, checked my identification, and took my fingerprints and scanned my palms. There was a locker provided for your belongings because nothing is allowed in the testing room. Once all that was done, I was offered earplugs. I took them, thinking it would be a good idea. Then I walked to a cubicle with a computer and headphones. The woman explained the instructions and left me to take the test. There were other students around, but everyone was focused on the test they were taking. The pacing man I saw outside was in the test room, taking his test.

I put in the earplugs, and I could hear my heart beating as clearly as I would have with a stethoscope. It was a big distraction, so I took them out. The first question was an easy, commonsense question just to give you an idea of the style of questions on the exam. After that, the test began. The first couple of questions were okay, but then there was a "Select all that apply" question. I was 100% sure I got it wrong. Then I had a few illustration questions that didn't seem as hard. My test had questions on content I didn't even remember studying. There were a lot of prioritizing and delegation questions.

Every now and then, a drug question came up, and I had no idea what the drug was and its effects. I felt unprepared, and I felt like I was guessing on every question. Other nursing students who took the test previously talked about how their test shut off at 85 questions. I was on my 85th question, waiting for the computer to shut off, and it didn't. My heart felt like it stopped. I couldn't help but think I was going to fail because my computer didn't shut off. I took a deep breath and kept answering questions. I got to question 130, and my computer was still giving me questions. I felt like I sat there forever. The administration woman walked over and asked if I would like a break. I simply said, "No, thank you." I was determined to finish this test. I prayed again and continued to answer each question the best I could.

I finally finished the test with all 205 questions. I walked out of that building wanting to cry. After all the stories I heard about people failing the test when given all 205 questions, I felt I failed, too. I called everyone announcing what a failure I was, even telling my teacher. I had so many people tell me they felt the same way but passed. The only difference was that I had all 205 questions. I kept thinking it's not possible to pass with that many questions. That day I cried and prayed, hoping for a good outcome. Food was not even appealing to me at the time. I stayed in bed all day and night. I would not know my results for 3 days, and all 3 days I was sick.

The day arrived when I would get my quick results. At 7:00 AM, I went to the website and tried to get my results, but they were not posted yet. Every hour I would check. Around 11:30 AM, I finally saw the option to get quick results. I argued with myself in my head about whether I was ready to know. I was tired of the headaches and the upset stomach feeling. I needed to see my results! After I hit the "Accept Payment" button, the next screen showed my results. There in big letters was the word PASS, with my name above it. I never felt so relieved. I was confused. All I could think was "How did I pass?" and then "Thank you!" I cried again, but this time they were tears of joy. I called everyone to tell them I had passed.

Getting ready for the NCLEX in my opinion is hard. It's that hurdle you have to jump over to win the race. There is so much preparation, but on test day it feels as if you studied nothing. Even though you feel you don't know anything, you will be proven wrong because you will pass. I doubted my ability to succeed due to having all 205 questions. What helped me pass was never giving up, and I kept on trying. I am proud to have passed NCLEX after receiving all the questions, so I am able to testify to others that you can still pass with 205 questions. All the material I used was helpful, but you have to trust what you know and not doubt yourself in order to succeed in passing the NCLEX.

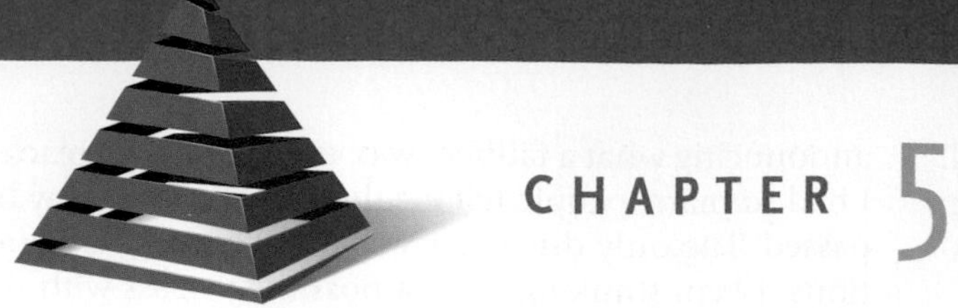

CHAPTER 5

Test-Taking Strategies

If you would like to read more about test-taking strategies after completing this chapter, *Saunders Strategies for Test Success: Passing Nursing School and the NCLEX® Exam* focuses on the test-taking strategies that will help you pass your nursing examinations while in nursing school and will prepare you for the NCLEX-PN® examination.

I. Key Test-Taking Strategies (Box 5-1)

II. How to Avoid Reading into the Question (Box 5-2)

A. Pyramid points
   1. Avoid asking yourself, "What if . . . ?" because this will lead you right into the "forbidden" act of reading into the question.
   2. Focus only on the information in the question, read every word, and make a decision regarding what the question is asking.
   3. Look for the strategic words in the question, such as *immediate, initial, first,* or *priority.* Strategic words make a difference with regard to what the question is asking about.
   4. For multiple-choice questions, multiple-response questions, or questions that require you to arrange nursing interventions or other data in order of priority, read every choice or option presented before answering.
   5. Always use the process of elimination when choices or options are presented. After you have eliminated options, reread the question before selecting your final choice or choices.
   6. With questions that require you to fill in the blank, focus on the information in the question, and determine what the question is asking. If the question requires you to calculate a medication dose, an intravenous flow rate, or intake and output amounts, recheck your work in calculating, and always use the on-screen calculator to verify the answer.

B. The Ingredients of a Question (Box 5-3)
   1. The ingredients of a question include the event, which is a client or clinical situation; the event query; and the options or answers.

BOX 5-1 Pyramid to Success

- Avoid asking yourself "What if . . . ?" because this will lead you right into reading into the question.
- Focus only on the information in the question, read every word, and make a decision regarding what the question is asking.
- Look for the strategic words in the question. Strategic words make a difference with regard to what the question is asking about.
- Always use the process of elimination when options are presented. After you have eliminated some options, reread the question before making your final choice or choices.
- Determine whether the question is a positive or negative event query.
- Use all your nursing knowledge, your clinical experiences, and your test-taking skills and strategies to answer the question.

BOX 5-2 Practice Question: Avoiding the "What If . . . ?" Syndrome and Reading into the Question

The nurse is changing the tapes on a tracheostomy tube. The client coughs, and the tube is dislodged. The nurse should take which **initial** action?

1. Cover the tracheostomy site with a sterile dressing.
2. Ventilate the client using a manual resuscitation bag.
3. Call the health care provider (HCP) to reinsert the tube.
4. Call the respiratory therapy department to reinsert the tracheostomy tube.

Answer: 2

Test-Taking Strategy: Now, you may immediately think, "The tube is dislodged, and I need the HCP." Read the question carefully, and note the **strategic word**, *initial.* Focus on the **subject** of the tube being dislodged. The question is asking you for a nursing action, so that is what you need to look for as you eliminate the incorrect options. Eliminate options 3 and 4 because they are **comparable or alike** and delay the initial intervention needed. Eliminate option 1, because this action will block the airway. If the tube is dislodged, the initial nursing action is to ventilate the client using a manual resuscitation bag. In addition, the use of the **ABCs—airway, breathing, and circulation**—will direct you to the correct option. Remember, avoid reading into the question!

BOX 5-3 Ingredients of a Question: Event, Event Query, and Options

Event: A client undergoes thoracic surgery and has two chest tubes inserted into the right pleural space that are attached to chest drainage systems.
Event Query: To promote optimal respiratory functioning, the nurse should implement which measure?
Options:

1. Milk and strip the chest tubes once per shift.
2. Position the client on the back and the right side.
3. Encourage the client to cough and deep breathe every hour.
4. Maintain the client on bed rest until the chest tubes are removed.

Answer: 3
Test-Taking Strategy: Focus on the **subject** of promoting optimal respiratory functioning. Option 1 is eliminated first, because milking and stripping a chest tube is done only with a health care provider's prescription or when allowed by agency policy. Bed rest (option 4) does not promote respiratory function and is eliminated next. From the remaining options, recalling that positioning is done according to surgeon preference directs you to option 3.

2. The event provides you with the content that you need to think about when answering the question.
3. The event query asks something specific about the content of the event.
4. The options are all of the answers provided with the question.
5. In a multiple-choice question, there will be four options, and you must select one. Read every option carefully, and think about the event and the event query as you use the process of elimination.
6. In a multiple-response question, there will be several options, and you must select all options that apply to the event in the question. Visualize the event, and use your nursing knowledge and clinical experiences to answer the question.
7. In a prioritizing (ordered-response)/drag-and-drop question, you will be required to arrange, in order of priority, nursing interventions or other data. Visualize the event, and use your nursing knowledge and clinical experiences to answer the question.
8. A fill-in-the-blank question will not contain options, and some figure/illustration questions and audio or video item formats may or may not contain options. A graphic option item will contain options in the form of a picture or graphic.
9. A chart/exhibit question will most likely contain options. Read the question carefully and all of the information in the chart/exhibit before selecting an answer.

III. The Strategic Words (Boxes 5-4 and 5-5)

A. Strategic words focus your attention on a critical point to consider when answering the question and will assist you with eliminating the incorrect options.
B. Some strategic words may indicate that all of the options are correct and that it will be necessary to prioritize to select the correct option; words that reflect the process of data collection are also important to note (see Box 5-4).
C. As you read the question, look for the strategic words; strategic words make a difference regarding the focus of the question. Throughout this book, *strategic words* presented in the question, such as those that indicate the need to prioritize, are **bolded.** If the test-taking strategy is to focus on *strategic words,* then ***strategic words*** is highlighted in blue where it appears in the test-taking strategy.

IV. The Subject of the Question (Box 5-6)

A. The subject of the question is the specific topic that the question is asking about.

BOX 5-4 Common Strategic Words and Data Collection Words

Words that Indicate the Need to Prioritize

- Best
- Early or late
- First
- Highest priority
- Immediate
- Initial
- Next
- Most
- Most appropriate or least appropriate
- Most important
- Most likely or least likely
- Primary
- Vital

Words that Reflect Data Collection

- Ascertain
- Assess
- Check
- Collect
- Determine
- Find out
- Gather
- Identify
- Monitor
- Observe
- Obtain information
- Recognize

B. Identifying the subject of the question will assist with eliminating the incorrect options and direct you to the correct option. Throughout this book, if the *subject* of the question is a specific strategy to use in answering the question correctly, it is highlighted in the test-taking strategy. Also, the specific content area to review—for example, *heart failure*—is in bold magenta.

C. The highlighting of the strategy and specific content areas will provide you with guidance on what topics to review for further remediation in *Saunders Strategies for Test Success: Passing Nursing School and the NCLEX® Exam* and *Saunders Comprehensive Review for the NCLEX-PN® Examination*.

BOX 5-5 Practice Question: Strategic Words

A client with a diagnosis of heart failure reports the occurrence of sudden shortness of breath and dyspnea. The nurse should take which **immediate** action?

1. Administer oxygen
2. Elevate the head of the bed
3. Call the health care provider
4. Prepare to administer furosemide (Lasix)

Answer: 2

Test-Taking Strategy: Note the **strategic word**, *immediate*. Focusing on this **strategic word** and the client's symptoms (shortness of breath and dyspnea) will direct you to the correct option. Note that the question is asking for an *immediate* nursing action, so that is what you need to look for as you eliminate each incorrect option. Although options 1, 3, and 4 are actions that will be taken, repositioning the client is a quick action that will assist to alleviate respiratory distress. Remember to look for **strategic words**!

BOX 5-6 Practice Question: The Subject of the Question

The nurse is planning to teach a client in skeletal leg traction about measures to increase bed mobility. Which item should be **most** helpful for this client?

1. Television
2. Fracture bedpan
3. Overhead trapeze
4. Reading materials

Answer: 3

Test-Taking Strategy: Focus on the **subject** of increasing bed mobility. Also note the **strategic word**, *most*. The use of an overhead trapeze is extremely helpful for assisting a client with moving about in bed and with getting on and off of the bedpan. Television and reading materials are helpful to reduce boredom and provide distraction. A fracture bedpan is useful for reducing discomfort with elimination. Remember to focus on the **subject**!

V. **Positive and Negative Event Queries (Boxes 5-7 and 5-8)**

A. A positive event query uses words that ask you to select an option that is correct. For example, the event query may read, "Which statement by a client

BOX 5-7 Practice Question: Positive Event Query

The nurse has reinforced discharge instructions regarding nitroglycerin therapy to the client with angina. Which statement by the client indicates an understanding of the home use of the nitroglycerin?

1. "If I use the nitroglycerin and the pain does not subside in 15 minutes, I should go to the hospital."
2. "When I have pain, I should lie down and place a tablet under my tongue. If unrelieved in 5 minutes, I should call for an ambulance."
3. "When I have chest pain, I should put a tablet under my tongue. If I have a burning sensation, I should call my doctor immediately."
4. "When I experience chest pain, I can continue what I'm doing. If it doesn't go away in 10 minutes, I should use a nitroglycerin tablet."

Answer: 2

Test-Taking Strategy: This question identifies an example of a positive event query. Focus on the **subject**, *client understanding of the use of nitroglycerin*. The client should call emergency medical services if relief is not obtained after 5 minutes. A burning sensation is a common side effect of nitroglycerin. The client taking sublingual nitroglycerin should recline after taking the medication because lightheadedness and dizziness may occur as a result of postural hypotension. Nitroglycerin should be taken with the onset of anginal pain. Remember, positive event queries ask you to select an option that is a correct item or statement!

BOX 5-8 Practice Question: Negative Event Query

The nurse has reinforced medication instructions to a client who will be taking warfarin sodium (Coumadin) indefinitely. Which statement by the client indicates a **need for further teaching**?

1. "I need to use a soft toothbrush."
2. "I need to use a straight razor for shaving."
3. "I need to avoid drinking alcohol while taking this medication."
4. "I need to carry identification about the medication being taken."

Answer: 2

Test-Taking Strategy: This question identifies an example of a **negative event query**. Note the **strategic words**, *need for further teaching*. These strategic words indicate that you need to select an option that identifies an incorrect client statement. Recalling that warfarin sodium is an anticoagulant and that the client is at risk for bleeding will direct you to the correct option. Remember that **negative event queries** ask you to select an option that is an incorrect item or statement!

indicates an understanding of the side effects of the prescribed medication?"

B. A negative event query uses strategic words that ask you to select an option that is an incorrect item or statement. For example, the event query may read, "Which statement by a client *indicates a need for further teaching* about the side effects of the prescribed medication?"

VI. Questions that Require Prioritizing

A. Many questions in the exam may require you to use the skill of prioritizing nursing actions.

B. Look for the strategic words in the question that indicate the need to prioritize (see Box 5-4).

C. Remember, when a question requires prioritization, all options may be correct, and you need to determine the correct order of action.

D. Strategies to use to prioritize include the ABCs—airway, breathing, and circulation; Maslow's Hierarchy of Needs theory; and the steps of the nursing process (clinical problem-solving process).

E. The ABCs (Box 5-9)

1. Use the ABCs—airway, breathing, and circulation—when selecting an answer or determining the order of priority.
2. Remember the order of priority: airway, breathing, and circulation.
3. Airway is always the first priority! Note that an exception is the performance of cardiopulmonary resuscitation; in this situation, the nurse follows the CAB (circulation, airway, breathing) guidelines.

F. Maslow's Hierarchy of Needs theory (Box 5-10 and Figure 5-1)

BOX 5-9 Practice Question: Use of the ABCs

A client with a compound (open) fracture of the radius has a cast applied in the emergency department. The nurse reinforces written home care instructions and tells the client to seek medical attention **immediately** if which occurs?

1. Numbness and tingling are felt in the fingers.
2. The cast feels heavy and damp 24 hours after application.
3. The entire cast feels warm during the first 24 hours after application.
4. Bloody drainage is noted on the cast during the first 6 hours after application.

Answer: 1

Test-Taking Strategy: Note the strategic word, *immediately*. Use the ABCs—airway, breathing, and circulation—as a guide to direct you to the correct option. A limb encased in a cast is at risk for nerve damage and diminished circulation from increased pressure caused by edema. Signs of increased pressure and diminished circulation from the cast include numbness, tingling, and increased pain. Remember to use the ABCs—airway, breathing, and circulation—to prioritize!

BOX 5-10 Practice Question: Maslow's Hierarchy of Needs Theory

The nurse is assigned to care for a client experiencing dystocia. When assisting with planning care, the nurse should consider which frequent action as the **highest priority**?

1. Position changes and providing comfort measures
2. Explanations to family members about what is happening to the client
3. Monitoring for changes in the physical condition of the mother and fetus
4. Reinforcement of breathing techniques learned in childbirth preparatory classes

Answer: 3

Test-Taking Strategy: All of the options presented are correct and would be implemented during the care of this client. However, note the strategic words, *highest priority*, and use Maslow's Hierarchy of Needs theory to prioritize, remembering that physiological needs come first. Using this guideline will direct you to options 1 and 3. Next, note that option 3 is the option that addresses the physical condition of both the mother and the fetus. Remember to use Maslow's Hierarchy of Needs theory to prioritize!

1. According to Maslow's Hierarchy of Needs theory, physiological needs are the priority, followed by safety and security needs, love and belonging needs, self-esteem needs, and finally, self-actualization needs. Therefore, select the option or determine the order of priority by addressing physiological needs first.
2. When a physiological need is not addressed in the question or noted in one of the options, continue to use Maslow's Hierarchy of Needs theory as a guide, and look for the option that addresses safety.

G. Steps of the nursing process (clinical problem-solving process)

1. Use the steps of the nursing process (clinical problem-solving process) to prioritize.
2. The steps include data collection, planning, implementation, and evaluation and are followed in this order.
3. Data collection
   - **a.** Data collection questions address the process of gathering subjective and objective data relative to the client, confirming the data, and communicating and documenting information gained during data collection.
   - **b.** Remember that data collection is the first step of the nursing process (clinical problem-solving process).
   - **c.** When you are asked to select your first, immediate, or initial nursing action, follow the steps of the nursing process to prioritize when selecting the correct option.

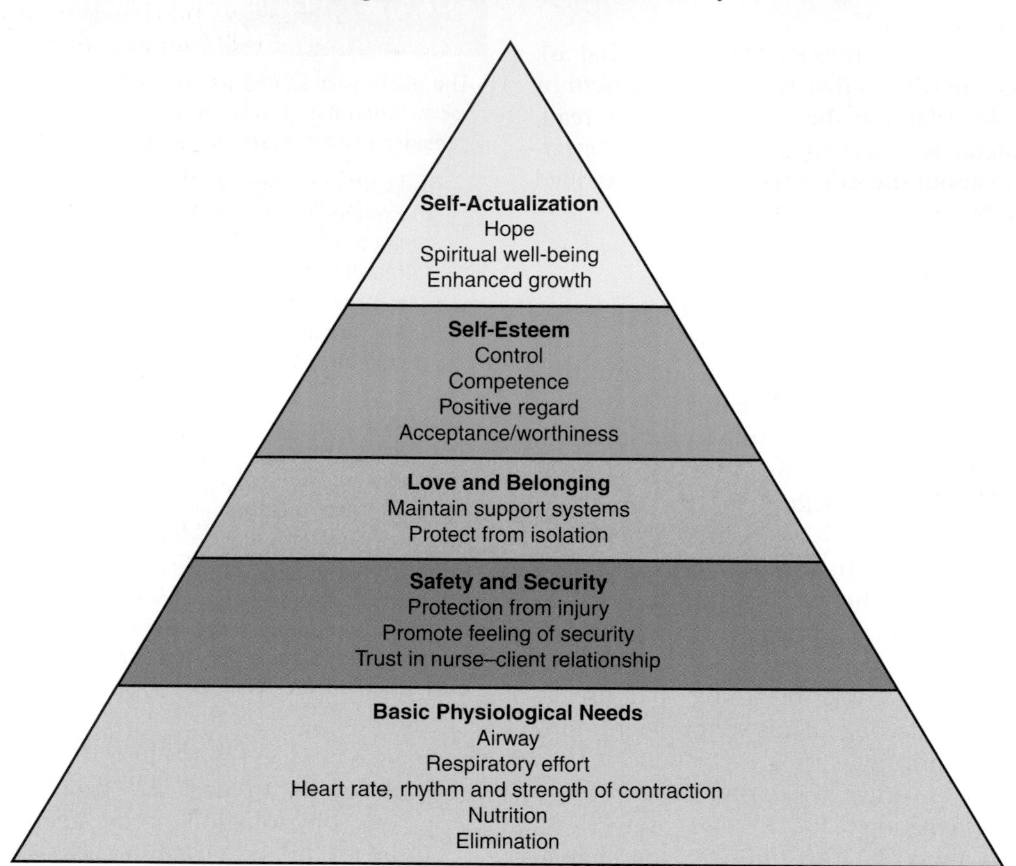

FIGURE 5-1 Using Maslow's Hierarchy of Needs theory to establish priorities. (From Harkreader H, Hogan MA, Thobaben M: Fundamentals of nursing: Caring and clinical judgment, ed 3, Philadelphia, 2007, Saunders.)

- **d.** Look for words in the options that reflect data collection (see Box 5-4).
- **e.** If an option contains the concept of collection of client data, the best choice is to select that option (Box 5-11).
- **f.** If a data-collection action is not one of the options, follow the steps of the nursing process (clinical problem-solving process) as your guide to select your first, immediate, or initial action.
- **g.** *Possible exception to the guideline:* If the question presents an emergency situation, read carefully. In an emergency situation, an intervention may be the priority.

4. Planning
   - **a.** Planning questions require prioritizing client problems, providing input into plan development, assisting with the formulation of the goals of care, and assisting with the development of a plan of care (Box 5-12).
   - **b.** Remember that existing client problems rather than potential client problems will most likely be the priority.

BOX 5-11 Practice Question: The Nursing Process/Data Collection

The nurse assists in developing a plan of care for an older client with diabetes mellitus. The nurse should plan to take which action **first**?

1. Structure menus for adherence to diet
2. Teach with videotapes showing insulin administration to ensure competence
3. Encourage dependence on others to prepare the client for the chronicity of the disease
4. Determine the client's ability to read markings on syringes and use blood glucose monitoring equipment

Answer: *4*

Test-Taking Strategy: Note the **strategic word**, *first*. Use the **steps of the nursing process** to answer the question, remembering that data collection is the first step. The only option that addresses data collection is option 4. Options 1, 2, and 3 address the implementation step of the nursing process. Remember, data collection is the first step in the **nursing process**.

BOX 5-12 Practice Question: The Nursing Process/Planning

The nurse reviews the plan of care for a client with a cataract and determines that which problem is the **priority**?

1. Concern about the loss of eyesight
2. Altered vision due to the opacity of the ocular lens
3. Difficulty moving around because of the need for glasses
4. Becoming lonely because of decreased community immersion

***Answer:* 2**
Test-Taking Strategy: This question relates to the planning of nursing care and asks you to identify the priority problem. Note the **strategic word**, *priority*. Use **Maslow's Hierarchy of Needs theory** to answer the question, remembering that physiological needs are the priority. Concern and becoming lonely are psychosocial needs and would be the last priorities. Note that the correct option directly addresses the client's problem. Remember that planning is the second step of the **nursing process**!

BOX 5-13 Practice Question: The Nursing Process/Implementation

The nurse is checking the fundus of a postpartum woman and notes that the uterus is soft and spongy. Which nursing action is appropriate **initially**?

1. Notify the health care provider
2. Encourage the mother to ambulate
3. Massage the fundus gently until it is firm
4. Document fundal position, consistency, and height

***Answer:* 3**
Test-Taking Strategy: Implementation questions address the process of organizing and managing care. Note the **strategic word**, *initially*. If the fundus is boggy (soft), it should be massaged gently until firm, and the nurse should observe for increased bleeding or clots. Remember that implementation is the third step of the **nursing process**!

5. Implementation (Box 5-13)
   a. Implementation questions address the process of assisting with organizing and managing care, providing care to achieve established goals, and communicating and documenting nursing interventions thoroughly and accurately.
   b. Focus on a nursing action rather than on a medical action when you are answering a question, unless the question is asking you what prescribed medical action is anticipated.
   c. On the NCLEX-PN, the only client that you need to be concerned about is the client in the question that you are answering. Avoid the "What if . . . ?" syndrome, and remember that the client in the question on the computer screen is your only assigned client.
   d. Answer the question from a textbook and ideal point of view; remember that the nurse has all the time and resources needed and readily available at the client's bedside; remember that you do not need to run to the treatment room to obtain, for example, sterile gauze or sterile gloves because these items will be at the client's bedside.
6. Evaluation (Box 5-14)
   a. Evaluation questions focus on comparing the actual outcomes of care with the expected outcomes and on communicating and documenting findings.
   b. These questions focus on assisting with determining the client's response to care and on identifying factors that may interfere with achieving expected outcomes.
   c. In an evaluation question, watch for negative event queries, because they are frequently used in evaluation-type questions.

VII. Client Needs

A. Safe and Effective Care Environment
   1. According to the National Council of State Boards of Nursing (NCSBN), these questions test the concepts that the nurse provides nursing care; collaborates with other health care team members to facilitate effective client care; and protects clients, significant others, and health care personnel from environmental hazards.
   2. Focus on safety with these types of questions, and remember the importance of hand washing, call bells, bed positioning, the appropriate use of side rails, asepsis, use of standard and other precautions, triage, and emergency response planning.

BOX 5-14 Practice Question: The Nursing Process/Evaluation

A client has just taken a dose of trimethobenzamide (Tigan). The nurse evaluates that the medication has been **effective** if the client states relief of which problem(s)?

1. Heartburn
2. Constipation
3. Abdominal pain
4. Nausea and vomiting

***Answer:* 4**
Test-Taking Strategy: Note the **strategic word**, *effective*. This word indicates that this is an evaluation-type question. Recalling that this medication is an antiemetic will direct you to option 4. Remember that evaluation is the fourth step of the **nursing process**!

B. Physiological Integrity

1. These questions test the concepts that the nurse provides comfort and assistance during the performance of activities of daily living; provides care related to the administration of medications; and monitors clients receiving parenteral therapies.
2. These questions also address the nurse's ability to reduce the client's potential for developing complications or health problems related to treatments, procedures, or existing conditions and the nurse's role in providing care to clients with acute, chronic, or life-threatening physical health conditions.
3. Focus on Maslow's Hierarchy of Needs theory for these types of questions, and remember that physiological needs are a priority and are addressed first.
4. Use the ABCs—airway, breathing, and circulation—and the steps of the nursing process (clinical problem-solving process) when selecting an option that addresses physiological integrity, unless the question addresses cardiopulmonary resuscitation (CPR). If the subject of the question relates to the performance of CPR, then the CAB (circulation, airway, breathing) guidelines are followed.

C. Psychosocial Integrity

1. The NCSBN notes that these questions test the concepts that the nurse provides nursing care that promotes and supports the emotional, mental, and social well-being of the client and significant others.
2. Content addressed in these questions relates to supporting and promoting the client's or significant others' abilities to cope, adapt, or problem-solve in situations involving illnesses, disabilities, or stressful events, including abuse, neglect, or violence.
3. In this Client Needs category, you may be asked communication-type questions that relate to how you would respond to a client, a client's family members or significant others, or other health care team members.
4. Use therapeutic communication techniques to answer communication questions because of their effectiveness in the communication process.
5. Remember to select the option that focuses on the thoughts, feelings, concerns, anxieties, and fears of the client; the client's family members'; or the client's significant others' (Box 5-15).

D. Health Promotion and Maintenance

1. According to the NCSBN, these questions test the concepts that the nurse provides and assists with directing nursing care to promote and maintain health.

BOX 5-15 Practice Question: Communication

A client with a diagnosis of depression says to the nurse, "I should have died. I've always been a failure." The nurse should make which therapeutic response to the client?

1. "I see a lot of positive things in you."
2. "You still have a great deal to live for."
3. "Feeling like a failure is part of your illness."
4. "You've been feeling like a failure for some time now?"

Answer: 4

Test-Taking Strategy: Use **therapeutic communication techniques** to answer this question. Address the client's feelings and concerns. Option 4 is the only option that is stated in the form of a question and that is open-ended; this will encourage the verbalization of feelings. Remember to use **therapeutic communication techniques** and focus on the client.

2. Content addressed in these questions relates to assisting the client and significant others during the normal expected stages of growth and development from conception through advanced old age and to providing client care related to the prevention and early detection of health problems.
3. Use the Teaching and Learning Theory if the question addresses client teaching, remembering that the client's willingness, desire, and readiness to learn are the first priorities.
4. Watch for negative event queries because they are frequently used in questions that address Health Promotion and Maintenance and client education.

VIII. Eliminate Comparable or Alike Options (Box 5-16)

A. When reading the options in multiple-choice questions, look for options that are comparable or alike;

BOX 5-16 Practice Question: Eliminate Comparable or Alike Options

The nurse instructs an adolescent with iron-deficiency anemia about the administration of oral iron preparations. The nurse should tell the adolescent that it is **best** to take the iron with which item?

1. Cola
2. Soda
3. Ginger ale
4. Tomato juice

Answer: 4

Test-Taking Strategy: Note the **strategic word**, *best*. Note that options 1, 2, and 3 are **comparable or alike** options in that they are carbonated beverages. Iron should be administered with vitamin C–rich fluids because vitamin C enhances the absorption of the iron preparation. Tomato juice contains a high content of ascorbic acid (vitamin C), whereas cola, soda, and ginger ale do not contain vitamin C. Remember to eliminate **comparable or alike** options!

these options will include a similar concept or nursing action.

B. Comparable or alike options can be eliminated as possible answers because it is not likely that both options will be correct.

IX. Eliminate Options that Contain Closed-Ended Words (Box 5-17)

A. Some closed-ended words include *all, always, every, must, none, never,* and *only.*

B. Eliminate options with closed-ended words because these words infer a fixed or extreme meaning; these types of options are usually incorrect.

C. Options that contain open-ended words such as *may, usually, normally, commonly,* or *generally* should be considered as possible correct options.

X. Look for the Umbrella Option (Box 5-18)

A. When answering a question, look for the umbrella option.

B. The umbrella option is one that is a broad or universal statement and that usually contains the concepts of the other options within it.

C. The umbrella option will be the correct answer.

XI. Use the Guidelines for Delegating and Assignment Making (Box 5-19)

A. You may be asked a question that will require you to decide how you will delegate a task or assign clients to other health care providers.

B. Focus on the information in the question and what task or assignment is to be delegated.

C. When you have determined what task or assignment is to be delegated, consider the client's needs, and match the client's needs with the scope of practice of the health care providers identified in the question.

D. The Nurse Practice Act and any practice limitations define which aspects of care can be delegated and which must be performed by an unlicensed assistive personnel (UAP), a licensed practical/vocational nurse, or a registered nurse.

E. In general, noninvasive interventions such as skin care, range-of-motion exercises, ambulation, grooming, and hygiene measures can be assigned to a UAP.

F. A licensed practical/vocational nurse can perform the tasks that a UAP can perform and can usually

BOX 5-17 Practice Question: Eliminate Options that Contain Closed-Ended Words

A client will undergo a barium swallow study, and the nurse reinforces preprocedure instructions to the client. The nurse should tell the client to take which action in the preprocedure period?

1. Avoid eating or drinking after midnight before the test.
2. Limit self to *only* two cigarettes on the morning of the test.
3. Have a clear-liquid breakfast *only* on the morning of the test.
4. Take *all* routine medications with a glass of water on the morning of the test.

Answer: *1*

Test-Taking Strategy: Note the closed-ended words, *only* in options 2 and 3 and *all* in option 4. Remember to eliminate options that contain closed-ended words, because these options are usually incorrect. In addition, note that options 2, 3, and 4 are comparable or alike in that they all involve taking in something on the morning of the examination. Remember to eliminate options that contain closed-ended words.

BOX 5-18 Practice Question: Look for the Umbrella Option

A client who is admitted to the hospital is diagnosed with urethritis caused by chlamydial infection. The nurse should implement which precaution to prevent contraction of the infection during care?

1. Enteric precautions
2. Contact precautions
3. Standard precautions
4. Wearing gloves and a mask

Answer: *3*

Test-Taking Strategy: Focus on the client's diagnosis and recall that this infection is sexually transmitted. Also, note that option 3 is the umbrella option. Remember, the umbrella option is a broad or universal option that includes the concepts of the other options in it!

BOX 5-19 Practice Question: Use the Guidelines for Delegating and Assignment Making

The nurse in charge of a long-term care facility is planning the client assignments for the day. Which client should be assigned to the unlicensed assistive personnel (UAP)?

1. A client on strict bed rest
2. A client with dyspnea who is receiving oxygen therapy
3. A client scheduled for transfer to the hospital for surgery
4. A client with a gastrostomy tube who requires tube feedings every 4 hours

Answer: *1*

Test-Taking Strategy: Note the subject of the question: *the assignment to be delegated to the UAP.* When asked questions related to delegation, think about the role description of the employee and the needs of the client. A client with dyspnea who is receiving oxygen therapy, a client scheduled for transfer to the hospital for surgery, or a client with a gastrostomy tube who requires tube feedings every 4 hours has both physiological and psychosocial needs that require care by a licensed nurse. The UAP has been trained to care for a client on bed rest. Remember to match the client's needs with the scope of practice of the health care provider!

perform certain invasive tasks such as dressings, suctioning, urinary catheterization, and administering oral, subcutaneous, or intramuscular medications; some selected piggyback (secondary) intravenous medications may also be administered (depending on state law and agency policy).

G. The registered nurse can perform the tasks that a licensed practical/vocational nurse can and is responsible for assessment and planning care, analyzing client data, implementing and evaluating care, supervising care, initiating teaching, and administering medications intravenously.

XII. Answering Pharmacology Questions (Box 5-20)

A. If you are familiar with the medication, use nursing knowledge to answer the question.

B. Note the name of the medication.

C. If the question identifies a medical diagnosis, then try to form a relationship between the medication and the diagnosis; for example, you can determine that cyclophosphamide (Neosar) is an antineoplastic medication if the question refers to a client with breast cancer who is taking this medication.

D. Try to determine the classification of the medication being addressed to assist with answering the question. Identifying the classification will assist in determining a medication's action or side effects or both; for example, diltiazem (*Card*izem) is a cardiac medication.

BOX 5-20 Practice Question: Answering Pharmacology Questions

The nurse is preparing to administer metoprolol ER (Toprol ER) to a client. The nurse should check which item as a **priority** before administering the medication?

1. Temperature
2. Blood pressure
3. Potassium level
4. Blood glucose level

Answer: 2

Test-Taking Strategy: Focus on the name of the medication and note the strategic word, *priority*. Recall that most β-blocker medication names end with the letters *-lol* and that these medications are used to treat hypertension. This will direct you to the correct option. Remember to focus on the medication name when answering pharmacology questions!

E. Recognize the common side effects associated with each medication classification and relate the appropriate nursing interventions to each side effect; for example, if a side effect is hypertension, the associated nursing intervention would be to monitor the blood pressure.

F. Focus on what the question is asking: intended effect, side effect, adverse effect, or toxic effect.

G. Learn medications that belong to a classification by commonalities in their names; for example, medications that are xanthine bronchodilators end with the letters *-line* (e.g., theophyl*line*).

H. Look at the medication name, and use medical terminology to assist with determining the medication action; for example, *Lopressor* lowers (*Lo*) the blood pressure (*pressor*).

I. If the question requires a medication calculation, remember that an on-screen calculator is available on the computer. Talk yourself through each step to be sure the answer makes sense, and recheck the calculation before answering the question, particularly if the answer seems like an unusual dosage.

J. Pharmacology: Pyramid Points to remember

1. In general, the client should not take an antacid with medication because the antacid will affect the absorption of the medication.
2. Enteric-coated and sustained-release tablets should not be crushed; also, capsules should not be opened.
3. The client should never adjust or change a medication dose or abruptly stop taking a medication.
4. The nurse never adjusts or changes the client's medication dosage and never discontinues a medication.
5. The client needs to avoid taking any over-the-counter medications or any other medications, such as herbal preparations, unless they are approved for use by the health care provider.
6. The client needs to avoid alcohol and smoking.
7. Medications are never administered if the prescription is difficult to read, is unclear, or identifies a medication dose that is not a normal one.
8. Additional strategies for answering pharmacology are presented in *Saunders Strategies for Test Success: Passing Nursing School and the NCLEX® Exam*.

UNIT II

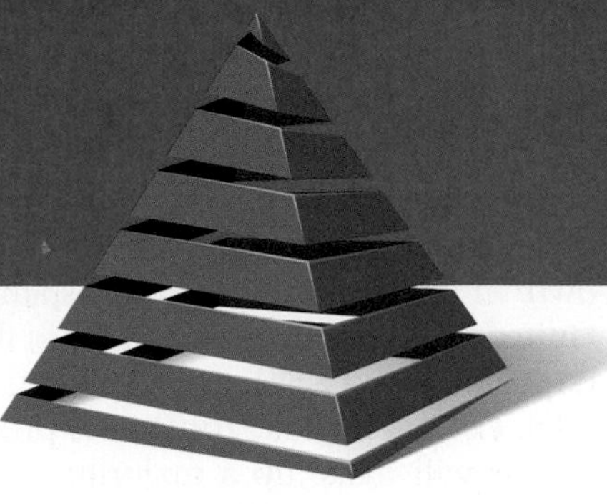

Issues in Nursing

PYRAMID TERMS

accountability Moral concept that involves acceptance by a professional nurse of the consequences of a decision or action.

advance directive Written document recognized by state law that provides directions concerning the provision of care when a client is unable to make his or her own treatment choices; the two basic types of advance directives include instructional directives such as a living wills and durable power of attorney for health care.

advocacy Acting on behalf of the client and protecting the client's right to make his or her own decisions.

Client's Bill of Rights The rights and responsibilities of clients receiving care.

confidentiality/information security In the health care system, refers to the protection of privacy of the client's personal health information.

consent Voluntary act whereby a person agrees to allow someone else to do something.

cultural awareness Learning about the culture, health care practices, and preferences of clients from different cultures.

cultural assimilation Process in which individuals from a minority group are absorbed by the dominant culture and take on the characteristics of the dominant culture.

cultural competence Acquisition of knowledge, understanding, and appreciation of a culture that facilitates provision of culturally appropriate health care.

cultural diversity Differences among groups of people that result from ethnic, racial, and cultural variables.

cultural imposition Tendency to impose one's own beliefs, values, and patterns of behavior on individuals from another culture.

culture Dynamic network of knowledge, beliefs, patterns of behavior, ideas, attitudes, values, and norms that are unique to a particular group of people.

delegation Process of transferring a selected nursing task in a situation to an individual who is competent to perform that specific task.

disaster Any human-made or natural event that causes destruction and devastation or a mass causality that cannot be alleviated without assistance; internal disasters are events that occur within a health care agency, whereas external disasters are events that occur outside the health care agency.

dominant culture Group whose values prevail within a society.

emergency response plan A health care agency's preparedness and response plan in the event of a disaster.

ethics The ideals of right and wrong; guiding principles that individuals may use to make decisions.

ethnic group People within a culture who share characteristics based on race, religion, color, national origin, or language.

ethnicity An individual's identification of self as part of an ethnic group.

evidence-based practice Approach to client care in which the nurse integrates the client's preferences, clinical expertise, and the best research evidence to deliver quality care.

informed consent A client's understanding of the reason for the proposed intervention, with its benefits and risks, and agreement with the treatment by signing a consent form. In most states, the nurse acts only as a witness to the client signing the informed consent form.

interprofessional collaboration Promotes sharing of expertise from health care professionals to create a plan of care that will restore and maintain a client's health.

leadership Interpersonal process that involves influencing others (followers) to achieve goals.

malpractice Type of negligence; failure to meet the standards of acceptable care, which results in harm to another person.

management Accomplishment of tasks or goals by oneself or by directing others.

negligence Conduct that falls below a standard of care; failure to meet a client's needs either willfully or by omission or failure to act.

prioritizing Deciding which needs or problems require immediate action and which ones could tolerate a delay in action until a later time because they are not urgent.

race A grouping of people based on biological similarities. Members of a racial group have similar physical characteristics, such as blood group; facial features; and color of skin, hair, and eyes.

racism Discrimination directed toward individuals or groups who are perceived to be inferior.

stereotyping Expectation that all people within the same racial, ethnic, or cultural group act alike and share the same beliefs and attitudes.

subculture Social group within a culture that has distinctive characteristics, such as patterns of behavior or beliefs.

triage Classifying procedure that ranks clients according to their need for medical care.

Pyramid to Success

Nurses often care for clients who come from ethnic, cultural, or religious backgrounds that are different from their own. In the past 10 years, the Hispanic population in the United States has increased by 43%; the African-American population by 12.3%; and the Asian population by 43% (U.S. Census Bureau, 2010). It is projected that minority groups will make up a majority of the U.S. population by 2042 (Perez and Hirschman, 2009). Awareness of and sensitivity to the unique health and illness beliefs and practices of people of different backgrounds are essential for the delivery of safe and effective care. Acknowledgment and acceptance of cultural differences with a nonjudgmental attitude are essential to providing culturally sensitive care. The NCLEX-PN® exam test plan is unique and individualized to the client's culture and beliefs. The nurse needs to avoid stereotyping and needs to be aware that there are several subcultures within cultures and several dialects within languages. In nursing practice, the nurse needs to assess the client's perceived needs before planning and implementing nursing care.

Across all settings in the practice of nursing, nurses frequently are confronted with ethical and legal issues related to client care. The professional nurse has the responsibility to be aware of the ethical principles, laws, and guidelines related to providing safe and quality care to clients. In the Pyramid to Success, focus on ethical practices; the Nurse Practice Act and clients' rights, particularly confidentiality, information security, and informed consent; advocacy, documentation, and advance directives; and cultural, religious, and spiritual issues. Knowledgeable use of information technology, such as an electronic health record, is also an important role of the nurse.

A nurse is a leader and a manager. As described in the NCLEX-RN exam test plan, a nurse needs to collaborate with other members of the interprofessional health care team. A primary Pyramid Point focuses on the skills required to prioritize client care activities. Pyramid Points also focus on concepts of leadership responsibilities, the process of delegation, an emergency response plan, and triaging clients.

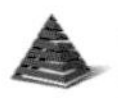

Client Needs

Safe and Effective Care Environment

Acting as a client advocate
Being familiar with the emergency response plan
Checking for advance directive documents
Checking for signed informed consent documents
Collaborating with members of the health care team about client care and referrals
Ensuring ethical practices are implemented
Ensuring legal rights and responsibilities are upheld
Establishing priorities related to client care activities
Maintaining confidentiality and information security issues related to the client's health care
Participating in the performance improvement (quality improvement) process
Providing continuity of care
Respecting the client's control of personal environment and property
Supervising the delivery of client care
Triaging clients
Upholding client rights
Using information technology in a confidential manner
Using resources appropriately

Health Promotion and Maintenance

Assisting with health screening and health promotion programs
Considering cultural issues related to family systems and family planning
Identifying changes related to the aging process
Identifying high-risk behaviors of the client
Performing data collection techniques
Promoting health and wellness and preventing disease
Promoting the client's ability to perform self-care
Respecting cultural preferences and lifestyle choices

Psychosocial Integrity

Addressing end-of-life care based on the client's preferences and beliefs
Identifying the use of effective coping mechanisms
Being aware of culture preferences and incorporating these preferences when planning and implementing care
Identifying abuse and neglect issues
Identifying chemical or other dependency issues
Identifying clients who do not speak or understand English and determining how language needs will be met, including the use of agency-approved interpreters
Identifying end-of-life care issues
Identifying family dynamics as they relate to the client's culture
Identifying support systems
Providing a therapeutic environment and building a relationship based on trust
Respecting religious and spiritual influences on health (see Box 6-1)

Physiological Integrity

Ensuring that emergencies are handled using a prioritization procedure
Identifying cultural differences for providing holistic client care
Identifying cultural issues related to alternative and complementary therapies
Identifying cultural issues related to receiving blood and blood products
Implementing therapeutic procedures considering cultural preferences
Providing nonpharmacological comfort interventions
Providing nutrition and oral hydration (see Box 6-1)
Ensuring that palliative and comfort care is provided to the client
Monitoring for alterations in body systems or unexpected responses to therapy

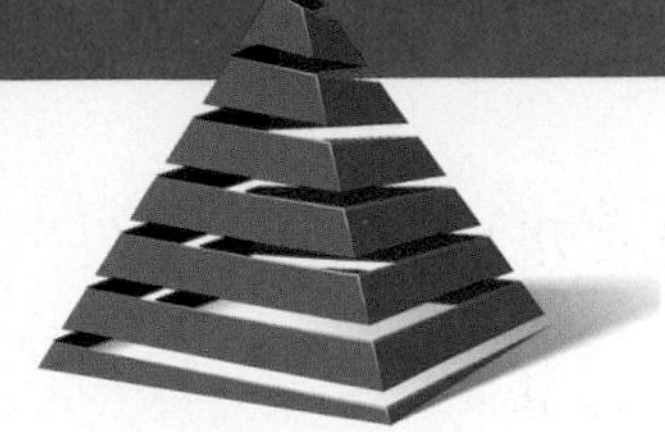

CHAPTER 6

Cultural Awareness and Health Practices

Fundamentals

CRITICAL THINKING What Should You Do?

The nurse is preparing a client for an echocardiogram and notes that the client is wearing a religious medal on a chain around the neck. What should the nurse do with regard to removing this personal item from the client?
Answer located on p. 43.

For reference throughout the chapter, see Figure 6-1 and Box 6-1.

Learn about the cultures of clients with whom you will be working; also, ask clients about their health care practices and preferences.

I. African Americans

A. Description: Citizens or residents of the United States who may have origins in any of the black populations in Africa.

B. Communication
1. Members are competent in standard English.
2. Head nodding does not always mean agreement.
3. Prolonged eye contact may be interpreted as rudeness or aggressive behavior.
4. Nonverbal communication may be important.
5. Personal questions asked on initial contact with a person may be viewed as intrusive.

C. Time orientation and personal space preferences
1. Time orientation varies according to age, socioeconomics, and **subcultures** and may include past, present, or future orientation.
2. Members may be late for an appointment because relationships and events that are occurring may be deemed more important than being on time.
3. Members are comfortable with close personal space when interacting with family and friends.

D. Social roles
1. Large extended family networks are important. Older adults are respected.
2. Many households may be headed by a single-parent woman.
3. Religious beliefs and church affiliation are sources of strength.

E. Health and illness
1. Religious beliefs profoundly affect ideas about health and illness.
2. Food preferences include such items as fried foods, chicken, pork, greens such as collard greens, and rice; some pregnant African-American women engage in pica.

F. Health risks
1. Sickle cell anemia
2. Hypertension
3. Heart disease
4. Cancer
5. Lactose intolerance
6. Diabetes mellitus
7. Obesity

G. Interventions
1. Assess the meaning of the client's verbal and nonverbal behaviors.
2. Be flexible and avoid rigidity in scheduling care.
3. Encourage family involvement.
4. Alternative modes of healing include herbs, prayer, and laying on of hands practices.

Assess each individual for cultural preferences because there are many individual and subculture variations.

II. Amish

A. Description
1. The Amish are known for simple living, plain dress, and reluctance to adopt modern convenience and can be considered a distinct **ethnic group**; the various Amish church fellowships are Christian religious denominations that form a very traditional subgrouping of Mennonite churches.
2. Cultural beliefs and preferences vary, depending on specific Amish community membership.
3. In general, they have fewer risk factors for disease than the general population because of their practice of manual labor, diet, and rare use of tobacco and alcohol; risk of certain genetic disorders is increased because of intermarriage (sexual abuse of women is a problem in some communities). 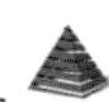

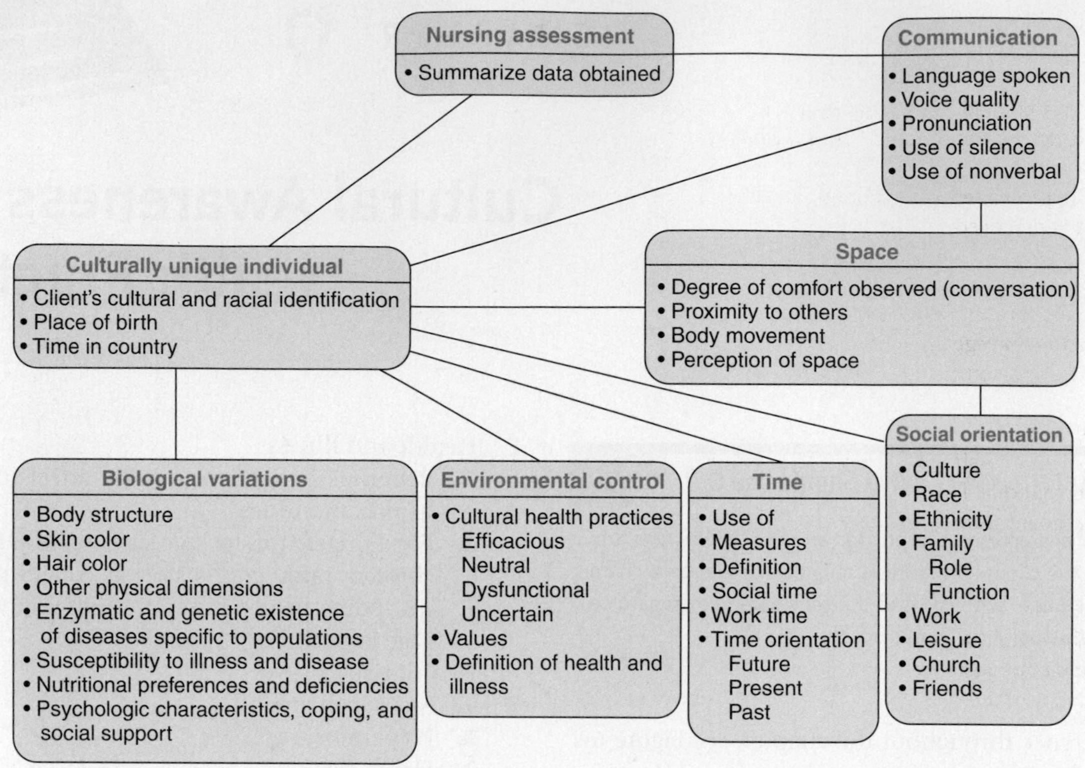

FIGURE 6-1 Giger and Davidhizar's Transcultural Assessment Model. (From Giger J: Transcultural nursing: Assessment and intervention, ed 6, St. Louis, 2013, Mosby.)

B. Communication: Usually speak a German dialect called Pennsylvania Dutch; German language is usually used during worship; and English is usually learned in school.

C. Time orientation and personal space preferences

1. Members generally remain separate from other communities, physically and socially.
2. They often work as farmers, builders, quilters, and homemakers.

D. Social roles

1. Women are not allowed to hold positions of power in the congregational organization.
2. Roles of women are considered equally important to those of men but are very unequal in terms of authority.
3. Family life has a patriarchal structure.
4. Marriage outside the faith is not usually allowed; unmarried women remain under the authority of their fathers.

E. Health and illness

1. Most Amish need to have church (bishop and community) permission to be hospitalized because the community will come together to help pay the costs.
2. Usually, Amish do not have health insurance because it is a "worldly product" and may show a lack of faith in God.
3. Some of the barriers to modern health care include distance, lack of transportation, cost, and language (most do not understand scientific jargon).

F. Health risks 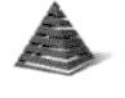

1. Genetic disorders because of intermarriage (inbreeding)
2. Nonimmunization
3. Sexual abuse of women

G. Interventions 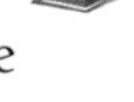

1. Speak to both the husband and the wife regarding health care decisions.
2. Health instructions must be given in simple, clear language.
3. Teaching should be focused on health implications associated with nonimmunization, intermarriage, and sexual abuse issues.

⚠ Be alert to cues regarding eye contact, personal space, time concepts, and understanding of the recommended plan of care.

III. Asian Americans

A. Description: Americans of Asian descent; can include ethnic groups such as Chinese Americans, Filipino Americans, Indian Americans, Vietnamese Americans, Korean Americans, Japanese Americans, and others whose national origin is from the Asian continent.

BOX 6-1 Religions and Dietary Preferences

Seventh-Day Adventist (Church of God)

Alcohol and caffeinated beverages are usually prohibited.

Many are lacto-ovo-vegetarians. Those who eat meat avoid pork.

Overeating is prohibited; 5 to 6 hours between meals without snacking is practiced.

Buddhism

Alcohol is usually prohibited.

Many are lacto-ovo-vegetarians.

Some eat fish, and some avoid only beef.

Roman Catholicism

They avoid meat on Ash Wednesday and Fridays during Lent.

They practice optional fasting during the Lenten season.

Children, pregnant women, and ill individuals are exempt from fasting.

Church of Jesus Christ of Latter-Day Saints (Mormon)

Alcohol, coffee, and tea are usually prohibited.

Consumption of meat may be limited.

The first Sunday of the month is optional for fasting.

Hinduism

Many are vegetarians. Those who eat meat do not eat beef or pork.

Fasting rituals vary.

Children are not allowed to participate in fasting.

Islam

Pork, birds of prey, alcohol, and any meat product not ritually slaughtered are prohibited.

During the month of Ramadan, fasting occurs during the daytime; some individuals may be exempt from fasting, such as pregnant women.

Jehovah's Witnesses

Any foods to which blood has been added are prohibited. They can eat animal flesh that has been drained.

Judaism

Orthodox believers need to adhere to dietary kosher laws:

- Meats allowed include animals that are vegetable eaters, cloven-hoofed animals, and animals that are ritually slaughtered.
- Fish that have scales and fins are allowed.
- Any combination of meat and milk is prohibited.
- During Yom Kippur, 24-hour fasting is observed.
- Pregnant women, children, and seriously ill individuals are exempt from fasting.
- During Passover, only unleavened bread is eaten.

Pentecostal (Assembly of God)

Alcohol is usually prohibited.

Members avoid consumption of anything to which blood has been added.

Some individuals avoid pork.

Eastern Orthodox

During Lent, all animal products, including dairy products, are forbidden.

Fasting occurs during Advent.

Exceptions from fasting include illness and pregnancy; children may also be exempt.

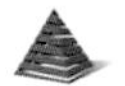

B. Communication
  1. Languages include Chinese, Japanese, Korean, Filipino, Vietnamese, and English.
  2. Silence is valued.
  3. Eye contact may be considered inappropriate or disrespectful (some Asian cultures interpret direct eye contact as a sexual invitation).
  4. Criticism or disagreement is not expressed verbally.
  5. Head nodding does not always mean agreement.
  6. The word "no" may be interpreted as disrespect for others.

C. Time orientation and personal space preferences
  1. Time orientation reflects respect for the past but includes emphasis on the present and future.
  2. Formal personal space is preferred, except with family and close friends.
  3. Members usually do not touch others during conversation.
  4. For some **cultures**, touching is unacceptable between members of the opposite gender.

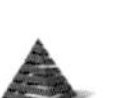

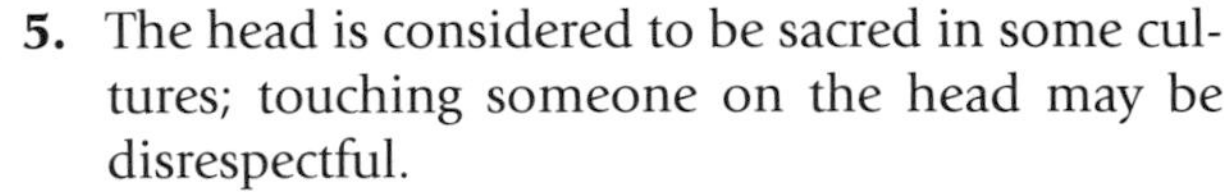

  5. The head is considered to be sacred in some cultures; touching someone on the head may be disrespectful.

D. Social roles
  1. Members are devoted to tradition.
  2. Large extended-family networks are common.
  3. Loyalty to immediate and extended family and honor are valued.
  4. The family unit is structured and hierarchical.
  5. Men have the power and authority, and women are expected to be obedient.
  6. Education is viewed as important.
  7. Religions include Taoism, Buddhism, Confucianism, Shintoism, Hinduism, Islam, and Christianity.
  8. Social organizations are strong within the community.

E. Health and illness
  1. Health is a state of physical and spiritual harmony with nature and a balance between positive and negative energy forces (yin and yang).
  2. A healthy body may be viewed as a gift from the ancestors.

3. Illness may be viewed as an imbalance between yin and yang.
4. Illness may also be attributed to prolonged sitting or lying or to overexertion.
5. Food preferences include raw fish, rice, and vegetables.

⚠ Yin foods are cold and yang foods are hot; one eats cold foods when one has a hot illness, and one eats hot foods when one has a cold illness.

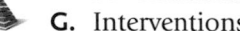

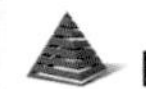
F. Health risks
1. Hypertension
2. Heart disease
3. Cancer
4. Lactose intolerance
5. Thalassemia

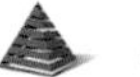
G. Interventions
1. Be aware of and respect physical boundaries; request permission to touch the client before doing so.
2. Limit eye contact.
3. Avoid gesturing with hands.
4. A female client usually prefers a female health care provider (HCP).
5. Clarify responses to questions and expectations of the HCP.
6. Be flexible and avoid rigidity in scheduling care.
7. Encourage family involvement.
8. Alternative modes of healing include herbs, acupuncture, restoration of balance with foods, massage, and offering of prayers and incense.

⚠ If health care recommendations, interventions, or treatments do not fit within the client's cultural values, they will not be followed.

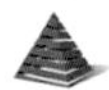
IV. Hispanic and Latino Americans

A. Description: Americans of origins in Latin countries; Mexican Americans, Cuban Americans, Colombian Americans, Dominican Americans, Puerto Rican Americans, Spanish Americans, and Salvadoran Americans are some Hispanic and Latino American subgroups.

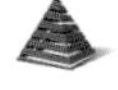
B. Communication
1. Languages include primarily English and Spanish.
2. Members tend to be verbally expressive, yet confidentiality is important.
3. Avoiding eye contact with a person in authority may indicate respect and attentiveness.
4. Direct confrontation is usually disrespectful, and the expression of negative feelings may be impolite.
5. Dramatic body language, such as gestures or facial expressions, may be used to express emotion or pain.

C. Time orientation and personal space preferences
1. Members are usually oriented more to the present.
2. Members may be late for an appointment because relationships and events that are occurring are valued more than being on time.
3. Members are comfortable in close proximity with family, friends, and acquaintances.
4. Members are very tactile and use embraces and handshakes.
5. Members value the physical presence of others.
6. Politeness and modesty are important.

D. Social roles
1. The nuclear family is the basic unit; also, large, extended-family networks are common.
2. The extended family is highly regarded.
3. Needs of the family take precedence over the needs of an individual family member.
4. Depending on age and acculturation factors, men are usually the decision makers and wage earners, and women are the caretakers and homemakers.
5. Religion usually is Catholicism but may vary, depending on origin.
6. Members usually have strong church affiliations.
7. Social organizations are strong within the community.

E. Health and illness
1. Health may be viewed as a reward from God or a result of good luck.
2. Some members believe that health results from a state of physical and emotional balance.
3. Illness may be viewed by some members to be a result of God's punishment for sins.
4. Some members may adhere to nontraditional health measures such as folk medicine.

F. Health risks
1. Hypertension
2. Heart disease
3. Diabetes mellitus
4. Obesity
5. Lactose intolerance
6. Parasites

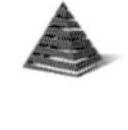

G. Interventions
1. Allow time for the client to discuss treatment options with family members.
2. Protect privacy.
3. Offer to call clergy because of the significance of religious preferences related to illnesses.
4. Ask permission before touching a child when planning to examine or care for him or her; some believe that touching the child is important when speaking to the child to prevent the "evil-eye."
5. Be flexible regarding time of arrival for appointments, and avoid rigidity in scheduling care.
6. Alternative modes of healing include herbs, consultation with lay healers, restoration of

balance with hot or cold foods, prayer, and religious medals.

⚠ Treat each client and individuals accompanying the client with respect, and appreciate the differences and diversity of beliefs about health, illness, and treatment modalities.

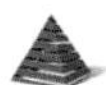

V. Native Americans

A. Description: Term that the U.S. government uses to describe indigenous peoples from the regions of North America encompassed by the continental United States, including parts of Alaska and the island state of Hawaii; comprise a large number of distinct tribes, states, and ethnic groups, many of which survive as intact political communities.

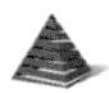

B. Communication
1. There is much linguistic diversity, depending on origin.
2. Silence indicates respect for the speaker for some groups.
3. Some members may speak in a low tone of voice and expect others to be attentive.
4. Eye contact may be viewed as a sign of disrespect.
5. Body language is important.

C. Time orientation and personal space preferences
1. Members are oriented primarily to the present.
2. Personal space is important.
3. Members may lightly touch another person's hand during greetings.
4. Massage may be used for newborn to promote bonding between the infant and mother.
5. Some groups may prohibit touching of a dead body.

D. Social roles
1. Members are family oriented.
2. The basic family unit is the extended family, which often includes persons from several households.
3. In some groups, grandparents are viewed as family leaders.
4. Elders are honored.
5. Children are taught to respect traditions.
6. The father usually does all the work outside the home, and the mother assumes responsibility for domestic duties.
7. Sacred myths and legends provide spiritual guidance for some groups.
8. Most members adhere to some form of Christianity, and religion and healing practices are usually integrated.
9. Community social organizations are important.

E. Health and illness
1. Health is usually considered a state of harmony between the individual, family, and environment.
2. Some groups believe that illness is caused by supernatural forces and disequilibrium between the person and environment.
3. Traditional health and illness beliefs may continue to be observed by some groups, including natural and religious folk medicine tradition.
4. For some groups, food preferences include cornmeal, fish, game, fruits, and berries.

F. Health risks
1. Alcohol abuse
2. Obesity
3. Heart disease
4. Diabetes mellitus
5. Tuberculosis
6. Arthritis
7. Lactose intolerance
8. Gallbladder disease

G. Interventions
1. Clarify communication.
2. Understand that the client may be attentive, even when eye contact is absent.
3. Be attentive to your own use of body language.
4. Obtain input from members of the extended family.
5. Encourage the client to personalize space in which health care is delivered; for example, encourage the client to bring personal items or objects to the hospital.
6. In the home, assess for the availability of running water, and modify infection control and hygiene practices as necessary.
7. Alternative modes of healing include herbs, restoration of balance between the person and the universe, and consultation with traditional healers

⚠ If language barriers pose a problem, seek a qualified medical interpreter; avoid using ancillary staff or family members as interpreters.

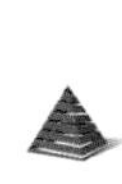

VI. White Americans

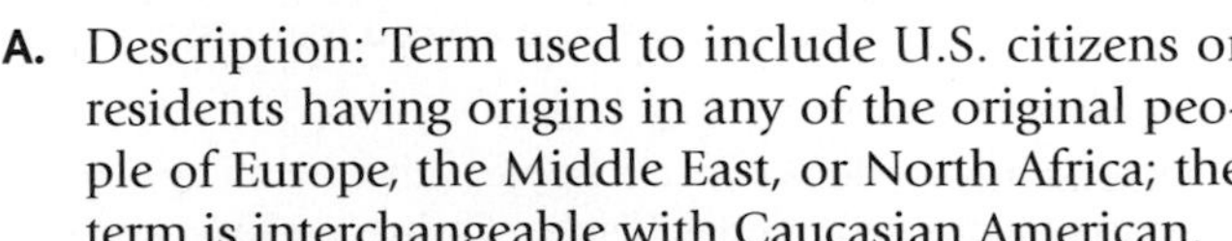

A. Description: Term used to include U.S. citizens or residents having origins in any of the original people of Europe, the Middle East, or North Africa; the term is interchangeable with Caucasian American.

B. Communication
1. Languages include language of origin (e.g., Italian, Polish, French, Russian) and English.
2. Silence can be used to show respect or disrespect for another, depending on the situation.
3. Eye contact is usually viewed as indicating trustworthiness in most origins.

C. Time orientation and personal space preferences
1. Members are usually future oriented.
2. Time is valued; members tend to be on time and to be impatient with people who are not on time.

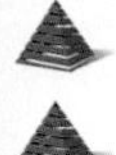

3. Some members may tend to avoid close physical contact.
4. Handshakes are usually used for formal greetings.

D. Social roles
1. The nuclear family is the basic unit; the extended family is also important.
2. The man is usually the dominant figure, but a variation of gender roles exists within families and relationships.
3. Religions are varied, depending on origin.
4. Community social organizations are important.

E. Health and illness
1. Health is usually viewed as an absence of disease or illness.
2. Many members usually have a tendency to be stoical when expressing physical concerns.
3. Members usually rely primarily on the modern Western health care delivery system.
4. Food preferences are based on origin; many members prefer foods containing carbohydrates and meat items.

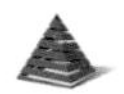

F. Health risks
1. Cancer
2. Heart disease
3. Diabetes mellitus
4. Obesity
5. Hypertension

G. Interventions
1. Assess the meaning of the client's verbal and nonverbal behaviors.
2. Respect the client's personal space and time.
3. Be flexible and avoid rigidity in scheduling care.
4. Encourage family involvement.

VII. End-of-Life Care (Box 6-2)

A. People in the Jewish faith generally oppose prolonging life after irreversible brain damage.

B. Some members of Eastern Orthodox religions, Muslims, and Orthodox Jews may prohibit, oppose, or discourage autopsy.

C. Muslims permit organ transplant for the purpose of saving human life.

D. The Amish permit organ donation, with the exception of heart transplants (the heart is the soul of the body).

E. Buddhists in the United States encourage organ donation and consider it an act of mercy.

BOX 6-2 Religion and End-of-Life Care

Christianity

Catholic and Orthodox

A priest anoints the sick.

Other sacraments before death include anointing of the sick and Holy Eucharist.

Protestant

No last rites are provided (anointing of the sick is accepted by some groups).

Prayers are given to offer comfort and support.

Church of Jesus Christ of Latter-Day Saints (Mormons)

A sacrament may be administered if the client requests.

Jehovah's Witnesses

Members do not believe in sacraments.

Members are not allowed to receive a blood transfusion.

Amish

Funerals are conducted in the home without a eulogy, flower decorations, or any other display. Caskets are plain and simple, without adornment.

At death, a woman is usually buried in her bridal dress.

One is believed to live on after death, either with eternal reward in heaven or punishment in hell.

Islam

Second-degree male relatives such as cousins or uncles should be the contact person and determine whether the client or family should be given information about the client.

The client may choose to face Mecca (west or southwest in the United States).

The head should be elevated above the body.

Discussions about death usually are not welcomed.

Stopping medical treatment is against the will of Allah (Arabic word for God).

Grief may be expressed through slapping or hitting the body.

If possible, only a same-gender Muslim should handle the body after death. If this is not possible, non-Muslims should wear gloves so as not to touch the body.

Judaism

Prolongation of life is important (a client on life support must remain so until death).

A dying person should not be left alone (a rabbi's presence is desired).

Autopsy and cremation are usually not allowed.

Hinduism

Rituals include tying a thread around the neck or wrist of the dying person, sprinkling the person with special water, and placing a leaf of basil on the tongue.

After death, the sacred threads are not removed, and the body is not washed.

Buddhism

A shrine to Buddha may be placed in the client's room.

Time for meditation at the shrine is important and should be respected.

Clients may refuse medications that may alter their awareness (e.g., opioids).

After death, a monk may recite prayers for 1 hour (need not be done in the presence of the body).

F. Some members of Mormon, Eastern Orthodox, Islamic, and Jewish (Conservative and Orthodox) faiths discourage, oppose, or prohibit cremation.
G. Hindus usually prefer cremation and cast the ashes in a holy river.
H. African Americans
   1. Members discuss issues with the spouse or older family member (elders are held in high respect).
   2. Family is highly valued and is central to the care of terminally ill members.
   3. Open displays of emotion are common and accepted.
   4. Members prefer to die at home.
I. Asian Americans
   1. Family members may make decisions about care and often do not tell the client the diagnosis or prognosis.
   2. Dying at home may be considered bad luck.
   3. Organ donation may not be allowed in some ethnic groups.
J. Hispanic and Latino groups
   1. The family generally makes decisions and may request to withhold the diagnosis or prognosis from the client.
   2. Extended-family members often are involved in end-of-life care (pregnant women may be prohibited from caring for dying clients or attending funerals).
   3. Several family members may be at the dying client's bedside.
   4. Vocal expression of grief and mourning is acceptable and expected.
   5. Members may refuse procedures that alter the body, such as autopsy.
   6. Dying at home may be considered bad luck.
K. Native Americans
   1. Family meetings may be held to make decisions about end-of-life care and the type of treatments that should be pursued.
   2. Some groups avoid contact with the dying (may prefer to die in the hospital).

⚠ Provide individualized end-of-life care to clients and families.

VIII. Complementary and Alternative Medicine (CAM)

A. Description
   1. Therapies are used in addition to conventional treatment to provide healing resources and focus on the mind–body connection.
   2. High-risk therapies (therapies that are invasive) and low-risk therapies (those that are noninvasive) are included in CAM.
   3. The National Center for Complementary and Alternative Medicine (NCCAM) has proposed a classification system that includes five categories of complementary and alternative types of therapy (Box 6-3).

BOX 6-3 Categories of Complementary and Alternative Medicine

- Whole medical systems
- Mind–body medicine
- Biologically based practices
- Manipulative and body-based practices
- Energy medicine

B. Whole medical systems
   1. Traditional Chinese medicine (TCM): Focuses on restoring and maintaining a balanced flow of vital energy; interventions include acupressure, acupuncture, herbal therapies, diet, meditation, tai chi, and qi gong (exercise that focuses on breathing, visualization, and movement).
   2. Ayurveda: Focuses on the balance of mind, body, and spirit; interventions include diet, medicinal herbs, detoxification, massage, breathing exercises, meditation, and yoga.
   3. Homeopathy: Focuses on healing and interventions consisting of small doses of specially prepared plant and mineral extracts that assist in the innate healing process of the body.
   4. Naturopathy: Focuses on enhancing the natural healing responses of the body; interventions include nutrition, herbology, hydrotherapy, acupuncture, physical therapies, and counseling.
C. Mind–body medicine
   1. Mind–body medicine focuses on the interactions among the brain, mind, body, and behavior and on the powerful ways in which emotional, mental, social, spiritual, and behavioral factors can directly affect health.
   2. Interventions include biofeedback, hypnosis, relaxation therapy, meditation, visual imagery, yoga, tai chi, qi gong, cognitive-behavioral therapies, group supports, autogenic training, and spirituality.
D. Biologically based practices (Box 6-4)
   1. Biologically based therapies in CAM use substances found in nature, such as herbs, foods, and vitamins.
   2. Therapies include botanicals, prebiotics and probiotics, whole-food diets, functional foods, animal-derived extracts, vitamins, minerals, fatty acids, amino acids, and proteins.
E. Manipulative and body-based practices
   1. Interventions involve manipulation and movement of the body by a therapist.
   2. Interventions include practices such as chiropractic and osteopathic manipulation, massage therapy, and reflexology.

BOX 6-4 Biologically Based Practices

Aromatherapy

The use of topical or inhaled oils (plant extracts) that promote and maintain health

Herbal Therapies

The use of herbs derived mostly from plant sources that maintain and restore balance and health

Macrobiotic Diet

Diet high in whole-grain cereals, vegetables, beans, sea vegetables, and vegetarian soups

Elimination of meat, animal fat, eggs, poultry, dairy products, sugars, and artificially produced food from the diet

Orthomolecular Therapy

Focus on nutritional balance, including use of vitamins, essential amino acids, essential fats, and minerals

F. Energy medicine
1. Energy therapies focus on energy originating within the body or on energy from other sources.
2. Interventions include sound energy therapy, light therapy, acupuncture, qi gong, Reiki and Johre, therapeutic touch, intercessory prayer, whole medical systems, and magnetic therapy.

IX. Herbal therapies (Box 6-5)

A. Herbal therapy is the use of herbs (plant or a plant part) for their therapeutic value in promoting health.
B. Some herbs have been determined to be safe, but some herbs, even in small amounts, can be toxic.
C. If the client is taking prescription medications, the client should consult with the health care provider regarding the use of herbs because serious herb–medication interactions can occur.
D. Client teaching points
1. Discuss herbal therapies with the health care provider (HCP) before use.
2. Contact the HCP if any side/adverse effects of the herbal substance occur.
3. Contact the HCP before stopping the use of a prescription medication.
4. Avoid using herbs to treat a serious medical condition such as heart disease.
5. Avoid taking herbs if pregnant or attempting to get pregnant or if nursing.
6. Do not give herbs to infants or young children.
7. Purchase herbal supplements only from a reputable manufacturer. The label should contain the scientific name of the herb, name and address of the manufacturer, batch or lot number, date of manufacture, and expiration date.
8. Adhere to the recommended dose. If herbal preparations are taken in high doses, they can be toxic.

BOX 6-5 Commonly Used Herbs and Health Products

Aloe: Anti-inflammatory and antimicrobial effect; accelerates wound healing

Angelica: Antispasmodic and vasodilator; balances the effects of estrogen

Bilberry: Improves microcirculation in the eyes

Black cohosh: Produces estrogen-like effects

Cat's claw: Antioxidant; stimulates the immune system, lowers blood pressure

Chamomile: Antispasmodic and anti-inflammatory; produces mild sedative effect

Dehydroepiandrosterone (DHEA): Converts to androgens and estrogen; slows the effects of aging; used for erectile dysfunction

Echinacea: Stimulates the immune system

Evening primrose: Assists with metabolism of fatty acid

Feverfew: Anti-inflammatory; used for migraine headaches, arthritis, and fever

Garlic: Antioxidant; used to lower cholesterol levels

Ginger: Antiemetic; used for nausea and vomiting

Ginkgo biloba: Antioxidant; used to improve memory

Ginseng: Increases physical endurance and stamina; used for stress and fatigue

Glucosamine: Amino acid that assists in the synthesis of cartilage

Goldenseal: Anti-inflammatory and antimicrobial used to stimulate the immune system; has an anticoagulant effect and may increase blood pressure

Kava: Antianxiety and skeletal muscle relaxant; produces a sedative effect

Melatonin: A hormone that regulates sleep; used for insomnia

Milk thistle: Antioxidant; stimulates the production of new liver cells, reduces liver inflammation; used for liver and gallbladder disease

Peppermint oil: Antispasmodic; used for irritable bowel syndrome

Saw palmetto: Antiestrogen activity; used for urinary tract infections and benign prostatic hypertrophy

St. John's wort: Antibacterial, antiviral, antidepressant

Valerian: Used to treat nervous disorders such as anxiety, restlessness, and insomnia

Zinc: Antiviral; stimulates the immune system

9. Moisture, sunlight, and heat may alter the components of herbal preparations.
10. If surgery is planned, the herbal therapy may need to be discontinued 2 to 3 weeks before surgery or as prescribed by the HCP.

⚠ Some herbs have been determined to be safe, but some herbs, even in small amounts, can be toxic. Inform the client to discuss herbal therapies with the health care provider before use.

X. Low-Risk Therapies

A. Low-risk therapies are therapies that have no adverse effects and, when implementing care, can be used by the nurse who has training and experience in their use.

B. Common low-risk therapies
1. Meditation
2. Relaxation techniques
3. Imagery
4. Music therapy
5. Massage
6. Touch
7. Laughter and humor
8. Spiritual measures, such as prayer

CRITICAL THINKING What Should You Do?

Answer: Before certain diagnostic procedures, it is typical to have a client remove personal objects that are worn on the body. The nurse should ask the client about the significance of such an item and its removal because it may have cultural or spiritual significance. The nurse should also determine whether the item will compromise client safety or the test results. If so, then the nurse should ask the client if the item can be either removed temporarily or placed on another part of the body during the procedure.

Reference(s): deWit, D. & Kumagai, C. (2013). *Medical-surgical nursing: Concepts & practice.* (2nd ed., pp. 9-10). St. Louis: Saunders.

PRACTICE QUESTIONS

1. A client is diagnosed with cancer and is told that surgery followed by chemotherapy will be necessary. The client states to the nurse, "I have read a lot about complementary therapies. Do you think I should try any?" The nurse should respond by making which appropriate statement?
1. "I would try anything that I could if I had cancer."
2. "You need to ask your health care provider about it."
3. "No, because it will interact with the chemotherapy."
4. "Let's talk more about the different forms of complementary therapies."

2. The nurse is preparing to assist a client of Orthodox Jewish faith with eating lunch. A kosher meal is delivered to the client. Which nursing action is appropriate when assisting the client with the meal?
1. Unwrapping the eating utensils for the client
2. Replacing the plastic utensils with metal utensils
3. Carefully transferring the food from paper plates to glass plates
4. Allowing the client to unwrap the utensils and prepare his own meal for eating

3. The nurse is caring for a group of clients who are taking herbal medications at home. Which client should be given instructions in regard to avoiding the use of herbal medications?
1. A 60-year-old male client with rhinitis
2. A 24-year-old male client with a lower back injury
3. A 10-year-old female client with a urinary tract infection
4. A 45-year-old female client with a history of migraine headaches

4. The client asks the nurse about various herbal therapies available for the treatment of insomnia. The nurse should encourage the client to discuss the use of which product with the health care provider?
1. Garlic
2. Valerian
3. Lavender
4. Glucosamine

5. The nurse is assisting with collecting data from an African-American client admitted to the ambulatory care unit who is scheduled for a hernia repair. Which information about the client is of **least priority** during the data collection?
1. Respiratory
2. Psychosocial
3. Neurological
4. Cardiovascular

6. The nurse is planning to reinforce nutrition instructions to an African-American client. When reviewing the plan, the nurse is aware that which food is a common dietary practice of clients with African-American heritage?
1. Raw fish
2. Red meat
3. Fried foods
4. Rice as the basis for all meals

7. The nurse consults with a dietitian regarding the dietary preferences of an Asian-American client. Which food should the nurse suggest to include in the diet plan?
1. Rice
2. Fruits
3. Red meat
4. Fried foods

8. An antihypertensive medication has been prescribed for a client with hypertension. The client tells the nurse that she would like to take an herbal substance to help lower her blood pressure. Which statement by the nurse is **most important** to provide to the client?
1. "Herbal substances are not safe and should never be used."
2. "I will teach you how to take your blood pressure so that it can be monitored closely."

3. "You will need to talk to your health care provider (HCP) before using an herbal substance."
4. "If you take an herbal substance, you will need to have your blood pressure checked frequently."

9. A Hispanic-American mother brings her child to the clinic for an examination. Which is **most important** when gathering data about the child?
1. Avoiding eye contact
2. Using body language only
3. Avoiding speaking to the child
4. Touching the child during the examination

❖ 10. A nursing student is asked to identify the practices and beliefs of the Amish society. Which should the student identify? **Select all that apply.**
- ❑ 1. Many choose not to have health insurance.
- ❑ 2. They believe that health is a gift from God.
- ❑ 3. The authority of women is equal to that of men.
- ❑ 4. They remain secluded and avoid helping others.
- ❑ 5. They use both traditional and alternative health care, such as healers, herbs, and massage.
- ❑ 6. Funerals are conducted in the home without a eulogy, flower decorations, or any other display. Caskets are plain and simple, without adornment.

ANSWERS

1. 4
Rationale: Complementary (alternative) therapies include a wide variety of treatment modalities that are used in addition to conventional treatment to treat a disease or illness. These therapies complement conventional treatment, but they should be approved by the person's health care provider (HCP) to ensure that the treatment does not interact with prescribed therapy. Although the HCP should approve the use of a complementary therapy, it is important for the nurse to explore the complementary therapies first with the client, which would eliminate option 2. The statement in option 3 is inappropriate. Similarly, option 1 is an inappropriate response to the client. Option 4 addresses the client's question and encourages discussion.
Test-Taking Strategy: Use therapeutic communication techniques. Eliminate options 1, 2, and 3, because they are nontherapeutic. Option 4 is the only option that addresses the client's question and encourages discussion. **Review:** **therapeutic communication techniques.**
Level of Cognitive Ability: Applying
Client Needs: Psychosocial Integrity
Integrated Process: Communication and Documentation
Content Area: Fundamental Skills: Cultural Awareness
Priority Concepts: Communication, Safety
Reference(s): deWit, Kumagai (2013), p. 166; Potter et al (2013), pp. 320–322.

2. 4
Rationale: Kosher meals arrive on paper plates and with plastic utensils sealed. Health care providers should not unwrap the utensils or transfer the food to another serving dish. Although the nurse may want to be helpful by assisting the client with the meal, the only appropriate option for this client is option 4.
Test-Taking Strategy: The focus of the subject is the rituals associated with kosher meals. Options 2 and 3 are comparable or alike and can be eliminated first. To choose from the remaining options, it is necessary to be familiar with kosher rituals. Review: **the dietary practices of the Orthodox Jewish client.**
Level of Cognitive Ability: Applying
Client Needs: Psychosocial Integrity
Integrated Process: Nursing Process/Implementation
Content Area: Fundamental Skills: Cultural Awareness
Priority Concepts: Culture, Nutrition
Reference(s): Jarvis (2012), p. 178; Nix (2013), pp. 266–267; Potter et al (2013), p. 111.

3. 3
Rationale: Children should not be given herbal therapies, especially in the home and without professional supervision. There are no general contraindications for the clients described in options 1, 2, and 4.
Test-Taking Strategy: Focus on the subject, safety and age developmental use of herbal therapies. Note the age in option 3 to direct you to this option. Options 1, 2, and 4 describe adult clients for which there are no contraindications and can thus be eliminated. **Review:** the indications and contraindications for **herbal therapies.**
Level of Cognitive Ability: Analyzing
Client Needs: Safe and Effective Care Environment
Integrated Process: Nursing Process/Data Collection
Content Area: Fundamental Skills: Cultural Awareness
Priority Concepts: Development, Safety
Reference(s): Hockenberry, Wilson (2013), p. 393.

4. 2
Rationale: Valerian has been used to treat insomnia, hyperactivity, and stress. It has also been used to treat nervous disorders such as anxiety and restlessness. Garlic is used as an antioxidant and to lower cholesterol levels. Lavender is used as an antiseptic and fragrance for a mild sedative effect. Glucosamine is an amino acid that assists with the synthesis of cartilage.
Test-Taking Strategy: Focus on the subject, a substance that may be used to treat insomnia. It is necessary to remember that valerian has been used to treat insomnia. **Review:** specific **herbal therapies.**
Level of Cognitive Ability: Applying
Client Needs: Physiological Integrity
Integrated Process: Nursing Process/Implementation
Content Area: Fundamental Skills: Hygiene/Sleep & Rest
Priority Concepts: Client Education, Safety
Reference(s): Potter et al (2013), p. 653.

5. 2
Rationale: The psychosocial data is the least priority during the initial admission data collection. In the African-American culture, it is considered intrusive to ask personal questions during the initial contact or meeting. Additionally, respiratory,

neurological, and cardiovascular data include physiological assessments that would be the priority.
Test-Taking Strategy: Note the strategic words, *least priority.* Use Maslow's Hierarchy of Needs theory to answer the question. Options 1, 3, and 4 address physiological needs. **Review:** the characteristics of the **African-American culture.**
Level of Cognitive Ability: Applying
Client Needs: Physiological Integrity
Integrated Process: Nursing Process/Data Collection
Content Area: Fundamental Skills: Cultural Awareness
Priority Concepts: Clinical Judgment, Culture
Reference(s): Lewis et al (2014), p. 23; Potter et al (2013), p. 318.

6. 3
Rationale: African-American food preferences include chicken, pork, greens, rice, and fried foods. Asian Americans eat raw fish, rice, and soy sauce. Hispanic Americans prefer beans, fried foods, spicy foods, chili, and carbonated beverages. European Americans prefer carbohydrates and red meat.
Test-Taking Strategy: Focus on the subject, dietary preferences for African-American heritage. This culture is at risk for hypertension and coronary artery disease. With this knowledge you will be directed to the correct option. **Review:** the food preferences of the **African-American culture.**
Level of Cognitive Ability: Applying
Client Needs: Physiological Integrity
Integrated Process: Teaching and Learning
Content Area: Fundamental Skills: Cultural Awareness
Priority Concepts: Culture, Nutrition
Reference(s): Nix (2013), pp. 270–272.

7. 1
Rationale: Asian-American food preferences include raw fish, rice, and soy sauce. African-American food preferences include chicken, pork, greens, rice, and fried foods. Hispanic Americans prefer beans, fried foods, spicy foods, chili, and carbonated beverages. European Americans prefer carbohydrates and red meat.
Test-Taking Strategy: Focus on the subject, dietary preferences of the Asian American. Correlating rice with Asian Americans will lead you to the correct option. **Review:** the food preferences associated with the **Asian-American culture.**
Level of Cognitive Ability: Applying
Client Needs: Physiological Integrity
Integrated Process: Nursing Process/Planning
Content Area: Fundamental Skills: Cultural Awareness
Priority Concepts: Culture, Nutrition
Reference(s): Nix (2013), pp. 273–274.

8. 3
Rationale: Although herbal substances may have some beneficial effects, not all herbs are safe to use. Clients who are being treated with conventional medication therapy should be advised to avoid herbal substances with similar pharmacological effects, because the combination may lead to an excessive reaction or unknown interaction effects. Therefore, the nurse would advise the client to discuss the use of the herbal substance with the HCP.
Test-Taking Strategy: Note the strategic words, *most important.* Eliminate option 1 first because of the closed-ended word, *never.* Next, eliminate options 2 and 4, because they are comparable or alike. **Review:** the limitations associated with the use of **herbal substances.**
Level of Cognitive Ability: Applying
Client Needs: Physiological Integrity
Integrated Process: Nursing Process/Implementation
Content Area: Fundamental Skills: Cultural Awareness
Priority Concepts: Client Education, Health Promotion
Reference(s): deWit, Kumagai (2013), p. 65; Lewis et al (2014), p. 81.

9. 4
Rationale: In the Hispanic-American culture, eye behavior is significant. It is believed that the "bad/evil eye" can be given to a child if a person looks at and admires a child without touching the child. Therefore, touching the child during the examination is very important. Although avoiding eye contact indicates respect and attentiveness, this is not the most important intervention. Avoiding speaking to the child and using body language only are not therapeutic interventions.
Test-Taking Strategy: Note the strategic words, *most important.* Eliminate options 2 and 3 first, because they are comparable or alike. From the remaining options, select the intervention that is most therapeutic, which is touch. **Review:** the characteristics of the **Hispanic-American culture.**
Level of Cognitive Ability: Applying
Client Needs: Psychosocial Integrity
Integrated Process: Nursing Process/Data Collection
Content Area: Fundamental Skills: Cultural Awareness
Priority Concepts: Culture, Professionalism
Reference(s): Giger (2013), pp. 212, 223.

❖ **10. 1, 2, 5, 6**
Rationale: The Amish society maintains a culture that is distinct and separate from the non-Amish society, and some members generally remain separate from the rest of the world, both physically and socially. Family life has a patriarchal structure, and although the roles of women are considered equally important to those of men, they are very unequal in terms of authority. Amish society rejects materialism and worldliness. Members value living simply, and they may choose to avoid technology, such as electricity and cars. They highly value responsibility, generosity, and helping others, and they often work as farmers, builders, quilters, and homemakers. The Amish use traditional health care and alternative health care, such as healers, herbs, and massage. They believe that health is a gift from God but that clean living and a balanced diet help maintain it. They may choose not to have health insurance and instead maintain mutual aid funds for those members who need help with medical costs. Funerals are conducted in the home without a eulogy, flower decorations, or any other display. Caskets are plain and simple, without adornment. At death, women are usually buried in their bridal dresses.
Test-Taking Strategy: Focus on the subject, beliefs and practices of the Amish society. Read each option, and think about the practices and beliefs of this society to answer the question. It is necessary to know these characteristics to answer correctly. **Review:** the characteristics of the **Amish society.**
Level of Cognitive Ability: Understanding
Client Needs: Psychosocial Integrity
Integrated Process: Teaching and Learning
Content Area: Fundamental Skills: Cultural Awareness
Priority Concepts: Culture, Family Dynamics
Reference(s): Lewis et al (2014), p. 27; http://www.religioustolerance.org/amish.htm.

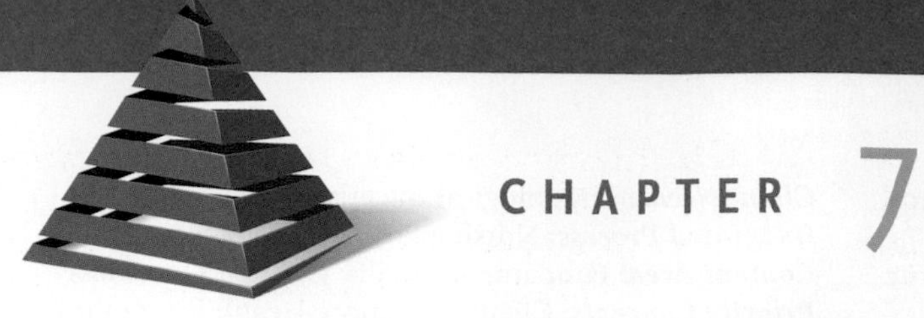

CHAPTER 7

Ethical and Legal Issues

Fundamentals

CRITICAL THINKING What Should You Do?

While preparing a client for surgery scheduled in 1 hour, the client states to the nurse, "I have changed my mind. I don't want this surgery." What should the nurse do?
Answer located on p. 56.

I. Ethics

A. Description: The branch of philosophy concerned with the distinction between right and wrong on the basis of a body of knowledge, not based only on the basis of opinions
B. Morality: Behavior in accordance with customs or traditions, usually reflecting personal or religious beliefs
C. Ethical principles: Codes that direct or govern nursing actions (Box 7-1)
D. Values: Beliefs and attitudes that may influence behavior and the process of decision making
E. Values clarification: Process of analyzing one's own values to understand oneself more completely regarding what is truly important

BOX 7-1 Ethical Principles

Autonomy	Respect for an individual's right to self-determination
Nonmaleficence	The obligation to do or cause no harm to another
Beneficence	The duty to do good to others and maintain a balance between benefits and harms. Paternalism is an undesirable outcome of beneficence, in which the health care provider decides what is best for the client and encourages the client to act against his or her own choices.
Justice	The equitable distribution of potential benefits and tasks determining the order in which clients should be provided care
Veracity	The obligation to tell the truth
Fidelity	The duty to do what one has promised

F. Ethical codes
1. Ethical codes provide broad principles for determining and evaluating client care.
2. These codes are not legally binding, but the board of nursing has authority in most states to reprimand nurses for unprofessional conduct that results from violation of the ethical codes.
3. Specific ethical codes are as follows:
   a. The Code of Ethics for Nurses developed by the International Council of Nurses website: http://www.icn.ch/about-icn/code-of-ethics-for-nurses/
   b. The American Nurses Association Code of Ethics can be viewed on the American Nurses Associate website: http://www.nursingworld.org/codeofethics.

G. Ethical dilemma
1. An ethical dilemma occurs when there is a conflict between two or more ethical principles.
2. No correct decision exists, and the nurse must make a choice between two alternatives that are equally unsatisfactory.
3. Such dilemmas may occur as a result of differences in cultural or religious beliefs.
4. Ethical reasoning is the process of thinking through what one should do in an orderly and systematic manner to provide justification for actions based on principles. The nurse should gather all information to determine whether an ethical dilemma exists, examine his or her own values, verbalize the problem, consider possible courses of action, negotiate the outcome, and evaluate the action taken.

H. Advocate
1. An advocate is a person who speaks up for or acts on the behalf of the client, protects the client's right to make his or her own decisions, and upholds the principle of fidelity.
2. An advocate represents the client's viewpoint to others.
3. An advocate avoids letting personal values influence **advocacy** for the client and supports the client's decision, even when it conflicts with the advocate's own preferences or choices.

I. Ethics committees

1. **Ethics** committees take an interprofessional approach to facilitate dialogue regarding ethical dilemmas.
2. These committees develop and establish policies and procedures to facilitate the prevention and resolution of dilemmas.

⚠ An important nursing responsibility is to act as a client advocate and protect the client's rights.

II. Regulation of Nursing Practice

A. Nurse practice act

1. A nurse practice act is a series of statutes that have been enacted by each state legislature to regulate the practice of nursing in that state. The nurse practice act is designed to protect the public.
2. Nurse practice acts set educational requirements for the nurse, distinguish between nursing practice and medical practice, and define the scope of nursing practice.
3. Additional issues covered by nurse practice acts include licensure requirements for protection of the public, grounds for disciplinary action, rights of the nurse licensee if a disciplinary action is taken, and related topics.
4. All nurses are responsible for knowing the provisions of the act of the state or province in which they work.

B. Standards of care

1. Standards of care are guidelines that identify what the client can expect to receive in terms of nursing care.
2. The guidelines determine whether nurses have performed duties in an appropriate manner.
3. If the nurse does not perform duties within accepted standards of care, the nurse places himself or herself in jeopardy of legal action.
4. If the nurse is named as a defendant in a **malpractice** lawsuit and proceedings show that the nurse followed neither the accepted standards of care outlined by the state or province nurse practice act nor the policies of the employing institution, the nurse's legal liability is clear. He or she is liable.

C. Employee guidelines

1. Respondent superior: The employer is held liable for any negligent acts of an employee if the alleged negligent act occurred during the employment relationship and was within the scope of the employee's responsibilities.
2. Contracts
   a. Nurses are responsible for carrying out the terms of a contractual agreement with the employing agency and the client.
   b. The nurse–employee relationship is governed by established employee handbooks and client care policies and procedures that create obligations, rights, and duties between those parties.
3. Institutional policies
   a. Written policies and procedures of the employing institution detail how nurses are to perform their duties.
   b. Policies and procedures are usually specific and describe the expected behavior on the part of the nurse.
   c. Although policies are not laws, courts generally rule against nurses who violate policies.
   d. If the nurse practices nursing according to client care policies and procedures established by the employer, functions within the job responsibility, and provides care consistently in a nonnegligent manner, the nurse minimizes the potential for liability.

⚠ The nurse must follow the guidelines identified in the nurse practice act and agency policies and procedures when delivering client care.

D. Hospital staffing

1. Charges of abandonment may be made against nurses who "walk out" when staffing is inadequate.
2. Nurses in short-staffing situations are obligated to make a report to the nursing administration.

E. Floating

1. Floating is an acceptable, legal practice used by health care facilities to alleviate understaffing and overstaffing.

2. Legally, the nurse cannot refuse to float unless a union contract guarantees that nurses can work only in a specified area or the nurse can prove lack of knowledge for the performance of assigned tasks.
3. Nurses in a floating situation must not assume responsibility beyond their level of experience or qualification.
4. Nurses who float should inform the supervisor of any lack of experience in caring for the type of clients on the new nursing unit.
5. The nurse should request and be given orientation to the new unit.

F. Disciplinary action

1. Boards of nursing may deny, revoke, or suspend any license to practice as a nurse, according to their statutory authority.
2. Some causes for disciplinary action are as follows:
   a. Unprofessional conduct

b. Conduct that could affect the health and welfare of the public adversely
c. Breach of client **confidentiality**
d. Failure to use sufficient knowledge, skills, or nursing judgment
e. Physically or verbally abusing a client
f. Assuming duties without sufficient preparation
g. Knowingly delegating to unlicensed personnel nursing care that places the client at risk for injury
h. Failure to maintain an accurate record for each client
i. Falsifying a client's record
j. Leaving a nursing assignment without properly notifying appropriate personnel

III. Legal Liability

A. Laws
1. Nurses are governed by civil and criminal law in roles as providers of services, employees of institutions, and private citizens.
2. The nurse has a personal and legal obligation to provide a standard of client care expected of a reasonably competent professional nurse.
3. Professional nurses are held responsible (liable) for harm resulting from their negligent acts or their failure to act.

B. Types of laws (Fig. 7-1)

C. **Negligence** and **malpractice** (Box 7-2)
1. Negligence is conduct that falls below the standard of care.
2. Negligence can include acts of commission and acts of omission.
3. The nurse who does not meet appropriate standards of care may be held liable.
4. Malpractice is negligence on the part of the nurse.
5. Malpractice is determined if the nurse owed a duty to the client and did not carry out the duty and the client was injured because the nurse failed to perform the duty.

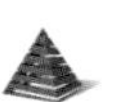

6. Proof of liability
   a. Duty: At the time of injury, a duty existed between the plaintiff and the defendant.
   b. Breach of duty: The defendant breached duty of care to the plaintiff.
   c. Proximate cause: The breach of the duty was the legal cause of injury to the client.
   d. Damage or injury: The plaintiff experienced injury or damages or both and can be compensated by law.

The nurse must meet appropriate standards of care when delivering care to the client; otherwise the nurse would be held liable if the client is harmed.

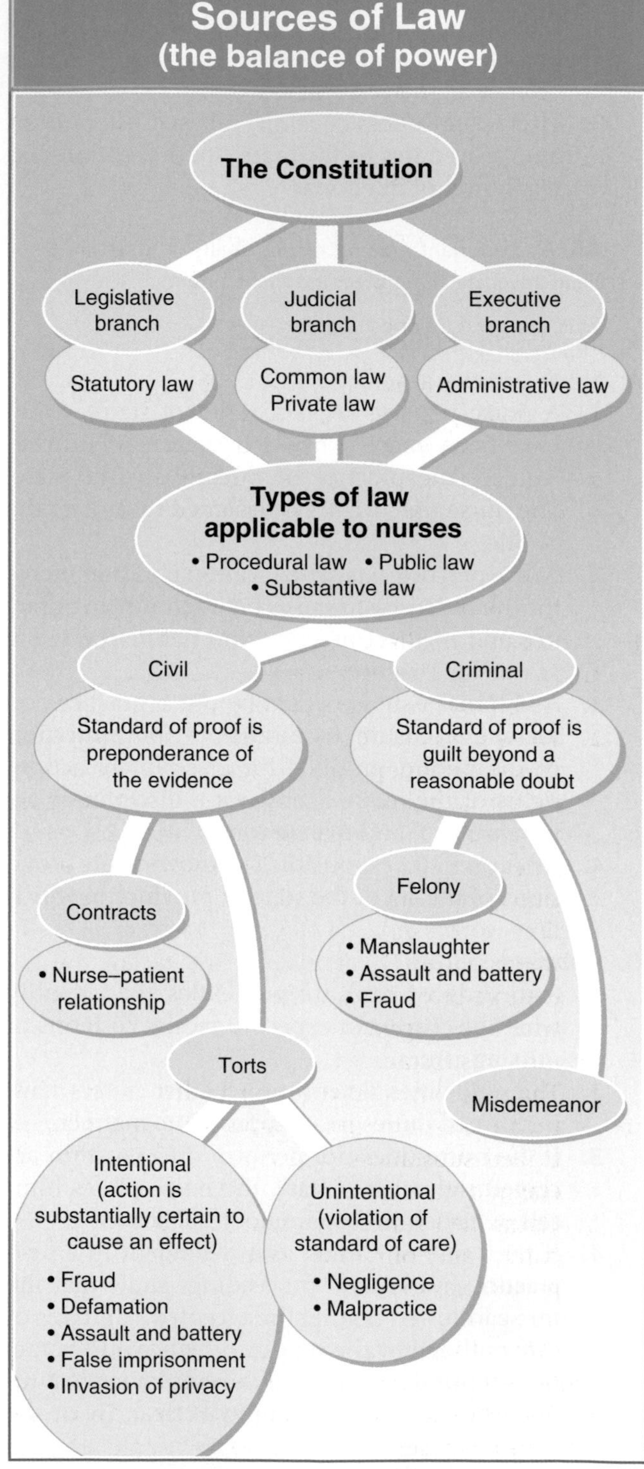

FIGURE 7-1 Sources of law for nursing practice. (From Harkreader H, Hogan MA, Thobaben M: Fundamentals of nursing: Caring and clinical judgment, ed 3, St. Louis, 2007, Saunders.)

D. Professional liability insurance
1. Nurses need their own liability insurance for protection against malpractice lawsuits. 
2. Having their own insurance provides nurses protection as individuals. This allows the nurse to have an attorney present who has only the nurse's interests in mind.

BOX 7-2 Examples of Negligent Acts

Medication errors that result in injury to the client
Intravenous administration errors such as incorrect flow rates or failure to monitor a flow rate that results in injury to the client
Falls that occur as a result of failure to provide safety to the client
Failure to use sterile technique when indicated
Failure to check equipment for proper functioning
Burns sustained by the client as a result of failure to monitor bath temperature or equipment
Failure to monitor a client's condition
Failure to report changes in the client's condition to the health care provider (HCP)
Failure to provide a complete report to the oncoming nursing staff

Adapted from Potter et al (2013), p. 302, St. Louis: Mosby.

E. Good Samaritan laws
   1. State legislatures pass Good Samaritan laws, which may vary from state to state.
   2. These laws encourage health care professionals to assist in emergency situations and limit liability and offer legal immunity for persons helping in an emergency, provided that they give reasonable care.
   3. Immunity from suit applies only when all conditions of the state law are met, such as the health care provider (HCP) receives no compensation for the care provided and the care given is not intentionally negligent.

F. Controlled substances
   1. The nurse should adhere to facility policies and procedures concerning administration of controlled substances, which are governed by federal and state laws.
   2. Controlled substances must be kept locked securely, and only authorized personnel should have access to them.

IV. Collective Bargaining

A. Collective bargaining is a formalized decision-making process between representatives of management and representatives of labor to negotiate wages and conditions of employment.

B. When collective bargaining breaks down because the parties cannot reach an agreement, the employees usually call a strike.

C. Striking presents a moral dilemma to many nurses because nursing practice is a service to people.

V. Legal Risk Areas

A. Assault
   1. Assault occurs when a person puts another person in fear of a harmful or offensive contact.
   2. The victim fears and believes that harm will result because of the threat.

B. Battery is an intentional touching of another's body without the other's **consent**.

C. Invasion of privacy includes violating confidentiality, intruding on private client or family matters, and sharing client information with unauthorized persons.

D. False imprisonment
   1. False imprisonment occurs when a client is not allowed to leave a health care facility when there is no legal justification to detain the client.
   2. False imprisonment occurs when restraining devices are used without an appropriate clinical need.
   3. A client can sign an Against Medical Advice form when the client refuses care and is competent to make decisions.
   4. The nurse should document circumstances in the medical record to avoid allegations by the client that cannot be defended.

E. Defamation is a false communication that causes damage to someone's reputation, either in writing (libel) or verbally (slander).

F. Fraud results from a deliberate deception intended to produce unlawful gains.

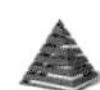

VI. Client's Rights

A. Description
   1. The client's rights document, also called the Patient's Bill of Rights, reflects acknowledgment of a client's right to participate in her or his health care with an emphasis on client autonomy.
   2. The document provides a list of the rights of the client and responsibilities that the hospital cannot violate (Box 7-3).
   3. The client's rights protect the client's ability to determine the level and type of care received. All health care agencies are required to have a **Client's Bill of Rights** posted in a visible area.
   4. Several laws and standards pertain to client's rights (Box 7-4).

B. Rights for the mentally ill (Box 7-5)
   1. The Mental Health Systems Act created rights for mentally ill people.
   2. The Joint Commission has developed policy statements on the rights of mentally ill people.
   3. Psychiatric facilities are required to have a Client's Bill of Rights posted in a visible area.

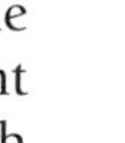

C. Organ donation and transplantation
   1. A client has the right to decide to become an organ donor and a right to refuse organ transplantation as a treatment option.
   2. An individual who is at least 18 years old may indicate a wish to become a donor on his or her driver's license (state-specific) or in an **advance directive**.

BOX 7-3 Client's Rights When Hospitalized

Right to considerate and respectful care
Right to be informed about diagnosis, possible treatments, likely outcome, and to discuss this information with the HCP
Right to know the names and roles of the persons who are involved in care
Right to consent or refuse a treatment
Right to have an advance directive
Right to privacy
Right to expect that medical records are confidential
Right to review the medical record and to have information explained
Right to expect that the hospital will provide necessary health services
Right to know if the hospital has relationships with outside parties that may influence treatment or care
Right to consent or refuse to take part in research
Right to be told of realistic care alternatives when hospital care is no longer appropriate
Right to know about hospital rules that affect treatment, and about charges and payment methods

From: Linton (2012). St. Louis: Saunders and adapted from American Hospital Association: *The patient care partnership: Understanding expectations, rights and responsibilities.* Available at http://www.aha.org/content/00-10/pcp_english_030730.pdf.

BOX 7-5 Rights for the Mentally Ill

Right to be treated with dignity and respect
Right to communicate with persons outside the hospital
Right to keep clothing and personal effects with them
Right to religious freedom
Right to be employed
Right to manage property
Right to execute wills
Right to enter into contractual agreements
Right to make purchases
Right to education
Right to habeas corpus (written request for release from the hospital)
Right to an independent psychiatric examination
Right to civil service status, including the right to vote
Right to retain licenses, privileges, or permits
Right to sue or be sued
Right to marry or divorce
Right to treatment in the least restrictive setting
Right not to be subject to unnecessary restraints
Right to privacy and confidentiality
Right to informed consent
Right to treatment and to refuse treatment
Right to refuse participation in experimental treatments or research

Adapted from deWit, Kumagai (2013). St. Louis: Saunders.

BOX 7-4 Laws and Standards

American Hospital Association: Issued Patient's Bill of Rights
American Nurses Association: Developed the Code for Nurses, which defines the nurse's responsibility for upholding the client's rights
Mental Health Systems Act: Developed rights for mentally ill clients
The Joint Commission: Developed policy statements on the rights of mentally ill individuals

3. The Uniform Anatomical Gift Act provides a list of individuals who can provide **informed consent** for the donation of a deceased individual's organs.
4. The United Network for Organ Sharing sets the criteria for organ donations.
5. Some organs, such as the heart, lungs, and liver, can be obtained only from a person who is on mechanical ventilation and has suffered brain death, whereas other organs or tissues can be removed several hours after death.
6. A donor must be free of infectious disease and cancer.
7. Requests to the deceased's family for organ donation usually are done by the HCP or nurse specially trained for making such requests.
8. Donation of organs does not delay funeral arrangements, no obvious evidence that the organs were removed from the body shows when the body is dressed, and the family incurs no cost for removal of the organs donated.

D. Religious beliefs: Organ donation and transplantation
   1. Catholic Church: Organ donation and transplants are acceptable.
   2. Orthodox Church: Church discourages organ donation.
   3. Islam (Muslim) beliefs: Body parts may not be removed or donated for transplantation.
   4. Jehovah's Witness: An organ transplant may be accepted, but the organ must be cleansed with a nonblood solution before transplantation.
   5. Orthodox Judaism
      a. All body parts removed during autopsy must be buried with the body because it is believed that the entire body must be returned to the earth; organ donation may not be considered by family members.
      b. Organ transplantation may be allowed with the rabbi's approval.
   6. Refer to Chapter 6 for additional information regarding end-of-life care.

VII. Informed Consent

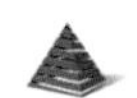

A. Description
   1. Informed consent is the client's approval (or that of the client's legal representative) to have his or her body touched by a specific individual.

BOX 7-6 Types of Consents

Admission Agreement

Admission agreements are obtained at the time of admission and identify the health care agency's responsibility to the client.

Immunization Consent

An immunization consent may be required before the administration of certain immunizations. The consent indicates that the client was informed of the benefits and risks of the immunization.

Blood Transfusion Consent

A blood transfusion consent indicates that the client was informed of the benefits and risks of the transfusion. Some clients hold religious beliefs that would prohibit them from receiving a blood transfusion, even in a life-threatening situation.

Surgical Consent

Surgical consent is obtained for all surgical or invasive procedures or diagnostic tests that are invasive. The HCP, surgeon, or anesthesiologist who performs the operative or other procedure is responsible for explaining the procedure, its risks and benefits, and possible alternative options.

Research Consent

The research consent obtains permission from the client regarding participation in a research study. The consent informs the client about the possible risks, consequences, and benefits of the research.

Special Consents

Special consents are required for the use of restraints, photographing the client, disposal of body parts during surgery, donating organs after death, or performing an autopsy.

2. **Consents**, or releases, are legal documents that indicate the client's permission to perform surgery, perform a treatment or procedure, or give information to a third party.
3. There are different types of consents (Box 7-6).
4. Informed consent indicates the client's participation in the decision regarding health care.
5. The client must be informed, in understandable terms, of the risks and benefits of the surgery or treatment, what the consequences are for not having the surgery or procedure performed, treatment options, and the name of the health care provider performing the surgery or procedure.
6. A client's questions about the surgery or procedure must be answered before signing the consent.
7. A consent must be signed freely by the client without threat or pressure and must be witnessed (witness must be an adult).

BOX 7-7 Mentally or Emotionally Incompetent Clients

Declared incompetent
Unconscious
Under the influence of chemical agents such as alcohol or drugs
Chronic dementia or other mental deficiency that impairs thought processes and ability to make decisions

8. A client who has been medicated with sedating medications or any other medications that can affect the client's cognitive abilities must not be asked to sign a consent form.
9. Legally, the client must be mentally and emotionally competent to give consent.
10. If a client is declared mentally or emotionally incompetent, the next of kin, appointed guardian (appointed by the court), or durable power of attorney for health care has legal authority to give consent (Box 7-7).
11. A competent client older than 18 years of age must sign the consent.
12. In most states, when the nurse is involved in the informed consent process, the nurse is witnessing only the signature of the client on the informed consent form.
13. An informed consent can be waived for urgent medical or surgical intervention as long as institutional policy so indicates.
14. A client has the right to refuse information and waive the informed consent and undergo treatment, but this decision must be documented in the medical record.
15. A client may withdraw consent at any time.

⚠ An informed consent is a legal document, and the client must be informed by the health care provider, in understandable terms, of the risks and benefits of surgery, treatments, procedures, and plan of care. The client needs to be a participant in decisions regarding health care.

B. Minors
1. A minor is a client under legal age as defined by state statute (usually younger than 18 years).
2. A minor may not give legal consent, and consent must be obtained from a parent or the legal guardian.
3. Parental or guardian consent should be obtained before treatment is initiated for a minor, except in the following cases: in an emergency; in situations in which the consent of the minor is sufficient, including treatment related to substance abuse, treatment of a sexually transmitted infection, human immunodeficiency virus (HIV)

testing and acquired immunodeficiency syndrome (AIDS) treatment, birth control services, pregnancy or psychiatric services; the minor is an emancipated minor; or a court order or other legal authorization has been obtained. Refer to the Guttmacher Report on Public Policy for additional information: http://www.guttmacher.org/pubs/tgr/03/4/gr030404.html.

C. Emancipated minor
  1. An emancipated minor has established independence from his or her parents through marriage, pregnancy, service in the armed forces, or by a court order.
  2. An emancipated minor is considered legally capable of signing an informed consent.

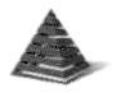

VIII. Health Insurance Portability and Accountability Act

A. Description
  1. The Health Insurance Portability and Accountability Act (HIPAA) describes how personal health information (PHI) may be used and how the client can obtain access to the information.
  2. PHI includes individually identifiable information that relates to the client's past, present, or future health; treatment; and payment for health care services.
  3. The act requires health care agencies to keep PHI private, provides information to the client about the legal responsibilities regarding privacy, and explains the client's rights with respect to PHI.
  4. The client has various rights as a consumer of health care under HIPAA, and any client requests may need to be placed in writing. A fee may be attached to certain client requests.
  5. The client may file a complaint if the client believes that privacy rights have been violated.

B. Client's rights include the right to do the following:
  1. Inspect a copy of PHI.
  2. Ask the health care agency to amend the PHI that is contained in a record if the PHI is inaccurate.
  3. Request a list of disclosures made regarding the PHI as specified by HIPAA.
  4. Request to restrict how the health care agency uses or discloses PHI regarding treatment, payment, or health care services, unless information is needed to provide emergency treatment.
  5. Request that the health care agency communicate with the client in a certain way or at a certain location. The request must specify how or where the client wishes to be contacted.
  6. Request a paper copy of the HIPAA notice.

C. Health care agency use and disclosure of PHI
  1. The health care agency obtains PHI in the course of providing or administering health insurance benefits.

BOX 7-8 Uses or Disclosures of Personal Health Information

Compliance with legal proceedings or for limited law enforcement purposes
To a family member or significant other in a medical emergency
To a personal representative appointed by the client or designated by law
For research purposes in limited circumstances
To a coroner, medical examiner, or funeral director about a deceased person
To an organ procurement organization in limited circumstances
To avert a serious threat to the client's health or safety or the health or safety of others
To a governmental agency authorized to oversee the health care system or government programs
To the Department of Health and Human Services for the investigation of compliance with the Health Insurance Portability and Accountability Act or to fulfill another lawful request
To federal officials for lawful intelligence or national security purposes
To protect health authorities for public health purposes
To appropriate military authorities if a client is a member of the armed forces
In accordance with a valid authorization signed by the client

Adapted from U.S. Department of Health and Human Services Office for Civil Rights: Health information privacy. Available at http://www.hhs.gov/ocr/privacy/.

  2. Use or disclosure of PHI may be done for the following:
    a. Health care payment purposes
    b. Health care operations purposes
    c. Treatment purposes
    d. Providing information about health care services
    e. Data aggregation purposes to make health care benefit decisions
    f. Administering health care benefits
  3. There are additional uses or disclosures of PHI (Box 7-8)

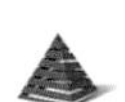

IX. Confidentiality/Information Security

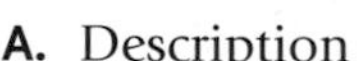

A. Description
  1. In the health care system, **confidentiality/information security** refers to the protection of privacy of the client's PHI.
  2. Clients have a right to privacy in the health care system.
  3. A special relationship exists between the client and the nurse, in which information discussed is not shared with a third party who is not directly involved in the client's care.
  4. Violations of privacy occur in various ways (Box 7-9).

BOX 7-9 Examples of Violations and Invasion of Client Privacy

Taking photographs of the client
Release of medical information to an unauthorized person, such as a member of the press, family, friend, or neighbor of the client, without the client's permission
Use of the client's name or picture for the health care agency's sole advantage
Intrusion by the health care agency regarding the client's affairs
Publication of information about the client or photographs of the client, including on a social networking site
Publication of embarrassing facts
Public disclosure of private information
Leaving the curtains or room door open while a treatment or procedure is being performed
Allowing individuals to observe a treatment or procedure without the client's consent
Leaving a confused or agitated client sitting in the nursing unit hallway
Interviewing a client in a room with only a curtain between clients or where conversation can be overheard
Accessing medical records when unauthorized to do so

B. Nurse's responsibility
 1. Nurses are bound to protect client confidentiality by most nurse practice acts, by ethical principles and standards, and by institutional and agency policies and procedures.
 2. Disclosure of confidential information exposes the nurse to liability for invasion of the client's privacy.
 3. The nurse needs to protect the client from indiscriminate disclosure of health care information that may cause harm (Box 7-10).

C. Social networks
 1. Specific social networking sites can be beneficial to HCPs and clients. Misuse of social networking sites by the HCP can lead to HIPAA violations and subsequent termination of the employee.
 2. Nurses need to adhere to the code of ethics, confidentiality rules, and social media rules. To access the American Nurses Association Social Media Guidelines, go to http://www.nursingworld.rg/FunctionalMenuCategories/AboutANA/Social-Media/Social-Networking-Principles-Toolkit.

BOX 7-10 Maintenance of Confidentiality

Not discussing client issues with other clients or staff uninvolved in the client's care
Not sharing health care information with others without the client's consent (includes family members or friends of the client)
Keeping all information about a client private, and not revealing it to someone not directly involved in care
Discussing client information only in private and secluded areas
Protecting the medical record from all unauthorized readers

 3. Standards of professionalism need to be maintained, and any information obtained through any nurse-client relationship cannot be shared.
 4. The nurse is responsible for reporting any breach of privacy or confidentiality.

D. Medical records
 1. Medical records are confidential.
 2. The client has the right to read the medical record and have copies of the record.
 3. Only staff members directly involved in care have legitimate access to a client's records. These may include HCPs and nurses caring for the client, technicians, therapists, social workers, unit secretaries, client advocates, and administrators (e.g., for statistical analysis, staffing, quality care review). Others must ask permission from the client to review a record.
 4. The medical record is sent to the records or the health information department after discharge of the client from the health care facility.

E. Information technology/computerized medical records
 1. Health care employees should have access only to the client's records in the nursing unit or work area.
 2. Confidentiality/information security can be protected by the use of special computer access codes to limit what employees have access to in computer systems.
 3. The use of a password or an identification code is needed to enter and sign off a computer system.
 4. A password or an identification code should never be shared with another person.
 5. Personal passwords should be changed periodically to prevent unauthorized computer access.

F. When conducting research, any information provided by the client is not to be reported in any manner that identifies the client and is not to be made accessible to anyone outside the research team.

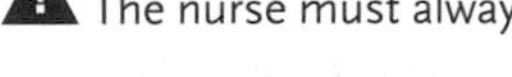

The nurse must always protect client confidentiality.

X. Legal Safeguards

A. Risk management
 1. Risk management is a planned method to identify, analyze, and evaluate risks, followed by a plan for reducing the frequency of accidents and injuries.
 2. Programs are based on a systematic reporting system for incidents or unusual occurrences.

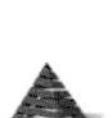

B. Incident reports (Box 7-11)
 1. The incident report is used as a means of identifying risk situations and improving client care.
 2. Follow specific documentation guidelines.
 3. Fill out the report completely, accurately, and factually.

BOX 7-11 Incidents That Need to Be Reported

Accidental omission of prescribed therapies
Circumstances that led to injury or a risk for client injury
Client falls
Medication administration errors
Needle-stick injuries
Procedure-related or equipment-related accidents
A visitor injury that occurred in the health care agency premises
A visitor who exhibits symptoms of a communicable disease

4. The report form should not be copied or placed in the client's record.
5. Make no reference to the incident report form in the client's record.
6. The report is not a substitute for a complete entry in the client's record regarding the incident.
7. If a client injury or error in care occurred, check the client frequently.

C. Safeguarding valuables

1. Client's valuables should be given to a family member or secured for safekeeping in a stored and locked designated location, such as the agency's safe. The location of the client's valuables should be documented per agency policy.
2. Many health care agencies require a client to sign a release to free the agency of the responsibility for lost valuables.
3. A client's wedding band can be taped in place unless a risk exists for swelling of the hands or fingers.
4. Religious items, such as medals, may be pinned to the client's gown if allowed by agency policy.

D. HCP's prescriptions

1. The nurse is obligated to carry out a HCP's prescription, except when the nurse believes a prescription to be inappropriate or inaccurate.
2. The nurse carrying out an inaccurate prescription may be legally responsible for any harm suffered by the client.
3. The nurse should clarify with the HCP an unclear or inappropriate prescription.
4. If no resolution occurs regarding the prescription in question, the nurse should contact the nurse manager or supervisor.
5. The nurse should follow specific agency guidelines for telephone prescriptions (Box 7-12).
6. The nurse should ensure that all components of a medication prescription are documented (Box 7-13).

E. Documentation

1. Documentation is legally required by accrediting agencies, state licensing laws, and state nurse and medical practice acts.
2. The nurse should follow agency guidelines and procedures (Box 7-14).

BOX 7-12 Telephone Prescriptions

Date and time the entry.
Repeat the prescription to the health care provider (HCP), and record the prescription.
Sign the prescription; begin with "t.o." (telephone order), write the HCP's name, and sign the prescription.
If another nurse witnessed the prescription, that nurse's signature follows.
The HCP needs to countersign the prescription within a time frame according to agency policy.
Note: The nurse always follows agency guidelines and procedures regarding HCP prescriptions.

BOX 7-13 Components of a Medication Prescription

Date and time prescription was written
Medication name
Medication dosage
Route of administration
Frequency of administration
Health care provider's signature

BOX 7-14 Do's and Don'ts Documentation Guidelines: Narrative and Information Technology

- Use a black-colored ink pen for narrative documentation.
- Date and time entries.
- Provide objective, factual, and complete documentation.
- Document care, medications, treatments, and procedures as soon as possible after completion.
- Document client responses to interventions.
- Document consent for or refusal of treatments.
- Document calls made to other health care providers.
- Use quotes as appropriate for subjective data.
- Use correct spelling, grammar, and punctuation.
- Sign and title each entry.
- Follow agency policies when an error is made (draw one line through the error, initial, and date).
- Follow agency guidelines regarding late entries.
- Use only the user identification code, name, or password for computerized documentation.
- Maintain privacy and confidentiality of documented information printed from the computer.
- Do not document for others or change documentation for other individuals.
- Do not use unacceptable abbreviations.
- Do not use judgmental or evaluative statements, such as "uncooperative client."
- Do not leave blank spaces on documentation forms.
- Do not lend access identification computer codes to another person; change password at regular intervals.

Note: The nurse always follows agency guidelines and procedures regarding documentation guidelines.

3. Refer to the Joint Commission website for acceptable abbreviations and documentation guidelines: http://www.jointcommission.org/standards_information/npsgs.aspx.

F. Client and family teaching
   1. Provide complete instructions in a language that the client or family can understand.
   2. Document client and family teaching, what was taught, evaluation of understanding, and who was present during the teaching.
   3. Inform the client of what could happen if information shared during teaching is not followed.

The nurse should never carry out a prescription if it is unclear or inappropriate. The HCP should be contacted immediately.

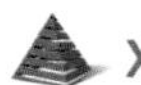

XI. Advance Directives

A. Patient Self-Determination Act
   1. The Patient Self-Determination Act is a law that indicates clients must be provided with information about their rights to identify written directions about the care they wish to receive in the event that they become incapacitated and are unable to make health care decisions.
   2. On admission to a health care facility, the client is asked about the existence of an advance directive, and if one exists, it must be documented and included as part of the medical record; if the client signs an advance directive at the time of admission, it must be documented in the client's medical record.
   3. The two basic types of advance directives include instructional directives and durable powers of attorney for health care (DPOAHC).
      a. Instructional directive: lists the medical treatment that a client chooses to omit or refuse if the client becomes unable to make decisions and is terminally ill.
      b. Durable powers of attorney for health care: appoints a person (health care proxy) chosen by the client to make health care decisions on the client's behalf when the client can no longer make decisions.

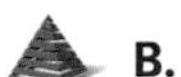

B. Do not resuscitate (DNR) orders
   1. The DNR is an order written by a HCP when a client has indicated a desire to be allowed to die if he or she suffers cardiac or respiratory arrest.
   2. The client or his or her legal representative must provide informed consent for the DNR status.
   3. The DNR order must be defined clearly so that other treatment, not refused by the client, will be continued.
   4. The DNR order must be reviewed regularly according to agency policy.
   5. All health care personnel must know whether a client has a DNR order.
   6. If a client does not have a DNR order, health care personnel need to make every effort to revive the client.
   7. DNR protocols may vary from state to state, and it is important for the nurse to know his or her state's protocols.

C. The nurse's role
   1. Discussing advance directives with the client opens the communication channel to establish what is important to the client and what the client may view as promoting life versus prolonging dying.
   2. The nurse needs to ensure that the client has been provided with information about the right to identify written directions about the care that the client wishes to receive.
   3. On admission to a health care facility, the nurse determines whether an advance directive exists and ensures that it is part of the medical record.
   4. The nurse ensures that the HCP is aware of the presence of an advance directive.
   5. All health care workers need to follow the directions of an advance directive to be safe from liability.
   6. Some agencies have specific policies that prohibit the nurse from signing as a witness to a legal document, such as a living will.
   7. If allowed by the agency, when the nurse acts as a witness to a legal document, the nurse must document the event and the factual circumstances surrounding the signing in the medical record. Documentation as a witness should include who was present, any significant comments made by the client, and the nurse's observations of the client's conduct during this process.

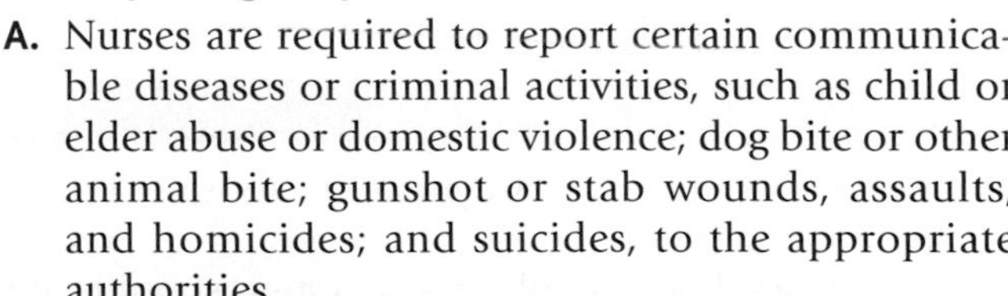

XII. Reporting Responsibilities

A. Nurses are required to report certain communicable diseases or criminal activities, such as child or elder abuse or domestic violence; dog bite or other animal bite; gunshot or stab wounds, assaults, and homicides; and suicides, to the appropriate authorities.

B. Impaired nurse
   1. If the nurse suspects that a co-worker is abusing chemicals and potentially jeopardizing a client's safety, the nurse must report the individual to the nursing administration in a confidential manner. (Client safety is always the first priority.)
   2. Nursing administration notifies the board of nursing regarding the nurse's behavior.

C. Occupational Safety and Health Act (OSHA)
   1. OSHA requires that an employer provide a safe workplace for employees according to regulations.

2. Employees can confidentially report working conditions that violate regulations.
3. An employee who reports unsafe working conditions cannot be retaliated against by the employer.

D. Sexual harassment
1. Sexual harassment is prohibited by state and federal laws.
2. Sexual harassment includes unwelcome conduct of a sexual nature.
3. Follow agency policies and procedures to handle reporting a concern or complaint.

CRITICAL THINKING What Should You Do?

Answer: If the client indicates that he or she does not want a prescribed therapy, treatment, or procedure such as surgery, then the nurse should further investigate the client's request. If the client indicates that he or she has changed his/her mind about surgery, the nurse should assess the client and explore with the client his or her concerns about not wanting the surgery. The nurse would then withhold further surgical preparation and contact the surgeon to report the client's request so that the surgeon can discuss the consequences of not having the surgery with the client. Under no circumstances would the nurse continue with surgical preparation if the client has indicated that he or she does not want the surgery. Further assessment and follow-up related to the client's request need to be done. In addition, it is the client's right to refuse treatment.

Reference(s): deWit, D. & Kumagai, C. (2013). *Medical-surgical nursing: Concepts & practice.* (2nd ed., p. 1108). St. Louis: Saunders.

Linton, A. (2012). *Introduction to medical-surgical nursing* (5th ed., p. 59). St. Louis: Saunders.

PRACTICE QUESTIONS

11. Which is a recommended guideline for safe computerized charting?
1. Passwords to the computer system should only be changed if lost.
2. Computer terminals may be left unattended during client-care activities.
3. Accidental deletions from the computerized file need to be reported to the nursing manager or supervisor.
4. Copies of printouts from computerized files should be kept on a clipboard at the nurses' station for other nurses to access.

12. The licensed practical nurse (LPN) enters a client's room and finds the client sitting on the floor. The LPN calls the registered nurse, who checks the client thoroughly and then assists the client back into bed. The LPN completes an incident report, and the nursing supervisor and health care provider (HCP) are notified of the incident. Which is the **next** nursing action regarding the incident?
1. Place the incident report in the client's chart.
2. Make a copy of the incident report for the HCP.
3. Document a complete entry in the client's record concerning the incident.
4. Document in the client's record that an incident report has been completed.

13. An unconscious client, bleeding profusely, is brought to the emergency department after a serious accident. Surgery is required immediately to save the client's life. With regard to informed consent for the surgical procedure, which is the **best** action?
1. Call the nursing supervisor to initiate a court order for the surgical procedure.
2. Try calling the client's spouse to obtain telephone consent before the surgical procedure.
3. Ask the friend who accompanied the client to the emergency department to sign the consent form.
4. Transport the client to the operating department immediately, as required by the health care provider, without obtaining an informed consent.

14. The nurse arrives at work and is told to report (float) to the pediatric unit for the day because the unit is understaffed and needs additional nurses to care for the clients. The nurse has never worked in the pediatric unit. Which is the appropriate nursing action?
1. Call the hospital lawyer.
2. Call the nursing supervisor.
3. Refuse to float to the pediatric unit.
4. Report to the pediatric unit and identify tasks that can be safely performed.

15. The nurse enters a client's room and notes that the client's lawyer is present and that the client is preparing a living will. The living will requires that the client's signature be witnessed, and the client asks the nurse to witness the signature. Which is the appropriate nursing action?
1. Decline to sign the will.
2. Sign the will as a witness to the signature only.
3. Call the hospital lawyer before signing the will.
4. Sign the will, clearly identifying credentials and employment agency.

16. The nurse finds the client lying on the floor. The nurse calls the registered nurse, who checks the client and then calls the nursing supervisor and the health care provider to inform them of the occurrence. The nurse completes the incident report for which purpose?

1. Providing clients with necessary stabilizing treatments
2. A method of promoting quality care and risk management
3. Determining the effectiveness of interventions in relation to outcomes
4. The appropriate method of reporting to local, state, and federal agencies

17. The nurse observes that a client received pain medication 1 hour ago from another nurse, but the client still has severe pain. The nurse has previously observed this same occurrence. Based on the nurse practice act, the observing nurse should plan to take which action?

1. Report the information to the police.
2. Call the impaired nurse organization.
3. Talk with the nurse who gave the medication.
4. Report the information to a nursing supervisor.

18. A client has died, and the nurse asks a family member about the funeral arrangements. The family member refuses to discuss the issue. Which is the appropriate nursing action?

1. Show acceptance of feelings.
2. Provide information needed for decision making.
3. Suggest a referral to a mental health professional.
4. Remain with the family member without discussing funeral arrangements.

19. A nurse lawyer provides an education session to the nursing staff regarding client rights. The nurse asks the lawyer to describe an example that may relate to invasion of client privacy. Which nursing action indicates a violation of client privacy?

1. Threatening to place a client in restraints
2. Performing a surgical procedure without consent
3. Taking photographs of the client without consent
4. Telling the client that he or she cannot leave the hospital

20. An older woman is brought to the emergency department. When caring for the client, the nurse notes old and new ecchymotic areas on both of the client's arms and buttocks. The nurse asks the client how the bruises were sustained. The client, although reluctant, tells the nurse in confidence that her daughter frequently hits her if she gets in the way. Which is the appropriate nursing response?

1. "I have a legal obligation to report this type of abuse."
2. "I promise I won't tell anyone, but let's see what we can do about this."
3. "Let's talk about ways that will prevent your daughter from hitting you."
4. "This should not be happening. If it happens again, you must call the emergency department."

ANSWERS

11. 3

Rationale: After any inadvertent deletions of permanent computerized records, the nurse should type an explanation into the computer file with the date, time, and his or her initials. The nurse should also contact the nursing manager or supervisor with a written explanation of the situation. Options 1, 2, and 4 represent unsafe charting actions. Only option 3 follows the guidelines for safe computer charting.

Test-Taking Strategy: Focusing on the **subject**, a safe guideline for computerized charting, will direct you to option 3. Eliminate option 1 because of the **closed-ended word**, *only*. Next, read each option and think about confidentiality and safety. Options 1, 2, and 4 represent unsafe charting actions. **Review:** the guidelines for **computerized documentation**.

Level of Cognitive Ability: Understanding

Client Needs: Safe and Effective Care Environment

Integrated Process: Nursing Process/Implementation

Content Area: Leadership/Management: Ethical/Legal

Priority Concepts: Health Care Law, Technology and Informatics

Reference(s): deWit, Kumagai (2013), p. 26; Linton (2012), p. 166; Potter et al (2013), p. 354.

12. 3

Rationale: The incident report is confidential and privileged information, and it should not be copied, placed in the chart, or have any reference made to it in the client's record. The incident report is not a substitute for a complete entry in the client's record concerning the incident.

Test-Taking Strategy: Note the **strategic word**, *next*. Eliminate options 1 and 4 first because they are **comparable or alike**. Recalling that incident reports should not be copied will direct you to the correct option. **Review:** the nursing responsibilities related to **incident reports**.

Level of Cognitive Ability: Applying

Client Needs: Safe and Effective Care Environment

Integrated Process: Communication and Documentation

Content Area: Leadership/Management: Ethical/Legal

Priority Concepts: Health Care Law, Health Policy

Reference(s): Huber (2014), pp. 318–319.

13. 4

Rationale: Generally there are only two instances in which the informed consent of an adult client is not needed. One instance is when an emergency is present and delaying treatment for the purpose of obtaining informed consent would result in injury or death to the client. The second instance is when the

client waives the right to give informed consent. Options 1, 2, and 3 are inappropriate.
Test-Taking Strategy: Note the **strategic word**, *best.* Option 3 can easily be eliminated first. Note the **subject**, *surgery is required immediately.* Options 1 and 2 would delay treatment and should be eliminated. **Review:** the issues surrounding **informed consent.**
Level of Cognitive Ability: Applying
Client Needs: Safe and Effective Care Environment
Integrated Process: Nursing Process/Implementation
Content Area: Leadership/Management: Ethical/Legal
Priority Concepts: Health Care Law, Health Policy
Reference(s): Dolan, Holt (2013), p. 446.

14. 4
Rationale: Floating is an acceptable legal practice used by hospitals to solve their understaffing problems. Legally the nurse cannot refuse to float unless a union contract guarantees that the nurse can only work in a specified area or the nurse can prove a lack of knowledge for the performance of assigned tasks. When faced with this situation, the nurse should identify potential areas of harm to the client.
Test-Taking Strategy: Options 1 and 2 can be eliminated first because they are **alike or comparable**. From the remaining options, eliminate option 3, because refusal is unacceptable behavior for a professional. **Review:** the nursing responsibilities related to accepting an assignment as a **float nurse**.
Level of Cognitive Ability: Applying
Client Needs: Safe and Effective Care Environment
Integrated Process: Nursing Process/Implementation
Content Area: Leadership/Management: Ethical/Legal
Priority Concepts: Health Care Organizations, Professionalism
Reference(s): Linton (2012), pp. 40–41.

15. 1
Rationale: Living wills are required to be in writing and signed by the client. The client's signature either must be witnessed by specified individuals or notarized. Many states prohibit any employee from being a witness, including the nurse in a facility in which the client is receiving care.
Test-Taking Strategy: Options 2 and 4 are **comparable or alike** and should be eliminated first. From the remaining options, option 1 is the appropriate action. **Review:** the legal implications associated with **living wills**.
Level of Cognitive Ability: Applying
Client Needs: Safe and Effective Care Environment
Integrated Process: Nursing Process/Implementation
Content Area: Leadership/Management: Ethical/Legal
Priority Concepts: Health Care Law, Health Policy
Reference(s): Hammond, Zimmermann (2013), p. 7.

16. 2
Rationale: Proper documentation of unusual occurrences, incidents, accidents, and the nursing actions taken as a result of the occurrence are internal to the institution or agency. Documentation on the incident report allows the nurse and administration to review the quality of care and determine any potential risks present. Options 1, 3, and 4 are incorrect.
Test-Taking Strategy: Focus on the **subject**, the purpose of completing incident reports. Eliminate options 1 and 3, because incident reports are not routinely filled out for interventions or treatment measures. Eliminate option 4, because incident reports are not used to report occurrences to other agencies; medical records are used for this purpose. **Review:** the purpose of **incident reports**.
Level of Cognitive Ability: Understanding
Client Needs: Safe and Effective Care Environment
Integrated Process: Nursing Process/Implementation
Content Area: Leadership/Management: Ethical/Legal
Priority Concepts: Evidence, Health Care Law
Reference(s): Potter et al (2013), pp. 305, 358.

17. 4
Rationale: Nurse practice acts require reporting the suspicion of impaired nurses. The state board of nursing has jurisdiction over the practice of nursing and may develop plans for treatment and supervision. This suspicion needs to be reported to the nursing supervisor, who will then report to the board of nursing. Options 1 and 2 are inappropriate. Option 3 may cause a conflict.
Test-Taking Strategy: Focus on the **subject**, following the channels of communication in a health care agency. By reporting the information, the nurse alerts the institution to the potential problem and sets the stage for further investigation and appropriate action. **Review:** the actions to take regarding reporting the suspicion of an **impaired nurse**.
Level of Cognitive Ability: Applying
Client Needs: Safe and Effective Care Environment
Integrated Process: Nursing Process/Planning
Content Area: Leadership/Management: Ethical/Legal
Priority Concepts: Communication, Health Care Law
Reference(s): deWit, Kumagai (2013), pp. 1–2, 1067; Linton (2012), p. 1341.

18. 4
Rationale: The family member is exhibiting the first stage of grief (denial), and the nurse should remain with the family member. Option 1 is an appropriate intervention for the acceptance or reorganization and restitution stage. Option 2 may be an appropriate intervention for the bargaining stage. Option 3 may be an appropriate intervention for depression.
Test-Taking Strategy: Use **therapeutic communication techniques** to direct you to option 4. Remember to address client and family feelings first. **Review:** the **grief** process and **therapeutic communication techniques**.
Level of Cognitive Ability: Applying
Client Needs: Psychosocial Integrity
Integrated Process: Caring
Content Area: Developmental Stages: End-of-Life Care
Priority Concepts: Communication, Coping
Reference(s): Linton (2012), pp. 377–378, 382; Potter et al (2013), p. 720.

19. 3
Rationale: Invasion of privacy takes place when an individual's private affairs are intruded on unreasonably. Threatening to place a client in restraints constitutes assault. Performing a surgical procedure without consent is an example of battery. Not allowing a client to leave the hospital constitutes false imprisonment.
Test-Taking Strategy: Note the **subject**, invasion of client privacy. These words should direct you to the correct option. Also reading each option carefully will direct you to the correct option.

Review: the situations that constitute the invasion of client privacy.
Level of Cognitive Ability: Understanding
Client Needs: Safe and Effective Care Environment
Integrated Process: Nursing Process/Implementation
Content Area: Leadership/Management: Ethical/Legal
Priority Concepts: Ethics, Health Care Law
Reference(s): Linton (2012), pp. 38–39.

20. 1

Rationale: Confidential issues are not to be discussed with nonmedical personnel or with the client's family or friends without the client's permission. Clients should be assured that information is kept confidential unless it places the nurse under a legal obligation. The nurse must report situations related to child, older adult abuse, and other types of abuse, depending on state laws; gunshot wounds; stabbings; and certain infectious diseases.
Test-Taking Strategy: Focus on the subject, elderly abuse. Option 4 can be eliminated first because this action does not protect the client from injury. Options 2 and 3 are comparable or alike and should be eliminated next. **Review:** the nursing responsibilities related to reporting obligations for abuse.
Level of Cognitive Ability: Applying
Client Needs: Psychosocial Integrity
Integrated Process: Nursing Process/Implementation
Content Area: Leadership/Management: Ethical/Legal
Priority Concepts: Health Care Law, Safety
Reference(s): deWit, Kumagai (2013), p. 1042.

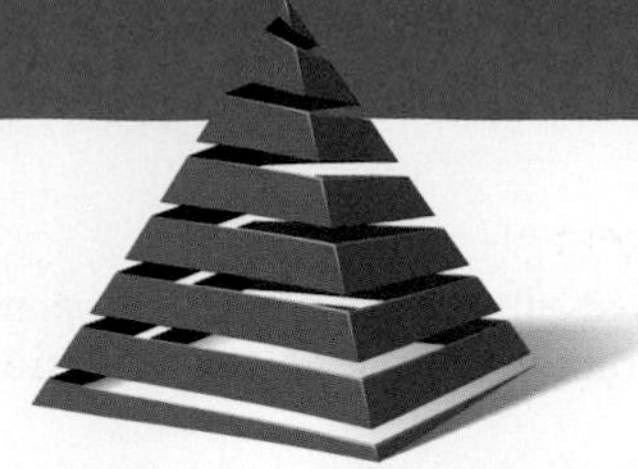

CHAPTER 8

Prioritizing Client Care: Leadership, Delegation, and Disaster Planning

CRITICAL THINKING What Should You Do?

The nurse notes that there has been an increase in the number of intravenous (IV) site infections that developed in the clients being cared for on the nursing unit. How should the nurse proceed to implement a quality improvement program?

Answer located on p. 70.

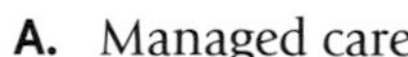

I. Health Care Delivery Systems

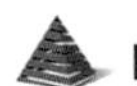

A. Managed care
1. *Managed care* is a broad term used to describe strategies used in the health care delivery system that reduce the costs of health care.
2. Client care is outcome driven and is managed by a case **management** process.
3. Managed care emphasizes the promotion of health, client education and responsible self-care, early identification of disease, and the use of health care resources.

B. Case management
1. Case management is a health care delivery strategy that supports managed care. It uses an interdisciplinary health care delivery approach that provides comprehensive client care throughout the client's illness using available resources to promote high-quality and cost-effective care.
2. Case management includes data collection and development of a plan of care, coordination of all services, referral, and follow-up.
3. Critical pathways are used, and variation analysis is conducted.

Case management involves collaboration with an interprofessional health care team.

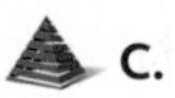

C. Case manager: A case manager is a professional nurse (often one with a master's degree) who assumes responsibility for coordinating the client's care at admission and after discharge.

D. Critical pathway
1. A critical pathway is a clinical management care plan for providing client-centered care and for planning and monitoring the client's progress within an established time frame; **interprofessional collaboration** and teamwork ensure shared decision making and quality client care.
2. Variation analysis is a continuous process that the case manager and other caregivers conduct by comparing the specific client outcomes with the expected outcomes described on the critical pathway.
3. The goal of a critical pathway is to anticipate and recognize negative variance (i.e., client problems) early so that appropriate action can be taken and positive client outcomes can result.

E. Nursing care plan
1. A nursing care plan is a written guideline and communication tool that identifies the client's pertinent assessment data, client problems, goals, interventions, and expected outcomes, which provides a framework for evaluation of the client's response to nursing actions.
2. The plan enhances continuity of care by identifying specific nursing actions necessary to achieve the goals of care.
3. The client and family are involved in developing the plan of care, and the plan identifies short- and long-term goals.

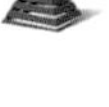

II. Nursing Delivery Systems

A. Functional nursing
1. Functional nursing involves a task approach to client care, with tasks being delegated to individual members of the team.
2. This type of system is task-oriented, and the team member focuses on the delegated task rather than the total client. This results in fragmentation of care and lack of **accountability** by the team member.

B. Team nursing
  1. The team generally is led by a registered nurse (team leader) who is responsible for assessing, developing client problem statements, planning, and evaluating each client's plan of care.
  2. The team leader determines the work assignment. Each staff member works fully within the realm of his or her educational and clinical expertise and job description.
  [illegible] staff member is accountable for client care [illegible] of care delivered in accordance with the licensing and practice scope as determined by health care agency policy and state law.
  4. Modular nursing is similar to team nursing, but it takes into account the structure of the unit. The unit is divided into modules, allowing nurses to care for a group of clients who are geographically close by.

C. Relationship-based practice
  1. Relationship-based practice (primary nursing) is concerned with keeping the nurse at the bedside, actively involved in client care, while planning goal-directed, individualized care.
  2. One (primary) nurse is responsible for managing and coordinating the client's care while in the hospital and for discharge, and an associate nurse cares for the client when the primary nurse is off-duty.

D. Client-focused care
  1. This is also known as the total care or case method; the registered nurse assumes total responsibility for planning and delivering care to a client.
  2. The client may have different nurses assigned during a 24-hour period. However, the nurse provides all necessary care needed for the assigned time period.

III. Professional Responsibilities

A. Accountability
  1. The process in which individuals have an obligation (or duty) to act and are answerable for their actions
  2. Involves assuming only the responsibilities that are within one's scope of practice and not assuming responsibility for activities in which competence has not been achieved
  3. Involves admitting mistakes rather than blaming others and evaluating the outcomes of one's own actions
  4. Includes a responsibility to the client to be competent, providing nursing care in accordance with standards of nursing practice, and adhering to the professional **ethics** codes

Accountability is accepting responsibility for one's actions. The nurse is always responsible for his or her actions when providing care to a client.

B. Leadership and management
  1. **Leadership** is the interpersonal process that involves influencing others (followers) to achieve goals.
  2. **Management** is the accomplishment of tasks or goals by oneself or by directing others.

C. Leader and manager approaches
  1. Autocratic
     a. The leader or manager is focused and maintains strong control, makes decisions, and addresses all problems.
     b. The leader or manager dominates the group and commands rather than seeks suggestions or input.
  2. Democratic
     a. This is also called *participative*.
     b. It is based on the belief that every group member should have input into the development of goals and problem solving.
     c. A democratic leader or manager acts primarily as a facilitator and resource person and is concerned for each member of the group.
     d. The democratic style is a more "talk with the members" style and much less authoritarian than the autocratic style.
  3. Laissez-faire
     a. A laissez-faire leader or manager assumes a passive, nondirective, and inactive approach and relinquishes part or all of the responsibilities to the members of the group.
     b. Decision making is left to the group, with the laissez-faire leader or manager providing little, if any, guidance, support, or feedback.
  4. Situational
     a. Situational style uses a combination of styles based on the current circumstances and events.
     b. Situational styles are assumed according to the needs of the group and the tasks to be achieved.
  5. Bureaucratic
     a. The leader or manager believes that individuals are motivated by external forces.
     b. The leader/manager relies on organizational policies and procedures for decision making.

D. Effective leader and manager behaviors and qualities (Box 8-1)

E. Problem-solving process and decision making
  1. Problem solving involves obtaining information and using it to reach an acceptable solution to a problem.
  2. Decision making involves identifying a problem and deciding which alternatives can best achieve objectives.
  3. Steps of the problem-solving process are similar to the steps of the nursing process (Table 8-1).

BOX 8-1 Effective Leader and Manager Behaviors and Qualities

Behaviors

Treats employees as unique individuals
Inspires employees and stimulates critical thinking
Shows employees how to think about old problems in new ways
Is visible to employees; is flexible; and provides guidance, assistance, and feedback
Communicates a vision, establishes trust, and empowers employees
Motivates employees to achieve goals

Qualities

Effective communicator
Credible
Critical thinker
Initiator of action
Risk taker
Is persuasive and influences employees

Potter, P., Perry, A. G., Stockert, P. A., & Hall, A. M. (2013). *Fundamentals of nursing.* (8th ed., p. 275). St. Louis: Mosby and Adapted from Huber, D., *Leadership and nursing care management,* ed 4, Philadelphia, 2010, Saunders.

TABLE 8-1 Similarities of the Problem-Solving Process and the Nursing Process

Problem-Solving Process	Nursing Process
Identifying a problem and collecting data about the problem	Data Collection
Deciding on a plan of action	Planning
Carrying out the plan	Implementation
Evaluating the plan	Evaluation

IV. Empowerment

A. Empowerment is an interpersonal process of enabling others to do for themselves.
B. Empowerment occurs when individuals are able to influence what happens to them more effectively.
C. Empowerment involves open communication, mutual goal setting, and decision making.
D. Nurses can empower clients through teaching and **advocacy**.

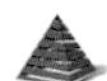

V. Formal Organizations

A. An organization's mission statement communicates in broad terms its reason for existence; the geographic area that the organization serves; and the attitudes, beliefs, and values from which the organization functions.
B. Goals and objectives are measurable activities specific to the development of designated services and programs of an organization.
C. The organizational chart depicts and communicates how activities are arranged, how authority relationships are defined, and how communication channels are established.
D. Policies, procedures, and protocols
   1. Policies are guidelines that define the organization's standpoint on courses of action.
   2. Procedures are based on policy and define methods for tasks.
   3. Protocols prescribe a specific course of action for a specific type of client or problem.
E. Centralization is the making of decisions by a few individuals at the top of the organization or by managers of a department or unit, and decisions are communicated thereafter to the employees.
F. Decentralization is the distribution of authority throughout the organization to allow for increased responsibility and **delegation** in decision making.

⚠ A nurse must follow policies, procedures, and protocols of the health care agency in which he or she is employed.

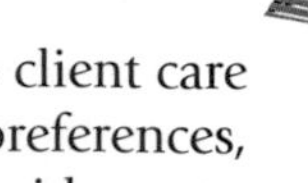

VI. Evidence-Based Practice

A. **Evidence-based practice** is an approach to client care in which the nurse integrates the client's preferences, clinical expertise, and the best research evidence to deliver quality care.
B. Determining the client's personal, social, cultural, and religious preferences ensures individualization and is a component of implementing evidence-based practice.
C. The nurse needs to be an observer and identify and question situations that require change or result in a less than desirable outcome.
D. Use of information technology such as online resources, including research publications, provides current research findings related to areas of practice.
E. The nurse needs to follow evidence-based practice protocols developed by the institution and question the rationale for nursing approaches identified in the protocols as necessary.

⚠ Evidence-based practice requires that the nurse base nursing practice on evidence from clinical research studies. The nurse should also be alert to clinical issues that warrant investigation and report these issues to the registered nurse.

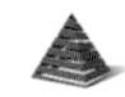

VII. Quality Improvement

A. Also known as *performance improvement,* quality improvement focuses on processes or systems that significantly contribute to client safety and effective client care outcomes. Criteria are used to monitor outcomes of care and to determine the need for change to improve the quality of care.

B. Quality improvement processes or systems may be named *quality assurance, continuous quality management,* or *continuous quality improvement.*

C. When quality improvement is part of the philosophy of a health care agency, every staff member becomes involved in ways to improve client care and outcomes.

D. A retrospective ("looking back") audit is an evaluation method used to inspect the medical record after the client's discharge for documentation of compliance with the standards.

E. A concurrent ("at the same time") audit is an evaluation method used to inspect compliance of nurses with predetermined standards and criteria while the nurses are providing care during the client's stay.

F. Peer review is a process in which nurses employed in an organization evaluate the quality of nursing care delivered to the client.

G. The quality improvement process is similar to the nursing process and involves an interprofessional approach.

H. An outcome describes the most positive response to care; comparison of client responses to the expected outcomes indicates whether the interventions are effective, whether the client has progressed, how well standards are met, and whether changes are necessary.

I. The nurse is responsible for recognizing trends in nursing practice, identifying recurrent problems, reporting these problems, and initiating opportunities to improve the quality of care.

Quality improvement processes improve the quality of care delivery to clients and the safety of health care agencies.

VIII. Conflict

A. Conflict arises from a perception of incompatibility or difference in beliefs, attitudes, values, goals, priorities, or decisions.

B. Types of conflict
1. Intrapersonal: Occurs within a person
2. Interpersonal: Occurs between and among clients, nurses, or other staff members
3. Organizational: Occurs when an employee confronts the policies and procedures of the organization

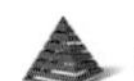

C. Modes of conflict resolution
1. Avoidance
   a. Avoiders are unassertive and uncooperative.
   b. Avoiders do not pursue their own needs, goals, or concerns, and they do not assist others to pursue theirs.
   c. Avoiders postpone dealing with the issue.
2. Accommodation
   a. Accommodators neglect their own needs, goals, or concerns (unassertive) while trying to satisfy those of others.
   b. Accommodators obey and serve others and often feel resentment and disappointment because they "get nothing in return."
3. Competition
   a. Competitors pursue their own needs and goals at the expense of others.
   b. Competitors also may stand up for rights and defend important principles.
4. Compromise
   a. Compromisers are assertive and cooperative.
   b. Compromisers work creatively and openly to find the solution that most fully satisfies all important goals and concerns to be achieved.

IX. Roles of Health Care Team Members

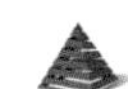

A. Nurse roles are as follows and are based on state nurse practice acts and agency policies and procedures:
1. Promote health and prevent disease
2. Provide comfort and care to clients
3. Make decisions
4. Act as client advocate
5. Manages client care
6. Communicate effectively
7. Reinforce teaching to clients, families, and communities and health care team members as appropriate
8. Act as a resource person
9. Use resources in a cost-effective manner

B. Health care provider (HCP): A HCP diagnoses and treats disease.

C. HCP assistant (physician's assistant, nurse practitioner)
1. The HCP assistant acts to a limited extent in the role of the HCP during the HCP's absence.
2. The HCP assistant conducts physical examinations, performs diagnostic procedures, assists in the operating room and emergency department, and performs treatments.
3. Certified and licensed HCP assistants in some states have prescriptive powers.

D. Physical therapist: A physical therapist assists in examining, testing, and treating physically disabled clients.

E. Occupational therapist: An occupational therapist develops adaptive devices that help chronically ill or handicapped clients perform activities of daily living.

F. Respiratory therapist: A respiratory therapist delivers treatments designed to improve the client's ventilation and oxygenation status.

G. Nutritionist: A nutritionist or dietitian assists in planning dietary measures to improve or maintain a client's nutritional status.
H. Continuing care nurse: This nurse coordinates discharge plans for the client.
I. Assistive personnel, including unlicensed assistive personnel (UAP), and client care technicians, help the nurse with specified tasks and functions.
J. Pharmacist: A pharmacist formulates and dispenses medications.
K. Social worker: A social worker counsels clients and families about home care services and assists the continuing care nurse with planning discharge.
L. Chaplain: A chaplain offers spiritual support and guidance to clients and families.
M. Administrative staff: Administrative or support staff members organize and schedule diagnostic tests and procedures and arrange for services needed by the client and family.

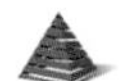

X. Interprofessional Collaboration

A. Client care planning can be accomplished through referrals to or consultations or interprofessional collaborations with other health care specialists and through client care conferences, which involve members from all health care disciplines. This approach helps ensure continuity of care.

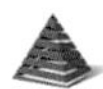

B. Reports
   1. Reports should be factual, accurate, current, complete, and organized.
   2. Reports should include essential background information, subjective data, objective data, any changes in the client's status, client problems, treatments and procedures, medication administration, client teaching, discharge planning, family information, the client's response to treatments and procedures, and the client's priority needs.
   3. Change of shift report
      a. The report facilitates continuity of care among nurses who are responsible for a client.
      b. The report may be written, oral, audiotaped, or provided during walking rounds at the client's bedside.
      c. The report describes the client's health status and informs the nurse on the next shift about the client's needs and priorities for care.
   4. Telephone reports
      a. Purposes include informing a health care provider of a client's change in status, communicating information about a client's transfer to or from another unit or facility, and obtaining results of laboratory or diagnostic tests.
      b. The telephone report should be documented and should include when the call was made, who made the call, who was called, to whom information was given, what information was given, and what information was received.
   5. Transfer reports
      a. Transferring nurse reports provide continuity of care and may be given by telephone or in person (Box 8-2).
      b. Receiving nurse should repeat transfer information to ensure client safety and ask questions to clarify information about the client's status.

BOX 8-2 Transfer Reports

Client's name, age, health care provider, and diagnoses
Current health status and plan of care
Client's needs and priorities for care
Any interventions that need to be performed after transfer, such as laboratory tests, medication administration, or dressing changes
Need for any special equipment
Additional considerations such as allergies, resuscitation status, precautionary considerations, or family issues

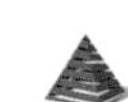

XI. Interprofessional Consultation

A. Consultation is a process in which a specialist is sought to identify methods of care or treatment plans to meet the needs of a client.
B. Consultation is needed when the nurse encounters a problem that cannot be solved using nursing knowledge, skills, and available resources.
C. Consultation also is needed when the exact problem remains unclear; a consultant can objectively and more clearly assess and identify the exact nature of the problem.
D. Rapid response teams are being developed within hospitals to provide nursing staff with internal consultative services provided by expert clinicians.
E. Rapid response teams are used to assist nursing staff with early detection and resolution of client problems.

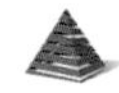

XII. Discharge Planning

A. Discharge planning begins when the client is admitted to the hospital or health care facility.
B. Discharge planning is an interprofessional process that ensures that the client has a plan for continuing care after leaving the health care facility and assists in the client's transition from one environment to another.
C. All caregivers need to be involved in discharge planning, and referrals to other health care professionals or agencies may be needed. A health care provider's

BOX 8-3 Discharge Teaching

How to administer prescribed medications
Side effects of medications that need to be reported to the health care provider (HCP)
Prescribed dietary and activity measures
Complications of the medical condition that need to be reported to the HCP
How to perform prescribed treatments
How to use special equipment prescribed for the client
Schedule for home care services that are planned
How to access available community resources
When to obtain follow-up care

(HCPs) prescription may be needed for the referral, and the referral needs to be approved by the client's health care insurer.

D. The nurse should anticipate the client's discharge needs and report these to the registered nurse so that referrals can be made as soon as possible (involving the client and family in the referral process is important).

E. The nurse needs to assist in teaching the client and family regarding care at home (Box 8-3).

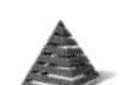

XIII. Delegation and Assignments

A. Delegation

1. Delegation is a process of transferring performance of a selected nursing task in a situation to an individual who is competent to perform that specific task.
2. Delegation involves achieving outcomes and sharing activities with other individuals who have the authority to accomplish the task.
3. The nurse practice act and any practice limitations define which aspects of care can be delegated.
4. Even though a task may be delegated to someone, the nurse who delegates retains accountability for the task.
5. Only the task, not the ultimate accountability, may be delegated to another.
6. The five rights of delegation are the right task, right circumstances, right person, right direction/communication, and right supervision/evaluation.

Delegate only tasks for which you are responsible. The nurse who delegates is accountable for the task; the person who assumes responsibility for the task is also accountable.

B. Principles and guidelines of delegating (Box 8-4)

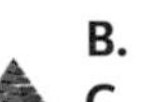

C. Assignments

1. Assignment is the transfer of performance of client care activities to specific staff members.
2. Guidelines for client care assignments
   a. Always ensure client safety.

BOX 8-4 Principles and Guidelines of Delegating

- Delegate the right task to the right delegatee. Be familiar with the experience of the delegatees, their scopes of practice, their job descriptions, agency policy and procedures, and the state nurse practice act.
- Provide clear directions about the task and ensure that the delegatee understands the expectations.
- Determine the degree of supervision that may be required.
- Provide the delegatee with the authority to complete the task. Provide a deadline for completion of the task.
- Evaluate the outcome of care that has been delegated.
- Provide feedback to the delegatee regarding his or her performance.
- In general, noninvasive interventions, such as skin care, range-of-motion exercises, ambulation, grooming, and hygiene measures, can be assigned to an unlicensed assistive personnel (UAP).
- In general, a licensed practical nurse (LPN) or licensed vocational nurse (LVN) can perform not only the tasks that a nursing assistant can perform but also certain invasive tasks, such as dressing changes, suctioning, urinary catheterization, and medication administration (oral, subcutaneous, intramuscular, and selected piggyback medications), according to the education and job description of the LPN or LVN. The LPN or LVN can also review teaching plans with the client that were initiated by the registered nurse.
- A registered nurse (RN) can perform the tasks that an LPN or LVN can perform and is responsible for assessment and planning care, initiating teaching, and administering medications intravenously.

   b. Be aware of individual variations in work abilities.
   c. Determine which tasks can be delegated and to whom.
   d. Match the task to the delegate on the basis of the nurse practice act and appropriate position descriptions.
   e. Provide directions that are clear, concise, accurate, and complete.
   f. Validate the delegatee's understanding of the directions.
   g. Communicate a feeling of confidence to the delegatee, and provide feedback promptly after the task is performed.
   h. Maintain continuity of care as much as possible when assigning client care.

XIV. Time Management

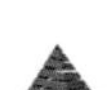

A. Description

1. Time management is a technique designed to assist in completing tasks within a definite time period.

2. Learning how, when, and where to use one's time and establishing personal goals and time frames are part of time management.
3. Time management requires an ability to anticipate the day's activities, to combine activities when possible, and not to be interrupted by nonessential activities.
4. Time management involves efficiency in completing tasks as quickly as possible and effectiveness in deciding on the most important task to do (i.e., **prioritizing**) and doing it correctly.

B. Principles and guidelines
1. Identify tasks, obligations, and activities and write them down.
2. Organize the work day; identify which tasks must be completed in specified time frames.
3. Prioritize client needs according to importance.
4. Anticipate the needs of the day and provide time for unexpected and unplanned tasks that may arise.
5. Focus on beginning the daily tasks, working on the most important first while keeping goals in mind. Look at the final goal for the day, which helps in the breakdown of tasks into manageable parts.
6. Begin client rounds at the beginning of the shift, collecting data on each assigned client.
7. Delegate tasks when appropriate.
8. Keep a daily hour-by-hour log to assist in providing structure to the tasks that must be accomplished, and cross tasks off the list as they are accomplished.
9. Use health care agency resources wisely, anticipating resource needs, and gather the necessary supplies before beginning the task.
10. Organize paperwork and continuously document task completion and necessary client data throughout the day (i.e., documentation should be concurrent with completion of a task or observation of pertinent client data).
11. At the end of the day, evaluate the effectiveness of time management.

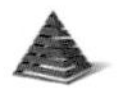

XV. Prioritizing Care

A. Prioritizing is deciding which needs or problems require immediate action and which ones could tolerate a delay in response until a later time because they are not urgent.

B. Guidelines for prioritizing (Box 8-5)

C. Setting priorities for client teaching
1. Determine the client's immediate learning needs.
2. Review the learning objectives established for the client.
3. Determine what the client perceives as important.
4. Assess the client's anxiety level and the time available to teach.

D. Prioritizing when caring for a group of clients (see Priority Nursing Actions)
1. Review the problems of each client.
2. Review nursing diagnoses.

PRIORITY NURSING ACTIONS!

Order of Priority in Assessing a Group of Clients

The nurse is assigned to the following clients. The order of priority in assessing these assigned clients is as follows:

1. A client with heart failure who has a 4-pound weight gain since yesterday and is experiencing shortness of breath
2. A 24-hour postoperative client who had a wedge resection of the lung and has a closed chest tube drainage system
3. A client admitted to the hospital for observation who has absent bowel sounds
4. A client who is undergoing surgery for a hysterectomy on the following day

The nurse determines the order of priority by considering the needs of the client. The nurse also uses guidelines for prioritizing, such as the ABCs—airway, breathing, and circulation—or the CAB—circulation, airway, breathing—guideline if cardiopulmonary resuscitation needs to be initiated; Maslow's Hierarchy of Needs theory; and the steps of the nursing process. Clients 1 and 2 have conditions that relate to the respiratory system or cardiac system. These clients are the high priorities. Client 1 is the first priority because this client is experiencing shortness of breath (life-threatening). There is no indication that client 3 is experiencing any difficulty. Because client 4 is scheduled for surgery on the following day, this client would be the last priority (low priority), and the nurse would assess this client and prepare this client for surgery after other clients are assessed. Because absent bowel sounds could be an indication of a bowel obstruction (intermediate priority), this client would be the third priority.

Reference(s): deWit, D. & Kumagai, C. (2013). *Medical-surgical nursing: Concepts & practice.* (2nd ed., pp. 26–27, 1023). St. Louis: Saunders.
Potter, P., Perry, A. G., Stockert, P. A., & Hall, A. M. (2013). *Fundamentals of nursing.* (8th ed., pp. 237–238). St. Louis: Mosby.

3. Determine which client problems are most urgent based on basic needs, the client's changing or unstable status, and complexity of the client's problems.
4. Anticipate the time that it may take to care for the priority needs of the clients.
5. Combine activities, if possible, to resolve more than one problem at a time.
6. Involve the client in his or her care as much as possible.

Use the ABCs—airway, breathing, and circulation—, Maslow's Hierarchy of Needs theory, and the steps of the nursing process (assessment is first) to prioritize. If cardiopulmonary resuscitation (CPR) needs to be initiated, use CAB—circulation, airway, and breathing—as the priority guideline.

XVI. Disasters and Emergency Response Plan

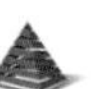

A. Description
1. A **disaster** is any human-made or natural event that causes destruction and devastation that cannot be alleviated without assistance (Box 8-6).

BOX 8-5 Guidelines for Prioritizing

- The nurse and the client mutually rank the client's needs in order of importance based on the client's preferences and expectations, safety, and physical and psychological needs. What the client sees as his or her priority needs may be different from what the nurse sees as the priority needs.
- Priorities are classified as high, intermediate, or low.
- Client needs that are life-threatening or that could result in harm to the client if they are left untreated are high priorities.
- Nonemergency and non-life-threatening client needs are intermediate priorities.
- Client needs that are not related directly to the client's illness or prognosis are low priorities.
- When providing care, the nurse needs to decide which needs or problems require immediate action and which ones could be delayed until a later time because they are not urgent.
- The nurse considers client problems that involve actual or life-threatening concerns before potential health-threatening concerns.
- When prioritizing care, the nurse must consider time constraints and available resources.
- Problems identified as important by the client must be given high priority.
- The nurse can use the ABCs—airway, breathing, and circulation—as a guide when determining priorities; client needs related to maintaining a patent airway are always the priority. If the nurse determines that cardiopulmonary resuscitation is necessary, then the nurse uses CAB—circulation, airway, and breathing—as a guide to prioritize actions.
- The nurse can use Maslow's Hierarchy of Needs theory as a guide to determine priorities and identify the levels of physiological needs, safety, love and belonging, self-esteem, and self-actualization. (Basic needs are met before moving to other needs in the hierarchy.)
- The nurse can use the steps of the nursing process as a guide to determine priorities, remembering that data collection is the first step of the nursing process.

BOX 8-6 Types of Disasters

Human-Made Disasters

Accidents involving release of radioactive material
Dam failures resulting in flooding
Hazardous substance accidents such as pollution, chemical spills, or toxic gas leaks
Mass transportation accidents
Resource shortages such as food, water, and electricity
Structural collapse, fire, or explosions
Terrorist attacks such as bombing, riots, and bioterrorism

Natural Disasters

Blizzards
Communicable disease epidemics
Cyclones
Droughts
Earthquakes
Floods
Forest fires
Hailstorms
Hurricanes
Landslides
Mudslides
Tidal waves (tsunami)
Tornadoes
Volcanic eruptions

2. Internal disasters are disasters that occur within a health care agency (e.g., health care agency fire, structural collapse, radiation spill), whereas external disasters are disasters that occur outside the health care agency.
3. An **emergency response plan** is a formal plan of action for coordinating the response of the health care agency staff in the event of a disaster in the health care agency or surrounding community.
4. A multicasualty event can usually be managed by the hospital with the assistance of local resources; a mass-casualty event requires multiple agencies and health care facilities, including state, regional, and national resources, to manage the event because the event is too overwhelming for local resources to manage.

B. American Red Cross (ARC)

1. The ARC has been given authority by the federal government to provide disaster relief.
2. All ARC disaster relief assistance is free, and local offices are located across the United States.
3. The ARC participates with the government in developing and testing community disaster plans.
4. The ARC identifies and trains personnel for emergency response.
5. The ARC works with businesses and labor organizations to identify resources and individuals for disaster work.
6. The ARC educates the public about ways to prepare for a disaster.
7. The ARC operates shelters, provides assistance to meet immediate emergency needs, and provides disaster health services, including crisis counseling.
8. The ARC handles inquiries from family members.
9. The ARC coordinates relief activities with other agencies.
10. Nurses are involved directly with the ARC and assume functions such as managers, supervisors, and educators of first aid; they also participate in emergency response plans and disaster relief programs and provide services, such as blood collection drives and immunization programs.

C. Phases of disaster management
   1. The Federal Emergency Management Agency (FEMA) identifies four disaster management phases: mitigation, preparedness, response, and recovery.
   2. Mitigation encompasses the following:
      a. Actions or measures that can prevent the occurrence of a disaster or reduce the damaging effects of a disaster
      b. Determination of the community hazards and community risks (actual and potential threats) before a disaster occurs
      c. Awareness of available community resources and community health personnel to facilitate mobilization of activities and minimize chaos and confusion if a disaster occurs
      d. Determination of the resources available for care to infants, older adults, disabled individuals, and individuals with chronic health problems
   3. Preparedness encompasses the following:
      a. Plans for rescue, evacuation, and caring for disaster victims
      b. Plans for training disaster personnel and gathering resources, equipment, and other materials needed for dealing with the disaster
      c. Identification of specific responsibilities for various emergency response personnel
      d. Establishment of a community emergency response plan and an effective public communication system
      e. Development of an emergency medical system and a plan for activation
      f. Verification of proper functioning of emergency equipment
      g. Collection of anticipatory provisions and creation of a location for providing food, water, clothing, shelter, other supplies, and needed medicine
      h. Inventory of supplies on a regular basis and replenishment of outdated supplies
      i. Practice of community emergency response plans (mock disaster drills)
   4. Response encompasses the following:
      a. Putting disaster planning services into action and the actions taken to save lives and prevent further damage
      b. Primary concerns include safety, physical health, and mental health of victims and members of the disaster response team
   5. Recovery encompasses the following:
      a. Actions taken to return to a normal situation after the disaster
      b. Preventing debilitating effects and restoring personal, economic, and environmental health and stability to the community

D. Levels of disaster
   1. FEMA identifies three levels of disaster with FEMA response (Box 8-7).
   2. When a federal emergency has been declared, the federal response plan may take effect and activate emergency support functions.
   3. The emergency support functions of the ARC include performing emergency first aid, sheltering, feeding, providing a disaster welfare information system, and coordinating bulk distribution of emergency relief supplies.
   4. Disaster medical assistant teams (teams of specially trained personnel) can be activated and sent to a disaster site to provide **triage** and medical care to victims until they can be transported to a hospital.

E. Nurse's role in disaster planning 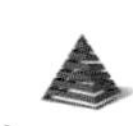
   1. Personal and professional preparedness (Box 8-8)

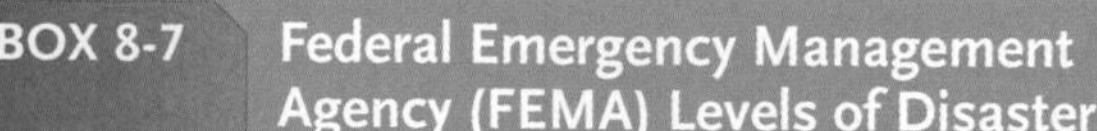

BOX 8-7 Federal Emergency Management Agency (FEMA) Levels of Disaster

Level I Disaster

Massive disaster that involves significant damage and results in a presidential disaster declaration, with major federal involvement and full engagement of federal, regional, and national resources

Level II Disaster

Moderate disaster that is likely to result in a presidential declaration of an emergency, with moderate federal assistance

Level III Disaster

Minor disaster that involves a minimal level of damage but could result in a presidential declaration of an emergency

BOX 8-8 Emergency Plans and Supplies

Plan a meeting place for family members.
Identify where to go if an evacuation is necessary.
Determine when and how to turn off water, gas, and electricity at main switches.
Locate the safe spots in the home for each type of disaster.
Replace stored water supply every 3 months and stored food supply every 6 months.
Include the following supplies:

- A 3-day supply of water (1 gallon per person per day)
- A 3-day supply of nonperishable food
- Clothing and blankets
- First-aid kit
- Adequate supply of prescription medication
- Battery-operated radio
- Flashlight and batteries
- Credit card, cash, or traveler's checks
- Extra set of car keys and a full tank of gas in the car
- Sanitation supplies for washing, toileting, and disposing of trash
- Extra pair of eyeglasses
- Special items for infants, older adults, or disabled individuals
- Items needed for a pet such as food, water, and leash
- Important documents in a waterproof case

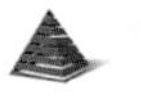

a. Make personal and family preparations (plan a meeting place for family members, identify where to go if evacuation is necessary, determine when and how to turn off water, gas, and electricity at main switches, locate the safe spots in the home for each type of disaster, have on hand needed pet supplies including a leash).
b. Be aware of the disaster plan at the place of employment and in the community.
c. Maintain certification in disaster training and in cardiopulmonary resuscitation.
d. Participate in mock disaster drills, including a bomb threat drill.
e. Prepare professional emergency response items, such as a copy of nursing license, personal health care equipment such as a stethoscope, cash, warm clothing, record-keeping materials, and other nursing care supplies.

2. Disaster response
   a. In the health care agency setting, if a disaster occurs, the agency disaster preparedness plan (emergency response plan) is activated immediately, and the nurse responds by following the directions identified in the plan.
   b. In the community setting, if the nurse is the first responder to a disaster, the nurse cares for the victims by attending to the victims with life-threatening problems first. When rescue workers arrive at the scene, immediate plans for triage should begin. (See Priority Nursing Actions.)

In the event of a disaster, activate the emergency response plan immediately.

F. Triage
   1. In a disaster or war, triage consists of brief assessment of victims that allows the nurse to classify victims according to the severity of the injury, urgency of treatment, and place for treatment.
   2. In an emergency department, triage consists of brief assessment of clients that allows the nurse to classify clients according to their need for care and establishing priorities of care; the type of illness or injury, the severity of the problem, and the resources available govern the process.

G. Emergency department triage system
   1. A commonly used rating system in an emergency department is a three-tier system that uses the categories of emergent, urgent, and nonurgent; these categories may be identified by color coding or numbers (Box 8-9).
   2. The nurse needs to be familiar with the triage system of the health care agency.
   3. When caring for a client who has died, the nurse needs to recognize the importance of family and religious rituals and provide support to loved ones.
   4. Organ donation procedures of the health care agency need to be addressed if appropriate.

H. Triage under mass casualty conditions: Includes a four-tier system that uses the categories of emergent (class I), urgent (class II), nonurgent (class III) as used in the emergency department rating system, and a fourth category of expectant or class IV (black tag and expected and allowed to die).

Think survivability. If you are the first responder to a scene of a disaster, such as a train crash, the priority victim is the one whose life can be saved.

PRIORITY NURSING ACTIONS!

Triaging Clients at the Site of an Accident

The nurse is the first responder at the scene of a school bus accident. The nurse triages the victims from highest to lowest priority as follows:

1. Confused child with bright red blood pulsating from a leg wound
2. Child with a closed head wound and multiple compound fractures of the arms and legs
3. Child with a simple fracture of the arm
4. Sobbing child with several minor lacerations on the face, arms, and legs

Triage systems identify which victims are the priority and should be treated first. Rankings are based on immediacy of needs, including victims with immediate threat to life requiring immediate treatment (emergent), victims whose injuries are not life-threatening provided that they are treated within 1 to 2 hours (urgent), and victims with sustained local injuries who do not have immediate complications and can wait several hours for medical treatment (nonurgent). Victim 1 has a wound that is pulsating bright red blood; this indicates arterial puncture. The child is also confused, which indicates the presence of hypoxia and shock (emergent). Victim 2 has sustained multiple traumas, so this victim is also classified as emergent and would require immediate treatment. Victim 1 is the higher priority because of the arterial puncture. Victim 3 sustained an injury that is not life-threatening provided that the injury can be treated in 1 to 2 hours (urgent). Victim 4 sustained minor injuries that can wait several hours for treatment (nonurgent).

Reference(s): deWit, D. & Kumagai, C. (2013). *Medical-surgical nursing: Concepts & practice.* (2nd ed., pp. 1001–1002). St. Louis: Saunders.
Ignatavicius, D., & Workman, M. (2013). *Medical-surgical nursing: Patient-centered collaborative care.* (7th ed., p. 157). St. Louis: Saunders.

BOX 8-9 Emergency Department Triage

Emergent (Red): Priority 1 (Highest)

This classification is assigned to clients who have life-threatening injuries and need immediate attention and continuous evaluation but have a high probability for survival when stabilized.

Such clients include trauma victims, clients with chest pain, clients with severe respiratory distress or cardiac arrest, clients with limb amputation, clients with acute neurological deficits, and clients who have sustained chemical splashes to the eyes.

Urgent (Yellow): Priority 2

This classification is assigned to clients who require treatment and whose injuries have complications that are not life-threatening, provided that they are treated within 1 to 2 hours. These clients require continuous evaluation every 30 to 60 minutes thereafter.

Such clients include clients with a simple fracture, asthma without respiratory distress, fever, hypertension, abdominal pain, or a renal stone.

Nonurgent (Green): Priority 3

This classification is assigned to clients with local injuries who do not have immediate complications and who can wait several hours for medical treatment. These clients require evaluation every 1 to 2 hours thereafter.

Such clients include clients with conditions such as a minor laceration, sprain, or cold symptoms.

Note: Some triage systems include tagging a client "black" if the victim is dead or who soon will be deceased because of severe injuries; these are victims who would not benefit from any care because of the severity of their injuries.

I. Client assessment in the emergency department
   1. Primary assessment
      a. The purpose of primary assessment is to identify any client problem that poses an immediate or potential threat to life.
      b. The nurse gathers information primarily through objective data and, on finding any abnormalities, immediately initiates interventions.
      c. The nurse uses the ABCs—airway, breathing, and circulation—as a guide in assessing a client's needs and assesses a client who has sustained a traumatic injury for signs of a head injury or cervical spine injury; CAB—circulation, airway, and breathing—is used if CPR needs to be initiated.
   2. Secondary assessment
      a. The nurse performs secondary assessment after the primary assessment and after treatment for any primary problems identified.
      b. Secondary assessment identifies any other life-threatening problems that a client might be experiencing.

CRITICAL THINKING What Should You Do?

Answer: Quality improvement, also known as performance improvement, focuses on processes or systems that significantly contribute to client safety and effective client care outcomes; criteria are used to monitor outcomes of care and to determine the need for change to improve the quality of care. If the nurse notes a particular problem, such as an increase in the number of intravenous site infections, the nurse should collaborate with the registered nurse and assist to collect data about the problem. This data should include information such as the primary and secondary diagnoses of the clients developing the infection, the type of IV catheters being used, the site of the catheter, IV site dressings being used, frequency of assessment and methods of care to the IV site, and length of time that the IV catheter was inserted. Once these data are collected and analyzed by the registered nurse, the nurse will assist to examine evidence-based practice protocols to identify the best practices for care to IV sites to prevent infection. These practices can then be implemented and followed by an evaluation of the results of the protocols used.

Reference(s): Potter, P., Perry, A. G., Stockert, P. A., & Hall, A. M. (2013). *Fundamentals of nursing.* (8th ed., pp. 60–62, 366). St. Louis: Mosby.

      c. The nurse obtains subjective and objective data, including a history, general overview, vital sign measurements, neurological assessment, pain assessment, and complete or focused physical assessment.

PRACTICE QUESTIONS

21. The nurse is recording a nursing hands-off (end-of-shift) report for a client. Which information needs to be included?
   1. As-needed medications given that shift
   2. Normal vital signs that have been normal since admission
   3. All of the tests and treatments the client has had since admission
   4. Total number of scheduled medications that the client received on that shift

22. The nurse is planning the client assignments for the day. Which is the **most appropriate** assignment for the unlicensed assistive personnel (UAP)?
   1. A client who requires wound irrigation
   2. A client who requires frequent ambulation
   3. A client who is receiving continuous tube feedings
   4. A client who requires frequent vital signs after a cardiac catheterization

23. The nurse employed in a long-term care facility is planning the client assignments for the shift. Which client should the nurse assign to the unlicensed assistive personnel (UAP)?
1. A client who requires a 24-hour urine collection
2. A client who requires twice-daily dressing changes
3. A client who is on a bowel management program and requires rectal suppositories and a daily enema
4. A client with diabetes mellitus who requires daily insulin and the reinforcement of dietary measures

24. The nurse is assigned to care for four clients. When planning client rounds, which client should the nurse check **first**?
1. A client on a ventilator
2. A client in skeletal traction
3. A postoperative client preparing for discharge
4. A client admitted on the previous shift who has a diagnosis of gastroenteritis

25. The nurse employed in an emergency department is assigned to assist with the triage of clients arriving to the emergency department. The nurse should assign **priority** to which client?
1. A client complaining of muscle aches, a headache, and malaise
2. A client who twisted her ankle when she fell while in-line skating
3. A client with a minor laceration on the index finger sustained while cutting an eggplant
4. A client with chest pain who states that he just ate pizza that was made with a very spicy sauce

❖ **26.** The nurse is educating a new nurse about mass casualty events (disasters). Which statement by the new nurse indicates a **need for further teaching**? **Select all that apply.**
- ❑ 1. "An event is termed a mass casualty when it overwhelms local medical capabilities."
- ❑ 2. "Mass casualty events do not require an increase in the number of staff that are needed."
- ❑ 3. "A mass casualty event occurs only within the heath care facility and could endanger staff."
- ❑ 4. "A mass casualty event occurs if a fight between visitors occurs in the emergency department."
- ❑ 5. "Mass casualty events may require the collaboration of many local agencies to handle the situation."

27. The nurse is attending an agency orientation meeting about the nursing model of practice implemented in the facility. The nurse is told that the nursing model is a team nursing approach. The nurse understands that which is a characteristic of this type of nursing model of practice?
1. A task approach method is used to provide care to clients.
2. Managed care concepts and tools are used when providing client care.
3. Nursing staff are led by the nurse when providing care to a group of clients.
4. A single registered nurse is responsible for providing nursing care to a group of clients.

28. A client experiences a cardiac arrest. The nurse leader quickly responds to the emergency and assigns clearly defined tasks to the work group. In this situation, the nurse is implementing which leadership style?
1. Autocratic
2. Situational
3. Democratic
4. Laissez-faire

29. The nurse has delegated several nursing tasks to staff members. Which is the nurse's **primary** responsibility after the delegation of the tasks?
1. Document that the task was completed.
2. Assign the tasks that were not completed to the next nursing shift.
3. Allow each staff member to make judgments when performing the tasks.
4. Perform follow-up with each staff member regarding the performance and outcome of the task.

30. The nurse is assigned to care for four clients. When planning client rounds, which client should the nurse collect data from **first**?
1. A client scheduled for a chest x-ray
2. A client requiring daily dressing changes
3. A postoperative client preparing for discharge
4. A client receiving oxygen who is having difficulty breathing

ANSWERS

21. 1

Rationale: The nursing hands-off (end-of-shift) report needs to be an efficient and accurate account of the client's condition during the last shift. It needs to include pertinent information about the client, such as tests and treatments; as-needed medications given or therapies performed during the past 24 hours, including the client's response to them; changes in the client's condition; scheduled tests and treatments; current problems; and any other special concerns. It is not necessary to include the total number of medications given or a list of all the tests and treatments that the client has had since admission. Only significant vital signs need to be included.
Test-Taking Strategy: Focus on the subject of the question, the end-of-shift report. The purpose of this report is to communicate accurate and significant information about the client. Think about the word "significant." Eliminate option 2 because of the word *normal.* Eliminate option 3 because of the closed-ended word, *all.* Eliminate option 4 because of the word *total* and *"scheduled medications."* **Review**: the information included in the **nursing hands-off (end-of-shift) report.**
Level of Cognitive Ability: Applying
Client Needs: Safe and Effective Care Environment
Integrated Process: Communication and Documentation
Content Area: Leadership/Management: Prioritizing
Priority Concepts: Communication, Health Policy
Reference(s): deWit, Kumagai (2013), p. 27; Potter et al (2013), pp. 244–245.

22. 2

Rationale: The nurse must determine the most appropriate assignment on the basis of the skills of the staff member and the needs of the client. In this case, the most appropriate assignment for the UAP would be to care for the client who requires frequent ambulation. The UAP is skilled in this task. The client who had a cardiac catheterization will require specific monitoring in addition to that of the vital signs. Wound irrigations and tube feedings are not performed by unlicensed personnel.
Test-Taking Strategy: Note the strategic words, *most appropriate,* and focus on the subject, an assignment to the UAP. Answer this question by recalling the principles of delegation and the supervision of work of others. Remember that work delegated to others must be done in a way that is consistent with the individual's level of expertise and that individual's licensure or lack of licensure. **Review: the principles of delegation.**
Level of Cognitive Ability: Applying
Client Needs: Safe and Effective Care Environment
Integrated Process: Nursing Process/Planning
Content Area: Leadership/Management: Delegating
Priority Concepts: Care Coordination, Leadership
Reference(s): Linton (2012), p. 53.

23. 1

Rationale: The nurse must determine the most appropriate assignment on the basis of the skills of the staff member and the needs of the client. The assignment of tasks needs to be implemented on the basis of the job description of the individual, the individual's level of clinical competence, and state law. Options 2, 3, and 4 involve care that requires the skill of a licensed nurse. A UAP is not licensed.
Test-Taking Strategy: Focus on the subject of the question, safe delegation of tasks to a UAP. Think about what an unlicensed person can perform for tasks. Eliminate options 2, 3, and 4, because these clients require care that needs to be provided by a licensed nurse. **Review: delegation principles.**
Level of Cognitive Ability: Applying
Client Needs: Safe and Effective Care Environment
Integrated Process: Nursing Process/Planning
Content Area: Leadership/Management: Delegating
Priority Concepts: Care Coordination, Leadership
Reference(s): deWit, Kumagai (2013), p. 26.

24. 1

Rationale: The airway is always a priority, and the nurse first checks the client on a ventilator. The clients described in options 2, 3, and 4 have needs that would be identified as intermediate priorities.
Test-Taking Strategy: Note the strategic word, *first.* Use ABCs—airway, breathing, and circulation—to answer the question. Remember that the airway is always the first priority. Review: the principles related to **prioritizing.**
Level of Cognitive Ability: Applying
Client Needs: Safe and Effective Care Environment
Integrated Process: Nursing Process/Planning
Content Area: Leadership/Management: Prioritizing
Priority Concepts: Care Coordination, Clinical Judgment
Reference(s): deWit, Kumagai (2013), pp. 25, 83.

25. 4

Rationale: In an emergency department, triage involves classifying clients according to their need for care, and it includes establishing priorities of care. The type of illness, the severity of the problem, and the resources available govern the process. Clients with trauma, chest pain, severe respiratory distress, cardiac arrest, limb amputation, or acute neurological deficits, and those who sustained a chemical splash to the eyes are classified as emergent, and these clients are the number 1 priority. Clients with conditions such as simple fractures, asthma without respiratory distress, fever, hypertension, abdominal pain, or renal stones have urgent needs, and these clients are classified as the number 2 priority. Clients with conditions such as minor lacerations, sprains, or cold symptoms are classified as nonurgent, and they are the number 3 priority.
Test-Taking Strategy: Note the strategic word, *priority.* Use the ABCs—airway, breathing, and circulation—to direct you to the correct option. A client who is experiencing chest pain is always classified as priority number 1 until a myocardial infarction has been ruled out. **Review**: the **triage classification** system commonly used in the hospital emergency department.
Level of Cognitive Ability: Applying
Client Needs: Safe and Effective Care Environment
Integrated Process: Nursing Process/Implementation
Content Area: Leadership/Management: Prioritizing
Priority Concepts: Care Coordination, Clinical Judgment
Reference(s): deWit, Kumagai (2013), pp. 25, 1022–1023.

❖ **26. 2, 3, 4**

Rationale: Mass casualty events, also known as disasters, overwhelm local medical capabilities and may require the

collaboration of multiple agencies and health care facilities to handle the crises. This type of event can occur in the health care facility or outside of it. Fights in the emergency department are not termed mass casualty events but are agency security and local enforcement issues. Mass casualty events almost always require an increase in staffing to ensure safe patient care.
Test-Taking Strategy: Note the strategic words, *need for further teaching*. These words indicate a negative event query and the need to select the incorrect statements. Think about what a mass casualty event or disaster is to assist in answering. Eliminate options 1 and 5 because they are correct statements and therefore do not indicate a need for further teaching. **Review:** **disasters.**
Level of Cognitive Ability: Evaluating
Client Needs: Safe and Effective Care Environment
Integrated Process: Nursing Process/Evaluation
Content Area: Leadership/Management-Disasters
Priority Concepts: Collaboration, Safety
Reference(s): deWit, Kumagai (2013), pp. 997–998; Ignatavicius, Workman (2013), p. 156.

27. 3
Rationale: In team nursing, nursing personnel are led by the nurse when providing care to a group of clients. Option 1 identifies functional nursing. Option 2 identifies a component of case management. Option 4 identifies primary nursing.
Test-Taking Strategy: Note that the subject relates to team nursing. Think about the meaning of the word *team*. Option 3 is the only option that identifies the concept of a team approach. **Review:** the various types of **nursing delivery systems.**
Level of Cognitive Ability: Understanding
Client Needs: Safe and Effective Care Environment
Integrated Process: Nursing Process/Implementation
Content Area: Leadership/Management: Delegating
Priority Concepts: Health Care Organization, Leadership
Reference(s): Linton (2012), pp. 5, 51–52.

28. 1
Rationale: Autocratic leadership is an approach in which the leader retains all authority and is primarily concerned with task accomplishment. It is an effective leadership style to implement in an emergency or crisis situation. The leader assigns clearly defined tasks and establishes one-way communication with the work group, and he or she makes all decisions independently. Situational leadership is a comprehensive approach that incorporates the leader's style, the maturity of the work group, and the situation at hand. Democratic leadership is a people-centered approach that is primarily concerned with human relations and teamwork. This leadership style facilitates goal accomplishment and contributes to the growth and development of the staff. Laissez-faire leadership is a permissive style in which the leader gives up control and delegates all decision making to the work group.
Test-Taking Strategy: Focus on the subject, identifying the type of leadership. Reviewing the nurse leader's actions described in the question and noting the words *assigns clearly defined tasks* will assist you in choosing the correct option. **Review:** the various **leadership styles.**
Level of Cognitive Ability: Applying
Client Needs: Safe and Effective Care Environment
Integrated Process: Nursing Process/Implementation
Content Area: Leadership/Management: Delegating
Priority Concepts: Clinical Judgment, Leadership
Reference(s): Linton (2012), pp. 45–46.

29. 4
Rationale: The ultimate responsibility for a task lies with the person who delegated it. Therefore, it is the nurse's primary responsibility to follow up with each staff member regarding the performance of the task and the outcomes related to implementing the task. Not all staff members have the education, knowledge, and ability to make judgments about tasks being performed. The nurse documents that the task has been completed, but this would not be done until follow-up was implemented and outcomes were identified. It is not appropriate to assign the tasks that were not completed to the next nursing shift.
Test-Taking Strategy: Note the strategic word, *primary*. Recalling that the ultimate responsibility for a task lies with the person who delegated it will direct you to the correct option. **Review:** the guidelines related to **delegating.**
Level of Cognitive Ability: Applying
Client Needs: Safe and Effective Care Environment
Integrated Process: Nursing Process/Implementation
Content Area: Leadership/Management: Delegating
Priority Concepts: Communication, Leadership
Reference(s): deWit, Kumagai (2013), pp. 3–4; Linton (2012), p. 53.

30. 4
Rationale: The airway is always a priority, and the nurse would attend to the client who has been experiencing an airway problem first. The clients described in options 1, 2, and 3 would have intermediate priority.
Test-Taking Strategy: Note the strategic word, *first*. Use the ABCs—airway, breathing, and circulation—to answer the question. Remember that the airway is always the first priority. **Review:** the principles related to **prioritizing.**
Level of Cognitive Ability: Applying
Client Needs: Safe and Effective Care Environment
Integrated Process: Nursing Process/Planning
Content Area: Leadership/Management: Prioritizing
Priority Concepts: Care Coordination, Clinical Judgment
Reference(s): deWit, Kumagai (2013), pp. 25, 83.

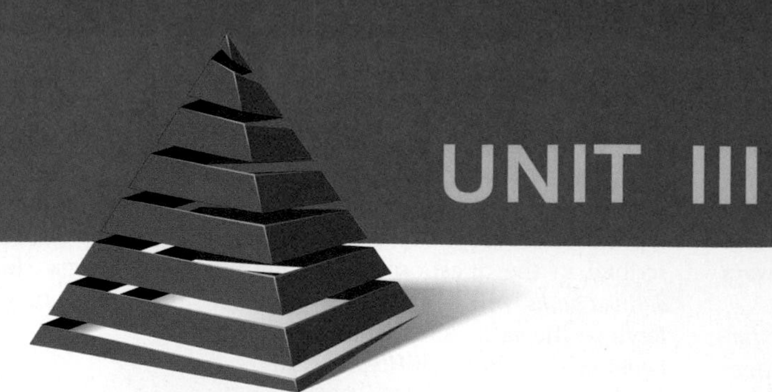

UNIT III

Nursing Sciences

PYRAMID TERMS

ABO A type of antigen system. The ABO type of the donor should be compatible with the recipient's. Type A can match with type A or O; type B can match with type B or O; type O can match only with type O; type AB can match with type A, B, AB, or O.

air embolism An obstruction caused by a bolus of air that enters the vein through an inadequately primed intravenous (IV) line, from a loose connection, during a tubing change, or during removal of an IV line.

Allen's test A test to assess for collateral circulation to the hand by evaluating the patency of the radial and ulnar arteries.

blood The liquid pumped by the heart through the arteries, veins, and capillaries. Blood is composed of a clear yellow fluid (plasma), formed elements, and cell types with various functions.

blood cell Any of the formed elements of the blood, including red cells (erythrocytes), white cells (leukocytes), and platelets (thrombocytes).

calcium A mineral element needed for the process of bone formation, coagulation of blood, excitation of cardiac and skeletal muscle, maintenance of muscle tone, conduction of neuromuscular impulses, and synthesis and regulation of the endocrine and exocrine glands. The normal adult level is 8.6 to 10 mg/dL.

catheter embolism An obstruction caused by breakage of the catheter tip during IV line insertion or removal.

circulatory overload A complication resulting from the infusion of blood at a rate too rapid for the size, age, cardiac status, or clinical condition of the recipient.

compatibility Matching of blood from two persons by two different types of antigen systems, ABO and Rh, present on the membrane surface of the red blood cells, to prevent a transfusion reaction.

compensation Compensation refers to the body processes that occur to counterbalance an acid-base disturbance. When compensation has occurred, the pH will be within normal limits.

crossmatching The testing of the donor's blood and the recipient's blood for compatibility.

enteral nutrition Administration of nutrition with liquefied foods into the gastrointestinal tract via a tube.

fat emulsion (lipids) A white, opaque solution administered intravenously during parenteral nutrition therapy to prevent fatty acid deficiency.

fluid volume deficit Dehydration in which the body's fluid intake is not sufficient to meet the body's fluid needs.

fluid volume excess Fluid intake or fluid retention that exceeds the body's fluid needs; also called overhydration or fluid overload.

homeostasis The tendency of biological systems to maintain relatively constant conditions in the internal environment while continuously interacting with and adjusting to changes originating within or outside of the system.

infiltration Seepage of IV fluid out of the vein and into the surrounding interstitial spaces.

magnesium An element concentrated in the bone, cartilage, and within the cell itself that is required for the use of adenosine triphosphate as a source of energy. It is necessary for the action of numerous enzyme systems, such as carbohydrate metabolism, protein synthesis, nucleic acid synthesis, and the contraction of muscular tissue. It also regulates neuromuscular activity and the clotting mechanism. The normal adult level is 1.6 to 2.6 mg/dL.

malnutrition Deficiency of the nutrients required for development and maintenance of the human body.

metabolic acidosis A total concentration of buffer base that is lower than normal, with a relative increase in the hydrogen ion concentration. This results from loss of buffer bases or retention of too many acids without sufficient bases, and occurs in conditions such as kidney failure and diabetic ketoacidosis, from the production of lactic acid, and from the ingestion of toxins, such as acetylsalicylic acid (aspirin).

metabolic alkalosis A deficit or loss of hydrogen ions or acids or an excess of base (bicarbonate) that results from the accumulation of base or from a loss of acid without a comparable loss of base in the body fluids. This occurs in conditions resulting in hypovolemia, the loss of gastric fluid, excessive bicarbonate intake, the massive transfusion of whole blood, and hyperaldosteronism.

metabolism Ongoing chemical process within the body that converts digested nutrients into energy for the functioning of body cells.

nutrients Carbohydrates, fats or lipids, proteins, vitamins, minerals, electrolytes, and water that must be supplied in adequate amounts to provide energy, growth, development, and maintenance of the human body.

packed red blood cells A blood product used to replace erythrocytes lost as a result of trauma or surgical interventions or in clients with bone marrow suppression.

parenteral nutrition (PN) Administration of a nutritionally complete formula through a central or peripheral intravenous (IV) catheter. In the clinical setting, the term *PN* may be used interchangeably with the term *total parenteral nutrition* (TPN) or *hyperalimentation.*

phlebitis An inflammation of the vein that can occur from mechanical or chemical (medication) trauma or from a local infection.

plasma The watery, straw-colored, fluid part of lymph and the blood in which the formed elements (blood cells) are suspended. Plasma is made up of water, electrolytes, protein, glucose, fats, bilirubin, and gases and is essential for carrying the cellular elements of the blood through the circulation.

platelet transfusion A blood product administered to clients with low platelet counts and to thrombocytopenic clients who are bleeding actively or are scheduled for an invasive procedure.

potassium A principal electrolyte of intracellular fluid and the primary buffer within the cell itself; it is needed for nerve conduction, muscle function, acid-base balance, and osmotic pressure. Along with calcium and magnesium, it controls the rate and force of contraction of the heart and, thus, cardiac output. The normal adult level is 3.5 to 5.0 mEq/L.

phosphorus An element needed for the generation of bony tissue; it functions in the metabolism of glucose and lipids, in the maintenance of acid-base balance, and in the storage and transfer of energy from one site in the body to another. Phosphorus levels are evaluated in relation to calcium levels because of their inverse relationship: when calcium levels are decreased, phosphorus levels are increased, and when phosphorus levels are decreased, calcium levels are increased. The normal adult level is 2.7 to 4.5 mg/dL.

respiratory acidosis A total concentration of buffer base that is lower than normal, with a relative increase in hydrogen ion concentration; thus a greater number of hydrogen ions is circulating in the blood than the buffer system can absorb. This is caused by primary defects in the function of the lungs or by changes in normal respiratory patterns as a result of secondary problems. Any condition that causes an obstruction of the airway or depresses respiratory status can cause respiratory acidosis.

respiratory alkalosis A deficit of carbonic acid or a decrease in hydrogen ion concentration that results from the accumulation of base or from a loss of acid without a comparable loss of base in the body fluids. This occurs in conditions that cause overstimulation of the respiratory system.

Rh factor Rh stands for rhesus factor. A person having the factor is Rh positive; a person lacking the factor is Rh negative. The presence or absence of Rh antigens on the surface of red blood cells determines the classification as Rh positive or Rh negative.

septicemia The presence of infective agents or their toxins in the bloodstream. Septicemia is a serious infection and must be treated promptly; otherwise, the infection leads to circulatory collapse, profound shock, and death.

serum The clear and thin fluid part of blood that remains after coagulation. Serum contains no blood cells, platelets, or fibrinogen.

sodium An abundant electrolyte that maintains osmotic pressure and acid-base balance and transmits nerve impulses. The normal adult level is 135 to 145 mEq/L.

transfusion reaction A hemolytic reaction caused by blood type or Rh incompatibility. An allergic transfusion reaction most often occurs in clients with a history of an allergy. A febrile transfusion reaction most commonly occurs in clients with antibodies directed against the transfused white blood cells. A bacterial transfusion reaction occurs after transfusion of contaminated blood products.

venipuncture Puncture into a vein to obtain a blood specimen for testing; the antecubital veins are the veins of choice because of ease of access.

Pyramid to Success

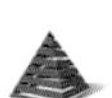

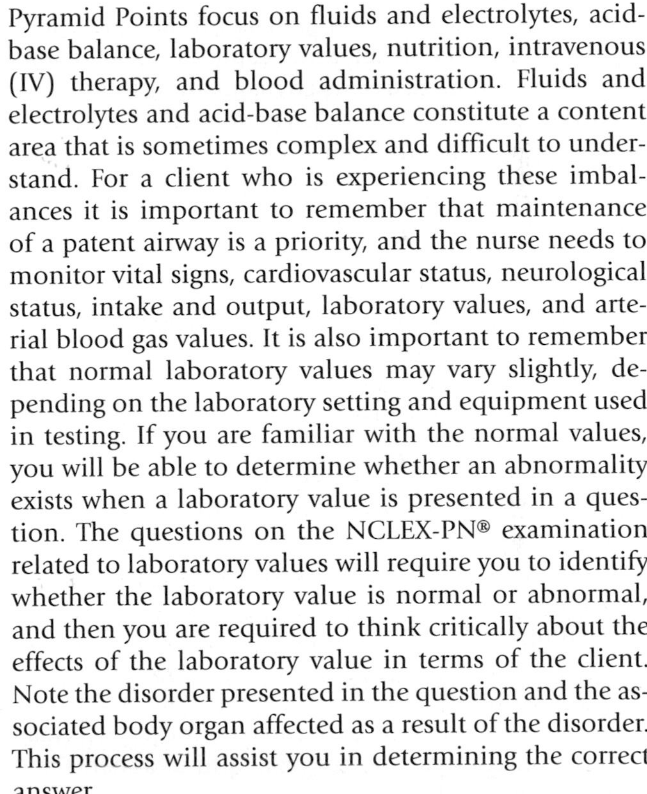

Pyramid Points focus on fluids and electrolytes, acid-base balance, laboratory values, nutrition, intravenous (IV) therapy, and blood administration. Fluids and electrolytes and acid-base balance constitute a content area that is sometimes complex and difficult to understand. For a client who is experiencing these imbalances it is important to remember that maintenance of a patent airway is a priority, and the nurse needs to monitor vital signs, cardiovascular status, neurological status, intake and output, laboratory values, and arterial blood gas values. It is also important to remember that normal laboratory values may vary slightly, depending on the laboratory setting and equipment used in testing. If you are familiar with the normal values, you will be able to determine whether an abnormality exists when a laboratory value is presented in a question. The questions on the NCLEX-PN® examination related to laboratory values will require you to identify whether the laboratory value is normal or abnormal, and then you are required to think critically about the effects of the laboratory value in terms of the client. Note the disorder presented in the question and the associated body organ affected as a result of the disorder. This process will assist you in determining the correct answer.

Nutrition is a basic need that must be met for all clients. The NCLEX-PN examination addresses the dietary measures required for basic needs and for particular body system alterations and addresses parenteral nutrition (PN). When presented with a question related to nutrition, consider the client's diagnosis and the particular requirement or restriction necessary for treatment of the disorder. With regard to IV therapy, data collection includes determining if client allergies exist, including latex sensitivity, before initiation of an IV line. Monitoring for complications is a critical nursing responsibility. Likewise, the procedure for administering blood components, the signs and symptoms of transfusion reaction, and the immediate interventions if a transfusion reaction occurs are a priority focus.

Client Needs

Safe and Effective Care Environment

Applying principles of infection control
Collaborating with members of the health care team
Ensuring that informed consent was obtained for invasive procedures
Establishing priorities for care
Handling hazardous and infectious materials safely to prevent injury to self and others
Identifying the client with at least two forms of identifiers (e.g., name and identification number) prior to administering care per agency procedures
Identifying the need for client referrals
Maintaining continuity of care and providing follow-up for client care issues
Maintaining medical and surgical asepsis and preventing infection in the client when samples for laboratory studies are obtained or when maintaining intravenous (IV) solutions or removing a peripheral IV catheter
Maintaining standard, transmission-based, and other precautions to prevent transmission of infection to self and others
Preventing accidents and ensuring safety of the client when a fluid or electrolyte imbalance exists, particularly when changes in cardiovascular, respiratory, gastrointestinal, neuromuscular, renal, or central nervous systems occur, or when the client is at risk for complications such as seizures, respiratory depression, or dysrhythmias
Providing information to the client about community classes for nutrition education
Providing safety for the client during implementation of treatments
Using equipment such as electronic IV infusion devices safely
Upholding client rights

Health Promotion and Maintenance

Collecting health history data and baseline physical data
Considering lifestyle choices related to treatments and procedures and home care needs
Determining the client's ability to perform self-care
Evaluating the client's home environment for necessary self-care modifications
Identifying clients at risk for an acid-base imbalance
Identifying community resources available for follow-up
Reinforcing client and family education regarding the administration of PN at home
Reinforcing education related to medication and diet management
Reinforcing education related to the potential risk for a fluid and electrolyte imbalance, measures to prevent an imbalance, signs and symptoms of an imbalance, and actions to take if signs and symptoms develop
Reporting the potential risk for a fluid and electrolyte imbalance

Psychosocial Integrity

Collecting data about the client's emotional response to treatment
Considering cultural preferences related to nutritional patterns and lifestyle choices
Discussing role changes related to the client's need to receive PN at home
Identifying coping mechanisms
Identifying and reporting religious, spiritual, and cultural considerations related to blood administration
Identifying support systems in the home to assist with caring for an IV and the administration of PN
Providing emotional support to the client during testing
Providing reassurance to the client who is experiencing a fluid or electrolyte imbalance
Providing support and continuously informing the client of the purposes for prescribed interventions

Physiological Integrity

Assisting with administering and monitoring medications, intravenous fluids, and other therapeutic interventions as appropriate
Assisting with obtaining an arterial blood gas specimen and reviewing the results with the registered nurse
Identifying clients who are at risk for a fluid or electrolyte imbalance
Managing medical emergencies if a transfusion reaction or other complication occurs
Monitoring for clinical manifestations associated with an abnormal laboratory value
Monitoring of enteral feedings and the client's ability to tolerate feedings
Monitoring for expected effects of pharmacological and parenteral therapies
Monitoring for expected and unexpected responses to therapeutic interventions and reporting and documenting findings
Monitoring laboratory values; determining the significance of an abnormal laboratory value and the need to report the findings
Monitoring of nutritional intake and oral hydration
Monitoring the administration of blood products and immediately reporting signs of a transfusion reaction
Monitoring IV therapy
Providing wound care when blood is obtained for an arterial blood gas study

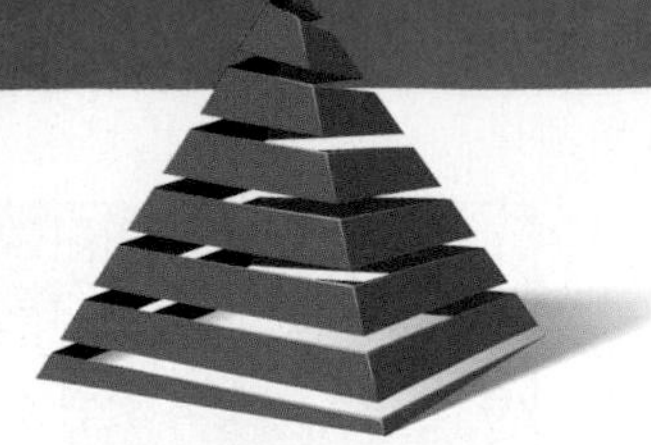

CHAPTER 9

Fluids and Electrolytes

CRITICAL THINKING What Should You Do?

The nurse looks at the client's monitor screen and notes that there is an additional prominent wave following each T wave. The nurse suspects the presence of U waves. What action(s) should the nurse take?

Answer located on p. 86.

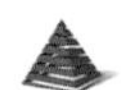

I. Concepts of Fluid and Electrolyte Balance

A. Electrolytes

1. An electrolyte is a substance that, on dissolving in solution, ionizes: that is, some of its molecules split or dissociate into electrically charged atoms or ions (Box 9-1)
2. Measurement

BOX 9-1 Cell Properties

Atom: The smallest part of an element that still has the properties of the element and that is composed of particles known as *protons* (positive charge), *neutrons* (neutral), and *electrons* (negative charge). Protons and neutrons are in the nucleus of the atom; therefore, the nucleus is positively charged. Electrons carry a negative charge and revolve around the nucleus. As long as the number of electrons is the same as the number of protons, there is no net charge on the atom—that is, it is neither positive nor negative. Atoms may gain, lose, or share electrons, and then they are no longer neutral.

Molecule: Two or more atoms that have combined to form a substance.

Ion: An atom that carries an electrical charge because it has either gained or lost electrons. Some ions carry a negative electrical charge, and some carry a positive charge.

Cation: An ion that has given away or lost electrons and therefore carries a positive charge. The result is fewer electrons than protons and a positive charge.

Anion: An ion that has gained electrons and therefore carries a negative charge. When an ion has gained or taken on electrons, it assumes a negative charge, and the result is a negatively charged ion.

   a. The metric system is used to measure volumes of fluids: liters (L) or milliliters (mL).
   b. The unit of measure that expresses the combining activity of an electrolyte is the milliequivalent (mEq).

B. Body fluid compartments (Box 9-2) (Fig. 9-1)

1. Fluid in each of the body compartments contains electrolytes.
2. Each compartment has a particular composition of electrolytes that differs from that of other compartments.
3. To function normally, body cells must have fluids and electrolytes in the right compartments and in the right amounts.
4. Whenever an electrolyte moves out of a cell, another electrolyte moves in to take its place.
5. The numbers of cations and anions must be the same for **homeostasis** to exist.
6. Compartments are separated by semipermeable membranes.

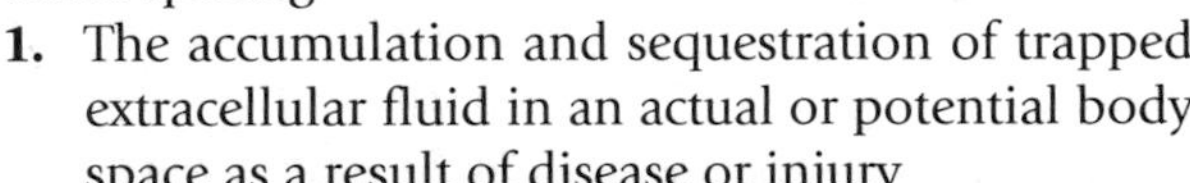

C. Third-spacing

1. The accumulation and sequestration of trapped extracellular fluid in an actual or potential body space as a result of disease or injury
2. The trapped fluid represents a volume loss and is unavailable for normal physiological processes.
3. Fluid may be trapped in body spaces such as the pericardial, pleural, peritoneal, or joint cavities; the bowel; the abdomen; or within soft tissues after trauma or burns.
4. Gathering data about intravascular fluid loss is difficult. It may not be reflected in weight

BOX 9-2 Body Fluid Compartments

Extracellular compartment: Refers to all fluid outside of the cells

Interstitial fluids: Fluid that is between the cells and the blood vessels

Intracellular compartment: Refers to all fluid inside the cells. Most body fluids are inside the cells.

Intravascular compartment: Fluid that is within blood vessels

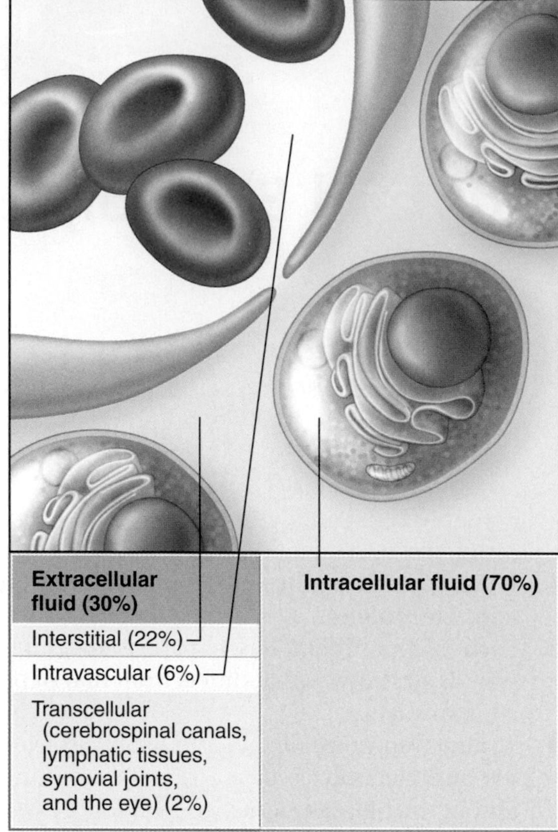

FIGURE 9-1 Distribution of fluid by compartments in the average adult. (From Harkreader H, Hogan MA: *Fundamentals of nursing: Caring and clinical judgment*, ed 3, St. Louis, 2007, Saunders.)

changes or intake and output (I&O) records, and it may not become apparent until after organ malfunction occurs.

D. Edema
1. An excess accumulation of fluid in the interstitial spaces; occurs as a result of alterations in oncotic pressure, hydrostatic pressure, capillary permeability, and lymphatic obstruction.
2. Localized edema occurs as a result of traumatic injury from accidents or surgery, local inflammatory processes, or burns.
3. Generalized edema, also called *anasarca*, is an excessive accumulation of fluid in the interstitial space throughout the body as a result of a condition such as cardiac, renal, or liver failure.

E. Body fluid
1. Description
   a. Provides the transportation of **nutrients** to the cells and carries waste products from the cells
   b. Total body fluid (intracellular and extracellular) amounts to about 60% of body weight in the adult, 55% in the older adult, and 80% in the infant.
   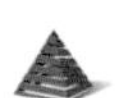
   c. Infants and older adults are at higher risk for fluid-related problems than younger adults; children have a greater proportion of body water than adults; and the older adult has the least proportion of body water.
2. Constituents of body fluids
   a. Body fluids consist of water and dissolved substances.
   b. The largest single fluid constituent of the body is water.

Infants and older adults need to be monitored closely for fluid imbalances.

F. Body fluid transport
1. Diffusion
   a. Diffusion is the process whereby a solute (substance that is dissolved) may spread through a solution or solvent (solution in which the solute is dissolved).
   b. Diffusion of a solute spreads the molecules from an area of higher concentration to an area of lower concentration.
   c. Diffusion occurs within fluid compartments and from one compartment to another if the barrier between the compartments is permeable to the diffusing substances.
2. Osmosis
   a. Osmosis is the movement of solvent molecules across a membrane in response to a concentration gradient, usually from a solution of lower to one of higher solute concentration.
   b. When a more concentrated solution is on one side of a selectively permeable membrane and a less concentrated solution is on the other side, a pull called *osmotic pressure* draws the water through the membrane to the more concentrated side, or the side with more solute.
3. Filtration
   a. Filtration is the movement of solutes and solvents by hydrostatic pressure.
   b. The movement is from an area of higher pressure to an area of lower pressure.
4. Hydrostatic pressure
   a. The force exerted by the weight of a solution
   b. When a difference exists in the hydrostatic pressure on two sides of a membrane, water and diffusible solutes move out of the solution that has the higher hydrostatic pressure by the process of filtration.
5. Osmolality
   a. Refers to the number of osmotically active particles per kilogram of water; it is the concentration of a solution.
   b. In the body, osmotic pressure is measured in milliosmols (mOsm).
   c. The normal osmolality of **plasma** is 270 to 300 (mOsm/kg) water.

G. Movement of body fluid

1. Description
   a. Cell membranes separate the interstitial fluid from the intravascular fluid.
   b. Cell membranes are selectively permeable; that is, the cell membrane and the capillary wall allow water and some solutes free passage through them.
   c. Several forces affect the movement of water and solutes through the walls of cells and capillaries; for example, the greater the number of particles within the cell, the more pressure that exists to force the water through the cell membrane and out of the cell.
   d. If the body loses more electrolytes than fluids, as can happen with diarrhea, then the extracellular fluid will contain fewer electrolytes or less solute than the intracellular fluid.
   e. Fluids and electrolytes must be kept in balance for health; when they remain out of balance, death can occur.
2. Isotonic solutions (Table 9-1)
   a. When the solutions on both sides of a selectively permeable membrane have established equilibrium or are equal in concentration, they are isotonic.
   b. Isotonic solutions are isotonic to human cells, and thus very little osmosis occurs; isotonic solutions have the same osmolality as body fluids.
3. Hypotonic solutions (see Table 9-1)
   a. When a solution contains a lower concentration of salt or solute than another more concentrated solution, it is considered hypotonic.
   b. A hypotonic solution has less salt or more water than an isotonic solution. These solutions have lower osmolality than body fluids.
   c. Hypotonic solutions are hypotonic to the cells; therefore, osmosis would continue in an attempt to bring about balance or equality.

TABLE 9-1 Tonicity of Intravenous Fluids

Solution	Tonicity
0.45% saline (½ normal saline [NS])	Hypotonic
0.9% saline (NS)	Isotonic
5% dextrose in water (D_5W)	Isotonic
5% dextrose in 0.225% saline (D_5/¼ NS)	Isotonic
Lactated Ringer's solution	Isotonic
5% dextrose in lactated Ringer's solution	Hypertonic
5% dextrose in 0.45% saline (D_5/½ NS)	Hypertonic
5% dextrose in 0.9% saline (D_5/NS)	Hypertonic
10% dextrose in water ($D_{10}W$)	Hypertonic

Fluid intake		Fluid output	
Ingested water	1200-1500 mL	Kidneys	1500 mL
Ingested food	800-1100 mL	Insensible loss through skin	600-800 mL
Metabolic oxidation	300 mL	Insensible loss through lungs	400-600 mL
		Gastrointestinal tract	100 mL
TOTAL	2300-2900 mL	TOTAL	2600-3000 mL

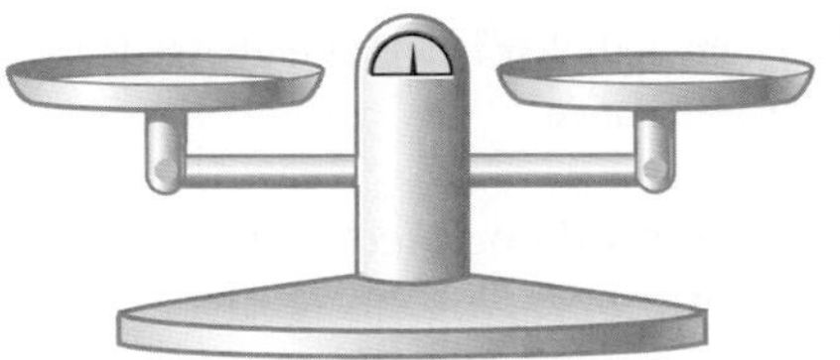

FIGURE 9-2 Sources of fluid intake and fluid output. (From Harkreader H, Hogan MA: *Fundamentals of nursing: Caring and clinical judgment*, ed 3, St. Louis, 2007, Saunders.)

4. Hypertonic solutions: A solution that has a higher concentration of solutes than another less concentrated solution is hypertonic. These solutions have a higher osmolality than body fluids (see Table 9-1).

H. Body fluid intake and output (Fig. 9-2) 

1. Body fluid intake
   a. Water enters the body through three sources—orally ingested liquids, water in foods, and water formed by oxidation of foods.
   b. About 10 mL of water is released by the **metabolism** of each 100 calories of fat, carbohydrates, or proteins.
2. Body fluid output
   a. Water lost through the skin is called *insensible loss* (the individual is unaware of losing that water).
   b. The amount of water lost by perspiration varies according to the temperature of the environment and of the body, but the average amount of loss by perspiration alone is 100 mL/day.
   c. Water lost from the lungs is called *insensible loss* and is lost through expired air that is saturated with water vapor.
   d. The amount of water lost from the lungs varies with the rate and the depth of respiration.
   e. Large quantities of water are secreted into the gastrointestinal tract, but almost all this fluid is reabsorbed.
   f. A large volume of electrolyte-containing liquids moves into the gastrointestinal tract and then returns again into the extracellular fluid.
   g. Severe diarrhea results in the loss of large quantities of fluids and electrolytes.
   h. The kidneys play a major role in regulating fluid and electrolyte balance and excrete the largest quantity of fluid.
   i. Normal kidneys can adjust the amount of water and electrolytes leaving the body.

j. The quantity of fluid excreted by the kidneys is determined by the amount of water ingested and the amount of waste and solutes excreted.
k. As long as all organs are functioning normally, the body is able to maintain balance in its fluid content.

The client with diarrhea is at high risk for a fluid and electrolyte imbalance.

I. Maintaining fluid and electrolyte balance
1. Description
a. **Homeostasis** is a term that indicates the relative stability of the internal environment.
b. Concentration and composition of body fluids must be nearly constant.
c. When one of the substances in a client is deficient—either fluid or electrolytes—the substance must be replaced normally by the intake of food and water or by therapy such as intravenous (IV) solutions and medications.
d. When the client has an excess of fluid or electrolytes, therapy is directed toward assisting the body with eliminating the excess.
2. The kidneys play a major role in controlling the balance of fluid and electrolytes.
3. The adrenal glands, through the secretion of aldosterone, also aid with controlling the extracellular fluid volume by regulating the amount of sodium reabsorbed by the kidneys.
4. Antidiuretic hormone from the pituitary gland regulates the osmotic pressure of extracellular fluid by regulating the amount of water reabsorbed by the kidney.

II. Fluid Volume Deficit

A. Description
1. Dehydration occurs when the body's fluid intake is not sufficient to meet the body's fluid needs.
2. The goal of treatment is to restore fluid volume, replace electrolytes as needed, and eliminate the cause of the **fluid volume deficit**.

B. Causes
1. Vomiting and/or diarrhea
2. Continuous gastrointestinal (GI) irrigation
3. GI suctioning
4. Ileostomy or colostomy drainage
5. Draining wounds, burns, or fistulas
6. Increased urine output from the use of diuretics

C. Data collection
1. Thirst
2. Poor skin turgor and dry mucous membranes
3. Increased heart rate, thready pulse, dyspnea, and postural hypotension
4. Weight loss
5. Flat neck or hand veins
6. Dizziness or weakness
7. Decrease in urine volume and dark, concentrated urine
8. Increased specific gravity of the urine
9. Confusion
10. Increased hematocrit level

D. Interventions
1. The cause of the fluid volume deficit is treated (for example antidiarrheal, antiemetic, antipyretic, antimicrobial medications may be prescribed), and fluids are replaced through administration of intravenous solutions as prescribed and oral rehydration.
2. Monitor vital signs and respiratory and neurological status closely.
3. Administer oxygen as prescribed.
4. Check mucous membranes and skin turgor.
5. Monitor weight daily.
6. Monitor intake and output.
7. Test urine for specific gravity.
8. Monitor hematocrit and electrolyte levels; prepare to correct electrolyte imbalance if needed.

III. Fluid Volume Excess

A. Description
1. Fluid intake or retention exceeds the body's fluid needs.
2. Also called *overhydration, fluid overload, or* **circulatory overload**.
3. The goals of treatment are to restore fluid balance; correct electrolyte imbalances, if present; and eliminate or control the underlying cause of the overload (impaired cardiac or renal function can lead to **fluid volume excess**).

B. Causes
1. Overhydration with IV fluids
2. Kidney damage
3. Heart failure
4. Long-term use of corticosteroids
5. Excessive sodium ingestion
6. Syndrome of inappropriate antidiuretic hormone secretion
7. Irrigation of wounds or body cavities with hypotonic fluids

C. Data collection 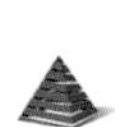
1. Cough and dyspnea
2. Lung crackles
3. Increased respirations and heart rate
4. Increased blood pressure and bounding pulse
5. Pitting edema
6. Weight gain
7. Neck and hand vein distention
8. Increased urine output if kidneys can compensate; decreased if kidney damage is the cause
9. Confusion
10. Decreased hematocrit level

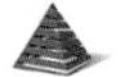

D. Interventions
1. Monitor vital signs and respiratory and neurological status closely.
2. Position the client in semi-Fowler's position.
3. Administer oxygen as prescribed.
4. Check for edema.
5. Monitor intake and output.
6. Monitor daily weight.
7. Administer diuretics as prescribed.
8. Monitor hematocrit and electrolyte levels.
9. Restrict fluids as prescribed.
10. Provide a low-sodium diet as prescribed.

⚠ A client with kidney damage or failure is at high risk for fluid volume excess.

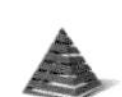

IV. Hypokalemia

A. Description (Box 9-3)
1. Hypokalemia is a serum **potassium** level lower than 3.5 mEq/L.
2. Potassium deficit is potentially life threatening because every body system is affected.

B. Causes and signs/symptoms (Table 9-2)

C. Interventions
1. Assist to monitor cardiovascular, respiratory, neuromuscular, gastrointestinal, and renal status; client is placed on a cardiac monitor.
2. Monitor vital signs closely.
3. Monitor intake and output.
4. Monitor electrolyte values.
5. Check for adequate renal function before administering prescribed potassium; monitor intake and output during administration.
6. Administer potassium supplements as prescribed (orally or monitor by IV).
7. Oral potassium supplements
   a. Oral potassium supplements may cause nausea and vomiting, and they should not be taken on an empty stomach; if the client complains of abdominal pain, distention, nausea, vomiting, diarrhea, or gastrointestinal bleeding, the supplement may need to be discontinued.
   b. Liquid potassium chloride has an unpleasant taste and should be taken with juice or another liquid.
8. Intravenously administered potassium
   a. The client receiving potassium by the intravenous route needs to be placed on a cardiac monitor and monitored closely, and the nurse should follow the RN's instructions regarding care.
   b. Monitor the IV site closely; if **phlebitis** or **infiltration** occurs, the IV should be stopped immediately, and the RN should be notified; the IV will be restarted at another site.
9. Institute safety measures for the client experiencing muscle weakness.
10. If the client is taking a potassium-depleting diuretic, it may be discontinued; a potassium-retaining diuretic may be prescribed.
11. Instruct the client about foods that are high in potassium content (see Box 9-3).

BOX 9-3 Potassium

Normal Value

3.5 to 5.0 mEq/L

Common Food Sources

Avocados
Bananas
Cantaloupe
Carrots
Fish
Mushrooms
Oranges
Potatoes
Pork, beef, and veal
Raisins
Spinach
Strawberries
Tomatoes

TABLE 9-2 Potassium Imbalances

Hypokalemia	Hyperkalemia
Causes	
Use of potassium-losing diuretics	Kidney failure
Diarrhea	Intestinal obstruction
Vomiting	Cell damage
Inadequate intake of potassium	Excessive oral or parenteral administration of potassium; potassium-retaining diuretics
Excessive gastric suction	Acidosis
Excessive fistula drainage	Addison's disease
Cushing's syndrome	Excessive use of potassium-based salt substitutes
Chronic use of corticosteroids or laxatives	Transfusion of stored blood (the breakdown of older red blood cells releases potassium)
Kidney disease	
Parenteral nutrition	
Uncontrolled diabetes	
Alkalosis	
Signs and Symptoms	
Leg and abdominal cramps	Muscle weakness
Lethargy and weakness	Paresthesias
Shallow respirations and thready pulse	Hypotension
Confusion	Diarrhea
Decreased or absent reflexes	Hyperactive bowel sounds
Hypoactive bowel sounds and ileus	Wide, flat P waves; widened QRS complex; prolonged PR interval; depressed ST segment; and narrow, peaked T waves
Postural hypotension	
Peaked P waves; flat T waves; depressed ST segment and U waves	

12. Reinforce instructions to the client not to use salt substitutes containing **potassium** unless prescribed by the health care provider.

⚠ Potassium is never administered by IV push, intramuscular, or subcutaneous routes. IV potassium is always diluted and administered using an infusion device.

V. Hyperkalemia

A. Description

1. Hyperkalemia is a serum potassium level that exceeds 5.0 mEq/L (see Box 9-3).
2. Pseudohyperkalemia: a condition that can occur due to methods of **blood** specimen collection and cell lysis; if an increased serum value is obtained in the absence of clinical symptoms, the specimen should be redrawn and evaluated.

B. Causes and signs/symptoms (see Table 9-2)

C. Interventions

1. Monitor cardiovascular, respiratory, neuromuscular, renal, and gastrointestinal status; the client is placed on a cardiac monitor.
2. If IV potassium is being administered, it is stopped immediately (however, the IV catheter is not removed and is kept patent); in addition, oral potassium supplements are withheld.
3. Assist to initiate a potassium-restricted diet.
4. Prepare to administer potassium-excreting diuretics as prescribed if kidney function is not impaired.
5. If kidney function is impaired, prepare to administer sodium polystyrene sulfonate (Kayexalate) as prescribed, a cation-exchange resin that promotes gastrointestinal sodium absorption and potassium excretion.
6. Dialysis may be prescribed if potassium levels are critically high.
7. Intravenous **calcium** may be prescribed if the hyperkalemia is severe to avert myocardial excitability.
8. Intravenous hypertonic glucose with regular insulin may be prescribed to move excess potassium into the cells.
9. Note that when blood transfusions are prescribed for a client with a potassium imbalance, the client should receive fresh blood, if possible; transfusions of stored blood may elevate the potassium level because the breakdown of older **blood cells** releases potassium.
10. Reinforce instructions to avoid foods high in potassium (see Box 9-3).
11. Reinforce instructions to avoid the use of salt substitutes or other potassium-containing substances.

⚠ Monitor the serum potassium level closely when a client is receiving a potassium-retaining diuretic!

VI. Hyponatremia

A. Description

1. Hyponatremia is a serum **sodium** level less than 135 mEq/L (Box 9-4).
2. Sodium imbalances are usually associated with fluid imbalances.

B. Causes and signs/symptoms (Table 9-3)

C. Interventions

1. Monitor cardiovascular, respiratory, neuromuscular, cerebral, renal, and gastrointestinal status.
2. If hyponatremia is accompanied by a fluid volume deficit (hypovolemia), IV sodium chloride infusions may be prescribed to restore sodium content and fluid volume.
3. If hyponatremia is accompanied by fluid volume excess (hypervolemia), osmotic diuretics may be prescribed to promote the excretion of water rather than sodium.
4. If caused by inappropriate or excessive secretion of antidiuretic hormone, medications that antagonize antidiuretic hormone may be prescribed.
5. Reinforce instructions about the need to increase oral sodium intake and inform the client about the foods to include in the diet (see Box 9-4).
6. If the client is taking lithium (Lithobid), monitor the lithium level, because hyponatremia can cause diminished lithium excretion, resulting in toxicity. 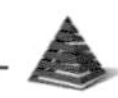

BOX 9-4 Sodium

Normal Value

135 to 145 mEq/L

Common Food Sources

Bacon
Butter
Canned foods
Cheese, such as American or cottage cheese
Hot dogs
Ketchup
Lunch meats
Milk
Mustard
Processed foods
Snack foods
Soy sauce
Table salt
White and whole-wheat bread

TABLE 9-3 Sodium Imbalances

Hyponatremia	Hypernatremia
Causes	
Inadequate sodium intake (nothing by mouth)	Decreased water intake
Gastrointestinal suction	Fever
Excessive intake of water	Excessive perspiration
Irrigation of gastrointestinal tubes with plain water	Dehydration
Diuretics	Hyperventilation
Increased perspiration	Watery diarrhea
Draining skin lesions	Enteral nutrition and parenteral nutrition deplete the cells of water
Burns	Diabetes insipidus
Nausea and vomiting	Cushing's syndrome
Diabetic ketoacidosis	Impaired kidney function
Syndrome of inappropriate antidiuretic hormone secretion	Use of corticosteroids
Retention of fluid, such as with kidney or heart failure	Excessive administration of sodium bicarbonate
Signs and Symptoms	
Rapid, thready pulse	Dry mucous membranes
Postural blood pressure changes	Loss of skin turgor
Weakness	Thirst
Abdominal cramping	Flushed skin
Poor skin turgor	Elevated temperature
Muscle twitching and seizures	Oliguria
Apprehension	Muscle twitching
	Fatigue
	Confusion
	Seizures

Hyponatremia precipitates lithium toxicity in a client taking lithium (Lithobid).

VII. Hypernatremia

A. Description: Hypernatremia is a serum sodium level that exceeds 145 mEq/L (see Box 9-4).

B. Causes and signs/symptoms (Table 9-3)

C. Interventions

1. Monitor cardiovascular, respiratory, neuromuscular, cerebral, renal, and integumentary status.
2. If the cause is fluid loss, IV fluids may be prescribed.
3. If the cause is inadequate renal excretion of sodium, diuretics that promote sodium loss may be prescribed.
4. Restrict sodium and fluid intake as prescribed (see Box 9-4).

VIII. Hypocalcemia

A. Description: Hypocalcemia is a serum calcium level less than 8.6 mg/dL (Box 9-5).

B. Causes and signs/symptoms (Table 9-4 and Fig. 9-3)

C. Interventions

BOX 9-5 Calcium

Normal Value

8.6 to 10 mg/dL

Common Food Sources

Cheese
Collard greens
Milk and soy milk
Rhubarb
Sardines
Spinach
Tofu
Yogurt

TABLE 9-4 Calcium Imbalances

Hypocalcemia	Hypercalcemia
Causes	
Inadequate dietary intake of calcium	Excessive intake of calcium supplements, milk, and antacid products that contain calcium
Inhibited absorption of calcium from the intestinal tract	Excessive intake of vitamin D
Inadequate vitamin D consumption	Increased bone resorption or destruction from conditions such as bone tumors, fractures, osteoporosis, and immobility
Diarrhea	Decreased excretion of calcium
Long-term immobilization and bone demineralization	Kidney disease
Excessive gastrointestinal losses from diarrhea or wound draining	Use of thiazide diuretics
End-stage kidney disease	Hyperparathyroidism
Calcium-excreting medications such as diuretics, caffeine, anticonvulsants, heparin, laxatives, and nicotine	Use of lithium
Decreased secretion of parathyroid hormone	Use of glucocorticoids
Acute pancreatitis	Adrenal insufficiency
Crohn's disease	
Excessive administration of blood	
Signs and Symptoms	
Tachycardia	Increased heart rate and blood pressure
Hypotension	Bounding pulse
Paresthesias	Bradycardia (late stage)
Twitching	Muscle weakness (hypotonicity)
Cramps	Diminished deep tendon reflexes
Tetany	Nausea and vomiting
Positive Chvostek's or Trousseau's sign	Constipation
Diarrhea	Abdominal distention
Hyperactive bowel sounds	Confusion, lethargy, and coma
Prolongation of QT interval	Shortened QT interval and widened T wave

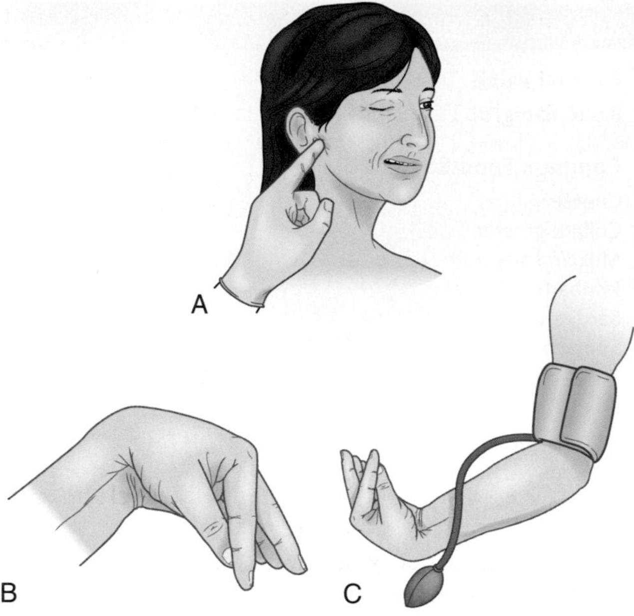

FIGURE 9-3 Tests for hypocalcemia. **A,** Chvostek's sign is a contraction of facial muscles in response to a light tap over the facial nerve in front of the ear. **B,** Trousseau's sign is a carpal spasm induced by inflating a blood pressure cuff (**C**) above the systolic pressure for a few minutes. (From Lewis S, Dirksen S, Heitkemper M, Bucher L: *Medical-surgical nursing: Assessment and management of clinical problems*, ed 9, St. Louis, 2014, Elsevier.)

1. Monitor cardiovascular, respiratory, neuromuscular, and gastrointestinal status; the client is placed on a cardiac monitor.
2. Assist to administer calcium supplements orally; calcium may be prescribed intravenously.
3. Assist to monitor the client receiving intravenous calcium; monitor for electrocardiographic changes, observe for infiltration, and monitor for hypercalcemia.
4. Medications that increase calcium absorption may be prescribed.
   a. Aluminum hydroxide reduces **phosphorus** levels, causing the countereffect of increasing calcium levels.
   b. Vitamin D aids in the absorption of calcium from the intestinal tract.
5. Provide a quiet environment to reduce environmental stimuli.
6. Initiate seizure precautions.
7. Keep 10% calcium gluconate available for treatment of acute calcium deficit.
8. Reinforce instructions regarding consuming foods high in calcium (see Box 9-5).

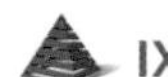

IX. Hypercalcemia

A. Description: Hypercalcemia is a **serum** calcium level that exceeds 10 mg/dL (see Box 9-5).

B. Causes and signs/symptoms (see Table 9-4)

C. Interventions

1. Monitor cardiovascular, respiratory, neuromuscular, renal, and gastrointestinal status; the client is placed on a cardiac monitor.
2. IV infusions of solutions containing calcium and oral medications containing calcium or vitamin D will be discontinued.
3. Thiazide diuretics may be discontinued and replaced with diuretics that enhance the excretion of calcium.
4. Assist to administer medications as prescribed that inhibit calcium resorption from the bone, such as phosphorus, calcitonin (Calcimar), bisphosphonates, and prostaglandin synthesis inhibitors (aspirin, nonsteroidal anti-inflammatory drugs).
5. Assist to prepare the client with severe hypercalcemia for dialysis if medications fail to reduce the serum calcium level.
6. Monitor for flank or abdominal pain, and strain the urine to check for the presence of urinary stones.
7. Reinforce instructions about the foods to avoid that are high in calcium (see Box 9-5).

A client with a calcium imbalance is at risk for a pathological fracture. Move the client carefully and slowly; assist the client with ambulation.

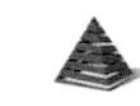

X. Hypomagnesemia

A. Description: Hypomagnesemia is a serum **magnesium** level less than 1.6 mg/dL (Box 9-6).

B. Causes and signs/symptoms (Table 9-5)

C. Interventions

1. Monitor cardiovascular, respiratory, gastrointestinal, neuromuscular, and central nervous system status; the client is placed on a cardiac monitor.

BOX 9-6 Magnesium

Normal Value

1.6 to 2.6 mg/dL

Common Food Sources

Avocados
Canned white tuna fish
Cauliflower
Oatmeal
Green leafy vegetables, such as spinach and broccoli
Yogurt
Milk
Peanut butter
Peas
Pork, beef, and chicken
Potatoes
Raisins

Fundamentals

TABLE 9-5 Magnesium Imbalances

Hypomagnesemia	Hypermagnesemia
Causes	
Malnutrition	Overuse of antacids or laxatives that contain magnesium
Diarrhea	Renal insufficiency and kidney failure
Celiac disease	Treatment of pre-eclampsia with magnesium
Crohn's disease	
Alcoholism	
Prolonged gastric suctioning	
Ileostomy, colostomy, or intestinal fistulas	
Acute pancreatitis	
Diabetic ketoacidosis	
Eclampsia	
Chemotherapy	
Sepsis	
Signs and Symptoms	
Twitching	Hypotension
Paresthesias	Bradycardia
Hyperactive reflexes	Weak pulse
Irritability	Sweating and flushing
Confusion	Respiratory depression
Positive Chvostek's or Trousseau's sign	Loss of deep tendon reflexes
Shallow respirations	Prolonged PR interval and widened QRS complexes
Tetany	
Seizures	
Tachycardia	
Tall T waves and depressed ST segment	

2. Because hypocalcemia frequently accompanies hypomagnesemia, interventions also aim to restore normal serum calcium levels.

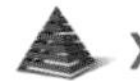

3. Oral preparations of magnesium may cause diarrhea and increase magnesium loss.
4. Magnesium sulfate by the IV route may be prescribed in severe cases (intramuscular injections cause pain and tissue damage); assist to monitor the client closely during administration; seizure precautions are initiated, serum magnesium levels are monitored frequently, and the client is monitored for diminished deep tendon reflexes that suggest hypermagnesemia.
5. Reinforce instructions to the client to eat food that is high in magnesium (see Box 9-6).

XI. Hypermagnesemia

A. Description: Hypermagnesemia is a serum magnesium level that exceeds 2.6 mg/dL (see Box 9-6).

B. Causes and signs/symptoms (see Table 9-5)

C. Interventions

1. Monitor cardiovascular, respiratory, neuromuscular, and central nervous system status; the client is placed on a cardiac monitor.
2. Diuretics are prescribed to increase renal excretion of magnesium.
3. Intravenously administered calcium chloride or calcium gluconate may be prescribed to reverse the effects of magnesium on cardiac muscle.
4. Reinforce instructions to restrict dietary intake of magnesium-containing foods (see Box 9-6).
5. Reinforce instructions to the client to avoid the use of laxatives and antacids that contain magnesium.

⚠ Calcium gluconate is the antidote for magnesium overdose!

XII. Hypophosphatemia

A. Description

1. Hypophosphatemia is a serum phosphorus level lower than 2.7 mg/dL (Box 9-7).
2. A decrease in the serum phosphorus level is accompanied by an increase in the serum calcium level. 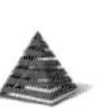

B. Causes and signs/symptoms (Table 9-6)

BOX 9-7 Phosphorus

Normal Value

2.7 to 4.5 mg/dL

Common Food Sources

Fish
Organ meats
Nuts
Pork, beef, and chicken
Whole-grain breads and cereals
Dairy products

TABLE 9-6 Phosphorus Imbalances

Hypophosphatemia	Hyperphosphatemia
Causes	
Decreased nutritional intake of phosphorus and malnutrition	Excessive dietary intake of phosphorus
Use of magnesium-based or aluminum-hydroxide–based antacids	Overuse of phosphate-containing laxatives or enemas
Kidney failure	Vitamin D intoxication
Hyperparathyroidism	Hypoparathyroidism
Malignancy	Renal insufficiency
Hypercalcemia	Chemotherapy
Alcohol withdrawal	
Diabetic ketoacidosis	
Respiratory alkalosis	
Signs and Symptoms	
Confusion	Neuromuscular irritability
Seizures	Muscle weakness
Weakness	Hyperactive reflexes
Decreased deep tendon reflexes	Tetany
Shallow respirations	Positive Chvostek's or Trousseau's sign
Increased bleeding tendency	
Immunosuppression	
Bone pain	

C. Interventions
1. Monitor cardiovascular, respiratory, neuromuscular, central nervous system, and hematological status.
2. Medications that contribute to hypophosphatemia will be discontinued.
3. Prepare to administer phosphorus orally along with a vitamin D supplement.
4. IV phosphorus may be prescribed when serum phosphorus levels fall below 1 mg/dL and when the client experiences critical clinical manifestations; assist with monitoring the client closely if IV phosphorus is prescribed.
5. Check for adequate renal function before administering phosphorus.
6. Move the client carefully, and monitor for signs of a pathological fracture.
7. Reinforce instructions to increase the intake of the phosphorus-containing foods while decreasing the intake of any calcium-containing foods (see Boxes 9-5 and 9-7).

A decrease in the serum phosphorus level is accompanied by an increase in the serum calcium level, and an increase in the serum phosphorus level is accompanied by a decrease in the serum calcium level.

XIII. Hyperphosphatemia

A. Description
1. Hyperphosphatemia is a serum phosphorus level that exceeds 4.5 mg/dL (see Box 9-7).
2. Most body systems tolerate elevated serum phosphorus levels well.
3. An increase in the serum phosphorus level is accompanied by a decrease in the serum calcium level.
4. The problems that occur in hyperphosphatemia center on the hypocalcemia that results when serum phosphorus levels increase.

B. Causes and signs/symptoms (see Table 9-6)

C. Interventions
1. Interventions entail the management of hypocalcemia.

2. Assist to administer phosphate-binding medications that increase fecal excretion of phosphorus by binding phosphorus from food in the gastrointestinal tract.

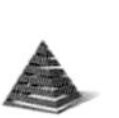

3. Reinforce instructions to avoid phosphate-containing medications, including laxatives and enemas.
4. Reinforce instructions to decrease the intake of food that is high in phosphorus (see Box 9-7).
5. Reinforce instructions in medication administration: take phosphate-binding medications, emphasizing that they should be taken with meals or immediately after meals.

CRITICAL THINKING What Should You Do?

Answer: Cardiac changes in hypokalemia include impaired repolarization, resulting in the emergence of prominent U waves. Therefore, the nurse should suspect hypokalemia. The incidence of potentially lethal ventricular dysrhythmias is increased in hypokalemia. The nurse should immediately notify the registered nurse and check the client's vital signs and cardiac status and for signs of hypokalemia. The nurse needs to stay with the client while the RN checks the client's most recent serum potassium level and contacts the health care provider to report the findings and obtain prescriptions to treat the hypokalemic state.

Reference(s): deWit, D. & Kumagai, C. (2013). *Medical-surgical nursing: Concepts & practice.* (2nd ed., pp. 42, 394). St. Louis: Saunders.

PRACTICE QUESTIONS

31. The nurse who is caring for a client with kidney failure notes that the client is dyspneic, and crackles are heard on auscultation of the lungs. Which additional signs/symptoms should the nurse expect to note in this client?
1. Rapid weight loss
2. Flat hand and neck veins
3. A weak and thready pulse
4. An increase in blood pressure

32. The nurse is reviewing the health records of assigned clients. The nurse should plan care knowing that which client is at risk for a potassium deficit?
1. The client with Addison's disease
2. The client with metabolic acidosis
3. The client with intestinal obstruction
4. The client receiving nasogastric suction

33. The nurse reviews a client's electrolyte results and notes a potassium level of 5.5 mEq/L. The nurse understands that a potassium value at this level would be noted with which condition?
1. Diarrhea
2. Traumatic burn
3. Cushing's syndrome
4. Overuse of laxatives

34. The nurse reviews a client's electrolyte results and notes that the potassium level is 5.4 mEq/L. Which should the nurse observe for on the cardiac monitor as a result of this laboratory value?
1. ST elevation
2. Peaked P waves

3. Prominent U waves
4. Narrow, peaked T waves

35. The nurse is reading the health care provider's (HCP's) progress notes in the client's record and sees that the HCP has documented "insensible fluid loss of approximately 800 mL daily." Which client is at risk for this loss?
   1. Client with a draining wound
   2. Client with a urinary catheter
   3. Client with a fast respiratory rate
   4. Client with a nasogastric tube to low suction

36. The nurse is reviewing the health records of assigned clients. The nurse should plan care knowing that which client is at the **least likely** risk for the development of third-spacing?
   1. The client with sepsis
   2. The client with cirrhosis
   3. The client with kidney failure
   4. The client with diabetes mellitus

37. The nurse is reviewing the health records of assigned clients. The nurse should plan care knowing that which client is at risk for fluid volume deficit?
   1. The client with cirrhosis
   2. The client with a colostomy
   3. The client with heart failure (HF)
   4. The client with decreased kidney function

38. The nurse is caring for a client who has been taking diuretics on a long-term basis. Which finding should the nurse expect to note as a result of this long-term use?
   1. Gurgling respirations
   2. Increased blood pressure
   3. Decreased hematocrit level
   4. Increased specific gravity of the urine

39. The nurse reviews electrolyte values and notes a sodium level of 130 mEq/L. The nurse expects that this sodium level would be noted in a client with which condition?
   1. The client with watery diarrhea
   2. The client with diabetes insipidus (DI)
   3. The client with an inadequate daily water intake
   4. The client with the syndrome of inappropriate secretion of antidiuretic hormone (SIADH)

40. The nurse is caring for a client with leukemia and notes that the client has poor skin turgor and flat neck and hand veins. The nurse suspects hyponatremia. Which additional signs/symptoms should the nurse expect to note in this client if hyponatremia is present?
   1. Intense thirst
   2. Slow bounding pulse
   3. Dry mucous membranes
   4. Postural blood pressure changes

41. The nurse is caring for a client with a diagnosis of hyperparathyroidism. Laboratory studies are performed, and the serum calcium level is 12.0 mg/dL. Based on this laboratory value, the nurse should take which action?
   1. Document the value in the client's record.
   2. Inform the registered nurse of the laboratory value.
   3. Place the laboratory result form in the client's record.
   4. Reassure the client that the laboratory result is normal.

42. The nurse reviews the client's serum calcium level and notes that the level is 8.0 mg/dL. The nurse understands that which condition would cause this serum calcium level?
   1. Prolonged bed rest
   2. Adrenal insufficiency
   3. Hyperparathyroidism
   4. Excessive ingestion of vitamin D

43. The nurse is caring for a client with a suspected diagnosis of hypercalcemia. Which signs/symptoms would be an indication of this electrolyte imbalance?
   1. Twitching
   2. Positive Trousseau's sign
   3. Hyperactive bowel sounds
   4. Generalized muscle weakness

44. The nurse is instructing a client on how to decrease the intake of calcium in the diet. The nurse should tell the client that which food item is **least likely** to contain calcium?
   1. Milk
   2. Butter
   3. Spinach
   4. Collard greens

45. The nurse is caring for a client with hyperparathyroidism and notes that the client's serum calcium level is 13 mg/dL. Which prescribed medication should the nurse prepare to assist in administering to the client?
   1. Calcium chloride
   2. Calcium gluconate
   3. Calcitonin (Miacalcin)
   4. Large doses of vitamin D

ANSWERS

31. 4

Rationale: Impaired cardiac or kidney function can result in fluid volume excess. Findings associated with fluid volume excess include cough, dyspnea, crackles, tachypnea, tachycardia, an elevated blood pressure, a bounding pulse, an elevated central venous pressure, weight gain, edema, neck and hand vein distention, an altered level of consciousness, and a decreased hematocrit level.

Test-Taking Strategy: Note that rapid weight loss; flat hand and neck veins; and weak, thready pulse are **comparable or alike** in that they all relate to a decrease in fluid volume. The correct option is the only option that reflects an increase in fluid volume. **Review:** signs/symptoms of **fluid volume excess.**

Level of Cognitive Ability: Analyzing
Client Needs: Physiological Integrity
Integrated Process: Nursing Process/Data Collection
Content Area: Fundamental Skills: Fluids & Electrolytes
Priority Concepts: Clinical Judgment, Fluid and Electrolyte Balance
Reference(s): Linton (2012), p. 208.

32. 4

Rationale: Potassium-rich gastrointestinal (GI) fluids are lost through GI suction, which places the client at risk for hypokalemia. The client with intestinal obstruction, Addison's disease, and metabolic acidosis is at risk for hyperkalemia.

Test-Taking Strategy: Focus on the **subject**, *potassium deficit (hypokalemia)*. Read the question carefully, and note that it asks for the client who is at risk for hypokalemia. Read each option, and think about the electrolyte loss that can occur with each condition. Nasogastric suction not only results in a loss of body fluid but also electrolytes. **Review:** causes of **hypokalemia**.

Level of Cognitive Ability: Analyzing
Client Needs: Physiological Integrity
Integrated Process: Nursing Process/Planning
Content Area: Fundamental Skills: Fluids & Electrolytes
Priority Concepts: Elimination, Fluid and Electrolyte Balance
Reference(s): Linton (2012), p. 209.

33. 2

Rationale: A serum potassium level that exceeds 5.0 mEq/L is indicative of hyperkalemia. Clients who experience the cellular shifting of potassium, as in the early stages of massive cell destruction (i.e., with trauma, burns, sepsis, or metabolic or respiratory acidosis), are at risk for hyperkalemia. The client with Cushing's syndrome or diarrhea and the client who has been overusing laxatives are at risk for hypokalemia.

Test-Taking Strategy: Eliminate diarrhea and overuse of laxatives first, because they are **comparable or alike** and reflect a gastrointestinal loss. From the remaining options, recalling that cell destruction that occurs with traumatic burns causes potassium shifts, will direct you to the correct option. Remember that Cushing's syndrome presents a risk for hypokalemia. **Review:** causes of **hyperkalemia**.

Level of Cognitive Ability: Analyzing
Client Needs: Physiological Integrity
Integrated Process: Nursing Process/Data Collection
Content Area: Fundamental Skills: Fluids & Electrolytes
Priority Concepts: Cellular Regulation, Fluid and Electrolyte Balance
Reference(s): deWit, Kumagai (2013), pp. 42, 982.

34. 4

Rationale: A serum potassium level of 5.4 mEq/L is indicative of hyperkalemia. Cardiac changes include a wide, flat P wave; a prolonged PR interval; a widened QRS complex; and narrow, peaked T waves.

Test-Taking Strategy: Focus on the **subject**, potassium level of 5.4 mEq/L. Determine next that this condition is a hyperkalemic one. From this point, it is necessary to know the cardiac changes that are expected when hyperkalemia exists. **Review: cardiac changes in hyperkalemia.**

Level of Cognitive Ability: Analyzing
Client Needs: Physiological Integrity
Integrated Process: Nursing Process/Data Collection
Content Area: Fundamental Skills: Fluids & Electrolytes
Priority Concepts: Fluid and Electrolyte Balance, Perfusion
Reference(s): Ignatavicius, Workman (2013), pp. 190–191; Lewis et al (2014), p. 296.

35. 3

Rationale: Sensible losses are those that the person is aware of, such as those that occur through wound drainage, GI tract losses, and urination. Insensible losses may occur without the person's awareness. Insensible losses occur daily through the skin and the lungs.

Test-Taking Strategy: Focus on the **subject**, insensible fluid loss. Note that wound drainage, urinary output, and gastric secretions are **comparable or alike** in that they represent visible losses. These types of losses can be measured for accurate output. Fluid loss through a fast respiratory rate cannot be accurately measured, only approximated. **Review: sensible and insensible fluid loss.**

Level of Cognitive Ability: Analyzing
Client Needs: Physiological Integrity
Integrated Process: Nursing Process/Data Collection
Content Area: Fundamental Skills: Fluids & Electrolytes
Priority Concepts: Elimination, Fluid and Electrolyte Balance
Reference(s): Lewis et al (2014), pp. 291, 293.

36. 4

Rationale: Fluid that shifts into the interstitial spaces and remains there is referred to as *third-space fluid*. Common sites for third-spacing include the abdomen, pleural cavity, peritoneal cavity, and pericardial sac. Third-space fluid is physiologically useless because it does not circulate to provide nutrients for the cells. Risk factors include liver or kidney disease, major trauma, burns, sepsis, wound healing, major surgery, malignancy, malabsorption syndrome, malnutrition, alcoholism, and older age.

Test-Taking Strategy: Note the **strategic words**, *least likely*. These words indicate a **negative event query** and ask you to select the client who is at least risk for third-spacing. Eliminate cirrhosis and kidney failure first, because it is likely that fluid balance disturbances will occur with these conditions. From the remaining options, sepsis is the option that is the most acute and therefore the most similar to cirrhosis and kidney failure. **Review:** risk factors associated with **third-spacing**.

Level of Cognitive Ability: Analyzing
Client Needs: Physiological Integrity

Integrated Process: Nursing Process/Planning
Content Area: Fundamental Skills: Fluids & Electrolytes
Priority Concepts: Clinical Judgment, Fluid and Electrolyte Balance
Reference(s): deWit, Kumagai (2013), p. 39; Lewis et al (2014), pp. 277, 289.

37. 2
Rationale: Causes of a fluid volume deficit include vomiting, diarrhea, conditions that cause increased respirations or increased urinary output, insufficient intravenous fluid replacement, draining fistulas, ileostomy, and colostomy. A client with cirrhosis, HF, or decreased kidney function is at risk for fluid volume excess.
Test-Taking Strategy: Focus on the **subject**, fluid volume deficit. Read the question carefully, and note that it asks for the client who is at risk for a deficit. Read each option, and think about the fluid imbalance that can occur in each client. Clients with cirrhosis, HF, and decreased kidney function all retain fluid. The only condition that can cause a fluid volume deficit is the condition noted in the correct option. **Review:** causes of **fluid volume deficit**.
Level of Cognitive Ability: Analyzing
Client Needs: Physiological Integrity
Integrated Process: Nursing Process/Planning
Content Area: Fundamental Skills: Fluids & Electrolytes
Priority Concepts: Elimination, Fluid and Electrolyte Balance
Reference(s): Lewis et al (2014), p. 292; Linton (2012), p. 206.

38. 4
Rationale: Clients taking diuretics on a long-term basis are at risk for fluid volume deficit. Findings of fluid volume deficit include increased respirations and heart rate, decreased central venous pressure, weight loss, poor skin turgor, dry mucous membranes, decreased urine volume, increased specific gravity of the urine, dark-colored and odorous urine, an increased hematocrit level, and an altered level of consciousness. Gurgling respirations, increased blood pressure, and decreased hematocrit as a result of hemodilution are seen in a client with fluid volume excess.
Test-Taking Strategy: Focus on the **subject**, long-term use of diuretics, and realize that this can lead to a fluid volume deficit. Eliminate gurgling respirations and increased blood pressure first because they would be noted in clients with fluid volume excess. Next, remember that the specific gravity of urine is increased in a client with a fluid volume deficit. **Review:** signs/symptoms of **fluid volume deficit**.
Level of Cognitive Ability: Analyzing
Client Needs: Physiological Integrity
Integrated Process: Nursing Process/Data Collection
Content Area: Fundamental Skills: Fluids & Electrolytes
Priority Concepts: Elimination, Fluid and Electrolyte Balance
Reference(s): Linton (2012), p. 205.

39. 4
Rationale: Hyponatremia is a serum sodium level less than 135 mEq/L. Hyponatremia can occur secondary to SIADH. The client with an inadequate daily water intake, watery diarrhea, or diabetes insipidus is at risk for hypernatremia.
Test-Taking Strategy: Focus on the **subject**, sodium level of 130 mEq/L, and determine that this represents hyponatremia. Knowledge regarding the normal sodium level and the causes of hyponatremia is required to answer the question. Remember that hyponatremia can occur secondary to SIADH. **Review:** causes of **hyponatremia**.
Level of Cognitive Ability: Analyzing
Client Needs: Physiological Integrity
Integrated Process: Nursing Process/Data Collection
Content Area: Fundamental Skills: Fluids & Electrolytes
Priority Concepts: Clinical Judgment, Fluid and Electrolyte Balance
Reference(s): deWit, Kumagai (2013), pp. 40–41, 838.

40. 4
Rationale: Postural blood pressure changes occur in the client with hyponatremia. Intense thirst and dry mucous membranes are seen in clients with hypernatremia. A slow, bounding pulse is not indicative of hyponatremia. In a client with hyponatremia, a rapid, thready pulse is noted.
Test-Taking Strategy: Focus on the **subject**, hyponatremia. Note the information provided in the question. Eliminate intense thirst and dry mucous membranes first, because they are **comparable or alike** (a client with dry mucous membranes is likely to have intense thirst). From the remaining options, it is necessary to recall the signs of hyponatremia. **Review:** signs/symptoms associated with **hyponatremia**.
Level of Cognitive Ability: Analyzing
Client Needs: Physiological Integrity
Integrated Process: Nursing Process/Data Collection
Content Area: Fundamental Skills: Fluids & Electrolytes
Priority Concepts: Clinical Judgment, Fluid and Electrolyte Balance
Reference(s): deWit, Kumagai (2013), p. 42.

41. 2
Rationale: The normal serum calcium level ranges from 8.6 to 10.0 mg/dL. The client is experiencing hypercalcemia, and the nurse would inform the registered nurse of the laboratory value. Because the client is experiencing hypercalcemia, the remaining options are incorrect actions.
Test-Taking Strategy: Focus on the laboratory value in the question to determine that the client is experiencing hypercalcemia. Note that options 1 and 3 are **comparable or alike** and indicate that no action would be taken to report the abnormal value. From the remaining options eliminate option 4 because the value is elevated. **Review:** normal serum **calcium** level.
Level of Cognitive Ability: Applying
Client Needs: Physiological Integrity
Integrated Process: Nursing Process/Implementation
Content Area: Fundamental Skills: Fluids & Electrolytes
Priority Concepts: Clinical Judgment, Fluid and Electrolyte Balance
Reference(s): deWit, Kumagai (2013), pp. 846–847.

42. 1
Rationale: The normal serum calcium level is 8.6 to 10.0 mg/dL. A client with a serum calcium level of 8.0 mg/dL is experiencing hypocalcemia. The excessive ingestion of vitamin D, adrenal insufficiency, and hyperparathyroidism are causative factors associated with hypercalcemia. Although immobilization can initially cause hypercalcemia, the long-term effect of prolonged bed rest is hypocalcemia.

Test-Taking Strategy: Focus on the subject, serum calcium level of 8.0 mg/dL. Knowledge regarding the normal serum calcium level will assist you with determining that the client is experiencing hypocalcemia. This should help you to eliminate excessive ingestion of vitamin D. Recalling the causative factors associated with hypocalcemia is necessary to select the correct option from those remaining. Remember that the long-term effect of prolonged bed rest is hypocalcemia. **Review:** causative factors associated with **hypocalcemia**.
Level of Cognitive Ability: Understanding
Client Needs: Physiological Integrity
Integrated Process: Nursing Process/Data Collection
Content Area: Fundamental Skills: Fluids & Electrolytes
Priority Concepts: Clinical Judgment, Fluid and Electrolyte Balance
Reference(s): deWit, Kumagai (2013), pp. 43–44.

43. 4
Rationale: Generalized muscle weakness is seen in clients with hypercalcemia. Twitching, positive Trousseau's sign, and hyperactive bowel sounds are signs of hypocalcemia.
Test-Taking Strategy: Recall the signs/symptoms of hypocalcemia and hypercalcemia. Note that twitching, positive Trousseau's sign, and hyperactive bowel sounds are comparable or alike, because they all reflect a hyperactivity of body systems. The option that is different is muscle weakness. Review: signs/symptoms of **hypercalcemia**.
Level of Cognitive Ability: Analyzing
Client Needs: Physiological Integrity
Integrated Process: Nursing Process/Data Collection
Content Area: Fundamental Skills: Fluids & Electrolytes
Priority Concepts: Clinical Judgment, Fluid and Electrolyte Balance
Reference(s): deWit, Kumagai (2013), p. 43.

44. 2
Rationale: Butter comes from milk fat and does not contain significant amounts of calcium. Milk, spinach, and collard greens are calcium-containing foods and should be avoided by the client on a calcium-restricted diet.
Test-Taking Strategy: Note the strategic words, *least likely.* These words indicate a negative event query and ask you to select the item that is lowest in calcium. Milk can be easily eliminated first. Eliminate spinach and collard greens next, because they are comparable or alike. **Review:** foods that are **high and low in calcium.**
Level of Cognitive Ability: Applying
Client Needs: Physiological Integrity
Integrated Process: Teaching and Learning
Content Area: Fundamental Skills: Fluids & Electrolytes
Priority Concepts: Fluid and Electrolyte Balance, Nutrition
Reference(s): deWit, Kumagai (2013), p. 133; Linton (2012), p. 120.

45. 3
Rationale: The normal serum calcium level is 8.6 to 10.0 mg/dL. This client is experiencing hypercalcemia. Calcium gluconate and calcium chloride are medications used for the treatment of tetany, which occurs as a result of acute hypocalcemia. In hypercalcemia, large doses of vitamin D need to be avoided. Calcitonin, a thyroid hormone, decreases the plasma calcium level by inhibiting bone resorption and lowering the serum calcium concentration.
Test-Taking Strategy: Focus on the subject, serum calcium level of 13 mg/dL. Recalling the normal serum calcium level will assist you with determining that the client is experiencing hypercalcemia. With this knowledge, you can easily eliminate calcium chloride and calcium gluconate, because you would not administer medication that adds calcium to the body. Remembering that excessive vitamin D is a causative factor of hypercalcemia will assist you with eliminating that option. Review: treatment of **hypercalcemia**.
Level of Cognitive Ability: Analyzing
Client Needs: Physiological Integrity
Integrated Process: Nursing Process/Planning
Content Area: Fundamental Skills: Fluids & Electrolytes
Priority Concepts: Clinical Judgment, Fluid and Electrolyte Balance
Reference(s): deWit, Kumagai (2013), p. 45.

CHAPTER 10

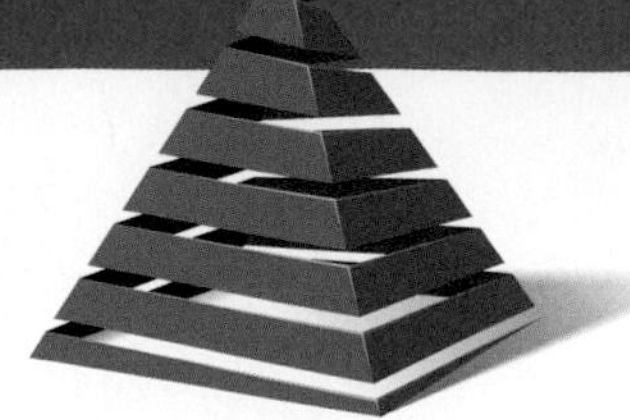

Acid–Base Balance

CRITICAL THINKING What Should You Do?

The nurse assists to perform an Allen's test on a client scheduled for an arterial blood gas draw from the radial artery. On release of pressure from the ulnar artery, color in the hand returns after 20 seconds. The nurse should take which actions?

Answer located on p. 97.

I. Hydrogen Ions, Acids, and Bases

A. Hydrogen (H^+) ions
   1. Vital to life, because H^+ ions determine the pH of the body, which must be maintained in a narrow range
   2. Expressed as pH; the pH scale is determined by the number of H^+ ions and goes from 1 to 14; 7 is considered neutral.
   3. The number of H^+ ions in the body fluid determines whether it is acid (acidic), alkaline (alkalosis), or neutral.
   4. The pH of body fluid is between 7.35 and 7.45.

B. Acids
   1. Produced as end products of **metabolism**
   2. Contain H^+ ions
   3. Are H^+ ion donors; they give up H^+ ions to neutralize or decrease the strength of an acid or to form a weaker base.

C. Bases
   1. Contain no H^+ ions
   2. Are H^+ ion acceptors; they accept H^+ ions from acids to neutralize or decrease the strength of a base or to form a weaker acid.
   3. Normal serum levels of bicarbonate (HCO_3^-) are 22 to 27 mEq/L.

II. Regulatory Systems for Hydrogen Concentration in the Blood

A. Buffers
   1. The fastest-acting regulatory system
   2. Provide immediate protection against changes in H^+ ion concentration in the extracellular fluid (i.e., absorb or release H^+ ions as needed)
   3. Serve as a transport mechanism that carries excess H^+ ions to the lungs
   4. Once the primary buffer systems react, they are consumed, and this leaves the body less able to withstand further stress until they are replaced.

B. Primary buffer systems in extracellular fluid
   1. Hemoglobin system
      a. Red **blood cells** contain hemoglobin.
      b. System maintains the acid–base balance by a process called *chloride shift.*
      c. Chloride shifts in and out of the red blood cells in response to the levels of oxygen (O_2) in the blood.
      d. For each chloride ion that leaves a red blood cell, a bicarbonate ion enters.
      e. For each chloride ion that enters a red blood cell, a bicarbonate ion leaves.
   2. Plasma proteins system
      a. Functions along with the liver to vary the amount of H^+ ions in the chemical structure of **plasma** proteins
      b. Plasma proteins have the ability to attract or release H^+ ions as the body needs them.
   3. Carbonic acid–bicarbonate (HCO_3^-) system 
      a. Primary buffer system in the body
      b. Maintains a pH of 7.4, with a ratio of 20 parts HCO_3^- to 1 part carbonic acid (H_2CO_3) (Fig. 10-1)
      c. This ratio (20:1) determines the concentration of H^+ ions in body fluid.
      d. The carbonic acid concentration is controlled by the excretion of carbon dioxide (CO_2) by the lungs. The rate and depth of respirations change in response to CO_2 levels.
      e. The kidneys control the bicarbonate (HCO_3^-) concentration and selectively retain or excrete HCO_3^- in response to bodily needs.
   4. Phosphate buffer system
      a. Present in the cells and body fluids and is especially active in the kidneys
      b. Acts like HCO_3^- and neutralizes excess hydrogen (H^+) ions

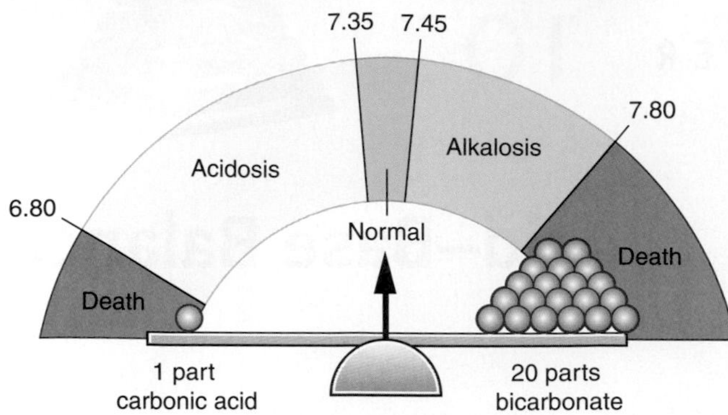

FIGURE 10-1 Acid–base balance. In the healthy state, a ratio of 1 part carbonic acid to 20 parts bicarbonate provides a normal serum pH between 7.35 and 7.45. Any deviation to the left of 7.35 results in an acidotic state. Any deviation to the right of 7.45 results in an alkalotic state. (From Harkreader H, Hogan MA: *Fundamentals of nursing: Caring and clinical judgment*, ed 3, St. Louis, 2007, Saunders.)

C. Lungs

1. The body's second defense and interact with the buffer system to maintain the acid–base balance
2. In acidosis, the pH decreases and the respiratory rate and depth increase in an attempt to exhale acids. The carbonic acid created by the neutralizing action of HCO_3^- can be carried to the lungs, where it is reduced to CO_2 and water and is exhaled. Thus, H^+ ions are inactivated and exhaled.
3. In alkalosis, the pH increases and the respiratory rate and depth decrease. CO_2 is retained, and carbonic acid increases to neutralize and decrease the strength of excess HCO_3.
4. The action of the lungs is reversible for controlling an excess or deficit.
5. The lungs can hold H^+ ions until the deficit is corrected or can inactivate H^+ ions, changing the ions to water molecules to be exhaled along with CO_2, thus correcting the excess.
6. The lungs can inactivate only H^+ ions carried by carbonic acid. Excess H^+ ions created by other problems must be excreted by the kidneys.

Monitor the client's respiratory status closely. In acidosis, the respiratory rate and depth increase in an attempt to exhale acids. In alkalosis, the respiratory rate and depth decrease. CO_2 is retained to neutralize and decrease the strength of excess bicarbonate.

D. Kidneys

1. The kidneys provide a more inclusive corrective response to acid–base disturbances than other corrective mechanisms, even though the renal excretion of acids and alkalis occurs more slowly.
2. **Compensation** requires a few hours to several days; however, it is a more thorough and selective process than that of other regulators, such as the buffer systems and the lungs.
3. In acidosis, the pH decreases and excess H^+ ions are secreted into the tubules and combine with buffers for excretion in the urine.
4. In alkalosis, the pH increases and excess HC_3^- ions move into the tubules, combine with sodium, and are excreted in the urine.
5. Selective regulation of HCO_3^- in the kidneys
   a. The kidneys restore HCO_3^- by excreting H^+ ions and retaining HCO_3^- ions.
   b. Excess H^+ ions are excreted in the urine in the form of phosphoric acid.
   c. The alteration of certain amino acids in the renal tubules results in the diffusion of ammonia into the kidneys. The ammonia combines with excess H^+ ions and is excreted into the urine.

E. Potassium (Fig. 10-2) 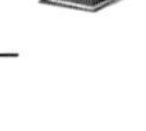

1. Plays an exchange role in maintaining the acid–base balance
2. The body changes the potassium (K) level by drawing H^+ ions into the cell or by pushing them out of the cells (potassium movement across cell membranes is facilitated by transcellular shifting in response to acid–base patterns).
3. In acidosis, the body protects itself from the acidic state by moving H^+ ions into the cell. Therefore, K moves out to make room for H^+ ions; the **serum** potassium level increases.
4. In alkalosis, the cells release H^+ ions into the blood in an attempt to increase the acidity of the blood; this forces the serum potassium into the cell and the serum potassium level decreases.

When the client experiences an acid–base imbalance, monitor the potassium level closely because the potassium moves in or out of the cells in an attempt to maintain acid–base balance.

III. Respiratory Acidosis

A. Description: The total concentration of buffer base is lower than normal, with a relative increase in H^+ ion concentration; thus, a greater number of H^+ ions are circulating in the blood than can be absorbed by the buffer system

B. Causes (Box 10-1)

If the client has a condition that causes an obstruction of the airway or depresses the respiratory system, monitor the client for respiratory acidosis.

C. Data collection: In an attempt to compensate, the respiratory rate and depth increase (Table 10-1). 

D. Interventions

1. Monitor for signs of respiratory distress.
2. Administer oxygen as prescribed.
3. Place the client in a semi-Fowler's position.

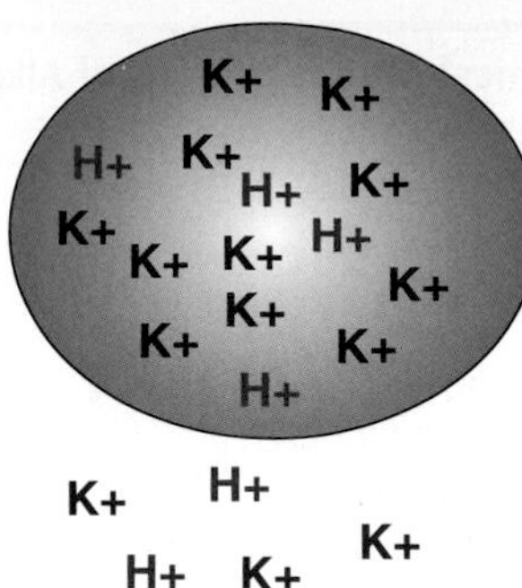

Under normal conditions, the intracellular potassium content is much greater than that of the extracellular fluid. The concentration of hydrogen ions is low in both compartments.

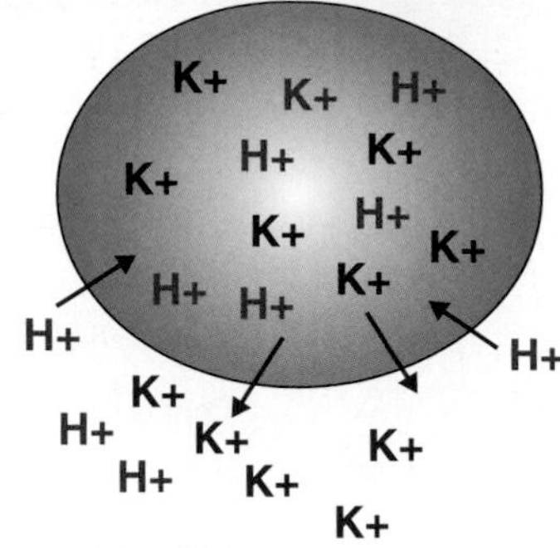

In acidosis, the extracellular hydrogen ion content increases, and the hydrogen ions move into the intracellular fluid. To keep the intracellular fluid electrically neutral, an equal number of potassium ions leave the cell, creating a relative hyperkalemia.

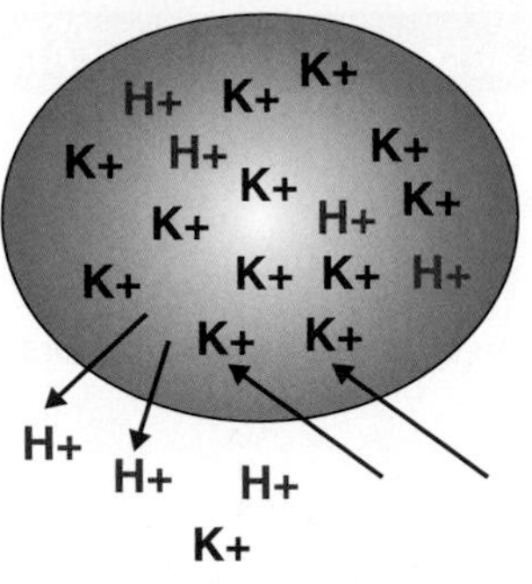

In alkalosis, more hydrogen ions are present in the intracellular fluid than in the extracellular fluid. Hydrogen ions move from the intracellular fluid into the extracellular fluid. To keep the intracellular fluid electrically neutral, potassium ions move from the extracellular fluid into the intracellular fluid, creating a relative hypokalemia.

FIGURE 10-2 Movement of potassium in response to changes in the extracellular fluid hydrogen ion concentration. (From Ignatavicius D, Workman ML: Medical-surgical nursing: Patient centered collaborative care, ed 7, Philadelphia, 2013, Saunders. Courtesy of M. Linda Workman.)

BOX 10-1 Causes of Respiratory Acidosis

- Asthma
- Atelectasis
- Brain trauma
- Bronchiectasis
- Bronchitis
- Central nervous system depressants
- Emphysema
- Hypoventilation
- Pneumonia
- Pulmonary edema
- Pulmonary emboli

4. Encourage and assist the client to turn, cough, and deep-breathe.
5. Prepare to assist to administer respiratory treatments as prescribed.
6. Encourage hydration to thin secretions.
7. Suction the client's airway, if necessary.
8. Reduce restlessness by improving ventilation rather than by administering tranquilizers, sedatives, or opioids because these medications further depress respirations.
9. Monitor electrolyte values, particularly the potassium level.
10. Assist to administer antibiotics for respiratory infection or other medications as prescribed.
11. Prepare for endotracheal intubation and mechanical ventilation if CO_2 levels rise above 50 mm Hg and if signs of acute respiratory distress are present.

TABLE 10-1 Clinical Manifestations of Acidosis

Respiratory (↑ Pco_2)	Metabolic (↓ HCO_3^-)
Neurological	
Drowsiness	Drowsiness
Disorientation	Confusion
Dizziness	Headache
Headache	Coma
Coma	
Cardiovascular	
Decreased blood pressure	Decreased blood pressure
Ventricular fibrillation (related to hyperkalemia from compensation)	Dysrhythmias (related to hyperkalemia from compensation)
Warm, flushed skin (related to peripheral vasodilation)	Warm, flushed skin (related to peripheral vasodilation)
Gastrointestinal	
No significant findings	Nausea, vomiting, diarrhea, abdominal pain
Neuromuscular	
Seizures	No significant findings
Respiratory	
Hypoventilation with hypoxia (lungs are unable to compensate when there is a respiratory problem)	Deep, rapid respirations (compensatory action by the lungs)

From Lewis S, Dirksen S, Heitkemper M, Bucher L, Camera I: *Medical-surgical nursing: Assessment and management of clinical problems*, ed 8, St. Louis, 2011, Mosby.

Fundamentals

BOX 10-2 Causes of Respiratory Alkalosis

- Fever
- Hyperventilation
- Hypoxia
- Hysteria
- Overventilation by mechanical ventilators
- Pain

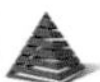

IV. Respiratory Alkalosis

A. Description: A deficit of carbonic acid and a decrease in H^+ ion concentration that results from the accumulation of base or the loss of acid without a comparable loss of base in the body fluids

B. Causes (Box 10-2)

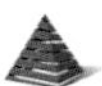 If the client has a condition that causes overstimulation of the respiratory system, monitor the client for respiratory alkalosis.

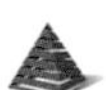

C. Data collection: In an attempt to compensate, the kidneys retain bicarbonate and excrete excess hydrogen ions into the urine (Table 10-2).

D. Interventions

1. Monitor for signs of respiratory distress.
2. Provide emotional support and reassurance to the client.
3. Assist with breathing techniques and breathing aids as prescribed.
   a. voluntary holding of the breath if appropriate
   b. use of a rebreathing mask as prescribed
   c. carbon dioxide breaths as prescribed (rebreathing into a paper bag)
4. Monitor ventilator clients to be sure that they are not forced to take breaths too deeply or rapidly.
5. 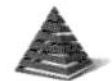 Monitor electrolyte values, particularly potassium and **calcium** levels.
6. Calcium gluconate may be prescribed for tetany; assist with administration.

V. Metabolic Acidosis

A. Description: A total concentration of buffer base that is lower than normal, with a relative increase in the H^+ ion concentration resulting from loss of too much base and/or retention of too much acid

B. Causes (Box 10-3)

An insufficient supply of insulin in a client with diabetes mellitus can result in metabolic acidosis known as diabetic ketoacidosis.

C. Data collection: To compensate for the acidosis, hyperpnea with Kussmaul's respiration occurs as the lungs attempt to exhale the excess CO_2 (see Table 10-1).

D. Interventions

1. Monitor for signs of respiratory distress.

TABLE 10-2 Clinical Manifestations of Alkalosis

Respiratory (↓ Pco_2)	Metabolic (↑ HCO_3^-)
Neurological	
Lethargy	Drowsiness
Lightheadedness	Dizziness
Confusion	Nervousness
	Confusion
Cardiovascular	
Tachycardia	Tachycardia
Dysrhythmias (related to hypokalemia from compensation)	Dysrhythmias (related to hypokalemia from compensation)
Gastrointestinal	
Nausea	Anorexia
Vomiting	Nausea
Epigastric pain	Vomiting
Neuromuscular	
Tetany	Tremors
Numbness	Hypertonic muscles
Tingling of extremities	Muscle cramps
Hyperreflexia	Tetany
Seizures	Tingling of extremities
	Seizures
Respiratory	
Hyperventilation (lungs are unable to compensate when there is a respiratory problem)	Hypoventilation (compensatory action by the lungs)

From Lewis S, Dirksen S, Heitkemper M, Bucher L, Camera I: *Medical-surgical nursing: Assessment and management of clinical problems*, ed 8, St. Louis, 2011, Mosby.

BOX 10-3 Causes of Metabolic Acidosis

- Diabetes mellitus or diabetic ketoacidosis
- Excessive ingestion of acetylsalicylic acid (aspirin)
- High-fat diet
- Insufficient metabolism of carbohydrates
- Malnutrition
- Renal insufficiency or failure
- Severe diarrhea

2. Check level of consciousness for central nervous system depression.
3. Monitor intake and output and assist with fluid and electrolyte replacement as prescribed.
4. Intravenous solutions that increase the buffer base may be prescribed.
5. Initiate safety and seizure precautions.
6. Monitor the potassium level closely; as **metabolic acidosis** resolves, potassium moves back into the cells and the potassium level decreases. 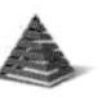

Monitor the client experiencing severe diarrhea for manifestations of metabolic acidosis.

E. Interventions for diabetes mellitus and diabetic ketoacidosis
  1. Give insulin as prescribed to hasten the movement of serum glucose into the cell, thereby decreasing the concurrent ketosis.
  2. When glucose is being properly metabolized, the body stops converting fats to glucose.
  3. Monitor for circulatory collapse caused by polyuria, which can result from the hyperglycemic state. Osmotic diuresis may lead to extracellular volume deficit and require fluid and electrolyte replacement.

F. Interventions for kidney failure
  1. Dialysis may be used to remove protein and waste products, thereby decreasing the acidosis.
  2. A diet low in protein and high in calories decreases the amount of protein waste products, which in turn lessens the acidosis.

VI. Metabolic Alkalosis

A. Description: A deficit of carbonic acid and a decrease in hydrogen ion concentration that results from the accumulation of base or from a loss of acid without a comparable loss of base in the body fluids

B. Causes (Box 10-4)

C. Data collection: To compensate, respiratory rate and depth decrease to conserve CO_2 (see Table 10-2).

Monitor the client experiencing excessive vomiting or the client with gastrointestinal suctioning for manifestations of metabolic alkalosis.

D. Interventions
  1. Monitor for signs of respiratory distress.
  2. Monitor potassium and calcium levels.
  3. Institute safety precautions.
  4. Medications and intravenous fluids to promote the kidney excretion of bicarbonate may be prescribed.
  5. Prepare to assist with potassium replacement as prescribed.
  6. The underlying cause of the alkalosis needs to be treated.

BOX 10-4 Causes of Metabolic Alkalosis

- Diuretics
- Excessive vomiting or gastrointestinal suctioning
- Hyperaldosteronism
- Ingestion and/or ingestion of excess sodium bicarbonate
- Massive transfusion of whole blood

VII. Arterial Blood Gases (Box 10-5)

A. Assisting with the collection of an arterial blood gas specimen
  1. Obtain vital signs
  2. **Allen's test** is performed to determine the presence of collateral circulation (see Priority Nursing Actions).

PRIORITY NURSING ACTIONS!

Actions Taken When an Allen's Test Is Performed Before Radial Artery Puncture

1. The procedure is explained to the client.
2. Pressure is applied over the ulnar and radial arteries simultaneously.
3. The client is asked to open and close the hand repeatedly.
4. Pressure is released from the ulnar artery while compressing the radial artery.
5. The color of the extremity distal to the pressure point is checked.
6. The findings are documented.

The Allen's test is performed before obtaining an arterial blood specimen from the radial artery to determine the presence of collateral circulation and the adequacy of the ulnar artery. Failure to determine the presence of adequate collateral circulation could result in severe ischemic injury to the hand if damage to the radial artery occurs with arterial puncture. The nurse assists to perform this test and first would explain the procedure to the client. To perform the test, the nurse applies direct pressure over the client's ulnar and radial arteries simultaneously. While applying pressure, the nurse asks the client to open and close the hand repeatedly; the hand should blanch. The nurse then releases pressure from the ulnar artery while compressing the radial artery and assesses the color of the extremity distal to the pressure point. If pinkness fails to return within 6 to 7 seconds, the ulnar artery is insufficient, indicating that the radial artery should not be used for obtaining a blood specimen. Finally, the nurse documents the findings. Other sites can be used if the radial artery is not deemed adequate, such as the brachial or femoral artery.

Reference(s): Pagana, K., & Pagana, T. (2013). *Mosby's diagnostic and laboratory tests reference* (11th ed., p. 117). St. Louis: Mosby.

Perry, A., Potter, P., & Ostendorf, W. (2014). *Clinical nursing skills & techniques* (8th ed., pp. 1091–1093). St. Louis: Mosby.

BOX 10-5 Normal Blood Gas Values

- pH: 7.35 to 7.45
- Pco_2: 35 to 45 mm Hg
- HCO_3^-: 22 to 27 mEq/L
- PO_2: 80 to 100 mm Hg

Fundamentals

TABLE 10-3 Acid–Base Imbalances: Significant Laboratory Value Changes That Normally Occur

Imbalance	pH	HCO_3^-	PaO_2	$PaCO_2$	K^+
Respiratory acidosis	Decreased	Normal or Increased	Decreased	Increased	Increased
Respiratory alkalosis	Increased	Normal or Decreased	Normal	Decreased	Decreased
Metabolic acidosis	Decreased	Decreased	Normal	Normal or decreased	Increased
Metabolic alkalosis	Increased	Increased	Normal	Normal or increased	Decreased

HCO_3^-, Bicarbonate; *K^+*, potassium; *Pao_2*, partial pressure of oxygen in arterial blood; *$Paco_2$*, partial pressure of carbon dioxide in arterial blood.

3. Identify factors that may affect the accuracy of the results, such as changes in the O_2 settings on respiratory assistive devices, suctioning within the past 20 minutes, and client activities.
4. Provide emotional support to the client.
5. Assist with the specimen draw by preparing a heparinized syringe (if not already prepackaged).
6. Apply pressure immediately to the puncture site following the blood draw; maintain pressure for 5 minutes or for 10 minutes if the client is taking anticoagulants.
7. Record the client's temperature and the type of supplemental O_2 that the client is receiving on the laboratory form.
8. Appropriately label the specimen, and transport it on ice to the laboratory.

C. Respiratory acid–base imbalances (Table 10-3)
1. Remember that the respiratory function indicator is the Pco_2.
2. In a respiratory imbalance, you will find an opposite relationship between the pH and the Pco_2. In other words, the pH will be elevated when the Pco_2 is decreased (alkalosis), or the pH will be decreased in the presence of an elevated Pco_2 (acidosis).
3. Look at the pH and the Pco_2 to determine whether the condition is a respiratory problem.
4. **Respiratory acidosis:** The pH is decreased; the Pco_2 is elevated.
5. **Respiratory alkalosis:** The pH is elevated; the Pco_2 is decreased.

D. Metabolic acid–base imbalances (see Table 10-3)
1. Remember that the metabolic function indicator is the HCO_3^-.
2. In a metabolic imbalance, you will find a corresponding relationship between the pH and the HCO_3^-. In other words, the pH will be elevated and the HCO_3^- will be elevated (alkalosis), or the pH will be decreased and the HCO_3^- will be decreased (acidosis).
3. Look at the pH and the HCO_3^- concentration to determine if the condition is a metabolic problem.
4. **Metabolic acidosis:** The pH is decreased; the HCO_3^- is decreased.
5. **Metabolic alkalosis:** The pH is elevated; the HCO_3^- is elevated.

In a respiratory imbalance, the arterial blood gas (ABG) result indicates an opposite relationship between the pH and the Pco_2. In a metabolic imbalance, the ABG result indicates a corresponding relationship between the pH and the HCO_3^-.

E. Steps for analyzing arterial blood gas results (Box 10-6).

BOX 10-6 Analyzing Arterial Blood Gas Results

If you can remember the following pyramid points and steps, you will be able to analyze any blood gas report.

Pyramid Points

In acidosis, the pH is down.
In alkalosis, the pH is up.
The respiratory function indicator is the partial pressure of carbon dioxide (Pco_2) value.
The metabolic function indicator is the bicarbonate (HCO_3^-) level.

Pyramid Steps

Pyramid Step 1

Look at the blood gas report. Look at the pH. Is the pH elevated or decreased? If the pH is elevated, it reflects alkalosis. If the pH is decreased, it reflects acidosis.

Pyramid Step 2

Look at the Pco_2. Is the Pco_2 elevated or decreased? If the Pco_2 reflects an opposite relationship to the pH, then the condition is a respiratory imbalance. If the Pco_2 does not reflect an opposite relationship to the pH, go to Pyramid Step 3.

Pyramid Step 3

Look at the HCO_3^-. Does the HCO_3^- reflect a corresponding relationship with the pH? If it does, then the condition is a metabolic imbalance.

CRITICAL THINKING What Should You Do?

Answer: Failure to determine the presence of adequate collateral circulation could result in severe ischemic injury to the hand if damage to the radial artery occurs with arterial puncture. Upon release of pressure on the ulnar artery, if pinkness fails to return within 6 to 7 seconds, the ulnar artery blood flow to the hand is insufficient, indicating that the radial artery should not be used for obtaining a blood specimen. Another site would need to be selected for the arterial puncture. The nurse would report this finding to the registered nurse, and the health care provider should also be notified of the finding.

Reference(s): Lewis, S., Dirksen, S., Heitkemper, M., & Bucher, L. (2014). *Medical-surgical nursing: Assessment and management of clinical problems* (9th ed., pp. 491, 1606). St. Louis: Mosby.

Pagana, K., & Pagana, T. (2013). *Mosby's diagnostic and laboratory tests reference* (11th ed., p. 117). St. Louis: Mosby.

PRACTICE QUESTIONS

46. A client has the following laboratory values: a pH of 7.55, an HCO_3^- level of 22 mm Hg, and a Pco_2 of 30 mm Hg. Which action should the nurse take?
1. Perform Allen's test.
2. Prepare the client for dialysis.
3. Administer insulin as prescribed.
4. Encourage the client to slow down breathing.

47. The nurse is told that the blood gas results indicate a pH of 7.50 and a Pco_2 of 32 mm Hg. The nurse determines that these results are indicative of which acid–base disturbance?
1. Metabolic acidosis
2. Metabolic alkalosis
3. Respiratory acidosis
4. Respiratory alkalosis

48. A client is scheduled for blood to be drawn from the radial artery for an arterial blood gas (ABG) determination. The nurse assists with performing Allen's test before drawing the blood to determine the adequacy of which?
1. Ulnar circulation
2. Carotid circulation
3. Femoral circulation
4. Brachial circulation

49. The nurse is caring for a client with a nasogastric tube that is attached to low suction. The nurse monitors the client closely for which acid–base disorder that is most likely to occur in this situation?
1. Metabolic acidosis
2. Metabolic alkalosis
3. Respiratory acidosis
4. Respiratory alkalosis

50. The nurse is caring for a client with severe diarrhea. The nurse monitors the client closely, understanding that this client is at risk for developing which acid–base disorder?
1. Metabolic acidosis
2. Metabolic alkalosis
3. Respiratory acidosis
4. Respiratory alkalosis

51. The nurse is caring for a client with diabetic ketoacidosis and observes that the client is experiencing abnormally deep, regular, rapid respirations. How should the nurse correctly document this observation in the medical record?
1. Apnea observed
2. Bradypnea noted
3. Cheyne stokes demonstrated
4. Kussmaul's respirations observed

52. The nurse is caring for a client with a diagnosis of chronic obstructive pulmonary disease (COPD). The nurse should monitor the client for which acid–base imbalance?
1. Metabolic acidosis
2. Metabolic alkalosis
3. Respiratory acidosis
4. Respiratory alkalosis

❖ **53.** When caring for the following group of clients, who does the nurse determine is at risk for development of metabolic alkalosis? **Select all that apply.**
- ❑ 1. Client with emphysema
- ❑ 2. Client who is hyperventilating
- ❑ 3. Client with chronic kidney disease
- ❑ 4. Client who has been vomiting for 2 days
- ❑ 5. Client receiving furosemide (Lasix) 40 mg daily
- ❑ 6. Client admitted with acetylsalicylic acid (aspirin) overdose

54. The nurse is caring for a client with respiratory insufficiency. The arterial blood gas results indicate a pH of 7.50 and a Pco_2 of 30 mm Hg, and the nurse is told that the client is experiencing respiratory alkalosis. Which additional laboratory value should the nurse expect to note?
   1. A sodium level of 145 mEq/L
   2. A potassium level of 3.2 mEq/L
   3. A magnesium level of 2.4 mg/dL
   4. A phosphorus level of 4.0 mg/dL

55. The registered nurse reviews the results of the arterial blood gases with the licensed practical nurse (LPN) and tells the LPN that the client is experiencing respiratory acidosis. The LPN should expect to note which on the laboratory result report?
   1. pH 7.50, Pco_2 52 mm Hg
   2. pH 7.35, Pco_2 40 mm Hg
   3. pH 7.25, Pco_2 50 mm Hg
   4. pH 7.50, Pco_2 30 mm Hg

ANSWERS

46. 4

Rationale: The client is in respiratory alkalosis based on the laboratory results of a high pH and a low Pco_2 level. Interventions for respiratory alkalosis are the voluntary holding of breath or slowed breathing and the rebreathing of exhaled CO_2 by methods such as using a paper bag or a rebreathing mask as prescribed. Performing Allen's test would be incorrect, because the blood specimen has already been drawn, and the laboratory results have been completed. Dialysis and insulin administration are interventions for metabolic acidosis.
Test-Taking Strategy: First determine the laboratory results. Because the pH is high and the Pco_2 level is low, a respiratory problem is occurring. Then, applying the ABCs—airway, breathing, and circulation—you can determine that only one intervention deals with respirations. **Review:** the interventions for **respiratory alkalosis**.
Level of Cognitive Ability: Analyzing
Client Needs: Physiological Integrity
Integrated Process: Nursing Process/Implementation
Content Area: Fundamental Skills: Acid–Base
Priority Concepts: Acid–Base Balance, Clinical Judgment
Reference(s): deWit, Kumagai (2013), pp. 47–49.

47. 4

Rationale: The normal pH is 7.35 to 7.45. In a respiratory condition, an opposite relationship will be seen between the pH and the Pco_2, as is seen in the correct option. In an alkalotic condition, the pH is increased. In an acidotic condition, the pH is decreased so both metabolic acidosis and respiratory acidosis can be eliminated. Metabolic alkalosis can also be eliminated because both pH and HCO_3^- are increased above normal values in this condition.
Test-Taking Strategy: First group together the comparable or alike options: respiratory imbalances and metabolic imbalances. Remember that with a respiratory condition, you will find an opposite relationship between the pH and the Pco_2 level. Recalling that pH is increased in an alkalotic condition helps direct you to select respiratory alkalosis and eliminate respiratory acidosis. In metabolic conditions pH and HCO_3^- are altered and either increase or decrease in the same direction.
Review: steps for **interpreting arterial blood gas (ABG) values.**
Level of Cognitive Ability: Analyzing
Client Needs: Physiological Integrity
Integrated Process: Nursing Process/Data Collection
Content Area: Fundamental Skills: Acid–Base
Priority Concepts: Acid–Base Balance, Clinical Judgment
Reference(s): deWit, Kumagai (2013), p. 47.

48. 1

Rationale: Before performing a radial puncture to obtain an arterial specimen for ABGs, Allen's test should be performed to determine adequate ulnar circulation. Failure to assess collateral circulation could result in severe ischemic injury to the hand if damage to the radial artery occurs with arterial puncture. The remaining options are not associated with this test.
Test-Taking Strategy: Focus on the subject, radial puncture. Visualize the location of each of the vessels in the options. First, eliminate carotid and femoral circulations, realizing their distance from the radial artery. From the remaining options, select the ulnar artery, realizing it runs parallel to the radial artery and supplies blood flow to the hand. **Review:** Allen's test.
Level of Cognitive Ability: Evaluating
Client Needs: Physiological Integrity
Integrated Process: Nursing Process/Evaluation
Content Area: Fundamental Skills: Diagnostic Tests
Priority Concepts: Perfusion, Safety
Reference(s): Pagana, Pagana (2013), p. 117.

49. 2

Rationale: The loss of gastric fluid via nasogastric suction or vomiting causes a metabolic condition. This also results in an alkalotic condition due to the loss of hydrochloric acid through gastrointestinal fluid losses. Also, the options denoting a respiratory problem—respiratory acidosis and respiratory alkalosis—can be easily eliminated.
Test-Taking Strategy: Focus on the subject, nasogastric tube to low suction. Remember that hydrochloric acid is lost when the client is receiving nasogastric suctioning. This will direct you to the options that identify an alkalotic condition. Because the question addresses a situation other than a respiratory one, the acid–base disorder would be a metabolic condition. **Review:** causes of **metabolic alkalosis.**
Level of Cognitive Ability: Analyzing
Client Needs: Physiological Integrity
Integrated Process: Nursing Process/Data Collection
Content Area: Fundamental Skills: Acid–Base
Priority Concepts: Acid–Base Balance, Elimination
Reference(s): deWit, Kumagai (2013), p. 47.
Lewis et al (2014), p. 304.

50. 1

Rationale: Intestinal secretions high in bicarbonate may be lost through enteric drainage tubes, an ileostomy, or diarrhea. The decreased bicarbonate level creates the actual base deficit of metabolic acidosis. The remaining options are unlikely to occur in a client with severe diarrhea.

Test-Taking Strategy: Focus on the **subject**, diarrhea. Knowing that this condition is a gastrointestinal disorder will direct you to think about a metabolic imbalance. Remembering that intestinal fluids are primarily alkaline will assist you with selecting the correct option. When excess bicarbonate is lost, acidosis will result. **Review:** causes of **metabolic acidosis.**

Level of Cognitive Ability: Analyzing
Client Needs: Physiological Integrity
Integrated Process: Nursing Process/Data Collection
Content Area: Fundamental Skills: Acid–Base
Priority Concepts: Acid–Base Balance, Elimination
Reference(s): deWit, Kumagai (2013), p. 48.

51. 4

Rationale: Abnormally deep, regular, and rapid respirations observed in the client with diabetic ketoacidosis are documented as Kussmaul's respirations. In apnea, respirations cease for several seconds. In bradypnea, respirations are regular but abnormally slow. Cheyne stokes respirations gradually become more shallow and are followed by periods of apnea (no breathing), with repetition of the pattern.

Test-Taking Strategy: Knowledge regarding the descriptions of alterations in breathing patterns is required to answer this question. Focus on options that are **comparable or alike**, such as apnea and Cheyne Stokes respirations, where there are periods of apnea to help you eliminate these two options. Next, note the client's diagnosis and remember that Kussmaul's respirations occur in clients with diabetic ketoacidosis. **Review:** data collection findings in **diabetic ketoacidosis.**

Level of Cognitive Ability: Applying
Client Needs: Physiological Integrity
Integrated Process: Communication and Documentation
Content Area: Fundamental Skills: Acid–Base
Priority Concepts: Acid–Base Balance, Glucose Regulation
Reference(s): deWit, Kumagai (2013), p. 871.

52. 3

Rationale: Respiratory acidosis most often occurs as a result of primary defects in the function of the lungs or changes in normal respiratory patterns from secondary problems. Chronic respiratory acidosis is most commonly caused by COPD. Acute respiratory acidosis also occurs in clients with COPD when superimposed respiratory infection or concurrent respiratory disease increases the work of breathing. The remaining options are not likely to occur unless other conditions complicate the COPD.

Test-Taking Strategy: Focus on the **subject**, chronic obstructive pulmonary disease, to assist with guiding you to select a respiratory acid–base balance. Then remembering that primary defects in the function of the lungs result in respiratory acidosis will direct you to the correct option. **Review:** causes of **respiratory acidosis.**

Level of Cognitive Ability: Analyzing
Client Needs: Physiological Integrity
Integrated Process: Nursing Process/Data Collection
Content Area: Fundamental Skills: Acid–Base
Priority Concepts: Acid–Base Balance, Clinical Judgment
Reference(s): deWit, Kumagai (2013), p. 48.

❖53. 4, 5

Rationale: Metabolic alkalosis is caused by any condition that creates the acid–base imbalance through either an increase in bases or a deficit of acids, such as the client who has been vomiting for 2 days and the client receiving furosemide daily. Recall that clients with emphysema and hyperventilation are at risk for a respiratory acid–base disturbance. Chronic kidney disease and aspirin overdose will result in metabolic acidosis.

Test-Taking Strategy: Focus on the **subject**, those at risk for metabolic alkalosis. Eliminate options that are **comparable or alike** and refer to respiratory conditions. From the remaining metabolic conditions, determine if there is an increase in bases or deficit of acids to answer correctly. **Review:** causes of **acid–base imbalances.**

Level of Cognitive Ability: Analyzing
Client Needs: Physiological Integrity
Integrated Process: Nursing Process/Data Collection
Content Area: Fundamental Skills: Acid–Base
Priority Concepts: Acid–Base Balance, Clinical Judgment
Reference(s): deWit, Kumagai (2013), pp. 47–48.

54. 2

Rationale: Signs/symptoms of respiratory alkalosis include tachypnea, mental status changes, dizziness, pallor around the mouth, spasms of the muscles of the hands, and hypokalemia. The remaining options identify normal laboratory results.

Test-Taking Strategy: Recalling the clinical manifestations of respiratory alkalosis and the normal laboratory values will assist you with answering this question. Eliminate options that are **comparable or alike** in that they reflect normal laboratory values. You can then determine that the only abnormal laboratory value is the potassium level. **Review:** signs/symptoms of **respiratory alkalosis.**

Level of Cognitive Ability: Analyzing
Client Needs: Physiological Integrity
Integrated Process: Nursing Process/Data Collection
Content Area: Fundamental Skills: Acid–Base
Priority Concepts: Acid–Base Balance, Clinical Judgment
Reference(s): deWit, Kumagai (2013), pp. 48–49.

55. 3

Rationale: The normal pH is 7.35 to 7.45, and the normal P_{CO_2} value is 35 to 45 mm Hg. In respiratory acidosis, the pH is down and the P_{CO_2} is up. Therefore, the option with the pH of 7.25 and the P_{CO_2} of 50 mm Hg is the only option that reflects an acidotic condition. Options with an elevated pH (options 1 and 4) indicate an alkalotic condition. Option 2 identifies normal values for pH and P_{CO_2}.

Test-Taking Strategy: Focus on the **subject**, respiratory acidosis. Remember that with a respiratory imbalance, you will find an opposite relationship between the pH and the P_{CO_2} value. In addition, remember that the pH is down in an acidotic condition. **Review: interpretation of arterial blood gases.**

Level of Cognitive Ability: Analyzing
Client Needs: Physiological Integrity
Integrated Process: Nursing Process/Data Collection
Content Area: Fundamental Skills: Acid–Base
Priority Concepts: Acid–Base Balance, Clinical Judgment
Reference(s): deWit, Kumagai (2013), pp. 47–48.

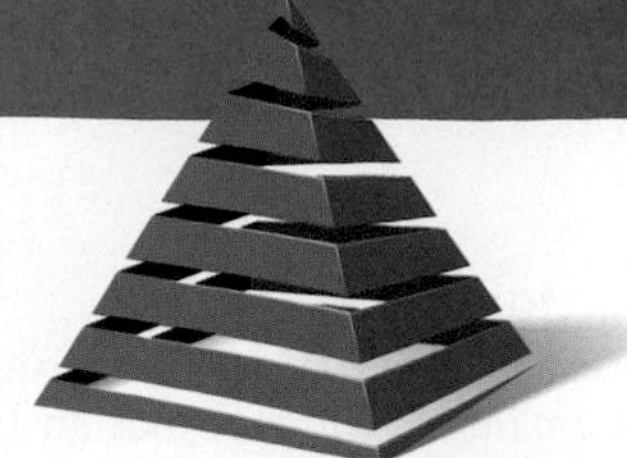

CHAPTER 11

Laboratory Values

CRITICAL THINKING What Should You Do?

The nurse notes that the client's alanine aminotransferase (ALT) level is 132 units/L and the aspartate aminotransferase (AST) level is 82 units/L. On the basis of these values, the nurse should collect which subjective data from the client? *Answer located on p. 109.*

For reference throughout the chapter, please see Figure 11-1 and Box 11-1, and Priority Nursing Actions Box.

⚠ Drawing blood specimens from an extremity in which an intravenous solution is infusing can produce an inaccurate result. Prolonged use of a tourniquet and clenching and unclenching the hand before venous sampling can increase the blood level of potassium, producing an inaccurate result.

I. Electrolytes

A. Serum sodium
  1. Description
    a. A major cation of extracellular fluid
    b. Maintains osmotic pressures and acid-base balance and assists with the transmission of nerve impulses
    c. Absorbed from the small intestine and excreted in the urine in amounts that depend on dietary intake
    d. Minimum daily requirement of sodium is approximately 15 mEq.
  2. Values: See Table 11-1

  3. Nursing consideration: Drawing **blood** samples in the extremity in which an intravenous (IV) solution of sodium chloride is infusing increases the serum sodium level.

⚠ Drawing blood specimens from an extremity in which an intravenous solution is infusing can produce an inaccurate result, depending on the test being performed and the type of solution infusing. Prolonged use of a tourniquet and clenching and unclenching the hand before venous sampling can increase the blood level of potassium, producing an inaccurate result.

B. Serum potassium
  1. Description
    a. A major intracellular cation; regulates cellular water balance, electrical conduction in muscle cells, and acid-base balance
    b. The body obtains potassium through dietary ingestion, and the kidneys either preserve or excrete potassium, depending on cellular need.
    c. Potassium levels are used to evaluate cardiac function, renal function, gastrointestinal function, and the need for IV replacement therapy.
  2. Values: See Table 11-1.
  3. Nursing considerations
    a. If the client is receiving potassium supplementation, note this on the laboratory form.
    b. Clients with elevated white **blood cell** (WBC) and platelet counts may have falsely elevated potassium levels.

II. Coagulation Studies

A. Activated partial thromboplastin time (aPTT)
  1. Description
    a. Evaluates how well the coagulation sequence is functioning by measuring the amount of time it takes in seconds for recalcified citrated plasma to clot after partial thromboplastin is added to it
    b. Screens for deficiencies and inhibitors of all factors except VII and XIII
    c. Most commonly used to monitor heparin therapy and to screen for coagulation disorders
  2. Value: 20 to 36 seconds, depending on the type of activator used
  3. Nursing considerations
    a. If the client is receiving intermittent heparin therapy, draw the blood sample 1 hour before the next scheduled dose.
    b. Do not draw samples from an arm into which heparin is infusing.
    c. Transport the specimen to the laboratory immediately.

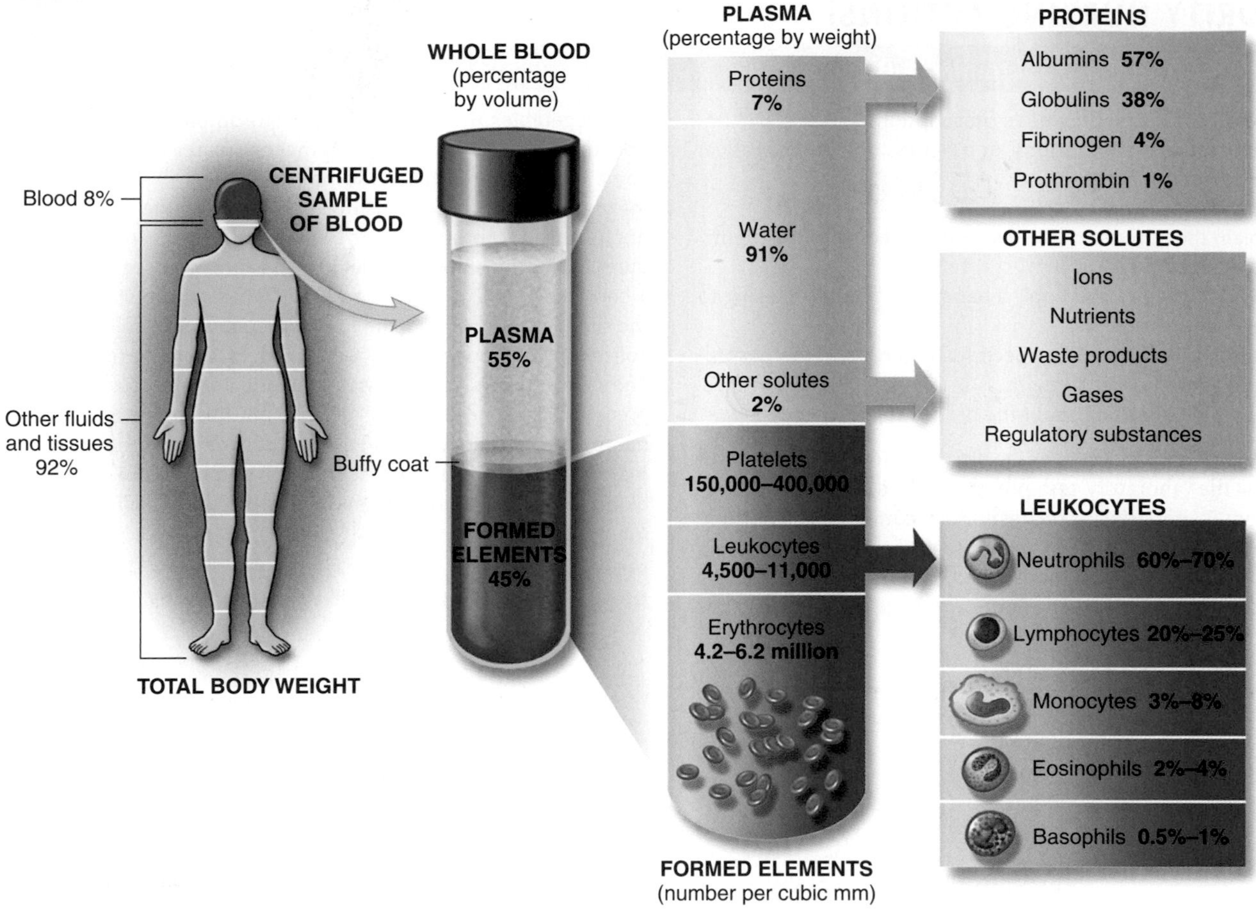

FIGURE 11-1 Approximate values for the components of blood in a normal adult. (Adapted from Thibodeau GA, Patton KT: *The human body in health and disease*, ed 6, St. Louis, 2014, Mosby.)

BOX 11-1 Pyramid Abbreviations

Abbreviation	Description
g/dL	Grams per deciliter
mcg/dL	Micrograms per deciliter
mcg/mL	Micrograms per milliliter
mg/dL	Milligrams per deciliter
mEq/L	Milliequivalents per liter
units/L or U/L	Units per liter
mm/hour	Millimeters per hour
IU/L	International units per liter
ng/mL	Nanograms per milliliter
microunits/mL	Microunits per milliliter
mL/kg	Milliliters per kilogram
mm^3	Millimeters cubed
μL	Microliters
pg/mL	Picogram per milliliter

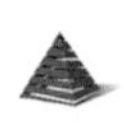

d. Provide pressure to the **venipuncture** site for 3 to 5 minutes.

e. The aPTT should be between 1.5 and 2.5 times normal when the client is receiving heparin therapy.

If the aPTT value is prolonged (longer than 90 seconds) in a client receiving IV heparin therapy, initiate bleeding precautions.

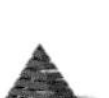

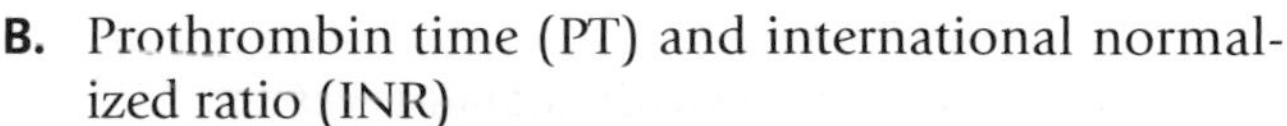

B. Prothrombin time (PT) and international normalized ratio (INR)

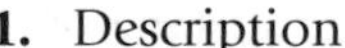

1. Description
   a. Prothrombin is a vitamin K–dependent glycoprotein produced by the liver that is necessary for firm fibrin clot formation.
   b. Each laboratory establishes a normal or control PT value based on the method used to perform the test.
   c. The PT measures the amount of time it takes for clot formation and is used to monitor response to warfarin sodium (Coumadin) therapy or screen for dysfunction of the extrinsic clotting system that results from liver disease, vitamin K deficiency, or disseminated intravascular coagulation.
   d. A PT value within 2 seconds (plus or minus) of the control value is considered normal.
   e. The INR is frequently used to measure the effects of oral anticoagulants.

PRIORITY NURSING ACTIONS!

Actions to Take When Obtaining a Blood Sample

1. Check health care provider's prescription.
2. Identify foods, medications, or other factors that may affect the procedure or results.
3. Identify the client.
4. Explain the purpose of the test and procedure to the client.
5. Draw the blood sample.
6. Provide pressure and apply a bandage or gauze dressing to the venipuncture site.
7. Maintain and deliver the specimen to the laboratory according to agency procedure.
8. Document specifics about the procedure.

The nurse should check the health care provider's prescription for the laboratory test prescribed and then ensure that the client is prepared for the test—for example, that a nothing by mouth status has been maintained if needed. The nurse would also identify any foods, medications, or other factors that may affect test results. For example, a diet high in fat or leafy vegetables may shorten the prothrombin time. In addition, there are many medications that can increase or decrease some test results. The nurse then identifies the client and makes sure that the test has been explained to the client. The nurse (or appropriate person as indicated by agency procedure) draws the blood sample, provides pressure, and applies a bandage or gauze dressing to the venipuncture site. Once the client is comfortable, the nurse maintains and delivers the specimen to the laboratory according to agency procedure. The nurse always follows standard and transmission-based precautions as necessary in performing this procedure. The nurse should also check agency guidelines and laboratory manuals regarding the procedure for obtaining the specific blood sample. The nurse then documents the specifics about the procedure.

Reference(s): Potter, P., Perry, A. G., Stockert, P. A., & Hall, A. M. (2013). *Fundamentals of nursing.* (8th ed., p. 420). St. Louis: Mosby.

TABLE 11-1 Normal Adult Electrolyte Values

Electrolyte	Value
Sodium	135–145 mEq/L
Potassium	3.5–5.0 mEq/L
Chloride	98–107 mEq/L
Bicarbonate (venous)	22–29 mEq/L

   f. The international normalized ratio (INR) was introduced in an attempt to standardize the PT.
2. Values
   a. PT: 9.6 to 11.8 seconds (adult male); 9.5 to 11.3 seconds (adult female)
   b. INR: 2 to 3 for standard warfarin sodium (Coumadin) therapy
   c. INR: 3 to 4.5 for high-dose warfarin sodium (Coumadin) therapy
3. Nursing considerations
   a. If a PT is prescribed, a baseline specimen should be drawn before anticoagulation therapy is started; note the time of collection on the laboratory form.
   b. Apply direct pressure to the venipuncture site for 3 to 5 minutes if a coagulation defect is present.
   c. Concurrent warfarin sodium (Coumadin) therapy with heparin therapy can lengthen the PT for up to 5 hours after dosing.

   d. Diets high in green leafy vegetables can increase the absorption of vitamin K, which shortens the PT.
   e. Oral anticoagulation therapy usually maintains the PT at 1.5 to 2 times the laboratory control value.

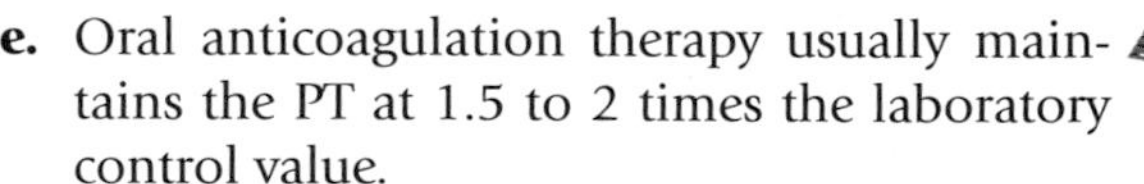

If the PT value is longer than 30 seconds in a client receiving warfarin therapy, initiate bleeding precautions.

C. Platelet count
1. Description
   a. Platelets function in hemostatic plug formation, clot retraction, and coagulation factor activation.
   b. Platelets are produced by the bone marrow to function in hemostasis.
2. Value: 150,000 to 400,000 cells/mm^3
3. Nursing considerations
   a. Monitor the venipuncture site for bleeding in clients with known thrombocytopenia.
   b. High altitudes, chronic cold weather, and exercise increase platelet counts.
   c. Bleeding precautions should be instituted in clients with low platelet counts.

Monitor the platelet count closely in clients receiving chemotherapy because of the risk for thrombocytopenia.

D. D-dimer test
1. A blood test that measures clot formation and lysis that results from the degradation of fibrin
2. Helps to diagnose (a positive test result) the presence of thrombus in conditions such as deep vein thrombosis, pulmonary embolism, or stroke; it is also used to diagnose disseminated intravascular coagulation (DIC) and to monitor the effectiveness of treatment.

III. Erythrocyte Studies

A. Erythrocyte sedimentation rate
  1. Description
    a. The rate at which erythrocytes settle out of anticoagulated blood in 1 hour
    b. A nonspecific test used to detect illnesses associated with acute and chronic infection, inflammation, advanced neoplasm, and tissue necrosis or infarction
  2. Value: 0 to 30 mm/hour, depending on the age of the client
  3. Nursing consideration: Fasting is not necessary, but a fatty meal may cause **plasma** alterations.

B. Hemoglobin and hematocrit
  1. Description
    a. Hemoglobin is the main component of erythrocytes and serves as the vehicle for the transportation of oxygen and carbon dioxide.
    b. Hemoglobin determinations are important for identifying anemia.
    c. Hematocrit represents red blood cell (RBC) mass and is an important measurement in the identification of anemia or polycythemia.
  2. Values: See Table 11-2
  3. Nursing consideration: Fasting is not required.

C. Serum iron
  1. Description
    a. Iron is found predominantly in hemoglobin.
    b. Iron acts as a carrier of oxygen from the lungs to the tissues and indirectly aids in the return of carbon dioxide to the lungs.
    c. Aids in diagnosing anemias and hemolytic disorders
  2. Values: See Table 11-2.
  3. Nursing consideration: Level of iron will be increased if the client has ingested iron before the test.

D. Red blood cell (RBC) count
  1. Description
    a. RBCs function in hemoglobin transport, which results in the delivery of oxygen to the body tissues.
    b. RBCs are formed by red bone marrow, have a life span of 120 days, and are removed from the blood by the liver, spleen, and bone marrow.
    c. Helps with diagnosing anemias and blood dyscrasias
    d. Evaluates the body's ability to produce RBCs in sufficient numbers
  2. Values: See Table 11-2.
  3. Nursing consideration: Fasting is not required.

TABLE 11-2 Normal Adult Hemoglobin, Hematocrit, Iron, and Red Blood Cell Levels

Blood Component	Normal Value
Hemoglobin	
Male adult	14–16.5 g/dL
Female adult	12–15 g/dL
Hematocrit	
Male adult	42%–52%
Female adult	35%–47%
Iron	
Male adult	65–175 mcg/dL
Female adult	50–170 mcg/dL
Red blood cells	
Male adult	4.5–6.2 million cells/μL
Female adult	4.0–5.5 million cells/μL

IV. Serum Enzymes and Cardiac Markers

A. Creatine kinase (CK)
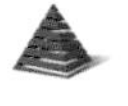
  1. Description
    a. An enzyme found in muscle and brain tissue; it reflects tissue breakdown resulting from cell trauma.
    b. The CK level begins to rise within 6 hours of muscle damage, peaks at 18 hours, and returns to normal in 2 to 3 days.
    c. The test is performed to detect myocardial or skeletal muscle damage or central nervous system damage; the normal CK value is 26 to 174 units/L.
    d. Isoenzymes include CK-MB (cardiac), CK-BB (brain), and CK-MM (muscle).
    e. CK-MB is found mainly in cardiac muscle, CK-BB is found mainly in brain tissue, and CK-MM is found mainly in skeletal muscle.
  2. Values: See Table 11-3
  3. Nursing considerations
    a. If the test is performed to evaluate skeletal muscle, instruct the client to avoid strenuous physical activity for 24 hours before the test.
    b. Instruct the client to avoid the ingestion of alcohol for 24 hours before the test.
    c. Invasive procedures and intramuscular injections may falsely elevate CK levels.

B. Troponins
  1. Description
    a. Troponins are regulatory proteins found in striated muscle (skeletal and myocardial).
    b. Increased amounts of troponins are released into the bloodstream when an infarction causes damage to the myocardium.
    c. Levels elevate as early as 3 hours after myocardial injury. Troponin I levels may remain elevated for 7 to 10 days and troponin T levels may remain elevated for up to 10 to 14 days.
    d. Serial measurements are important to compare with a baseline test.

TABLE 11-3 Normal Adult Serum Enzyme and Cardiac Marker Values

Serum Enzyme	Normal Value
Creatine kinase (CK)	26–174 units/L
CK Isoenzymes	
CK-MB	0%–5% of total
CK-MM	95%–100% of total
CK-BB	0%
Troponins	
Troponin I	<0.6 ng/mL; >1.5 ng/mL indicates myocardial infarction
Troponin T	>0.1–0.2 ng/mL; an elevation indicates myocardial infarction
Myoglobin	<90 mcg/L; an elevation could indicate myocardial infarction
Natriuretic peptides	ANP: 22 to 27 pg/mL BNP: Less than 100 pg/mL CNP: Reference range provided with results should be reviewed

2. Values: See Table 11-3.
3. Nursing considerations:
   a. Testing is repeated after 12 hours or as prescribed, and followed by daily testing for 3 to 5 days
   b. Rotate venipuncture sites

D. Myoglobin
1. Description
   a. An oxygen-binding protein found in striated (cardiac and skeletal) muscle that releases oxygen at very low tensions
   b. Any injury to skeletal muscle will cause a release of myoglobin into the blood.
2. Values: See Table 11-3.
3. Nursing considerations
   a. The level can rise as early as 2 hours after a myocardial infarction, with a rapid decline in the level seen after 7 hours.
   b. Because the myoglobin level is not cardiac specific and rises and falls so rapidly, its use for diagnosing myocardial infarction may be limited.

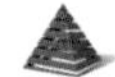

E. Natriuretic peptides
1. Natriuretic peptides are neuroendocrine peptides that are used to identify clients with heart failure (HF).
2. There are three major peptides: atrial natriuretic peptides (ANP) synthesized in cardiac atrial muscle, brain natriuretic peptides (BNP) synthesized primarily in cardiac ventricle muscle (although originally BNP was identified in extracts of porcine brain), and C-type natriuretic peptides (CNP) synthesized by endothelial cells.
3. BNP is the primary marker for identifying heart failure as the cause of dyspnea.
4. Values: See Table 11-3.
5. Nursing consideration: Fasting is not required.

The higher the BNP level, the more severe the heart failure. If the BNP is elevated, the dyspnea is a result of heart failure. If it is normal, the dyspnea is a result of a pulmonary problem.

V. Serum Gastrointestinal Studies

A. Albumin
1. Description
   a. A main plasma protein of blood
   b. Maintains oncotic pressure and transports bilirubin, fatty acids, medications, hormones, and other substances that are insoluble in water
   c. Increased in conditions such as dehydration, diarrhea, and metastatic carcinoma; decreased in conditions such as acute infection, ascites, and alcoholism
   d. The presence of detectable albumin or protein in the urine is indicative of abnormal renal function.
2. Value: 3.4 to 5 g/dL
3. Nursing considerations: Fasting is not required.

B. Ammonia
1. Description
   a. Ammonia is a by-product of protein catabolism; most of it is created by bacteria acting on proteins present in the gut.
   b. Ammonia is metabolized by the liver and excreted by the kidneys as urea.
   c. Elevated levels resulting from hepatic dysfunction may lead to encephalopathy.
   d. Venous ammonia levels are not a reliable indicator of hepatic coma.
2. Value: 10 to 80 mcg/dL
3. Nursing considerations
   a. Instruct the client to fast, except for water, and to refrain from smoking for 8 to 10 hours before the test; smoking increases ammonia levels.
   b. Place the specimen on ice and transport to the laboratory immediately.

C. Alanine aminotransferase (ALT) 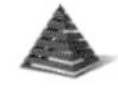
1. Description: Used to identify hepatocellular injury and inflammation of the liver and to monitor improvement or worsening of disease.
2. Value: 10 to 40 units/L.

3. Nursing considerations
   a. Previous intramuscular injections may cause elevated levels.
   b. No fasting is required.

D. Aspartate aminotransferase (AST)
1. Description: Used to evaluate a client with suspected hepatocellular disease, injury, or inflammation (may also be used along with cardiac markers to evaluate coronary artery occlusive disease)
2. Value: 10 to 30 units/L
3. Nursing considerations
   a. Previous intramuscular injections may cause elevated levels.
   b. No fasting is required.

E. Amylase
1. Description
   a. This enzyme, produced by the pancreas and salivary glands, aids in the digestion of complex carbohydrates and is excreted by the kidneys.
   b. In acute pancreatitis, the amylase level may exceed five times the normal value; the level starts rising 6 hours after the onset of pain, peaks at about 24 hours, and returns to normal in 2 to 3 days after the onset of pain.
   c. In chronic pancreatitis, the rise in **serum** amylase usually does not exceed three times the normal value.
2. Value: 25 to 151 units/L
3. Nursing considerations
   a. On the laboratory form, list the medications that the client has taken during the previous 24 hours before the test.
   b. Note that many medications may cause false-positive or false-negative results.
   c. Results are invalidated if the specimen was obtained less than 72 hours after cholecystography with radiopaque dyes.

F. Lipase
1. Description
   a. This pancreatic enzyme converts fats and triglycerides into fatty acids and glycerol.
   b. Elevated lipase levels occur in pancreatic disorders; elevations may not occur until 24 to 36 hours after the onset of illness and may remain elevated for up to 14 days.
2. Value: 10 to 140 units/L
3. Nursing considerations: Endoscopic retrograde cholangiopancreatography (ERCP) may increase lipase activity.

G. Bilirubin
1. Description
   a. Bilirubin is produced by the liver, spleen, and bone marrow and is also a by-product of hemoglobin breakdown.
   b. Total bilirubin levels can be broken down into direct bilirubin, which is excreted primarily via the intestinal tract, and indirect bilirubin, which circulates primarily in the bloodstream.
   c. Total bilirubin levels increase with any type of jaundice; direct and indirect bilirubin levels help differentiate the cause of the jaundice.
2. Values
   a. Bilirubin, direct (conjugated): 0 to 0.3 mg/dL
   b. Bilirubin, indirect (unconjugated): 0.1 to 1 mg/dL
   c. Bilirubin, total: Lower than 1.5 mg/dL
3. Nursing consideration
   a. Instruct the client to eat a diet low in yellow foods, avoiding foods such as carrots, yams, yellow beans, and pumpkin, for 3 to 4 days before the blood is drawn.
   b. Instruct the client to fast for 4 hours before the blood is drawn.
   c. Note that results will be elevated with the ingestion of alcohol or the administration of morphine sulfate, theophylline, ascorbic acid (vitamin C), or acetylsalicylic acid (aspirin).
   d. Note that results are invalidated if the client has received a radioactive scan within 24 hours before the test.

H. Lipids
1. Description
   a. Blood lipids consist primarily of cholesterol, triglycerides, and phospholipids.
   b. Lipid assessment includes total cholesterol, high-density lipoprotein (HDL), low-density lipoprotein (LDL), and triglycerides.
   c. Cholesterol is present in all body tissues and is a major component of LDLs, brain and nerve cells, cell membranes, and some gallbladder stones.
   d. Triglycerides constitute a major part of very low-density lipoproteins (VLDLs) and a small part of LDLs.
   e. Triglycerides are synthesized in the liver from fatty acids, protein, and glucose, and they are obtained from the diet.
   f. Increased cholesterol, LDL, and triglyceride levels place the client at risk for coronary artery disease.
   g. HDLs help protect against the risk of coronary artery disease.
2. Values
   a. Total cholesterol: Lower than 200 mg/dL
   b. LDLs: Lower than 130 mg/dL (near ideal); lower than 100 mg/dL for those at risk for heart disease; lower than 70 mg/dL for those at very high risk for heart disease
   c. HDLs: 60 mg/dL and higher
   d. Triglycerides: Less than 150 mg/dL
3. Nursing considerations
   a. Oral contraceptives may increase the lipid level.

TABLE 11-4 Normal Adult Glucose Values

Point of Measurement	Normal Value
Glucose, fasting	70–100 mg/dL (without diabetes); 70–130 mg/dL (with diabetes)
Glucose Tolerance Test, Oral (Nonpregnant Client)	
Baseline fasting	60–100 mg/dL
60-minute fasting	lower than 200 mg/dL
120-minute fasting	70–120 mg/dL
Glucose, 2-hour postprandial	lower than 140 mg/dL (without diabetes); lower than 180 mg/dL (with diabetes)

b. Instruct the client to abstain from foods and fluid, except for water, for 12 to 14 hours before the test and from alcohol for 24 hours before the test.
c. Instruct the client to avoid consuming high-cholesterol foods with the evening meal before the test.

I. Protein
1. Description
a. Reflects the total amount of albumin and globulins in the plasma.
b. Regulates osmotic pressure and is necessary for the formation of many hormones, enzymes, and antibodies. It is a major source of building material for blood, skin, hair, nails, and internal organs.
c. Increased in conditions such as Addison's disease, autoimmune collagen disorders, chronic infection, and Crohn's disease
d. Decreased in conditions such as burns, cirrhosis, edema, and severe hepatic disease
2. Value: 6 to 8 g/dL
3. Nursing considerations: No special preparation is necessary.

Clients with liver disease often have prolonged clotting times; therefore, provide prolonged pressure at the venipuncture site and monitor the site closely for bleeding.

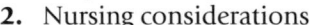

VI. Glucose Studies

A. Fasting blood glucose
1. Description
a. Glucose is a monosaccharide found in fruits and formed from the digestion of carbohydrates and the conversion of glycogen by the liver.
b. Glucose is the body's main source of cellular energy, and it is essential for brain and erythrocyte function.
c. Fasting blood glucose levels are used to help diagnose diabetes mellitus and hypoglycemia (Table 11-4).
2. Nursing considerations
a. Instruct the client to fast for 8 to 12 hours before the test.
b. Instruct a client with diabetes mellitus to withhold morning insulin or oral hypoglycemic medication until after the blood is drawn.

B. Glucose tolerance test (see Table 11-4)
1. Description
a. Aids in the diagnosis of diabetes mellitus
b. If the glucose levels peak at higher than normal at 1 to 2 hours after the injection or ingestion of glucose and are slower than normal to return to fasting levels, then diabetes mellitus is confirmed.
2. Nursing considerations
a. Instruct the client to eat a high-carbohydrate (200 to 300g) diet for 3 days before the test.
b. Instruct the client to avoid alcohol, coffee, and smoking for 36 hours before the test.
c. Instruct the client to fast for 10 to 16 hours before the test.
d. Instruct the client to avoid strenuous exercise for 8 hours before and after the test.
e. Instruct the client that the test will take 3 to 5 hours, requires the IV or oral administration of glucose, and the taking of multiple blood samples.

C. Glycosylated hemoglobin 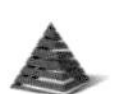
1. Description
a. Glycosylated hemoglobin is blood glucose that is bound to hemoglobin.
b. Hemoglobin A (HbA_{1c}) is a reflection of how well blood glucose levels have been controlled for up to the past 3 to 4 months.
c. Hyperglycemia in clients with diabetes is usually a cause of an increase in the HbA_{1c} level.
2. Values
a. Values are expressed as a percentage of the total hemoglobin.
b. Without diabetes: 4.5% to 6%
c. Prediabetes (indicating high risk): 5.7% to 6.4%
d. 6.5% or above on 2 separate tests indicates diabetes
3. Nursing considerations: Fasting is not required before the test. 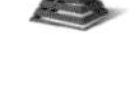

D. Diabetes mellitus autoantibody panel
1. Description: Used to evaluate insulin resistance and to identify type 1 diabetes and clients with a suspected allergy to insulin
2. Value: Less than 1:4 titer with no antibody detected

3. Nursing considerations
   a. Radioactive scans within 7 days before the test may interfere with test results.
   b. No fasting is required.

VII. Renal Function Studies

A. Serum creatinine
   1. Description
      a. Very specific indicator of renal function
      b. Increased levels indicate a slowing of the glomerular filtration rate.
   2. Value: 0.6 to 1.3 mg/dL
   3. Nursing considerations: Instruct the client to avoid excessive exercise for 8 hours before the test and excessive red meat intake for 24 hours before the test.

B. Blood urea nitrogen
   1. Description
      a. Urea nitrogen is the nitrogen portion of urea, a substance formed in the liver through an enzymatic protein breakdown process.
      b. Urea is normally freely filtered through the renal glomeruli, with a small amount reabsorbed in the tubules and the remainder excreted into the urine.
      c. Elevated levels indicate a slowing of the glomerular filtration rate.
   2. Value: 8 to 25 mg/dL
   3. Nursing considerations: BUN and creatinine levels should be analyzed when renal function is evaluated.

VIII. Elements

A. Calcium
   1. Description
      a. A cation that is absorbed into the bloodstream from dietary sources and functions in bone formation, nerve impulse transmission, and the contraction of myocardial and skeletal muscles
      b. Aids in blood clotting by converting prothrombin to thrombin
   2. Value: 8.6 to 10 mg/dL
   3. Nursing considerations
      a. Instruct the client to eat a diet with normal calcium levels (800 mg/day) for 3 days before the test.
      b. Instruct the client that fasting may be required for 8 hours before the test.
      c. Note that calcium levels can be affected by decreased protein levels and the use of anticonvulsant medications.

B. Magnesium
   1. Description
      a. Used as an index to determine metabolic activity and renal function
      b. Magnesium is needed for the blood-clotting process, regulates neuromuscular activity, acts as a cofactor that modifies the activity of many enzymes, and has an effect on the metabolism of calcium.
   2. Value: 1.6 to 2.6 mg/dL
   3. Nursing considerations
      a. Prolonged use of magnesium products will cause increased levels of magnesium.
      b. Long-term parenteral nutrition therapy or excessive loss of body fluids may decrease serum levels.

C. Phosphorus
   1. Description
      a. Important in bone formation, energy storage and release, urinary acid–base buffering, and carbohydrate metabolism
      b. Absorbed from food and excreted by the kidneys
      c. High concentrations of phosphorus are stored in bone and skeletal muscle.
   2. Value: 2.7 to 4.5 mg/dL
   3. Nursing considerations: Instruct the client to fast before the test.

IX. Thyroid Studies

A. Description
   1. Performed if a thyroid disorder is suspected
   2. Helps to differentiate primary thyroid disease from secondary causes and abnormalities in thyroxine-binding globulin levels
   3. Thyroid peridoxidase antibodies test may be done to identify the presence of autoimmune conditions involving the thyroid gland.

B. Values
   1. Thyroid-stimulating hormone (thyrotropin): 0.2 to 5.4 microunits/mL
   2. Thyroxine (T4): 5 to 12 mcg/dL
   3. Thyroxine, free (FT4): 0.8 to 2.4 ng/dL
   4. Triiodothyronine (T3): 80 to 230 ng/dL

C. Nursing considerations: Test results may be invalid if the client has undergone a radionuclide scan within 7 days before the test.

X. White Blood Cell (WBC) Count

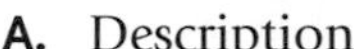

A. Description
   1. WBCs function in the body's immune defense system.
   2. The WBC count assesses leukocyte distribution.

B. Value: 4500 to 11,000 cells/mm^3 (Table 11-5)

C. Nursing considerations
   1. A "shift to the left" means there is an increased number of immature neutrophils in the peripheral blood.
   2. A low total WBC count with a left shift indicates a recovery from bone marrow depression or an infection of such intensity that the demand for

TABLE 11-5 Normal Adult White Blood Cell Differential Count

Cell Type	Count
Neutrophils	1800–7800 cells/mm³
Bands	0–700 cells/mm³
Eosinophils	0–450 cells/mm³
Basophils	0–200 cells/mm³
Lymphocytes	1000–4800 cells/mm³
Monocytes	0–800 cells/mm³

neutrophils in the tissue is greater than the capacity of the bone marrow to release them into the circulation.

3. A high total WBC count with a left shift indicates an increased release of neutrophils by the bone marrow in response to an overwhelming infection or inflammation.
4. An increased neutrophil count with a left shift is usually associated with bacterial infection.
5. A "shift to the right" means that cells have more than the usual number of nuclear segments. This is found with liver disease, Down syndrome, and megaloblastic and pernicious anemia.

Monitor the WBC count and differential closely in clients receiving chemotherapy because of the risk for neutropenia.

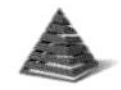

XI. Hepatitis Tests

A. Description
1. Tests include radioimmunoassay, enzyme-linked immunosorbent assay (ELISA), and microparticle enzyme immunoassay.
2. Serologic tests for specific hepatitis virus markers assist with defining the specific type of hepatitis.

B. Values
1. The presence of immunoglobulin M (IgM) antibody to hepatitis A virus and the presence of total antibody (IgG and IgM) to hepatitis A virus suggests recent or current hepatitis A virus infection.
2. Detection of hepatitis B core antigen (HBcAg), envelope antigen (HbeAg), and surface antigen (HbsAg) or their corresponding antibodies constitutes hepatitis B assessment.
3. Hepatitis C is confirmed by the presence of antibodies to hepatitis C.
4. Serologic hepatitis D virus (HDV) determination is made by the detection of the hepatitis D antigen (HDAg) early in the course of the infection and anti-HDV antibody in later disease stages.
5. Specific serologic tests for hepatitis E virus include the detection of IgM and immunoglobulin G antibodies to hepatitis E.
6. Hepatitis G virus (HGV) has been found in some blood donors (donated blood), IV drug users, hemodialysis clients, and clients with hemophilia; however, HGV does not appear to cause significant liver disease.

C. Nursing considerations: If the radioimmunoassay technique is being used, the injection of radionuclides within 1 week before the blood test may falsely elevate results.

XII. Human Immunodeficiency Virus (HIV) and Acquired Immunodeficiency Syndrome (AIDS) Testing

A. Description
1. Detects HIV, which is the cause of AIDS
2. Common tests used to determine the presence of antibodies to HIV include ELISA, Western blot (WB), and immunofluorescence assay (IFA).
3. A single reactive ELISA test by itself cannot be used to diagnose HIV and should be repeated in duplicate with the same blood sample. If the result is repeatedly reactive, follow-up tests using WB or IFA should be performed.
4. A positive WB or IFA is considered confirmatory for HIV.
5. A positive ELISA that fails to be confirmed by WB or IFA should not be considered negative, and repeat testing should take place in 3 to 6 months.

B. CD4 T-cell counts
1. Monitors the progression of HIV
2. As the disease progresses, there is usually a decrease in the $CD4^+$ T-cell count and a resultant decrease in immunity.
3. The normal $CD4^+$ T-cell count is between 500 and 1600 cells/mm³.
4. In general, the immune system remains healthy with $CD4^+$ T-cell counts greater than 500 cells/mm³.
5. Immune system problems occur when the $CD4^+$ T-cell count is between 200 and 499 cells/mm³.
6. Severe immune system problems occur when the $CD4^+$ T-cell count is less than 200 cells/mm³.

C. $CD4^+$ to $CD8^+$ ratio
1. Monitors the progression of the disease
2. The normal ratio is approximately 2:1.

D. Viral culture involves placing the infected client's blood cells in a culture medium and measuring the amount of reverse transcriptase activity over a specified period of time.

E. Viral load testing measures the presence of HIV viral genetic material (RNA) or other viral protein in the client's blood.

F. The p24 antigen assay quantifies the amount of HIV viral core protein in the client's serum.

G. Oral testing for HIV
   1. Uses a device that is placed against the gum and cheek for 2 minutes
   2. Fluid (not saliva) is drawn into an absorbable pad. This fluid contains antibodies in an HIV-positive individual.
   3. The pad is placed in a solution, and a specified observable change is noted if the test is positive.
   4. If the result is positive, a blood test is needed to confirm the results.

H. Home test kits for HIV
   1. Various kits are available; in one at-home test kit, a drop of blood is placed on a test card with a special code number. The card is mailed to the laboratory for testing for HIV antibodies.
   2. The individual receives the results by calling a special telephone number and entering the special code number. Test results are then given.

I. Nursing considerations
   1. Maintain issues of confidentiality surrounding HIV and AIDS testing.
   2. Follow prescribed state regulations and protocols related to reporting positive test results.

XIII. Urine Tests (Table 11-6)

TABLE 11-6 Normal Adult Values Urine Tests

Name of Test	Value
Color	Pale yellow
Odor	Specific aromatic odor similar to ammonia
Turbidity	Clear
pH	4.5–7.8
Specific gravity	1.016–1.022
Glucose	<0.5 g/day
Ketones	None
Protein	None
Bilirubin	None
Casts	None to few
Crystals	None
Bacteria	None or <1000 colonies/mL
Red blood cells	<3 cells/HPF
White blood cells	≤4 cells/HPF
Chloride	110–250 mEq/24 hours
Magnesium	7.3–12.2 mg/dL per day
Potassium	25–125 mEq/24 hours
Sodium	40–220 mEq/24 hours
Uric acid	250–750 mg/24 hours

HPF, High-powered field.

TABLE 11-7 Therapeutic Serum Medication Levels

Medication	Therapeutic Range
Acetaminophen (Tylenol)	10–20 mcg/mL
Carbamazepine (Tegretol)	5–12 mcg/mL
Digoxin (Lanoxin)	0.5–2 ng/mL
Gentamicin	5–10 mcg/mL
Lithium (Lithobid)	0.5–1.2 mEq/L
Magnesium sulfate	4–7 mg/dL
Phenytoin (Dilantin)	10–20 mcg/mL
Salicylates	100–250 mcg/mL
Theophylline	10–20 mcg/mL
Tobramycin (Nebcin)	5–10 mcg/mL
Valproic acid (Depakene)	50–100 mcg/mL

XIV. Therapeutic Serum Medication Levels (Table 11-7)

A. If the result is below the therapeutic level, the client may not be compliant with the medicine regimen, or the dose may need to be increased. Notify the registered nurse (RN) or health care provider (HCP).

B. If the result is within the range, the medication can be administered as prescribed.

C. If the result is above the therapeutic level (toxic), the dose is too high. The client may not understand the medicine regimen and may be taking too much or may have organ dysfunction, leading to poor metabolism/elimination of the medication. Withhold the dose and notify the RN or HCP.

CRITICAL THINKING What Should You Do?

Answer: The normal ALT level is 10 to 40 units/L. The normal AST level is 10 to 30 units/L. These tests are used to identify hepatocellular disease, injury to the liver, and liver inflammation and to monitor improvement or worsening of disease. If the client's levels are elevated, the nurse should collect subjective data about factors that could affect the liver. The nurse should ask the client about consumption of alcohol or hepatotoxic medications such as acetaminophen (Tylenol). The nurse should also collect subjective data about signs of infection such as an elevated temperature, which could be an indication of liver inflammation (hepatitis, liver abscess, or other infectious process).

Reference(s): deWit, D. & Kumagai, C. (2013). *Medical-surgical nursing: Concepts & practice.* (2nd ed., pp. 17–18). St. Louis: Saunders.

PRACTICE QUESTIONS

56. The nurse is told that the laboratory result for the serum digoxin level is 2.4 ng/mL. Which action should the nurse take?
1. Withhold the medication.
2. Check the client's last respiratory rate.
3. Record the normal value on the client's flow sheet.
4. Administer the next dose of the medication as scheduled.

57. A client with atrial fibrillation who is receiving maintenance therapy with warfarin sodium (Coumadin) has a prothrombin time (PT) of 30 seconds. The nurse anticipates that which will be prescribed?
1. Adding a dose of heparin
2. Increasing the next dose of warfarin sodium
3. Withholding the next dose of warfarin sodium
4. Administering the next dose of warfarin sodium

58. A client having preadmission testing before surgery has blood drawn for the determination of serum electrolyte levels. The nurse determines that which result warrants a call to the health care provider by the nurse?
1. Sodium, 148 mEq/L
2. Chloride, 101 mEq/L
3. Potassium, 3.8 mEq/L
4. Bicarbonate, 26 mEq/L

59. The nurse determines that sodium polystyrene sulfonate (Kayexalate) has been **effective** in a client if which laboratory result is noted?
1. Serum sodium is 148 mEq/L
2. Serum glucose is 110 mg/dL
3. Serum chloride is 110 mEq/L
4. Serum potassium is 4.9 mEq/L

60. A client with a history of cardiac disease is scheduled for a dose of furosemide (Lasix). Which serum potassium level warrants a call to the health care provider by the nurse before administering the furosemide?
1. 3.2 mEq/L
2. 3.8 mEq/L
3. 4.2 mEq/L
4. 5.2 mEq/L

61. A client with diabetes mellitus has a blood sample drawn for the determination of a fasting blood glucose level. When reviewing the client's results, the nurse determines that which requires a call to the health care provider for intervention?
1. 75 mg/dL
2. 92 mg/dL
3. 120 mg/dL
4. 240 mg/dL

62. A client with a history of gastrointestinal bleeding has a platelet count of 300,000 cells/mL. Which action by the nurse is **most appropriate** after reading this report?
1. Report the abnormally low count.
2. Report the abnormally high count.
3. Place the client on bleeding precautions.
4. Place the normal report in the client's medical record.

❖**63.** The nurse is reviewing the serum magnesium results for a group of clients. Which results warrant a call to the health care provider by the nurse? **Select all that apply.**
- ❑ 1. 1.2 mg/dL
- ❑ 2. 2.0 mg/dL
- ❑ 3. 2.6 mg/dL
- ❑ 4. 3.0 mg/dL
- ❑ 5. 4.2 mg/dL

64. A client has a history of mild renal insufficiency. Which serum creatinine level should the nurse determine is consistent with this problem?
1. 0.6 mg/dL
2. 1.1 mg/dL
3. 1.9 mg/dL
4. 3.5 mg/dL

65. A client with a seizure disorder is taking phenytoin (Dilantin). A sample for a serum phenytoin level is drawn, and the nurse determines that the next dose of the medication may be administered if which laboratory result is noted?
1. 17 mcg/mL
2. 21 mcg/mL
3. 24 mcg/mL
4. 27 mcg/mL

66. A client with hepatic cirrhosis has been consuming a diet with optimal amounts of protein. The nurse determines that the client's consumption of dietary protein has been **most effective** if the total protein level is which value?
1. 0.4 g/dL
2. 3.7 g/dL
3. 5.4 g/dL
4. 6.8 g/dL

67. A client was diagnosed with acute pancreatitis 10 days ago. The nurse interprets that the episode of acute pancreatitis is fully resolved if the serum lipase level drops to which value?
1. 135 units/L
2. 175 units/L
3. 200 units/L
4. 250 units/L

68. A client arrives in the emergency department complaining of chest pain that began 4 hours ago. A troponin T blood specimen is obtained, and the results indicate a level of 0.6 ng/mL. How should the nurse correctly interpret these results?
1. It is a normal level
2. It is a low value that may be indicative of gastritis
3. The level is indicative of a myocardial infarction
4. The level indicates the presence of possible angina

69. A client has a hemoglobin level of 10.8 g/dL. The nurse interprets that this result is **most likely** the result of which factor in the client's history?
1. Heart failure
2. Dehydration
3. Iron deficiency anemia
4. Chronic obstructive pulmonary disease (COPD)

70. The nurse determines that an adult male client admitted with dehydration and a hematocrit level of 56% has received adequate fluid volume replacement if which repeat hematocrit level is noted?
1. 48%
2. 54%
3. 60%
4. 64%

ANSWERS

56. 1

Rationale: The normal therapeutic range for digoxin is 0.5 to 2 ng/mL. A value of 2.4 ng/mL exceeds the therapeutic range and could be toxic to the client. The nursing action is to hold further doses of digoxin. Because the value is not normal, option 3 can be eliminated. Administration of the next dose would cause the client to become more toxic. Checking the client's respiratory rate is not applicable at this time.
Test-Taking Strategy: Focus on the subject, a serum digoxin level of 2.4 ng/mL. Recall that the normal therapeutic range for digoxin is 0.5 to 2 ng/mL. Noting that the value is high will direct you to the correct option. **Review: digoxin levels.**
Level of Cognitive Ability: Applying
Client Needs: Physiological Integrity
Integrated Process: Nursing Process/Implementation
Content Area: Fundamental Skills: Laboratory Values
Priority Concepts: Clinical Judgment, Safety
Reference(s): deWit, Kumagai (2013), p. 1123; Linton (2012), p. 679.

57. 3

Rationale: The normal PT is 9.6 to 11.8 seconds for the adult male and 9.5 to 11.3 seconds for the adult female. The goal of oral anticoagulation with warfarin sodium therapy is to achieve a PT at 1.5 to 2 times the laboratory control value. A PT of 30 seconds places the client at risk for bleeding, so the nurse should anticipate that the client would not receive further doses at this time. If the level is too high, the antidote (vitamin K) may be prescribed. The remaining options would make the client even more prone to bleeding.
Test-Taking Strategy: Focus on the subject, the PT is 30 seconds. Noting that the PT value is high will direct you to the correct option. Also note that the incorrect options are comparable or alike and indicate administering medication. **Review:** therapeutic range for **warfarin sodium** therapy.
Level of Cognitive Ability: Analyzing
Client Needs: Physiological Integrity
Integrated Process: Nursing Process/Planning
Content Area: Fundamental Skills: Laboratory Values
Priority Concepts: Clotting, Safety
Reference(s): Linton (2012), pp. 494, 735; Pagana, Pagana (2013), p. 769.

58. 1

Rationale: The normal serum electrolyte ranges for adults are as follows: sodium, 135 to 145 mEq/L; potassium, 3.5 to 5.0 mEq/L; chloride, 98 to 107 mEq/L; and bicarbonate (venous), 22 to 29 mEq/L. The only abnormal value identified is the serum sodium level.
Test-Taking Strategy: Focus on the subject, the need to contact the *HCP*. Recalling the normal serum electrolyte values will direct you to the correct option. **Review: electrolyte values.**
Level of Cognitive Ability: Applying
Client Needs: Physiological Integrity
Integrated Process: Nursing Process: Implementation
Content Area: Fundamental Skills: Laboratory Values
Priority Concepts: Collaboration, Fluid and Electrolyte Balance
Reference(s): deWit, Kumagai (2013), p. 41.

59. 4

Rationale: The normal serum potassium level in the adult is 3.5 to 5.0 mEq/L. Sodium polystyrene (Kayexalate) is a medication that is used to treat hyperkalemia. The laboratory values in the remaining options are slightly elevated; in addition, this medication would have no effect on these other electrolytes.
Test-Taking Strategy: Note the strategic word, *effective*. Knowing that this medication is administered to treat elevated potassium levels will direct you to the correct option. Also, look at the medication *Kayexalate* to assist in determining that the medication assists to excrete potassium. **Review:** expected outcome of **sodium polystyrene**.
Level of Cognitive Ability: Evaluating
Client Needs: Physiological Integrity
Integrated Process: Nursing Process/Evaluation
Content Area: Fundamental Skills: Laboratory Values

Priority Concepts: Clinical Judgment, Fluid and Electrolyte Balance
Reference(s): deWit, Kumagai (2013), pp. 41, 804.

60. 1

Rationale: The normal adult serum potassium level is 3.5 to 5.0 mEq/L. A serum potassium level of 3.2 mEq/L is the only value that falls below the therapeutic range. Administering furosemide (Lasix) to a client with a low potassium level and a cardiac history could precipitate ventricular dysrhythmias in the client. Even though a result of 5.2 mEq/L is high, administration of the furosemide can only assist with excretion of the excess potassium.
Test-Taking Strategy: First, eliminate comparable or alike options—serum potassium of 3.8 mEq/L and 4.2 mEq/L—because they are both within the normal range. Recall that furosemide leads to potassium loss, so a client with a serum potassium level of 3.2 mEq/L is already depleted. **Review:** normal adult **serum potassium** levels.
Level of Cognitive Ability: Applying
Client Needs: Physiological Integrity
Integrated Process: Nursing Process/Implementation
Content Area: Fundamental Skills: Laboratory Values
Priority Concepts: Collaboration, Fluid and Electrolyte Balance
Reference(s): deWit, Kumagai (2013), pp. 41, 402.

61. 4

Rationale: The normal fasting blood glucose level is 70 to 100 mg/dL in the adult client without diabetes and 70 to 130 in the client with diabetes. Values above the normal range should be evaluated to determine if further intervention is needed. The most critical value is 240 mg/dL.
Test-Taking Strategy: First, eliminate options that are comparable or alike—75 mg/dL and 92 mg/dL—because they are both within the normal fasting blood glucose range. Next, consider the blood glucose level of 120 mg/dL, and realize it is just above normal range and can be eliminated. A fasting blood glucose of 240 mg/dL would require a call to the health care provider for further prescriptions. **Review:** normal **fasting blood glucose** levels.
Level of Cognitive Ability: Applying
Client Needs: Physiological Integrity
Integrated Process: Nursing Process: Implementation
Content Area: Fundamental Skills: Laboratory Values
Priority Concepts: Collaboration, Glucose Regulation
Reference(s): deWit, Kumagai (2013), pp. 868, 872;
Pagana, Pagana (2013), p. 478.

62. 4

Rationale: A normal platelet count ranges from 150,000 to 400,000 cells/mm^3. The nurse should place the report that contains the normal laboratory value into the client's medical record. The remaining options are incorrect and unnecessary.
Test-Taking Strategy: Focus on the strategic words, *most appropriate.* Remember that options that are comparable or alike are not likely to be correct. With this in mind, eliminate reporting the abnormally low count and instituting bleeding precautions. From the remaining options, recalling the normal range for this laboratory test will direct you to the correct option. **Review:** the normal **platelet count**.
Level of Cognitive Ability: Applying
Client Needs: Physiological Integrity
Integrated Process: Nursing Process/Implementation
Content Area: Fundamental Skills: Laboratory Values
Priority Concepts: Cellular Regulation, Clinical Judgment
Reference(s):
Pagana, Pagana (2013), p. 726.

❖ **63. 1, 4, 5**

Rationale: The normal magnesium level in an adult client is 1.6 to 2.6 mg/dL. Magnesium levels that are below or above the normal range should be reported to the health care provider.
Test-Taking Strategy: Focus on options that are comparable or alike in that they represent normal magnesium levels—magnesium level of 2.0 and 2.6 mg/dL. Therefore, these can be easily eliminated. A call to the health care provider would be warranted for results that are too low or too high. **Review: serum magnesium** levels.
Level of Cognitive Ability: Analyzing
Client Needs: Physiological Integrity
Integrated Process: Nursing Process: Implementation
Content Area: Fundamental Skills: Laboratory Values
Priority Concepts: Collaboration, Fluid and Electrolyte Balance
Reference(s): deWit, Kumagai (2013), pp. 41, 43;
Pagana, Pagana (2013), p. 626.

64. 3

Rationale: The normal serum creatinine level is 0.6 to 1.3 mg/dL. The client with mild renal insufficiency would have a slightly elevated level, which would be the value of 1.9 mg/dL. Creatinine levels of 3.5 mg/dL may be associated with acute kidney injury or chronic kidney disease.
Test-Taking Strategy: Focus on the subject, mild renal insufficiency. This tells you that the correct option will be an abnormal value but perhaps not the most abnormal of all the values in the options. Use your knowledge of the normal serum creatinine level to direct you to the correct option. Options 1 and 2 are comparable or alike and are normal values. Option 4 is an extremely high value, which is not indicative of a "mild" condition. **Review:** normal **serum creatinine** values.
Level of Cognitive Ability: Analyzing
Client Needs: Physiological Integrity
Integrated Process: Nursing Process/Data Collection
Content Area: Fundamental Skills: Laboratory Values
Priority Concepts: Clinical Judgment, Fluid and Electrolyte Balance
Reference(s): deWit, Kumagai (2013), p. 769.
Pagana, Pagana (2013), p. 313.

65. 3

Rationale: The therapeutic range for serum phenytoin (Dilantin) level is 10 to 20 mcg/mL, so the next dose of phenytoin should be given if the level is 17 mcg/mL. If the level is too high, such as in the remaining options, the client could experience phenytoin toxicity.
Test-Taking Strategy: Focus on the subject, administration of the next phenytoin dose. Remember that the therapeutic range for serum phenytoin (Dilantin) level is 10 to 20 mcg/mL. This will direct you to the correct option. **Review:** therapeutic **serum phenytoin** levels.
Level of Cognitive Ability: Evaluating

Client Needs: Physiological Integrity
Integrated Process: Nursing Process/Evaluation
Content Area: Fundamental Skills: Laboratory Values
Priority Concepts: Clinical Judgment, Intracranial Regulation
Reference(s): Hodgson, Kizior (2014), p. 947.

66. 4
Rationale: The normal range for the protein level in the adult client is 6 to 8 g/dL, which makes the value of 6.8 g/dL the correct choice. The remaining options are all low levels and do not indicate that the diet has been most effective.
Test-Taking Strategy: Note the **strategic words**, *most effective.* Recalling the normal protein levels will direct you to the correct option. Also note that options 1, 2, and 3 are **comparable or alike** and are below the normal level. **Review:** normal protein levels.
Level of Cognitive Ability: Evaluating
Client Needs: Physiological Integrity
Integrated Process: Nursing Process/Evaluation
Content Area: Fundamental Skills: Laboratory Values
Priority Concepts: Clinical Judgment, Nutrition
Reference(s): deWit, Kumagai (2013), pp. 701–702; Pagana, Pagana (2013), p. 762.

67. 1
Rationale: The normal serum lipase level is 10 to 140 units/L. The client who is recovering from acute pancreatitis usually has elevated lipase levels for approximately 10 days after the onset of symptoms. This makes lipase a valuable test for monitoring the client's pancreatic function. The serum lipase level of 135 units/L indicates resolution of the acute pancreatitis because it is a normal value. The remaining options identify elevated lipase levels.
Test-Taking Strategy: Focus on the **subject**, resolution of acute pancreatitis. Recalling that lipase levels rise in acute pancreatitis and stay elevated for approximately 10 days will direct you to select the normal value of 135 units/L. **Review: lipase** levels and **acute pancreatitis.**
Level of Cognitive Ability: Evaluating
Client Needs: Physiological Integrity
Integrated Process: Nursing Process/Evaluation
Content Area: Fundamental Skills: Laboratory Values
Priority Concepts: Cellular Regulation, Nutrition
Reference(s): deWit, Kumagai (2013), pp. 708–709; Pagana, Pagana (2013), p. 595.

68. 3
Rationale: Troponins are regulatory proteins that are found in striated muscle. The troponins function together in the contractile apparatus for striated muscle in the skeletal muscle and the myocardium. Increased amounts of troponins are released into the bloodstream when an infarction causes damage to the myocardium. A troponin T level greater than 0.1 to 0.2 ng/mL is consistent with a myocardial infarction. A normal troponin I level is less than 0.6 ng/mL, whereas a level greater than 1.5 ng/mL is consistent with a myocardial infarction. A troponin T level of 0.6 is not normal, so that option can be eliminated. Troponin T does not test for gastritis or angina, so those options can also be eliminated.
Test-Taking Strategy: Focus on the **subject**, troponin T level of 0.6 ng/mL. Recalling that a level greater than 0.1 to 0.2 ng/mL is consistent with a myocardial infarction will direct you to the correct option. **Review: Troponin** T levels.
Level of Cognitive Ability: Analyzing
Client Needs: Physiological Integrity
Integrated Process: Nursing Process/Data Collection
Content Area: Fundamental Skills: Laboratory Values
Priority Concepts: Clinical Judgment, Perfusion
Reference(s): deWit, Kumagai (2013), pp. 383, 459.

69. 3
Rationale: The normal hemoglobin level for an adult female client is 12 to 15 g/dL and 14 to 16.5 for a male client. A low hemoglobin level usually indicates anemia. Iron deficiency anemia can result in lower hemoglobin levels. Heart failure and COPD may increase the hemoglobin level as a result of the body's need for more oxygen-carrying capacity. Dehydration may increase the hemoglobin level by hemoconcentration.
Test-Taking Strategy: Note the **strategic words**, *most likely*. Apply knowledge of normal values to help you determine that this level is low. Evaluate each condition presented in the options with regard to whether it is likely to raise or lower the hemoglobin level. **Review:** the normal **hemoglobin level** and the causes of a low level.
Level of Cognitive Ability: Analyzing
Client Needs: Physiological Integrity
Integrated Process: Nursing Process/Data Collection
Content Area: Fundamental Skills: Laboratory Values
Priority Concepts: Clinical Judgment, Perfusion
Reference(s): deWit, Kumagai (2013), p. 353; Pagana, Pagana (2013), p. 507.

70. 1
Rationale: The normal hematocrit level for an adult male is 42% to 52%. Thus, 48% is the only correct choice. The client who is dehydrated has an elevated level as a result of hemoconcentration. The client's level may be expected to drift back down to within the normal range after the fluid volume has been adequately restored. The remaining options are too high and indicate fluid replacement is still indicated.
Test-Taking Strategy: Focus on the **subject**, adequate fluid volume replacement in dehydration. Recalling that dehydration causes hematocrit to rise and fluid replacement helps it to normalize will direct you to the only normal hematocrit level. **Review: dehydration** and **hematocrit levels.**
Level of Cognitive Ability: Evaluating
Client Needs: Physiological Integrity
Integrated Process: Nursing Process/Evaluation
Content Area: Fundamental Skills: Laboratory Values
Priority Concepts: Clinical Judgment; Fluid and Electrolyte Balance
Reference(s): Pagana, Pagana (2013), p. 504.

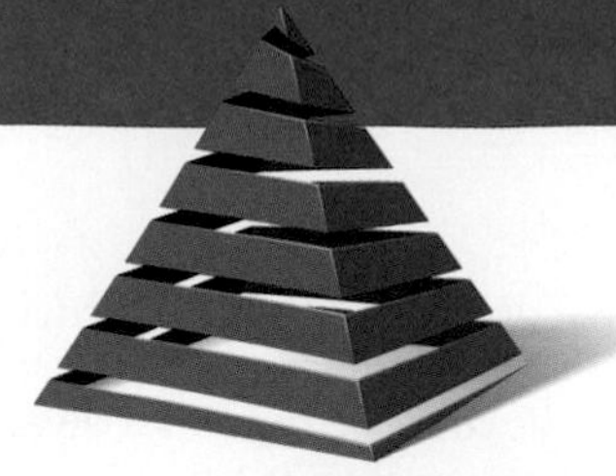

CHAPTER 12

Nutritional Components of Care

CRITICAL THINKING What Should You Do?

A client has been placed on a fluid restriction due to acute kidney injury. The client complains of thirst and asks what can be done to relieve this discomfort. What measures can the nurse tell the client to take to relieve thirst while adhering to the fluid restriction?

Answer located on p. 123.

I. Nutrients

A. Carbohydrates (Box 12-1)

1. Carbohydrates are the preferred source of energy and provide 4 cal/g.
2. Carbohydrates promote normal fat **metabolism**, spare protein, and enhance lower gastrointestinal (GI) function.
3. Major food sources of carbohydrates include milk, grains, fruits, and vegetables.
4. Inadequate carbohydrate intake affects metabolism.

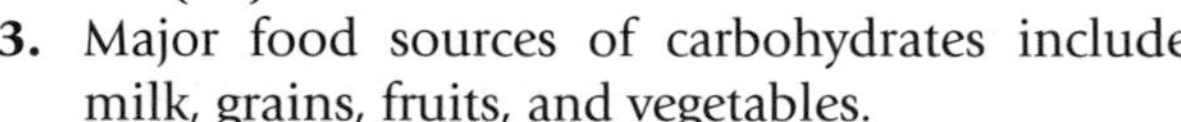

B. Fats (Box 12-2)

1. Fats provide a concentrated source and a stored form of energy and 9 cal/g.
2. Fats protect internal organs and maintain body temperature.
3. Fats enhance the absorption of the fat-soluble vitamins.
4. Inadequate intake of essential fatty acids leads to clinical manifestations of sensitivity to cold, skin lesions, increased risk of infection, and amenorrhea in women.
5. Diets high in fat can lead to obesity and increase the risk of cardiovascular disease and some cancers.

C. Proteins (Box 12-3)

1. Amino acids, which make up proteins, are critical to all aspects of the growth and development of body tissues and provide 4 cal/g.
2. Proteins build and repair body tissues, regulate fluid balance, maintain acid-base balance, produce antibodies, provide energy, and produce enzymes and hormones.

3. Essential amino acids (EAAs) are required in the diet because the body cannot manufacture them. 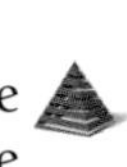
4. Complete proteins contain all essential amino acids; incomplete proteins lack some of the essential fatty acids.
5. Inadequate protein intake can cause protein energy **malnutrition** and severe wasting of fat and muscle tissue.

D. Vitamins (Box 12-4)

1. Vitamins facilitate metabolism of proteins, fats, and carbohydrates and act as catalysts for metabolic functions.
2. Vitamins promote life and growth processes, and maintain and regulate body functions.
3. Fat-soluble vitamins A, D, E, and K can be stored in the body, so an excess can cause toxicity.
4. The B vitamins and vitamin C are water soluble, are not stored in the body, and can be excreted in the urine.

E. Minerals (Box 12-5)

1. Minerals are components of hormones, cells, tissues, and bones.
2. Minerals act as catalysts for chemical reactions and enhancers of cell function.
3. Almost all foods contain some form of minerals.
4. A deficiency of minerals can develop in chronically ill or hospitalized clients.

⚠ Always check the client's ability to eat and swallow and promote independence in eating as much as is possible.

II. MyPlate (Fig. 12-1)

A. Provides a description of a balanced diet that includes grains, vegetables, fruits, dairy products, and protein foods (refer to http://www.choosemyplate.gov/).

B. A nutritionist should be consulted for individualized dietary recommendations.

C. Guidelines

1. Avoid eating oversized portions of foods.
2. Fill half of the plate with fruits and vegetables.
3. Vary the type of vegetables and fruits eaten.

BOX 12-1 Food Sources of Carbohydrates

Cellulose
Apples
Beans
Bran
Cab bage

Fructose
Fruits
Honey

Glucose
Carrots
Corn
Dates
Grapes
Oranges

Lactose
Milk

Starch
Barley
Beets, carrots, and peas
Corn
Oats
Potatoes and pasta
Rye
Wheat

Sucrose
Apricots
Granulated table sugar
Honeydew and cantaloupe
Molasses
Peaches
Peas and corn
Plums

BOX 12-2 Food Sources of Fat

Cholesterol
Animal products
Egg yolks
Liver and organ meats
Shellfish

Monounsaturated Fats
Duck and goose
Eggs
Olive and peanut oils

Polyunsaturated Fats
Safflower oil
Corn oil
Sunflower oil

Saturated Fats
Beef
Butter
Hard yellow cheeses
Luncheon meats

Trans Fats
Cookies, cakes, candy
Chips and crackers
Fried foods
Frozen pies, pot pies, waffles, pizza
Margarine
Packaged cake mixes and other mixes
Soups

BOX 12-3 Food Sources of Protein

Bread and cereal products
Dairy products
Dried beans
Eggs
Meats, fish, and poultry

4. Select at least half of the grains as whole grains.
5. Ensure that foods from the dairy group are high in **calcium**.
6. Drink milk that is fat-free or low fat (1%).
7. Eat protein foods that are lean.
8. Select fresh foods over frozen or canned foods.
9. Drink water rather than liquids that contain sugar.

BOX 12-4 Food Sources of Vitamins

Water Soluble
- Folic acid: Green, leafy vegetables; liver, beef, and fish; legumes; grapefruit and oranges
- Niacin: Meats, poultry, fish, beans, peanuts, grains
- Vitamin B_1 (thiamine): Pork, nuts, whole-grain cereals, legumes
- Vitamin B_2 (riboflavin): Milk, lean meats, fish, grains
- Vitamin B_6 (pyridoxine): Yeast, corn, meat, poultry, fish
- Vitamin B_{12} (cobalamin): Meat, liver (only found in animal products)
- Vitamin C (ascorbic acid): Citrus fruits, tomatoes, broccoli, cabbage

Fat Soluble
- Vitamin A: Liver, egg yolk, whole milk, green or orange vegetables, fruits
- Vitamin D: Fortified milk, fish oils, cereals
- Vitamin E: Vegetable oils; green, leafy vegetables; cereals; apricots; apples; peaches
- Vitamin K: Green, leafy vegetables; cauliflower; cabbage

⚠ Always consider the client's cultural and personal choices when planning nutritional intake.

III. Therapeutic Diets

A. Clear liquid diet
1. Indications
   a. Serves the primary function of providing fluids and electrolytes to prevent dehydration
   b. Initial feeding after complete bowel rest
   c. Used initially to feed a malnourished person or a person who has not had any oral intake for some time
   d. Clear liquid diet is used for bowel preparation for surgery or tests, as well as postoperatively and in clients with fever, vomiting, or diarrhea.
   e. Clear liquid diet is used in gastroenteritis.
2. Nursing considerations
   a. Is deficient in energy (calories) and many nutrients
   b. The body digests and absorbs clear liquids easily
   c. Contributes to little or no residue in the GI tract
   d. Can be unappetizing and boring
   e. As a transition diet, clear liquids are intended for short-term use only. 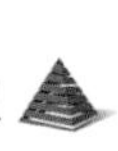
   f. Clear liquids and foods that are relatively transparent to light and are liquid at body temperature are considered "clear liquids," such as water, bouillon, clear broth, carbonated

BOX 12-5 Food Sources of Minerals

Calcium
Broccoli
Carrots
Cheese
Collard greens
Green beans
Milk
Rhubarb
Spinach
Tofu
Yogurt

Chloride
Salt

Iron
Breads and cereals
Dark green vegetables
Dried fruits
Egg yolk
Legumes
Liver
Meats

Magnesium
Avocados
Canned white tuna
Cauliflower
Cooked rolled oats
Green, leafy vegetables
Milk
Peanut butter
Peas
Pork, beef, chicken
Potatoes
Raisins
Yogurt

Phosphorus
Fish
Nuts
Organ meats
Pork, beef, chicken
Whole-grain breads and cereals

Potassium
Avocados
Bananas
Cantaloupe
Carrots
Fish
Mushrooms
Oranges
Pork, beef, veal
Potatoes
Raisins
Spinach
Strawberries
Tomatoes

Sodium
Bacon
Butter
Canned food
Cheese
Cottage cheese
Cured pork
Hot dogs
Ketchup
Lunch meat
Milk
Mustard
Processed food
Snack food
Soy sauce
Table salt
White and whole-wheat bread

Zinc
Eggs
Green, leafy vegetables
Meats
Protein-rich foods

beverages, gelatin, hard candy, lemonade, ice pops, and regular or decaffeinated coffee or tea.
- **g.** By limiting caffeine intake, upset stomach and sleeplessness may be prevented.
- **i.** Client may have salt or sugar.
- **j.** Dairy products and fruit juices with pulp are not clear liquids.

Monitor the client's hydration status by checking intake and output, checking weight, monitoring for edema, and monitoring for signs of dehydration.

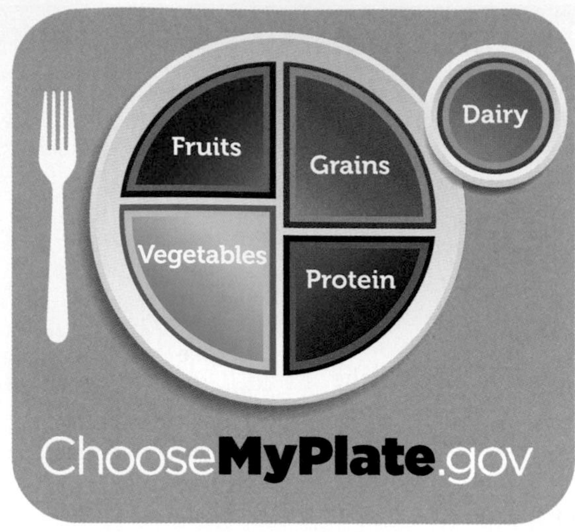

FIGURE 12-1 MyPlate. (From U.S. Department of Agriculture. http://www.choosemyplate.gov.)

B. Full liquid diet
- **1.** Indication: May be used as a transition diet after clear liquids after surgery or for clients who have difficulty chewing, swallowing, or tolerating solid foods
- **2.** Nursing considerations
  - **a.** A full liquid diet is nutritionally deficient in energy (calories) and many nutrients.
  - **b.** The diet includes both clear and opaque liquid foods and those that are liquid at body temperature.
  - **c.** Foods include all clear liquids and items such as plain ice cream, sherbet, breakfast drinks, milk, pudding and custard, soups that are strained, refined cooked cereals, fruit juices, and strained vegetable juices. 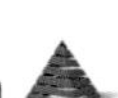
  - **d.** Use of a complete nutritional liquid supplement is often necessary to meet nutrient needs for clients on a full liquid diet for more than 3 days.

Provide nutritional supplements such as those high in protein, as prescribed for the client on a liquid diet.

C. Mechanically diet
- **1.** Indications
  - **a.** Provides foods that have been mechanically altered in texture to require minimal chewing
  - **b.** Used for clients who have difficulty chewing but who can tolerate more variety in texture than a liquid diet offers
  - **c.** Used for clients who have dental problems, have undergone surgery of the head or neck, or have dysphagia (requires swallowing evaluation and may require thickened liquids if the client has swallowing difficulties)

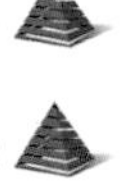

2. Nursing considerations
   a. Degree of texture modification depends on individual need, including puréed, mashed, ground, or chopped.
   b. Foods to be avoided in mechanically altered diets include nuts; dried fruit; raw fruits and vegetables; fried foods; chocolate candy; tough, smoked, or salted meats; and foods with coarse textures.

D. Soft diet
1. Indications
   a. Used for clients with difficulty chewing or swallowing
   b. Used for clients with ulcerations of the mouth or gums, broken jaws, or dysphagia and for those who have experienced oral surgery, plastic surgery of the head or neck, or stroke
2. Nursing considerations
   a. Clients with mouth sores should be served foods at cooler temperatures.
   b. Clients who have difficulty chewing and swallowing because of the reduced flow of saliva can increase salivary flow by sucking on sour candy.
   c. Encourage the client to eat a variety of foods.
   d. Provide plenty of fluids with meals to ease chewing and swallowing of foods.
   e. Drinking fluids through a straw may be easier than drinking from a cup or glass.
   f. All foods and seasonings are permitted; however, liquid, chopped, or puréed foods or regular foods with a soft consistency are tolerated best.
   g. Foods that contain nuts or seeds, which can easily become trapped in the mouth and cause discomfort, should be avoided.
   h. Raw fruits and vegetables, fried foods, and whole grains should be avoided.

⚠ Consider the client's disease or illness and how it may affect his or her nutritional status.

E. Low-residue, low-fiber diet
1. Indications
   a. Supplies foods that are least likely to form an obstruction when the intestinal tract is narrowed by inflammation or scarring or when GI motility is slowed
   b. Used for inflammatory bowel disease, partial obstructions of the intestinal tract, gastroenteritis, diarrhea, or other GI disorders
2. Nursing considerations
   a. Foods that are low in residue include white bread, refined cooked cereals, cooked potatoes without skins, white rice, and refined pasta.
   b. Foods to limit or avoid are raw fruits (except bananas), vegetables, nuts and seeds, plant fiber, and whole grains.
   c. Dairy products should be limited to two servings a day.

F. High-residue, high-fiber diet
1. Indications: Used for clients with constipation; irritable bowel syndrome, when the primary symptom is alternating constipation and diarrhea; and asymptomatic diverticular disease
2. Nursing considerations
   a. Provides 20 to 35 g of dietary fiber daily
   b. Adds volume and weight to the stool and speeds the movement of undigested materials through the intestine
   c. Consists of fruits, vegetables, and whole-grain products
   d. Increase fiber gradually and provide adequate fluids to reduce possible undesirable side effects such as abdominal cramps, bloating, diarrhea, and dehydration.
   e. Gas-forming foods should be limited (Box 12-6).

G. Cardiac diet (see Box 12-2 and Box 12-7)
1. Indications
   a. Indicated for atherosclerosis, diabetes mellitus, hyperlipidemia, hypertension, myocardial infarction, nephrotic syndrome, and kidney failure
   b. Reduces the risk of heart disease
2. Nursing consideration: Restricts total amounts of fat, including saturated, trans, polyunsaturated, and monounsaturated; cholesterol; and **sodium**

H. Fat-restricted diet
1. Indications
   a. Used to reduce symptoms of abdominal pain, steatorrhea, flatulence, and diarrhea associated with high intakes of dietary fat, and to decrease nutrient losses caused by the

BOX 12-6 Gas-Forming Foods

- Apples
- Artichokes
- Barley
- Beans
- Bran
- Broccoli
- Brussels sprouts
- Cabbage
- Celery
- Cherries
- Coconuts
- Eggplant
- Figs
- Honey
- Melons
- Milk
- Molasses
- Nuts
- Onions
- Radishes
- Soybeans
- Wheat
- Yeast

BOX 12-7 Sodium-Free Spices and Flavorings

- Allspice
- Almond extract
- Bay leaves
- Caraway seeds
- Cinnamon
- Curry powder
- Garlic and garlic powder
- Ginger
- Lemon extract
- Maple extract
- Marjoram
- Mustard powder
- Nutmeg

ingestion of dietary fat in individuals with malabsorption disorders

b. Used for clients with malabsorption disorders, pancreatitis, gallbladder disease, and gastroesophageal reflux

2. Nursing considerations
   a. Restricts the total amount of fat, including saturated fats, trans fats, polyunsaturated fats, and monounsaturated fats
   b. Clients with malabsorption may also have difficulty tolerating fiber and lactose.
   c. Vitamin and mineral deficiencies may occur in clients with diarrhea or steatorrhea.
   d. A fecal-fat test indicates fat malabsorption with the excretion of more than 6 to 8 g of fat (or more than 10% of the fat consumed) per day during the 3 days of specimen collection.

I. High-calorie, high-protein diet
1. Indications: Severe stress, burns, cancer, human immunodeficiency virus infection, acquired immunodeficiency syndrome, chronic obstructive pulmonary disease, respiratory failure, or any other type of debilitating disease
2. Nursing considerations
   a. Encourage nutrient-dense, high-calorie, high-protein foods such as whole milk and milk products, peanut butter, nuts, seeds, beef, chicken, fish, pork, and eggs.
   b. Some high-calorie foods include sugar, cream, gravy, oil, butter, mayonnaise, dried fruit, avocados, and honey.
   c. Encourage snacks between meals, such as milkshakes, instant breakfasts, and nutritional supplements.

Calorie counts assist in determining the client's total nutritional intake and can identify a deficit or excess intake.

J. Carbohydrate-consistent diet
1. Indications: Diabetes mellitus, hypoglycemia, hyperglycemia, and obesity
2. Nursing considerations
   a. The Exchange System for Meal Planning, developed by the Academy of Nutrition and Dietetics and the American Diabetes Association, is a food guide that may be recommended.
   b. The Exchange System groups foods according to the amounts of carbohydrates, fats, and proteins that they contain.
   c. Major food groups include the carbohydrate group, the meat and meat substitute group, and the fat group.
   d. The MyPlate diet may also be recommended.

K. Sodium-restricted diet
1. Indications: Hypertension, heart failure, kidney disease, cardiac disease, and liver disease 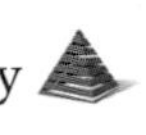
2. Nursing considerations (see Box 12-7)
   a. Individualized; can include 4 g of sodium daily (no-added-salt diet), 2 to 3 g of sodium daily (moderate restriction), 1 g of sodium daily (strict restriction), or 500 mg of sodium daily (severe and seldom prescribed)
   b. Encourage the intake of fresh rather than processed foods, which contain higher amounts of sodium.
   c. Canned, frozen, instant, smoked, pickled, and boxed items usually contain higher amounts of sodium. Lunch meats, soy sauce, salad dressings, fast foods, soups, and snacks such as potato chips and pretzels also contain large amounts of sodium.
   d. Certain medications contain significant amounts of sodium.
   e. Salt substitutes may be used to improve palatability. Most salt substitutes contain large amounts of potassium and should not be used by clients with kidney disease.

L. Protein-restricted diet
1. Indications: Used for kidney disease and liver disease
2. Nursing considerations
   a. Provides enough protein to maintain nutritional status but not an amount that will allow the buildup of waste products from protein metabolism (40 to 60 g of protein daily)
   b. The less protein allowed, the more important it becomes that all protein in the diet be of high biological value (contain all essential amino acids in recommended proportions). 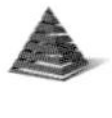
   c. An adequate total energy intake from foods is critical for clients on protein-restricted diets. (Protein will be used for energy rather than for protein synthesis.)
   d. Special low-protein products, such as pastas, bread, cookies, wafers, and gelatin made with wheat starch, can improve energy intake and add variety to the diet.
   e. Carbohydrates in powdered or liquid form can also provide additional energy.

f. Vegetables and fruits contain some protein. For very low-protein diets, these foods must be calculated into the diet.

g. Foods from the milk, meat, bread, and starch groups are limited.

M. Gluten-free diet: See Chapter 33 for information on this diet.

N. Renal diet (see Box 12-3 and Box 12-5)

1. Indications: Acute kidney injury and chronic kidney disease, and those clients requiring hemodialysis or peritoneal dialysis
2. Nursing considerations
   a. Controlled amounts of protein, sodium, phosphorus, calcium, potassium, and fluids may be prescribed; may also require modifications of the amounts of fiber, cholesterol, and fat based on individual requirements
   b. Most clients who are receiving dialysis need to restrict fluids (Box 12-8).

Initial data collection includes identifying food and medication interactions.

O. Potassium-modified diet (see Box 12-5)

1. Indications
   a. A low-potassium diet is indicated for hyperkalemia, which may be the result of impaired renal function, hypoaldosteronism, Addison's disease, angiotensin-converting enzyme inhibitor medications, immunosuppressive medications, potassium-retaining diuretics, and chronic hyperkalemia.
   b. A high-potassium diet is indicated for hypokalemia, which may be the result of renal tubular acidosis, GI losses (diarrhea, vomiting), intracellular shifts, potassium-wasting diuretics, antibiotics, mineralocorticoid or glucocorticoid excess caused by primary or secondary aldosteronism, Cushing's syndrome, or exogenous corticosteroid use.

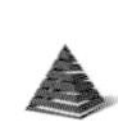

2. Nursing considerations
   a. Foods that are low in potassium include applesauce, green beans, cabbage, lettuce, peppers, grapes, blueberries, cooked summer squash, cooked turnip greens, fresh pineapple, and raspberries.
   b. Refer to Box 12-5 for foods that are high in potassium.

BOX 12-8 Measures to Relieve Thirst

Chew gum or suck hard candy.
Freeze fluids so that they take longer to consume.
Add lemon juice to water to make it more refreshing.
Gargle with refrigerated mouthwash.

P. High-calcium diet

1. Indications: Calcium is needed during bone growth and in adulthood to prevent osteoporosis and facilitate vascular contraction and vasodilation, muscle contraction, and nerve transmission.
2. Nursing considerations
   a. Primary dietary sources of calcium are dairy products (see Box 12-5 for food items high in calcium).
   b. Clients with lactose intolerance need to incorporate sources of calcium other than dairy products into their dietary patterns regularly.

Q. Low-purine diet

1. Indications: Gout, kidney stones, and elevated uric acid levels
2. Nursing considerations
   a. Purine is a precursor of uric acid, which forms stones and crystals.
   b. Foods to restrict include anchovies, herring, mackerel, sardines, scallops, glandular meats, gravies, meat extracts, wild game, goose, and sweetbreads.

R. High-iron diet

1. Indication: Anemia
2. Nursing considerations
   a. The high-iron diet replaces an iron deficit caused by inadequate intake or loss.
   b. The diet includes organ meats; meat; egg yolks; whole-wheat products; dark green, leafy vegetables; dried fruit; and legumes (see Box 12-5).

S. Miscellaneous diets: See Chapter 9 (Boxes 9-3, 9-4, 9-5, 9-6, and 9-7) for foods high in potassium, sodium, calcium, magnesium, and phosphorus.

IV. Vegetarian and Flexitarian (Semivegetarian) Diets

A. Types (Box 12-9)

B. Nursing considerations

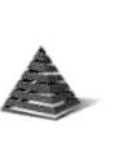

1. Ensure that the client eats a sufficient amount of varied foods to meet normal nutrient and energy needs.
2. Reinforce to clients about consuming complementary proteins over the course of each day to ensure that all essential amino acids are provided.
3. Potential deficiencies in vegetarian diets include protein, vitamin B_{12}, zinc, iron, calcium, omega-3 fatty acids, and vitamin D (if limited exposure to sunlight).
4. To enhance the absorption of iron, vegetarians should include a good source of iron and vitamin C with each meal.
5. Foods commonly eaten include tofu, tempeh, soy milk and soy products, meat analogues,

BOX 12-9 Types of Vegetarian and Semivegetarian Diets

Pescatarian

Abstains from eating all meat and animal flesh with the exception of fish

Flexitarian/Semivegetarian

Consumes mostly a vegetarian diet, but occasionally eats meat

Vegetarian (Lacto-Ovo Vegetarian)

Does not consume beef, pork, poultry, fish, shellfish, or animal flesh of any kind, but does eat eggs and dairy products

A lacto-vegetarian does not eat eggs, but does eat dairy products.

An ovo-vegetarian does not eat meat or dairy products, but does eat eggs.

Vegan

Does not consume meat of any kind and also does not eat eggs, dairy products, or processed foods containing these or other animal-derived ingredients such as gelatin

Raw Vegan/Raw Food Diet

Consumes unprocessed vegan foods that have not been heated above 115° F (46° C)

Macrobiotic

Consumes unprocessed vegan foods, such as whole grains and fruits and vegetables, and occasionally consumes fish; also consumes Asian vegetables, such as daikon, and sea vegetables, such as seaweed

legumes, nuts, seeds, sprouts, and a variety of fruits and vegetables.

6. Soy protein is considered equivalent in quality to animal proteins.

Body mass index (BMI) can be calculated by dividing the client's weight in kilograms by height in meters squared. For example, a client who weighs 82 kg (180 pounds) and is 1.9 m (6 feet 1 inch tall) has a BMI of 22.7 (82 divided by 1.9^2 [3.61] = 22.7).

V. Enteral Nutrition

A. Description: Provides liquefied foods to the GI tract via a tube

B. Indications
   1. When the GI tract is functional but oral intake is not meeting estimated nutrient needs
   2. Used for clients with swallowing problems, burns, major trauma, liver or other organ failure, or severe malnutrition

C. Nursing considerations
   1. Clients with lactose intolerance (diarrhea, bloating, cramping) need to be placed on lactose-free formulas.
   2. See Chapter 19 for information regarding the administration of gastrointestinal tube feedings and associated complications.

VI. Parenteral Nutrition (PN)

A. Description
   1. **Parenteral nutrition** (also termed total parenteral nutrition or TPN) supplies nutrients via the veins.
   2. Supplies carbohydrates in the form of dextrose; fats in a special emulsified form; proteins in the form of amino acids; vitamins; minerals; electrolytes; and water
   3. Prevents subcutaneous fat and muscle protein from being catabolized by the body for energy

B. Indications
   1. Clients with severely dysfunctional or nonfunctional GI tracts who are unable to process nutrients may benefit from PN.
   2. Clients who can take some oral nutrition (but not enough to meet their nutrient requirements) may benefit from PN.
   3. Clients with multiple GI surgeries, GI trauma, severe intolerance to enteral feedings, intestinal obstructions, or those who need to rest the bowel for healing may benefit from PN.
   4. Clients with severe nutritionally deficient conditions such as acquired immunodeficiency syndrome, cancer, burn injuries, or malnutrition, or clients receiving chemotherapy, may benefit from PN.

PN is a form of nutrition and is used when there is no other nutritional alternative. Other forms of administering nutrition, such as orally or via a gastrointestinal tube, are initiated first.

C. Administration of PN
   1. Central vein
      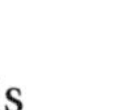
      a. PN is administered through a central vein when the client requires larger concentrations of carbohydrates (>10% glucose concentration).
      b. The subclavian or internal jugular vein is used when PN is a short-term intervention (less than 4 weeks).
      c. When PN is anticipated for an extended period (longer than 4 weeks), a more permanent catheter (e.g., a peripherally inserted central catheter [PICC] line), a tunneled catheter, or an implanted vascular access device is used.
   2. Peripheral vein

      a. PN can be administered through a peripheral vein, typically in the arm through a traditional intravenous catheter, or through a midline catheter, which is placed in an upper arm vein

such as the brachial or cephalic vein with the tip ending below the level of the axillary line.
   b. PN administered through a peripheral vein delivers isotonic or mildly hypertonic solutions as compared to the solutions administered through a central vein.

The delivery of hypertonic solutions into peripheral veins can cause sclerosis, phlebitis, or swelling. Monitor closely for these complications.

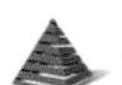

D. Fat emulsion (lipids)
   1. Lipids provide up to 30% of calorie (energy) needs and nonprotein calories and prevent or correct fatty-acid deficiency.
   2. Lipid solutions are isotonic and therefore can be administered through a peripheral or central vein.
   3. Most fat emulsions are prepared from soybean or safflower oil with egg yolk to provide emulsification. The primary components are linoleic, oleic, palmitic, linolenic, and stearic acids.
   4. Glucose-intolerant clients or those with diabetes mellitus may benefit from receiving a larger percentage of their PN from lipids. This can help control blood glucose levels and lower insulin requirements as a result of decreased infused dextrose.
   5. The bottle is examined for the separation of the emulsion into layers, fat globules, and the accumulation of froth. If observed, it is not used and is returned to the pharmacy.
   6. Additives should not be put into the **fat emulsion** solution.
   7. Monitor vital signs every 10 minutes, and observe for adverse reactions for the first 30 minutes of administration. If signs of an adverse reaction occur, stop the infusion and notify the registered nurse (Box 12-10).

BOX 12-10 Signs of an Adverse Reaction to Lipids

- Chest and back pain
- Chills
- Cyanosis
- Diaphoresis
- Dyspnea
- Fever
- Flushing
- Headache
- Nausea and vomiting
- Pressure over the eyes
- Rash
- Thrombophlebitis
- Vertigo

   8. Serum lipids are checked 4 hours after discontinuing the infusion.

Fat emulsions (lipids) contain egg yolk phospholipids and should not be given to clients with egg allergies.

E. Additional additives to PN solutions
   1. Vitamins are usually added to meet needs and prevent deficiencies.
   2. Minerals and trace elements may be added to promote normal metabolism.
   3. Electrolytes may be added to correct losses related to organ dysfunction and disease processes.
   4. Water amounts in PN are determined by electrolyte balance and fluid requirements.
   5. Insulin may be added to control blood glucose level because of the high concentration of glucose in the PN solution.
   6. Heparin may be added to reduce the buildup of fibrinous clot at the tip of centrally inserted catheters.

VII. Complications of Parenteral Nutrition and Nursing Considerations

A. See Table 12-1
B. Always check the **PN** solution with the health care provider's (HCP's) prescription to ensure that the prescribed components are contained in the solution.
C. To prevent infection and solution incompatibility, intravenous medications and blood are not given through the PN line.
D. Monitor partial thromboplastin time and prothrombin time for clients receiving anticoagulants.
E. Monitor electrolyte and albumin levels and liver and renal function studies, as well as any other prescribed laboratory studies.
F. In severely dehydrated clients, the albumin level may drop initially after initiating PN, because the treatment restores hydration.
G. With severely malnourished clients, monitor for "refeeding syndrome" (a rapid drop in potassium, magnesium, and phosphate serum levels).
H. Abnormal liver function values may indicate intolerance to or an excess of fat emulsion or problems with the metabolism of glucose and protein.
I. Abnormal renal function tests may indicate an excess of amino acids.
J. PN solutions should be refrigerated and administered within 24 hours from the time that they were prepared (remove from the refrigerator 0.5 to 1 hour before use).
K. PN solutions that are cloudy or darkened should not be used and should be returned to the pharmacy.
L. Additions to PN solutions should be made in the pharmacy and not in the nursing unit.

TABLE 12-1 Complications of Parenteral Nutrition

Complication	Possible Cause	Signs/Symptoms	Intervention	Prevention
Air embolism	■ Catheter system is opened or IV tubing is disconnected ■ Air entry occurs on IV tubing changes	■ Apprehension ■ Chest pain ■ Dyspnea ■ Hypotension ■ Loud churning sound heard over the pericardium on auscultation ■ Rapid and weak pulse ■ Respiratory distress	■ Clamp the catheter ■ Place the client in a left-side-lying position with the head lower than the feet ■ Notify the RN and HCP ■ Administer oxygen	■ Make sure all catheter connections are secure ■ Clamp the catheter when not in use ■ Instruct the client in Valsalva's maneuver for tubing and cap changes ■ For tubing and cap changes, place the client in Trendelenburg's position (if not contraindicated) with the head turned in the opposite direction of the insertion site
Hyperglycemia	■ Client is receiving solution too quickly ■ Not enough insulin	■ Restlessness ■ Weakness ■ Confusion ■ Diaphoresis ■ Elevated blood glucose level (>200 mg/dL) ■ Excessive thirst ■ Fatigue ■ Kussmaul's respirations	■ Notify the RN and HCP ■ May need to slow the infusion rate. ■ Administer regular insulin as prescribed. ■ Monitor blood glucose levels	■ Check the client for a history of glucose intolerance. ■ Check the client's medication history.
Hypervolemia	■ Excessive fluid administration or administration of fluid too rapidly. ■ Renal dysfunction ■ Heart failure ■ Hepatic failure	■ Bounding pulse ■ Crackles on lung auscultation ■ Headache ■ Increased blood pressure ■ Jugular vein distention ■ Weight gain greater than desired	■ Slow or stop the IV infusion ■ Restrict fluids ■ Diuretics ■ Dialysis (in extreme cases)	■ Check the client's history for risk for hypervolemia ■ Ensure proper function of the electronic infusion device ■ Monitor weight daily and intake and output
Hypoglycemia	■ PN abruptly discontinued ■ Too much insulin is being administered	■ Anxiety ■ Diaphoresis ■ Hunger ■ Low blood glucose level (<70 mg/dL) ■ Shakiness ■ Weakness	■ The RN and HCP is notified ■ Assist to administer IV dextrose ■ Monitor blood glucose level	■ PN solution is gradually decreased when discontinuing it. ■ 10% dextrose is infused at the same rate as the PN to prevent hypoglycemia when the PN solution is discontinued. ■ Monitor glucose levels when insulin is being given.
Infection	■ Poor aseptic technique ■ Catheter contamination ■ Contamination of solution	■ Chills ■ Fever ■ Elevated white blood cell count ■ Redness or drainage at the insertion site	■ Notify the RN and HCP ■ Assist the HCP with removal of catheter ■ Send the catheter tip to the laboratory for culture ■ Prepare to assist to obtain blood cultures ■ Prepare to assist antibiotic administration	■ Use strict aseptic technique ■ Monitor temperature ■ Check the IV site for signs of infection ■ Assist to change site dressing, solution, and tubing as specified by agency policy ■ Avoid disconnecting tubing unnecessarily
Pneumothorax	■ Inexact catheter placement	■ Chest or shoulder pain ■ Sudden shortness of breath ■ Tachycardia ■ Cyanosis ■ Absence of breath sounds on affected side	■ The RN and HCP are notified ■ Prepare to obtain a chest x-ray ■ Small pneumothorax may resolve ■ Larger pneumothorax may require chest tube	■ Monitor for signs of pneumothorax ■ A chest x-ray is obtained after the insertion of the catheter to ensure proper placement ■ PN is not initiated until correct catheter placement is verified and the absence of pneumothorax is confirmed

HCP, Health care provider; *IV*, intravenous; *PN*, parenteral nutrition; *RN*, registered nurse.

Adapted from Ignatavicius D, Workman M: *Medical-surgical nursing: Patient-centered collaborative care*, ed 7, St. Louis, 2013, Saunders.

M. Consultation with the nutritionist should be done on a regular basis (as prescribed or per agency protocol).

N. Discontinuing PN therapy
1. Evaluation of nutritional status by a nutritionist is done before PN is discontinued.
2. If discontinuation is prescribed, the flow rate is gradually decreased for 1 to 2 hours while increasing oral intake (this assists in preventing hypoglycemia).
3. After the IV catheter is removed, the dressing is changed daily until the insertion site heals.
4. Encourage oral nutrition.
5. Record oral intake, body weight, and laboratory results of serum electrolyte and glucose levels.

⚠ Abrupt discontinuation of a PN solution can result in hypoglycemia. The flow rate should be decreased gradually when the PN is discontinued.

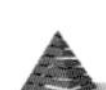

IX. Reinforcement of Home-Care Instructions (Box 12-11)

BOX 12-11 Home-Care Instructions

Reinforce to the client and caregiver how to administer and maintain parenteral nutrition fluids.

Reinforce to the client and the caregiver how to change a sterile dressing.

Obtain a daily weight at the same time of day in the same clothes.

Stress that weight gain of more than 3 lb/week may indicate excessive fluid intake and should be reported.

Monitor the blood glucose level, and report abnormalities immediately.

Check for signs and symptoms of infection, thrombosis, air embolism, and catheter displacement.

Teach the client and caregiver about the signs and symptoms of side or adverse effects such as infection, thrombosis, air embolism, and catheter displacement.

Teach the client and caregiver the actions to take if a complication arises and about the importance of reporting complications to the health care provider.

For symptoms of thrombosis, the client should report edema of the arm or at the catheter insertion site, neck pain, and jugular vein distention.

The leakage of fluid from the insertion site or pain or discomfort as the fluids are infused may indicate the displacement of the catheter. This must be reported immediately.

Reinforce to the client and caregiver about the importance of follow-up care.

Teach the client to keep electronic infusion devices fully charged in case of electrical power failure.

CRITICAL THINKING What Should You Do?

Answer: The client with acute kidney injury may be placed on fluid restriction because of decreased renal function and glomerular filtration rate, resulting in fluid volume excess. To allow the kidneys to rest, decreased fluid consumption may be indicated. When a client is placed on this restriction, increased thirst may be a problem. The nurse should instruct the client in measures to relieve thirst in order to promote adherence to the fluid restriction. These measures include chewing gum or sucking hard candy, freezing fluids so they take longer to consume, adding lemon juice to water to make it more refreshing, and gargling with refrigerated mouthwash.

Reference(s): deWit, D. & Kumagai, C. (2013). *Medical-surgical nursing: Concepts & practice.* (2nd ed., pp. 809–810). St. Louis: Saunders.

Ignatavicius, D., & Workman, M. (2013). *Medical-surgical nursing: Patient-centered collaborative care.* (7th ed., p. 175). St. Louis: Saunders.

PRACTICE QUESTIONS

71. A client is having problems with blood clotting. Which food item should the nurse encourage the client to eat?
1. Legumes
2. Citrus fruits
3. Vegetable oils
4. Green, leafy vegetables

72. When reinforcing instructions to a client with acute diverticulitis, which should the nurse include?
1. Avoid whole-grain products
2. Limit fluids to 1000 mL daily
3. Increase intake of seeds and nuts
4. Increase intake of raw fruits and vegetables

73. A client is a lacto-vegetarian. Which food item should the nurse remove from the tray?
1. Eggs
2. Milk
3. Cheese
4. Broccoli

74. A low-sodium diet has been prescribed for a client with hypertension. Which food selected from the menu by the client indicates an understanding of this diet?
1. Baked turkey
2. Tomato soup
3. Boiled shrimp
4. Chicken gumbo

75. The nurse is providing dietary instructions to a client with gout. The nurse should tell the client to avoid which food item?
1. Scallops
2. Chocolate
3. Cornbread
4. Macaroni products

76. A clear liquid diet has been prescribed for a client with gastroenteritis. Which item is appropriate to offer to the client?
1. Soft custard
2. Orange juice
3. Clam chowder
4. Fat-free beef broth

77. A client with heart disease is instructed regarding a low-fat diet. The nurse determines that the client understands the diet if the client states to avoid which food item?
1. Apples
2. Cheese
3. Oranges
4. Skim milk

78. The nurse reinforces instructions to a client to increase the amount of riboflavin in the diet. The nurse should tell the client to select which food item that is high in riboflavin?
1. Milk
2. Tomatoes
3. Citrus fruits
4. Green, leafy vegetables

79. A client with a burn injury is transferred to the nursing unit and a regular diet has been prescribed. The nurse encourages the client to eat which dietary items to promote wound healing?
1. Veal, potatoes, gelatin, and orange juice
2. Chicken breast, broccoli, strawberries, and milk
3. Peanut butter and jelly sandwich, cantaloupe, and tea
4. Spaghetti with tomato sauce, garlic bread, and ginger ale

80. The nurse has completed diet teaching for a client who has been prescribed a low-sodium diet to treat hypertension. The nurse determines that there is a **need for further teaching** when the client makes which statement?
1. "This diet will help lower my blood pressure."
2. "Fresh foods such as fruits and vegetables are high in sodium."
3. "This diet is not a replacement for my antihypertensive medications."
4. "The reason I need to lower my salt intake is to reduce fluid retention."

ANSWERS

71. 4

Rationale: Green, leafy vegetables are high in vitamin K, which acts as a catalyst for facilitating blood-clotting factors. Legumes are high in folic acid and thiamine. Citrus fruits are high in vitamin C, which helps with wound healing. Vegetable oil is high in vitamin E, which acts as an antioxidant.
Test-Taking Strategy: First, focus on the subject, problems with blood clotting, and recall that vitamin K is involved in the clotting process. Next, determine the food sources that are high in vitamin K. **Review:** functions of **vitamin K.**
Level of Cognitive Ability: Applying
Client Needs: Physiological Integrity
Integrated Process: Teaching and Learning
Content Area: Fundamental Skills: Nutrition
Priority Concepts: Clotting, Nutrition
Reference(s): deWit, Kumagai (2013), p. 696; Nix (2013), pp. 103–105.

72. 1

Rationale: Diet therapy for acute diverticulitis involves allowing the bowel to rest by avoiding high-fiber foods, such as whole-grain products and raw fruits and vegetables. Fluids are encouraged rather than restricted. Seeds and nuts are to be avoided so that they do not become trapped in the diverticula and cause irritation. In non-acute stages, a high-fiber diet may be prescribed.
Test-Taking Strategy: Focus on the subject, acute diverticulitis. Think about the pathophysiology associated with this diagnosis and that gastrointestinal inflammation occurs. Think about the food items that would increase inflammation to direct you to the correct option. **Review:** diet therapy for **acute diverticulitis.**
Level of Cognitive Ability: Applying
Client Needs: Physiological Integrity
Integrated Process: Teaching and Learning
Content Area: Fundamental Skills: Nutrition
Priority Concepts: Inflammation, Nutrition
References(s): deWit, Kumagai (2013), p. 668. Nix (2013), p. 366.

73. 1

Rationale: Eggs are not consumed by lacto-vegetarians. Other dairy and plant products are eaten by lacto-vegetarians.
Test-Taking Strategy: Focus on the subject, lacto-vegetarian. With that in mind immediately eliminate broccoli. From the remaining three options note that milk and cheese are dairy products, making them comparable or alike, so they can be eliminated. Eggs are the food items that are not consumed by lacto-vegetarians; however, they are eaten by lacto-ovo vegetarians. **Review: vegetarian diets.**
Level of Cognitive Ability: Applying
Client Needs: Physiological Integrity
Integrated Process: Nursing Process/Implementation
Content Area: Fundamental Skills: Nutrition
Priority Concepts: Adherence, Nutrition
Reference(s): Linton (2012), pp. 122–123; Nix (2013), p. 53.

74. 1

Rationale: Regular soup (1 cup) contains 900 mg of sodium. Fresh shellfish (1 oz) contains 50 mg of sodium. Poultry (1 oz) contains 25 mg of sodium.
Test-Taking Strategy: Eliminate tomato soup and chicken gumbo first, because they are comparable or alike. Also, recall that canned foods are high in sodium. From the remaining options, select baked turkey, remembering that shellfish is also high in sodium, even if it is boiled. **Review:** foods high in **sodium**.
Level of Cognitive Ability: Evaluating
Client Needs: Physiological Integrity
Integrated Process: Nursing Process/Evaluation
Content Area: Fundamental Skills: Nutrition
Priority Concepts: Fluid and Electrolyte Balance, Nutrition
Reference(s): deWit, Kumagai (2013), pp. 41, 405.
Nix (2013), pp. 136–137, 389.

75. 1

Rationale: Scallops should be omitted from the diet of a client who has gout because of the high purine content. The food items identified in the remaining options have negligible purine content and may be consumed by the client with gout.
Test-Taking Strategy: Focus on the subject, the food item to avoid. Note the client's diagnosis of gout, and think about the pathophysiology associated with this condition. Recalling the food items that are high in purine will direct you to the correct option. **Review: high-purine foods.**
Level of Cognitive Ability: Applying
Client Needs: Physiological Integrity
Integrated Process: Teaching and Learning
Content Area: Fundamental Skills: Nutrition
Priority Concepts: Client Education, Nutrition
Reference(s): deWit, Kumagai (2013), p. 755; Linton (2012), pp. 952–953.

76. 4

Rationale: A clear liquid diet consists of foods that are relatively transparent. Soft custard and orange juice would be included in a full liquid diet because they are opaque, not clear. Clam chowder is opaque and also includes pieces of clams, thus eliminating it from a full liquid diet.
Test-Taking Strategy: Focus on the subject, clear liquid diet. Remember that a clear liquid diet consists of foods that are relatively transparent. This will direct you to fat-free beef broth, because this is the only food item that is transparent. **Review:** clear liquid and full **liquid diets.**
Level of Cognitive Ability: Applying
Client Needs: Physiological Integrity
Integrated Process: Nursing Process/Implementation
Content Area: Fundamental Skills: Nutrition
Priority Concepts: Inflammation, Nutrition
Reference(s): Potter et al (2013), p. 1017.

77. 2

Rationale: Fruits, vegetables, and skim milk contain minimal amounts of fat. Cheese is high in fat.
Test-Taking Strategy: Focus on the subject, the food item to avoid. First note that apples and oranges are comparable or alike in that they are both fruits so they can be eliminated. From the remaining options recall that skim milk has minimal fat when compared to cheese, which is high in fat. **Review:** foods high in fat.
Level of Cognitive Ability: Evaluating
Client Needs: Physiological Integrity
Integrated Process: Nursing Process/Evaluation
Content Area: Fundamental Skills: Nutrition
Priority Concepts: Client Education, Nutrition
Reference(s): Nix (2013), p. 38.

78. 1

Rationale: Food sources of riboflavin include milk, lean meats, fish, and grains. Tomatoes and citrus fruits are high in vitamin C. Green leafy vegetables are high in folic acid.
Test-Taking Strategy: Focus on the subject, food sources high in riboflavin. Knowledge regarding food items that are high in riboflavin is required to answer this question. Remember that milk is a food source of riboflavin, so this will help you to eliminate the remaining options. **Review:** foods high in **riboflavin** content.
Level of Cognitive Ability: Applying
Client Needs: Physiological Integrity
Integrated Process: Teaching and Learning
Content Area: Fundamental Skills: Nutrition
Priority Concepts: Client Education, Nutrition
Reference(s): Nix (2013), pp. 110, 119.

79. 2

Rationale: Protein and vitamin C are necessary for wound healing. Poultry and milk are good sources of protein. Broccoli and strawberries are good sources of vitamin C. Peanut butter is a source of niacin. Gelatin and jelly have no nutrient value. Spaghetti is a complex carbohydrate.
Test-Taking Strategy: Focus on the subject, promoting wound healing, and recall that protein and vitamin C are necessary for wound healing. Eliminate options containing gelatin and jelly first, because they have no nutrient value related to healing. From the remaining options, select chicken breast, broccoli, strawberries, and milk over the remaining option because of the greater nutrient value of the foods. **Review:** foods high in **protein and vitamin C.**
Level of Cognitive Ability: Applying
Client Needs: Physiological Integrity
Integrated Process: Nursing Process/Implementation
Content Area: Fundamental Skills: Nutrition
Priority Concepts: Nutrition, Tissue Integrity
Reference(s): deWit, Kumagai (2013), p. 89; Nix (2013), pp. 449–450.

80. 2

Rationale: A low-sodium diet is used as an adjunct to antihypertensive medications for the treatment of hypertension. Sodium retains fluid, which leads to hypertension secondary to increased fluid volume. Fresh foods such as fruits and vegetables are low in sodium.
Test-Taking Strategy: Note the strategic words, *need for further teaching.* These words indicate a negative event query and ask you to select an option that is an incorrect statement. Remember that fresh foods are low in sodium, so they should be incorporated in the diet. Eliminate the remaining options because these are accurate statements related to management of hypertension. **Review:** purpose of a **low-sodium diet.**
Level of Cognitive Ability: Evaluating
Client Needs: Physiological Integrity
Integrated Process: Teaching and Learning
Content Area: Fundamental Skills: Nutrition
Priority Concepts: Fluid and Electrolyte Balance, Nutrition
Reference(s): Linton (2012), p. 686; Nix (2013), p. 389.

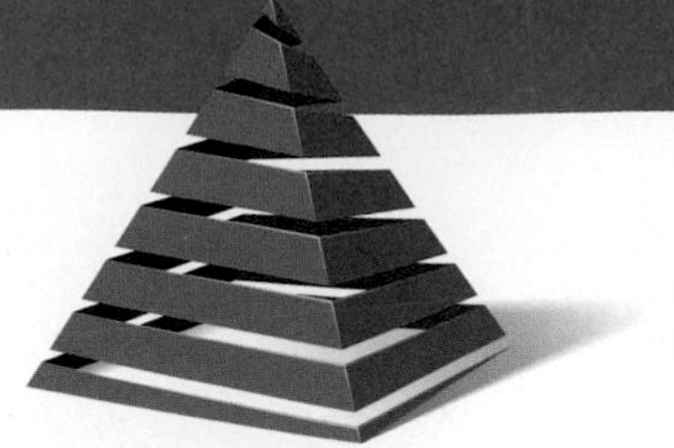

CHAPTER 13

Intravenous Therapy and Blood Administration

CRITICAL THINKING What Should You Do?

The nurse is monitoring a client receiving packed red blood cells (PRBCs) who has never received a blood transfusion. The client suddenly becomes apprehensive and complains of back pain after the first 10 minutes of administration. What should the nurse do?

Answer is located on p. 135.

I. Intravenous Therapy (see Chapter 9 and Table 9-1)

A. Used to sustain clients who are unable to take substances orally
B. Replaces water, electrolytes, and nutrients more rapidly than oral administration
C. Provides immediate access to the vascular system for the rapid delivery of specific solutions without the time required for gastrointestinal tract absorption
D. Provides a vascular route for the administration of medication or blood components

II. Intravenous (IV) Devices

A. IV cannulas
   1. Butterfly sets
      a. Wing-tipped needle with a metal cannula and plastic wings; the needle is 0.5 to 1.5 inches in length with needle gauge sizes from 16 to 26
      b. Infiltration is more common with these devices as a result of their stiffness.
      c. May commonly be used with children and older clients, whose veins are likely to be small or fragile.
   2. Plastic cannulas
      a. Used primarily for short-term therapy, especially if rapid infusion is necessary; more comfortable for the client
      b. Can cause a catheter embolism if the tip of the cannula breaks
B. IV gauges
   1. The gauge refers to the diameter of the lumen of the needle or cannula.
   2. The smaller the gauge number, the larger the outside diameter of the cannula.
   3. The gauge size used depends on the solution to be administered and the diameter of the available vein.
   4. Large-diameter lumens (smaller gauge numbers) allow a higher fluid rate than smaller diameter lumens and allow the administration of higher concentrations of solutions.
   5. For rapid emergency fluid administration, blood products, or anesthetics, a large needle (e.g., 14-, 16-, 18-, or 19-gauge) is used.
   6. For standard IV fluid infusion, a 20- or 22-gauge needle is used.
   7. If the client has very small veins, a 24- to 25-gauge needle is used.
C. IV containers
   1. May be glass or plastic
   2. Squeeze the plastic bag to ensure that it is intact. Check the glass bottle for any punctures or cracks.
   3. The expiration date of IV fluid and all supplies should be checked.

Do not write on a plastic IV bag with a marking pen because the ink may be absorbed through the plastic into the solution. Use a label and a ballpoint pen for marking the bag, placing the label onto the bag.

D. IV tubing (Fig. 13-1)
   1. Contains a spike end for the bag or bottle, a drop (drip) chamber, a roller clamp, a Y site, and an adapter end for attachment to the cannula or needle that is inserted into the client's vein
   2. Shorter secondary tubing is used for piggyback solutions, connecting them to the injection sites nearest to the drop chamber (Fig. 13-2).
   3. Special tubing is used for medication that absorbs into plastic. (Check specific medication administration guidelines.)
   4. Vented and nonvented tubing are available. 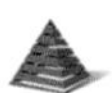
      a. A vent allows air to enter the IV container as the fluid leaves.

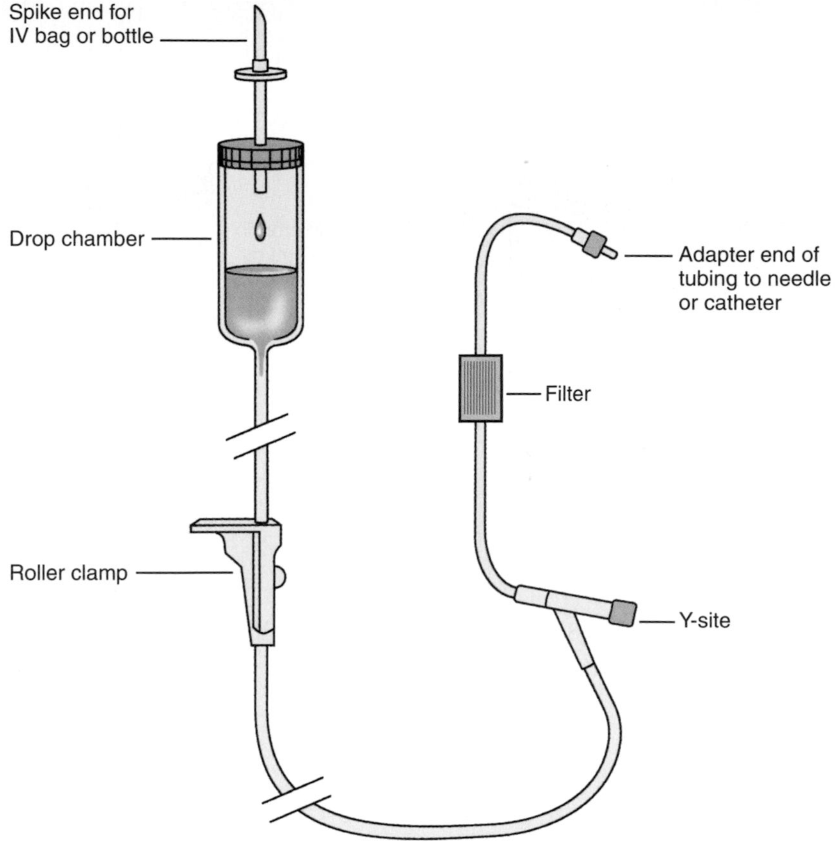

FIGURE 13-1 Intravenous tubing. (From Kee J, Marshall S: *Clinical calculations: With applications to general and specialty areas*, ed 7, St. Louis, 2013, Saunders.)

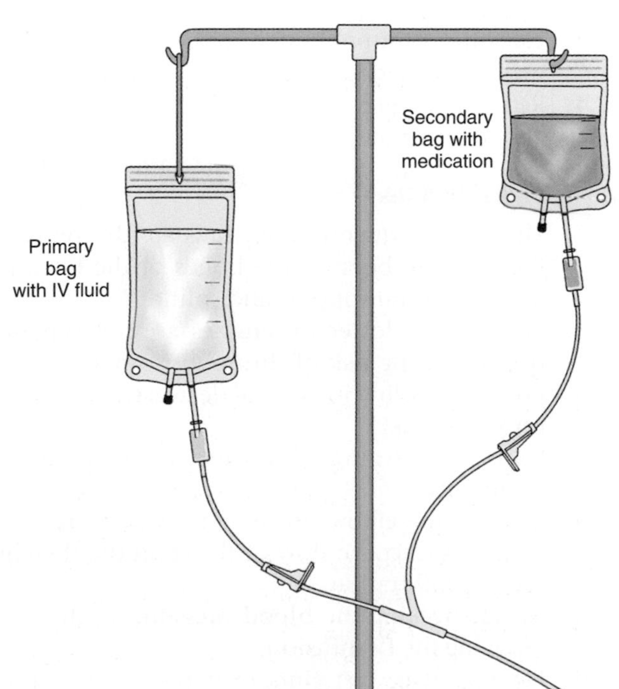

FIGURE 13-2 Secondary bag with medication. (From Kee J, Marshall S: *Clinical calculations: With applications to general and specialty areas*, ed 7, St. Louis, 2013, Saunders.)

b. A vented adapter can be used to add a vent to a nonvented IV tubing system.

c. Use nonvented tubing for flexible containers.

d. Use vented tubing for glass or rigid plastic containers to allow air to enter and displace the fluid as it leaves. Fluid will not flow from a rigid IV container unless it is vented. 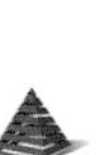

 Extension tubing can be added to an IV tubing set to provide extra length to the tubing. Add extension tubing to the IV tubing set for children, clients who are restless, or clients who have special mobility needs.

E. Drip chambers (Fig. 13-3)

1. Microdrip chamber

a. Normally has a short, vertical, metal piece where the drop forms

b. Delivers about 60 drops (gtt)/mL

c. Read the tubing package to determine how many drops per milliliter are delivered (drop factor).

d. Used if fluid will be infused at a slow rate (less than 50 mL/hour), or if the solution contains a potent medication that needs to be titrated, such as in a critical care setting or in the pediatric client

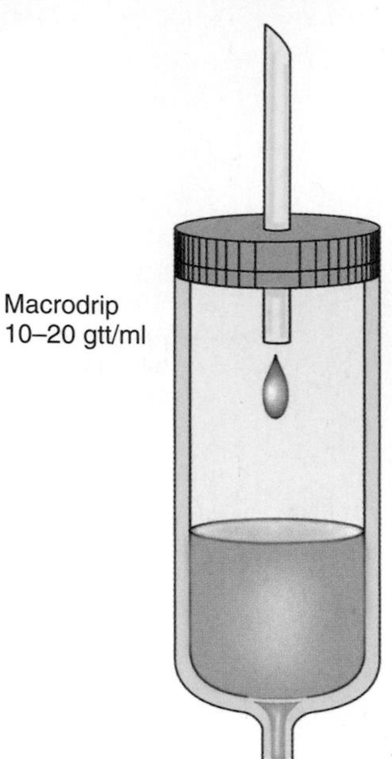

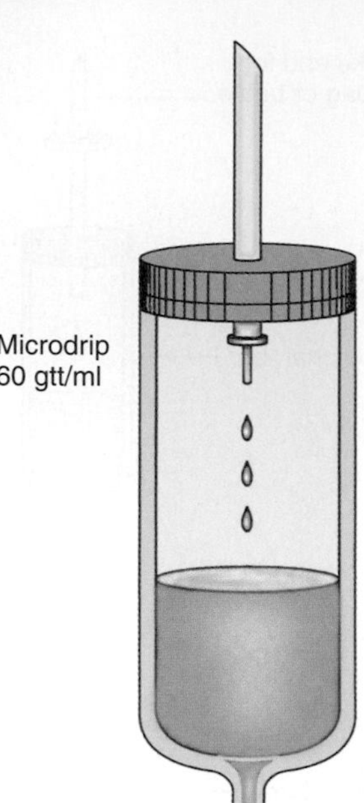

FIGURE 13-3 Macrodrip and microdrip sizes. (From Kee J, Marshall S: *Clinical calculations: With applications to general and specialty areas*, ed 7, St. Louis, 2013, Saunders.)

2. Macrodrip chamber
   a. Used if the solution is thick or needs to infuse rapidly
   b. Drop factor varies from 10 to 20 gtt/mL, depending on the manufacturer
   c. Read the tubing package to determine how many drops per milliliter are delivered (drop factor).

F. Filters: May be used in IV lines to trap small particles and provide protection by preventing particles from entering the client's veins

G. Needleless infusion devices: Include recessed needles, plastic cannulas, or one-way valves; these devices decrease exposure to contaminated needles

H. Intermittent infusion sets: Used when intravascular accessibility is desired for the intermittent administration of medications or solutions
   1. Require periodic flushing with normal saline as well as before and after medication administration to maintain patency.
   2. Normal saline is typically used to flush intermittent infusion sets. Hospital policy should be reviewed regarding amount of flush solution to instill.

I. Electronic infusion devices: Control the amount of fluid or medication infusing (for example, an infusion pump or controller, syringe pump, or patient-controlled analgesia [PCA]).

▲ Check electronic IV infusion devices frequently. Although these devices are electronic, this does not ensure that they are infusing solutions and medications accurately.

III. Latex Allergy

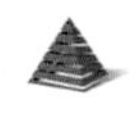

1. Ask the client about an allergy to latex.
2. IV supplies that may contain latex include IV catheters, IV tubing, IV ports (particularly IV rubber injection ports), rubber stoppers on multidose vials, and adhesive tape. Manufacturers typically label packaging when the item is latex-free.
3. Latex-free IV supplies need to be used for clients with latex allergy.
4. Refer to Chapter 61 for additional information about latex allergy.

IV. Peripheral IV Sites

1. The most frequently used sites are the veins of the forearm, because the bones of the forearm act as a natural support and splint.
2. Veins in the lower extremities are not suitable because of the risk of thrombus formation and possible pooling in areas of decreased venous return (Box 13-1).
3. Veins in the scalp and feet may be suitable sites for infants.
4. Bending the elbow on the arm with an IV may easily obstruct the flow of the solution, thereby causing infiltration.
5. Avoid checking the blood pressure on the arm receiving the IV infusion.
6. Do not place restraints over the venipuncture site.
7. An orphan may be prescribed when the venipuncture site is located in an area of flexion.

BOX 13-1 Peripheral Intravenous Sites to Avoid

- Edematous extremity
- The lower extremities
- An arm that is weak, traumatized, or paralyzed
- The arm on the same side as a mastectomy
- An arm that has an arteriovenous fistula or a shunt for dialysis
- A skin area that is infected

In an adult, the most frequently used sites for inserting an IV cannula/needle are the veins of the forearm because the bones of the forearm act as a natural support and splint.

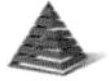

V. Administering IV Solutions

A. The IV solution should be checked against the health care provider's (HCP's) prescription for the type, amount, percentage of solution, and rate of flow.

B. Check the health status and medical disorders of the client and identify client conditions that contraindicate use of a particular IV solution or IV equipment such as an allergy to cleansing solution, adhesive materials, or latex.

C. Wash hands thoroughly and use sterile technique when working with an IV.

D. When preparing a new solution for administration, clamp the tubing, attach the spike end of the tubing to the IV bag, and then prime the tubing to remove air from the tubing and IV system.

E. The venipuncture site is changed every 72 to 96 hours in accordance with Centers for Disease Control and Prevention (CDC) recommendations and agency policy.

F. The IV dressing is changed when the dressing is wet or contaminated, or as specified by the agency policy and the IV tubing is changed every 96 hours in accordance with CDC recommendations and agency policy or with change of venipuncture site.

G. Do not let an IV bag or bottle of solution hang for more than 24 hours to diminish the potential for bacterial contamination and possibly sepsis.

H. Do not allow the IV tubing to touch the floor to prevent potential bacterial contamination.

I. See Priority Nursing Actions for instructions on removing an IV.

VI. Precautions for IV Lines

A. On insertion, can cause initial pain and discomfort for the client

B. An IV puncture provides a route of entry for microorganisms into the body.

PRIORITY NURSING ACTIONS!

Steps for Removing a Peripheral Intravenous (IV) Line

1. Check the HCP's prescription and explain the procedure to the client. Ask the client to hold the extremity still during cannula/needle removal.
2. Turn the IV tubing clamp off and remove the dressing and tape covering the site while stabilizing the catheter.
3. Apply light pressure with sterile gauze or other material as specified by agency procedure over the site and withdraw the catheter using a slow steady movement keeping the hub parallel to the skin.
4. Apply pressure for 2 to 3 minutes using dry sterile gauze (apply pressure for a longer period of time if the client has a bleeding disorder or is taking anticoagulant medication).
5. Inspect the site for redness, drainage, or swelling and check the catheter for intactness.
6. Document the procedure and the client's response.

The nurse checks for a HCP's prescription to remove the IV line and then explains the procedure to the client. The nurse asks the client to hold the extremity still during removal. The IV tubing clamp is placed in the off position and the dressing and tape is removed. The nurse is careful to stabilize the catheter so that it is not pulled, resulting in vein trauma. Light pressure is applied over the site to stabilize the catheter and it is removed using a slow steady movement keeping the hub parallel to the skin. Pressure is applied until hemostasis occurs. The site is inspected for redness, drainage, or swelling and the catheter is checked for intactness to ensure that any part of it has not broken off. Finally the nurse documents the procedure and the client's response.

Reference(s): Perry, A., Potter, P., & Elkin, M. (2012). *Nursing interventions & clinical skills* (5th ed., pp. 678–679). St. Louis: Mosby.

C. Fluid (circulatory) overload or electrolyte imbalances can occur from an excessive or too-rapid infusion of fluids. An IV infusion should be checked at least once per hour in an adult client.

D. Incompatibilities between certain solutions can occur.

A client with heart failure usually is not given a solution containing saline because this type of fluid promotes the retention of water and would therefore exacerbate heart failure by increasing the fluid overload.

VII. Complications (Table 13-1)

A. Air embolism

1. Description: A bolus of air enters the vein through an inadequately primed IV line, from a loose connection, during a tubing change, or the removal of the IV.

TABLE 13-1 Signs of Complications of IV Therapy

Complication	Signs
Air embolism	Tachycardia Chest pain and dyspnea Hypotension Cyanosis Decreased level of consciousness
Catheter embolism	Decrease in blood pressure Pain along the vein Weak, rapid pulse Cyanosis of the nail beds Loss of consciousness
Circulatory overload	Increased blood pressure Distended jugular veins Rapid breathing Dyspnea Moist cough and crackles
Electrolyte overload	Signs depend on the specific electrolyte overload imbalance
Infection	Local—redness, swelling, and drainage at the site Systemic—chills, fever, malaise, headache, nausea, vomiting, backache, tachycardia
Infiltration	Edema, pain, and coolness at the site; may or may not have a blood return
Phlebitis	Heat, redness, tenderness at the site Not swollen or hard Intravenous infusion sluggish
Thrombophlebitis	Hard and cordlike vein Heat, redness, tenderness at site Intravenous infusion sluggish

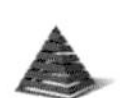

2. Prevention and interventions
   a. Prime the tubing with fluid before use, and monitor for any air bubbles in the tubing.
   b. Secure all connections.
   c. Replace IV fluid before the bag or bottle is empty.
   d. If an air embolism is suspected, the registered nurse (RN) is notified immediately, the tubing is clamped, the client is turned on his or her left side with the head of the bed lowered (Trendelenburg position) to trap the air in the right atrium, and the HCP is notified.

B. Catheter embolism
1. Description: An obstruction that results from the breakage of the catheter tip during IV insertion or removal
2. Prevention and interventions
   a. Inspect the catheter before insertion.
   b. Remove the IV catheter carefully, and inspect the catheter when removed.
   c. If the catheter tip has broken off, the RN notifies the HCP immediately. A tourniquet is placed high on the limb of the IV site as prescribed, an x-ray study is obtained, and the client may require surgery to remove the catheter pieces.

C. Circulatory overload
1. Description: Also known as *fluid overload;* results from the administration of fluids too rapidly or in a client who is at risk for fluid overload
2. Prevention and interventions
   a. Identify clients at risk for circulatory overload.
   b. Calculate and monitor the drip (flow) rate frequently.
   c. Use an electronic IV infusion device and frequently check the drip rate or setting (at least every hour for an adult).
   d. Monitor for signs of circulatory overload. If circulatory overload occurs, decrease the flow rate to a minimum, at a keep-vein-open rate; elevate the head of the bed; keep the client warm; check lung sounds; assess for edema; and the RN and HCP are notified immediately.

Clients with respiratory, cardiac, renal, or liver disease, older clients, and very young persons are at risk for circulatory overload and cannot tolerate an excessive fluid volume.

D. Electrolyte overload
1. Description: An electrolyte imbalance caused by too-rapid or excessive infusion or use of an inappropriate IV solution

2. Prevention and interventions
   a. Review laboratory value reports.
   b. Verify the correct solution and additives with the HCP prescriptions.
   c. Calculate and monitor the flow rate closely
   d. Use an electronic infusion device and frequently check the settings.

Lactated Ringer's solution contains potassium and should not be administered to clients with acute kidney injury or chronic kidney disease.

E. Infection
1. Description
   a. The entry of microorganisms into the body through the venipuncture site
   b. Venipuncture interrupts the integrity of the skin, which is the first line of defense against infection.

c. The longer the therapy continues, the greater the risk of infection.
d. Infection can occur locally at the IV insertion site or systemically from the entry of microorganisms into the body.

2. At-risk clients
   a. Clients who are immunocompromised as a result of diseases such as cancer or acquired immunodeficiency syndrome
   b. Clients receiving treatments such as chemotherapy who have an altered or lowered white blood cell count
   c. Older clients, because aging alters the effectiveness of the immune system
   d. Clients with diabetes mellitus are at risk for infection

A client with diabetes mellitus usually does not receive dextrose (glucose) solutions because the solution can increase the blood glucose level.

3. Prevention and interventions
   a. Determine is the client is at risk for infection.
   b. Maintain strict asepsis when caring for the IV site.
   c. Monitor for signs of local or systemic infection.
   d. Monitor white blood cell counts.
   e. Check fluid containers for cracks, leaks, cloudiness, or other evidence of contamination.
   f. IV tubing is changed no more frequently than every 96 hours per CDC recommendations and agency policy; the IV site dressing is changed when soiled or contaminated and according to agency policy.
   g. Ensure that the IV site, bag or bottle, and tubing are labeled with the date and time to ensure that these are changed on time according to agency policy.
   h. Ensure that the IV solution is not hanging for more than 24 hours.
   i. If signs of infection occurs, the RN and HCP is notified; the IV is discontinued, and the venipuncture device is placed in a sterile container for possible culture.
   j. Assist to obtain blood cultures as prescribed if infection occurs.
   k. The IV is restarted in the opposite arm to differentiate sepsis (systemic infection) from local infection at the IV site.

F. Infiltration
1. Description
   a. Seepage of the IV fluid out of the vein and into the surrounding tissues
   b. Occurs when an IV device has become dislodged or perforates the wall of the vein
   c. *Extravasation* is a form of tissue damage caused by the seepage of vesicant or irritant solutions into the tissues; this occurrence requires immediate HCP notification so that treatment can be prescribed to prevent tissue necrosis.
2. Prevention and interventions
   a. Avoid venipuncture over an area of flexion.
   b. Anchor the cannula and loop of tubing securely with tape.
   c. Use an armboard or splint as prescribed if the client is restless or active.
   d. Monitor the IV rate for a decrease or cessation of flow.
   e. If **infiltration** has occurred, the IV device is removed immediately; the extremity is elevated, and compresses (warm or cool, depending on the IV solution that was infusing and the HCP's prescription) are applied over the affected area.
   f. Do not rub an infiltrated area because this can cause the development of a hematoma.

G. Phlebitis and thrombophlebitis
1. Description
   a. Phlebitis is an inflammation of the vein that can occur from mechanical or chemical (medication) trauma or local infection
   b. Phlebitis can cause the development of a clot (thrombophlebitis).
2. Prevention and interventions
   a. An IV cannula smaller than the vein is used. Very small veins are avoided when administering irritating solutions. Veins over an area of flexion are avoided.
   b. Anchor the cannula and loop of tubing securely with tape.
   c. Use an armboard or splint as prescribed if the client is restless or active.
   d. If phlebitis occurs, the IV device is removed immediately.
   e. The RN and HCP are notified if phlebitis is suspected, and warm, moist compresses are applied as prescribed. 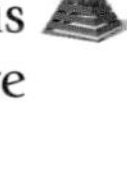

Always document the occurrence of a complication, data collection findings, actions taken, and the client's response.

VIII. Central Venous Catheters (Fig. 13-4)

A. Description
1. Used to deliver hyperosmolar solutions, measure central venous pressure, and infuse parenteral nutrition and multiple IV infusions or medications
2. Catheter position is determined by x-ray study after insertion. 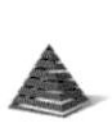
3. May have a single, double, or triple lumen

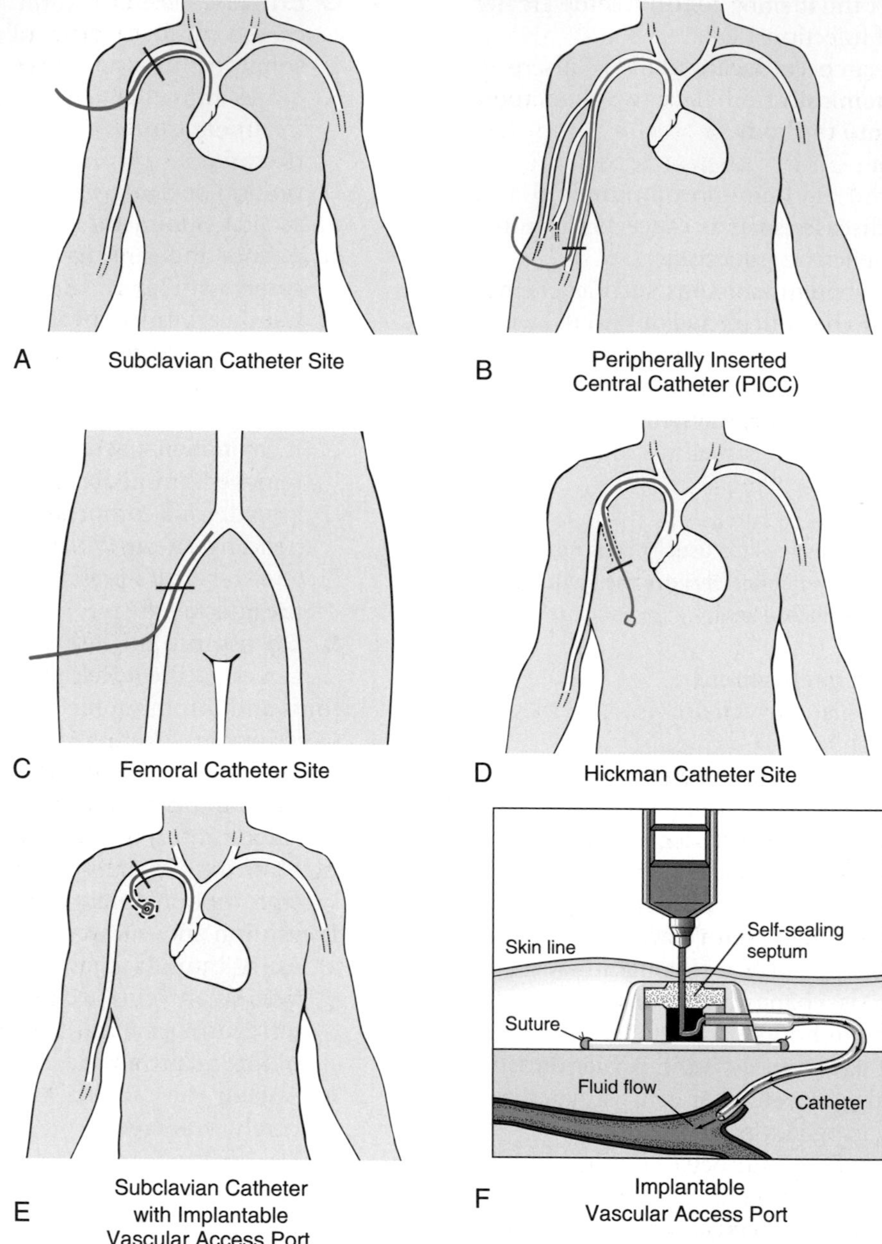

FIGURE 13-4 Central venous access sites. **A,** Subclavian catheter. **B,** Peripherally inserted central catheter (PICC). **C,** Femoral catheter. **D,** Hickman catheter. **E,** Subclavian catheter with implantable vascular access port. **F,** Implantable vascular access port. (**A–E,** From Kee J, Marshall S: *Clinical calculations: With applications to general and specialty areas,* ed 7, St. Louis, 2013, Saunders; **F,** redrawn from Winters B: Implantable vascular access devices. *Oncology Nursing Forum* 11, 25–30, 1984.)

4. May be inserted peripherally and threaded through the basilic or cephalic vein into the superior vena cava, inserted centrally through the internal jugular or subclavian veins, or surgically tunneled through subcutaneous tissue into the cephalic vein.
5. With multilumen catheters, more than one medication can be administered at the same time without incompatibility problems, and there is only one insertion site for care.

⚠ For central line insertion, tubing change, and line removal, the client is placed in the Trendelenburg's position if not contraindicated or in the supine position, and instruct the client to perform the Valsalva maneuver to increase pressure in the central veins when the IV system is open.

B. Tunneled central venous catheters
1. A more permanent type of catheter (e.g., Hickman, Broviac, Groshong) used for long-term IV therapy
2. May be single or multilumen
3. Inserted in the operating room. The catheter is threaded into the lower part of the vena cava at the entrance of the right atrium.

4. The catheter will be fitted with an intermittent infusion device to allow access as needed and to keep the system closed and intact.
5. Patency is maintained by flushing with a diluted heparin solution or a normal saline solution, depending on the type of catheter and according to agency policy.

C. Vascular access ports (implantable ports)
1. Surgically implanted under the skin (e.g., Port-a-Cath, Mediport, Infusaport); used for the long-term administration of repeated IV therapy
2. For access, the port requires palpation and injection through the skin into the self-sealing port with a noncoring needle, such as a Huber-point needle.
3. Patency is maintained by periodic flushing with a diluted heparin solution as prescribed and per agency policy.

D. Peripherally inserted central catheter line (PICC)
1. Used for long-term IV therapy, frequently in the home
2. The basilic vein is usually used, but the median cubital and cephalic veins in the antecubital area can also be used.
3. Threaded so that the catheter tip may terminate in the subclavian vein or the superior vena cava
4. A small amount of bleeding may occur at the time of insertion and continue for 24 hours, but bleeding thereafter is not expected.
5. Phlebitis is a common complication.
6. Insertion is below the heart level; therefore air embolism is not common.

IX. Blood Administration

A. Types of blood components
1. Red blood cells (RBCs) transfusion
   a. Used to replace erythrocytes; infusion time for 1 unit is usually between 2 and 4 hours
   b. Evaluation of an effective response is based on the resolution of the symptoms of anemia and an increase of the erythrocyte count.

! Washed red blood cells (depleted of plasma, platelets, and leukocytes) may be prescribed for a client with a history of allergic transfusion reactions or those who underwent hematopoietic stem cell transplant.

2. Platelet transfusion
   a. Platelets are used to treat thrombocytopenia and platelet dysfunctions.
   b. Crossmatching is not required but is usually done (platelet concentrates contain few RBCs).
   c. Platelets are administered rapidly usually over 15 to 30 minutes.
   d. Evaluation of an effective response is based on the improvement of the platelet count.
3. Fresh-frozen plasma
   a. May be used to provide clotting factors or volume expansion; contains no platelets
   b. Rh factor and ABO **compatibility** are required for the transfusion of plasma products
   c. Fresh frozen plasma is infused after thawing and administered rapidly, usually over 15 to 30 minutes.
   d. Evaluation of an effective response is assessed by monitoring coagulation studies, particularly the prothrombin time and the partial thromboplastin time, and resolution of hypovolemia.

B. Compatibility (Table 13-2)
1. Client (the recipient) blood samples are drawn and labeled at the bedside at the time the blood sample is drawn. The client is asked to state his or her name, which is compared with the identification band or bracelet.
2. The recipient's ABO and Rh factor are identified.
3. An antibody screen is done to determine the presence of antibodies other than anti-A and anti-B.
4. To determine compatibility, crossmatching is done, in which donor red blood cells are combined with the recipient's serum and Coombs' serum; the crossmatch is compatible if no red blood cell agglutination occurs.
5. The universal RBC donor is O negative. The universal recipient is AB positive. 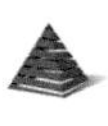
6. Clients with Rh-positive blood can receive RBC transfusion from an Rh-negative donor if necessary; however, an Rh-negative client should not receive Rh-positive blood. 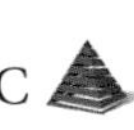

! The donor's blood and the recipient's blood must be tested for compatibility. If the blood is not compatible, a life-threatening transfusion reaction can occur.

TABLE 13-2 Compatibility Chart for Red Blood Cell Transfusions

	Recipient			
Donor	**A**	**B**	**AB**	**O**
A	X		X	
B		X	X	
AB			X	
O	X	X	X	X

The ABO type of the donor should be compatible with the recipient's. Type A can receive from type A or O; type B from type B or O; type AB can receive from type A, B, AB, or O; type O only from type O.

From Ignatavicius D, Workman ML: *Medical-surgical nursing: Patient centered collaborative care,* ed 7, Philadelphia, 2013, Saunders.

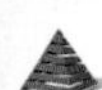

C. Precautions and nursing responsibilities (Box 13-2)

⚠ Stay with the client for the first 15 minutes of the infusion of the blood and monitor the client for signs and symptoms of a transfusion reaction. The first 15 minutes of the transfusion are the most critical, and the nurse must stay with the client.

D. Transfusion reactions

1. Immediate transfusion reaction
   a. Chills and diaphoresis
   b. Muscle aches, back pain, or chest pain
   c. Rashes, hives, itching, and swelling
   d. Rapid, thready pulse
   e. Dyspnea, cough, or wheezing

BOX 13-2 Blood Administration Precautions and Nursing Responsibilities

General Precautions

- A large volume of refrigerated blood infused rapidly through a central venous catheter into the ventricle of the heart can cause cardiac dysrhythmias.
- Medications are never added to blood components or piggybacked into a blood transfusion; no solution other than normal saline should be added to blood components.
- To avoid the risk of septicemia, infusions (1 unit) should not exceed the prescribed time for administration (2 to 4 hours for PRBCs); the blood administration set should also be changed with each unit. Follow evidence-based practice guidelines and agency procedure.
- Always check the blood bag for the date of expiration; components expire at midnight on the day marked on the bag unless otherwise specified.
- Inspect the blood bag for leaks, abnormal color, clots, and bubbles.
- Blood must be administered as soon as possible, within 20 to 30 minutes—the maximum allowable time out of monitored storage—from its being received from the blood bank. If the blood is not administered within that time, return it to the blood bank.
- Never refrigerate blood in refrigerators other than those used in blood banks.
- The recommended rate of infusion varies with the blood component being transfused and depends on the client's condition; generally, blood is infused as quickly as the client's condition allows; caution should be taken to avoid circulatory overload.
- The nurse should measure vital signs and check the lung sounds before the transfusion and again after the first 15 minutes and every hour until 1 hour after the transfusion is completed.

Blood Bank Precautions

- Blood will be released from the blood bank only to personnel specified by agency policy.
- The name and identification number of the intended recipient must be provided to the blood bank, and a documented permanent record of this information must be maintained.
- Blood should be transported from the blood bank to only one client at a time to prevent blood delivery to the wrong client.

Client Identity and Compatibility

- The most critical phase of the transfusion is confirming product compatibility and verifying client identity.
- Two licensed nurses (follow agency policy) need to check the health care provider's (HCP's) prescription. At bedside, check the client's identity—asking the client to state his/her name—and compare the name to the client's identification band or bracelet and number, verifying that the name and number are identical to those on the blood component tag.
- The nurse checks the blood bag tag, label, and blood requisition form to ensure that ABO and Rh types are compatible.
- If the nurse notes any inconsistencies when verifying client identity and compatibility, the nurse notifies the blood bank immediately.

Client Assessment

- Determine any cultural or religious beliefs regarding blood transfusions (e.g., a Jehovah's Witness cannot receive blood or blood products; this group believes that blood transfusions have eternal consequences).
- Ensure that an informed consent has been obtained.
- Explain the procedure to the client and determine whether the client has ever received a blood transfusion or experienced any previous reactions to blood transfusions.
- Check the client's vital signs and check renal, circulatory, and respiratory status and the client's ability to tolerate intravenously administered fluids.
- If the client's temperature is elevated, the HCP is notified before beginning the transfusion; a fever may be a cause for delaying the transfusion in addition to masking a possible symptom of an acute transfusion reaction.

Administration of the Transfusion

- Maintain standard and transmission-based precautions and surgical asepsis as necessary.
- Assist the registered nurse in administering the blood.
- Always check the bag for the volume of the blood component.
- Blood products should be infused through administration sets designed specifically for blood; use a Y-tubing or straight tubing blood administration set that contains a filter designed to trap fibrin clots and other debris that accumulate during blood storage.
- Premedicate the client with acetaminophen (Tylenol) or diphenhydramine (Benadryl), as prescribed, if the client has a history of adverse reactions; if prescribed, oral medications should be administered 30 minutes before the transfusion is started, and intravenously administered medications may be given immediately before the transfusion is started.
- Reinforce instructions to the client to report anything unusual immediately.
- Determine the rate of infusion by the HCP's prescription or, if not specified, by agency policy.

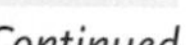

Continued

BOX 13-2 Blood Administration Precautions and Nursing Responsibilities—Cont'd

- Begin the transfusion slowly under close supervision; stay with the client and monitor for signs and symptoms of a transfusion reaction. If no reaction is noted within the first, most critical, 15 minutes, the flow can be increased to the prescribed rate.
- If a major ABO incompatibility exists or a severe allergic reaction occurs, the reaction is usually evident within the first 50 mL of the transfusion.
- Document the client's tolerance to the administration of the blood product.
- Monitor appropriate laboratory values and document effectiveness of treatment related to the specific type of blood product.

Reactions to the Transfusion

- If a transfusion reaction occurs, stop the transfusion, change the IV tubing down to the IV site, keep the IV line open with normal saline, the HCP is notified immediately; the blood bank is notified and the blood bag and tubing is returned the blood bank. (Refer to Priority Nursing Actions.)
- Do not leave the client alone, and monitor the client for any life-threatening symptoms.
- Obtain appropriate laboratory samples according to agency policies, such as blood and urine samples (free hemoglobin indicates that red blood cells were hemolyzed).

f. Pallor and cyanosis
g. Apprehension
h. Tingling and numbness
i. Headache
j. Nausea, vomiting, abdominal cramping, and diarrhea

2. Delayed transfusion reaction
   a. Reactions can occur days to years after a transfusion
   b. Signs include fever, mild jaundice, and a decreased hematocrit level.
3. Refer to Priority Nursing Actions for caring for a client experiencing a transfusion reaction.

CRITICAL THINKING What Should You Do?

Answer: Signs of an immediate transfusion reaction include the following: chills and diaphoresis; muscle aches, back pain, or chest pain; rash, hives, itching, and swelling; rapid, thready pulse; dyspnea, cough, or wheezing; pallor and cyanosis; apprehension; tingling and numbness; headache; and nausea, vomiting, abdominal cramping, and diarrhea. In the event that a transfusion reaction is suspected, the nurse immediately calls for the registered nurse and stops the infusion. The nurse should then assist to change the intravenous (IV) tubing down to the IV site and keep the IV line open with normal saline. The health care provider is notified, as is the blood bank, and the blood bag and the tubing are returned to the blood bank. The nurse should also collect a urine specimen. The nurse should assist to implement prescriptions and always stays with the client and monitors the client closely until the client is stabilized.

Reference(s): deWit, D. & Kumagai, C. (2013). *Medical-surgical nursing: Concepts & practice.* (2nd ed., pp. 364–365). St. Louis: Saunders.

PRIORITY NURSING ACTIONS!

Steps to Take in the Care of a Client Experiencing a Transfusion Reaction

1. Stop the transfusion.
2. Assist to change the intravenous (IV) tubing down to the IV site and keep the IV line open with normal saline.
3. Notify the health care provider and blood bank.
4. Stay with the client, observing signs and symptoms and monitoring vital signs as often as every 5 minutes.
5. Assist to administer emergency medications as prescribed.
6. Obtain a urine specimen for laboratory studies (and perform any other laboratory studies as prescribed).
7. Return blood bag, tubing, attached labels, and transfusion record to the blood bank.
8. Document the occurrence, actions taken, and the client's response.

If the client exhibits signs of a transfusion reaction, the nurse immediately stops the transfusion and changes the IV tubing down to the IV site to prevent the entrance of additional blood solution into the client. Normal saline solution is hung and infused to keep the IV line open in the event that emergency medications need to be administered. The registered nurse and health care provider are notified. The nurse also notifies the blood bank of the occurrence. The nurse stays with the client and monitors the client closely while other personnel obtain needed supplies to treat the client. As prescribed by the health care provider, the nurse assists to administer emergency medications. The nurse then obtains a urine specimen for laboratory studies and performs any other laboratory studies as prescribed to check for free hemoglobin indicating that red blood cells were hemolyzed. The blood bag, tubing, attached labels, and transfusion record are returned to the blood bank so that the blood bank can check the items to determine the reason that the reaction occurred. Finally the nurse documents the occurrence, the actions taken, and the client's response.

Reference(s): Potter, P., Perry, A. G., Stockert, P. A., & Hall, A. M. (2013). *Fundamentals of nursing.* (8th ed., p. 912). St. Louis: Mosby.

PRACTICE QUESTIONS

81. The nurse is assisting with caring for a client who will receive a unit of blood. Just before the infusion, it is **most important** for the nurse to check which item?
1. Vital signs
2. Skin color
3. Oxygen saturation
4. Latest hematocrit level

82. A client who is receiving a blood transfusion rings the call bell for the nurse. When entering the room, the nurse notes that the client is flushed, dyspneic, and complaining of generalized itching. How should the nurse correctly interpret these findings?
1. Bacteremia
2. Fluid overload
3. Hypovolemic shock
4. Transfusion reaction

83. A client who was receiving a blood transfusion has experienced a transfusion reaction. The nurse sends the blood bag that was used for the client to which area?
1. The pharmacy
2. The laboratory
3. The blood bank
4. The risk-management department

84. The nurse takes a client's temperature before giving a blood transfusion. The temperature is 100°F orally. The nurse reports the finding to the registered nurse (RN) and anticipates that which action will take place?
1. The transfusion will begin as prescribed.
2. The blood will be held, and the health care provider will be notified.
3. The transfusion will begin after the administration of an antihistamine.
4. The transfusion will begin after the administration of 650 mg of acetaminophen (Tylenol).

❖ **85.** Which of these clients are **most likely** to develop fluid (circulatory) overload? **Select all that apply.**
- ☐ 1. A premature infant
- ☐ 2. A 101-year-old man
- ☐ 3. A client on renal dialysis
- ☐ 4. A client with heart failure
- ☐ 5. A client with diabetes mellitus
- ☐ 6. A 29-year-old client with pneumonia

86. A client has a prescription to receive 1000 mL of 5% dextrose in 0.45% sodium chloride. After gathering the appropriate equipment, the nurse takes which action **first** before spiking the IV bag with the tubing?
1. Uncaps the distal end of the tubing
2. Uncaps the spike portion of the tubing
3. Opens the roller clamp on the IV tubing
4. Closes the roller clamp on the IV tubing

87. The nurse is doing a routine assessment of a client's peripheral intravenous (IV) site. The nurse notes that the site is cool, pale, and swollen and that the IV has stopped running. The nurse determines that which has probably occurred?
1. Phlebitis
2. Infection
3. Infiltration
4. Thrombosis

88. The nurse is assigned to care for a client with a peripheral intravenous (IV) infusion. The nurse is providing hygiene care to the client and should avoid which while changing the client's hospital gown?
1. Using a hospital gown with snaps at the sleeves
2. Disconnecting the IV tubing from the catheter in the vein
3. Checking the IV flow rate immediately after changing the hospital gown
4. Putting the bag and tubing through the sleeve, followed by the client's arm

89. The nurse is making a worksheet and listing the tasks that need to be performed for assigned adult clients during the shift. The nurse writes on the plan to check the intravenous (IV) of an assigned client who is receiving fluid replacement therapy how frequently?
1. Every hour
2. Every 2 hours
3. Every 3 hours
4. Every 4 hours

90. The nurse is checking the insertion site of a peripheral intravenous (IV) catheter. The nurse notes the site to be reddened, warm, painful, and slightly edematous in the area of the vein proximal to the IV catheter. The nurse interprets that this is likely the result of which?
1. Phlebitis of the vein
2. Infiltration of the IV line
3. Hypersensitivity to the IV solution
4. An allergic reaction to the IV catheter material

91. The nurse has been instructed to remove an intravenous (IV) line. The nurse removes the catheter by withdrawing the catheter while applying pressure to the site with which item?
1. Band-Aid
2. Alcohol swab
3. Betadine swab
4. Sterile 2×2 gauze

92. The nurse is preparing an intravenous (IV) solution and tubing for a client who requires IV fluids. While preparing to prime the tubing, the tubing drops and hits the top of the medication cart. The nurse should plan to take which action?

1. Change the IV tubing.
2. Wipe the tubing with Betadine.
3. Scrub the tubing with an alcohol swab.
4. Scrub the tubing before attaching it to the IV bag.

93. A client is going to be transfused with a unit of packed red blood cells (PRBCs). The nurse understands that it is necessary to remain with the client for what time period after the transfusion is started?

1. 5 minutes
2. 15 minutes
3. 30 minutes
4. 45 minutes

94. The nurse is assisting with caring for a client who is receiving a unit of packed red blood cells (PRBCs). The nurse should tell the client that it is **most important** to report which sign(s) **immediately**?

1. Sore throat or earache
2. Chills, itching, or rash
3. Unusual sleepiness or fatigue
4. Mild discomfort at the catheter site

95. The nurse is assisting with caring for a client who has received a transfusion of platelets. The nurse determines that the client is benefiting **most** from this therapy if the client exhibits which finding?

1. An increased hematocrit level
2. An increased hemoglobin level
3. A decline of the temperature to normal
4. A decrease in oozing from puncture sites and gums

ANSWERS

81. 1

Rationale: A change in the vital signs may indicate that a transfusion reaction is occurring. The nurse assesses the client's vital signs before the procedure to obtain a baseline every 15 minutes for the first half hour after beginning the transfusion and every half hour thereafter. Skin color, oxygen saturation, and most recent hematocrit may be checked but are not the most important.

Test-Taking Strategy: Note the strategic words, *most important.* This tells you that more than one option may be partially or totally correct. Recalling the signs of a blood transfusion reaction will direct you to vital signs. In addition, vital signs are the umbrella option. **Review: blood administration** procedure.

Level of Cognitive Ability: Applying

Client Needs: Physiological Integrity

Integrated Process: Nursing Process/Data Collection

Content Area: Critical Care: Blood Administration

Priority Concepts: Clinical Judgment, Safety

Reference(s): Linton (2012), p. 614.

82. 4

Rationale: The signs and symptoms exhibited by the client are consistent with a transfusion reaction. With bacteremia, the client would have a fever, which is not part of the clinical picture presented. With fluid (circulatory) overload, the client would have crackles in addition to dyspnea. There is no correlation between the signs mentioned in the question and hypovolemic shock. The signs identified in the question are indicative of an allergic reaction, which is one type of blood transfusion reaction.

Test-Taking Strategy: Focus on the subject, interpretation of the client findings. Focus on this data. Recalling signs and symptoms of transfusion reaction will direct you to the correct option. **Review: transfusion reaction.**

Level of Cognitive Ability: Analyzing

Client Needs: Physiological Integrity

Integrated Process: Nursing Process/Data Collection

Content Area: Critical Care: Blood Administration

Priority Concepts: Clinical Judgment, Perfusion

Reference(s): deWit, Kumagai (2013), pp. 364–365; Perry, Potter, Elkin (2012), p. 687.

83. 3

Rationale: The nurse prepares to return the blood transfusion bag containing any remaining blood to the blood bank. This allows the blood bank to complete any follow-up testing procedures that are needed after a transfusion reaction has been documented. The remaining options are incorrect.

Test-Taking Strategy: Focus on the subject, actions to take if a blood transfusion reaction occurs. Recalling that blood is obtained from the blood bank will help you to eliminate each of the incorrect options. **Review:** procedures to follow for **blood transfusion reaction.**

Level of Cognitive Ability: Applying

Client Needs: Physiological Integrity

Integrated Process: Nursing Process/Implementation

Content Area: Critical Care: Blood Administration

Priority Concepts: Clinical Judgment, Health Policy

Reference(s): Linton (2012), p. 614.

84. 2

Rationale: If the client has a temperature of 100°F or more, the unit of blood should be held until the health care provider is notified and has the opportunity to give further prescriptions. The other options are incorrect actions.

Test-Taking Strategy: Eliminate the options that are comparable or alike in that they all involve initiation of the transfusion. Remember that if the temperature is elevated, the health care provider needs to be notified before a blood transfusion is initiated. **Review: administration of a blood transfusion.**

Level of Cognitive Ability: Applying
Client Needs: Physiological Integrity
Integrated Process: Nursing Process/Implementation
Content Area: Critical Care: Blood Administration
Priority Concepts: Clinical Judgment, Safety
Reference(s): Lewis, Dirksen, Heitkemper, Bucher (2014), p. 677.

❖85. 1, 2, 3, 4
Rationale: Clients with cardiac, respiratory, renal, or liver diseases and older and very young clients cannot tolerate an excessive fluid volume. The risk of fluid (circulatory) overload exists with these clients.
Test-Taking Strategy: Note the strategic words, *most likely.* Focus on the subject, those at risk for fluid (circulatory) overload. Thinking about the physiology associated with each client described in the options will assist you with answering correctly. **Review:** risk factors for **fluid overload.**
Level of Cognitive Ability: Analyzing
Client Needs: Physiological Integrity
Integrated Process: Nursing Process/Data Collection
Content Area: Fundamental Skills: Fluids & Electrolytes
Priority Concepts: Fluid and Electrolyte Balance, Perfusion
Reference(s): Lewis, Dirksen, Heitkemper, Bucher (2014), p. 678; Linton (2012), p. 615.

86. 4
Rationale: The nurse should first clamp the tubing to prevent the solution from running freely through the tubing after it is attached to the IV bag. The nurse should next uncap the proximal (spike) portion of the tubing and attach it to the IV bag. The IV bag is elevated and the roller clamp is then opened slowly, and the fluid is allowed to flow through the tubing in a controlled fashion to prevent air from remaining in parts of the tubing.
Test-Taking Strategy: Note the strategic word, *first.* This question tests a specific procedure related to IV therapy. Visualize this procedure to answer the question correctly. **Review:** preparation of the **intravenous infusion.**
Level of Cognitive Ability: Applying
Client Needs: Physiological Integrity
Integrated Process: Nursing Process/Implementation
Content Area: Fundamental Skills: Safety
Priority Concepts: Clinical Judgment, Safety
Reference(s): deWit, Kumagai (2013), p. 53.

87. 3
Rationale: An infiltrated IV is one that has dislodged from the vein and is lying in subcutaneous tissue. The pallor, coolness, and swelling are the result of IV fluid being deposited into the subcutaneous tissue. When the pressure in the tissues exceeds the pressure in the tubing, the flow of the IV solution will stop. The other three options identify complications that are likely to be accompanied by warmth at the site rather than coolness.
Test-Taking Strategy: Focus on the data in the question, and note the word *cool.* Recalling that coolness occurs at the site of IV infiltration will direct you to the correct option. Also note that options 1, 2, and 4 are comparable or alike and are accompanied by warmth at the IV site. **Review:** signs/symptoms of **infiltration.**
Level of Cognitive Ability: Analyzing
Client Needs: Physiological Integrity
Integrated Process: Nursing Process/Data Collection
Content Area: Critical Care: Medications and Intravenous Therapy
Priority Concepts: Clinical Judgment, Tissue Integrity
Reference(s): deWit, Kumagai (2013), p. 54.

88. 2
Rationale: The tubing should not be removed from the IV catheter. With each break in the system, there is an increased chance of introducing bacteria into the system, which can lead to infection. Using gowns with snaps and inserting the IV bag and tubing through the sleeve of the gown first are appropriate. The flow rate should be checked immediately after changing the hospital gown, because the position of the roller clamp may have been affected during the change.
Test-Taking Strategy: Focus on the subject, the action to avoid. This word asks you to select an incorrect action. Visualize this procedure, and use your knowledge of the basic principles related to IV therapy and asepsis to direct you to the correct option. **Review:** hygiene when receiving **intravenous therapy.**
Level of Cognitive Ability: Applying
Client Needs: Safe and Effective Care Environment
Integrated Process: Nursing Process/Implementation
Content Area: Fundamental Skills: Safety
Priority Concepts: Infection, Safety
Reference(s): deWit, Kumagai (2013), p. 53.

89. 1
Rationale: Safe nursing practice includes monitoring an IV infusion at least once per hour for an adult client. The remaining options do not provide time frames that are safe or acceptable.
Test-Taking Strategy: Focus on the subject, frequency of observation of the IV infusion. To answer this question accurately, it is necessary to be familiar with the specific time frames indicated for this nursing procedure. For questions similar to this one, it is best to select the most frequently occurring time frame. **Review:** safety related to **intravenous therapy.**
Level of Cognitive Ability: Applying
Client Needs: Physiological Integrity
Integrated Process: Nursing Process/Implementation
Content Area: Fundamental Skills: Safety
Priority Concepts: Clinical Judgment, Safety
Reference(s): deWit, Kumagai (2013), p. 54.

90. 1
Rationale: Phlebitis at an IV site results in discomfort at the site and redness, warmth, and swelling proximal to the IV catheter. The IV catheter should be removed, and a new IV line should be inserted at a different site. The remaining options are incorrect; the signs and symptoms in the question are not associated with these conditions.
Test-Taking Strategy: Remember that comparable or alike options are not likely to be correct. In this case, hypersensitivity to the IV solution and an allergic reaction to the IV catheter material are comparable or alike and are therefore eliminated. Recalling that warmth occurs at the site of phlebitis directs you to the correct option. **Review:** signs/symptoms of **phlebitis.**
Level of Cognitive Ability: Analyzing
Client Needs: Physiological Integrity
Integrated Process: Nursing Process/Data Collection

Content Area: Critical Care: Medications and Intravenous Therapy
Priority Concepts: Clotting, Tissue Integrity
Reference(s): deWit, Kumagai (2013), p. 54.

91. 4
Rationale: A dry, sterile dressing such as sterile 2×2 gauze is used to apply pressure to the site while the catheter is discontinued and removed. This material is absorbent, sterile, and nonirritating to the site. A Band-Aid may be used to cover the site after hemostasis has occurred. An alcohol swab or Betadine would irritate the opened puncture site and would not stop the blood flow.
Test-Taking Strategy: Focus on the subject, the procedure for removing an IV. Visualize this procedure, and think about each of the items identified in the options to answer the question. Noting the word *sterile* will assist with directing you to the correct option. **Review:** **discontinuation of a intravenous line.**
Level of Cognitive Ability: Applying
Client Needs: Safe and Effective Care Environment
Integrated Process: Nursing Process/Implementation
Content Area: Critical Care: Medications and Intravenous Therapy
Priority Concepts: Infection, Tissue Integrity
Reference(s): Perry, Potter, Elkin (2012), p. 678.

92. 1
Rationale: The nurse should change the IV tubing. The tubing has become contaminated, and, if used, it could result in a systemic infection in the client. Wiping or scrubbing the tubing is insufficient to prevent systemic infection.
Test-Taking Strategy: Use your knowledge of basic infection control measures and IV therapy concepts to answer this question. Note that three of the options are comparable or alike in that they involve wiping the end of the tubing. **Review:** aseptic technique and **intravenous therapy.**
Level of Cognitive Ability: Applying
Client Needs: Safe and Effective Care Environment
Integrated Process: Nursing Process/Implementation
Content Area: Fundamental Skills: Infection Control
Priority Concepts: Clinical Judgment, Infection
Reference(s): deWit, Kumagai (2013), p. 56.

93. 2
Rationale: The nurse must remain with the client for the first 15 minutes of a transfusion, which is the most likely time that a transfusion reaction will occur. This enables the nurse to detect a reaction and intervene quickly. The nurse engages in safe nursing practice by obtaining coverage for the other clients during this time. Five minutes is too short of a time period, while 30 and 45 minutes are lengthy time periods.
Test-Taking Strategy: Focus on the subject, length of time to remain with the client after initiation of a transfusion. Use knowledge regarding blood transfusion procedures to answer this question. Remember, the client must be directly monitored for the first 15 minutes of the transfusion. **Review:** monitoring during **blood transfusion.**
Level of Cognitive Ability: Applying
Client Needs: Physiological Integrity
Integrated Process: Nursing Process/Implementation
Content Area: Critical Care: Blood Administration
Priority Concepts: Clinical Judgment, Safety
Reference(s): Lewis, Dirksen, Heitkemper, Bucher (2014), p. 677.

94. 2
Rationale: The client is told to report chills, itching, or rash immediately, because these could be signs of a possible transfusion reaction. Mild discomfort at the catheter site may be indicative of a problem, or it could result from the size of the IV catheter required to infuse the blood product. Sore throat, earache, sleepiness, and fatigue are unrelated to a transfusion reaction.
Test-Taking Strategy: Note the strategic words, *most important* and *immediately.* These tell you that more than one or all of the options may be partially or totally correct. With the knowledge that a transfusion reaction is of greatest concern to the nurse, prioritize and select the option that characterizes this problem. **Review:** signs/symptoms of **transfusion reaction.**
Level of Cognitive Ability: Applying
Client Needs: Physiological Integrity
Integrated Process: Nursing Process/Implementation
Content Area: Critical Care: Blood Administration
Priority Concepts: Clinical Judgment, Safety
Reference(s): deWit, Kumagai (2013), pp. 364–365; Linton (2012), p. 614.

95. 4
Rationale: Platelets are necessary for proper blood clotting. The client with insufficient platelets may exhibit frank bleeding or the oozing of blood from puncture sites, wounds, and mucous membranes. The client's temperature would decline to normal after the infusion of granulocytes if those transfused cells were then instrumental in fighting infection in the body. Increased hemoglobin and hematocrit levels would be seen when the client has received a transfusion of red blood cells.
Test-Taking Strategy: Focus on the subject, expected outcome, and note the strategic word, *most.* Recalling that bleeding is a concern when the platelets are low will direct you to the correct option. **Review:** function of **platelets.**
Level of Cognitive Ability: Evaluating
Client Needs: Physiological Integrity
Integrated Process: Nursing Process/Evaluation
Content Area: Critical Care: Blood Administration
Priority Concepts: Clotting, Evidence
Reference(s): Lewis, Dirksen, Heitkemper, Bucher (2014), p. 676; Linton (2012), p. 614.

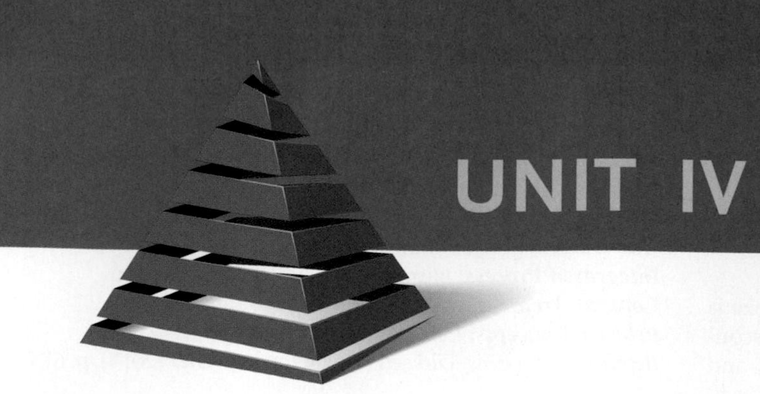

UNIT IV

Fundamental Skills

PYRAMID TERMS

abdominal thrust maneuver Method to relieve a foreign body airway obstruction.

automated external defibrillator (AED) Machine that converts ventricular fibrillation into a perfusing rhythm and allows for early defibrillation by first responders.

basic life support (BLS) Provision of oxygen to the brain, heart, and other vital organs until help arrives.

body mechanics The coordinated efforts of the musculoskeletal and nervous systems to maintain balance, posture, and body alignment during lifting, bending, and moving to perform activities safely.

cardiopulmonary resuscitation (CPR) An interchangeable term for basic life support.

chest tube Tube that returns negative pressure to the intrapleural space; used to remove abnormal accumulations of air and fluid from the pleural space.

conversion The first step in the calculation of a medication problem.

endotracheal tube Tube used to maintain a patent airway; indicated when a client needs mechanical ventilation.

ergonomic principles The anatomical, physiological, psychological, and mechanical principles affecting the efficient and safe use of an individual's energy.

extended postoperative stage The period of at least 1 to 4 days after surgery.

Fowler's position The client is supine, and the head of the bed is elevated to 45 to 60 degrees.

generic name Also known as the nonproprietary name of a medication, or the U.S. adopted name; each medication has only one generic name.

health care–associated (nosocomial) infections Infections acquired in the hospital or other health care facility that were not present or incubating at the time of the client's admission; also referred to as "hospital-acquired" infections.

high Fowler's position The client is supine, and the head of the bed is elevated to 90 degrees.

immediate postoperative stage The period of 1 to 4 hours after surgery.

intermediate postoperative stage The period of 4 to 24 hours after surgery.

lateral (side-lying) position The client is lying on the side, and the head and shoulders are aligned with the hips and the spine and are parallel to the edge of the mattress. The head, neck, and upper arm are supported by a pillow. The lower shoulder is pulled forward slightly and, along with the elbow, flexed at 90 degrees. The legs are flexed or extended. A pillow is placed to support the back.

lithotomy position The client is lying on the back with the hips and knees flexed at right angles and the feet in stirrups.

medication reconciliation An organized process to avoid medication errors by comparing the client's medication prescriptions with all the medications that the client was previously taking.

parenteral Given by injection, such as by the intravenous, intramuscular, subcutaneous, or intradermal route.

perioperative care Nursing care given before (preoperative), during (intraoperative), and after surgery (postoperative).

physical hazard Any situation or event that places the client at risk for accident, injury, or death.

poison Any substance that impairs health or destroys life when ingested, inhaled, or otherwise absorbed by the body.

prone position The client is lying on the abdomen with the head turned to the side.

restraints (safety devices) Physical devices (that the client is unable to remove) applied to restrict a client's movement are known as physical restraints. Medications given to inhibit a specific behavior or movement are known as chemical restraints.

reverse Trendelenburg's position The bed is tilted so that the client's foot of the bed is down.

semi-Fowler's position (low Fowler's) The client is supine, and the head of the bed is elevated about 30 degrees.

Sims' position The client is lying on the side with the body turned prone at 45 degrees. The lower leg is extended, with the upper leg flexed at the hip and knee to a 45- to 90-degree angle.

standard precautions Guidelines used by all health care providers with all clients to reduce the risk of infection for both clients and caregivers.

supine position The client is lying on the back. The head and shoulders usually are elevated slightly (depending on the client's condition) with a small pillow. The arms and legs are extended, and the legs are slightly abducted.

tracheostomy An opening made surgically directly into the trachea to establish an airway. A tracheostomy tube is inserted into the opening and the tube attaches to the mechanical ventilator or another type of oxygen delivery device.

trade name Also known as the proprietary or brand name of a medication. The trade name is the name under which a medication is marketed. A medication can have many trade names; therefore, trade names must be approved by the U.S. Food and Drug Administration (FDA) to ensure that no two trade names are alike.

transmission-based precautions Guidelines that are used in addition to standard precautions; used for specific syndromes that are highly suggestive of infection until a diagnosis is confirmed.

Trendelenburg's position The bed is tilted so the head of the bed is lower. This position is contraindicated in clients with head injuries, increased intracranial pressure, spinal cord injuries, and certain respiratory and cardiac disorders.

unit A measurement of a medication in terms of its action, not its physical weight.

warfare agent Substance that may be biological, chemical, or radioactive in nature that can cause mass destruction and fatality.

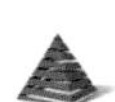

Pyramid to Success

On the NCLEX-PN®, safety and infection control concepts, including standard precautions and transmission-based precautions and the measures required to handle hazardous or infectious materials, are a priority focus. The pyramid points also focus on maintaining environmental safety, preventing accidents, the medication reconciliation process, using restraints, and the emergency response plan in the event of a disaster.

Medication or intravenous (IV) flow rate questions are also a focus on the NCLEX-PN examination. Fill-in-the-blank questions may require that you calculate a medication dose or an intravenous (IV) flow rate. Use the on-screen calculator for these medication and IV problems and then recheck the calculation before selecting an option or typing the answer.

The Pyramid to Success also focuses on emergency care guidelines and procedures performed by the health care provider (HCP), such as cardiopulmonary resuscitation (CPR), the abdominal thrust maneuver, and use of the automated external defibrillator (AED). Perioperative nursing care and monitoring for postoperative complications are priorities. Client safety, related to positioning and ambulation, and care to the client with a tube such as a gastrointestinal tube or chest tube, is an important concept addressed on the NCLEX. Because many surgical procedures are performed through ambulatory care units (1-day-stay units), Pyramid Points also focus on preparing the client for discharge, teaching related to the prescribed treatments and medications, follow-up care, and the mobilization of home care support services.

Client Needs

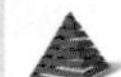

Safe and Effective Care Environment

Acting as an advocate regarding the client's wishes
Collaborating with health care members in other disciplines
Ensuring environmental, personal, and home safety
Ensuring that client's rights are upheld, including informed consent
Ensuring that the client is informed of the surgical process and that informed consent was obtained
Establishing priorities for client care
Following advance directives regarding the client's documented requests
Following guidelines regarding the use of safety devices
Handling hazardous and infectious materials safely
Knowing the emergency response plan and actions to take for exposure to biological and chemical warfare agents
Maintaining confidentiality
Maintaining continuity of care and suggesting referrals to home care and other support services
Maintaining precautions to prevent errors, accidents, and injury
Positioning the client appropriately and safely
Preparing and administering medications, using rights of medication administration
Preventing a surgical infection
Protecting the medicated client from injury
Using equipment safely
Using ergonomic principles and body mechanics when moving a client
Using standard and transmission-based precautions and surgical asepsis procedures

Health Promotion and Maintenance

Assisting clients and families to identify environmental hazards in the home
Assisting to perform home safety assessments
Assisting the registered nurse (RN) with health and wellness teaching to prevent complications
Performing the techniques of data collection specific to the client's condition
Reinforcing teaching to clients and families about accident prevention
Reinforcing teaching to clients and families about measures to be implemented in an emergency or disaster
Reinforcing teaching to clients and families about preventing the spread of infection and preventing diseases
Reinforcing teaching to the client about prescribed medication(s) or therapy
Reinforcing teaching to significant others to perform Lay Rescuer CPR and the abdominal thrust maneuver
Respecting lifestyle choices

Psychosocial Integrity

Caring for the client with sensory and perception alterations
Discussing expected body image changes and situational role changes
Facilitating client and family coping
Identifying support systems
Identifying the cultural, religious, and spiritual factors influencing health
Keeping the family informed of client progress
Promoting an environment that will allow the client to express concerns
Providing emotional support to significant others
Providing end-of-life care

Physiological Integrity

Administering medications safely
Assisting the client with activities of daily living
Assisting with medical emergencies
Calculating medication doses and intravenous flow rates
Checking the mobility and immobility level of the client
Documenting the client's response to basic life support (BLS) measures
Identifying client allergies/sensitivities
Identifying the adverse effects of and contraindications to medication or IV therapy
Implementing priority nursing actions in an emergency or disaster
Monitoring for alterations in body systems
Monitoring for expected and unexpected effects of pharmacological therapy
Monitoring for surgical complications and initiating nursing interventions when surgical complications arise
Monitoring for wound infection
Performing CPR or the abdominal thrust maneuver
Preparing for diagnostic tests to confirm accurate placement of a tube
Preventing the complications of immobility
Providing care to clients with infectious diseases
Providing comfort and assistance to the client
Providing nutrition and oral intake
Providing personal hygiene as needed
Recognizing changes in the client's condition that indicate a potential complication and reporting these changes immediately to the RN
Using assistive devices to prevent injury

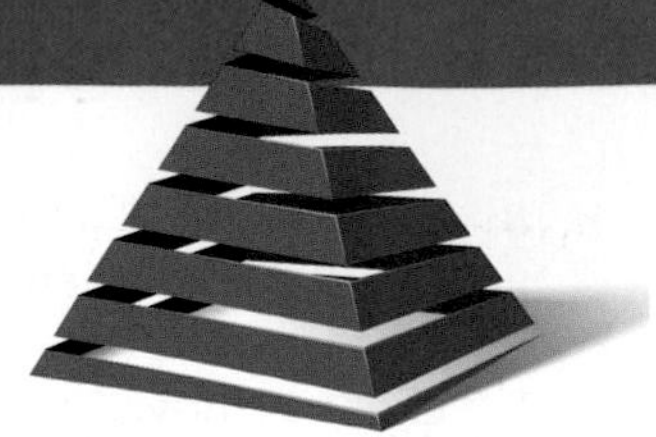

CHAPTER 14

Hygiene and Safety

CRITICAL THINKING What Should You Do?

The nurse is working in a long-term care facility that has a "no restraint policy." An assigned client is disoriented and unsteady and continually attempts to climb out of bed. What should the nurse do with regard to instituting safety precautions for this client?

Answer located on p. 150.

I. Hygiene

A. Description
1. The activity of providing care or promoting self-care, which includes bathing and grooming.
2. Includes care of the skin, hair, nails, mouth, teeth, eyes, ears, nasal cavities, and perineal and genital areas.
3. Personal hygiene is the activity of self-care, including bathing and grooming.

B. General principles
1. Ensure privacy.
2. Wash hands and wear gloves.
3. Explain procedures to the client.
4. Determine and treat pain.
5. Determine the client's health status and readiness for hygiene procedures.
6. Determine the client's routine hygiene practices.
7. Use proper body mechanics during bathing and hygiene activities.
8. Use time spent with client as an opportunity to determine the client's mental health status and implement communication and teaching.
9. Maintain and encourage independence as much as possible.

II. Environmental Safety

A. Fire safety (See Priority Nursing Actions)
1. Keep open spaces free of clutter.
2. Clearly mark fire exits.
3. Know the locations of all fire alarms, exits, and extinguishers (Table 14-1).
4. Know the telephone number for reporting fires.
5. Know the agency's fire drill and evacuation plan.
6. Never use the elevator in the event of a fire.
7. Turn off oxygen and appliances in the vicinity of the fire.

PRIORITY NURSING ACTIONS!

Actions to Take in the Event of a Fire

1. Rescue clients and remove those in immediate danger.
2. Activate the fire alarm.
3. Confine the fire.
4. Extinguish the fire: obtain the fire extinguisher.
5. Pull the pin on the fire extinguisher.
6. Aim at the base of the fire.
7. Squeeze the extinguisher handle.
8. Sweep extinguisher from side to side to coat the area of the fire evenly.

Remember the mnemonic *RACE* to prioritize in the event of a fire. *R* is rescue clients in immediate danger, *A* is alarm (sound the alarm), *C* is confine the fire by closing all doors, and *E* is extinguish or evacuate. To properly use the fire extinguisher, remember the mnemonic *PASS* to prioritize in the use of a fire extinguisher. *P* is pull the pin, *A* is aim at the base of the fire, *S* is squeeze the handle, and *S* is sweep from side to side to coat the area evenly.

Reference(s): Potter, P., Perry, A. G., Stockert, P. A., & Hall, A. M. (2013). *Fundamentals of nursing.* (8th ed., pp. 386–387). St. Louis: Mosby.

TABLE 14-1 Types of Fire Extinguishers

Type	Class of Fires
A	Wood, cloth, upholstery, paper, rubbish, and plastic
B	Flammable liquids or gases, grease, tar, and oil-based paint
C	Electrical equipment

Note: Certain extinguishers may be appropriate for more than one type of fire.

Fundamentals

8. In the event of a fire, if a client is on life support, maintain the client's respiratory status manually with an Ambu bag (resuscitation bag) until the client is moved away from the threat of the fire and placed back on life support.
9. In the event of a fire, ambulatory clients can be directed to walk by themselves to a safe area. In some cases, they may be able to assist with moving clients who are in wheelchairs.
10. Bedridden clients are generally moved from the scene of a fire by stretcher, bed, or wheelchair.
11. If a client must be carried from the area of a fire, appropriate transfer techniques should be used; **ergonomic principles** and good body mechanics should be instituted to prevent injury.
12. If fire department personnel are at the scene of the fire, they can help evacuate clients.

Remember the mnemonic RACE to set priorities in the event of a fire and the mnemonic PASS to use a fire extinguisher.

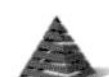

B. Electrical safety
   1. Electrical equipment must be maintained in good working order and should be grounded; otherwise, it is a **physical hazard**.
   2. Use a three-pronged electrical cord.
   3. In a three-pronged electrical cord, the third, longer prong of the cord is the ground. The other two prongs carry the power to the piece of electrical equipment.
   4. Check electrical cords and outlets for exposed, frayed, or damaged wires.
   5. Avoid overloading any circuit.
   6. Read warning labels on all equipment. Never operate unfamiliar equipment.
   7. Use safety extension cords only when absolutely necessary, and tape them to the floor with electrical tape.
   8. Never run electrical wiring under carpets.
   9. Never pull a plug by using the cord. Always grasp the plug itself.
   10. Never use electrical appliances near sinks, bathtubs, or other water sources.
   11. Always disconnect a plug from the outlet before cleaning equipment or appliances.
   12. If a client receives an electrical shock, turn off the electricity before touching the client.

Any electrical equipment that the client brings into the health care facility must be inspected for safety before use.

C. Radiation safety
   1. Know the health care agency's protocols and guidelines.
   2. Label potentially radioactive material.
   3. To reduce exposure to radiation:
      a. The time spent near the source should be limited (30 minutes per care provider per shift).
      b. The distance from the source should be as great as possible.
      c. A shielding device such as a lead apron should be used.
      d. A pregnant person and children younger than 16 years should not enter the room
      e. Limit visits from visitors to 30 minutes. Visitors should be at least 6 feet from the client.
   4. Monitor radiation exposure with a film (dosimeter) badge.
   5. Place the client who has a radiation implant in a private room.
   6. Keep all linens and dressings in the client's room until the implant is removed.
   7. Never touch dislodged implants.

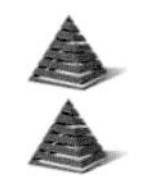

D. Disposal of infectious wastes
   1. Handle all infectious materials as a hazard.
   2. Dispose of waste in designated areas only, and use proper containers for disposal.
   3. Ensure that infectious material is properly labeled.
   4. Dispose of all sharps immediately after use in closed, puncture-resistant disposal containers that are leakproof and labeled or color coded.

Needles (sharps) should not be recapped, bent, or broken because of the risk of accidental injury (needle-stick).

E. Physiological changes in the older client that increase the risk of accidents (Box 14-1)
F. Falls (Box 14-2 lists measures to prevent falls)
G. Measures to promote safety in ambulation for the client
   1. Gait belt may be used to keep the center of gravity midline.
      a. Place the belt on the client prior to ambulation.
      b. Encircle the client's waist with the belt.
      c. Hold onto the side or back of the belt so that the client does not lean to one side.
      d. Return the client to bed or a nearby chair if the client develops dizziness or becomes unsteady.

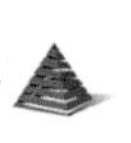

H. Steps to prevent injury to the health care worker (Box 14-3)
I. National Patient Safety Goals (Box 14-4)
J. **Restraints (safety devices)**
   1. Protective devices used to limit the physical activity of a client or immobilize a client or an extremity; state and agency policy must be followed with regard to their use
   2. Physical restraints: Restrict client movement through the application of a device.

BOX 14-1 Physiological Changes in the Older Client That Increase the Risk of Accidents

Musculoskeletal Changes

- Strength and function of muscles decrease.
- Joints become less mobile and bones become brittle.
- Postural changes and limited range of motion occur.

Nervous System Changes

- Voluntary and autonomic reflexes become slower.
- Decreased ability to respond to multiple stimuli occurs.
- Decreased sensitivity to touch occurs.

Sensory Changes

- Decreased vision and lens accommodation and cataracts develop.
- Delayed transmission of hot and cold impulses occurs.
- Impaired hearing develops, with high-frequency tones less perceptible.

Genitourinary Changes

- Increased nocturia and occurrences of incontinence may occur.

Adapted from Potter A, Perry P, Stockert P, Hall A: *Fundamentals of nursing*, ed 8, St. Louis, 2013, Mosby; and Touhy T, Jett K: *Ebersole and Hess' Toward healthy aging*, ed 8, St. Louis, 2012, Mosby.

BOX 14-2 Measures to Prevent Falls

- Determine the client's risk for falling.
- Ensure that the client at risk for falling is in a room near the nurses' station.
- Be alert to clients who are at risk for falling.
- Check to see if there is a notation on the door to the room indicating a fall risk.
- Orient the client to his or her physical surroundings.
- Instruct the client to seek assistance when getting up.
- Explain the use of the call-bell system.
- Keep the bed in the low position; the use of siderails is based on state and agency policies and procedures and must be followed
- Lock all beds, wheelchairs, and stretchers.
- Keep personal items within reach.
- Eliminate clutter and obstacles in the client's room.
- Provide adequate lighting, including subdued lighting at night.
- Reduce bathroom hazards.
- Maintain the client's toileting schedule throughout the day.

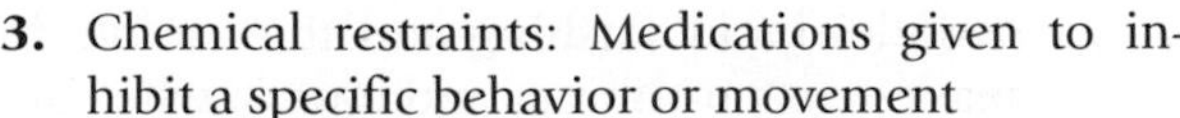

3. **Chemical restraints:** Medications given to inhibit a specific behavior or movement

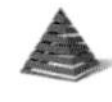

4. Interventions
   a. Use alternative devices whenever possible, such as pressure-sensitive beds or chair pads with alarms or other types of bed or chair alarms.
   b. If safety devices are necessary, the health care provider's (HCP's) prescriptions should state the type of restraint, identify specific client behaviors for which restraints are to be used, and identify a limited time frame for use.
   c. HCP's prescriptions for safety devices should be renewed within a specific time frame according to the policy of the agency.
   d. Safety devices are not to be prescribed PRN—that is, as needed.
   e. The reason for the safety device should be given to the client and the family, and their permission should be sought.
   f. Safety devices should not interfere with any treatments or affect the client's health problem.
   g. Use a half-bow or safety knot (quick release tie) to secure the device to the bed frame or chair, not to the side rails.
   h. Ensure that enough slack is on the straps to allow some movement of the body part.
   i. Assess skin integrity and neurovascular and circulatory status every 30 minutes and remove the safety device at least every 2 hours to permit muscle exercise and to promote circulation (follow agency policies).
   j. Continually assess and document the need for safety devices (Box 14-5).

BOX 14-3 Steps to Prevent Injury to the Health Care Worker

- Keep the weight to be lifted as close to the body as possible.
- Bend at the knees.
- Tighten abdominal muscles and tuck the pelvis.
- Maintain the trunk erect and knees bent so that multiple muscle groups work together in a coordinated manner.

Adapted from Potter A, Perry P, Stockert P, Hall A: *Fundamentals of nursing*, ed 8, St. Louis, 2013, Mosby.

BOX 14-4 National Patient Safety Goals

- Identify patient's correctly
- Improve staff communication
- Use medicines safely
- Use alarms safely
- Prevent infection
- Identify patient safety risks
- Prevent mistakes in surgery

From The Joint Commission. http://www.jointcommission.org/assets/1/6/2014_HAP_NPSG_E.pdf

⚠ A health care provider's (HCP's) prescription for use of a safety device is needed. Alternative measures for safety devices should always be used first.

BOX 14-5 Documentation Points with the Use of a Restraint (Safety Device)

- Reason for safety device
- Method of safety device
- Date and time of the application of safety device
- Duration of use of safety device and the client's response
- Release from safety device with periodic exercise and circulatory, neurovascular, and skin assessment
- Determination of the continued need for safety device
- Evaluation of the client's response

6. Alternatives to restraints
   a. Orient the client and family to surroundings.
   b. Explain all procedures and treatments to the client and family.
   c. Encourage family and friends to stay with the client, and use sitters for clients who need supervision.
   d. Assign confused and disoriented clients to rooms near the nurses' station.
   e. Provide appropriate visual and auditory stimuli to the client (e.g., clock, calendar, television, radio).
   f. Place familiar items (e.g., family pictures) near the client's bedside.
   g. Maintain toileting routines.
   h. Eliminate bothersome treatments (e.g., tube feedings) as soon as possible.
   i. Evaluate all medications that the client is receiving.
   j. Use relaxation techniques with the client.
   k. Institute exercise and ambulation schedules as the client's condition allows.

K. Poisons

1. Any substance that impairs health or destroys life when ingested, inhaled, or otherwise absorbed by the body
2. Specific antidotes or treatments are available for only some types of poisons.
3. The capability of body tissue to recover from a poison determines the reversibility of the effect.
4. Poison can impair the respiratory, circulatory, central nervous, hepatic, gastrointestinal, and renal systems of the body.
5. Toddlers, preschoolers, and young school-age children must be protected from accidental poisoning.
6. In older adults, diminished eyesight and impaired memory may result in the accidental ingestion of poisonous substances or an overdose of prescribed medications.

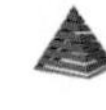

7. A poison control center phone number should be visible on the telephone in homes with small children. In all cases of suspected poisoning, the number should be called immediately.
8. Interventions
   a. Remove any obvious materials from the mouth, eye, or body area immediately.
   b. Identify the type and amount of substance ingested.
   c. Call the poison control center before attempting an intervention.
   d. If the victim vomits or vomiting is induced, save the vomitus if requested to do so, and deliver it to the poison control center.
   e. If instructed by the poison control center to take the poisoned person to the emergency department, call an ambulance.
   f. Vomiting is never induced after the ingestion of lye, household cleaners, grease, or petroleum products.
   g. Vomiting is never induced in an unconscious victim.

The poison control center should be called first before attempting an intervention.

III. Health Care–Associated (Nosocomial) Infections

A. **Health care–associated (nosocomial) infections** also are referred to as hospital-acquired infections.

B. These infections are infections acquired in a hospital or other health care facility that were not present or incubating at the time of a client's admission.

C. *Clostridium difficile* is spread mainly by hand-to-hand contact in a health care setting. Clients taking multiple antibiotics for a prolonged period are most at risk.

D. Common drug-resistant infections: Vancomycin-resistant enterococci, methicillin-resistant *Staphylococcus aureus,* multidrug-resistant tuberculosis

E. Illness impairs the normal defense mechanisms of the body.

F. The hospital environment provides exposure to a variety of virulent organisms that the client has not been exposed to in the past; therefore, the client has not developed resistance to these organisms.

G. Infections can be transmitted by health care personnel who fail to practice proper hand washing procedures or fail to change gloves between client contacts.

IV. Standard Precautions

A. Description

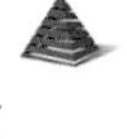

1. Must be practiced with all clients in any setting, regardless of the diagnosis or presumed infectiousness
2. Includes hand washing and the use of gloves, masks, eye protection, and gowns, when appropriate, during client contact
3. These precautions apply to blood, all body fluids, secretions, and excretions (whether or not

they contain blood), nonintact skin, or mucous membranes.

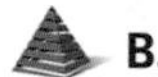

B. Interventions

1. Wash hands between client contacts; after contact with blood, body fluids, secretions or excretions, nonintact skin, or mucous membranes; after contact with equipment or contaminated articles; and immediately after removing gloves.
2. Wear gloves when touching blood, body fluids, secretions, excretions, nonintact skin, mucous membranes, or contaminated items; remove gloves and wash hands between client care contacts.
3. For routine decontamination of hands, alcohol-based hand rubs may be used when hands are not visibly soiled, but the use of alcohol-based hand rubs is controversial. For more information on hand hygiene from the Centers for Disease Control and Prevention, please see www.cdc.gov/nceh/vsp/cruiselines/hand_hygiene_general.htm.
4. Wear masks, eye protection, or face shields if client care activities may generate splashes or sprays of blood or body fluid.
5. Wear gowns if soiling of clothing is likely from blood or body fluid; wash hands after removing a gown.
6. Clean and reprocess client care equipment properly and discard single-use items.
7. Place contaminated linen in leakproof bags and limit handling to prevent skin and mucous membrane exposure.
8. Use needleless devices or special needle safety devices whenever possible to reduce the risk of needle sticks and sharps injuries to health care workers.
9. Discard all sharp instruments and needles in a puncture-resistant container; dispose of needles uncapped or use a mechanical device for recapping the needle, if necessary and available.
10. Clean spills of blood or body fluids with a solution of bleach and water (diluted 1:10) or agency-approved disinfectant.

⚠ Handle all blood and body fluids from all clients as if they were contaminated.

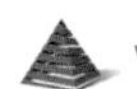

V. Transmission-Based Precautions

A. Transmission-based precautions include airborne, droplet, and contact precautions.

B. Airborne precautions

1. Diseases
   - **a.** Measles
   - **b.** Chickenpox (varicella)
   - **c.** Disseminated varicella zoster
   - **d.** Tuberculosis
2. Barrier protection for airborne precautions
   - **a.** Single room maintained under negative pressure; door kept closed except when someone is entering or exiting the room
   - **b.** Negative airflow pressure in the room, with a minimum of 6 to 12 air exchanges per hour, depending on the health care agency
   - **c.** Use of ultraviolet germicide irradiation or a high-efficiency particulate air filter in the room
   - **d.** Health care workers wear a mask or personal respiratory protection device.
   - **e.** Place a mask on the client when the client needs to leave the room. The client leaves the room only if necessary.

C. Droplet precautions

1. Diseases
   - **a.** Adenovirus
   - **b.** Diphtheria (pharyngeal)
   - **c.** Epiglottitis
   - **d.** Influenza (flu)
   - **e.** Meningitis
   - **f.** Mumps
   - **g.** Mycoplasmal pneumonia or meningococcal pneumonia
   - **h.** Parvovirus B19
   - **i.** Pertussis
   - **j.** Pneumonia
   - **k.** Pneumonic plague
   - **l.** Rubella
   - **m.** Scarlet fever
   - **n.** Sepsis
   - **o.** Streptococcal pharyngitis
2. Barrier protection for droplet precautions
   - **a.** Private room or cohort client (a client whose body culture(s) contain the same organism)
   - **b.** Wear a surgical mask when within 3 feet of a client.
   - **c.** Place a mask on the client when the client needs to leave the room.

D. Contact precautions

1. Diseases
   - **a.** Colonization or infection with a multidrug-resistant organism
   - **b.** Enteric infections such as *Clostridium difficile*
   - **c.** Respiratory infections such as respiratory syncytial virus
   - **d.** Influenza: Infection can occur by touching something with flu viruses on it and then touching the mouth or nose.
   - **e.** Wound infections
   - **f.** Skin infections, such as cutaneous diphtheria, herpes simplex, impetigo, pediculosis, scabies, staphylococci, and varicella zoster
   - **g.** Eye infections, such as conjunctivitis
   - **h.** Indirect contact transmission may occur when contaminated object or instrument, or hands, are encountered.

2. Barrier protection
   a. Private room or cohort client
   b. Use of gloves and a gown when in contact with the client

VI. Emergency Response Plan and Disasters

A. Know the emergency response plan of the agency
B. Internal disasters are those in which the agency is in danger.
C. External disasters occur in the community, and victims will be brought to the health care facility for care.
D. When the health care agency is notified of a disaster, the nurse should follow the guidelines specified in the agency's emergency response plan.
E. See Chapter 8 for additional information about disaster planning.

In the event of a disaster, the emergency response plan is immediately activated.

VII. Biological Warfare Agents

A. A **warfare agent** is a biological or chemical substance that can cause mass casualty destruction or fatality.
B. Anthrax (Fig. 14-1)
   1. Caused by *Bacillus anthracis;* can be contracted through the digestive system, abrasions in the skin, or inhalation
   2. Transmitted by direct contact with the bacteria and its spores; spores are dormant encapsulated bacteria that become active when they enter a living host (no person-to-person spread; Box 14-6)
   3. Carried to the lymph nodes and then spread to the rest of the body via the blood and lymph; high levels of toxins lead to shock and death
   4. In the lungs, anthrax can cause a buildup of fluid, tissue decay, and death. It is fatal if untreated.
   5. A blood test is available to detect anthrax (detects and amplifies *Bacillus anthracis* DNA if present in the blood sample).

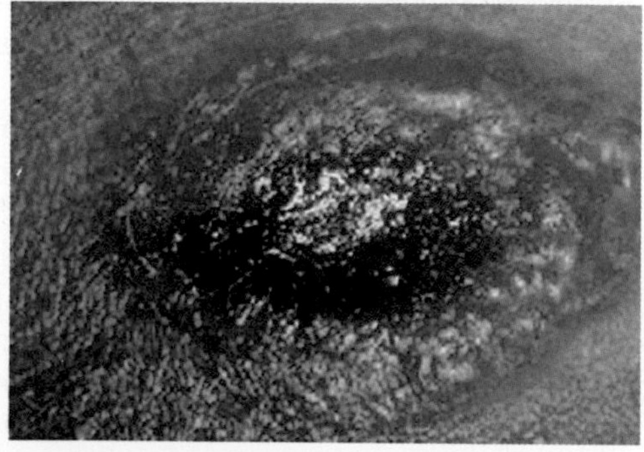

FIGURE 14-1 Anthrax. (From Swartz M: *Textbook of physical diagnosis*, ed 6, Philadelphia, 2010, Saunders.)

BOX 14-6 Transmission and Symptoms of Anthrax

Skin

Spores enter the skin through cuts and abrasions and are contracted by handling contaminated animal skin products.
The infection starts with an itchy bump like a mosquito bite that progresses to a small, liquid-filled sac.
The sac becomes a painless ulcer with an area of black, dead tissue in the middle.
Toxins destroy the surrounding tissue.

Gastrointestinal System

Infection occurs after the ingestion of contaminated, undercooked meat.
Symptoms begin with nausea, loss of appetite, and vomiting.
The infection progresses to severe abdominal pain, the vomiting of blood, and severe diarrhea.

Inhalation

Infection is caused by the inhalation of bacterial spores, which multiply in the alveoli.
Symptoms begin with the same symptoms as influenza, including fever, muscle aches, and fatigue.
Symptoms suddenly become more severe with the development of breathing problems and shock.
Toxins cause hemorrhage and the destruction of lung tissue.

   6. Anthrax is usually treated with antibiotics such as ciprofloxacin (Cipro), doxycycline, or penicillin.
   7. The vaccine for anthrax has limited availability.

Anthrax is transmitted by direct contact with bacteria and spores and can be contracted through the digestive system, abrasions in the skin, or inhalation through the lungs.

C. Smallpox (Fig. 14-2)
   1. Smallpox is transmitted in air droplets and by handling contaminated materials and is highly contagious. 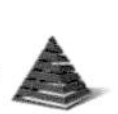

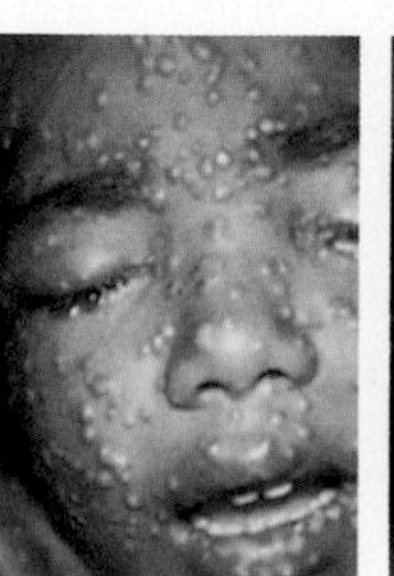
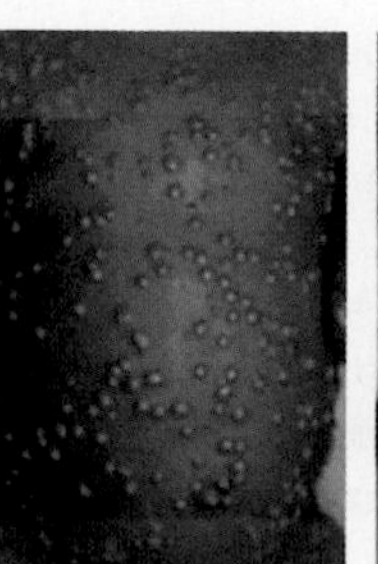
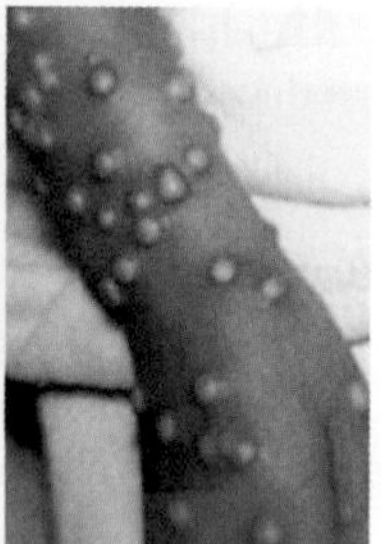

FIGURE 14-2 Smallpox. (Courtesy of Centers for Disease Control and Prevention [CDC]: *Evaluating patients for smallpox.* Atlanta, 2002, CDC. Available at http://www.bt.cdc.gov/agent/smallpox/diagnosis/evalposter.asp)

2. Symptoms begin 7 to 17 days after exposure and include fever, back pain, vomiting, malaise, and headache.
3. Papules develop 2 days after symptoms develop and progress to pustular vesicles that are abundant on the face and extremities initially.
4. A vaccine is available to those at risk for exposure to smallpox.

D. Botulism
1. Serious paralytic illness caused by a nerve toxin that is produced by the bacterium *Clostridium botulinum*. An infected client can die within 24 hours.
2. Spores are found in the soil and can spread through the air or food (particularly improperly canned food) or via a contaminated wound.
3. Cannot be spread from person to person.
4. Symptoms include abdominal cramps, diarrhea, nausea, vomiting, double vision, blurred vision, drooping eyelids, difficulty swallowing or speaking, dry mouth, and muscle weakness.
5. Neurological symptoms begin 12 to 36 hours after ingestion of food-borne botulism and 24 to 72 hours after inhalation and can progress to paralysis of the arms, legs, trunk, or respiratory muscles (mechanical ventilation is necessary).
6. If diagnosed early, food-borne and wound botulism can be treated with an antitoxin that blocks the action of toxin circulating in the blood.
7. Other treatments include induction of vomiting, enemas, and penicillin.
8. No vaccine is available.

E. Plague
1. Caused by *Yersinia pestis,* which is a bacteria found in rodents and fleas.
2. Contracted by being bitten by a rodent or flea carrying the plague bacterium, the ingestion of contaminated meat, or the handling of an animal infected with the bacteria.
3. Transmitted by direct person-to-person spread
4. Forms include bubonic (most common), pneumonic, and septicemic (most deadly).
5. Symptoms usually begin within 1 to 3 days and include fever, chest pain, lymph node swelling, and a productive cough (hemoptysis).
6. The disease rapidly progresses to dyspnea, stridor, and cyanosis; death occurs from respiratory failure, shock, and bleeding.
7. Antibiotics are effective only if administered immediately; the usual medications of choice include streptomycin or gentamicin.
8. A vaccine is available.

F. Tularemia
1. Infectious disease of animals caused by the bacillus *Francisella tularensis;* also called deerfly fever or rabbit fever
2. Transmitted by ticks, deerflies, or contact with an infected animal
3. Symptoms include fever, headache, ulcerated skin lesion with localized lymph node enlargement, eye infection, gastrointestinal ulceration, and pneumonia.
4. Treated with antibiotics
5. Recovery produces lifelong immunity (a vaccine is available).

G. Hemorrhagic fever
1. Caused by several viruses, including Marburg, Lassa, Junin, and Ebola

2. Virus is carried by rodents and mosquitoes.
3. Can be transmitted by direct person-to-person spread via body fluids
4. Symptoms include fever, headache, malaise, conjunctivitis, nausea, vomiting, hypotension, hemorrhage of tissues and organs, and organ failure.
5. No known specific treatment is available; treatment is symptomatic.

VIII. Chemical Warfare Agents

A. Sarin
1. A highly toxic nerve gas that can cause death within minutes of exposure
2. Enters the body through the eyes and skin; acts by paralyzing the respiratory muscles

B. Phosgene: Colorless gas normally used in chemical manufacturing; if inhaled at high concentrations for a long-enough period, it leads to severe respiratory distress, pulmonary edema, and death

C. Mustard gas: Yellow to brown in color and has a garlic-like odor that irritates the eyes and causes skin burns and blisters

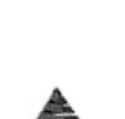

D. Ionizing radiation
1. Acute radiation poisoning develops after substantial exposure to radiation.
2. Can occur from external radiation or internal absorption
3. Symptoms depend on the amount of exposure to the radiation; range from nausea and vomiting, diarrhea, fever, electrolyte imbalances, and neurological and cardiovascular impairment to leukopenia, purpura, hemorrhage, and death.

IX. Nursing Role in Exposure to Warfare Agents

A. Be aware that initially, a bioterrorism attack may resemble a naturally occurring outbreak of an infectious disease.

B. Nurses and other health care workers must be prepared to assess and determine what type of event occurred, the number of clients who may be affected, and how and when clients will be expected to arrive at the health care agency.

C. It is essential to determine any changes in the microorganism that may increase its virulence or make it resistant to conventional antibiotics or vaccines.

D. See Chapter 8 for additional information on disasters and emergency response planning.

CRITICAL THINKING What Should You Do?

Answer: Many facilities implement a "no restraint policy," which requires health care workers to implement other safety strategies for clients who pose a risk for falls. These strategies include orienting the client and family to the surroundings; explaining all procedures and treatments to the client and family; encouraging family and friends to stay with the client as appropriate and using sitters for clients who need supervision; assigning confused and disoriented clients to rooms near the nurses' station; providing appropriate visual and auditory stimuli to the client, such as clocks, calendars, a television, and a radio; maintaining toileting routines; eliminating bothersome treatments, such as tube feedings, as soon as possible; evaluating all medications that the client is receiving; using relaxation techniques with the client; and instituting exercise and ambulation schedules as the client's condition allows.

Reference(s): deWit, D. & Kumagai, C. (2013). *Medical-surgical nursing: Concepts & practice.* (2nd ed., pp. 184–185). St. Louis: Saunders.

PRACTICE QUESTIONS

96. A mother calls a neighborhood nurse and tells the nurse that her 3-year-old child has just ingested liquid furniture polish. Which action should the nurse instruct the mother to take **first**?

1. Induce vomiting.
2. Call an ambulance.
3. Call the poison control center.
4. Bring the child to the emergency department.

97. The emergency department nurse receives a telephone call and is informed that a tornado has hit a local residential area and numerous casualties have occurred. The victims will be brought to the emergency department. Which should be the **initial** nursing action?

1. Prepare the triage rooms.
2. Activate the agency emergency response plan.
3. Obtain additional supplies from the central supply department.
4. Obtain additional nursing staff to assist with treating the casualties.

98. The nurse is caring for a client with a health care–associated infection caused by methicillin-resistant *Staphylococcus aureus* who is on contact precautions. The nurse prepares to provide colostomy care to the client. Which protective items will be required to perform this procedure?

1. Gloves and a gown
2. Gloves and goggles
3. Gloves, a gown, and goggles
4. Gloves, a gown, and shoe protectors

99. The nurse should institute which type of precaution for a client diagnosed with *Clostridium difficile*?

1. Droplet
2. Contact
3. Airborne
4. Neutropenic

100. The nurse enters a client's room and finds that the wastebasket is on fire. The nurse immediately assists the client out of the room. Which is the **next** nursing action?

1. Call for help.
2. Extinguish the fire.
3. Activate the fire alarm.
4. Confine the fire by closing the room door.

❖ **101.** The community health nurse has completed a teaching session about anthrax with members of the community. The licensed practical nurse (LPN) reinforcing the teaching tells those attending that anthrax can be transmitted via which routes? **Select all that apply.**

- ❑ 1. Skin
- ❑ 2. Kissing
- ❑ 3. Inhalation
- ❑ 4. Gastrointestinal
- ❑ 5. Direct contact with an infected individual
- ❑ 6. Sexual contact with an infected individual

102. The nurse obtains a prescription from the health care provider (HCP) to restrain a client using a jacket (safety) restraint and instructs the unlicensed assistive personnel (UAP) to apply the restraint. Which observation, if made by the nurse, should indicate unsafe application of the restraint?

1. A safety knot is made in the restraint strap.
2. The restraint straps are safely secured to the side rails.
3. The jacket restraint strap does not tighten when force is applied against it.
4. The jacket restraint is secure, and two fingers can easily slide between the restraint and the client's skin.

103. The nurse is caring for a client who has hand restraints. How often should the nurse assess the skin integrity of the restrained hands?

1. Every 2 hours
2. Every 3 hours
3. Every 4 hours
4. Every 30 minutes

❖**104.** The nurse is assisting with planning care for a client with an internal radiation implant. Which should be included in the plan of care? **Select all that apply.**

- ❑ 1. Wearing gloves when emptying the client's bedpan
- ❑ 2. Keeping all linens in the room until the implant is removed
- ❑ 3. Wearing a film (dosimeter) badge when in the client's room
- ❑ 4. Wearing a lead apron when providing direct care to the client
- ❑ 5. Placing the client in a semiprivate room at the end of the hallway

105. The nurse enters the nursing lounge and discovers that a chair is on fire. The nurse activates the alarm, closes the lounge door, and obtains the fire extinguisher to extinguish the fire. The nurse pulls the pin on the fire extinguisher. Which is the **next** action the nurse should perform?

1. Aim at the base of the fire.
2. Squeeze the handle on the extinguisher.
3. Sweep the fire from side to side with the extinguisher.
4. Sweep the fire from top to bottom with the extinguisher.

ANSWERS

96. 3

Rationale: If a poisoning occurs, the poison control center should be contacted immediately. Vomiting should not be induced without instructions to do so if the victim is unconscious or the substance ingested is a strong corrosive or petroleum product. Bringing the child to the emergency department or calling an ambulance would not be the initial action because this would delay treatment. The poison control center may advise the mother to bring the child to the emergency department; if this is the case, the mother should call an ambulance.

Test-Taking Strategy: Note the strategic word, *first* in the question. Eliminate options 2 and 4, because these options will delay treatment. Recalling that vomiting should not be induced if a corrosive substance was ingested will assist you with eliminating option 1. **Review: poison control** measures.

Level of Cognitive Ability: Applying

Client Needs: Physiological Integrity

Integrated Process: Nursing Process/Implementation

Content Area: Critical Care: Emergency Situations

Priority Concepts: Clinical Judgment, Safety

Reference(s): deWit, Kumagai (2013), pp. 1028–1029.

97. 2

Rationale: During a widespread disaster, many people will be brought to the emergency department for treatment. Although options 1, 3, and 4 may be components of preparing for the casualties, the initial nursing action should be to activate the emergency response plan.

Test-Taking Strategy: Note the strategic word, *initial,* and note that option 2 is the umbrella option. **Review:** the procedures related to the management of a disaster.

Level of Cognitive Ability: Applying

Client Needs: Safe and Effective Care Environment

Integrated Process: Nursing Process/Implementation

Content Area: Leadership/Management: Disasters

Priority Concepts: Collaboration, Safety

Reference(s): deWit, Kumagai (2013), pp. 999–1001.

98. 3

Rationale: Goggles are worn to protect the mucous membranes of the eye during interventions that may produce splashes of blood, body fluids, secretions, and excretions. In addition, contact precautions require the use of gloves, and a gown should be worn if direct client contact is anticipated. Shoe protectors are not necessary.

Test-Taking Strategy: Focus on the subject, protective items needed for performing colostomy care. Visualize the procedure for performing colostomy care to determine the items required to care for this client. **Review: contact precautions.**

Level of Cognitive Ability: Applying

Client Needs: Safe and Effective Care Environment

Integrated Process: Nursing Process/Implementation

Content Area: Fundamental Skills: Infection Control

Priority Concepts: Infection, Safety

Reference(s): deWit, Kumagai (2013), pp. 109, 967.

99. 2

Rationale: Contact precautions are necessary for colonization or infection with a multidrug-resistant organism. This includes enteric infection with *Clostridium difficile.* Droplet or airborne precautions are not necessary because the organism is not transferred via the respiratory route. Neutropenic precautions are used when the client needs protection from contracting an infection from others.

Test-Taking Strategy: Focus on the subject, route of transmission of the infection. Options 1 and 3 are comparable or alike and should be eliminated. Recalling the purpose of neutropenic precautions will assist in eliminating option 4. **Review:** care of a client with *Clostridium difficile.*

Level of Cognitive Ability: Applying

Client Needs: Safe and Effective Care Environment

Integrated Process: Nursing Process/Implementation

Content Area: Fundamental Skills: Infection Control
Priority Concepts: Infection, Safety
Reference(s): deWit, Kumagai (2013), p. 109.

100. 3
Rationale: The order of priority in the event of a fire is to rescue the clients who are in immediate danger. The next step is to activate the fire alarm. The fire is then confined by closing all doors. Finally, the fire is extinguished.
Test-Taking Strategy: Note the **strategic word**, *next*. Remember the mnemonic *RACE* to help you to prioritize in the event of a fire: *R* = *R*escue clients who are in immediate danger; *A* = *A*larm, activate the alarm; *C* = *C*onfine the fire by closing all doors; *E* = *E*xtinguish or evacuate. **Review: fire safety procedures.**
Level of Cognitive Ability: Applying
Client Needs: Safe and Effective Care Environment
Integrated Process: Nursing Process/Implementation
Content Area: Fundamental Skills: Safety
Priority Concepts: Clinical Judgment, Safety
Reference(s): Perry, Potter, Elkin (2012), pp. 53–54.

❖ **101. 1, 3, 4**
Rationale: Anthrax is caused by *Bacillus anthracis,* and it can be contracted through the digestive system, abrasions in the skin, or inhalation. It cannot be spread from person to person.
Test-Taking Strategy: Focus on the **subject**, methods of contracting anthrax. Remembering that it is not spread by person-to-person contact will assist in answering. Also note that the incorrect options are **comparable or alike** and identify person-to-person contact. **Review:** information related to anthrax infection.
Level of Cognitive Ability: Applying
Client Needs: Safe and Effective Care Environment
Integrated Process: Teaching and Learning
Content Area: Fundamental Skills: Infection Control
Priority Concepts: Infection, Safety
Reference(s): deWit, Kumagai (2013), pp. 1011–1012.

102. 2
Rationale: A half-bow or safety knot should be used when applying a restraint, because it does not tighten when force is applied against it and allows for the quick and easy removal of the restraint in case of an emergency. The restraint strap is secured to the bed frame (never to the side rail) to avoid accidental injury in case the side rail is released. The jacket restraint should be secure, and one to two fingers should easily slide between the restraint and the client's skin.
Test-Taking Strategy: Focus on the **subject**, an unsafe action. This indicates that you are looking for an option that identifies an inaccurate measure related to the application of restraints. The words *secured to the side rails* in option 2 should direct you to this option as an unsafe action. **Review:** the guidelines related to the application of **restraints.**
Level of Cognitive Ability: Evaluating
Client Needs: Safe and Effective Care Environment
Integrated Process: Teaching and Learning
Content Area: Fundamental Skills: Safety
Priority Concepts: Health Care Quality, Safety
Reference(s): Linton (2012), pp. 324–326; Perry, Potter, Elkin (2012), p. 47.

103. 4
Rationale: The nurse needs to assess restraints and skin integrity every 30 minutes. Therefore, options 1, 2, and 3 are incorrect. Agency guidelines regarding the use of restraints should always be followed.
Test-Taking Strategy: Note the **subject**, frequency of time to check skin integrity. In this situation, it is best to select the option that identifies the most frequent time frame. **Review:** the guidelines related to the use of **restraints.**
Level of Cognitive Ability: Applying
Client Needs: Safe and Effective Care Environment
Integrated Process: Nursing Process/Implementation
Content Area: Fundamental Skills: Safety
Priority Concepts: Safety, Tissue Integrity
Reference(s): Perry, Potter, Elkin (2012), p. 48.

❖ **104. 1, 2, 3, 4**
Rationale: A private room with a private bath is essential if a client has an internal radiation implant. This is necessary to prevent the accidental exposure of other clients to radiation. The remaining options identify interventions that are necessary for a client with a radiation device.
Test-Taking Strategy: Focus on the **subject**, interventions to be included in the plan of care for a client with an internal radiation implant. Read each option carefully and think about the concerns related to exposure. Noting the word *semiprivate* will assist in eliminating this option. **Review: radiation safety** principles.
Level of Cognitive Ability: Analyzing
Client Needs: Safe and Effective Care Environment
Integrated Process: Nursing Process/Planning
Content Area: Fundamental Skills: Safety
Priority Concepts: Cellular Regulation, Safety
Reference(s): deWit, Kumagai (2013), pp. 160–161.

105. 1
Rationale: A fire can be extinguished by using a fire extinguisher. To use the extinguisher, the pin is pulled first. The extinguisher should then be aimed at the base of the fire. The handle of the extinguisher is squeezed, and the fire is extinguished by sweeping from side to side to coat the area evenly.
Test-Taking Strategy: Note the **strategic word**, *next.* Remember the mnemonic *PASS* to prioritize in the use of a fire extinguisher: *P* = *P*ull the pin; *A* = *A*im at the base of the fire; *S* = *S*queeze the handle; *S* = *S*weep from side to side to coat the area evenly. **Review:** the procedures related to the use of a **fire extinguisher.**
Level of Cognitive Ability: Applying
Client Needs: Safe and Effective Care Environment
Integrated Process: Nursing Process/Implementation
Content Area: Fundamental Skills: Safety
Priority Concepts: Clinical Judgment, Safety
Reference(s): Perry, Potter, Elkin (2012), pp. 53–54.

CHAPTER 15

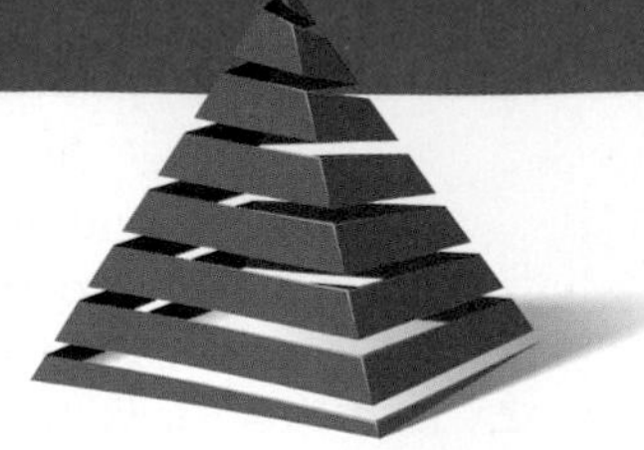

Fundamentals

Medication and Intravenous Administration

CRITICAL THINKING What Should You Do?

The nurse is preparing to administer 30 mL of a liquid medication to an assigned client. What should the nurse do when preparing this medication?
Answer can be located on p. 158.

I. Medication Administration (Box 15-1)

II. Drug-Measurement Systems

A. Metric system (Box 15-2)
  1. The basic units of metric measurement are meter, liter, and gram.
  2. Meter measures length; liter measures volume; gram measures mass.

BOX 15-1 Medication Administration

Check the medication prescription.
Compare the client's medication prescription with all the medications that the client was previously taking (medication reconciliation).
Ask the client about a history of allergies.
Determine the client's current condition and the purpose of the prescribed medication or intravenous solution.
Determine the client's understanding regarding the purpose of the prescribed medication or intravenous solution.
Plan to reinforce teaching to the client about the medication and about self-administration at home.
Identify and address social, cultural, and religious concerns that the client may have about taking the medication.
Determine the need for conversion when preparing a dose of medication for administration to the client.
Check the six rights: right medication, right dose, right client, right route, right time and frequency, and right documentation.
Check the client's vital signs, check significant laboratory results, and identify any potential interactions (food or medication interactions) before administering medication, when appropriate.
Identify any food or medication interactions before administering the medication.
Document the administration of the prescribed therapy and client's response to the therapy.

B. Apothecary and household systems (Box 15-3)
  1. Apothecary measures such as dram, grains, and minim are not commonly used in the clinical setting.
  2. Commonly used household measures include drop, teaspoon, tablespoon, ounce, pint, and cup.

C. Additional common drug measures
  1. Milliequivalent (mEq)
    a. The milliequivalent is an expression of the number of grams of a medication contained in 1 mL of a solution.
    b. For example: the measure of potassium is given in milliequivalents, such as 5 mEq of potassium
  2. Unit
    a. Measures a medication in terms of its action rather than its physical weight
    b. For example: penicillin, heparin sodium, and insulin are measured in units

III. Conversions

A. Conversion between metric units (Box 15-4)
  1. The metric system is a decimal system; therefore, conversions between the units in this system can 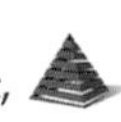

BOX 15-2 Metric System

Abbreviations

meter: m
liter: L
milliliter: mL
kilogram: kg
gram: g
milligram: mg
microgram: mcg

Equivalents

1 mcg = 0.000001 g
1 mg = 1000 mcg or 0.001 g
1 g = 1000 mg
1 kg = 1000 g
1 kg = 2.2 lb
1 mL = 0.001 L

be done by either dividing or multiplying by 1000 or by moving the decimal point three places to the right or three places to the left.

2. In the metric system, to convert larger to smaller, multiply by 1000 or move the decimal point three places to the right; for example, 1 g = 1000 mg.
3. In the metric system, to convert smaller to larger, divide by 1000 or move the decimal point three places to the left; for example, 1000 mg = 1 g.

BOX 15-3 Apothecary and Household Systems

Abbreviations

Apothecary (Weight)

grain: gr
ounce: oz

Household (Volume)

drops: gtt
teaspoon: t or tsp
tablespoon: T or tbs
fluid ounce: fl oz
cup: C
pint: pt
quart: qt

Household (Weight)

pound: lb

Equivalents

1 gr = 60 or 65 mg
5 gr = 300 or 325 mg
15 gr = 1000 mg or 1 g
$^{1}/_{150}$ gr = 0.4 mg
1 fl oz = 30 mL
1 T = 15 mL or 3 tsp
1 t or tsp = 5 mL
1 C = 8 fl oz
1 qt = 946 mL or 0.946 L
1 qt = 2 pt or 32 fl oz
1 pt = 16 fl oz
16 oz = 1 lb
1 kg = 2.2 lb

BOX 15-4 Conversion Between Metric Units

Problem 1

Convert 2 g to milligrams.

Solution

Change a larger unit to a smaller unit.
2 g = 2000 mg (moving decimal point three places to right)

Problem 2

Convert 250 mL to liters.

Solution

Change a smaller unit to a larger unit.
250 mL = 0.25 L (moving decimal point three places to left)

B. Conversion between household and metric systems

1. Conversions between the metric and household systems are equivalent—not equal—measures.
2. Conversion to equivalent measures between systems is necessary when a medication prescription is written in one system but the medication label is given in another.
3. Medications are not always prescribed and prepared in the same system of measurement. Therefore, it is necessary to convert units from one system to another.
4. Calculating equivalents between two systems may be done by using the method of ratio and proportion (Boxes 15-5 and 15-6).

BOX 15-5 Ratio and Proportion

Ratio: The relationship between two numbers, separated by a colon; for example, 1:2 (1 to 2).

Proportion: The relationship between two ratios, separated by a double colon (::) or an equal sign (=).

Formula: H (on hand): V (vehicle):: (=) desired dose: X (unknown)

To solve a ratio and proportion problem: The middle numbers (means) are multiplied and the end numbers (extremes) are multiplied.

Sample Problem

H = 1
V = 2
Desired dose = 3
X = unknown
Set up the formula: 1: 2:: 3: X
Solve: Multiply means and extremes.
1X = 6
X = 6

BOX 15-6 Calculating Equivalents Between Two Systems by Ratio and Proportion

Calculating equivalents between two systems may be done by using the method of ratio and proportion.

Problem

The health care provider prescribes nitroglycerin, grain (gr) $^{1}/_{150}$. The medication label reads 0.4 milligram (mg) per tablet. The nurse prepares to administer how many tablets to the client?

If you know that $^{1}/_{150}$ gr is equal to 0.4 mg, you know that you need to administer 1 tablet. Otherwise, use the ratio and proportion formula.

Ratio and Proportion Formula

H (on hand): V (vehicle):: (=) desired dose: X
1 gr: 60 mg:: $^{1}/_{150}$ gr: X mg
$60 \times {}^{1}/_{150} = {}^{60}/_{150} = X$
X = 0.4 mg (1 tablet)

Conversion is the first step in the calculation of dosages.

IV. Celsius and Fahrenheit Temperatures (Box 15-7)

A. To convert Fahrenheit to Celsius, first subtract 32, and then divide the result by 1.8.

B. To convert Celsius to Fahrenheit, first multiply by 1.8, and then add 32.

V. Medication Labels

A. A medication label will usually contain both the **generic name** and the **trade name** of the medication.

B. Always check the expiration dates on medication labels.

VI. Medication Prescriptions (Box 15-8)

A. In a medication prescription, the name of the medication is written first, followed by the dosage, route, and frequency (depending on the frequency of the prescription, times of administration are usually established by the health care agency and written in an agency policy).

B. Medication prescriptions are written according to the accepted abbreviations identified by The Joint Commission; also follow agency guidelines.

If the nurse has any questions about or sees inconsistencies in the written prescription, the nurse must contact the person who wrote the prescription immediately and must verify the prescription.

BOX 15-7 Celsius and Fahrenheit Temperature Conversion

Fahrenheit (F) to Celsius (C)

To convert Fahrenheit to Celsius, subtract 32 and divide the result by 1.8.

Formula:

$$C = \frac{F - 32}{1.8}$$

Celsius to Fahrenheit

To convert Celsius to Fahrenheit, multiply by 1.8 and add 32.

Formula:

$$F = (1.8 \times C) + 32$$

BOX 15-8 Medication Prescriptions

Name of client
Date and time when prescription is written
Name of medication to be given
Dosage of medication
Medication route
Time and frequency of administration
Signature of person who wrote the prescription

VII. Oral Medications

A. Scored tablets contain an indented mark to be used for breaking the tablet into partial dosages. When necessary, scored tablets (those marked for division) can be divided into halves or quarters.

B. Enteric-coated tablets and sustained-released capsules delay absorption until the medication reaches the small intestine. These medications should not be crushed.

C. Capsules contain a powdered or oily medication in a gelatin cover.

D. Oral liquids are supplied in solution form and contain a specific amount of medication in a given amount of solution, as stated on the label.

E. The medicine cup

1. The medicine cup has a capacity of 30 mL or 1 oz and is used for orally administered liquids.
2. The medicine cup is calibrated to measure teaspoons, tablespoons, and ounces.
3. To pour accurately, place the medication cup on a level surface at eye level and then pour the liquid while reading the measuring markings.
4. Volumes of less than 5 mL are measured by using a syringe with the needle removed.

A calibrated dropper is used for giving medicine to children.

VIII. Parenteral Medications

A. *Parenteral* always means injection route, and parenteral medications are administered by IV, intramuscular, intradermal, or subcutaneous routes (Fig. 15-1, angles of injection).

B. Parenteral medications are packaged in single-use ampules, single- and multiple-use rubber-stoppered vials, and premeasured syringes and cartridges.

C. The nurse should not administer more than 3 mL per intramuscular injection site or 1 mL per subcutaneous injection site; larger volumes are difficult for an injection site to absorb and, if prescribed, need to be verified. Variations for pediatric clients are discussed in the pediatric sections of this book.

D. The standard 3-mL syringe is used to measure most injectable medications. It is calibrated in tenths (0.1) of a milliliter.

E. The syringe is filled by drawing in solution until the top ring on the plunger (i.e., the ring closest to the needle), not the middle section and not the bottom ring of the plunger, is aligned with the desired calibration (Fig. 15-2).

F. Prefilled medication cartridge

1. The medication cartridge slips into the cartridge holder, which provides a plunger for the injection of the medication.
2. Designed to provide sufficient capacity to allow for the addition of a second medication when combined dosages are prescribed

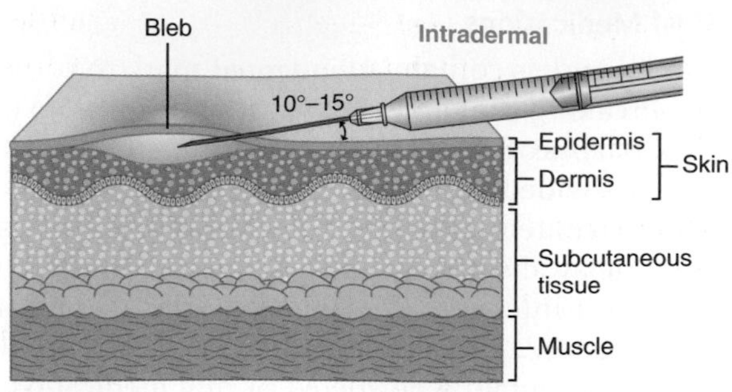

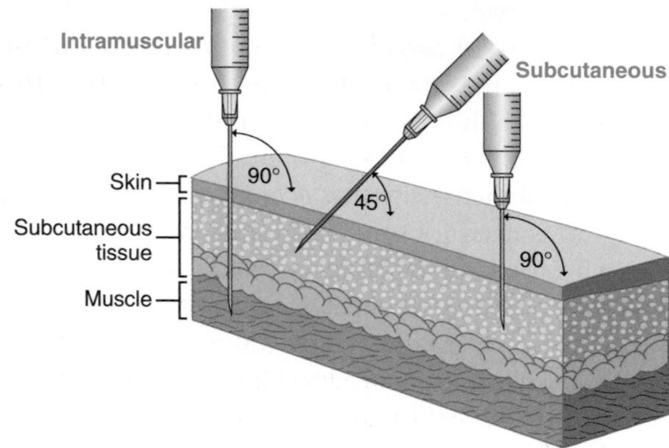

FIGURE 15-1 Angles of injection. (From Kee J, Marshall S: *Clinical calculations: With applications to general and specialty areas*, ed 7, St. Louis, 2013, Saunders.)

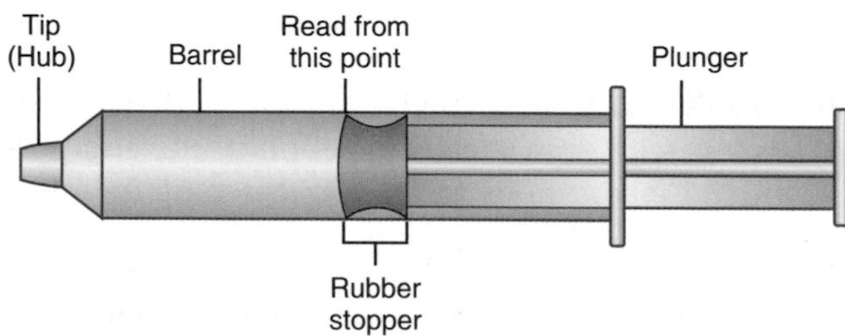

FIGURE 15-2 Parts of a syringe. (From Kee J, Marshall S: *Clinical calculations: With applications to general and specialty areas*, ed 7, St. Louis, 2013, Saunders.)

3. The prefilled medication cartridge is to be used once and discarded. If the nurse is to give less than the full single dose provided, he or she needs to discard the extra amount before giving the client the injection, in accordance with agency policies and procedures.

Always question and verify excessively large or small volumes of medication.

G. In general, standard medication doses for adults are to be rounded to the nearest tenth (0.1) of a milliliter and measured on the milliliter scale; for example, 1.26 mL is rounded to 1.3 mL (follow agency policy for rounding medication doses).
H. When volumes of more than 3 mL are required, a 5-mL syringe may be used. These syringes are calibrated in fifths (0.2 mL) (Fig. 15-3).
I. Other syringes that may be available are 10-, 20-, and 50-mL and may be used for medication administration requiring dilution.
J. Tuberculin syringe (Fig. 15-4)
   1. Holds a total capacity of 1 mL; used to measure small or critical amounts of medication, such as allergen extract, vaccine, or a child's medication.
   2. It is calibrated in hundredths (0.01) of a milliliter, with each one tenth (0.1) marked on the metric scale.
K. Insulin syringe (Fig. 15-5)
   1. The standard unit-100 insulin syringe is used to measure unit-100 insulin only. It is calibrated for a total of 100 units or 1 mL. Low-dose insulin syringes (½-mL sizes) may be used when administering smaller doses.
   2. Insulin should not be measured in any other type of syringe.

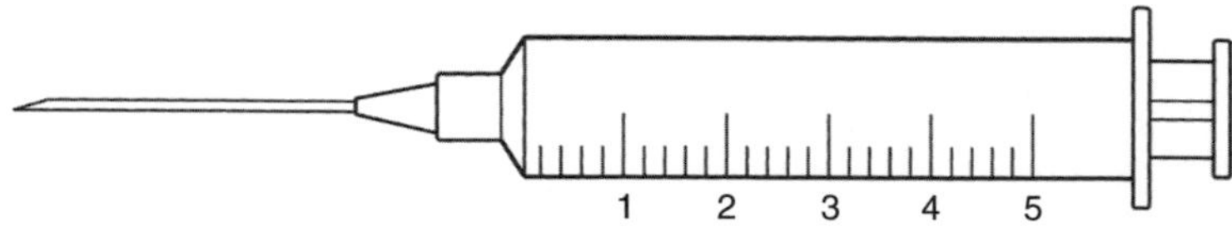

FIGURE 15-3 Five-milliliter syringe. (From Kee J, Marshall S: *Clinical calculations: With applications to general and specialty areas*, ed 7, St. Louis, 2013, Saunders.)

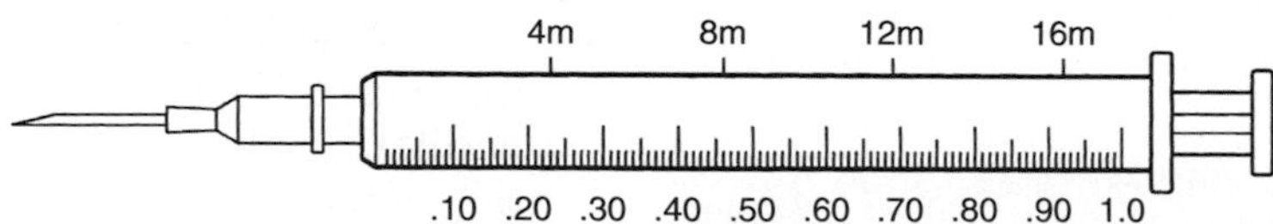

FIGURE 15-4 Tuberculin syringe. (From Kee J, Marshall S: *Clinical calculations: With applications to general and specialty areas*, ed 7, St. Louis, 2013, Saunders.)

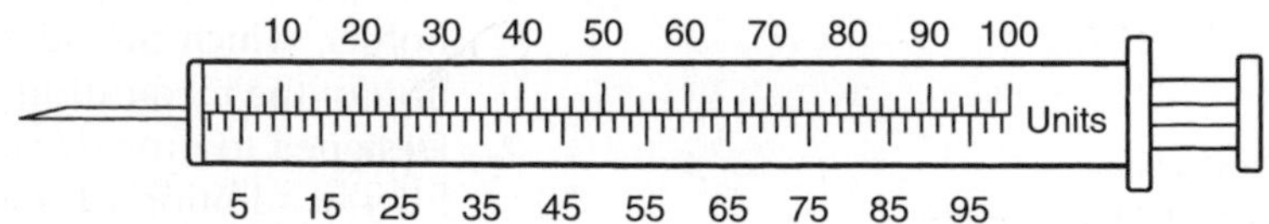

FIGURE 15-5 Insulin syringe. (From Kee J, Marshall S: *Clinical calculations: With applications to general and specialty areas*, ed 7, St. Louis, 2013, Saunders.)

If the insulin prescription states to administer regular and NPH insulin, combine both types of insulin in the same syringe. Use the mnemonic RN: draw Regular insulin into the insulin syringe first, and then draw the NPH insulin.

L. Safety needles contain shielding devices that are attached to the syringe and slipped over the needle; their use reduces the incidence of needle stick injuries.

IX. Injectable Medications in Powder Form

A. Some medications become unstable when stored in solution form and are therefore packaged in powder form.

B. Powders must be dissolved with a sterile diluent before use. Usually sterile water or normal saline is used. The dissolving procedure is called "reconstitution" (Box 15-9).

X. Calculating the Correct Dosage (Box 15-10)

A. When calculating dosages of oral medications, check the calculation, and question the prescription if the calculation calls for more than three tablets.

BOX 15-9 Reconstitution

When reconstituting a medication, locate the instructions on the label or in the vial package insert, and read and follow the directions carefully.

The instructions will state the volume of diluent to be used and the resulting volume of the reconstituted medication.

Often a powdered medication adds volume to the solution in addition to the amount of diluent added.

The total volume of the prepared solution will always exceed the volume of the diluent added.

When reconstituting a multiple-dose vial, label the medication vial with the date and time of preparation, your initials, and the date of expiration.

Indicating the strength per volume on the medication label also is important.

BOX 15-10 Standard Formula for Calculating a Medication Dosage

$$\frac{D}{A} \times Q = X$$

D (desired) is the dosage that the HCP prescribed.

A (available) is the dosage strength as stated on the medication label.

Q (quantity) is the volume or form in which the dosage strength is available, such as tablets, capsules, or milliliters.

B. When calculating dosages of parenteral medications, check the calculation, and question the prescription if the amount to be given is too large a dose.

C. Be sure that all measures are in the same system and that all units are in the same size, converting them when necessary. Carefully consider the reasonable amount of the medication that should be administered.

D. Round standard adult injection doses to tenths, and measure in a 3-mL syringe (follow agency policy).

E. Round small, critical, or children's doses to hundredths, and measure in a 1-mL tuberculin syringe (follow agency policy).

F. In addition to using the standard formula (see Box 15-10), calculations can be done through the use of dimensional analysis; the required elements of a dimensional analysis equation include the desired answer units, conversion formula that includes the desired answer units and the units that need to be converted, and the original factors to convert including quantity and units.

Regardless of the source of the error, if the nurse gives an incorrect dose, he or she is legally responsible for the action.

XI. Intravenous Flow Rates (Box 15-11 and Figure 15-6)

A. Monitor intravenous (IV) flow rate frequently even if the IV solution is being administered through an electronic infusion device (follow agency policy regarding frequency).

B. If an IV is running behind schedule, collaborate with the health care provider (HCP) to determine the client's ability to tolerate an increased flow rate, particularly if the client has cardiac, pulmonary, renal, or neurological conditions.

BOX 15-11 Formulas for Intravenous Calculations

Flow Rates

$$\frac{\text{Total volume} \times \text{drop factor}}{\text{Time in minutes}} = \text{drops per minute}$$

Infusion Time

$$\frac{\text{Total volume to infuse}}{\text{Milliliters per hour being infused}} = \text{infusion time}$$

Number of Milliliters per Hour

$$\frac{\text{Total volume in milliliters}}{\text{Number of hours}} = \text{number of milliliters per hour}$$

Fundamentals

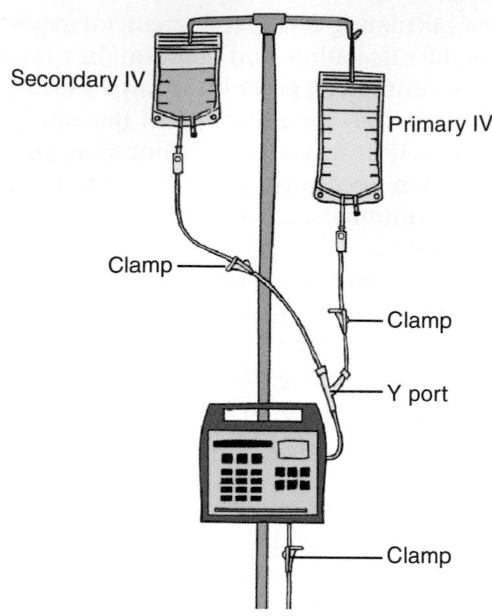

FIGURE 15-6 Infusion pump. (From Kee J, Marshall S: *Clinical calculations: With applications to general and specialty areas*, ed 7, St. Louis, 2013, Saunders.)

CRITICAL THINKING What Should You Do?

Answer: When preparing to administer a liquid medication, the nurse should use a medicine cup, pouring liquids into it after placing it on a flat surface at eye level, with the thumbnail at the medicine cup line indicating the desired amount. Liquids should not be mixed with tablets or with other liquids in the same container. The nurse should be sure not to return poured medication to its container and should properly discard poured medication if not used. The nurse should pour liquids from the side opposite the bottle's label to avoid spilling medicine on the label. Medications that irritate the gastric mucosa, such as potassium products, should be diluted or be taken with meals. Ice chips should be offered before administering unpleasant-tasting medications in order to numb the client's taste buds.

Reference(s): Potter, P., Perry, A. G., Stockert, P. A., & Hall, A. M. (2013). *Fundamentals of nursing.* (8th ed., pp. 614–615). St. Louis: Mosby.

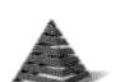

C. Whenever a prescribed IV rate is increased, the nurse should monitor the client for increased heart rate, increased respirations, or increased lung congestion, which could indicate fluid overload.

D. IV fluids are most frequently prescribed on the basis of milliliters (mL) per hour to be administered.

E. The volume per hour prescribed is administered by adjusting the rate at which the IV infuses, which is counted in drops (gtt) per minute.

F. Most flow-rate calculations involve changing mL/hour into gtt/minute.

⚠ The nurse should never increase (speed up) the rate of an IV infusion to catch up if the infusion is running behind schedule.

G. IV tubing

1. Calibrated in gtts/mL. This calibration is needed for calculating flow rates.
2. A standard or macrodrip set is used for routine adult IV administrations. Depending on the manufacturer and type of tubing, it requires 10, or 15 gtts to equal 1 mL.
3. A minidrip or microdrip set is used when more exact measurements are needed, such as in intensive care and pediatric units.
4. In a minidrip or microdrip set, 60 gtts is equal to 1 mL.
5. The calibration, in gtts/mL, is written on the IV tubing package.

PRACTICE QUESTIONS

❖**106.** The medication prescribed is hydromorphone hydrochloride (Dilaudid), 3 mg intramuscularly, every 4 hours as needed. The medication label reads hydromorphone hydrochloride (Dilaudid), 4 mg/1 mL. The nurse should prepare to administer how many mL to the client? **Fill in the blank.**
Answer: _____ mL

❖**107.** The medication prescribed is digoxin (Lanoxin), 0.25 mg orally, daily. The medication label reads digoxin (Lanoxin), 0.125 mg/tablet. The nurse should prepare how many tablet(s) to administer the dose? **Fill in the blank.**
Answer: _____ tablet(s)

❖**108.** The medication prescribed is heparin sodium 650 units subcutaneously, every 12 hours. The medication vial reads heparin sodium 1000 units/mL. The nurse prepares how many milliliters to administer one dose? **Fill in the blank.**
Answer: _____ mL

❖**109.** The medication prescribed is metoclopramide hydrochloride (Reglan) 10 mg intramuscularly times one dose. The medication label reads metoclopramide hydrochloride (Reglan), 5 mg/mL. The nurse prepares how much medication to administer the dose? **Fill in the blank.**
Answer: _____ mL

❖**110.** The medication prescribed is meperidine hydrochloride (Demerol), 35 mg intramuscularly. The medication label states meperidine hydrochloride (Demerol), 50 mg/mL. The nurse plans to prepare how much medication to administer the dose? **Fill in the blank.**

Answer: _____ mL

❖**111.** The medication prescribed is prochlorperazine 5 mg intramuscularly, every 4 hours as needed. The medication label states prochlorperazine 10 mg/mL. The nurse prepares how much medication to administer the dose? **Fill in the blank.**

Answer: _____ mL

❖**112.** The medication prescribed is atropine sulfate, 0.4 mg intramuscularly, immediately. The medication label states atropine sulfate, 0.3 mg/0.5 mL. The nurse prepares how much medication to administer the dose? **Fill in the blank and round answer to one decimal place.**

Answer: _____ mL

❖**113.** The medication prescribed is levodopa 1 g orally, daily. The medication label states levodopa, 500-mg tablets. The nurse prepares to administer how many tablets at the evening dose? **Fill in the blank.**

Answer: _____ tablet(s)

❖**114.** The medication prescribed is zidovudine (Retrovir), 0.2 g orally, three times daily. The medication label states zidovudine, 100-mg tablets. The nurse prepares to administer how many tablets for one dose? **Fill in the blank.**

Answer: _____ tablet(s)

❖**115.** The medication prescribed is atropine sulfate, 0.4 mg. The medication label states atropine sulfate, 0.5 mg/0.5 mL. How many milliliters will the nurse prepare to administer to the client? **Fill in the blank.**

Answer: _____ mL

116. The medication prescription states to administer acetaminophen (Tylenol), 650 mg orally for a temperature of more than 38 °C. The medication bottle states Tylenol (acetaminophen), 325 mg tablets. The nurse takes the client's temperature and notes that it is 101° F. The nurse plans to take which action?

1. Administer two Tylenol tablets.
2. Administer three Tylenol tablets.
3. Do not administer the Tylenol at this time.
4. Check the client's temperature in 30 minutes.

❖**117.** The medication prescription reads phenytoin (Dilantin), 0.2 g orally, twice daily. The medication label states 100-mg capsules. The nurse prepares how many capsule(s) to administer one dose? **Fill in the blank.**

Answer: _____ capsule(s)

❖**118.** The intravenous prescription is 1000 mL of 0.9% NaCl (normal saline) to run over 12 hours. The drop factor is 15 gtts/1 mL. The nurse plans to adjust the flow rate to how many gtts/minute? **Fill in the blank and record the answer to the nearest whole number.**

Answer: _____ gtts/minute

❖**119.** The medication is an intramuscular dose of 400,000 units of penicillin G benzathine (Bicillin). The medication label reads penicillin G benzathine (Bicillin) 300,000 units/mL. The nurse prepares how much medication to administer the correct dose? **Fill in the blank and record the answer using one decimal place.**

Answer: _____ mL

❖**120.** The intravenous prescription is 3000 mL of 5% dextrose (D5W) to run over a 24-hour period. The drop factor is 10 gtts/1 mL. The nurse plans to adjust the flow rate to how many gtts/minute? **Fill in the blank and record the answer to the nearest whole number.**

Answer: _____ gtts/minute

Fundamentals

ANSWERS

❖**106. 0.75**

Rationale: Follow the formula for dosage calculation.
Formula:

$$\frac{Desired \times mL}{Available} = mL \ per \ dose$$

$$\frac{3 \ mg \times 1 \ mL}{4 \ mg} = 0.75 \ mL$$

Test-Taking Strategy: Focus on the **subject**, a dosage calculation. Follow the formula for the calculation of the correct medication dose. Once you have performed the calculation, verify your answer using a calculator and make sure that the answer makes sense. **Review: medication calculations.**
Level of Cognitive Ability: Applying
Client Needs: Physiological Integrity
Integrated Process: Nursing Process/Planning
Content Area: Fundamental Skills: Medication/IV Calculations
Priority Concepts: Clinical Judgment, Safety
Reference(s): Cooper, Gosnell (2015), pp. 566–567.

❖**107. 2**

Rationale: Follow the formula for dosage calculation.
Formula:

$$\frac{Desired \times tablet(s)}{Available} = tablet(s) \ per \ dose$$

$$\frac{0.25 \ mg \times 1 \ tablet}{0.125 \ mg} = 2 \ tablets$$

Test-Taking Strategy: Focus on the **subject**, a dosage calculation. Follow the formula for the calculation of the correct medication dose. Once you have performed the calculation, verify your answer using a calculator and make sure that the answer makes sense. **Review: medication calculations.**
Level of Cognitive Ability: Applying
Client Needs: Physiological Integrity
Integrated Process: Nursing Process/Planning
Content Area: Fundamental Skills: Medication/IV Calculations
Priority Concepts: Clinical Judgment, Safety
Reference(s): Cooper, Gosnell (2015), pp. 566–567.

❖**108. 0.65**

Rationale: Follow the formula for dosage calculation.
Formula:

$$\frac{Desired \times mL}{Available} = mL \ per \ dose$$

$$\frac{650 \ units \times 1 \ mL}{1000 \ units} = 0.65 \ mL$$

Test-Taking Strategy: Focus on the **subject**, a dosage calculation. Follow the formula for the calculation of the correct medication dose. Once you have performed the calculation, verify your answer using a calculator and make sure that the answer makes sense. **Review: medication calculations.**
Level of Cognitive Ability: Applying
Client Needs: Physiological Integrity
Integrated Process: Nursing Process/Planning
Content Area: Fundamental Skills: Medication/IV Calculations
Priority Concepts: Clinical Judgment, Safety
Reference(s): Cooper, Gosnell (2015), pp. 566–567.

❖**109. 2**

Rationale: Follow the formula for dosage calculation.
Formula:

$$\frac{Desired \times mL}{Available} = mL \ per \ dose$$

$$\frac{10 \ mg \times 1 \ mL}{5 \ mg} = 2 \ mL$$

Test-Taking Strategy: Focus on the **subject**, a dosage calculation. Follow the formula for the calculation of the correct medication dose. Once you have performed the calculation, verify your answer using a calculator and make sure that the answer makes sense. **Review: medication calculations.**
Level of Cognitive Ability: Applying
Client Needs: Physiological Integrity
Integrated Process: Nursing Process/Planning
Content Area: Fundamental Skills: Medication/IV Calculations
Priority Concepts: Clinical Judgment, Safety
Reference(s): Cooper, Gosnell (2015), pp. 566–567.

❖**110. 0.7**

Rationale: Follow the formula for dosage calculation.
Formula:

$$\frac{Desired \times mL}{Available} = mL \ per \ dose$$

$$\frac{35 \ mg \times 1 \ mL}{50 \ mg} = 0.7 \ mL$$

Test-Taking Strategy: Focus on the **subject**, a dosage calculation. Follow the formula for the calculation of the correct medication dose. Once you have performed the calculation, verify your answer using a calculator and make sure that the answer makes sense. Review: **medication calculations.**
Level of Cognitive Ability: Applying
Client Needs: Physiological Integrity
Integrated Process: Nursing Process/Planning
Content Area: Fundamental Skills: Medication/IV Calculations
Priority Concepts: Clinical Judgment, Safety
Reference(s): Cooper, Gosnell (2015), pp. 566–567.

❖**111. 0.5**

Rationale: Follow the formula for dosage calculation.
Formula:

$$\frac{Desired \times mL}{Available} = mL \ per \ dose$$

$$\frac{5 \ mg \times 1 \ mL}{10 \ mg} = 0.5 \ mL$$

Test-Taking Strategy: Focus on the subject, a dosage calculation. Follow the formula for the calculation of the correct medication dose. Once you have performed the calculation, verify your answer using a calculator and make sure that the answer makes sense. **Review: medication calculations.**
Level of Cognitive Ability: Applying
Client Needs: Physiological Integrity
Integrated Process: Nursing Process/Planning
Content Area: Fundamental Skills: Medication/IV Calculations
Priority Concepts: Clinical Judgment, Safety
Reference(s): Cooper, Gosnell (2015), pp. 566–567.

❖112. 0.7
Rationale: Follow the formula for dosage calculation.
Formula:

$$\frac{Desired \times mL}{Available} = mL\ per\ dose$$

$$\frac{0.4\ mg \times 0.5\ mL}{0.3\ mg} = 0.66,\ or\ 0.7\ mL$$

Test-Taking Strategy: Focus on the subject, a dosage calculation. Follow the formula for the calculation of the correct medication dose. Once you have performed the calculation, verify your answer using a calculator and make sure that the answer makes sense. Remember to round the answer and record to one decimal place. **Review: medication calculations.**
Level of Cognitive Ability: Applying
Client Needs: Physiological Integrity
Integrated Process: Nursing Process/Planning
Content Area: Fundamental Skills: Medication/IV Calculations
Priority Concepts: Clinical Judgment, Safety
Reference(s): Perry, Potter, Elkin (2012), pp. 494–495.

❖113. 2
Rationale: Convert 1 g to milligrams. In the metric system, to convert larger to smaller, multiply by 1000, or move the decimal three places to the right; therefore, 1 g = 1000 mg.
Formula:

$$\frac{Desired \times tablet(s)}{Available} = tablet(s)\ per\ dose$$

$$\frac{1000\ mg \times 1\ tablet}{500\ mg} = 2\ tablets$$

Test-Taking Strategy: Focus on the subject, a medication calculation. For this medication calculation problem, it is necessary to first convert grams to milligrams. Follow the formula for conversion, and read the question carefully. After you have performed the calculation, verify your answer using a calculator. **Review: medication calculations and conversions.**
Level of Cognitive Ability: Applying
Client Needs: Physiological Integrity
Integrated Process: Nursing Process/Planning
Content Area: Fundamental Skills: Medication/IV Calculations
Priority Concepts: Clinical Judgment, Safety
Reference(s): Potter, Perry, Stockert, Hall (2013), pp. 573–574.

❖114. 2
Rationale: Convert 0.2 g to mg. In the metric system, to convert larger to smaller, multiply by 1000, or move the decimal three places to the right; therefore, 0.2 g = 200 mg.
Formula:

$$\frac{Desired \times tablet(s)}{Available} = tablet(s)\ per\ dose$$

$$\frac{200\ mg \times 1\ tablet}{100\ mg} = 2\ tablets$$

Test-Taking Strategy: Focus on the subject, a medication calculation. For this medication calculation problem, it is necessary to first convert grams to milligrams. Follow the formula for conversion, and read the question carefully. After you have performed the calculation, verify your answer using a calculator.
Review: medication calculations and conversions.
Level of Cognitive Ability: Applying
Client Needs: Physiological Integrity
Integrated Process: Nursing Process/Planning
Content Area: Fundamental Skills: Medication/IV Calculations
Priority Concepts: Clinical Judgment, Safety
Reference(s): Potter, Perry, Stockert, Hall (2013), pp. 573–574.

❖115. 0.4
Rationale: Follow the formula for dosage calculation.
Formula:

$$\frac{Desired \times mL}{Available} = mL\ per\ dose$$

$$\frac{0.4\ mg \times 0.5\ mL}{0.5\ mg} = 0.4\ mL$$

Test-Taking Strategy: Focus on the subject, a dosage calculation. Follow the formula for the calculation of the correct medication dose. Once you have performed the calculation, verify your answer using a calculator and make sure that the answer makes sense. **Review: medication calculations.**
Level of Cognitive Ability: Applying
Client Needs: Physiological Integrity
Integrated Process: Nursing Process/Planning
Content Area: Fundamental Skills: Medication/IV Calculations
Priority Concepts: Clinical Judgment, Safety
Reference(s): Cooper, Gosnell (2015), pp. 566–567.

116. 1
Rationale: Convert Fahrenheit to Celsius, and then calculate the dose to be administered.
Step 1: Conversion of Fahrenheit to Celsius
Formula: To convert Fahrenheit to Celsius, subtract 32, and divide the result by 1.8:
C = (101 − 32) = 69, divided by 1.8 = 38.3°
Step 2: Dosage calculation
Formula:

$$\frac{Desired \times tablet(s)}{Available} = tablet(s)\ per\ dose$$

$$\frac{650\ mg \times 1\ tablet}{325\ mg} = 2\ tablets$$

Therefore, option 1 is the correct option.
Test-Taking Strategy: Focus on the subject, a medication calculation. For this medication calculation problem, it is necessary to convert Fahrenheit to Celsius. Follow the formula for conversion, and then perform the medication calculation. After you have performed the calculation, verify the calculation using a calculator. This will direct you to the correct option of administering two Tylenol tablets. **Review: medication calculations and conversions.**
Level of Cognitive Ability: Applying
Client Needs: Physiological Integrity
Integrated Process: Nursing Process/Planning
Content Area: Fundamental Skills: Medication/IV Calculations
Priority Concepts: Clinical Judgment, Safety
Reference(s): Cooper, Gosnell (2015), pp. 566–567; Potter, Perry, Stockert, Hall (2013), pp. 446–447.

❖ 117. 2
Rationale: You must convert 0.2 g to milligrams. In the metric system, to convert larger to smaller, multiply by 1000 or move the decimal three places to the right. Therefore, 0.2 g equals 200 mg. After conversion from grams to milligrams, use the formula to calculate the correct dose.
Formula:

$$\frac{Desired \times capsule(s)}{Available} = capsule(s)\ per\ dose$$

$$\frac{200\ mg \times 1\ capsule}{100\ mg} = 2\ capsules$$

Test-Taking Strategy: Focus on the subject, a medication calculation. In this medication calculation problem, first you must convert grams to milligrams. Once you have done the conversion and reread the medication calculation problem, you will know that 2 capsules is the correct answer. Recheck your work using a calculator and make sure that the answer makes sense. **Review: medication calculations** and **conversions.**
Level of Cognitive Ability: Applying
Client Needs: Physiological Integrity
Integrated Process: Nursing Process/Planning
Content Area: Fundamental Skills: Medication/IV Calculations
Priority Concepts: Clinical Judgment, Safety
Reference(s): Cooper, Gosnell (2015), pp. 566-567; Potter, Perry, Stockert, Hall (2013), pp. 573–574.

❖ 118. 21
Rationale: Use the intravenous (IV) flow rate formula.
Formula:

$$\frac{Total\ volume \times drop\ factor}{Time\ in\ minutes} = drops\ per\ minute$$

$$\frac{1000\ mL \times 15\ gtt}{720\ minutes} = \frac{15,000}{720} = 20.8, or\ 21\ gtts / minute$$

Test-Taking Strategy: Focus on the subject, an IV calculation. Follow the formula for calculating an infusion rate for an IV. Be sure to change 12 hours to minutes. After you have performed the calculation, verify your answer using a calculator and remember to record the answer to the nearest whole number. **Review: intravenous calculations.**
Level of Cognitive Ability: Applying
Client Needs: Physiological Integrity
Integrated Process: Nursing Process/Planning
Content Area: Fundamental Skills: Medication/IV Calculations
Priority Concepts: Clinical Judgment, Safety
Reference(s): deWit, Kumagai (2013), pp. 53–55.

❖ 119. 1.3
Rationale: Follow the formula for dosage calculation.
Formula:

$$\frac{Desired \times mL}{Available} = mL\ per\ dose$$

$$\frac{400,000\ units \times 1\ mL}{300,000\ units} = 1.3\ mL$$

Test-Taking Strategy: Focus on the subject, a dosage calculation. Follow the formula for the calculation of the correct medication dose. Once you have performed the calculation, verify your answer using a calculator and make sure that the answer makes sense. Remember to record the answer using one decimal place. **Review: medication calculations.**
Level of Cognitive Ability: Applying
Client Needs: Physiological Integrity
Integrated Process: Nursing Process/Planning
Content Area: Fundamental Skills: Medication/IV Calculations
Priority Concepts: Clinical Judgment, Safety
Reference(s): Cooper, Gosnell (2015), pp. 566–567.

❖ 120. 21
Rationale: Use the intravenous (IV) flow rate formula.
Formula:

$$\frac{Total\ volume \times drop\ factor}{Time\ in\ minutes} = gtts / minute$$

$$\frac{3,000\ mL \times 10\ gtt}{1440\ minutes} = \frac{30,000}{1440} = 20.8, or\ 21\ gtts / minute$$

Test-Taking Strategy: Focus on the subject, an IV calculation. Follow the formula for calculating the infusion rate for an IV. Be sure to change 24 hours to minutes. After you have performed the calculation, verify your answer using a calculator, and remember to record the answer to the nearest whole number. **Review: intravenous calculations.**
Level of Cognitive Ability: Applying
Client Needs: Physiological Integrity
Integrated Process: Nursing Process/Planning
Content Area: Fundamental Skills: Medication/IV Calculations
Priority Concepts: Clinical Judgment, Safety
Reference(s): Cooper, Gosnell (2015), pp. 566–567.

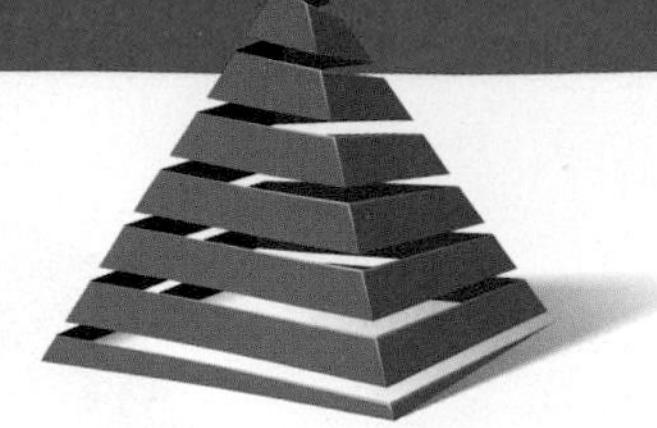

CHAPTER 16

Basic Life Support

CRITICAL THINKING What Should You Do?

The nurse working in the long-term care facility enters a client's room and finds the client unconscious, not breathing, and without a pulse. What should the nurse do?
Answer is located on p. 168.

I. **Basic Life Support (BLS)** (Box 16-1)

A. BLS provides oxygen to the brain, heart, and other vital organs until help arrives.

B. It is also known as cardiopulmonary resuscitation (CPR).

II. General CAB Guidelines

A. Description: **Cardiopulmonary resuscitation**, known by most as **CPR**, is the process of providing oxygen, with the use of chest compressions, to the brain, heart, and other vital organs in a victim who cannot do so for himself or herself.

B. Rescuers should follow the C-A-B formula:
C: compressions
A: airway
B: breathing

C. Basic steps include immediate recognition of the sudden cardiac arrest (unresponsiveness and absence of normal breathing) and activation of the emergency response system, early CPR, and rapid defibrillation with a defibrillator or **automated external defibrillator (AED)**.

D. Chest compressions (Figs. 16-1 and 16-2)
Description: Chest compressions are used to keep blood moving through the victim's body, delivering oxygen to crucial areas, such as the brain.

⚠ When performing chest compressions, push hard and fast and avoid interrupted compressions.

1. Nursing considerations
   a. Stand or kneel beside the victim's chest; ensure that the victim is lying supine on a firm surface (if possible); air-filled mattresses should be deflated and a backboard should be used.

PRIORITY NURSING ACTIONS!

Actions for the Health Care Provider for Performing Adult CPR

1. Determine unresponsiveness.
2. Check for pulse at carotid artery.
3. Perform chest compressions.
4. Open the airway, using the head tilt–chin lift method.
5. Check breathing and deliver breaths.

The sequence for basic CPR for health care providers (HCPs) follows the CAB—compressions, airway, breathing—sequence and is as follows. After determining unresponsiveness, the HCP assesses the carotid artery for the presence of a pulse. In the absence of any pulse, chest compressions are provided at an adequate rate and depth that will allow adequate chest recoil, with minimal interruptions in chest compressions. The HCP next opens the airway and checks for breathing. In the absence of breathing, the HCP delivers breaths.

Reference(s): deWit, D. & Kumagai, C. (2013). *Medical-surgical nursing: Concepts & practice.* (2nd ed., p. 1034). St. Louis: Saunders.
Potter, P., Perry, A. G., Stockert, P. A., & Hall, A. M. (2013). *Fundamentals of nursing.* (8th ed., p. 594). St. Louis: Mosby.

BOX 16-1 The CABs of Basic Life Support for the Health Care Provider

C: Compressions
A: Airway
B: Breathing

Note: Each step of the CABs of basic life support begins with assessment.

   b. Place the heel of one hand on the lower half of the sternum, which is the center or middle part of the victim's chest, with the heel of the other hand on top of the first so that the hands are overlapped and parallel.
   c. The adult chest is compressed to a depth of at least 2 inches, and compressions should be hard and fast at a rate of at least 100 per minute. If there is difficulty pushing deeply during chest compressions, one hand should be placed on the breastbone

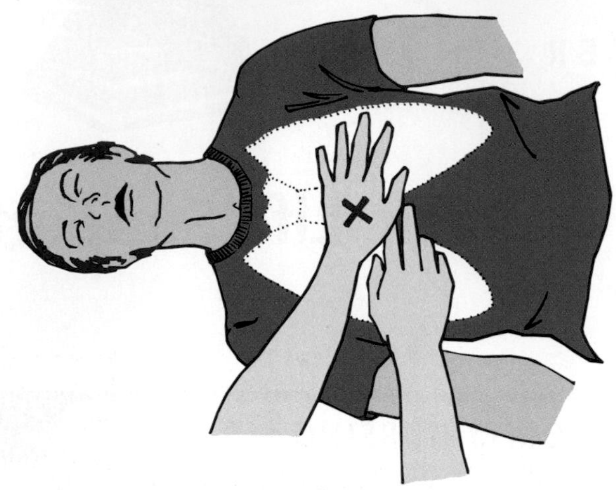

FIGURE 16-1 Chest compressions: Proper hand position for an adult. (From Potter A, Perry P: *Clinical nursing skills & techniques*, ed 7, St. Louis, 2010, Mosby.)

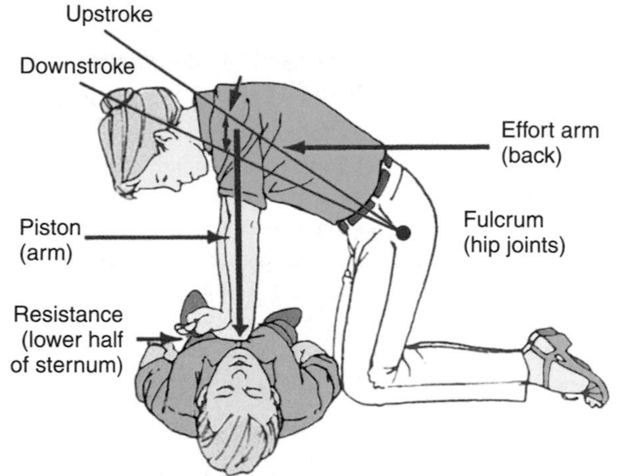

FIGURE 16-2 Positioning for proper compression techniques. (From Christensen B, Kockrow E: *Foundations of adult health nursing*, ed 6, St. Louis, 2010, Mosby.)

and the other should grasp the wrist of that hand to support the first hand to deliver compressions.

d. Allow complete recoil of the chest after each compression to allow the heart to fill completely before the next compression.

e. A compression-to-ventilation ratio of 30:2 is recommended.

f. If two rescuers are present, to prevent rescuer fatigue, rescuers may switch positions (compressor and ventilator) after approximately 2 minutes (or after 5 cycles of compression and ventilation at a ratio of 30:2).

g. Interruptions in chest compressions need to be minimized.

h. Chest compressions and ventilations are continued until spontaneous circulation returns or resuscitative efforts are terminated.

⚠ To produce as much blood flow as possible, allow the chest to recoil (return to normal position) completely after delivery of each breath and each compression. At least 23 out of 30 compressions should be allowed to completely recoil.

E. Airway

1. Description: Before effective rescue breathing can be administered, a patent airway must be confirmed or, if it is not present, opened manually.
2. Nursing considerations
   - **a.** After delivering 30 compressions, the rescuer opens the victim's airway (after donning gloves and a face shield, if they are available).
   - **b.** The head tilt–chin lift is the preferred method of opening the airway.
   - **c.** To perform the head tilt–chin lift, one hand is placed on the client's forehead, and firm pressure is applied to tilt the head backward; using the first and second fingers of the other hand, pressure is applied under the bony part of the jaw, taking care not to block the airway and ensuring that the tongue is not obstructing the airway (Fig. 16-3).
   - **d.** The jaw thrust maneuver is performed by placing the first and second fingers of both hands on the corner-point of the mandible and both thumbs on the chin, then pushing the mandible upward; this prevents obstruction of the airway by the tongue (Fig. 16-4).

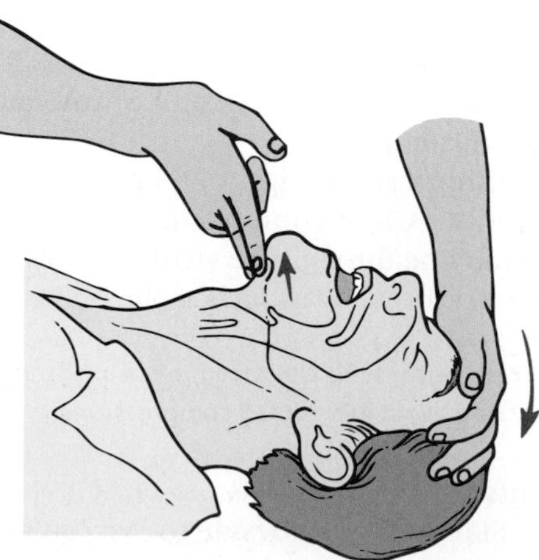

FIGURE 16-3 Opening the airway using the head tilt–chin lift maneuver. (From Lewis SM, Heitkemper MM, Dirksen SR: *Medical-surgical nursing: Assessment and management of clinical problems*, ed 7, St. Louis, 2007, Mosby.)

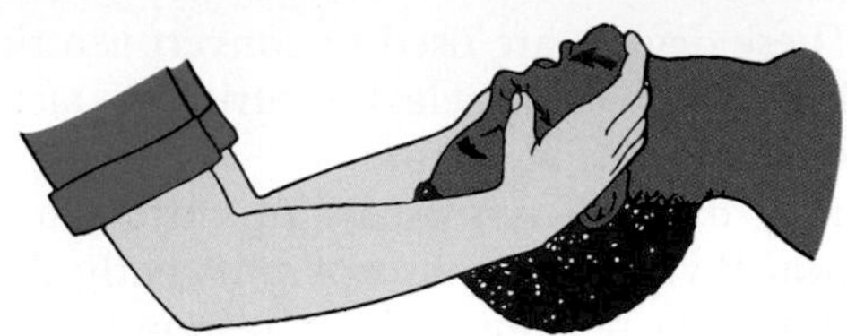

FIGURE 16-4 Opening the airway using the jaw thrust maneuver. (Perry A, Potter P: *Nursing Interventions and Clinical Skills*, ed 5, St. Louis, 2012, Mosby.)

If a head, neck, or spinal cord injury is suspected, the jaw thrust maneuver is used to open the victim's airway.

F. Breathing

1. Description: Once the airway has been secured, the rescuer delivers breaths to keep oxygen moving through the victim's body. A healthcare worker should not deliver mouth-to-mouth breaths in the workplace without a barrier device, and should continue delivering chest compressions until a barrier device arrives.
2. Nursing considerations
   a. A victim who is breathing is log-rolled onto his or her side as a unit (without twisting) with the lower arm in front of the body (recovery position) to help maintain an open airway; if a spinal cord injury is suspected, however, the victim should not be moved.
   b. Occasional gasps from a victim may not result in adequate ventilation, and this victim should be treated as if he or she is not breathing.
   c. If the victim is not breathing but has a pulse, give rescue breathing (mouth-to-barrier device, or bag mask if available ensuring an adequate air seal); allow the victim to exhale between breaths (avoid excessive ventilation).
   d. Each rescue breath is delivered over 1 second; ventilations are delivered at a rate of 1 breath every 6 to 8 seconds (8 to 10 ventilations per minute).

When performing CPR, if you are unsuccessful at giving a breath, reposition the victim's head and try again (improper chin and head position is a common cause of difficulty in ventilating a victim).

   e. While giving ventilations, watch for a visible chest rise; be alert to gastric distention, which indicates that the airway has not been properly opened and air from ventilations is entering the stomach rather than the lungs; this can result in regurgitation and aspiration. If a client is receiving feedings, the feeding tube should be attached to a suction device and any feedings in the stomach should be suctioned out to prevent aspiration.

BOX 16-2 Alternative Breathing Methods

- Mouth-to-nose breathing may be used when it is impossible to ventilate a victim through the mouth (e.g., the mouth cannot be opened, the mouth is seriously injured, or a tight mouth-to-mouth seal is difficult to achieve).
- Mouth-to-stoma breathing is used for the victim who has a tracheal stoma; a round pediatric face mask is used to create an adequate seal.

   f. A sufficient tidal volume is needed when delivering breaths to produce a visible chest rise.
   g. If compressions are needed, a compression-to-ventilation ratio of 30:2 is recommended until an advanced airway is placed.
   h. In special situations, an alternative breathing method may be used (Box 16-2).

III. Guidelines for the Adult

A. Description: Adult CPR consists of life-support measures that include early recognition of cardiac arrest and activation of the emergency response system, early CPR using the CAB procedure, rapid defibrillation if necessary, advanced life support, and post–cardiac arrest care.

B. Nursing considerations

1. The rescuer should ensure that the scene is safe before approaching the victim.
2. The health care provider (HCP) should first determine if the victim is unresponsive with no breathing or not breathing normally (by tapping the victim at the shoulder and shouting "Are you OK?"); activate the emergency response system; obtain the crash cart or AED if alone and if one is easily accessible, attach and use the AED; and then begin CPR (using C-A-B procedures). If two rescuers are present then one can obtain the crash cart or AED while the other begins CPR.
3. Checking for a pulse: the carotid artery is used for a pulse check in an adult; if a pulse is not felt within 10 seconds, the rescuer should start CPR, beginning with chest compressions at a ratio of 30:2 (compressions to ventilations) (see Fig. 16-1).
4. If a pulse is definitely felt, the rescuer should give one breath every 6 to 8 seconds if the victim is not breathing and recheck the pulse every 2 minutes.

IV. Variations in CPR

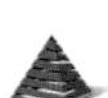

A. Child

1. Description
   a. A child is defined as a person between 1 and 8 years of age.
   b. The procedure is basically the same as that done for an adult; variations are listed below under nursing considerations.

2. Nursing considerations
   a. The health care provider can use the femoral artery for a pulse check in a child.
   b. If the rescuer is alone, five cycles of compressions and breaths (which will take about 2 minutes) are done before activating the emergency response system and obtaining the crash cart or AED.
   c. One hand is used for chest compressions, and ventilations are delivered more gently than in an adult.
   d. Adjust chest compressions to the child's age and size; compression–breath ratio is 30:2 for a single rescuer.
   e. If the child is breathing, ensure that the airway stays open.
   f. If the child is not breathing, take the appropriate measures (ventilation with a barrier device).
   g. After 5 cycles of CPR, if there is no response and an AED is available, apply it and follow the AED prompts. Use pediatric pads if available; if pediatric pads are not available, use adult pads.
   h. Continue CPR until the child moves or help arrives.

B. Infant
1. Description: A person who is younger than 1 year of age.
2. Nursing considerations
   a. Determine unresponsiveness; stroke the infant and watch for a response, such as movement, but don't shake the infant.
   b. If there is no response, follow the CAB procedures.
   c. The health care provider can use the brachial or femoral artery for a pulse check in an infant.
   d. If the rescuer is alone, five cycles of compressions and breaths (which will take about 2 minutes) are done before activating emergency response system and obtaining an AED. If a second rescuer is present, that person activates the emergency response system while the first attends to the infant.
   e. Compression–breath ratio is 30:2 for a single rescuer.
   f. The breastbone is compressed 1.5 inches at a rate of 100 times per minute with the use of two or three fingers.
   g. In an infant, provide mouth-to-nose ventilation when delivering breaths.

⚠ The chest compression landmark for a child is in the center of the chest between the nipples. For the infant, the landmark is just below the nipple line.

V. Defibrillator or Automated External Defibrillator Used by the HCP

A. Description
1. These devices are used to convert ventricular fibrillation or pulseless ventricular tachycardia into a perfusing rhythm.
2. The AED differentiates nonventricular fibrillation rhythms and also permits early defibrillation by laypersons and first responders.

⚠ When using the AED on an adult, do not use the child pads; these pads will not provide an effective shock.

B. Nursing considerations for an AED
1. Attach the AED leads to the victim per the AED instructions.
2. Turn on the AED and follow the AED prompts.
3. Ensure that no one is touching the victim when the shock is delivered.
4. Shockable rhythm: resume CPR immediately after the shock so as to minimize interruptions.
5. Nonshockable rhythm: resume CPR immediately for 2 minutes and check rhythm every 2 minutes.

VI. Foreign Body Airway Obstruction

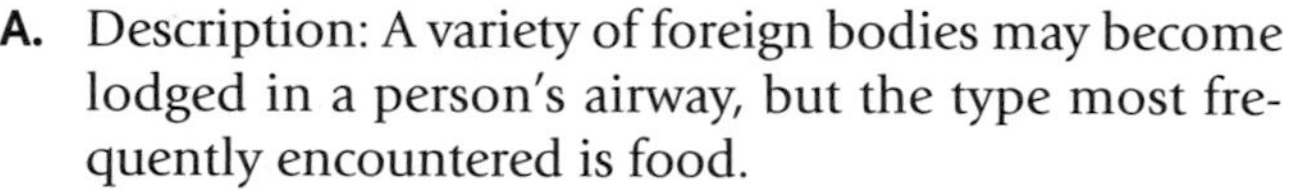

A. Description: A variety of foreign bodies may become lodged in a person's airway, but the type most frequently encountered is food.

⚠ Blind finger sweeps in the mouth of a victim with a foreign body airway obstruction (FBAO) should not be performed because of the risk of pushing the object further into the airway.

B. Nursing considerations for the adult
1. Ask the victim, "Are you choking?" The victim will not be able to speak or cough if he or she is choking and may place both hands on the neck (the universal sign for choking) or nod "yes."
2. If the victim's airway is partially obstructed, a crowing sound is heard; encourage the victim to cough.
3. If the victim is having difficulty breathing, activate the emergency response system.
4. Relieve the obstruction with the use of the **abdominal thrust maneuver** (Fig. 16-5 and Box 16-3).
5. Perform the abdominal thrust maneuver in rapid sequence until the object is dislodged or victim becomes unconscious.
6. If the victim becomes unconscious, place in a supine position, and begin CPR for 2 minutes and then activate emergency response system; if a second rescuer is present, that person should immediately activate the emergency response system.

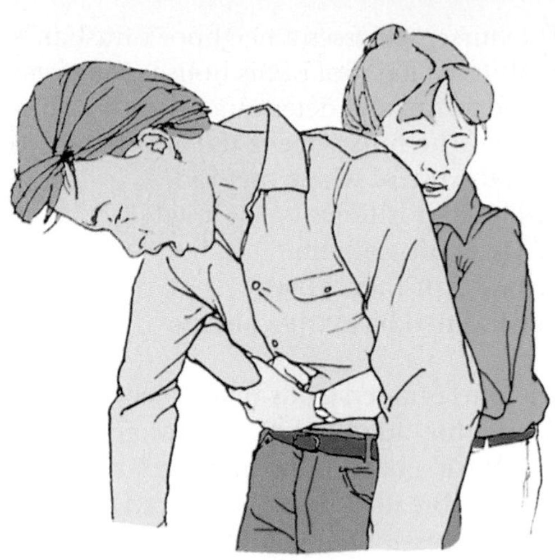

FIGURE 16-5 Abdominal thrusts. (From Christensen B, Kockrow E: *Foundations of adult health nursing,* ed 6, St. Louis, 2010, Mosby.)

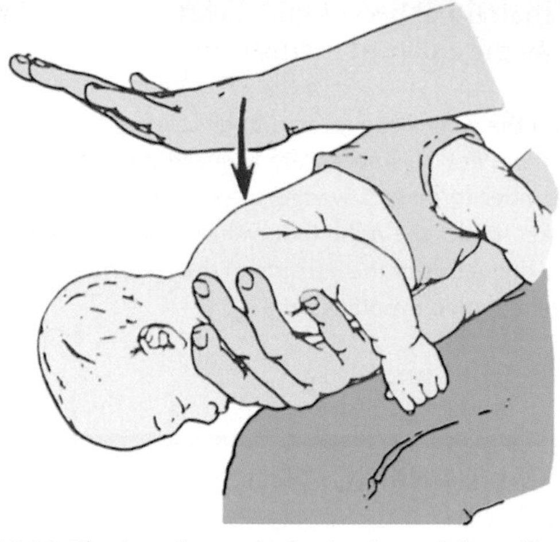

FIGURE 16-6 Clearing airway obstruction in an infant. (From Christensen B, Kockrow E: *Foundations of adult health nursing,* ed 6, St. Louis, 2010, Mosby.)

BOX 16-3 Abdominal Thrusts

1. Stand behind the victim.
2. Place your arms around the victim's waist.
3. Make a fist.
4. Place the thumb side of your fist just above the umbilicus (belly button) and well below the xiphoid process.
5. Perform five quick in and up abdominal thrusts (between the umbilicus and the xiphoid process).
6. Use chest thrusts for the obese victim or for the victim in the late stages of pregnancy.

7. Each time the airway is opened during CPR, the rescuer should look in the victim's mouth, and if an object is easily removable, remove it with two fingers.

⚠ To perform the abdominal thrust maneuver on an adult, straddle the victim's thighs, place the heel of one hand on top of the other, between the umbilicus and xiphoid process, and give five abdominal thrusts in and up with the heel of the bottom hand.

C. Nursing considerations for the child
1. Choking is suspected in a child or an infant experiencing acute respiratory distress associated with coughing, gagging, or stridor (high-pitched, noisy breathing).
2. Allow the victim to continue coughing if the cough is forceful.
3. If the cough is ineffective or the victim demonstrates increased respiratory difficulty accompanied by a high-pitched noise while inhaling, help is needed.
4. In a conscious child, the abdominal thrust maneuver should be performed until the obstruction is dislodged.

D. Nursing considerations for the infant
1. Assess the victim for obstruction, and note breathing problems.
2. Place the infant over an arm or on the lap, position the head lower than the trunk, and support the head firmly, holding the jaw.
3. Deliver five back slaps with the heel of the hand between the shoulder blades (Fig. 16-6).
4. Turn the infant over, positioning the head lower than the trunk.
5. Deliver five chest thrusts at the same location used for chest compressions.
6. Check for a foreign object and remove it only if seen; blind finger sweeps are avoided because the object can be forced back further into the throat.
7. Repeat the sequence until the object has been removed.

⚠ In an infant, deliver five back slaps and then five chest thrusts to remove the foreign body from the airway.

E. Pregnant or obese victim
1. Chest thrusts are used for obese victims or a victim in the late stage of pregnancy.
2. The rescuer places his or her arms under the victim's axillae and across the chest.
3. The thumb side of a clenched fist is placed against the middle of the sternum, and the other hand is placed over the fist.
4. Backward chest thrusts are performed until the foreign body is expelled or the victim loses consciousness.
5. The rescuer then attempts ventilations; if ventilation is unsuccessful, the rescuer positions the hands as for chest compressions and delivers firm chest thrusts to remove the obstruction.
6. If defibrillation is needed in a pregnant victim, the paddles are placed one rib interspace higher

than usual because the heart is displaced slightly by the enlarged uterus.

⚠ If the victim of a foreign body airway obstruction is pregnant, and it is necessary to place the client supine, remember to place a wedge, such as a pillow or rolled blanket, under the right abdominal flank and hip to displace the uterus to the left side of the abdomen. This will prevent supine hypotension.

CRITICAL THINKING What Should You Do?

Answer: In an unwitnessed event, after determining unconsciousness and no pulse or breathing, the nurse should begin chest compressions at a compression-to-ventilation ratio of 30:2. To produce as much blood flow as possible, allow the chest to recoil (return to normal position) completely after delivery of each breath and each compression. Since the nurse is working in a long-term care facility, assistance should be obtained in activating the emergency response system, obtaining a crash cart or automated external defibrillator, and performing cardiopulmonary resuscitation.

Reference(s): deWit, D. & Kumagai, C. (2013). *Medical-surgical nursing: Concepts & practice.* (2nd ed., p. 1034). St. Louis: Saunders.

PRACTICE QUESTIONS

121. The nursing instructor asks a nursing student to describe the procedure for relieving an airway obstruction on an unconscious pregnant woman at 8 months' gestation. How should the student describe the procedure correctly?
1. Place the hands in the pelvis to perform the thrusts.
2. Perform abdominal thrusts until the object is dislodged.
3. Perform left lateral abdominal thrusts until the object is dislodged.
4. Place a rolled blanket under the right abdominal flank and hip area.

122. The nurse on the day shift walks into a client's room and finds the client unresponsive. The client is not breathing and does not have a pulse, and the nurse immediately calls out for help. The **next** nursing action is which?
1. Deliver breaths.
2. Give the client oxygen.
3. Start chest compressions.
4. Ventilate with a mouth-to-mask device.

123. The nurse witnesses a neighbor's husband sustain a fall from the roof of his house. The nurse rushes to the victim and determines the need to open the airway. The nurse opens the airway in this victim with the use of which method?
1. Flexed position
2. Head tilt–chin lift
3. Jaw thrust maneuver
4. Modified head tilt–chin lift

124. The nurse understands that which is a correct guideline for adult cardiopulmonary resuscitation (CPR) for a health care provider?
1. One breath should be given for every five compressions.
2. Two breaths should be given for every 15 compressions.
3. Initially, two quick breaths should be given as rapidly as possible.
4. Each rescue breath should be given over 1 second and should produce a visible chest rise.

125. The nurse attempts to relieve an airway obstruction on a 6-year-old conscious child. Which location is the correct placement of the hands to perform this maneuver?
1. Between the groin and the abdomen
2. Between the umbilicus and the groin
3. Between the lower abdomen and the chest
4. Between the umbilicus and the xiphoid process

126. The nurse is performing cardiopulmonary resuscitation (CPR) on an adult. The nurse should deliver how many breaths per minute to the client?
1. 6
2. 10
3. 18
4. 20

127. The nurse is performing cardiopulmonary resuscitation (CPR) on an infant. When performing chest compressions, which is the compression rate for an infant?
1. 60 times per minute
2. 80 times per minute
3. 100 times per minute
4. 160 times per minute

128. Which is the **most appropriate** location for assessing the pulse of an infant who is less than 1 year old?
1. Radial
2. Carotid
3. Brachial
4. Popliteal

129. The nurse educator is teaching principles of cardiopulmonary resuscitation to a group of nursing students. The nurse asks a student to describe the reason why blind finger sweeps are avoided in infants. The nurse determines that the student understands the reason if the student makes which statement?

1. "The object may have been swallowed."
2. "The infant may bite down on the finger."
3. "The mouth is too small to see the object."
4. "The object may be forced back further into the throat."

130. The nurse is performing cardiopulmonary resuscitation (CPR) on an adult client. How far should the sternum be depressed in an adult client for effective chest compressions?

1. 1 inch
2. ¾ inch
3. 2 inches
4. 3 inches

ANSWERS

121. 4

Rationale: To relieve an airway obstruction on an unconscious woman in an advanced stage of pregnancy, the woman is placed on her back. A wedge, such as a pillow or rolled blanket, is placed under the right abdominal flank and hip to displace the uterus to the left side of the abdomen. Options 1, 2, and 3 are incorrect and can cause harm to the woman and the fetus.

Test-Taking Strategy: Focus on the subject, an unconscious pregnant woman at 8 months' gestation. Recalling the complications associated with the supine position in a pregnant client (supine hypotension) will direct you to the correct option. Review: the principles associated with relieving an airway obstruction on a pregnant woman.

Level of Cognitive Ability: Evaluating

Client Needs: Physiological Integrity

Integrated Process: Nursing Process/Evaluation

Content Area: Critical Care: Basic Life Support/Cardiopulmonary

Priority Concepts: Gas Exchange, Perfusion

Reference(s): Lowdermilk, Perry, Cashion, Alden (2012), p. 719; McKinney, James, Murray, Nelson, Ashwill (2013), pp. 237–238).

122. 3

Rationale: The nurse would follow CAB—compressions, airway, and breathing. Therefore, the next nursing action would be to start chest compressions.

Test-Taking Strategy: Focus on the strategic word, *next.* Recalling CAB—compressions, airway, breathing—will assist with directing you to option 3. Also note that options 1, 2, and 4 are comparable or alike options and address the airway. Review: CPR guidelines.

Level of Cognitive Ability: Applying

Client Needs: Physiological Integrity

Integrated Process: Nursing Process/Implementation

Content Area: Critical Care: Basic Life Support/Cardiopulmonary Resuscitation

Priority Concepts: Clinical Judgment, Gas Exchange

Reference(s): Cooper, Gosnell (2015), pp. 419–420; deWit, Kumagai (2013), p. 1034.

123. 3

Rationale: If a neck injury is suspected, the jaw thrust maneuver is used to open the airway. The head tilt–chin lift produces hyperextension of the neck and could cause complications if a neck injury is present. A flexed position is an inappropriate position for opening the airway.

Test-Taking Strategy: Focus on the subject, basic life support and opening the airway if a head or neck injury is suspected. Eliminate options 1, 2, and 4 because they are comparable or alike options. Review: Cardiopulmonary resuscitation (CPR) guidelines.

Level of Cognitive Ability: Applying

Client Needs: Physiological Integrity

Integrated Process: Nursing Process/Implementation

Content Area: Critical Care: Basic Life Support/Cardiopulmonary Resuscitation

Priority Concepts: Gas Exchange, Safety

Reference(s): deWit, Kumagai (2013), p. 1024.

124. 4

Rationale: During adult CPR, each rescue breath should be given over 1 second and should produce a visible chest rise. Excessive ventilation (too many breaths per minute or breaths that are too large or forceful) may be harmful and should not be performed. Health care providers should employ a 30 compressions-to-2 ventilations ratio for the adult victim. Options 1, 2, and 3 are incorrect.

Test-Taking Strategy: Focus on the subject, rescue breathing. Read each option carefully. Noting the words *visible chest rise* in the correct option will direct you to this option. Review: cardiopulmonary resuscitation guidelines.

Level of Cognitive Ability: Understanding

Client Needs: Physiological Integrity

Integrated Process: Nursing Process/Implementation

Content Area: Critical Care: Basic Life Support/Cardiopulmonary Resuscitation

Priority Concepts: Clinical Judgment, Gas Exchange

Reference(s): Perry, Potter, Ostendorf (2014), pp. 658, 688.

125. 4

Rationale: To relieve an airway obstruction in a child, the rescuer stands behind the victim and places the arms directly under the victim's axillae and around the victim. The rescuer places the thumb side of one fist against the victim's abdomen in the midline slightly above the umbilicus and well below the tip of the xiphoid process. The rescuer grasps the fist with the other hand and delivers up to five thrusts. One must take care not to touch the xiphoid process or the lower margins of the rib cage, because force applied to these structures may damage the internal organs. Options 1, 2, and 3 are incorrect hand placements.

Test-Taking Strategy: Focus on the subject, airway obstruction in a child. Eliminate options 1 and 2 first, because they are comparable or alike options. From the remaining options, considering the anatomic location and the effect of the maneuver for dislodging an obstruction will direct you to option 4. **Review:** the correct hand placement for relieving an **airway obstruction.**
Level of Cognitive Ability: Applying
Client Needs: Physiological Integrity
Integrated Process: Nursing Process/Implementation
Content Area: Critical Care: Basic Life Support/Cardiopulmonary Resuscitation
Priority Concepts: Clinical Judgment, Gas Exchange
Reference(s): Hockenberry, Wilson (2013), p. 759; McKinney, James, Murray, Nelson, Ashwill (2013), pp. 851–852.

126. 2
Rationale: Each rescue breath is delivered over 1 second at a rate of 1 breath every 8 seconds (8 to 10 ventilations per minute). Options 1, 3, and 4 are incorrect.
Test-Taking Strategy: Focus on the subject, breaths per minute. It is necessary to know that the client receives 8 to 10 ventilations per minute. **Review: cardiopulmonary resuscitation guidelines.**
Level of Cognitive Ability: Applying
Client Needs: Physiological Integrity
Integrated Process: Nursing Process/Implementation
Content Area: Critical Care: Basic Life Support/Cardiopulmonary Resuscitation
Priority Concepts: Gas Exchange, Perfusion
Reference(s): Perry, Potter, Ostendorf (2014), p. 685.

127. 3
Rationale: For an infant, the rate of chest compressions is at least 100 per minute. Options 1 and 2 identify rates that are too low, and option 4 identifies a rate that is too high.
Test-Taking Strategy: Focus on the subject, normal heart rate of an infant. Eliminate options 1 and 2 because of the low rates identified in the options. Eliminate option 4 because this rate would be much too rapid for an infant. **Review: cardiopulmonary resuscitation guidelines for an infant.**
Level of Cognitive Ability: Applying
Client Needs: Physiological Integrity
Integrated Process: Nursing Process/Implementation
Content Area: Critical Care: Basic Life Support/Cardiopulmonary Resuscitation
Priority Concepts: Gas Exchange, Perfusion
Reference(s): Hockenberry, Wilson (2013), p. 756.

128. 3
Rationale: To assess a pulse in an infant (i.e., a child younger than 1 year old), the pulse is checked at the brachial artery (femoral artery can also be used). The infant's relatively short, fat neck makes palpation of the carotid artery difficult. The popliteal and radial pulses are also difficult to palpate in an infant.
Test-Taking Strategy: Note the strategic words, *most appropriate,* and focus on the subject, the location for a pulse check in an infant. Considering the body structure of an infant will assist with directing you to the correct option. **Review: cardiopulmonary resuscitation guidelines for an infant.**
Level of Cognitive Ability: Applying
Client Needs: Physiological Integrity
Integrated Process: Nursing Process/Data Collection
Content Area: Critical Care: Basic Life Support/Cardiopulmonary Resuscitation
Priority Concepts: Development, Perfusion
Reference(s): Hockenberry, Wilson (2013), p. 757.

129. 4
Rationale: Blind finger sweeps are not recommended for infants and children because of the risk of forcing the object further down into the airway. Options 1, 2, and 3 are not related directly to the subject of the question.
Test-Taking Strategy: Focus on the subject, the reason for avoiding blind finger sweeps. Note that the correct option addresses the airway. **Review:** the management of an **obstructed airway in an infant or a child.**
Level of Cognitive Ability: Evaluating
Client Needs: Physiological Integrity
Integrated Process: Teaching and Learning
Content Area: Critical Care: Basic Life Support/Cardiopulmonary Resuscitation
Priority Concepts: Gas Exchange, Safety
Reference(s): Hockenberry, Wilson (2013), p. 758.

130. 3
Rationale: When performing CPR on an adult client, the sternum is depressed 2 inches. Options 1 and 2 identify compression depths that would be ineffective for an adult, and option 4 identifies a depth that could cause injury to the client.
Test-Taking Strategy: Note the subject, depth of chest compressions for an adult. Consider the normal body structure of an adult to assist with directing you to option 3. **Review: cardiopulmonary resuscitation guidelines.**
Level of Cognitive Ability: Applying
Client Needs: Physiological Integrity
Integrated Process: Nursing Process/Implementation
Content Area: Critical Care: Basic Life Support/Cardiopulmonary Resuscitation
Priority Concepts: Gas Exchange, Perfusion
Reference(s): Perry, Potter, Ostendorf (2014), p. 685.

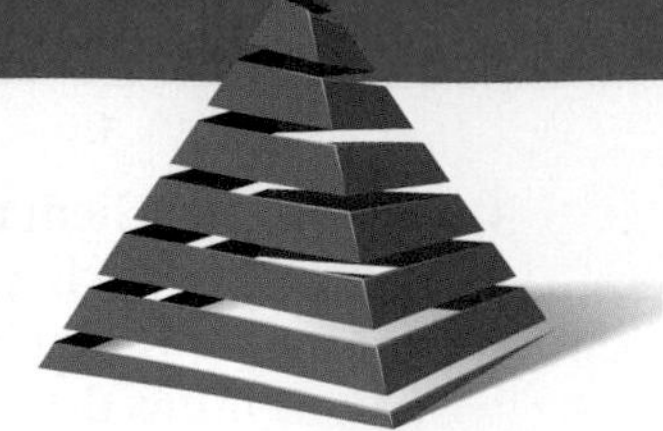

CHAPTER 17

Perioperative Nursing Care

CRITICAL THINKING What Should You Do?

The nurse is present when a surgeon is obtaining informed consent from a client for a scheduled surgical procedure. The client signs the consent, and after the surgeon leaves the nursing unit, the client informs the nurse that he is unclear about certain aspects of the surgical procedure. What should the nurse do?

Answer is located on p. 181.

I. Preoperative Care

A client may return home shortly after having a surgical procedure because many surgical procedures are done through ambulatory care or 1-day-stay surgical units. Perioperative care procedures apply even if the client returns home the same day of the surgical procedure.

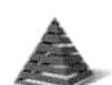

A. Obtaining informed consent
   1. The surgeon is responsible for obtaining the informed consent for surgery.
   2. Minors (clients younger than 18 years old) may need a parent or legal guardian to sign the informed consent form.
   3. Older clients may need a legal guardian to sign the informed consent form.
   4. Psychiatric clients have a right to refuse treatment until a court has legally determined that they are unable to make decisions for themselves.
   5. No sedation should be administered to the client before he or she signs the informed consent form.
   6. The nurse may witness the client signing the informed consent form, but the nurse must be sure that the client has understood the surgeon's explanation of the surgery.
   7. The nurse needs to document the witnessing of the signing of the operative consent form after the client acknowledges understanding the procedure.

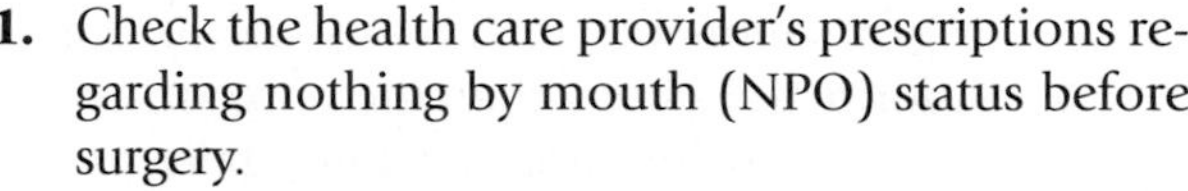

B. Nutrition
   1. Check the health care provider's prescriptions regarding nothing by mouth (NPO) status before surgery.
   2. Solid foods and liquids are generally withheld for 6 to 8 hours before general anesthesia and for 3 hours before surgery with local anesthesia to avoid aspiration.
   3. Monitor intravenous (IV) fluids, if prescribed.
   4. Note that parenteral nutrition may be prescribed for clients who are malnourished, have protein or metabolic deficiencies from underlying disease, or cannot ingest foods.

C. Elimination
   1. If the client is to have intestinal or abdominal surgery, the surgeon may prescribe an enema, laxative, or both the day or evening before surgery.
   2. The client should void immediately before surgery. 
   3. Prepare to insert a Foley catheter, if prescribed; if there is a Foley catheter in place, it should be emptied immediately before surgery, and the amount and quality of urine output should be documented.

D. Surgical site
   1. Prepare to clean the surgical site with a mild antiseptic soap the night before surgery, as prescribed.
   2. Inform the client about the procedure for shaving the operative site; shaving may be done in the operative area.

The hair on the head or face is shaved only if it will interfere with the surgical procedure and only if prescribed.

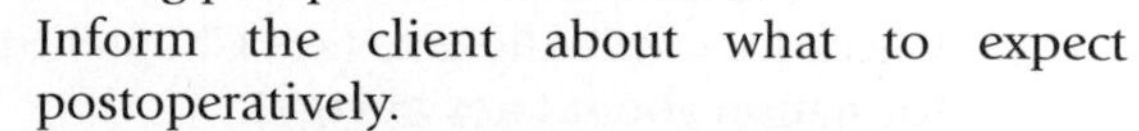

E. Reinforcing preoperative instructions
   1. Inform the client about what to expect postoperatively.
   2. Tell the client to notify the nurse if he or she experiences any postoperative pain and that pain medication will be prescribed to be given as the client requests.

3. Instruct the client to use noninvasive pain relief techniques such as relaxation or guided imagery before the pain occurs and as soon as the pain is noticed.
4. Reinforce instructions about the use of a patient-controlled analgesia pump if its use is prescribed.
5. Inform the client that requesting an opioid after surgery will not make the client a drug addict, and explain the difference between analgesic need and psychological dependence.
6. The client should be instructed not to smoke for at least 24 hours before surgery; discuss smoking cessation and treatments and programs.
7. Inform the client that the surgeon will need to be consulted about taking daily prescribed medications, aspirin, selected vitamins, and herbal products before surgery and when these products need to be stopped.

8. Instruct the client in deep breathing and coughing techniques, the use of incentive spirometry, and the importance of performing the techniques after surgery to prevent the development of pneumonia and atelectasis (Box 17-1 and Fig. 17-1).
9. Instruct the client in leg and foot exercises to prevent venous stasis of blood and facilitate venous blood return (Fig. 17-2; also see Box 17-1).
10. Instruct the client about how to splint an incision and how to turn and reposition (Fig. 17-3; also see Box 17-1).
11. Inform the client of any invasive devices that may be needed after surgery, such as tubes, drains, Foley catheters, or IV lines.
12. Tell the client not to pull on any of the invasive devices. They will be removed as soon as possible.

F. Psychosocial preparation
1. Be alert to the client's anxiety level.
2. Encourage the client to talk about feelings.
3. Answer questions or address concerns that the client may have regarding surgery.
4. Allow time for privacy for the client to prepare psychologically for surgery.
5. Provide support and assistance as needed.
6. Consider any cultural aspects when providing care (Box 17-2).

G. Preoperative checklist
1. Ensure that the client is wearing an identification bracelet.
2. Check for client allergies (see Chapter 61 for information about latex allergy).
3. Review the preoperative checklist to be sure that each item is addressed before the client is transported to surgery.
4. Follow agency policies regarding preoperative procedures, including informed consents, preoperative checklists, prescribed laboratory or radiological tests, or any other preoperative procedure.
5. Ensure that consent forms have been signed for the operative procedure, anesthesia, any blood transfusions, the disposal of a limb, or surgical sterilization procedures.
6. Ensure that a history and physical examination were completed and documented in the client's record (Box 17-3).
7. Ensure that any consultation reports that were prescribed are completed and documented in the client's record.

BOX 17-1 Preoperative Instructions

Deep Breathing and Coughing Exercises

Instruct the client that a sitting position provides the best lung expansion for coughing and deep breathing exercises.

Instruct the client to breathe deeply three times by inhaling through the nostrils and exhaling slowly through pursed lips.

Instruct the client that the third breath should be held for 3 seconds; then the client should cough deeply three times splinting the operative site if necessary.

The client should perform this exercise every 2 hours.

Incentive Spirometry

Instruct the client to assume a sitting or upright position.

Instruct the client to place the mouth tightly around the mouthpiece.

Instruct the client to inhale slowly to raise and maintain the flow rate indicator between the 600 and 900 marks.

Instruct the client to hold his or her breath for 5 seconds and then to exhale through pursed lips.

Instruct the client to repeat this process 10 times every hour.

Leg and Foot Exercises

Gastrocnemius (calf) pumping: Instruct the client to move both ankles by pointing the toes up and then down.

Quadriceps (thigh) setting: Instruct the client to press the back of the knees against the bed and then to relax the knees. This contracts and relaxes the thigh and calf muscles to prevent thrombus formation.

Foot circles: Instruct the client to rotate each foot in a circle.

Hip and knee movements: Instruct the client to flex the knee and thigh, straighten the leg, and hold the position for 5 seconds before lowering. (This should not be performed if the client is having abdominal surgery or has a back problem.)

Splinting the Incision

If the surgical incision is abdominal or thoracic, instruct the client to place a pillow or one hand with the other hand on top over the incisional area.

During deep breathing and coughing, the client presses gently against the area of the incision to splint or support it.

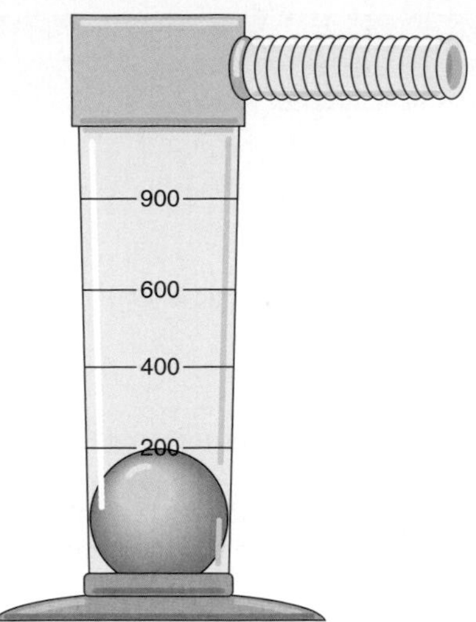

FIGURE 17-1 Incentive spirometer. (From Monahan F, Sands J, Neighbors M, Marek J, Green C: *Phipps' medical-surgical nursing: Health and illness perspectives,* ed 8, St. Louis, 2007, Mosby.)

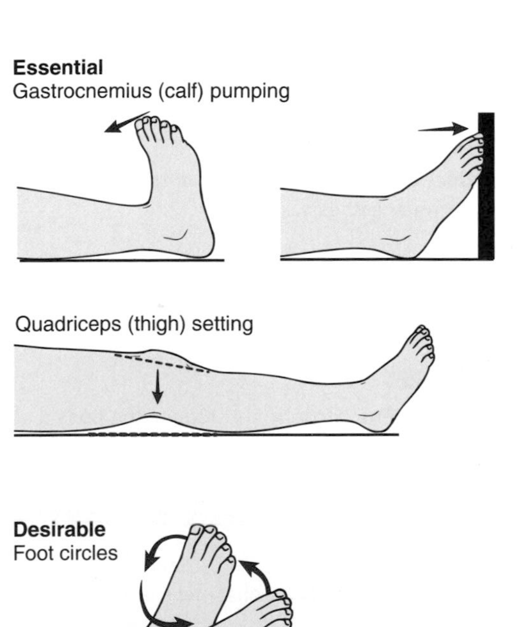

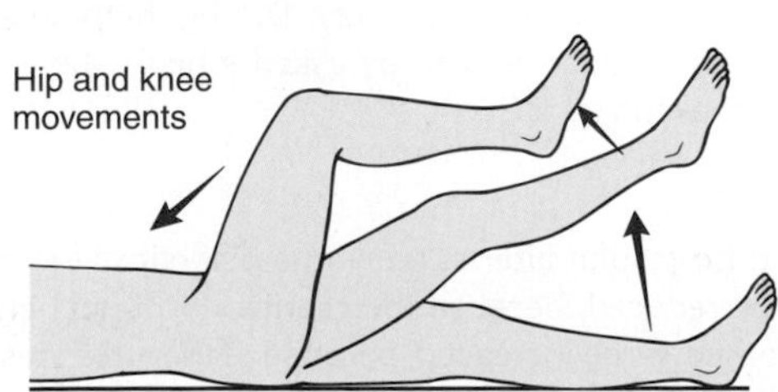

FIGURE 17-2 Postoperative leg exercises. (From Lewis S, Heitkemper M, Dirksen S: *Medical-surgical nursing: Assessment and management of clinical problems,* ed 6, St. Louis, 2004, Mosby.)

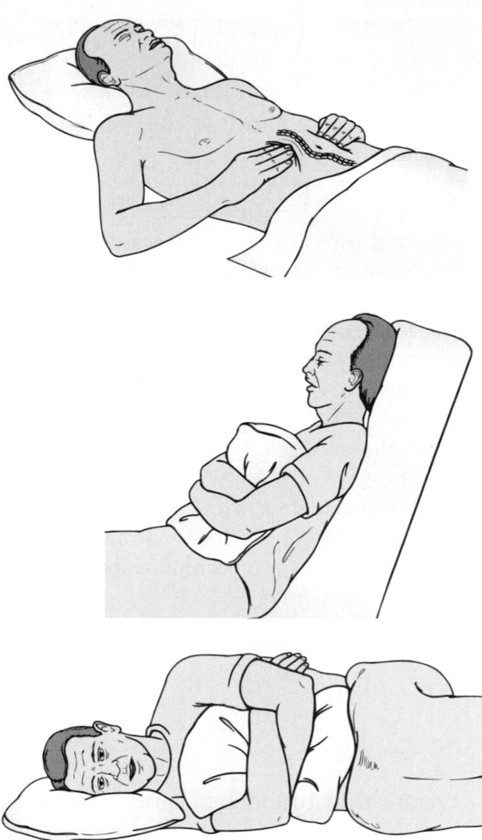

FIGURE 17-3 Techniques for splinting a wound when coughing. (From Lewis S, Dirksen S, Heitkemper M, Bucher L, Camera I: *Medical-surgical nursing: Assessment and management of clinical problems,* ed 8, St. Louis, 2011, Mosby.)

BOX 17-2 Cultural Aspects of Perioperative Nursing Care

Cultural assessment includes questions related to:

- Primary language spoken and cultural practices
- Feelings related to surgery and pain
- Pain management
- Expectations
- Support systems
- Feelings toward self

Allow a family member to be present, if appropriate.

Secure the help of a professional interpreter to communicate with non-English-speaking clients.

Use pictures or phrase cards to communicate and assess the non-English-speaking client's perception of pain or other feelings.

Provide preoperative and postoperative educational materials in the appropriate language.

Adapted from Potter P, Perry A, Stockel P, Hall A: *Fundamentals of Nursing,* ed 8, St. Louis, 2013, Mosby.

8. Ensure that the prescribed laboratory test results are documented in the client's rec ord.
9. Ensure that any prescribed electrocardiography and chest radiography reports are noted in the client's record.

BOX 17-3 Medical Conditions That Increase the Risk of Surgery

- Bleeding disorders, such as thrombocytopenia and hemophilia
- Diabetes mellitus
- Chronic pain
- Heart disease, such as a recent myocardial infarction, dysrhythmia, congestive heart failure, and peripheral vascular disease
- Obstructive sleep apnea
- Upper respiratory infection
- Liver disease
- Fever
- Chronic respiratory disease, such as emphysema, bronchitis, or asthma
- Immunological disorders, such as leukemia, acquired immunodeficiency syndrome, bone marrow depression, and the use of chemotherapy or immunosuppressive agents
- The abuse of street drugs

Adapted from Potter P, Perry A, Stockel P, Hall A: *Fundamentals of Nursing*, ed 8, St. Louis, 2013, Mosby.

10. Ensure that blood type and screen and cross-match are noted in the client's record.
11. Remove according to the agency's policy the client's jewelry, makeup, dentures, hairpins, nail polish, and any prostheses.
    a. Hearing aids or glasses may be removed at the last possible moment before surgery.
    b. Clients with language or hearing concerns need to have access to agency-approved translators until anesthesia induction.
12. Document that valuables were given to the client's family members or locked in the hospital safe.
13. Monitor and document the client's vital signs.
14. Document the last time that the client ate or drank.
15. Document that the client has voided before surgery.
16. Document that the prescribed preoperative medication was given (Box 17-4).

H. Preoperative medications
1. Prepare to assist to administer preoperative medications as prescribed or to have them be administered in the operating room immediately before the surgery.
2. Instruct the client that he or she will feel drowsy after the medications are given.

⚠ After administering the preoperative medications, keep the client in bed with the side rails up (per agency policy). Place the call bell next to the client; instruct the client not to get out of bed and to call for assistance if needed.

BOX 17-4 Substances That Can Affect the Surgical Client

Antibiotics

These potentiate the action of anesthetic agents.

Anticholinergics

Medications with anticholinergic effects increase the potential for confusion.

Anticoagulants

These alter normal clotting factors and increase the risk of hemorrhage.

Aspirin (acetylsalicylic acid) and nonsteroidal anti-inflammatory drugs are commonly used medications that can alter clotting mechanisms.

Complementary remedies such as garlic and ginseng may also alter normal clotting factors.

These medications should be discontinued at least 48 hours before surgery or as prescribed.

Anticonvulsants

The long-term use of certain anticonvulsants can alter the metabolism of anesthetic agents.

Antidepressants

These may lower the blood pressure during anesthesia.

Complementary remedies such as St. John's wort may also lower blood pressure.

Antidysrhythmics

These reduce cardiac contractility and impair cardiac conduction during anesthesia.

Antihypertensives

These can interact with anesthetic agents and cause bradycardia, hypotension, and impaired circulation.

Corticosteroids

These cause adrenal atrophy and reduce the body's ability to withstand stress.

Before and during surgery, dosages may be temporarily increased.

Diuretics

These potentiate electrolyte imbalances after surgery.

Herbal Substances

These can interact with anesthesia and cause a variety of adverse effects. These substances may need to be stopped at a specific time before surgery. During the preoperative period, the client needs to be asked if he or she is taking any herbal substances.

Insulin

The need for insulin after surgery in a diabetic client may either be reduced, because the client's nutritional intake is decreased, or be increased, because of the stress response and the intravenous administration of glucose solutions.

Adapted from Potter P, Perry A, Stockel P, Hall A: *Fundamentals of Nursing*, ed 8, St. Louis, 2013, Mosby.

I. Arrival in the operating room
   1. Guidelines to eliminate wrong site and wrong procedure surgery
      a. The surgeon meets with the client in the preoperative area and uses indelible ink to mark the operative site.
      b. In the operating room, the nurse and surgeon ensure and reconfirm that the operative site has been appropriately marked.
      c. Just before starting the surgical procedure, a time-out is conducted with all members of the operative team present to identify the appropriate surgical site again.
   2. When the client arrives in the operating room, the operating room nurse will verify the identification bracelet with the client's verbal response and will review the client's chart.
   3. The client's chart will be checked for completeness and reviewed for informed consent forms, history and physical examination, and allergic reaction information.
   4. HCPs' prescriptions will be verified and implemented.
   5. The IV line may be initiated at this time (or in the preoperative area), if prescribed.
   6. The anesthesia team will administer the prescribed anesthesia.

Verification of the client and the surgical operative site is critical.

II. Postoperative Care

A. Description:
   1. **Immediate postoperative stage:** the period of 1 to 4 hours after surgery
   2. **Intermediate postoperative stage:** the period of 4 to 24 hours after surgery
   3. **Extended postoperative stage:** the period of at least 1 to 4 days after surgery

B. Respiratory system

Monitor breath sounds. Stridor, wheezing, or a crowing sound can indicate partial obstruction, bronchospasm, or laryngospasm; crackles or rhonchi may indicate pulmonary edema.

   1. Monitor vital signs.
   2. Monitor airway patency and ensure adequate ventilation (prolonged mechanical ventilation during anesthesia may affect postoperative lung function).
   3. Remember that extubated clients who are lethargic may not be able to maintain an airway.
   4. Monitor for secretions; if the client is unable to clear the airway by coughing, suction the secretions from the client's airway.
   5. Observe chest movement for symmetry and the use of accessory muscles.
   6. Monitor oxygen administration if prescribed.
   7. Monitor pulse oximetry.
   8. Encourage deep breathing and coughing exercises and the use of the incentive spirometer as soon as possible after surgery.
   9. Note the rate, depth, and quality of respirations; the respiratory rate should be higher than 10 and lower than 30 breaths/minute.
   10. Monitor for signs of respiratory distress, atelectasis, or other respiratory complications.

C. Cardiovascular system
   1. Monitor circulatory status, such as skin color, peripheral pulses, capillary refill, and the absence of edema, numbness, and tingling.
   2. Monitor for bleeding.
   3. Check the pulse for rate and rhythm (a bounding pulse may indicate hypertension, fluid overload, or client anxiety).
   4. Monitor for cardiac dysrhythmias.
   5. Monitor for signs of thrombophlebitis, particularly in clients who were in the lithotomy position during surgery.
   6. Encourage the use of antiembolism stockings, if prescribed, to promote venous return, strengthen muscle tone, and prevent pooling of blood in the extremities.

D. Musculoskeletal system
   1. Monitor the client for movement of the extremities.
   2. Review surgeon's prescriptions regarding client positioning or restrictions.
   3. Encourage ambulation if prescribed; before ambulation, instruct the client to sit at the edge of the bed with his or her feet supported to assume balance.
   4. Unless contraindicated, place the client in a low **Fowler's position** after surgery to increase the size of the thorax for lung expansion.

   5. Avoid positioning the postoperative client in a supine position until pharyngeal reflexes have returned; if the client is comatose or semicomatose, position on the side (in addition, an oral airway may be needed).
   6. If the client is unable to get out of bed, turn the client every 1 to 2 hours.

E. Neurological system
   1. Monitor level of consciousness.
   2. Frequent periodic attempts to awaken the client should continue until the client awakens.

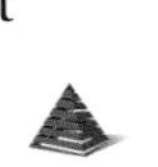

   3. Orient the client to the environment.
   4. Speak in a soft tone; filter out extraneous noises in the environment.
   5. Maintain body temperature and prevent heat loss by providing the client with warm blankets and raising the room temperature as necessary.

F. Temperature control
   1. Monitor temperature.

2. Monitor for signs of hypothermia that may result from anesthesia, a cool operating room, or exposure of the skin and internal organs during surgery.
3. Apply warm blankets and continue oxygen as prescribed if the client experiences shivering.

G. Integumentary system
1. Check the surgical site, drains, and wound dressings (serous drainage may occur from an incision, but if excessive bleeding occurs from the site, the surgeon is notified).
2. Check the skin for redness, abrasions, or breakdown that may have resulted from surgical positioning.
3. Monitor body temperature and wound for signs of infection.
4. Maintain a dry, intact dressing.
5. Change dressings as prescribed, noting the amount of bleeding or drainage, odor, and intactness of sutures or staples.
6. Wound drains should be patent; prepare to assist with the removal of drains (as prescribed by the surgeon) when the drainage amount becomes insignificant.
7. An abdominal binder may be prescribed for obese and debilitated individuals to prevent dehiscence of the incision (Fig. 17-4).

H. Fluid and electrolyte balance
1. Monitor IV fluid administration as prescribed.
2. Record intake and output.
3. Monitor for signs of fluid or electrolyte imbalances.

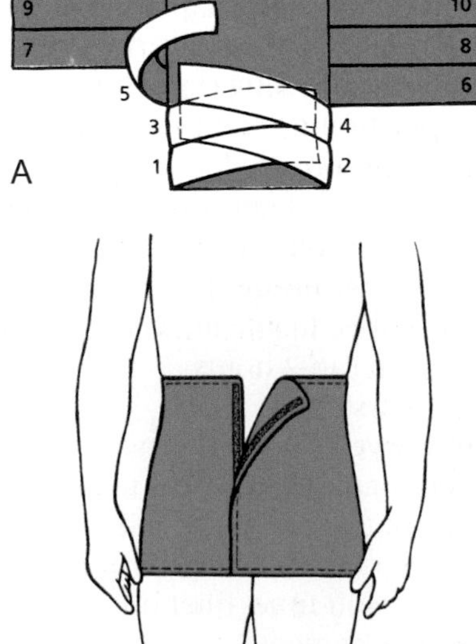

FIGURE 17-4 Abdominal binders. **A,** Scultetus: binder with flaps that wrap over each other. **B,** Straight binder with Velcro. (From Elkin M, Perry A, Potter P: *Nursing interventions and clinical skills*, ed 4, St. Louis, 2008, Mosby.)

I. Gastrointestinal system
1. Monitor intake and output and for nausea and vomiting.
2. Maintain patency of the nasogastric tube if present.
3. Monitor for abdominal distention.
4. Monitor for passage of flatus and return of bowel sounds. 
5. Administer frequent oral care, at least every 2 hours.
6. Maintain the NPO status until the gag reflex and peristalsis return. 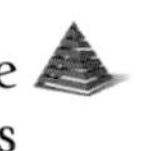
7. When oral fluids are permitted, start with ice chips and water.
8. Ensure that the client advances to clear liquids and then to a regular diet, as prescribed and as the client can tolerate.

To prevent aspiration, turn the client to a side-lying position if vomiting occurs and have suctioning equipment available and ready to use.

J. Renal system
1. Assess the bladder for distention.
2. Monitor urine output (urinary output should be at least 30 mL/hr). 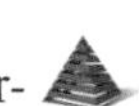
3. If the client does not have a Foley catheter, the client is expected to void within 6 to 8 hours postoperatively, depending on the type of anesthesia administered; ensure that the amount is at least 200 mL. 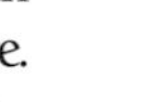

K. Pain management
1. Assess the type of anesthetic used and preoperative medication that the client received, and note whether the client received any pain medications in the postanesthesia period.
2. Assess for pain and inquire about the type and location of pain; ask the client to rate the degree of pain on a scale of 1 to 10, with 10 being the most severe.
3. If the client is unable to rate the pain with a numerical pain scale, then use a descriptor scale that lists words that describe different levels of pain intensity, such as *no pain, mild pain, moderate pain*, and *severe pain*.
4. Monitor for objective data related to pain, such as facial expressions, body gestures, increased pulse rate, increased blood pressure, and increased respirations.
5. Inquire about the effectiveness of the last pain medication.
6. Administer pain medication as prescribed.
7. Ensure that the client with a patient-controlled analgesia pump understands how to use it; reinforce instructions as needed.
8. If an opioid has been prescribed, during the initial administration, assess the client every 30 minutes for respiratory rate and pain relief.

9. Use noninvasive measures to relieve postoperative pain, including distraction, comfort measures, positioning, backrubs, and providing a quiet and restful environment.
10. Document effectiveness of the pain medication and noninvasive pain relief measures.

⚠ Consider cultural practices and beliefs when planning pain management.

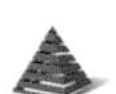

III. Pneumonia and Atelectasis (Fig. 17-5 and Box 17-5)

A. Description
   1. Pneumonia, which is an inflammation of the alveoli caused by an infectious process, may develop 3 to 5 days after the surgical procedure because of infection, aspiration, or immobility.
   2. Atelectasis, which is a collapse of the alveoli with retained mucous secretions, is the most common postoperative complication. It usually occurs 1 to 2 days after the surgical procedure.

B. Data collection
   1. Dyspnea and increased respiratory rate
   2. Elevated temperature
   3. Productive cough and chest pain
   4. Crackles over involved lung area

C. Interventions
   1. Monitor lung and breath sounds and temperature.
   2. Encourage fluid intake and ambulation.
   3. Reposition the client every 1 to 2 hours.
   4. Encourage the client to deep breathe, cough, and use an incentive spirometer.
   5. Suction to clear secretions if the client is unable to cough.

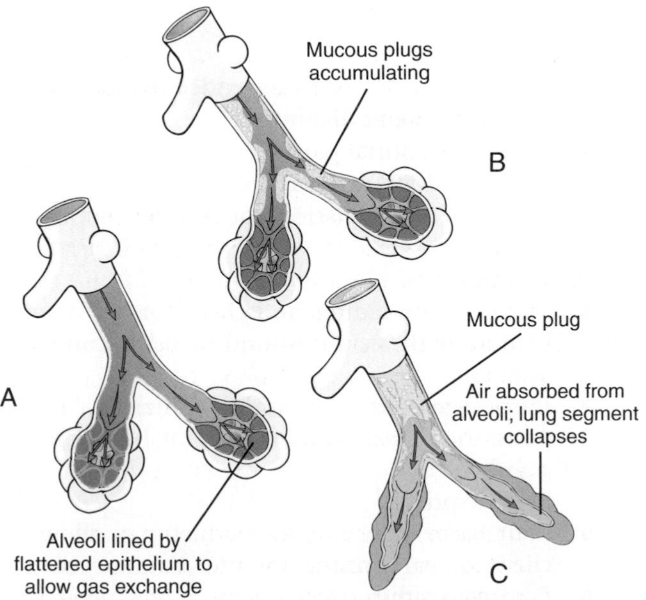

FIGURE 17-5 Postoperative atelectasis. **A,** Normal bronchiole and alveoli. **B,** Mucous plug in bronchiole. **C,** Collapse of alveoli as a result of atelectasis after the absorption of air. (From Lewis S, Dirksen S, Heitkemper M, Bucher L, Camera I: *Medical-surgical nursing: Assessment and management of clinical problems,* ed 8, St. Louis, 2011, Mosby.)

BOX 17-5 Postoperative Complications

- Constipation
- Hemorrhage
- Hypoxia
- Paralytic ileus
- Pneumonia and atelectasis
- Pulmonary embolism
- Shock
- Thrombophlebitis
- Urinary retention
- Wound dehiscence
- Wound evisceration
- Wound infection

Note: The licensed practical/vocational nurse always notifies the registered nurse and/or the surgeon if signs of complications are noted.

IV. Hypoxia (see Box 17-5)

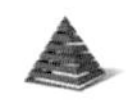

A. Description: An inadequate concentration of oxygen in arterial blood; in the postoperative client, hypoxemia can be due to shallow breathing from the effects of anesthesia or medications.

B. Data collection
   1. Restlessness
   2. Dyspnea
   3. Diaphoresis
   4. Tachycardia
   5. Hypertension
   6. Cyanosis

C. Interventions
   1. Monitor for signs of hypoxia, eliminate the cause of hypoxia, and notify the registered nurse and/or surgeon immediately.
   2. Monitor lung and breath sounds and pulse oximetry.
   3. Administer oxygen, as prescribed.
   4. Encourage coughing, deep breathing, and the use of incentive spirometry.
   5. Turn and reposition the client frequently; encourage ambulation.

V. Pulmonary Embolism (see Box 17-5)

A. Description: An embolus blocking the pulmonary artery and disrupting the blood flow to one or more lobes of the lung

B. Data collection
   1. Sudden dyspnea
   2. Sudden sharp chest or upper abdominal pain
   3. Cyanosis
   4. Tachycardia
   5. A drop in blood pressure

C. Interventions
   1. Notify the registered nurse and/or surgeon immediately because pulmonary embolism may be life-threatening and requires emergency action.
   2. Monitor vital signs.
   3. Administer oxygen, as prescribed.

VI. Hemorrhage (see Box 17-5)

A. Description: The loss of a large amount of blood externally or internally during a short period of time

B. Data collection
1. Restlessness
2. Weak, rapid pulse and hypotension
3. Tachypnea
4. Cool, clammy skin
5. Reduced urine output

C. Interventions
1. Apply pressure to the site of bleeding.
2. Notify the registered nurse and/or surgeon immediately.
3. Administer oxygen, as prescribed.

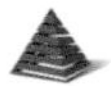

VII. Shock (see Box 17-5)

A. Description: A loss of circulatory fluid volume that is usually caused by hemorrhage

B. Data collection: Similar to data collection findings of hemorrhage

C. Interventions
1. If shock develops, elevate the legs.
2. If the client has had spinal anesthesia, do not elevate the legs any higher than placing them on a pillow; otherwise, diaphragm muscles could be impaired.
3. Notify the registered nurse and/or surgeon immediately.
4. Administer oxygen, as prescribed.
5. Monitor the level of consciousness.
6. Monitor vital signs for an increased pulse and decreased blood pressure.
7. Monitor color, temperature, turgor, and moisture of the skin and mucous membranes.
8. Assist with the administration of medications as prescribed.

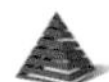

VIII. Thrombophlebitis (see Box 17-5)

A. Description
1. An inflammation of a vein, often accompanied by clot formation
2. Veins in the legs are most commonly affected.

B. Data collection
1. Aching or cramping leg pain
2. Vein inflammation; vein feels hard and cord-like and is tender to touch.
3. Elevated temperature

C. Interventions
1. Monitor legs for swelling, inflammation, cyanosis, pain, tenderness, and venous distention; the registered nurse is notified immediately.
2. Elevate the extremity 30 degrees without allowing any pressure on the popliteal area as prescribed.

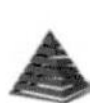

3. Encourage the use of antiembolism stockings as prescribed; remove stockings twice a day to wash and inspect the legs.

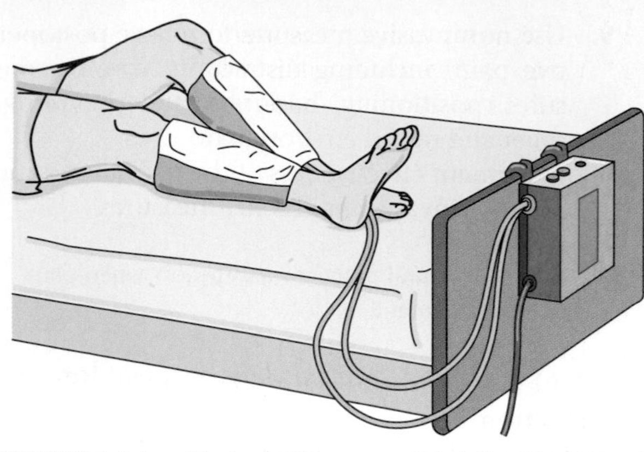

FIGURE 17-6 Intermittent pulsatile compression device. (From Monahan F, Sands J, Neighbors M, Marek J, Green C: *Phipps' medical-surgical nursing: Health and illness perspectives*, ed 8, St. Louis, 2007, Mosby.)

4. Use an intermittent pulsatile compression device as prescribed (Fig. 17-6).
5. Prepare to perform passive range-of-motion exercises every 2 hours if the client is confined to bed rest.
6. Encourage early ambulation, as prescribed.
7. Do not allow the client to dangle the legs.
8. Instruct the client not to sit in one position for an extended period of time.
9. Anticoagulants such as heparin sodium or warfarin (Coumadin) may be prescribed.

IX. Urinary Retention (see Box 17-5)

A. Description
1. The involuntary accumulation of urine in the bladder from a loss of muscle tone
2. Occurs as a result of the effects of anesthetics and opioid analgesics and appears about 6 to 8 hours after surgery

B. Data collection
1. Inability to void and a distended bladder
2. Restlessness and diaphoresis
3. Lower abdominal pain
4. Elevated blood pressure
5. Note that on percussion, the bladder sounds like a drum.

C. Interventions
1. Monitor for voiding, and check for a distended bladder with an ultrasound bladder scanner, if available.
2. Encourage fluid intake unless contraindicated.
3. Assist the client to void by helping him or her to stand.
4. Provide privacy.
5. Pour warm water over the perineum or allow the client to hear running water to promote voiding.
6. Prepare to catheterize the client, as prescribed, after all noninvasive techniques have been attempted.

X. Constipation (see Box 17-5)

A. Description

1. The abnormal and infrequent passage of stool
2. When the client resumes a solid diet after surgery, failure to pass stool within 48 hours is a cause for concern.

B. Data collection
1. Absence of bowel movements
2. Abdominal distention
3. Anorexia, headache, and nausea

C. Interventions
1. Check bowel sounds.
2. Encourage fluid intake up to 3000 mL/day unless contraindicated.
3. Encourage early ambulation.
4. Encourage the consumption of fiber-rich foods unless contraindicated.
5. Provide privacy and adequate time for bowel elimination.
6. Administer stool softeners and laxatives, as prescribed.

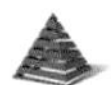

XI. Paralytic Ileus (see Box 17-5)

A. Description
1. A failure of the appropriate forward movement of bowel contents
2. May occur as a result of anesthetic medications or the manipulation of the bowel during the surgical procedure

B. Data collection
1. Postoperative nausea and vomiting
2. Abdominal distention
3. Absence of bowel sounds, bowel movement, or flatus

C. Interventions
1. Maintain NPO status until bowel sounds return.
2. Maintain the patency of the nasogastric tube, if present.
3. Encourage ambulation.
4. Monitor IV fluids, as prescribed.
5. Assist to administer medications, as prescribed, to increase gastrointestinal motility and secretions.
6. If ileus occurs, it is usually first treated nonsurgically with bowel decompression by the insertion of a nasogastric tube attached to intermittent or constant suction.

Vomiting postoperatively, abdominal distention, and absence of bowel sounds may be signs of paralytic ileus.

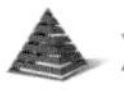

XII. Wound Infection (see Box 17-5)

A. Description
1. Wound infection may be caused by poor aseptic technique or a contaminated wound before surgical exploration; existing client conditions such as diabetes mellitus or immunocompromise may place the client at risk.
2. Infection usually occurs 3 to 6 days after surgery.
3. Purulent material may exit from the drains or separated wound edges.

B. Data collection
1. Fever and chills
2. Warm, tender, painful, and inflamed incision site
3. Edematous skin at the incision and tight skin sutures
4. Elevated white blood cell count

C. Interventions
1. Monitor the temperature.
2. Monitor the incision site for approximation of the suture line, edema, bleeding, and signs of infection (*REEDA*: Redness, Edema, Ecchymosis, Drainage, and Approximation of the wound edges); the registered nurse and surgeon are notified if signs of infection are present
3. Maintain patency of drains, and assess drainage amount, color, and consistency.
4. Maintain asepsis and change the dressing, as prescribed.
5. Assist to administer antibiotics, as prescribed.

XIII. Wound Dehiscence and Evisceration (Fig. 17-7; also see Box 17-5)

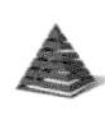

A. Description
1. Wound dehiscence is separation of the wound edges at the suture line; it usually occurs 6 to 8 days after surgery.
2. Wound evisceration is protrusion of the internal organs through an incision; it usually occurs 6 to 8 days after surgery.
3. Evisceration is most common among obese clients, clients who have had abdominal surgery, or those who have poor wound-healing ability.
4. Wound evisceration is an emergency. 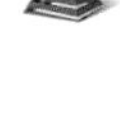

B. Data collection: Dehiscence
1. Increased drainage
2. Opened wound edges
3. The appearance of underlying tissues through the wound

C. Data Collection: Evisceration
1. Discharge of serosanguineous fluid from a previously dry wound
2. The appearance of loops of bowel or other abdominal contents through the wound
3. Client reports feeling a popping sensation after coughing or turning.

D. Interventions (see Priority Nursing Actions)
1. Notify the registered nurse and/or surgeon immediately.
2. Place the client in a low Fowler's position with the knees bent to prevent abdominal tension on abdominal wounds.
3. Cover the wound with a sterile normal saline dressing.
4. Prevent wound infection through strict asepsis.
5. Assist to administer antiemetics as prescribed to prevent vomiting and further strain on the abdominal incision.

Fundamentals

PRIORITY NURSING ACTIONS!

Actions to Take If Evisceration Occurs

1. Call for help; the registered nurse will contact the surgeon and ask that needed supplies be brought to the client's room.
2. Stay with the client.
3. While waiting for supplies to arrive, place the client in a low Fowler's position with the knees bent.
4. Cover the wound with a sterile normal saline dressing and keep the dressing moist.
5. Take vital signs and monitor the client closely for signs of shock.
6. Prepare the client for surgery as necessary.
7. Document the occurrence, the actions taken, and the client's response.

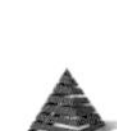

Wound evisceration is protrusion of the internal organs through an incision; it usually occurs 6 to 8 days after surgery. Evisceration is most common among obese clients, clients who have had abdominal surgery, or those who have poor wound-healing ability. Wound evisceration is an emergency. The nurse immediately calls the registered nurse for help, and the surgeon will be notified. Needed supplies (vital sign measurement devices, sterile normal saline and dressings) should be brought to the client's room by another health care provider. The nurse stays with the client and while waiting for supplies to arrive places the client in a low Fowler's position with the knees bent to prevent abdominal tension on an abdominal suture line. The nurse covers the wound with a sterile normal saline dressing as soon as supplies are available and keeps the dressing moist. Vital signs are monitored closely, and the client is monitored for signs of shock. The client is prepared for surgery if prescribed. The nurse also documents the occurrence, the actions taken, and the client's response.

Reference(s): deWit, D. & Kumagai, C. (2013). *Medical-surgical nursing: Concepts & practice.* (2nd ed., pp. 91–93). St. Louis: Saunders.

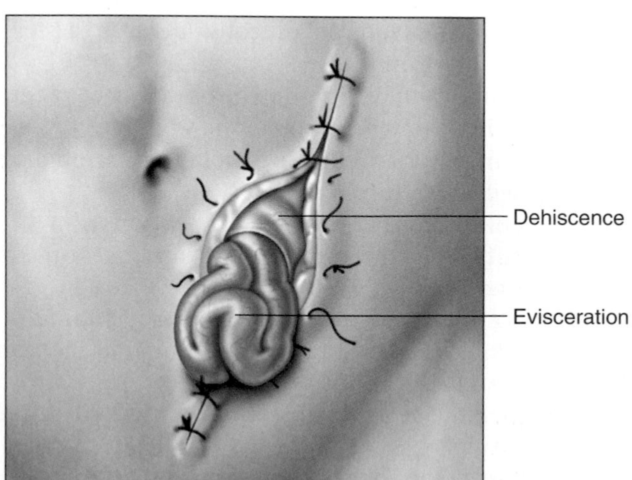

FIGURE 17-7 Complications of wound healing. (From Ignatavicius D, Workman ML: *Medical-surgical nursing: Patient centered collaborative care,* ed 7, Philadelphia, 2013, Saunders.)

6. Instruct the client to splint the abdominal incision when coughing; this action assists in preventing or worsening these complications.
7. Assist to prepare the client for surgery as necessary.

XV. Ambulatory Surgery

A. General criteria for client discharge
1. Is alert and oriented
2. Has voided
3. Has no respiratory distress
4. Vital signs and oxygen saturation are within normal limits.
5. Is able to ambulate, swallow, and cough
6. Has minimal pain
7. Is not vomiting
8. Has minimal (if any) bleeding from the incision site
9. A responsible adult is available to drive the client home.
10. The surgeon has signed a release form.

B. Reinforcing discharge instructions (Box 17-6).
1. Should be performed before the date of the scheduled procedure

BOX 17-6 Reinforcing Discharge Instructions

Determine the client's readiness to learn, educational level, and desire to change or modify his or her lifestyle.
Determine the need for resources for home care.
Demonstrate the care of the incision and how to change the dressing.
Instruct the client to cover the incision with plastic as prescribed if showering is allowed.
Be sure that the client is provided with a 48-hour supply of dressings for home use.
Instruct the client about the importance of returning to the surgeon's office for follow-up visits.
Instruct the client that sutures and staples are usually removed in the surgeon's office 7 to 10 days after surgery and that the skin may become slightly reddened when they are ready to be removed.
Sterile adhesive strips (e.g., Steri-Strips) may be applied to provide extra support after the sutures are removed. Instruct the client to not remove the strips until they are close to falling off.
Instruct the client regarding the use of medications and their purposes, doses, administration, and side effects.
Instruct the client regarding proper diet and to drink 6 to 8 glasses of liquid per day.
Instruct the client regarding activity levels and to resume normal activities gradually.
Instruct the client to avoid lifting for 6 weeks if a major surgical procedure was performed.
Instruct the client with an abdominal incision to not lift anything weighing 10 lb or more and to not engage in any activities that involve pushing or pulling.
Clients usually can return to work after 6 to 8 weeks, as prescribed by the surgeon.
Instruct the client regarding the signs and symptoms of complications and when to call the surgeon.

2. Provide written instructions to the client and family regarding the specifics of care.
3. Instruct the client and family about postoperative complications that can occur.
4. Suggest appropriate resources for home-care support.
5. Instruct the client not to drive for 24 hours if he or she has had a general anesthetic.
6. Inform the client to call the surgeon, ambulatory center, or emergency department if postoperative problems occur.
7. Instruct the client to keep follow-up appointments with the surgeon.

CRITICAL THINKING What Should You Do?

Answer: With regard to informed consent for a surgical procedure, the nurse can act as a witness to the client's signing of the consent form, but the nurse must be sure that the client has understood the surgeon's explanation of the surgery. The nurse needs to document the witnessing of the signing of the consent form after the client acknowledges understanding of the procedure. If the client informs the nurse that the explanation was not fully understood, the nurse must notify the surgeon, and the surgeon will need to clarify anything that was not understood by the client.

Reference(s): deWit, D. & Kumagai, C. (2013). *Medical-surgical nursing: Concepts & practice.* (2nd ed., pp. 68, 70). St. Louis: Saunders.

PRACTICE QUESTIONS

131. The nurse is developing a plan of care for a client who is scheduled for surgery. The nurse should include which activity in the nursing care plan for the client on the day of surgery?
1. Have the client void immediately before surgery.
2. Avoid oral hygiene and rinsing with mouthwash.
3. Verify that the client has not eaten for the last 24 hours.
4. Report immediately any slight increase in blood pressure or pulse.

132. The nurse is caring for a client who is scheduled for surgery. The client is concerned about the surgical procedure. Which action should alleviate the client's fears and misconceptions about surgery?
1. Tell the client that preoperative fear is normal.
2. Explain all nursing care and possible discomfort that may result.
3. Ask the client to discuss information known about the planned surgery.
4. Provide explanations about the procedures involved in the planned surgery.

133. The nurse is collecting data from a client who is scheduled for surgery in 1 week in the ambulatory care surgical center. The nurse notes that the client has a history of arthritis and has been taking acetylsalicylic acid (aspirin). The nurse reports the information to the health care provider and anticipates that the provider will prescribe which?
1. Discontinue the aspirin immediately.
2. Continue to take the aspirin as prescribed.
3. Discontinue the aspirin 48 hours before the scheduled surgery.
4. Decrease the dose of the aspirin to half of what is normally taken.

134. The nurse obtains the vital signs on a postoperative client who just returned to the nursing unit. The client's blood pressure (BP) is 100/60 mm Hg, the pulse is 90 beats per minute, and the respiration rate is 20 breaths per minute. On the basis of these findings, which nursing action should be performed?
1. Shake the client gently to arouse.
2. Continue to monitor the vital signs.
3. Call the registered nurse immediately.
4. Cover the client with a warm blanket.

135. A client arrives to the surgical nursing unit after surgery. What should be the **initial** nursing action after surgery?
1. Patency of the airway
2. Dressing for bleeding
3. Tubes or drains for patency
4. Vital signs to compare with preoperative measurements

136. The nurse is monitoring an adult client for postoperative complications. Which is **most** indicative of a potential postoperative complication that requires further observation?
1. A urinary output of 20 mL/hour
2. A temperature of 37.6 °C (99.6 °F)
3. A blood pressure of 100/70 mm Hg
4. Serous drainage on the surgical dressing

137. The nurse monitors the postoperative client frequently, knowing that accumulated secretions can lead to which problem?
1. Pneumonia
2. Fluid imbalance
3. Pulmonary edema
4. Carbon dioxide retention

138. The nurse is caring for a postoperative client who has a drain inserted into the surgical wound. Which action should the nurse avoid in the care of the drain?

1. Check the drain for patency.
2. Observe for bright red, bloody drainage.
3. Maintain aseptic technique when emptying.
4. Secure the drain by curling or folding it and taping it firmly to the body.

139. The nurse checks the client's surgical incision for signs of infection. Which is indicative of a potential infection?

1. The presence of serous drainage
2. The presence of purulent drainage
3. A temperature of 98.8°F (37.1°C)
4. The client complaining of feeling cold

140. The nurse is checking a client's surgical incision and notes an increase in the amount of drainage, a separation of the incision line, and the appearance of underlying tissue. Which should be the **initial** action by the nurse?

1. Cover the wound with a Betadine-soaked dressing.
2. Apply a sterile dressing soaked with normal saline to the wound.
3. Leave the incision open to the air to assist with drying the drainage.
4. Clean the wound using aseptic technique, and apply a sterile, dry dressing.

ANSWERS

131. 1

Rationale: The nurse should assist the client with voiding immediately before surgery so that the bladder will be empty. Oral hygiene is allowed, but the client should not swallow any water. The client usually has a restriction of food and fluids for 8 hours before surgery rather than 24 hours. A slight increase in blood pressure and pulse is common during the preoperative period; this is generally the result of anxiety.

Test-Taking Strategy: Focus on the subject, preoperative care. Eliminate option 3, knowing that the client should receive nothing by mouth for 8 hours before surgery. Eliminate option 4 because of the words *immediately* and *slight*. Oral hygiene may make the client feel more comfortable. **Review:** preoperative care.

Level of Cognitive Ability: Applying

Client Needs: Physiological Integrity

Integrated Process: Nursing Process/Planning

Content Area: Fundamental Skills: Perioperative Care

Priority Concepts: Clinical Judgment, Elimination

Reference(s): deWit, Kumagai (2013), p. 70.

132. 3

Rationale: Explanations should begin with the information that the client knows. Option 1 is a block to communication, and options 2 and 4 may produce additional anxiety in the client.

Test-Taking Strategy: Use therapeutic communication techniques and focus on the client's feelings first. Additionally, option 3 is the only option that addresses data collection, which is the first step of the nursing process. **Review:** the psychosocial aspects related to the preoperative care.

Level of Cognitive Ability: Applying

Client Needs: Psychosocial Integrity

Integrated Process: Caring

Content Area: Fundamental Skills: Perioperative Care

Priority Concepts: Caregiving, Communication

Reference(s): deWit, Kumagai (2013), p. 68; Linton (2012), pp. 266–267.

133. 3

Rationale: Anticoagulants alter normal clotting factors and increase the risk of bleeding after surgery. Aspirin has properties that can alter the clotting mechanism and should be discontinued at least 48 hours before surgery. However, the client should always check with his or her health care provider regarding when to stop taking the aspirin when a surgical procedure is scheduled. Therefore, the remaining options are incorrect.

Test-Taking Strategy: Focus on the subject, the effect of aspirin and surgery. Recalling that aspirin has anticoagulant properties and can alter the normal clotting mechanism will assist in answering correctly. Also, use of general medication guidelines will assist in answering correctly. **Review:** the medications that affect the preoperative client.

Level of Cognitive Ability: Analyzing

Client Needs: Physiological Integrity

Integrated Process: Nursing Process/Planning

Content Area: Fundamental Skills: Perioperative Care

Priority Concepts: Clotting, Safety

Reference(s): deWit, Kumagai (2013), p. 65.

134. 2

Rationale: A slightly lower-than-normal BP and an increased pulse rate are common after surgery. The level of consciousness can be determined by checking the client's response to light touch and verbal stimuli rather than by shaking the client. Warm blankets are applied to maintain the client's body temperature. There is no reason to contact the registered nurse immediately.

Test-Taking Strategy: Focus on the ABCs—airway, breathing, and circulation. Noting that the vital signs are within normal limits will direct you to the correct option. **Review:** expected postoperative care findings.

Level of Cognitive Ability: Applying

Client Needs: Physiological Integrity

Integrated Process: Nursing Process/Implementation

Content Area: Fundamental Skills: Perioperative Care

Priority Concepts: Clinical Judgment, Gas Exchange

Reference(s): deWit, Kumagai (2013), pp. 83, 94; Perry, Potter, Elkin (2012), pp. 88–89.

135. 1

Rationale: If the airway is not patent, immediate measures must be taken for the survival of the client. After checking the client's airway, the nurse would then check the client's vital signs, and this would be followed by checking the dressings, tubes, and drains.

Test-Taking Strategy: Note the strategic word, *initial.* Use the ABCs—airway, breathing, and circulation. Maintaining the airway patency is the first action to be taken. Options 2, 3, and 4 are all nursing actions that should be performed after a patent airway has been established. **Review: postoperative care.**
Level of Cognitive Ability: Applying
Client Needs: Physiological Integrity
Integrated Process: Nursing Process/Implementation
Content Area: Fundamental Skills: Perioperative Care
Priority Concepts: Clinical Judgment, Gas Exchange
Reference(s): deWit, Kumagai (2013), pp. 83–84.

136. 1
Rationale: Urine output is maintained at a minimum of at least 30 mL/hour for an adult. An output of less than 30 mL/hour for each of 2 consecutive hours should be reported to the surgeon. A temperature more than 37°C (100°F) or less than 36.1°C (97°F) and a falling systolic blood pressure less than 90 mm Hg are to be reported. The client's preoperative or baseline blood pressure is used to make informed postoperative comparisons. Moderate or light serous drainage from the surgical site is considered normal.
Test-Taking Strategy: Note the strategic word, *most.* Focus on the subject, normal assessment data in a postoperative client. Use knowledge of normal expected postoperative ranges to determine that the urinary output is the only finding that is not within normal range. **Review: expected postoperative care findings.**
Level of Cognitive Ability: Analyzing
Client Needs: Physiological Integrity
Integrated Process: Nursing Process/Data Collection
Content Area: Fundamental Skills: Perioperative Care
Priority Concepts: Clinical Judgment, Safety
Reference(s): deWit, Kumagai (2013), p. 86.

137. 1
Rationale: The most common postoperative respiratory problems are atelectasis, pneumonia, and pulmonary emboli. Pneumonia is the inflammation of lung tissue that causes a productive cough, dyspnea, and crackles. Fluid imbalance can be a deficit or excess related to fluid loss or overload. Pulmonary edema usually results from left-sided heart failure, and it can be caused by medications, fluid overload, and smoke inhalation. Carbon dioxide retention results from the inability to exhale carbon dioxide in clients with conditions such as chronic obstructive pulmonary disease.
Test-Taking Strategy: Note the subject, presence of accumulated secretions in the lungs of the postoperative client. This will direct you to the correct option. Options 2, 3, and 4 most commonly occur with other conditions. **Review: postoperative complications.**
Level of Cognitive Ability: Analyzing
Client Needs: Physiological Integrity
Integrated Process: Nursing Process/Data Collection
Content Area: Fundamental Skills: Perioperative Care
Priority Concepts: Clinical Judgment, Gas Exchange
Reference(s): deWit, Kumagai (2013), p. 84.

138. 4
Rationale: Aseptic technique must be used when emptying the drainage container or changing the dressing to avoid contamination of the wound. Usually drainage from the wound is pale, red, and watery, whereas active bleeding will be bright red in color. The drain should be checked for patency to provide an exit for the fluid or blood to promote healing. The nurse needs to ensure that drainage flows freely and that there are no kinks in the drains. Curling or folding the drain prevents the flow of the drainage.
Test-Taking Strategy: Focus on the subject, caring for a surgical drain. Note the word *avoid.* Remember that the nurse needs to ensure that drainage flows freely from a drain. **Review:** the care of the **postoperative client with a drain.**
Level of Cognitive Ability: Applying
Client Needs: Physiological Integrity
Integrated Process: Nursing Process/Implementation
Content Area: Fundamental Skills: Perioperative Care
Priority Concepts: Safety, Tissue Integrity
Reference(s): deWit, Kumagai (2013), p. 90.

139. 2
Rationale: Signs and symptoms of a wound infection include warm, red, and tender skin around the incision. The client may have fever and chills. Purulent material may exit from drains or from separated wound edges. Infection may be caused by poor aseptic technique or a wound that was contaminated before surgical exploration; it appears 3 to 6 days after surgery. Serous drainage is not indicative of a wound infection. A temperature of 98.8°F is not an abnormal finding in a postoperative client. The fact that a client feels cold is not indicative of an infection, although chills and fever are signs of infection.
Test-Taking Strategy: Focus on the subject, infection. Noting the word *purulent* will direct you to the correct option. **Review:** the signs of a **wound infection.**
Level of Cognitive Ability: Understanding
Client Needs: Physiological Integrity
Integrated Process: Nursing Process/Data Collection
Content Area: Fundamental Skills: Perioperative Care
Priority Concepts: Clinical Judgment, Infection
Reference(s): deWit, Kumagai (2013), pp. 89–90; Linton (2012), p. 283.

140. 2
Rationale: Wound dehiscence is the separation of the wound edges at the suture line. Signs and symptoms include increased drainage and the appearance of underlying tissues. It usually occurs as a complication 6 to 8 days after surgery. The client should be instructed to remain quiet and avoid coughing or straining, and he or she should be positioned to prevent further stress on the wound. Sterile dressings soaked with sterile normal saline should be used to cover the wound. The surgeon needs to be notified.
Test-Taking Strategy: Note the strategic word, *initial,* and the subject, the postoperative complication of wound dehiscence. Eliminate option 3 first, because this action would expose the open wound and the underlying tissues to infection. Eliminate options 1 and 4 next, because a dressing soaked with Betadine and a dry dressing will irritate the exposed body tissues. Review: emergency care for **dehiscence or evisceration.**
Level of Cognitive Ability: Applying
Client Needs: Physiological Integrity
Integrated Process: Nursing Process/Implementation
Content Area: Fundamental Skills: Perioperative Care
Priority Concepts: Clinical Judgment, Tissue Integrity
Reference(s): deWit, Kumagai (2013), p. 93.

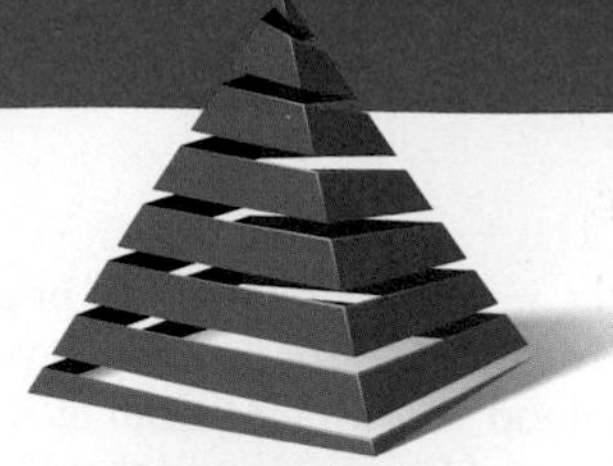

CHAPTER 18

Positioning Clients

CRITICAL THINKING What Should You Do?

The nurse is caring for a client who is receiving intermittent tube feedings via a nasogastric tube. In maintaining proper positioning for this client, what actions should the nurse take?
Answer is located on p. 189.

For reference throughout the chapter, please see Figures 18-1, 18-2, 18-3, and 18-4.

I. Guidelines for Positioning

A. Principles of body movement for clients
   1. Body movement and alignment are important for clients. Many clients are unable to change position or move in bed independently.
   2. Basic principles include maintaining correct anatomical position and changing the position frequently.

B. Position in a safe and appropriate manner to provide safety, alignment, and comfort.

C. Select a position that will prevent the development of complications related to an existing condition, a prescribed treatment, or a medical or surgical procedure.

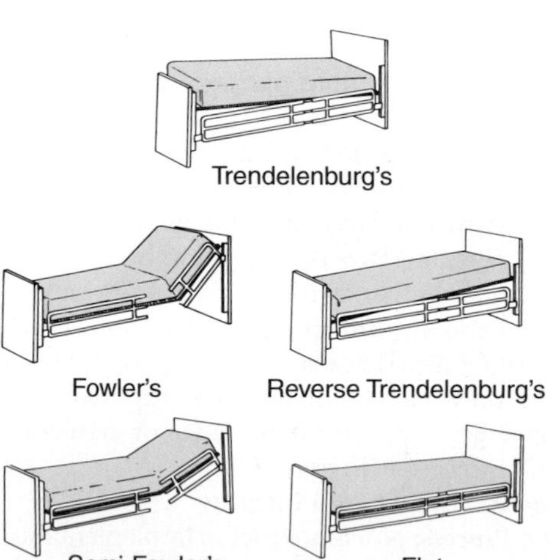

FIGURE 18-1 Common bed positions. (From Potter P, Perry A, Stockert P, Hall A: *Fundamentals of nursing*, ed 8, St. Louis, 2013, Mosby.)

Always review the health care provider's (HCP's) prescription, especially after treatments or procedures, and take note of instructions regarding positioning and mobility.

II. Ergonomic Principles Related to Body Mechanics (Box 18-1) 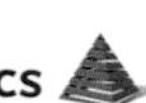

III. Positions to Ensure Safety and Comfort

A. Integumentary system
   1. Autograft: After surgery, the site is immobilized for approximately 3 to 7 days to provide the time needed for the graft to adhere and attach to the wound bed.
   2. Burns of the face and head: Elevate the head of the bed to prevent or reduce facial, head, and tracheal edema.
   3. Circumferential burns of the extremities: Elevate the extremities above the level of the heart to prevent or reduce dependent edema.
   4. Skin graft: Elevate and immobilize the graft site to prevent the movement and shearing of the graft and the disruption of tissue; avoid weight bearing.

B. Reproductive system
   1. Mastectomy
      a. Position the client with the head of the bed elevated at least 30 degrees (semi-Fowler's position), with the affected arm elevated on a pillow to promote lymphatic fluid return after the removal of axillary lymph nodes.
      b. Turn the client only to the back and the unaffected side.
   2. Perineal and vaginal procedures: Place the client in the **lithotomy position**.

C. Endocrine system
   1. Hypophysectomy: Elevate the head of the bed to prevent increased intracranial pressure.
   2. Thyroidectomy
      a. Place the client in the **semi-Fowler's** or **Fowler's position** to reduce swelling and edema in the neck area.
      b. Sandbags or pillows may be used to support the client's head or neck.

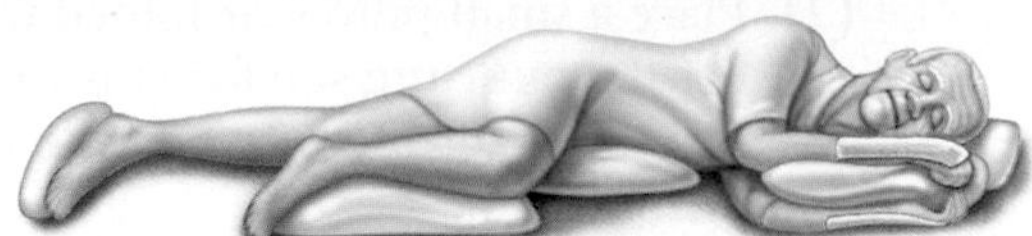
Lateral (side-lying) position

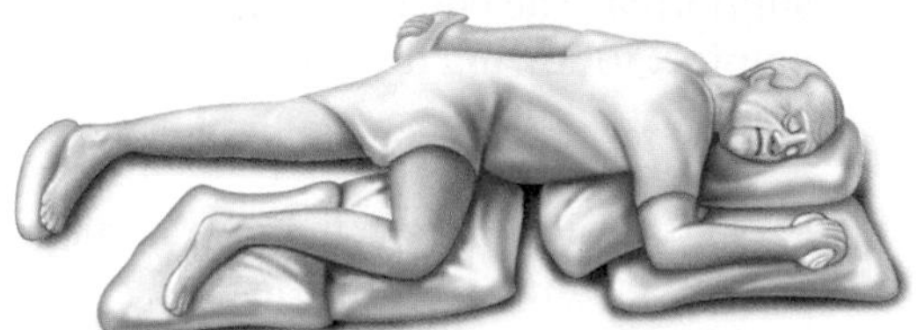
Semiprone (Sims' or forward side-lying) position

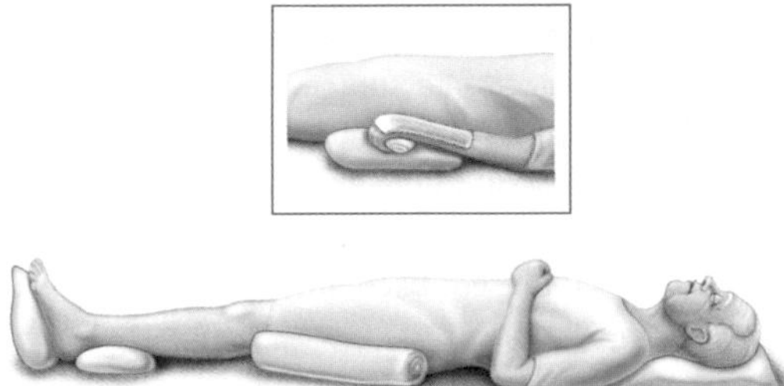
Supine position

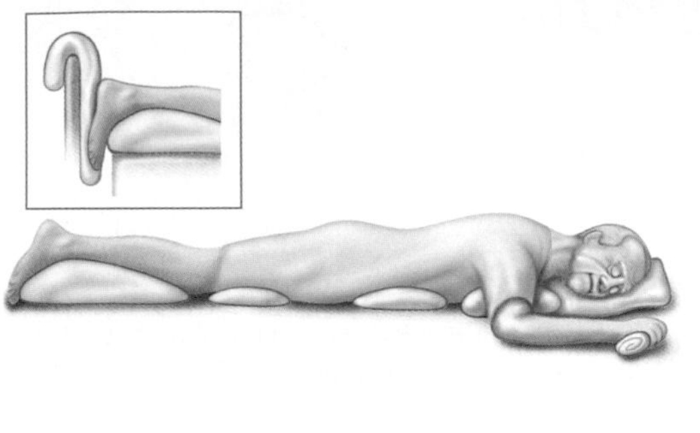

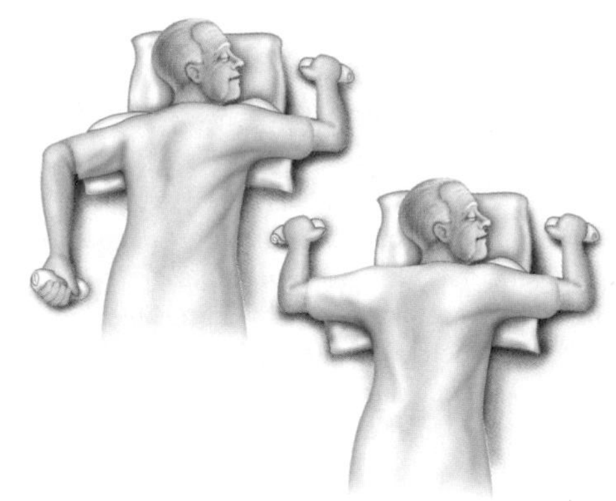
Prone position. The client's arms and shoulders may be positioned in internal or external rotation.

FIGURE 18-2 Common client positions. (From Harkreader H, Hogan MA: *Fundamentals of nursing: Caring and clinical judgment,* ed 3, St. Louis, 2007, Saunders.)

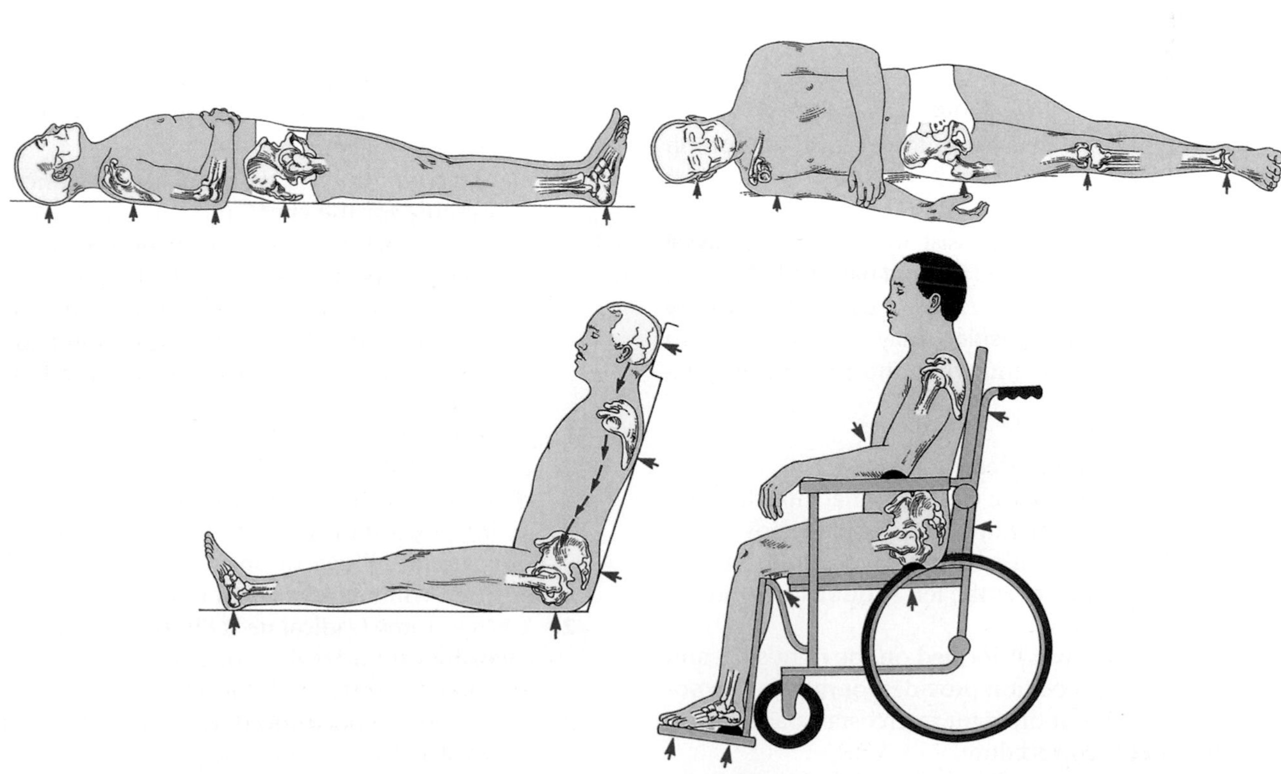

FIGURE 18-3 Pressure points of lying and sitting positions. (From Perry A, Potter P, Elkin M: *Nursing interventions & clinical skills*, ed 5, St. Louis, 2012, Mosby.)

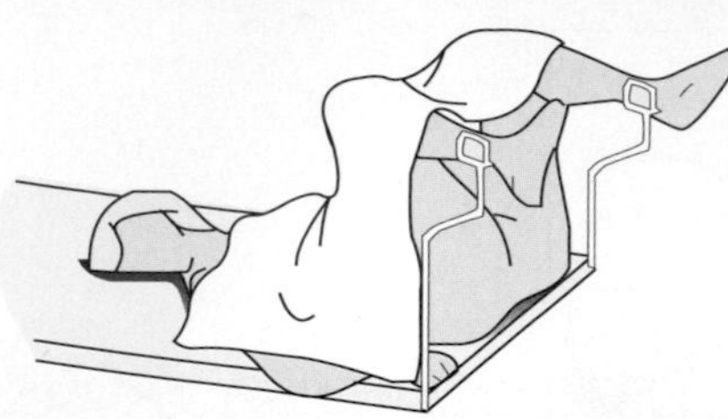

FIGURE 18-4 Lithotomy position for examination. (From Potter P, Perry A, Stockert P, Hall A: *Fundamentals of nursing*, ed 8, St. Louis, 2013, Mosby.)

BOX 18-1 Body Mechanics for Health Care Workers

When planning to move a client, arrange for adequate help. Use mechanical aids as much as possible.
Encourage the client to assist as much as possible.
Keep your back, neck, pelvis, and feet aligned. Avoid twisting.
Flex your knees, and keep your feet wide apart.
Position yourself close to the client or to the object being lifted.
Use your arms and legs rather than your back.
Slide the client toward yourself using a pull sheet. When transferring a client onto a stretcher, a slide board is more appropriate.
Set (tighten) your abdominal and gluteal muscles in preparation for the move.
The person with the heaviest load should coordinate the efforts of the team involved by counting to three.

Adapted from Potter P, Perry A, Stockert P, Hall A: *Fundamentals of nursing*, ed 8, St. Louis, 2013, Mosby.

c. Avoid neck extension to decrease tension on the suture line.

D. Gastrointestinal system
1. Hemorrhoidectomy: Assist the client to a **lateral (side-lying) position** to prevent pain and bleeding.
2. Gastroesophageal reflux disease: **Reverse Trendelenburg's position** may be prescribed to promote gastric emptying and prevent esophageal reflux.

3. Liver biopsy
   a. During the procedure
      (1) Position the client supine with the right side of the upper abdomen exposed.
      (2) The client's right arm is raised and extended over the left shoulder behind the head.
      (3) The liver is located on the right side, and this position provides for maximal exposure of the right intercostal spaces.
   b. After the procedure
      (1) Assist the client into a right lateral (side-lying) position.
      (2) Place a small pillow or folded towel under the puncture site for at least 3 hours to provide pressure to the site and prevent bleeding.
4. Paracentesis: The client is positioned in a semi-Fowler's position in bed, or sitting upright on the side of the bed or in a chair with the feet supported. The client is assisted to a position of comfort following the procedure.
5. Nasogastric tube
   a. Insertion
      (1) Position the client in a **high Fowler's position** with the head tilted forward.
      (2) This position will help close the trachea and open the esophagus.

⚠ If the client receiving a continuous tube feeding needs to be placed in a supine position when providing care, such as when giving a bed bath or changing linens, shut the feeding off to prevent aspiration. Remember to turn the feeding back on and check the rate of flow when the client is placed back into the semi-Fowler's or Fowler's position.

   b. Irrigations and tube feedings
      (1) Keep the head of the bed elevated 30 degrees (semi-Fowler's position) to prevent aspiration.
      (2) Maintain head elevation for 1 hour after an intermittent feeding.
      (3) The head of the bed should remain elevated for continuous feedings.
6. Rectal enemas or irrigations: Place the client in left **Sims' position** to allow the solution to flow by gravity in the natural direction of the colon.
7. Sengstaken-Blakemore
   a. Not commonly used because they are uncomfortable for the client and can cause complications, but their use may be necessary when other interventions are not feasible.
   b. If prescribed, maintain elevation of the head of the bed to enhance lung expansion and reduce portal blood flow, permitting effective esophagogastric balloon tamponade.

E. Respiratory system

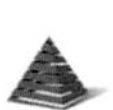

1. Chronic obstructive pulmonary disease: For the client with advanced disease, place the client in a sitting position, leaning forward, with the arms over several pillows or on an overbed table. This position will help the client to breathe easier.
2. Laryngectomy (radical neck dissection): Place the client in a semi-Fowler's or Fowler's position to maintain a patent airway and minimize edema.
3. Bronchoscopy postprocedure: Place the client in a semi-Fowler's position to prevent choking or aspiration resulting from an impaired ability to swallow.

4. Postural drainage: The lung segment to be drained should be in the uppermost position. **Trendelenburg's position** may be used.
5. Thoracentesis
   a. During the procedure: To facilitate the removal of fluid from the pleural space, position the client sitting on the edge of the bed and leaning over the bedside table with the feet supported on a stool or lying in bed on the unaffected side with the head of the bed elevated approximately 45 degrees (Fowler's position).
   b. After the procedure: Assist the client to a position of comfort.
6. Thoracotomy: Check the HCP's prescriptions regarding positioning.

Always check the HCP's prescription regarding positioning for the client who had a thoracotomy, lung wedge resection, lobectomy of the lung, or pneumonectomy.

F. Cardiovascular system
1. Abdominal aneurysm resection
   a. After surgery, limit the elevation of the head of the bed to 45 degrees (Fowler's position) to avoid flexion of the graft.
   b. The client may be turned from side to side.
2. Amputation of the lower extremity
   a. During the first 24 hours after amputation, elevate the foot of the bed to reduce edema. The stump is supported with pillows but not elevated because of the risk of flexion contractures.
   b. Consult with the health care provider (HCP) and, if prescribed, position the client in a **prone position** twice a day for a 20- to 30-minute period to stretch muscles and prevent flexion contractures of the hip.
3. Arterial vascular grafting of an extremity
   a. To promote graft patency after the procedure, bed rest is usually maintained for approximately 24 hours, and the client's affected extremity is kept straight.
   b. Limit movement and avoid flexion of the client's hip and knee.
4. Cardiac catheterization
   a. If the femoral artery was used, the client is maintained on bed rest for approximately 3 to 4 hours. The client may turn from side to side.
   b. The client's affected extremity is kept straight and the head elevated no more than 30 degrees until hemostasis is adequately achieved.
5. Heart failure and pulmonary edema: Position the client upright (high Fowler's position), preferably with the bed in a chair-sitting position, to decrease venous return and lung congestion.

Most often, clients with respiratory and cardiac disorders should be positioned with the head of the bed elevated.

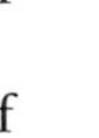

6. Peripheral arterial disease
   a. Obtain the HCP's prescription for positioning.
   b. Because swelling can prevent arterial blood flow, clients may be advised to elevate their feet when at rest. They should not raise their legs above the level of the heart, because extreme elevation slows arterial blood flow. Some clients may be advised to maintain a slightly dependent position to promote perfusion.
7. Deep vein thrombosis
   a. If the extremity is red, edematous, and painful and traditional heparin therapy is initiated, bed rest with leg elevation may be prescribed for the client.
   b. Clients receiving low-molecular-weight heparin can usually be out of bed after 24 hours, if the pain level permits.
8. Varicose veins: Leg elevation above the level of the heart is usually prescribed. The client is also advised to minimize prolonged sitting or standing during daily activities.
9. Venous insufficiency and leg ulcers: Leg elevation is usually prescribed.

G. Sensory system

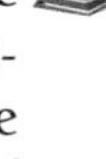

1. Cataract surgery: Postoperatively, elevate the head of the bed (semi-Fowler's to Fowler's position), and position the client on the back or the nonoperative side to prevent the development of edema at the operative site.
2. Retinal detachment
   a. If the detachment is large, bed rest and bilateral eye patching may be prescribed to minimize eye movement and prevent the extension of the detachment.
   b. Restrictions in activity and positioning after the repair of the detachment depend on the HCP's preference and the surgical procedure performed.

H. Neurological system

1. Autonomic dysreflexia: Elevate the head of the bed to a high Fowler's position to help with adequate ventilation and prevent hypertensive stroke.

If autonomic dysreflexia occurs, immediately place the client in a high Fowler's position.

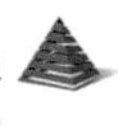

2. Cerebral aneurysm: Bed rest is maintained with the head of the bed elevated 30 to 45 degrees (semi-Fowler's to Fowler's position) to prevent pressure on the aneurysm site.

3. Cerebral angiography
   a. Maintain bed rest for the length of time, as prescribed.
   b. The extremity into which the contrast medium is injected is kept straight and immobilized for approximately 8 hours.
4. Stroke (brain attack)
   a. In clients with hemorrhagic strokes, the head of the bed is usually elevated 30 degrees to reduce intracranial pressure and facilitate venous drainage.
   b. For clients with ischemic strokes, the head of the bed is usually kept flat.
   c. Maintain the client's head in a midline, neutral position to facilitate venous drainage from the head.
   d. Avoid extreme hip and neck flexion; extreme hip flexion may increase intrathoracic pressure, whereas extreme neck flexion prohibits venous drainage from the brain.
5. Craniotomy
   a. The client should not be positioned on the site that was operated on, especially if the bone flap has been removed, because the brain has no bony covering over the affected site.
   b. Elevate the head of the bed 30 to 45 degrees (semi-Fowler's to Fowler's position), and maintain the head in a midline, neutral position to facilitate venous drainage from the head.
   c. Avoid extreme hip and neck flexion.
6. Laminectomy
   a. Logroll the client.
   b. When the client is out of bed, the client's back is kept straight (the client is placed in a straight-backed chair) with the feet resting comfortably on the floor.
7. Increased intracranial pressure
   a. Elevate the head of the bed 30 to 45 degrees (semi-Fowler's to Fowler's position), and maintain the head in a midline, neutral position to facilitate venous drainage from the head.
   b. Avoid extreme hip and neck flexion.

⚠ Do not place a client with a head injury in a flat or Trendelenburg position because of the risk of increased intracranial pressure.

8. Lumbar puncture
   a. During the procedure: Assist the client to the lateral (side-lying) position, with the back bowed at the edge of the examining table, the knees flexed up to the abdomen, and the head bent so that the chin is resting on the chest.
   b. After the procedure: Place the client in the supine position for 4 to 12 hours, as prescribed.
9. Spinal cord injury
   a. Immobilize the client on a spinal backboard with the head in a neutral position to prevent an incomplete injury from becoming complete.
   b. Prevent head flexion, rotation, or extension. The head is immobilized with a firm, padded cervical collar.
   c. Logroll the client. No part of the body should be twisted or turned, and the client should not be allowed to assume a sitting position.

I. Musculoskeletal system
1. Total hip replacement
   a. Positioning depends on the surgical techniques used, the method of implantation, and the prosthesis. Also follow the surgeon's prescriptions and agency procedures.
   b. Avoid extreme internal and external rotation.
   c. Avoid adduction; in most cases side-lying is permittable as long as an abduction pillow is in place; some surgeons allow turning to only one side.
   d. Maintain abduction when the client is in a **supine position** or positioned on the nonoperative side.
   e. Place a pillow between the client's legs to maintain abduction; instruct the client not to cross the legs (Box 18-2).

BOX 18-2 Devices Used for Proper Positioning

Bed Boards

These plywood boards are placed under the entire surface area of the mattress. They are useful for increasing back support and body alignment.

Foot Boots

Foot boots are made of rigid plastic or heavy foam, and they keep the foot flexed at the proper angle. They should be removed two or three times a day to assess skin integrity and joint mobility.

Hand Rolls

Hand rolls maintain the fingers in a slightly flexed and functional position, and they keep the thumb slightly adducted in opposition to the fingers.

Hand–Wrist Splints

These splints are individually molded for the client to maintain the proper alignment of the thumb in slight adduction and the wrist in slight dorsiflexion.

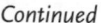

Continued

BOX 18-2 Devices Used for Proper Positioning—cont'd

Pillows

Pillows provide support, elevate body parts, splint incisional areas, and reduce postoperative pain during activity, coughing, or deep breathing. They should be the appropriate size for the body part to be positioned.

Sandbags

Sandbags are soft devices filled with a substance that can be shaped to body contours to provide support. They immobilize extremities and maintain specific body alignment.

Side Rails

These bars, positioned along the sides of the length of the bed, ensure client safety and are useful for increasing mobility. They also provide assistance in rolling from side to side or sitting up in bed. Agency policies regarding the use of side rails should always be followed.

Trapeze Bar

This bar descends from a securely fastened overhead bar attached to the bed frame. It allows the client to use the upper extremities to raise the trunk off of the bed, to assist with transfer from the bed to a wheelchair, and to perform upper-arm strengthening exercises.

Trochanter Rolls

These rolls prevent the external rotation of the legs when the client is in the supine position. To form a roll, use a cotton bath blanket or a sheet folded lengthwise to a width that extends from the greater trochanter of the femur to the lower border of the popliteal space.

Wedge Pillow

This triangular-shaped pillow is made of heavy foam, and it is used to maintain the legs in abduction after total hip replacement surgery.

Adapted from Potter P, Perry A, Stockert P, Hall A: *Fundamentals of nursing*, ed 8, St. Louis, 2013, Mosby.

f. Check the HCP's prescriptions regarding elevation of the head of the bed and hip flexion.

2. Devices used to promote proper positioning (see Box 18-2)

CRITICAL THINKING What Should You Do?

Answer: For the client receiving intermittent tube feedings via a nasogastric tube, the nurse should position the client in an upright (semi-Fowler's or high Fowler's) position during the feeding and for 1 hour following the feeding, per agency policy. Positioning the client in an upright position prevents aspiration of the formula. For the client receiving a continuous tube feeding, an upright position should be maintained at all times.

Reference(s): deWit, D. & Kumagai, C. (2013). *Medical-surgical nursing: Concepts & practice.* (2nd ed., p. 660). St. Louis: Saunders.

PRACTICE QUESTIONS

141. The nurse is preparing to reposition a dependent client who weighs more than 250 pounds. Which intervention is **best** for the nurse to consider when moving this client?

1. Find someone who can help.
2. Place the client in Trendelenburg's position.
3. Keep elbows close and work close to the body.
4. Administer oral pain medication 5 minutes before moving the client.

142. The nurse is assigned to assist with caring for a client after cardiac catheterization. The nurse should plan to maintain bed rest for this client in which position?

1. High Fowler's position
2. Lateral (side-lying) position
3. Head elevation of 45 degrees
4. Head elevation of no more than 30 degrees

143. The nurse is reinforcing home-care instructions to a client and family regarding care after cataract removal from the right eye. Which statement made by the client indicates an understanding of the instructions?

1. "I should not sleep on my left side."
2. "I should not sleep on my right side."
3. "I will take aspirin if I have any pain."
4. "I should not wear my glasses until my surgeon says it is okay."

144. After a liver biopsy, the nurse should place the client in which position?

1. Trendelenburg and on the left side
2. Prone with the head of the bed in a flat position
3. Supine with the head of the bed at a 30-degree angle
4. A right side-lying position with a small pillow or folded towel under the puncture site

145. The nurse is administering a cleansing enema to a client with a fecal impaction. Before administering the enema, the nurse should assist the client to which position?

1. Left Sims' position, with the head of the bed flat
2. Right Sims' position, with the head of the bed elevated 15 to 30 degrees

3. On the left side of the body, with the head of the bed elevated 45 degrees
4. On the right side of the body, with the head of the bed elevated 45 degrees

146. A client is being prepared for a thoracentesis. The nurse should assist the client to which position for the procedure?
1. Sims' position, with the head of the bed flat
2. Prone, with the head turned to the side supported by a pillow
3. Lying in bed on the affected side, with the head of the bed elevated 45 degrees
4. Lying in bed on the unaffected side, with the head of the bed elevated 45 degrees

147. The nurse is assisting with the insertion of a nasogastric tube into a client. The nurse should place the client in which position for insertion?
1. Right side
2. Low Fowler's position
3. High Fowler's position
4. Supine, with the head flat

148. The nurse is assisting with caring for a client after a craniotomy. Which is the **best** position for the client to be placed?
1. Prone position
2. Supine position
3. Semi-Fowler's position
4. Dorsal recumbent position

149. The nurse is caring for a client following a supratentorial craniotomy, in which a large tumor was removed from the left side. In which position can the nurse safely place the client? **Refer to Figures 1 to 4.**

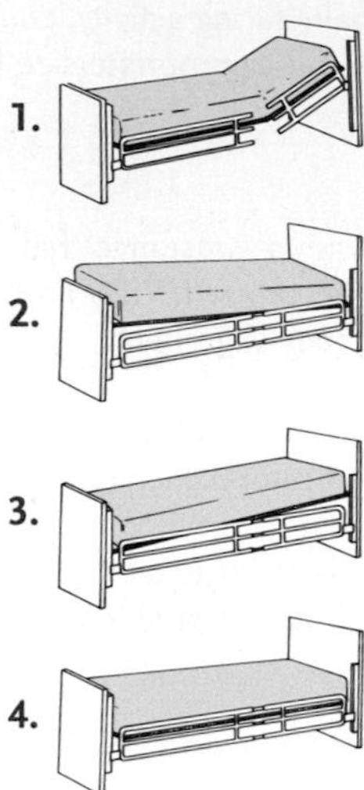

(Figures from Potter P, Perry A, Stockert P, Hall A: *Fundamentals of nursing*, ed 8, St. Louis, 2013, Mosby.)

150. The nurse is turning a postoperative client who had extensive spinal surgery on the previous day. Which turning intervention or position would be **best** for repositioning this client?
1. Logrolling
2. Semi-Fowler's
3. Sims' (semi-prone)
4. 30-degree lateral (side-lying)

ANSWERS

141. 1

Rationale: Although it is possible to move and position clients independently, getting help is the best intervention. Lower back strain is a common injury among health care workers. In addition, the shearing of the client's skin over bony prominences may occur when health care workers move clients independently. Placing the client in Trendelenburg is not a useful technique for repositioning and could be harmful to the client because of the pressure this position places on the diaphragm. Keeping the elbows close and working close to the body are useful techniques, but they would not be enough when independently moving a 250-pound client. This client is dependent, so he or she is probably not able to help much, if any. Administering oral pain medication is necessary, but oral medications need to be given at least 30 to 45 minutes before clients are moved.

Test-Taking Strategy: Focus on the strategic word, *best.* Next, focus on the data in the question. This client's dependent condition and weight make him or her too difficult for one person to move. **Review:** the procedures and interventions for moving and positioning clients.

Level of Cognitive Ability: Applying
Client Needs: Physiological Integrity
Integrated Process: Nursing Process/Planning
Content Area: Fundamental Skills: Safety
Priority Concepts: Health Promotion, Safety
Reference(s): Perry, Potter, Elkin (2012), p. 367; Perry, Potter, Ostendorf (2014), p. 199.

142. 4

Rationale: After cardiac catheterization, the extremity into which the catheter was inserted is kept straight for the prescribed time period. The client may turn from side to side. The client is placed in the supine position and the head of the bed is not elevated to more than 30 degrees to keep the affected leg straight at the groin and prevent arterial occlusion. Bathroom privileges are not allowed during the immediate postcatheterization period. For the high Fowler's position, the head of the bed is elevated 90 degrees.

Test-Taking Strategy: Focus on the subject, positioning after cardiac catheterization. Recalling that concerns after this procedure are bleeding and arterial occlusion will direct you to the correct option. **Review:** the care of the client after cardiac catheterization.

Level of Cognitive Ability: Applying
Client Needs: Physiological Integrity
Integrated Process: Nursing Process/Planning
Content Area: Adult Health: Cardiovascular
Priority Concepts: Perfusion, Safety
Reference(s): Ignatavicius, Workman (2013), p. 705.

143. 2
Rationale: After cataract surgery, the client should not sleep on the side of the body that was operated on. Clients should be instructed not to take aspirin or any medications that contain aspirin because of their antiplatelet properties that can increase the risk of bleeding. Acetaminophen (Tylenol) can be taken as needed for pain. Clients may wear their glasses.
Test-Taking Strategy: Focus on the **subject**, cataract surgery and positioning. Think about the effect of gravity and the development of edema after a surgical procedure. After cataract surgery the client should stay off the operative side. **Review:** the care of the client after cataract surgery.
Level of Cognitive Ability: Evaluating
Client Needs: Physiological Integrity
Integrated Process: Nursing Process/Evaluation
Content Area: Adult Health: Eye
Priority Concepts: Client Education, Safety
Reference(s): deWit, Kumagai (2013), p. 600.

144. 4
Rationale: After a liver biopsy, the client is assisted with assuming a right side-lying position with a small pillow or folded towel under the puncture site for at least 3 hours. Options 1, 2, and 3 are incorrect positions.
Test-Taking Strategy: Focus on the **subject**, liver biopsy. Think about the anatomical location of the liver. Remember that the liver is on the right side of the body and that the application of pressure on the right side will minimize the escape of blood or bile through the puncture site. **Review:** the care of the client after a liver biopsy.
Level of Cognitive Ability: Applying
Client Needs: Physiological Integrity
Integrated Process: Nursing Process/Implementation
Content Area: Adult Health: Gastrointestinal
Priority Concepts: Clinical Judgment, Safety
Reference(s): deWit, Kumagai (2013), pp. 628–629; Pagana, Pagana (2013), p. 604.

145. 1
Rationale: When administering an enema, the client is placed in a left Sims' position so that the enema solution can flow by gravity in the natural direction of the colon. The head of the bed is not elevated.
Test-Taking Strategy: Focus on the **subject**, enema administration. Recalling the anatomy of the bowel will assist you with selecting the correct option. Also note that the incorrect options are **comparable or alike** and address head elevation. **Review:** the procedure for enema administration.
Level of Cognitive Ability: Applying
Client Needs: Physiological Integrity
Integrated Process: Nursing Process/Implementation
Content Area: Fundamental Skills: Elimination
Priority Concepts: Elimination, Safety
Reference(s): Perry, Potter, Elkin (2012), p. 463.

146. 4
Rationale: To facilitate the removal of fluid from the chest, the client is positioned sitting on the edge of the bed, leaning over a bedside table, with the feet supported on a stool or lying in bed on the unaffected side, with the head of the bed elevated 45 degrees (Fowler's position). Options 1, 2, and 3 are incorrect.
Test-Taking Strategy: Focus on the **subject**, thoracentesis. Option 3 can be eliminated because if the client was lying on the affected side, it would be very difficult to perform the procedure. Option 1 can be eliminated because the Sims' position is primarily used for rectal enemas or irrigations. In the prone position, the client is lying on his or her abdomen, which is not an appropriate position for this procedure. **Review: thoracentesis.**
Level of Cognitive Ability: Applying
Client Needs: Physiological Integrity
Integrated Process: Nursing Process/Implementation
Content Area: Adult Health: Respiratory
Priority Concepts: Gas Exchange, Safety
Reference(s): deWit, Kumagai (2013), p. 267.

147. 3
Rationale: During the insertion of a nasogastric tube, the client is placed in a sitting or high Fowler's position to reduce the risk of pulmonary aspiration if the client should vomit. Options 1, 2, and 4 do not facilitate the insertion of the tube or prevent aspiration.
Test-Taking Strategy: Focus on the **subject**, insertion of a nasogastric tube. Visualize this procedure. Use the **ABCs—airway, breathing, and circulation**—since pulmonary aspiration is a concern with insertion of a nasogastric tube. **Review:** the procedure for inserting a nasogastric tube.
Level of Cognitive Ability: Applying
Client Needs: Physiological Integrity
Integrated Process: Nursing Process/Implementation
Content Area: Adult Health: Gastrointestinal
Priority Concepts: Gas Exchange, Safety
Reference(s): Perry, Potter, Elkin (2012), p. 270.

148. 3
Rationale: After a craniotomy, the head of the bed is elevated 30 to 45 degrees (semi-Fowler's to Fowler's position), and the client's head is maintained in a midline, neutral position to facilitate venous drainage. Options 1, 2, and 4 are incorrect positions.
Test-Taking Strategy: Focus on the **strategic word**, *best.* Also note the **subject**, positioning after craniotomy. Use knowledge about the effects of gravity and the development of edema to answer correctly. **Review:** the care of the client after a craniotomy.
Level of Cognitive Ability: Applying
Client Needs: Physiological Integrity
Integrated Process: Nursing Process/Implementation
Content Area: Adult Health: Neurological
Priority Concepts: Intracranial Regulation, Safety
Reference(s): Lewis, Dirksen, Heitkemper, Bucher (2014), p. 1380.

149. 1
Rationale: Clients who have undergone supratentorial surgery should have the head of the bed elevated 30 degrees to promote venous drainage from the head. The client is positioned to avoid extreme hip or neck flexion and the head is maintained in a midline neutral position. If a large tumor has been removed, the client should be placed on the nonoperative side

to prevent displacement of the cranial contents. A flat position or Trendelenburg's position would increase intracranial pressure. A reverse Trendelenburg's position would not be helpful and may be uncomfortable for the client.
Test-Taking Strategy: Focus on the subject, positioning following a supratentorial craniotomy. Remember that a primary concern is the risk for increased intracranial pressure. Therefore, use concepts related to preventing increased intracranial pressure to answer this question. In addition, remember that with "supra" tentorial surgery, the head is kept "up," and the client is placed on the nonoperative side. ***Review:*** the positioning of a client after **supratentorial craniotomy.**
Level of Cognitive Ability: Analyzing
Client Needs: Physiological Integrity
Integrated Process: Nursing Process/Implementation
Content Area: Adult Health: Neurological
Priority Concepts: Intracranial Regulation, Safety
Reference(s): Ignatavicius, Workman (2013), p. 1034.

150. 1
Rationale: Logrolling is used to maintain neck and spinal alignment after injury or surgery. A minimum of three to four staff members is recommended to prevent injury to the client, and a draw or pull sheet is also suggested. Options 2, 3, and 4 do not maintain proper spinal alignment and could be harmful.
Test-Taking Strategy: Note the strategic word, *best.* Options 2, 3, and 4 are positions and are comparable or alike and do not maintain proper spinal alignment. This will direct you to the correct option. **Review:** the care of the client after **spinal surgery.**
Level of Cognitive Ability: Applying
Client Needs: Physiological Integrity
Integrated Process: Nursing Process/Implementation
Content Area: Fundamental Skills: Safety
Priority Concepts: Clinical Judgment, Safety
Reference(s): deWit, Kumagai (2013), p. 519.

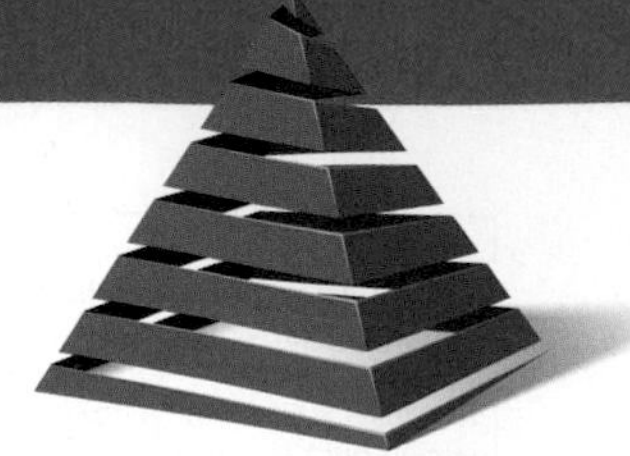

CHAPTER 19

Care of a Client with a Tube

Fundamentals

CRITICAL THINKING What Should You Do?

The nurse is assisting in monitoring a client with a closed chest tube drainage system. On inspection, the nurse notes that the system is cracked. What should the nurse do?
Answer is located on p. 204.

I. Nasogastric Tubes

A. Description
1. Short tubes used to intubate the stomach
2. Inserted from the nose to the stomach

B. Purpose
1. To decompress the stomach by removing fluids or gas to promote abdominal comfort
2. To allow surgical anastomoses to heal without distention
3. To decrease the risk of aspiration
4. To administer medications in clients who are unable to swallow
5. To provide nutrition by acting as a temporary feeding tube
6. To irrigate the stomach and remove toxic substances, such as in poisonings

C. Types of tubes and routes (Fig. 19-1)
1. Levin: Single-lumen nasogastric (NG) tube used to remove gastric contents via intermittent suction or to provide tube feedings
2. Salem sump tube: A Salem sump is a double-lumen nasogastric tube with air vent (pigtail) used for decompression with intermittent continuous suction.

⚠ The air vent on a Salem sump tube is not to be clamped and is to be kept above the level of the stomach. If leakage occurs through the air vent, instill 30 mL of air into the air vent and irrigate the main lumen with normal saline (NS).

D. Intubation procedures (Box 19-1)

E. Irrigation
1. Check placement before irrigating (see Box 19-1).
2. Perform irrigation every 4 hours to monitor and maintain the patency of the tube.
3. Gently instill 30 to 50 mL of water or NS (depending on agency policy) with an irrigation syringe.
4. Pull back on the syringe plunger to withdraw the fluid to check patency; repeat if the tube flow is sluggish.

F. Removal of a nasogastric tube: Ask the client to take a deep breath and hold; remove the tube slowly and evenly over the course of 3 to 6 seconds (coil the tube around the hand while removing it).

II. Gastrointestinal Tube Feedings

A. Tubes (Fig. 19-2)

B. Types of administration
1. Bolus
   a. Resembles normal meal feeding patterns
   b. Formula is administrated over a 30- to 60-minute period every 3 to 6 hours; the amount of formula is prescribed by the health care provider (HCP).
2. Continuous
   a. Administered continuously for 24 hours
   b. An infusion pump regulates the flow
3. Cyclical
   a. Administered either during the daytime or nighttime for 8 to 16 hours
   b. An infusion pump regulates the flow
   c. Feedings at night allow for more freedom during the day.

C. Administering feedings
1. Check the HCP's prescription and agency policy regarding residual amounts; usually, if the residual is less than 100 mL, feeding is administered; large-volume aspirates indicate delayed gastric emptying and place the client at risk for aspiration.
2. Check bowel sounds; hold the feeding and notify the registered nurse if bowel sounds are absent.
3. Position the client in a high Fowler's position; if comatose, place in high Fowler's and on the right side.
4. Check tube placement by aspirating gastric contents and measuring the pH (should be 3.5 or lower).

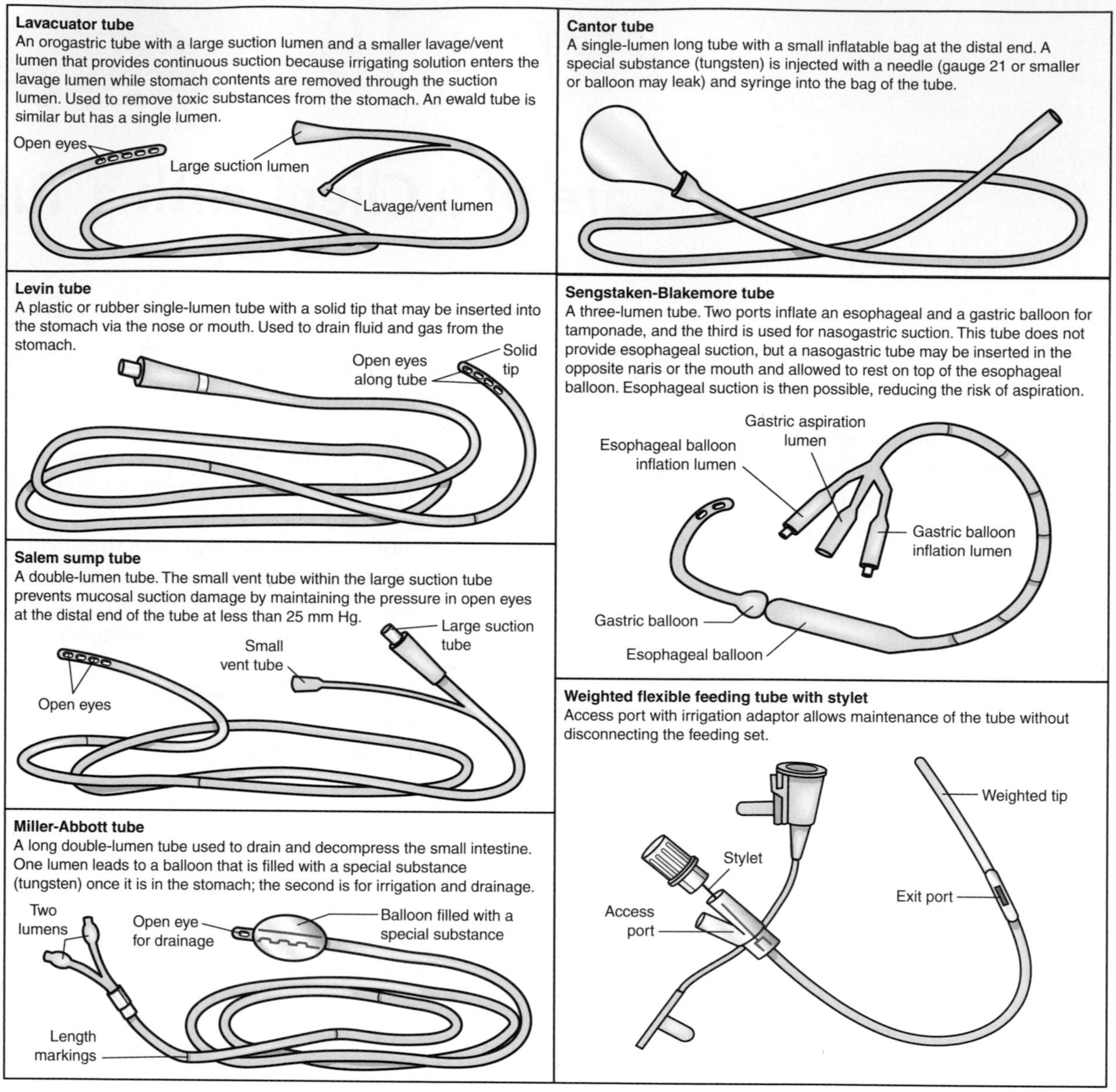

Lavacuator tube
An orogastric tube with a large suction lumen and a smaller lavage/vent lumen that provides continuous suction because irrigating solution enters the lavage lumen while stomach contents are removed through the suction lumen. Used to remove toxic substances from the stomach. An ewald tube is similar but has a single lumen.

Open eyes
Large suction lumen
Lavage/vent lumen

Cantor tube
A single-lumen long tube with a small inflatable bag at the distal end. A special substance (tungsten) is injected with a needle (gauge 21 or smaller or balloon may leak) and syringe into the bag of the tube.

Levin tube
A plastic or rubber single-lumen tube with a solid tip that may be inserted into the stomach via the nose or mouth. Used to drain fluid and gas from the stomach.

Open eyes along tube
Solid tip

Sengstaken-Blakemore tube
A three-lumen tube. Two ports inflate an esophageal and a gastric balloon for tamponade, and the third is used for nasogastric suction. This tube does not provide esophageal suction, but a nasogastric tube may be inserted in the opposite naris or the mouth and allowed to rest on top of the esophageal balloon. Esophageal suction is then possible, reducing the risk of aspiration.

Esophageal balloon inflation lumen
Gastric aspiration lumen
Gastric balloon inflation lumen
Gastric balloon
Esophageal balloon

Salem sump tube
A double-lumen tube. The small vent tube within the large suction tube prevents mucosal suction damage by maintaining the pressure in open eyes at the distal end of the tube at less than 25 mm Hg.

Open eyes
Small vent tube
Large suction tube

Weighted flexible feeding tube with stylet
Access port with irrigation adaptor allows maintenance of the tube without disconnecting the feeding set.

Stylet
Access port
Weighted tip
Exit port

Miller-Abbott tube
A long double-lumen tube used to drain and decompress the small intestine. One lumen leads to a balloon that is filled with a special substance (tungsten) once it is in the stomach; the second is for irrigation and drainage.

Two lumens
Open eye for drainage
Balloon filled with a special substance
Length markings

FIGURE 19-1 Comparison of design and function of selected gastrointestinal tubes.

5. Aspirate all stomach contents (residual), measure the amount, and return the contents to the stomach to prevent electrolyte imbalances.
6. Warm the feeding to room temperature to prevent diarrhea and cramps.
7. Use an infusion feeding pump for continuous or cyclic feedings.
8. For bolus feeding, maintain the client in a high Fowler's position for 30 minutes after the feeding.
9. For a continuous feeding, keep the client in a semi-Fowler's position at all times.

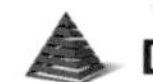

D. Precautions

⚠ Always check the placement of a gastrointestinal tube before instilling feeding solutions, medications, or any other solution. If the tube is incorrectly placed, the client is at risk for aspiration.

1. Change the feeding container and tubing every 24 hours.
2. Do not hang more solution than required for a 4-hour period; this prevents bacterial growth.
3. Check the expiration date on the formula before administering it.
4. Shake the formula well before pouring it into the feeding bag.
5. Always check the bowel sounds. Feedings cannot be administered if bowel sounds are absent.
6. Administer the feeding at the prescribed rate or via gravity flow (intermittent bolus feedings) with a 50- to 60-mL syringe with the plunger removed.
7. Gently flush with 30 to 50 mL of water or normal saline (depending on agency policy) with the irrigation syringe after the feeding.

BOX 19-1 Nasogastric Tubes: Intubation Procedures

1. Follow agency procedures.
2. Explain the procedure and its potential discomfort to the client.
3. Position the client with pillows behind the shoulders.
4. Determine which nostril is more patent.
5. Measure the length of the tube from the bridge of the nose to the earlobe to the xiphoid process and indicate this length with a piece of tape on the tube.
6. If the client is conscious and alert, have him or her swallow or drink water (follow agency procedure).
7. Lubricate the tip of the tube with water-soluble lubricant.
8. Gently insert the tube into the nasopharynx and advance the tube.
9. When the tube nears the back of the throat (first black measurement on the tube) instruct the client to swallow or drink sips of water (unless contraindicated). If resistance is met, then slowly rotate and aim the tube downward and toward the closer ear; in the intubated or semiconscious client, flex the head toward the chest while passing the tube.
10. Immediately withdraw the tube if any change is noted in the client's respiratory status.
11. Following insertion, obtain an abdominal x-ray study to confirm placement of the tube.
12. Connect the tube to suction, to either the intermittent or continuous suction setting, as prescribed.
13. Secure the tube to the client's nose with adhesive tape and to the client's gown (follow agency procedure and check for client allergy to tape).
14. Observe the client for nausea, vomiting, abdominal fullness, or distention, and monitor output.
15. Check residual volumes every 4 hours, before each feeding, and before giving medications. Aspirate all stomach contents (residual) and measure the amount. Reinstill residual contents to prevent excessive fluid and electrolyte losses, unless the residual contents appear abnormal and the volume is large (follow agency procedure). Withhold the feeding if the amount is more than 100 mL or according to agency or nutritional consult recommendations.
16. Before the instillation of any substance through the tube (i.e., irrigation solution, feeding, medications), aspirate stomach contents and test the pH (a pH of 3.5 or lower indicates that the tip of the tube is in a gastric location).
17. If irrigation is indicated, use normal saline solution (check agency procedure).
18. Observe the client for fluid and electrolyte balance.
19. Instruct the client about movement to prevent nasal irritation and dislodgment of the tube.
20. On a daily basis, remove the adhesive tape that is securing the tube to the nose and clean and dry the skin, assessing for excoriation; then reapply the tape.

Note: Gastrostomy or jejunostomy tubes are surgically inserted. A dressing is placed at the site of insertion. The dressing needs to be removed, the skin needs to be cleansed (with a solution determined by the health care provider or agency procedure), and a new sterile dressing needs to be applied every 8 hours (or as specified by agency policy). The skin at the insertion site is checked for signs of excoriation, infection, or other abnormalities, such as leakage of the feeding solution.

Potter, P., Perry, A. G., Stockert, P. A., & Hall, A. M. (2013). *Fundamentals of nursing.* (8th ed., p. 594). St. Louis: Mosby.

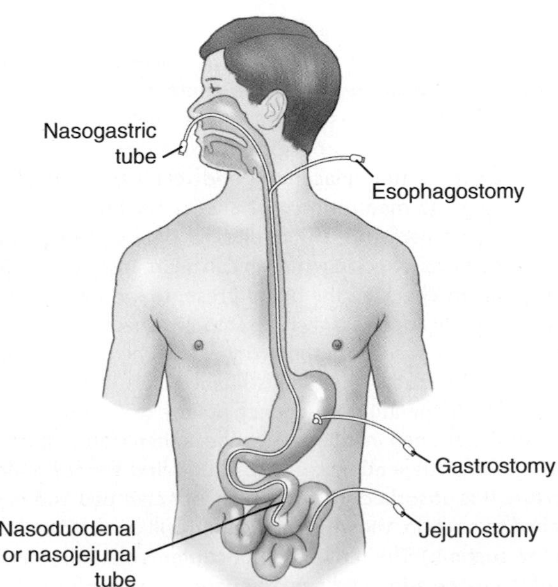

FIGURE 19-2 Diagram of the placement of enteral feeding tubes. (From Leonard P: *Building a medical vocabulary: With Spanish translations*, ed 7, St. Louis, 2009, Mosby.)

E. Prevention of complications 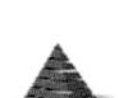
  1. Diarrhea
    a. Check the client for lactose intolerance.
    b. Fiber-containing feedings may be prescribed.
    c. Administer feeding slowly and at room temperature.
  2. Aspiration
    a. Verify tube placement.
    b. Do not administer the feeding if residual is more than 100 mL (check with the registered nurse and HCP's prescription and agency policy).
    c. Keep the head of the bed elevated.
    d. If aspiration occurs, suction as needed, monitor respiratory rate, auscultate lung sounds, monitor temperature for aspiration pneumonia, and prepare to obtain chest radiograph.
  3. Clogged tube
    a. Use liquid forms of medication, if possible; if liquid forms cannot be used, medications need to be crushed.

b. Flush the tube with 30 to 50 mL of water or NS (depending on agency policy) before and after medication administration and before and after bolus feeding.

c. Flush with water every 4 hours for continuous feeding.

4. Vomiting

⚠ If the client vomits, stop the tube feeding and place the client in a side-lying position; suction the client as needed.

a. Administer feedings slowly and, for bolus feedings, make feeding last for at least 30 minutes.

b. Measure abdominal girth.

c. Do not allow the feeding bag to empty.

d. Do not allow air to enter the tubing.

e. Administer the feeding at room temperature.

f. Elevate the head of the bed.

g. Administer antiemetics as prescribed.

⚠ If the client vomits, stop the tube feeding and place the client in a side-lying position; suction the client as needed.

F. Administration of medications (see Priority Nursing Actions)

III. Intestinal Tubes

A. Description

1. Passed nasally into the small intestine
2. Used to decompress the bowel or to remove intestinal contents
3. Designed to enter the small intestine through the pyloric sphincter with the use of the weight of a small bag containing a special substance (tungsten) at the end

B. Types of tubes include the Cantor tube (single lumen) and the Miller-Abbott tube (double lumen) (see Fig. 19-1).

C. Interventions 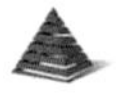

1. Check the HCP's prescriptions and agency policy for advancement and removal of the tube and tungsten; assist the registered nurse.
2. Position the client on the right side to facilitate passage of the weighted bag in the tube through the pylorus of the stomach and into the small intestine.

PRIORITY NURSING ACTIONS!

Steps for Administering Medications via a Nasogastric or Gastrostomy Tube

1. Check the HCP's prescription.
2. Prepare the medication for administration.
3. Ensure that the medication prescribed can be crushed or (if it is a capsule) that it can be opened; use elixir forms of medications if available.
4. Dissolve crushed medication or capsule contents in 15 to 30 mL of water.
5. Verify the client's identity and explain the procedure to the client.
6. Check tube placement and residual contents before instilling the medication; check for bowel sounds.
7. Draw up the medication into a catheter tip syringe, clear excess air from the syringe, and insert the medication into the tube.
8. Flush with 30 to 50 mL of water or NS (depending on agency policy).
9. Clamp the tube for 30 to 60 minutes (depending on medication and agency policy).
10. Document the administration of the medication and any other appropriate information.

The nurse always checks the HCP's prescription before administering any medication to a client. Once the prescription is verified, the medication is prepared for administration. The nurse determines the reason for administration and checks for any contraindications to administering the medication and for any potential interactions. When preparing medications for administration through a nasogastric or gastrostomy tube, the nurse needs to ensure that the medication prescribed can be crushed or (if it is a capsule) that it can be opened. Whole tablets or capsules cannot be administered through a tube because they can cause a tube blockage. Elixir forms of medications can also be used if available. The nurse then dissolves the crushed medication or capsule contents in 15 to 30 mL of water. Client identity is always verified before medication administration, and the procedure is explained to the client. The nurse checks tube placement and residual contents before instilling the medication and checks for bowel sounds. The nurse also performs any additional data collection procedures, such as checking the apical heart rate for cardiac medications or checking the blood pressure for antihypertensives. The medication is drawn up into a catheter tip syringe, excess air is removed from the syringe, and the medication is inserted into the tube. The tube is flushed with 30 to 50 mL of water or NS (depending on agency policy) to ensure that all medication has been instilled. The tube is then clamped for 30 to 60 minutes (depending on medication and agency policy) to ensure it is absorbed. (If the tube is not clamped and is reattached to suction, then the medication will be aspirated out with the suction.) The nurse then documents the administration of the medication and any other appropriate information.

Reference(s): Cooper, K. & Gosnell, K. (2015). *Foundations and adult health nursing* (7th ed., pp. 583–584). St. Louis, Elsevier.

3. Do not secure the tube to the face with tape until it has reached final placement (may take several hours) in the intestines.
4. Check the abdomen during the procedure by monitoring drainage from the tube and the abdominal girth.
5. If the tube becomes blocked, notify registered nurse and the HCP.
6. When the tube is removed, the tungsten is removed from the balloon portion of the tube with a syringe; the tube is removed gradually (6 inches every hour) as prescribed by the HCP.

IV. Esophageal and Gastric Tubes

A. Description
  1. May be used to apply pressure against bleeding esophageal veins to control the bleeding when other interventions are not effective or they are contraindicated.
  2. Not used if the client has ulceration or necrosis of the esophagus or has had previous esophageal surgery because of the risk of rupture.
  3. Examples are the Sengstaken-Blakemore tube or Minnesota tube (a modified Sengstaken-Blakemore tube with an additional lumen for aspirating esophagopharyngeal secretions). These tubes are uncomfortable for the client and can cause complications, but their use may be necessary when other interventions are not feasible (see Fig. 19-1).

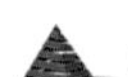
B. Interventions
  1. The patency and integrity of all balloons are checked before insertion, and each lumen is labeled.
  2. The client is placed in an upright or Fowler's position for insertion.
  3. Prepare the client for an x-ray study immediately after insertion to verify placement.
  4. Maintain head elevation after the tube is in place.
  5. The balloon ports are double-clamped to prevent air leaks.
  6. Scissors are kept at the bedside at all times.
  7. The client is monitored for respiratory distress. If it occurs, notify the registered nurse immediately. The tubes will be cut to deflate the balloons.
  8. Monitor for increased bloody drainage that may indicate persistent bleeding.
  9. Monitor for signs of esophageal rupture, including a drop in blood pressure, increased heart rate, and back and upper abdominal pain. (Esophageal rupture is an emergency and must be reported immediately.)

V. Lavage Tubes

A. Description: Used to remove toxic substances from the stomach

B. Types of tubes
  1. Lavacuator (see Fig. 19-1)
    a. The Lavacuator is an orogastric tube with a large suction lumen and a smaller lavage–vent lumen that provides continuous suction.
    b. Irrigation solution enters the lavage lumen while stomach contents are removed through the suction lumen.
  2. Ewald tube: A single-lumen large tube used for rapid one-time irrigation and evacuation

VI. Urinary and Renal Tubes

A. Types of urinary catheters (Fig. 19-3)
  1. Single lumen is used for straight catheterizations: Usually used for straight catheterization to empty the client's bladder, obtain sterile urine specimens, or to check the residual amount of urine after the client voids.
  2. Double lumen: Used when an indwelling catheter is needed for continuous bladder drainage; one lumen is for drainage and the other is for balloon inflation.
  3. Triple lumen: Used when bladder irrigation and drainage is necessary; one lumen is for instilling the bladder irrigant solution, one lumen is for continuous bladder drainage, and one lumen is for balloon inflation.
  4. Strict aseptic technique is necessary for insertion and care of the catheter.

B. Routine urinary catheter care
  1. Use gloves, and wash the perineal area with warm, soapy water.
  2. With the nondominant hand, pull back the labia or foreskin to expose the meatus (in the adult male, return the foreskin to its normal position).
  3. Clean along the catheter with soap and water.
  4. Anchor the catheter to the thigh according to agency policy.
  5. Maintain the catheter bag below the level of the bladder.

C. Ureteral and nephrostomy tubes
  1. Never clamp the tubes.
  2. Maintain patency.
  3. Monitor output closely.
  4. Tube irrigation may be prescribed by the HCP and will be done by the registered nurse per prescription

D. Catheter insertion and removal (Box 19-2)

⚠ If the client has a ureteral or nephrostomy tube, monitor output closely. Urine output of less than 30 mL/hour or lack of output for more than 15 minutes should be reported to the HCP immediately.

VII. Respiratory System Tubes

A. **Endotracheal tubes** (Fig. 19-4)
  1. Description
    a. Used to maintain a patent airway

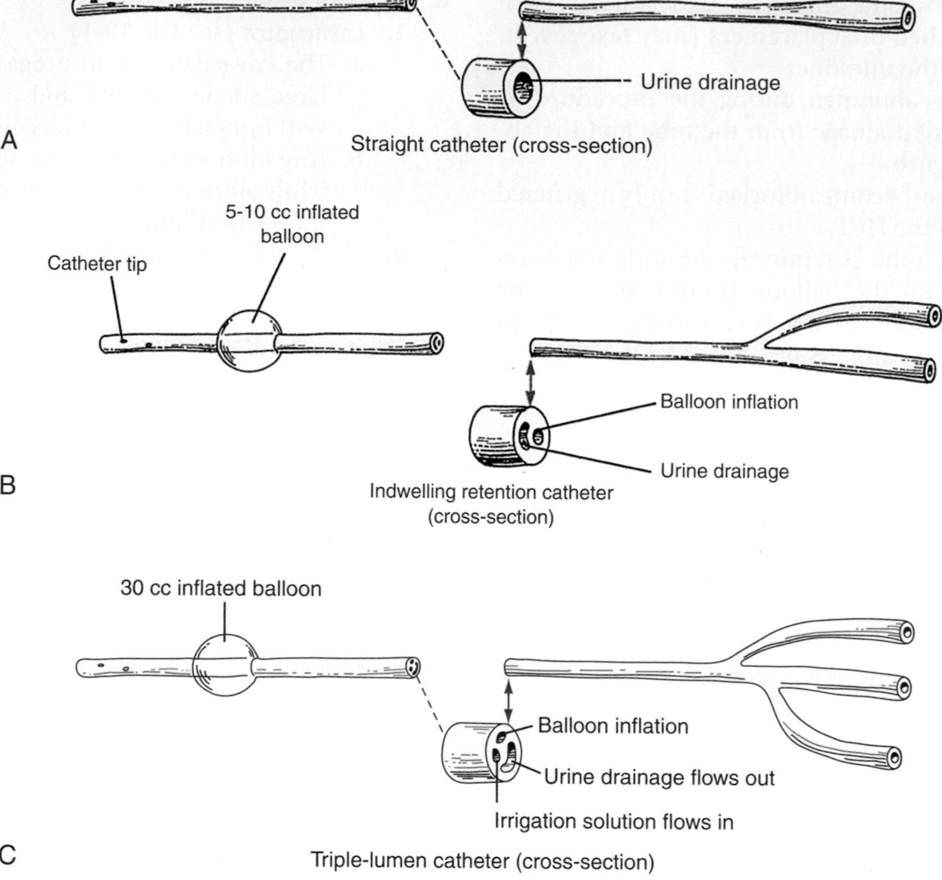

FIGURE 19-3 Types of urinary catheters: **A,** Straight catheter (cross-section). **B,** Indwelling retention catheter (cross-section). **C,** Triple-lumen catheter (cross-section). (From Perry A, Potter P, Elkin M: *Nursing interventions and clinical skills*, ed 5, St. Louis, 2012, Mosby.)

b. Indicated when the client needs mechanical ventilation

c. If the client requires an artificial airway for longer than 10 to 14 days, a tracheostomy may be created to avoid the mucosal and vocal cord damage that can be caused by the endotracheal tube.

d. Types of tubes: Orotracheal and nasotracheal

2. Orotracheal

a. Inserted through the mouth; allows for the use of a larger-diameter tube and reduces the work of breathing

b. Indicated when the client has a nasal obstruction or a predisposition to epistaxis

c. Uncomfortable for the client and can be manipulated by the tongue, thus causing airway obstruction; an oral airway may be needed to prevent the client from biting on the tube

3. Nasotracheal

a. Inserted through the nose; this smaller tube increases both resistance and the client's work of breathing

b. Use of this type of tube is avoided in clients with bleeding disorders

c. More comfortable for the client; he or she is unable to manipulate the tube with the tongue

4. Interventions

a. Placement is confirmed by a chest x-ray study (correct placement is 1 to 2 cm above the carina) and by auscultating both sides of chest while manually ventilating with resuscitation (Ambu) bag. If breath sounds and chest wall movement are absent on the left side, the tube may be in the right main stem bronchus.

b. If the tube is in the stomach, louder breath sounds will be heard over the stomach than over the chest, and abdominal distention will be present.

c. The tube is secured immediately after intubation with adhesive tape.

d. Monitor the position of the tube at the lip or nose.

e. Monitor the skin and mucous membranes.

f. Suction the tube only when needed.

g. The oral tube needs to be moved to the opposite side of the mouth daily to prevent pressure and necrosis of the lip and mouth area,

BOX 19-2 Urinary Catheters: Insertion and Removal Procedures

Urinary Catheters: Insertion Procedure

1. Follow agency procedures.
2. Explain the procedure and its potential discomfort to the client.
3. Place in position for catheterization:
   Female: Assist to dorsal recumbent position (supine with knees flexed). Support legs with pillows to reduce muscle tension and promote comfort.
   Male: Assist to supine position with thighs slightly abducted.
4. Wearing clean gloves, wash perineal area with soap and water as needed; dry thoroughly. Remove and discard gloves; perform hand hygiene.
5. Open outer wrapping of the catheter kit, remembering that all components of the catheterization tray are sterile (all supplies are arranged in the box in order of sequence of use).
6. Apply waterproof sterile drape (when packed as first item in tray).
7. Foley catheter procedure with specifics for male and female:
   a. Place sterile drape with plastic side down under the client's buttocks.
   b. Don sterile gloves.
   c. Pick up fenestrated drape out of tray. Allow it to unfold without touching nonsterile surface. Apply drape over perineum, exposing labia or penis.
   d. Catheter insertion
   Female: With nondominant hand, fully expose urethral meatus by spreading labia. Using forceps in sterile dominant hand, pick up cotton ball or swab sticks saturated with antiseptic solution, wiping from front to back (from clitoris toward anus). Using a new cotton ball or swab for each area you clean, wipe far labial fold, near labial fold, and directly over center of urethral meatus. Open packet containing lubricant and lubricate catheter tip. Advance catheter a total of 7.5 cm (3 inches) in adult or until urine flows out of catheter end. When urine appears, advance catheter another 2.5 to 5 cm (1 to 2 inches). Do not use force to insert catheter.
   Male: Use of square sterile drape is optional; you may apply fenestrated drape with fenestrated slit resting over penis. Open package of sterile antiseptic solution. Pour solution over sterile cotton balls. Grasp penis at shaft just below glans. (If client is not circumcised, retract foreskin with nondominant hand.) With dominant hand pick up antiseptic-soaked cotton ball with forceps or swab stick and clean penis. Move cotton ball or swab in circular motion from urethral meatus down to base of glans. Repeat cleaning 3 more times, using clean cotton ball/stick each time. Pick up catheter with gloved dominant hand and insert catheter by lifting penis to position perpendicular to patient's body and apply light traction. Advance catheter 17 to 22.5 cm (7 to 9 inches) in adult or until urine flows out of catheter end. Lower penis, and hold catheter securely in nondominant hand.
8. Inflate balloon fully per manufacturer's directions.
9. Secure catheter tubing to inner thigh with strip of nonallergenic tape (use paper tape if allergic to silk tape or a multipurpose tube holder with a Velcro strap).
10. Record type and size of catheter inserted, amount of fluid used to inflate the balloon, characteristics and amount of urine, specimen collection if appropriate, client's response to procedure, and that teaching is completed.

Urinary Catheters: Removal Procedure

1. Follow agency procedures.
2. Explain the procedure and its potential discomfort to the client.
3. Position the client in the same position as during catheterization.
4. Remove the tape and place the towel between a female client's thighs or over a male client's thighs.
5. Insert a 10-mL syringe into the balloon injection port. Slowly withdraw all of the solution to deflate the balloon totally.
6. After deflation, explain to the client that they may feel a burning sensation as the catheter is withdrawn. Pull the catheter out smoothly and slowly.
7. Monitor the client's urinary function by noting the first voiding after catheter removal and documenting the time and amount of voiding for the next 24 hours.

From Potter P, Perry A, Stockert P, Hall A: *Fundamentals of nursing*, ed 8, St. Louis, 2013, Mosby.

prevent nerve damage, and facilitate the inspection and cleaning of the mouth. Moving the tube to the opposite side of the mouth should be done by two health care providers.

h. Prevent dislodgment and pulling or tugging on the tube. Suction, coughing, and speaking attempts by the client place extra stress on the tube and can cause dislodgment.

i. Cuff inflation is maintained to create a seal and to allow for the complete mechanical control of respirations.

A resuscitation (Ambu) bag needs to be kept at the bedside of a client with an endotracheal tube or tracheostomy tube at all times.

5. Extubation 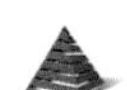

a. Hyperoxygenate the client, and suction the endotracheal tube and the oral cavity.
b. Place the client in semi-Fowler's position.
c. The cuff is deflated. The client is asked to inhale. At peak inspiration, the tube is removed and the airway is suctioned through the tube as it is pulled out.
d. After removal, instruct the client to cough and deep breathe to assist with the removal of accumulated secretions from the throat.
e. Apply oxygen therapy, as prescribed.
f. Monitor for respiratory difficulty. Contact the registered nurse and HCP if respiratory difficulty occurs.

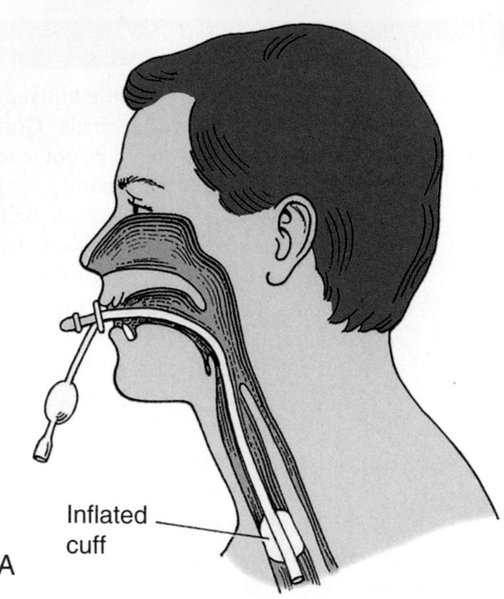

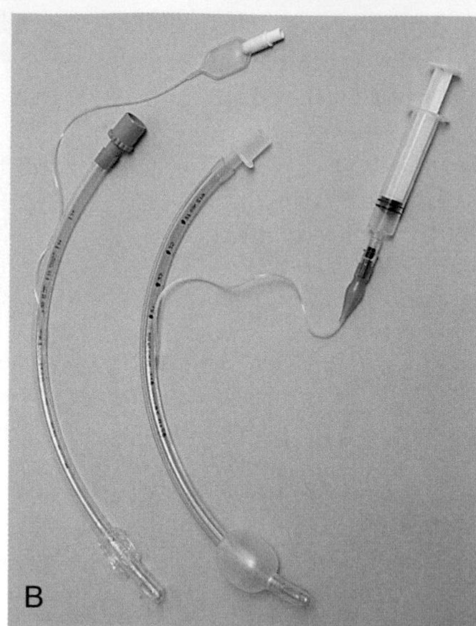

FIGURE 19-4 **A,** Endotracheal (ET) tube with inflated cuff. **B,** ET tubes with uninflated and inflated cuffs and syringe for inflation. (From Perry A, Potter P, Elkin M: *Nursing interventions and clinical skills*, ed 5, St. Louis, 2012, Mosby.)

g. Inform the client that hoarseness or a sore throat is normal and that he or she should limit talking if it occurs.

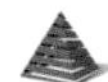

B. Tracheostomy

1. Description
   a. A tracheostomy is an opening made surgically directly into the trachea to establish an airway; a tracheostomy tube is inserted into the opening and the tube attaches to the mechanical ventilator or another type of oxygen delivery device.
   b. The tracheostomy can be temporary or permanent.
2. Single-cannula tube: Has an outer but no inner cannula; used for a client with a thick neck or longer trachea in whom a standard tube will not enter the trachea
3. Cuffed tube: Has an outer and inner cannula, an obturator, and a cuff
4. Cuffless tube
   a. Has an outer cannula, an open and plugged inner cannula, and an obturator
   b. Used long term for the client who is no longer at risk for aspiration

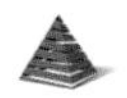

5. Fenestrated tube (Fig. 19-5)
   a. Has an opening along the posterior wall of the outer cannula
   b. When the tube is capped, the client can breathe through the upper airway and speak.
   c. The cuff is always deflated before the tube is capped.

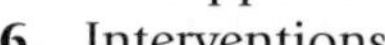

6. Interventions
   a. Monitor the respirations and for bilateral breath sounds.
   b. Monitor the pulse oximetry; arterial blood gas results are also monitored.

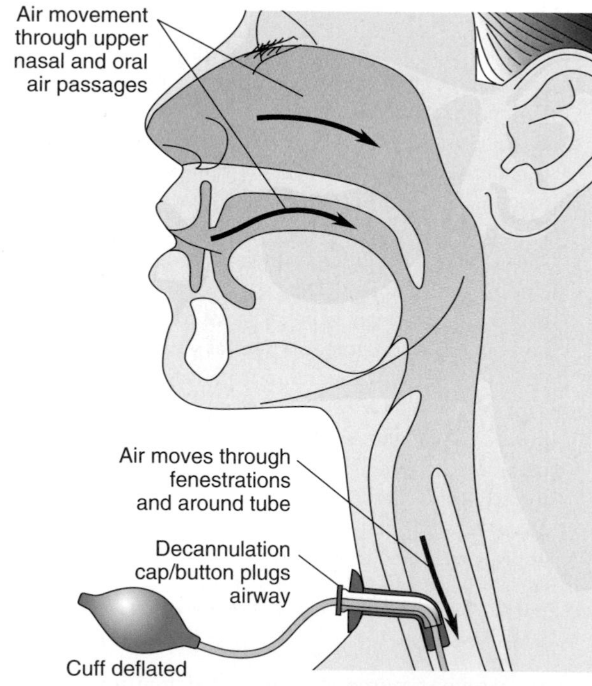

FIGURE 19-5 Breathing through a fenestrated tracheostomy tube with a cap in place and the cuff deflated. (From Ignatavicius D, Workman M: *Medical-surgical nursing: Patient-centered collaborative care*, ed 6, St. Louis, 2010, Saunders.)

   c. Encourage coughing and deep breathing.
   d. Maintain a semi-Fowler's to high Fowler's position.
   e. Monitor for bleeding, difficulty breathing (pneumothorax), and crepitus (subcutaneous emphysema), which are indications of hemorrhage or pneumothorax.

f. Provide respiratory treatments, as prescribed.
g. Suction as needed; hyperoxygenate the client before suction (see Chapter 49 for the suctioning procedure).
h. If the client is allowed to eat, sit him or her up for meals, and ensure that the cuff is inflated (if the tube is not capped) for meals and for 1 hour after meals.
i. Check the stoma and secretions for blood or purulent drainage.
j. Follow the HCP's prescriptions and agency policy for cleaning the tracheostomy site and inner cannula (many inner cannulas are disposable); usually, half-strength hydrogen peroxide is used.
k. Administer humidified oxygen, as prescribed. The normal humidification process is bypassed in a client with a tracheostomy.
l. Obtain assistance with changing the tracheostomy ties. After placing the new ties, cut and remove the old ties that are holding the tracheostomy tube in place (some securing devices are soft and made with Velcro to hold the tube in place).
m. Keep a resuscitation (Ambu) bag, an obturator, clamps, and a spare tracheotomy set at the bedside.
n. Provide frequent mouth care, to reduce the risk of pneumonia.

7. Complications of a tracheostomy (Table 19-1)

TABLE 19-1 Complications of a Tracheostomy

Complications and Description	Manifestations	Management	Prevention
Tracheomalacia: Constant pressure exerted by the cuff causes tracheal dilation and erosion of cartilage.	An increased amount of air is required in the cuff to maintain the seal. A larger tracheostomy tube is required to prevent an air leak at the stoma. Food particles are seen in tracheal secretions. The client does not receive the set tidal volume on the ventilator.	No special management is needed unless bleeding or airway problems occur.	Use an uncuffed tube as soon as possible. Monitor cuff pressure and air volume closely to detect changes.
Tracheal stenosis: Narrowed tracheal lumen is the result of scar formation from irritation of tracheal mucosa by the cuff.	Stenosis is usually seen after the cuff is deflated or the tracheostomy tube is removed. The client has increased coughing, inability to expectorate secretions, or difficulty in breathing and talking.	Tracheal dilation or surgical intervention is used.	Prevent pulling of and traction on the tracheostomy tube. Properly secure the tube in the midline position. Maintain cuff pressure. Minimize oronasal intubation time.
Tracheoesophageal fistula (TEF): Excessive cuff pressure causes erosion of the posterior wall of the trachea. A hole is created between the trachea and the anterior esophagus. The client at highest risk also has a nasogastric tube present.	Similar to tracheomalacia: ■ Food particles are seen in tracheal secretions. ■ Increased air in cuff is needed to achieve a seal. ■ The client has increased coughing and choking while eating. ■ The client does not receive the set tidal volume on the ventilator.	Manually administer oxygen by mask to prevent hypoxemia. Use a small, soft feeding tube instead of a nasogastric tube for tube feedings. A gastrostomy or jejunostomy may be performed. Monitor the client with a nasogastric tube closely; assess for TEF and aspiration.	Maintain cuff pressure. Monitor the amount of air needed for inflation to detect changes. Progress to a deflated or cuffless tube as soon as possible.
Trachea–innominate artery fistula: A malpositioned tube causes its distal tip to push against the lateral wall of the trachea. Continued pressure causes necrosis and erosion of the innominate artery. *This is a medical emergency.*	The tracheostomy tube pulsates in synchrony with the heartbeat. There is heavy bleeding from the stoma. *This is a life-threatening complication.*	Remove the tracheostomy tube immediately. Apply direct pressure to the innominate artery at the stoma site. Prepare the client for immediate repair surgery.	Use the correct tube size and length, and maintain the tube in midline position. Prevent pulling or tugging of the tracheostomy tube. Immediately notify the health care provider of a pulsating tube.
Tube obstruction	■ Difficulty in breathing ■ Noisy respirations ■ Difficulty in inserting the suction catheter ■ Thick, dry secretions ■ Unexplained peak pressures if client is on a mechanical ventilator	The health care provider repositions or replaces the tube if obstruction occurs as a result of cuff prolapse over the end of the tube.	Assist the client to cough and deep breathe. Provide humidification and suctioning. Clean the inner cannula regularly.

Continued

TABLE 19-1 Complications of a Tracheostomy—cont'd

Complications and Description	Manifestations	Management	Prevention
Tube dislodgment	■ Difficulty in breathing ■ Noisy respirations ■ Restlessness ■ Excessive coughing ■ Audible wheeze or stridor	Be familiar with institutional policy regarding replacement of a tracheostomy tube as a nursing procedure. During the first 72 hr following surgical placement of the tracheostomy, the nurse manually ventilates the client by using a manual resuscitation (Ambu) bag, while another nurse calls the Rapid Response team for help. 72 hr following surgical placement of the tracheostomy: ■ Extend the client's neck and open the tissues of the stoma to secure the airway. ■ Grasp the retention sutures (if they are present) to spread the opening. ■ Use a tracheal dilator (curved clamp) to hold the stoma open. ■ Prepare to insert a tracheostomy tube; place the obturator into the tracheostomy tube, replace the tube, and remove the obturator. ■ Maintain ventilation by resuscitation (Ambu) bag. ■ Assess airflow and bilateral breath sounds. ■ If unable to secure an airway, call the Rapid Response team and the anesthesiologist.	Secure the tube in place. Minimize manipulation and traction on the tube. Ensure that the client does not pull on the tube. Ensure that a tracheostomy tube of the same type and size is at the client's bedside.

Adapted from Ignatavicius D, Workman ML: *Medical-surgical nursing: Patient centered collaborative care*, ed 7, Philadelphia, 2013, Saunders.

Never insert a decannulation plug into a tracheostomy tube until the cuff is deflated and the inner cannula is removed. Prior insertion prevents airflow to the client.

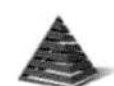

VIII. Chest-tube Drainage System (Fig. 19-6)

A. Description
1. Returns negative pressure to the intrapleural space
2. Used to remove abnormal accumulations of air and fluid from the pleural space
3. Chest-tube placement (Fig. 19-7)

B. Drainage collection chamber (see Fig. 19-6)
1. Located where the chest tube from the client connects to the system
2. Drainage from the tube drains into and collects in a series of calibrated columns in this chamber.

C. Water-seal chamber (see Fig. 19-6)
1. The tip of the tube is underwater, allowing fluid and air to drain from the pleural space and preventing air from entering the pleural space.
2. Water oscillates (i.e., moves up as the client inhales and moves down as the client exhales).
3. Continuous bubbling indicates an air leak in the chest-tube system.

D. Suction-control chamber (see Fig. 19-6)
1. Provides suction, which can be controlled to provide negative pressure to the chest.
2. Filled with various levels of water to achieve the desired level of suction; without this control, lung tissue could be sucked into the chest tube
3. Gentle bubbling indicates that there is suction. It does not indicate that air is escaping from the pleural space.

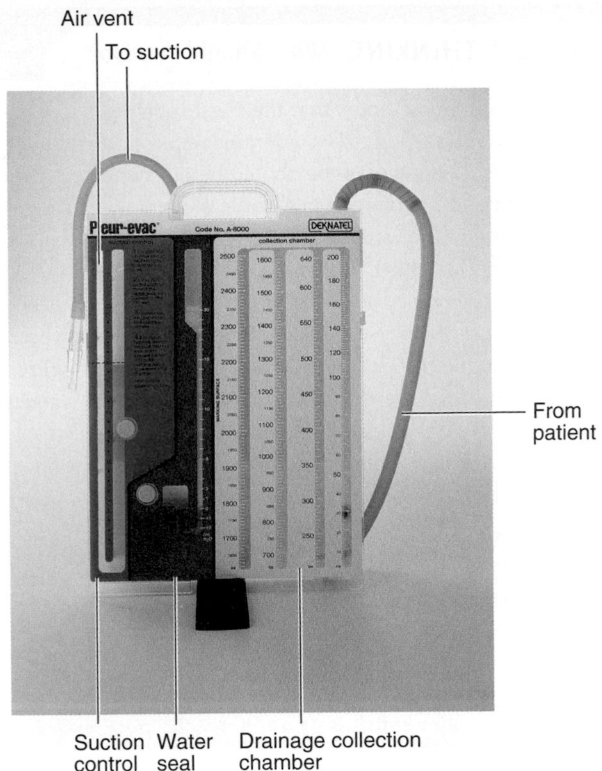

FIGURE 19-6 The Pleur-Evac drainage system, a commercial three-bottle chest drainage device. (From Ignatavicius D, Workman ML: *Medical-surgical nursing: Patient centered collaborative care*, ed 7, Philadelphia, 2013, Saunders. Courtesy of M. Linda Workman.)

E. Dry-suction system
  1. This is another type of chest drainage system, and because this is a dry suction system, absence of bubbling is noted in the suction control chamber.
  2. A knob on the collection device is used to set the prescribed amount of suction; then the wall suction source dial is turned until a small orange floater valve appears in the window on the device (when the orange floater valve is in the window, the correct amount of suction is applied).

F. Portable chest drainage system
  1. Small and portable chest drainage systems are also available and are dry systems that use a control flutter valve to prevent the backflow of air into the client's lung.
  2. Principles of gravity and pressure, and the nursing care involved, are the same for all types of systems, and these systems allow greater ambulation and allow the client to go home with the chest tubes in place.

G. Interventions
  1. Collection chamber
    a. Monitor the drainage. The HCP is notified if the drainage is more than 70 to 100 mL/hour or the drainage becomes bright red or increases suddenly.

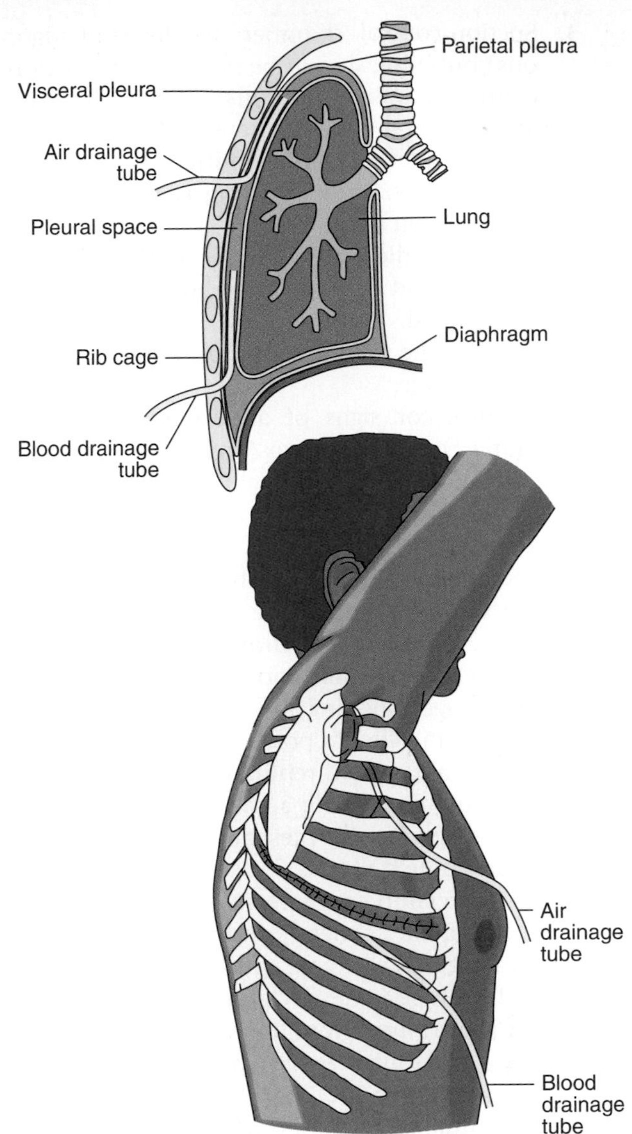

FIGURE 19-7 Chest tube placement. (From Ignatavicius D, Workman ML: *Medical-surgical nursing: Patient centered collaborative care*, ed 7, Philadelphia, 2013, Saunders.)

    b. Mark the chest-tube drainage in the collection chamber at 1- to 4-hour intervals with the use of a piece of tape.
  2. Water-seal chamber
    a. Monitor for the fluctuation of the fluid level in the water-seal chamber.
    b. Fluctuation in the water-seal chamber stops if the tube is obstructed, a dependent loop exists, the suction is not working properly, or the lung has reexpanded.
    c. If the client has a known pneumothorax, intermittent bubbling in the water-seal chamber is expected as air is drained from the chest. Continuous bubbling indicates an air leak in the system.
    d. Notify the registered nurse and HCP if there is continuous bubbling in the water-seal chamber.

3. Suction-control chamber: Gentle (not vigorous) bubbling should be noted in the suction-control chamber. Vigorous bubbling indicates an air leak, and the registered nurse and health care provider should be notified.
4. An occlusive sterile dressing is maintained at the insertion site.
5. A chest radiograph assesses the position of the tube and determines whether the lung has reexpanded.
6. Monitor the respiratory status and listen to the lung sounds.
7. Monitor for signs of an extended pneumothorax or hemothorax (respiratory distress, crepitus [subcutaneous emphysema], increase in bloody drainage or a change to bright red drainage).
8. Keep the drainage system below the level of the chest and the tubes free of kinks, dependent loops, or other obstructions.
9. Ensure that all connections are secure.
10. Encourage coughing and deep breathing.
11. Change the client's position frequently to promote drainage and ventilation.
12. Stripping or milking a chest tube is not done unless specifically prescribed by a HCP and agency policy allows.
13. Keep a clamp (may be needed if the system needs to be changed) and a sterile occlusive dressing at the bedside at all times.
14. A chest tube is never clamped without a written prescription from the health care provider. Also, determine agency policy for clamping chest tubes.
15. If the drainage system cracks or breaks, the registered nurse is notified immediately and the chest tube is inserted into a bottle of sterile water. The cracked or broken system is removed and replaced with a new system.
16. When the chest tube is to be removed, the client is asked to take a deep breath and hold it, and the tube is removed. A dry sterile dressing, petroleum gauze dressing, or Telfa dressing (depending on the HCP's preference) is taped in place after the removal of the chest tube.
17. Depending on the HCP's preference, when the chest tube is removed, the client may be asked to take a deep breath, exhale, and bear down (i.e., Valsalva's maneuver).

⚠ If the chest tube is pulled out of the chest accidentally, pinch the skin opening together, apply an occlusive sterile dressing, cover the dressing with overlapping pieces of 2-inch tape, and call the registered nurse and health care provider immediately.

CRITICAL THINKING What Should You Do?

Answer: If the nurse notes that the chest tube drainage system is cracked, the nurse should immediately notify the registered nurse. The chest tube should be disconnected from the system and submerged in a bottle of sterile water in order to maintain the water seal. The system will then need to be replaced, and this can be done by the registered nurse, depending on agency policy. A clamp should be kept at the bedside in case the system needs to be changed. However, the nurse should never clamp a chest tube without a written prescription from the health care provider and per agency policy. The drainage system (chest tube and bottle of sterile water) should also be maintained below the level of the chest if this complication occurs.

Reference(s): Ignatavicius, D., & Workman, M. (2013). *Medical-surgical nursing: Patient-centered collaborative care.* (7th ed., p. 637). St. Louis: Saunders.

PRACTICE QUESTIONS

151. The nurse is preparing to administer an intermittent tube feeding to a client. The nurse aspirates 90 mL of residual from the tube. What should the nurse do with the aspirated residual?
1. Hold the feeding.
2. Place it into a container for laboratory analysis.
3. Reinstill the residual and administer the feeding.
4. Deduct the amount of the residual from the new feeding and administer that amount to the client.

152. The nurse is providing endotracheal suctioning to a client who is mechanically ventilated when the client becomes restless and tachycardic. Which action should the nurse take?
1. Notify the Rapid Response Team.
2. Finish the suctioning as quickly as possible.
3. Contact the respiratory department to suction the client.
4. Discontinue suctioning until the client is stabilized and monitor vital signs.

153. The nurse is checking a client for the correct placement of a nasogastric (NG) tube. The nurse aspirates the client's stomach contents and checks its pH level. Which pH value indicates the correct placement of the tube?
1. 3.5
2. 4.5
3. 6.0
4. 7.35

154. A licensed practical nurse (LPN) is preparing to assist a registered nurse (RN) with removing a nasogastric (NG) tube from the client. The LPN should reinforce instructing the client to perform which action?
1. Exhale
2. Inhale and exhale quickly
3. Take and hold a deep breath
4. Perform Valsalva's maneuver

❖ **155.** The nurse is assisting with monitoring the functioning of a chest-tube drainage system in a client who just returned from the recovery room after a thoracotomy with wedge resection. Which findings should the nurse expect to note? **Select all that apply.**
❑ 1. Excessive bubbling in the water-seal chamber.
❑ 2. Vigorous bubbling in the suction-control chamber.
❑ 3. 50 mL of drainage in the drainage-collection chamber.
❑ 4. The drainage system is maintained below the client's chest.
❑ 5. An occlusive dressing is in place over the chest-tube insertion site.
❑ 6. Fluctuation of water in the tube of the water-seal chamber during inhalation and exhalation.

156. The nurse is assigned to assist with caring for a client with esophageal varices who had a Sengstaken-Blakemore tube inserted because other treatment measures were unsuccessful. The nurse should check the client's room to ensure that which **priority** item is at the bedside?
1. An obturator
2. A Kelly clamp
3. An irrigation set
4. A pair of scissors

157. The nurse is inserting an indwelling urinary catheter into a male client. As the catheter is inserted into the urethra, urine begins to flow into the tubing. The nurse should take which step **next**?
1. Immediately inflate the balloon.
2. Insert the catheter 2.5 to 5 cm and inflate the balloon.
3. Insert the catheter until resistance is met and inflate the balloon.
4. Withdraw the catheter approximately 1 inch and inflate the balloon.

158. The nurse is assigned to assist with caring for a client who has a chest tube. The nurse notes fluctuations of the fluid level in the water-seal chamber. Based on this observation, which action would be appropriate?
1. Empty the drainage.
2. Encourage the client to deep breathe.
3. Continue to monitor, because this is an expected finding.
4. Encourage the client to hold his or her breath periodically.

159. The nurse is assigned to assist the health care provider with the removal of a chest tube. The nurse should reinforce instructing the client to do which during this process?
1. Stay very still
2. Exhale forcefully
3. Inhale and exhale quickly
4. Perform Valsalva's maneuver

160. The nurse is preparing to begin a continuous tube feeding on a client with a nasogastric tube. In which position should the nurse place the client for safe administration of the tube feeding?
1. Supine
2. Supine on the right side
3. With the head elevated 15 degrees
4. With the head elevated 45 degrees

161. The nurse is preparing to administer an intermittent tube feeding to a client with a nasogastric tube. The nurse checks the residual and obtains an amount of 200 mL. Which action should the nurse take?
1. Hold the feeding.
2. Administer the feeding.
3. Flush the tubing with 30 mL of water.
4. Elevate the head of the bed to 90 degrees and administer the feeding.

❖ **162.** The nurse is assisting in planning care for a client with a chest tube. The nurse should suggest to include which interventions in the plan? **Select all that apply.**
❑ 1. Pin the tubing to the bed linens.
❑ 2. Be sure all connections remain airtight.
❑ 3. Be sure all connections are taped and secure.
❑ 4. Empty the drainage from the drainage collection chamber daily.
❑ 5. Monitor closely for tubing that is kinked or obstructed by the weight of the client.

163. The nurse is assigned to care for a client who has a chest tube. The nurse is told to monitor the client for crepitus (subcutaneous emphysema). Which method should be used to monitor the client for crepitus?
1. Asking the client about pain
2. Checking the respirations hourly
3. Checking the blood pressure every 2 hours
4. Palpating for the leakage of air into the subcutaneous tissues

164. The nurse is told that an assigned client will have a fenestrated tracheostomy tube inserted. The nurse should provide the client with which information about this type of tube?

1. Enables the client to speak
2. Prevents the client from speaking
3. Is necessary for mechanical ventilation
4. Prevents air from being inhaled through the tracheostomy opening

165. The nurse is preparing to administer medication through a nasogastric (NG) tube that is connected to suction. Which indicates the accurate procedure for medication administration?

1. Position the client supine to assist with medication absorption.
2. Clamp the NG tube for 30 minutes after medication administration.
3. Aspirate the NG tube after medication administration to maintain patency.
4. Change the suction setting to low intermittent suction for 30 minutes after medication administration.

ANSWERS

151. 3

Rationale: Unless otherwise instructed or if the residual contents appear abnormal, an amount of less than 100 mL may be reinstituted; then a normal amount of prescribed tube feeding is administered. It is important to return the contents to the stomach to prevent electrolyte imbalances. Therefore, options 1, 2, and 4 are incorrect.

Test-Taking Strategy: Note the subject, residual from a nasogastric tube. Option 1 could cause an electrolyte and nutritional imbalance. There is no data in the question that indicates that laboratory analysis is necessary. To prevent dehydration, clients need to get the correct amount of feeding prescribed. **Review:** **tube-feeding administration.**

Level of Cognitive Ability: Applying
Client Needs: Physiological Integrity
Integrated Process: Nursing Process/Implementation
Content Area: Fundamental Skills: Nutrition
Priority Concepts: Fluid and Electrolyte Balance, Nutrition
Reference(s): Cooper, Gosnell (2015), p. 527.

152. 4

Rationale: If a client becomes cyanotic or restless or develops tachycardia, bradycardia, or another abnormal heart rhythm, the nurse must discontinue suctioning until the client is stabilized. The nurse would also notify the registered nurse. It is also important to monitor the vital signs and the pulse oximetry. If the client's condition continues to deteriorate, then the respiratory department and health care provider may need to be notified. There is no data in the question that indicates that the rapid response team needs to be notified.

Test-Taking Strategy: Focus on the subject, the client becomes restless and tachycardic during suctioning. Use the ABCs—airway, breathing, circulation—to direct you to the correct option. **Review:** endotracheal **suctioning.**

Level of Cognitive Ability: Applying
Client Needs: Physiological Integrity
Integrated Process: Nursing Process/Implementation
Content Area: Adult Health: Respiratory
Priority Concepts: Fluid and Electrolyte Balance, Gas Exchange
Reference(s): Cooper, Gosnell (2015), pp. 660–661.

153. 1

Rationale: If the NG tube is in the stomach, the pH of the contents will be acidic. Options 2 and 3 indicate a slightly acidic pH. Option 4 indicates a neutral pH.

Test-Taking Strategy: Focus on the subject, the pH value of gastric contents. Recalling that gastric contents are acidic and recalling the pH values of acidity and alkalinity will direct you to the correct option. **Review:** **the procedure for checking nasogastric tube placement.**

Level of Cognitive Ability: Understanding
Client Needs: Physiological Integrity
Integrated Process: Nursing Process/Data Collection
Content Area: Adult Health: Gastrointestinal
Priority Concepts: Acid-Base Balance, Clinical Judgment
Reference(s): Cooper, Gosnell (2015), pp. 679–681.

154. 3

Rationale: When the NG tube is removed, the client is instructed to take and hold a deep breath. This will close the epiglottis, and the airway will be temporarily obstructed during the tube removal. This allows for the easy withdrawal of the tube through the esophagus into the nose. The tube is removed with one very smooth, continuous pull. Options 1, 2, and 4 are incorrect.

Test-Taking Strategy: Focus on the subject, the procedure for removing an NG tube. Think about the procedure and consider what each client action identified in the options would produce. This will help direct you to the correct option. **Review:** **the removal of a nasogastric tube.**

Level of Cognitive Ability: Applying
Client Needs: Physiological Integrity
Integrated Process: Nursing Process/Implementation
Content Area: Adult Health: Gastrointestinal
Priority Concepts: Clinical Judgment, Gas Exchange
Reference(s): Cooper, Gosnell (2015), p. 683; Potter, Perry, Stockert, Hall (2013), p. 1120.

155. 3, 4, 5, 6 

Rationale: The bubbling of water in the water-seal chamber indicates air drainage from the client. This is usually seen when intrathoracic pressure is greater than atmospheric pressure, and it may occur during exhalation, coughing, or sneezing. Excessive bubbling in the water-seal chamber may indicate an

air leak, which is an unexpected finding. The fluctuation of water in the tube in the water-seal chamber during inhalation and exhalation is expected. An absence of fluctuation may indicate that the chest tube is obstructed, the lung has reexpanded, or no more air is leaking into the pleural space. Gentle (not vigorous) bubbling should be noted in the suction-control chamber. A total of 50 mL of drainage is not excessive in a client returning to the nursing unit from the recovery room; however, drainage of more than 70 to 100 mL/hour is considered excessive and requires registered nurse and health care provider notification. The chest-tube insertion site is covered with an occlusive (airtight) dressing to prevent air from entering the pleural space. Positioning the drainage system below the client's chest allows gravity to drain the pleural space.
Test-Taking Strategy: Focus on the **subject**, expected findings in a chest-tube drainage system. The words *excessive bubbling* and *vigorous bubbling* in options 1 and 2 are **comparable or alike** and should be eliminated. Also, think about the physiology associated with chest tube drainage systems to answer correctly.
Review: the care of the client with a **chest-tube drainage** system.
Level of Cognitive Ability: Analyzing
Client Needs: Physiological Integrity
Integrated Process: Nursing Process/Data Collection
Content Area: Adult Health: Respiratory
Priority Concepts: Clinical Judgment, Gas Exchange
Reference(s): deWit, Kumagai (2013), pp. 316–317; Lewis, Dirksen, Heitkemper, Bucher (2014), pp. 546–547.

156. 4
Rationale: When the client has a Sengstaken-Blakemore tube, a pair of scissors must be kept at the client's bedside at all times. The client needs to be observed for sudden respiratory distress, which occurs if the gastric balloon ruptures and the entire tube moves upward. If this occurs, the registered nurse is notified immediately and the balloon lumens will be cut. An obturator and a Kelly clamp are kept at the bedside of a client with a tracheostomy. An irrigation set may also be kept at the bedside, but it is not the priority item.
Test-Taking Strategy: Note the **strategic word**, *priority.* Use your knowledge of the structure, function, and placement of a Sengstaken-Blakemore tube to assist you in answering this question. ***Review:*** the care of a client with a **Sengstaken-Blakemore tube**.
Level of Cognitive Ability: Applying
Client Needs: Safe and Effective Care Environment
Integrated Process: Nursing Process/Implementation
Content Area: Fundamental Skills: Safety
Priority Concepts: Gas Exchange, Safety
Reference(s): Lewis, Dirksen, Heitkemper, Bucher (2014), p. 1026.

157. 2
Rationale: The catheter's balloon is behind the opening at the insertion tip. The catheter is inserted 2.5 to 5 cm after urine begins to flow to provide sufficient space to inflate the balloon. Inserting the catheter the extra distance will ensure that the balloon is inflated inside the bladder and not in the urethra, which could produce trauma. Inserting the catheter until resistance is met could cause trauma to the bladder wall.
Test-Taking Strategy: Note the **strategic word**, *next.* Visualize the proper procedure for inserting an indwelling urinary catheter. Recalling that the catheter's balloon is behind the opening of the tip will assist in answering correctly. **Review: bladder catheterization.**
Level of Cognitive Ability: Applying
Client Needs: Physiological Integrity
Integrated Process: Nursing Process/Implementation
Content Area: Fundamental Skills: Elimination
Priority Concepts: Elimination, Safety
Reference(s): Cooper, Gosnell (2015), pp. 666–667.

158. 3
Rationale: The presence of fluctuations in the fluid level in the water-seal chamber indicates a patent drainage system. With normal breathing, the water level rises with inspiration and falls with expiration. The apparatus and all connections must remain airtight at all times, and the drainage is never emptied because of the risk of disruption in the closed system, which can result in lung collapse. Encouraging the client to deep breathe is unrelated to this observation. The client is not told to hold his or her breath.
Test-Taking Strategy: Focus on the **subject**, the fluctuation of the fluid level in the water-seal chamber. Eliminate option 1 first because drainage is not emptied. Options 2 and 4 are **comparable or alike** and can be eliminated. **Review:** the expected and unexpected findings when caring for a client with a **chest tube**.
Level of Cognitive Ability: Applying
Client Needs: Physiological Integrity
Integrated Process: Nursing Process/Implementation
Content Area: Adult Health: Respiratory
Priority Concepts: Gas Exchange, Safety
Reference(s): Cooper, Gosnell (2015), pp. 1645–1646.

159. 4
Rationale: When the chest tube is removed, the client is asked to perform Valsalva's maneuver (i.e., take a deep breath, exhale, and bear down), the tube is quickly withdrawn, and an airtight dressing is taped in place. An alternative instruction is to ask the client to take a deep breath and hold the breath while the tube is removed. Options 1, 2, and 3 are incorrect client instructions.
Test-Taking Strategy: Focus on the **subject**, removal of a chest tube. Visualize the procedure, client instructions, and the effect of each of the actions in the options to answer correctly. **Review: Chest tube removal.**
Level of Cognitive Ability: Applying
Client Needs: Physiological Integrity
Integrated Process: Nursing Process/Implementation
Content Area: Adult Health: Respiratory
Priority Concepts: Gas Exchange, Safety
Reference(s): Perry, Potter, Ostendorf (2014), p. 670.

160. 4
Rationale: When a tube feeding is administered, the client is placed in a high Fowler's position for a bolus feeding and in a semi-Fowler's position (30 to 45 degrees) for a continuous

feeding to allow gravity to help the flow of formula and to prevent reflux and aspiration. Options 1, 2, and 3 are inappropriate positions during a tube feeding.
Test-Taking Strategy: Focus on the subject, positioning for tube feeding administration. Eliminate options 1 and 2 first, because they are comparable or alike. Next, recalling the associated risk of aspiration when a tube feeding is administered will assist in directing you to the correct option. **Review: tube feedings.**
Level of Cognitive Ability: Applying
Client Needs: Physiological Integrity
Integrated Process: Nursing Process/Implementation
Content Area: Fundamental Skills: Safety
Priority Concepts: Gas Exchange, Safety
Reference(s): deWit, Kumagai (2013), p. 660.

161. 1
Rationale: When 200 mL of residual formula are obtained, the feeding is held and the registered nurse is notified because this is an indication that the feeding is not being absorbed. If the residual is less than 100 mL, the feeding is usually administered. Large-volume aspirates indicate delayed gastric emptying and place the client at risk for aspiration. In addition, the nurse should always check the health care provider's prescriptions and agency policy regarding residual amounts. Elevating the head of the bed to 90 degrees and flushing the tubing are not appropriate actions.
Test-Taking Strategy: Focus on the subject, the action to take with a residual of 200 mL. Eliminate options 2 and 4 first because they are comparable or alike. Recalling that the feeding is held when more than 100 mL of residual are obtained will direct you to the correct option. **Review: tube feedings.**
Level of Cognitive Ability: Applying
Client Needs: Physiological Integrity
Integrated Process: Nursing Process/Implementation
Content Area: Fundamental Skills: Safety
Priority Concepts: Clinical Judgment, Safety
Reference(s): Cooper, Gosnell (2015), p. 527.

❖ **162. 2, 3, 5**
Rationale: Chest-tube tubing is never pinned to the bed linens because this presents the risk of accidental dislodgment of the tube when the client moves. The chest tube system is not opened and emptied because a closed system must be maintained; if the system is opened, lung collapse can occur. Options 2, 3, and 5 are appropriate interventions for the plan of care for a client with a chest tube.
Test-Taking Strategy: Focus on the subject, interventions for the client with a chest tube. Think about the principles associated with a closed chest-tube drainage system and its purpose. Opening the system can cause a lung collapse. **Review:** the care of the client with a **chest tube.**
Level of Cognitive Ability: Analyzing
Client Needs: Physiological Integrity
Integrated Process: Nursing Process/Planning
Content Area: Adult Health: Respiratory
Priority Concepts: Gas Exchange, Safety
Reference(s): deWit, Kumagai (2013), p. 317.

163. 4
Rationale: Subcutaneous emphysema is also known as crepitus. It presents as a "puffed-up" appearance that is caused by the leakage of air into the subcutaneous tissues. It is monitored by palpating, and it feels like bubble wrap when palpated. Although options 1, 2, and 3 may be components of the plan of care for a client with a chest tube, these actions will not identify subcutaneous emphysema.
Test-Taking Strategy: Note the subject, monitoring for subcutaneous emphysema. Think about what this condition entails to answer correctly. Also note the word *subcutaneous* in the question and in the correct option. **Review: subcutaneous emphysema.**
Level of Cognitive Ability: Applying
Client Needs: Physiological Integrity
Integrated Process: Nursing Process/Data Collection
Content Area: Adult Health: Respiratory
Priority Concepts: Gas Exchange, Tissue Integrity
Reference(s): deWit, Kumagai (2013), p. 317.

164. 1
Rationale: A fenestrated tube has a small opening in the outer cannula that allows some air to escape through the larynx; this type of tube enables the client to speak. Options 2, 3, and 4 are incorrect with regard to this type of tube.
Test-Taking Strategy: Focus on the subject, a fenestrated tracheostomy tube. Knowledge regarding the design and purpose of a fenestrated tracheostomy tube will direct you to the correct option.
Review: the purpose of a **fenestrated tube.**
Level of Cognitive Ability: Applying
Client Needs: Physiological Integrity
Integrated Process: Nursing Process/Implementation
Content Area: Adult Health: Respiratory
Priority Concepts: Client Education, Gas Exchange
Reference(s): deWit, Kumagai (2013), pp. 285–286.

165. *Answer:* 2
Rationale: If a client has an NG tube connected to suction, the nurse should wait up to 30 minutes before reconnecting the tube to the suction apparatus to allow adequate time for medication absorption. Aspirating the NG tube will remove the medication that has just been administered. Low intermittent suction will also remove the medication. The client should not be placed in the supine position because of the risk for aspiration.
Test-Taking Strategy: Focus on the subject, medication administration to a client with a nasogastric tube. Eliminate options 3 and 4 first, because these actions are comparable or alike and will produce the same effect of removing the medication administered. Eliminate option 1 because placing the client supine places the client at risk for aspiration **Review:** the administration of medications through a **nasogastric tube.**
Level of Cognitive Ability: Applying
Client Needs: Physiological Integrity
Integrated Process: Nursing Process/Implementation
Content Area: Fundamental Skills: Safety
Priority Concepts: Clinical Judgment, Safety
Reference(s): Cooper, Gosnell (2015), pp. 583–584.

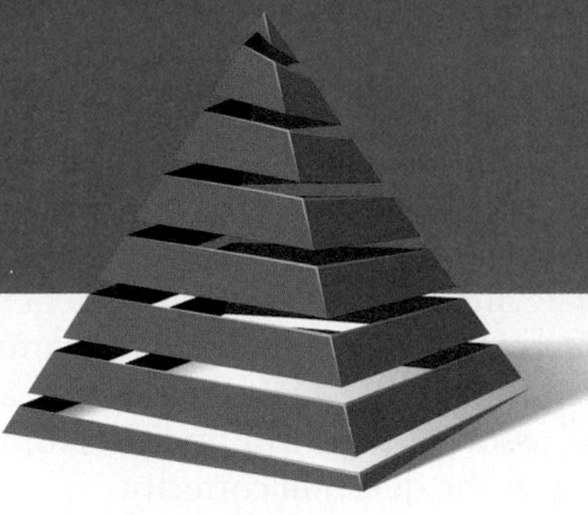

UNIT V

Growth and Development Across the Life Span

PYRAMID TERMS

abuse The willful infliction of pain, injury, mental anguish, or unreasonable confinement. Abuse can include verbal assaults, the demand to perform demeaning tasks, theft, or the mismanagement of personal belongings (exploitation). Abuse inflicted can be physical, emotional, or sexual.

aging The biopsychosocial process of change that occurs between birth and death.

auscultation The physical assessment (data collection) technique that involves listening to sounds within the body. Special equipment such as a stethoscope may be needed to perform this technique.

dementia An organic syndrome identified by a gradual and progressive deterioration in intellectual functioning. Long- and short-term memory losses occur with impairment in judgment, abstract thinking, problem-solving ability, and behavior resulting in a self-care deficit. A common type of dementia is Alzheimer's disease.

depression A mood disorder that can be identified by feelings of sadness, hopelessness, worthlessness, and a decreased interest in activities.

health history The collection of subjective data when interviewing the client. It includes information such as the client's current state of health, the medications taken, previous illnesses and surgeries, family histories, and a review of systems.

inspection The first physical assessment (data collection) technique; begins the moment that the examiner meets the client. It involves a visual assessment of the client during the health history and making observations during the physical examination of specific body systems.

neglect The failure to provide services necessary for physical or mental health, including a failure to prevent injury.

objective data Information about the client that is obtained by the examiner through the physical examination and review of the results of laboratory, radiological, or other diagnostic studies.

palpation A physical assessment (data collection) technique that involves using the hands to feel certain parts of the client's body, including some organs. The examiner uses this technique to collect data about texture, size, and consistency of the body part being examined.

percussion A physical assessment (data collection) technique that involves tapping the body to check the size, borders, and consistency of some organs, as well as to check for the presence of fluid within body cavities. Direct percussion is performed by striking the fingers directly on the body surface. Indirect percussion is performed by striking a finger of one hand on a finger of the other hand as it is placed on the body surface, such as over an organ.

play An activity that is spontaneous or organized and provides entertainment or diversion. It is a part of childhood that is necessary for the development of a normal personality and social, physical, and intellectual skills.

polypharmacy Taking multiple prescription and/or over-the-counter medications together.

safety measures Interventions that ensure protection of the client and the prevention of an accident or injury.

self-neglect The choice to avoid medical care or other services that could improve one's optimal function. Unless an individual has been declared legally incompetent, he or she has the right to refuse care.

subjective data Information obtained from the client during history-taking. It is what the client says about himself or herself.

Pyramid to Success

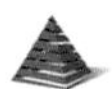

Normal growth and development proceed in an orderly, systematic, and predictable pattern that provides a basis for identifying and assessing an individual's abilities. Understanding the path of growth and development across the life span assists the nurse with identifying appropriate and expected human behavior. The Pyramid to Success focuses on Sigmund Freud's theory of psychosexual development, Jean Piaget's theory of cognitive development, Erik Erikson's psychosocial theory, and Lawrence Kohlberg's theory of moral development. Growth and development concepts also focus on the health and physical assessment of the adult client; on the aging process; and on physical characteristics, nutritional behaviors, skills, play, and specific safety measures relevant to a particular age-group that will ensure a safe and hazard-free environment. When a question is presented on the NCLEX-PN® examination, if an age is identified in the question, note the age and think about the associated growth and developmental concepts to answer the question correctly.

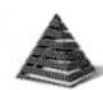

Client Needs

Safe and Effective Care Environment

Acting as a client advocate
Consulting with members of the health care team
Ensuring home safety and security plans
Establishing priorities
Maintaining confidentiality
Preventing errors and accidents
Providing care in accordance with ethical and legal standards
Providing care using a nonjudgmental approach
Respecting client and family needs on the basis of their preferences
Upholding client's rights
Using standard precautions, transmission-based precautions, and surgical asepsis

Health Promotion and Maintenance

Discussing high-risk behaviors and lifestyle choices
Identifying changes that occur as a result of the aging process
Identifying developmental stages and transitions
Maintaining health and wellness and self-care measures
Monitoring growth and development
Performing the data collection techniques associated with the health and physical assessment of the client
Reinforcing client and family education
Respecting health care beliefs and preferences

Psychosocial Integrity

Assessing for abuse and neglect
Considering grief and loss issues and end-of-life care
Identifying coping mechanisms
Identifying cultural practices and beliefs of the client and appropriate support systems
Identifying the loss of the quantity and quality of relationships with the older client
Monitoring for adjustment to potential deteriorations in physical and mental health and well-being in the older client
Monitoring for changes in and adjustment to role functioning in the older client (i.e., threats to independent functioning)
Monitoring for sensory and perceptual alterations
Providing resources for the client and family

Physiological Integrity

Administering medications safely and reinforcing teaching to the client about prescribed medications
Identifying practices or restrictions related to procedures and treatments
Monitoring for alterations in body systems and the related risks associated with the client's age
Providing basic care and comfort needs
Providing interventions that are compatible with the client's age; cultural, religious, and health care beliefs; education level; and language

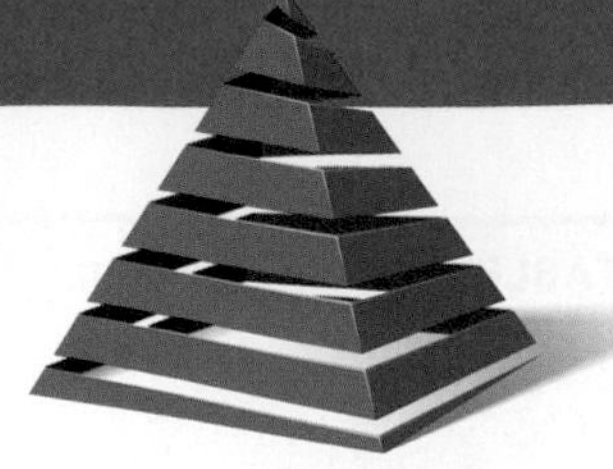

CHAPTER 20

Theories of Growth and Development

CRITICAL THINKING What Should You Do?

The nurse employed in a day care center notes that a 5-year-old child does not recognize that objects exist even when outside of the visual field. What should the nurse do?

Answer is located on p. 215.

I. Psychosocial Development and Erik Erikson

A. The theory

1. Erikson's theory of psychosocial development describes the human life cycle as a series of eight ego developmental stages from birth to death.
2. Each stage presents a psychosocial crisis, the goal of which is to integrate physical, maturational, and societal demands.
3. The result of one stage may not be permanent, but it can be changed by experience(s) later in life.
4. The theory focuses on psychosocial tasks that are accomplished throughout the life cycle.

B. Psychosocial development: Occurs through a lifelong series of crises affected by social and cultural factors.

According to Erikson's theory of psychosocial development, each psychosocial crisis must be resolved for the child or adult to progress emotionally. Unsuccessful resolution may leave the person emotionally disabled.

C. Stages of psychosocial development (Table 20-1)

D. Interventions to assist the client in achieving Erikson's stages of development (Box 20-1)

II. Cognitive Development and Jean Piaget

A. The theory

1. Piaget's theory defines cognitive acts as the ways in which the mind organizes and adapts to its environment (i.e., "mental mapping").
2. Schema: Refers to an individual's cognitive structure or framework of thought.
3. Schemata
   - **a.** Schemata are categories that an individual forms in his or her mind to organize and understand the world.
   - **b.** A young child has only a few schemata with which to understand the world; gradually these are increased.
   - **c.** Adults use a wide variety of schemata to understand the world.
4. Assimilation
   - **a.** Assimilation is the ability to incorporate new ideas, objects, and experiences into the framework of one's thoughts.
   - **b.** The growing child will perceive and give meaning to new information according to what is already known and understood.
5. Accommodation
   - **a.** Accommodation is the ability to change a schema to introduce new ideas, objects, or experiences.
   - **b.** Accommodation changes the mental structure so that new experiences can be added.

B. Stages of cognitive development 

1. Sensorimotor stage
   - **a.** Birth to 2 years
   - **b.** Development proceeds from reflex activity to imagining and solving problems through the senses and movement.
   - **c.** The infant or toddler learns about reality and how it works.
   - **d.** The infant or toddler does not recognize that objects continue to exist, even if out of the visual field.
2. Preoperational stage
   - **a.** 2 to 7 years
   - **b.** The child learns to think in terms of past, present, and future.
   - **c.** The child moves from knowing the world through sensation and movement to prelogical thinking and finding solutions to problems.
   - **d.** The child is egocentric.
   - **e.** The child is unable to conceptualize and requires concrete examples.

TABLE 20-1 Erik Erikson's Stages of Psychosocial Development

			Resolution of Crisis	
Age	**Psychosocial Crisis**	**Task**	**Successful**	**Unsuccessful**
Infancy (birth to 18 months)	Trust vs. mistrust	Attachment to the mother	Trust in other people; faith and hope about the environment and the future	General difficulties relating to others effectively; suspicion; trust/fear conflict; fear of the future
Early childhood (18 months to 3 years)	Autonomy vs. shame and doubt	Gaining some basic control over the self and the environment	Sense of self-control and adequacy; will power	Independence/fear conflict; severe feelings of self-doubt
Late childhood (3 to 6 years)	Initiative vs. guilt	Becoming purposeful and directive	Ability to initiate one's own activities; sense of purpose	Aggression/fear conflict; sense of inadequacy or guilt
School age (6 to 12 years)	Industry vs. inferiority	Developing social, physical, and learning skills	Competence; ability to learn and work	Sense of inferiority; difficulty learning and working
Adolescence (12 to 20 years)	Identity vs. role confusion	Developing a sense of identity	Sense of personal identity	Confusion about who one is; identity submerged in relationships or group memberships
Early adulthood (20 to 35 years)	Intimacy vs. isolation	Establishing intimate bonds of love and friendship	Ability to love deeply and commit oneself	Emotional isolation; egocentricity
Middle adulthood (35 to 65 years)	Generativity vs. stagnation	Fulfilling life goals that involve family, career, and society	Ability to give and care for others	Self-absorption; inability to grow as a person
Later (65 years to death)	Integrity vs. despair	Looking back over one's life and accepting its meaning	Sense of integrity and fulfillment	Dissatisfaction with life

Adapted from Halter MJ: *Varcarolis' Foundations of Psychiatric Mental Health Nursing*, ed 7, St. Louis, 2014, Saunders.

BOX 20-1 Interventions to Assist the Client in Achieving Erikson's Stages of Development

Infancy

Hold the infant often.
Offer comfort after painful procedures.
Meet the infant's needs for food and hygiene.
Encourage parents to room in while infant is hospitalized.

Early Childhood

Allow self-feeding opportunities.
Encourage child to remove and put on own clothes.
Allow for choice.

Late Childhood

Offer medical equipment for play.
Accept the child's choices and expressions of feelings.

School Age

Encourage the child to continue schoolwork while hospitalized.
Encourage the child to bring favorite leisure activities, such as board games, electronic games, or books to the hospital.

Adolescence

Take the health history and perform examinations without parents present.
Introduce the adolescent to other teens with the same health condition.

Early Adulthood

Include support from client's partner or significant other.
Assist with rehabilitation needed before returning to work.

Middle Adulthood

Assist in choosing creative ways to foster social development.
Encourage volunteer activities.

Later Adulthood

Listen attentively to reminiscent stories about their life's accomplishments.
Assist with making changes to living arrangements.

3. Concrete operational
   a. 7 to 11 years
   b. The child is able to classify, order, and sort facts.
   c. The child moves from prelogical thought to solving concrete problems through logic.
4. Formal operations
   a. 11 years to adulthood
   b. The person is able to think abstractly and logically.
   c. Logical thinking is expanded to include solving abstract and concrete problems.

III. Moral Development and Lawrence Kohlberg

A. Moral development
   1. Moral development is a complicated process involving the acceptance of the values and rules of society in a way that shapes behavior.
   2. Moral development is classified into a series of levels and behaviors.
   3. Moral development is sequential, but people do not automatically go from one stage or level to the next as they mature.
   4. Stages or levels of moral development cannot be skipped.

B. Levels of moral development (Box 20-2)

IV. Psychosexual Development: Sigmund Freud

A. Components of the theory (Box 20-3)

B. Levels of awareness
   1. Unconscious level of awareness
      a. The unconscious is not logical and is governed by the pleasure principle, which refers to seeking immediate tension reduction.
      b. Memories, feelings, thoughts, and wishes are repressed and not available to the conscious mind.
      c. These repressed memories, thoughts, or feelings, if made prematurely conscious, can cause anxiety.
   2. Preconscious level of awareness
      a. The preconscious is also called the *subconscious.*
      b. Preconscious includes experiences, thoughts, feelings, or desires that might not be in an individual's immediate awareness but that can be recalled to consciousness.
      c. The subconscious can help repress unpleasant thoughts or feelings and examine and censor certain wishes and thinking.
   3. Conscious level of awareness
      a. The conscious mind is logical and regulated by the reality principle.
      b. Consciousness includes all experiences that are within an individual's awareness and that the individual is able to control and includes all information that is easily remembered and immediately available to an individual.

BOX 20-2 Moral Development and Lawrence Kohlberg

Level One: Preconventional Morality

Stage 0 (Birth to 2 Years): Egocentric Judgment

The infant has no awareness of right or wrong.

Stage 1 (2 to 3 Years): Punishment–Obedience Orientation

At this stage, children cannot reason as mature members of society.

Children view the world in a selfish way, with no real understanding of right or wrong.

The child obeys rules and demonstrates acceptable behavior to avoid punishment and to avoid displeasing those who are in power, and because he or she fears punishment from a superior force, such as a parent.

A toddler typically is at the first substage of the preconventional stage. This involves a punishment–obedience orientation in which the toddler makes judgments on the basis of avoiding punishment or obtaining a reward.

Physical punishment and withholding privileges tend to give the toddler a negative view of morals.

Withdrawing love and affection as punishment leads to feelings of guilt in the toddler.

Appropriate discipline includes providing simple explanations of why certain behaviors are not acceptable, praising appropriate behavior, and using distractions when the toddler is headed for danger.

Stage 2 (4 to 7 Years): Instrumental Relativist Orientation

The child conforms to rules to obtain rewards or have favors returned.

The child's moral standards are those of others, and the child observes them to avoid punishment or obtain rewards.

A preschooler is in the preconventional stage of moral development.

During this stage, the conscience emerges, and the emphasis is on external control.

Level Two: Conventional Morality

The child conforms to rules to please others.

The child has an increased awareness of others' feelings.

A concern for social order begins to emerge.

A child views good behavior as that of which those in authority will approve.

If the behavior is not acceptable, the child feels guilty.

Continued

BOX 20-2 Moral Development and Lawrence Kohlberg—*cont'd*

Stage 3 (7 to 10 Years): Good Boy–Nice Girl Orientation

Conformity occurs to avoid disapproval or dislike by others.

This stage involves living up to what is expected by individuals close to the child or what individuals generally expect of others in their roles as son, brother, friend, and so on.

Being good is important and is interpreted as having good motives and showing concern about others.

It also means maintaining mutual relationships with the use of such characteristics as trust, loyalty, respect, and gratitude.

Stage 4 (10 to 12 Years): Law and Order Orientation

The child has more concern with society as a whole.

The emphasis is on obeying laws to maintain social order.

Moral reasoning develops as the child shifts the focus of living to society.

The school-age child is at the conventional level of the role-conformity stage and has an increased desire to please others.

The child observes and to some extent internalizes the standards of others.

The child wants to be considered "good" by those individuals whose opinions matter to him or her.

Level Three: Postconventional Morality

The individual focuses on individual rights and principles of conscience.

The focus is a concern regarding what is best for all.

Stage 5 (12 Years and Older): Social Contract and Legalistic Orientation

The adolescent is aware that people hold a variety of values and opinions and most values and rules are relative to the group.

The adolescent in this stage gives as well as takes and does not expect to get something without paying for it.

Stage 6: Universal Ethical Principles Orientation

Conformity is based on universal principles of justice and occurs to avoid self-condemnation.

This stage involves following self-chosen ethical principles.

The development of the postconventional level of morality occurs in the adolescent at about the age of 13 years. It is marked by the development of an individual conscience and a defined set of moral values.

The adolescent can now acknowledge a conflict between two socially accepted standards and try to decide between them.

The control of conduct is now internal, both in standards observed and in reasoning about right and wrong.

BOX 20-3 Psychosexual Development and Sigmund Freud: Components of the Theory

- Levels of awareness
- Agencies of the mind: id, ego, and superego
- Concept of anxiety and defense mechanisms
- Psychosexual stages of development

C. Agencies of the mind: id, ego, and superego

⚠ The id, ego, and superego are the three systems of personality. These psychological processes follow different operating principles. In a mature and well-adjusted personality, they work together as a team under the leadership of the ego.

1. The id
   - **a.** Source of all drives, present at birth, operates according to the Pleasure Principle
   - **b.** Does not tolerate uncomfortable states and seeks to discharge the tension and return to a more comfortable, constant level of energy
   - **c.** Acts immediately in an impulsive, irrational way and pays no attention to the consequences of its actions; therefore, often behaves in ways harmful to self and others
   - **d.** The primary process is a psychological activity in which the id attempts to reduce tension.
   - **e.** The primary process by itself is not capable of reducing tension; therefore, a secondary psychological process must develop if the individual is to survive. When this occurs, the structure of the second system of the personality, the ego, begins to take form.
2. The ego
   - **a.** Functions include reality testing and problem solving; follows the Reality Principle
   - **b.** Begins its development during the fourth or fifth month of life
   - **c.** Emerges out of the id and acts as an intermediary between the id and the external world
   - **d.** Emerges because the needs, wishes, and demands of the id require appropriate exchanges with the outside world of reality
   - **e.** Distinguishes between things in the mind and things in the external world

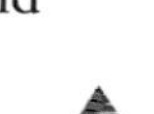

3. The superego
   - **a.** Necessary part of socialization that develops during the phallic stage of 3 to 6 years of age
   - **b.** Develops from the interactions with one's parents during the extended period of childhood dependency
   - **c.** Includes the internalization of the values, ideals, and moral standards of society
   - **d.** The superego consists of the conscience and the ego ideal.
   - **e.** The conscience refers to the capacity for self-evaluation and criticism. When moral codes are violated, the conscience punishes the individual by instilling guilt.

BOX 20-4 Freud's Psychosexual Stages of Development

Oral Stage (Birth to 1 Year)

During this stage, the infant is concerned with his or her own gratification.

The infant is all id, operating on the pleasure principle and striving for the immediate gratification of his or her needs.

When the infant experiences the gratification of basic needs, a sense of trust and security begins.

The ego begins to emerge as the infant begins to see himself or herself as separate from the mother. This marks the beginning of the development of a sense of self.

Anal Stage (1 to 3 Years)

Toilet training occurs during this period, and the child gains pleasure from both the elimination and retention of feces.

The conflict of this stage is between demands from society and parents and the sensations of pleasure associated with the anus.

The child begins to gain a sense of control over instinctive drives and learns to delay immediate gratification to gain a future goal.

Phallic Stage (3 to 6 Years)

The child experiences both pleasurable and conflicting feelings associated with the genital organs.

The pleasures of masturbation and the fantasy life of children set the stage for the Oedipus complex.

The child's unconscious sexual attraction to and wish to possess the parent of the opposite sex, the hostility toward and desire to remove the parent of the same sex, and the subsequent guilt regarding these wishes comprise the conflict that the child faces.

The conflict is resolved when the child identifies with the parent of the same sex.

The emergence of the superego is both the solution to and the result of these intense impulses.

Latency Stage (6 to 12 Years)

During this stage, there is a tapering off of conscious biological and sexual urges.

The sexual impulses are channeled and elevated into a more culturally accepted level of activity.

The growth of ego functions and the ability to care about and relate to others outside of the home are the tasks of this stage of development.

Genital Stage (12 Years and Beyond)

This emerges at adolescence with the onset of puberty, when the genital organs mature.

The individual gains gratification from his or her own body.

During this stage, the individual develops satisfying sexual and emotional relationships with members of the opposite sex.

The individual plans life goals and gains a strong sense of personal identity.

D. Anxiety and defense mechanisms

1. The ego develops defenses or defense mechanisms to fight off anxiety.
2. Defense mechanisms operate on an unconscious level (except for suppression), so the individual is not aware of their operation.
3. Defense mechanisms deny, falsify, or distort reality to make it less threatening.
4. An individual cannot survive without defense mechanisms; however, if they become too extreme in distorting reality, then interference in healthy adjustment and personal growth may occur.

E. Psychosexual stages of development (Box 20-4)

1. Human development proceeds through a series of stages from infancy to adulthood.
2. Each stage is characterized by the inborn tendency of all individuals to reduce tension and seek pleasure.
3. Each stage is associated with a particular conflict that must be resolved before the child can move successfully to the next stage.

4. Experiences during the early stages determine an individual's adjustment patterns and the personality traits that the individual has as an adult.

CRITICAL THINKING What Should You Do?

Answer: According to Jean Piaget's theory of cognitive development, if a 5-year-old child does not recognize that objects still exist even when outside the visual field, the child is not progressing normally through the developmental stages. The nurse should report this finding to the health care provider. It is normal for the infant or toddler not to recognize that objects continue to be in existence, even if out of the visual field; however, this is abnormal for the 5-year-old.

Reference(s): Hockenberry, M., & Wilson, D. (2013). *Wong's: Essentials of pediatric nursing* (9th ed., pp. 72–73, 460). St. Louis: Mosby.

PRACTICE QUESTIONS

166. Which statement by a nursing student about Kohlberg's theory of moral development indicates the **need for further teaching** about the theory?

1. "Individuals move through all six stages in a sequential fashion."
2. "Moral development progresses in relation to cognitive development."

3. "A person's ability to make moral judgments develops over a period of time."
4. "It provides a framework for understanding how individuals determine a moral code to guide his or her behavior."

167. The parents of an 8-year-old child tell the nurse that they are concerned about the child because the child seems to be more attentive to friends than anyone else. Which is the appropriate nursing response?
1. "You need to be concerned."
2. "You need to monitor the child's behavior closely."
3. "At this age, the child is developing his or her own personality."
4. "You need to praise the child more often to stop this behavior."

168. The parents of a 4-year-old child tell the nurse that they are concerned because the child has been masturbating. Which is the appropriate response by the nurse?
1. "This is a normal behavior at this age."
2. "Children usually begin this behavior at the age of 8 years."
3. "This is not normal behavior. The child should be brought to the mental health clinic."
4. "The child is very young to begin this behavior and should be brought to the mental health clinic."

169. The nurse is providing instructions to a new parent regarding the psychosocial development of the infant. Using Erikson's psychosocial development theory, which instruction should the nurse reinforce to the parents?
1. Allow the infant to signal a need.
2. Anticipate all of the needs of the infant.
3. Attend to the crying infant immediately.
4. Avoid the infant during the first 10 minutes of crying.

170. The parent of a 3-year-old tells the nurse that the child is constantly rebelling and having temper tantrums. Which instruction should the nurse reinforce to the parent?
1. Set limits on the child's behavior.
2. Ignore the child when this behavior occurs.
3. Allow the behavior, because this is normal at this age period.
4. Punish the child every time the child says "no" to change the behavior.

171. The nurse is caring for an older client who is reminiscing about past life experiences in a positive manner. The nurse plans care with the understanding that this behavior indicates which?
1. A mental status alteration
2. A normal psychosocial response
3. A need for psychiatric consultation
4. A sensory deficit requiring social activities

❖ **172.** Which are components of Kohlberg's theory of moral development? **Select all that apply.**
- ❑ 1. Individuals move through all six stages in a sequential fashion.
- ❑ 2. Moral development progresses in relation to cognitive development.
- ❑ 3. A person's ability to make moral judgments develops over a period of time.
- ❑ 4. The theory provides a framework for understanding how individuals determine a moral code to guide their behavior.
- ❑ 5. In stage 1 (punishment–obedience orientation), children are expected to reason as mature members of society.
- ❑ 6. In stage 2 (instrumental relativist orientation), the child conforms to rules to obtain rewards or to have favors returned.

173. The nursing instructor asks a nursing student to describe the formal operations stage of Piaget's cognitive developmental theory. The appropriate response by the nursing student is which?
1. "The child has the ability to think abstractly."
2. "The child develops logical thought patterns."
3. "The child begins to understand the environment."
4. "The child has difficulty separating fantasy from reality."

174. According to Kohlberg's theory of moral development, at the preconventional level, moral development is thought to be motivated by which factor?
1. Peer pressure
2. Social pressures
3. The parents' behavior
4. Punishment and reward

175. The nursing student is preparing a conference on Freud's psychosexual stages of development, specifically the anal stage. Which appropriately relates to this stage?
1. Gratification of self
2. Beginning of toilet training
3. Tapering off of conscious biological and sexual urges
4. Association with pleasurable and conflicting feelings about the genital organs

ANSWERS

166. 1

Rationale: Kohlberg's theory states that individuals move through the six stages of development in a sequential fashion but that not everyone reaches stages 5 or 6 as part of their development of personal morality. Options 2, 3, and 4 are correct statements regarding Kohlberg's theory.

Test-Taking Strategy: Note the strategic words, *need for further teaching.* These words indicate a negative event query and ask you to select an option that is an incorrect statement. Also, note the closed-ended word, *all* in option 1. **Review:** Kohlberg's theory.

Level of Cognitive Ability: Evaluating

Client Needs: Health Promotion and Maintenance

Integrated Process: Teaching and Learning

Content Area: Developmental Stages: Infancy to Adolescence

Priority Concepts: Cognition, Development

Reference(s): McKinney et al (2013), pp. 74–75.

167. 3

Rationale: According to Erikson, at ages 7 to 12 years, the child begins to move toward receiving support from peers and friends and away from that of parents. The child also begins to develop special interests that reflect his or her own developing personality instead of those of the parents. Therefore, the other options identify incorrect responses.

Test-Taking Strategy: Note the subject, Erikson's psychosocial development for a school-age child, and remember the importance of peer groups. You can eliminate options 1 and 2 because there is no reason to be concerned or to monitor the child's behavior. Eliminate option 4 next; although praising the child for accomplishments is important at this age, the behavior that the child is exhibiting is normal. **Review:** Erikson's psychosocial development.

Level of Cognitive Ability: Applying

Client Needs: Health Promotion and Maintenance

Integrated Process: Nursing Process/Implementation

Content Area: Developmental Stages: Infancy to Adolescence

Priority Concepts: Development, Family Dynamics

Reference(s): Hockenberry, Wilson (2013), p. 459.

168. 1

Rationale: According to Freud's psychosexual stages of development, the child is in the phallic stage between the ages of 3 and 6 years. At this time, the child devotes much energy to examining his or her genitalia, masturbating, and expressing interest in sexual concerns. Therefore, the other options are incorrect.

Test-Taking Strategy: Note the subject, Freud's psychosexual stage of development for a 4-year-old. Eliminate options 3 and 4 because they are comparable or alike. From the remaining options, use Freud's psychosexual stages of development to direct you to the correct option. **Review:** Freud's psychosexual stages of development.

Level of Cognitive Ability: Applying

Client Needs: Health Promotion and Maintenance

Integrated Process: Nursing Process/Implementation

Content Area: Developmental Stages: Infancy to Adolescence

Priority Concepts: Development, Sexuality

Reference(s): McKinney et al (2013), p. 74.

169. 1

Rationale: According to Erikson, the caregiver should not try to anticipate the infant's needs at all times but rather allow the infant to signal his or her needs. If an infant is not allowed to signal a need, he or she will not learn how to control the environment. Erikson believed that a delayed or prolonged response to an infant's signal would inhibit the development of trust and lead to the mistrust of others. Therefore, the remaining options are incorrect.

Test-Taking Strategy: Note the subject, Erikson's stage of development for an infant. This stage is to develop trust. Eliminate options 3 and 4 first because of the words *immediately* and *avoid.* Additionally, option 2 can be eliminated because of the closed-ended word, *all.* **Review:** Erikson's psychosocial development.

Level of Cognitive Ability: Applying

Client Needs: Health Promotion and Maintenance

Integrated Process: Teaching and Learning

Content Area: Developmental Stages: Infancy to Adolescence

Priority Concepts: Development, Functional Ability

Reference(s): Hockenberry, Wilson (2013), p. 318.

170. 1

Rationale: According to Erikson, the child focuses on independence between the ages of 1 and 3 years. Gaining independence often means that the child has to rebel against the parents' wishes. Saying things like "no" and "mine" and having temper tantrums are common during this period of development. Being consistent and setting limits on the child's behavior are necessary elements. Punishing the child every time the child says "no" is likely to produce a negative response.

Test-Taking Strategy: Note the subject, actions to take for "temper tantrums." Options 2 and 3 can be eliminated first because they are comparable or alike. Eliminate option 4 next because this action is likely to produce a negative response during this normal developmental pattern. **Review:** the psychosocial development of the toddler.

Level of Cognitive Ability: Applying

Client Needs: Health Promotion and Maintenance

Integrated Process: Teaching and Learning

Content Area: Developmental Stages: Infancy to Adolescence

Priority Concepts: Development, Functional Ability

Reference(s): Hockenberry, Wilson (2013), p. 380.

171. 2

Rationale: According to Erikson, the later years of life are from 65 years of age until death. The adult reminisces about past life experiences, often viewing them in a positive way. The adult needs to feel good about his or her accomplishments, see successes in his or her life, and feel that he or she has made a contribution to society.

Test-Taking Strategy: Use your knowledge of the subject, Erikson's theory of psychosocial development in regard to late adulthood, to answer the question. Note that options 1, 3, and 4 are comparable or alike; this will direct you to the correct option. **Review:** Erikson's theory of psychosocial development.

Level of Cognitive Ability: Applying

Client Needs: Psychosocial Integrity

Integrated Process: Nursing Process/Planning

Content Area: Developmental Stages: Early Adulthood to Later Adulthood
Priority Concepts: Cognition, Development
Reference(s): Potter et al (2013), p. 187.

❖172. 2, 3, 4, 6
Rationale: Kohlberg's theory states that individuals move through the six stages of development in a sequential fashion, but not everyone reaches stages 5 and 6 during his or her development of personal morality. The theory provides a framework for understanding how individuals determine a moral code to guide their behavior. It also states that moral development progresses in relation to cognitive development and a person's ability to make moral judgments develops over a period of time. In stage 1 (ages 2 to 3 years; punishment–obedience orientation), children cannot reason as mature members of society because they are too young to do so. In stage 2 (ages 4 to 7 years; instrumental relativist orientation), the child conforms to rules to obtain rewards or have favors returned.
Test-Taking Strategy: Focus on the subject, Kohlberg's theory of moral development. Recall the ages associated with each stage and that the theory provides a framework for understanding how individuals determine a moral code to guide their behavior. **Review:** Kohlberg's theory.
Level of Cognitive Ability: Understanding
Client Needs: Psychosocial Integrity
Integrated Process: Nursing Process/Planning
Content Area: Developmental Stages: Infancy to Adolescence
Priority Concepts: Cognition, Development
Reference(s): Hockenberry, Wilson (2013), p. 71; McKinney et al (2013), pp. 74–75.

173. 1
Rationale: In the formal operations stage, the child has the ability to think abstractly and solve problems. Option 2 identifies the concrete operations stage. Option 3 identifies the sensorimotor stage. Option 4 identifies the preoperational stage.
Test-Taking Strategy: Focus on the subject, Piaget's theory. Use knowledge regarding the characteristics of cognitive developmental theory for a child in the formal stage. Remember, in the formal operations stage, the child has the ability to think abstractly and solve problems. **Review:** Piaget's cognitive developmental theory.
Level of Cognitive Ability: Evaluating
Client Needs: Health Promotion and Maintenance
Integrated Process: Teaching and Learning
Content Area: Developmental Stages: Infancy to Adolescence
Priority Concepts: Development, Functional Ability
Reference(s): Hockenberry, Wilson (2013), p. 73.

174. 4
Rationale: In the preconventional level, morals are thought to be motivated by punishment and reward. If the child is obedient and not punished, then he or she is being moral. The child sees actions as either good or bad. If the child's actions are good, then the child is praised. If the child's actions are bad, then the child is punished.
Test-Taking Strategy: Eliminate options 1 and 2 because they are comparable or alike. Knowledge that the preconventional stage occurs between the ages of 2 and 7 years will assist with directing you to option 4. **Review:** Kohlberg's theory of moral development.
Level of Cognitive Ability: Understanding
Client Needs: Psychosocial Integrity
Integrated Process: Nursing Process/Planning
Content Area: Developmental Stages: Infancy to Adolescence
Priority Concepts: Development, Functional Ability
Reference(s): Hockenberry, Wilson (2013), p. 409; McKinney et al (2013), p. 24.

175. 2
Rationale: Toilet training generally occurs during this period. According to Freud, the child gains pleasure from both the elimination and retention of feces. Option 1 relates to the oral stage. Option 3 relates to the latency period. Option 4 relates to the phallic stage.
Test-Taking Strategy: Focus on the subject, Freud's stages of psychosexual development. Note the relationship between the words *anal* in the question and *toilet training* in the correct option. **Review:** Freud's psychosocial stages of development.
Level of Cognitive Ability: Applying
Client Needs: Health Promotion and Maintenance
Integrated Process: Nursing Process/Planning
Content Area: Developmental Stages: Infancy to Adolescence
Priority Concepts: Development, Elimination
Reference(s): McKinney et al (2013), p. 74.

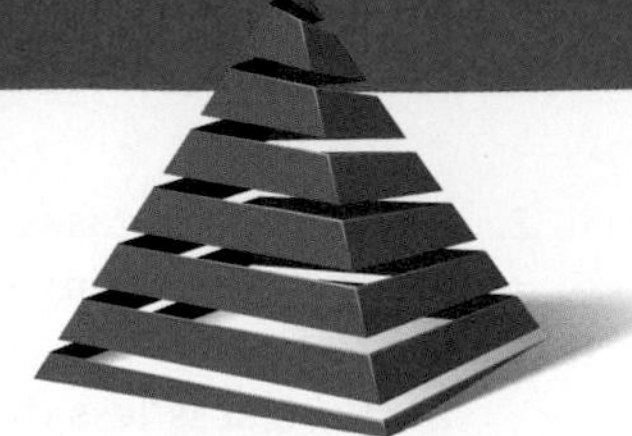

CHAPTER 21

Developmental Stages

> **CRITICAL THINKING What Should You Do?**
>
> The nurse is caring for a hospitalized preschool child who is very apprehensive. What should the nurse do to assist in promoting comfort in the child?
>
> *Answer is located on p. 230.*

I. The Hospitalized Infant and Toddler

A. Separation anxiety
   1. Protest
      a. Cries, screams, searches for a parent; avoids and rejects contact with strangers
      b. Verbal attacks on others
      c. Physical fighting: kicks, fights, hits, and pinches
   2. Despair
      a. Withdrawn, depressed, and uninterested in the environment
      b. Loss of newly learned skills
   3. Detachment
      a. Detachment is uncommon and occurs only after lengthy separations from the parent.
      b. Superficially, the toddler appears to have adjusted to the loss.
      c. During the detachment phase, the toddler again becomes more interested in the environment, **plays** with others, and seems to form new relationships. This behavior is a form of resignation and is not a sign of contentment.
      d. The toddler detaches from the parents in an effort to escape the emotional pain of desiring the parent's presence.
      e. The toddler copes by forming shallow relationships with others, becoming increasingly self-centered, and attaching primary importance to material objects.
      f. Detachment is the most serious phase, because the reversal of the potential adverse effects is less likely to occur after detachment is established. In most situations, the temporary separation imposed by hospitalization does not cause such prolonged parental absence that the toddler enters into detachment.

B. Fear of injury and pain: Affected by previous experiences, separation from parents, and preparation for the experience

C. Loss of control
   1. Hospitalization with its own set of rituals and routines can severely disrupt the life of a toddler.
   2. The lack of control is often exhibited in behaviors related to feeding, toileting, playing, and bedtime.
   3. The toddler may demonstrate regression.

D. Interventions
   1. Provide cuddling and touch and talk softly to the infant.
   2. Provide opportunities for sucking and oral stimulation for the infant using a pacifier if the infant is not to receive anything by mouth.
   3. Provide stimulation for the infant, if appropriate, with the use of objects of contrasting colors and textures.
   4. Provide as many choices to the toddler as possible to enable him or her to have some control.
   5. Approach the toddler with a positive attitude.
   6. Allow the toddler to express feelings of protest.
   7. Encourage the toddler to talk about parents or others in his or her life.
   8. Accept regressive behavior without ridiculing the toddler.
   9. Provide the toddler with favorite and comforting objects.
   10. Allow the toddler as much mobility as possible.
   11. Anticipate temper tantrums from the toddler, and maintain a safe environment for physical acting out.
   12. Employ pain-reduction techniques, as appropriate.

⚠ For the hospitalized toddler, provide routines and rituals as close to possible to what he or she is used to at home.

II. The Hospitalized Preschooler

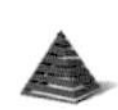

A. Separation anxiety
   1. Separation anxiety is generally less obvious and less serious than in the toddler.

2. As stress increases, the preschooler's ability to separate from the parents decreases.
3. Protest
   a. Protest is less direct and aggressive than seen in the toddler.
   b. The preschooler may displace feelings onto others.
4. Despair
   a. The preschooler reacts in a manner similar to the toddler.
   b. The preschooler is quietly withdrawn, depressed, and uninterested in the environment.
   c. The child exhibits loss of newly learned skills.
   d. The preschooler becomes generally uncooperative, refusing to eat or take medication.
   e. The preschooler repeatedly asks when the parents will be visiting.
5. Detachment: Similar to the toddler

B. Fear of injury and pain
1. The preschooler has a general lack of understanding of body integrity.
2. The child fears invasive procedures and mutilation.
3. The child imagines things to be much worse than they are.
4. Preschoolers believe they are ill because of something they did or thought.

C. Loss of control
1. The preschooler likes familiar routines and rituals, and may show regression if not allowed to maintain some control.
2. Preschoolers' egocentric and magical thinking limits their ability to understand events because they view all experiences from their own self-referenced (egocentric) perspective.
3. The child has attained a good deal of independence and self-care at home. He or she may expect that to continue in the hospital.

D. Interventions
1. Provide a safe and secure environment.
2. Take time for communication.
3. Allow the preschooler to express anger.
4. Acknowledge fears and anxieties.
5. Accept regressive behavior. Assist the preschooler to move from regressive to appropriate behaviors according to age.
6. Encourage rooming-in or leaving a favorite toy.
7. Allow mobility, and provide play and diversional activities.
8. Place the preschooler with other children of the same age if possible.
9. Encourage the preschooler to be independent.
10. Explain procedures simply, on the preschooler's level.
11. Avoid intrusive procedures when possible.
12. Allow for the wearing of underpants.

III. The Hospitalized School-Age Child

A. Separation anxiety
1. The school-age child is accustomed to periods of separation from the parents, but as stressors are added, the separation becomes more difficult.
2. The child is more concerned with missing school and the fear that friends will forget him or her.
3. Usually, the stages of behavior of protest, despair, and detachment do not occur with the school-age child.

B. Fear of injury and pain
1. The school-age child fears bodily injury and pain.
2. The child fears illness itself, disability, death, and intrusive procedures in genital areas.
3. The child is uncomfortable with any type of sexual examination.
4. The child groans or whines, holds rigidly still, and communicates about pain.

C. Loss of control
1. The child is usually highly social, independent, and involved with activities.
2. The child seeks information and asks relevant questions about tests, procedures, and the illness.
3. The child associates his or her actions with the cause of the illness.
4. The child may feel helpless and dependent if physical limitations occur.

D. Interventions
1. Encourage rooming-in.
2. Focus on the school-age child's abilities and needs.
3. Encourage the school-age child to become involved with his or her own care.
4. Accept regression but encourage independence.
5. Provide choices to the school-age child.
6. Allow for the expression of feelings, both verbally and nonverbally.
7. Acknowledge fears and concerns and allow for discussion.
8. Explain all procedures with the use of body diagrams or outlines.
9. Provide privacy.
10. Avoid intrusive procedures, if possible.
11. Allow the school-age child to wear underpants.
12. Involve the school-age child in activities that are appropriate to his or her developmental level and illness.
13. Encourage the school-age child to contact friends.
14. Provide for educational needs.
15. Employ appropriate interventions to relieve pain.

IV. The Hospitalized Adolescent

A. Separation anxiety 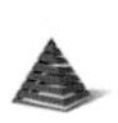
1. Adolescents are not sure whether they want their parents with them when they are hospitalized.

2. Adolescents become upset if friends go on with their lives, excluding them.

⚠ For the hospitalized adolescent, separation from friends is a source of anxiety.

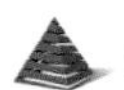

B. Fear of injury and pain
   1. Adolescents fear being different from others and their peers.
   2. Adolescents may give the impression that they are not afraid, although they are terrified.
   3. Adolescents become guarded when any areas related to sexual development are examined.

C. Loss of control
   1. Behaviors exhibited include anger, withdrawal, and uncooperativeness.
   2. Adolescents seek help and then reject it.

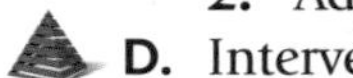

D. Interventions
   1. Encourage questions about appearance and the effects of the illness on the future.
   2. Explore feelings about the hospital and the significance that the illness might have with regard to relationships.
   3. Encourage the adolescent to wear his or her own clothes and perform normal grooming activities.
   4. Allow favorite foods to be brought in to the hospital, if possible.
   5. Provide privacy.
   6. Use body diagrams to prepare for procedures.
   7. Introduce to other adolescents in the nursing unit.
   8. Encourage the maintenance of contact with peer groups.
   9. Provide for educational needs.
   10. Identify the formation of future plans.
   11. Help develop positive coping mechanisms.

V. Communication Approaches

A. General guidelines (Box 21-1)

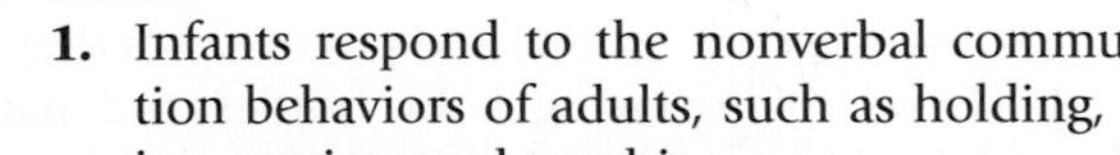

B. Infant
   1. Infants respond to the nonverbal communication behaviors of adults, such as holding, rocking, patting, and touching.

BOX 21-1 General Guidelines for Communication

Allow the child time to feel comfortable with the nurse.
Communicate through the use of objects.
Allow the child to express fears and concerns.
Speak clearly and in a quiet, unhurried voice.
Offer choices when possible.
Be honest with the child.
Set limits with the child as appropriate.

   2. Use a slow approach; allow the infant to get to know the nurse.
   3. Use a calm, soft, soothing voice.
   4. Be responsive to cries.
   5. Talk and read to infants.
   6. Allow security objects such as blankets and pacifiers, if the infant has them.

C. Toddler
   1. Approach the toddler cautiously.
   2. Remember that toddlers accept the verbal communications of others literally.
   3. Learn the toddler's words for common items and use them in conversations.
   4. Use short, concrete terms.
   5. Prepare the toddler for procedures immediately before the event.

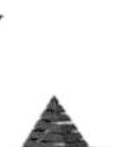

   6. Repeat explanations and descriptions.
   7. Use play for demonstrations.
   8. Use visual aids such as picture books, puppets, and dolls.
   9. Allow the toddler to handle the equipment or instruments. Explain what the equipment or instrument does and how it feels.
   10. Encourage the use of comfort objects.

D. Preschooler
   1. Seek opportunities to offer choices.
   2. Speak in simple sentences.
   3. Be concise. Limit the length of explanations.
   4. Allow for the asking of questions.
   5. Describe the procedures as they are about to be performed.
   6. Use play to explain procedures and activities.
   7. Allow the handling of equipment or instruments, which will ease fear and help answer questions.

E. School-age child
   1. Establish limits.
   2. Provide reassurance to help with alleviating fears and anxieties.
   3. Engage in conversations that encourage thinking.
   4. Use medical play techniques.
   5. Use photographs, books, dolls, DVDs, and videos to explain procedures.
   6. Explain in clear terms.
   7. Allow time for composure and privacy.

F. Adolescent
   1. Remember that the adolescent may be preoccupied with body image.
   2. Encourage and support independence.
   3. Provide privacy.
   4. Use photographs, books, CDs, DVDs, videos, and the Internet to explain procedures.
   5. Engage in conversations about the adolescent's interests.
   6. Avoid becoming too abstract, too detailed, and too technical.

7. Avoid responding to less-than-desirable social behaviors by prying, confrontation, or judgmental attitudes.

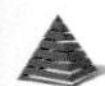

VI. Car Safety Seats and Guidelines

A. The safest place for all children to ride, regardless of age, is in the backseat of the car.
B. Lock the car doors; four-door cars should be equipped with child safety locks on the back doors.
C. There are different types of car safety seats and the manufacturer's guidelines need to be followed.
D. For specific information regarding car safety, refer to *Car Safety Seats: Information for Families for 2014* at http://www.healthychildren.org/English/safety-prevention/on-the-go/Pages/Car-Safety-Seats-Information-for-Families.aspx.

VII. Developmental Characteristics

A. Infant
   1. Physical
      a. Height increases by 1 inch per month in the first 6 months, and by 1 year, the length has increased by 50%.
      b. Weight is doubled at 5 to 6 months and tripled at 12 months.
      c. At birth, head circumference is 33 to 35 cm (13.2 to 14 inches), approximately 2 to 3 cm more than chest circumference.
      d. By 1 to 2 years of age, head circumference and chest circumference are equal.

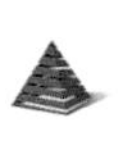

      e. The anterior fontanel (soft and flat in a normal infant) closes by 12 to 18 months.

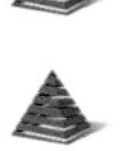

      f. The posterior fontanel (soft and flat in a normal infant) closes by the end of the second month.
      g. The first primary teeth to erupt are the lower central incisors at approximately 6 to 10 months of age.
      h. Sleep patterns vary among infants; in general, by 3 to 4 months of age, most infants have developed a nocturnal pattern of sleep that lasts 9 to 11 hours.
   2. Vital signs (Box 21-2)

BOX 21-2 Vital Signs: The Newborn and 1-Year-Old Infant

Newborn

Temperature: Axillary, 98.6° to 99°F
Apical rate: 120 to 160 beats per minute
Respirations: 30 to 60 (average 40) breaths per minute
Blood pressure: 80-90/40-50 mm Hg

1-Year-Old Infant

Temperature: Axillary, 97° to 99°F
Apical rate: 90 to 130 beats per minute
Respirations: 20 to 40 breaths per minute
Blood pressure: Average, 90/56 mm Hg

   3. Nutrition
      a. The infant may breastfeed or bottle-feed (with iron-fortified formula), depending on the mother's choice; however, human milk is the preferred form of nutrition for all infants, especially during the first 6 months.
      b. Exclusively breastfed infants and infants ingesting less than 1000 mL of vitamin D–fortified formula or milk per day should receive daily vitamin D supplementation (400 IU) starting in the first few days of life to prevent rickets and vitamin D deficiency.
      c. Iron stores from birth are depleted by 4 months; if the infant is being only breastfed, iron supplementation usually with iron-fortified cereal is needed.
      d. Whole milk, low-fat milk, skim milk, other animal milk, or imitation milk should not be given to infants as a primary source of nutrition because these food sources lack the necessary components needed for growth and have limited digestibility.
      e. Fluoride supplementation may be needed at about 6 months of age, depending on the infant's intake of fluoridated tap water.
      f. Solid foods (strained, pureed, or finely mashed) are introduced at about 5 to 6 months of age. Introduce solid foods one at a time, usually at intervals of 4 to 5 days, to identify food allergens.
      g. The sequence of introduction of solid foods varies depending on the health care provider's preference and usually is first, iron-fortified rice cereal, then fruits and vegetables, and then meats.
      h. At 12 months of age, eggs can be given (introduce egg whites in small quantities to detect an allergy); cheese may be used as a substitute for meat.
      i. Avoid solid foods that place the infant at risk for choking, such as nuts, foods with seeds, raisins, popcorn, grapes, and pieces of hot dog.
      j. Avoid microwaving baby bottles and baby food.
      k. Never mix food and/or medications with formula.
      l. Avoid adding honey to formula, water, or other fluids (risk of botulism).
      m. Offer fruit juice from a cup (12 to 13 months or at a prescribed age) rather than a bottle to prevent nursing (bottle-mouth) caries; fruit juice is limited because of its high sugar content.
   4. Skills (Table 21-1)
   5. **Play**
      a. Solitary
      b. Birth to 3 months: Verbal, visual, and tactile stimuli

TABLE 21-1 Infant Skills

Age	Skills
2 to 3 Months	Smiles Turns head from side to side Cries Follows objects Holds head in midline
4 to 5 Months	Grasps objects Switches objects from hand to hand Rolls over for the first time Enjoys social interaction Begins to show memory Aware of unfamiliar surroundings
6 to 7 Months	Creeps Sits with support Imitates Exhibits fear of strangers Holds arms out Frequent mood swings Waves "bye-bye"
8 to 9 Months	Sits steadily unsupported Crawls May stand while holding on Begins to stand without help
10 to 11 Months	Can change from a prone to a sitting position Walks while holding onto furniture Stands securely Entertains self for periods of time
12 to 13 Months	Walks with one hand held Can take a few steps without falling Can drink from a cup
14 to 15 Months	Walks alone Can crawl up stairs Shows emotions such as anger and affection Will explore away from his or her mother in familiar surroundings

c. 4 to 6 months: Initiates actions and recognizes new experiences
d. 6 to 12 months: Aware of self, imitates, and repeats pleasurable actions
e. Enjoys soft stuffed animals, crib mobiles with contrasting colors, squeeze toys, rattles, musical toys, water toys during the bath, large picture books, and push toys after he or she begins to walk

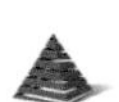

6. Safety

The parents need to be instructed to keep the poison control number available and to contact the poison control center immediately in the event of a poisoning.

a. Parents must baby-proof the home.
b. Guard the infant when on a bed or changing table.
c. Use gates to protect the infant from stairs.
d. Be sure that bathwater is not hot. Do not leave the infant unattended in the bath.
e. Do not hold the infant while drinking or working near hot liquids.
f. Cool vaporizers should be used rather than steam vaporizers to prevent burn injuries.
g. Avoid offering food that is round and similar in size to the airway to prevent choking.
h. Be sure that toys have no small pieces.
i. Hanging toys or mobiles over the crib should be well out of reach to prevent strangulation.
j. Avoid placing large toys in the crib. An older infant may use them as steps to climb out.
k. Cribs should be positioned away from curtains and blind cords.
l. Cover electrical outlets.
m. Remove hazardous objects from low, reachable places.
n. Remove chemicals, medications, poisons, and plants from the infant's reach.

Never shake an infant because of the risk of causing a closed head injury known as shaken baby syndrome.

B. Toddler

1. Physical
   a. Height and weight increase in phases, reflecting growth spurts and lags.
   b. The head circumference increases about 1 inch between the ages of 1 and 2 years. Thereafter, head circumference increases about ½ inch per year until the age of 5 years.
   c. Anterior fontanel closes between ages 12 and 18 months.
   d. Weight gain is slower than in infancy. By 2 years of age, the average weight is 22 to 27 pounds.
   e. Normal height changes include a growth of about 3 inches per year. The average height of a toddler is 34 inches at 2 years old.
   f. Lordosis, also known as a potbelly, is evident.
   g. The toddler should see a dentist soon after the first teeth erupt (usually around 1 year of age), and oral hygiene measures should be instituted. Regular dental care is essential, and the toddler will require assistance with brushing and flossing the teeth. (Fluoride supplements may be necessary if the water is not fluoridated.)
   h. A toddler should never be allowed to fall asleep with a bottle containing milk, juice, soda, or sweetened water because of the risk of nursing (bottle-mouth) caries.
   i. A toddler typically sleeps through the night. He or she has one daytime nap, which is usually discontinued at about the age of 3.
   j. A consistent bedtime ritual helps prepare the toddler for sleep.
   k. Security objects at bedtime may assist in sleep.

BOX 21-3 The Toddler's Vital Signs

Temperature: Axillary, 97.5° to 98.6°F
Apical rate: 80 to 120 beats per minute
Respirations: 20 to 30 breaths per minute
Blood pressure: Average, 92/55 mm Hg

2. Vital signs (Box 21-3)
3. Nutrition
   a. The MyPlate food guide (see Fig. 12-1) provides dietary guidelines and applies to children as young as 2 years of age (see www.choosemyplate.gov).
   b. The toddler should average an intake of two to three servings of milk daily (24 to 30 oz) to ensure an adequate amount of calcium and phosphorus (low-fat milk may be given after 2 years of age).
   c. Trans-fatty acids and saturated fats need to be restricted; otherwise, fat restriction is not appropriate for a toddler (mothers should be taught about the types of food that contain fat that should be selected).
   d. Iron-fortified cereal and a high-iron diet, adequate amounts of calcium and vitamin D, and vitamin C (4 to 6 oz of juice daily) are essential components for the toddler's diet.
   e. Most toddlers prefer to feed themselves.
   f. The toddler generally does best by eating several small nutritious meals each day rather than three large meals.
   g. Offer a limited number of foods at any one time.
   h. Offer finger foods and avoid concentrated sweets and empty calories.

   i. The toddler is at risk for aspiration of small foods that are not chewed easily, such as nuts, foods with seeds, raisins, popcorn, grapes, and hot dog pieces.
   j. Physiological anorexia may occur and is normal because of the alternating stages of fast and slow growth.
   k. Sit the toddler in a high chair at the family table for meals.
   l. Allow sufficient time to eat, but remove food when the toddler begins to play with it.
   m. The toddler drinks well from a cup held with both hands.
   n. Avoid using food as a reward or punishment.
4. Skills
   a. The toddler begins to walk with one hand held by the age of 12 to 13 months.
   b. The toddler runs by the age of 2 years and walks backward and hops on one foot by the age of 3 years.
   c. The toddler usually cannot alternate feet when climbing stairs.
   d. The toddler begins to master fine motor skills for building, undressing, and drawing lines.
   e. The young toddler often uses the word "no," even when he or she means "yes," to assert independence.
   f. The toddler begins to use short sentences and has a vocabulary of about 300 words by the age of 2 years.
5. Bowel and bladder control
   a. Certain signs indicate a toddler is ready for toilet training (Box 21-4).
   b. Bowel control develops before bladder control.
   c. By age 3, the toddler achieves fairly good bowel and bladder control.
   d. The toddler may stay dry during the day but may need a diaper at night until about age 4.
6. Play
   a. The major socializing mechanism is parallel play. Therapeutic play can begin at this age.
   b. The toddler has a short attention span that causes him or her to change toys often.
   c. The toddler explores the body parts of self and others.
   d. Typical toys include push-pull toys, blocks, sand, finger paints, bubbles, large balls, crayons, trucks, dolls, Play-Doh, toy telephones, cloth books, and wooden puzzles.
7. Safety

⚠ Toddlers are eager to explore the world around them. They need to be supervised at play to ensure safety.

   a. Use back burners on the stove to prepare a meal, and turn pot handles inward and toward the middle of the stove.
   b. Keep dangling cords from small appliances away from the toddler.
   c. Place inaccessible locks on windows and doors, and keep furniture away from windows.
   d. Secure screens on all windows.
   e. Place safety gates at stairways.

BOX 21-4 Signs of Readiness for Toilet Training

- Able to stay dry for 2 hours
- Waking dry from a nap
- Able to sit, squat, and walk
- Able to remove clothing
- Recognizes urge to defecate or urinate
- Expresses willingness to please parent
- Able to sit on toilet for 5 to 10 minutes without fussing or getting off

Data from Hockenberry M, Wilson D: *Nursing care of infants and children*, ed 9, St. Louis, 2011, Mosby.

f. Do not allow the toddler to sleep or play in an upper bunk bed.
g. Never leave the toddler alone near a bathtub, pail of water, swimming pool, or any other body of water.
h. Keep toilet lids closed.
i. Keep all medicines, poisons, household plants, and toxic products high and locked out of reach.

C. Preschooler
1. Physical
a. Grows 2½ to 3 inches per year
b. Average height is 37 inches at age 3, 40½ inches at age 4, and 43 inches at age 5.
c. Gains 5 pounds per year; average weight of 35 to 40 pounds at age 5
d. Requires about 12 hours of sleep each day
e. A security object and a nightlight help with sleeping.
f. At the beginning of the preschool period, the eruption of the deciduous (primary) teeth is complete.
g. Regular dental care is essential, and the preschooler requires assistance with the brushing and flossing of teeth. Fluoride supplements may be necessary if the water is not fluoridated.
2. Vital signs (Box 21-5)
3. Nutrition
a. Nutritional needs are similar to those required for the toddler, although the daily amounts of minerals, vitamins, and protein may increase with age.
b. The MyPlate food guide is appropriate for preschoolers (see www.choosemyplate.gov).
c. The preschooler exhibits food fads and certain taste preferences and may exhibit finicky eating.
d. By 5 years old, the child tends to focus on social aspects of eating, table conversations, manners, and willingness to try new foods.
4. Skills
a. Has good posture
b. Develops fine motor coordination
c. Can hop, skip, and run more smoothly
d. Athletic abilities begin to develop
e. Demonstrates increased balancing skills
f. Alternates feet when climbing stairs
g. Can tie shoelaces by age 6
h. May talk continuously and ask many "why" questions

BOX 21-5 The Preschooler's Vital Signs

Temperature: Axillary, 97.5° to 98.6°F
Apical rate: 70 to 110 beats per minute
Respirations: 16 to 22 breaths per minute
Blood pressure: Average, 95/57 mm Hg

i. Vocabulary increases to about 900 words by age 3 and to about 2100 words by age 5.
j. By age 3, the preschooler usually talks in three- or four-word sentences and speaks in short phrases.
k. By age 4, the preschooler uses five- or six-word sentences. By age 5, the preschooler speaks in longer sentences that contain all parts of speech.
l. The preschooler can be readily understood by others and can clearly understand what others are saying.
5. Bowel and bladder control
a. By age 4, the preschooler has daytime control of bowel and bladder, but may experience bed-wetting accidents at night.
b. By age 5, the preschooler achieves both bowel and bladder control, although accidents may occur in stressful situations.
6. Play
a. Cooperative
b. Imaginary playmates
c. Likes to build and create things; play is simple and imaginative
d. Understands sharing and is able to interact with peers
e. Requires regular socialization with children of the same age
f. Play activities include a large space for running and jumping
g. Likes dress-up clothes, paints, paper, and crayons for creative expression
h. Swimming and sports aid with growth and development.
i. Puzzles and toys aid with fine motor development.

7. Safety
a. Preschoolers are active and inquisitive.
b. Because of their magical thinking, they may believe that daring feats seen in cartoons are possible and may attempt them.
c. Preschoolers can learn simple safety practices, because they can follow simple and verbal directions, and their attention span is longer.
d. Reinforce instructions to the preschooler basic safety rules to ensure safety when playing in a playground near swings and ladders.
e. Reinforce instructions to the preschooler never to play with matches or lighters.
f. The preschooler should be taught what to do in the event of a fire or if his or her clothes catch fire. Fire drills should be practiced with the preschooler.
g. Guns should be stored unloaded and secured under lock and key, regardless of the age of the child (ammunition should be locked in a separate place).

h. Reinforce instructions to the preschooler regarding his or her full name, address, parents' names, and telephone number.
i. Reinforce instructions to the preschooler how to dial 911 in an emergency situation.

Teach a preschooler and school-age child to leave an area immediately if a gun is visible and to tell an adult. The child should also be taught never to point a toy gun at another person.

D. School-age child
1. Physical
a. Girls usually grow faster than boys.
b. Growth of about 2 inches per year between the ages of 6 and 12 years
c. Height ranges from 45 inches at age 6 to 59 inches at age 12.
d. Weight gain of 4½ to 6½ pounds per year
e. Average weight of 46 pounds at age 6 and 88 pounds at age 12
f. The first permanent (secondary) teeth erupt around age 6, and the deciduous teeth are gradually lost.
g. Regular dentist visits are necessary, and the school-age child needs to be supervised during the brushing and flossing of teeth. Fluoride supplements may be necessary if the water is not fluoridated.
h. For school-age children with primary and permanent dentition, the best toothbrush is one with soft nylon bristles and an overall length of about 6 inches.
i. Sleep requirements range from 10 to 12 hours per night.
2. Vital signs (Box 21-6)
3. Nutrition
a. School-age children have increased growth needs.
b. Children require a balanced diet from foods in the MyPlate food guide; healthy snacks should continue to be emphasized to prevent childhood obesity (see www.choosemyplate.gov).
c. School-age children may still be picky eaters but are willing to try new foods.
4. Skills
a. School-age children exhibit refinement of fine motor skills.
b. Development of gross motor skills continues.
c. Strength and endurance increase.

BOX 21-6 The School-Age Child's Vital Signs

Temperature: Oral, 97.5° to 98.6°F
Apical rate: 60 to 100 beats per minute
Respirations: 18 to 20 breaths per minute
Blood pressure: Average, 107/64 mm Hg

5. Play
a. Play is more competitive.
b. Rules and rituals are important aspects of play and games.
c. The school-age child enjoys drawing, collecting items, dolls, pets, guessing games, board games, listening to the radio, television, reading, videos or DVDs, and computer games.
d. The child participates in team sports.
e. The child participates in secret clubs, peer-group activities, and scout organizations.
6. Safety
a. The school-age child experiences less fear during play activities. He or she frequently imitates real life with the use of tools and household items.
b. Major causes of injuries include bicycles, skateboards, and team sports as the child increases motor abilities and independence.
c. Children should always wear a helmet when riding a bike or using inline skates or skateboards.
d. Reinforce instructions to the school-age child regarding water safety rules.
e. Reinforce instructions to the school-age child to avoid teasing or playing roughly with animals.
f. Reinforce instructions to the school-age child never to play with matches or lighters.
g. The school-age child should be taught what to do in the event of a fire or if clothes catch fire. Fire drills should be practiced with the school-age child.
h. Guns should be stored unloaded and secured under lock and key, regardless of the age of the child (ammunition should be locked in a separate place).
i. Reinforce instructions to the school-age child regarding traffic safety rules.
j. Reinforce instructions to the school-age child how to dial 911 in an emergency situation.
k. Reinforce instructions to the preschooler and school-age child that if another person touches his or her body in an inappropriate way, an adult should be told. Also teach the child to avoid speaking to strangers and never to accept a ride, toys, or gifts from a stranger.

E. Adolescent
1. Physical
a. Puberty: The maturational, hormonal, and growth process that occurs when the reproductive organs begin to function and the secondary sex characteristics develop
b. Body mass increases to adult size.
c. Sebaceous and sweat glands become active and fully functional.
d. Body hair distribution occurs.
e. Increase in height, weight, breast development, and pelvic girth occur in girls.

f. Menstrual periods usually occur about 2½ years after the onset of puberty.
g. In boys, an increase in height, weight, muscle mass, and penis and testicle size occur.
h. The voice deepens in boys.
i. Normal weight gain during puberty: Girls gain 15 to 55 pounds, and boys gain 15 to 65 pounds.
j. Careful brushing and care of the teeth are important, and many adolescents need to wear braces.
k. Sleep patterns include a tendency to stay up late; therefore, in an attempt to catch up on missed sleep, adolescents sleep late whenever possible. An overall average of 8 hours per night is recommended.

2. Vital signs (Box 21-7)
3. Nutrition
   a. Reinforcing instructions about the MyPlate food guide is important (see www.choosemyplate.gov).
   b. Adolescents typically eat whenever they have a break in activities.
   c. Calcium, zinc, iron, folic acid, and protein are especially important nutritional needs.
   d. Adolescents tend to snack on empty calories, and the importance of adequate and healthy nutrition needs to be stressed.
   e. Body image is important.
4. Skills
   a. Gross and fine motor skills are well developed.
   b. Strength and endurance increase.
5. Play
   a. Games and athletics are the most common forms of play.
   b. Competition and strict rules are important.
   c. Adolescents enjoy activities such as sports, videos, movies, reading, parties, dancing, hobbies, computer games, music, communicating via the Internet and other social media platforms, and experimenting, such as with makeup, hairstyles, tattoos, and piercings.
   d. Friends are important. Adolescents like to gather in small groups.
6. Safety
   a. Adolescents are risk takers.
   b. Adolescents have a natural urge to experiment and be independent.
   c. Reinforce instructions to the adolescents regarding the dangers related to drugs, alcohol, cigarettes, caffeine ingestion, and motor vehicles of any type.
   d. Help adolescents to recognize that there are choices when difficult or potentially dangerous situations arise.
   e. Ensure that the adolescent uses a seat belt.
   f. Reinforce instructions to the adolescents regarding the consequences of the injuries that motor vehicle crashes can cause.
   g. Reinforce instructions to the adolescents regarding water safety. Emphasize that they should enter the water feet first, as opposed to diving, especially when the depth of the water is unknown.
   h. Reinforce instructions to the adolescents about the dangers associated with guns, violence, and gangs.
   i. Reinforce instructions to the adolescents about the complications associated with body piercing, tattooing, and suntanning.

BOX 21-7 The Adolescent's Vital Signs

Temperature: Oral, 97.5° to 98.6°F
Apical rate: 55 to 90 beats per minute
Respirations: 12 to 20 breaths per minute
Blood pressure: Average, 121/70 mm Hg

Discuss issues such as date rape, sexual relationships, and transmission of sexually transmitted infections with the adolescent. Also discuss the dangers of the Internet and other social media platforms related to communicating and setting up meetings (dates) with unknown persons.

F. Early adulthood
1. Description: Period between the late teens and the mid- to late 30s
2. Physical changes
   a. The person has completed physical growth by the age of 20 years.
   b. The person is quite active.
   c. Severe illnesses are less common than those seen among older age groups.
   d. The person tends to ignore physical symptoms and postpones seeking health care.
   e. Lifestyle habits such as smoking, stress, lack of exercise, poor personal hygiene, and family history of disease increase the risk of future illness.
3. Cognitive changes
   a. The person has rational thinking habits.
   b. Conceptual, problem-solving, and motor skills increase.
   c. The person identifies preferred occupational areas.
4. Psychosocial changes
   a. The person separates from the family of origin.
   b. The person gives much attention to occupational and social pursuits to improve socioeconomic status. 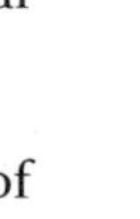

c. The person makes decisions regarding career, marriage, and parenthood.
d. The person needs to adapt to new situations.
5. Sexuality
a. The person has the emotional maturity to develop mature sexual relationships.
b. The person is at risk for sexually transmitted infections.

G. Middle adulthood
1. Description: Period between the mid- to late 30s and the mid-60s
2. Physical changes
a. Occur between the ages of 40 and 65 years
b. The individual becomes aware that changes in reproductive and physical abilities signify the beginning of another stage in life.
c. Menopause occurs in women; climacteric occurs in men.
d. Physiological changes often have an impact on self-concept and body image.
e. Physiological concerns include stress, level of wellness, and the formation of positive health habits.
3. Cognitive changes
a. The person may be interested in learning new skills.
b. The person may become involved with educational or vocational programs for entering the job market or changing careers.
4. Psychosocial changes
a. These may include expected events, such as children moving away from home (postparental family stage), or unexpected events, such as the death of a close friend.
b. Time and financial demands decrease as children move away from home and the couple face redefining their relationship.
c. Adults may become grandparents.
d. Adults are achieving generativity.
5. Sexuality
a. Many couples renew their relationships and find increased marital and sexual satisfaction.
b. The onset of menopause and climacteric may affect sexual health.
c. Stress, health, and medications can affect sexuality.

H. Later adulthood (period between 65 years to death): refer to Chapter 22.

VIII. End-of-Life Care

A. Description: End-of-life care relates to death and dying.

B. Cultural and religious issues (see Chapter 6 and Box 6-2 for information regarding cultural and religious issues)

C. Legal and ethical issues
1. Outcomes related to care during illness and the dying experience should be based on the client's wishes.
2. Issues for consideration may include organ and tissue donations, advance directives or other legal documents, withholding or withdrawing treatment, and cardiopulmonary resuscitation.

D. Palliative care
1. Palliative care focuses on caring interventions and symptom management rather than cure for diseases or conditions that no longer respond to treatment.
2. Pain and symptoms are controlled; the dying client should be as pain-free and as comfortable as possible.
3. Hospice care provides support and care for clients in the last phases of incurable diseases so that they might live as fully and as comfortably as possible; client and family needs are the focus of any intervention.

E. Near-death physiological manifestations
1. As death approaches, metabolism is reduced, and the body gradually slows down until all functions end.
2. Sensory: The client experiences blurred vision, decreased sense of taste and smell, decreased pain and touch perception, loss of blink reflex, and appears to stare (hearing is believed to be the last sense lost).
3. Respirations
a. Respirations may be rapid or slow, shallow, and irregular.
b. Respirations may be noisy and wet sounding (death rattle).
c. Cheyne-Stokes respiration is alternating periods of apnea and deep, rapid breathing.
4. Circulation
a. Heart rate slows, and blood pressure falls progressively.
b. Skin is cool to touch, and the extremities become pale, mottled, and cyanotic.
c. Skin is waxlike very near death.
5. Urinary output decreases; incontinence may occur.
6. Gastrointestinal motility and peristalsis diminish, leading to constipation, gas accumulation, and distention; incontinence may occur.
7. Musculoskeletal system: The client gradually loses ability to move, has difficulty speaking and swallowing, and loses the gag reflex.

F. Death
1. Death occurs when all vital organs and body systems cease to function.
2. In general, respirations cease first, and then the heartbeat stops a few minutes thereafter.

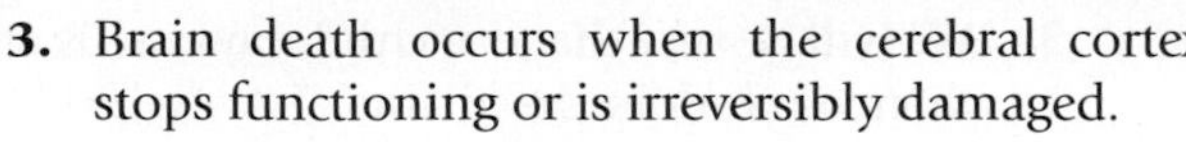

3. Brain death occurs when the cerebral cortex stops functioning or is irreversibly damaged.

G. Nursing care
1. Frequency of assessment depends on the client's stability (at least every 4 hours); as changes occur, assessment needs to be done more frequently.
2. Physical care (Box 21-8)
3. Psychosocial care
   a. Monitor for anxiety and depression.
   b. Monitor for fear (Box 21-9).
   c. Encourage the client and family to express feelings.

BOX 21-8 Physical Care of the Dying Client

Pain

Administer pain medication.
Do not delay or deny pain medication.

Dyspnea

Elevate the head of the bed or position the client on his or her side.
Administer supplemental oxygen.
Suction fluids from the airway as needed.

Skin

Assess color and temperature.
Assess for breakdown.
Implement measures to prevent breakdown.

Dehydration

Maintain regular oral care.
Encourage taking ice chips and sips of fluid.
Do not force the client to eat or drink.
Use moist cloths to provide moisture to the mouth.
Apply lubricant to the lips and oral mucous membranes.

Anorexia, Nausea, and Vomiting

Provide antiemetics before meals.
Have family members provide the client's favorite foods.
Provide frequent small portions of favorite foods.

Elimination

Monitor urinary and bowel elimination.
Place absorbent pads under the client and check frequently.

Weakness and Fatigue

Provide rest periods.
Assess tolerance for activities.
Provide assistance and support as needed for maintaining bed or chair positions.

Restlessness

Maintain a calm, soothing environment.
Do not restrain.
Limit the number of visitors at the client's bedside (consider cultural practices).
Allow a family member to stay with the client.

BOX 21-9 Fear Associated with Dying

Fear of Pain

Fear of pain may occur, based on anxieties related to dying.
Do not delay or deny pain relief measures to a terminally ill client.

Fear of Loneliness and Abandonment

Allow family members to stay with the client.
Holding hands, touching (if culturally acceptable), and listening to the client are important.

Fear of Being Meaningless

Client may feel hopeless and powerless.
Encourage life reviews and focus on the positive aspects of the client's life.

Adapted from Lewis S, Dirksen S, Heitkemper M, Bucher L: *Medical-surgical nursing: Assessment and management of clinical problems*, ed 9, St. Louis, 2014, Mosby.

BOX 21-10 General Postmortem Procedures

Close the client's eyes.
Replace dentures.
Wash the body.
Place pads under the perineum.
Remove tubes and dressings.
Straighten the body and place a pillow under the head in preparation for family viewing.

   d. Provide support and advocacy for the client and family.
   e. Provide privacy for the client and family.
   f. Provide a private room for the client.
4. Postmortem care (Box 21-10)
   a. Maintain respect and dignity for the client.
   b. Determine whether the client is an organ donor; if so, follow appropriate procedures related to the donation.
   c. Consider cultural rituals, state laws, and agency procedures when performing postmortem care.
   d. Prepare the body for immediate viewing by the family.
   e. Provide privacy and time for the family to be with the deceased person.
   f. Medical examiner jurisdiction guidelines are determined by each state and usually include nonnatural, traumatic, or question of criminal involvement deaths; any forensic evidence is preserved, and the body is not cleaned or prepared prior to transfer to the morgue.

CRITICAL THINKING What Should You Do?

Answer: When caring for a child who is apprehensive, the nurse should provide a safe and secure environment. The nurse should also take time for communication with the child; allow the child to express feelings such as anxiety, fear, or anger; accept any regressive behavior and assist the preschooler in moving from regressive to appropriate behaviors. Additional interventions include encouraging rooming-in with the parents or leaving a favorite toy; allowing mobility and providing play and diversional activities; placing the preschooler with other children of the same age if possible; and encouraging the preschooler to be independent. The nurse should also explain procedures simply on the preschooler's level, avoid intrusive procedures when possible, and allow the child to wear underpants.

Reference(s): McKinney, E., James, S., Murray, S., Nelson, K. & Ashwill, J. (2013). *Maternal-child nursing* (4th ed., p. 884). St. Louis: Elsevier.

PRACTICE QUESTIONS

176. The parents of a 16-year-old child tell the nurse that they are concerned because the child sleeps until noon every weekend. Which is the **most appropriate** nursing response?
1. "Adolescents love to sleep late in the morning."
2. "The child shouldn't be staying up so late at night."
3. "If the child eats properly, that shouldn't be happening."
4. "The child should have a blood test to check for anemia."

177. A 16-year-old child is admitted to the hospital for acute appendicitis, and an appendectomy is performed. Which intervention is **most appropriate** to facilitate normal growth and development?
1. Encourage the child to rest and read.
2. Encourage the parents to room-in with the child.
3. Allow the family to bring in favorite computer games.
4. Allow the child to participate in activities with other individuals in the same age group when the condition permits.

178. The emergency department nurse is reinforcing discharge instructions to the parents of a 2-year-old child who sustained accidental burns from a hot cup of coffee. The nurse determines that the parents have correctly understood the teaching when they make which statement?
1. "We will be sure not to leave hot liquids unattended."
2. "I guess my child needs to understand what the word 'hot' means."
3. "We will be sure that our child stays in his room when we work in the kitchen."
4. "We will install a safety gate as soon as we get home so that our child can't get into the kitchen."

❖ **179.** Which interventions are appropriate for the care of an infant? **Select all that apply.**
- ❑ **1.** Provide swaddling.
- ❑ **2.** Talk in a loud voice.
- ❑ **3.** Provide the infant with a bottle of juice at naptime.
- ❑ **4.** Hang mobiles with black-and-white contrast designs.
- ❑ **5.** Caress the infant while bathing or during diaper changes.
- ❑ **6.** Allow the infant to cry for at least 10 minutes before responding.

❖ **180.** The nurse is preparing to care for a dying client, and several family members are at the client's bedside. Which therapeutic techniques should the nurse use when communicating with the family? **Select all that apply.**
- ❑ **1.** Discourage reminiscing.
- ❑ **2.** Make the decisions for the family.
- ❑ **3.** Encourage expression of feelings, concerns, and fears.
- ❑ **4.** Explain everything that is happening to all family members.
- ❑ **5.** Touch and hold the client's or family member's hand if appropriate.
- ❑ **6.** Be honest and let the client and family know that they will not be abandoned by the nurse.

181. The parents of a 2-year-old arrive at the hospital to visit their child. The child is in the play room and ignores the parents during the visit. The nurse tells the parents that this behavior in a 2-year-old child indicates which?
1. The child is withdrawn.
2. The child is upset with the parents.
3. The child is exhibiting a normal pattern.
4. The child has adjusted to the hospitalized setting.

182. When caring for a 3-year-old child, the nurse should provide which toy for the child?
1. A puzzle
2. A wagon
3. A golf set
4. A farm set

183. Upon palpation of the fontanel of a 3-month-old newborn, the nurse notes that the anterior fontanel has not closed and is soft and flat. Which action should the nurse take?
1. Increase oral fluids.
2. Document the findings.

3. Notify the registered nurse.
4. Elevate the head of the bed to 90 degrees.

184. The nurse is caring for a 5-year-old child who has been placed in traction after a fracture of the femur. Which is the **most appropriate** activity for this child?
1. Blocks
2. A puzzle
3. A music video
4. Large picture books

185. The parent of a 4-year-old child expresses concern because her hospitalized child has started sucking his thumb. The mother states that this behavior began 2 days after hospital admission. Which is the appropriate nursing response?
1. "It is best to ignore the behavior."
2. "Your child is acting like a baby."
3. "The doctor will need to be notified."
4. "A 4-year-old is too old for this type of behavior."

ANSWERS

176. 1

Rationale: The sleep patterns of the adolescent vary some according to individual needs. However, in general, adolescents love to sleep late in the morning, but they should be encouraged to be responsible for waking themselves, particularly in time to get ready for school. Options 2, 3, and 4 are incorrect.
Test-Taking Strategy: Focus on the subject, adolescent sleep patterns, and note the strategic words, *most appropriate.* Options 2 and 3 can be eliminated first because they are inappropriate responses and are not helpful or therapeutic. From the remaining options, there is no indication that a physiological alteration is present; therefore, option 1 is most appropriate. **Review: adolescent sleep patterns.**
Level of Cognitive Ability: Applying
Client Needs: Physiological Integrity
Integrated Process: Nursing Process/Implementation
Content Area: Developmental Stages: Infancy to Adolescence
Priority Concepts: Development, Functional Ability
References(s): Hockenberry, Wilson (2013), p. 490.

177. 4

Rationale: Adolescents are not often sure they want their parents with them when they are hospitalized. Because of the importance of the peer group, separation from friends is a source of anxiety. Ideally, the peer group will support the ill friend. Options 1, 2, and 3 isolate the child from the peer group.
Test-Taking Strategy: Note the strategic words, *most appropriate.* Consider the psychosocial needs of the adolescent when answering the question. Options 1, 2, and 3 are comparable or alike in that they isolate the child from their own peer group. **Review:** the psychosocial needs of the **adolescent.**
Level of Cognitive Ability: Applying
Client Needs: Psychosocial Integrity
Integrated Process: Nursing Process/Implementation
Content Area: Developmental Stages: Infancy to Adolescence
Priority Concepts: Development, Functional Ability
Reference(s): McKinney et al (2013), p. 884.

178. 1

Rationale: Toddlers, with their increased mobility and developing motor skills, can reach hot water, open fires, or hot objects placed on counters and stoves above their eye level. Parents should be encouraged to remain in the kitchen when preparing a meal and reminded to use the back burners on the stove. Pot handles should be turned inward and toward the middle of the stove. Hot liquids should never be left unattended, and the toddler should always be supervised. Options 2, 3, and 4 do not reflect an adequate understanding of the principles of safety.
Test-Taking Strategy: Option 2 can be easily eliminated considering the development level of the 2-year-old. Options 3 and 4 are comparable or alike in that they isolate the child from the environment. **Review: safety principles for the toddler.**
Level of Cognitive Ability: Evaluating
Client Needs: Safe and Effective Care Environment
Integrated Process: Nursing Process/Evaluation
Content Area: Fundamental Skills: Safety
Priority Concepts: Development, Safety
Reference(s): Hockenberry, Wilson (2013), pp. 347, 349.

❖ **179. 1, 4, 5**

Rationale: Holding, caressing, and swaddling provide warmth and tactile stimulation for the infant. To provide auditory stimulation, the nurse should talk to the infant in a soft voice and should instruct the mother to do so also. Additional interventions include playing a music box, radio, or television or having a ticking clock or metronome nearby. Hanging a bright, shiny object within 20 to 25 cm of the infant's face in the midline and hanging mobiles with contrasting colors (e.g., black and white) provide visual stimulation. Crying is an infant's way of communicating; therefore, the nurse would respond to the infant's crying. The mother is taught to do so also. An infant or child should never be allowed to fall asleep with a bottle containing milk, juice, soda, or sweetened water because of the risk of nursing (bottle-mouth) caries.
Test-Taking Strategy: Focus on the subject, the care of the infant. Noting the word *loud* in option 2 and the words *at least 10 minutes before responding* in option 6 will assist you with eliminating these interventions. Recalling the concerns related to dental caries will assist you with eliminating option 3. **Review:** the guidelines related to the care of an **infant.**
Level of Cognitive Ability: Analyzing
Client Needs: Psychosocial Integrity
Integrated Process: Nursing Process/Implementation
Content Area: Development Stages: Infancy to Adolescence
Priority Concepts: Development, Family Dynamics
Reference(s): McKinney et al (2013), p. 523.

❖ **180. 3, 5, 6**
Rationale: The nurse must determine whether there is a spokesperson for the family and how much the client and family want to know. The nurse needs to allow the family and client the opportunity for informed choices and assist with the decision-making process if asked. The nurse should encourage expression of feelings, concerns, and fears and reminiscing. The nurse needs to be honest and let the client and family know that they will not be abandoned. The nurse should touch and hold the client's or family member's hand, if appropriate.
Test-Taking Strategy: Use therapeutic communication techniques, and recall client and family rights to assist in directing you to the correct options. **Review:** end-of-life care.
Level of Cognitive Ability: Analyzing
Client Needs: Psychosocial Integrity
Integrated Process: Caring
Content Area: Developmental Stages: End-of-Life Care
Priority Concepts: Family Dynamics; Palliation
Reference(s): deWit, Kumagai (2013), pp. 174, 1135–1136.

181. 3
Rationale: The toddler is particularly vulnerable to separation. A toddler often shows anger at being left by ignoring the parent or pretending to be more interested in play than in going home. The parents of hospitalized toddlers are frequently distressed by such behavior. The toddler normally engages in parallel play and plays alongside (but not with) other children. Options 1, 2, and 4 are incorrect.
Test-Taking Strategy: Focus on the subject, separation anxiety, and use the concepts of growth and development. Option 4 can be easily eliminated first because there is no indication that the child has adjusted. There is no information in the question to support option 1, so eliminate this option. From the remaining options, knowledge regarding separation anxiety in the toddler will direct you to the correct option. **Review:** concepts of separation anxiety.
Level of Cognitive Ability: Applying
Client Needs: Psychosocial Integrity
Integrated Process: Nursing Process/Implementation
Content Area: Developmental Stages: Infancy to Adolescence
Priority Concepts: Coping, Family Dynamics
Reference(s): Hockenberry, Wilson (2013), p. 613.

182. 2
Rationale: Toys for the toddler must be strong, safe, and too large to swallow or place in the ear or nose. Toddlers need supervision at all times. Push-pull toys, large balls, large crayons, trucks, and dolls are some appropriate toys. A puzzle with large pieces only may be appropriate. A farm set and a golf set may contain items that the child could swallow.
Test-Taking Strategy: Focus on the subject, appropriate toys for a 3-year-old. Options 3 and 4 can be easily eliminated because they contain items that could be swallowed by the child. From the remaining options, the appropriate toy is a wagon. Remember that large and strong toys are safest for the toddler. Review: safety measures for the toddler.
Level of Cognitive Ability: Applying
Client Needs: Safe and Effective Care Environment
Integrated Process: Nursing Process/Implementation
Content Area: Developmental Stages: Infancy to Adolescence
Priority Concepts: Development, Safety
Reference(s): Hockenberry, Wilson (2013), pp. 384–385.

183. 2
Rationale: The anterior fontanel is diamond shaped and located on the top of the head. It should be soft and flat in a normal infant, and it normally closes by 12 to 18 months of age. The posterior fontanel closes by 2 to 3 months of age. Therefore, because the findings are normal, the nurse should document the findings.
Test-Taking Strategy: Note the subject, assessment findings for an infant's fontanelles. Since they are "soft and flat," this should provide you with the clue that this is a normal finding. A bulging or tense fontanel may result from crying or increased intracranial pressure. **Review: fontanelles in the infant.**
Level of Cognitive Ability: Applying
Client Needs: Physiological Integrity
Integrated Process: Nursing Process/Implementation
Content Area: Developmental Stages: Health Assessment/Physical Exam
Priority Concepts: Development, Tissue Integrity
Reference(s): Cooper, Gosnell (2015), pp. 801.

184. 2
Rationale: In the preschooler, play is simple and imaginative, and it includes activities such as dressing up, paints, crayons, and simple board and card games. Puzzles are also appropriate and aid with fine motor development. Blocks are most appropriate for the toddler. A music video is most appropriate for the adolescent. Large picture books are most appropriate for the infant.
Test-Taking Strategy: Note the strategic words, *most appropriate*. Also note the subject, play activity and the age of the child, and then think about the age-related activity that would be appropriate. Eliminate option 3, knowing that it is most appropriate for the adolescent. From the remaining options, the word *blocks* in option 1 and *large* in option 4 should provide you with the clue that these activities would be more appropriate for a child who is less than 5 years old. **Review:** the appropriate play activities for a **preschooler**.
Level of Cognitive Ability: Applying
Client Needs: Psychosocial Integrity
Integrated Process: Nursing Process/Implementation
Content Area: Developmental Stages: Infancy to Adolescence
Priority Concepts: Development, Functional Ability
Reference(s): McKinney et al (2013), pp. 126–127, 1345.

185. 1
Rationale: In the hospitalized preschooler, it is best to accept regression if it occurs, because it is most often caused by the stress of the hospitalization. Parents may be overly concerned about regression and should be told that their child may continue the behavior at home. There is no need to call the health care provider. Options 2 and 4 are inappropriate.
Test-Taking Strategy: Focus on the subject, regression because of hospitalization. Options 2, 3, and 4 will cause additional stress and concern in the parent. **Review:** the psychosocial issues related to the hospitalized **preschool child**.
Level of Cognitive Ability: Applying
Client Needs: Psychosocial Integrity
Integrated Process: Nursing Process/Implementation
Content Area: Developmental Stages: Infancy to Adolescence
Priority Concepts: Development, Stress
Reference(s): Hockenberry, Wilson (2013), p. 390.

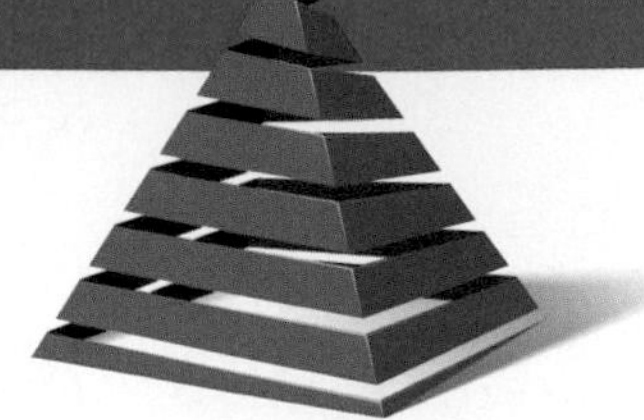

CHAPTER 22

Care of the Older Client

Fundamentals

CRITICAL THINKING What Should You Do?

The home care nurse is caring for an older female client who lives with her son and is physically and financially dependent on her son. The nurse notes multiple bruises on the client's arms and asks the client how these bruises occurred. The client confides in the nurse that her son takes out his anger on her sometimes. What should the nurse do?

Answer is located on p. 236.

I. Aging and Gerontology

A. **Aging** is the biopsychosocial process of change that occurs in a person between birth and death.

B. Gerontology is the study of the aging process.

II. Physiological Changes

A. Integumentary system
   1. Loss of pigment in hair and skin
   2. Wrinkling of the skin
   3. Thinning of the epidermis; easy bruising and tearing of the skin
   4. Decreased skin turgor, elasticity, and subcutaneous fat
   5. Increased nail thickness and decreased nail growth
   6. Decreased perspiration
   7. Dry, itchy, and scaly skin
   8. Seborrheic dermatitis and keratosis formation (overgrowth and thickening of the skin)

B. Neurological system
   1. Slowed reflexes
   2. Slight tremors and difficulty with fine motor movement
   3. Loss of balance
   4. An increased incidence of awakening after sleep onset
   5. Increased susceptibility to hypothermia and hyperthermia
   6. Short-term memory may decline.
   7. Long-term memory usually maintained.

C. Musculoskeletal system
   1. Muscle mass and strength decrease; muscles atrophy 
   2. Decreased mobility, range of motion, flexibility, coordination, and stability
   3. Change of gait, with a shortened step and a wider base
   4. Posture and stature changes that cause a decrease in height (Fig. 22-1)
   5. Increased brittleness of the bones
   6. Deterioration of joint capsule components
   7. Kyphosis of the dorsal spine (increased convexity in the curvature of the spine)

The older client is at risk for falls because of the changes that occur in the neurological and musculoskeletal systems.

D. Cardiovascular system
   1. Diminished energy and endurance, with lowered tolerance to exercise
   2. Decreased compliance of the heart muscle; heart valves become thicker and more rigid
   3. Decreased cardiac output; decreased efficiency of blood return to the heart
   4. Decreased compensatory response, so less able to respond to increased demands on the cardiovascular system
   5. Decreased resting heart rate
   6. Weak peripheral pulses
   7. Increased blood pressure but susceptible to postural hypotension

E. Respiratory system
   1. Decreased stretch and compliance of the chest wall
   2. Decreased strength and function of the respiratory muscles
   3. Decreased size and number of alveoli
   4. The respiratory rate usually remains unchanged.
   5. Decreased depth of respirations and oxygen intake
   6. Decreased ability to cough and expectorate sputum

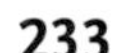

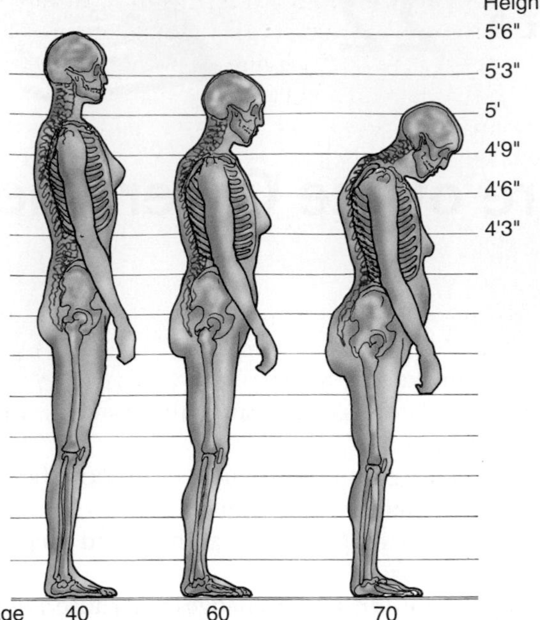

FIGURE 22-1 A normal spine at age 40 years of age and osteoporotic changes at 60 and 70 years of age. These changes can cause a loss of as much as 6 inches in height and can result in the so-called dowager's hump *(far right)* in the upper thoracic vertebrae. (From Ignatavicius D, Workman ML: *Medical-surgical nursing: Patient-centered collaborative care,* ed 7, Philadelphia, 2013, Saunders.)

F. Hematological system
   1. Hemoglobin and hematocrit levels average toward the low end of normal.
   2. Prone to increased blood clotting
   3. Decreased protein available for protein-bound medications.

G. Immune system
   1. Tendency for lymphocyte counts to be low with altered immunoglobulin production
   2. Decreased resistance to infection and disease

H. Gastrointestinal system
   1. Decreased need for calories because of lowered basal metabolic rate
   2. Decreased appetite, thirst, and oral intake
   3. Decreased lean body mass
   4. Decreased stomach-emptying time
   5. Increased tendency toward constipation
   6. Increased susceptibility to dehydration
   7. Tooth loss
   8. Difficulty with chewing and swallowing food

I. Endocrine system
   1. Decreased secretion of hormones, with specific changes related to each hormone function
   2. Decreased metabolic rate
   3. Decreased glucose tolerance, with resistance to insulin in the peripheral tissues

J. Renal system
   1. Decreased kidney size, function, and ability to concentrate urine
   2. Decreased glomerular filtration rate
   3. Decreased capacity of the bladder
   4. Increased residual urine; increased incidence of infection and possibly incontinence
   5. Impaired medication excretion

K. Reproductive system
   1. Decreased testosterone production and size of testes
   2. Changes in the prostate gland, leading to urinary problems
   3. Decreased secretion of hormones, with the cessation of menses
   4. Vaginal changes, including decreased muscle tone and lubrication
   5. Impotence or sexual dysfunction for both genders; sexual function varies and depends on general physical condition, mental health status, and medications.

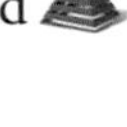

L. Special senses
   1. Decreased visual acuity
   2. Decreased accommodation in eyes, which requires increased time for adjustment to changes in light
   3. Decreased peripheral vision and increased sensitivity to glare
   4. Presbyopia and cataract formation
   5. Possible loss of hearing ability; low-pitched tones are more easily heard
   6. Inability to discern taste of food
   7. Decreased sense of smell
   8. Changes in touch sensation
   9. Decreased pain awareness

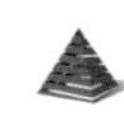

III. Psychosocial Concerns

A. Adjustment to deterioration in physical and mental health and well-being
B. Threat to independent functioning; fear of becoming a burden to loved ones
C. Adjustment to retirement and loss of income
D. Loss of skills and competencies developed early in life
E. Coping with changes in role function and social life
F. Diminished quantity and quality of relationships and coping with loss
G. Dependence on governmental and social systems
H. Access to social support systems
I. Costs of health care and medications

IV. Mental Health Concerns

A. **Depression:** The increased dependency that older adults may experience can lead to hopelessness, helplessness, a lowered sense of self-control, and decreased self-esteem and self-worth. These changes can interfere with daily functioning and lead to depression.
B. Grief: Client reacts to the perception of loss, including physical, psychological, social, and spiritual aspects.

C. Isolation: Client is alone and desires contact with others but is unable to make that contact.

D. Suicide: Depression can lead to thoughts of self-harm.

E. Depression differs from delirium and **dementia** (Table 22-1).

Any suicide threat from an older client should be taken seriously.

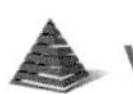

V. Pain

A. Description

1. Pain can come about from numerous causes and most often occurs from degenerative changes in the musculoskeletal system.
2. The failure to alleviate pain in the older client can lead to functional limitations that affect the client's ability to function independently.

B. Data collection

1. Restlessness
2. Verbal reporting of pain
3. Agitation
4. Moaning
5. Crying

C. Interventions

1. Monitor the client for signs of pain.
2. Identify the pattern of pain.
3. Identify the precipitating factor(s) for the pain.
4. Monitor the impact of the pain on the client's activities of daily living.
5. Provide pain relief through measures such as distraction, relaxation, massage, and biofeedback.
6. Administer pain medications, as prescribed. Instruct the client in their use.
7. Evaluate the effects of pain-reducing measures.

VI. Infection

A. Confusion is a common sign of infection in the older adult, especially infection of the urinary tract.

B. Carefully monitor the older adult with an infection because of diminished and altered immune response.

C. Nonspecific symptoms may indicate illness or infection (Box 22-1).

VII. Medications

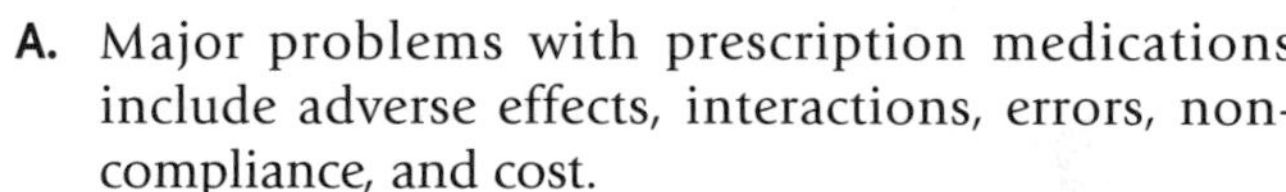

A. Major problems with prescription medications include adverse effects, interactions, errors, noncompliance, and cost.

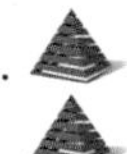

B. Determine the use of over-the-counter medications.

C. **Polypharmacy**

1. Routinely monitor the number of prescription and nonprescription medications used and determine if any can be eliminated or combined.

TABLE 22-1 Differentiating Delirium, Depression, and Dementia

Characteristic	Delirium	Depression	Dementia
Onset	Sudden, abrupt	Recent; may relate to life change	Insidious, slow, over years and often unrecognized until deficits obvious
Course over 24 hr	Fluctuating, often worse at night	Fairly stable; may be worse in the morning	Fairly stable; may see changes with stress
Consciousness	Reduced	Clear	Clear
Alertness	Increased, decreased, or variable	Normal	Generally normal
Psychomotor activity	Increased, decreased, or mixed Sometimes increased, other times decreased	Variable, agitation, or retardation	Normal; may have apraxia or agnosia
Duration	Hours to weeks	Variable and may be chronic	Years
Attention	Disordered, fluctuates	Little impairment	Generally normal but may have trouble focusing
Orientation	Usually impaired, fluctuates	Usually normal; may answer "I don't know" to questions or may not try to answer	Often impaired; may make up answers or answer close to the right thing, or may confabulate but tries to answer
Speech	Often incoherent, slow or rapid; may call out repeatedly or repeat the same phrase	May be slow	Difficulty finding word, perseveration
Affect	Variable but may look disturbed, frightened	Flat	Slowed response; may be labile

Modified from Rapp CG, Mentes J, Titler M: Acute confusion/delirium protocol, *J Gerontol Nurse* 27(4):21–33, 2001. Reprinted with permission from SLACK, Inc, Thorofare, NJ.

BOX 22-1 Nonspecific Symptoms That May Indicate Illness or Infection

- Anorexia
- Apathy
- Changes in functional status
- Confusion
- Dyspnea
- Falling
- Fatigue
- Incontinence
- Self-neglect
- Shortness of breath
- Tachypnea
- Vital sign changes

2. Keep the use of medications to a minimum.
3. Overprescribing medications leads to increased problems with more side effects, increased interaction among medications, replication of medication treatment, diminished quality of life, and increased costs.

D. Medication dosages normally are prescribed at one third to one half of the normal adult doses.

E. Closely monitor the client for side effects and adverse effects and response to therapy because of the increased risk for medication toxicity.

F. Check for medication interactions in the client who is taking multiple medications.

G. Advise the client to use one pharmacy and notify the consulting health care providers of the medications taken.

A common sign of an adverse reaction to a medication in the older client is an acute change in mental status.

H. Administration of medications
1. Place the client in a sitting position when administering medication.
2. Check for mouth dryness, because medication may stick and dissolve in the mouth.
3. Administer liquid preparations if the client has difficulty swallowing tablets.
4. Crush tablets, if necessary, and give with textured food (e.g., applesauce) if not contraindicated.
5. Enteric-coated tablets are not crushed and capsules are not opened.
6. If administering a suppository, avoid inserting the suppository immediately after removing it from the refrigerator. A suppository may take a while to dissolve because of a decreased body core temperature.
7. When administering parenteral medication, monitor the site, because it may ooze medication or bleed as a result of decreased tissue elasticity. An immobile limb is not used for administering parenteral medication.
8. Monitor client compliance with the taking of prescribed medications.
9. Monitor the client for **safety** with regard to correctly taking medications, including an assessment of the client's ability to read the instructions and discriminate among the pills and their color and shape.
10. Use a medication cassette to facilitate the proper administration of medication.

VIII. Abuse of the Older Adult

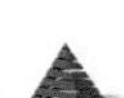

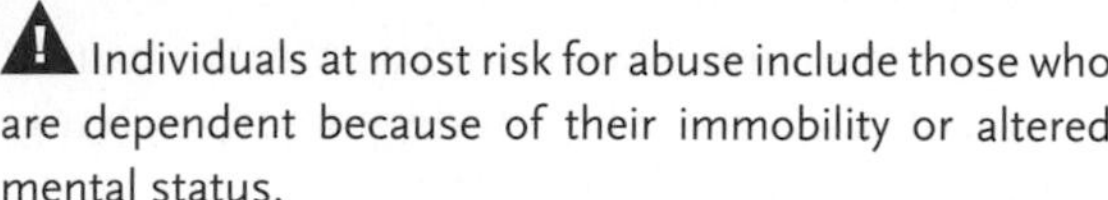

Individuals at most risk for abuse include those who are dependent because of their immobility or altered mental status.

A. Domestic mistreatment takes place in the home of the older adult and is usually carried out by a family member or significant other; this can include physical maltreatment, **neglect**, or abandonment.

B. Institutional mistreatment takes place when an older adult experiences **abuse** when hospitalized or living somewhere other than home (e.g., long-term care facility).

C. **Self-neglect** is the choice by a mentally competent individual to avoid medical care or other services that could improve optimal function, not to care for oneself, and engage in actions that negatively affect his or her personal safety; unless declared legally incompetent, an individual has the right to refuse care.

D. For additional information about abuse of the older client, see Chapter 66.

CRITICAL THINKING What Should You Do?

Answer: If the nurse suspects or knows for certain that elder abuse is occurring, the nurse should report this abuse to the appropriate authorities and follow state and agency guidelines in doing so. The nurse should then perform a thorough assessment of physical injuries, while providing confidentiality during the assessment with an empathetic and nonjudgmental approach. The nurse should reassure the victim that she or he has done nothing wrong. The nurse should also assist the victim in developing self-protective and problem-solving skills. Even if the victim is not ready to leave the situation, encourage the victim to develop a specific safety plan (a fast escape if the violence returns) and where to obtain help (hotlines, safe houses, and shelters); an abused person is usually reluctant to call the police.

Reference(s): deWit, D. & Kumagai, C. (2013). *Medical-surgical nursing: Concepts & practice.* (2nd ed., p. 1042). St. Louis: Saunders.

PRACTICE QUESTIONS

186. An older client has been prescribed digoxin (Lanoxin). The nurse understands that which age-related change would place the client at risk for digoxin toxicity?
1. Decreased cough efficiency and vital capacity
2. Decreased salivation and gastrointestinal motility
3. Decreased muscle strength and loss of bone density
4. Decreased lean body mass and glomerular filtration rate

187. The nurse should plan which to encourage autonomy in the client who is a resident in a long-term care facility?
1. Choosing his meals
2. Decorating his room
3. Scheduling his barber appointments
4. Allowing the client to choose social activities

188. Which data indicate to the nurse that a client may be experiencing ineffective coping following the loss of her spouse?
1. Constantly neglects personal grooming
2. Visits her husband's grave once a month
3. Visits the senior citizens' center once a month
4. Frequently looks at snapshots of her husband and family

189. The nurse is preparing to communicate with an older client who is hearing impaired. Which intervention should be implemented **initially**?
1. Stand in front of the client.
2. Exaggerate the lip movements.
3. Obtain a sign-language interpreter.
4. Pantomime and write the client notes.

190. Which intervention should be implemented for the older client with presbycusis who has a hearing loss?
1. Speak louder
2. Speak more slowly
3. Use low-pitched tones
4. Use high-pitched tones

❖ **191.** When the nurse is collecting data from the older adult, which findings should be considered normal physiological changes? **Select all that apply.**
- ❑ 1. Increased heart rate
- ❑ 2. Decline in visual acuity
- ❑ 3. Decreased respiratory rate
- ❑ 4. Decline in long-term memory
- ❑ 5. Increased susceptibility to urinary tract infections
- ❑ 6. Increased incidence of awakening after sleep onset

192. The nurse is planning to feed an older client who is at risk for aspiration of food. During the meal, how should the nurse position the client?
1. Upright in a chair
2. On the left side in bed
3. On the right side in bed
4. In a low-Fowler's position, with the legs elevated

193. The nurse is providing an education class to healthy older adults. Which exercise will **best** promote health maintenance?
1. Gardening every day for an hour
2. Sculpting once a week for 40 minutes
3. Cycling three times a week for 20 minutes
4. Walking three to five times a week for 30 minutes

194. The nurse should implement which activity to promote reminiscence among older clients?
1. Having storytelling hours
2. Setting up pet therapy sessions
3. Displaying calendars and clocks
4. Encouraging client participation in a pottery class

195. Which client is **most likely** at risk to become a victim of elder abuse?
1. A 75-year-old man with moderate hypertension
2. A 68-year-old man with newly diagnosed cataracts
3. A 90-year-old woman with advanced Parkinson's disease
4. A 70-year-old woman with early diagnosed Lyme disease

ANSWERS

186. 4

Rationale: The older client is at risk for medication toxicity because of decreased lean body mass and an age-associated decreased glomerular filtration rate. Although options 1, 2, and 3 identify age-related changes that occur in the older client, they are not specifically associated with this risk.

Test-Taking Strategy: Focus on the subject, age-related body change that could place the client at risk for medication toxicity. Note that option 4 is the only choice that addresses renal excretion. **Review:** the physiological changes associated with **aging**.

Level of Cognitive Ability: Analyzing

Client Needs: Physiological Integrity

Integrated Process: Nursing Process/Data Collection

Content Area: Developmental Stages: Early Adulthood to Later Adulthood

Priority Concepts: Development, Safety

Reference(s): Cooper, Gosnell (2015), p. 610; deWit, Kumagai (2013), p. 718.

187. 4

Rationale: Autonomy is the personal freedom to direct one's own life as long as it does not impinge on the rights of others. An autonomous person is capable of rational thought. This individual can identify problems, search for alternatives, and choose solutions that allow for continued personal freedom as long as the rights and property of others are not harmed. The loss of autonomy—and, therefore, independence—is a very real fear among older clients. Option 4 is the only choice that allows the client to be a decision maker.

Test-Taking Strategy: Focus on the subject, encouraging autonomy. Recalling the definition of autonomy will direct you to the correct option. Remember that to promote independence in clients, it is essential to give the client choices. **Review:** the concept of **autonomy**.

Level of Cognitive Ability: Applying

Client Needs: Safe and Effective Care Environment

Integrated Process: Caring

Content Area: Developmental Stages: Early Adulthood to Later Adulthood

Priority Concepts: Caregiving, Coping

Reference(s): Cooper, Gosnell (2015), p. 34.

188. 1

Rationale: Coping mechanisms are behaviors that are used to decrease stress and anxiety. In response to a death, ineffective coping is manifested by an extreme behavior that in some instances may be harmful to the individual physically, psychologically, or both. Option 1 is indicative of a behavior that identifies an ineffective coping behavior as part of the grieving process. The remaining options identify effective coping behaviors.

Test-Taking Strategy: Focus on the subject, an indication of ineffective coping behavior. Eliminate options 2, 3, and 4 because they are comparable or alike and are positive activities that the individual is engaging in to get on with her life. **Review:** the coping mechanisms for dealing with **grief and loss**.

Level of Cognitive Ability: Analyzing

Client Needs: Psychosocial Integrity

Integrated Process: Nursing Process/Data Collection

Content Area: Mental Health

Priority Concepts: Coping, Mood and Affect

Reference(s): Cooper, Gosnell (2015), pp. 1116–1117.

189. 1

Rationale: The nurse would ensure that the hearing-impaired client can see the nurse when the nurse is speaking by providing adequate lighting and standing in front of the client. The nurse should enunciate words clearly but not exaggerate lip movements. If the client is profoundly hearing impaired and uses signing, a sign-language interpreter should be obtained. If a client cannot understand by reading lips, the nurse would try using gestures, pantomiming, or writing notes.

Test-Taking Strategy: Note the strategic word, *initially*. To communicate effectively with a hearing-impaired client, the nurse first makes sure that the client can see him or her. **Review:** the nursing interventions for the **hearing-impaired client**.

Level of Cognitive Ability: Applying

Client Needs: Physiological Integrity

Integrated Process: Communication and Documentation

Content Area: Adult Health: Ear

Priority Concepts: Communication, Sensory Perception

Reference(s): deWit, Kumagai (2013), p. 587.

190. 3

Rationale: Presbycusis refers to the age-related, irreversible, degenerative changes of the inner ear that lead to decreased hearing acuity. As a result of these changes, the older client has a decreased response to high-frequency sounds. Low-pitched tones of voice are more easily heard and interpreted by the older client. Speaking softly or slowly is not helpful.

Test-Taking Strategy: Focus on the subject, interventions for a client with hearing loss. Recalling that the client with a hearing loss responds better to low-pitched tones will direct you to the correct option. **Review:** the characteristics associated with **presbycusis and hearing loss**.

Level of Cognitive Ability: Applying

Client Needs: Physiological Integrity

Integrated Process: Nursing Process/Implementation

Content Area: Adult Health: Ear

Priority Concepts: Communication, Sensory Perception

Reference(s): deWit, Kumagai (2013), p. 589.

❖ **191. 2, 5, 6**

Rationale: Anatomical changes to the eye affect the individual's visual ability, which leads to potential problems with activities of daily living. Light adaptation and visual fields are reduced. Respiratory rates are usually unchanged. The heart rate decreases, and the heart valves thicken. Age-related changes that affect the urinary tract increase an older client's susceptibility to urinary tract infections. Short-term memory may decline with age, but long-term memory is usually maintained. Changes in sleep patterns are consistent, age-related changes. Older persons experience an increased incidence of awakening after sleep onset.

Test-Taking Strategy: Focus on the subject, normal physiological changes. Read each characteristic carefully, and think about the physiological changes that occur with aging to select the correct items. **Review:** normal **age-related changes**.

Level of Cognitive Ability: Analyzing

Client Needs: Health Promotion and Maintenance

Integrated Process: Nursing Process/Data Collection
Content Area: Developmental Stages: Early Adulthood to Later Adulthood
Priority Concepts: Development, Functional Ability
Reference(s): Cooper, Gosnell (2015), pp. 729–730.

192. 1

Rationale: It is preferable to get clients out of bed and sitting in a chair for meals. This position facilitates chewing and swallowing and prevents the reflux of stomach contents and aspiration. Options 2, 3, and 4 do not identify positions that will reduce the risk of aspiration.
Test-Taking Strategy: Focus on the **subject**, reducing the risk of aspiration. Read each option and think about how the position can affect swallowing. This should direct you to the correct option. **Review:** the measures that will prevent **aspiration**.
Level of Cognitive Ability: Applying
Client Needs: Safe and Effective Care Environment
Integrated Process: Nursing Process/Implementation
Content Area: Fundamental Skills: Safety
Priority Concepts: Clinical Judgment, Safety
Reference(s): Potter et al (2013), p. 1026.

193. 4

Rationale: Exercise and activity are essential for health promotion and maintenance in the older adult and for achieving an optimal level of functioning. Approximately half of the physical deterioration of the older client is caused by disuse rather than by the aging process or disease. One of the best exercises for an older adult is walking, with the goal of progressing to 30-minute sessions three to five times each week. Swimming and dancing are also beneficial.
Test-Taking Strategy: Note the **strategic word**, *best.* Options 1, 2, and 3, although possible, are not the best activities. Remember that walking is one of the best forms of exercise. **Review:** health promotion activities for the **older client**.
Level of Cognitive Ability: Applying
Client Needs: Health Promotion and Maintenance
Integrated Process: Teaching and Learning
Content Area: Developmental Stages: Early Adulthood to Later Adulthood
Priority Concepts: Development, Health Promotion
Reference(s): Cooper, Gosnell (2015), pp. 731, 1086.

194. 1

Rationale: Clients who like to retell stories or to describe past events need to be provided with the opportunity to do so. This phenomenon is called life review or reminiscence. In a sense, it is a way for the older client to relive and restructure life experiences, and it is a part of achieving ego identity. Option 3 indicates reality orientation techniques. Options 2 and 4 indicate socialization and physical activity.
Test-Taking Strategy: Focusing on the **subject**, reminiscence, and recalling its definition will direct you to option 1. **Review:** this form of activity for the **older client**.
Level of Cognitive Ability: Applying
Client Needs: Psychosocial Integrity
Integrated Process: Caring
Content Area: Developmental Stages: Early Adulthood to Later Adulthood
Priority Concepts: Coping, Development
Reference(s): Potter et al (2013), p. 187.

195. 3

Rationale: Elder abuse is widespread and occurs among all subgroups of the population. It includes physical and psychological abuse, the misuse of property, and the violation of rights. The typical abuse victim is a woman of advanced age with few social contacts and at least one physical or mental impairment that limits her ability to perform activities of daily living. In addition, the client usually lives alone or with the abuser and depends on the abuser for care.
Test-Taking Strategy: Focus on the **strategic words**, *most likely,* and read each option carefully to identify the client who is most defenseless as a result of the disease process. **Review:** the characteristics of **elder abuse**.
Level of Cognitive Ability: Analyzing
Client Needs: Psychosocial Integrity
Integrated Process: Nursing Process/Data Collection
Content Area: Mental Health
Priority Concepts: Caregiving, Interpersonal Violence
Reference(s): deWit, Kumagai (2013), p. 1042.

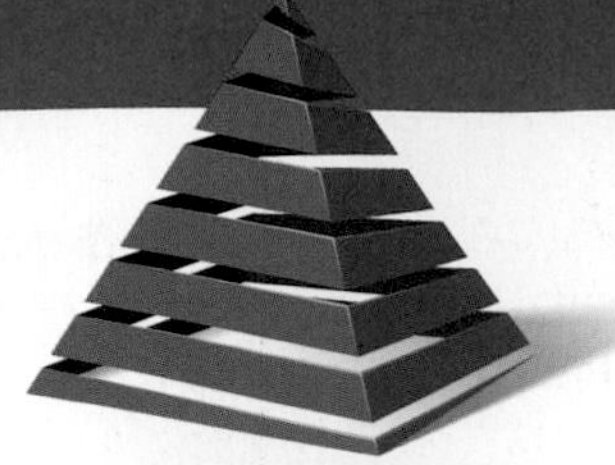

CHAPTER 23

Health and Physical Assessment of the Adult Client

CRITICAL THINKING What Should You Do?

The nurse is collecting cardiovascular data from a client. The nurse notes an irregular beat when auscultating the heart rate. What should the nurse do?

Answer is located on p. 256.

Health and physical assessment techniques that can be performed by the licensed practical nurse/licensed vocational nurse may vary depending on the scope of practice defined by the employment agency and state board of nursing practice act.

I. Environment/Setting

A. Establish a relationship and explain the procedure to the client.

B. Ensure privacy and make the client feel comfortable (provide a comfortable room temperature and sufficient lighting; remove distractions such as noise or objects; and avoid interruptions).

C. Sit down for the interview (avoid barriers such as a desk), maintain an appropriate social distance, and maintain eye level.

D. Use therapeutic communication techniques and open-ended questions to obtain information about the client's symptoms and concerns. Allow time for the client to ask questions.

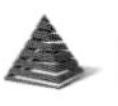

E. Consider religious and cultural characteristics such as language (the need for an interpreter), values and beliefs, health practices, eye contact, and touch.

F. Keep note-taking to a minimum so the client is the focus of attention.

G. Types of health and physical assessments (Box 23-1)

II. Health History

A. General state of health: Body features and physical characteristics, body movements, body posture, level of consciousness, nutritional status, speech

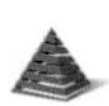

B. Chief complaint and history of present illness (direct client quotes) that directs the client to seek care

BOX 23-1 Types of Health and Physical Data Collections

Complete data collection: Includes a complete health history and physical examination and forms a baseline database

Focused data collection: Focuses on a limited or short-term problem, such as the client's complaint

Episodic/follow-up data collection: Focuses on evaluating a client's progress

Emergency data collection: Involves the rapid collection of data, often during the provision of lifesaving measures

Adapted from Jarvis C: *Physical examination & health assessment*, ed 6, St. Louis, 2012, Saunders.

C. Family history: The health status of direct blood relatives, as well as the client's spouse

D. Social history

1. Data about the client's lifestyle, with a focus on factors that may affect health
2. Information about alcohol, drug, and tobacco use; sexual practices; tattoos; body piercing; travel history; and work setting to identify occupational hazards

E. Domestic violence screening

1. Done to determine whether the client is experiencing any form of domestic violence
2. Conducted during a one-to-one interview with client while obtaining the health history

III. Mental Status Exam

A. The mental status can be checked while obtaining subjective data from the client during the health history interview.

B. Appearance

1. Note appearance, including posture, body movements, dress, hygiene, and grooming.
2. An inappropriate appearance and poor hygiene may be indicative of **depression**, manic disorder, **dementia**, organic brain disease, or another disorder.

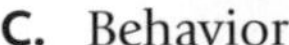

C. Behavior

1. Level of consciousness: Check alertness and awareness and the client's ability to interact appropriately with the environment.

BOX 23-2 The Mental-Status Examination: Cognitive Level of Functioning

Orientation: Assess the client's orientation to person, place, and time.
Attention span: Assess the client's ability to concentrate.
Recent memory: This is assessed by asking the client to recall a recent occurrence (e.g., the means of transportation used to get to the health care agency for the physical assessment).
Remote memory: This is assessed by asking the client about a verifiable past event (e.g., a vacation).
New learning: This is used to assess the client's ability to recall unrelated words identified by the examiner. The examiner selects four words and asks the client to recall the words 5, 10, and 30 minutes later.
Judgment: This determines whether the client's actions or decisions regarding discussions during the interview are realistic.
Thought processes and perceptions: The way the client thinks and what the client says should be logical, coherent, and relevant. The client should be consistently aware of reality.

2. Facial expression and body language: Check for appropriate eye contact and determine whether facial expression and body language are appropriate to the situation. This data collection technique also provides information regarding the client's mood and affect.
3. Speech: Check speech pattern for articulation and appropriateness of conversation.

D. Cognitive level of functioning (Box 23-2)

IV. Physical Exam

A. Overview
1. Gather equipment needed for the examination.
2. Use the senses of sight, smell, touch, and hearing to collect data.
3. Data collection includes inspection, palpation, percussion, and auscultation. These skills are performed one at a time, in this order (except for the abdominal assessment).

B. Data collection techniques

Data collection techniques primarily used by the licensed practical nurse/licensed vocational nurse include inspection, some palpation procedures, and auscultation.

1. **Inspection**
   a. The first data collection technique uses vision and smell senses while observing the client.
   b. Requires good lighting, adequate exposure, and possibly the use of certain instruments by the registered nurse (RN) or health care provider (HCP) (examiners), such as an otoscope or ophthalmoscope.
2. **Palpation**
   a. Uses the sense of touch
   b. Warm the hands before touching the client.
   c. Identify tender areas and palpate them last.
   d. The examiner will start with light palpation to detect surface characteristics and then perform deeper palpation.
   e. Check texture, temperature, and moisture of the skin, as well as organ location and size.
   f. Check for swelling, vibration or pulsation, rigidity or spasticity, and crepitation.
   g. Check for the presence of lumps or masses, as well as the presence of tenderness or pain.
3. **Percussion**
   a. The examiner will tap the client's skin to check underlying structures and determine the presence of vibrations and sounds, and if present, their intensity, duration, pitch, quality, and location.
   b. Provides information related to the presence of air, fluid, or solid masses, as well as organ size, shape, and position.
4. **Auscultation**: Involves listening to sounds produced by the body, such as heart, lung, or bowel sounds

C. Vital signs
1. Includes temperature, radial pulse (apical pulse may be measured during the cardiovascular data collection process), respirations, blood pressure, pulse oximetry, and presence of pain
2. Height and weight and nutritional status are also checked.

V. Body Systems: Data Collection Process

A. Integumentary system: Involves **inspection** and palpation of skin, hair, and nails.
1. **Subjective data**: Self-care behaviors, history of skin disease, medications being taken, environmental or occupational hazards and exposure to toxic substances, changes in skin color or pigmentation, change in a mole or a sore that does not heal, presence of tattoos
2. **Objective data**: Color, temperature (hypothermia or hyperthermia); excessive dryness or moisture; skin turgor; texture (smoothness, firmness); excessive bruising, itching, rash; hair loss (alopecia) or nail abnormalities such as pitting; lesions (may be inspected by the examiner with a magnifier and light or with the use of a wood's lamp [ultraviolet light used in a darkened room]); scars or birthmarks; edema; capillary filling time (Boxes 23-3 and 23-4, and Table 23-1)

BOX 23-3 Characteristics of Skin Color

Cyanosis: Mottled bluish coloration
Erythema: Redness
Pallor: Pale, whitish coloration
Jaundice: Yellow coloration

BOX 23-4 Assessing Capillary Filling Time

Depress the nail bed to produce blanching.
Release and observe for the return of color.
Color will return within 3 seconds if arterial capillary perfusion is normal.

To test skin turgor, gently pinch a large fold of skin and check the ability of the skin to return to its place when released. (Poor turgor occurs in severe dehydration or extreme weight loss.)

3. Dark-skinned client
   a. Cyanosis: Check lips and tongue for a gray color; nailbeds, palms, and soles for a blue color; and conjunctivae for pallor.
   b. Jaundice: Check oral mucous membranes for a yellow color; check the sclera nearest to the iris for a yellow color.
   c. Bleeding: Look for skin swelling and darkening, and compare the affected side with the unaffected side.
   d. Inflammation: Check for warmth, a shiny or taut and pitting skin area, and compare with the unaffected side.

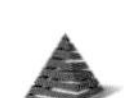

4. Reinforce client teaching
   a. Provide information about factors that can be harmful to the skin, such as the sun.
   b. Encourage performing self-examination of the skin monthly.

B. Head, neck, and lymph nodes: Involves inspection and palpation of the head, neck, and lymph nodes
   1. Ask the client about headaches; episodes of dizziness (lightheadedness) or vertigo (spinning sensation); history of head injury; loss of consciousness; seizures; episodes of neck pain; limitations of range of motion; numbness or tingling in the shoulders, arms, or hands; lumps or swelling in the neck; difficulty swallowing; medications being taken; history of surgery in the head/neck region.
   2. Head
      a. Inspect and palpate: Size, shape, masses or tenderness, and symmetry of the skull
      b. The temporal arteries, located above the cheekbone between the eye and the top of the ear, will be palpated.
      c. Temporomandibular joint: The client is asked to open his or her mouth. The examiner will look for any crepitation, tenderness, or limited range of motion.
      d. Face: Inspect facial structures for shape, symmetry, involuntary movements, or swelling such as periorbital edema (swelling around the eyes).
   3. Neck
      a. Inspected for symmetry of accessory neck muscles.
      b. Check the range of motion.
      c. Cranial nerve XI (spinal accessory nerve) is tested to check muscle strength. The client is asked to rotate the head forcibly against resistance applied to the side of the chin. Also is asked to shrug the shoulders against resistance.

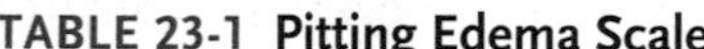

TABLE 23-1 Pitting Edema Scale

Scale	Description	"Measurement"*
1+	A barely perceptible pit	2 mm (3/32 in)
2+	A deeper pit, rebounds in a few seconds	4 mm (5/32 in)
3+	A deep pit, rebounds in 10-20 seconds	6 mm (1/4 in)
4+	A deeper pit, rebounds in >30 seconds	8 mm (5/16 in)

*"Measurement" is in quotation marks because depth of edema is rarely actually measured but is included as a frame of reference.

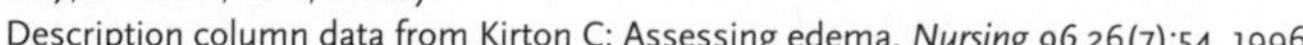

Data from Wilson AF, Giddens JF: *Health assessment for nursing practice*, ed 5, St. Louis, 2013, Mosby. Illustration from Seidel HM et al.: *Mosby's guide to physical examination*, ed 7, St. Louis, 2011, Mosby.
Description column data from Kirton C: Assessing edema, *Nursing 96* 26(7):54, 1996.

d. The trachea is palpated: It should be midline, without any deviations.

e. Thyroid gland: The neck is inspected as the client takes a sip of water and swallows (thyroid tissue moves up with a swallow). Palpation is done using an anterior-and-posterior approach. (Usually the normal adult thyroid cannot be palpated. If it is enlarged, the examiner will auscultate for a bruit.)

4. Lymph nodes
   a. The examiner will palpate using a gentle pressure and a circular motion of the finger pads.
   b. The examiner will begin with the preauricular lymph nodes (in front of the ear). Then the examiner moves to the posterior auricular lymph nodes and then downward toward the supraclavicular lymph nodes.
   c. Palpated with both hands, comparing the two sides for symmetry
   d. If nodes are palpated, their size, shape, location, mobility, consistency, and tenderness are noted.
5. Reinforce client teaching: The client is instructed to notify the health care provider if persistent headache, dizziness, or neck pain occurs; swelling or lumps are noted in the head/neck region; or a neck or head injury occurs.

Neck movements are never performed if the client has sustained a neck injury or a neck injury is suspected.

C. Eyes: Includes inspection, palpation, vision-testing procedures, and the use of an ophthalmoscope
   1. Subjective data: Difficulty with vision (e.g., decreased acuity, double vision, blurring, blind spots); pain, redness, swelling, watery or other discharge from the eye; use of glasses or contact lenses; medications being taken; history of eye problems
   2. Objective data
      a. The external eye structures are inspected, including eyebrows, for symmetry; eyelashes for even distribution; eyelids for ptosis (drooping); eyeballs for exophthalmos (protrusion) or enophthalmos (sunken or recession into the orbit).
      b. Structures inspected include the conjunctiva (should be clear), sclera (should be white), and lacrimal apparatus (check for excessive tearing, redness, tenderness, or swelling), cornea and lens (should be smooth and clear), iris (should be flat, with a round, regular shape and even coloration), eyelids, and pupils (Box 23-5).
   3. Snellen eye chart
      a. A simple tool to measure distance vision
      b. The client is positioned in a well-lit spot 20 feet from the chart, with the chart at eye level, and asked to read the smallest line he or she can discern. (The client is instructed to leave glasses on or contact lenses in. If the glasses are for reading only, they are removed because they blur distant vision.)
      c. One eye at a time is tested.
      d. Results are recorded using the fraction at the end of the last line successfully read on the chart. Normal visual acuity is 20/20 (distance in feet at which the client is standing from the chart/distance in feet at which a normal eye could have read that particular line).
   4. Near vision
      a. Tested using a handheld vision screener (held about 14 inches from the eye) that contains various sizes of print, or the client is asked to read from a magazine
      b. Each eye is tested separately with the client's glasses on or contact lenses in; normal result is 14/14 (distance in inches at which the subject holds the card from the eye/distance in inches at which a normal eye could have read that particular line)
   5. Confrontation test
      a. Used to measure peripheral vision and compare the client's peripheral vision with the examiner's (under the assumption that the examiner's peripheral vision is normal)
      b. The client covers one eye and looks straight ahead. The examiner, positioned 2 feet away, covers his or her eye opposite the client's covered eye.

BOX 23-5 Checking and Documenting Pupillary Responses

Pupillary Light Reflex

Darken the room (to dilate the client's pupils) and ask the client to look forward.

Test each eye.

Advance a light in from the side to note constriction of the same-side pupil (direct light reflex) and simultaneous constriction of the other pupil (consensual light reflex).

Accommodation

Ask the client to focus on a distant object (dilates the pupil).

Ask the client to shift gaze to a near object held about 3 inches from the nose.

Normal response includes pupillary constriction and convergence of the axes of the eye.

Documenting Normal Findings: PERRLA

P=pupils
E=equal
R=round
RL=reactive to light
A=reactive to accommodation

c. The examiner advances a finger or other small object in from the periphery from several directions. The client should see the object at the same time the examiner does.
6. Corneal light reflex
 a. Used to check for parallel alignment of the axes of the eye
 b. The client is asked to gaze straight ahead as the examiner holds a light about 12 inches from the client.
 c. The examiner looks for reflection of the light on the corneas in exactly the same spot in each eye.
7. Cover/Uncover test
 a. Used to check for slight degrees of deviated alignment
 b. Each eye is tested separately.
 c. The examiner asks the client to gaze straight ahead and cover one eye.
 d. The examiner observes the uncovered eye, expecting to note a steady, fixed gaze.
8. Six cardinal positions of gaze (Fig. 23-1)
 a. The six muscles that attach the eyeball to its orbit and serve to direct the eye to points of interest are tested.
 b. Client holds head still and is asked to move his or her eyes and follow a small object.
 c. The examiner notes any parallel movements of the eye or nystagmus, an involuntary, rhythmic, rapid twitching of the eyeballs.
9. Color vision
 a. Tests for color vision involve picking numbers or letters out of a complex and colorful picture.
 b. The Ishihara chart is used for testing and consists of numbers composed of colored dots located within a circle of colored dots.
 c. The client is asked to read the numbers on the chart.
 d. Each eye is tested separately.
 e. Reading the numbers correctly indicates normal color vision.
 f. The test is sensitive for the diagnosis of red-green blindness but cannot detect discrimination of blue.

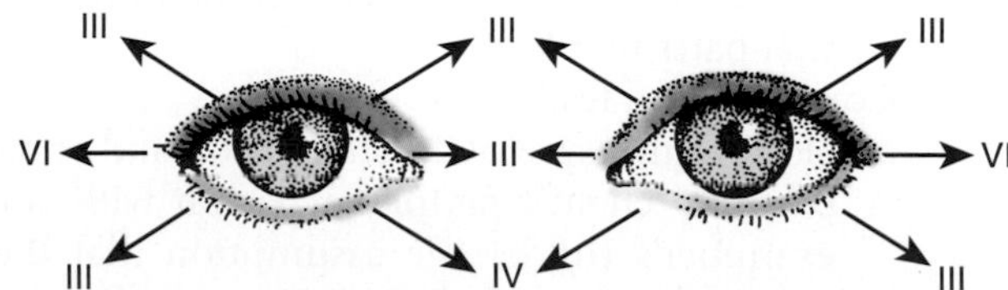

FIGURE 23-1 Checking extraocular muscles in the six cardinal positions. This indicates the functioning of cranial nerves III, IV, and VI. (From Ignatavicius D, Workman ML: *Medical-surgical nursing: Patient-centered collaborative care*, ed 7, Philadelphia, 2013, Saunders.)

The first slide on the Ishihara chart is one that everyone can discriminate; failure to identify numbers on this slide suggests a problem with performing the test, not a problem with color vision.

10. Pupils (see Box 23-5)
 a. The pupils are round and of equal size.
 b. Increasing light causes pupillary constriction.
 c. Decreasing light causes pupillary dilation.
 d. Constriction of both pupils is a normal response to direct light.
11. Sclera and cornea
 a. Normal sclera color is white.
 b. A yellow color to the sclera may indicate jaundice or systemic problems.
 c. In a dark-skinned person, the sclera may normally appear yellow; pigmented dots may be present.
 d. The cornea is transparent, smooth, shiny, and bright.
 e. Cloudy areas or specks on the cornea may be the result of an accident or eye injury.
12. Ophthalmoscopy
 a. The ophthalmoscope is an instrument used to examine the external structures and the interior of the eye.
 b. The room is darkened so that the pupil will dilate.
 c. The examiner inspects the size, color, and clarity of the disc; the integrity of the vessels; and the appearance of the macula and fovea; and looks for retinal lesions.
13. Reinforce client teaching
 a. Instruct the client to notify the health care provider if alterations in vision occur or any redness, swelling, or drainage from the eye is noted.
 b. Inform the client of the importance of regular eye examinations.

D. Ears: Includes inspection, palpation, hearing tests, vestibular assessment, and the use of an otoscope
1. Subjective data: Difficulty hearing, earaches, drainage from the ears, dizziness, ringing in the ears, exposure to environmental noise, use of a hearing aid, medications being taken, history of ear problems or infections
2. Objective data
 a. Inspect and palpate the external ear, noting size, shape, symmetry, skin color, and the presence of pain.
 b. Inspect the external auditory meatus for size, swelling, redness, discharge, and foreign bodies. Some cerumen (ear wax) may be present.
3. Auditory assessment
 a. Sound is transmitted by air conduction and bone conduction.

b. Air conduction takes two or three times longer than bone conduction.
c. Hearing loss is categorized as conductive, sensorineural, or mixed conductive and sensorineural.
d. Conductive hearing loss is caused by any physical obstruction to the transmission of sound waves.
e. Sensorineural hearing loss is caused by a defect in the cochlea, eighth cranial nerve, or the brain itself.
f. A mixed conductive-sensorineural hearing loss results in profound hearing loss.
g. Pure-tone audiometry testing: Provides a precise quantitative measure of hearing by assessing the client's ability to hear sounds of varying frequencies (done by a person skilled in performing audiometry testing)

4. Voice test
a. Used to determine whether hearing loss has occurred
b. One ear is tested at a time. (The ear not being tested is occluded by the client.)
c. The examiner stands 1 to 2 feet from the client, covers his or her mouth so that the client cannot read the lips, exhales fully, and softly whispers two-syllable words in the direction of the unoccluded ear. The client points a finger up during the test when the examiner's voice is heard. (A ticking watch may also be used to test hearing acuity.)

5. Watch test
a. A ticking watch is used to test for high-frequency sounds.
b. The examiner holds a ticking watch about 5 inches from each ear and asks the client if the ticking is heard.

6. Tuning fork tests
a. Used to measure hearing on the basis of air conduction or bone conduction; includes the Weber and Rinne tests
b. To activate the tuning fork, the nurse holds the base and lightly taps the tines against the other hand, setting the fork in vibration.

7. Weber test
a. Stem of the vibrating tuning fork is placed in the midline of the client's skull, and the client is asked if the tone sounds the same in both ears or better in one ear.
b. The client hears the tone by bone conduction, and the sound should be heard equally in both ears.

8. Rinne test
a. Stem of the vibrating tuning fork is placed on the client's mastoid process.
b. When the client no longer hears the sound, the tuning fork is quickly inverted and placed near the ear canal; the client should still hear a sound.
c. Normally the sound is heard twice as long by way of air conduction (near the ear canal) than by way of bone conduction (at the mastoid process).

9. Vestibular assessment (Box 23-6)

10. Otoscopic exam
a. An otoscope is used. For best visualization, the largest speculum that fits comfortably into the client's ear canal should be used.
b. The examiner asks the client to tilt the head slightly away, to the opposite shoulder. Next the nurse pulls the pinna up and back

BOX 23-6 Vestibular Assessment

Test for Falling

1. The examiner asks the client to stand with the feet together, arms hanging loosely at the sides, and eyes closed.
2. The client normally remains erect, with only slight swaying.
3. A significant sway is a positive Romberg sign.

Test for Past Pointing

1. The client sits in front of the examiner.
2. The client closes the eyes and extends the arms in front, pointing both index fingers at the examiner.
3. The examiner holds and touches his or her own extended index fingers under the client's extended index fingers to give the client a point of reference.
4. The client is instructed to raise both arms and then lower them, attempting to return to the examiner's extended index fingers.
5. The normal test response is that the client can easily return to the point of reference.
6. The client with a vestibular function problem lacks a normal sense of position and cannot return the extended fingers to the point of reference; instead, the fingers deviate to the right or left of the reference point.

Gaze Nystagmus Evaluation

1. The client's eyes are examined as the client looks straight ahead, 30 degrees to each side, upward and downward.
2. Any spontaneous nystagmus—an involuntary, rhythmic, rapid twitching of the eyeballs—represents a problem with the vestibular system.

Dix-Hallpike Maneuver

1. The client starts in a sitting position; the examiner lowers the client to the exam table and rather quickly turns the client's head to the 45 degrees position.
2. If after about 30 seconds there is no nystagmus, the client is returned to a sitting position and the test is repeated on the other side.

(on an adult or older child), holds the otoscope upside down, and inserts the speculum slightly down and forward, approximately half an inch, into the ear canal.

c. The normal tympanic membrane is translucent, shiny, and pearly gray.

Before performing an otoscopic exam and inserting the speculum, the examiner checks the auditory canal for foreign bodies. The client is instructed not to move the head during the examination to avoid damage to the canal and tympanic membrane.

11. Reinforce client teaching

a. Instruct the client to notify the health care provider if an alteration in hearing or ear pain or ringing in the ears occurs, or redness, swelling, or drainage from the ear is noted.

b. Instruct the client in the proper method of cleaning the ear canal.

c. The client should cleanse the ear canal with the corner of a moistened washcloth and should never insert sharp objects or cotton-tipped applicators into the ear canal.

E. Nose, mouth, and throat: Includes inspection and palpation

1. Subjective data

a. Nose: Check for discharge or nosebleed (epistaxis), facial or sinus pain, history of frequent colds, altered sense of smell, allergies, medications being taken, history of nose trauma or surgery.

b. Mouth and throat: Check for the presence of sores or lesions, bleeding from the gums or elsewhere, altered sense of taste, toothaches, use of dentures or other appliances, tooth- and mouth-care hygiene habits, at-risk behaviors (e.g., smoking, alcohol consumption), history of infection, trauma, or surgery.

2. Objective data

a. External nose should be midline and in proportion to other facial features.

b. Patency of the nostrils can be tested by pushing each nasal cavity closed and asking the client to sniff inward through the other nostril.

c. The examiner uses a nasal speculum and penlight or a short, wide-tipped speculum attached to an otoscope head to inspect for redness, swelling, discharge, bleeding, or foreign bodies. The nasal septum is checked for deviation.

d. The examiner presses the frontal sinuses (below the eyebrows) and over the maxillary sinuses (below the cheekbones). The client should feel firm pressure but no pain.

e. The external and inner surfaces of the lips are checked for color, moisture, cracking, or lesions.

f. The teeth are inspected for condition and number (should be white, spaced evenly, straight, and clean, free of debris and decay).

g. The alignment of the upper and lower jaw is checked by having the client bite down.

h. The gums are inspected for swelling, bleeding, discoloration, and retraction of gingival margins (gums normally appear pink).

i. The tongue is inspected for color, surface characteristics, moisture, white patches, nodules, and ulcerations (dorsal surface is normally rough; ventral surface is smooth and glistening, with visible veins).

j. The examiner retracts the cheek with a tongue depressor to check the buccal mucosa and checks the color and for the presence of nodules or lesions. Normal mucosa is glistening, pink, soft, moist, and smooth.

k. Using a penlight and tongue depressor, the examiner inspects the hard and soft palates for color, shape, texture, and defects. The hard palate (roof of the mouth), which is located anteriorly, should be white and dome-shaped; the soft palate, which extends posteriorly, should be light pink and smooth. The pharyngeal (gag) reflex can also be tested.

l. The uvula is inspected for midline location. The examiner asks the client to say "ahhh" and watches for the soft palate and uvula to rise in the midline. (This tests one function of cranial nerve X, the vagus nerve.)

m. Using a penlight and tongue depressor, the examiner inspects the throat for color, presence of tonsils, and the presence of exudate or lesions; cranial nerve XII is tested (the hypoglossal nerve) by asking the client to stick out the tongue (should protrude in the midline).

3. Reinforce client teaching 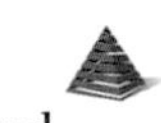

a. Emphasize the importance of hygiene and tooth care, as well as regular dental examinations and the use of fluoridated water or fluoride supplements.

b. Encourage the client to avoid at-risk behaviors (e.g., smoking, alcohol consumption).

c. Stress the importance of reporting pain or abnormal occurrence (e.g., nodules, lesions, signs of infection).

F. Lungs

1. Subjective data: Cough; expectoration of sputum; shortness of breath or dyspnea; chest pain on breathing; environmental exposure to pollution or chemicals; medications being taken; history of respiratory disease or infection; last tuberculosis test; chest x-ray; pneumonia and any influenza immunizations, including the H1N1 vaccine (H and N, which refer to the surface antigens

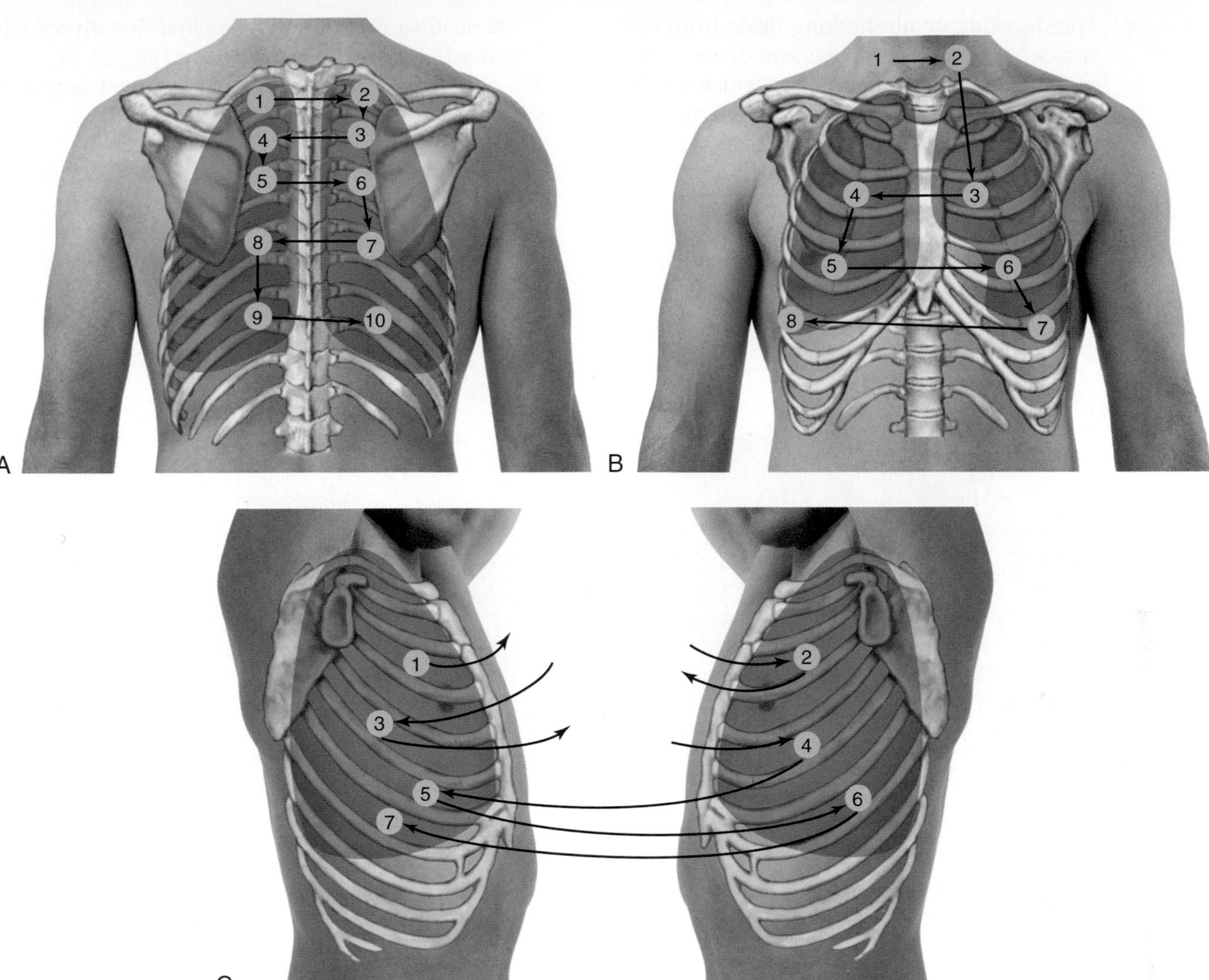

FIGURE 23-2 Landmarks for chest auscultation and percussion. **A,** Posterior view. **B,** Anterior view. **C,** Lateral view. (From Wilson AF, Giddens JF: *Health assessment for nursing practice*, ed 5, St. Louis, 2013, Mosby.)

hemagglutinin and *neuroaminidase,* respectively; the number 1 refers to the specific subtype of those antigens). Record the smoking history in pack/years (the number of packs per day times the number of years smoked). For example, a client who has smoked one half pack a day for 20 years has a 10 pack/year smoking history.

2. Objective data: Includes inspection, palpation, percussion, and auscultation
3. Inspection of the anterior and posterior chest: Note skin color and condition and the rate and quality of respirations, look for lumps or lesions, note the shape and configuration of the chest wall, note the position the client takes to breathe.
4. Palpation: The examiner will palpate the entire chest wall, noting skin temperature and moisture and looking for areas of tenderness and lumps, lesions, masses, or tenderness; chest excursion and tactile or vocal fremitus are assessed.
5. Percussion
   - **a.** The examiner starts at the apices, percusses across the top of the shoulders, moving to the interspaces, making a side-to-side comparison all the way down the lung area (Fig. 23-2).
   - **b.** The examiner will determine the predominant note. Resonance is noted in healthy lung tissue.
   - **c.** Hyperresonance is noted when excessive air is present, and a dull note indicates lung density.
6. Auscultation
   - **a.** Use the flat diaphragm end piece of the stethoscope and hold it firmly against the chest wall and listen to at least one full respiration in each location (anterior, posterior, and lateral).
   - **b.** Posterior: Start at the apices and move side to side for comparison (see Fig. 23-2).

c. Anterior: Auscultate the lung fields from the apices in the supraclavicular area down to the sixth rib. Avoid auscultation over female breast tissue (displace this tissue) because sounds will not be heard clearly (see Fig. 23-2).
d. Compare findings on each side
7. Normal breath sounds: Three types of breath sounds are considered normal in certain parts of the thorax. These include vesicular, bronchovesicular, and bronchial. Breath sounds should be clear to auscultation (Fig. 23-3).
8. Abnormal breath sounds: Also known as adventitious sounds (Table 23-2)
9. Voice sounds (Box 23-7)
   a. Performed when a pathological lung condition is suspected
   b. The examiner will auscultate the spoken word over the chest wall.

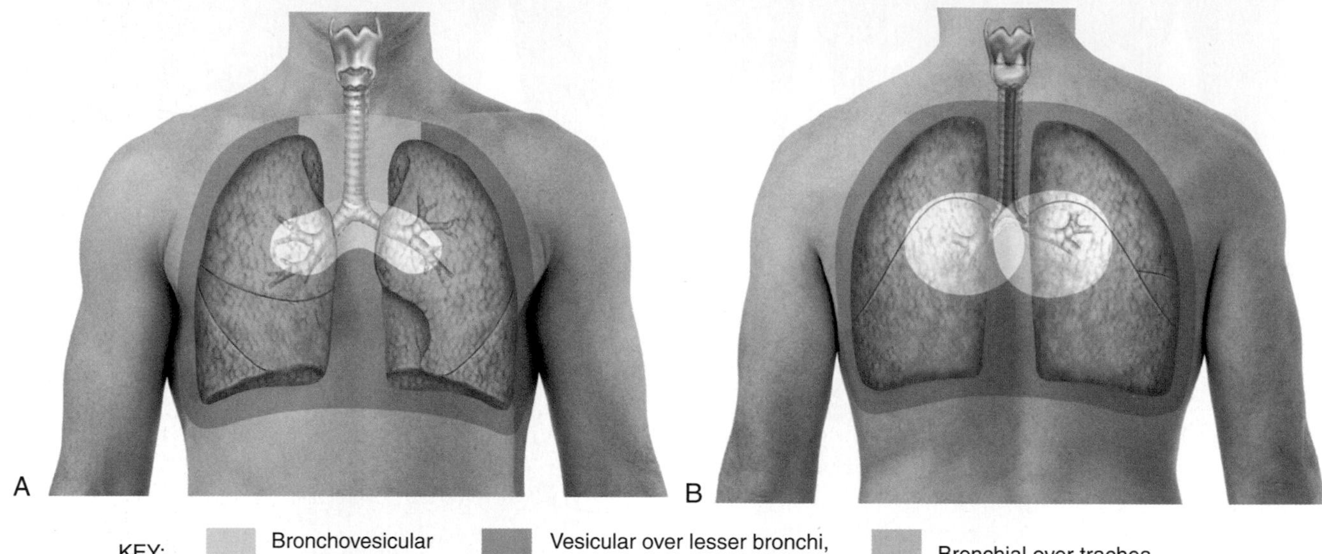

FIGURE 23-3 Auscultatory sounds. **A,** Anterior thorax. **B,** Posterior thorax. (From Wilson AF, Giddens JF: *Health assessment for nursing practice,* ed 5, St. Louis, 2013, Mosby.)

TABLE 23-2 Characteristics of Adventitious Sounds

Adventitious Sounds	Characteristics	Clinical Examples
Crackles (previously called *rales*) fine crackles	Fine: high-pitched crackling and popping noises (discontinuous sounds) heard during the end of inspiration. Not cleared by cough. Medium: medium-pitched moist sound heard about halfway through inspiration; not cleared by cough. Coarse: Low-pitched, bubbling or gurgling sounds that start early in inspiration and extend into the first part of expiration.	Fine: may be heard in pneumonia, heart failure, asthma, and restrictive pulmonary diseases. Medium: same as fine, but condition is worse. Coarse: same as fine and medium as noted above; may be heard in terminally ill clients with diminished gag reflex and in individuals with pulmonary edema or pulmonary fibrosis.
Wheeze (also called *sibilant* wheeze)	High-pitched, musical sound similar to a squeak. Heard more commonly during expiration, but may also be heard during inspiration. Occurs in small airways.	Heard in narrowed airway diseases such as asthma.
Rhonchi (also called *sonorous* wheeze)	Low-pitched, coarse, loud, low snoring or moaning tone. Actually sounds like snoring. Heard primarily during expiration, but may also be heard during inspiration. Coughing may clear.	Heard in disorders causing obstruction of the trachea or bronchus, such as chronic bronchitis.
Pleural friction rub	A superficial, low-pitched, coarse rubbing or grating sound. Sounds like two surfaces rubbing together. Heard throughout inspiration and expiration. Loudest over the lower anterolateral surface. Not cleared by cough.	Heard in individuals with pleurisy (inflammation of the pleural surfaces).

Data from Wilson AF, Giddens JF: *Health assessment for nursing practice,* ed 4, St. Louis, 2009, Mosby.

BOX 23-7 Voice Sounds on Lung Auscultation

Bronchophony

Ask the client to repeat the words "ninety-nine."
Normal voice transmission is soft, muffled, and indistinct.

Egophony

Ask the client to repeat a long "ee-ee-ee" sound.
Normally the nurse would hear the "ee-ee-ee" sound.

Whispered Pectoriloquy

Ask the client to whisper the word "ninety-nine."
Normal voice transmission is faint, muffled, and almost inaudible.

c. The client is asked to repeat a phrase while the examiner listens to the chest.
d. Normal voice transmission is soft and muffled. The examiner can hear the sound but is unable to distinguish exactly what is being said.

When auscultating breath sounds, instruct the client to breathe through the mouth, and monitor the client for dizziness.

10. Reinforce client teaching
    a. Encourage the client to avoid exposure to environmental hazards, including smoking. (Discuss smoking-cessation programs as appropriate.)
    b. The client should undergo periodic examinations as prescribed (e.g., chest x-ray, tuberculosis skin testing).
    c. Encourage the client to obtain pneumonia and influenza immunizations.
    d. The health care provider should be notified if the client experiences persistent cough, shortness of breath, or other respiratory symptoms.

G. The heart and peripheral vascular system
1. Subjective data: Chest pain, dyspnea, cough, fatigue, edema, nocturia, leg pain or cramps (claudication), changes in skin color, obesity, medications being taken, cardiovascular risk factors, family history of cardiac or vascular problems, personal history of cardiac or vascular problems
2. Objective data: May include inspection, palpation, percussion, and auscultation
3. Inspection: The examiner will inspect the anterior chest for pulsations (apical impulse) created as the left ventricle rotates against the chest wall during systole; not always visible.
4. Palpation
    a. The examiner will palpate the apical impulse at the fourth or fifth interspace, or medial to the midclavicular line (not palpable in obese clients or clients with thick chest walls).
    b. The examiner will palpate the apex, left sternal border, and base for pulsations; normally none are present.
5. Percussion: This may be performed by the examiner to outline the heart's borders and check for cardiac enlargement (denoted by resonance over the lung and dull notes over the heart).
6. Auscultation
    a. Auscultation areas of the heart (Fig. 23-4)
    b. Auscultate heart rate and rhythm. Check for a pulse deficit (auscultate the apical heartbeat while palpating an artery) if an irregularity is noted.
    c. Check for S1 ("lub") and S2 ("dub") sounds. If abnormalities such as irregularities in the beat, extra heart sounds, or the presence of gentle blowing or swooshing noises (murmurs) are noted, the registered nurse or health care provider is notified.
7. Peripheral vascular system
    a. Check for adequacy of blood flow to the extremities by palpating arterial pulses for equality and symmetry and checking the condition of the skin and nails.
    b. Check for pretibial edema and measure calf circumference (see Table 23-1).
    c. Measure blood pressure.
    d. The examiner will palpate superficial inguinal nodes (using firm but gentle pressure), beginning in the inguinal area and moving down toward the inner thigh.
    e. An ultrasonic stethoscope may be needed to amplify the sounds of a pulse wave if the pulse cannot be palpated.

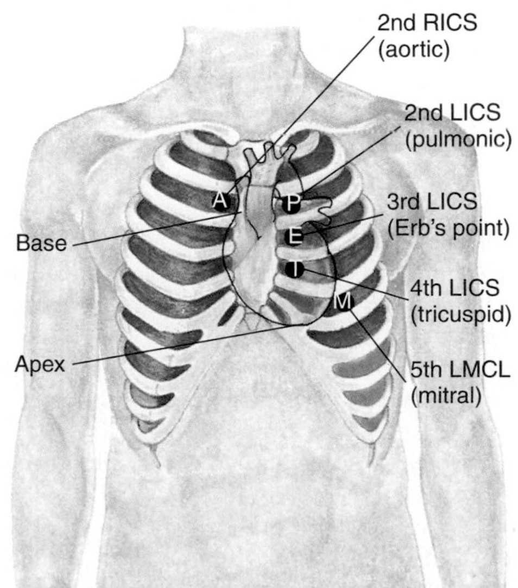

FIGURE 23-4 Auscultation areas of the heart. *LMCL*, left midclavicular line; *RICS*, right intercostal space; *LICS*, left intercostal space. (From Wilson AF, Giddens JF: *Health assessment for nursing practice*, ed 4, St. Louis, 2009, Mosby.)

f. Carotid artery: Located in the groove between the trachea and sternocleidomastoid muscle, medial to and alongside the muscle
g. The examiner will palpate one carotid artery at a time to avoid compromising blood flow to the brain. The examiner will also auscultate each carotid artery for the presence of a bruit (a blowing, swishing sound, which indicates blood-flow turbulence). Normally a bruit is not present.
h. Palpate the arteries in the extremities (Box 23-8).

8. Reinforce client teaching
   a. Advise the client to modify lifestyle for risk factors associated with heart and vascular disease.
   b. Encourage the client to seek regular physical examinations.
   c. Client should seek medical assistance for signs of heart or vascular disease.

H. The breasts
1. Subjective data: Pain or tenderness, lumps or thickening, swollen axillary lymph nodes, nipple discharge, rash or swelling, medications being taken, personal or family history of breast disease, trauma or injury to the breasts, previous surgery on the breasts, breast self-examination compliance, mammograms as prescribed
2. Objective data: Includes inspection and palpation

An important role of the nurse is to teach the client how to perform the breast self-examination (BSE), which involves inspection and palpation.

BOX 23-8 Arterial Pulse Points and Grading the Force of Pulses

Arteries in the Arms and Hands

Radial pulse: Located at the radial side of the forearm at the wrist
Ulnar pulse: Located on the opposite side of the location of the radial pulse at the wrist
Brachial pulse: Located above the elbow at the antecubital fossa, between the biceps and triceps muscles

Arteries in the Legs

Femoral pulse: Located below the inguinal ligament, midway between the symphysis pubis and the anterosuperior iliac spine
Popliteal pulse: Located behind the knee
Dorsalis pedis pulse: Located at the top of the foot, in line with the groove between the extensor tendons of the great and first toes
Posterior tibial pulse: Located inside of the ankle, behind and below the medial malleolus (ankle bone)

Grading the Force

4 + = strong and bounding
3 + = full pulse, increased
2 + = normal, easily palpable
1 + = weak, barely palpable

3. Inspection
   a. Performed with the client's arms raised above the head, the hands pressed against the hips, and the arms extended straight ahead while the client sits and leans forward
   b. The client is taught to check size and symmetry (one breast is often larger than the other); masses, flattening, retraction, or dimpling; color and venous pattern; size, color, shape, and discharge in the nipple and areola; and the direction in which nipples point.
4. Palpation
   a. Client lies supine, with the arm on the side being examined behind the head and a small pillow under the shoulder.
   b. The client is taught to use the pads of the first three fingers to compress the breast tissue gently against the chest wall, noting tissue consistency.
   c. Palpation is performed systematically, ensuring that the entire breast and tail are palpated.
   d. The client is taught to note the consistency of the breast tissue, which normally feels dense, firm, and elastic.
   e. The client is taught to gently palpate the nipple and areola and compress the nipple, noting any discharge.
5. Axillary lymph nodes
   a. The examiner faces the client and stands on the side being examined, supporting the client's arm in a slightly flexed position, and abducts the arm away from the chest wall.
   b. The examiner places the free hand against the client's chest wall and high in the axillary hollow; then, with the fingertips, gently presses down, rolling soft tissue over the surface of the ribs and muscles.
   c. Lymph nodes are normally not palpable.
6. Reinforce client teaching
   a. Encourage and teach the client to perform breast self-examination (BSE). (Refer to Chapter 43 for information on performing the BSE.)
   b. Breast self-examination should be performed 7 to 10 days after the menses. Postmenopausal clients or those who have had a hysterectomy should select a specific day of the month and perform BSE monthly on that day.
   c. Regular physical examinations and mammograms should be obtained as prescribed.
   d. The client should report lumps or masses to the health care provider immediately.

I. The abdomen
1. Subjective data: Changes in appetite or weight, difficulty swallowing, dietary intake, intolerance to certain foods, nausea or vomiting, pain, bowel habits, medications being taken, history of abdominal problems or abdominal surgery

2. Objective data
   a. The client is asked to empty the bladder.
   b. Be sure to warm the hands and the end piece of the stethoscope.
   c. Painful areas are examined last.

When performing an abdominal assessment, the specific order for assessment techniques is inspection, auscultation, percussion, and palpation.

3. Inspection
   a. Contour: The examiner will look down at the abdomen and then across the abdomen from the rib margin to the pubic bone; described as flat, rounded, concave, or protuberant.
   b. Symmetry: Note any bulging or masses.
   c. Umbilicus: Should be midline and inverted
   d. Skin surface: Should be smooth and even
   e. Pulsations from the aorta may be noted in the epigastric area, and peristaltic waves may be noted across the abdomen.
4. Auscultation
   a. The examiner will perform auscultation before percussion and palpation, which can increase peristalsis.
   b. Hold the stethoscope lightly against the skin and listen for bowel sounds in all four quadrants. Begin in the right lower quadrant (as bowel sounds are normally heard here).
   c. Note the character and frequency of normal bowel sounds: high-pitched gurgling sounds occurring irregularly from 5 to 30 times a minute.
   d. Identify as normal, hypoactive, or hyperactive (borborygmus).
   e. Absent sounds: Auscultate for 5 minutes before determining that sounds are absent.
5. Percussion
   a. All four quadrants are percussed lightly by the examiner.
   b. Borders of the liver and spleen are percussed.
   c. Tympany should predominate over the abdomen with dullness over the liver and spleen.
   d. Percussion over the kidney at the 12th rib (costovertebral angle) should produce no pain.
6. Palpation
   a. The examiner will begin with light palpation of all four quadrants, using the fingers to depress the skin about 1 cm. Next, deep palpation is performed.
   b. The examiner will palpate the liver and spleen (which may not be palpable).
   c. The aortic pulsation is palpated in the upper abdomen slightly to the left of midline. Normally it pulsates in a forward direction. (Pulsation expands laterally if an aneurysm is present.)
7. Reinforce client teaching
   a. Encourage the client to consume a balanced diet.
   b. Substances that can cause gastric irritation should be avoided.
   c. The regular use of laxatives is discouraged.
   d. Lifestyle behaviors that can cause gastric irritation (e.g., smoking, spicy foods) should be avoided.
   e. Regular physical examinations are important.
   f. The client should report gastrointestinal problems to the health care provider.

J. Musculoskeletal system
1. Subjective data: Joint pain or stiffness; redness, swelling, or warm joints; limited motion of joints; muscle pain, cramps, or weakness; bone pain; limitations in activities of daily living; exercise patterns; exposure to occupational hazards (e.g., heavy lifting, prolonged standing or sitting); medications being taken; history of joint, muscle, or bone injuries; history of surgery of the joints, muscles, or bones
2. Objective data: Can include inspection and palpation
3. Inspection: Inspect gait and posture and for cervical, thoracic, and lumbar curves (Box 23-9).
4. Palpation: The examiner will palpate all bones, joints, and surrounding muscles.
5. Range of motion
   a. The examiner will perform active and passive range-of-motion exercises of each major joint.
   b. Check for pain, limited mobility, spastic movement, joint instability, stiffness, and contractures.
   c. Normally joints are nontender, without swelling, and move freely.

6. Muscle tone and strength
   a. This will be checked during measurement of range of motion
   b. The client is asked to flex the muscle to be examined and then to resist while applying opposing force against the flexion.
   c. Check for increased tone (hypertonicity) or little tone (hypotonicity).
7. Grading muscle strength (Table 23-3)
8. Reinforce client teaching

   a. The client should consume a balanced diet, including foods high in calcium and vitamin D.

BOX 23-9 Common Postural Abnormalities

Lordosis (swayback): Increased lumbar curvature
Kyphosis (hunchback): Exaggeration of the posterior curvature of the thoracic spine
Scoliosis: Lateral spinal curvature

TABLE 23-3 Criteria for Grading and Recording Muscle Strength

Functional Level	Lovett Scale	Grade	Percent of Normal
No evidence of contractility	Zero (0)	0	0
Evidence of slight contractility	Trace (T)	1	10
Complete range of motion with gravity eliminated	Poor (P)	2	25
Complete range of motion with gravity	Fair (F)	3	50
Complete range of motion against gravity with some resistance	Good (G)	4	75
Complete range of motion against gravity with full resistance	Normal (N)	5	100

Data from Wilson AF, Giddens JF: *Health assessment for nursing practice*, ed 4, St. Louis, 2009, Mosby.

b. Activities that cause muscle strain or stress to the joints should be avoided.

c. Encourage the client to maintain a normal weight.

d. Participation in a regular exercise program is beneficial.

e. The client should contact the health care provider if joint or muscle pain or problems occur or if limitations in range of motion or muscle strength develop.

K. Neurological system (refer to Chapter 57 for additional information)

1. Subjective data: Headaches, dizziness or vertigo, tremors, weakness, incoordination, numbness or tingling in any area of the body, difficulty speaking or swallowing, medications being taken, history of seizures, history of head injury or surgery, exposure to environmental or occupational hazards (e.g., chemicals, alcohol, drugs)
2. Objective data: Include assessment of cranial nerves, level of consciousness, pupils, motor function, cerebellar function, coordination, sensory function, and reflexes.
3. Note mental and emotional status, behavior and appearance, language ability, and intellectual functioning, including memory, knowledge, abstract thinking, association, and judgment.
4. Vital signs: Check temperature, pulse, respirations, and blood pressure; monitor for blood pressure or pulse changes, which may indicate increased intracranial pressure (ICP). (See Chapter 57 for abnormal respiratory patterns.)
5. Cranial nerves: Assessed by the examiner (Table 23-4)

TABLE 23-4 Assessment of the Cranial Nerves

Cranial Nerve	Function of Nerve	Testing the Nerve
Cranial nerve I: Olfactory	Sensory: Controls the sense of smell	The client is asked to close the eyes and occlude one nostril with a finger. Then, the client is asked to identify nonirritating and familiar odors (e.g., coffee, tea, cloves, soap, chewing gum, peppermint). The test is repeated on the other nostril.
Cranial nerve II: Optic	Sensory: Controls vision	Visual acuity is assessed with a Snellen chart and an ophthalmoscopic exam. Peripheral vision is checked by confrontation. Color vision is checked.
Cranial nerves III, IV, and VI		
Cranial nerve III: Oculomotor	Motor: Controls pupillary constriction, upper-eyelid elevation, and most eye movement	The motor functions of these nerves overlap; therefore, they should be tested together. The eyelids are inspected for ptosis (drooping); then ocular movements are assessed, noting any eye deviation.
Cranial nerve IV: Trochlear	Motor: Controls downward and inward eye movement	Accommodation and direct and consensual light reflexes are tested.
Cranial nerve VI: Abducens	Motor: Controls lateral eye movement	

Continued

TABLE 23-4 Assessment of the Cranial Nerves—*cont'd*

Cranial Nerve	Function of Nerve	Testing the Nerve
Cranial nerve V: Trigeminal	Sensory and motor: Controls sensation in the cornea, nasal and oral mucosa, and facial skin, as well as mastication	To test motor function, the client is asked to clench the teeth, and the muscles of mastication are assessed; then the examiner tries to open the client's jaws after asking client to keep them tightly closed. The corneal reflex is tested by lightly touching the client's cornea with a cotton wisp. (This test may be omitted if the client is alert and blinking normally.) Sensory function is checked by asking the client to close the eyes; the examiner lightly touches forehead, cheeks, and chin, noting whether the touch is felt equally on the two sides.
Cranial nerve VII: Facial	Sensory and motor: Controls movement of the face and taste sensation	Taste perception is tested on the anterior two thirds of the tongue; the client should be able to taste salty and sweet tastes. The client is asked to smile, frown, and show the teeth, and asked to puff out the cheeks. The examiner attempts to close the client's eyes against resistance.
Cranial nerve VIII: Acoustic or vestibulocochlear	Sensory: Controls hearing and vestibular function	Assessing the client's ability to hear tests the cochlear portion. Assessing the client's sense of equilibrium tests the vestibular portion. The client's hearing is checked using acuity tests. Observe the client's balance and watch for swaying when he or she is walking or standing. Assessment of sensorineural hearing loss may be done by the examiner with the Weber or Rinne test.
Cranial nerve IX: Glossopharyngeal	Sensory and motor: Controls swallowing ability, sensation in the pharyngeal soft palate and tonsillar mucosa, taste perception on the posterior third of the tongue, and salivation	Usually cranial nerves IX and X are tested together. The client's taste perception is tested on the posterior one third of the tongue or pharynx; the client should be able to taste bitter and sour tastes. The soft palate is inspected, and the examiner watches for symmetrical elevation when the client says "aaah."
Cranial nerve X: Vagus	Sensory and motor: Controls swallowing and phonation, sensation in the exterior ear's posterior wall, and sensation behind the ear Controls sensation in the thoracic and abdominal viscera	The posterior pharyngeal wall is touched with a tongue depressor to elicit the gag reflex.
Cranial nerve XI: Spinal accessory	Motor: Controls strength of neck and shoulder muscles	The examiner palpates and inspects the sternocleidomastoid muscle as the client pushes the chin against the examiner's hand. The examiner palpates and inspects the trapezius muscle as the client shrugs the shoulders against the examiner's resistance.
Cranial nerve XII: Hypoglossal	Motor: Controls tongue movements involved in swallowing and speech	The examiner observes the tongue for asymmetry, atrophy, deviation to one side, and fasciculations (uncontrollable twitching). The client is asked to push the tongue against a tongue depressor, and then the client is asked to move the tongue rapidly in and out and from side to side.

6. Level of consciousness
  a. Check the client's behavior to determine level of consciousness (e.g., alertness, confusion, delirium, unconsciousness, stupor, coma). The data collection process becomes increasingly invasive as the client is less responsive.
  b. Speak to client.
  c. Determine appropriateness of behavior and conversation.
  d. Lightly touch the client (as culturally appropriate).

7. Pupils
  a. Check size, equality, and reaction to light (brisk, slow, or fixed), and note any unusual eye movements (check direct light and consensual light reflex).
  b. This component of the neurological examination may be performed during the data collection process of the eye.

8. Motor function
  a. Check muscle tone, including strength and equality.

b. Monitor for voluntary and involuntary movements and purposeful and nonpurposeful movements.
c. This component of the neurological examination may be performed during the data collection process of the musculoskeletal system.

9. Cerebellar function
   a. Monitor gait as the client walks in a straight line, heel to toe (tandem walking).
   b. Romberg test: The client is asked to stand with the feet together and the arms at the sides and to close the eyes and hold the position. Normally the client can maintain posture and balance.
   c. If appropriate, the client is asked to perform a shallow knee bend or hop in place on one leg and then the other.
10. Coordination
    a. This is checked by asking the client to perform rapid alternating movements of the hands (e.g., turning the hands over and patting the knees continuously).
    b. The examiner asks the client to touch the examiner's finger, then his or her own nose. The client keeps the eyes open, and the examiner moves the finger to different spots to ensure that the client's movements are smooth and accurate.
    c. Heel-to-shin test: The client is assisted into a supine position, then asked to place the heel on the opposite knee and run it down the shin. Normally the client moves the heel down the shin in a straight line.
11. Sensory function
    a. Pain: Checked by applying an object with a sharp point and one with a dull point to the client's body in random order; the client is asked to identify the sharp and dull feelings.
    b. Light touch: A piece of cotton is brushed over the client's skin at various locations in a random order, and the client is asked to say when the touch is felt.
    c. Vibration: A tuning fork is used to test the client's ability to feel vibrations over bony prominences. The client is asked to announce when the vibration starts and stops.
    d. Position sense (kinesthesia): The client's finger or toe is moved up or down, and the client is asked which way it has been moved. This tests the client's ability to perceive passive movement.
    e. Stereognosis: Tests the client's ability to recognize objects placed in his or her hand
    f. Graphesthesia: Tests the client's ability to identify a number traced on the client's hand
    g. Two-point discrimination: Tests the client's ability to discriminate two simultaneous pinpricks on the skin
12. Deep tendon reflexes
    a. Includes testing the following reflexes: biceps, triceps, brachioradialis, patella, Achilles
    b. Limb should be relaxed.
    c. The tendon is tapped quickly with a reflex hammer, which should cause contraction of muscle.
    d. Scoring deep tendon reflex activity (Box 23-10)
13. Plantar reflex
    a. A cutaneous (superficial) reflex; is tested with a pointed but not sharp object
    b. The sole of the client's foot is stroked from the heel, up the lateral side, and then across the ball of the foot to the medial side.
    c. The normal response is plantar flexion of all toes.

⚠ Dorsiflexion of the great toe and fanning of the other toes (Babinski's sign) are abnormal in anyone older than 2 years and indicate the presence of central nervous system disease.

14. Testing for meningeal irritation
    a. A positive Brudzinski's sign or Kernig's sign indicates meningeal irritation.
    b. Brudzinski's sign is tested with the client in the supine position. The nurse flexes the client's head (gently moves the head to the chest), and there should be no reports of pain or resistance to the neck flexion; a positive Brudzinski's sign is observed if the client passively flexes the hip and knee in response to neck flexion and reports pain in the vertebral column.
    c. Kernig's sign is positive when the client flexes the legs at the hip and knee and complains of pain along the vertebral column when the leg is extended.
15. Reinforce client teaching
    a. The client should avoid exposure to environmental hazards (e.g., insecticides, lead).

BOX 23-10 Scoring Deep Tendon Reflex Activity

0 = No response
1+ = Sluggish or diminished
2+ = Active or expected response
3+ = Slightly hyperactive, more brisk than normal; not necessarily pathologic
4+ = Brisk, hyperactive with intermittent clonus associated with disease

Adapted from Wilson AF, Giddens JF: *Health assessment for nursing practice*, ed 4, St. Louis, 2009, Mosby.

b. High-risk behaviors that can result in head and spinal cord injuries should be avoided.
c. Protective devices (e.g., a helmet, body pads) should be worn when participating in high-risk behaviors.

L. Female genitalia and reproductive tract
1. Subjective data: Urinary difficulties or symptoms such as frequency, urgency, or burning; vaginal discharge; pain; menstrual and obstetric histories; onset of menopause; medications being taken; sexual activity and the use of contraceptives; history of sexually transmitted infections
2. Objective data
a. Use a calm and relaxing approach. The examination is embarrassing for many women and may be a difficult experience for an adolescent.
b. Consider the client's cultural background and her beliefs with regard to examination of the genitalia.
c. A complete examination will include the external genitalia and a vaginal examination.
d. The nurse's role is to prepare the client for the examination and assist the health care provider.
e. The client is asked to empty her bladder before the examination.
f. The client is placed in the lithotomy position, and a drape is placed across the client.
3. External genitalia
a. Quantity and distribution of hair
b. Characteristics of labia majora and minora (no inflammation, edema, lesions, or lacerations should be noted)
c. Urethral orifice is observed for color and position.
d. Vaginal orifice (introitus) is inspected for inflammation, edema, discoloration, discharge, and lesions.
e. The examiner may check Skene's and Bartholin's glands for tenderness or discharge (if discharge is present, color, odor, and consistency are noted and a culture of the discharge is obtained).
f. The client is checked for the presence of a cystocele (a portion of the vaginal wall and bladder prolapse or fall into the orifice anteriorly) or a rectocele (bulging of the posterior wall of the vagina caused by prolapse of the rectum).
4. Speculum examination of the internal genitalia
a. Performed by the health care provider
b. Permits visualization of the cervix and vagina

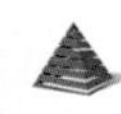

c. Papanicolaou smear: A painless screening test for cervical cancer is done; the specimen is obtained during the speculum examination, and the nurse helps prepare the specimen for laboratory analysis.
5. Reinforce client teaching
a. Stress the importance of personal hygiene.
b. Explain the purpose and recommended frequency of Papanicolaou (Pap) tests.
c. Explain the signs of sexually transmitted infections.
d. Educate the client on the measures to prevent a sexually transmitted infection.
e. Inform the client with a sexually transmitted infection that she must inform her sexual partner of the need for an examination.

M. Male genitalia
1. Subjective data: Urinary difficulty (e.g., frequency, urgency, hesitancy or straining, dysuria, nocturia); pain, lesions, or discharge on or from the penis; pain or lesions in the scrotum; medications being taken; sexual activity and the use of contraceptives; history of sexually transmitted infections
2. Objective data
a. Includes assessment (inspection and palpation) by the examiner of the external genitalia and inguinal ring and canal
b. The client may stand or lie down for this examination.
c. Genitalia are manipulated gently to avoid causing erection or discomfort.
d. Sexual maturity is checked by noting the size and shape of the penis and testes, the color and texture of the scrotal skin, and the character and distribution of pubic hair.
e. The penis is checked for the presence of lesions or discharge. A culture is obtained if a discharge is present.
f. The scrotum is inspected for size, shape, and symmetry (normally the left testicle hangs lower than the right) and palpated for the presence of any lumps.
g. Inguinal ring and canal: Inspection (asking the client to bear down) and palpation are performed by the health care provider to check for the presence of a hernia.
3. Reinforce client teaching
a. Stress the importance of personal hygiene.
b. Teach the client how to perform testicular self-examination (TSE). A day of the month is selected, and the exam is performed on the same day each month after a shower or bath when the hands are warm and soapy and the scrotum is warm. (Refer to Chapter 43 for information on performing the TSE.)
c. Explain the signs of sexually transmitted infections.
d. Educate the client on measures to prevent sexually transmitted infections.

e. Inform the client with a sexually transmitted infection that he must inform his sexual partner of the need for an examination.

N. Rectum and anus

1. Subjective data: Usual bowel pattern; any change in bowel habits; rectal pain, bleeding from the rectum, or black or tarry stools; dietary habits; problems with urination; previous screening for colorectal cancer; medications being taken; history of rectal or colon problems; family history of rectal or colon problems
2. Objective data
   a. Examination can detect colorectal cancer in its early stages. In men, the rectal examination can also detect prostate tumors.
   b. Women may be examined in the lithotomy position after examination of the genitalia.
   c. A man is best examined by having the client bend forward with his hips flexed and upper body resting over the examination table.
   d. A nonambulatory client may be examined in the left lateral (Sims') position.
   e. The external anus is inspected for lumps or lesions, rashes, inflammation or excoriation, scars, or hemorrhoids.
   f. Digital examination is performed by the health care provider to assess sphincter tone; check for tenderness, irregularities, polyps, masses, or nodules in the rectal wall; and assess the prostate gland.
   g. The prostate gland is normally firm, without bogginess, tenderness, or nodules. (Hardness or nodules may indicate the presence of a cancerous lesion.)
3. Reinforce client teaching
   a. The diet should include high-fiber and low-fat foods and plenty of liquids.
   b. The client should obtain regular digital examinations.
   c. The client should be able to identify the symptoms of colorectal cancer or prostatic cancer (men).
   d. The client should follow the American Cancer Society's guidelines for screening for colorectal cancer.

VI. Documenting Health and Physical Assessment Findings

A. Documentation findings may be recorded either written or electronically (depending on agency protocol).

B. Whether written or electronic, the documentation is a legal document and permanent record of the client's health status.

C. Principles of documentation need to be followed, and data need to be recorded accurately, concisely, completely, legibly, and objectively without bias or opinions. Also, always follow agency protocol for documentation.

D. Documentation findings serve as a source of client information for other HCPs.

E. Record findings about the client's health history and physical examination as soon as possible after completion of the health assessment.

F. Refer to Chapter 7 for additional information about documentation guidelines.

CRITICAL THINKING What Should You Do?

Answer: If the nurse notes an irregular beat when auscultating the heart rate, the nurse should be sure to listen for 1 full minute to obtain adequate information. The nurse should also note the client's appearance and notify the registered nurse. The registered nurse will then perform a complete cardiac assessment and notify the health care provider. The nurse should also document the findings.

Reference(s): dеWit, D. & Kumagai, C. (2013). *Medical-surgical nursing: Concepts & practice.* (2nd ed., p. 386). St. Louis: Saunders.

Lewis, S., Dirksen, S., Heitkemper, M., & Bucher, L. (2014). *Medical-surgical nursing: Assessment and management of clinical problems* (9th ed., pp. 41–42). St. Louis: Mosby.

PRACTICE QUESTIONS

❖ **196.** The clinic nurse is assisting to perform a focused data collection process on a client who is complaining of symptoms of a cold, a cough, and lung congestion. Which should the nurse include for this type of data collection? **Select all that apply.**

- ☐ 1. Auscultating lung sounds
- ☐ 2. Obtaining the client's temperature
- ☐ 3. Checking the strength of peripheral pulses
- ☐ 4. Obtaining information about the client's respirations
- ☐ 5. Performing a musculoskeletal and neurological examination
- ☐ 6. Asking the client about a family history of any illness or disease

197. A client with a diagnosis of asthma is admitted to the hospital with respiratory distress. Which type of adventitious lung sounds should the nurse expect to note documented in the health record when collecting data related to the respiratory system for this client?

1. Stridor
2. Wheezes
3. Diminished
4. Pleural friction rub

198. The nurse is reviewing the client's health record and notes that the client elicited a positive Romberg sign. The nurse understands that this indicates which finding?
1. An involuntary rhythmic, rapid, twitching of the eyeballs
2. A dorsiflexion of the ankle and great toe with fanning of the other toes
3. A significant sway when the client stands erect with feet together, arms at the side, and the eyes closed
4. A lack of normal sense of position when the client is unable to return extended fingers to a point of reference

199. The nurse notes documentation that a client is exhibiting Cheyne-Stokes respirations. On data collection of the client, the nurse expects to note which finding?
1. Rhythmic respirations with periods of apnea
2. Regular rapid and deep, sustained respirations
3. Totally irregular respiration in rhythm and depth
4. Irregular respirations with pauses at the end of inspiration and expiration

200. The nurse notes documentation that a client has conductive hearing loss. The nurse understands that which is a cause of this type of hearing loss?
1. A defect in the cochlea
2. A defect in the 8th cranial nerve
3. A physical obstruction to the transmission of sound waves
4. A defect in the sensory fibers that lead to the cerebral cortex

201. While collecting data related to the cardiac system on a client diagnosed with an incompetent heart valve, the nurse auscultates a murmur. Which **best** describes the sound of a heart murmur?
1. Lubb-dubb sounds
2. Scratchy, leathery heart noise
3. Gentle, blowing or swooshing noise
4. Abrupt, high-pitched snapping noise

202. The nurse is preparing to assist the health care provider to test the extraocular movements in a client for muscle weakness in the eyes. The nurse anticipates that which physical assessment technique will be done to assess for muscle weakness in the eye?
1. Testing sensory function
2. Testing the corneal reflexes
3. Testing the six cardinal positions of gaze
4. Testing visual acuity using a Snellen eye chart

203. The nurse is reinforcing instructions for a client in how to perform a testicular self-examination (TSE). The nurse explains that which is the **best** time to perform this exam?
1. After a shower or bath
2. While standing to void
3. After having a bowel movement
4. While lying in bed before arising

204. The nurse notes that the physical assessment findings for a client with meningeal irritation indicate a positive Brudzinski's sign. The nurse understands that which observation was made?
1. The client rigidly extends the arms with pronated forearms and plantar flexion of the feet.
2. The client flexes a leg at the hip and knee and reports pain in the vertebral column when the leg is extended.
3. The client passively flexes the hip and knee in response to neck flexion and reports pain in the vertebral column.
4. The client's upper arms are flexed and held tightly to the sides of the body and the legs are extended and internally rotated.

205. A Spanish-speaking client arrives at the triage desk in the emergency department and states to the nurse, "No speak English, need interpreter." Which is the **best** action for the nurse to take?
1. Have one of the client's family members interpret.
2. Have the Spanish-speaking triage receptionist interpret.
3. Seek an interpreter from the hospital's interpreter services.
4. Obtain a Spanish-English dictionary and attempt to triage the client.

ANSWERS

❖196. 1, 2, 4

Rationale: A focused data collection process focuses on a limited or short-term problem, such as the client's complaint. Because the client is complaining of symptoms of a cold, a cough, and lung congestion, the nurse would focus on the respiratory system and the presence of an infection. A complete data collection includes a complete health history and physical examination and forms a baseline database. Checking the strength of peripheral pulses relates to a vascular assessment, which is not related to this client's complaints. A musculoskeletal and neurological examination also is not related to this client's complaints. However, strength of peripheral pulses and a musculoskeletal and neurological examination would be included in a complete data collection. Likewise, asking the client about a family history of any illness or disease would be included in a complete assessment.

Test-Taking Strategy: Focus on the data in the question. Noting the **subject**, how the client's symptoms relate to the respiratory system, and the presence of an infection will direct you to options 1, 2, and 4. **Review:** the **types of health and physical assessments.**

Level of Cognitive Ability: Analyzing

Client Needs: Health Promotion and Maintenance

Integrated Process: Nursing Process/Data Collection

Content Area: Developmental Stages: Health Assessment/ Physical Exam

Priority Concepts: Health Promotion, Infection

Reference(s): deWit, Kumagai (2013), p. 20.

197. 2

Rationale: Asthma is a respiratory disorder characterized by recurring episodes of dyspnea, constriction of the bronchi, and wheezing. Wheezes are described as high-pitched musical sounds heard when air passes through an obstructed or narrowed lumen of a respiratory passageway. Stridor is a harsh sound noted with an upper airway obstruction and often signals a life-threatening emergency. Diminished lung sounds are heard over lung tissue where poor oxygen exchange is occurring. A pleural friction rub is heard in individuals with pleurisy (inflammation of the pleural surfaces).

Test-Taking Strategy: Focus on the **subject**, asthma and adventitious breath sounds. Think about the pathophysiology that occurs in this disorder. Recalling that bronchial constriction occurs will assist in directing you to option 2. Also, thinking about the definition of each adventitious lung sound identified in the choices will direct you to the correct option. **Review:** the characteristics of **adventitious breath sounds.**

Level of Cognitive Ability: Analyzing

Client Needs: Physiological Integrity

Integrated Process: Nursing Process/Data Collection

Content Area: Developmental Stages: Health Assessment/ Physical Exam

Priority Concepts: Gas Exchange, Health Promotion

Reference(s): deWit, Kumagai (2013), pp. 305–306.

198. 3

Rationale: In the Romberg test, the client is asked to stand with the feet together, the arms at the sides and to close the eyes and hold the position. Normally the client can maintain posture and balance. A positive Romberg is a vestibular neurological sign that is found when a client elicits a loss of balance when closing the eyes. This may occur with cerebellar ataxia, loss of proprioception, and loss of vestibular function. A positive gaze nystagmus evaluation results in an involuntary rhythmic, rapid, twitching of the eyeballs. A positive Babinski test results with dorsiflexion of the ankle and great toe with fanning of the other toes. If this occurs in anyone older than 2 years, it indicates the presence of central nervous system disease. A lack of normal sense of position coupled with an inability to return extended fingers to a point of reference is a finding in a past pointing test.

Test-Taking Strategy: Focus on the **subject**, the Romberg test. Specific knowledge regarding the technique for performing the Romberg test is needed to answer this question. You can easily answer this question if you can recall that the client's balance is tested in this test. **Review:** the procedure for performing the **Romberg test** and the purpose of the test.

Level of Cognitive Ability: Evaluating

Client Needs: Physiological Integrity

Integrated Process: Nursing Process/Data Collection

Content Area: Developmental Stages: Health Assessment/ Physical Exam

Priority Concepts: Health Promotion, Intracranial Regulation

Reference(s): deWit, Kumagai (2013), p. 585.

199. 1

Rationale: Cheyne-Stokes respirations are rhythmic respirations with periods of apnea and can indicate a metabolic dysfunction in the cerebral hemisphere or basal ganglia. Neurogenic hyperventilation is a regular, rapid and deep, sustained respiration that can indicate a dysfunction in the low midbrain and middle pons. Ataxic respirations are totally irregular in rhythm and depth and indicate a dysfunction in the medulla. Apneustic respirations are irregular respirations with pauses at the end of inspiration and expiration and can indicate a dysfunction in the middle or caudal pons.

Test-Taking Strategy: Focus on the **subject**, the characteristics of Cheyne-Stokes respirations. If you can recall that periods of apnea occur with this type of respiration, you will be able to answer this question correctly. **Review:** the characteristics of **Cheyne-Stokes respirations.**

Level of Cognitive Ability: Evaluating

Client Needs: Physiological Integrity

Integrated Process: Nursing Process/Data Collection

Content Area: Developmental Stages: Health Assessment/ Physical Exam

Priority Concepts: Gas Exchange, Health Promotion

Reference(s): deWit, Kumagai (2013), pp. 273, 507.

200. 3

Rationale: A conductive hearing loss occurs as a result of a physical obstruction to the transmission of sound waves. A sensorineural hearing loss occurs as a result of a pathological process in the inner ear, a defect in the 8th cranial nerve, or a defect of the sensory fibers that lead to the cerebral cortex.

Test-Taking Strategy: Focus on the **subject**, a conductive hearing loss. Noting the relationship of the word *conductive* in the question and *transmission* in option 3 will direct you to this option. **Review:** the causes of a conductive and a sensorineural **hearing loss.**

Level of Cognitive Ability: Understanding

Client Needs: Physiological Integrity

Integrated Process: Nursing Process/Data Collection

Content Area: Developmental Stages: Health Assessment/ Physical Exam

Priority Concepts: Health Promotion, Sensory Perception

Reference(s): deWit, Kumagai (2013), p. 581.

201. 3

Rationale: A heart murmur is an abnormal heart sound and is described as a gentle, blowing, swooshing sound. Lubb-dubb sounds are normal and represent the S1 (first heart sound) and S2 (second heart sound), respectively. A pericardial friction rub is described as a scratchy, leathery heart sound. A click is described as an abrupt, high-pitched snapping sound.

Test-Taking Strategy: Focus on the subject, characteristics of a murmur, and note the strategic word, *best*. Eliminate option 1 because it describes normal heart sounds. Next, recall that a murmur occurs as a result of the manner in which the blood is flowing through the cardiac chambers and valves. This will direct you to the correct option. **Review:** the characteristics of a murmur.

Level of Cognitive Ability: Understanding
Client Needs: Physiological Integrity
Integrated Process: Nursing Process/Data Collection
Content Area: Developmental Stages: Health Assessment/Physical Exam
Priority Concepts: Health Promotion, Perfusion
Reference(s): Potter et al (2013), p. 530.

202. 3

Rationale: Testing the six cardinal positions of gaze is done to check for muscle weakness in the eyes. The client is asked to hold the head steady, then to follow movement of an object through the positions of gaze. The client should follow the object in a parallel manner with the two eyes. A Snellen eye chart checks visual acuity and Cranial nerve II (optic). Testing sensory function by having the client close his or her eyes and then lightly touching areas of the face and testing the corneal reflexes check Cranial nerve V (trigeminal).

Test-Taking Strategy: Focus on the subject, checking for muscle weakness in the eyes. Note the relationship between the words *extraocular* movements in the question and *positions of gaze* in the correct option. **Review:** the physical assessment technique for checking for **muscle weakness in the eyes.**

Level of Cognitive Ability: Applying
Client Needs: Physiological Integrity
Integrated Process: Nursing Process/Planning
Content Area: Developmental Stages: Health Assessment/Physical Exam
Priority Concepts: Health Promotion, Sensory Perception
Reference(s): deWit, Kumagai (2013), p. 487; Ignatavicius, Workman (2013), p. 1047.

203. 1

Rationale: The nurse needs to teach the client how to perform a testicular self-examination (TSE). The nurse should instruct the client to select a day of the month and perform the exam on the same day each month. The nurse should also instruct the client that the best time to perform a TSE is after a shower or bath when the hands are warm and soapy and the scrotum is warm. This will provide ease in palpating, and the client will be better able to identify any abnormalities. The client would stand to perform the exam, but it would be difficult to perform the exam while voiding. Having a bowel movement is unrelated to performing the TSE.

Test-Taking Strategy: Note the strategic word, *best.* Think about the subject, the best time to perform TSE, and visualize this data collection technique. Eliminate option 3 because having a bowel movement is unrelated to performing the TSE. Next, eliminate options 2 and 4 because it would be difficult to perform this self-exam lying down or during voiding. **Review: testicular self-examination.**

Level of Cognitive Ability: Applying
Client Needs: Health Promotion and Maintenance
Integrated Process: Teaching and Learning
Content Area: Developmental Stages: Health Assessment/Physical Exam
Priority Concepts: Client Education, Health Promotion
Reference(s): deWit, Kumagai (2013), pp. 921–922, 933.

204. 3

Rationale: Brudzinski's sign is tested with the client in the supine position. The examiner flexes the client's head, and there should be no reports of pain or resistance to the neck flexion. A positive Brudzinski's sign is observed if the client passively flexes the hip and knee in response to neck flexion and reports pain in the vertebral column. Kernig's sign also tests for meningeal irritation and is positive when the client flexes the legs at the hip and knee and complains of pain along the vertebral column when the leg is extended. Decerebrate posturing is abnormal extension and occurs when the arms are fully extended, forearms pronated, wrists and fingers flexed, jaws clenched, neck extended, and feet plantar-flexed. Decorticate posturing is abnormal flexion and is noted when the client's upper arms are flexed and held tightly to the sides of the body and the legs are extended and internally rotated.

Test-Taking Strategy: Focus on the subject, a positive Brudzinski's sign. Recalling that a positive sign is elicited if the client reports pain will assist in eliminating options 1 and 4. Next, it is necessary to know that a positive Brudzinski's sign is observed if the client passively flexes the hip and knee in response to neck flexion and reports pain in the vertebral column. **Review:** the findings in a positive **Brudzinski's sign.**

Level of Cognitive Ability: Analyzing
Client Needs: Physiological Integrity
Integrated Process: Nursing Process/Data Collection
Content Area: Developmental Stages: Health Assessment/Physical Exam
Priority Concepts: Intracranial Regulation, Pain
Reference(s): deWit, Kumagai (2013), p. 542.

205. 3

Rationale: The best action is to have a professional hospital-based interpreter translate for the client. English-speaking family members may not appropriately understand what is asked of them and may paraphrase what the client is actually saying. Also, client confidentiality as well as accurate information may be compromised when a family member or a non-health care provider acts as interpreter. Using a Spanish-English dictionary is not the best action; accurate interpretation is best done by a professional hospital-based interpreter.

Test-Taking Strategy: Note the strategic word, *best.* Initially focus on what the client needs. In this case the client needs and asks for an interpreter. Next keep in mind the issue of confidentiality and making sure that information is obtained in the most efficient and accurate way. This will assist in eliminating options 1, 2, and 4. **Review:** the best nursing actions to take to obtain data from a **non-English-speaking** client.

Level of Cognitive Ability: Applying
Client Needs: Psychosocial Integrity
Integrated Process: Communication and Documentation
Content Area: Fundamental Skills: Cultural Awareness
Priority Concepts: Communication; Culture
Reference(s): Cooper, Gosnell (2015), pp. 69–70, 98.

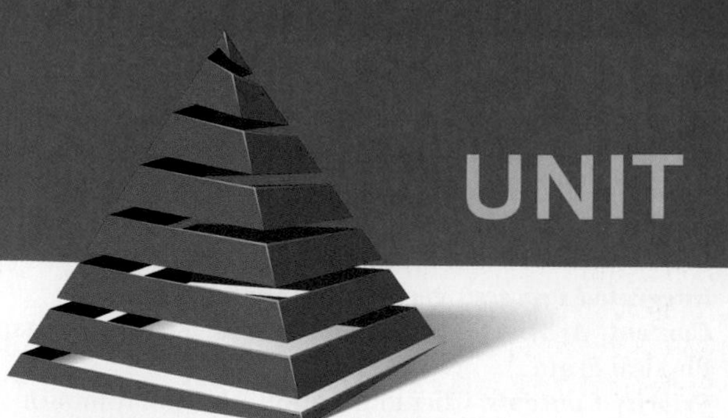

UNIT VI

Maternity Nursing

PYRAMID TERMS

amniotic fluid The pale, straw-colored fluid that surrounds and protects the fetus. The fetus floats in the amniotic fluid, which serves as a cushion against injury from sudden blows or movements. It also helps maintain a constant body temperature for the fetus. The fetus modifies the amniotic fluid through the processes of swallowing, urinating, and movement through the respiratory tract.

ballottement The rebounding of the fetus against the examiner's finger on palpation, beginning at 16 to 18 weeks of gestation. When the cervix is tapped, the fetus floats upward in the amniotic fluid. A rebound is felt by the examiner when the fetus falls back.

Chadwick's sign The violet-bluish coloration of the vaginal mucous membranes that is visible from about 4 weeks' gestation and presents as a result of increased vascularity. This is considered a probable sign of pregnancy.

delivery The actual event of birth. The expulsion or extraction of the neonate and the fetal membranes at birth.

fertilization The union of an ovum and sperm. Fertilization occurs within 12 hours of ovulation and within 2 to 3 days of insemination, the average duration of viability of the ovum and the sperm.

Goodell's sign The softening of the cervix. This occurs at the beginning of the second month of gestation and is considered a probable sign of pregnancy.

gravida A pregnant woman. The woman is called gravida I (or primigravida) during the first pregnancy, gravida II during the second, and so on.

Hegar's sign The compressibility and softening of the lower uterine segment. This occurs at about 6 weeks' gestation, and it is considered a probable sign of pregnancy.

implantation The embedding of the fertilized ovum in the uterine mucosa, which occurs 6 to 10 days after conception.

infant A human born alive; also, a human from 28 days of age until the first birthday.

labor A coordinated sequence of rhythmic, involuntary uterine contractions that result in the effacement and dilation of cervix. This is followed by the expulsion of the products of conception.

lecithin-to-sphingomyelin (L/S) ratio Ratio of two components of amniotic fluid, used for predicting fetal lung maturity; normal L/S ratio in amniotic fluid is 2:1 or greater when the fetal lungs are mature.

lochia Vaginal discharge from the uterus that consists of blood from the vessels of the placental site, tissue debris from the decidua, and mucus. Lochia lasts for 2 to 6 weeks postpartum and is differentiated by color: rubra, serosa, or alba.

Nägele's rule A way to determine the estimated date of birth that works on the premise that the woman has a 28-day menstrual cycle. Subtract 3 months from the first day of the last menstrual period, add 7 days, and then adjust the year.

newborn; neonate A human offspring from the time of birth to day 28 of life.

parity The number of pregnancies that have reached viability, regardless of whether the infants were alive or stillborn.

placenta The organ that provides for the exchange of nutrients and waste products between the fetus and the mother and that produces hormones to maintain pregnancy. It develops by the third month of gestation and is also called the afterbirth.

quickening The maternal perception of fetal movement, which usually appears around 16 to 20 weeks' gestation.

surfactant Phospholipid that is necessary to keep the fetal lung alveoli from collapsing; amount is usually sufficient after 32 weeks' gestation.

uterus Organ located behind the symphysis pubis, between the bladder and the rectum. It has four parts: fundus (upper part), corpus (body), isthmus (lower segment), and cervix.

vagina Tubular structure located behind the bladder and in front of the rectum; it extends from the cervix to the vaginal opening in the perineum. It functions as the outflow tract for menstrual fluid and for vaginal and cervical secretions, as the birth canal, and as the organ for coitus.

Pyramid to Success

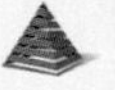

The Pyramid to Success focuses on the physiological and psychosocial aspects related to the experience of pregnancy. The pyramid points begin with reinforcement of teaching the pregnant client with regard to measures that will promote a healthy environment for both the mother and the fetus. Focus on the importance of antenatal follow-up care, nutrition, and the interventions for common discomforts that occur during pregnancy.

Review the purpose of the commonly prescribed diagnostic tests and procedures during the antenatal period. Focus on disorders that can occur during pregnancy, particularly gestational hypertension and diabetes. Review the labor and delivery process and the immediate interventions when the mother or fetal status is compromised, such as a prolapsed cord or altered fetal heart rate. Review the fetal effects that result from the mother with acquired immunodeficiency syndrome or the mother who abuses substances. Focus on the normal expectations of the postpartum period and the complications that can occur. The pyramid points also focus on the normal physical assessment findings of the newborn and the early identification of disorders of the newborn. The last pyramid point focuses on maternity and newborn medications.

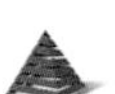

Client Needs

Safe and Effective Care Environment

Collaborating with other members of the health care team
Ensuring that informed consent for diagnostic tests and procedures has been obtained
Establishing priorities of care
Handling hazardous and infectious materials safely
Maintaining confidentiality
Providing continuity of care
Upholding parent rights
Using standard, transmission-based, and other precautions when delivering care
Using surgical asepsis when providing care

Health Promotion and Maintenance

Monitoring growth and development
Discussing expected body-image changes
Discussing family planning and birthing and parenting issues
Identifying at-risk clients during pregnancy
Identifying health and wellness concepts and providing health care screening
Identifying lifestyle choices and high-risk behaviors
Performing techniques of data collection
Providing antepartum, intrapartum, postpartum, and newborn care

Psychosocial Integrity

Considering cultural, spiritual, and religious influences regarding birth and motherhood
Discussing situational role changes in the family
Ensuring therapeutic interactions within the family
Identifying available support systems
Identifying coping mechanisms

Physiological Integrity

Monitoring for normal expectations during pregnancy
Monitoring for side effects and adverse effects related to prescribed pharmacological and parenteral therapies
Monitoring the client during the labor and delivery process
Providing information to the client about prescribed diagnostic tests and procedures
Providing interventions for unexpected events during pregnancy
Providing nonpharmacological comfort interventions and pharmacological pain management during labor
Reinforcing client teaching about nutrition during pregnancy and the postpartum period
Reinforcing client teaching about the physiological changes that occur during pregnancy

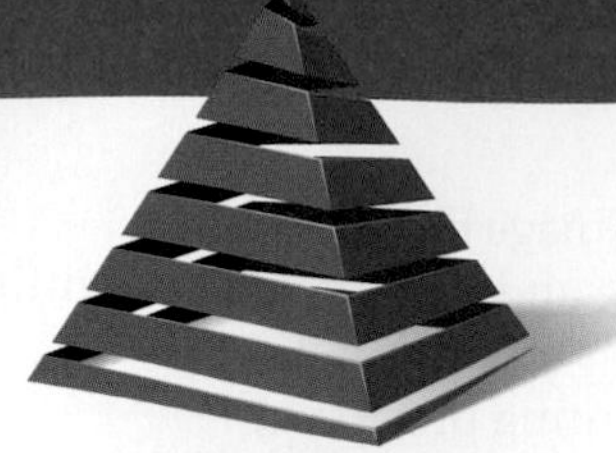

CHAPTER 24

Reproductive System

CRITICAL THINKING What Should You Do?

The nurse is collecting data for the first time from a pregnant adolescent who reports consuming small amounts of alcohol on a daily basis. On the basis of the information provided, what should the nurse do?

Answer is located on p. 266.

I. Female Reproductive Structures

A. Ovaries
   1. Form and expel ova
   2. Primary source of estrogen and progesterone

B. Fallopian tubes
   1. Muscular tubes (oviducts) lying near the ovaries and that connect into the uterus
   2. Provide transportation for the ova from the ovaries to the uterus

C. **Uterus** (womb)
   1. Muscular pear-shaped cavity that holds the fetus during development and produces rhythmic contractions for expulsion of fetus
   2. Cavity from which menstruation occurs

D. Cervix
   1. Internal os of the cervix opens into the body of the uterine cavity.
   2. Cervical canal is located between the internal cervical os and the external cervical os.
   3. External cervical os opens into the vagina.

E. Vagina
   1. A muscular tube that extends from the cervix to the vaginal opening in the perineum
   2. Known as the birth canal
   3. Passageway for menstrual blood flow, for penis for intercourse, and for the fetus

II. Male Reproductive Structures

A. Penis
   1. Structures include the body or shaft, glans penis, and urethra.
   2. Primary functions include pathway for urination and is the organ for intercourse.

B. Scrotum
   1. Structures include the testes, epididymis, and van deferens.
   2. Normal temperature within the scrotum is slightly cooler than body temperature for optimum sperm production.

C. Prostate gland
   1. Secretes a milky alkaline fluid
   2. Enhances sperm movement and neutralizes acidic vaginal secretions

III. Menstrual Cycle (Box 24-1)

A. Ovarian hormones
   1. Ovarian hormones, released by the anterior pituitary gland, include follicle-stimulating hormone (FSH) and luteinizing hormone (LH).
   2. The hormones produce changes in the ovaries and in the endometrium.
   3. The menstrual cycle, the regularly recurring physiological changes in the endometrium that culminate in its shedding, may vary in length, with the average length being about 28 days.

B. Ovarian and uterine phases (see Box 24-1)

IV. Female Pelvis

A. True pelvis
   1. Lies below the pelvic brim (the lower, curved, bony canal)
   2. Consists of the pelvic inlet, the mid pelvis, and the pelvic outlet

B. False pelvis
   1. Shallow portion above the pelvic brim
   2. Supports the abdominal viscera

C. Types of pelvis
   1. Gynecoid
      a. Normal female pelvis
      b. Transversely rounded or blunt

⚠ The gynecoid pelvis is most favorable for successful labor and birth.

   2. Android
      a. Heart-shaped or angulated

BOX 24-1 Menstrual Cycle

Ovarian Changes

Preovulatory Phase

- The hypothalamus releases gonadotropin-releasing hormone through the portal system to the anterior pituitary system.
- Secretion of follicle-stimulating hormone (FSH) by the anterior lobe of the pituitary gland stimulates growth of follicles.
- Most follicles die, leaving one to mature into a large graafian follicle.
- Estrogen produced by the follicle stimulates increased secretions of luteinizing hormone (LH) by the anterior lobe of the pituitary gland.
- The follicle ruptures and releases an ovum into the peritoneal cavity.

Luteal Phase

- The luteal phase begins with ovulation.
- Body temperature drops and then rises by 0.5° to 1°F around the time of ovulation.
- Corpus luteum is formed from follicle cells that remain in the ovary following ovulation.
- Corpus luteum secretes estrogen and progesterone during the remaining 14 days of the cycle.
- Corpus luteum degenerates if the ovum is not fertilized, and secretion of estrogen and progesterone declines.
- The decline of estrogen and progesterone stimulates the anterior pituitary to secrete more FSH and LH, initiating a new reproductive cycle.

Uterine Changes

Menstrual Phase

- The menstrual phase consists of 4 to 6 days of bleeding as the endometrium breaks down because of the decreased levels of estrogen and progesterone.
- The level of FSH increases, enabling the beginning of a new cycle.

Proliferative Phase

- The proliferative phase lasts about 9 days.
- Estrogen stimulates proliferation and growth of the endometrium.
- As estrogen increases, it suppresses secretion of FSH and increases secretion of LH.
- Secretion of LH stimulates ovulation and the development of the corpus luteum.
- Ovulation occurs between days 12 and 16.
- The estrogen level is high and the progesterone level is low.

Secretory Phase

- The secretory phase lasts about 12 days and follows ovulation.
- This phase is initiated in response to the increase in LH level.
- The graafian follicle is replaced by the corpus luteum.
- The corpus luteum secretes progesterone and estrogen.
- Progesterone prepares the endometrium for pregnancy if a fertilized ovum is implanted.

b. Resembles a male pelvis
c. Not favorable for **labor** and birth
d. Narrow pelvic planes can cause slow descent and midpelvis arrest

3. Anthropoid
   a. Oval shape
   b. The outlet is adequate, with a normal or moderately narrow pubic arch.
4. Platypelloid
   a. Flat shape with an oval inlet
   b. The transverse diameter is wide, but the anteroposterior diameter is short, thus making labor and birth difficult.

V. Fertilization and Implantation

A. Fertilization

1. Fertilization occurs in the ampulla of the fallopian (uterine) tube when sperm and ova unite.
2. When fertilized, the membrane of the ovum undergoes changes that prevent entry of other sperm.
3. Each reproductive cell carries 23 chromosomes.
4. Sperm carry an X or a Y chromosome—XY, male; XX, female.

B. Implantation

1. The zygote is propelled toward the uterus and implants 6 to 8 days after ovulation.
2. The blastocyst secretes chorionic gonadotropin to ensure that the corpus luteum remains viable and secretes estrogen and progesterone for the first 2 to 3 months of gestation.

VI. Fetal Development (Box 24-2)

A. Preembryonic period: First 2 weeks after conception
B. Embryonic stage: Begins on day 15 and continues through approximately the eighth week after conception
C. Fetal period: Begins the ninth week after conception and ends with birth

VII. Fetal Environment

A. Amnion
1. Encloses the amniotic cavity
2. Inner cell membrane that forms about the second week of embryonic development
3. Forms a fluid-filled sac that surrounds the embryo and later the fetus

B. Chorion
1. Outer membrane enclosing the amniotic cavity
2. Becomes vascularized and forms the fetal part of the placenta

C. Amniotic fluid

1. Consists of 800 to 1200 mL by end of pregnancy
2. Surrounds, cushions, and protects the fetus and allows for fetal movement

BOX 24-2 Fetal Development

Preembryonic Period
First 2 weeks after conception

Embryonic Period
Beginning day 15 through approximately week 8 after conception

Fetal Period
Week 9 after conception to birth

Week 1
Blastocyst is free-floating.

Weeks 2 to 3
Embryo is 1.5 to 2 mm in length.
Lung buds appear.
Blood circulation begins.
Heart is tubular and begins to beat.
Neural plate becomes brain and spinal cord.

Week 5
Embryo is 0.4 to 0.5 cm in length.
Embryo is 0.4 g.
Double heart chambers are visible.
Heart is beating.
Limb buds form.

Week 8
Embryo is 3 cm in length.
Embryo is 2 g.
Eyelids begin to fuse.
Circulatory system through umbilical cord is well established.
Every organ system is present.

Week 12
Fetus is 6 to 9 cm in length.
Fetus is 19 g.
Face is well formed
Limbs are long and slender.
Kidneys begin to form urine.
Spontaneous movements occur.
Heartbeat is detected by Doppler transducer between 10 and 12 weeks.
Gender is visually recognizable.

Week 16
Fetus is 11.5 to 13.5 cm in length.
Fetus is 100 g.
Active movements are present.
Fetal skin is transparent.
Lanugo hair begins to develop.
Skeletal ossification occurs.

Week 20
Fetus is 16 to 18.5 cm in length.
Fetus is 300 g.
Lanugo covers the entire body.
Fetus has nails.
Muscles are developed.
Enamel and dentin are depositing.
Heartbeat is detected by regular (nonelectronic) fetoscope.

Week 24
Fetus is 23 cm in length.
Fetus is 600 g.
Hair on head is well formed.
Skin is reddish and wrinkled.
Reflex hand grasp functions.
Vernix caseosa covers entire body.
Fetus has ability to hear.

Week 28
Fetus is 27 cm in length.
Fetus is 1100 g.
Limbs are well flexed.
Brain is developing rapidly.
Eyelids open and close.
Lungs are developed sufficiently to provide gas exchange (lecithin forming).
If born, neonate can breathe at this time.

Week 32
Fetus is 31 cm in length.
Fetus is 1800 to 2100 g.
Bones are fully developed.
Subcutaneous fat has collected.
The L/S (lecithin-to-sphingomyelin) ratio is 1.2:1.

Week 36
The fetus is 35 cm in length.
The fetus is 2200 to 2900 g.
The skin is pink and the body is rounded.
The skin is less wrinkled.
Lanugo is disappearing.
The L/S ratio is higher than 2:1.

Week 40
The fetus is 40 cm in length.
The fetus is 3200 + g.
The skin is pinkish and smooth.
Lanugo is present on upper arms and shoulders.
Vernix caseosa decreases.
Fingernails extend beyond fingertips.
Sole (plantar) creases run down to the heel.
The testes are in the scrotum.
The labia majora are well developed.

3. Maintains the body temperature of the fetus
4. Consists largely of fetal urine and is therefore a measure of fetal kidney function
5. The fetus modifies the amniotic fluid through the processes of swallowing, urinating, and movement of fluid through the respiratory tract.

D. Placenta

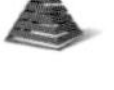

1. The placenta provides for exchange of nutrients and waste products between the fetus and the mother.
2. Begins to form at **implantation**; structure is complete by week 12.

3. It produces hormones to maintain pregnancy and assumes full responsibility for the production of these hormones by the twelfth week of gestation.
4. In the third trimester, transfer of maternal immunoglobulin provides the fetus with passive immunity to certain diseases for the first few months after birth.
5. By week 10 and 12, genetic testing can be done via chorionic villus sampling (CVS).

Large particles such as bacteria cannot pass through the placenta, but nutrients, drugs, antibodies, and viruses can pass through the placenta.

VIII. Fetal Circulation (Fig. 24-1)

A. Umbilical cord
   1. Contains two arteries and one vein
   2. Arteries carry deoxygenated blood and waste products from the fetus
   3. Vein carries oxygenated blood and provides oxygen and nutrients to the fetus

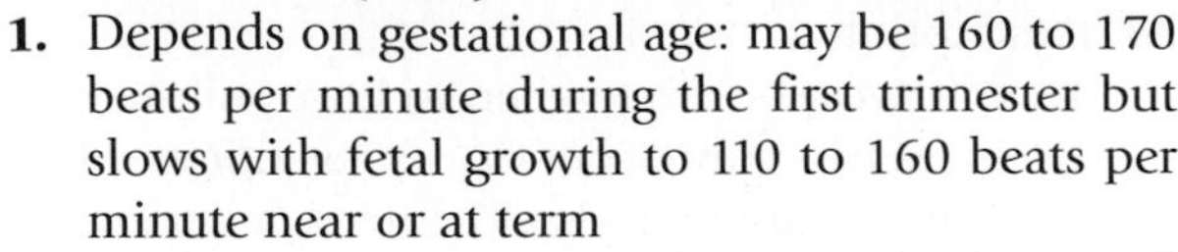

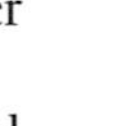

B. Fetal heart rate (FHR)
   1. Depends on gestational age: may be 160 to 170 beats per minute during the first trimester but slows with fetal growth to 110 to 160 beats per minute near or at term
   2. The FHR is approximately twice the maternal heart rate.

C. Fetal circulation bypass
   1. Present as a result of nonfunctioning lungs
   2. Bypasses must close after birth to allow blood to flow through the lungs and the liver.
   3. Ductus arteriosus connects the pulmonary artery to the aorta, bypassing the lungs.
   4. Ductus venosus connects the umbilical vein and the inferior vena cava, bypassing the liver.
   5. Foramen ovale is the opening between the right and left atria of heart, bypassing the lungs.

The fetal heart is 160 to 170 beats/min in the first trimester but slows with fetal growth to 120 to 160 beats/min near or at term. The health care provider (HCP) must be notified if the fetal heart rate is outside these parameters.

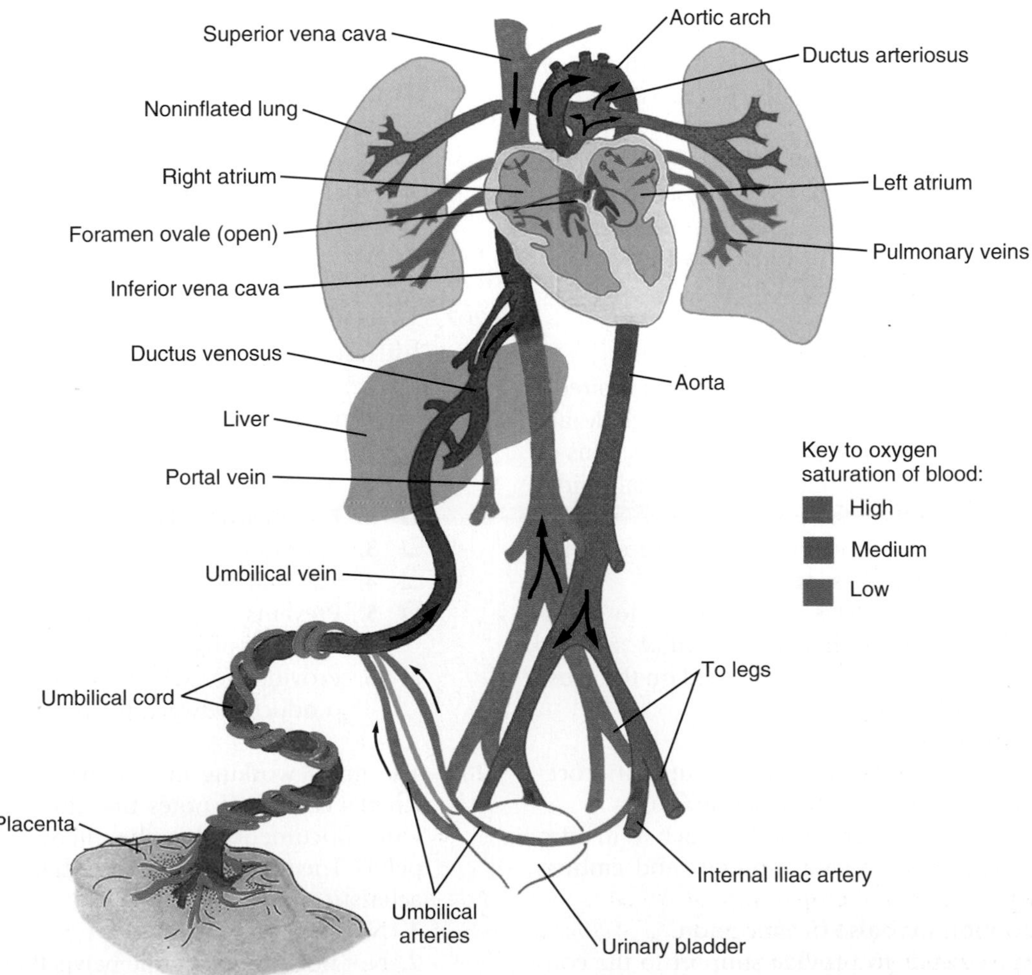

FIGURE 24-1 Fetal circulation. Three shunts (ductus venosus, ductus arteriosus, and foramen ovale) allow most blood from the placenta to bypass the fetal lungs and liver. (From McKinney E, James S, Murray S, Ashwill J: *Maternal-child nursing*, ed 4, St. Louis, 2013, Saunders.)

IX. Family Planning

A. Description
1. Involves choosing when to have children
2. Includes contraception, prevention of pregnancy, and methods to achieve pregnancy

B. Birth control
1. The focus of counseling on contraception must meet the needs and feelings of the woman and her partner.
2. Several factors should be considered when choosing a method of birth control, including effectiveness, safety, and personal preference.
3. The woman's preferences are most important, and cultural practices and beliefs and religious or other personal beliefs may affect the choice of contraceptives.
4. Other factors that bear on selection of a contraceptive method include family-planning goals, age, frequency of intercourse, and the individual's capacity for compliance.
5. If planning goals have already been met, sterilization of either the male or female partner may be desirable (it is important for the couple to understand that tubal reconstruction may be unsuccessful).
6. For women who frequently engage in coitus, oral contraceptives or a long-term method such as implants or an intrauterine device (IUD) may be considered.
7. When sexual activity is limited, use of spermicide, condoms, or a diaphragm may be most appropriate.
8. Because some methods have adverse effects, a signed informed consent form may be needed.
9. For additional information on the use of contraceptives, see Chapter 46.

C. Infertility
1. Involuntary inability to conceive when desired
2. Some contributing factors in men include abnormalities of the sperm, abnormal erections or ejaculations, or abnormalities of seminal fluid.
3. Some contributing factors in women include disorders of ovulation or abnormalities of the uterus, fallopian tubes, or cervix
4. Several diagnostic tests are available to determine the probable cause of infertility, and the therapy recommended may depend on the cause of the infertility.
5. Infertility options
   a. Options include medication, surgical procedures, and therapeutic insemination.
   b. Other therapies are available, such as in vitro **fertilization**, surrogate mothers, and embryo hosts.
   c. Adoption may also be an option.
6. The nurse needs to provide support to the couple in their decision-making process and during therapy.

CRITICAL THINKING What Should You Do?

Answer: Adolescent pregnancies are considered high risk due to the immaturity of the reproductive system, as well as the high-risk behaviors that some adolescents engage in. The nurse should provide information to the adolescent regarding the risks associated with drug and alcohol consumption during pregnancy. The nurse should explain to the adolescent that large particles such as bacteria cannot pass through the placenta, but nutrients, drugs, antibodies, and viruses can pass through; therefore, measures should be taken to minimize exposure to substances that can cross the placental barrier and affect the health of the fetus. Follow-up regarding this high-risk behavior is also necessary.

Reference(s): McKinney, E., James, S., Murray, S., Nelson, K. & Ashwill, J. (2013). *Maternal-child nursing* (4th ed., pp. 552, 558). St. Louis: Elsevier.

PRACTICE QUESTIONS

206. The nurse is collecting data from a pregnant client when the client asks the nurse about the purpose of the fallopian tubes. Which is the accurate response the nurse should make?
1. The organ of copulation
2. Where the fetus develops
3. Where fertilization occurs
4. Secrete estrogen and progesterone

❖ **207.** The nursing instructor asks a nursing student to list the functions of the amniotic fluid. The student responds correctly by stating that which are functions of amniotic fluid? **Select all that apply.**
- ❑ 1. Allows for fetal movement
- ❑ 2. Is a measure of kidney function
- ❑ 3. Surrounds, cushions, and protects the fetus
- ❑ 4. Maintains the body temperature of the fetus
- ❑ 5. Prevents large particles such as bacteria from passing to the fetus
- ❑ 6. Provides an exchange of nutrients and waste products between the mother and the fetus

208. The nurse working in a prenatal clinic reviews a client's chart and notes that the health care provider documents that the client has a gynecoid pelvis. The nurse understands that which is a characteristic of this type of pelvis?
1. Not favorable for labor
2. Not normally a female pelvis type
3. A wide pelvis with a short diameter
4. The most favorable for labor and birth

209. The client asks the nurse about the purpose of the placenta. The nurse plans to respond to the client knowing which about the placenta?
1. Cushions and protects the fetus
2. Maintains the body temperature of the fetus
3. Surrounds the fetus and allows for fetal movement
4. Provides an exchange of nutrients and waste products between the mother and the fetus

210. The nurse is describing the process of fetal circulation to a client during a prenatal visit. The nurse should tell the client that fetal circulation consists of which?
1. Two umbilical veins and one umbilical artery
2. Two umbilical arteries and one umbilical vein
3. Arteries that carry oxygenated blood to the fetus
4. Veins that carry deoxygenated blood to the fetus

211. A nursing student is assigned to a client in labor. The nursing instructor asks the student to describe fetal circulation, specifically the ductus venosus. The instructor determines that the student understands the structure of the ductus venosus if the student states which about the ductus venosus?
1. Connects the pulmonary artery to the aorta
2. Is an opening between the right and left atria
3. Connects the umbilical vein to the inferior vena cava
4. Connects the umbilical artery to the inferior vena cava

212. During a prenatal visit, the nurse checks the fetal heart rate (FHR) of a client in the third trimester of pregnancy. The nurse determines that the FHR is normal if which heart rate is noted?
1. 80 beats per minute
2. 100 beats per minute
3. 150 beats per minute
4. 180 beats per minute

213. The nurse is reinforcing teaching to a pregnant woman about the physiological effects and hormone changes that occur during pregnancy. The woman asks the nurse about the purpose of estrogen. The nurse bases the response on which purpose of estrogen?
1. It maintains the uterine lining for implantation.
2. It stimulates the metabolism of glucose and converts glucose to fat.
3. It stimulates uterine development to provide an environment for the fetus and stimulates the breasts to prepare for lactation.
4. It prevents the involution of the corpus luteum and maintains the production of progesterone until the placenta is formed.

214. The nursing student is asked to describe the size of the uterus in a nonpregnant client. Which response indicates an understanding of the anatomy of this structure?
1. "The uterus weighs about 2 ounces."
2. "The uterus weighs about 2.2 pounds."
3. "The uterus has a capacity of about 50 milliliters."
4. "The uterus is round in shape and weighs approximately 1000 grams."

215. A couple comes to the family planning clinic and asks about sterilization procedures. Which question by the nurse would determine whether this method of family planning would be appropriate?
1. "Have either of you ever had surgery?"
2. "Do you plan to have any other children?"
3. "Do either of you have diabetes mellitus?"
4. "Do either of you have problems with high blood pressure?"

ANSWERS

206. 3

Rationale: Each fallopian tube is a hollow muscular tube that transports a mature oocyte for final maturation and fertilization. Fertilization typically occurs near the boundary between the ampulla and the isthmus of the tube. The vagina is the organ of copulation, and the fetus develops in the uterus. Estrogen is a hormone that is produced by the ovarian follicles, the corpus luteum, the adrenal cortex, and the placenta during pregnancy. Progesterone is a hormone that is secreted by the corpus luteum of the ovary, the adrenal glands, and the placenta during pregnancy.

Test-Taking Strategy: Focus on the subject, anatomy and physiology of the female reproductive system, which will direct you to the correct option. Remember that fertilization occurs in the fallopian tube. **Review:** **the female reproductive system.**

Level of Cognitive Ability: Applying
Client Needs: Physiological Integrity
Integrated Process: Nursing Process/Implementation
Content Area: Maternity: Antepartum
Priority Concepts: Client Education, Reproduction
Reference(s): deWit, Kumagai (2013), p. 881.

❖ **207. 1, 2, 3, 4**

Rationale: The amniotic fluid surrounds, cushions, and protects the fetus. It allows the fetus to move freely, it maintains the body temperature of the fetus, and it helps to measure kidney function, because the amount of fluid is based on the

amount of urination from the fetus. The placenta prevents large particles such as bacteria from passing to the fetus, and it provides an exchange of nutrients and waste products between the mother and the fetus.
Test-Taking Strategy: Focus on the subject, the functions of the amniotic fluid. Visualizing the anatomical location of the amniotic fluid will direct you to the correct options. **Review:** the function of the **amniotic fluid**.
Level of Cognitive Ability: Understanding
Client Needs: Physiological Integrity
Integrated Process: Teaching and Learning
Content Area: Adult Health: Reproductive
Priority Concepts: Development, Reproduction
Reference(s): McKinney et al (2013), pp. 228–229.

208. 4
Rationale: A gynecoid pelvis is a normal female pelvis, and it is the most favorable for successful labor and birth. An android pelvis would not be favorable for labor because of the narrow pelvic planes. An anthropoid pelvis has an outlet that is adequate, with a normal or moderately narrow pubic arch. The platypelloid pelvis has a wide transverse diameter, but the anteroposterior diameter is short, thus making the outlet inadequate.
Test-Taking Strategy: Focus on the subject, knowledge regarding pelvic types, to answer this question. Remember that the gynecoid pelvis is the normal female pelvis. **Review: pelvic types.**
Level of Cognitive Ability: Understanding
Client Needs: Physiological Integrity
Integrated Process: Nursing Process/Data Collection
Content Area: Maternity: Antepartum
Priority Concepts: Clinical Judgment, Reproduction
Reference(s): McKinney et al (2013), p. 642.

209. 4
Rationale: The placenta provides an exchange of nutrients and waste products between the mother and the fetus. The amniotic fluid surrounds, cushions, and protects the fetus and allows for fetal movement. The amniotic fluid also maintains the body temperature of the fetus.
Test-Taking Strategy: Focus on the subject, the purpose of the placenta. This knowledge is required to answer this question. Remember that the placenta provides nutrients. **Review:** the structure and function of the **placenta** and the **amniotic fluid**.
Level of Cognitive Ability: Applying
Client Needs: Physiological Integrity
Integrated Process: Nursing Process/Planning
Content Area: Maternity: Antepartum
Priority Concepts: Client Education, Reproduction
Reference(s): McKinney et al (2013), p. 225.

210. 2
Rationale: Blood pumped by the fetus's heart leaves the fetus through two umbilical arteries. After the blood is oxygenated, it is then returned by one umbilical vein. Arteries carry deoxygenated blood and waste products from the fetus, and veins carry oxygenated blood and provide oxygen and nutrients to the fetus.
Test-Taking Strategy: Focus on the subject, anatomy of fetal circulation. Remember that there are three umbilical vessels within an umbilical cord (two arteries and one vein). **Review: fetal circulation.**
Level of Cognitive Ability: Applying
Client Needs: Physiological Integrity
Integrated Process: Teaching and Learning
Content Area: Maternity: Antepartum
Priority Concepts: Perfusion, Reproduction
Reference(s): McKinney et al (2013), p. 365.

211. 3
Rationale: The ductus venosus connects the umbilical vein to the inferior vena cava. The foramen ovale is a temporary opening between the right and left atria. The ductus arteriosus joins the aorta and the pulmonary artery.
Test-Taking Strategy: Focus on the subject, fetal circulation. Recall the anatomy of the fetal circulation to answer this question. Remember that the ductus venosus connects the umbilical vein to the inferior vena cava. **Review: fetal circulation.**
Level of Cognitive Ability: Evaluating
Client Needs: Physiological Integrity
Integrated Process: Teaching and Learning
Content Area: Maternity: Antepartum
Priority Concepts: Perfusion, Reproduction
Reference(s): McKinney et al (2013), pp. 468–469.

212. 3
Rationale: Fetal heart rate depends on gestational age. It is normally 160 to 170 beats per minute during the first trimester, but it slows with fetal growth to 110 to 160 beats per minute near or at term.
Test-Taking Strategy: Focus on the subject, the fetal heart rate in the third trimester of pregnancy. Think about the physiology associated with cardiac structures in fetal development to answer correctly. **Review: fetal heart rate.**
Level of Cognitive Ability: Evaluating
Client Needs: Physiological Integrity
Integrated Process: Nursing Process/Data Collection
Content Area: Maternity: Antepartum
Priority Concepts: Perfusion, Reproduction
Reference(s): McKinney et al (2013), p. 368.

213. 3
Rationale: Estrogen stimulates uterine development to provide an environment for the fetus, and it stimulates the breasts to prepare for lactation. Progesterone maintains the uterine lining for implantation and relaxes all smooth muscle. Human placental lactogen stimulates the metabolism of glucose and converts the glucose to fat. Human chorionic gonadotropin prevents the involution of the corpus luteum and maintains the production of progesterone until the placenta is formed.
Test-Taking Strategy: Focus on the subject, functions of various hormones related to pregnancy. Remember that estrogen stimulates uterine development to provide an environment for the fetus and that it stimulates the breasts to prepare for lactation. **Review:** these various **hormones**.
Level of Cognitive Ability: Applying
Client Needs: Physiological Integrity
Integrated Process: Teaching and Learning
Content Area: Maternity: Antepartum
Priority Concepts: Client Education, Reproduction
Reference(s): McKinney et al (2013), pp. 238, 241.

214. 1

Rationale: Before conception, the uterus is a small, pear-shaped organ that is contained entirely in the pelvic cavity. Before pregnancy, the uterus weighs approximately 60 g (2 oz), and it has a capacity of about 10 mL (⅓ oz). At the end of pregnancy, the uterus weighs approximately 1000 g (2.2 lb), and it has a capacity that is sufficient for the fetus, the placenta, and the amniotic fluid.

Test-Taking Strategy: Focus on the subject, size of the uterus, and note the word, *nonpregnant*. Visualizing each of the items identified in the options will direct you to the correct answer. Review: the anatomy of the uterus.

Level of Cognitive Ability: Evaluating

Client Needs: Physiological Integrity

Integrated Process: Teaching and Learning

Content Area: Adult Health: Reproductive

Priority Concepts: Client Education, Reproduction

Reference(s): Mosby (2013), p. 1850.

215. 2

Rationale: Sterilization is a method of contraception for couples who have completed their families. It should be considered a permanent end to fertility because reversal surgery is not always successful. The nurse would ask the couple about their plans for having children in the future. Options 1, 3, and 4 are unrelated to this procedure.

Test-Taking Strategy: Focus on the subject, sterilization procedure. Noting the relationship between the word *sterilization* and the correct option will direct you to this answer. **Review:** effects of sterilization.

Level of Cognitive Ability: Applying

Client Needs: Health Promotion and Maintenance

Integrated Process: Nursing Process/Data Collection

Content Area: Maternity: Antepartum

Priority Concepts: Health Promotion, Reproduction

Reference(s): McKinney et al (2013), pp. 742–743.

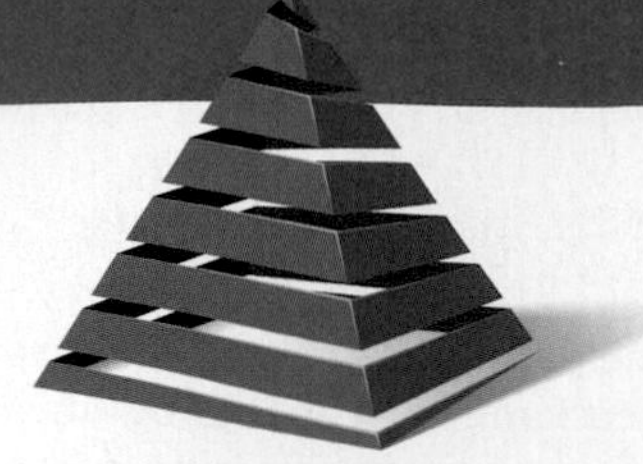

CHAPTER 25

Obstetrical Assessment

CRITICAL THINKING What Should You Do?

The nurse is assisting in collecting data from a pregnant client suspected of substance (drug) abuse. What signs should the nurse assess for?

Answer is located on p. 273.

I. Gestation

A. Time from the **fertilization** of the ovum until the estimated date of birth
B. Lasts approximately 280 days or 40 weeks
C. First trimester lasts from week 1 through 13; second trimester lasts from weeks 14 through 26; third trimester lasts from weeks 27 through 40
D. **Nägele's rule** for estimating date of birth: To be accurate, the woman must have a regular 28-day menstrual cycle. The rule must be adjusted if woman's cycle is longer or shorter than 28 days (Box 25-1).

II. Gravidity and Parity

A. Gravidity
  1. **Gravida**: A woman who is pregnant
  2. Gravidity: Number of pregnancies
  3. Nulligravida: A woman who has never been pregnant
  4. Primigravida: A woman who is pregnant for the first time
  5. Multigravida: A woman who has had two or more pregnancies

B. **Parity**
  1. Parity: The number of births (not the number of fetuses [e.g., twins]) carried past 20 weeks' gestation, whether or not the fetus was born alive
  2. Nullipara: A woman who has not had a birth at more than 20 weeks' gestation
  3. Primipara: A woman who has had one birth that occurred after 20 weeks' gestation
  4. Multipara: A woman who has had two or more pregnancies that resulted in viable offspring

C. Use of GTPAL: Pregnancy outcomes can be described with the GTPAL acronym (Box 25-2).
  1. G = Gravidity; number of pregnancies, including the present one
  2. T = Term births; number of children born at term (i.e., longer than 37 weeks' gestation)
  3. P = Preterm births; number of children born before 37 weeks' gestation
  4. A = Abortions or miscarriages; number of abortions/miscarriages (included in gravida if

BOX 25-1 Nägele's Rule for Determining the Estimated Date of Birth

Take the first day of the last menstrual period: September 12, 2016

Subtract 3 months:
June 12, 2016

Add 7 days:
June 19, 2016

Add 1 year:
June 19, 2017

Estimated date of confinement (delivery):
June 19, 2017

BOX 25-2 GTPAL Acronym

G = Gravidity
T = Term births
P = Preterm births
A = Abortions/miscarriages
L = Live births

Example: A woman is pregnant for the fourth time. She had one elective abortion during the first trimester, a daughter who was born at 40 weeks' gestation, and a son who was born at 36 weeks' gestation. Therefore, she is gravida (G) = 4; term (T) = 1 (the daughter born at 40 weeks' gestation). She is also preterm (P) = 1 (the son born at 36 weeks' gestation); abortion (A) = 1 (the abortion is counted in the gravida because it occurred before 20 weeks' gestation); and live births (L) = 2. Therefore, she would be considered GTPAL = 4, 1, 1, 1, 2.

before 20 weeks' gestation; included in parity if past 20 weeks' gestation). Note that a termination of the pregnancy after 20 weeks is referred to as a "therapeutic termination."

5. L = Live births; number of live births or living children

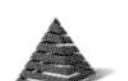

III. Pregnancy Signs

A. Presumptive signs
  1. Amenorrhea
  2. Nausea and vomiting
  3. Increased size and fullness in breasts; pronounced nipples
  4. Urinary frequency
  5. Fatigue
  6. **Quickening**: First perception of fetal movement appearing usually in the sixteenth to twentieth week of gestation
  7. Discoloration of vaginal mucosa

B. Probable signs
  1. Uterine enlargement
  2. **Goodell's sign**: Softening of the cervix that occurs at the beginning of the second month of pregnancy
  3. **Chadwick's sign**: Violet coloration of the mucous membranes of the cervix, **vagina**, and vulva that occurs at about week 4
  4. **Hegar's sign**: Compressibility and softening of the lower uterine segment that occurs at about week 6
  5. **Ballottement**: The rebounding of the fetus against the examiner's fingers on palpation
  6. Braxton Hicks contractions: Irregular contractions that occur intermittently throughout pregnancy and do not increase in intensity or duration or cause cervical dilation
  7. Positive pregnancy test for determination of human chorionic gonadotropin

C. Positive signs (diagnostic)
  1. Outline of the fetus via radiography or ultrasound
  2. Fetal heart rate (approximately 120 to 160 beats per minute) detected by electronic devices at 10 to 12 weeks' gestation, and by nonelectronic device (fetoscope) at 20 weeks' gestation
  3. Active fetal movements palpated by the examiner

IV. Fundal Height (Box 25-3)

A. Measured to evaluate the gestational age of the fetus (Fig. 25-1)

BOX 25-3 Measuring Fundal Height

1. Place the client in a supine position.
2. Place the end of the tape measure at the level of the symphysis pubis.
3. Stretch the tape to the top of the uterine fundus.
4. Note and record the measurement.

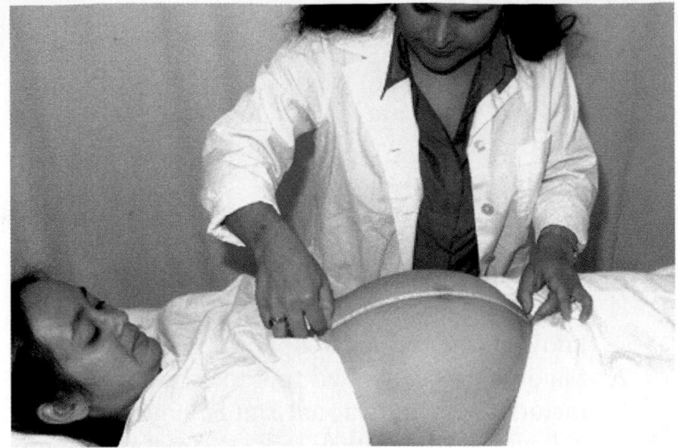

FIGURE 25-1 Measurement of fundal height. (From Perry S, Hockenberry M, Lowdermilk D, Wilson D: *Maternal-child nursing care*, ed 4, St. Louis, 2010, Mosby. Courtesy of Chris Rozales, San Francisco, CA.)

B. During the second and third trimesters (weeks 18 to 30), the fundal height in centimeters approximately equals the fetus's age in weeks, plus or minus 2 cm (Fig. 25-2).

C. At 16 weeks, the fundus can be found approximately halfway between the symphysis pubis and the umbilicus.

D. At 20 to 22 weeks, the fundus is approximately at the location of the umbilicus.

E. At 36 weeks, the fundus is at the xiphoid process.

When assessing fundal height, monitor the client closely for supine hypotension when placed in the supine position.

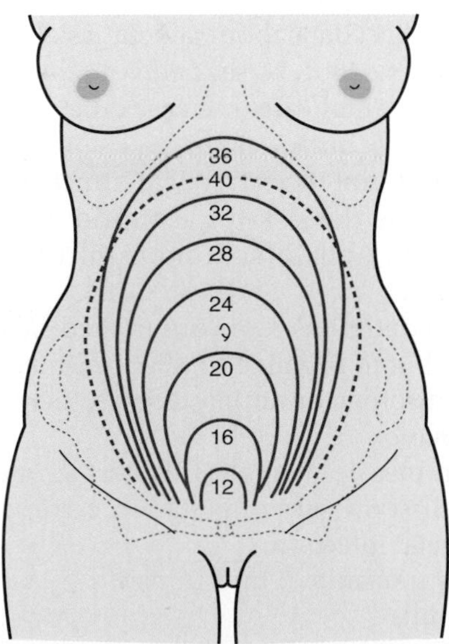

FIGURE 25-2 Height of fundus by weeks of normal gestation with a single fetus. *Dashed line*, Height after lightening. (From Perry S, Hockenberry M, Lowdermilk D, Wilson D: *Maternal-child nursing care*, ed 4, St. Louis, 2010, Mosby.)

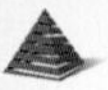

V. Maternal Risk Factors

A. Maternal age
   1. Women younger than 20 years and older than 35 years are at risk for adverse perinatal outcomes.

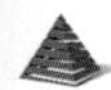

B. Adolescent pregnancy
   1. Factors that result in adolescent pregnancy include the early onset of menarche, changing sexual behaviors in this age group, problems with family relationships, poverty, and a lack of knowledge of reproduction and birth control.
   2. Major concerns related to adolescent pregnancy include poor nutritional status, emotional and behavioral difficulties, lack of support systems, increased risk of stillbirth, low birth weight, fetal mortality, cephalopelvic disproportion, and increased risks of maternal complications such as hypertension, anemia, prolonged **labor**, and infections.
   3. The role of the nurse in reducing the risks and consequences of adolescent pregnancy is twofold: first, to encourage early and continued prenatal care, and second, to refer the adolescent, if necessary, for appropriate assistance, which can help counter the effects of a negative socioeconomic environment.

C. Nutrition: Adequate nutrition is necessary for normal fetal growth and development.

⚠ Women of childbearing age should take folic acid supplements to prevent neural tube defects and orofacial clefts in the fetus.

D. Genetic considerations: Genetic abnormalities such as defective genes or transmissible inherited disorders can result in congenital anomalies; the nurse should collect data about genetic risks.

E. Health care: Failure to seek and obtain prenatal care, including dental care, increases the risk of preterm birth and low birth weight.

F. Abuse and violence: Physical abuse and violence can increase the risk for abruptio placentae, preterm birth, and infections from unwanted and forced sex.

G. Medical conditions: Concurrent medical conditions, such as, but not limited to, diabetes mellitus, hypertensive disorder, or cardiac disease, increase the risks in pregnancy.

H. German measles (rubella): Maternal infection during the first 8 weeks of gestation carries the highest rate of fetal infection.

I. Sexually transmitted infections
   1. Syphilis
      a. Organism may cross the **placenta**
      b. Infection usually leads to spontaneous abortions and increases the incidence of mental subnormality and physical deformities
   2. Condylomata acuminata (human papillomavirus)
      a. Transmission may occur during vaginal birth.
      b. Infection is associated with the development of epithelial tumors of the mucous membranes of the larynx in children.
   3. Gonorrhea
      a. Fetus is contaminated at the time of **delivery**.
      b. Maternal infection may result in postpartum infection in the **newborn**.
      c. Risks to the **neonate** include ophthalmia neonatorum, pneumonia, and sepsis.
   4. Chlamydial infection
      a. Transmission may occur during vaginal birth and can result in neonatal conjunctivitis or pneumonitis.
      b. Infection can cause premature rupture of the membranes, premature labor, and postpartum endometritis.
   5. Trichomoniasis: Associated with premature rupture of the membranes and postpartum endometritis
   6. Genital herpes simplex virus
      a. Characterized by painful lesions, fever, chills, malaise, and severe dysuria and may last 2 to 3 weeks
      b. Assessment includes questioning all women about symptoms and inspecting the vulvar, perineal, and vaginal areas for vesicles or areas of ulceration or crusting; this is done during pregnancy and at the onset of labor.
      c. Vaginal birth may be acceptable; cesarean birth is recommended if visible lesions are present.
      d. Infants who are born through an infected vagina should be carefully observed, and samples should be taken for culture.

J. Human immunodeficiency virus (HIV)
   1. HIV is transmitted via blood, blood products, and other body fluids such as urine, semen, and vaginal secretions; the virus is also transmitted through exposure to infected secretions during birth and via breast milk.
   2. Repeated exposure to the virus during pregnancy through unsafe sex practices and/or intravenous drug use can increase the risk of transmission to the fetus.
   3. Perinatal administration of zidovudine may be recommended to decrease risk of transmission of HIV from mother to fetus.

K. Substance abuse
   1. Substance abuse threatens normal fetal growth and the successful term completion of the pregnancy.
   2. Substance abuse places the pregnancy at risk for fetal growth restriction, abruptio placentae, and fetal bradycardia.

3. Many substances cross the placenta and can be teratogenic; no drugs, including tobacco and over-the-counter medications, should be taken unless prescribed by the health care provider.
4. Smoking (tobacco) can lead to low birth weight, a higher incidence of birth defects, and stillbirths.
5. Physical signs of drug abuse may include dilated or contracted pupils, fatigue, track (needle) marks, skin abscesses, inflamed nasal mucosa, and inappropriate behavior by the mother.
6. The consumption of alcohol during pregnancy may lead to fetal alcohol syndrome and can cause jitteriness, physical abnormalities, congenital anomalies, and growth deficits.

L. Viral hepatitis (see Chapter 26 for information regarding hepatitis B infection)

CRITICAL THINKING What Should You Do?

Answer: Physical signs of drug abuse may include dilated or contracted pupils, fatigue, track (needle) marks, skin abscesses, inflamed nasal mucosa, and inappropriate behavior by the mother. If these are noted, the nurse should report the findings to the registered nurse and health care provider so that appropriate assistance can be planned to protect the mother and fetus.

Reference(s): McKinney, E., James, S., Murray, S., Nelson, K. & Ashwill, J. (2013). *Maternal-child nursing* (4th ed., p. 561). St. Louis: Elsevier.

PRACTICE QUESTIONS

216. The client arrives at the prenatal clinic for her first prenatal assessment. The client tells the nurse that the first day of her last menstrual period (LMP) was October 20, 2016. Using Nägele's rule, the nurse determines the estimated date of birth is which?

1. July 12, 2017
2. July 27, 2017
3. August 12, 2017
4. August 27, 2017

217. A pregnant client asks the nurse in the clinic when she will be able to start feeling the fetus move. The nurse responds by telling the mother that fetal movements will be noted between which weeks of gestation?

1. 6 and 8 weeks' gestation
2. 8 and 10 weeks' gestation
3. 10 and 12 weeks' gestation
4. 16 and 20 weeks' gestation

218. The nurse is collecting data from a client who is pregnant with twins. The client has a healthy 5-year-old child who was delivered at 38 weeks, and she tells the nurse that she does not have a history of any type of abortion or fetal demise. The nurse should document the GTPAL for this client as which?

1. G = 3, T = 2, P = 0, A = 0, L = 1
2. G = 2, T = 1, P = 0, A = 0, L = 1
3. G = 1, T = 1, P = 1, A = 0, L = 1
4. G = 2, T = 0, P = 0, A = 0, L = 1

219. The nurse is collecting data from a client who is pregnant with triplets. The client also has a 3-year-old child who was born at 39 weeks' gestation. The nurse should document which gravida and para status on this client?

1. Gravida I, para I
2. Gravida II, para I
3. Gravida II, para II
4. Gravida III, para II

220. The nurse is reviewing the record of a client who has just been told that her pregnancy test is positive. The nurse notes that the health care provider has documented the presence of Goodell's sign. The nurse determines that this sign is indicative of which?

1. A softening of the cervix
2. The presence of fetal movement
3. The presence of human chorionic gonadotropin in the urine
4. A soft blowing sound that corresponds with the maternal pulse that is heard while auscultating the uterus

221. A primipara is being evaluated in the clinic during her second trimester of pregnancy. Which indicates an abnormal physical finding that necessitates further testing?

1. Quickening
2. Braxton Hicks contractions
3. Consistent increase in fundal height
4. Fetal heart rate of 180 beats per minute

222. The nurse is collecting data from a pregnant client who is at 28 weeks' gestation. The nurse measures the fundal height in centimeters and should expect which finding?

1. 22 cm
2. 28 cm
3. 36 cm
4. 40 cm

223. A pregnant client is seen in the health care clinic for a regular prenatal visit. The client tells the nurse that she is experiencing irregular contractions.

The nurse determines that the client is experiencing Braxton Hicks contractions. Based on this finding, which nursing action is appropriate?

1. Contact the health care provider.
2. Instruct the client to maintain bed rest for the remainder of the pregnancy.
3. Tell the client that these are common and they may occur throughout the pregnancy.
4. Call the maternity unit and inform them that the client will be admitted in a prelabor condition.

❖ **224.** The nurse is collecting data from a client who suspects she is pregnant. The nurse is checking the client for probable signs of pregnancy. Which are the probable signs of pregnancy that the nurse should note? **Select all that apply.**

- ❑ 1. Ballottement
- ❑ 2. Chadwick's sign
- ❑ 3. Uterine enlargement
- ❑ 4. Braxton Hicks contractions
- ❑ 5. Outline of fetus via radiography or ultrasound
- ❑ 6. Fetal heart rate detected by a nonelectronic device

225. The nursing instructor asks a nursing student to describe the process of quickening. Which statement indicates an understanding of this term?

1. "It is the fetal movement that is felt by the mother."
2. "It is the compressibility of the lower uterine segment."
3. "It is the irregular, painless contractions that occur throughout pregnancy."
4. "It is the soft blowing sound that can be heard when the uterus is auscultated."

ANSWERS

216. 2

Rationale: The accurate use of Nägele's rule requires that the woman have a regular 28-day menstrual cycle. Subtract 3 months from the first day of the last menstrual period, add 7 days, and then adjust the year as appropriate. In this case, the first day of the LMP was October 20, 2016. When you subtract 3 months, you get July 20, 2016. If you add 7 days, you get July 27, 2016. Add 1 year to this, and you get the estimated date of birth: July 27, 2017.

Test-Taking Strategy: Follow the subject, Nägele's rule, to answer this question. Read all of the options carefully, and use this rule. Then, note the dates and years in the options before selecting an answer. **Review: Nägele's rule.**

Level of Cognitive Ability: Applying

Client Needs: Health Promotion and Maintenance

Integrated Process: Nursing Process/Data Collection

Content Area: Maternity: Antepartum

Priority Concepts: Clinical Judgment, Reproduction

Reference(s): McKinney et al (2013), p. 247.

217. 4

Rationale: Quickening is fetal movement that usually first occurs between 16 and 20 weeks' gestation. The expectant mother first notices subtle fetal movements during this time, and these gradually increase in intensity. Options 1, 2, and 3 are incorrect; these gestational time frames are too early for quickening.

Test-Taking Strategy: Focus on the subject, the occurrence of quickening. In this situation, it is best to select the option that indicates the greatest length of gestational time. **Review:** the process of quickening.

Level of Cognitive Ability: Applying

Client Needs: Health Promotion and Maintenance

Integrated Process: Teaching and Learning

Content Area: Maternity: Antepartum

Priority Concepts: Client Education, Reproduction

Reference(s): McKinney et al (2013), p. 244.

218. 2

Rationale: Pregnancy outcomes can be described with the GTPAL acronym: G = gravidity (number of pregnancies); T = term births (number born after 37 weeks); P = preterm births (number born before 37 weeks' gestation); A = abortions/miscarriages (number of abortions/miscarriages); L = live births (number of live births or living children). Therefore, a woman who is pregnant with twins and who already has a child has a gravida of 2. Because the child was delivered at 38 weeks, the number of preterm births is 0, and the number of term births is 1. The number of abortions is 0, and the number of live births is 1.

Test-Taking Strategy: Specific knowledge about the subject, GTPAL, is needed to answer this question. Your knowledge and understanding will direct you to the correct option. **Review:** the GTPAL method of describing pregnancy outcomes.

Level of Cognitive Ability: Applying

Client Needs: Health Promotion and Maintenance

Integrated Process: Nursing Process/Data Collection

Content Area: Maternity: Antepartum

Priority Concepts: Clinical Judgment, Reproduction

Reference(s): McKinney et al (2013), pp. 246–247.

219. 2

Rationale: *Gravida* is a term that refers to a woman who is or who has been pregnant, regardless of the duration of the pregnancy. *Parity* is a term that means the number of births after 20 weeks' gestation; it does not reflect the number of fetuses or infants. Options 1, 3, and 4 are incorrect on the basis of these definitions.

Test-Taking Strategy: Focus on the subject, the terms gravida and parity, which are necessary to answer this question correctly. Remember that *gravida* refers to a woman who is or has been pregnant, regardless of the duration of the pregnancy. *Parity* means the number of births past 20 weeks' gestation. Review: the definitions of gravida and parity.

Level of Cognitive Ability: Applying

Client Needs: Physiological Integrity

Integrated Process: Nursing Process/Implementation

Content Area: Maternity: Antepartum

Priority Concepts: Clinical Judgment, Reproduction

Reference(s): McKinney et al (2013), pp. 246–247.

220. 1

Rationale: During the early weeks of pregnancy, the cervix becomes softer as a result of pelvic vasoconstriction, which

causes Goodell's sign. Cervical softening is noted by the examiner during a pelvic examination. Goodell's sign does not indicate the presence of fetal movement. Human chorionic gonadotropin is noted in maternal urine with a positive urine pregnancy test. A soft blowing sound that corresponds with the maternal pulse may be auscultated over the uterus; it is the result of blood circulating through the placenta.
Test-Taking Strategy: Focus on the subject, the physiological findings of Goodell's sign. Remember that Goodell's sign refers to a softening of the cervix. **Review: Goodell's sign** that occurs during pregnancy.
Level of Cognitive Ability: Evaluating
Client Needs: Health Promotion and Maintenance
Integrated Process: Nursing Process/Data Collection
Content Area: Maternity: Antepartum
Priority Concepts: Clinical Judgment, Reproduction
Reference(s): McKinney et al (2013), pp. 235, 244.

221. 4
Rationale: The fetal heart rate depends on the gestational age. It is 160 to 170 beats per minute during the first trimester, and it slows with fetal growth to approximately 120 to 160 beats per minute. Options 1, 2, and 3 are normal expected findings.
Test-Taking Strategy: Focus on the subject, an abnormal physical finding. Recalling the normal fetal heart rate will direct you to the correct option. **Review:** the normal **assessment findings of pregnancy**.
Level of Cognitive Ability: Analyzing
Client Needs: Physiological Integrity
Integrated Process: Nursing Process/Data Collection
Content Area: Maternity: Antepartum
Priority Concepts: Perfusion, Reproduction
Reference(s): McKinney et al (2013), p. 251.

222. 2
Rationale: During the second and third trimesters (18 to 30 weeks' gestation), the fundal height in centimeters approximately equals the fetus's age in weeks plus or minus 2 cm. At 14 to 16 weeks' gestation, the fundus can be located halfway between the symphysis pubis and the umbilicus. At 20 to 22 weeks' gestation, the fundus is at the umbilicus, and at term, the fundus is at the xiphoid process.
Test-Taking Strategy: Focus on the subject, expected fundal height at 28 weeks gestation. Remember that during the second and third trimesters, the fundal height in centimeters approximately equals the fetus's age in weeks plus or minus 2 cm. **Review: fundal height**.
Level of Cognitive Ability: Understanding
Client Needs: Health Promotion and Maintenance
Integrated Process: Nursing Process/Data Collection
Content Area: Maternity: Antepartum
Priority Concepts: Clinical Judgment, Reproduction
References: McKinney et al (2013), pp. 250–251.

223. 3
Rationale: Braxton Hicks contractions are irregular, painless contractions that may occur intermittently throughout pregnancy. Because Braxton Hicks contractions may occur and are normal in some pregnant women during pregnancy, options 1, 2, and 4 are unnecessary and inappropriate actions.
Test-Taking Strategy: Options 1 and 4 are comparable or alike and can thus be eliminated first. From the remaining options, knowing that Braxton Hicks contractions are common and can occur throughout pregnancy will assist with directing you to the correct option. **Review:** the physiology associated with **Braxton Hicks** contractions.
Level of Cognitive Ability: Applying
Client Needs: Health Promotion and Maintenance
Integrated Process: Nursing Process/Implementation
Content Area: Maternity: Antepartum
Priority Concepts: Client Education, Reproduction
Reference(s): McKinney et al (2013), pp. 235, 244.

❖ **224. 1, 2, 3, 4**
Rationale: The probable signs of pregnancy include uterine enlargement; Hegar's sign (the compressibility and softening of the lower uterine segment that occurs at about week 6); Goodell's sign (the softening of the cervix that occurs at the beginning of the second month of pregnancy); Chadwick's sign (the violet coloration of the mucous membranes of the cervix, vagina, and vulva that occurs at about week 4); ballottement (the rebounding of the fetus against the examiner's fingers on palpation); Braxton Hicks contractions; and a positive pregnancy test that measures for human chorionic gonadotropin. Positive signs of pregnancy include a fetal heart rate that is detected by an electronic device (Doppler transducer) at 10 to 12 weeks' gestation and by a nonelectronic device (fetoscope) at 20 weeks' gestation; active fetal movements that are palpable by the examiner; and an outline of the fetus via radiography or ultrasound.
Test-Taking Strategy: Focusing on the subject, the probable signs of pregnancy, will assist you with answering this question. Remember that the detection of the fetal heart rate and an outline of the fetus via radiography or ultrasound are positive signs of pregnancy. **Review:** the **probable signs of pregnancy**.
Level of Cognitive Ability: Evaluating
Client Needs: Health Promotion and Maintenance
Integrated Process: Nursing Process/Data Collection
Content Area: Maternity: Antepartum
Priority Concepts: Clinical Judgment, Reproduction
Reference(s): McKinney et al (2013), p. 244.

225. 1
Rationale: Quickening is fetal movement that appears usually at weeks 16 to 20, when the expectant mother first notices subtle fetal movements that gradually increase in intensity. A compressibility of the lower uterine segment occurs at about 6 weeks' gestation and is called *Hegar's sign*. Braxton Hicks contractions are irregular, painless contractions that may occur throughout pregnancy. A soft blowing sound that corresponds with the maternal pulse may be auscultated over the uterus; this is known as *uterine souffle*. This sound is the result of blood circulation to the placenta, and it corresponds with the maternal pulse.
Test-Taking Strategy: Focus on the subject, a description of quickening. Remember that *quickening* is fetal movement. **Review: quickening**.
Level of Cognitive Ability: Understanding
Client Needs: Health Promotion and Maintenance
Integrated Process: Teaching and Learning
Content Area: Maternity: Antepartum
Priority Concepts: Perfusion, Reproduction
Reference(s): McKinney et al (2013), p. 244.

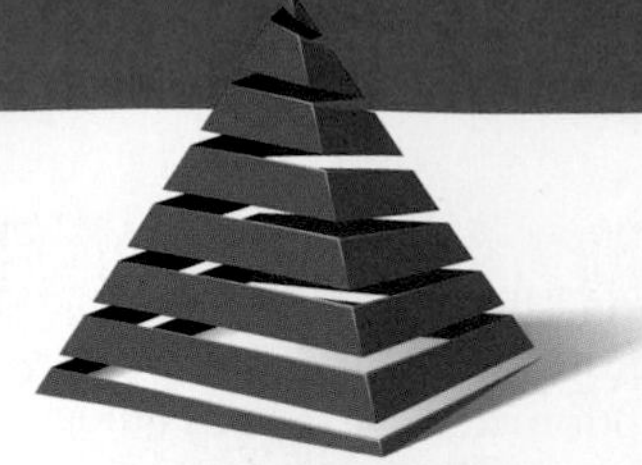

CHAPTER 26

Prenatal Period and Risk Conditions

CRITICAL THINKING What Should You Do?

The pregnant client tells the nurse that she is experiencing morning sickness. What information should the nurse provide to the client to assist in relief of this problem?

Answer is located on p. 297.

I. Physiological Maternal Changes

A. Cardiovascular system
   1. Circulating blood volume increases by approximately 40% to 50%; physiological anemia may occur as the plasma increase exceeds the increase in the production of red blood cells.
   2. Heart size is increased, and the heart is elevated upward and to the left because of displacement of the diaphragm as the **uterus** enlarges (Fig. 26-1).
   3. There is an increase in the body's demand for iron.
   4. Sodium and water retention may occur, which can lead to weight gain.

B. Respiratory system
   1. Oxygen consumption increases by approximately 15% to 20%
   2. Diaphragm is elevated as a result of the enlarged uterus (see Fig. 26-1).
   3. Shortness of breath may be experienced.

⚠ During pregnancy, a woman's pulse rate may increase about 10 to 15 beats/minute, the blood pressure slightly decreases in the second trimester, and the respiratory rate remains unchanged or slightly increases.

C. Gastrointestinal (GI) system
   1. Nausea and vomiting may occur as a result of the secretion of human chorionic gonadotropin (hCG), which usually subsides by the third month.
   2. Lack of appetite may occur because of decreased gastric motility.
   3. Alterations in taste and smell may occur.
   4. Constipation may occur because of an increase in progesterone production or pressure of the uterus, resulting in decreased gastrointestinal motility.
   5. Flatulence and heartburn may occur because of decreased gastrointestinal motility and slowed emptying of the stomach caused by an increase in progesterone production.
   6. Hemorrhoids may occur as a result of increased venous pressure.
   7. Gum tissue may become swollen and easily bleed because of increasing levels of estrogen.
   8. Ptyalism (excessive secretion of saliva) may occur because of increasing levels of estrogen.

D. Renal system
   1. Frequency of urination increases in the first and third trimesters because of increased bladder sensitivity and pressure of the enlarging uterus on the bladder.
   2. Decreased bladder tone may occur and is caused by an increase in progesterone and estrogen levels; bladder capacity increases in response to increasing levels of progesterone.
   3. The renal threshold for glucose may be reduced.

E. Endocrine system
   1. Basal metabolic rate and metabolic function increases.
   2. Anterior lobe of pituitary gland enlarges.
   3. Thyroid gland enlarges slightly and thyroid activity increases.
   4. Parathyroid gland increases in size.
   5. Aldosterone levels gradually increase.
   6. Body weight increases.
   7. Water retention is increased, which can contribute to weight gain.

F. Reproductive system
   1. Uterus
      a. Uterus enlarges, increasing in mass from approximately 60 to 1000 g as a result of hyperplasia (influence of estrogen) and hypertrophy.
      b. Size and number of blood vessels and lymphatics increase.
      c. Irregular contractions occur.

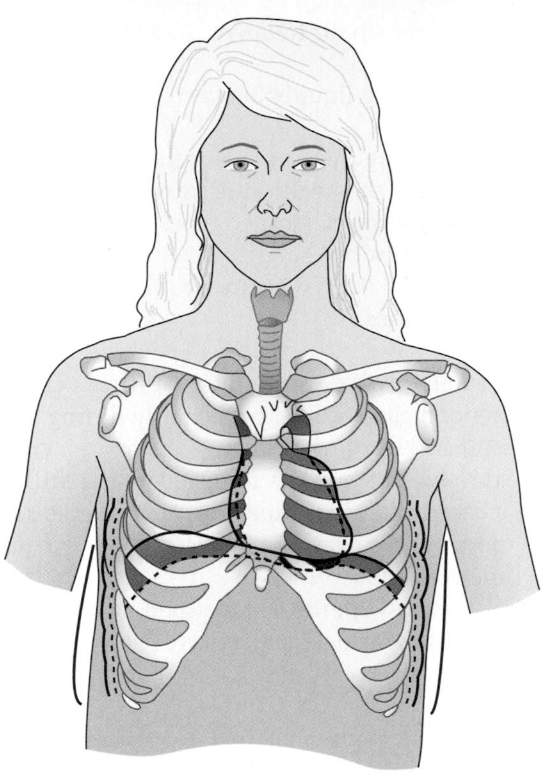

FIGURE 26-1 Changes in position of the heart, lungs, and thoracic cage in pregnancy. *Broken line*, nonpregnant state; *solid line*, change that occurs during pregnancy. (From Perry S, Hockenberry M, Lowdermilk D, Wilson D: *Maternal-child nursing care*, ed 4, St. Louis, 2010, Mosby.)

2. Cervix
   a. Cervix becomes shorter, more elastic, and larger in diameter.
   b. Endocervical glands secrete a thick mucus plug, which is expelled from the canal when dilation begins.
   c. Increased vascularization and an increase in estrogen causes a softening and a violet discoloration (**Chadwick's sign**), which occurs at about week 4.
3. Ovaries
   a. Secrete progesterone for first 6 to 7 weeks of pregnancy
   b. Block maturation of new follicles
   c. Cease ovum production
4. Vagina
   a. Hypertrophy and thickening of the muscle occurs.
   b. Increase in vaginal secretions is experienced; secretions are usually thick, white, and acidic.
5. Breasts
   a. Breast size increases, and breasts may be tender.
   b. Nipples become more pronounced, and the areolae become darker, with an increase in ductal growth.
   c. Superficial veins become prominent.

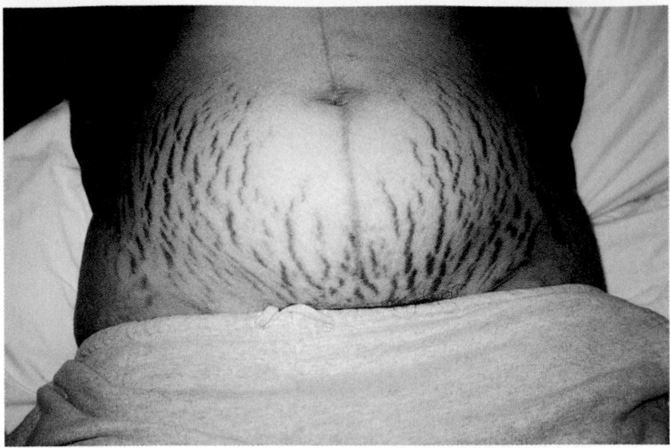

FIGURE 26-2 Striae gravidarum and linea nigra in a dark-skinned person. (From Perry S, Hockenberry M, Lowdermilk D, Wilson D: *Maternal-child nursing care*, ed 4, St. Louis, 2010, Mosby. Courtesy Shannon Perry, Phoenix, AZ).

   d. Montgomery's follicles become hypertrophied.
   e. Colostrum may leak from the breasts.

G. Skin
1. Changes in skin occur because of increased levels of melanocyte-stimulating hormone, which increase secondary to increases in estrogen and progesterone; these changes include the following:
   a. Increased pigmentation
   b. A dark streak down the midline of the abdomen may appear (linea nigra; (Fig. 26-2).
   c. Chloasma (mask of pregnancy), which is a blotchy, brownish hyperpigmentation, may occur over the forehead, cheeks, and nose.
   d. Reddish-purple stretch marks (striae) may occur on the abdomen, breasts, thighs, and upper arms. (See Fig. 26-2.)
2. Vascular spider nevi may occur on neck, chest, face, arms, and legs.
3. The rate of hair growth may increase.

H. Musculoskeletal system
1. Changes in center of gravity begin in the second trimester and are caused by the hormones relaxin and progesterone.
2. The lumbrosacral curve increases.
3. Aching, numbness, and weakness may result; walking becomes more difficult, and the woman develops a waddling gait and is at risk for falls.
4. Relaxation and increased mobility of pelvic joints occurs, which permit enlargement of pelvic dimensions.
5. Abdominal wall stretches with loss of tone throughout pregnancy, regained postpartum.
6. Umbilicus flattens or protrudes.

During pregnancy, postural changes occur as the increased weight of uterus causes a forward pull of the bony pelvis. It is important for the nurse to encourage the client to implement measures that maintain correct posture to prevent a backache.

II. Psychological Maternal Changes

A. Ambivalence
1. May occur early in pregnancy, even when the pregnancy is planned
2. Mother may experience a dependence–independence conflict and ambivalence related to role changes.
3. Partner may experience ambivalence related to assuming a new role, increased financial responsibilities, and having to share attention with the child.

B. Acceptance: Factors that may be related to the acceptance of the pregnancy are the woman's readiness for the experience and her identification with the motherhood role.

C. Emotional ability
1. Manifested by frequency in the change of emotional states or extremes in emotional states caused by hormone changes
2. These emotional changes are common, but the mother may believe that these changes are abnormal.

D. Body image changes
1. The changes in a woman's perception of her image during pregnancy occur gradually and may be positive or negative.
2. Physical changes and symptoms that the woman experiences during pregnancy contribute to her body image.

E. Relationship with the fetus
1. The woman may daydream to prepare for motherhood and think about the maternal qualities she would like to possess.
2. The woman first accepts the biological fact that she is pregnant.
3. The woman next accepts the growing fetus as distinct from herself and a person to nurture.
4. Finally, the woman prepares realistically for the birth and parenting of the child.

III. Discomforts of Pregnancy

A. Nausea and vomiting
1. Occurs during the first trimester and subsides by the third month
2. Caused by elevated hCG levels and changes in carbohydrate metabolism
3. Interventions
   a. Eating dry crackers before rising
   b. Avoiding brushing the teeth immediately after rising
   c. Eating small, frequent, low-fat meals during the day
   d. Drinking liquids between meals rather than at meals
   e. Avoiding fried and spicy foods
   f. Asking the health care provider (HCP) about acupressure (some types may require a prescription)
   g. Asking the HCP about the use of herbal remedies

B. Syncope
1. Usually occurs during the first trimester; supine hypotension occurs, particularly during the second and third trimesters
2. May be hormonally triggered or caused by increased blood volume, anemia, fatigue, sudden position changes, or lying supine
3. Interventions
   a. Sitting with the feet elevated
   b. Changing positions slowly because of the risk for falls

The nurse needs to inform the pregnant client to avoid lying in the supine position, particularly in the second and third trimesters. The supine position places the woman at risk for supine hypotension, which occurs as a result of pressure of the uterus on the inferior vena cava.

C. Urinary urgency and frequency
1. Usually occurs during the first and third trimesters
2. Caused by the pressure of the uterus on the bladder
3. Interventions
   a. Drinking no less than 2000 mL of fluid during the day
   b. Limiting fluid intake during the evening
   c. Voiding at regular intervals
   d. Sleeping on the side at night
   e. Wearing perineal pads, if necessary
   f. Performing Kegel exercises

D. Breast tenderness
1. Can occur from the first through the third trimesters
2. Caused by increased levels of estrogen and progesterone
3. Interventions
   a. Encouraging wearing a supportive bra
   b. Avoiding the use of soap on the nipples and areolae to prevent drying

E. Increased vaginal discharge
1. Can occur from the first through the third trimesters
2. Caused by hypertrophy and thickening of the vaginal mucosa and increased mucus production

3. Interventions
   a. Using proper cleansing and hygiene techniques
   b. Wearing cotton underwear
   c. Avoiding douching
   d. Informing the client of the signs of infection and to consult the HCP if an infection is suspected

F. Nasal stuffiness or nosebleeds
1. Occur during the first through the third trimesters
2. Occur as a result of increased estrogen that causes swelling of the nasal tissues and dryness
3. Interventions
   a. Encouraging the use of a humidifier
   b. Avoiding the use of nasal sprays or antihistamines (the HCP should always be consulted regarding their use)

G. Fatigue
1. Occurs usually during the first and third trimesters
2. Is usually the result of hormonal changes
3. Interventions
   a. Arranging frequent rest periods throughout the day
   b. Using correct body mechanics
   c. Engaging in regular exercise with HCP approval
   d. Performing muscle relaxation and strengthening exercises for the legs and hip joints
   e. Avoiding eating and drinking foods that contain stimulants throughout the pregnancy

H. Heartburn
1. Occurs during the second and third trimesters
2. Results from increased progesterone levels, decreased GI motility, esophageal reflux, and the displacement of the stomach by the enlarging uterus
3. Interventions
   a. Eating small, frequent meals and avoid fatty and spicy food
   b. Sitting upright for 30 minutes after a meal
   c. Drinking milk between meals
   d. Performing tailor-sitting exercises
   e. Consulting with the HCP about the use of antacids

I. Ankle edema
1. Usually occurs during the second and third trimesters
2. Occurs as a result of vasodilation, venous stasis, and increased venous pressure below the uterus
3. Interventions
   a. Elevating the legs at least twice a day and when resting
   b. Sleeping in a side-lying position
   c. Wearing supportive stockings
   d. Avoiding sitting or standing in one position for long periods

J. Varicose veins
1. Usually occur during the second and third trimesters
2. Occur because of weakening walls of the veins or valves and venous congestion
3. Interventions
   a. Wearing supportive stockings or hose
   b. Elevating the feet when sitting
   c. Lying with the feet and hips elevated
   d. Avoiding long periods of standing or sitting
   e. Moving about while standing to improve circulation
   f. Avoiding leg crossing
   g. Avoiding constricting articles of clothing such as knee-high stockings
4. Thrombophlebitis is rare, but it may occur.
   a. Teaching leg exercises
   b. Avoiding airline travel if possible

K. Headaches
1. Usually occur during the second and third trimesters
2. Occur as a result of changes in blood volume and vascular tone
3. Interventions
   a. Changing position slowly
   b. Applying a cool cloth to the forehead
   c. Eating a small snack
   d. Using acetaminophen (Tylenol) only if prescribed by the HCP

L. Hemorrhoids
1. Usually occur during the second and third trimesters
2. Occur as a result of increased venous pressure and constipation
3. Interventions
   a. Soaking in a warm sitz bath
   b. Sitting on a soft pillow
   c. Eating high-fiber foods and drinking sufficient fluids to avoid constipation
   d. Increasing exercise, such as walking
   e. Applying ointments, suppositories, or compresses as prescribed by the HCP

M. Constipation
1. Usually occurs during the second and third trimesters
2. Results from an increase in progesterone production, decreased intestinal motility, displacement of the intestines, pressure of the uterus, and taking iron supplements
3. Interventions
   a. Eating high-fiber foods such as whole grains, fruits, and vegetables
   b. Drinking no less than 2000 mL per day
   c. Exercising regularly, such as a daily 20-minute walk
   d. Consulting with the health care provider about interventions such as the use of stool softeners, laxatives, or enemas

N. Backache
1. Usually occurs during the second and third trimesters
2. Occurs as a result of the exaggerated lumbosacral curve, resulting from an enlarged uterus
3. Risk for falls; teach to move about slowly
4. Interventions
a. Obtaining rest
b. Using correct posture and body mechanics
c. Wearing low-heeled, comfortable, and supportive shoes
d. Performing pelvic tilt (rock) exercises and conscious relaxation exercises
e. Sleeping on a firm mattress

O. Leg cramps
1. Usually occur during the second and third trimesters
2. Occur as a result of an altered calcium–phosphorus balance, the pressure of the uterus on nerves, or from fatigue
3. Interventions
a. Getting regular exercise, such as walking
b. Dorsiflexing the foot of the affected leg
c. Increasing calcium intake

P. Shortness of breath
1. Can occur during the second and third trimesters
2. Occurs as a result of pressure on the diaphragm from the enlarged uterus
3. Interventions
a. Taking frequent rest periods and avoiding overexertion
b. Sitting and sleeping with the head elevated or on the side

IV. Antepartum Diagnostic Testing

⚠ The usual schedule for antepartum health care visits is every 4 weeks for the first 28 to 32 weeks, every 2 weeks from 32 to 36 weeks, and every week from 36 to 40 weeks.

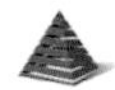

A. Blood type and Rh factor
1. ABO typing is performed to determine the woman's blood type in the ABO antigen system.
2. Rh typing is done to determine the woman's blood type in the rhesus antigen system (Rh positive indicates the presence of the antigen; Rh negative indicates the absence of the antigen).
3. If the client is Rh negative and has a negative antibody screen, the client will need repeat antibody screens and should receive Rh_o(D) immune globulin (RhoGAM) at 28 weeks' gestation.

B. Rubella titer
1. If the client has a negative titer (less than 1:8), this indicates susceptibility to the rubella virus. The client should receive the appropriate immunization postpartum.
2. The client must be using effective birth control at the time of the immunization. She must be counseled not to become pregnant for 1 to 3 months after immunization (as specified by the HCP) and to avoid contact with anyone who is immunocompromised.
3. If the rubella vaccine is administered at the same time as the Rh_o(D) immune globulin, it may not be effective.

⚠ Rubella vaccine is not given during pregnancy because the live attenuated virus may cross the placenta and present a risk to the developing fetus.

C. Hemoglobin and hematocrit levels
1. Hemoglobin and hematocrit levels decline during gestation as a result of increased plasma volume.
2. A decrease in the hemoglobin level below 10 g/dL or a decrease in the hematocrit level below 30% indicates anemia.

D. Papanicolaou (Pap) smear: Done during the initial prenatal examination to screen for cervical neoplasia

E. Sexually transmitted infections (Table 26-1)

F. Sickle cell screening
1. Indicated for clients who are at risk for sickle cell disease
2. A positive test result may indicate a need for further screening.

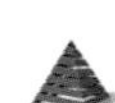

G. Tuberculin skin test
1. The HCP may prefer to perform this skin test after **delivery**.
2. A positive skin test indicates the need for a chest radiograph (using an abdominal lead shield) to rule out active disease. In a pregnant client, a chest radiograph will not be performed until after 20 weeks' gestation (after the fetal organs are formed).
3. Those who convert to positive may be referred for treatment with medication after delivery.

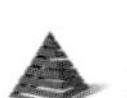

H. Hepatitis B surface antigen
1. Recommended for all women because of the prevalence of the disease in the general population
2. Vaccination for hepatitis B antigen may be specifically indicated for the following:
a. Health care workers
b. Intravenous (IV) drug abusers
c. Clients born in high-risk countries such as Asia, Africa, Haiti, or the Pacific islands
d. Clients with previously undiagnosed jaundice or chronic liver disease
e. Clients with tattoos
f. Clients with histories of blood transfusions
g. Clients with histories of multiple episodes of sexually transmitted infections

TABLE 26-1 Monitoring for Sexually Transmitted Infections

Disease	Laboratory Test
Gonorrhea	A vaginal culture is performed during the initial prenatal examination to screen for gonorrhea; it may be repeated during the third trimester for high-risk clients.
Syphilis	A culture of lesions (if present) is performed during the initial prenatal examination to screen for syphilis. Diagnosis is dependent on the microscopic examination of primary and secondary lesion tissue and serology (Venereal Disease Research Laboratory [VDRL] or rapid plasma reagin test) during latency and late infection. The culture may be repeated during the third trimester for high-risk clients.
Condyloma acuminatum (human papillomavirus)	Culture is indicated for clients with positive history or with active lesions. Test is performed to determine route of delivery. Weekly cultures may be done at weeks 35 or 36 of pregnancy until delivery.
Chlamydia	Vaginal culture is indicated for all pregnant clients if client is in a high-risk group or if infants from previous pregnancies have developed neonatal conjunctivitis or pneumonia.
Trichomoniasis	Normal saline wet smear of vaginal secretions is checked for presence of protozoa. Associated with premature rupture of membranes and postpartum endometritis.
Genital herpes simplex virus (HSV-2)	Culture is done of lesions (if present) during initial prenatal examination to screen for HSV. Microscopic examination is done to determine presence of virus. Additional screening may be necessary as pregnancy progresses.
HIV	Testing may be done for high-risk client. Common tests to determine the presence of antibodies include ELISA, Western blot, and immunofluorescence assay (IFA).
Bacterial vaginosis	Microscopic examination of vaginal secretions identifies the infection.
Vaginal candidiasis	Diagnosis is by identifying the spores of *Candida albicans* in the vagina.

ELISA, Enzyme-linked immunosorbent assay; *HIV*, human immunodeficiency virus.

h. Clients who have been rejected previously as blood donors
i. Clients with histories of dialysis or renal transplantation
j. Clients from households having hepatitis B–infected members or hemodialysis clients

3. Hepatitis B vaccine is not contraindicated during pregnancy and may be recommended by the HCP.
4. See Chapter 47 for additional information about hepatitis.

I. Urinalysis and urine culture
1. A urine specimen for glucose and protein determinations should be obtained at every prenatal visit.
2. Glycosuria is a common result of decreased renal threshold that occurs during pregnancy.
3. If glycosuria persists, this may indicate diabetes mellitus.
4. White blood cells in the urine may indicate infection.
5. Ketonuria may result from insufficient food intake or vomiting.
6. Protein levels of 2+ to 4+ in the urine may indicate infection or preeclampsia.

J. Ultrasonography
1. Outlines and identifies fetal and maternal structures
2. Assists in confirming gestational age and estimated date of delivery and evaluating **amniotic fluid** volume (amniotic fluid index), which is done via special measurements
3. May be done abdominally or transvaginally during pregnancy
4. Interventions
a. If an abdominal ultrasound is being performed, the woman may be asked to drink water to fill the bladder before the procedure to obtain a better image of the fetus.
b. If a transvaginal ultrasound is being performed, a lubricated probe is inserted into the **vagina**.
c. Inform the client that the test presents no known risks to the client or the fetus.

K. Biophysical profile
1. Noninvasive assessment of the fetus that includes fetal breathing movements, fetal movements, fetal tone, amniotic fluid index, and fetal heart rate patterns via a nonstress test
2. Normal fetal biophysical activities indicate that the central nervous system is functional and the fetus is not hypoxemic.

L. Doppler blood flow analysis; noninvasive (ultrasonography) method of studying blood flow in the fetus and **placenta**

M. Percutaneous umbilical blood sampling
1. Performed if fetal blood sampling is necessary
2. Involves insertion of needle directly into fetal umbilical vessel under ultrasound guidance

3. Fetal heart rate monitoring is necessary for 1 hour after procedure, and a follow-up ultrasound to check for bleeding or hematoma formation is done 1 hour after the procedure.

N. Alpha-fetoprotein (AFP) screening
1. Assesses the quantity of fetal serum proteins; abnormal protein levels are associated with open neural tube and abdominal wall defects.
2. Can detect spina bifida and Down syndrome
3. If abnormal, the test is repeated; a false-positive test result is common.
4. Interventions
   a. The AFP level is determined by a maternal blood sample drawn between 16 and 18 weeks' gestation.
   b. If the level is abnormal and the gestation is less than 18 weeks, a second sample is drawn and screened.
   c. An ultrasound is performed for elevated levels to rule out fetal abnormalities or multiple gestation.

O. Chorionic villus sampling (CVS)
1. Performed for the purpose of detecting genetic abnormalities; the HCP aspirates a small sample of chorionic villus tissue at 10 to 13 weeks' gestation.
2. Interventions
   a. The client may need to drink water to fill the bladder before the procedure to aid in visualizing the uterus for catheter insertion.
   b. Obtain baseline vital signs and fetal heart rate; monitor frequently after the procedure.
   c. Rh-negative women may be given Rh_o(D) immune globulin (RhoGAM), because chorionic villus sampling increases the risk of Rh sensitization.

⚠ The nurse needs to ensure that an informed consent has been obtained for any procedure that is invasive, such as a chorionic villus sampling or amniocentesis.

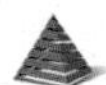 **P.** Amniocentesis
1. Aspiration of amniotic fluid; best performed between 15 and 20 weeks of pregnancy because amniotic fluid volume is adequate and many viable fetal cells are present in the fluid by this time
2. Performed to determine genetic disorders, metabolic defects, and fetal lung maturity
3. Risks
   a. Maternal hemorrhage
   b. Infection
   c. Rh isoimmunization
   d. Abruptio placentae
   e. Amniotic fluid emboli
   f. Premature rupture of the membranes
4. Interventions
   a. If less than 20 weeks' gestation, the woman should have a full bladder to support the uterus. If more than 20 weeks' gestation, the woman should have an empty bladder to minimize the chance of puncture.
   b. Prepare the client for ultrasonography, which is performed to locate the placenta and avoid puncture of it.
   c. Obtain baseline vital signs and fetal heart rate. Monitor every 15 minutes.
   d. Position the client supine during the procedure and on the left side after the procedure.

⚠ After chorionic villus sampling and amniocentesis, instruct the client that if chills, fever, bleeding, leakage of fluid at the needle insertion site, decreased fetal movement, uterine contractions, or cramping occurs, she must notify the HCP.

Q. Kick counts (fetal movement counting)
1. The client is instructed to sit quietly or lie down on her side and counts fetal kicks for a period of time, as instructed.
2. Instruct the client to notify the HCP if there are fewer than 10 kicks in two consecutive 2-hour periods or as instructed by her HCP.

R. Fern test
1. A microscopic slide test to determine the presence of amniotic fluid leakage
2. Using sterile technique, a specimen is obtained from the external os of the cervix and vaginal pool and examined on a slide under a microscope.
3. A fernlike pattern that results from the salts of amniotic fluid indicates the presence of amniotic fluid.
4. Interventions
   a. Position the client in the dorsal lithotomy position.
   b. Instruct the client to cough. This causes the fluid to leak from the uterus if the membranes are ruptured.

S. Nitrazine test
1. A Nitrazine test strip is used to detect the presence of amniotic fluid in vaginal secretions.
2. Vaginal secretions have a pH of 4.5 to 5.5. They do not affect the yellow color of the Nitrazine strip or swab.
3. Amniotic fluid has a pH of 7.0 to 7.5 and turns the yellow Nitrazine strip or swab blue in color.
4. Interventions
   a. Position the client in the dorsal lithotomy position.
   b. Touch the test tape to the fluid.
   c. Check the test tape for a blue-green, blue-gray, or deep blue color, which indicates that the membranes are probably ruptured.

Maternity

T. Fibronectin test
   1. Sampling of cervical and vaginal secretions for fetal fibronectin is done (a protein present in fetal tissues normally found in cervical and vaginal secretions until 16 to 20 weeks' gestation and again at or near term)
   2. Positive results indicate the onset of labor in 1 to 3 weeks.
   3. Test is used if the client is at risk for preterm labor, before 37 weeks' gestation.
   4. Interventions
      a. Client is placed in lithotomy position for a sterile speculum exam.
      b. Cervical secretions are obtained with a cotton swab.
      c. Laboratory tests are done for the presence of fibronectin.

U. Nonstress test (Box 26-1)

V. Contraction stress test (Box 26-2)

BOX 26-1 Nonstress Test

Description

- Performed to assess placental function and oxygenation
- Determines fetal well-being
- Evaluates fetal heart rate (FHR) in response to fetal movement

Interventions

- An external ultrasound transducer and tocodynamometer are applied to the mother, and a tracing of at least 20 minutes' duration is obtained so that the FHR and the uterine activity can be observed.
- Obtain a baseline blood pressure reading, and monitor the blood pressure frequently.
- Position the mother in the left lateral position to avoid vena cava compression.
- The mother may be asked to press a button every time she feels fetal movement. The monitor records a mark at each point of fetal movement, and this is used as a reference point to assess FHR response.

Results

Reactive Nonstress Test (Normal, Negative)

"Reactive" indicates a healthy fetus.

The result requires two or more FHR accelerations of at least 15 beats per minute and lasting at least 15 seconds from the beginning of the acceleration to the end, in association with fetal movement, during a 20-minute period.

Nonreactive Nonstress Test (Abnormal)

No accelerations or accelerations of less than 15 beats per minute or lasting less than 15 seconds in duration during a 40-minute observation

Unsatisfactory

The result cannot be interpreted because of the poor quality of the FHR tracing.

BOX 26-2 Contraction Stress Test

Description

- Assesses placental oxygenation and function
- Determines fetal ability to tolerate labor and determines fetal well-being
- Fetus is exposed to the stress of contractions to assess the adequacy of placental perfusion under simulated labor conditions
- Performed if the nonstress test is abnormal

Interventions

- The external fetal monitor is applied to the mother, and a 20- to 30-minute baseline strip is recorded.
- The uterus is stimulated to contract, either by the administration of a dilute dose of oxytocin (Pitocin) or by having the mother use nipple stimulation, until three palpable contractions with a duration of 40 seconds or more during a 10-minute period have been achieved.
- Frequent maternal blood pressure readings are obtained, and the mother is monitored closely while increasing doses of oxytocin are given.

Results

Negative Contraction Stress Test (Normal)

Represented by no late decelerations of the fetal heart rate (FHR)

Positive Contraction Stress Test (Abnormal)

Represented by late decelerations of the FHR with 50% or more of the contractions in the absence of hyperstimulation of the uterus

Equivocal

Contains decelerations but with less than 50% of the contractions, or uterine activity shows a hyperstimulated uterus

Unsatisfactory

Adequate uterine contractions cannot be achieved, or the FHR tracing is not of sufficient quality for adequate interpretation.

V. Nutrition

A. General guidelines
   1. Guidelines for health and nutrition information for breastfeeding and pregnant women are located at the U.S. Department of Agriculture ChooseMyPlate website at http://www.choosemyplate.gov/pregnancy-breastfeeding.html. The woman should be assisted with accessing this site and preparing a nutritional plan.
   2. The average expected weight gain during pregnancy is 25 to 35 pounds for women with a normal prepregnancy weight, depending on HCP preference.
   3. An increase of about 300 calories per day is needed during pregnancy.
   4. Calorie needs are greater during the last two trimesters than in the first.

5. An increase of about 500 calories per day is needed during lactation.
6. A diet high in folic acid and folic acid supplements is recommended.
7. A diet high in folic acid is necessary for all women of childbearing age to prevent neural tube defects and orofacial clefts in the fetus.
8. Encourage the consumption of at least 8 to 10 (8-oz) glasses of fluid each day, of which 4 to 6 glasses should be water.
9. Sodium is not restricted unless specifically prescribed by the HCP.

B. Vegetarianism (See Box 12-9.)
1. Ensure that the client eats a sufficient amount of varied foods to meet normal nutrient and energy needs.
2. Clients should be educated about consuming complementary proteins over the course of each day to ensure that all essential amino acids are provided.
3. Potential deficiencies in vegetarian diets include energy, protein, vitamin B_{12}, zinc, iron, calcium, omega-3 fatty acids, and vitamin D (if limited exposure to sunlight).
4. Protein intake can be increased by consumption of a variety of vegetable protein sources based on whole grains, legumes, seeds, nuts, and vegetables combined to provide essential amino acids.
5. To enhance absorption of iron, vegetarians should include a good source of iron and vitamin C with each meal.
6. Foods commonly eaten include tofu, tempeh, soy milk and soy products, meat analogues, legumes, nuts, seeds, sprouts, and a variety of fruits and vegetables.

C. Lactose intolerance
1. Lactose consumed by an individual with lactose intolerance can cause abdominal distention, discomfort, nausea, vomiting, cramps, and loose stools.
2. Clients who experience lactose intolerance need to regularly incorporate sources of calcium (other than dairy products) into their dietary patterns.
3. Milk may be tolerated in cooked form (e.g., custards, fermented dairy products).
4. Cheese and yogurt are sometimes tolerated.
5. Lactase, which is an enzyme, may be prescribed and taken before ingesting milk or milk products.
6. Lactase-treated milk and lactose-free products are also available commercially.

D. Pica
1. Definition: Eating nonfood substances such as dirt, clay, starch, and freezer frost
2. The cause is unknown. Cultural values, such as beliefs regarding a material's effect on the mother or fetus, may make pica a common practice.
3. Iron-deficiency anemia may occur as a result of pica.

E. Cultural considerations: See Chapter 6 for information about cultural considerations and nutrition.

VI. Abortion

A. Description: A pregnancy that ends before 20 weeks' gestation, either spontaneously or electively

B. Types (Box 26-3)

C. Data collection
1. Spontaneous vaginal bleeding with the passage of clots and tissue through the vagina
2. Low uterine cramping and contractions
3. Hemorrhage and shock can result if bleeding is excessive.

D. Interventions
1. Maintain bed rest as prescribed.
2. Monitor the vital signs.
3. Monitor for cramping and bleeding.
4. Count perineal pads to evaluate blood loss. Save expelled tissues and clots.
5. Maintain IV fluids as prescribed. Monitor for the signs of hemorrhage or shock.
6. Prepare the client for dilation and curettage, as prescribed, for incomplete abortion.
7. Prepare to administer Rh_o(D) immune globulin (RhoGAM) to an Rh-negative women.

VII. Anemia

A. Description
1. Develops as a result of an inadequate amount of serum iron

2. Predisposes the client to postpartum infection

B. Data collection
1. Fatigue
2. Headache
3. Pallor
4. Tachycardia
5. Hemoglobin value usually less than 10 g/dL and hematocrit value usually less than 30%

BOX 26-3 Types of Abortions

Spontaneous Pregnancy ends because of natural causes.
Induced Therapeutic or elective reasons exist for terminating pregnancy.
Threatened Spotting and cramping without cervical change occur.
Inevitable Spotting and cramping occur, and cervix begins to dilate and efface.
Incomplete Loss of some of the products of conception occurs, with part of the products retained (most often placenta is retained).
Complete Loss of all products of conception occurs.
Missed Products of conception are retained in utero after fetal death.
Habitual Spontaneous abortions occur in three or more successive pregnancies.

C. Interventions

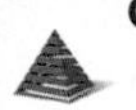

1. Hemoglobin and hematocrit levels are monitored every 2 weeks.
2. Administer and reinforce instructions about iron and folic acid supplements.
3. Instruct the client to take iron with a source of vitamin C to increase its absorption and to avoid taking iron with tea or milk products; absorbed best if taken between meals.
4. Instruct the client to eat foods high in iron, folic acid, and protein.
5. Teach the client to monitor for signs and symptoms of infection.
6. Prepare to assist to administer parenteral iron or blood transfusions, which may be prescribed for severe anemia.
7. Prepare to assist in the administration of oxytocic medications during the postpartum period if excessive bleeding is a concern.

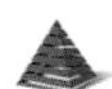

VIII. Cardiac Disease

A. Description: A pregnant client with cardiac disease may be unable physiologically to cope with the added plasma volume and increased cardiac output that occur during pregnancy; blood volume is at a maximum during the last weeks of the second trimester.

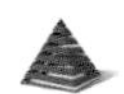

B. Data collection
1. Signs and symptoms of cardiac decompensation
   a. Cough and respiratory congestion
   b. Dyspnea and fatigue
   c. Palpitations and tachycardia
   d. Peripheral edema
   e. Chest pain
2. Signs of respiratory infection
3. Signs of heart failure and pulmonary edema

C. Interventions
1. Monitor the vital signs, fetal heart rate, and condition of fetus.
2. Limit physical activities, and stress the need for sufficient rest.
3. Monitor for signs of cardiac stress and decompensation.
4. Encourage adequate nutrition to prevent anemia, which would worsen the cardiac status; in addition, a low-sodium diet may be prescribed to prevent fluid retention and heart failure.
5. Avoid excessive weight gain.
6. During **labor**, prepare to assist with the following:
   a. Monitor the vital signs frequently.
   b. Place the client on a cardiac monitor and an external fetal monitor.
   c. Maintain bed rest, with the mother lying on her side and her head and shoulders elevated.
   d. Administer oxygen and pain medication, as prescribed.
   e. Manage pain early in labor.
   f. Use controlled pushing efforts to decrease cardiac stress.

Excessive weight gain places stress on the heart. In addition, obesity places the client at increased risk for complications of pregnancy.

IX. Chorioamnionitis

A. Description
1. A bacterial infection of the amniotic cavity that can result from the premature rupture of the membranes, vaginitis, amniocentesis, or intrauterine procedures
2. It may result in the development of postpartum endometritis and neonatal sepsis.

B. Data collection
1. Uterine tenderness
2. Elevated temperature
3. Maternal or fetal tachycardia
4. Foul odor to amniotic fluid
5. Leukocytosis

C. Interventions
1. Monitor maternal vital signs and fetal heart rate.
2. Monitor for uterine tenderness, contractions, and fetal activity.
3. Monitor the results of blood cultures.
4. Prepare for amniocentesis to obtain amniotic fluid for analysis (Gram stain and leukocyte count).
5. Administer antibiotics, as prescribed, after cultures are obtained.
6. Oxytocic medications may be prescribed to increase uterine tone.
7. Prepare to obtain neonatal cultures after delivery, as prescribed.

X. Diabetes Mellitus

A. Description
1. Pregnancy places demands on carbohydrate metabolism and causes insulin requirements to change.
2. Maternal glucose crosses the placenta, but insulin does not.
3. During the first trimester, maternal insulin needs decrease.
4. The fetus produces its own insulin and pulls glucose from the mother, which predisposes the mother to hypoglycemic reactions.
5. The **newborn** of a diabetic mother may be large in size but will have functions related to gestational age rather than size.
6. The newborn of a diabetic mother is at risk for hypoglycemia, hyperbilirubinemia, respiratory distress syndrome, hypocalcemia, and congenital anomalies.

During the first trimester, maternal insulin needs decrease. During the second and third trimesters, increases in placental hormones cause an insulin-resistant state, requiring an increase in the client's insulin dose. After placental delivery, placental hormone levels abruptly decrease and insulin requirements decrease.

B. Gestational diabetes mellitus
1. Occurs during pregnancy (during the second or third trimester) among clients not previously diagnosed as diabetic. Occurs when the pancreas cannot respond to the demand for more insulin.
2. Pregnant women should be screened for gestational diabetes between 24 and 28 weeks' gestation.
3. An oral glucose tolerance test may be prescribed to confirm gestational diabetes mellitus.
4. Gestational diabetes frequently can be treated by diet alone; however, some clients may need insulin.
5. Most gestational diabetics convert to a euglycemic state after delivery; however, these individuals have an increased risk for developing diabetes mellitus during their lifetimes.

Many oral hypoglycemic agents are unsafe for use during pregnancy; usually insulin is prescribed.

C. Predisposing conditions for gestational diabetes
1. Older than 35 years old
2. Obese
3. Multiple gestations
4. Family history of diabetes mellitus
5. Large for gestational age fetus

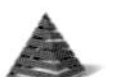

D. Data collection
1. Excessive thirst
2. Hunger
3. Weight loss
4. Frequent urination
5. Blurred vision
6. Recurrent urinary tract infections and vaginal yeast infections
7. Glycosuria and ketonuria
8. Signs of gestational hypertension
9. Polyhydramnios
10. Large for gestational age fetus

E. Interventions
1. Include diet, insulin (if diet cannot control blood glucose levels), prescribed exercise, and blood glucose determinations to maintain blood glucose levels between 65 and 130 mg/dL.
2. Observe for signs of hyperglycemia, glycosuria, ketonuria, and hypoglycemia.
3. Monitor weight.
4. Increase calorie intake, as prescribed, with adequate insulin therapy so that glucose will move into the cells.
5. Monitor for signs of maternal complications, such as preeclampsia (hypertension and proteinuria).
6. Monitor for signs of infection.
7. Instruct the client to report burning and pain on urination, vaginal discharge or itching, or any other signs of infection to the HCP.
8. Monitor the fetal status and for signs of fetal compromise.

F. Interventions during labor
1. Monitor the fetal status continuously for signs of distress; if noted, assist to prepare the client for immediate cesarean section.
2. Assist to carefully regulate insulin and provide IV glucose, as prescribed, because labor depletes glycogen.

G. Interventions during the postpartum period
1. Observe the client closely for a hypoglycemic reaction, because a precipitous drop in insulin requirements normally occurs. The client may not require insulin for the first 24 hours.
2. Reregulate insulin needs, as prescribed, after the first day, according to blood glucose testing and HCP's prescriptions.
3. Determine dietary needs on the basis of blood glucose and insulin requirements.
4. Monitor for signs of infection or postpartum hemorrhage.

XI. Disseminated Intravascular Coagulation (DIC)

A. Description: DIC is a maternal condition in which the clotting cascade is activated, resulting in the formation of clots in the microcirculation

The rapid and extensive formation of clots that occurs in DIC causes the platelets and clotting factors to be depleted. This results in bleeding and the potential vascular occlusion of organs from thromboembolus formation.

B. Predisposing conditions (Box 26-4)

C. Data collection
1. Uncontrolled bleeding
2. Bruising, purpura, petechiae, and ecchymosis
3. Presence of occult blood in excretions, such as stool (melena)

BOX 26-4 Predisposing Conditions for Disseminated Intravascular Coagulation

- Abruptio placentae
- Amniotic fluid embolism
- Gestational hypertension
- Intrauterine fetal death
- Liver disease
- Sepsis

4. Hematuria, hematemesis, or vaginal bleeding
5. Signs of shock
6. Decreased fibrinogen level, platelet count, and hematocrit level
7. Increased prothrombin time, partial thromboplastin time, clotting time, and fibrin degradation products

D. Interventions
1. Eliminate by treating the underlying cause.
2. Monitor the vital signs and for bleeding and signs of shock.
3. Assist in preparing to administer oxygen therapy, volume replacement, blood-component therapy, and possibly heparin therapy.
4. Monitor for complications associated with fluid and blood replacement and heparin therapy.
5. Monitor the urine output, and maintain it at 30 mL/hr (kidney failure is a complication of DIC).

XII. Ectopic Pregnancy (Fig. 26-3)

A. Description: Pregnancy that occurs in a site other than a uterine site, with **implantation** usually occurring in the ampulla of the fallopian tube

B. Data collection
1. Missed period
2. Abdominal pain
3. Vaginal spotting to bleeding that is dark red or brown
4. Rupture: Increased pain, referred shoulder pain, and signs of shock

C. Interventions
1. Obtain vital signs.
2. Monitor bleeding and prepare to assist to initiate measures to prevent rupture and shock.
3. Methotrexate (a folic acid antagonist) may be prescribed to inhibit cell division in the developing embryo.
4. Prepare the client for laparotomy and the removal of the pregnancy and tube, if necessary, or repair of the tube.
5. Assist to administer antibiotics. Rh_o(D) immune globulin is prescribed for Rh-negative women.

XIII. Endometritis

A. Description
1. Infection of the lining of the uterus occurring in the postpartum period; caused by bacteria that invade the uterus at the placental site
2. The infection may spread, involve the entire endometrium, and cause peritonitis or pelvic thrombophlebitis.

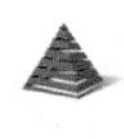

B. Data collection
1. Chills and fever
2. Increased pulse
3. Decreased appetite
4. Headache
5. Backache
6. Prolonged, severe afterpains
7. Tender, large uterus
8. Foul odor to **lochia** or reddish-brown lochia
9. Ileus
10. Elevated white blood cell count

C. Interventions
1. Monitor the vital signs.
2. Place the mother in Fowler's position to facilitate the drainage of lochia.
3. Provide a private room for the mother.
4. Inform the mother that it is not necessary to isolate the newborn from the mother.

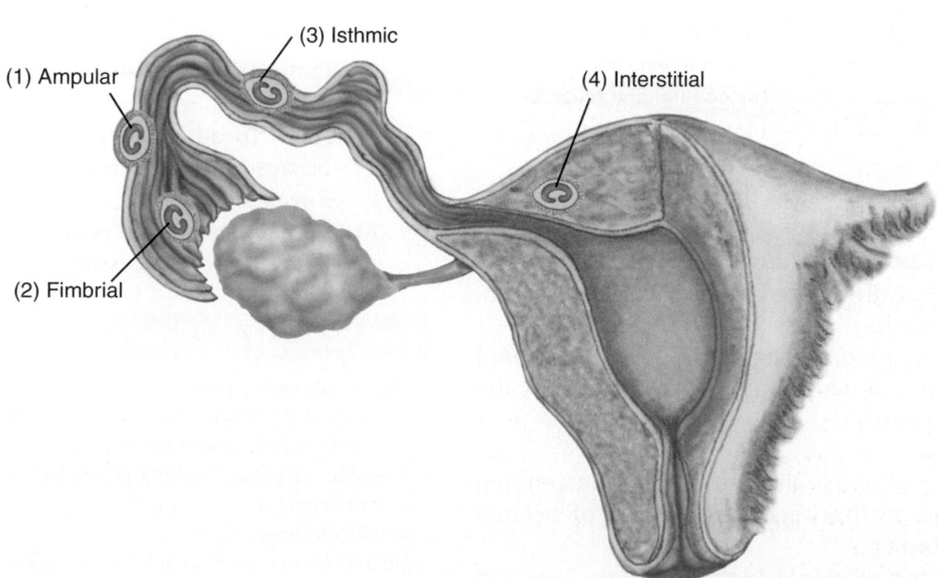

FIGURE 26-3 Sites of tubal ectopic pregnancy. The numbers indicate the order of prevalence. (From Lowdermilk D, Cashion MC, Perry S, Alden K: *Maternity & women's health care*, ed 10, St. Louis, 2012, Mosby.)

5. Instruct the mother in proper hand-washing techniques.
6. Initiate contact precautions, as necessary.
7. Monitor intake and output (I&O), and encourage fluid intake.
8. Intravenous antibiotics may be prescribed.
9. Administer comfort measures, such as back rubs, position changes, and pain medications, as prescribed, and provide emotional support.
10. Oxytocic medications may be prescribed to improve uterine tone.

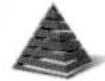

XIV. Fetal Death in Utero

A. Description
1. Death of a fetus after 20 weeks' gestation and before birth
2. Disseminated intravascular coagulation can develop if the dead fetus is retained in the uterus for 3 to 4 weeks or longer.

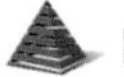

B. Data collection
1. Absence of fetal movement
2. Absence of fetal heart tones
3. Maternal weight loss
4. Lack of fetal growth or decrease in fundal height
5. Lack of cardiac activity and other characteristics suggestive of fetal death noted on the ultrasound

C. Interventions
1. Prepare for the delivery of the fetus.
2. Support the client's decision about labor, birth, and the postpartum period.
3. Facilitate the grieving process as appropriate considering cultural practices and beliefs.
4. Accept behaviors such as anger and hostility from the parents.
5. Refer parents to an appropriate support group.

Cultural and religious practices and beliefs are important to consider when caring for the parents of a fetus who has died. Be aware of the cultural and religious practices and beliefs of the client.

XV. Hepatitis B

A. Description
1. The risks of prematurity, low birth weight, and neonatal death increase if the mother has hepatitis B infection.

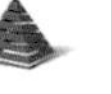

2. It is transmitted through blood, saliva, vaginal secretions, semen, breast milk, and across the placental barrier.

B. Interventions
1. Minimize the risk for intrapartum ascending infections by limiting the number of vaginal examinations.
2. Remove the maternal blood from the neonate immediately after birth.
3. Suction the neonate immediately after birth.
4. Bathe the neonate before any invasive procedures.
5. Clean and dry the face and eyes of the neonate before instilling eye prophylaxis.
6. Infection of the neonate can be prevented by the administration of hepatitis B immune globulin and hepatitis B vaccine soon after birth.
7. Discourage the mother from kissing the neonate until the neonate has received the vaccine.
8. Inform the mother that the hepatitis B vaccine will be administered to the neonate and that the second dose will be administered at 1 month (obtain consent for the administration of a vaccine). The third dose is administered at 6 months.

Support breastfeeding after neonatal treatment for hepatitis B; breastfeeding is not contraindicated if the neonate has been vaccinated.

XVI. Hematoma

A. Description
1. Occurs after the escape of blood into the maternal tissue after the delivery
2. Predisposing conditions include operative delivery with forceps or injury to a blood vessel.

B. Data collection (Box 26-5)

C. Interventions
1. Monitor the vital signs.
2. Monitor the client for abnormal pain, especially when forceps delivery has been performed.
3. Apply ice to the hematoma site.
4. Administer analgesics, as prescribed.
5. Monitor intake and output.
6. Encourage fluids and voiding. Prepare for urinary catheterization if the client is unable to void.
7. Prepare to assist in administering blood replacements, as prescribed.
8. Monitor for signs of infection, such as increased temperature, pulse rate, and white blood cell count.
9. Assist to administer antibiotics, as prescribed, because infection is common after hematoma formation.
10. Prepare for the incision and evacuation of the hematoma, if necessary.

BOX 26-5 Hematoma: Data Collection Findings

Abnormal, severe pain
Pressure in perineal area (client states that she feels like she has to have a bowel movement)
Palpable, sensitive swelling in the perineal area, with discolored skin
Inability to void
Decreased hemoglobin and hematocrit levels
Signs of shock, such as pallor, tachycardia, and hypotension, if significant blood loss has occurred

XVII. Human Immunodeficiency Virus (HIV) and Acquired Immunodeficiency Syndrome (AIDS)

A. Description

1. The human immunodeficiency virus (HIV) is the causative factor of the development of acquired immunodeficiency syndrome (AIDS).
2. Women infected with the HIV virus may first demonstrate symptoms at the time of pregnancy or possibly develop life-threatening infections, because normal pregnancy involves some suppression of the maternal immune system.
3. Repeated exposure to the virus during pregnancy through unsafe sex practices or intravenous drug use can increase the risk of transmission to the fetus.
4. Zidovudine (Retrovir) is recommended for the prevention of maternal–fetal HIV transmission. It is administered orally beginning after 14 weeks' gestation, intravenously during labor, and in the form of syrup to the neonate for 6 weeks after birth.

B. Transmission

1. Sexual exposure to genital secretions of an infected person
2. Parenteral exposure to infected blood and tissue
3. Perinatal exposure of a newborn to infected maternal secretions through the birth process or breastfeeding

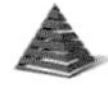

C. Risks to the mother: The mother with HIV is managed as high risk because she is vulnerable to infections.

D. Diagnosis

1. Tests used to determine the presence of antibodies to HIV include enzyme-linked immunosorbent assay (ELISA), Western blot (WB), and immunofluorescence assay (IFA).
2. A single reactive ELISA test result by itself cannot be used to diagnose HIV and should be repeated in duplicate with the same blood sample. If the result is repeatedly reactive, follow-up tests using WB or IFA should be performed.
3. A positive WB or IFA is considered confirmatory for HIV.
4. A positive ELISA that fails to be confirmed by WB or IFA should not be considered negative for HIV. Repeat testing should take place in 3 to 6 months.
5. See Chapter 11 for additional laboratory tests.

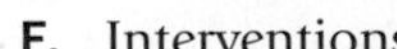

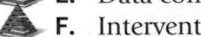

E. Data collection (Box 26-6)

F. Interventions

1. Prenatal period
   a. Prevent opportunistic infections.
   b. Procedures that increase the risk of perinatal transmission are avoided, such as amniocentesis and fetal scalp sampling.

BOX 26-6 Stages of Acquired Immunodeficiency Syndrome

Stage 1
- Fever
- Headache
- Myalgia
- Lymphadenopathy

Stage 2
- Active infection but asymptomatic; may remain so for years
- May experience an outbreak of herpes zoster (shingles)
- May experience a transient thrombocytopenia

Stage 3
- Symptomatic
- Evidence of immune dysfunction
- All body systems can present with signs of immune dysfunction
- Integumentary and gynecological problems are common

Stage 4
- Advanced human immunodeficiency virus infection
- Vulnerable to common bacterial infections
- Development of opportunistic infections
- Serious immune compromise

2. Intrapartum period
   a. If the fetus has not been exposed to HIV in utero, the highest risk exists during delivery through the birth canal.
   b. The use of scalp electrodes is avoided.
   c. Episiotomy is avoided to decrease the amount of maternal blood in and around the birth canal.
   d. The administration of oxytocin (Pitocin) is avoided, because oxytocin contractions can be strong, thus inducing vaginal tears or necessitating the need for an episiotomy.
   e. Place heavy absorbent pads under the mother's hips to absorb amniotic fluid and maternal blood.
   f. Minimize the neonate's exposure to maternal blood and body fluids. Promptly remove the neonate from the mother's blood after delivery.
   g. Suction fluids from the newborn promptly.
   h. Prepare to assist to administer zidovudine (Retrovir) as prescribed to the mother during labor and delivery.
3. Postpartum period
   a. Monitor for signs of infection.
   b. Place the mother in protective isolation if she is immunosuppressed.
   c. Breastfeeding is usually restricted.
   d. Instruct the mother to monitor for signs of infection and report any signs if they occur.

G. The neonate and HIV
1. Description
a. Neonates born to HIV-positive clients may test positive because the mother's positive antibodies may persist for as long as 18 months after birth. All neonates acquire maternal antibody to HIV infection, but not all acquire infection.
b. The use of antiviral medication, the reduction of neonate exposure to maternal blood and body fluids, and the early identification of HIV during pregnancy reduce the risk of transmission to the neonate.
2. Interventions
a. Bathe the neonate carefully before any invasive procedure, such as the administration of vitamin K, heel sticks, or venipunctures. The umbilical cord stump is cleaned meticulously every day until it is healed.
b. The neonate can room with the mother.
c. Prepare to assist to administer zidovudine (Retrovir) to the newborn, as prescribed, for the first 6 weeks of life.
d. All HIV-exposed newborns should be treated with medication to prevent infection with *Pneumocystis jiroveci*.
e. Note that an HIV culture is recommended at the age of 1 month and 4 months of age. Infants at risk for HIV infection should be seen by the HCP at birth and at 1 week, 2 weeks, 1 month, 2 months, and 4 months of age.
f. The child may be asymptomatic for the first several years of life. He or she needs to be monitored for early signs of immunodeficiency.

Infants at risk for HIV infection need to receive all recommended immunizations at the regular schedule; however, no live vaccines should be administered.

XVIII. Hydatidiform Mole

A. Description
1. A form of gestational trophoblastic disease that occurs when the trophoblasts, which are the peripheral cells that attach the fertilized ovum to the uterine wall, develop abnormally.
2. Presents as an edematous, grapelike cluster that may be nonmalignant or may develop into choriocarcinoma

B. Data collection
1. Fetal heart rate not detectable
2. Vaginal bleeding, which may occur as early as the fourth week or as late as the second trimester; it is usually bright red or dark brown in color, and it may be slight, profuse, or intermittent.
3. Signs of gestational hypertension, such as an elevated blood pressure and proteinuria, may be present before gestational week 20.
4. Fundal height is greater than expected for date.
5. Elevated hCG levels
6. Ultrasound shows a characteristic snowstorm pattern.

C. Interventions
1. Assist to prepare the mother for uterine evacuation (before evacuation, diagnostic tests are done to detect metastatic disease).
2. Evacuation of the mole is done by vacuum aspiration. Oxytocin (Pitocin) is administered after evacuation to contract the uterus.
3. Tissue is sent to the laboratory for evaluation. Follow-up is important to detect changes that are suggestive of malignancy. 
4. Monitor for postprocedure hemorrhage and infection.
5. Human chorionic gonadotropin levels are monitored every 1 to 2 weeks until normal prepregnancy levels are attained. The levels are then checked every 1 to 2 months for 1 year.
6. Instruct the parents regarding birth control measures so that pregnancy can be prevented during the 1-year follow-up.

XIX. Hyperemesis Gravidarum

A. Description: Intractable nausea and vomiting that persists beyond the first trimester and causes disturbances in nutrition and fluid and electrolyte balance

B. Data collection
1. Nausea is most pronounced on arising; however, it can occur at other times during the day. 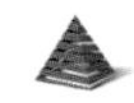
2. Persistent vomiting and weight loss
3. Signs of dehydration and electrolyte imbalances

C. Interventions
1. Measures to alleviate nausea, including medication therapy, are initiated. If this is unsuccessful and weight loss and fluid and electrolyte imbalances occur, the administration of IV fluid and electrolyte replacement or parenteral nutrition may be necessary.
2. Monitor the vital signs, intake, output, weight, and calorie count.
3. Monitor the laboratory data and for signs of dehydration and electrolyte imbalances.
4. Monitor the urine for ketones.
5. Monitor the fetal heart rate, fetal activity, and fetal growth.
6. Encourage the intake of small portions of food (low-fat, easily digestible carbohydrates, such as cereals, rice, and pasta).
7. Liquids should be taken between meals to avoid distending the stomach and triggering vomiting.
8. Encourage the client to sit upright after meals.

XX. Gestational Hypertension (GH)

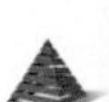

A. Description and types (Table 26-2): Hypertension can be mild or severe, leading to preeclampsia and then eclampsia (seizures).

Maternity

TABLE 26-2 Classification of Hypertensive States of Pregnancy

Type	Description
Gestational Hypertensive Disorders	
Gestational hypertension	Blood pressure elevation detected first time after midpregnancy without proteinuria
Transient hypertension	Gestational hypertension with no signs of preeclampsia present at time of birth and hypertension resolves by 12 wk after birth
Preeclampsia	Pregnancy-specific syndrome that usually occurs after 20 wk of gestation and is determined by gestational hypertension plus proteinuria
Eclampsia	Occurrence of seizures in a preeclamptic woman
Chronic Hypertensive Disorders	
Chronic hypertension	Hypertension that is present and observable before pregnancy or that is diagnosed before week 20 of gestation
Preeclampsia superimposed on chronic hypertension	Chronic hypertension with new proteinuria or exacerbation of hypertension (previously well controlled) or proteinuria, thrombocytopenia, or increases in hepatocellular enzymes

From Lowdermilk D, Perry S, Cashion K, Alden K: *Maternity & women's health care*, ed 10, St. Louis, 2012, Mosby.

Signs of preeclampsia are hypertension and proteinuria.

B. Data collection (Table 26-3)
C. Predisposing conditions
  1. Primigravida
  2. Age younger than 19 years or older than 40 years
  3. Chronic kidney disease
  4. Chronic hypertension
  5. Diabetes mellitus
  6. Rh incompatibility
  7. History of or family history of gestational hypertension
D. Complications of gestational hypertension
  1. Abruptio placentae
  2. Disseminated intravascular coagulation
  3. Thrombocytopenia
  4. Placental insufficiency
  5. Intrauterine growth restriction
  6. Intrauterine fetal death
  7. HELLP syndrome, a laboratory diagnosis for severe preeclampsia characterized by *h*emolysis, *el*evated *l*iver enzyme levels, and *l*ow *p*latelet count

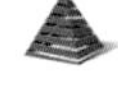

E. Interventions for mild hypertension
  1. Monitor blood pressure.
  2. Monitor fetal activity and fetal growth.

TABLE 26-3 Mild Versus Severe Preeclampsia

Parameter Evaluated	Mild	Severe
Systolic blood pressure	≥140 but <160 mm Hg	≥160 mm Hg (two readings, 6 hours apart, while on bed rest)
Diastolic blood pressure	≥90 but <110 mm Hg	≥110 mm Hg
Proteinuria (a 24-hour specimen is preferred to eliminate hour-to-hour variations)	≥0.3 g but <2 g in a 24-hour specimen (1+ on a random dipstick test)	≥5 g in a 24-hour specimen (≥3+ on a random dipstick test)
Creatinine, serum (renal function)	Normal	Elevated (>1.2 mg/dL)
Platelets	Normal	Decreased (<100,000 cells/mm^3)
Liver enzymes (alanine aminotransferase or aspartate aminotransferase)	Normal or minimal increase in levels	Elevated levels
Urine output	Normal	Oliguria common, often <500 mL/day
Severe, unrelenting headache not attributable to other cause; mental confusion (cerebral edema)	Absent	Often present
Persistent right upper quadrant or epigastric pain or pain penetrating to the back (distention of the liver capsule); nausea and vomiting	Absent	May be present and often precedes seizure
Visual disturbances (spots or "sparkles," temporary blindness; photophobia)	Absent to minimal	Common
Pulmonary edema, heart failure, and cyanosis	Absent	May be present
Fetal growth restriction	Normal growth	Growth restriction; reduced amniotic fluid volume

From Lowdermilk D, Cashion MC, Perry S: *Maternity & women's health care*, ed 10, St. Louis, 2012, Mosby.

3. Encourage frequent rest periods. Instruct the client to lie in the lateral position.
4. Assist to administer antihypertensive medications, as prescribed. Teach the client about the importance of the medications.
5. Monitor intake and output.
6. Evaluate renal function through prescribed studies such as blood urea nitrogen, serum creatinine, and 24-hour urine levels for creatinine clearance and protein.

F. Interventions for mild preeclampsia
1. Provide bed rest, and place the client in a lateral position.
2. Monitor the blood pressure and weight.
3. Monitor the neurological status, because changes can indicate cerebral hypoxia or impending seizure.
4. Monitor the deep tendon reflexes and for the presence of clonus, because hyperreflexia indicates increased central nervous system irritability (Box 26-7).
5. Provide adequate fluids.
6. Monitor intake and output. A urinary output of 30 mL/hour indicates adequate renal perfusion.
7. Increase dietary protein and carbohydrates with no added salt, if prescribed.
8. Assist to administer medications, as prescribed, to lower the blood pressure. Blood pressure should not be lowered drastically, because placental perfusion can be compromised.
9. Monitor for HELLP syndrome.

G. Interventions for severe preeclampsia
1. Maintain bed rest.
2. Magnesium sulfate (always administered with a controlled infusion device) may be prescribed to prevent seizures. This may be continued for 24 to 48 hours postpartum.
3. Monitor for signs of magnesium toxicity, including flushing, sweating, hypotension, depressed deep tendon reflexes, and central nervous system depression, including respiratory depression. Keep the antidote (calcium gluconate) available for immediate use, if needed.
4. Assist to administer antihypertensives, as prescribed.
5. Prepare for the induction of labor.

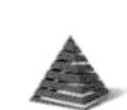

H. Eclampsia
1. Data collection: Characterized by generalized seizures (Box 26-8)
2. Interventions (see Priority Nursing Actions)

BOX 26-8 Eclampsia

1. Seizure typically begins with twitching around the mouth.
2. Body then becomes rigid in a state of tonic muscular contractions that last 15 to 20 seconds.
3. Facial muscles and then all body muscles alternately contract and relax in rapid succession (clonic phase may last about 1 minute).
4. Respiration ceases during seizure because diaphragm tends to remain fixed (breathing resumes shortly after the seizure).
5. Postictal sleep occurs.

BOX 26-7 Checking Reflexes

Biceps Reflex

The thumb is placed over the client's biceps tendon, and the client's elbow is supported with the palm of the hand.
The examiner strikes a downward blow over the thumb with the percussion hammer.
Normal Response: Flexion of the arm at the elbow

Patellar Reflex

The client is positioned with the legs dangling over the edge of the examining table, or lying on her back, with the legs slightly flexed.
The examiner strikes the patellar tendon just below the kneecap with the percussion hammer.
Normal Response: Extension or kicking out of the leg

Clonus Reflex

The client is positioned with the legs dangling over the edge of the examining table.
The leg is supported with one hand, and the client's foot is sharply dorsiflexed with the other hand.
The dorsiflexed position is maintained for a few seconds; then the foot is released.
Normal Response (Negative Clonus Response):
The foot will remain steady in the dorsiflexed position.
No rhythmic oscillations or jerking of the foot will be felt.
When released, the foot will drop to a plantarflexed position, with no oscillations.
Abnormal Response (Positive Clonus Response):
Rhythmic oscillations will occur when the foot is dorsiflexed.
Similar oscillations will be noted when the foot drops to the plantarflexed position.

Grading the Response

0 = Reflex absent
1+ = Reflex present but hypoactive
2+ = Normal reflex
3+ = Hyperactive reflex
4+ = Hyperactive reflex with clonus present

PRIORITY NURSING ACTIONS!

Actions to Take in the Event of Eclampsia

1. Remain with the client and call for help.
2. Ensure an open airway, turn the client on her side, and administer oxygen by face mask at 8 to 10 L/minute.
3. Monitor fetal heart rate patterns.
4. Assist in administering medications to control the seizures as prescribed.
5. After the seizure has ended, insert an oral airway and suction the client's mouth as needed.
6. Prepare for the delivery of the fetus after stabilization of the client, if warranted.
7. Document the occurrence, the client's response, and outcome.

Eclampsia refers to the occurrence of a seizure. It is a potentially preventable extension of severe preeclampsia; early identification of preeclampsia in a pregnant client allows intervention before the condition reaches the seizure state. If eclampsia occurs, the nurse remains with the client and calls for help. The nurse ensures an open airway. If the client is not on her side already, the nurse attempts to turn the client on her side. The side-lying position permits greater circulation through the placenta and may help prevent aspiration. The nurse administers oxygen by face mask at 8 to 10 L/minute to ensure adequate placental oxygenation. The nurse also notes the time the seizure began and the duration of the seizure and protects the client from injury during the event. The nurse monitors fetal heart rate patterns closely and assists to administer medications as prescribed (magnesium sulfate may be prescribed). After the seizure has ended, the nurse inserts an oral airway to maintain airway patency and suctions the client's mouth as needed. If warranted, the nurse prepares for the delivery of the fetus after stabilization of the client. The nurse documents the occurrence, the client's response, and the outcome.

Reference(s): McKinney, E., James, S., Murray, S., Nelson, K. & Ashwill, J. (2013). *Maternal-child nursing* (4th ed., p. 597). St. Louis: Elsevier.

XXI. Incompetent Cervix

A. Description
1. Premature dilation of the cervix, which occurs most often during the fourth or fifth month of pregnancy and is associated with structural or functional defects of the cervix
2. Treatment involves surgical placement of a cervical cerclage.

B. Data collection
1. Vaginal bleeding
2. Fetal membranes are visible through the cervix.

C. Interventions
1. Provide bed rest, hydration, and assist with tocolysis, as prescribed, to inhibit uterine contractions.
2. Prepare for cervical cerclage (at 10 to 14 weeks' gestation), in which a band of fascia or nonabsorbable ribbon is placed around the cervix beneath the mucosa to constrict the internal os of the cervix.
3. After cervical cerclage, the woman is told to refrain from intercourse and avoid prolonged standing and heavy lifting.
4. The cervical cerclage is removed at 37 weeks' gestation or left in place, and a cesarean delivery is performed. If removed, the cerclage must be repeated with each successive pregnancy.
5. After the procedure, monitor for contractions, rupture of the membranes, and signs of infection.
6. Instruct the woman to report any postprocedure vaginal bleeding or increased uterine contractions immediately to the HCP.

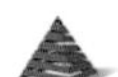

XXII. Infections

A. Toxoplasmosis
1. Caused by infection with the protozoan intracellular parasite *Toxoplasma gondii*
2. Produces a rash and symptoms of acute, flu-like infection in the mother
3. Transmitted to the mother through the consumption of raw meat or the handling of the cat litter of infected cats
4. Organism is transmitted to the fetus across the placenta.
5. Can cause spontaneous abortion in the first trimester

B. Rubella (German measles)
1. Extremely teratogenic during the first trimester
2. Transmitted to the fetus across the placenta
3. Causes congenital defects of the eyes, heart, ears, and brain
4. If not immune (titer of 1:8 or less), the mother should be vaccinated during the postpartum period. She must then wait 1 to 3 months (as specified by HCP) before becoming pregnant again.

C. Cytomegalovirus
1. The organism is transmitted through close personal contact or across the placenta to the fetus, or the fetus may be infected through the birth canal.
2. The mother may be asymptomatic, and most infants are asymptomatic at birth.
3. Cytomegalovirus causes low birth weight, intrauterine growth retardation, enlarged liver and spleen, jaundice, mental retardation, blindness, hearing loss, and seizures.
4. Antiviral medications may be prescribed for severe infections in the mother, but these medications are toxic and may only temporarily suppress the shedding of the virus.

D. Herpes simplex virus (see Table **26-1**)
1. Herpes simplex virus affects the external genitalia, vagina, and cervix and causes draining, painful vesicles.

2. Acyclovir (Zovirax) can be used to treat recurrent outbreaks during pregnancy or used as suppressive therapy late in pregnancy to prevent an outbreak during labor and birth.
3. Virus usually is transmitted to the fetus during birth through the infected vagina or via an ascending infection after rupture of the membranes.
4. No vaginal examinations are done in the presence of active vaginal herpetic lesions.
5. Herpes can cause death or severe neurological impairment in the newborn.
6. Delivery of the fetus is usually by cesarean section if active lesions are present in the vagina; delivery may be performed vaginally if the lesions are in the anal, perineal, or inner thigh area (strict precautions are necessary to protect the fetus during delivery).
7. Maintain contact precautions.

E. Group B *Streptococcus* (GBS)
1. A leading cause of life-threatening perinatal infections
2. The gram-positive bacterium colonizes the rectum, vagina, cervix, and urethra of pregnant and nonpregnant women.
3. Meningitis, fasciitis, and intraabdominal abscess can occur in the pregnant client if she is infected at the time of birth.
4. Transmission occurs during vaginal delivery.
5. Early-onset newborn GBS occurs within the first week after birth, usually within 48 hours. It can include infections such as sepsis, pneumonia, or meningitis, and permanent neurological disability can result.
6. Diagnosis of the mother is done via vaginal and rectal cultures between 35 and 37 weeks' gestation.
7. Antibiotics such as penicillin may be prescribed for the mother during labor and birth. IV antibiotics may be prescribed for infected infants.

XXIII. Multiple Gestation

A. Description
1. Results from the **fertilization** of two ova (fraternal or dizygotic) or a splitting of one of the fertilized ovum (identical or monozygotic)
2. Complications in pregnancy can occur and include spontaneous abortion, anemia, congenital anomalies, hyperemesis gravidarum, intrauterine growth restriction, gestational hypertension, polyhydramnios, postpartum hemorrhage, premature rupture of membranes, and preterm labor and delivery.

B. Data collection
1. Excessive fetal activity
2. Uterus large for gestational age
3. Palpation of three or four large fetal parts in the uterus
4. Auscultation of more than one fetal heart rate
5. Excessive weight gain

C. Interventions
1. Monitor the vital signs.
2. Monitor the fetal heart rates, fetal activity, and fetal growth.
3. Monitor for cervical changes.
4. Prepare the client for ultrasound, as prescribed.
5. Monitor for anemia. Administer supplemental vitamins, as prescribed.
6. Monitor for preterm labor and assist to treat it promptly.
7. Prepare for cesarean section for abnormal presentations.
8. Prepare to administer oxytocic medications after delivery to prevent postpartum hemorrhage from uterine overdistention.

XXIV. Pyelonephritis

A. Description
1. Results from bacterial infections that extend upward from the bladder through the blood vessels and lymphatics
2. Frequently follows untreated urinary tract infections and is associated with increased incidence of anemia, low birth weight, gestational hypertension, preterm labor and delivery, and premature rupture of the membranes

B. Assessment and Interventions (refer to Chapter 53).

XXV. Sexually Transmitted Infections (see Table 26-1)

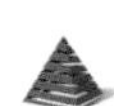

A. Gonorrhea
1. Description
   a. An infection caused by *Neisseria gonorrhoeae*, which causes inflammation of the mucous membranes of the genital and urinary tracts
   b. Transmission of the organism is by sexual intercourse.
   c. Infection may be transmitted to the newborn's eyes during delivery, causing blindness (ophthalmia neonatorum).
2. Data collection: Usually asymptomatic. Vaginal discharge, urinary frequency, and lower abdominal pain in the mother are possible.
3. Interventions
   a. Obtain a vaginal culture for gonorrhea on the first prenatal visit. Prepare to repeat the culture during the third trimester in high-risk clients.
   b. Instruct the client that the treatment of her partner is necessary if infection is present.

B. Syphilis
1. Description
   a. Chronic infectious disease caused by the organism *Treponema pallidum*
   b. Transmission is by intimate physical contact with syphilitic lesions, which are usually

BOX 26-9 Stages of Syphilis

Primary Stage

- Most infectious stage
- Appearance of ulcerative, painless lesions produced by spirochetes at the point of entry into the body

Secondary Stage

- Highly infectious stage
- Lesions appear about 6 weeks to 6 months after the primary stage and may occur anywhere on the skin and mucous membranes.
- Generalized lymphadenopathy occurs

Tertiary Stage

- Spirochetes enter the internal organs and cause permanent damage; symptoms may occur 10 to 30 years after the occurrence of an untreated primary lesion.
- Disease invades the central nervous system, causing meningitis, ataxia, general paresis, and progressive mental deterioration.
- Affects the aortic valve and the aorta

found on the skin, mucous membranes of the mouth, and genitals.

c. Infection may cause abortion or preterm labor. Passed to the fetus after the fourth month of pregnancy as congenital syphilis.

2. Data collection (Box 26-9)
3. Interventions
   a. Prepare to assist with the culture of lesions (if present) during the initial prenatal examination to screen for syphilis. Diagnosis is dependent on the microscopic examination of primary and secondary lesion tissue and serology (Venereal Disease Research Laboratory [VDRL] or rapid plasma reagin test) during latency and late infection. The culture may be repeated during the third trimester for high-risk clients.
   b. If the test result is positive, treatment with an antibiotic such as penicillin may be necessary.
   c. Instruct the client that the treatment of her partner is necessary if an infection is present.

C. Condylomata acuminata *(human papillomavirus)*
1. Description
   a. Caused by *human papillomavirus* (HPV). Affects the cervix, urethra, anus, penis, and scrotum.
   b. A culture is indicated for clients with a positive history or with active lesions, and weekly cultures may be done at weeks 35 or 36 of pregnancy until delivery. The test is performed to determine the route of delivery.
2. Data collection
   a. Small to large wartlike growths on the genitals
   b. Cervical cell changes may be noted, because HPV is associated with cervical malignancies.
3. Interventions
   a. Lesions are removed with the use of cytotoxic agents, cryotherapy, electrocautery, and laser.
   b. Encourage a yearly Papanicolaou (Pap) smear.
   c. Sexual contact is avoided until the lesions are healed. (Condoms reduce transmission.)

D. Chlamydia
1. Description
   a. Sexually transmitted pathogen associated with an increased risk of preterm birth, stillbirth, neonatal conjunctivitis, and newborn chlamydial pneumonia
   b. Can cause salpingitis, pelvic abscesses, ectopic pregnancy, chronic pelvic pain, and infertility
   c. Diagnostic test is a vaginal culture for *Chlamydia trachomatis.*
2. Data collection
   a. Usually asymptomatic
   b. Bleeding between periods or after coitus
   c. Mucoid or purulent cervical discharge
   d. Dysuria and pelvic pain
3. Interventions
   a. Screen the client to determine whether the client is at high risk. A vaginal culture is indicated for all pregnant clients if the client is in a high-risk group or infants from previous pregnancies have developed neonatal conjunctivitis or pneumonia.
   b. Instruct the client about the importance of rescreening, because reinfection can occur as the client nears term.
   c. Ensure that the sexual partner is treated.

E. Trichomoniasis
1. Description
   a. Caused by *Trichomonas vaginalis.*
   b. Normal saline wet smear of vaginal secretions is checked for the presence of protozoa.
   c. Infection is associated with premature rupture of membranes and postpartum endometritis.
2. Data collection
   a. Yellowish to greenish, frothy, mucopurulent, copious, and malodorous vaginal discharge
   b. Inflammation of the vulva, vagina, or both may be present.
3. Interventions
   a. Metronidazole (Flagyl) may be prescribed.
   b. Sexual partner may need to be treated.

F. Bacterial vaginosis
1. Description
   a. Caused by *Haemophilus vaginalis* (*Gardnerella vaginalis*)
   b. Associated with preterm labor and birth

2. Data collection
    a. Client complains of "fishy odor" to vaginal secretions and increased odor after intercourse.
    b. Microscopic examination of vaginal secretions identifies the infection.
3. Interventions
    a. Treatment with oral metronidazole (Flagyl) may be prescribed.
    b. Sexual partner may need to be treated

G. Vaginal candidiasis
1. Description
    a. *Candida albicans* is the most common causative organism.
    b. Predisposing factors include the use of antibiotics, diabetes mellitus, and obesity.
    c. Diagnosis is by identifying the spores of *Candida albicans.*
2. Data collection
    a. Vulvar and vaginal pruritus
    b. White, lumpy, and cottage cheese–like discharge from the vagina
3. Interventions
    a. An antifungal vaginal preparation such as miconazole (Monistat) may be prescribed.
    b. For extensive irritation and swelling, sitz baths may be prescribed.
    c. Sexual partner may need to be treated.

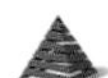

XXVI. Tuberculosis

A. Description
1. A highly communicable disease caused by *Mycobacterium tuberculosis*
2. Transmitted by the airborne route

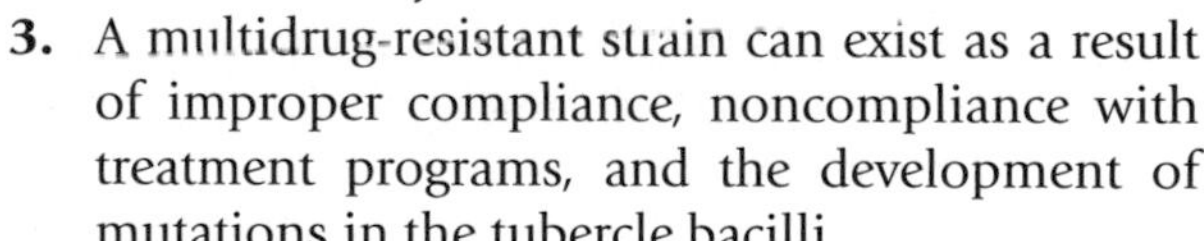

3. A multidrug-resistant strain can exist as a result of improper compliance, noncompliance with treatment programs, and the development of mutations in the tubercle bacilli.

B. Transmission
1. Transplacental transmission is rare.
2. Can occur during birth through the aspiration of infected amniotic fluid.
3. Newborn can become infected from contact with infected individuals.

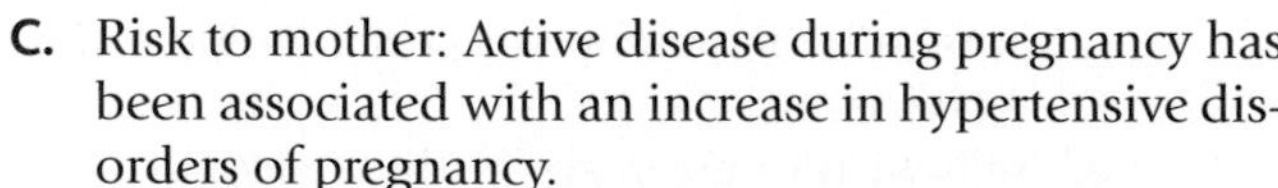

C. Risk to mother: Active disease during pregnancy has been associated with an increase in hypertensive disorders of pregnancy.

D. Diagnosis: If a chest radiograph is required for the mother, it is obtained only after 20 weeks' gestation, and a lead shield for the abdomen is required.

Tuberculin skin testing is safe during pregnancy; however, the HCP may want to delay testing until after delivery.

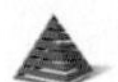

E. Data collection
1. Mother
    a. May be asymptomatic
    b. Fever and chills
    c. Night sweats
    d. Weight loss
    e. Fatigue
    f. Cough, hemoptysis, or green or yellow sputum
    g. Dyspnea
    h. Pleural pain
2. Neonate
    a. Fever
    b. Lethargy
    c. Poor feeding
    d. Failure to thrive
    e. Respiratory distress
    f. Hepatosplenomegaly
    g. Meningitis
    h. Disease may spread to all major organs.

F. Interventions
1. Pregnant client
    a. Administer isoniazid, pyrazinamide, and rifampin (Rifadin) daily for 9 months, as prescribed. Ethambutol (Myambutol) is added if medication resistance is probable.
    b. Pyridoxine (vitamin B_6) should be administered along with isoniazid to pregnant women to prevent fetal neurotoxicity caused by the isoniazid.
    c. Promote breastfeeding only if the mother is noninfectious and per health care provider prescription.
2. Newborn
    a. Management focuses on preventing disease and treating early infection.
    b. The newborn is skin tested at birth and may be placed on isoniazid therapy. The skin test is repeated in 3 to 4 months, and the isoniazid may be stopped if the skin test results remain negative.
    c. If the skin test result is positive, the newborn should receive isoniazid for at least 6 months.
    d. If the mother's sputum is free of organisms, the newborn does not need to be isolated from the mother while in the hospital.

XXVII. Urinary Tract Infection

A. Description: A urinary tract infection can occur during pregnancy (pregnancy is a predisposing factor); if untreated, the client can develop pyelonephritis.

B. Predisposing conditions
1. History of urinary tract infections
2. Sickle cell trait
3. Poor hygiene
4. Anemia
5. Diabetes mellitus

C. Data Collection and Interventions (refer to Chapter 53).

CRITICAL THINKING What Should You Do?

Answer: Interventions for nausea and vomiting in the pregnant client include eating dry crackers before arising; avoiding brushing teeth immediately after arising; eating small, frequent, low-fat meals during the day; drinking liquids between meals rather than at meals; avoiding fried foods and spicy foods; asking the health care provider (HCP) about acupressure (some types may require a prescription); and asking the HCP about the use of herbal remedies.

Reference(s): McKinney, E., James, S., Murray, S., Nelson, K. & Ashwill, J. (2013). *Maternal-child nursing* (4th ed., pp. 252–253). St. Louis: Elsevier.

PRACTICE QUESTIONS

226. The client is undergoing an amniocentesis at 16 weeks' gestation to detect the presence of biochemical or chromosomal abnormalities. Which instructions should the nurse reinforce to the client?
1. The bladder must be full during the exam.
2. The bladder must be empty during the exam.
3. She will be given RhoGAM because she is Rh positive.
4. Do not eat or drink anything 4 to 6 hours before the exam.

227. The client at 28 weeks' gestation is Rh negative and Coombs antibody negative. The nurse determines that the client understands what the nurse has taught her about Rh sensitization when the client makes which statement?
1. "I know I can never have another child."
2. "I am glad I won't have to have these shots if I have another child."
3. "I will have to have an injection once a month until the baby is born."
4. "I will tell the nurse at the hospital that I had RhoGAM during pregnancy."

228. While assisting with the measurement of fundal height, the client at 36 weeks' gestation states that she is feeling lightheaded. On the basis of the nurse's knowledge of pregnancy, the nurse determines that this is **most likely** a result of which?
1. A full bladder
2. Emotional instability
3. Insufficient iron intake
4. Compression of the vena cava

229. A contraction stress test is scheduled for the client. The woman asks the nurse about the test. Which response describes the **most** accurate description of the test?
1. "Uterine contractions are stimulated by Leopold's maneuvers."
2. "An internal fetal monitor is attached, and you will walk on a treadmill until contractions begin."
3. "The uterus is stimulated to contract by either small amounts of oxytocin (Pitocin) or by nipple stimulation."
4. "Small amounts of oxytocin (Pitocin) are administered during internal fetal monitoring to stimulate uterine contractions."

230. The client at 38 weeks' gestation is admitted to the birthing center in early labor. The client is carrying twins, and one of the fetuses is in a breech presentation. The nurse assists with planning care for the client and identifies which as **least likely** necessary for the care of this client?
1. Measuring the fundal height
2. Attaching electronic fetal monitoring
3. Preparing the client for a possible cesarean section
4. Gathering equipment for starting an intravenous line

231. The perinatal client is admitted to the obstetric unit during an exacerbation of a heart condition. When planning for the nutritional requirements of the client, the nurse should consult with the dietitian to ensure which dietary measure?
1. A low-calorie diet to ensure the absence of weight gain
2. A diet that is high in fluids and fiber to decrease constipation
3. A diet that is low in fluids and fiber to decrease blood volume
4. Unlimited sodium intake to increase the circulating blood volume

232. The nurse caring for a client with abruptio placentae is monitoring the client for signs of disseminated intravascular coagulopathy (DIC). The nurse would suspect DIC if which is observed?
1. Rapid clotting times
2. Pain and swelling of the calf of one leg
3. Laboratory values that indicate increased platelets
4. Petechiae, oozing from injection sites, and hematuria

233. The nurse has a teaching session with a malnourished client regarding iron supplementation to prevent anemia during pregnancy. Which would indicate successful learning?
1. "Iron supplements will give me diarrhea."
2. "The iron is needed for the red blood cells."
3. "Meat does not provide iron and should be avoided."
4. "My body has all the iron it needs, and I don't need to take supplements."

234. During a prenatal visit, the nurse is explaining dietary management to a client with diabetes mellitus. The nurse determines that the teaching has been effective when the client makes which statement?

1. "I can eat more sweets now because I need more calories."
2. "I need more fat in my diet so that the baby can gain enough weight."
3. "I need to eat a high-protein, low-carbohydrate diet now to control my blood glucose."
4. "I need to increase the fiber in my diet to control my blood glucose and prevent constipation."

235. The nurse is assigned to assist with caring for a client who is at risk for eclampsia. If the client progresses from preeclampsia to eclampsia, the nurse should take which **first** action?

1. Administer oxygen by face mask.
2. Clear and maintain an open airway.
3. Check the blood pressure and the fetal heart tones.
4. Prepare for the administration of intravenous magnesium sulfate.

236. The client is in her second trimester of pregnancy. She complains of frequent low back pain and ankle edema at the end of the day. The nurse should recommend which measure to help relieve both discomforts?

1. Lie on the left side with the feet dorsiflexed.
2. Soak the feet in hot water after performing 10 pelvic tilt exercises.
3. Lie on the right side with the feet elevated on a pillow and a heating pad on the back.
4. Lie on the floor with the legs elevated onto a couch or padded chair, with the hips and knees at a right angle.

237. The pregnant woman complains of being awakened frequently by leg cramps. The nurse reinforces instructions to the client's partner and should tell the client to perform which measure?

1. Dorsiflex the client's foot while flexing the knee.
2. Plantarflex the client's foot while flexing the knee.
3. Dorsiflex the client's foot while extending the knee.
4. Plantarflex the client's foot while extending the knee.

238. The nurse is reinforcing instructions to a pregnant client regarding measures to prevent heartburn. The nurse should instruct the client to take which **best** measure?

1. Eliminate between-meal snacks.
2. Drink decaffeinated coffee and tea.
3. Lie down for 30 minutes after eating.
4. Substitute salt in cooking for other spices.

239. The nurse is doing a 48-hour postpartum check on a client with mild gestational hypertension (GH). Which data indicate that the GH is a concern?

1. Urinary output has increased.
2. There is no evidence of proteinuria.
3. The client complains of a headache and blurred vision.
4. The blood pressure reading has returned to the prenatal baseline.

❖**240.** The nurse is monitoring a pregnant client with gestational hypertension (GH) who is at risk for preeclampsia. The nurse should check the client for which signs of preeclampsia? **Select all that apply.**

- ❑ **1.** Proteinuria
- ❑ **2.** Hypertension
- ❑ **3.** Low-grade fever
- ❑ **4.** Increased pulse rate
- ❑ **5.** Increased respiratory rate

ANSWERS

226. 1

Rationale: Before 20 weeks' gestation, the bladder must be kept full during amniocentesis to support the weight of the uterus. After 20 weeks' gestation, the bladder should be emptied to minimize the chance of puncturing the placenta or fetus. Rh_o(D) immune globulin (RhoGAM) is administered to Rh-negative women because of the risk of contact with the fetal blood during the exam. There are no fluid or food restrictions. Monitoring the fetal heart tones and the vital signs throughout and after the exam is an important intervention.

Test-Taking Strategy: Focus on the subject, an amniocentesis at 16 weeks' gestation. Remember that before 20 weeks' gestation, the bladder must be kept full to support the weight of the uterus. **Review:** client instructions for **amniocentesis.**

Level of Cognitive Ability: Applying
Client Needs: Physiological Integrity
Integrated Process: Nursing Process/Implementation
Content Area: Maternity: Antepartum

Priority Concepts: Client Education, Reproduction
Reference(s): Pagana, Pagana (2013), p. 53.

227. 4
Rationale: As described in the question, it is accepted practice to administer Rh_o(D) immune globulin (RhoGAM) to an Rh-negative woman at 28 weeks' gestation, with a second injection within 72 hours of delivery. This prevents sensitization, which could jeopardize a future pregnancy. For subsequent pregnancies or abortions, the injections must be repeated, because the immunity is passive. Options 1, 2, and 3 are inaccurate information.
Test-Taking Strategy: Note the subject, an understanding of Rh sensitization. Recalling the guidelines regarding the administration of RhoGAM will direct you to the correct option. Review: **Rh sensitization.**
Level of Cognitive Ability: Evaluating
Client Needs: Physiological Integrity
Integrated Process: Nursing Process/Evaluation
Content Area: Maternity: Antepartum
Priority Concepts: Client Education, Reproduction
Reference(s): McKinney et al (2013), pp. 439, 603.

228. 4
Rationale: Compression of the inferior vena cava and aorta by the uterus may cause supine hypotension syndrome during pregnancy. Having the woman turn onto her left side or elevating the right buttock during fundal height measurement will prevent or correct the problem. Options 1, 2, and 3 are not the cause of the problem described in the question.
Test-Taking Strategy: Note the strategic words, *most likely.* Focus on the data in the question, and recall the complications associated with pregnancy. Use the ABCs—airway, breathing, and circulation—to direct you to the correct option. **Review:** the interventions for **supine hypotension syndrome.**
Level of Cognitive Ability: Analyzing
Client Needs: Physiological Integrity
Integrated Process: Nursing Process/Data Collection
Content Area: Maternity: Antepartum
Priority Concepts: Perfusion, Reproduction
Reference(s): McKinney et al (2013), p. 237.

229. 3
Rationale: A contraction stress test assesses placental oxygenation and function and determines the fetus's ability to tolerate labor, as well as its well-being. The test is performed if the nonstress test result is abnormal. During the stress test, the fetus is exposed to the stressor of contractions to assess the adequacy of placental perfusion under simulated labor conditions. An external fetal monitor is applied to the mother, and a 20- to 30-minute baseline strip is recorded. The uterus is stimulated to contract, either by the administration of a dilute dose of oxytocin (Pitocin) or by having the mother use nipple stimulation, until three palpable contractions with a duration of 40 seconds or more during a 10-minute period have occurred. Frequent maternal blood pressure readings are performed, and the client is monitored closely while increasing doses of oxytocin are given. Leopold's maneuvers are performed to locate the position of the fetus.
Test-Taking Strategy: Note the strategic word, *most,* and focus on the subject, the contraction stress test. Remember that during both the nonstress test and the contraction stress test, external monitoring is performed; therefore, eliminate options 2 and 4 because they are comparable or alike. Next, recalling the purpose of Leopold's maneuvers will assist in eliminating option 1. **Review:** the **contraction stress test.**
Level of Cognitive Ability: Applying
Client Needs: Physiological Integrity
Integrated Process: Nursing Process/Implementation
Content Area: Maternity: Antepartum
Priority Concepts: Client Education, Reproduction
Reference(s): Pagana, Pagana (2013), pp. 432–434.

230. 1
Rationale: Option 1 is a low priority because fundal height should be measured at each antepartal clinic visit; it is not a priority of care during the intrapartum period. Options 2, 3, and 4 are all high priorities. The twins should be monitored by dual electronic fetal monitoring, and any signs of distress should be reported. Many health care providers choose to perform a cesarean birth if either of the twins is breech. The mother should have an intravenous line in place in case fluid or blood replacement is required.
Test-Taking Strategy: Note the strategic words, *least likely.* Use the Maslow's Hierarchy of Needs theory and the ABCs—airway, breathing, and circulation—to prioritize and direct you to the correct option. **Review: breech presentation.**
Level of Cognitive Ability: Analyzing
Client Needs: Physiological Integrity
Integrated Process: Nursing Process/Planning
Content Area: Maternity: Intrapartum
Priority Concepts: Perfusion, Reproduction
Reference(s): McKinney et al (2013), pp. 325, 640–641.

231. 2
Rationale: Constipation causes the client to use Valsalva's maneuver. This causes blood to rush to the heart and overload the cardiac system. The absence of weight gain is not recommended during pregnancy. Diets that are low in fluid and fiber cause a decrease in blood volume, which in turn deprives the fetus of nutrients. Too much sodium could cause an overload to the circulating blood volume and contribute to the cardiac condition.
Test-Taking Strategy: Focus on the subject, nutritional requirements for the pregnant client with a heart condition. Try to relate the situation to something with which you are familiar. Look for options that would apply to any heart condition, and think about the needs of a pregnant client. **Review:** dietary measures for the client with **cardiac disease.**
Level of Cognitive Ability: Applying
Client Needs: Physiological Integrity
Integrated Process: Nursing Process/Planning
Content Area: Maternity: Antepartum
Priority Concepts: Nutrition, Reproduction
Reference(s): McKinney et al (2013), pp. 253, 620–621.

232. 4
Rationale: DIC is a state of diffuse clotting in which clotting factors are consumed, which leads to widespread bleeding. Platelet counts are decreased, because they are consumed by the process. Coagulation studies show no clot formation (clotting times are thus prolonged), and fibrin plugs may clog the microvasculature diffusely rather than in an isolated area.
Test-Taking Strategy: Focus on the subject, the signs/symptoms of DIC. Eliminate option 2 on the basis of the knowledge

that DIC is a widespread problem rather than a localized one. Eliminate options 1 and 3 next, because they are comparable or alike. **Review:** the signs/symptoms related to disseminated intravascular coagulation.
Level of Cognitive Ability: Analyzing
Client Needs: Physiological Integrity
Integrated Process: Nursing Process/Data Collection
Content Area: Maternity: Antepartum
Priority Concepts: Clotting, Reproduction
Reference(s): McKinney et al (2013), p. 578.

233. 2
Rationale: A nutritional supplement that is commonly needed during pregnancy for the red blood cells is iron. Anemia in pregnancy is primarily caused by iron deficiency. Iron supplements usually cause constipation. Meats are an excellent source of iron. Iron for the fetus comes from the maternal serum.
Test-Taking Strategy: Note the subject, iron supplementation. Eliminate options 3 and 4 because of the closed-ended words, *not* and *all.* Knowledge regarding the effects of iron supplements will assist you with eliminating option 1. **Review:** anemia and iron supplements.
Level of Cognitive Ability: Evaluating
Client Needs: Physiological Integrity
Integrated Process: Nursing Process/Evaluation
Content Area: Maternity: Antepartum
Priority Concepts: Client Education, Nutrition
Reference(s): McKinney et al (2013), pp. 282, 621.

234. 4
Rationale: An increase in calories is needed during pregnancy, but concentrated sugars should be avoided because they may cause hyperglycemia. Per health care provider recommendations, fat intake should be 20% to 30% of the total calories. In addition, the client with diabetes needs about 50% to 60% of her caloric intake from carbohydrates and about 12% to 20% from protein. High-fiber foods will control blood glucose levels and prevent constipation.
Test-Taking Strategy: Note the subject, teaching has been effective. Use knowledge regarding diabetes mellitus and diet therapy to direct you to the correct option. **Review:** diabetes and pregnancy.
Level of Cognitive Ability: Evaluating
Client Needs: Health Promotion and Maintenance
Integrated Process: Nursing Process/Evaluation
Content Area: Maternity: Antepartum
Priority Concepts: Glucose Regulation, Reproduction
Reference(s): McKinney et al (2013), pp. 612, 614–616.

235. 2
Rationale: The first actions are to maintain an open airway and to prevent injuries to the client. The client should be turned to the side and monitored for airway compromise. Options 1, 3, and 4 may be components of care, but they are not the first actions.
Test-Taking Strategy: Note the strategic word, *first.* Use the ABCs—airway, breathing, and circulation—to answer this question. Airway is the first priority. **Review:** the care of the client with eclampsia.
Level of Cognitive Ability: Applying
Client Needs: Physiological Integrity
Integrated Process: Nursing Process/Implementation
Content Area: Critical Care: Emergency Situations
Priority Concepts: Gas Exchange, Reproduction
Reference(s): McKinney et al (2013), p. 597.

236. 4
Rationale: The position described in option 4 will produce the posture of the pelvic tilt while countering gravity as the force that leads to the edema of the lower extremities. Although the other options may seem useful, options 2 and 3 identify heat, which should be prescribed by the health care provider (HCP). Option 1 will not relieve back pain and ankle edema.
Test-Taking Strategy: Focus on the subject, measures to alleviate back pain and ankle edema. Eliminate options 2 and 3, because the application of heat needs to be prescribed by the HCP. From the remaining options, focus on the subject to direct you to the correct option. **Review:** the measures that will reduce discomforts of pregnancy.
Level of Cognitive Ability: Applying
Client Needs: Physiological Integrity
Integrated Process: Nursing Process/Implementation
Content Area: Maternity: Antepartum
Priority Concepts: Pain, Reproduction
Reference(s): McKinney et al (2013), pp. 252–253.

237. 3
Rationale: Leg cramps often occur when the pregnant woman stretches her leg and plantarflexes her foot. Dorsiflexion of the foot while extending the knee stretches the gastrocnemius muscle, prevents the muscle from contracting, and halts the cramping. Therefore, the remaining options are incorrect.
Test-Taking Strategy: Focus on the subject, the measure that will alleviate muscle cramps. Visualize each of the descriptions in the options to help direct you to the correct option. **Review:** the measures to alleviate muscle cramps.
Level of Cognitive Ability: Applying
Client Needs: Health Promotion and Maintenance
Integrated Process: Teaching and Learning
Content Area: Maternity: Antepartum
Priority Concepts: Pain, Reproduction
Reference(s): McKinney et al (2013), pp. 253–254.

238. 2
Rationale: Caffeine, like spices, may cause heartburn and needs to be avoided. Spices tend to trigger heartburn. Eating smaller, more frequent portions is preferable to eating three large meals to control heartburn. Lying down after meals is likely to lead to the reflux of stomach contents and cause heartburn. Salt leads to the retention of fluid.
Test-Taking Strategy: Note the strategic word, *best,* and focus on the subject, measures to prevent heartburn. This will direct you to the correct option. **Review:** the measures that prevent and alleviate heartburn.
Level of Cognitive Ability: Applying
Client Needs: Health Promotion and Maintenance
Integrated Process: Teaching and Learning
Content Area: Maternity: Antepartum
Priority Concepts: Client Education, Nutrition
Reference(s): McKinney et al (2013), pp. 252–253.

239. 3

Rationale: Options 1, 2, and 4 are all signs that gestational hypertension is not present. Option 3 is a symptom of the worsening of the gestational hypertension and is a concern that needs to be reported.

Test-Taking Strategy: Focus on the subject, a concern associated with gestational hypertension. Recalling the signs and symptoms associated with gestational hypertension will direct you to the correct option. **Review:** gestational hypertension.

Level of Cognitive Ability: Evaluating

Client Needs: Physiological Integrity

Integrated Process: Nursing Process/Evaluation

Content Area: Maternity: Antepartum

Priority Concepts: Perfusion, Reproduction

Reference(s): McKinney et al (2013), p. 593.

❖ **240. 1, 2, 4**

Rationale: Signs of preeclampsia are hypertension and proteinuria. A low-grade fever, increased pulse rate, and increased respiratory rate are not associated with preeclampsia.

Test-Taking Strategy: Focus on the subject, signs of preeclampsia. Thinking about the pathophysiology associated with this disorder will direct you to the correct options. Remember that the signs of preeclampsia are hypertension and proteinuria. **Review:** the signs of preeclampsia.

Level of Cognitive Ability: Analyzing

Client Needs: Physiological Integrity

Integrated Process: Nursing Process/Data Collection

Content Area: Maternity: Antepartum

Priority Concepts: Clinical Judgment, Reproduction

Reference(s): McKinney et al (2013), p. 594.

Maternity

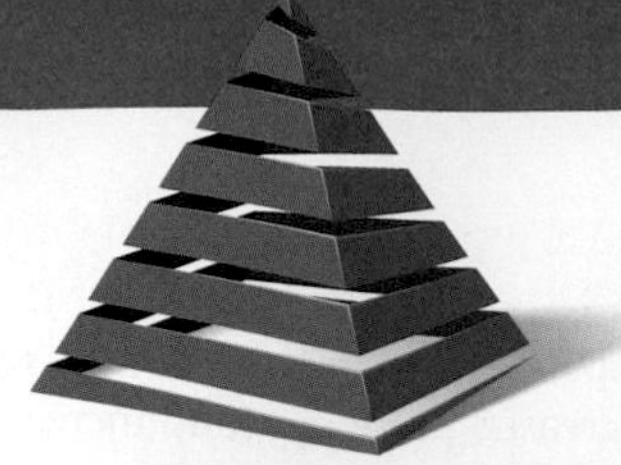

CHAPTER 27

Labor and Delivery and Associated Complications

CRITICAL THINKING What Should You Do?

A client is in active labor. The nurse is monitoring the fetal heart rate and notes that the heart rate is 180 beats/minute, lasting for longer than 10 minutes. What should the nurse do?
Answer is located on p. 315.

I. The Process of Labor: "the Four *P*s"

A. Description
1. **Labor**: A coordinated sequence of rhythmic involuntary uterine contractions
2. **Delivery**: The actual event of birth

B. Four major factors (four *P*s) interact during normal childbirth; the four *P*s are interrelated and depend on one another for a safe delivery and include *powers, passageway, passenger,* and *psyche.*

C. Powers: Uterine contractions
1. The forces acting to expel the fetus and **placenta**
2. Effacement: The shortening and thinning of the cervix during the first stage of labor
3. Dilation: The enlargement of the cervical os and cervical canal during the first stage of labor
4. Pushing efforts of the mother during the second stage

D. Passageway: Composed of the mother's rigid bony pelvis and the soft tissues of the cervix, pelvic floor, **vagina**, and introitus (external opening to the vagina)

E. Passenger: The fetus, membranes, and placenta

F. Psyche: A woman's emotional structure that can determine her entire response to labor and influence physiological and psychological functioning; the mother may experience anxiety or fear.

G. Attitude
1. The relationship of the fetal body parts with one another
2. The normal intrauterine attitude is flexion, in which the fetal back is rounded, the head is forward on the chest, and the arms and legs are flexed in against the body. The other attitude, known as extension, tends to present larger fetal diameters.

H. Fetal lie
1. Relationship of the spine of the fetus to the spine of the mother
2. Longitudinal or vertical: Fetal spine is parallel to the mother's spine. The fetus is in either a cephalic or breech presentation (Fig. 27-1).
3. Transverse or horizontal: Fetal spine is at a right angle, or perpendicular, to the mother's spine. The presenting part is usually the shoulder, and delivery is by cesarean section (see Fig. 27-1).

I. Presentation
1. Portion of the fetus that enters the pelvis first
2. Cephalic: The most common presentation; fetal head presents first.
3. Breech: Buttocks present first.
   a. Delivery by cesarean section may be required, although vaginal birth is often possible.

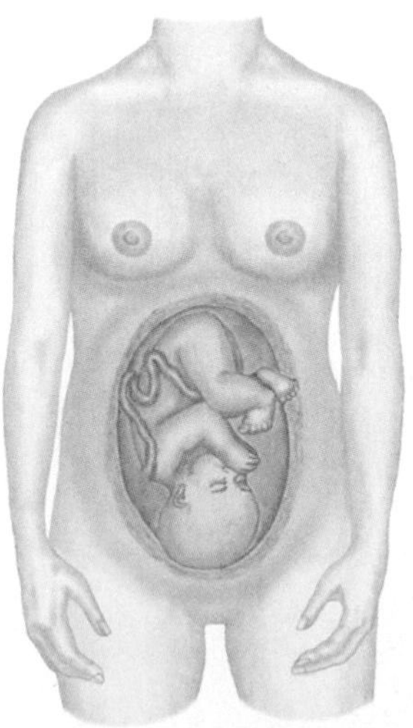

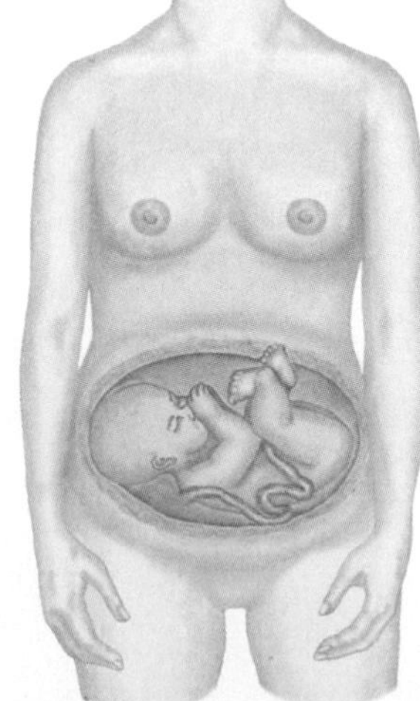

FIGURE 27-1 Fetal lie. **A,** In a longitudinal lie, the long axis of the fetus is parallel to the long axis of the mother. **B,** In a transverse lie, the long axis of the fetus is at a right angle to the long axis of the mother. The mother's abdomen has a wide, short appearance. (From McKinney E, James S, Murray S, Ashwill J: *Maternal-child nursing*, ed 4, St. Louis, 2013, Saunders.)

b. Breech presentation has three variations: frank, full (complete), and footling.
4. Shoulder: Fetus is in a transverse lie; the arm, back, abdomen, or side could present. If the fetus does not spontaneously rotate or it is not possible to turn the fetus manually, a cesarean section may be performed.

J. Presenting part: The specific fetal structure lying nearest to the cervix

K. Position: The relationship of the assigned area of the presenting part or landmark to the maternal pelvis (Box 27-1 and Fig. 27-2)

BOX 27-1 Fetal Positions

Vertex Presentations

- See Figure 27-2.

Face Presentations

- RMA: Right mentoanterior
- LMA: Left mentoanterior
- RMP: Right mentoposterior

Breech Presentations

- LSA: Left sacroanterior
- LSP: Left sacroposterior

Other Presentations

- Brow presentation
- Shoulder presentation

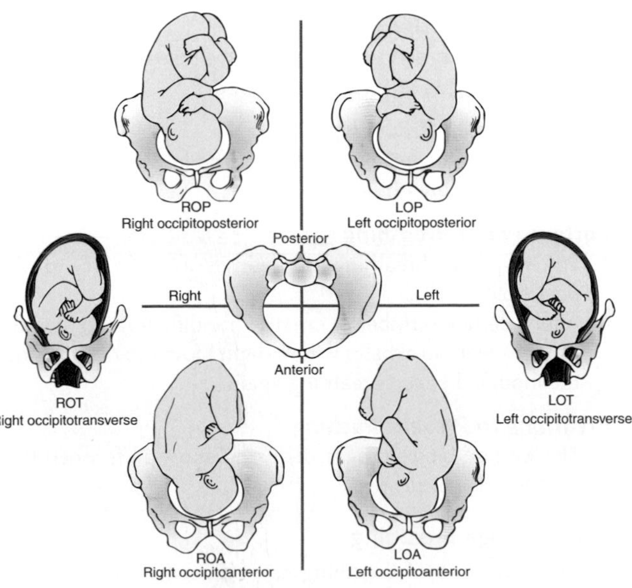

FIGURE 27-2 Fetal vertex (occiput) presentations in relation to the front, back, or side of the maternal pelvis. (From Perry S, Hockenberry M, Lowdermilk D, Wilson D: *Maternal-child nursing care*, ed 4, St. Louis, 2010, Mosby.)

L. Station
1. The measurement of the progress of descent in centimeters above or below the midplane from the presenting part to the ischial spine
2. Station 0: At the ischial spine
3. Minus station: Above the ischial spine
4. Plus station: Below the ischial spine
5. Engagement: When the widest part of the presenting part has passed the inlet; usually corresponds to a 0 station

II. Mechanisms of Labor (Box 27-2)

A. Data collection
1. Lightening or dropping: Is also known as engagement and occurs when the fetus descends into the pelvis about 2 weeks before delivery. Lightening or dropping is most noticeable in

BOX 27-2 Mechanisms of Labor

Engagement

Engagement is the mechanism by which the fetus nestles into the pelvis. It also is called *lightening* or *dropping*.

Descent

Descent is the process that the fetal head undergoes as it begins its journey through the pelvis. It is a continuous process from the time of engagement until birth, and is assessed by the measurement called *station*.

Flexion

Flexion is the process of the fetal head's nodding forward toward the fetal chest.

Internal Rotation

The internal rotation of the fetus occurs most commonly from the occipitotransverse position, which is assumed at engagement into the pelvis, to the occipitoanterior position while continuously descending.

Extension

Extension enables the head to emerge when the fetus is in a cephalic position, and it begins after the head crowns. Extension is complete when the head passes under the symphysis pubis and occiput and the anterior fontanel, brow, face, and chin pass over the sacrum and coccyx and are over the perineum.

Restitution

Restitution is the realignment of the fetal head with the body after the head emerges.

External Rotation

The shoulders externally rotate after the head emerges and restitution occurs, so that the shoulders are in the anteroposterior diameter of the pelvis.

Expulsion

Expulsion is the birth of the entire body.

first pregnancies; may not occur until the onset of true labor in the multigravida.
2. Braxton Hicks contractions increase.
3. Vaginal mucosa congested. Vaginal discharge increases.
4. Brownish or blood-tinged cervical mucus is passed.
5. Cervix ripens and becomes soft and partly effaced; it may begin to dilate.
6. Sudden burst of energy experienced by the mother. This is also known as "nesting" and occurs 24 to 48 hours before the onset of labor.
7. Loss of 1 to 3 pounds from water loss resulting from fluid shifts produced by changes in progesterone and estrogen levels
8. Spontaneous rupture of the membranes occurs.

B. True labor: Contractions may manifest as back pain in some women; contractions often resemble menstrual cramps during early labor (Box 27-3).
C. False labor: Also known as prodromal labor, contractions are felt in the abdomen and groin and may be more annoying than painful (see Box 27-3).

In true labor, contractions increase in duration and intensity. In false labor, contractions are irregular and do not produce dilation, effacement, or descent.

III. Leopold's Maneuvers

A. Description: A method of palpation for determining the presentation and position of the fetus; an aid for locating fetal heart sounds
B. If the head is in the fundus, a hard, round, movable object is felt. The buttocks feel soft and have an irregular shape, and they are more difficult to move.
C. The fetus's back, which is a smooth, hard surface, should be felt on one side of the abdomen.
D. Irregular knobs and lumps, which may be the hands, feet, elbows, and knees, are felt on the opposite side of the abdomen.

IV. Breathing Techniques (Box 27-4)

A. Provide a focus during contractions, thus interfering with pain sensory transmission
B. Promote relaxation and oxygenation
C. Begin with simple breathing patterns and progress to more complex ones as needed

V. Fetal Monitoring

A. Description
1. Displays fetal heart rate (FHR) and uterine activity
2. Monitors the uterine activity, frequency, and duration of contractions
3. Monitors the FHR in relation to maternal contractions
4. Baseline FHR is measured between contractions. The normal FHR at term is 110 to 160 beats per minute.

BOX 27-3 True Labor and False Labor

True Labor

Contractions occur regularly. They become stronger, last longer, and occur closer together.
Cervical dilation and effacement are progressive.
The fetus usually becomes engaged in the pelvis and begins to descend.

False Labor

False labor does not produce dilation, effacement, or descent.
Contractions are irregular and without progression.
Activity, such as walking, often relieves false labor.

Example:
If a woman has been sleeping and wakes up with contractions, gets up, and moves around, and her contractions become stronger and closer together, this is true labor. If the contractions go away, this is false labor.

BOX 27-4 Breathing Techniques

First-Stage Breathing

Cleansing Breath
- Each contraction begins and ends with a deep inspiration and expiration.

Slow-Paced Breathing
- A slow, deep breathing that promotes relaxation
- Used as long as possible during labor

Modified-Paced Breathing
- Used when slow-paced breathing is no longer effective
- Shallow, fast breathing

Pattern-Paced Breathing
- Pattern-paced breathing sometimes is referred to as *pant-blow*.
- After a certain number of breaths (modified-paced breathing), the woman exhales with a slight blow and then begins the modified-paced breathing again.

Breathing to Prevent Pushing
- The woman blows repeatedly using short puffs when the urge to push is strong.

Second-Stage Breathing

Several variations of breathing can be used in the pushing stage of labor, and the woman may grunt, groan, sigh, or moan as she pushes. Prolonged breath holding while pushing with a closed glottis may result in a decrease in cardiac output. If breath holding while pushing is used, the open glottis method or limiting breath holding to less than 6 to 8 seconds should be done.

B. External fetal monitoring
  1. Noninvasive; performed with the use of a tocotransducer or a Doppler ultrasonic transducer
  2. Leopold's maneuvers are performed to determine on which side the fetal back is located, and the ultrasound transducer is then placed over this area and fastened with a belt.
  3. The tocotransducer is placed over the fundus of the **uterus**, where contractions feel the strongest, and fastened with a belt.
  4. Allow the client to assume a comfortable position, avoiding vena cava compression (maternal supine hypotensive syndrome).
  5. The preferred maternal position is to have her lie on her side to increase placental perfusion.

C. Internal fetal monitoring
  1. Invasive; requires rupturing the membranes and attaching an electrode to the presenting part of the fetus
  2. Mother must be dilated 2 to 3 cm before internal monitoring can be performed.

D. Periodic patterns in the FHR
  1. Fetal bradycardia and tachycardia
    a. Bradycardia: FHR is less than 110 beats per minute for 10 minutes or longer.
    b. Tachycardia: FHR is greater than 160 beats per minute for 10 minutes or longer.

! If fetal bradycardia or tachycardia occurs, change the position of the mother, administer oxygen, and check the mother's vital signs. Notify the registered nurse immediately. The health care provider (HCP) is also notified.

  2. Variability
    a. Fluctuations in the baseline FHR
    b. Absence of variability or undetected variability is considered nonreassuring.
    c. Decreased variability can result from fetal hypoxemia, acidosis, or certain medications.
    d. A temporary decrease in variability can occur when the fetus is in a sleep state. (Sleep states do not usually last more than 30 minutes.)
  3. Accelerations
    a. Brief, temporary increases in the FHR of at least 15 beats above the baseline and lasting at least 15 seconds
    b. Usually a reassuring sign that reflects a responsive, nonacidotic fetus
    c. Usually occur with fetal movement or stimulation
    d. May be nonperiodic (having no relation to contractions) or periodic (with contractions)
    e. May occur with uterine contractions, vaginal examinations, mild cord compression, or when the fetus is in a breech presentation
  4. Early decelerations
    a. Decrease in FHR below baseline. The rate at the lowest point of the deceleration usually remains greater than 100 beats/min.
    b. Occur during contractions as the fetal head is pressed against the woman's pelvis or soft tissues, such as the cervix, and return to baseline FHR by the end of the contraction
    c. Not associated with fetal compromise and require no intervention
  5. Late decelerations
    a. Nonreassuring patterns that reflect impaired placental exchange or uteroplacental insufficiency
    b. Degree of the fall in the heart rate from baseline is not related to the amount of uteroplacental insufficiency.

! Interventions for late decelerations include immediately improving placental blood flow and fetal oxygenation.

  6. Variable decelerations
    a. Caused by conditions that restrict flow through the umbilical cord
    b. May be nonperiodic, occurring at times that are unrelated to contractions
    c. One considers the baseline rate and variability when evaluating variable decelerations.
    d. Are significant when the FHR repeatedly decreases to less than 70 beats per minute and persists at that level for at least 60 seconds before returning to baseline

! If variable decelerations occur, the nurse should change the position of the mother, administer oxygen, discontinue oxytocin (Pitocin) if infusing, and check the mother's vital signs. The registered nurse will notify the HCP immediately. Amnioinfusion (intrauterine instillation of warmed saline to decrease compression on the umbilical cord) may be prescribed.

  7. Hypertonic uterine activity
    a. Checking uterine activity includes frequency, duration, intensity of contractions, and uterine resting tone; assessment is performed either by palpating by hand or with an internal uterine pressure catheter (IUPC).
    b. Uterus should relax between contractions for 60 seconds or more.
    c. Uterine contraction intensity is about 50 to 75 mm Hg (with intrauterine catheter) during labor and may reach 110 mm Hg with pushing during the second stage.
    d. Average resting tone is 5 to 15 mm Hg.

Maternity

BOX 27-5 Nonreassuring FHR Patterns

Bradycardia
Tachycardia
Late decelerations
Prolonged decelerations
Hypertonic uterine activity
Decreased or absent variability
Variable decelerations falling to less than 70 beats/min for longer than 60 seconds

e. In hypertonic uterine activity, the uterine resting tone between contractions is high, reducing uterine blood flow and decreasing fetal oxygen supply.

8. Nonreassuring FHR patterns (Box 27-5)
9. Interventions for nonreassuring patterns (see Priority Nursing Actions)

VI. Four Stages of Labor (Table 27-1)

A. Stage 1: Latent phase
 1. Description: Stage 1 is the longest.
 2. Data collection
  a. Cervical dilation of up to 1 to 4 cm
  b. Uterine contractions every 15 to 30 minutes, 15 to 30 seconds in duration, and of mild intensity
 3. Interventions
  a. Encourage the mother and partner to participate in care.
  b. Assist with comfort measures, changes of position, and ambulation.
  c. Keep the mother and partner informed of progress.
  d. Offer fluids and ice chips.
  e. Encourage voiding every 1 to 2 hours.

PRIORITY NURSING ACTIONS!

Actions to Take for a Nonreassuring Fetal Heart Rate Pattern

1. Call the registered nurse and stay with the client.
2. Identify the cause.
3. Stop the oxytocin (Pitocin) infusion.
4. Change the mother's position.
5. Administer oxygen by face mask at 8 to 10 L/min and infuse intravenous fluids as prescribed.
6. Prepare to assist to initiate continuous electronic fetal monitoring with internal devices if not contraindicated.
7. Prepare for cesarean delivery if necessary.
8. Document the event, actions taken, and the mother's response.

Nonreassuring fetal heart rate patterns include bradycardia, tachycardia, late decelerations, prolonged decelerations, hypertonic uterine activity, decreased or absent variability, or variable decelerations falling to less than 70 beats/min for longer than 60 seconds. If a nonreassuring fetal heart rate pattern is noted, the registered nurse is called, who will then contact the HCP as soon as possible. (The nurse stays with the client and asks another nurse to contact the registered nurse.) The nurse needs to identify the cause of the pattern immediately. This includes checking for a prolapsed umbilical cord and checking maternal vital signs to identify hypotension, hypertension, or fever that can contribute to the fetal response associated with the nonreassuring pattern. If the mother is receiving an oxytocin (Pitocin) infusion, it is stopped because oxytocin causes uterine stimulation, which can worsen the nonreassuring pattern. A tocolytic may be prescribed. The mother is repositioned because this may improve placental perfusion (avoid the supine position). Oxygen is administered by face mask at 8 to 10 L/min to increase maternal blood oxygen saturation making more oxygen available to the fetus, and intravenous fluids are infused to expand the mother's blood volume and improve placental perfusion. If not contraindicated, the nurse prepares to initiate continuous electronic fetal monitoring with internal devices. Cesarean delivery may be necessary, and the nurse should prepare for this procedure. Birth preparation should also include neonatal resuscitation. The nurse documents the event, actions taken, the mother's response, and any other pertinent data.

References: McKinney, E., James, S., Murray, S., Nelson, K. & Ashwill, J. (2013). *Maternal-child nursing* (4th ed., p. 377). St. Louis: Elsevier.

TABLE 27-1 Four Stages of Labor

First Stage	Second Stage	Third Stage	Fourth Stage
Effacement and dilation of the cervix	Expulsion of the fetus	Separation of the placenta	Physical recovery
Divided into three stages: latent, active, and transition	Pushing stage	Expulsion of the placenta	1 to 4 hours after the expulsion of the placenta
Woman is sociable, talkative, and excited in the latent phase; becoming tired, restless, and anxious as labor intensifies and contractions become stronger	Woman has intense concentration on pushing with contractions; may fall asleep between contractions	Woman is relieved after baby's birth; usually very tired	Woman is tired but may find it difficult to rest because of excitement; eager to become acquainted with her newborn

B. Stage 1: Active phase
   1. Data collection
      a. Cervical dilation of 4 to 7 cm
      b. Uterine contractions every 3 to 5 minutes, 30 to 60 seconds in duration, and of moderate intensity
   2. Interventions
      a. Encourage the maintenance of effective breathing patterns.
      b. Provide a quiet environment.
      c. Keep the mother and partner informed of progress.
      d. Promote comfort with back rubs, sacral pressure, pillow support, frequent position changes, and oral care; fluids and ice chips, as prescribed; and ointment for dry lips.
      e. Instruct the partner in effleurage (light stroking of abdomen).
      f. Encourage voiding every 1 to 2 hours.

C. Stage 1: Transition phase
   1. Data collection
      a. Cervical dilation of 8 to 10 cm
      b. Uterine contractions every 2 to 3 minutes, 45 to 90 seconds in duration, and of strong intensity
   2. Interventions
      a. Encourage rest between contractions.
      b. Wake mother at beginning of contraction so she can begin breathing pattern.
      c. Keep the mother and partner informed of progress.
      d. Provide privacy.
      e. Offer fluids, ice chips, and ointment for dry lips.
      f. Encourage voiding every 1 to 2 hours.

D. Interventions throughout stage 1
   1. Monitor maternal vital signs.
   2. Monitor FHR via ultrasound Doppler, fetoscope, or electronic fetal monitor.
   3. Check the FHR before, during, and after a contraction, noting that the normal FHR is 110 to 160 beats per minute.
   4. Assist with monitoring uterine contractions by palpation or tocodynamometer, and determine frequency, duration, and intensity.
   5. Assist with monitoring the status of cervical dilation and effacement.
   6. Assist with monitoring fetal station, presentation, and position by Leopold's maneuvers.
   7. Assist with pelvic examinations and prepare for a fern test to check for the rupture of membranes.

⚠ If the membranes rupture, the priority is to check the fetal heart rate because of the risk of collapsed umbilical cord. Then, check the color of the amniotic fluid because meconium-stained fluid can indicate fetal distress.

E. Stage 2
   1. Data collection
      a. Cervical dilation is complete.
      b. Progress of labor is measured by the descent of the fetal head through the birth canal (change in fetal station).
      c. Uterine contractions occur every 2 to 3 minutes and last 60 to 75 seconds, and are of strong intensity.
      d. Increase in bloody show occurs.
      e. The mother feels the urge to bear down. Assist the mother with pushing efforts.
   2. Interventions
      a. Perform assessments every 5 minutes.
      b. Monitor maternal vital signs.
      c. Monitor FHR via ultrasound Doppler, fetoscope, or electronic fetal monitor.
      d. Monitor the FHR before, during, and after a contraction, noting that normal FHR is 110 to 160 beats per minute.
      e. Monitor the uterine contractions with palpation or monitoring device, determining the frequency, duration, and intensity.
      f. Provide the mother with encouragement and praise, and provide for rest between contractions.
      g. Keep the mother and partner informed of progress.
      h. Maintain privacy.
      i. Provide ice chips and ointment for dry lips.
      j. Assist mother into a position that promotes comfort and facilitates pushing efforts, such as lithotomy, semi-sitting, kneeling, side-lying, or squatting.
      k. Monitor for signs of approaching birth, such as perineal bulging or visualization of the fetal head.
      l. Prepare for birth (expulsion of fetus).

F. Stage 3
   1. Data collection
      a. Contractions occur until the placenta is expelled.
      b. Placental separation and expulsion occur.
      c. Expulsion of the placenta occurs 5 to 30 minutes after the birth of the baby.
      d. Schultze mechanism: Center portion of placenta separates first, and its shiny fetal surface emerges from vagina.
      e. Duncan mechanism: Margin of the placenta separates, and the dull, red, rough maternal surface emerges from the vagina first.
   2. Interventions
      a. Monitor maternal vital signs and uterine status.
      b. Provide the parents with explanation regarding expulsion of the placenta.
      c. After the expulsion of the placenta, the uterine fundus remains firm and is located approximately two fingerbreadths below the umbilicus.

d. Examine the placenta for cotyledons and membranes to verify that it is intact. Examine the umbilical cord for the presence of one vein and two arteries.
e. Monitor the mother for shivering. Provide warmth.
f. Promote parental–neonatal attachment.

G. Stage 4
1. Description: The period of time from 1 to 4 hours after delivery
2. Data collection
a. Blood pressure returns to prelabor level.
b. Pulse is slightly lower than during labor.
c. Fundus remains contracted, in the midline, 1 or 2 fingerbreadths below the umbilicus.

⚠ Monitor lochia discharge. Lochia may be moderate in amount and red in color in stage 4.

3. Interventions
a. Maternal assessments are performed every 15 minutes for 1 hour, every 30 minutes for 1 hour, and hourly for 2 hours (or as per agency policy).
b. Provide warm blankets.
c. Apply ice packs to the perineum.
d. Massage the fundus, if needed, if the fundus is flaccid (boggy).
e. Provide breastfeeding support, as needed.
f. See Chapter 29 for information about caring for the **newborn**.

VII. Anesthesia

A. Local anesthesia
1. Used for blocking the pain during episiotomy
2. Administered just before the birth of the baby
3. No effect on the fetus

B. Lumbar epidural block
1. Injection site in the epidural space at L3-L4
2. Administered after labor is established or just before a scheduled cesarean birth
3. Relieves pain from contractions and numbs the vagina and perineum
4. May cause hypotension, bladder distention, and a prolonged second stage
5. Does not cause headache, because the dura mater is not penetrated
6. Monitor maternal blood pressure and assess bladder frequently.
7. IV fluids are administered, as prescribed. Increase fluids, as prescribed, if hypotension occurs.
8. Observe for any adverse effects from opioid epidurals, such as nausea and vomiting, pruritus, or respiratory depression.

C. Intrathecal opioid analgesics
1. Medication is injected into the subarachnoid space and has a rapid onset of action.
2. May be used in combination with a lumbar epidural block

D. Subarachnoid (spinal) block
1. Injection site is in the spinal subarachnoid space at L3-L5
2. The block is administered just before birth
3. Relieves uterine and perineal pain and numbs the vagina, perineum, and lower extremities
4. Usually causes maternal hypotension
5. Observe for postspinal headache—a headache that is worse when woman is upright and that may disappear when she is lying flat. Notify anesthesia provider if it occurs (a blood patch may be done).
6. IV fluids are administered, if prescribed.

E. General anesthesia
1. May be used for some surgical interventions
2. The mother is not awake.

⚠ General anesthesia presents a danger of respiratory depression, vomiting, and aspiration.

VIII. Obstetrical Procedures

A. Bishop score (Table 27-2)
1. Used to determine maternal readiness for labor induction and evaluates cervical status and fetal position
2. Indicated before the induction of labor
3. The five factors are assigned a score of 0 to 3, and the total score is calculated.
4. A score of 6 or more indicates a readiness for labor induction.

TABLE 27-2 Factors of the Bishop Score

Score	0	1	2	3
Dilation of cervix (cm)	0	1 to 2 cm	3 to 4 cm	>5 cm
Effacement of cervix (%)	0% to 30%	40% to 50%	60% to 70%	>80%
Consistency of cervix	Firm	Medium	Soft	
Position of cervix	Posterior	Midposition	Anterior	
Station of presenting part	−3	−2	−1	+1, +2

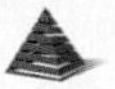

B. Induction

1. Induction is a deliberate initiation of uterine contractions that stimulates labor.
2. Elective induction may be accomplished by oxytocin (Pitocin) infusion.
3. Baseline tracing of uterine contractions and FHR is obtained.
4. The IV dosage of oxytocin may be increased, as prescribed; contractions, FHR, and maternal blood pressure and pulse are assessed by the registered nurse before increasing the dose.
5. The rate of oxytocin is not increased when the desired contraction pattern is obtained (contraction frequency of 2 to 3 minutes and lasting 60 seconds).

An oxytocin (Pitocin) infusion is discontinued if uterine contraction frequency is less than 2 minutes or duration is longer than 90 seconds, or if fetal distress is noted.

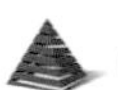

C. Amniotomy

1. Artificial rupture of membranes (AROM); performed by the HCP to stimulate labor
2. Performed if the fetus is at 0 or a plus station
3. Increases the risk of prolapsed cord and infection
4. Monitor the FHR before and after amniotomy.
5. Record the time of amniotomy, FHR, and characteristics of the fluid.
6. Meconium-stained **amniotic fluid** may be associated with fetal distress.
7. Bloody amniotic fluid may indicate abruptio placentae or fetal trauma.
8. An unpleasant odor to the amniotic fluid is associated with infection.
9. Polyhydramnios is associated with maternal diabetes and certain congenital disorders.
10. Oligohydramnios is associated with intrauterine growth restriction and congenital disorders.
11. More variable decelerations are likely to occur after the rupture of the membranes as a result of cord compression during contractions.
12. Limit client activity, if prescribed.

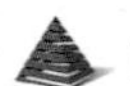

D. External version

1. External manipulation of the fetus from an abnormal presentation into a normal presentation
2. Indicated for an abnormal presentation that exists after 34 weeks' gestation
3. Monitor vital signs.
4. If the mother is Rh-negative, ensure that Rh_o(D) immune globulin (RhoGAM) was given at 28 weeks' gestation.
5. Prepare for a nonstress test to evaluate fetal well-being.
6. IV fluids and tocolytic therapy may be administered to relax the uterus and permit easier manipulation of the fetus.
7. Ultrasound is used during the procedure to evaluate fetal position and placental placement and guide direction of the fetus.
8. The abdominal wall is manipulated to direct the fetus into a cephalic presentation if possible.
9. Monitor blood pressure to identify vena cava syndrome (supine hypotensive syndrome).
10. Monitor for unusual pain.
11. After the procedure, the following is performed:
    a. A nonstress test to evaluate fetal well-being
    b. Monitoring for uterine activity, bleeding, ruptured membranes, and decreased fetal activity
    c. With Rh-negative clients, a Kleihauer-Betke test is performed as prescribed to detect the presence and amount of fetal blood in the maternal circulation and to identify clients who need additional Rh_o(D) immune globulin.

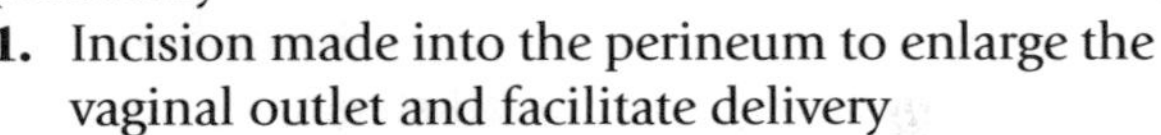

E. Episiotomy

1. Incision made into the perineum to enlarge the vaginal outlet and facilitate delivery
2. Check episiotomy site.
3. Institute measures to relieve pain.
4. Provide an ice pack during the first 24 hours.
5. Instruct the client in the use of an ice pack for the first 24 hours, and then sitz baths thereafter.
6. Apply analgesic spray or ointment, as prescribed.
7. Provide perineal care, using clean technique.
8. Instruct the client regarding the proper care of the incision.
9. Instruct the client to dry the perineal area from front to back and to blot the area rather than wipe it.
10. Instruct the client to shower rather than bathe in a tub.
11. Apply a perineal pad without touching the inside surface of the pad.
12. Report any bleeding or discharge from the episiotomy site to the registered nurse.

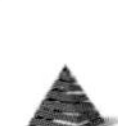

F. Forceps delivery

1. Two double-crossed, spoonlike articulated blades are used to assist in the delivery of the fetal head.
2. Reassure the mother and explain the need for the forceps.
3. Monitor the mother and fetus during delivery.
4. Check the **neonate** and mother after delivery for any possible injury.
5. Assist with the repair of any lacerations.

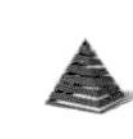

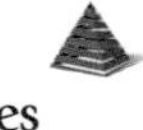

G. Vacuum extraction

1. A cap-like suction device is applied to the fetal head to facilitate extraction.
2. Suction is used to assist with the delivery of the fetal head.
3. Traction is applied during uterine contractions until the descent of the fetal head is achieved.
4. The suction device should not be kept in place any longer than 25 minutes.

5. Monitor the FHR every 5 minutes if external fetal monitoring is not used.
6. Check the newborn at birth and monitor him or her throughout the postpartum period for signs of cerebral trauma.
7. Monitor for developing cephalhematoma.
8. Caput succedaneum is normal and will resolve in 24 hours.

H. Cesarean delivery
1. Birth of the fetus usually through a transabdominal incision of the uterus
2. Preoperative
   a. If planned, prepare the mother and partner.
   b. If an emergency, quickly explain the need and procedure to the mother and partner.
   c. Obtain informed consent.
   d. Make sure that the preoperative diagnostic tests are done, including Rh factor determination.
   e. Prepare the mother for the insertion of an IV line and a Foley catheter.
   f. Prepare the abdomen, as prescribed.
   g. Monitor the mother and fetus continuously.
   h. Provide emotional support.
   i. Administer preoperative medications, as prescribed.
3. Postoperative
   a. Monitor vital signs.
   b. Perform a fundal assessment; evaluate incision.
   c. Provide pain relief.
   d. Encourage turning, coughing, and deep breathing.
   e. Encourage ambulation.
   f. Encourage bonding/attachment with newborn.
   g. Provide psychological support.
   h. Monitor for signs of infection and bleeding.
   i. Burning and pain on urination may indicate a bladder infection.
   j. A tender uterus and foul-smelling **lochia** may indicate endometritis.
   k. A productive cough or chills may indicate pneumonia.
   l. Pain, redness, or edema of an extremity may indicate thrombophlebitis.

IX. Placental Abnormalities

A. Description: Placenta accreta is an abnormally adherent placenta. Placenta increta occurs when the placenta penetrates the uterine muscle itself. Placenta percreta occurs when the placenta goes all the way through the uterus.

B. Data collection: May cause hemorrhage immediately after birth because the placenta does not separate cleanly

C. Intervention

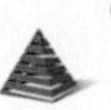

1. Monitor for hemorrhage and shock.
2. Prepare the client for a hysterectomy if a large portion of the placenta is abnormally adherent.

X. Placenta Previa (Fig. 27-3)

A. Description
1. The placenta is improperly implanted in the lower uterine segment near or over the internal cervical os.
2. Total: The internal cervical os is covered entirely by the placenta when the cervix is dilated fully.
3. Partial: The lower border of the placenta is within 3 cm of the internal cervical os, but does not fully cover it.
4. Marginal: The placenta is implanted in the lower uterus, but its lower border is more than 3 cm from the internal cervical os.
5. Management depends on the classification of the placenta previa and gestational age of the fetus.

B. Data collection
1. Sudden onset of painless, bright-red vaginal bleeding occurs during the last half of pregnancy.

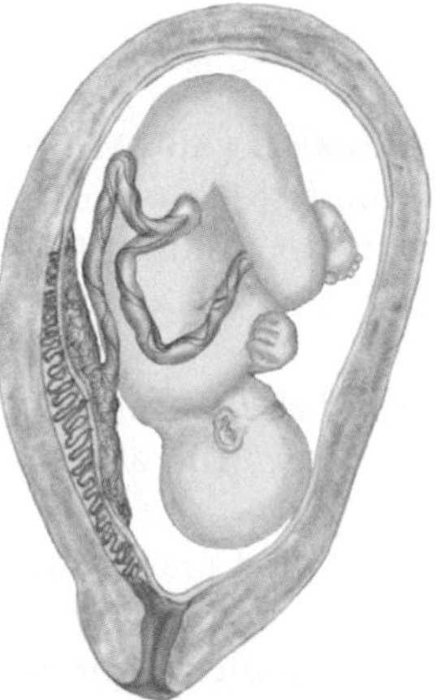

Marginal
Placenta is implanted in lower uterus but its lower border is >3 cm from internal cervical os.

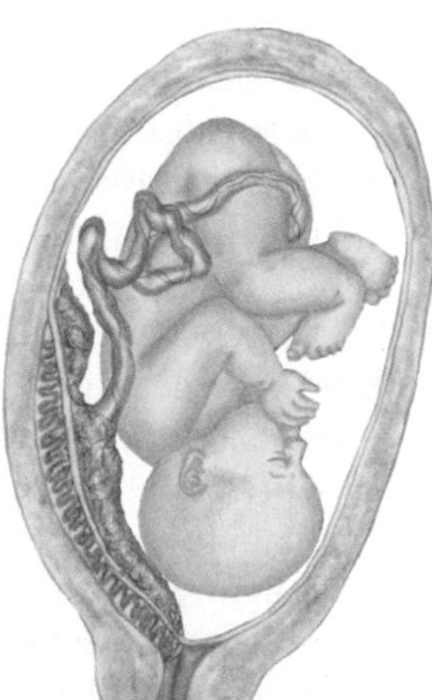

Partial
Lower border of placenta is within 3 cm of internal cervical os but does not fully cover it.

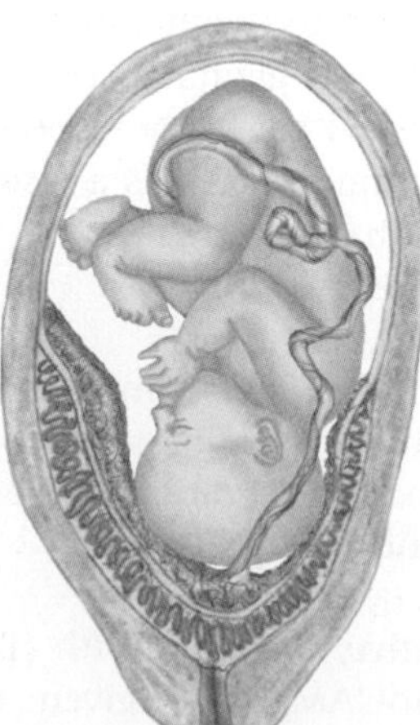

FIGURE 27-3 The three classifications of placenta previa. (From McKinney E, James S, Murray S, Ashwill J: *Maternal-child nursing*, ed 4, St. Louis, 2013, Saunders.)

2. Soft, relaxed, nontender uterus
3. Fundal height may be greater than expected for gestational age.

C. Interventions
1. Monitor maternal vital signs, FHR, and fetal activity.
2. Prepare for ultrasound to confirm diagnosis.
3. Vaginal examination or any other action that would stimulate uterine activity is avoided.
4. Maintain bed rest in a side-lying position as prescribed.
5. Monitor the amount of bleeding; treat signs of shock.
6. IV fluids, blood products, or tocolytic medications may be prescribed; Rh_o(D) immune globulin (RhoGAM) may be prescribed.
7. If bleeding is heavy, a cesarean section may be performed.

Vaginal exams are contraindicated if the client is suspected of having or has a known placenta previa.

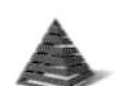

XI. Abruptio Placentae (Fig. 27-4)

A. Description: Premature separation of the placenta from the uterine wall after 20 weeks' gestation and before the birth of the baby

B. Data collection
1. Dark red vaginal bleeding; however, if the bleeding is high in the uterus or minimal, there can be an absence of visible blood.
2. Uterine pain or tenderness or both
3. Uterine rigidity
4. Severe abdominal pain
5. Signs of fetal distress
6. Signs of maternal shock if bleeding is excessive

C. Interventions
1. Monitor maternal vital signs and FHR.
2. Assess for excessive vaginal bleeding, abdominal pain, and an increase in fundal height.
3. Maintain bed rest; administer oxygen, IV fluids, and blood products, as prescribed.
4. Place the mother in Trendelenburg's position, if indicated, to decrease the pressure of the fetus on the placenta, or in the lateral position with the head of the bed flat if there are signs of hypovolemic shock caused by blood loss.
5. Monitor and report any uterine activity.
6. Prepare for the delivery of the fetus as quickly as possible, with vaginal delivery preferable if the fetus is healthy and stable and the presenting part is in the pelvis. Emergency cesarean section is performed if the fetus is alive but shows signs of distress.
7. Monitor for signs of disseminated intravascular coagulopathy (DIC) in the postpartum period.

Know the differences between placenta previa and abruptio placentae. In placenta previa, there is painless, bright red vaginal bleeding, and the uterus is soft, relaxed, and nontender. In abruptio placentae, there is dark red vaginal bleeding; uterine pain or tenderness, or both; and uterine rigidity.

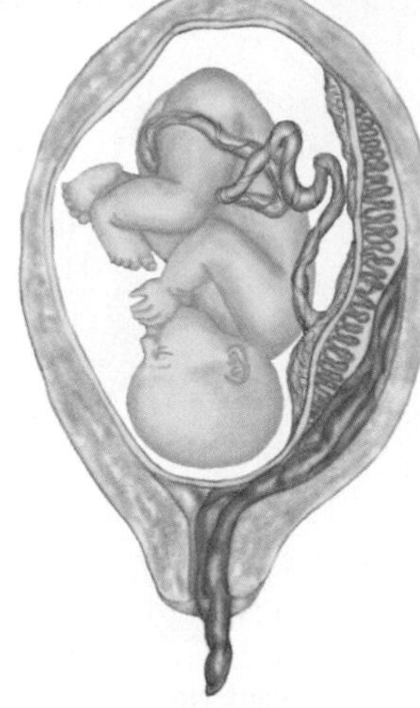

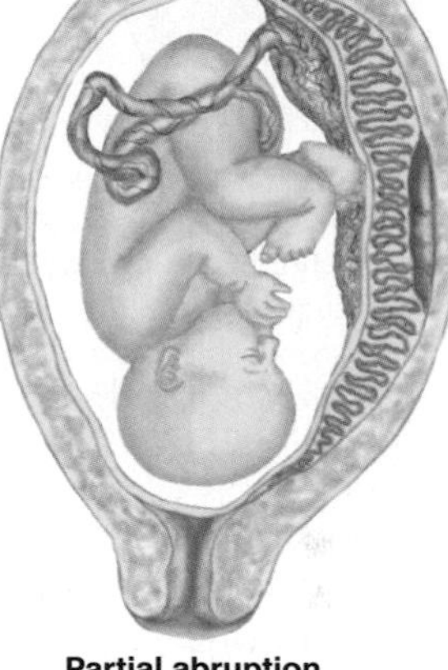

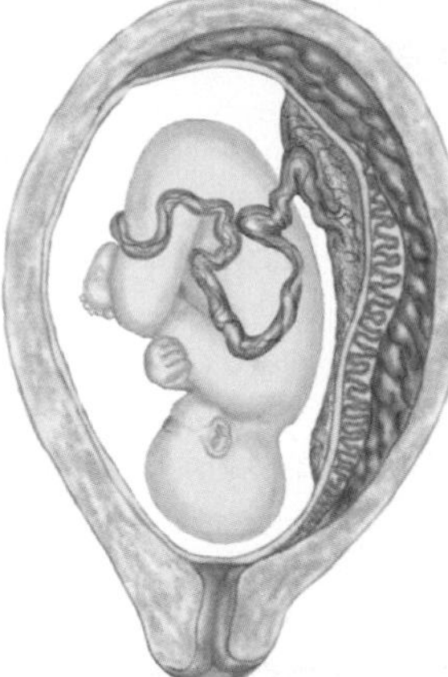

FIGURE 27-4 Types of abruptio placentae. (From Murray S, McKinney E: *Foundations of maternal-newborn nursing*, ed 6, St. Louis, 2014, Saunders.)

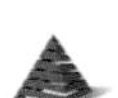

XII. Premature Rupture of the Membranes

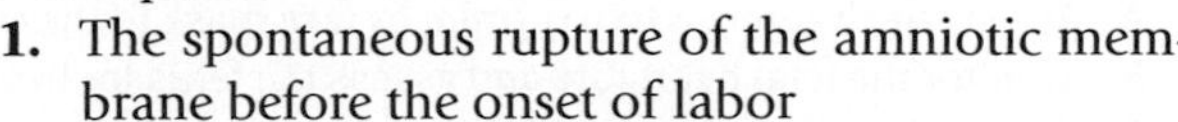

A. Description
1. The spontaneous rupture of the amniotic membrane before the onset of labor
2. Gestational age usually determines the plan and intervention.
3. When the rupture of membranes is before term and delivery will be delayed, infection becomes a risk.

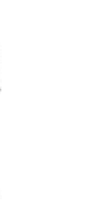

B. Data collection
1. Evidence of fluid pooling in the vaginal vault. The Nitrazine test or Fern test is positive.
2. Amount, color, consistency, and odor of fluid needs to be assessed.
3. Vital signs are monitored; elevated temperature may indicate the presence of infection.

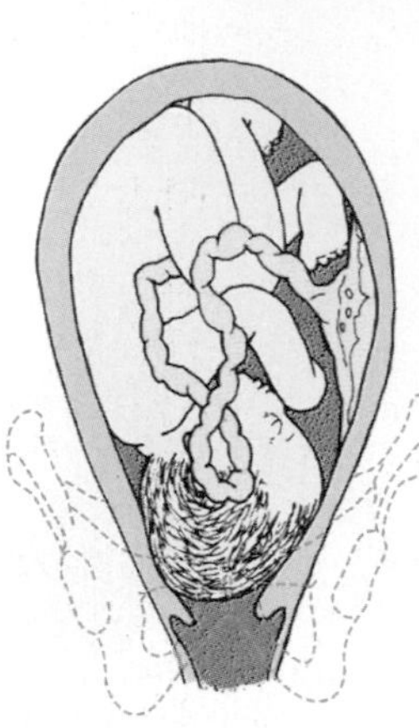
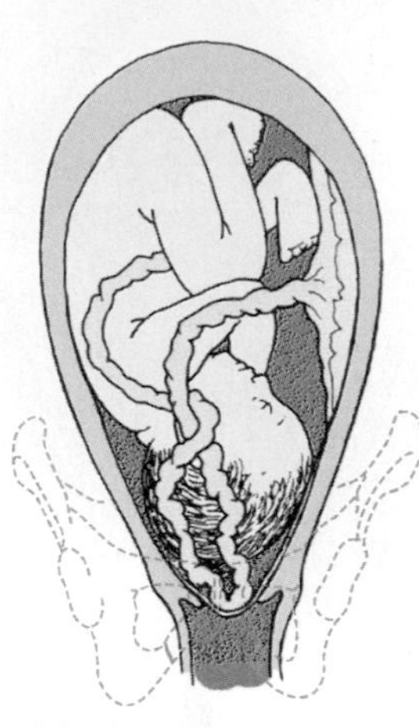
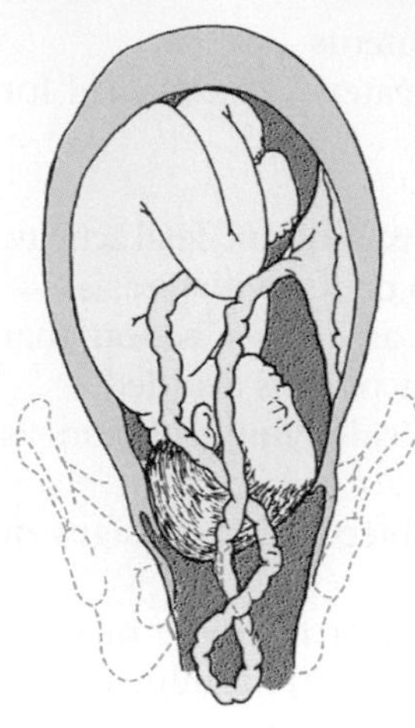
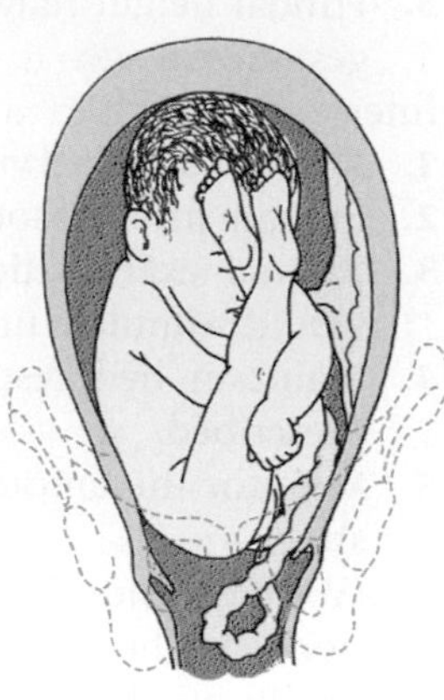

FIGURE 27-5 Prolapse of the umbilical cord. Note the pressure of the presenting part on the umbilical cord; this endangers fetal circulation. **A,** Occult (hidden) prolapse of the cord. **B,** Complete prolapse of the cord. **C,** Cord presenting in front of the fetal head may be seen in the vagina. **D,** Frank breech presentation with prolapsed cord. (From Perry S, Hockenberry M, Lowdermilk D, Wilson D: *Maternal-child nursing care*, ed 4, St. Louis, 2010, Mosby.)

4. Fetal monitoring is necessary; tachycardia may indicate infection.

C. Interventions
1. Assist with tests to assess gestational age.
2. Avoid vaginal examinations because of the risk of infection.
3. Monitor maternal and fetal status for signs of compromise or infection.
4. Assist to administer antibiotics, as prescribed.

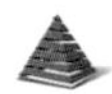

XIII. Prolapsed Umbilical Cord (Fig. 27-5)

A. Description: The umbilical cord is displaced between the presenting part and the amnion, or it is protruding through the cervix, causing compression of the cord and compromising fetal circulation.

B. Data collection
1. The client has a feeling that something is coming through the vagina.
2. The umbilical cord is visible or palpable.
3. The FHR is irregular and slow.
4. The fetal heart monitor will show variable deceleration or bradycardia after the rupture of the membranes.
5. If fetal hypoxia is severe, violent fetal activity may occur and then cease.

C. Interventions (see Priority Nursing Actions)

PRIORITY NURSING ACTIONS!

Steps to Take if Umbilical Cord Prolapse Is Suspected

1. Call the registered nurse and stay with the client.
2. Elevate the fetal presenting part that is lying on the cord by applying finger pressure on the fetal part with a gloved hand.
3. Place the client into extreme Trendelenburg's or modified Sims' position or a knee-chest position.
4. Administer oxygen, 8 to 10 L/min, by face mask to the client.
5. Monitor the fetal heart rate and assess the fetus for hypoxia.
6. Prepare to start intravenous fluids or increase the rate of an existing solution.
7. Prepare for immediate birth.
8. Document the event, actions taken, and the client's response.

If umbilical cord prolapse occurs, the cord is lying alongside or below the presenting part of the fetus and can be seen or felt in or protruding from the vagina. The nurse stays with the client and asks another nurse to call the registered nurse, who will contact the HCP immediately. The nurse must relieve cord pressure immediately so that the fetus receives adequate oxygenation. The nurse can relieve cord pressure by elevating the fetal presenting part that is lying on the cord. The nurse does this by quickly gloving the hand and inserting two fingers into the vagina to the cervix and exerting upward pressure on the presenting part. The nurse also relieves cord pressure by placing the client into extreme Trendelenburg's or modified Sims' position or a knee-chest position (a rolled towel is placed under the client's hip). The nurse administers oxygen, 8 to 10 L/min, by face mask to the client; monitors the fetal heart rate and fetal heart rate patterns; and assesses the fetus for hypoxia. The client is prepared for immediate birth (vaginal or cesarean). The nurse documents the event, actions taken, the client's response, and any additional pertinent information. The nurse never attempts to push the cord into the uterus. If the umbilical cord is protruding from the vagina, the cord is wrapped loosely in a sterile towel saturated with warm sterile normal saline.

Reference(s): McKinney, E., James, S., Murray, S., Nelson, K. & Ashwill, J. (2013). *Maternal-child nursing* (4th ed., pp. 412, 658–660). St. Louis: Elsevier.

XIV. Supine Hypotension (Vena Cava Syndrome)

A. Description
1. Occurs when the venous return to the heart is impaired by the weight of the uterus
2. Results from the partial occlusion of the vena cava and the descending aorta and causes reduced cardiac return, cardiac output, and blood pressure

B. Data collection
1. Faintness, dizziness, and breathlessness
2. Pallor, clammy (damp, cool) skin, and sweating
3. Hypotension and tachycardia
4. Fetal distress

C. Interventions
1. Position the client on her side to shift the weight of the fetus off the inferior vena cava until signs and symptoms subside and vital signs stabilize.
2. Monitor the vital signs and the FHR.

To prevent supine hypotension, avoid the supine position; position the client by placing a pillow or wedge under the client's hip to displace the gravid uterus off the vena cava.

XV. Preterm Labor

A. Description
1. Preterm labor occurs after week 20 but before week 37 of gestation.
2. Risk factors include a history of medical conditions; present and past obstetric problems; infection; and social and environmental factors, including substance abuse.
3. Additional risk factors include a multifetal pregnancy, which contributes to overdistention of uterus; anemia, which decreases oxygen supply to uterus; and age younger than 18 years, or first pregnancy and older than 40 years.

B. Data collection
1. Uterine contractions (painful or painless)
2. Abdominal cramping (may be accompanied by diarrhea)
3. Low back pain
4. Pelvic pressure or heaviness
5. Change in the character and amount of usual discharge; may be thicker or thinner, bloody, brown or colorless, odorous
6. Rupture of amniotic membranes

C. Interventions
1. Focus is on stopping the labor: identify and treat infection, restrict activity, and ensure hydration.
2. Maintain bed rest and a lateral position.
3. Monitor the fetal status.
4. Administer fluids as prescribed.
5. Tocolytic medications may be prescribed to suppress labor.

XVI. Precipitous Labor and Delivery

A. Description: Labor that lasts less than 3 hours

B. Interventions
1. Have a precipitous delivery tray available (hemostats, scissors, and cord clamp).
2. Stay with the mother at all times.
3. Provide emotional support and keep the mother calm.
4. Encourage the mother to pant between contractions.
5. Prepare for the rupturing of the membranes when the head crowns, if they are not already ruptured.
6. Do not try to keep the fetus from being delivered.
7. If delivery is necessary before the arrival of the HCP, assist with the following:
   a. Apply gentle pressure to the fetal head upward toward the vagina to prevent damage to the fetal head and vaginal lacerations.
   b. Support the newborn's body during delivery.
   c. Deliver the newborn between contractions, checking for the cord around the neck.
   d. Restitution is used to deliver the posterior shoulder.
   e. Gentle downward pressure is used to move the anterior shoulder under the pubic symphysis.
   f. Suction the newborn's mouth first and then suction each naris.
   g. Dry and cover the newborn to keep the body warm.
   h. Allow the placenta to separate naturally.
   i. Place the newborn on the mother's abdomen or breast to induce uterine contractions.

XVII. Dystocia

A. Description
1. Difficult labor that is prolonged or more painful
2. Occurs as a result of problems caused by uterine contractions, the fetus, or the bones and tissues of the maternal pelvis
3. The fetus may be excessively large, malpositioned, or in an abnormal position.
4. Contractions may be hypotonic or hypertonic.
5. Hypotonic contractions are short, irregular, and weak. Amniotomy and oxytocin (Pitocin) infusion may be treatment measures.
6. Hypertonic contractions are painful, occur frequently, and are uncoordinated. Treatment depends on cause and includes pain relief measures and rest.
7. Dystocia can result in maternal dehydration, infection, fetal injury, or death.

B. Data collection 
1. Excessive abdominal pain
2. Abnormal contraction pattern
3. Fetal distress
4. Maternal or fetal tachycardia
5. Lack of progress of labor

C. Interventions
1. Check FHR; monitor for fetal distress.
2. Monitor uterine contractions.
3. Monitor maternal temperature and heart rate.
4. Assist with pelvic examination, measurements, ultrasound, and other procedures.
5. Prophylactic antibiotics may be prescribed to prevent infection.
6. IV fluids may be prescribed.
7. Monitor intake and output.
8. Monitor for dehydration.
9. Instruct the mother in breathing techniques and relaxation exercises.
10. Fetal monitoring is needed if oxytocin (Pitocin) is prescribed (oxytocin is not prescribed for hypertonic uterine contractions).
11. Monitor the color of the amniotic fluid.
12. Provide rest and comfort as with a normal delivery, such as back rubs and position changes.
13. Assess the mother's fatigue and pain. Administer sedatives and pain medications, as prescribed.
14. Monitor for prolapse of the cord after the rupture of the membranes.

XVIII. Amniotic Fluid Embolism

A. Description
1. Amniotic fluid embolism is the escape of amniotic fluid into the maternal circulation.
2. The debris-containing amniotic fluid deposits in the pulmonary arterioles and is usually fatal to the mother.

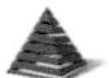
B. Data collection
1. Abrupt onset of respiratory distress and chest pain
2. Cyanosis
3. Fetal bradycardia and distress if delivery has not occurred at the time of the embolism

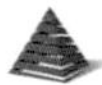
C. Interventions
1. Institute emergency measures to maintain life.
2. Administer oxygen at 8 to 10 L/min by face mask or resuscitation bag delivering 100% oxygen, as prescribed.
3. Prepare the client for intubation and mechanical ventilation.
4. Position the woman on her side.
5. IV fluids, blood products, and medications may be prescribed to correct coagulation failure.
6. Monitor the fetal status.
7. Prepare for emergency delivery after the woman is stabilized.
8. Provide emotional support to the woman, the partner, and the family.

XIX. Fetal Distress

A. Data collection
1. FHR of less than 110 or more than 160 beats per minute
2. Meconium-stained amniotic fluid
3. Fetal hyperactivity
4. Progressive decrease in baseline variability
5. Severe variable decelerations
6. Late decelerations

B. Interventions
1. Place the mother in a lateral position.
2. Administer oxygen at 8 to 10 L/min via face mask, as prescribed.
3. Oxytocin (Pitocin), if infusing, is discontinued.
4. Monitor the maternal and fetal status.

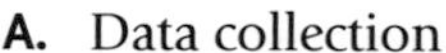
In the event of fetal distress, prepare the client for emergency cesarean delivery.

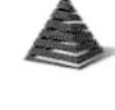

XX. Intrauterine Fetal Demise

A. Data collection
1. Loss of fetal movement
2. Absence of fetal heart tones
3. DIC screen: Monitor for coagulation abnormalities, because DIC is a complication that is related to intrauterine fetal demise.
4. Low hemoglobin and hematocrit levels; low platelet count; prolonged bleeding and clotting times
5. Bleeding from puncture sites (which could be indicative of DIC)

B. Interventions
1. Encourage the mother and her family to verbalize their feelings; provide emotional support.
2. Incorporate religious and cultural health care beliefs and practices into the plan of care.
3. Allow the mother choices related to labor and delivery.
4. Assist to administer intravenous fluids, medications, and blood and blood products as prescribed if DIC occurs.

XXI. Rupture of the Uterus

A. Description
1. Complete or incomplete separation of the uterine tissue as a result of a tear in the wall of the uterus from the stress of labor
2. Complete: Direct communication between the uterine and peritoneal cavities
3. Incomplete: Rupture into the peritoneum covering the uterus, but not into the peritoneal cavity
4. Manifestations vary with the extent of the rupture.
5. Risk factors: Labor after cesarean section, overdistended uterus (e.g., multiple fetuses or hydramnios) after cesarean section, abdominal trauma

B. Data Collection
1. Abdominal pain or tenderness

2. Chest pain
3. Contractions may stop or fail to progress.
4. Rigid abdomen
5. Absent fetal heart rate
6. Signs of maternal shock
7. Fetus palpated outside of the uterus (complete rupture)

C. Interventions
1. Monitor for and assist with treating signs of shock (oxygen, IV fluids, and blood products may be prescribed).
2. Prepare the client for cesarean section (hysterectomy may be necessary).
3. Provide emotional support for the mother and partner.

XXII. Uterine Inversion

A. Description
1. Uterus completely or partly turns inside out.
2. This can occur during delivery or after delivery of the placenta.
3. Risk factors: Fundal implantation of the placenta, manual extraction of the placenta, short umbilical cord, uterine atony, leiomyomas, and abnormally adherent placental tissue

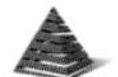
B. Data collection
1. A depression in the fundal area of the uterus is noted.
2. Interior of the uterus may be seen through the cervix or protruding through the vagina.
3. Severe pain
4. Hemorrhage
5. Signs of shock

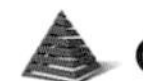
C. Interventions
1. Monitor for hemorrhage and signs of shock, and treat shock.
2. Prepare the client for a return of the uterus to the correct position via the vagina. If unsuccessful, laparotomy with replacement to the correct position is done.

CRITICAL THINKING What Should You Do?

Answer: Near or at term, the normal fetal heart rate is 110 to 160 beats/minute. If fetal tachycardia or bradycardia occurs, the nurse should change the position of the mother, administer oxygen, and check the mother's vital signs. In addition, the nurse should notify the registered nurse immediately so that further assessment can be done regarding the cause of the tachycardia. The health care provider is also notified.

Reference(s): McKinney, E., James, S., Murray, S., Nelson, K. & Ashwill, J. (2013). *Maternal-child nursing* (4th ed., p. 377). St. Louis: Elsevier.

PRACTICE QUESTIONS

241. The nurse is assigned to care for a client who is in early labor. When collecting data from the client, which should the nurse check **first**?
1. Baseline fetal heart rate
2. Intensity of contractions
3. Maternal blood pressure
4. Frequency of contractions

242. Leopold's maneuvers will be performed on a pregnant client. The client asks the nurse about the procedure. Which information should the nurse provide to the client about Leopold's maneuvers?
1. The maneuvers measure the height of the maternal fundus.
2. The maneuvers determine the "lie" and "attitude" of the fetus.
3. The maneuvers are a systematic method for palpating the fetus through the maternal back.
4. The maneuvers are a systematic method for palpating the fetus through the maternal abdominal wall.

243. The nurse is caring for a client who is in labor. The nurse rechecks the client's blood pressure and notes that it has dropped. To decrease the incidence of supine hypotension, the nurse should encourage the client to remain in which position?
1. Squatting
2. Side-lying
3. Tailor sitting
4. Semi-Fowler's

244. After a precipitous delivery, the nurse notes that the new mother is passive and only touches her newborn briefly with her fingertips. The nurse should do which to help the woman process what has happened?
1. Encourage the mother to breastfeed soon after birth.
2. Support the mother in her reaction to the newborn.
3. Tell the mother that it is important to hold the newborn.
4. Document a complete account of the mother's reaction in the birth record.

245. A primigravida's membranes rupture spontaneously. Which action should the nurse take **first**?
1. Determine the fetal heart rate.
2. Prepare for immediate delivery.
3. Monitor the contraction pattern.
4. Note the amount, color, and odor of the amniotic fluid.

246. After the client vaginally delivers a viable newborn, the nurse sees the umbilical cord lengthen and observes a spurt of blood from the vagina. The nurse recognizes these findings as signs of which condition?
1. Uterine atony
2. Placenta previa
3. Abruptio placentae
4. Placental separation

247. The nurse is assigned to assist with caring for a client who has been admitted to the labor unit. The client is 9 cm dilated and is experiencing precipitous labor. Which is the **priority** nursing action?
1. Prepare for an oxytocin infusion.
2. Keep the client in a side-lying position.
3. Prepare the client for epidural anesthesia.
4. Encourage the client to start pushing with the contractions.

248. The client is admitted to the labor suite complaining of painless vaginal bleeding. The nurse assists with the examination of the client, knowing that which routine labor procedure is contraindicated?
1. Leopold's maneuvers
2. A manual pelvic examination
3. Hemoglobin and hematocrit evaluation
4. External electronic fetal heart rate monitoring

249. The nurse is assigned to assist with caring for a client with abruptio placentae who is experiencing vaginal bleeding. The nurse collects data from the client, knowing that abruptio placentae is accompanied by which additional finding?
1. Soft abdomen on palpation
2. Uterine tenderness on palpation
3. No complaints of abdominal pain
4. Lack of uterine irritability or tetanic contractions

❖ **250.** The nurse is collecting data from a client who has been diagnosed with placenta previa. Which findings should the nurse expect to note? **Select all that apply.**
- ❑ 1. Uterine rigidity
- ❑ 2. Uterine tenderness
- ❑ 3. Severe abdominal pain
- ❑ 4. Bright red vaginal bleeding
- ❑ 5. Soft, relaxed, nontender uterus

251. The nurse is assisting with caring for a client with abruptio placentae. While caring for the client, the nurse notes that the client begins to develop signs of shock. The nurse should take which action **first**?
1. Monitor the urinary output.
2. Monitor the maternal pulse.
3. Turn the client onto her side.
4. Monitor the maternal blood pressure.

252. The client who is being prepared for a cesarean delivery is brought to the delivery room. To maintain the optimal perfusion of oxygenated blood to the fetus, the nurse should place the client in which position?
1. Prone position
2. Semi-Fowler's position
3. Trendelenburg's position
4. Supine position with a wedge under the right hip

253. A woman in active labor has contractions every 2 to 3 minutes that last for 45 seconds. The fetal heart rate between contractions is 100 beats per minute. On the basis of these findings which is the **priority** nursing action?
1. Monitor the maternal vital signs.
2. Notify the registered nurse (RN) immediately.
3. Continue monitoring labor and the fetal heart rate.
4. Encourage relaxation and breathing techniques between contractions.

254. The nurse is assigned to assist with caring for a client who is being admitted to the birthing center in early labor. On admission, which action should the nurse take **initially**?
1. Estimate the fetal size.
2. Check pelvic adequacy.
3. Administer an analgesic.
4. Determine the maternal and fetal vital signs.

255. The nurse is assigned to work in the delivery room and is assisting with caring for a client who has just delivered a newborn. The nurse is monitoring for signs of placental separation knowing that which indicates that the placenta has separated?
1. A change in the uterine contour
2. Sudden and sharp abdominal pain
3. A shortening of the umbilical cord
4. A decrease in blood loss from the introitus

ANSWERS

241. 1

Rationale: The nurse should first determine the baseline fetal heart rate. Although options 2, 3, and 4 are components of the data collection process, the fetal heart rate is the priority.

Test-Taking Strategy: Note the strategic word, *first.* Use the ABCs—airway, breathing, and circulation—when selecting an answer. Fetal heart rate reflects the use of the ABCs. **Review:** the client in labor.

Level of Cognitive Ability: Analyzing

Client Needs: Physiological Integrity

Integrated Process: Nursing Process/Implementation

Content Area: Maternity: Intrapartum

Priority Concepts: Gas Exchange, Reproduction

Reference(s): McKinney et al (2013), pp. 345–346.

242. 4

Rationale: Leopold's maneuvers comprise a systematic method for palpating the fetus through the maternal abdominal wall. Options 1, 2, and 3 are incorrect descriptions.

Test-Taking Strategy: Note the subject, the purpose of and procedure for Leopold's maneuvers. Visualizing this procedure will assist with directing you to the correct option. **Review:** Leopold's maneuvers.

Level of Cognitive Ability: Applying

Client Needs: Physiological Integrity

Integrated Process: Nursing Process/Implementation

Content Area: Maternity: Intrapartum

Priority Concepts: Client Education, Reproduction

Reference(s): McKinney et al (2013), pp. 25, 342–343.

243. 2

Rationale: Pressure from the enlarged uterus on the aorta and the vena cava when the woman is supine can result in hypotension. This can be relieved by having the woman lie on her side. Options 1, 3, and 4 are incorrect because they would not prevent hypotension.

Test-Taking Strategy: Focus on the subject, measures to decrease the incidence of supine hypotension. Think about the anatomy of the pregnant uterus and the physiological response caused by pressure on the large abdominal vessels. Note that options 1, 3, and 4 are all comparable or alike in that the client would be upright. **Review:** nursing measures for the hypotensive pregnant client.

Level of Cognitive Ability: Applying

Client Needs: Physiological Integrity

Integrated Process: Nursing Process/Implementation

Content Area: Maternity: Intrapartum

Priority Concepts: Perfusion, Safety

Reference(s): McKinney et al (2013), p. 237.

244. 2

Rationale: Women who have experienced precipitous labor and delivery often describe feelings of disbelief that their labor has progressed so rapidly. To assist the woman with understanding what has happened, it is best to support the mother in her reaction to the newborn. Options 1, 3, and 4 do not acknowledge the mother's feelings.

Test-Taking Strategy: Use therapeutic communication techniques. Option 2 is the only choice that acknowledges the mother's feelings. **Review:** care of the mother after a precipitous birth.

Level of Cognitive Ability: Applying

Client Needs: Psychosocial Integrity

Integrated Process: Caring

Content Area: Maternity: Intrapartum

Priority Concepts: Coping, Reproduction

Reference(s): McKinney et al (2013), pp. 642–643.

245. 1

Rationale: When the membranes rupture, the nurse immediately assesses the fetal heart rate to detect changes associated with prolapse or the compression of the umbilical cord. Monitoring the contraction pattern and noting the amount, color, and odor of the amniotic fluid may be performed, but these would not be the first actions. There is no information in the question that indicates the need to prepare the client for immediate delivery.

Test-Taking Strategy: Note the strategic word, *first.* Use the ABCs—airway, breathing, and circulation. Fetal heart rate is associated with fetal circulation. **Review:** initial nursing interventions for ruptured membranes.

Level of Cognitive Ability: Analyzing

Client Needs: Physiological Integrity

Integrated Process: Nursing Process/Implementation

Content Area: Maternity: Intrapartum

Priority Concepts: Gas Exchange, Perfusion

Reference(s): McKinney et al (2013), pp. 413, 644–645.

246. 4

Rationale: As the placenta separates, it settles downward into the lower uterine segment, the umbilical cord lengthens, and a sudden trickle or spurt of blood appears. The clinical manifestations identified in the question are not related to options 1, 2, and 3.

Test-Taking Strategy: Note that options 1, 2, and 3 are comparable or alike in that they represent complications associated with pregnancy. Option 4 indicates a normal finding after the vaginal delivery of the newborn. **Review:** stages of labor.

Level of Cognitive Ability: Understanding

Client Needs: Physiological Integrity

Integrated Process: Nursing Process/Data Collection

Content Area: Maternity: Intrapartum

Priority Concepts: Clinical Judgment, Reproduction

Reference(s): McKinney et al (2013), p. 333.

247. 2

Rationale: Precipitous labor progresses quickly, with frequent contractions and short periods of relaxation between them. This does not allow for the maximal reperfusion of the placenta with oxygenated blood. Priority care of this client includes the promotion of fetal oxygenation. A side-lying position can assist with providing blood flow to the uterus by preventing vena cava and abdominal aorta compression. Further stimulation with oxytocin is contraindicated. There may not be enough time to administer epidural anesthesia before delivery with such quick progression. Pushing with contractions is not indicated, especially with this type of labor. The controlled delivery of the fetus is essential to prevent maternal and fetal injury.

Test-Taking Strategy: Note the strategic word, *priority.* Use the ABCs—airway, breathing, and circulation—and consider the

baby's as well as the mother's needs. Option 2 will promote fetal oxygenation. **Review:** the client with **precipitous labor.**
Level of Cognitive Ability: Analyzing
Client Needs: Physiological Integrity
Integrated Process: Nursing Process/Implementation
Content Area: Maternity: Intrapartum
Priority Concepts: Gas Exchange, Perfusion
Reference(s): Lowdermilk et al (2012), p. 794; McKinney et al (2013), pp. 642–643.

248. 2
Rationale: Painless vaginal bleeding is a sign of possible placenta previa. Digital examination of the cervix is contraindicated because it can lead to maternal and fetal hemorrhage. Leopold's maneuvers can reveal a nonengaged presenting part or malpresentation, both of which often accompany placenta previa because of the placenta filling the lower uterine segment. Hemoglobin and hematocrit values help estimate the amount of blood loss. External electronic fetal monitoring is crucial for evaluating the status of the fetus, which is at risk for severe hypoxia. Options 1, 3, and 4 are procedures that would not place the client at further risk.
Test-Taking Strategy: Focus on the **subject**, the procedure that is contraindicated. Option 2 is the only procedure that is invasive to the pregnancy and that endangers the physiological safety of the client and fetus. **Review: placenta previa.**
Level of Cognitive Ability: Analyzing
Client Needs: Physiological Integrity
Integrated Process: Nursing Process/Data Collection
Content Area: Maternity: Intrapartum
Priority Concepts: Reproduction, Safety
Reference(s): McKinney et al (2013), p. 584.

249. 2
Rationale: Vaginal bleeding in a pregnant client is most often caused by placenta previa or a placental abruption. Uterine tenderness accompanies abruptio placentae, especially with a central abruption and trapped blood behind the placenta. The abdomen will feel hard and boardlike on palpation as the blood penetrates the myometrium and causes uterine irritability. A sustained tetanic contraction can occur if the client is in labor and the uterine muscle cannot relax.
Test-Taking Strategy: Note the **subject**, abruptio placentae. It can be easy to confuse a placenta previa and abruption. Remember, the difference involves the presence of uterine pain and tenderness with an abruptio placentae, as opposed to painless bleeding with a placenta previa. Options 1, 3, and 4 describe the absence of a sign or symptom of abruptio placentae, whereas option 2 is the only one that describes the presence of one. **Review:** the signs of **abruptio placentae.**
Level of Cognitive Ability: Analyzing
Client Needs: Physiological Integrity
Integrated Process: Nursing Process/Data Collection
Content Area: Maternity: Intrapartum
Priority Concepts: Perfusion, Reproduction
Reference(s): McKinney et al (2013), pp. 585–586.

❖250. 4, 5
Rationale: Painless bright red vaginal bleeding during the second or third trimester of pregnancy is a sign of placenta previa. The client will have a soft and relaxed nontender uterus. In clients with abruptio placentae, severe abdominal pain is present. Uterine tenderness accompanies placental abruption. Additionally, with abruptio placentae, the abdomen will feel hard and boardlike on palpation as the blood penetrates the myometrium and causes uterine irritability.
Test-Taking Strategy: Focus on the **subject**, the difference between placenta previa and abruptio placentae. Abruptio placentae involves the presence of uterine pain and tenderness as opposed to painless bleeding with a previa. **Review:** the signs of placenta previa and **abruptio placentae.**
Level of Cognitive Ability: Analyzing
Client Needs: Physiological Integrity
Integrated Process: Nursing Process/Data Collection
Content Area: Maternity: Intrapartum
Priority Concepts: Perfusion, Reproduction
Reference(s): McKinney et al (2013), pp. 583–584.

251. 3
Rationale: With a pregnant client who is in shock, the nurse would want to increase perfusion to the placenta. A simple way to do this that requires no equipment is to turn the mother on her side. This would increase blood flow to the placenta by relieving pressure from the gravid uterus on the great vessels. The nurse would immediately contact the registered nurse, who would then contact the health care provider. The other options would follow quickly.
Test-Taking Strategy: Note the **strategic word**, *first.* Eliminate options 2 and 4, because they are **comparable or alike.** Recalling that positioning will affect the status of blood flow will assist with directing you to the correct option from the remaining options. **Review: abruptio placentae.**
Level of Cognitive Ability: Analyzing
Client Needs: Physiological Integrity
Integrated Process: Nursing Process/Implementation
Content Area: Critical Care: Emergency Situations
Priority Concepts: Perfusion, Reproduction
Reference(s): McKinney et al (2013), pp. 588–589.

252. 4
Rationale: Vena cava and descending aorta compression by the pregnant uterus impede blood return from the lower trunk and extremities, thereby decreasing cardiac return, cardiac output, and blood flow to the uterus and subsequently to the fetus. The best position to prevent this would be side-lying, with the uterus displaced off the abdominal vessels. Positioning for abdominal surgery necessitates a supine position; however, a wedge placed under the right hip provides for the displacement of the uterus. A prone or semi-Fowler's position is not practical for this type of abdominal surgery. Trendelenburg's position places pressure from the pregnant uterus on the diaphragm and lungs, thus decreasing respiratory capacity and oxygenation.
Test-Taking Strategy: Note the **subject**, maintaining optimal perfusion to the fetus. Visualize each of the positions in the options and think about their effect on the fetus. **Review:** vena cava syndrome.
Level of Cognitive Ability: Applying
Client Needs: Physiological Integrity
Integrated Process: Nursing Process/Implementation
Content Area: Maternity: Intrapartum
Priority Concepts: Perfusion, Safety
Reference(s): McKinney et al (2013), p. 428.

253. 2

Rationale: Fetal bradycardia between contractions may indicate the need for immediate medical management. The nurse would immediately contact the RN, who would then contact the health care provider. Options 1, 3, and 4 will delay necessary and immediate interventions.
Test-Taking Strategy: Note the **strategic word**, *priority*. Use the **ABCs—airway, breathing, and circulation**. Note that the woman is in active labor and the fetal heart rate is below normal. It is imperative that the circulation in the fetus be restored to normal limits. **Review:** the care of the client in active labor.
Level of Cognitive Ability: Analyzing
Client Needs: Physiological Integrity
Integrated Process: Nursing Process/Implementation
Content Area: Critical Care: Emergency Situations
Priority Concepts: Perfusion, Reproduction
Reference(s): McKinney et al (2013), pp. 377–378.

254. 4

Rationale: To evaluate a woman's physical well-being, her temperature, pulse, respirations, and blood pressure (as well as the fetal heartbeat) are checked. Option 3 is incorrect because it would be too premature for an analgesic; medication given too early tends to slow or stop labor contractions. Options 1 and 2 are incorrect. These assessments should be performed by the health care provider during prenatal visits.
Test-Taking Strategy: Note the **strategic word**, *initially*, and use the **ABCs—airway, breathing, and circulation**; this will direct you to the correct option. Remember, measuring the vital signs is the priority. **Review:** care of the client in labor.
Level of Cognitive Ability: Applying
Client Needs: Physiological Integrity
Integrated Process: Nursing Process/Implementation
Content Area: Maternity: Intrapartum
Priority Concepts: Perfusion, Reproduction
Reference(s): McKinney et al (2013), p. 344.

255. 1

Rationale: Signs of placental separation include the lengthening of the umbilical cord, a sudden gush of dark blood from the introitus, a firmly contracted uterus, and the uterus changing from a discoid to a globular shape. The client may experience vaginal fullness but not sudden and sharp abdominal pain.
Test-Taking Strategy: Focus on the **subject**, indications that the placenta has separated. Thinking about what one would expect to occur when the placenta separates will assist you to eliminate options 3 and 4. Option 2 is eliminated because of the words *sudden and sharp*. **Review:** the signs of placental separation.
Level of Cognitive Ability: Applying
Client Needs: Physiological Integrity
Integrated Process: Nursing Process/Data Collection
Content Area: Maternity: Intrapartum
Priority Concepts: Clinical Judgment, Reproduction
Reference(s): Lowdermilk et al (2012), p. 472; McKinney et al (2013), p. 333.

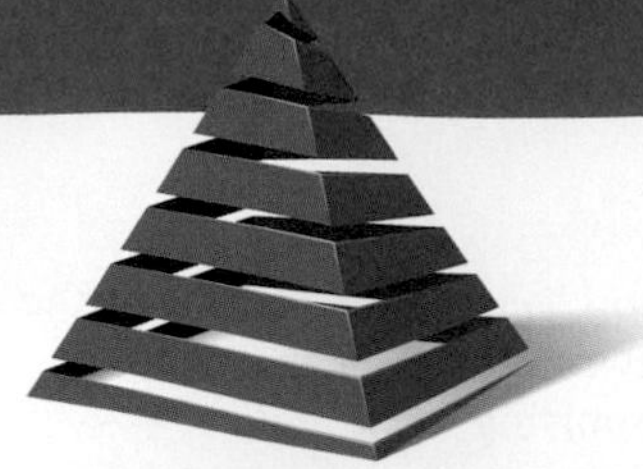

CHAPTER 28

The Postpartum Period and Associated Complications

CRITICAL THINKING What Should You Do?

The nurse is caring for a postpartum client and is preparing to measure the amount of lochial flow. What should the nurse do to obtain an accurate assessment?
Answer is located on p. 327.

I. Postpartum

A. Description: Period when the reproductive tract returns to the normal, nonpregnant state
B. Postpartum period: Starts immediately after **delivery** and is usually completed by week 6 after delivery

II. Physiological Maternal Changes

A. Involution (Fig. 28-1)
 1. Description
  a. The rapid decrease in the size of the **uterus** as it returns to the nonpregnant state
  b. Clients who breastfeed may experience a more rapid involution due to the release of oxytocin during breastfeeding.
 2. Data collection
  a. Weight of the uterus decreases from 2 lb to 2 oz in 6 weeks
  b. Endometrium regenerates
  c. Fundus steadily descends into the pelvis. The fundal height decreases about 1 fingerbreadth (1 cm) per day.
  d. By 10 days postpartum, the uterus cannot be palpated abdominally.
  e. A flaccid fundus indicates uterine atony and should be massaged until firm.
  f. A tender fundus indicates an infection.
  g. Afterpains decrease in frequency after the first few days.
B. **Lochia** (Fig. 28-2)
 1. Description: Discharge from the uterus that consists of blood from the vessels of the placental site and debris from the decidua
 2. Data collection (Box 28-1)
  a. Rubra: Bright red discharge that occurs from delivery day to day 3 postpartum
  b. Serosa: Brownish-pink discharge that occurs from days 4 to 10 postpartum
  c. Alba: White discharge that occurs from days 11 to 14 postpartum
  d. Normally the discharge smells like normal menstrual flow.
  e. Discharge decreases daily in amount.
  f. Discharge increases with ambulation.

⚠ To determine most accurately the amount of lochial flow, weigh the perineal pad before and after use and identify the amount of time between pad changes.

C. Cervix: Cervical involution occurs. After 1 week, the muscle begins to regenerate.
D. **Vagina**: Vaginal distention decreases, although muscle tone is never restored completely to the pregravid state.
E. Ovarian function and menstruation
 1. Ovarian function depends on the rapidity with which pituitary function is restored.
 2. Menstrual flow resumes within 1 to 2 months in nonbreastfeeding mothers.
 3. Menstrual flow usually resumes within 3 to 6 months in breastfeeding mothers.
 4. Breastfeeding mothers may experience amenorrhea during the entire period of lactation.

⚠ Woman may ovulate without menstruating, so breastfeeding should not be considered a form of birth control.

F. Breasts
 1. Breasts continue to secrete colostrum for the first 48 to 72 hours after delivery.
 2. A decrease of estrogen and progesterone levels after delivery stimulates increased prolactin levels, which promote breast milk production.
 3. Breasts become distended with milk on the third day.

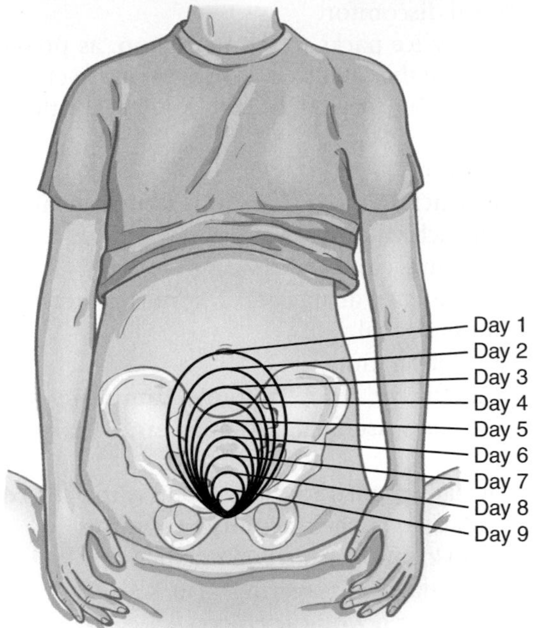

FIGURE 28-1 Involution of the uterus. The height of uterine fundus decreases by approximately 1 cm/day. (From McKinney E, James S, Murray S, Ashwill J: *Maternal-child nursing*, ed 4, St. Louis, 2013, Saunders.)

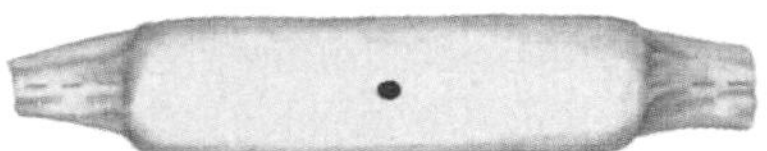

Scant: <2.5-cm (1-inch) stain

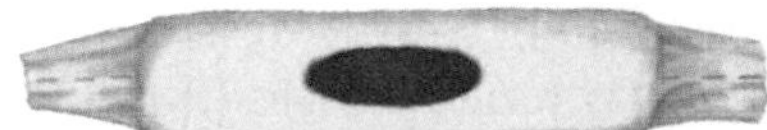

Light: 2.5- to 10-cm (1- to 4-inch) stain

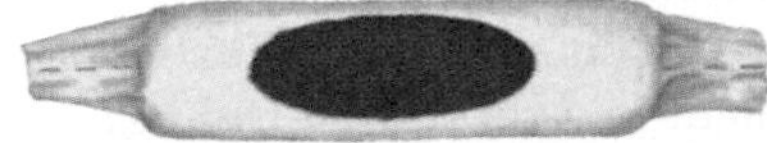

Moderate: 10- to 15-cm (4- to 6-inch) stain

Heavy: Saturated in 1 hour

FIGURE 28-2 Guidelines for assessing the amount of lochia on the perineal pad. (From McKinney E, James S, Murray S, Ashwill J: *Maternal-child nursing*, ed 3, St. Louis, 2009, Saunders.)

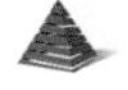

4. Engorgement occurs on approximately day 4 in both breastfeeding and nonbreastfeeding mothers.
5. Breastfeeding relieves engorgement.

Non-breastfeeding mothers should avoid nipple stimulation and apply a breast binder, wear a snug-fitting bra, apply ice packs, or take a mild analgesic for engorgement. Engorgement usually resolves within 24 to 36 hours after it begins.

BOX 28-1 Amount of Lochia

Scant
Less than 2.5 cm (<1 inch) on menstrual pad in 1 hour

Light
Less than 10 cm (<4 inches) on menstrual pad in 1 hour

Moderate
Less than 15 cm (<6 inches) on menstrual pad in 1 hour

Heavy
Saturated menstrual pad in 1 hour

Excessive
Menstrual pad saturated in 15 minutes

From Murray S, McKinney E: *Foundations of maternal-newborn and women's health nursing*, ed 5, Philadelphia, 2010, Saunders.

G. Urinary tract
  1. May have urinary retention because of a loss of elasticity, tone, and sensation in the bladder from trauma, medications, anesthesia, and lack of privacy
  2. Diuresis usually begins within the first 12 hours after delivery.

H. Gastrointestinal tract
  1. Women are usually hungry after delivery.
  2. Constipation can occur, with bowel movement (soft, formed stool) by the second or third postpartum day.
  3. Hemorrhoids are common.

I. Vital signs (Table 28-1)

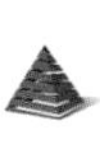

III. Postpartum Interventions

A. Data collection
  1. Monitor the vital signs.
  2. Monitor pain level.

TABLE 28-1 Normal Postpartum Vital Signs

Vital Sign	Description
Temperature	May rise to 100.4°F during the first 24 hours postpartum as a result of the dehydrating effects of labor; any higher elevation may be caused by infection and must be reported.
Pulse	May decrease to 50 beats per minute (normal puerperal bradycardia); a pulse rate of >100 beats per minute may indicate excessive blood loss or infection.
Blood pressure	Should be normal; suspect hypovolemia if it decreases.
Respirations	Rarely changes; if respirations increase significantly, suspect pulmonary embolism, uterine atony, or hemorrhage.

3. Monitor the height, consistency, and location of the fundus.
4. Monitor the color, amount, and odor of the lochia.
5. Check the breasts for engorgement.
6. Monitor the perineum for swelling or discoloration.
7. Monitor for perineal lacerations or episiotomy for healing.
8. Check the incisions or dressings of the client who had a cesarean birth.
9. Monitor the intake and output (I&O).
10. Encourage frequent voiding.
11. Monitor the bowel status.
12. Encourage ambulation.
13. Check the extremities for thrombophlebitis (redness, tenderness, or warmth of legs).

14. Rh_o(D) immune globulin (RhoGAM) is prescribed to be administered within 72 hours postpartum to the Rh-negative client who has given birth to an Rh-positive **newborn**.

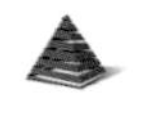

15. Monitor parent–newborn bonding.
16. Monitor the mother's emotional status.

B. Client teaching
1. Demonstrate newborn care skills as necessary.
2. Provide the opportunity for the mother to bathe the newborn.
3. Reinforce instructions to the mother regarding feeding technique.
4. Reinforce instructions to the mother to avoid heavy lifting for at least 3 weeks.
5. Reinforce instructions to the mother to plan at least one rest period per day.
6. Reinforce instructions to the mother that contraception should begin after delivery or with the initiation of intercourse.
7. Reinforce instructions to the mother regarding the importance of follow-up care, which should be scheduled at 4 to 6 weeks postpartum.
8. Reinforce instructions to the mother to report immediately any signs of chills, fever, increased lochia, or depressed feelings to the health care provider (HCP).

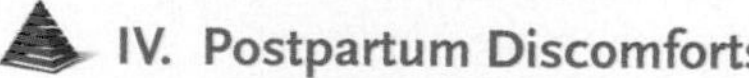

IV. Postpartum Discomforts

A. Afterbirth pains
1. Occur as a result of contractions of the uterus
2. Are more common among multiparas, breastfeeding mothers, clients treated with oxytocin (Pitocin), and clients who had an overdistended uterus during pregnancy (e.g., those who carried twins)

⚠ The nurse should consult with the registered nurse and check the HCP's prescriptions regarding treatment measures for postpartum discomforts.

B. Perineal discomfort
1. Apply ice packs to the perineum, as prescribed, during the first 24 hours to reduce swelling.
2. After the first 24 hours, apply warmth by sitz baths.

C. Episiotomy
1. Instruct the client to administer perineal care after each voiding.
2. Encourage the use of analgesic spray.
3. Administer analgesics if comfort measures are unsuccessful.

D. Perineal lacerations
1. Care as for an episiotomy. Administer perineal care and use analgesic spray and analgesics for comfort.
2. Rectal suppositories and enemas may be contraindicated (to avoid injury to sutures).

E. Breast discomfort from engorgement
1. Encourage the wearing of a support bra at all times, even while sleeping.
2. Encourage the use of ice packs.
3. Encourage the use of warm soaks before feeding for the breastfeeding mother.
4. Administer analgesics if comfort measures are unsuccessful.

F. Constipation
1. Encourage adequate intake of fluids (2000 mL/day).
2. Encourage a diet high in fiber.
3. Encourage ambulation.
4. Administer stool softener or laxative if needed.

G. Postpartum emotional changes (Box 28-2)
1. Acknowledge the client's feelings and demonstrate a caring attitude.
2. Determine availability of family support and other support systems, and encourage and assist the client to verbalize her feelings.
3. Monitor the newborn for appropriate growth and development expectations.
4. Assist significant other and other appropriate family members to discuss feelings and identify ways to assist client.

⚠ All clients should be assessed for depression during pregnancy and in the postpartum period.

V. Nutritional Counseling

A. Discuss caloric intake for breastfeeding and nonbreastfeeding mothers.

B. Nutritional needs depend on prepregnancy weight, ideal weight for height, and whether the mother is breastfeeding (check the HCP's prescription).

C. If the mother is breastfeeding, calorie needs increase by approximately 200 to 500 cal/day, and the mother may require increased fluids and the continuance of prenatal vitamins and minerals.

BOX 28-2 Signs and Symptoms of Emotional Changes

Postpartum Blues

- Anger
- Anxiety
- Cries easily for no apparent reason
- Emotionally labile
- Expresses a let-down feeling
- Fatigue
- Headache
- Insomnia
- Restlessness
- Sadness

Postpartum Depression

- Anxiety
- Appetite changes
- Crying, sadness
- Difficulty concentrating or making decisions
- Fatigue, unable to sleep
- Feelings of guilt
- Irritability and agitation
- Lack of energy
- Less responsive to the infant
- Loss of pleasure in normal activities
- Suicidal thoughts

Postpartum Psychosis

- Break with reality
- Confusion
- Delirium
- Delusions
- Hallucinations
- Panic

Data from: Lowdermilk D, Cashion MC, Perry S: *Maternity & women's health care*, ed 9, St. Louis, 2011, Mosby; Lowdermilk D, Cashion MC, Perry S: *Maternity & women's health care*, ed 10, St. Louis, 2012, Mosby; Perry S, Hockenberry M, Lowdermilk D, Wilson D: *Maternal-child nursing care*, ed 4, St. Louis, 2013.

VI. Breastfeeding

A. Interventions

1. Put the baby to the mother's breast as soon as the mother's and baby's conditions are stable (on the delivery table, if possible).
2. Stay with the mother each time she nurses until she feels secure and confident with the baby and her feelings.
3. Monitor LATCH (L=*l*atch achieved by newborn; A=*a*udible swallowing; T=*t*ype of nipple; C=*c*omfort of mother; H=*h*old or position of the newborn).
4. Uterine cramping may occur during the first day after delivery while the mother is nursing, when oxytocin stimulation causes the uterus to contract.
5. Instruct the client in general hygiene and to wash the breasts once daily.
6. The mother should not use soap on the breasts because it tends to remove natural oils, which increases the chance of cracked nipples.
7. If engorgement occurs, have the mother breastfeed frequently, apply warm packs before feeding, apply ice packs after feedings, and massage the breasts.
8. If cracked nipples develop, expose the nipples to air for 10 to 20 minutes after feeding, rotate the position of the baby for each feeding, and be sure that the baby is latched onto the areola and not just the nipple.
9. Bra should be well fitted and supportive; avoid an underwire bra.
10. Breasts may leak between feedings or during coitus. Place a breast pad in the bra.
11. Calories should be increased by 200 to 500 cal/day, and the diet should include additional fluids. Prenatal vitamins should be taken, as prescribed.
12. Baby's stools are usually light yellow, seedy, watery, and frequent.
13. Medications, including over-the-counter medications, need to be avoided, unless prescribed because they may be unsafe when breastfeeding.
14. Gas-producing foods and caffeine should be avoided.
15. Hormonal contraceptives may cause a decrease in the milk supply and are best avoided during the first 6 weeks after birth.
16. Oral contraceptives that contain estrogen are not recommended for breastfeeding mothers. Progestin-only birth control pills are less likely to interfere with the milk supply.
17. The baby will develop his or her own feeding schedule.

B. Breastfeeding procedure for mother (Box 28-3)

BOX 28-3 Breastfeeding Procedure for the Mother

1. Wash hands and assume a comfortable position.
2. Start with the breast with which the last feeding ended.
3. Brush the newborn's lower lip with nipple.
4. Tickle the lips to have the newborn open the mouth wide.
5. Guide the nipple and surrounding areola into the newborn's mouth.
6. Encourage the newborn to nurse on each breast for 15 to 20 minutes.
7. Listen for audible sucking and swallowing.
8. After the newborn has nursed, release suction by depressing the newborn's chin or inserting a clean finger into the newborn's mouth.
9. Burp the newborn after the first breast.
10. Repeat the procedure on the second breast until the newborn stops nursing.
11. Burp the newborn again.

VII. Cystitis

A. Description: Infection of the bladder can occur in the postpartum period, and the postpartum woman should be encouraged to consume adequate fluids and void frequently to avoid bladder distension.

B. Data collection and interventions: Refer to Chapter 53 for information.

If cystitis is suspected, obtain a urine specimen for culture and sensitivity before initiating antibiotic therapy.

VIII. Hematoma

A. Description
1. Localized collection of blood into the tissues of the reproductive sac after delivery. Vulvar hematomas are the most common (Fig. 28-3).
2. Predisposing conditions include operative delivery with forceps or injury to a blood vessel.
3. Can be a life-threatening condition

B. Data collection
1. Abnormal severe pain
2. Pressure in the perineal area
3. Sensitive, bulging mass in the perineal area with discolored skin
4. Inability to void
5. Decreased hemoglobin and hematocrit levels
6. Signs of shock (e.g., pallor, tachycardia, hypotension) if significant blood loss has occurred

C. Interventions
1. Monitor the vital signs.
2. Monitor the client for abnormal pain, especially when a forceps delivery has occurred.
3. Place ice on the hematoma site as prescribed.
4. Assist to administer analgesics as prescribed.
5. Monitor intake and output.
6. Encourage fluids and voiding.
7. Prepare for urinary catheterization if the client is unable to void.
8. Assist to administer blood products as prescribed.
9. Monitor for signs of infection, such as increased temperature, pulse rate, and white blood cell (WBC) count.
10. Assist to administer antibiotics as prescribed because infection is common after hematoma formation.
11. Prepare the client for the incision and evacuation of the hematoma, if necessary.

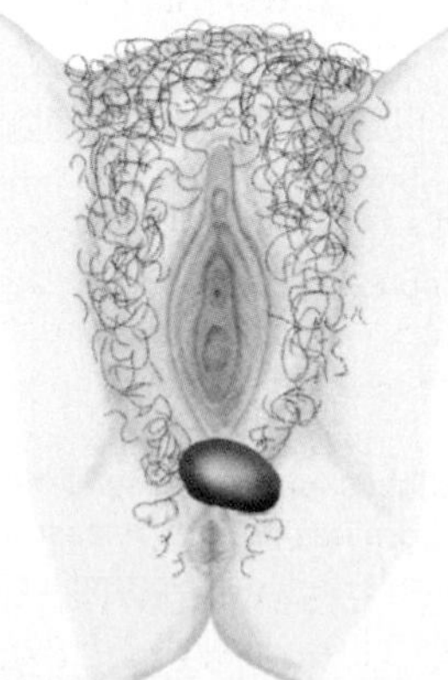

FIGURE 28-3 A vulvar hematoma is caused by rapid bleeding into soft tissue. It causes severe pain and feelings of pressure. (From Murray S, McKinney E: *Foundations of maternal-newborn and women's health nursing,* ed 5, Philadelphia, 2010, Saunders.)

IX. Hemorrhage (Box 28-4)

A. Description
1. Bleeding of 500 mL or more after delivery
2. Primary cause of maternal mortality that demands prompt recognition and intervention

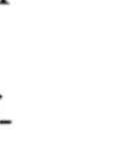

B. Data collection
1. Early: Hemorrhage occurs during the first 24 hours after delivery.
2. Late: Hemorrhage occurs more than 24 hours after delivery.

C. Interventions
1. Massage the fundus for uterine atony (Fig. 28-4).
2. Remain with the client and ask another nurse to notify the registered nurse (RN), who will then contact the HCP.
3. Monitor vital signs and fundus every 5 to 15 minutes; monitor for early signs of hemorrhaging and shock, including restlessness and increased pulse rate (a decrease in blood pressure is a later sign of hemorrhage).
4. Assess and estimate blood loss by pad count.
5. Turn the client to check for pooled blood underneath her.
6. Monitor level of consciousness.
7. Administer fluids, as prescribed, and monitor intake and output.
8. Monitor hemoglobin and hematocrit levels.

BOX 28-4 Postpartum Hemorrhage

Causes
- Uterine atony
- Laceration of the cervix or vagina
- Hematoma development in the cervix, perineum, or labia
- Retained placental fragments

Predisposing Factors
- Previous history of postpartum hemorrhage
- Placenta previa
- Abruptio placentae
- Overdistention of the uterus—polyhydramnios, multiple gestation, large neonate
- Infection
- Multiparity
- Dystocia or labor that is prolonged
- Operative delivery—cesarean or forceps delivery, intrauterine manipulation

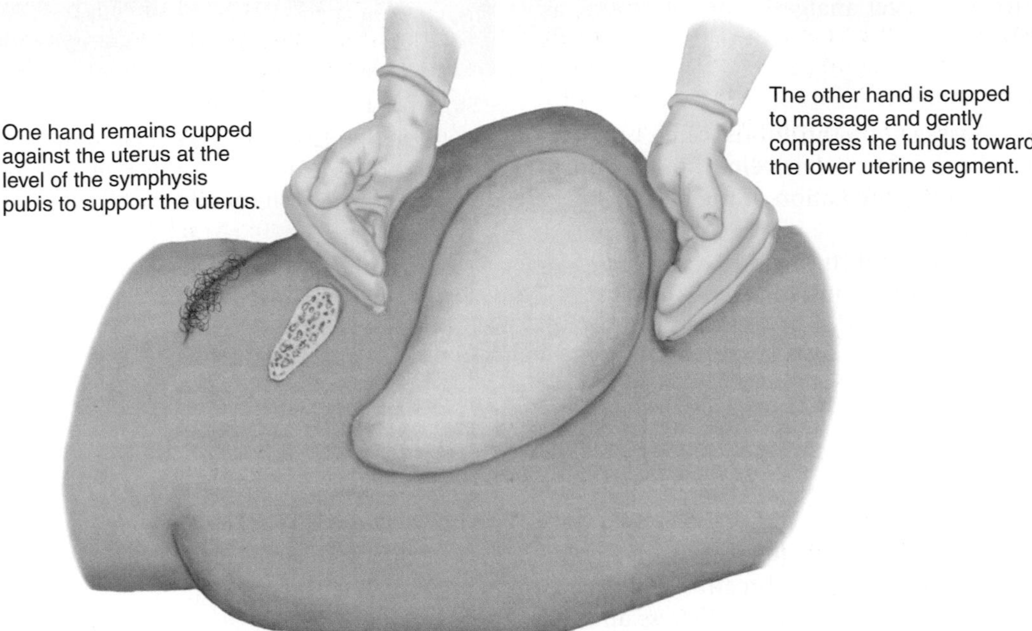
One hand remains cupped against the uterus at the level of the symphysis pubis to support the uterus.
The other hand is cupped to massage and gently compress the fundus toward the lower uterine segment.

FIGURE 28-4 Technique for fundal massage. One hand remains cupped against the uterus at the level of the symphysis pubis to support the uterus. The other hand is cupped to massage and compress the fundus gently toward the lower uterine segment. (From McKinney E, James S, Murray S, Ashwill J: *Maternal-child nursing*, ed 4, St. Louis, 2013, Saunders.)

9. Maintain asepsis because hemorrhage predisposes infection.
10. Assist to prepare for administration of oxytocin (Pitocin) if prescribed.
11. Assist to prepare for administration of IV fluids and blood transfusions if prescribed.
12. Assist to prepare for surgical intervention (e.g., dilation and curettage or hysterectomy).

X. Infection

A. Description: Any infection of the reproductive organs that occurs within 28 days of delivery or abortion

B. Data collection
1. Fever
2. Chills
3. Anorexia
4. Pelvic discomfort or pain
5. Vaginal discharge that is malodorous. Normal vaginal discharge has a fleshy odor or an odor similar to a menstrual period.
6. Elevated WBC count

A temperature of 100.4°F is normal during the first 24 hours postpartum because of dehydration; a temperature of 100.4°F or greater after 24 hours postpartum indicates infection.

C. Interventions
1. Monitor the vital signs and temperature every 2 to 4 hours.
2. Make the mother as comfortable as possible. Position her for comfort and to promote vaginal drainage.
3. Keep the mother warmed if she is chilled.
4. Isolate the baby from the mother only if the mother can infect the baby. 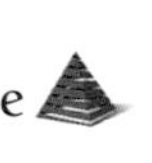
5. Provide a nutritious, high-calorie, high-protein diet.
6. Encourage fluids of 3000 to 4000 mL/day, if not contraindicated.
7. Encourage frequent voiding; monitor the intake and output.
8. Monitor culture results if cultures were prescribed.
9. Assist to administer antibiotics, as prescribed.

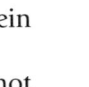

XI. Mastitis

A. Description
1. Inflammation of the breast as a result of infection
2. Primarily occurs in breastfeeding mothers 2 to 3 weeks after delivery but may occur at any time during lactation

B. Data collection
1. Localized heat and swelling
2. Pain; tender axillary lymph nodes
3. Elevated temperature
4. Complaints of flu-like symptoms

C. Interventions 
1. Instruct the mother in good hand-washing and breast hygiene techniques.
2. Promote comfort.
3. Apply heat or cold to the site, as prescribed.
4. Maintain lactation in breastfeeding mothers.
5. Encourage the manual expression of breast milk or the use of a breast pump every 4 hours.
6. Encourage the mother to support the breasts with a supportive, nonunderwire bra.

7. Assist to administer analgesics or antibiotics, as prescribed.

XII. Pulmonary Embolism

A. Description: Passage of a thrombus, often originating in a uterine or other pelvic vein, into the lungs, where it disrupts the circulation of the blood

B. Data collection

1. Sudden dyspnea and chest pain
2. Tachypnea and tachycardia
3. Cough and lung crackles
4. Hemoptysis
5. Feeling of impending doom

C. Interventions

1. Administer oxygen.
2. Position the client with the head of the bed elevated.
3. Monitor the vital signs frequently, especially respiratory and heart rate and breath sounds.
4. Monitor for signs of respiratory distress and for signs of increasing hypoxemia, such as tachypnea, tachycardia, restlessness, cool and clammy skin, cyanosis, and the use of accessory muscles for breathing.
5. Assist to administer intravenous fluids and anticoagulants as prescribed.
6. Prepare to assist the HCP to administer medications to dissolve the clot if prescribed.

XIII. Subinvolution

A. Description: Incomplete involution or the failure of the uterus to return to its normal size and condition

B. Data collection

1. Uterine pain on palpation
2. Uterus is larger than expected
3. More than normal vaginal bleeding

C. Interventions

1. Monitor the vital signs.
2. Check the uterus and fundus.
3. Monitor for uterine pain and vaginal bleeding.
4. Elevate the legs to promote venous return.
5. Encourage frequent voiding.
6. Monitor the hemoglobin and hematocrit levels.
7. Prepare to assist to administer methylergonovine maleate (Methergine), which provides sustained contraction of the uterus, as prescribed.

XIV. Thrombophlebitis

A. Description

1. A condition in which a clot forms in a vessel wall as a result of the inflammation of the vessel wall.
2. A partial obstruction of the vessel can occur.
3. Increased blood-clotting factors during the postpartum period place the client at risk.
4. Early ambulation in the postoperative period after cesarean section is a preventive action.

BOX 28-5 Data Collection: Types of Thrombophlebitis

Superficial

- Palpable thrombus that feels bumpy and hard
- Tenderness and pain in the affected lower extremity
- Warm and pinkish-red color over the thrombus area

Femoral

- Malaise
- Chills and fever
- Diminished peripheral pulses
- Shiny, white skin over the affected area
- Pain, stiffness, and swelling of the affected leg

Pelvic

- Severe chills
- Dramatic body temperature changes
- Occurrence of pulmonary embolism may be the first sign

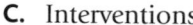

B. Data Collection: Types of thrombophlebitis (Box 28-5) 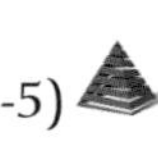

C. Interventions

1. Specific therapies may depend on the location of the thrombophlebitis.
2. Check the lower extremities for edema, tenderness, varices, and increased skin temperature.
3. Maintain bed rest, if prescribed.
4. Elevate the affected leg.
5. Apply a bed cradle, and keep bedclothes off the affected leg.
6. Never massage the leg.
7. Monitor for manifestations of pulmonary embolism.
8. Apply hot packs or moist heat to the affected site as prescribed to alleviate discomfort.
9. Apply elastic stockings (support hose) if prescribed.
10. Assist to administer analgesics and antibiotics as prescribed.
11. Intravenous heparin sodium may be prescribed for femoral or pelvic thrombophlebitis to prevent further thrombus formation.

D. Reinforcement of client teaching (Box 28-6)

BOX 28-6 Client Education for Thrombophlebitis

Never massage the leg.
Avoid crossing the legs.
Avoid prolonged sitting.
Avoid constrictive clothing.
Avoid pressure behind the knees.
Know how to apply elastic stockings (support hose) if prescribed.
Understand the importance of anticoagulant therapy if prescribed.
Understand the importance of follow-up with the HCP.

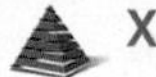

XV. Perinatal Loss

A. Description

1. Perinatal loss is associated with miscarriage, neonatal death, stillbirth, and therapeutic abortion.
2. Loss and grief may also coincide with the birth of a preterm **infant**, an infant who has suffered complications, or an infant with congenital anomalies. It may also occur within a family who is giving up a child for adoption.

B. Interventions

Not all interventions are appropriate for every woman and her significant family. It is crucial to consider religious and cultural health care practices and beliefs when planning care for a woman and family who have experienced perinatal loss.

1. Communicate therapeutically and actively listen, providing parents with time to grieve.
2. Notify the hospital chaplain or other religious person.
3. Discuss with the parents about options such as seeing, holding, bathing, and/or dressing the deceased infant; visitation by other family members or friends; religious or cultural rituals; and funeral arrangements.
4. Prepare a special memories box with keepsakes such as footprints, handprints, locks of hair, and pictures.
5. Admit the mother to a private room. If possible, mark the door to the room with a special card (per agency procedure and maintaining confidentiality) that denotes to hospital staff that this family has experienced a loss.
6. See Chapter 26 for additional information on fetal demise.

CRITICAL THINKING What Should You Do?

Answer: To determine most accurately the amount of lochial flow, the nurse should weigh the perineal pad before and after use and identify the amount of time between pad changes. This information is then documented according to agency procedures. The nurse should also note the color, odor, and the presence and characteristics of clots if any are noted.

Reference(s): McKinney, E., James, S., Murray, S., Nelson, K. & Ashwill, J. (2013). *Maternal-child nursing* (4th ed., pp. 434–435). St. Louis: Elsevier.

PRACTICE QUESTIONS

256. The client received epidural anesthesia during labor and had a forceps delivery after pushing for 2 hours. At 6 hours postpartum, the client's systolic blood pressure (BP) dropped 20 points, the diastolic BP dropped 10 points, and her pulse is 120 beats per minute. The client is very anxious and restless. The nurse is told that the client has a vulvar hematoma. Based on this diagnosis, the nurse should plan which action?

1. Reassuring the client
2. Applying perineal pressure
3. Monitoring the fundal height
4. Preparing the client for surgery

❖257. The nurse is preparing a list of self-care instructions for a postpartum client who has been diagnosed with mastitis. Which instructions should be included on the list? **Select all that apply.**

- ❑ 1. Rest during the acute phase.
- ❑ 2. Wear a supportive, nonunderwire bra.
- ❑ 3. Maintain a fluid intake of at least 3000 mL.
- ❑ 4. Continue to breastfeed if the breasts are not too sore.
- ❑ 5. Take the prescribed antibiotics until the soreness subsides.
- ❑ 6. Avoid decompression of the breasts by breastfeeding or breast pump.

258. A postpartum client is getting ready for discharge. The nurse suspects that the client **needs further teaching** related to breastfeeding when she makes which statement?

1. "I don't need birth control because I will be breastfeeding."
2. "I need to increase my caloric intake by 500 calories a day."
3. "I shouldn't use soap to wash my breasts because I will be breastfeeding."
4. "I need to be sure that I increase my fluid intake and take my prenatal vitamins while breastfeeding."

259. The nurse is caring for a postpartum client with a diagnosis of thrombophlebitis. The client suddenly complains of chest pain and dyspnea. The nurse should **initially** check which item?

1. Vital signs
2. Fundal height
3. Presence of calf pain
4. Level of consciousness (LOC)

260. The nurse suspects that the client has a pulmonary embolism. Which is the **most important** nursing action?

1. Monitor the vital signs.
2. Elevate the head of the bed.
3. Increase the intravenous flow rate.
4. Administer oxygen by face mask, as prescribed.

261. The nurse notes that the 4-hour postpartum client has cool, clammy skin and that she is restless and excessively thirsty. The nurse immediately notifies the registered nurse and then performs which action?

1. Checks the vital signs
2. Begins fundal massage
3. Encourages ambulation
4. Encourages the client to drink fluids

262. The nurse is assisting with caring for a postpartum client who is experiencing uterine hemorrhage. When planning to meet the psychosocial needs of the client, the nurse should plan which action?

1. Maintaining strict bed rest
2. Monitoring the vital signs every 2 hours
3. Performing firm fundal massage every 2 hours
4. Keeping the client and her family members informed of her progress

263. The nurse palpates the fundus and checks the character of the lochia of a postpartum client who is in the fourth stage of labor. Which lochia characteristic should the nurse expect to note?

1. Red
2. Pink
3. White
4. Serosanguineous

264. After episiotomy and the delivery of a newborn, the nurse performs a perineal check on the mother. The nurse notes a trickle of bright red blood coming from the perineum. The nurse checks the fundus and notes that it is firm. Which determination should the nurse make?

1. This is a normal expectation after episiotomy.
2. The mother should be allowed bathroom privileges only.
3. The bright red bleeding is abnormal and should be reported.
4. The perineal assessment should be performed more frequently.

265. The nurse is assigned to care for the client during the postpartum period. The client asks the nurse what the term *involution* means. Which description should the nurse give to the client?

1. The inverted uterus returning to normal
2. The gradual reversal of the uterine muscle into the abdominal cavity
3. The descent of the uterus into the pelvic cavity, which occurs at a rate of 2 cm/day
4. The progressive descent of the uterus into the pelvic cavity, which occurs at a rate of approximately 1 cm/day

266. A mother is breastfeeding her newborn baby and experiences breast engorgement. The nurse should encourage the mother to do which to provide relief of the engorgement?

1. Breastfeed only during the daytime hours.
2. Apply cold compresses to the breast before feeding.
3. Avoid the use of a bra while the breasts are engorged.
4. Massage the breasts before feeding to stimulate let-down.

267. After delivery the nurse checks the height of the uterine fundus. Which position of the fundus should the nurse expect to note?

1. To the right of the abdomen
2. At the level of the umbilicus
3. About 4 cm above the level of the umbilicus
4. One fingerbreadth above the symphysis pubis

268. The nurse is caring for a postpartum client. At 4 hours postpartum, the client's temperature is 102 °F (38.9 °C). Which is the appropriate nursing action?

1. Apply cool packs to the abdomen.
2. Continue to monitor the temperature.
3. Remove the blanket from the client's bed.
4. Notify the registered nurse, who will then contact the health care provider (HCP).

269. The nurse is assisting with planning care for a postpartum woman who has small vulvar hematomas. To assist with reducing the swelling, the nurse should perform which action?

1. Check the vital signs every 4 hours.
2. Measure the fundal height every 4 hours.
3. Prepare a heat pack for application to the area.
4. Prepare an ice pack for application to the area.

270. The nurse is assigned to care for the client after a cesarean section. To prevent thrombophlebitis, the nurse should encourage the woman to take which **priority** action?

1. Ambulate frequently.
2. Wear support stockings.
3. Apply warm, moist packs to the legs.
4. Remain on bed rest, with the legs elevated.

ANSWERS

256. 4

Rationale: The information provided in the question indicates that the client is experiencing blood loss. Surgery would be indicated for this complication to stop the bleeding. Options 1, 2, and 3 would not assist with controlling the bleeding in this emergency situation.

Test-Taking Strategy: Focus on the information provided in the question and note that the subject of the question is that the client has a vulvar hematoma. Note that the signs and symptoms in the question indicate the presence of bleeding; this should direct you to the correct option. **Review:** the nursing interventions related to **vulvar hematomas**.

Level of Cognitive Ability: Analyzing
Client Needs: Physiological Integrity
Integrated Process: Nursing Process/Planning
Content Area: Maternity: Postpartum
Priority Concepts: Clotting, Reproduction
Reference(s): McKinney (2013), pp. 669–670.

❖ **257. 1, 2, 3, 4**

Rationale: Mastitis is an infection of the lactating breast. Client instructions include resting during the acute phase, maintaining a fluid intake of at least 3000 mL per day, and taking analgesics to relieve discomfort. Antibiotics may be prescribed and are taken until the complete prescribed course is finished. They are not stopped when the soreness subsides. Additional supportive measures include the use of moist heat or ice packs and the wearing of a supportive bra. Continued decompression of the breast by breastfeeding or breast pump is important to empty the breast and prevent the formation of an abscess.

Test-Taking Strategy: Think about the pathophysiology associated with the subject, mastitis. Recalling that supportive measures include rest, moist heat or ice packs, antibiotics, analgesics, increased fluid intake, breast support, and the decompression of the breasts will assist you with answering the question. **Review:** the treatment of **mastitis**.

Level of Cognitive Ability: Analyzing
Client Needs: Physiological Integrity
Integrated Process: Teaching and Learning
Content Area: Maternity: Postpartum
Priority Concepts: Client Education, Inflammation
Reference(s): McKinney et al (2013), pp. 680–681.

258. 1

Rationale: Amenorrhea may occur during breastfeeding, but the client can still ovulate without menstruating. The use of soap on the breasts is avoided because it tends to remove natural oils, which can lead to cracked nipples. The caloric intake should be increased by 200 to 500 cal/day (per health care provider's prescription), and the diet should include additional fluids and prenatal vitamins, as prescribed.

Test-Taking Strategy: Note the strategic words, *needs further teaching*. These words indicate a negative event query and the need to select the incorrect statement. Recalling the physiology related to amenorrhea and ovulation during breastfeeding will direct you to the correct option. **Review:** teaching points for the woman who is **breastfeeding**.

Level of Cognitive Ability: Evaluating
Client Needs: Health Promotion and Maintenance
Integrated Process: Teaching and Learning
Content Area: Maternity: Postpartum
Priority Concepts: Client Education, Reproduction
Reference(s): McKinney et al (2013), pp. 242, 753.

259. 1

Rationale: Pulmonary embolism is a complication of thrombophlebitis. Changes in the vital signs are one of the first things to occur with pulmonary embolism, because pulmonary blood flow is compromised. Fundal height is unrelated to the subject of the question. Calf pain is an indicator of thrombophlebitis. Level of consciousness may change as the condition worsens; worsening would indicate hypoxia.

Test-Taking Strategy: Note the strategic word, *initially*. Use the ABCs—airway, breathing, and circulation—to direct you to the correct option. **Review:** the complications of **thrombophlebitis**.

Level of Cognitive Ability: Analyzing
Client Needs: Physiological Integrity
Integrated Process: Nursing Process/Data Collection
Content Area: Critical Care: Emergency Situations
Priority Concepts: Pain, Perfusion
Reference(s): McKinney et al (2013), p. 677.

260. 4

Rationale: Because pulmonary circulation is compromised in the presence of an embolus, cardiorespiratory support is initiated by oxygen administration. Options 1 and 2 may be components of the plan of care, but they are not the most important actions. The nurse would not increase the intravenous rate without a prescription from the health care provider to do so.

Test-Taking Strategy: Note the strategic words, *most important*, and use the ABCs—airway, breathing, and circulation. This will direct you to the correct option: *oxygen is the priority.* **Review:** the care of the client in the event of a **pulmonary embolism**.

Level of Cognitive Ability: Applying
Client Needs: Physiological Integrity
Integrated Process: Nursing Process/Implementation
Content Area: Critical Care: Emergency Situations
Priority Concepts: Gas Exchange, Perfusion
Reference(s): McKinney et al (2013), p. 677.

261. 1

Rationale: Symptoms of hypovolemia include cool, clammy, and pale skin; feelings of anxiety and restlessness; and thirst. The nurse would check the vital signs. The nurse would not ambulate the client or encourage fluids until specific prescriptions are given to do so. There is no information in the question to indicate the need for fundal massage.

Test-Taking Strategy: Focus on the subject, the symptoms in the question. Use the ABCs—airway, breathing, and circulation—to direct you to the correct option. **Review:** the nursing care of the client with **hypovolemia**.

Level of Cognitive Ability: Applying
Client Needs: Physiological Integrity
Integrated Process: Nursing Process/Implementation
Content Area: Critical Care: Emergency Situations
Priority Concepts: Clotting, Perfusion
Reference(s): McKinney et al (2013), pp. 670–671.

262. 4

Rationale: Keeping the client and her family informed about her condition will help minimize fear and apprehension. Options 1, 2, and 3 identify physiological interventions.

Test-Taking Strategy: Focus on the subject, meeting psychosocial needs. The correct option is the only option that addresses psychosocial needs. **Review:** the interventions that will meet the psychosocial needs of the client.

Level of Cognitive Ability: Applying
Client Needs: Psychosocial Integrity
Integrated Process: Caring
Content Area: Maternity: Postpartum
Priority Concepts: Caregiving, Coping
Reference(s): McKinney et al (2013), pp. 670, 672–673.

263. 1

Rationale: The color of the lochia during the fourth stage of labor is bright red, and this may last from 1 to 3 days. The color of the lochia then changes to a pinkish-brown and occurs from day 4 to 10 postpartum. Finally, the lochia changes to a creamy white color that occurs from day 10 to 14 postpartum.

Test-Taking Strategy: Focus on the subject, fourth stage of labor; this will direct you to the correct option. In the immediate postpartum period, the lochia is red in color. **Review:** the expected postpartum findings for lochia.

Level of Cognitive Ability: Applying
Client Needs: Physiological Integrity
Integrated Process: Nursing Process/Data Collection
Content Area: Maternity: Postpartum
Priority Concepts: Reproduction, Tissue Integrity
Reference(s): McKinney et al (2013), p. 360.

264. 3

Rationale: Lochial flow should be distinguished from bleeding that originates from a laceration or an episiotomy, which is usually brighter red than lochia and presents as a continuous trickle of bleeding, even though the fundus of the uterus is firm. This bright red bleeding is abnormal and needs to be reported. Therefore, the other options are incorrect interpretations.

Test-Taking Strategy: Note the subject, trickle of bright red blood. This should be an indication that the flow is not normal. **Review:** the lochial flow and the complications associated with episiotomy.

Level of Cognitive Ability: Analyzing
Client Needs: Physiological Integrity
Integrated Process: Nursing Process/Data Collection
Content Area: Maternity: Postpartum
Priority Concepts: Clotting, Reproduction
Reference(s): McKinney et al (2013), pp. 360, 434–435.

265. 4

Rationale: Involution is the progressive descent of the uterus into the pelvic cavity. After birth, descent occurs at a rate of approximately 1 fingerbreadth or 1 cm per day. The other options do not accurately describe involution.

Test-Taking Strategy: Focus on the subject, a description of involution. Use your knowledge of medical terminology to help you to define *involution*. This will assist with directing you to the correct option. **Review:** the process of involution.

Level of Cognitive Ability: Applying
Client Needs: Health Promotion and Maintenance
Integrated Process: Nursing Process/Implementation
Content Area: Maternity: Postpartum
Priority Concepts: Client Education, Reproduction
Reference(s): McKinney et al (2013), p. 433–434.

266. 4

Rationale: Comfort measures for breast engorgement include massaging the breasts before feeding to stimulate let-down, wearing a supportive and well-fitting bra at all times, taking a warm shower or applying warm compresses just before feeding, and alternating breasts during feeding.

Test-Taking Strategy: Focus on the subject, engorgement. Eliminate option 1 because of the closed-ended word, *only*. From the remaining options, recalling the self-care measures that promote the comfort of the mother with breast engorgement will direct you to the correct option. **Review:** the measures to take if engorgement occurs.

Level of Cognitive Ability: Applying
Client Needs: Health Promotion and Maintenance
Integrated Process: Nursing Process/Implementation
Content Area: Maternity: Postpartum
Priority Concepts: Inflammation, Pain
Reference(s): McKinney et al (2013), pp. 542–543.

267. 2

Rationale: After delivery, the uterine fundus should be at the level of the umbilicus or 1 to 3 fingerbreadths below it and in the midline of the abdomen. If the fundus is 4 cm above the umbilicus, this may indicate that there are blood clots in the uterus that need to be expelled by fundal massage. If the fundus is noted to the right of the abdomen, it may indicate a full bladder. By about 10 days postpartum, the uterus will be in the symphysis pubis area.

Test-Taking Strategy: Note the subject, height of the fundus after delivery, and visualize the process of involution. Remember that after delivery, the uterine fundus should be at the level of the umbilicus or 1 to 3 fingerbreadths below it and in the midline of the abdomen. **Review:** expected postpartum findings.

Level of Cognitive Ability: Applying
Client Needs: Physiological Integrity
Integrated Process: Nursing Process/Data Collection
Content Area: Maternity: Postpartum
Priority Concepts: Reproduction, Tissue Integrity
Reference(s): McKinney et al (2013), pp. 357, 360, 441.

268. 4

Rationale: During the first 24 hours postpartum, the mother's temperature may be elevated as a result of dehydration. However, if the temperature is more than 2°F above normal, this may indicate infection, and the HCP will need to be notified. Applying cool packs to the abdomen is an inappropriate action, and, additionally, this action requires a prescription. The remaining options may be a component of care but are not the most appropriate based on the data in the question.

Test-Taking Strategy: Focus on the subject, a temperature of 102°F 4 hours after delivery. Noting that this temperature is extreme as compared with the normal temperature will direct you to the correct option. **Review:** the expected postpartum findings.

Level of Cognitive Ability: Applying
Client Needs: Physiological Integrity
Integrated Process: Nursing Process/Implementation
Content Area: Maternity: Postpartum
Priority Concepts: Reproduction, Thermoregulation
Reference(s): McKinney et al (2013), pp. 440, 682–683.

269. 4
Rationale: The application of ice will reduce the swelling caused by hematoma formation in the vulvar area. Options 1, 2, and 3 will not reduce swelling.
Test-Taking Strategy: Focus on the subject, the reduction of swelling. This will assist you with eliminating options 1 and 2. Recalling the principles related to heat and cold will direct you to the correct option. **Review:** the nursing care of the client with a **hematoma.**
Level of Cognitive Ability: Applying
Client Needs: Physiological Integrity
Integrated Process: Nursing Process/Implementation
Content Area: Maternity: Postpartum
Priority Concepts: Reproduction, Tissue Integrity
Reference(s): McKinney et al (2013), pp. 360, 443–444.

270. 1
Rationale: Stasis is believed to be a major predisposing factor for the development of thrombophlebitis. Because cesarean delivery poses a risk factor, the client should ambulate early and frequently to promote circulation and prevent stasis. Options 2, 3, and 4 are implemented if thrombophlebitis occurs.
Test-Taking Strategy: Focus on the subject, the prevention of thrombophlebitis, and note the strategic word, *priority.* Options 3 and 4 are implemented if thrombophlebitis occurs. Although wearing support stockings may be prescribed in the postoperative period to promote venous return, ambulating frequently (option 1) is the priority preventive measure. **Review:** prevention of **thrombophlebitis** during the postoperative period.
Level of Cognitive Ability: Applying
Client Needs: Physiological Integrity
Integrated Process: Nursing Process/Implementation
Content Area: Maternity: Postpartum
Priority Concepts: Clotting, Reproduction
Reference(s): McKinney et al (2013), pp. 674–675.

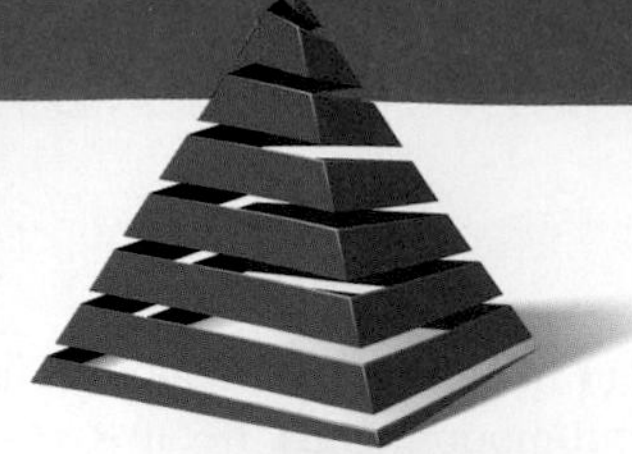

Maternity

CHAPTER 29

Care of the Newborn

CRITICAL THINKING What Should You Do?

The nurse is assisting in collecting data on a newborn who just arrived to the newborn nursery and notes that the newborn is experiencing tremors. What should the nurse do?

Answer is located on p. 346.

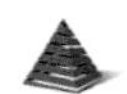

I. Initial Care of the Newborn

A. Data collection

1. Observe or assist with the initiation of respirations.
2. Determine Apgar score.
3. Note characteristics of cry.
4. Monitor for nasal flaring, grunting, retractions, and abnormal respirations, such as a seesaw respiratory pattern (rise and fall of the chest and abdomen do not occur together).
5. Check for central cyanosis and acrocyanosis.
6. Obtain vital signs.
7. Observe for signs of hypothermia or hyperthermia.
8. Check for gross anomalies.

B. Interventions

1. Suction the mouth first and then the nares with a bulb syringe.
2. Dry the baby and stimulate crying by rubbing.
3. Maintain temperature stability; wrap the baby in warm blankets and place a stockinette cap on the **newborn's** head.
4. Keep the baby with the mother to facilitate bonding.
5. Place the baby at the mother's breast if breastfeeding is planned, or place the baby on the mother's abdomen.
6. Place the baby in a radiant warmer.
7. Position the newborn on the side with a rolled blanket at the back to facilitate drainage of mucus.
8. Ensure proper identification.
9. Footprint the newborn and fingerprint the mother on the identification sheet per agency policies and procedures; initiate other agency identification and safety procedures.
10. Place matching identification bracelets on the mother and the newborn.

C. Apgar scoring system

1. Assess each of the five items to be scored, and add the points assessed for each item to determine the newborn's total score.
2. Five vital indicators (Table 29-1)
3. Interventions: Apgar score (Table 29-2)

⚠ The newborn's Apgar score is assessed and recorded at 1 minute and 5 minutes after birth, and at 10 minutes if needed.

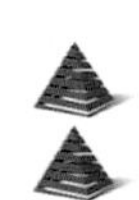

II. Initial Physical Examination

A. General guidelines

1. Keep the newborn warm during the examination.
2. Begin with general observations; then first perform the assessments that are the least disturbing to the newborn.
3. Initiate nursing interventions for abnormal findings and document findings.
4. The Ballard Scale may be used for gestational age assessment; in this scale, scores are assigned to physical and neurological criteria.

⚠ The phases of newborn instability occur during the first 6 to 8 hours after birth and are known as the transition period between intrauterine and extrauterine existence. These phases include the first period of reactivity, period of decreased responsiveness, and second period of reactivity.

B. Vital signs

1. Heart rate (resting): 120 to 160 beats/minute (apical), 80 to 100 beats/minute (if sleeping), up to 180 beats/minute (if crying); auscultate at the fourth intercostal space for 1 full minute to detect abnormalities.
2. Respirations: 30 to 60 breaths per minute. Check for a full minute.
3. Assess heart rate and respiratory rate first before assessing other vital signs while the newborn is resting or sleeping.
4. Axillary temperature: 96.8° to 99°F

TABLE 29-1 The Five Vital Indicators of the Apgar Score

Indicator	0 Points	1 Point	2 Points
Heart rate	Absent	Less than 100 beats/minute	More than 100 beats/minute
Respiratory rate/Effort	Absent	Slow, irregular breathing, weak cry	Good rate and effort, vigorous cry
Muscle tone	Flaccid, limp	Minimal flexion of the extremities	Good flexion, active motion
Reflex irritability	No response	Minimal response (grimace) to suction or the gentle slap on the soles	Responds promptly with a cry or active movement
Skin color	Pallor or cyanosis	Body skin color normal, extremities blue	Body and extremity skin color normal

TABLE 29-2 Apgar Score Interventions

Score	Intervention
8-10	No intervention except support the newborn's spontaneous efforts
4-7	Gently stimulate Rub the newborn's back Administer oxygen to the newborn
0-3	Newborn requires full resuscitation; rescore at specific intervals

Note: The newborn's Apgar score obtained at 5 minutes of age reflects the efficacy of any initial resuscitation efforts.

TABLE 29-3 Fontanels

Location	Characteristics	Closure
Anterior	Soft, flat, and diamond-shaped; 3-4 cm wide by 2-3 cm long	Between the ages of 12 and 18 months
Posterior	Triangular, 0.5-1 cm wide; located between the occipital and parietal bones	Between birth and the age of 2 or 3 months

5. Blood pressure: Usually not done in term newborn, 80-90/40-50 mm Hg

C. Body measurements (approximate)
   1. Length: 45 to 55 cm (18 to 22 inches)
   2. Weight: 2500 to 4000 g (5.5 to 8.75 pounds)
   3. Head circumference: 33 to 35 cm (13.2 to 14 inches)

D. Head
   1. One fourth of the body length (cephalocaudal development)
   2. Bones of the skull are not fused.
   3. Palpable sutures (connective tissue between the skull bones) are palpable and may be overlapping because of head molding, but should not be widened.
   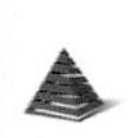
   4. Fontanels: Unossified membranous tissue at the junction of the sutures (Table 29-3)
   5. Molding: Asymmetry of the head as a result of pressure in the birth canal; disappears in about 72 hours (Fig. 29-1)
   6. Masses from birth trauma
      a. Caput succedaneum: Edema of the soft tissue over bone (crosses over the suture line); subsides within a few days
      b. Cephalhematoma: Swelling caused by bleeding into an area between the bone and its periosteum (does not cross over the suture line); usually absorbed within 6 weeks with no treatment

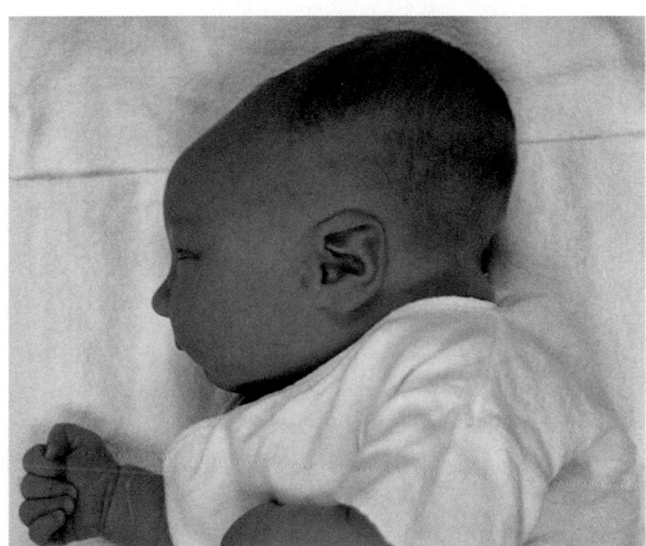

FIGURE 29-1 Significant molding after vaginal birth. (From Perry S, Hockenberry M, Lowdermilk D, Wilson D: *Maternal-child nursing care*, ed 4, St. Louis, 2010, Mosby. Courtesy of Kim Molloy, Knoxville, IA.)

   7. Head lag
      a. Common when pulling the newborn to a sitting position
      b. When prone, the newborn should be able to lift the head slightly and turn the head from side to side.

E. Eyes
   1. Slate gray (light skin), dark blue, or brown-gray (dark skin)
   2. Symmetrical and clear

3. Pupils are equal and round; react to light by accommodation.
4. Blink reflex is present.
5. Eyes cross because of weak extraocular muscles.
6. Able to track and fixate momentarily
7. Red reflex is present.
8. Eyelids often edematous as a result of pressure during the birth process and the effects of eye medication.

F. Ears
1. Symmetrical
2. Firm cartilage with recoil
3. Top of pinna on or above line drawn from outer canthus of eye
4. Low-set ears are associated with many syndromes and genetic abnormalities, such as Down syndrome.

G. Nose
1. Flat, broad, and located in the center of the face
2. Obligatory nose breathing
3. Occasional sneezing to remove obstructions
4. Nares are patent and should not flare (flaring is an indication of respiratory distress).

H. Mouth
1. Gums pink and moist
2. Soft and hard palates intact
3. Epstein's pearls (small, white cysts) may be present on the hard palate.
4. Uvula in midline
5. Tongue is symmetrical and moves freely, with a short frenulum.
6. Sucking and crying movements are symmetrical.
7. Able to swallow
8. Root and gag reflexes present.

When assessing the newborn's mouth, look for the presence of thrush (*Candida albicans*), which are white patchy areas on the tongue or gums that cannot be removed with a washcloth; these may be painful.

I. Neck
1. Short and thick
2. Head held in midline
3. Trachea in midline
4. Good range of motion and ability to flex and extend
5. Check for torticollis (head inclined to one side as a result of contraction of muscles on that side of the neck).

J. Chest
1. Circular appearance because anteroposterior and lateral diameters are about equal (approximately 30 to 33 cm [12 to 13.2 inches] at birth)
2. Respirations are diaphragmatic—chest and abdomen should rise and fall in synchrony, not in a seesaw pattern.
3. Bronchial sounds on auscultation
4. Nipples are prominent and often edematous; milky secretion (witch's milk) common.
5. Breast tissue present.
6. Clavicles are palpated to check for fractures.

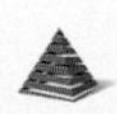

K. Skin
1. Pinkish-red (light-skinned newborn) to pinkish-brown or pinkish-yellow (dark-skinned newborn)
2. Vernix caseosa, a cheesy white substance, on entire body in preterm newborns, but is more prominent between folds closer to term; may be absent after 42 weeks of gestation.
3. Lanugo, fine body hair, might be seen, especially on the back.
4. Milia, small white sebaceous glands, appear on the forehead, nose, and chin.
5. Dry, peeling skin, increased in postmature newborns
6. Dark red color (plethoric) common in premature newborns
7. Cyanosis may be noted with hypothermia, infection, and hypoglycemia and with cardiac, respiratory, or neurological abnormalities.
8. Acrocyanosis (peripheral cyanosis of hands and feet) is normal in the first few hours after birth and may be noted intermittently for the next 7 to 10 days (Fig. 29-2).
9. Check for ecchymosis and petechiae as a result of the trauma of birth.
10. Check the skin turgor over the abdomen to determine hydration status.
11. Observe for forceps marks.
12. Harlequin sign
    a. Deep pink or red color develops over one side of the newborn's body, while the other side remains pale or of normal color
    b. May indicate shunting of blood that occurs with a cardiac problem or may indicate sepsis
13. Birthmarks (Table 29-4)

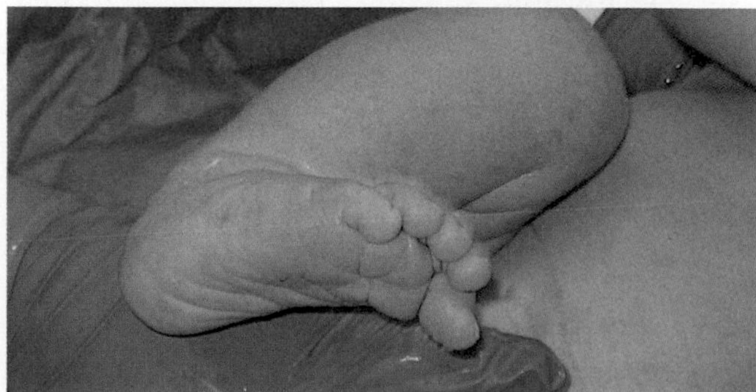

FIGURE 29-2 Acrocyanosis. (From McKinney E, James S, Murray S, Ashwill J: *Maternal-child nursing*, ed 4, St. Louis, 2013, Saunders. Courtesy of Todd Shiros, Santa Fe Springs, CA.)

TABLE 29-4 Birthmarks

Birthmark	Characteristics
Telangiectatic nevi (stork bites)	Pale pink or red, flat, dilated capillaries On eyelids, nose, lower occipital bone, and nape of neck Blanch easily More noticeable during crying periods Disappear by age 2 yr
Nevus flammeus (port-wine stain)	Capillary angioma directly below epidermis Nonelevated, sharply demarcated, red to purple, dense areas of capillaries Commonly appear on face No fading with time May require future surgery
Nevus vasculosus (strawberry mark)	Capillary hemangioma Raised, clearly delineated, dark red, with rough surface Common in head region Disappears by age 7-9 yr
Mongolian spots	Bluish-black pigmentation On lumbar dorsal area and buttocks Gradually fade during first and second years of life Common in Asian and dark-skinned individuals

L. Abdomen
1. Umbilical cord
   a. There are three vessels (two arteries and one vein) in the cord. If fewer than three vessels are noted, notify the health care provider (HCP).
   b. A small, thin cord may be associated with poor fetal growth.
   c. Check for an intact cord, and ensure that the clamp is secured.
   d. The cord should be clamped for at least the first 24 hours after birth. The clamp can be removed when the cord is dried and occluded and no longer bleeding.
   e. Note any bleeding or drainage from the cord.
   f. Hospital protocol and HCP's preference determine the technique for cord care. Protocols may include the use of antibiotic ointment, triple dye, soap and water, sterile water, povidone-iodine, alcohol, or another treatment.
   g. If symptoms of infection (e.g., moistness, oozing, discharge, reddened base) occur, notify the HCP; usually an antibiotic treatment is prescribed.
2. Gastrointestinal
   a. Monitor the cord for meconium staining.
   b. The newborn will be checked for the presence of an umbilical hernia.
   c. Note abdominal depression that may be associated with diaphragmatic hernia.
   d. Assess for abdominal distention associated with obstruction, mass, or sepsis.
   e. Monitor bowel sounds (present within the first hour after birth).
3. Anus
   a. Ensure that anal opening is present.
   b. First stool (meconium) should pass within the first 24 hours.

M. Genitals
1. Female
   a. Labia edematous and clitoris enlarged
   b. Smegma present (thick, white mucus discharge)
   c. Pseudomenstruation, caused by the withdrawal of the maternal hormone estrogen, is possible (blood-tinged mucus).
   d. Hymen tag may be visible.
   e. First voiding should occur within 24 hours.
2. Male
   a. Prepuce (foreskin) covers glans penis.
   b. Scrotum edematous
   c. Verify meatus at tip of penis.
   d. Testes descended but may retract with cold
   e. The newborn is checked for hernia or hydrocele.
   f. First voiding should occur within 24 hours.

N. Spine
1. Straight
2. Posture flexed
3. Supports head momentarily when prone
4. Chin flexed on upper chest
5. Sporadic movements that are well coordinated
6. A degree of hypotonicity or hypertonicity is indicative of central nervous system damage, and this finding needs to be reported.
7. Check for hair tufts and dimples along the spinal column (may be indicative of a possible opening).

O. Extremities
1. Flexed
2. Full range of motion and symmetrical movements
3. Fists clenched
4. Should be 10 fingers and 10 toes, all separate
5. Legs bowed
6. Major gluteal folds are even.
7. Creases on soles of feet
8. The newborn will be checked for fractures (especially clavicle) or dislocations (hip).
9. The newborn will be checked for developmental dysplasia of the hip; when the thighs are rotated outward, no clicks should be heard. (Ortolani's sign and Barlow's sign are two assessment tools that the HCP may use to assess for developmental dysplasia of hip.)
10. Pulses palpable (radial, brachial, and femoral)

Slight tremors in the newborn may be a common finding, but they could also be a sign of hypoglycemia or drug withdrawal.

III. Body Systems: Data Collection and Interventions

A. Cardiovascular system
1. Keep the newborn warm.
2. Take the apical heart rate for 1 full minute.
3. The HCP will listen for murmurs; check oxygen saturation via pulse oximetry if a murmur is heard.
4. Palpate pulses.
5. Check for cyanosis; blanch the skin on the trunk and extremities to check circulation.
6. Observe for cardiac distress when the newborn is feeding.

B. Respiratory system
1. Suction the airway as necessary. Use a bulb syringe for upper airway suctioning (compress bulb before insertion) and a French catheter for deeper suctioning.
2. Observe for respiratory distress and hypoxemia.
   a. Nasal flaring
   b. Increasingly severe retractions
   c. Grunting
   d. Cyanosis
   e. Bradycardia and periods of apnea that last more than 15 seconds
3. Administer oxygen via hood if necessary and as prescribed.

C. Hepatic system
1. Normal or physiological jaundice appears after the first 24 hours in full-term neonates and after the first 48 hours in premature neonates. Jaundice occurring before this time (pathological jaundice) may indicate the early hemolysis of red blood cells and must be reported to the HCP.
2. Physiological jaundice peaks about the fifth day of life (indirect bilirubin levels: 6 to 7 mg/dL).
3. Feed early to stimulate intestinal activity and to keep the bilirubin level low.
4. Prevent chilling, because hypothermia can cause acidosis, which interferes with bilirubin conjugation and excretion.
5. The newborn's liver stores iron that was passed from the mother for 5 to 6 months.
6. Glycogen storage occurs in the liver.

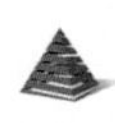

7. The **neonate** is at risk for hemorrhagic disorders. Coagulation factors synthesized in the liver are dependent on vitamin K, which is not synthesized until intestinal bacteria are present.
8. Handle the neonate carefully and monitor for any bruising or bleeding episodes.
9. Watch for meconium stool and subsequent stools.

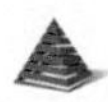

10. Intramuscular vitamin K will be prescribed for the neonate to prevent hemorrhagic disorders; administer in the lateral aspect of the middle third of the vastus lateralis muscle.
11. Check the newborn's hemoglobin and blood glucose levels per facility protocol.

D. Renal system
1. The immature kidneys cannot concentrate urine.
2. A weight loss of approximately 5% to 10% occurs as a result of water loss and limited intake; birth weight should be regained by 10 to 14 days after birth.
3. Weigh the newborn daily.
4. Monitor intake and output; weigh diapers if necessary (1 g of diaper weight equals 1 mL of urine).
5. If the diaper requires weighing, record the weight before putting it on the newborn; after the newborn voids, reweigh the diaper and subtract the prevoided weight.
6. Monitor for signs of dehydration (dry mucous membranes, sunken eyeballs, poor skin turgor, sunken fontanels).

E. Immune system
1. The newborn receives passive immunity via the **placenta** (immunoglobulin G).
2. The newborn receives passive immunity from the colostrum (immunoglobulin A).
3. Elevations in immunoglobulin M indicate infection in utero.
4. Use aseptic technique and standard precautions when caring for the newborn.
5. Ensure meticulous hand washing.
6. Ensure that infection-free staff members care for the newborn.
7. Monitor the newborn's temperature.
8. Observe for any cracks or openings in the skin.
9. Administer eye medication within 1 hour after birth to prevent ophthalmia neonatorum; agent used varies depending on agency protocols, but usually ophthalmic forms of erythromycin (0.5%) or tetracycline (1%) are prescribed because they are bacteriostatic and bactericidal and provide prophylaxis against *Neisseria gonorrhoeae* and *Chlamydia trachomatis*.
10. Provide cord care.
    a. Umbilical clamp can be removed after 24 hours if cord is dried and occluded and is not bleeding.
    b. Reinforce instructions to the mother how to perform cord care.
    c. Keep the cord clean and dry; soap and water may be prescribed for cleaning the cord.
    d. Keep the diaper from covering the cord; fold the diaper below the cord.
    e. Monitor the cord for odor, swelling, or discharge.
    f. The newborn is washed via a sponge bath until the cord falls off (within 2 weeks).

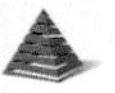

11. Provide circumcision care.
    a. Apply petroleum jelly gauze to the penis, except when a PlastiBell is used.
    b. Remove the petroleum jelly gauze, if applied, after the first voiding following the circumcision.
    c. Observe for swelling, infection, or bleeding from the circumcision site.
    d. Reinforce instructions to the mother how to care for the circumcision site.
    e. Clean the penis after each voiding by squeezing warm water over it.
    f. A milky covering over the glans penis is normal and should not be disrupted.
    g. Monitor for urinary retention.

F. Thermal regulatory system
1. Prevent cold stress (Fig. 29-3).
2. Newborns do not shiver to produce heat.
3. Newborns have brown fat deposits, which produce heat.
4. Prevent heat loss that results from evaporation by keeping the newborn dry and well wrapped with a blanket.
5. Prevent heat loss that results from radiation by keeping the newborn away from cold objects and outside walls.
6. Prevent heat loss that results from convection by shielding the newborn from drafts.

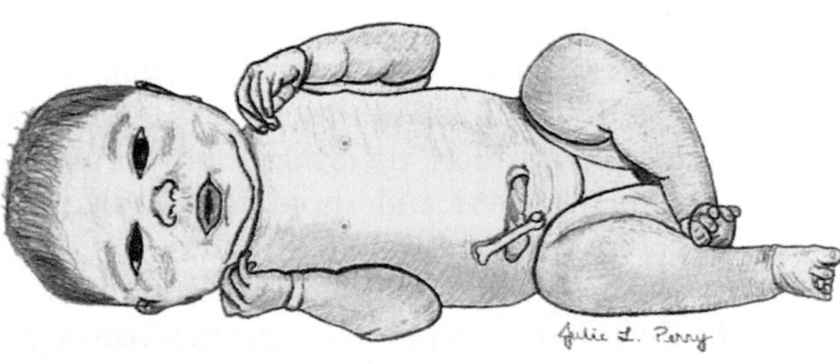

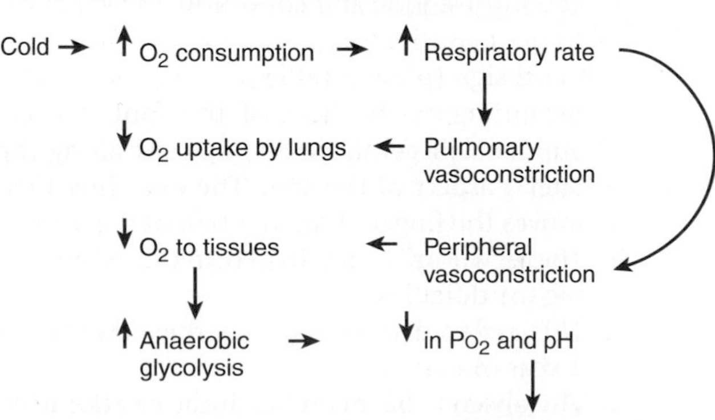

FIGURE 29-3 Effects of cold stress. When a newborn is stressed by cold, oxygen consumption increases, and pulmonary and peripheral vasoconstriction occur, decreasing oxygen uptake by the lungs and oxygen delivery to the tissues; anaerobic glycolysis increases; and there is a decrease in PO_2 and pH, leading to metabolic acidosis. (From Perry S, Hockenberry M, Lowdermilk D, Wilson D: *Maternal-child nursing care*, ed 4, St. Louis, 2010, Mosby.)

7. Prevent heat loss that results from conduction by performing all treatments on a warm, padded surface.
8. Keep the room temperature warm.
9. Take the newborn's axillary temperature every hour for the first 4 hours of life, every 4 hours for the remainder of the first 24 hours, and then every shift (as per agency protocol).

Cold stress causes oxygen consumption and energy to be diverted from maintaining normal brain cell function and cardiac function, resulting in serious metabolic and physiological conditions.

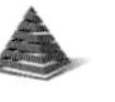

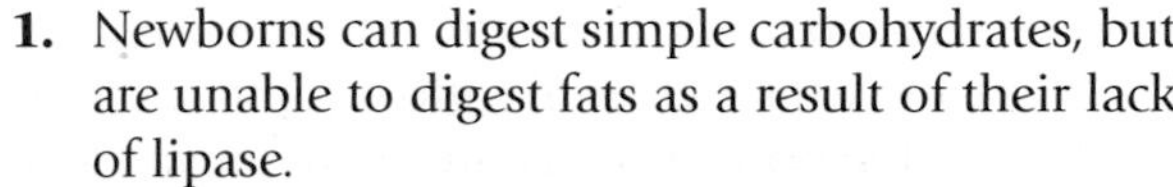

G. Metabolic system and gastrointestinal system
1. Newborns can digest simple carbohydrates, but are unable to digest fats as a result of their lack of lipase.
2. Proteins may be only partially broken down, so they may serve as antigens and provoke an allergic reaction.
3. The newborn has a small stomach capacity (about 90 mL) with rapid intestinal peristalsis (bowel emptying time is 2.5 to 3 hours).
4. Breastfeeding usually can begin immediately after birth; based on HCP preference and agency protocols, bottle-fed newborns may be initially offered no more than 30 mL of formula.

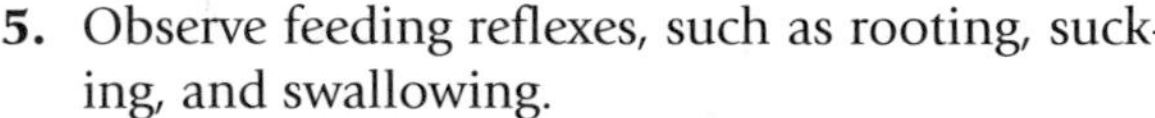

5. Observe feeding reflexes, such as rooting, sucking, and swallowing.
6. Assist the mother with breastfeeding or formula feeding; breastfeeding should be done every 2 to 3 hours, and formula feeding (minimum of 30 mL, or 1 oz) should be done every 3 to 4 hours (or per HCP preference or agency protocols).
7. Burp the newborn during and after feeding.
8. Monitor for regurgitation or vomiting.
9. Position the newborn on the right side after feeding; however, the side-lying position is not recommended for sleep because this position makes it easy for the newborn to roll to the prone position (prone position is contraindicated because the prone position increases the risk of sudden infant death syndrome).
10. Observe for normal stool and the passage of meconium.
    a. Meconium stool, which is greenish-black with a thick, sticky, tar-like consistency, is usually passed within the first 24 hours of life.
    b. Transitional stool, which is the second type of stool excreted by the newborn, is greenish-brown and of looser consistency than meconium.
    c. Seedy, yellow stools are usually noted in breastfed newborns; pale yellow to light brown stools are usually seen in formula-fed newborns.

11. Newborn: A screening test is performed (includes the test for phenylketonuria) before discharge after sufficient protein intake occurs. The newborn should be on formula or breast milk for a minimum of 24 hours before screening.

H. Neurological system
1. The newborn's head size is proportionally larger than that of adults as a result of cephalocaudal development.
2. Myelinization of the nerve fibers is incomplete, so primitive reflexes are present.
3. Fontanels are open to allow for brain growth.
4. Check for an abnormal head size and a bulging or depressed anterior fontanel.
5. Measure and graph the head circumference in relation to the chest circumference and length.
6. Check the newborn's movements, noting symmetry, posture, and abnormal movements.
7. Observe for jitteriness, marked tremors, and seizures.
8. The newborn's reflexes will be tested.
9. Check for lethargy.
10. Monitor the pitch of the cry. A high-shrill cry can indicate increased intracranial pressure.

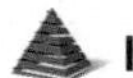
I. Reflexes
1. Sucking and rooting
   a. The newborn's lip, cheek, or the corner of the mouth is touched with a nipple.
   b. The newborn turns his or her head toward the nipple, opens the mouth, takes hold of the nipple, and sucks.
   c. The rooting reflex usually disappears after 3 to 4 months but may persist for up to 1 year.
2. Swallowing reflex
   a. Occurs spontaneously after sucking and obtaining fluids
   b. The newborn swallows in coordination with sucking without gagging, coughing, or vomiting.
3. Tonic neck or fencing position
   a. While the newborn is falling asleep or sleeping, the head is turned gently and quickly to one side.
   b. As the newborn faces the left side, the left arm and leg extend outward, while the right arm and leg flex.
   c. When the head is turned to the right side, the right arm and leg extend outward, while the left arm and leg flex.
   d. Usually disappears within 3 to 4 months
4. Palmar–plantar grasp
   a. The examiner's finger is placed in the palm of the newborn's hand, and then another finger is placed at the base of the toes.
   b. The newborn's fingers curl around the examiner's fingers, and the newborn's toes curl downward.
   c. Palmar response lessens within 3 to 4 months.
   d. Plantar response lessens within 8 months.
5. Moro reflex
   a. The newborn is held in a semi-sitting position, and then the head and trunk are allowed to fall backward to at least a 30-degree angle.
   b. The newborn assumes sharp extension and abduction of the arms with the thumbs and forefingers in a "C" position; this is followed by flexion and adduction to an "embrace" position (legs following a similar pattern).
   c. Present at birth and is absent by 6 months of age if neurological maturation is not delayed.
   d. A body jerk motion may be the response between 8 to 18 weeks.
   e. A persistent response lasting more than 6 months may indicate pregnancy neurological abnormality.
6. Startle reflex
   a. The response is best elicited if the newborn is at least 24 hours old.
   b. The examiner makes a loud noise or claps the hands to elicit the response.
   c. The newborn's arms adduct, while the elbows flex.
   d. The hands stay clenched.
   e. The reflex should disappear within 4 months.
7. Pull to sit response
   a. The newborn is pulled up from the wrist while he or she is in the flat position.
   b. The head will lag until the newborn is in an upright position; then the head will be level with the chest and shoulders momentarily before falling forward.
   c. The head will then lift for a few minutes.
   d. The response depends on the newborn's general muscle tone and condition, as well as his or her maturity level.
8. Babinski sign (plantar reflex)
   a. Beginning at the heel of the foot, the examiner will gently stroke upward along the lateral aspect of the sole. The examiner then moves the finger along the ball of the foot.
   b. The newborn's toes hyperextend, while the big toe dorsiflexes.
   c. This reflex disappears after the newborn is 1 year old.
   d. The absence of this reflex indicates the need for a neurological examination.
9. Stepping or walking
   a. The newborn is held in a vertical position, allowing one foot to touch a table surface.
   b. The newborn simulates walking, alternately flexing and extending the feet.
   c. The reflex is usually present for 3 to 4 months.

10. Crawling
   a. The newborn is placed on his or her abdomen.
   b. The newborn begins making crawling movements with the arms and legs.
   c. The reflex usually disappears after about 6 weeks.

IV. Newborn Safety

A. Newborn identification
   1. Information bracelets are applied to the mother and the newborn immediately after birth and before the mother and the newborn are separated; in addition, identification pictures of the newborn and footprints from the newborn may be obtained before the newborn leaves the mother's side in the **delivery** room. (Agency policies and protocols are always followed.)
   2. Identification bracelets include name, sex, date, time of birth, and identification numbers.
   3. Some agencies use identification bracelets that have radiofrequency transmitters that set off alarms if the newborn is removed from a certain area.
   4. Agencies also conduct unit- and hospital-wide drills to prevent newborn abductions.

B. Newborn abduction
   1. The mother is taught to check the identification of any person who comes to remove the baby from her room and is taught other precautions to prevent newborn abduction (nurses must be wearing photo identification or some other security badge) (Box 29-1).
   2. Closed-circuit televisions, code-alert bands, or computer monitoring systems may be used on some units.
   3. The newborn is wheeled in a bassinette rather than carried in a staff member's arms.

BOX 29-1 Precautions to Prevent Infant Abductions

All personnel must wear identification that is easily visible at all times.
Teach the parents to only allow hospital staff with proper identification to take their newborn from them.
Question anyone with a newborn near an exit or in an unusual part of the facility.
Never leave newborns unattended.
Teach the parents that the newborn must be observed at all times.
When the newborn is in the mother's room, position the crib away from the doorway.
Teach the parents home safety precautions: suggest that the parents do not place announcements in the paper or signs in their yard that may alert an abductor that a new baby is in the home.

V. Reinforce Parent Teaching

A. Formula feeding
   1. Teach sterilization techniques if the water supply is from an area where the purification process of the water is questionable.
   2. Remind the mother not to heat the bottle of formula in a microwave oven.
   3. Inform the mother that formula is a sufficient diet for the first 4 to 6 months.
   4. Assess the mother's ability to burp the newborn.

B. Breastfeeding
   1. Monitor the newborn's ability to properly attach to the mother's breast and suck (Fig. 29-4).
   2. Teach the mother about engorgement.
   3. Teach the mother how to pump her breasts and how to store breast milk properly.
   4. Inform the mother that breast milk is a sufficient diet for the first 4 to 6 months.
   5. Give the mother the phone numbers of local organizations that offer support to breastfeeding mothers.

C. Bathing
   1. Bathe the newborn in a warm room before feeding.
   2. Have all equipment for bathing available.
   3. Use a mild soap (not on the face).
   4. Proceed from the cleanest area to the dirtiest area.
   5. Clean the eyes from the inner canthus outward.
   6. Special care should be taken to clean under the folds of the neck, the underarms, groin, and genital area.
   7. Make bath time enjoyable for both the newborn and the mother.

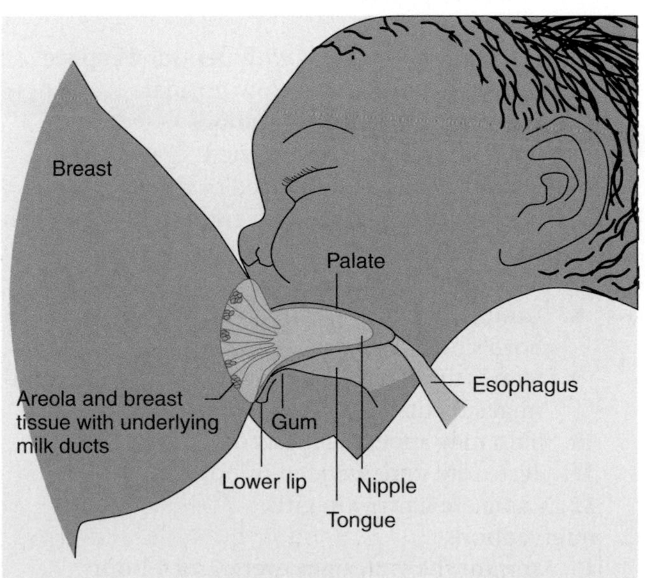

FIGURE 29-4 Correct attachment (latch-on) of an infant at the breast. (From Perry S, Hockenberry M, Lowdermilk D, Wilson D: *Maternal-child nursing care*, ed 4, St. Louis, 2010, Mosby.)

D. Clothing
 1. Assess diaper and clothing needs for the newborn with the mother.
 2. Instruct the mother that the newborn's head should be covered during cold weather to prevent heat loss.
 3. Instruct the mother to layer the newborn's clothing in cooler weather.
 4. To be comfortable, the newborn should be dressed in one more layer of clothing than what the parents are wearing.

E. Cord care: See II. Initial Physical Examination L. Abdomen

F. Circumcision: See earlier for circumcision care, "Body Systems: Data Collection and Interventions."

G. Uncircumcised newborn
 1. Inform the mother that the foreskin and glans are two similar layers of cells that separate from each other and that the separation process is normally complete by 3 years of age but can remain adhered until puberty.
 2. Instruct the mother not to pull back the foreskin but rather to allow for the natural separation to occur.
 3. Inform the mother that, as the process of separation occurs, sterile sloughed cells build up between the layers of the foreskin and the glans. When retraction occurs, daily gentle washing of the glans with soap and water is sufficient to maintain adequate cleanliness.

VI. Preterm Newborn

A. Description
 1. An **infant** born before 37 weeks' gestation
 2. The primary concern relates to the immaturity of all body systems.

B. Data collection
 1. Respirations irregular with periods of apnea
 2. Body temperature is below normal.
 3. Poor suck and swallow reflexes
 4. Bowel sounds are diminished.
 5. Urinary output is increased or decreased.
 6. Extremities are thin, with minimal creasing on the soles and palms.
 7. Extremities extend but do not maintain flexion.
 8. Lanugo, on the skin and in the hair on the newborn's head, is present in woolly patches.
 9. Skin is thin, with visible blood vessels and minimal subcutaneous fat pads.
 10. Skin may appear jaundiced.
 11. Testes are undescended in boys.
 12. Labia are narrow in girls.

C. Interventions
 1. Monitor the vital signs every 2 to 4 hours.
 2. Maintain airway and cardiopulmonary function.
 3. Administer oxygen and humidification, as prescribed.
 4. Monitor intake and output and electrolyte balance.
 5. Monitor the weight daily.
 6. Maintain the newborn in a warming device.
 7. Avoid exposing the newborn to infections.
 8. Provide the newborn with appropriate stimulation, such as touch and cuddling.

VII. Postterm Newborn

A. Description: An infant born after 42 weeks'

B. Data collection
 1. Hypoglycemia
 2. Parchment-like skin (dry and cracked) without lanugo
 3. Fingernails long, extended over the ends of the fingers
 4. Profuse scalp hair
 5. Long and thin body
 6. Extremities show wasting of fat and muscle.
 7. Meconium staining may be present on nails and umbilical cord.

C. Interventions
 1. Provide normal newborn care, including stimulation such as touching and cuddling.
 2. Monitor for hypoglycemia.
 3. Maintain newborn's temperature.
 4. Monitor for meconium aspiration.

VIII. Small for Gestational Age

A. Description: A neonate who is plotted at or below the 10th percentile on the intrauterine growth curve

B. Data collection
 1. Fetal distress
 2. Decreased or elevated body temperature
 3. Physical abnormalities
 4. Hypoglycemia
 5. Signs of polycythemia: ruddy appearance, cyanosis, jaundice
 6. Signs of infection
 7. Signs of meconium aspiration

C. Interventions
 1. Maintain airway and cardiopulmonary function; observe for signs of respiratory distress.
 2. Maintain body temperature.
 3. Monitor for infection; initiate measures to prevent sepsis.
 4. Monitor the blood glucose levels and for signs of hypoglycemia.
 5. Initiate early feedings. Monitor for signs of aspiration.
 6. Provide stimulation, such as touch and cuddling.

IX. Large for Gestational Age

A. Description: A neonate who is plotted at or above the 90th percentile on the intrauterine growth curve

Maternity

B. Data collection
1. Respiratory distress
2. Birth trauma or injury
3. Hypoglycemia

C. Interventions
1. Maintain airway; observe for signs of respiratory distress.
2. Monitor the blood glucose levels and for signs of hypoglycemia.
3. Initiate early feedings.
4. Monitor for infection; initiate measures to prevent sepsis.
5. Provide stimulation, such as touch and cuddling.

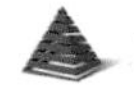

X. Respiratory Distress Syndrome

A. Description: A serious lung disorder caused by immaturity and the inability to produce **surfactant**, resulting in hypoxia and acidosis

B. Data collection
1. Respiratory distress; can include tachypnea, nasal flaring, expiratory grunting, retractions, seesaw respirations, decreased breath sounds, apnea
2. Pallor and cyanosis
3. Hypothermia
4. Poor muscle tone

C. Interventions
1. Monitor color, respiratory rate, and degree of effort in breathing.
2. Maintain airway and cardiopulmonary function and support respirations as prescribed.
3. Monitor the arterial blood gases (ABGs) and the oxygen saturation levels (ABGs from umbilical artery) as prescribed.
4. Monitor the ABGs so that oxygen administered to the newborn is at the lowest possible concentration necessary to maintain adequate arterial oxygenation.
5. Any premature newborn who required oxygen support should be scheduled for an eye examination before discharge to assess for retinal damage.
6. Suction every 2 hours or more often, as necessary.
7. As prescribed, position the newborn on his or her side or back, with the neck slightly extended.
8. Administer respiratory therapy (percussion and vibration), as prescribed. Use a padded small plastic cup or a small oxygen mask for percussion. Use a padded electric toothbrush for vibration.
9. Provide nutrition.
10. Support bonding.
11. Prepare parents for a short- to long-term period of oxygen dependency, if necessary.
12. Encourage the mother to pump her breasts for future breastfeeding, if she so desires.
13. Encourage as much parental participation in the newborn's care as the condition allows.

⚠ Prepare to assist to administer surfactant replacement (instilled into endotracheal tube) to a newborn with respiratory distress syndrome.

XI. Meconium Aspiration Syndrome

A. Description
1. Occurs in term or postterm infants
2. Exact etiology is unknown, but the release of meconium into the **amniotic fluid** is thought to be related to a stressful fetal event initiating a biochemical chain of events.
3. Aspiration can occur in utero or with the first breath.

B. Data collection
1. Respiratory distress is present at birth. Tachypnea, cyanosis, retractions, nasal flaring, grunting, crackles, and rhonchi may be present.
2. The newborn's nails, skin, and umbilical cord may be stained a yellow-green color.

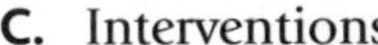

C. Interventions
1. Suctioning must be done immediately after the head is delivered before the first breath is taken; vocal cords should be viewed to see if the airway is clear before stimulation and crying.
2. Newborns with severe meconium aspiration syndrome may benefit from extracorporeal membrane oxygenation; this therapy uses a modified heart-lung machine and provides oxygen to the circulation, allowing the lungs to rest and decreasing pulmonary hypertension and hypoxemia in some conditions, such as meconium aspiration.

XII. Bronchopulmonary Dysplasia

A. Description
1. A chronic pulmonary condition that affects newborns who have experienced respiratory failure or who have been oxygen dependent for more than 28 days
2. X-ray findings are abnormal, indicating areas of overinflation and atelectasis.

B. Data collection
1. Tachypnea and tachycardia
2. Retractions, nasal flaring, and labored breathing
3. Crackles, decreased air movement, and occasional expiratory wheezing

C. Interventions
1. Monitor airway and cardiopulmonary status and provide oxygen as prescribed.
2. Medications may include surfactant, diuretics, corticosteroids, and bronchodilators.

XIII. Transient Tachypnea of the Newborn

A. Description
1. Respiratory condition that results from the incomplete reabsorption of the fetal lung fluid in full-term infants
2. Usually disappears within 24 to 48 hours

B. Data collection
   1. Tachypnea
   2. Nasal flaring, expiratory grunting, and retractions
   3. Fluid breath sounds heard during auscultation
   4. Cyanosis

C. Interventions
   1. Supportive care (based on manifestations)
   2. Oxygen is administered as prescribed

XIV. Intraventricular Hemorrhage

A. Description
   1. Bleeding within the ventricles of the brain
   2. Risk factors include prematurity, respiratory distress syndrome, trauma, or asphyxia.

B. Data collection
   1. Diminished or absent Moro reflex, lethargy, apnea, poor feeding, high-pitched and shrill cry, and seizure activity

C. Interventions: Treatment is supportive.

XV. Retinopathy of Prematurity

A. Description
   1. A vascular disorder that involves the gradual replacement of the retina by fibrous tissue and blood vessels.
   2. Primarily caused by prematurity and the use of supplemental oxygen in the newborn for more than 30 days

B. Data collection: Leukcoria (white tissue on the retrolental space), vitreous hemorrhage, myopia, strabismus, and cataracts (check for red reflex)

C. Interventions: Laser photocoagulation surgery

XVI. Necrotizing Enterocolitis

A. Description
   1. An acute inflammatory disease of the gastrointestinal tract
   2. Usually occurs 4 to 10 days after birth, and is most frequently seen in preterm newborns

B. Data collection: Increased abdominal girth, decreased or absent bowel sounds, bowel loop distension, vomiting, bile-stained emesis, abdominal tenderness, and occult blood in the stools

C. Interventions
   1. Oral feedings are held and a gastric tube is used to decompress the abdomen.
   2. Intravenous antibiotics and intravenous fluids may be prescribed.
   3. Surgery may be indicated.

XVII. Hyperbilirubinemia

A. Description
   1. Elevated serum bilirubin level
   2. Evaluation is indicated when serum bilirubin levels are more than 12 mg/dL in the term newborn.
   3. Therapy is aimed at preventing kernicterus, which results in permanent neurological damage as a result of the deposition of bilirubin in the brain cells.

B. Data collection
   1. Jaundice
   2. Elevated serum bilirubin levels
   3. Enlarged liver
   4. Poor muscle tone
   5. Lethargy
   6. Poor sucking reflex

C. Interventions
   1. Monitor for the presence of jaundice; assess skin and sclera for jaundice.
      a. Examine the newborn's skin color in natural light.
      b. Press a finger over a bony prominence or the tip of the newborn's nose to press out capillary blood from the tissues.
      c. Note that jaundice starts at the head first and then spreads to the chest, the abdomen, the arms and legs, and the hands and feet, which are the last to be jaundiced.
   2. Keep the newborn well hydrated to maintain blood volume.
   3. Facilitate early, frequent feeding to hasten the passage of meconium and to encourage the excretion of bilirubin.
   4. Report any signs of jaundice that presents during the first 24 hours and any abnormal signs and symptoms to the registered nurse and HCP.
   5. Prepare for phototherapy, and monitor the newborn closely during the treatment.

At any serum bilirubin level, the appearance of jaundice during the first day of life indicates a pathological process.

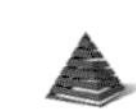

D. Phototherapy
   1. Description
      a. Use of light to reduce serum bilirubin levels in the newborn
      b. Injury from treatment (e.g., eye damage, dehydration, sensory deprivation) can occur.
   2. Interventions
      a. Expose as much of the newborn's skin as possible.
      b. Cover the genital area, and monitor the genital area for skin irritation or breakdown.
      c. Cover the newborn's eyes with shields or patches; make sure the eyelids are closed when shields or patches are applied.
      d. Remove the shields or patches at least once per shift (during a feeding) to inspect the eyes for infection or irritation and to allow for eye contact and bonding with the parents.

e. Measure the lamp energy output to ensure efficacy of the treatment (done with a special device known as a photometer).
f. Monitor the skin temperature closely.
g. Increase fluids to compensate for water loss.
h. Expect loose green stools.
i. Monitor the newborn's skin color with the light turned off every 4 to 8 hours.
j. Monitor the skin for bronze baby syndrome, which is a grayish-brown discoloration of the skin; notify the registered nurse and HCP because this may indicate a complication of phototherapy.
k. Reposition the newborn every 2 hours; monitor the newborn closely.
l. Provide stimulation
m. After treatment, continue monitoring for signs of hyperbilirubinemia, because rebound elevations can occur after therapy is discontinued.
n. Turn off phototherapy lights before drawing a blood specimen for serum bilirubin levels and do not leave blood specimen uncovered under the lights (to prevent breakdown of bilirubin in blood specimen).

XVIII. Erythroblastosis Fetalis

A. Description
1. Destruction of the red blood cells that result from an antigen–antibody reaction.
2. Characterized by hemolytic anemia or hyperbilirubinemia
3. Exchange of fetal and maternal blood takes place primarily when the placenta separates at birth (Fig. 29-5).
4. Antibodies are harmless to the mother but attach to the erythrocytes in the fetus and cause hemolysis.
5. Sensitization is rare with the first pregnancy.
6. ABO incompatibility is usually less severe.

B. Data collection
1. Anemia
2. Jaundice that develops rapidly after birth and before 24 hours
3. Edema

C. Interventions
1. $Rh_o(D)$ immune globulin (RhoGAM) is administered to the mother during the first 72 hours after delivery if the Rh-negative mother delivers an Rh-positive fetus but remains unsensitized.
2. Assist with exchange transfusion after birth or intrauterine transfusion, as prescribed.
3. The newborn's blood is replaced with Rh-negative blood to stop the destruction of the baby's red blood cells. The Rh-negative blood is gradually replaced with the baby's own blood.
4. Reassure the mother that the newborn will experience no untoward effects as a result of the condition.

XIX. Sepsis

A. Description: Generalized infection resulting from the presence of bacteria in the blood, such as Group B *Streptococcus* infection

B. Data Collection
1. Pallor
2. Tachypnea, tachycardia
3. Poor feeding
4. Abdominal distention
5. Temperature instability

C. Interventions
1. Monitor for periods of apnea or irregular respirations.
2. If apnea is present, stimulate by gently rubbing the chest or foot.
3. Administer oxygen as prescribed.
4. Monitor vital signs; check for fever.

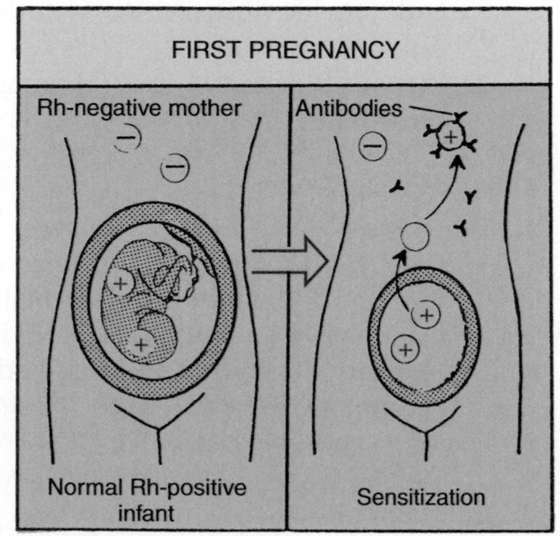

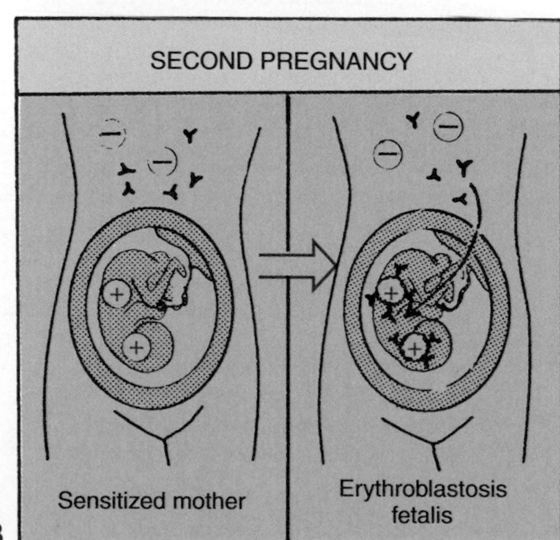

FIGURE 29-5 Development of maternal sensitization to Rh antigens. **A,** Fetal Rh-positive erythrocytes enter the maternal system. Maternal anti-Rh antibodies are formed. **B,** Anti-Rh antibodies cross placenta and attack fetal erythrocytes. (Modified from Seeley RR, Stephens TD, Tate P: *Anatomy and physiology*, ed 3, St. Louis, 1995, Mosby.)

5. Maintain warmth in a radiant warmer.
6. Provide isolation as necessary.
7. Monitor intake and output, and obtain daily weight.
8. Monitor for diarrhea.
9. Check feeding and sucking reflex, which may be poor.
10. Monitor for jaundice.
11. Observe for irritability and lethargy.
12. Assist to administer antibiotics as prescribed, and observe carefully for toxicity because a newborn's liver and kidneys are immature.

XX. TORCH Syndrome

A. Description (Table 29-5)
1. TORCH infections are infections that occur in the fetus or newborn
2. Caused by one of the following:
   a. Toxoplasmosis
   b. Other infections
   c. Rubella
   d. Cytomegalovirus
   e. Herpes simplex virus

TABLE 29-5 Infections Included in TORCH Syndrome

Infection	Characteristics and Description
Toxoplasmosis	Caused by protozoan infection Produces no serious effects in mother Organism can be transmitted to fetus Infection can result in severe physical, developmental abnormalities Common carriers include cat feces, raw beef
Other infections	Can include syphilis, gonorrhea, varicella, hepatitis B, HIV, human parvovirus B19
Rubella	Systemic viral infection Rubella causes congenital rubella syndrome—includes congenital heart disease, cataracts, growth retardation, and pneumonia if mother becomes infected within first trimester Deafness and some learning disabilities can occur if mother becomes infected during first trimester
Cytomegalovirus	Viral infection that persists in the body indefinitely; has periods of reactivation without symptoms Can infect fetus or newborn during delivery or after birth through breast milk, blood transfusions, or contact with infected secretions May cause microcephaly, blindness, deafness, mental and motor retardation
Herpes simplex virus	Sexually transmitted infection Has periods of reactivation Newborn commonly infected during delivery by direct contact with lesions in genital tract Can cause neurological impairment or death

HIV, Human immunodeficiency virus.

XXI. Syphilis

A. Description
1. Sexually transmitted infection
2. Congenital syphilis can result in premature delivery, skin lesions, and abnormal skeletal development.
3. The organism *Treponema pallidum*, a spirochete, can cross the placenta throughout pregnancy and infect the fetus, usually after 18 weeks' gestation.
4. Risks include preterm birth, stillbirth, and low birth weight.
5. Congenital effects are irreversible and may include central nervous system damage and hearing loss.

B. Data collection
1. Hepatosplenomegaly
2. Joint swelling
3. Palmar rash and lesions
4. Anemia
5. Jaundice
6. Snuffles
7. Ascites
8. Pneumonitis
9. Cerebrospinal fluid changes

C. Interventions
1. Monitor the newborn for signs of syphilis.
2. Prepare the newborn for serological testing, if prescribed.
3. Assist to administer antibiotic therapy, as prescribed.
4. Use standard precautions and drainage and secretion (contact) precautions with suspected congenital syphilis.
5. Wear gloves when handling the neonate until antibiotic therapy has been administered for 24 hours.

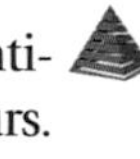

6. Provide psychological support to the mother, and provide instructions regarding follow-up care of the newborn.
7. Refer to Chapter 26 for additional information on syphilis.

XXII. Addicted Newborn

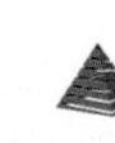

A. Description

1. A newborn who has become passively addicted to drugs that have passed through the placenta
2. Data collection findings and withdrawal times may vary, depending on specific addicting drugs.

3. See also XXIII. Fetal Alcohol Syndrome

B. Data collection

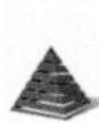

1. Irritability
2. Tremors
3. Hyperactivity and hypertonicity
4. Respiratory distress

5. Vomiting
6. High-pitched cry
7. Sneezing
8. Fever
9. Diarrhea
10. Excessive sweating
11. Poor feeding
12. Extreme sucking of fists
13. Seizures

C. Interventions
1. Monitor the respiratory and cardiac status frequently.
2. Monitor vital signs.
3. Hold the newborn firm and close to the body during feeding and when giving care. Swaddle the newborn.
4. Initiate seizure precautions (pad the sides of the crib).
5. Provide small frequent feedings and allow a longer period for feeding.
6. Monitor intake and output.
7. Assist with administering intravenous hydration, as prescribed.
8. Protect the neonate's skin from injury, which can be caused by constant rubbing from hyperactive jitters.
9. Place the newborn in a quiet room and reduce stimulation.
10. Allow the mother to express feelings such as anxiety and guilt.
11. Refer the mother for treatment of her substance abuse problem.

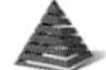

XXIII. Fetal Alcohol Syndrome

A. Description
1. Caused by maternal alcohol use during pregnancy
2. Most serious cause of teratogenesis
3. Causes mental and physical retardation

B. Data collection
1. Facial changes
   a. Short palpebral fissures
   b. Hypoplastic philtrum
   c. Short, upturned nose
   d. Flat midface
   e. Thin upper lip
   f. Low nasal bridge
2. Abnormal palmar creases
3. Respiratory distress (apnea, cyanosis)
4. Congenital heart disorders
5. Irritability and hypersensitivity to stimuli
6. Tremors
7. Poor feeding
8. Seizures

C. Interventions
1. Monitor for respiratory distress.
2. Position the newborn on the side to facilitate drainage of secretions; have a nasal aspirator or suction available.
3. Keep resuscitation equipment at the bedside.
4. Monitor for hypoglycemia.
5. Check the suck and swallow reflex.
6. Administer small feedings and burp the newborn well.
7. Suction as necessary.
8. Monitor intake and output.
9. Monitor the weight and head circumference.
10. Decrease environmental stimuli.

XXIV. Newborn of a Mother with Human Immunodeficiency Virus (HIV)

A. Description
1. The fetus of a mother who is positive for HIV antibody should be monitored closely throughout the pregnancy.
2. Serial ultrasound screenings should be done during pregnancy to identify intrauterine growth restriction.
3. Weekly nonstress testing after 32 weeks of gestation and biophysical profiles may be necessary during pregnancy.
4. Neonates born to HIV-positive clients may test positive because the mother's positive antibodies may persist for as long as 18 months after birth.
5. The use of antiviral medication, the reduction of neonate exposure to maternal blood and body fluids, and the early identification of HIV during pregnancy reduce the risk of transmission to the newborn.
6. All neonates born to HIV-positive mothers acquire maternal antibody to HIV infection, but not all acquire the infection.
7. The neonate may be asymptomatic for the first several years of life.

B. Transmission
1. Across placental barrier
2. During **labor** and **delivery**
3. Via breast milk; breastfeeding usually is not allowed if the mother is HIV-positive, unless specifically recommended and prescribed.

C. Data collection
1. Possibly no outward signs at birth
2. Signs of immunodeficiency
3. Hepatomegaly
4. Splenomegaly
5. Lymphadenopathy
6. Impairment in growth and development

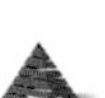

D. Interventions
1. Cleanse the newborn's skin carefully before any invasive procedure, such as the administration of vitamin K, heel sticks, or venipunctures.

2. Circumcisions are not done on newborns with HIV-positive mothers until the newborn's status is determined.
3. Newborn can room with mother.
4. All HIV-exposed newborns should be treated with medication to prevent infection by *Pneumocystis jiroveci*.
5. Antiretroviral medication may be administered for the first 6 weeks of life or longer, if prescribed.
6. Monitor for early signs of immunodeficiency, such as enlarged spleen or liver, lymphadenopathy, and impairment in growth and development.
7. Newborns at risk for HIV infection should be seen by the HCP at birth and at 1 week, 2 weeks, 1 month, and 2 months of life.
8. Inform the mother that an HIV culture is recommended at the ages of 1 month and 4 months.

E. Immunizations
1. Immunizations with live vaccines, such as measles–mumps–rubella, should not be done until the newborn's, infant's, or child's HIV status is confirmed.
2. If infected, live vaccine will not be given.

Newborns at risk for HIV infection need to receive all recommended immunizations according to the regular schedule; live vaccines are not administered until HIV status is determined.

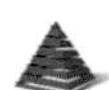

XXV. Newborn of a Diabetic Mother

A. Description
1. A neonate born to a mother with insulin-dependent diabetes or gestational diabetes
2. Hypoglycemia, hyperbilirubinemia, respiratory distress syndrome, hypocalcemia, birth trauma, and congenital anomalies may be present.

B. Data collection
1. Excessive size and weight as a result of excess fat and glycogen in tissues
2. Edema or puffiness in the face and cheeks
3. Signs of hypoglycemia, such as twitching, difficulty feeding, lethargy, apnea, seizures, and cyanosis
4. Hyperbilirubinemia
5. Signs of respiratory distress, such as tachypnea, cyanosis, retractions, grunting, and nasal flaring

C. Interventions
1. Monitor for signs of respiratory distress, birth trauma, and congenital anomalies.
2. Monitor the bilirubin and blood glucose levels.
3. Monitor the weight.
4. Feed the newborn soon after birth with glucose in water, breast milk, or formula, as prescribed.
5. Prepare to assist in administering intravenous glucose to treat hypoglycemia, if necessary and as prescribed.
6. Monitor for edema.
7. Monitor for apnea, tremors, and seizures.

XXVI. Hypoglycemia

A. Description
1. Abnormally low levels of glucose in the blood (<40 mg/dL during the first 72 hours or <45 mg/dL after the first 3 days of life)
2. Normal blood glucose level is 40 to 60 mg/dL in a 1-day-old newborn and 50 to 90 mg/dL in a newborn who is older than 1 day old.

B. Data collection
1. Increased respiratory rate
2. Twitching, nervousness, tremors, or poor muscle tone
3. Unstable temperature
4. Lethargy, apnea, seizures, or cyanosis

C. Interventions
1. Prevent low blood glucose through early feedings.
2. Administer formula orally or assist to administer glucose intravenously, as prescribed.
3. Monitor the blood glucose levels, as prescribed.
4. Monitor for feeding problems.
5. Monitor for apneic periods.
6. Monitor for shrill or intermittent cries.
7. Evaluate lethargy and poor muscle tone.

XXVII. Hypothyroidism

A. Description: Hypothyroidism is a decrease in the production of thyroid hormone.

B. Assessment
1. Protruding or thick tongue
2. Dull look
3. Swollen face
4. Decreased muscle tone

C. Interventions: Focus on thyroid replacement

CRITICAL THINKING What Should You Do?

Answer: Slight tremors noted in the newborn may be a common finding but could also be a sign of hypoglycemia, hypocalcemia, or drug withdrawal. The nurse should notify the registered nurse immediately. Determination of the cause of the tremors is necessary so that treatment can be initiated immediately. This finding should also be immediately reported to the health care provider.

Reference(s): Hockenberry, M., & Wilson, D. (2013). *Wong's: Essentials of pediatric nursing* (9th ed., p. 289). St. Louis: Mosby.

McKinney, E., James, S., Murray, S., Nelson, K. & Ashwill, J. (2013). *Maternal-child nursing* (4th ed., pp. 493–494). St. Louis: Elsevier.

PRACTICE QUESTIONS

271. The nurse administers erythromycin ointment (0.5%) to the newborn's eyes, and the mother asks the nurse why this is done. The nurse should give which response to the client?
1. Prevents cataracts in the neonate born to a woman who is susceptible to rubella
2. Protects the neonate's eyes from possible infections acquired while hospitalized
3. Minimizes the spread of microorganisms to the neonate from invasive procedures during labor
4. Prevents ophthalmia neonatorum from occurring after delivery to a neonate born to a woman with an untreated gonococcal infection

272. A client asks the nurse why her newborn baby needs an injection of vitamin K. The nurse should make which statement to the client?
1. "Your newborn needs vitamin K to develop immunity."
2. "The vitamin K will protect your newborn from becoming jaundiced."
3. "Newborns are deficient in vitamin K. This injection prevents your baby from abnormal bleeding."
4. "Newborns have sterile bowels. The vitamin K will colonize the bowel with the necessary bacteria."

273. The nurse is assigned to assist with caring for a neonate born to a mother who is human immunodeficiency virus (HIV)-positive. The nurse understands that which should be included in the plan of care?
1. Monitoring the neonate's vital signs routinely
2. Maintaining standard precautions at all times while caring for the neonate
3. Instructing breastfeeding mothers regarding the treatment of their nipples with an antifungal cream
4. Initiating a referral to evaluate for blindness, deafness, learning, or behavioral problems in the neonate

274. The nurse in the newborn nursery receives a telephone call to prepare for the admission of a neonate born at 43 weeks' gestation with Apgar scores of 1 and 4. When planning for the admission of this infant which is the nurse's **highest priority**?
1. Turning on the apnea and cardiorespiratory monitor
2. Connecting the resuscitation bag to the oxygen outlet
3. Setting up the intravenous line with 5% dextrose in water
4. Setting the radiant warmer control temperature at 36.5°C (97.6°F)

275. The nurse is assisting in caring for a postterm neonate immediately after admission to the nursery. The **priority** nursing action should be to monitor which?
1. Urinary output
2. Blood glucose levels
3. Total bilirubin levels
4. Hemoglobin and hematocrit level

276. The nurse is reinforcing instructions to a new mother about cord care and how to monitor for infection. The nurse should tell the mother that which is a sign of infection?
1. A darkened drying stump
2. A moist cord with discharge
3. A purple stump that shows pinkness around the base
4. A purple stump that shows some moistness at the base

277. The nurse is reinforcing measures regarding the care of the newborn with a mother. To bathe the newborn, the mother should be taught which intervention?
1. Begin with the eyes and face.
2. Start with the dirtiest area first.
3. Begin with the feet and work upward.
4. Only wash the diaper area, because this is the only part of the baby that gets soiled.

278. After birth the nurse prevents hypothermia as a result of evaporation by performing which action?
1. Warming the crib pad
2. Closing the doors of the room
3. Drying the baby with a warm blanket
4. Turning on the overhead radiant warmer

❖ **279.** The nurse is preparing to care for a newborn who is receiving phototherapy. Which measures should be implemented? **Select all that apply.**
- ❑ 1. Avoid stimulation.
- ❑ 2. Decrease fluid intake.
- ❑ 3. Expose all of the newborn's skin.
- ❑ 4. Monitor the skin temperature closely.
- ❑ 5. Reposition the newborn every 2 hours.
- ❑ 6. Cover the newborn's eyes with shields or patches.

280. A newborn has just been circumcised. Which describes how the nurse should expect the surgical site to appear?
1. Pink, without drainage
2. Reddened, with a small amount of bloody drainage
3. Reddened, with a small amount of yellow exudate on the glans
4. Reddened, with a large amount of bloody drainage that requires a dressing change every 30 minutes

281. The nurse should monitor for which signs associated with respiratory distress syndrome (RDS) in a preterm newborn?

1. Tachypnea and retractions
2. Acrocyanosis and grunting
3. Hypotension and bradycardia
4. The presence of a barrel chest with acrocyanosis

282. The nurse notes hypotonia, irritability, and a poor sucking reflex in a full-term newborn after admission to the nursery. The nurse suspects fetal alcohol syndrome (FAS) and is aware that which additional sign is consistent with FAS?

1. A length of 19 inches
2. Abnormal palmar creases
3. A birth weight of 6 pounds and 14 ounces
4. A head circumference that is appropriate for gestational age

283. A pregnant human immunodeficiency virus (HIV)-positive woman delivers a baby. The nurse provides guidance to help the client make decisions regarding newborn care. Which statement by the woman indicates that **additional guidance is needed**?

1. "I will be sure to wash my hands before feeding the newborn."
2. "I will breastfeed, especially for the first 6 weeks postpartum."
3. "I will be sure to wash my hands before and after bathroom use."
4. "I will administer the prescribed antiviral medication to the newborn for the first 6 weeks after delivery."

284. A pregnant woman has a positive history of genital herpes, but she has not had lesions during her pregnancy. The nurse plans to provide which information to the client?

1. "You will be isolated from your newborn after delivery."
2. "There is little risk to your baby during your pregnancy, birth, and after delivery."
3. "Vaginal deliveries can reduce neonatal infection risks, even if you have an active lesion at birth."
4. "You will be evaluated at the time of delivery for herpetic genital tract lesions. If they are present, a cesarean delivery will be needed."

285. The nurse is planning to reinforce instructions about cord care to a new mother. The nurse should plan to tell the mother which about cord care?

1. Alcohol is the only agent used to clean the cord.
2. It takes 21 days for the cord to dry up and fall off.
3. Cord care is done only at birth to control bleeding.
4. The process of keeping the cord clean and dry will decrease bacterial growth.

ANSWERS

271. 4

Rationale: Erythromycin ophthalmic ointment 0.5% is used as a prophylactic treatment for ophthalmia neonatorum, which is caused by the bacteria *Neisseria gonorrhoeae*. The preventive treatment of gonorrhea is required by law. Options 1, 2, and 3 are not the purposes of administering this medication to the newborn.

Test-Taking Strategy: Focus on the subject, the purpose of administering erythromycin ophthalmic ointment to the newborn. Remember that erythromycin ophthalmic ointment 0.5% is used as a prophylactic treatment of ophthalmia neonatorum in newborns. **Review:** the initial care of the newborn.

Level of Cognitive Ability: Applying
Client Needs: Safe and Effective Care Environment
Integrated Process: Nursing Process/Implementation
Content Area: Maternity: Newborn
Priority Concepts: Infection, Safety
Reference(s): McKinney et al (2013), pp. 509–510.

272. 3

Rationale: Vitamin K is necessary for the body to synthesize coagulation factors, and it is administered to the newborn infant to prevent abnormal bleeding. It promotes the liver's formation of the clotting factors II, VII, IX, and X. Newborn infants are deficient in vitamin K because the bowel does not have the bacteria necessary for synthesizing this fat-soluble vitamin. The normal flora in the intestinal tract produces vitamin K, but the newborn's bowel does not support the normal production of vitamin K until bacteria have adequately colonized it. The bowel becomes colonized by bacteria as food is ingested. Vitamin K does not promote the development of immunity or prevent the infant from becoming jaundiced.

Test-Taking Strategy: Focus on the subject, the purpose of administering vitamin K to a newborn. Because jaundice and immunity are not related to the action of vitamin K, eliminate options 1 and 2. From the remaining options, recall the action of vitamin K to direct you to option 3. **Review:** the purpose of vitamin K injection.

Level of Cognitive Ability: Applying
Client Needs: Physiological Integrity
Integrated Process: Nursing Process/Implementation
Content Area: Maternity: Newborn
Priority Concepts: Clotting, Immunity
Reference(s): McKinney et al (2013), pp. 509–510.

273. 2

Rationale: The neonate born to a mother who is HIV-positive must be cared for with strict attention to standard precautions. This prevents the transmission of the infection from the neonate, if he or she is infected, to others, and it prevents the

transmission of other infectious agents to the possibly immunocompromised neonate. The mother should not breastfeed, unless the health care provider has specific recommendations about doing so. Options 1 and 4 are not specifically associated with the care of a potentially AIDS-infected neonate.
Test-Taking Strategy: Focus on the subject, the care of a neonate infant born to a woman who is HIV-positive. Eliminate options 1 and 4 first because they are not specifically associated with the care of a potentially infected neonate. Recalling that mothers who are HIV-positive should not breastfeed will direct you to the correct option. **Review:** the care of a neonate born to a woman who is human immunodeficiency virus positive.
Level of Cognitive Ability: Analyzing
Client Needs: Safe and Effective Care Environment
Integrated Process: Nursing Process/Planning
Content Area: Maternity: Newborn
Priority Concepts: Infection, Safety
Reference(s): Hockenberry, Wilson (2013), p. 897.

274. 2
Rationale: The highest priority during the admission to the nursery of a newborn with low Apgar scores is airway support, which would involve preparing respiratory resuscitation equipment. The remaining options are also important, although they are of lower initial priority. The newborn infant will be placed on a cardiorespiratory monitor. Setting up an intravenous line with 5% dextrose in water would provide circulatory support and may be prescribed. The radiant warmer will provide an external heat source, which is necessary to prevent further respiratory distress.
Test-Taking Strategy: Note the strategic words, *highest priority.* This question asks you to prioritize care on the basis of information about a newborn's condition. Use the ABCs—airway, breathing, and circulation. A method of planning for airway support is to have the resuscitation bag connected to an oxygen source. **Review:** the care of the newborn infant with low Apgar scores.
Level of Cognitive Ability: Analyzing
Client Needs: Physiological Integrity
Integrated Process: Nursing Process/Planning
Content Area: Critical Care: Basic Life Support/Cardiopulmonary Resuscitation
Priority Concepts: Gas Exchange, Perfusion
Reference(s): Hockenberry, Wilson (2013), p. 189.

275. 2
Rationale: The most common metabolic complication in the postterm newborn is hypoglycemia, which can produce central nervous system abnormalities and mental retardation if it is not corrected immediately. Urinary output, although important, is not the highest priority action. The polycythemia contributes to increased bilirubin levels, usually beginning on the second day after delivery. Hemoglobin and hematocrit levels are monitored, because the postterm neonate may exhibit polycythemia; however, this also does not require immediate attention.
Test-Taking Strategy: Note the strategic word, *priority.* Think about the characteristics of a postterm newborn. Recalling that hypoglycemia is a primary concern in the postterm newborn will direct you to the correct option. **Review:** the care of the postterm newborn.
Level of Cognitive Ability: Analyzing
Client Needs: Physiological Integrity
Integrated Process: Nursing Process/Data Collection
Content Area: Maternity: Newborn
Priority Concepts: Cellular Regulation, Glucose Regulation
Reference(s): McKinney et al (2013), p. 711.

276. 2
Rationale: Signs of infection of the umbilical cord are moistness, oozing, discharge, and a reddened base. If signs of infection occur, the health care provider is notified. Antibiotic treatment may be necessary.
Test-Taking Strategy: Focus on the subject, signs of infection. Options 1 and 3 identify normal signs and are eliminated first. From the remaining options, noting the word *discharge* will direct you to this option. **Review:** the signs and symptoms of infection.
Level of Cognitive Ability: Applying
Client Needs: Physiological Integrity
Integrated Process: Teaching and Learning
Content Area: Maternity: Newborn
Priority Concepts: Client Education, Infection
Reference(s): Hockenberry, Wilson (2013), p. 211.

277. 1
Rationale: Bathing should start at the eyes and face, which are usually the cleanest areas. Next, the external of the ears and behind the ears are cleansed. The newborn's neck should be washed, because formula, breast milk, or lint will often accumulate in the folds of the neck. The hands and arms are then washed. The baby's legs are washed, with the diaper area being washed last.
Test-Taking Strategy: Focus on the subject, bathing a newborn. Remember, when bathing an adult or a baby, start with the cleanest part of the body and proceed to the dirtiest part. Options 2, 3, and 4 are incorrect. **Review:** the techniques for bathing a newborn.
Level of Cognitive Ability: Applying
Client Needs: Health Promotion and Maintenance
Integrated Process: Teaching and Learning
Content Area: Maternity: Newborn
Priority Concepts: Client Education, Caregiving
Reference(s): McKinney et al (2013), p. 522.

278. 3
Rationale: Evaporation occurs when moisture from the newborn's wet body surface dissipates heat along with moisture. By keeping the newborn dry (and by drying the wet newborn at birth), evaporation is prevented. Conduction occurs when the newborn is on a cold surface, such as a cold pad or mattress. Convection occurs as air moves across the newborn's skin from an open door and heat is transferred to the air. Radiation occurs when heat from the newborn radiates to a colder surface.
Test-Taking Strategy: Recalling the methods of preventing heat loss in a newborn and focusing on the subject, evaporation, and thinking about the definition of evaporation will direct you to the correct option. **Review:** the methods of heat loss.
Level of Cognitive Ability: Applying
Client Needs: Physiological Integrity

Integrated Process: Nursing Process/Implementation
Content Area: Maternity: Newborn
Priority Concepts: Thermoregulation, Safety
Reference(s): Hockenberry, Wilson (2013), p. 207.

❖279. 4, 5, 6
Rationale: Phototherapy is the use of intense fluorescent lights to reduce serum bilirubin levels in the newborn. Injury from treatment (e.g., eye damage, dehydration, sensory deprivation) can occur. Interventions include exposing as much of the newborn's skin as possible; however, the genital area is covered. The newborn's eyes are also covered with shields or patches to ensure that the eyelids are closed. The shields or patches are removed at least once per shift to inspect the eyes for infection or irritation and to allow for eye contact. The nurse measures the quantity of light every 8 hours, monitors the skin temperature closely, and increases fluids to compensate for water loss. The newborn will have loose green stools and green-colored urine. The newborn's skin color is monitored with the fluorescent light turned off every 4 to 8 hours, and he or she is monitored for bronze baby syndrome, which is a grayish-brown discoloration of the skin. The newborn is repositioned every 2 hours, and stimulation is provided. After treatment, the newborn is monitored for signs of hyperbilirubinemia, because rebound elevations are normal after therapy is discontinued.
Test-Taking Strategy: Focus on the subject, phototherapy. Recalling that injury from treatment and sensory deprivation can occur will assist you with determining the correct interventions. **Review:** the interventions for the newborn who is receiving phototherapy.
Level of Cognitive Ability: Applying
Client Needs: Safe and Effective Care Environment
Integrated Process: Nursing Process/Implementation
Content Area: Maternity: Newborn
Priority Concepts: Sensory Perception, Tissue Integrity
Reference(s): McKinney et al (2013), pp. 723–724.

280. 2
Rationale: The glans penis is normally dark red. After circumcision, a small amount of bloody drainage is expected. During the normal healing process, the glans becomes covered with a yellow exudate. If excessive bleeding is noted from the circumcision, the nurse applies gentle pressure to the site of bleeding with a sterile gauze pad. If the bleeding is not controlled, the health care provider is notified because a blood vessel may need to be ligated.
Test-Taking Strategy: Focus on the subject, the expected appearance following circumcision. Remember that a small amount of bloody drainage is expected. **Review:** the expected findings after circumcision.
Level of Cognitive Ability: Understanding
Client Needs: Physiological Integrity
Integrated Process: Nursing Process/Data Collection
Content Area: Maternity: Newborn
Priority Concepts: Clotting, Tissue Integrity
Reference(s): McKinney et al (2013), p. 523.

281. 1
Rationale: The newborn infant with RDS may present with clinical signs of cyanosis, tachypnea, apnea, nasal flaring, chest wall retractions, or audible grunts. Acrocyanosis is a bluish discoloration of the hands and feet that is associated with immature peripheral circulation, and it is not uncommon during the first few hours of life. Options 2, 3, and 4 do not indicate clinical signs of RDS.
Test-Taking Strategy: Focus on the subject, signs of respiratory distress syndrome. Recalling that acrocyanosis may be a normal sign in a newborn infant will assist you with eliminating options 2 and 4. From the remaining options, it is necessary to be familiar with the signs of RDS. In addition, note the relationship between the diagnosis and the signs noted in option 1. **Review:** the signs of respiratory distress syndrome.
Level of Cognitive Ability: Analyzing
Client Needs: Physiological Integrity
Integrated Process: Nursing Process/Data Collection
Content Area: Maternity: Newborn
Priority Concepts: Gas Exchange, Perfusion
Reference(s): Hockenberry, Wilson (2013), p. 269.

282. 2
Rationale: Features of newborn infants who are diagnosed with FAS include craniofacial abnormalities, intrauterine growth restriction, cardiac abnormalities, abnormal palmar creases, and respiratory distress. Options 1, 3, and 4 are normal findings in the full-term newborn infant.
Test-Taking Strategy: Focus on the subject, signs of fetal alcohol syndrome. Use your knowledge regarding the normal findings in the full-term newborn infant to answer this question. Note that options 1, 3, and 4 are comparable or alike and that they represent normal findings. **Review:** the content related to normal newborn infant findings and fetal alcohol syndrome.
Level of Cognitive Ability: Analyzing
Client Needs: Physiological Integrity
Integrated Process: Nursing Process/Data Collection
Content Area: Maternity: Newborn
Priority Concepts: Addiction, Tissue Integrity
Reference(s): Hockenberry, Wilson (2013), p. 289.

283. 2
Rationale: The mode of perinatal transmission of HIV to the fetus or neonate of an HIV-positive woman can occur during the antenatal, intrapartal, or postpartum periods. HIV transmission can occur during breastfeeding; thus, HIV-positive clients need to bottle-feed their neonates. Antiviral medications will be prescribed for the neonate for the first 6 weeks of life. The principles related to hand washing need to be taught to the mother.
Test-Taking Strategy: Note the strategic words, *additional guidance is needed.* These words indicate a negative event query and ask you to select an option that is an incorrect statement. Options 1 and 3 can be eliminated first because they are comparable or alike. From the remaining options, recalling the modes of transmission of HIV from the mother to the newborn will direct you to the correct option. **Review:** the modes of human immunodeficiency virus transmission.
Level of Cognitive Ability: Evaluating
Client Needs: Safe and Effective Care Environment
Integrated Process: Teaching and Learning
Content Area: Maternity: Newborn
Priority Concepts: Infection, Safety
Reference(s): McKinney et al (2013), p. 628.

284. 4

Rationale: If herpetic genital lesions are present at the time of delivery, a cesarean delivery will be necessary to reduce the risk of infecting the neonate. In the absence of herpetic genital lesions, a vaginal delivery may be indicated, unless there are other reasons for performing a cesarean delivery. Maternal isolation is not necessary, but potentially exposed neonates should be cultured on the day of delivery.

Test-Taking Strategy: Focusing on the subject, a positive history of genital herpes. Recalling the risks to the neonate associated with this infection will direct you to the correct option. **Review:** the methods of transmission of genital herpes to the neonate.

Level of Cognitive Ability: Applying

Client Needs: Safe and Effective Care Environment

Integrated Process: Nursing Process/Implementation

Content Area: Fundamental Skills: Infection Control

Priority Concepts: Client Education, Infection

Reference(s): McKinney et al (2013), p. 425.

285. 4

Rationale: The cord should be kept clean and dry to decrease bacterial growth; this includes keeping the diaper folded below the cord to keep urine away from the cord. The cord should be cleansed two to three times a day. It usually falls off within 7 to 14 days. Agents other than alcohol may be prescribed to clean the cord.

Test-Taking Strategy: Eliminate options 1 and 3, noting the closed-ended word, *only.* Recall that cord care is required until the cord dries up and falls off and that agents other than alcohol may be prescribed for cord care. Option 2 is incorrect because the cord should fall off between 7 and 14 days after birth. **Review:** the concepts of cord care.

Level of Cognitive Ability: Applying

Client Needs: Physiological Integrity

Integrated Process: Teaching and Learning

Content Area: Maternity: Newborn

Priority Concepts: Client Education, Infection

Reference(s): McKinney et al (2013), p. 522.

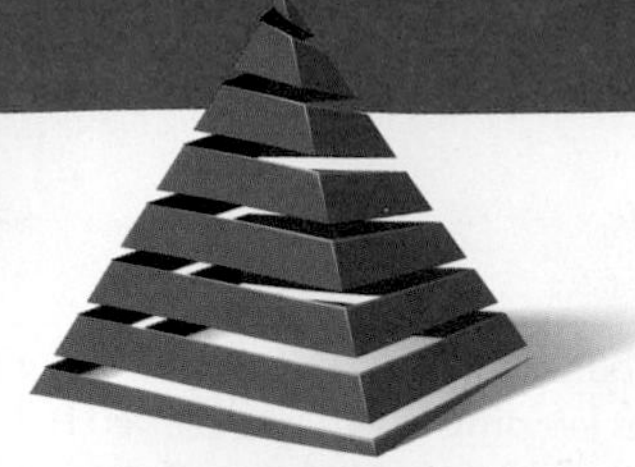

CHAPTER 30

Maternity and Newborn Medications

CRITICAL THINKING What Should You Do?

The nurse notes that a pregnant client who has undergone amniocentesis is Rh negative. What should the nurse do?
Answer is located on p. 358.

I. Tocolytics

A. Description: Tocolytics are medications that produce uterine relaxation and suppress uterine activity (Box 30-1 and Table 30-1).

B. Uses: To halt uterine contractions and prevent preterm birth

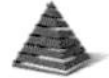

C. Adverse effects and contraindications

1. See Table 30-1 for a description of adverse effects.
2. Maternal contraindications include severe preeclampsia and eclampsia, active vaginal bleeding, intrauterine infection, cardiac disease, and a medical or obstetric condition that contraindicates continuation of pregnancy.
3. Fetal contraindications include estimated gestational age greater than 37 weeks, cervical dilation greater than 4 cm, fetal demise, lethal fetal anomaly, chorioamnionitis, acute fetal distress, and chronic intrauterine growth restriction.

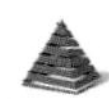

D. Interventions for the client receiving tocolytic therapy

1. Position the client on her side to enhance placental perfusion and reduce pressure on the cervix.
2. Monitor maternal vital signs, fetal status, and **labor** status frequently according to agency protocol.
3. Monitor for signs of adverse effects to the medication.
4. Monitor daily weight and input and output (I&O) status and provide fluid intake as prescribed.
5. Offer comfort measures and provide psychosocial support to the client and family.
6. See Table 30-1 for interventions specific to each tocolytic medication.

BOX 30-1 Tocolytics

Indomethacin (Indocin): prostaglandin inhibitor
Magnesium sulfate: central nervous system depressant; anticonvulsant
Nifedipine (Procardia, Adalat, Nifedical): calcium channel blocker
Terbutaline: β_2 selective adrenergic agonist

II. Magnesium Sulfate

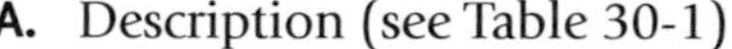

A. Description (see Table 30-1)

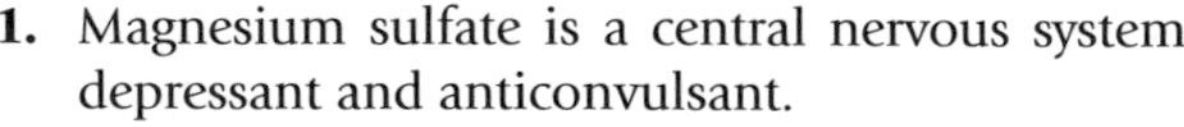

1. Magnesium sulfate is a central nervous system depressant and anticonvulsant.

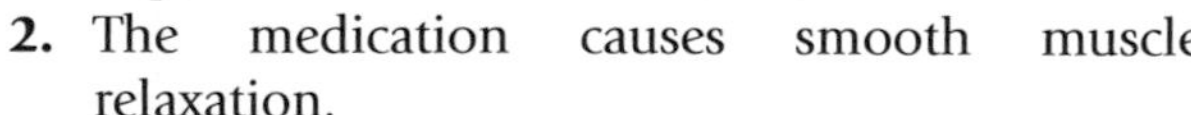

2. The medication causes smooth muscle relaxation.
3. The antidote is calcium gluconate.

B. Uses

1. Stopping preterm labor to prevent preterm birth
2. Preventing and controlling seizures in preeclamptic and eclamptic clients

C. Adverse effects and contraindications

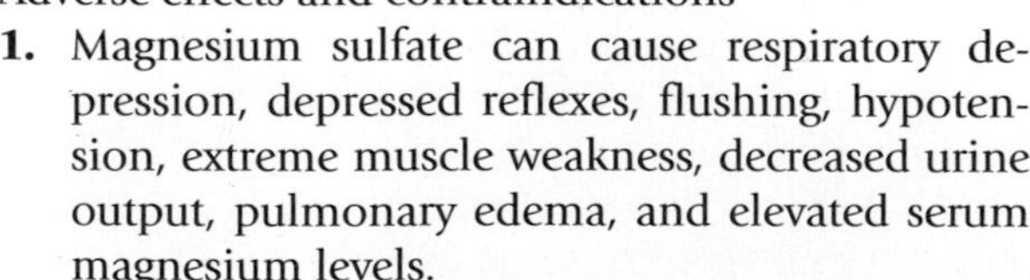

1. Magnesium sulfate can cause respiratory depression, depressed reflexes, flushing, hypotension, extreme muscle weakness, decreased urine output, pulmonary edema, and elevated serum magnesium levels.
2. Continuous IV infusion increases the risk of magnesium toxicity in the **newborn**.
3. Intravenous administration should not be used for 2 hours preceding **delivery**.
4. Magnesium sulfate may be prescribed for the first 12 to 24 hours postpartum if it is used for preeclampsia.
5. High doses can cause loss of deep tendon reflexes, heart block, respiratory paralysis, and cardiac arrest.

TABLE 30-1 Tocolytics

Medication, Classification, and Actions	Adverse Effects	Nursing Interventions
Indomethacin (Indocin)—prostaglandin inhibitor; relaxes uterine smooth muscle	*Maternal*—Nausea and vomiting, dyspepsia, dizziness *Fetal*—Premature closure of ductus arteriosus *Newborn*—Bronchopulmonary dysplasia, respiratory distress syndrome, intracranial pressure, necrotizing enterocolitis, hyperbilirubinemia	Used when other methods fail, depending on gestational age. Not used in women with bleeding potential, peptic ulcer disease, or oligohydramnios. Agency protocol for administration is followed. Amniotic fluid volume and function of ductus arteriosus is determined before therapy and within 48 hours of discontinuing therapy.
Magnesium sulfate—central nervous system depressant; relaxes smooth muscle, including the uterus; used to stop preterm labor contractions; used for preeclamptic clients to prevent seizures	*Maternal*—Depressed respirations, depressed deep tendon reflexes (DTRs), hypotension, extreme muscle weakness, flushing, decreased urine output, pulmonary edema, serum magnesium levels >9 mg/dL *Newborn*—Hypotonia and sleepiness	An IV controller pump is used for administration. Agency protocol for administration is followed. Infusion is discontinued and the HCP is notified if adverse effects occur. Monitor for respirations <12/min, urine output <100 mL/4 hr (30 mL/hr). DTRs are monitored. Magnesium levels are monitored and values outside therapeutic range are reported (4 to 7.5 mEq/L or 5 to 8 mg/dL). Keep calcium gluconate available (antidote).
Nifedipine (Procardia, Adalat, Nifedical)—calcium channel blocker; relaxes smooth muscles, including the uterus, by blocking calcium entry	*Maternal*—Tachycardia, hypotension, dizziness, headache, nervousness, facial flushing, fatigue, nausea *Newborn*—Hypotension	Agency protocol for administration is followed. The use of this medication is avoided or used cautiously with magnesium sulfate because severe hypotension can occur. Monitor for adverse effects.
Terbutaline —β-adrenergic agonist; relaxes smooth muscles, inhibiting uterine activity and causing bronchodilation	*Maternal*—Tachycardia, palpitations, pulmonary edema, chest pain, myocardial ischemia, hypotension, tremors, hypokalemia, hyperglycemia *Newborn*—Tachycardia, hypotension, ileus, hypocalcemia, hyperbilirubinemia, hyperinsulinemia with hypoglycemia	Monitor for adverse effects and the HCP is notified if they occur. Teach woman and family to monitor for adverse effects and when to notify the HCP.

DTRs, Deep tendon reflexes.

6. The medication is contraindicated in the client with heart block, myocardial damage, or kidney failure.
7. The medication is used with caution in the client with severe kidney impairment.

D. Interventions
1. Monitor maternal vital signs, especially respirations, every 30 to 60 minutes.
2. Monitor renal function (output and renal function laboratory values) and cardiac function (electrocardiogram).
3. Monitor magnesium levels—the target range is 4 to 7.5 mEq/L (5 to 8 mg/dL); if a rise in the magnesium level occurs, the health care provider (HCP) is notified immediately.
4. It is always administered by IV infusion via an infusion monitoring device such as a controller pump. The dose being administered is closely and carefully monitored and agency protocol for administration is always followed.
5. Calcium gluconate is always kept on hand in case of a magnesium sulfate overdose, because calcium gluconate antagonizes the effect of magnesium sulfate.
6. Deep tendon reflexes are monitored hourly for signs of developing toxicity.
7. The patellar reflex or knee jerk reflex is tested before administration of a repeat parenteral dose (used as an indicator of central nervous system depression); suppressed reflex may be a sign of impending respiratory arrest (Table 30-2).
8. Patellar reflex must be present, and respiratory rate must be greater than 16 breaths/min (or as designated by agency protocol) before each parenteral dose.

TABLE 30-2 Assessing Deep Tendon Reflexes

Grade	Deep Tendon Reflex Response
0	No response
1	Sluggish or diminished
2	Active or expected response
3	More brisk than expected, slightly hyperactive
4	Brisk, hyperactive, with intermittent or transient clonus

Data from Seidel H, Ball J, Dains J, Flynn J, Solomon B, Stewart R: *Mosby's guide to physical examination*, ed 6, St. Louis, 2011, Mosby.

9. Monitor intake and output hourly; output should be maintained at 30 mL/hr because the medication is eliminated through the kidneys.

The client receiving magnesium sulfate intravenously is monitored closely for signs of toxicity. The HCP is contacted if respirations are less than 12 breaths/min, which indicate respiratory depression, or if any other adverse effects occur.

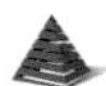

III. Betamethasone and Dexamethasone

A. Description: Corticosteroid that increases the production of **surfactant** to accelerate fetal lung maturity and reduce the incidence or severity of respiratory distress syndrome
B. Use: For the client in preterm labor between 28 and 32 weeks' gestation whose labor can be inhibited for 48 hours without jeopardizing the mother or fetus
C. Adverse effects and contraindications
   1. May decrease the mother's resistance to infection
   2. Pulmonary edema secondary to sodium and fluid retention can occur.
   3. Elevated blood glucose levels in a woman with diabetes mellitus can occur.
D. Interventions

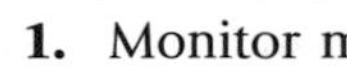

   1. Monitor maternal vital signs, lung sounds, and check for edema.
   2. Monitor mother for signs of infection.
   3. Monitor white blood cell count.
   4. Monitor blood glucose levels.
   5. Administered by deep intramuscular injection

IV. Opioid Analgesics

A. Description
   1. Used to relieve moderate to severe pain associated with labor
   2. Administered by the intramuscular or intravenous (IV) route
   3. Regular use of opioids during pregnancy may produce withdrawal symptoms in the newborn (irritability, excessive crying, tremors, hyperactive reflexes, fever, vomiting, diarrhea, yawning, sneezing, and seizures).
   4. Antidotes for opioids
      a. Naloxone (Narcan) is usually the treatment of choice because it rapidly reverses the opioid toxicity; the dose may need to be repeated every few hours until opioid concentrations have dropped to nontoxic levels.
      b. These medications can cause withdrawal in opioid-dependent clients.
B. Meperidine hydrochloride (Demerol) and hydromorphone hydrochloride (Dilaudid)
   1. Can cause dizziness, nausea, vomiting, sedation, decreased blood pressure, decreased respirations, diaphoresis, flushed face, urinary retention
   2. May be prescribed to be administered with an antiemetic such as promethazine (Phenergan) to prevent nausea
   3. High dosages may result in respiratory depression, skeletal muscle flaccidity, cold clammy skin, cyanosis, extreme somnolence progressing to seizures, stupor, and coma.
   4. Used cautiously in clients delivering preterm newborns
   5. Not administered in early labor because it may slow the labor process
   6. Not administered in advanced labor (within 1 hour of expected delivery); if the medication is not adequately removed from the fetal circulation, respiratory depression can occur
C. Fentanyl (Duragesic) and sufentanil (Sufenta): Can cause respiratory depression, dizziness, drowsiness, hypotension, urinary retention, fetal narcosis and distress
D. Butorphanol tartrate and nalbuphine
   1. Can cause confusion, sedation, sweating, nausea, vomiting, hypotension, sinusoidal-like fetal heart rhythm
   2. Use with caution in a woman with preexisting opioid dependency because these medications can precipitate withdrawal symptoms in the woman and newborn.
E. Interventions
   1. Monitor vital signs, particularly respiratory status; if respirations are 12 breaths/min or fewer, withhold the medication and notify the registered nurse (RN).
   2. Monitor the fetal heart rate and characteristics of uterine contractions.
   3. Monitor for blood pressure changes (hypotension); maintain the woman in a recumbent position (elevate the hip with a wedge pillow or other device).
   4. Record the woman's response and level of pain relief.
   5. Monitor the bladder for distention and urinary retention.
   6. The antidote naloxone should be available, especially if delivery is going to occur during peak drug absorption time.

A drug history is obtained before the administration of an opioid analgesic. Some medications may be contraindicated if the woman has a history of opioid dependency because these medications can precipitate withdrawal symptoms in the woman and newborn.

V. Prostaglandins

A. Description

1. Two common types are Prostaglandin E1: Misoprostol (Cytotec) intravaginal tablet and Prostaglandin E_2: Dinoprostone (Cervidil vaginal insert, Prepidil gel).
2. Ripen the cervix, making it softer and causing it to begin to dilate and efface
3. Stimulate uterine contractions
4. Administered vaginally

B. Uses

1. Preinduction cervical ripening (ripening of the cervix before the induction of labor when the Bishop score is 4 or less)
2. Induction of labor
3. Induction of abortion (abortifacient agent)

C. Adverse effects and contraindications

1. Gastrointestinal effects, including diarrhea, nausea, vomiting, and stomach cramps
2. Fever, chills, flushing, headache, hypotension
3. Tachysystole (12 or more uterine contractions in 20 minutes without an alteration in the fetal heart rate pattern)
4. Hyperstimulation of the **uterus**
5. Fetal passage of meconium
6. Contraindications (Box 30-2)

D. Interventions

1. Maternal vital signs, fetal heart rate pattern, and status of pregnancy, including indications for cervical ripening or the induction of labor, signs of labor or impending labor, and the Bishop score, are monitored (see Table 27-2 for information about the Bishop score).
2. Monitor for adverse effects to the medication.
3. Assist in the administration of the medication; have the woman void before administration of the medication and then have her maintain a supine with lateral tilt or side-lying position for 30 to 60 minutes (gel form) up to 2 hours (insert form) after administration, depending on the medication administered.
4. Treatment is discontinued when the Bishop score is 8 or more (cervix ripens) or an effective contraction pattern is established (three or more contractions in a 10-minute period). Additionally, signs of adverse effects indicate that the treatment needs to be discontinued.
5. Agency protocol is followed for the induction of labor if cervical ripening has occurred and labor has not begun; oxytocin (Pitocin) may be prescribed if needed 6 to 12 hours after discontinuation of prostaglandin therapy.

BOX 30-2 Contraindications to the Use of Prostaglandins

Active cardiac, hepatic, pulmonary, or kidney disease
Acute pelvic inflammatory disease
Clients whom vaginal delivery is not indicated
Fetal malpresentation
History of cesarean section or major uterine surgery
History of difficult labor or traumatic labor
Hypersensitivity to prostaglandins
Maternal fever or infection
Nonreassuring fetal heart rate pattern
Placenta previa or unexplained vaginal bleeding
Regular progressive uterine contractions
Significant cephalopelvic disproportion

VI. Uterine Stimulants (Oxytocics): Oxytocin (Pitocin)

A. Description

1. Oxytocin stimulates the smooth muscle of the uterus and increases the force, frequency, and duration of uterine contractions.
2. Oxytocin also promotes milk let-down.
3. For the induction of labor, oxytocin is administered by the IV route.
4. Minimal cervical change usually is noted until the active phase of labor is achieved.

B. Uses

1. Induces or augments labor
2. Controls postpartum bleeding
3. Promotes milk let-down and facilitates breast-feeding (intranasal route)
4. Manages an incomplete abortion

C. Adverse effects and contraindications

1. Adverse effects may include allergies, dysrhythmias, changes in blood pressure, uterine rupture, and water intoxication; intranasal administration may cause nasal vasoconstriction.
2. Oxytocin may produce uterine hypertonicity, resulting in fetal or maternal adverse effects.
3. High doses may cause hypotension, with rebound hypertension.
4. Postpartum hemorrhage can occur and should be monitored for because the uterus may become atonic when the medication wears off.
5. Oxytocin should not be used in a client who cannot deliver vaginally or in a client with hypertonic uterine contractions; it is also contraindicated in a client with active genital herpes.

D. Interventions

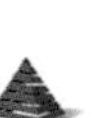

1. Monitor maternal vital signs (every 15 minutes), especially the blood pressure and heart rate, weight, intake and output, level of consciousness, and lung sounds.

Maternity

2. Frequency, duration, force of contractions, and resting uterine tone is monitored every 15 minutes.
3. The fetal heart rate is monitored every 15 minutes. The HCP is notified if significant changes occur; use of an internal fetal scalp electrode may be prescribed.
4. The medication is administered by IV infusion via an infusion monitoring device; the prescribed additive solution is piggybacked at the port nearest the point of venous insertion (prescribed additive solution may be normal saline, lactated Ringer's, or D5W).
5. The dose being administered is carefully monitored; the client is not left unattended while the oxytocin is infusing.
6. Administer oxygen if prescribed.
7. The client is monitored for hypertonic contractions or a nonreassuring fetal heart rate (FHR). The HCP is notified if these occur (see Priority Nursing Actions).
8. The medication is stopped if uterine hyperstimulation or a nonreassuring FHR occurs; the client is turned on her side, the IV rate of the normal saline will be increased, and oxygen will be administered via face mask.
9. Monitor for signs of water intoxication.
10. Have emergency equipment available.
11. The dose of the medication and the time the medication was started, increased, maintained, and discontinued is documented. The client's response is documented.
12. Keep the client and family informed of the client's progress.

VII. Medications Used to Manage Postpartum Hemorrhage (Box 30-3)

A. Ergot alkaloids
1. Description
   a. Ergonovine maleate or ergometrine and methylergonovine maleate are ergot alkaloids.
   b. These medications directly stimulate uterine muscle, increase the force and frequency of contractions, and produce a firm tetanic contraction of the uterus
   c. Can produce arterial vasoconstriction and vasospasm of the coronary arteries 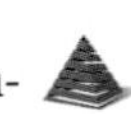
   d. Ergot alkaloids are administered postpartum and are not administered before the delivery of the **placenta**.
2. Uses
   a. Postpartum hemorrhage
   b. Postabortal hemorrhage resulting from atony or involution
3. Adverse effects and contraindications 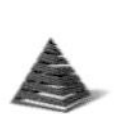

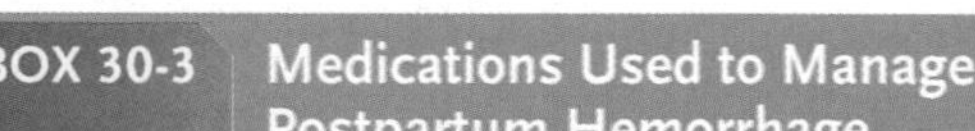

BOX 30-3 Medications Used to Manage Postpartum Hemorrhage

Ergonovine maleate
Methylergonovine
Oxytocin (Pitocin)
Prostaglandin $F_{2\alpha}$ (Carboprost tromethamine [Hemabate])

PRIORITY NURSING ACTIONS!

Steps to Take if Hypertonic Contractions or a Nonreassuring Fetal Heart Rate Occurs During Oxytocin (Pitocin) Infusion

1. Stop the oxytocin (Pitocin) infusion and notify the registered nurse (RN) immediately, who in turn will contact the health care provider (HCP).
2. Turn the woman on her side and stay with the woman.
3. Increase the flow rate of the IV additive solution as directed by the RN.
4. Administer oxygen by snug facemask at 8 to 10 L/min.
5. Monitor maternal vital signs; fetal heart rate (FHR) and patterns; and frequency, duration, and force of contractions.
6. The event, actions taken, and the response are documented.

Oxytocin (Pitocin) is a uterine stimulant and stimulates the smooth muscle of the uterus and increases the force, frequency, and duration of uterine contractions. It is administered to induce or augment labor. The presence of hypertonic contractions or a nonreassuring FHR indicates the need to institute emergency measures to reduce uterine stimulation and increase fetal oxygenation. The nurse would always follow the agency's protocol regarding the procedure to take in this event. Keeping the emergency goals of care in mind (to reduce uterine stimulation and increase fetal oxygenation) will assist in guiding your actions. The oxytocin infusion needs to be stopped in order to reduce uterine contractions. The RN is notified immediately and will then contact the HCP. The nurse turns the woman to her side to increase placental oxygenation. The nurse never leaves a client if an emergency situation is present. The flow rate of the IV additive solution is increased and oxygen is administered. These actions will also facilitate the goals of care. Once these emergency actions are taken, the nurse continuously monitors maternal vital signs, FHR and patterns, and frequency, duration, and force of contractions. The nurse also assists in implementing any additional prescriptions and documents the event, actions taken, and the response.

Reference(s): McKinney, E., James, S., Murray, S., Nelson, K. & Ashwill, J. (2013). *Maternal-child nursing* (4th ed., pp. 366, 416–417). St. Louis: Elsevier.

a. Can cause nausea, uterine cramping, bradycardia, dysrhythmias, myocardial infarction, and severe hypertension
b. High doses are associated with peripheral vasospasm or vasoconstriction, angina, miosis, confusion, respiratory depression, seizures, or unconsciousness; uterine tetany can occur
c. Contraindicated during pregnancy and in clients with significant cardiovascular disease, peripheral vascular disease, or hypertension

4. Interventions
   a. Monitor maternal vital signs, weight, intake and output, level of consciousness, and lung sounds.
   b. Monitor the blood pressure closely; the medication produces vasoconstriction and, if a rise in blood pressure is noted, the medication is withheld; the RN is notified as is the HCP.
   c. Uterine contractions are monitored (frequency, strength, and duration).
   d. Monitor for chest pain, headache, shortness of breath, itching, pale or cold hands or feet, nausea, diarrhea, or dizziness.
   e. Monitor the extremities for color, warmth, movement, and pain.
   f. Monitor for vaginal bleeding.
   g. Notify the RN who will then notify the HCP, if chest pain or other adverse effects occur.
   h. Analgesics are administered as prescribed; they may be required because the medication produces painful uterine contractions.

The woman's blood pressure is checked before administration of an ergot alkaloid. These medications can cause severe hypertension and are therefore contraindicated in a client with hypertension.

B. Prostaglandin $F_{2\alpha}$ (carboprost tromethamine [Hemabate])
1. Description: Contracts the uterus
2. Uses: Postpartum hemorrhage
3. Adverse effects and contraindications
   a. Can cause headache, nausea, vomiting, diarrhea, fever, tachycardia, hypertension
   b. Contraindicated if the client has asthma
4. Interventions
   a. Monitor vital signs.
   b. Monitor for vaginal bleeding (uterine tone is also monitored).

C. Oxytocin (Pitocin): See section on uterine stimulants

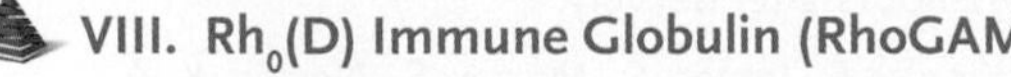

VIII. Rh_0(D) Immune Globulin (RhoGAM)

A. Description
1. Prevention of anti-Rh_0(D) antibody formation is most successful if the medication is administered twice, at 28 weeks of gestation and again within 72 hours after delivery.

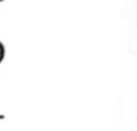

2. The immune globulin also should be administered within 72 hours after potential or actual exposure to Rh-positive blood and must be given with each subsequent exposure or potential exposure to Rh-positive blood.

B. Use: To prevent isoimmunization in Rh-negative clients who are exposed or potentially exposed to Rh-positive red blood cells by amniocentesis, chorionic villus sampling (CVS), transfusion, termination of pregnancy, abdominal trauma, or bleeding during pregnancy or birth process

C. Adverse effects and contraindications
1. Adverse effects include elevated temperature and tenderness at the injection site
2. Contraindicated for Rh-positive women and in clients with a history of systemic allergic reactions to preparations containing human immunoglobulins
3. Not administered to a newborn

D. Interventions
1. Administer to the mother by intramuscular injection at 28 weeks' gestation and within 72 hours after delivery; it is never administered by the intravenous (IV) route.
2. Monitor for temperature elevation.
3. Monitor injection site for tenderness.

Rh_0(D) immune globulin (RhoGAM) is of no benefit once the client has developed a positive antibody titer to the Rh antigen.

IX. Rubella Vaccine

A. Given subcutaneously before hospital discharge to a nonimmune postpartum client

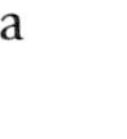

B. Administered if the rubella titer is less than 1:8
C. Adverse effects: Transient rash, hypersensitivity
D. Contraindicated in a client with an allergy to duck eggs
E. Interventions
1. Ask the client about an allergy to duck eggs; the HCP is notified before administration if an allergy exists.
2. The vaccine is not administered if the client or other family members are immunocompromised.

The client should avoid pregnancy for 1 to 3 months (or as prescribed) after immunization with rubella vaccine. Inform the client about the need for using a contraception method during this time.

X. Lung Surfactants (Box 30-4)

A. Description
1. Lung surfactants replenish surfactant and restore surface activity to the lungs to prevent and treat respiratory distress syndrome.
2. Lung surfactants are administered by the intratracheal route.

Maternity

BOX 30-4 Lung Surfactant Replacement Therapy

Beractant (Survanta)
Calfactant (Infasurf)
Poractant alfa (Curosurf)
Lucinactant (Surfaxin)

B. Use: To prevent or treat respiratory distress syndrome in preterm newborns
C. Adverse effects and contraindications
 1. Adverse effects include transient bradycardia and oxygen desaturation; pulmonary hemorrhage, mucus plugging, and endotracheal tube reflex can also occur.
 2. Surfactants are administered with caution in newborns at risk for circulatory overload.

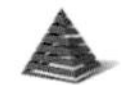
D. Interventions
 1. The surfactant is instilled through the catheter inserted into the newborn's endotracheal tube; suctioning is avoided for at least 2 hours after administration.
 2. Monitor for bradycardia and decreased oxygen saturation during administration.
 3. Monitor respiratory status and lung sounds and for signs of adverse effects.

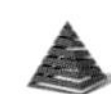
XI. Eye Prophylaxis for the Newborn

A. Description
 1. Preventive eye treatment against ophthalmia neonatorum in the newborn is required by law in the United States.
 2. The agent used varies, depending on agency protocols, but usually ophthalmic forms of erythromycin 0.5% (Ilotycin) is prescribed because it is bacteriostatic and bactericidal and provides prophylaxis against *Neisseria gonorrhoeae* and *Chlamydia trachomatis*.

B. Use: A prophylactic measure to protect against *Neisseria gonorrhoeae* and *Chlamydia trachomatis*

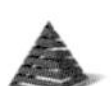
C. Interventions
 1. Cleanse the newborn's eyes before instilling the medication.
 2. Do not flush the eyes after instillation.

Instillation of eye medication can be delayed for up to 1 hour after birth to facilitate eye contact and parent-newborn attachment and bonding.

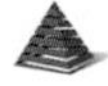
XII. Vitamin K (Phytonadione)

A. Description
 1. The newborn is at risk for hemorrhagic disorders; coagulation factors synthesized in the liver depend on vitamin K, which is not synthesized until intestinal bacteria are present.
 2. Newborns are deficient in vitamin K for the first 5 to 8 days of life because of the lack of intestinal bacteria.

B. Use: Prophylaxis and treatment of hemorrhagic disease of the newborn

C. Adverse effect: Vitamin K can cause hyperbilirubinemia in the newborn.

D. Interventions
 1. Protect the medication from light.
 2. Administer during the early newborn period.
 3. Administer in the lateral aspect of the middle third of the vastus lateralis muscle of the thigh.
 4. Monitor for bruising at the injection site and for bleeding from the cord.
 5. Monitor for jaundice and monitor the bilirubin level because the medication can cause hyperbilirubinemia in the newborn.

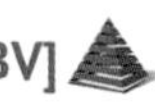
XIII. Recombivax HB Pediatric (Hepatitis B Virus [HBV] Vaccine)

A. Description: Given intramuscularly to the newborn before discharge from the agency

B. Use: Recommended for all newborns to prevent hepatitis B

C. Adverse effect: Rash, fever, erythema, and pain at injection site

D. Interventions
 1. Parental consent must be obtained.
 2. Administer in the lateral aspect of the middle third of the vastus lateralis muscle.
 3. If the **infant** was born to a mother positive for hepatitis B surface antigen, hepatitis B immune globulin (HBIG) is usually given within 12 hours of birth in addition to the hepatitis B vaccine. Then, the regularly scheduled HBV vaccination schedule is followed.
 4. Document immunization administration on a vaccination card for the parents to have a record that it was administered.

CRITICAL THINKING What Should You Do?

Answer: The nurse should report this finding to the registered nurse, and a prescription from the health care provider for the administration of Rh_0(D) immune globulin (RhoGAM) should be obtained. Rh_0(D) immune globulin is administered to prevent isoimmunization in Rh-negative clients who are negative for Rh antibodies and exposed or potentially exposed to Rh-positive red blood cells from the fetus by amniocentesis or chorionic villus sampling, transfusion, termination of pregnancy, abdominal trauma, or bleeding during pregnancy or the birth process. It is administered to the Rh-negative client by intramuscular injection at 28 weeks' gestation and within 72 hours after delivery.

Reference(s): McKinney, E., James, S., Murray, S., Nelson, K. & Ashwill, J. (2013). *Maternal-child nursing* (4th ed., pp. 249, 603–604). St. Louis: Elsevier.

PRACTICE QUESTIONS

286. Methylergonovine is prescribed for a woman to treat postpartum hemorrhage. Before the administration of methylergonovine, the nurse should check which **priority** item?
1. Uterine tone
2. Blood pressure
3. Amount of lochia
4. Deep tendon reflexes

❖ **287.** The nurse is monitoring a preterm labor client who is receiving magnesium sulfate intravenously. The nurse should monitor for which adverse effects of this medication? **Select all that apply.**
- ☐ 1. Flushing
- ☐ 2. Hypertension
- ☐ 3. Increased urine output
- ☐ 4. Depressed respirations
- ☐ 5. Extreme muscle weakness
- ☐ 6. Hyperactive deep tendon reflexes

288. A pregnant client is receiving magnesium sulfate for the management of preeclampsia. The nurse determines that the client is experiencing toxicity from the medication if which is noted on data collection?
1. Proteinuria of 3+
2. Presence of deep tendon reflexes
3. Serum magnesium level of 6 mEq/L
4. Respirations of 10 breaths per minute

289. Epidural analgesia is administered to a woman for pain relief after a cesarean birth. The nurse assigned to care for the woman ensures that which medication is readily available if respiratory depression occurs?
1. Betamethasone
2. Morphine sulfate
3. Naloxone (Narcan)
4. Meperidine hydrochloride (Demerol)

290. Rh_0(D) immune globulin (RhoGAM) is prescribed for a woman after the delivery of a newborn infant, and the nurse provides information to the woman about the purpose of the medication. The nurse determines that the woman understands the purpose of the medication if the woman states that it will protect her next baby from which condition?
1. Having Rh-positive blood
2. Developing a rubella infection
3. Developing physiological jaundice
4. Being affected by Rh incompatibility

291. A woman with preeclampsia is receiving magnesium sulfate. Which indicates to the nurse that the magnesium sulfate therapy is **effective**?
1. Scotomas are present.
2. Seizures do not occur.
3. Ankle clonus is noted.
4. The blood pressure decreases.

292. Methylergonovine is prescribed for a client with postpartum hemorrhage. Before administering the medication, the nurse should question administration of the medication if which condition is documented in the client's medical history?
1. Hypotension
2. Hypothyroidism
3. Diabetes mellitus
4. Peripheral vascular disease

293. The nursing instructor asks a nursing student to describe the procedure for administering erythromycin ointment to the eyes of a neonate. The instructor determines that the student **needs to research** this procedure further if the student makes which statement?
1. "I will flush the eyes after instilling the ointment."
2. "I will cleanse the neonate's eyes before instilling the ointment."
3. "The administration of the eye ointment is within 1 hour after delivery."
4. "I will instill the eye ointment into each of the neonate's conjunctival sacs."

294. A 31-week preterm labor client dilated to 4 centimeters has been started on magnesium sulfate. Her contractions have stopped. If the client's labor can be inhibited for the next 48 hours, which medication does the nurse anticipate will be prescribed?
1. Nalbuphine
2. Betamethasone
3. Misoprostol (Cytotec)
4. Rh_0(D) immune globulin (RhoGAM)

295. The nurse is caring for a client who is receiving oxytocin (Pitocin) to induce labor. The nurse should discontinue the oxytocin infusion and notify the registered nurse if which is noted on data collection of the client?
1. Fatigue
2. Drowsiness
3. Uterine hyperstimulation
4. Early decelerations of the fetal heart rate

ANSWERS

286. 2

Rationale: Methylergonovine, which is an ergot alkaloid, is an agent that is used to prevent or control postpartum hemorrhage by contracting the uterus. Methylergonovine causes continuous uterine contractions and may elevate the blood pressure. A priority before the administration of the medication is to check the blood pressure. The health care provider should be notified if hypertension is present. Although options 1, 3, and 4 may be components of the postpartum data collection procedures, option 2 is related specifically to the administration of this medication.
Test-Taking Strategy: Note the strategic word, *priority.* Eliminate options 1 and 3 first, because they are comparable or alike and related to one another. From the remaining options, use the ABCs—airway, breathing, and circulation. Obtaining the blood pressure is a method of checking circulation. Review: the adverse effects of **methylergonovine**.
Level of Cognitive Ability: Analyzing
Client Needs: Physiological Integrity
Integrated Process: Nursing Process/Data Collection
Content Area: Pharmacology: Reproductive/Maternity/Newborn Medications
Priority Concepts: Clinical Judgment, Perfusion
Reference(s): McKinney et al (2013), p. 668.

❖287. 1, 4, 5

Rationale: Magnesium sulfate is a central nervous system depressant, and it relaxes smooth muscle, including the uterus. It is used to stop preterm labor contractions, and it is used for preeclamptic clients to prevent seizures. Adverse effects include flushing, depressed respirations, depressed deep tendon reflexes, hypotension, extreme muscle weakness, decreased urine output, pulmonary edema, and elevated serum magnesium levels.
Test-Taking Strategy: Focus on the subject, adverse effects of magnesium sulfate. Recalling that this medication is a central nervous system depressant will assist you with answering correctly. Review: the adverse effects of **magnesium sulfate**.
Level of Cognitive Ability: Analyzing
Client Needs: Physiological Integrity
Integrated Process: Nursing Process/Data Collection
Content Area: Pharmacology: Reproductive/Maternity/Newborn Medications
Priority Concepts: Clinical Judgment, Intracranial Regulation
Reference(s): Skidmore-Roth (2014), p. 767.

288. 4

Rationale: Magnesium toxicity can occur as a result of magnesium sulfate therapy. Signs of magnesium sulfate toxicity relate to the central nervous system depressant effects of the medication and include respiratory depression (respiratory rate less than 12 breaths per minute), a loss of deep tendon reflexes, and a sudden drop in the fetal heart rate, maternal heart rate, and blood pressure. Therapeutic serum levels of magnesium are 4 to 7.5 mEq/L or 5 to 8 mg/dL. Proteinuria of 3+ is likely to be noted in a client with preeclampsia.
Test-Taking Strategy: Focus on the subject, signs of toxicity from magnesium sulfate. Eliminate option 2 first because it is a normal finding. Next, eliminate option 3, knowing that the therapeutic serum level of magnesium is between 4 and 7.5 mEq/L. From the remaining options, recalling that proteinuria of 3+ would be noted in a client with preeclampsia will direct you to the correct option. Review: the adverse effects of **magnesium sulfate**.
Level of Cognitive Ability: Analyzing
Client Needs: Physiological Integrity
Integrated Process: Nursing Process/Data Collection
Content Area: Pharmacology: Reproductive/Maternity/Newborn Medications
Priority Concepts: Clinical Judgment, Intracranial Regulation
Reference(s): McKinney et al (2013), p. 595.

289. 3

Rationale: Opioids are used for epidural analgesia. An adverse effect of epidural analgesia is a delayed respiratory depression. Naloxone (Narcan) is an opioid antagonist, which reverses the effects of opioids and is given for respiratory depression. Morphine sulfate and meperidine hydrochloride are opioid analgesics. Betamethasone is a corticosteroid that is administered to enhance fetal lung maturity.
Test-Taking Strategy: Focus on the subject, the antidote for respiratory depression. Eliminate options 2 and 4 first, knowing that these medications are opioid analgesics. Next, eliminate option 1, knowing that this medication is a corticosteroid. Review: the purposes and actions of **naloxone**.
Level of Cognitive Ability: Applying
Client Needs: Physiological Integrity
Integrated Process: Nursing Process/Planning
Content Area: Pharmacology: Reproductive/Maternity/Newborn Medications
Priority Concepts: Gas Exchange, Safety
Reference(s): Hodgson, Kizior (2014), pp. 813–814.

290. 4

Rationale: Rh incompatibility can occur when an Rh-negative mother becomes sensitized to the Rh antigen. Sensitization may develop when an Rh-negative woman becomes pregnant with a fetus that is Rh positive. During pregnancy and at delivery, some of the baby's Rh-positive blood can enter the maternal circulation, thus causing the woman's immune system to form antibodies against the Rh-positive blood. The administration of Rh_0(D) immune globulin prevents the woman from developing antibodies against Rh-positive blood by providing passive antibody protection against the Rh antigen.
Test-Taking Strategy: Focus on the subject, the purpose of Rh_0(D) immune globulin. Note the relationship between the name of the medication, Rh_0(D) immune globulin, and the word *incompatibility* in the correct option. Review: the purpose of **Rh_0(D) immune globulin**.
Level of Cognitive Ability: Evaluating
Client Needs: Physiological Integrity
Integrated Process: Teaching and Learning
Content Area: Pharmacology: Reproductive/Maternity/Newborn Medications
Priority Concepts: Client Education, Immunity
Reference(s): Hodgson, Kizior (2014), pp. 1031–1032.

291. 2

Rationale: For a client with preeclampsia, the goal of care is directed at preventing eclampsia (seizures). Magnesium sulfate is an anticonvulsant rather than an antihypertensive agent. Although a decrease in blood pressure may be noted initially,

this effect is usually transient. Scotomas are areas of complete or partial blindness. Visual disturbances, such as scotomas, often precede an eclamptic seizure. Ankle clonus indicates hyperreflexia and may precede the onset of eclampsia.
Test-Taking Strategy: Note the strategic word, *effective*, and the subject, that magnesium sulfate is effective. Knowing that magnesium sulfate is an anticonvulsant will direct you to the correct option. **Review:** the actions and uses of **magnesium sulfate.**
Level of Cognitive Ability: Evaluating
Client Needs: Physiological Integrity
Integrated Process: Nursing Process/Evaluation
Content Area: Pharmacology: Reproductive/Maternity/Newborn Medications
Priority Concepts: Clinical Judgment, Intracranial Regulation
Reference(s): McKinney et al (2013), pp. 594–595; Skidmore-Roth (2014), p. 767.

292. 4
Rationale: Methylergonovine is an ergot alkaloid that is used to treat postpartum hemorrhage. Ergot alkaloids are avoided in clients with significant cardiovascular disease, peripheral vascular disease, hypertension, eclampsia, or preeclampsia because these conditions are worsened by the vasoconstrictive effects of the ergot alkaloids. Options 1, 2, and 3 are not contraindications related to the use of ergot alkaloids.
Test-Taking Strategy: Focus on the subject, a contraindication associated with methylergonovine. Recalling that ergot alkaloids produce vasoconstriction will direct you to the correct option. **Review:** the effects of **ergot alkaloids** and the associated contraindications.
Level of Cognitive Ability: Analyzing
Client Needs: Physiological Integrity
Integrated Process: Nursing Process/Implementation
Content Area: Pharmacology: Reproductive/Maternity/Newborn Medications
Priority Concepts: Clinical Judgment, Safety
Reference(s): Hodgson, Kizior (2014), pp. 756–757.

293. 1
Rationale: Eye prophylaxis protects the neonate against *Neisseria gonorrhoeae* and *Chlamydia trachomatis*. The eyes are not flushed after the instillation of the medication because the flush will wash away the administered medication. Options 2, 3, and 4 are correct statements regarding the procedure for administering eye medication to the neonate.
Test-Taking Strategy: Note the strategic words, *needs to research*. These words indicate a negative event query and ask you to select an option that is an incorrect statement. Visualize the effect of each statement. This will direct you to the correct option. **Review:** the procedure for administering **eye medication to the newborn.**
Level of Cognitive Ability: Evaluating
Client Needs: Physiological Integrity
Integrated Process: Teaching and Learning
Content Area: Pharmacology: Reproductive/Maternity/Newborn Medications
Priority Concepts: Infection, Sensory Perception
Reference(s): Hodgson, Kizior (2014), p. 433; McKinney et al (2013), pp. 509–510.

294. 2
Rationale: Betamethasone, which is a glucocorticoid, is given to stimulate fetal lung maturation. It is used for clients in preterm labor between 28 and 32 weeks' gestation if the labor can be inhibited for 48 hours. Nalbuphine is an opioid analgesic. Misoprostol (Cytotec) is a prostaglandin that is given to ripen and soften the cervix and to stimulate uterine contractions. Rh_0(D) immune globulin (RhoGAM) is given to RH-negative clients to prevent sensitization.
Test-Taking Strategy: Note the subject, a 31-week preterm labor client. Recalling that betamethasone is used to stimulate surfactant release will direct you to the correct option. **Review:** the purpose and actions of **bethamethasone.**
Level of Cognitive Ability: Analyzing
Client Needs: Physiological Integrity
Integrated Process: Nursing Process/Planning
Content Area: Pharmacology: Reproductive/Maternity/Newborn Medications
Priority Concepts: Development, Reproduction
Reference(s): McKinney et al (2013), pp. 652–653.

295. 3
Rationale: Oxytocin stimulates uterine contractions, and it is one of the common pharmacological methods used to induce labor. An adverse effect associated with the administration of the medication is the hyperstimulation of uterine contractions. Therefore, oxytocin infusion must be stopped when any signs of uterine hyperstimulation are present. Fatigue and drowsiness may be caused by the labor experience. Early decelerations of the fetal heart rate are a reassuring sign and do not indicate fetal distress.
Test-Taking Strategy: Focus on the subject, an adverse effect to oxytocin. Options 1 and 2 can be eliminated first because they are comparable or alike. From the remaining options, recalling that early decelerations of the fetal heart rate are a reassuring sign will direct you to the correct option. **Review:** the nursing responsibilities associated with **oxytocin.**
Level of Cognitive Ability: Analyzing
Client Needs: Physiological Integrity
Integrated Process: Nursing Process/Implementation
Content Area: Pharmacology: Reproductive/Maternity/Newborn Medications
Priority Concepts: Perfusion, Reproduction
Reference(s): McKinney et al (2013), pp. 416–417.

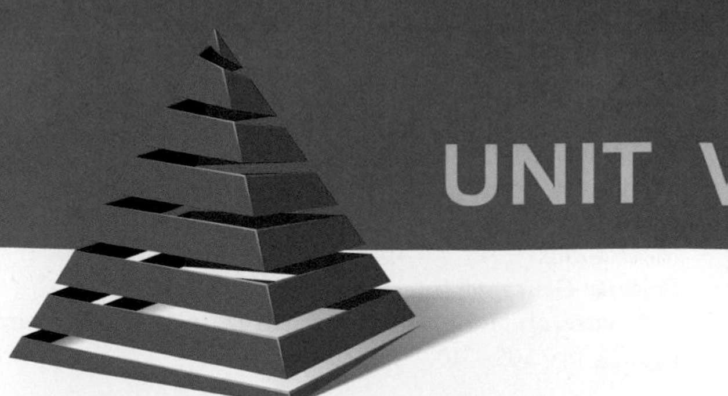

UNIT VII

Pediatric Nursing

PYRAMID TERMS

abuse Nonaccidental physical injury or the nonaccidental act of omission of care by a parent or person responsible for a child; includes neglect and physical, sexual, or emotional maltreatment.

atresia The congenital absence or closure of a body orifice.

chronological age Age in years.

crackles Audible high-pitched crackling or popping sounds heard during lung auscultation; result from fluid in the airways and are not cleared by coughing.

cyanosis The bluish color that results in tissues, nail beds, and mucous membranes when tissues are deprived of adequate amounts of oxygen.

developmental age Age based on a child's maturational progress. It is determined by standardized resources such as body size, physical and psychological functioning, motor skills, and aptitude tests.

growth Measurable physical and physiological body changes that occur over time.

grunting The sound made by forced expiration, which is the body's attempt to improve oxygenation when hypoxemia is present.

hereditary Refers to the transmission of genetic characteristics from parent to offspring.

nasal flaring A widening of the nares to enable an infant or child to take in more oxygen; a serious indicator of air hunger.

passive immunity A form of acquired immunity that occurs artificially through injection or is acquired naturally as the result of antibody transfer through the placenta to a fetus or through colostrum to an infant; is not permanent and does not last as long as active immunity.

prodromal Pertaining to early symptoms that mark the onset of a disease.

puberty The period of time during which the adolescent experiences a growth spurt, develops secondary sex characteristics, and achieves reproductive maturity.

regurgitation An abnormal backward flow of body fluid.

retraction An abnormal movement of the chest wall during inspiration in which the skin appears to be drawn in between the ribs and above and/or below the clavicle and scapula; this condition indicates respiratory difficulty.

shunt The movement of blood or body fluid through an abnormal anatomical or surgically created opening.

stenosis The narrowing or constriction of an opening.

stridor A shrill, harsh sound heard during inspiration, expiration, or both that is produced by the flow of air through a narrowed segment of the respiratory tract.

vaccine A suspension of attenuated or killed microorganisms administered to induce active immunity to an infectious disease.

wheezing A high-pitched musical whistling sound that is heard with or without a stethoscope as air is compressed through narrowed or obstructed airways because of swelling, secretions, or tumors.

Pyramid to Success

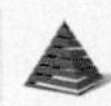

The pyramid points focus on growth and development, safety, and the age-appropriate measures to ensure a safe and hazard-free environment for the child, protection of the child, prevention of accidents, and acute disorders that occur in children. The focus is on nutrition, specific feeding techniques, positioning techniques, and interventions that will provide and maintain adequate airway, breathing, and circulation patterns in the child. In addition, neglect and abuse of a child are emphasized. On the NCLEX-PN® examination, be alert to the age of the child if the age is presented in the question. If an age is presented in the question, think about the specific growth and development characteristics of that age-group to answer the question correctly.

Client Needs

Safe and Effective Care Environment

Considering issues related to informed consent for minors

Ensuring environmental and personal safety, including home safety, related to the developmental age of the child

Establishing priorities

Instituting measures related to the spread and control of infectious agents, particularly communicable diseases

Maintaining confidentiality

Preventing accidents

Providing continuity of care

Providing protective measures

Protecting the child and other contacts to prevent illness
Upholding parents' and child's rights

Health Promotion and Maintenance

Ensuring that immunization schedules are up to date
Focusing on developmental stages when planning care
Performing data collection techniques specific to the pediatric client
Preventing disease in the pediatric population
Providing health-promotion programs for the pediatric client
Reinforcing child and parent teaching regarding care at home

Psychosocial Integrity

Assessing for child abuse and neglect
Communicating with the pediatric client
Considering concepts of family dynamics when planning care
Considering cultural, religious, and spiritual beliefs when planning care
Considering end-of-life issues, grief, and loss in the pediatric population
Identifying family and support systems for the child
Providing play therapies

Physiological Integrity

Following medication administration procedures
Following nutritional guidelines for the pediatric population
Identifying comfort measures that are appropriate for the child
Maintaining sensitivity during intrusive procedures that are required for the pediatric client
Managing childhood illnesses
Monitoring elimination patterns
Monitoring for age-appropriate normal body structure and function
Monitoring for infectious diseases of the pediatric client
Monitoring for potential alterations in body systems as a result of disease
Monitoring for responses to treatments
Providing for consistent rest and sleep patterns
Responding to medical emergencies

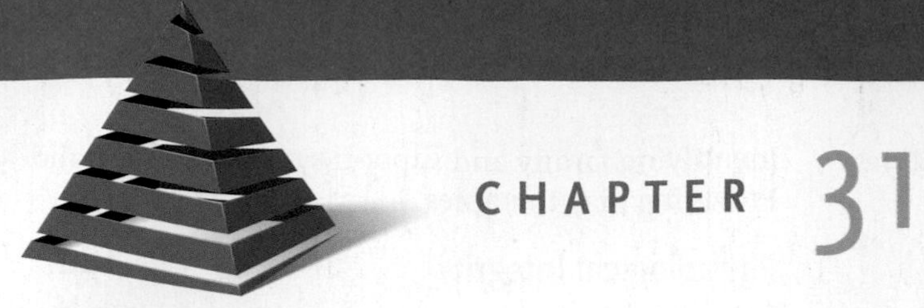

CHAPTER 31

Integumentary Disorders

CRITICAL THINKING What Should You Do?

A child, being admitted to the pediatric unit, is suspected of having impetigo. In order to prevent the spread of this infectious disease, what should the nurse do?

Answer is located on p. 368.

I. Atopic Dermatitis (Eczema)

A. Description

1. A superficial inflammatory process that primarily involves the epidermis and that is characterized by pruritic lesions
2. Associated with family history of the disorder, allergies, asthma, or allergic rhinitis

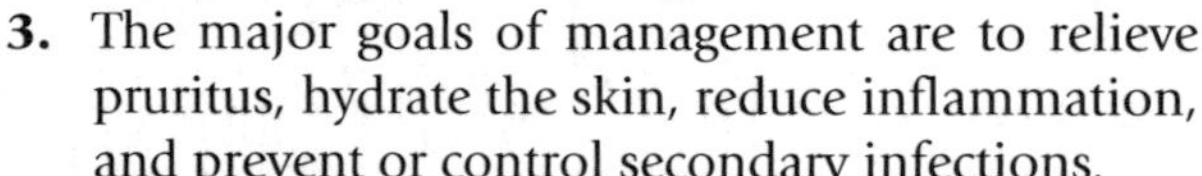

3. The major goals of management are to relieve pruritus, hydrate the skin, reduce inflammation, and prevent or control secondary infections.

B. Forms of eczema (Box 31-1)

C. Data collection (Box 31-2)

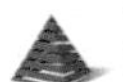

D. Interventions

1. Avoid exposure to skin irritants such as soaps, detergents, fabric softeners, diaper wipes, and powder.
2. Avoid excessive bathing and washing of affected areas; bathing water should be tepid, and the skin should be lubricated immediately after the bath.
3. Intermittently apply cool, wet compresses for short periods to soothe the skin and alleviate itching; pat the skin dry between cooling treatments.
4. Administer antihistamines and topical corticosteroids, as prescribed. Corticosteroids are applied in a thin layer and rubbed into the area thoroughly.
5. Immunomodulator medications may be prescribed.
6. Antibiotics may be prescribed if secondary infections occur.
7. Prevent or minimize scratching. Keep the nails short and clean, and place gloves or cotton socks over the hands.
8. Eliminate conditions that increase itching, such as wet diapers, excessive bathing, ambient heat, woolen clothes or blankets, and proximity to rough fabrics or furry stuffed animals; exposure to latex should also be avoided.
9. Reinforce instructions to the parents to wash the child's clothing in a mild detergent and rinse it thoroughly. Putting the clothes through a second complete wash cycle without detergent will minimize the amount of residue remaining on the fabric.
10. Reinforce instructions to the parents in the measures to prevent skin infections.

BOX 31-1 Forms of Eczema

Infantile

Usually begins at 2 to 6 months of age; generally undergoes spontaneous remission by 3 years of age

Childhood

May follow the infantile form; occurs at 2 to 3 years of age

Preadolescent and Adolescent

Begins at about 12 years of age; may continue into the early adult years or indefinitely

BOX 31-2 Data Collection Findings: Atopic Dermatitis (Eczema)

- Redness
- Scaliness
- Itching
- Minute papules (firm elevated circumscribed lesions smaller than 1 cm in diameter) and vesicles (similar to papules but fluid-filled)
- Weeping, oozing, and crusting of lesions
- Adolescent and early adult forms commonly occur in antecubital and popliteal areas.

11. Reinforce instructions to the parents to monitor the lesions for signs of infection (i.e., honey-colored crusts with surrounding erythema) and to seek immediate medical intervention if such signs are noted.

A child with an integumentary disorder needs to be monitored for signs of either a skin infection or a systemic infection.

II. Impetigo

A. Description
1. A highly contagious bacterial infection of the skin caused by β-hemolytic streptococci, *Staphylococcus aureus,* or both.
2. Impetigo can occur because of poor hygiene. It can be a primary infection or occur secondarily at a site that has been injured or sustained an insect bite, or at a site that was originally a rash, such as atopic dermatitis or poison ivy or poison oak.
3. The most common sites of infection are the face, around the mouth, the hands, the neck, and the extremities.
4. The lesions begin as vesicles or pustules surrounded by edema and redness (a pustule is similar to a vesicle except that its fluid content is purulent).
5. After the crusting of the lesions, the initially serous vesicular fluid becomes cloudy, and the vesicle ruptures, leaving a honey-colored crust that covers an ulcerated base.

B. Data collection (Fig. 31-1)
1. Lesions
2. Erythema
3. Pruritus
4. Burning
5. Secondary lymph node involvement

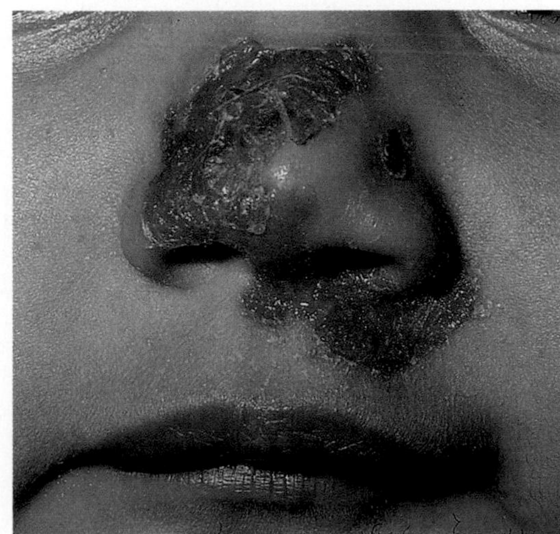

FIGURE 31-1 Impetigo contagiosa. (From Hockenberry M, Wilson D: *Wong's: Nursing care of infants and children*, ed 9, St. Louis, 2012, Mosby.)

C. Interventions
1. Contact isolation. Use standard precautions and implement agency-specific isolation procedures for the hospitalized child. Strict hygiene practices are important because it is a highly contagious condition.
2. Allow lesions to dry by air exposure.
3. Assist the child with daily bathing with antibacterial soap, as prescribed.
4. Apply warm saline or other prescribed compresses to the lesions two or three times daily, followed by a mild soap and water to remove crusts and allow for healing; Burow's solution may also be prescribed to soften the crusts.
5. Apply topical antibiotic ointments with a clean/sterile cotton swab without touching the tube opening with fingers or skin and instruct parents in their use; the infection is still communicable for 48 hours beyond initiation of antibiotic treatment.
6. Administer oral antibiotics, which may be prescribed if there is no response to topical antibiotic treatment. It is extremely important to comply with the prescribed antibiotic regimen because secondary infections such as glomerulonephritis may result if the infectious agent is of a streptococcal type that can affect the nephrons.
7. Apply and instruct the parents in the use of emollients, as prescribed, to prevent skin cracking.
8. Reinforce instructions to the parents in the methods of preventing the spread of the infection, especially careful hand washing.
9. Inform the parents that the child needs to use separate towels, linens, and dishes.
10. Inform parents that all linens and clothing used by the child should be washed with detergent in hot water separately from linens and clothing of other household members.

III. Pediculosis Capitis (Lice)

A. Description
1. An infestation of the hair and scalp with lice
2. The most common sites of involvement are the occipital area, behind the ears, at the nape of the neck, and, occasionally, the eyebrows and eyelashes.
3. The female louse lays her eggs (nits) on the hair shaft, close to the scalp. The incubation period is 7 to 10 days.

4. Head lice live and reproduce only on humans and are transmitted by direct and indirect contact, such as the sharing of brushes, hats, towels, and bedding.
5. All contacts of the infested child should be examined for lice infestation and referred for treatment as appropriate.

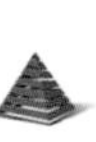

B. Data collection (Box 31-3)

BOX 31-3 Data Collection Findings: Pediculosis Capitis

- Child scratches the scalp excessively.
- Pruritis is caused by the crawling insect and insect saliva on the skin.
- Nits (white eggs) are observable on the hair shaft (it is important to differentiate nits from lint or dandruff, which flakes away easily).
- Adult lice are difficult to see and appear as small tan or grayish specks, which may crawl fast.

C. Interventions
1. Use a pediculicide product as prescribed; follow package instructions for timing the application and for contraindications for their use in children.
2. Daily removal of nits with an extra-fine-tooth metal nit comb should be done as a control measure after use of the pediculicide product. Gloves should be worn for removal of nits. Hairbrushes or combs should be discarded or soaked in boiling water for 10 minutes or in a commercially available lice-killing product for 1 hour.
3. Reinforce instructions to the parents that siblings may also need treatment; grooming items are not to be shared, and a single comb or brush should be used for each individual child.
4. Reinforce instructions to the parents that bedding and clothing used by the child should be changed daily, laundered in hot water with detergent, and dried in a hot dryer for 20 minutes; this process should continue for 1 week.
5. Reinforce instructions to the parents that nonessential bedding and clothing can be stored in a tightly sealed bag for 2 weeks and then washed.
6. Reinforce instructions to the parents to seal toys that cannot be washed or dry-cleaned in a plastic bag for 2 weeks.
7. Reinforce instructions to the parents that furniture and carpets need to be vacuumed frequently and that the dust bag from the vacuum should be discarded after vacuuming.
8. Reinforce teaching the parents and the child not to share clothing, headwear, brushes, and combs.
9. Lice of the eyelashes or eyebrows may need to be removed manually.

IV. Scabies

A. Description
1. A parasitic skin disorder caused by an infestation of *Sarcoptes scabiei* (itch mite)
2. Endemic among schoolchildren and institutionalized populations as a result of close personal contact
3. Incubation period
   a. Female mite burrows into the epidermis, lays eggs, and dies in the burrow after 4 to 5 weeks.
   b. The eggs hatch in 3 to 5 days, and the larvae migrate to the skin to mature and complete their life cycle.
4. Infectious period: During the course of the infestation

B. Data collection (Box 31-4 and Fig. 31-2)

Scabies is transmitted by close personal contact with an infected person. Household members and contacts of an infected child need to be treated simultaneously.

C. Interventions
1. Topical application of a scabicide such as permethrin (Elimite) kills the mites.
2. Lindane, an alternative product that may be prescribed, should not be used in children younger than 2 years because of the risk of neurotoxicity and seizures.
3. Reinforce instructions to the parents in the application of the scabicide.
4. When permethrin is used, it is applied to cool, dry skin at least 30 minutes after bathing; the cream is massaged thoroughly and gently into all skin surfaces (not just the areas that have the rash) from the head to the soles of the feet (avoid contact with the eyes); left on the skin for 8 to 14 hours; and then removed by bathing. A repeat treatment may be necessary.
5. Household members and contacts of the infected child need to be treated at the same time.

BOX 31-4 Data Collection Findings: Scabies

- Pruritic papular rash
- Burrows on the skin (fine grayish-red lines that may be difficult to see)

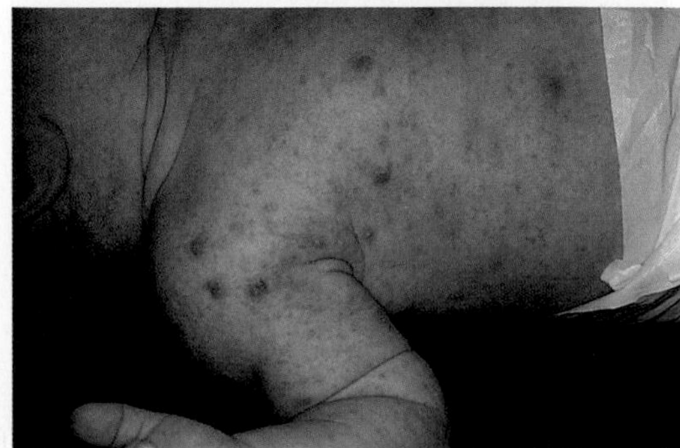

FIGURE 31-2 Scabies rash on an infant. (From Calen JP, Greer KE, Hood AF, Paller AS, Swinyer LJ: *Color atlas of dermatology,* Philadelphia, 1993, Saunders. Courtesy of Dr. Steve Estes.)

6. Reinforce instructions to the parents about the importance of frequent hand washing.
7. Reinforce instructions to the parents that all clothing, bedding, and pillowcases used by the child need to be changed daily; washed in hot water with detergent; dried in a hot dryer; and ironed before reuse; this process should continue for 1 week.
8. Reinforce instructions to the parents that nonwashable toys and other items should be sealed in plastic bags for 4 days.
9. Anti-itch topical treatment may be necessary, and antibiotics may be prescribed if a secondary infection develops.

V. The Burned Child (see Priority Nursing Actions)

A. Pediatric differences (see Chapter 41 for additional information about burns)
   1. Very young children who have been severely burned have a higher mortality rate than older children and adults with comparable burns.
   2. Lower burn temperatures and shorter exposure to heat can cause a more severe burn in a child than an adult because a child's skin is thinner.
   3. The degree of pain experienced by the child and the ability to communicate it will be different than in an adult with the same exposure.
   4. Severely burned children are at increased risk for fluid and heat loss, dehydration, and metabolic acidosis than an adult.
   5. The higher proportion of body fluid to mass in children increases the risk of cardiovascular problems.
   6. Burns involving more than 10% of the total body surface area require some form of fluid resuscitation.
   7. Infants and children are at increased risk for protein and calorie deficiency because they have smaller muscle mass and less body fat than adults.
   8. Scarring is more severe in a child; disturbed body image will be a distinct issue for a child or adolescent, especially as **growth** continues.
   9. An immature immune system presents an increased risk of infection for infants and young children.
   10. A delay in growth may occur following a burn.

B. Extent of burn injury
   1. The rule of nines, used for an adult with a burn injury, gives an inaccurate estimate in children because of the difference in body proportions between children and adults.
   2. In the pediatric client, the extent of the burn is expressed as a percentage of the total body surface area (TBSA) using specific age-related charts. 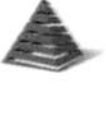 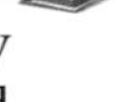

C. Fluid replacement therapy 

To determine adequacy of fluid resuscitation, vital signs (especially heart rate), urine output, adequacy of capillary filling, and sensorium status are assessed.

   1. Fluid replacement is necessary during the initial 24-hour period following the burn injury because of the fluid shifts that occur as a result of the injury.
   2. Several formulas are available to calculate the child's fluid needs, and the formula used depends on the health care provider's preference.
   3. Crystalloid solutions are used during the initial phase of therapy; colloid solutions such as albumin, Plasma-Lyte (combined electrolyte solution), or fresh-frozen plasma are useful in maintaining plasma volume.
   4. See Chapter 41 for additional information related to burns and their management.

PRIORITY NURSING ACTIONS

Actions to Take in the Event of a Major Burn Injury

1. Stop the burning process.
2. Check circulation, airway, and breathing status.
3. Begin resuscitation if necessary.
4. Remove burned clothing and jewelry.
5. Cover the wound with a clean cloth.
6. Keep the child warm.
7. Transport the child to the emergency department.

The initial management of the burn injury begins at the scene of the injury. The first priority is to stop the burning process; this must be done before other interventions. To stop the burning process, flames should be smothered. The child should be placed in a horizontal position because a vertical position may cause the hair to ignite or the inhalation of flames, heat, or smoke. The child should be rolled in a blanket or other article, taking care not to cover the face and head because of the danger of inhaling smoke and fumes. As soon as the flames are extinguished, the child's circulation, airway, and breathing are checked. Measures are taken immediately if resuscitation is necessary. Burned clothing and jewelry are removed to prevent further burning of the skin and disruption of skin integrity, and then the burn is covered with a clean cloth, which prevents contamination of the wound, reduces pain by eliminating air contact, and prevents hypothermia. The child is also kept warm to prevent hypothermia and is immediately transported to the nearest emergency facility.

Reference(s): Hockenberry, M., & Wilson, D. (2013). *Wong's: Essentials of pediatric nursing* (9th ed., p. 1040). St. Louis: Mosby.

CRITICAL THINKING What Should You Do?

Answer: For a child suspected of having impetigo, the nurse should institute strict contact precautions and use standard precautions. The nurse should also implement agency-specific isolation procedures for the hospitalized child. Strict hygiene practices are important because impetigo is a highly contagious condition. The nurse should ensure that all health care workers and visitors are aware of the necessary precautions in order to prevent the spread of infection.

Reference(s): Hockenberry, M., & Wilson, D. (2013). *Wong's: Essentials of pediatric nursing* (9th ed., pp. 1018–1019). St. Louis: Mosby.

PRACTICE QUESTIONS

296. The school nurse prepares a list of home care instructions for the parents of school children who have been diagnosed with pediculosis capitis (head lice). Which should be included in the list?

1. Use anti-lice sprays on all bedding and furniture.
2. Use a pediculicide shampoo and repeat treatment in 14 days.
3. Launder all the bedding and clothing in cold water and dry on low heat.
4. Vacuum floors, play areas, and furniture to remove any hairs that may carry live nits.

297. A mother of a 3-year-old child tells the nurse that the child has been continuously scratching the skin and has developed a rash. On data collection, which finding indicates that the child may have scabies?

1. Fine, grayish-red lines
2. Purple-colored lesions
3. Thick, honey-colored crusts
4. Clusters of fluid-filled vesicles

298. Permethrin (Elimite) is prescribed for a 4-year-old child with a diagnosis of scabies. The nurse reinforces instructions to the mother regarding the use of this treatment. Which instruction is appropriate?

1. Apply the lotion and leave it on for 4 hours.
2. Apply the lotion to the hair, the face, and the entire body.
3. The child should wear no clothing while the lotion is in place.
4. Apply the lotion to cool, dry skin at least half an hour after bathing.

299. A corticosteroid cream is prescribed by a health care provider for a child with atopic dermatitis (eczema). The nurse reinforces instructions to the mother regarding how to apply the cream. Which instruction is appropriate?

1. Apply the cream over the entire body.
2. Apply a thick layer of cream to affected areas only.
3. Avoid cleansing the area before applying the cream.
4. Apply a thin layer of cream, and rub it into the area thoroughly.

300. The nurse assists in planning care for a child who sustained a burn injury. The nurse plans care based on which accurate statement?

1. Scarring is not as severe in a child as in an adult.
2. Children are at a lower risk of infection than adults because of their strong immune systems.
3. Lower burn temperatures and shorter exposure to heat can cause a more severe burn in a child than an adult because a child's skin is thinner.
4. Infants and children are at decreased risk for protein and calorie deficiency because they have smaller muscle mass and less body fat than adults.

ANSWERS

296. 4

Rationale: Thorough home cleaning is necessary to remove any remaining lice or nits. Anti-lice sprays are unnecessary. Additionally, they should never be used on bedding, furniture, or a child. The pediculicide product needs to be used as prescribed, and the parents are instructed to follow package instructions for timing the application and for contraindications for their use in children. Bedding and linens should be washed with hot water and dried on a hot setting.

Test-Taking Strategy: Focus on the subject, home care instructions for pediculosis capitis. Eliminate option 1, knowing that anti-lice sprays should not be used. The pediculicide product needs to be used based on the manufacturer's instructions. Knowing that bedding and linens should be washed in hot water and dried on a high heat setting will eliminate option 3.

Review: the home care instructions for the child with pediculosis capitis.

Level of Cognitive Ability: Applying

Client Needs: Safe and Effective Care Environment

Integrated Process: Teaching and Learning

Content Area: Child Health: Infectious and Communicable Diseases

Priority Concepts: Infection, Safety

Reference(s): Hockenberry, Wilson (2013), p. 1028; McKinney et al (2013), pp. 1315–1316.

297. 1

Rationale: Scabies appears as burrows or fine, grayish-red lines. They may be difficult to see if they are obscured by excoriation and inflammation. Purple-colored lesions may be indicative of various disorders, including systemic conditions. Thick, honey-colored crusts are characteristic of impetigo. Clusters of fluid-filled vesicles are seen in clients with herpes virus.
Test-Taking Strategy: Focus on the **subject**, characteristics of scabies infestation. Recalling that scabies infestation produces burrows will direct you to the correct option. **Review:** the characteristics of scabies.
Level of Cognitive Ability: Understanding
Client Needs: Physiological Integrity
Integrated Process: Nursing Process/Data Collection
Content Area: Child Health: Infectious and Communicable Diseases
Priority Concepts: Infection, Tissue Integrity
Reference(s): Hockenberry, Wilson (2013), pp. 1024, 1026; Jarvis (2012), p. 248.

298. 4

Rationale: Permethrin is applied from the neck downward, with care taken to ensure that the soles of the feet, the areas behind the ears, and the areas under the toenails and fingernails are covered. The lotion should be kept on for 8 to 14 hours, and then the child should be given a bath. The lotion should be applied at least 30 minutes after bathing, and it should be applied only to cool, dry skin. The child should be clothed during treatment.
Test-Taking Strategy: Focus on the **subject**, application of permethrin. Reading options 2 and 3 carefully and noting the words *entire* and *no* will assist you with eliminating these options. From the remaining options, recalling the treatment time for this medication will direct you to the correct option. Review: permethrin treatment.
Level of Cognitive Ability: Applying
Client Needs: Physiological Integrity
Integrated Process: Teaching and Learning
Content Area: Child Health: Infectious and Communicable Diseases
Priority Concepts: Client Education, Safety
Reference(s): McKinney et al (2013), p. 1317.

299. 4

Rationale: Corticosteroid cream should be applied sparingly and rubbed into the area thoroughly. The affected area should be cleansed gently before application. The cream should not be applied over extensive areas. Systemic absorption is more likely to occur with extensive application.
Test-Taking Strategy: Focus on the **subject**, application of a corticosteroid cream for eczema. Eliminate option 1 because the cream should be applied only to the area that is affected. Eliminate option 2 because of the words *thick* and *only*. Eliminate option 3 because it does not make sense to avoid cleansing an affected area. **Review:** treatment for eczema.
Level of Cognitive Ability: Applying
Client Needs: Physiological Integrity
Integrated Process: Teaching and Learning
Content Area: Child Health: Infectious and Communicable Diseases
Priority Concepts: Safety, Tissue Integrity
Reference(s): Lilley et al (2014), p. 908; McKinney et al (2013), p. 1304.

300. 3

Rationale: Lower burn temperatures and shorter exposure to heat can cause a more severe burn in a child than an adult because a child's skin is thinner. Scarring is more severe in a child; additionally, disturbed body image will be a distinct issue for a child or adolescent, especially as growth continues. An immature immune system presents an increased risk of infection for infants and young children. Infants and children are at increased risk for protein and calorie deficiency because they have smaller muscle mass and less body fat than adults.
Test-Taking Strategy: Focus on the **subject**, the effect of a burn injury in a child. Read each option carefully. Thinking about the anatomy and physiology of an infant and child will assist in selecting the correct option. **Review:** **pediatric burn injury.**
Level of Cognitive Ability: Applying
Client Needs: Physiological Integrity
Integrated Process: Nursing Process/Planning
Content Area: Critical Care: Emergency Situations
Priority Concepts: Development, Tissue Integrity
Reference(s): McKinney et al (2013), p. 1323.

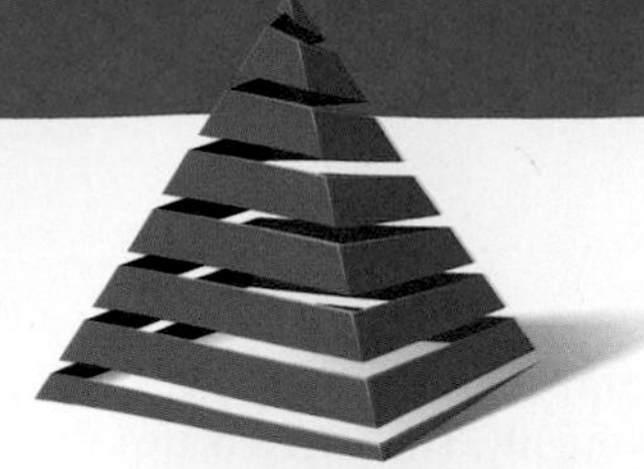

CHAPTER 32

Hematological and Oncological Disorders

CRITICAL THINKING What Should You Do?

A child with hemophilia who has been in a motor vehicle crash is admitted to the pediatric unit. What should the nurse do in the care of this child?

Answer located on p. 379.

I. Sickle Cell Anemia

A. Description

1. Sickle cell anemia constitutes a group of diseases termed *hemoglobinopathies,* in which hemoglobin A is partly or completely replaced by abnormal sickle hemoglobin S.
2. It is caused by the inheritance of a gene for a structurally abnormal portion of the hemoglobin chain.
3. Risk factors include having parents heterozygous for hemoglobin S or being of African-American descent.
4. For screening purposes the sickle-turbidity test (Sickledex) is frequently used because it can be performed on blood from a finger stick and yields accurate results in 3 minutes. However, if the test result is positive, hemoglobin (Hgb) electrophoresis is necessary to distinguish between children with the trait and those with the disease.
5. Hemoglobin S is sensitive to changes in the oxygen content of the red blood cell.
6. Insufficient oxygen causes the cells to assume a sickle shape, and the cells become rigid and clumped together, obstructing capillary blood flow (Fig. 32-1).
7. The clinical manifestations occur primarily as a result of obstruction caused by sickled red blood cells and increased red blood cell destruction.

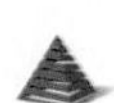

8. Situations that precipitate sickling include fever, dehydration, and emotional or physical stress; any condition that increases the need for oxygen or alters the transport of oxygen can result in sickle cell crisis (acute exacerbation).
9. Sickle cell crises are acute exacerbations of the disease, which vary considerably in severity and frequency; these include vaso-occlusive crisis, splenic sequestration, hyperhemolytic crisis, and aplastic crisis.
10. The sickling response is reversible under conditions of adequate oxygenation and hydration; after repeated sickling, the cell becomes permanently sickled.
11. A multidisciplinary approach to care is needed, and care focuses on the prevention (preventing exposure to infection and maintaining normal hydration) and treatment (hydration, oxygen, pain management, and bed rest) of the crisis.

B. Sickle cell crisis: Data collection (see Box 32-1)

C. Interventions

1. Maintain adequate hydration and blood flow with oral and intravenous (IV) administered fluids. Electrolyte replacement is also provided as needed; without adequate hydration pain will not be controlled.
2. Administer oxygen, as prescribed, to increase tissue perfusion; blood transfusions may also be prescribed.
3. Assist to administer analgesics as prescribed (around the clock).
4. Assist the child with assuming a comfortable position so that the child keeps the extremities extended to promote venous return; elevate the head of the bed no more than 30 degrees, avoid putting strain on painful joints, and do not raise the knee gatch of the bed.
5. Encourage the consumption of a high-calorie, high-protein diet with folic acid supplementation.
6. Assist to administer antibiotics, as prescribed, to prevent infection.
7. Monitor for complications, including increasing anemia, decreased perfusion, and shock (i.e., mental status changes, pallor, and vital sign changes).

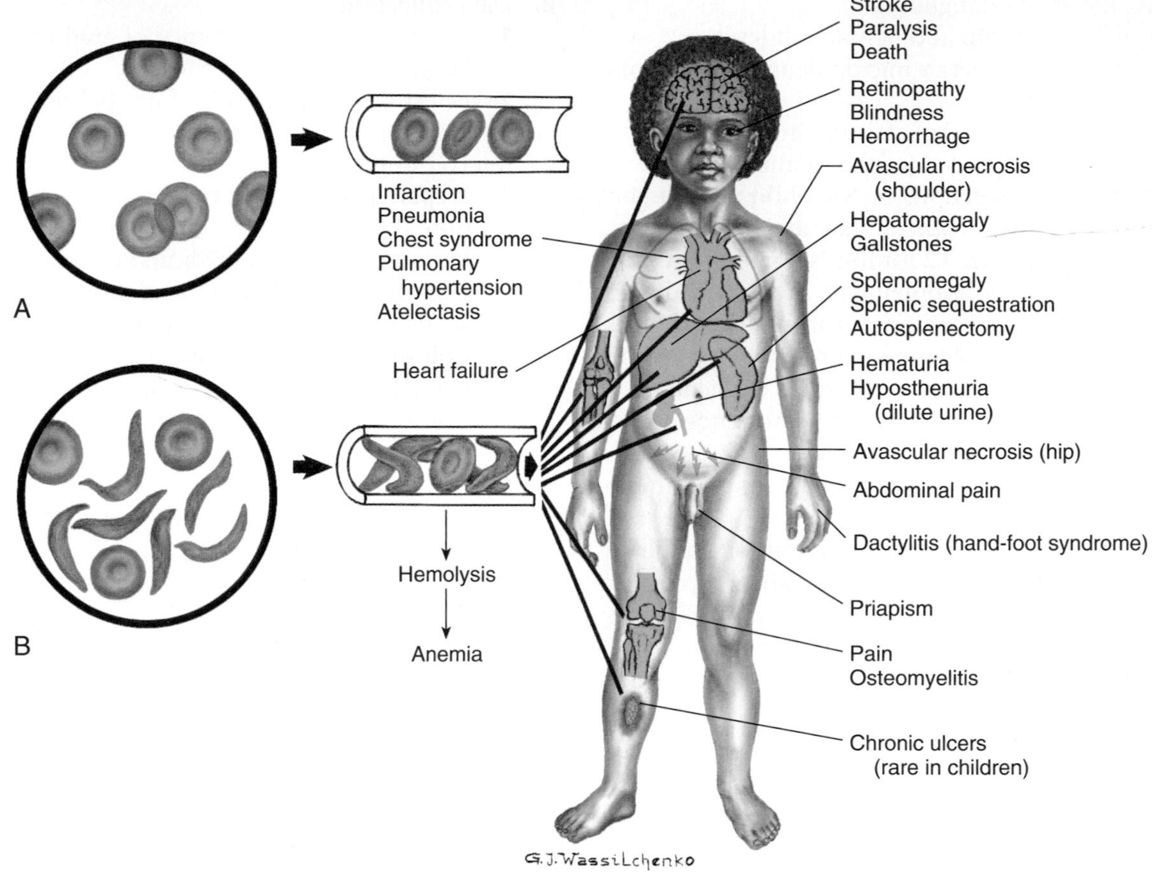

FIGURE 32-1 Differences between **A**, normal red blood cells and **B**, sickled red blood cells in circulation with related complications. (From Hockenberry M, Wilson D: *Nursing care of infants and children,* ed 9, St. Louis, 2013, Mosby.)

BOX 32-1 Sickle Cell Crisis

Vaso-occlusive Crisis

Caused by stasis of blood with clumping of cells in the microcirculation, ischemia, and infarction

Manifestations: Fever; painful swelling of hands, feet, and joints; and abdominal pain

Splenic Sequestration

Caused by pooling and clumping of blood in the spleen (hypersplenism)

Manifestations: Profound anemia, hypovolemia, and shock

Hyperhemolytic Crisis

An accelerated rate of red blood cell destruction

Manifestations: Anemia, jaundice, and reticulocytosis

Aplastic Crisis

Caused by diminished production and increased destruction of red blood cells, triggered by viral infection or depletion of folic acid

Manifestations: Profound anemia and pallor

8. Reinforce instructions to the child and parents about the early signs and symptoms of crisis and the measures to prevent a crisis.
9. Emphasize the need to maintain strict adherence to immunization schedules; ensure that the child receives pneumococcal and meningococcal **vaccines** and an annual influenza vaccine because of the susceptibility to infection from functional asplenia.
10. A splenectomy may be necessary for those who experience recurrent splenic sequestration.
11. Inform the parents of the **hereditary** aspects of the disorder.

Administration of meperidine (Demerol) for pain is avoided because of the risk of normeperidine-induced seizures.

II. Iron Deficiency Anemia

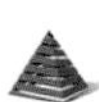

A. Description
1. Iron stores are depleted, which results in a decreased supply of iron for the manufacture of hemoglobin in RBCs.
2. Commonly results from blood loss, increased metabolic demands, syndromes of gastrointestinal (GI) malabsorption, and dietary inadequacy

B. Data collection
1. Pallor

2. Weakness and fatigue
3. Low hemoglobin and hematocrit levels
4. Red blood cells that are microcytic and hypochromic

C. Interventions
1. Increase oral intake of iron; iron-fortified formula will be needed for the infant.
2. Reinforce instructions to the child and parents regarding food choices that are high in iron. (Refer to Chapter 12 for foods high in iron.)
3. Administer iron supplements as prescribed.
4. Intramuscular injections of iron (using Z-track method) or intravenous administration of iron may be prescribed in severe cases of anemia.
5. Reinforce teaching the parents about how to administer the iron supplements.
    a. Give them between meals for maximum absorption.
    b. Give them with a multivitamin or fruit juice, because vitamin C increases absorption.
    c. Do not give them with milk or antacids, because these items decrease absorption.
    d. Reinforce instructions to the child and parents about the side effects of iron supplements (i.e., black stools, constipation, foul aftertaste).
    e. Emphasize the importance of keeping the medication in a safe place out of reach of the child (iron overdose can result if an excess amount is consumed).

Liquid iron preparation stains the teeth. Teach the parents and child that liquid iron should be taken through a straw and that the teeth should be brushed after administration.

III. Aplastic Anemia

A. Description
1. A deficiency of circulating erythrocytes and all other formed elements of blood, resulting from the arrested development of cells within the bone marrow
2. It can be primary (present at birth) or secondary (acquired).
3. Several possible causes exist, including chronic exposure to myelotoxic agents, viruses, infection, autoimmune disorders, and allergic states.
4. The definitive diagnosis is determined by bone marrow aspiration, which shows the conversion of red bone marrow to yellow fatty bone marrow.
5. Therapeutic management focuses on restoring function to the bone marrow and involves immunosuppressive therapy and bone marrow transplantation (treatment of choice if a suitable donor exists).
6. If the cause is a myelotoxic medication that is being administered for another purpose, the medication may be discontinued to improve bone marrow function.

B. Data collection
1. Pancytopenia (a deficiency of erythrocytes, leukocytes, and thrombocytes)
2. Petechiae, purpura, bleeding, pallor, weakness, tachycardia, and fatigue

C. Interventions
1. Prepare the child for bone marrow transplantation, if planned.
2. Immunosuppressive medications: Antilymphocyte globulin or antithymocyte globulin may be prescribed to suppress the autoimmune response.
3. Colony-stimulating factors may be prescribed to enhance bone marrow production.
4. Corticosteroids and cyclosporine (Sandimmune) may be prescribed.
5. Blood or platelet transfusions may be prescribed.
6. Advise the parents to obtain a Medic-Alert bracelet for the child.

IV. Hemophilia

A. Description
1. Refers to a group of bleeding disorders resulting from a deficiency of specific coagulation proteins
2. Identifying the specific coagulation deficiency is important so that definitive treatment with the specific replacement agent can be implemented; aggressive replacement therapy is initiated to prevent the chronic crippling effects from joint bleeding.
3. The most common types include factor VIII deficiency (hemophilia A or classic hemophilia) and factor IX deficiency (hemophilia B or Christmas disease).
4. Hemophilia is transmitted as an X-linked recessive disorder (it may also occur as a result of a gene mutation).
5. Carrier females pass on the defect to affected males; female offspring are rarely born with the disorder but may be if they inherit an affected gene from their mother and are offspring of a father with hemophilia.
6. The primary treatment is the replacement of the missing clotting factor; additional medications, such as those to relieve pain, may be prescribed, depending on the source of bleeding.

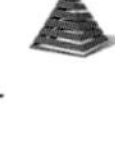

B. Data collection
1. Abnormal bleeding in response to trauma or surgery (sometimes is detected after circumcision)
2. Joint bleeding that causes pain, tenderness, swelling, and a limited range of motion
3. Tendency to bruise easily
4. Results of tests that measure platelet function are normal; results of tests that measure clotting factor function may be abnormal.

C. Interventions
1. Monitor for bleeding and maintain bleeding precautions.

2. Prepare to assist to administer replacement factors as prescribed.
3. DDAVP (1-deamino-8-D-arginine vasopressin), a synthetic form of vasopressin, increases plasma factor VIII and may be prescribed to treat mild hemophilia.
4. Monitor for joint pain; immobilize the affected extremity if joint pain occurs.
5. Monitor the neurological status; the child is at risk for intracranial hemorrhage.
6. Monitor the urine for hematuria.
7. Control bleeding by immobilization, elevation, and the application of ice; in addition, apply pressure (15 minutes) for superficial bleeding.
8. Reinforce instructions to the child and parents about the signs of internal bleeding and how to control bleeding if it occurs.
9. Reinforce instructions to the parents regarding activities for the child, emphasizing the avoidance of contact sports and the need for protective devices while learning to walk; assist in developing an appropriate exercise plan.
10. Reinforce instructions to the child to wear protective devices such as helmets and knee and elbow pads when participating in sports such as bicycling and skating.

V. von Willebrand's Disease

A. Description

1. A hereditary bleeding disorder characterized by a deficiency of or a defect in the protein called von Willebrand's factor (vWF)
2. The disorder causes platelets to adhere to damaged endothelium; the vWF protein also serves as a carrier protein for factor VIII.
3. It is characterized by an increased tendency to bleed from the mucous membranes.

B. Data collection

1. Epistaxis
2. Gum bleeding
3. Easy bruising
4. Excessive menstrual bleeding

C. Interventions

1. Treatment and care are similar to those measures implemented for hemophilia, including the administration of clotting factors.
2. Provide emotional support to the child and parents, especially if the child is experiencing an episode of bleeding.

A child with a bleeding disorder needs to wear a Medic-Alert bracelet.

VI. β-Thalassemia Major (Box 32-2)

A. Description

1. An autosomal-recessive disorder characterized by the reduced production of one of the globin chains in the synthesis of hemoglobin (both parents must be carriers to produce a child with β-thalassemia major)

BOX 32-2 Types of β-Thalassemia

Thalassemia minor: Asymptomatic silent carrier case
Thalassemia trait: Produces a mild microcytic anemia
Thalassemia intermedia: Manifested as splenomegaly and moderate to severe anemia
Thalassemia major: Results in severe anemia requiring transfusion support to sustain life (also known as Cooley's anemia)

2. The incidence is highest in individuals of Mediterranean descent, such as Italians, Greeks, Syrians, and their offspring.
3. Treatment is supportive; the goal of therapy is to maintain normal hemoglobin levels by the administration of blood transfusions.
4. Bone marrow transplantation may be offered as an alternative therapy.
5. A splenectomy may be performed in a child with severe splenomegaly who requires repeated transfusions (assists in relieving abdominal pressure and may increase the life span of supplemental red blood cells).

B. Data collection 

1. Frontal bossing
2. Maxillary prominence
3. Wide-set eyes with a flattened nose
4. Greenish-yellow skin tone
5. Hepatosplenomegaly
6. Severe anemia
7. Microcytic, hypochromic RBCs

C. Interventions

1. Blood transfusions may be prescribed.
2. Monitor for iron overload, and administer chelation therapy, which may be prescribed to treat iron overload and to prevent organ damage from the elevated levels of iron caused by the multiple transfusion therapy.
3. If the child has had a splenectomy, instruct the parents to report any signs of infection because of the risk of sepsis.
4. Ensure that parents understand the importance of the child receiving pneumococcal and meningococcal vaccines in addition to an annual influenza vaccine and the regularly scheduled vaccines.
5. Provide resources for genetic counseling.

VII. Leukemia 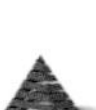

A. Description (also refer to Chapter 43)

1. Malignant increase in the number of leukocytes, usually at an immature stage, in the bone marrow

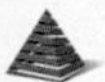

2. In leukemia, proliferating immature white blood cells (WBCs) depress the bone marrow, causing anemia from decreased erythrocytes, infection from neutropenia, and bleeding from decreased platelet production (thrombocytopenia).
3. The cause is unknown and appears to involve the gene damage of cells, thus leading to the transformation of cells from a normal state to a malignant state.
4. Risk factors include genetic, viral, immunological, and environmental factors and exposure to radiation, chemicals, and medications.
5. Acute lymphocytic leukemia is the most frequent type of cancer in children.
6. Leukemia is more common among boys than girls after 1 year of age.
7. Prognosis depends on various factors such as age at diagnosis, initial white blood cell count, type of cell involved, and sex of the child.
8. Treatment involves chemotherapy and possibly radiation and hematopoietic stem cell transplantation.

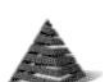

B. Data collection
1. Infiltration of the bone marrow causes fever, pallor, fatigue, anorexia, hemorrhage (usually petechiae), and bone and joint pain; pathological fractures can occur as a result of bone marrow invasion with leukemic cells.
2. Signs of infection as a result of neutropenia
3. Hepatosplenomegaly and lymphadenopathy
4. Normal, elevated, or low white blood cell count, depending on the presence of infection or of immature versus mature white blood cells
5. Decreased hemoglobin and hematocrit levels
6. Decreased platelet count
7. Positive bone marrow biopsy identifying leukemic blast (immature) phase cells
8. Signs of increased intracranial pressure occur as a result of central nervous system involvement (Refer to XII. Brain Tumors)
9. Signs of cranial nerve (cranial nerve VII, the facial nerve, is most commonly affected) or spinal nerve involvement; signs and symptoms relate to the area involved
10. Signs and symptoms that indicate the invasion of leukemic cells in the kidneys, testes, prostate, ovaries, GI tract, and lungs

C. Infection (Box 32-3)
1. Infection can occur through self-contamination or cross-contamination.
2. Most common sites of infection are the skin (any break in the skin is a potential site of infection), respiratory tract, and gastrointestinal (GI) tract.

D. Bleeding (Box 32-4)
1. Platelet transfusions are generally reserved for active bleeding episodes that do not respond to local treatment and that may occur during induction or relapse therapy.
2. Packed red blood cells may be prescribed for a child with severe blood loss.

E. Fatigue and nutrition
1. Assist the child with selecting a well-balanced diet.

BOX 32-3 Protecting the Child from Infection

Initiate protective isolation procedures.
Maintain frequent and thorough hand washing.
Maintain the child in a private room with high-efficiency particulate air filtration or laminar airflow system, if possible.
Be sure that the child's room is cleaned daily.
Use strict aseptic technique for all nursing procedures.
Limit the number of caregivers entering the child's room, and ensure that anyone entering the child's room is wearing a mask.
Keep supplies for the child separate from supplies for other children.
Reduce exposure to environmental organisms by eliminating raw fruits and vegetables and fresh flowers and by not leaving standing water in the child's room.
Assist the child with daily bathing with the use of antimicrobial soap.
Assist the child with performing oral hygiene frequently.
Monitor for signs and symptoms of infection.
Monitor the temperature, pulse, and blood pressure.
Change wound dressings daily, and inspect wounds for redness, swelling, or drainage.
Monitor the urine for color and cloudiness.
Monitor the skin and oral mucous membranes for signs of infection.
Check the lung sounds.
Encourage the child to cough and deep breathe.
Monitor the white blood cell and the neutrophil count.
Notify the health care provider (HCP) if signs of infection are present; prepare to obtain specimens for the culture of open lesions, urine, and sputum.
Initiate a bowel program to prevent constipation and rectal trauma.
Avoid invasive procedures, such as injections, rectal temperatures, and urinary catheterization.
Assist to administer antibiotic, antifungal, and antiviral medication, as prescribed.
Assist to administer granulocyte colony-stimulating factor, as prescribed.
Reinforce instructions to the parents to keep the child away from crowds and those with infections.
Reinforce instructions to the parents that the child should not receive immunization with a live virus (measles, mumps, rubella, polio) because if the immune system is depressed, the attenuated virus can result in a life-threatening infection; also, the child should not receive the varicella vaccine. The Salk (inactivated) vaccine for poliomyelitis may be administered.
Reinforce instructions to the parents to inform the teacher that they should be notified immediately if a case of a communicable disease occurs in another child at school.

BOX 32-4 Protecting the Child from Bleeding

Examine the child for signs and symptoms of bleeding.
Handle the child gently.
Measure the abdominal girth, which can indicate internal hemorrhage.
Reinforce instructions to the child to use a soft toothbrush and to avoid dental floss.
Provide soft foods that are cool to warm in temperature.
Avoid injections, if possible, to prevent trauma to the skin and bleeding.
Apply firm and gentle pressure to a needle-stick site for at least 10 minutes.
Pad side rails and sharp corners of the bed and other furniture.
Discourage the child from engaging in activities that involve the use of objects that can be harmful.
Reinforce instructions to the child to avoid constrictive or tight clothing.
Use caution when taking the blood pressure to prevent skin injury.
Reinforce instructions to the child to avoid blowing his or her nose.
Avoid rectal suppositories, enemas, and rectal thermometers; initiate a bowel program to prevent constipation and rectal trauma.
Examine all body fluids and excrement for the presence of blood.
Count the number of pads or tampons used if the adolescent girl is menstruating.
Reinforce instructions to the child regarding the signs and symptoms of bleeding.
Reinforce instructions to the parents to avoid administering nonsteroidal anti-inflammatory drugs and products that contain aspirin to the child.

2. Provide small meals that require little chewing and will not be irritating to the oral mucosa.
3. If the child cannot take oral feedings, parenteral nutrition or enteral feedings may be prescribed.
4. Assist the child with self-care and mobility activities.
5. Allow for adequate rest periods during care.
6. Avoid performing nursing care activities unless they are essential.

F. Chemotherapy
1. Monitor for severe bone marrow suppression; during the period of greatest bone marrow suppression (the nadir), blood counts will be extremely low.
2. Monitor for infection and bleeding.
3. Protect the child from life-threatening infections.
4. Monitor for nausea, vomiting, and alterations in bowel function.
5. Administer stool softeners as prescribed and if needed to prevent straining and resultant bleeding if constipation occurs.
6. Provide rectal hygiene gently as needed.
7. Assist to administer antiemetics before beginning chemotherapy as prescribed.
8. Monitor for signs of dehydration.
9. Monitor for signs of hemorrhagic cystitis.
10. Monitor for signs of peripheral neuropathy.
11. Check oral mucous membranes for mucositis; administer frequent mouth rinses per agency procedure and as prescribed to promote healing and/or prevent infection (local oral anesthetics may also be prescribed).
12. Reinforce instructions to the parents regarding the signs and symptoms to monitor after chemotherapy and when to notify the health care provider (HCP).
13. Inform the parents that hair loss may occur from chemotherapy; the hair will regrow in 3 to 6 months and may be a slightly different color or texture.
14. Reinforce instructions to the parents about the care of a central venous access device, as necessary. (Refer to Chapter 13 for information on central venous access devices.)
15. Listen to the child and family, and encourage them to verbalize their feelings and express their concerns.
16. Introduce the family to other families of children with cancer if appropriate.
17. Consult social services and chaplains, as necessary.

Monitor a child receiving chemotherapy closely for signs of infection. Infection is a major cause of death in the immunosuppressed child.

VIII. Hodgkin's Disease

A. Description
1. A malignancy of the lymph nodes that originates in a single lymph node or a single chain of nodes (Fig. 32-2).
2. It predictably metastasizes to nonnodal or extralymphatic sites, especially the spleen, liver, bone marrow, lungs, and mediastinum.
3. Characterized by the presence of Reed-Sternberg cells in the lymph nodes 
4. Peak incidence is in midadolescence.
5. Possible causes include viral infections and previous exposure to alkylating chemical agents.
6. The prognosis is excellent, with long-term survival rates depending on the stage of the disease.
7. The primary treatment modalities are radiation and chemotherapy; each may be used alone or in combination, depending on the clinical staging of the disease.

B. Data collection 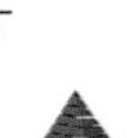
1. Painless enlargement of the lymph nodes
2. Enlarged, firm, nontender, movable nodes in the supraclavicular area; in children, the sentinel node located near the left clavicle may be the first enlarged node.
3. Nonproductive cough as a result of mediastinal lymphadenopathy

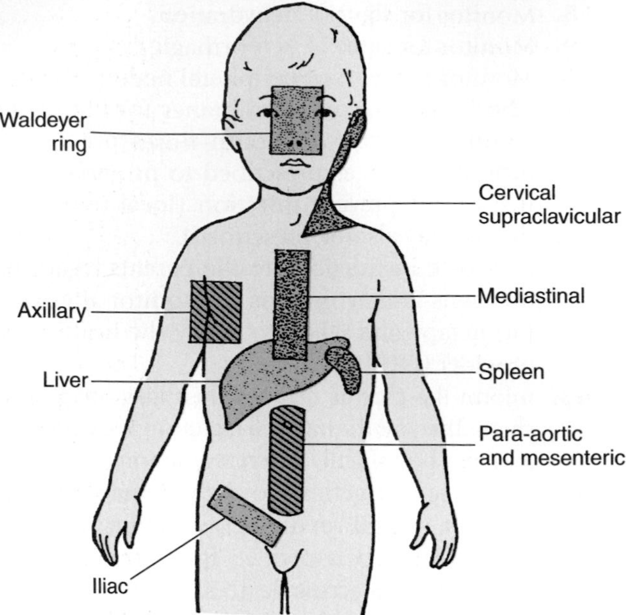

FIGURE 32-2 Main areas of lymphadenopathy and organ involvement in Hodgkin's disease. (From Hockenberry M, Wilson D: *Wong's: Essentials of pediatric nursing*, ed 9, St. Louis, 2013, Mosby.)

4. Abdominal pain as a result of enlarged retroperitoneal nodes
5. Advanced lymph node and extralymphatic involvement may cause systemic symptoms, such as low-grade and/or intermittent fever, anorexia, nausea, weight loss, night sweats, and pruritus.

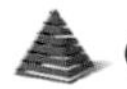

6. Positive biopsy of a lymph node (presence of Reed-Sternberg cells) and positive bone marrow biopsy
7. Computed tomography scan of the liver, spleen, and bone marrow may be done to detect metastasis.

C. Interventions
1. For early stages without mediastinal node involvement, the treatment of choice is usually extensive external radiation of the involved lymph node regions.
2. With more extensive disease, radiation in combination with multiagent chemotherapy is used.
3. Monitor for drug-induced pancytopenia, which increases the risk for infection, bleeding, and anemia.
4. Protect the child from infection.
5. Provide a safe, hazard-free environment.
6. Monitor for side effects related to chemotherapy or radiation; the most common side effect of extensive irradiation is malaise, which can be difficult for older children and adolescents to tolerate both physically and psychologically (Table 32-1).
7. Monitor for nausea and vomiting; administer antiemetics, as prescribed.

TABLE 32-1 Side Effects of Radiation Therapy and Nursing Interventions

Body Area and Side Effects	Interventions
Gastrointestinal Tract	
Anorexia	Encourage fluids and foods as best tolerated. Provide small, frequent meals. Monitor for weight loss.
Nausea, vomiting	Administer antiemetics around the clock. Monitor for dehydration.
Mucosal ulceration	Provide soothing oral hygiene and prescribed mouth rinses. Topical anesthetic may be prescribed.
Diarrhea	Administer antispasmodics and antidiarrheal preparations as prescribed. Monitor for dehydration.
Skin	
Alopecia (hair loss)	Introduce idea of a wig. Provide scalp hygiene. Stress the need for head covering in cold weather.
Dry or moist desquamation	Keep the skin clean. Wash the skin daily, using a mild soap sparingly. Do not remove skin markings for radiation. Avoid exposure to the sun and other extreme temperature changes. For dryness, apply lubricant as prescribed.
Urinary Bladder	
Cystitis	Encourage fluid intake and frequent voiding. Monitor for hematuria.
Bone Marrow	
Myelosuppression	Monitor for fever. Administer antibiotics as prescribed. Avoid the use of suppositories, enemas, and rectal temperatures. Institute neutropenic or bleeding precautions as needed. Monitor for signs of anemia.

Adapted from Hockenberry M, Wilson D: *Wong's: Nursing care of infants and children*, ed 9, St. Louis, 2013, Mosby; and McKinney E, James S, Murray S, Ashwill J: *Maternal-child nursing*, ed 4, St. Louis, 2013, Saunders.

IX. Nephroblastoma (Wilms' Tumor)

A. Description
1. Wilms' tumor is the most common intraabdominal and kidney tumor of childhood; it may present unilaterally and localized or bilaterally, sometimes with metastasis to other organs.
2. The peak incidence is at 3 years of age.
3. Occurrence is associated with a genetic inheritance and with several congenital anomalies.

4. Therapeutic management includes a combination treatment of surgery (partial to total nephrectomy) and chemotherapy with or without radiation, depending on the clinical stage and histologic pattern of the tumor.

B. Data collection
1. A swelling or mass within the abdomen; the mass is characteristically firm, nontender, confined to one side, and deep within the flank.
2. Urinary retention and/or hematuria
3. Anemia caused by hemorrhage within the tumor
4. Pallor, anorexia, and lethargy resulting from anemia
5. Hypertension, caused by the secretion of excess amounts of renin by the tumor
6. Weight loss and fever
7. Symptoms of lung involvement, such as dyspnea, shortness of breath, and pain in the chest, if metastasis has occurred

C. Preoperative interventions
1. Monitor the vital signs, particularly the blood pressure.
2. Avoid the palpation of the abdomen; place a sign at the bedside that reads as follows: "Do not palpate abdomen."
3. Measure the abdominal girth at least once daily.

D. Postoperative interventions
1. Monitor the temperature and blood pressure closely.
2. Monitor for signs of hemorrhage and infection.
3. Monitor strict intake and output closely.
4. Monitor for abdominal distention, bowel sounds, and other signs of GI activity because of the risk for intestinal obstruction.

Avoid palpation of the abdomen in a child with Wilms' tumor and be cautious when bathing, moving, or handling the child. It is important to keep the encapsulated tumor intact. Rupture of the tumor can cause the cancer cells to spread throughout the abdomen, lymph system, and bloodstream.

X. Neuroblastoma

A. Description
1. A tumor that originates from the embryonic neural crest cells that normally give rise to the adrenal medulla and the sympathetic ganglia.
2. Most tumors develop in the adrenal gland or the retroperitoneal sympathetic chain; other sites may be within the head, neck, chest, or pelvis.
3. Most children present with the tumor before 10 years of age. Most presenting signs are caused by the tumor compressing adjacent normal tissue and organs.
4. Diagnostic evaluation is aimed at locating the primary site of the tumor.
5. The prognosis is poor because of the frequency of invasiveness of the tumor and because, in most cases, the diagnosis is not made until after metastasis has occurred; the younger the child at diagnosis, the better the survival rate.
6. Surgery is performed to remove as much of the tumor as possible and to obtain samples for biopsy; in early stages, complete surgical removal of the tumor is the treatment of choice.
7. Surgery is usually limited to biopsy in the later stages because of the extensive metastasis.
8. Radiation is commonly used with late-stage disease and provides palliation for metastatic lesions in the bones, lungs, liver, or brain.
9. Chemotherapy is used for treatment for extensive local or disseminated disease.

B. Data collection: Signs and symptoms depend on the location of the primary tumor.
1. Firm, nontender, irregular mass in the abdomen that crosses the midline
2. Urinary frequency or retention from the compression of the kidney, ureter, or bladder
3. Lymphadenopathy, especially in the cervical and supraclavicular area
4. Bone pain if skeletal involvement occurs
5. Supraorbital ecchymosis (raccoon eyes), periorbital edema, and exophthalmos as a result of the invasion of retrobulbar soft tissue
6. Pallor, weakness, irritability, anorexia, weight loss
7. Signs of respiratory impairment (thoracic lesion)
8. Signs of neurological impairment (intracranial lesion)
9. Paralysis from the compression of the spinal cord

C. Preoperative interventions
1. Monitor for signs and symptoms related to the location of the tumor.
2. Provide emotional support to the child and parents.

D. Postoperative interventions
1. Monitor for postoperative complications related to the location (organ) of the surgery.
2. Monitor for complications related to chemotherapy or radiation, if prescribed.
3. Provide support for the parents, and encourage them to express their feelings; many parents feel guilt for not having recognized signs in the child earlier.
4. Refer the parents to appropriate community services.

XI. Osteosarcoma (Osteogenic Sarcoma)

A. Description
1. The most common bone cancer in children 

Pediatric

2. Usually found in the metaphysis of the long bones, especially in the lower extremities, with most tumors occurring in the femur
3. Peak age of incidence is between 10 and 25 years.
4. Symptoms during the earliest stage are almost always attributed to extremity injury or normal growing pains.
5. Treatment may include surgical resection to save a limb or to remove affected tissue, or amputation.
6. Chemotherapy is used to treat the cancer and may be used before and after surgery.

B. Data collection
1. Localized pain at the affected site (may be severe or dull) that may be attributed to trauma or the vague complaint of "growing pains"; pain is often relieved by a flexed position.
2. Palpable mass
3. Limping if weight-bearing limb is affected
4. Progressively limited range of motion; child curtails physical activity.
5. Child may be unable to hold heavy objects because of their weight and resultant pain in the affected extremity.
6. Pathological fractures at the tumor site

C. Interventions
1. Prepare the child and family for prescribed treatment modalities, which may include surgical resection to remove affected tissue, amputation, and chemotherapy.
2. Communicate honesty and provide support to the child and family.
3. Prepare for prosthetic fitting, as necessary.
4. Assist the child with dealing with self-image problems.
5. Reinforce instructions to the child and parents about the potential development of phantom limb pain that may occur after amputation, characterized by tingling, itching, and a painful sensation in the area where the limb was amputated.

XII. Brain Tumors

A. Description
1. An infratentorial (below the tentorium cerebelli) tumor, the most common brain tumor, is located in the posterior third of the brain (primarily in the cerebellum or brainstem) and accounts for the frequency of symptoms resulting from increased intracranial pressure (ICP).
2. A supratentorial tumor is located within the anterior two thirds of the brain—mainly the cerebrum.
3. The signs and symptoms of a brain tumor depend on its anatomical location and size and, to some extent, the age of the child; a number of tests may be used in the neurological evaluation, but the most common diagnostic procedure is magnetic resonance imaging (MRI), which determines the location and extent of the tumor.
4. Therapeutic management includes surgery, radiation, and chemotherapy; the treatment of choice is the total removal of the tumor without residual neurological damage.

B. Data collection
1. Headache that is worse on awakening and that improves during the day
2. Vomiting that is unrelated to feeding or eating
3. Behavioral changes
4. Clumsiness; awkward gait or difficulty walking
5. Facial weakness
6. Signs of increased intracranial pressure (see Box 32-5)

Monitor for signs of increased ICP in a child with a brain tumor and after a craniotomy. If signs of increased ICP occur, notify the HCP immediately.

C. Preoperative interventions
1. Monitor the neurological status.
2. Institute seizure precautions and safety measures.
3. Monitor the weight and nutritional status.
4. The child's head will be shaved (provide a favorite cap or hat for the child); shaving the head may also be done in the surgical suite.
5. Prepare the child as much as possible; tell the child that he or she will wake up with a large head dressing.

D. Postoperative interventions
1. Monitor the neurological and motor function and the level of consciousness.
2. Monitor the temperature closely because it may be elevated as a result of hypothalamus or brainstem involvement during surgery; maintain a cooling blanket by the bedside.
3. Monitor for signs of respiratory infection.
4. Monitor for signs of meningitis (opisthotonos, Kernig's and Brudzinski's signs).
5. Monitor for signs of increased ICP (see Box 32-5) or hemorrhage; check the back of the head dressing for the posterior pooling of blood.
6. Monitor the pupillary response; sluggish, dilated, or unequal pupils are reported immediately, because they may indicate increased ICP and potential brainstem herniation.
7. Monitor for colorless drainage on the dressing or from the ears or nose; this is indicative of cerebrospinal fluid and should be reported immediately. Assess for the presence of glucose in the drainage (dipstick).

BOX 32-5 Manifestations of Increased Intracranial Pressure in Infants and Children

Infants

Tense, bulging fontanel
Separated cranial sutures
Macewen's sign (cracked pot sound on percussion)
Irritability
High-pitched cry
Increased head circumference
Distended scalp veins
Poor feeding
Crying when disturbed
Setting sun sign (eyes appear to look only downward, with the sclera prominent over the iris)

Children

Headache
Nausea
Forceful vomiting
Diplopia; blurred vision
Seizures

Personality and Behavior Signs

Irritability, restlessness
Indifference, drowsiness
Decline in school performance
Diminished physical activity and motor performance
Increased sleeping
Inability to follow simple commands
Lethargy

Late Signs

Bradycardia
Decreased motor response to command
Decreased sensory response to painful stimuli
Alterations in pupil size and reaction
Decerebrate or decorticate posturing
Cheyne-Stokes respirations
Papilledema
Decreased consciousness
Coma

From Perry S, Hockenberry M, Lowdermilk D, Wilson D: *Maternal child nursing care*, ed 4, St. Louis, 2010, Elsevier.

8. Check the HCP's prescription for positioning, including the degree of neck flexion. (Refer to Chapter 57 for additional information on craniotomy.)
9. Monitor IV fluids closely to prevent volume overload.
10. Promote measures that prevent vomiting; vomiting increases ICP and the risk for incisional rupture.
11. Provide a quiet environment.
12. Administer analgesics, as prescribed.
13. Provide emotional support to the child and parents, and promote maximum functioning in the child.

CRITICAL THINKING What Should You Do?

Answer: The child with hemophilia is at risk for bleeding. If the child experienced recent trauma, the nurse should place the child on bleeding precautions and monitor for bleeding. This is the priority intervention. The nurse should monitor vital signs and monitor for joint pain. Joint bleeding should be controlled by immobilization, elevation, and application of ice. Pressure should be applied for 15 minutes for any superficial bleeding. The neurological status should be checked because the child is at risk for intracranial hemorrhage, and the nurse should monitor the urine for hematuria. Blood replacement factors may be prescribed.

Reference(s): Hockenberry, M., & Wilson, D. (2013). *Wong's: Essentials of pediatric nursing* (9th ed., pp. 885–886). St. Louis: Mosby.

PRACTICE QUESTIONS

301. The nurse reinforces instructions to the mother of a child with sickle cell disease regarding the precipitating factors related to pain crisis. Which, if identified by the mother as a precipitating factor, indicates the **need for further teaching**?

1. Stress
2. Trauma
3. Infection
4. Fluid overload

❖ **302.** The nurse is reviewing a health care provider's prescription for a child with sickle cell anemia who was admitted to the hospital for the treatment of vaso-occlusive crisis. Which prescriptions documented in the child's record should the nurse question? **Select all that apply.**

- ❑ 1. Restrict fluid intake.
- ❑ 2. Position for comfort.
- ❑ 3. Avoid strain on painful joints.
- ❑ 4. Apply nasal oxygen at 2 L per minute.
- ❑ 5. Provide a high-calorie, high-protein diet.
- ❑ 6. Administer meperidine (Demerol) 25 mg for pain.

303. The nurse, caring for a child with aplastic anemia, is reviewing the laboratory results and notes a white blood cell (WBC) count of 6000 cells/mm^3 and a platelet count of 20,000 cells/mm^3. Which nursing intervention should be incorporated into the plan of care?

1. Encourage naps.
2. Encourage a diet high in iron.
3. Encourage quiet play activities.
4. Maintain strict isolation precautions.

304. The nurse reinforces home-care instructions to the parents of a 3-year-old child who has been hospitalized with hemophilia. Which statement by a parent indicates the **need for further teaching**?
1. "I will supervise my child closely."
2. "I will pad the corners of the furniture."
3. "I will remove household items that can easily fall over."
4. "I will avoid immunizations and dental hygiene treatments for my child."

305. The nurse reinforces instructions to the parents of a child with leukemia regarding measures related to monitoring for infection. Which statement by the parents indicates the **need for further teaching**?
1. "I need to use proper hand-washing techniques."
2. "I need to take my child's rectal temperature daily."
3. "I need to inspect my child's skin daily for redness."
4. "I need to inspect my child's mouth daily for lesions."

306. The nurse is reviewing the health record of a 14-year-old child who is suspected of having Hodgkin's disease. Which is the **primary** characteristic of this disease?
1. Fever and malaise
2. Anorexia and weight loss
3. Painful, enlarged inguinal lymph nodes
4. Painless, firm, and movable lymph nodes in the cervical area

307. A 4-year-old child is hospitalized with a suspected diagnosis of Wilms' tumor. The nurse reviews the plan of care and should question which intervention that is written in the plan?
1. Palpate the abdomen for a mass.
2. Check the urine for the presence of hematuria.
3. Monitor the blood pressure for the presence of hypertension.
4. Monitor the temperature for the presence of a kidney infection.

308. The nursing instructor asks a student nurse to describe osteogenic sarcoma. Which statement by the student indicates the **need to further research** the disease?
1. "The femur is the most common site of this sarcoma."
2. "The child does not experience pain at the primary tumor site."
3. "If a weight-bearing limb is affected, then limping is a clinical manifestation."
4. "The symptoms of the disease during the early stage are almost always attributed to normal growing pains."

309. The nurse is monitoring for bleeding in a child after surgery to remove a brain tumor. The nurse checks the head dressing for the presence of blood and notes a colorless drainage on the back of the dressing. Which nursing action is appropriate?
1. Reinforce the dressing.
2. Notify the registered nurse (RN).
3. Document the findings and continue to monitor.
4. Circle the area of drainage and continue to monitor.

310. Oral iron supplements are prescribed for a 6-year-old child with iron deficiency anemia. The nurse reinforces instructions to the mother and tells the mother to administer the iron with which **best** food item?
1. Milk
2. Water
3. Apple juice
4. Orange juice

ANSWERS

301. 4
Rationale: Pain crisis may be precipitated by infection, dehydration, hypoxia, trauma, or general stress. The mother of a child with sickle cell disease should encourage a fluid intake of 1.5 to 2 times the daily requirement to prevent dehydration.
Test-Taking Strategy: Note the strategic words, *need for further teaching*. These words indicate a negative event query and ask you to select an option that is an incorrect statement. Recalling that fluid administration is a main component of the treatment of sickle cell disease to prevent dehydration and pain crisis will direct you to the correct option. **Review:** sickle cell disease.
Level of Cognitive Ability: Evaluating
Client Needs: Physiological Integrity
Integrated Process: Teaching and Learning
Content Area: Child Health: Hematological
Priority Concepts: Fluid and Electrolyte Balance, Perfusion
Reference(s): Hockenberry, Wilson (2013), pp. 879–880.

❖ **302.** 1, 6
Rationale: Sickle cell anemia is one of a group of diseases called hemoglobinopathies in which hemoglobin A is partly or completely replaced by abnormal sickle hemoglobin S. It is caused by the inheritance of a gene for a structurally abnormal portion of the hemoglobin chain. Hemoglobin S is sensitive to changes in the oxygen content of the red blood cell, and insufficient oxygen causes the cells to assume a sickle shape; the cells become rigid and clumped together, thus

obstructing capillary blood flow. Oral and intravenous fluids are important parts of treatment. Meperidine (Demerol) is not recommended for the child with sickle cell disease because of the risk for normeperidine-induced seizures. Normeperidine, which is a metabolite of meperidine, is a central nervous system stimulant that produces anxiety, tremors, myoclonus, and generalized seizures when it accumulates with repetitive dosing. Therefore, the nurse would question the prescriptions for restricted fluids and meperidine for pain control. Positioning for comfort, avoiding strain in painful joints, oxygen, and a high-calorie, high-protein diet are important parts of the treatment plan.

Test-Taking Strategy: Focus on the subject, pathophysiology that occurs with sickle cell anemia, to assist you with identifying the prescriptions that need to be questioned. Recalling that fluids are an important component of the treatment plan will help you to identify that a fluid-restriction prescription would need to be questioned. Next, recalling the effects of meperidine will assist you with identifying that this prescription needs to be questioned. **Review: sickle cell anemia.**

Level of Cognitive Ability: Analyzing
Client Needs: Safe and Effective Care Environment
Integrated Process: Nursing Process/Implementation
Content Area: Child Health: Hematological
Priority Concepts: Clinical Judgment, Safety
Reference(s): Hockenberry, Wilson (2013), pp. 875–876.

303. 3

Rationale: Precautionary measures to prevent bleeding should be taken when a child has a low platelet count. These include no injections, no rectal temperatures, the use of a soft toothbrush, and abstinence from contact sports or activities that could cause an injury. Strict isolation would be required if the WBC count was low. Naps and a diet high in iron are unrelated to the risk of bleeding.

Test-Taking Strategy: Focus on the subject, the intervention that should be incorporated into the plan of care. Note that the WBC count is normal and that the platelet count is low. Recall that a low platelet count places the client at risk for bleeding. This will assist you with eliminating the incorrect options. **Review: aplastic anemia and bleeding precautions.**

Level of Cognitive Ability: Analyzing
Client Needs: Physiological Integrity
Integrated Process: Nursing Process/Planning
Content Area: Child Health: Hematological
Priority Concepts: Clinical Judgment, Safety
Reference(s): McKinney et al (2013), pp. 1260–1261.

304. 4

Rationale: The nurse needs to stress the importance of immunizations, dental hygiene, and routine well-child care. Options 1, 2, and 3 are appropriate statements. The parents are also provided instructions regarding measures to take in the event of blunt trauma (especially trauma that involves the joints), and they are instructed to apply prolonged pressure to superficial wounds until the bleeding has stopped.

Test-Taking Strategy: Note the strategic words, *need for further teaching.* These words indicate a negative event query and ask you to select an option that is an incorrect statement. Recalling that bleeding is a concern among clients with this disorder will assist you with eliminating options 1, 2, and 3, because they include measures of protection and safety for the child. **Review: hemophilia.**

Level of Cognitive Ability: Evaluating
Client Needs: Safe and Effective Care Environment
Integrated Process: Teaching and Learning
Content Area: Child Health: Hematological
Priority Concepts: Immunity, Safety
Reference(s): McKinney et al (2013), p. 1255.

305. 2

Rationale: The risk of injury to the fragile mucous membranes is so great in the child with leukemia that only oral, axillary, or temporal or tympanic temperatures should be taken. Rectal abscesses can easily occur in damaged rectal tissue, so no rectal temperatures should be taken. In addition, oral temperatures should be avoided if the child has oral ulcers. Options 1, 3, and 4 are appropriate teaching measures.

Test-Taking Strategy: Note the strategic words, *need for further teaching.* These words indicate a negative event query and ask you to select an option that is an incorrect statement. Options 1, 3, and 4 are reasonable measures and can be easily eliminated. Also, note the word *rectal* in option 2. Recalling that rectal temperatures should be avoided because of the risk for bleeding will direct you to this option. **Review: leukemia.**

Level of Cognitive Ability: Evaluating
Client Needs: Safe and Effective Care Environment
Integrated Process: Teaching and Learning
Content Area: Child Health: Oncological
Priority Concepts: Cellular Regulation, Infection
Reference(s): Hockenberry, Wilson (2013), p. 892.

306. 4

Rationale: Signs and symptoms specifically associated with Hodgkin's disease include painless, firm, and movable adenopathy in the cervical and supraclavicular areas. Hepatosplenomegaly is also noted. Although anorexia, weight loss, fever, and malaise are associated with Hodgkin's disease, these manifestations are not the primary characteristics and are seen with many disorders.

Test-Taking Strategy: Note the subject, primary characteristic of Hodgkin's disease, and note the strategic word, *primary.* Eliminate options 1 and 2 first because these symptoms are general and vague. Recalling that painless adenopathy is associated with Hodgkin's disease will direct you to the correct option. **Review: Hodgkin's disease.**

Level of Cognitive Ability: Understanding
Client Needs: Physiological Integrity
Integrated Process: Nursing Process/Data Collection
Content Area: Child Health: Oncological
Priority Concepts: Cellular Regulation, Immunity
Reference(s): McKinney et al (2013), p. 1285.

307. 1

Rationale: Wilms' tumor is an intraabdominal and kidney tumor. If Wilms' tumor is suspected, the mass should not be palpated. Excessive manipulation can cause seeding of the tumor and thus cause the spread of the cancerous cells. Hematuria, hypertension, and fever are signs and symptoms that are associated with Wilms' tumor.

Test-Taking Strategy: Focus on the subject, the intervention that the nurse should question. This means that you need to

select an option that is an incorrect intervention. Knowledge that Wilms' tumor is an intraabdominal and kidney tumor will assist you with eliminating options 2, 3, and 4 because of the relationship of these options to renal function. **Review:** Wilms' tumor.
Level of Cognitive Ability: Analyzing
Client Needs: Safe and Effective Care Environment
Integrated Process: Nursing Process/Implementation
Content Area: Child Health: Oncological
Priority Concepts: Cellular Regulation, Safety
Reference(s): Hockenberry, Wilson (2013), pp. 917–918.

308. 2
Rationale: Osteogenic sarcoma is the most common bone tumor in children. A clinical manifestation of osteogenic sarcoma is progressive, insidious, intermittent pain at the tumor site. By the time these children receive medical attention, they may be in considerable pain from the tumor. Options 1, 3, and 4 are accurate regarding osteogenic sarcoma.
Test-Taking Strategy: Note the strategic words, *need to further research.* These words indicate a negative event query and the need to select the incorrect student statement. Recalling that osteogenic sarcoma is a malignant tumor of the bone will direct you to the correct option. **Review:** osteogenic sarcoma.
Level of Cognitive Ability: Evaluating
Client Needs: Physiological Integrity
Integrated Process: Teaching and Learning
Content Area: Child Health: Oncological
Priority Concepts: Cellular Regulation, Pain
Reference(s): McKinney et al (2013), pp. 1287–1288.

309. 2
Rationale: Colorless drainage on the dressing would indicate the presence of cerebrospinal fluid and should be reported to the RN immediately; the RN would then contact the health care provider. The colorless drainage should also be checked for evidence of cerebrospinal fluid; one method is to check for the presence of glucose using a dipstick. Options 1, 3, and 4 are incorrect and delay required immediate interventions.
Test-Taking Strategy: Note the subject, colorless drainage following surgery for a brain tumor. This should quickly alert you to the possibility of the presence of cerebrospinal fluid. Therefore, eliminate options 1, 3, and 4. **Review:** brain tumors.
Level of Cognitive Ability: Applying
Client Needs: Physiological Integrity
Integrated Process: Nursing Process/Implementation
Content Area: Child Health: Oncological
Priority Concepts: Clinical Judgment, Intracranial Regulation
Reference(s): Hockenberry, Wilson (2013), p. 948; McKinney et al (2013), p. 1282.

310. 4
Rationale: Vitamin C increases the absorption of iron by the body. The mother should be instructed to administer the medication with a citrus fruit or a juice that is high in vitamin C. Milk may affect absorption of the iron. Water will not assist in absorption. Orange juice contains a greater amount of vitamin C than apple juice.
Test-Taking Strategy: Note the strategic word, *best.* Recalling that vitamin C increases the absorption of iron will assist you with eliminating milk and water. From the remaining options, select orange juice, because this food item contains the highest amount of vitamin C. **Review:** iron supplements.
Level of Cognitive Ability: Applying
Client Needs: Physiological Integrity
Integrated Process: Teaching and Learning
Content Area: Pharmacology: Hematological Medications
Priority Concepts: Health Promotion, Nutrition
Reference(s): Hockenberry, Wilson (2013), p. 872.

CHAPTER 33

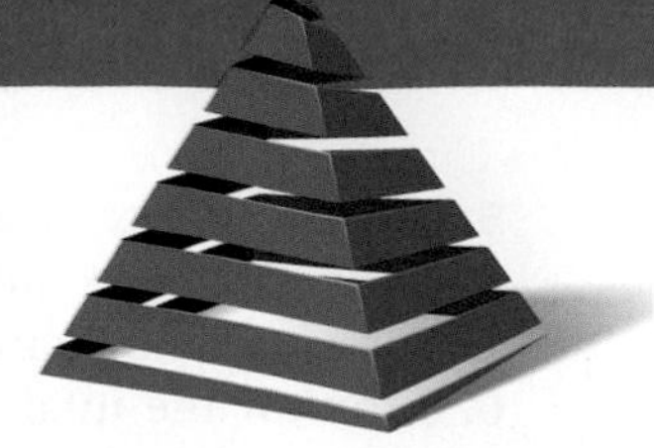

Metabolic, Endocrine, and Gastrointestinal Disorders

CRITICAL THINKING What Should You Do?

A child suddenly vomits. What should the nurse do to prevent aspiration?

Answer located on p. 402.

I. Fever

A. Description
1. An abnormal body temperature elevation.
2. A child's temperature can vary, depending on activity, emotional stress, the type of clothing that the child is wearing, and the temperature of the environment.
3. Data collection findings associated with the fever provide important indications of its seriousness.

B. Data collection
1. Temperature elevation: Normal temperature range for a child is 36.4°C to 37°C (97.5°F to 98.6°F); 38°C (100.4°F) is considered to be fever.
2. Flushed skin; warm to touch
3. Diaphoresis
4. Chills
5. Restlessness or lethargy

C. Interventions
1. Monitor vital signs. Take the temperature via the electronic route or per agency procedures.
2. Remove excess clothing and blankets, reduce the room temperature, and increase the air circulation. Use other cooling measures, such as the application of a cool compress to the forehead if appropriate.
3. Administer a sponge bath with tepid water for 20 to 30 minutes, and gently squeeze water from a facecloth over the back and chest; recheck the temperature 30 minutes after the bath; do not use alcohol because it can cause peripheral vasoconstriction.
4. Administer antipyretics such as ibuprofen (Motrin), as prescribed.
5. Aspirin (acetylsalicylic acid) should not be administered, unless specifically prescribed, because of the risk of Reye's syndrome. 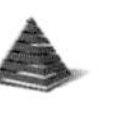
6. Retake the temperature 30 to 60 minutes after the antipyretic is administered. 
7. Provide adequate fluid intake, as tolerated and prescribed.
8. Monitor for signs and symptoms that indicate dehydration and electrolyte imbalances; monitor laboratory values.
9. Reinforce instructions to the parents regarding how to take the child's temperature, how to safely medicate the child, and when it is necessary to call the health care provider (HCP).

II. Vomiting

A. Description
1. The major concerns when a child is vomiting are the risk of dehydration, the loss of fluid and electrolytes, and the development of metabolic alkalosis.
2. Additional concerns include aspiration, atelectasis, and the development of pneumonia.
3. Causes of vomiting include acute infectious diseases, increased intracranial pressure, toxic ingestions, food intolerance, mechanical obstruction of the gastrointestinal tract, metabolic disorders, and psychogenic disorders.

B. Data collection
1. Signs of aspiration 
2. Character of vomitus
3. Pain and abdominal cramping
4. Signs of dehydration
5. Signs of fluid and electrolyte imbalances
6. Signs of metabolic alkalosis

C. Interventions
1. Maintain a patent airway.
2. Position the child on his or her side to prevent aspiration. 
3. Monitor the vital signs.
4. Monitor the character, amount, and frequency of vomiting.

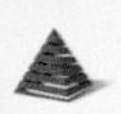

5. Note the force of the vomiting, because projectile vomiting is indicative of pyloric **stenosis** or increased intracranial pressure.
6. Monitor the intake and output (I&O) and for signs of dehydration, such as a sunken fontanel (age-appropriate), nonelastic skin turgor, dry mucous membranes, decreased tear production, and oliguria.
7. Monitor the electrolyte levels.
8. Provide oral rehydration therapy, as tolerated and as prescribed. Start feeding slowly, with small amounts of fluid at frequent intervals (intravenous [IV] fluids may need to be prescribed).
9. Monitor for diarrhea or abdominal pain.
10. Tell the parents to contact the HCP when signs of dehydration, blood in the vomitus, forceful vomiting, or abdominal pain is present.

III. Diarrhea

A. Description
1. Acute diarrhea is a cause of dehydration, particularly in children younger than 5 years.
2. Some causes of acute diarrhea include acute infectious disorders of the gastrointestinal tract, antibiotic therapy, and parasitic infestation.
3. Some causes of chronic diarrhea include rotavirus, malabsorption syndromes, inflammatory bowel disease, immune deficiencies, food intolerances, and nonspecific factors.
4. Rotavirus is a cause of serious gastroenteritis and is a nosocomial (hospital-acquired) pathogen that is most severe in children ages 3 to 24 months; children younger than 3 months of age have some protection because of maternally acquired antibodies.

B. Data collection
1. Character of stools
2. Pain and abdominal cramping
3. Signs of dehydration and fluid and electrolyte imbalances
4. Signs of metabolic acidosis

C. Interventions
1. Monitor the character, amount, and frequency of diarrhea.
2. Provide enteric isolation as required; instruct the parents in effective hand-washing technique (the child should be taught this technique also).
3. Monitor skin integrity.
4. Monitor strict intake and output.
5. Monitor electrolyte levels.
6. Monitor for signs and symptoms of dehydration.
7. For mild to moderate dehydration, oral rehydration therapy with Pedialyte or a similar rehydration solution may be prescribed; avoid carbonated beverages because they are gas-producing, as well as fluids that contain high amounts of sugar, such as apple juice.
8. For severe dehydration, an NPO status may be prescribed to place the bowel at rest and fluid and electrolyte replacement by the intravenous (IV) route may be prescribed; if potassium is prescribed for IV administration, ensure that the child has voided before its administration and has adequate kidney function.
9. Reintroduce a normal diet once rehydration is achieved.

The major concerns when a child is having diarrhea are the risk of dehydration, the loss of fluid and electrolytes, and the development of metabolic acidosis.

IV. Dehydration

A. Description
1. Dehydration is a common fluid and electrolyte imbalance in infants and children.
2. In infants and children, the organs that conserve water are immature, thus placing them at risk for fluid volume deficit.
3. The causes can include decreased fluid intake, diaphoresis, vomiting, diarrhea, diabetic ketoacidosis, and extensive burns or other serious injuries.

Infants and children are more vulnerable to fluid volume deficit because more of their body water is in the extracellular fluid compartment.

B. Data collection (Table 33-1)

C. Interventions
1. The cause of the dehydration is treated. Monitor the vital signs.

2. Monitor the weight and for weight changes, including fluid gains and losses.
3. Monitor the I&O and the urine for specific gravity.
4. Monitor the level of consciousness.
5. Monitor the skin turgor and mucous membranes for dryness.
6. Fluid replacement therapy is the same as for the child with vomiting or diarrhea.
7. Reinforce instructions to the parents about the types and amounts of fluid to encourage, the signs of dehydration, and indications of the need to notify the HCP.

V. Phenylketonuria (PKU)

A. Description
1. A genetic disorder (autosomal recessive disorder) that results in central nervous system damage from toxic levels of phenylalanine (an essential amino acid) in the blood.
2. Characterized by blood phenylalanine levels greater than 20 mg/dL. (A normal level is 1.2 to 3.4 mg/dL in newborns and 0.8 to 1.8 mg/dL thereafter.)

TABLE 33-1 Evaluating the Extent of Dehydration

	LEVEL OF DEHYDRATION		
Clinical Signs	**Mild**	**Moderate**	**Severe**
Weight loss—infants	3% to 5%	6% to 9%	≥10%
Weight loss—children	3% to 4%	6% to 8%	10%
Pulse	Normal	Slightly increased	Very increased
Respiratory rate	Normal	Slight tachypnea (rapid)	Hyperpnea (deep and rapid)
Blood pressure	Normal	Normal to orthostatic (>10 mm Hg change)	Orthostatic to shock
Behavior	Normal	Irritable, more thirsty	Hyperirritable to lethargic
Thirst	Slight	Moderate	Intense
Mucous membranes*	Normal	Dry	Parched
Tears	Present	Decreased	Absent; sunken eyes
Anterior fontanel	Normal	Normal to sunken	Sunken
External jugular vein	Visible when supine	Not visible except with supraclavicular pressure	Not visible even with supraclavicular pressure
Skin*	Capillary refill >2 sec	Slowed capillary refill (2-4 sec [decreased turgor])	Very delayed capillary refill (>4 sec) and tenting; skin cool, acrocyanotic or mottled
Urine specific gravity	>1.020	>1.020; oliguria	Oliguria or anuria

*These signs are less prominent in the child who has hypernatremia.
Data from Jospe N, Forbes G: Fluids and electrolytes—clinical aspects, *Pediatr Rev* 17:395–403, 1996; and Steiner MJ, DeWalt DA, Byerley JS: Is this child dehydrated? *JAMA* 291:2746–2754, 2004. Table from Perry S, Hockenberry M, Lowdermilk D, Wilson D: *Maternal-child nursing care*, ed 4, St. Louis, 2010, Mosby.

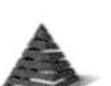

3. All 50 states require routine screening of all newborn infants for PKU.

B. Data collection

1. In all children:
   - **a.** Digestive problems and vomiting
   - **b.** Seizures
   - **c.** Musty odor of the urine
   - **d.** Mental retardation
2. In older children
   - **a.** Eczema
   - **b.** Hypertonia
   - **c.** Hypopigmentation of the hair, skin, and irises
   - **d.** Hyperactive behavior

C. Interventions

1. Screening of newborn infants for phenylketonuria: The infant should have begun formula or breast milk feeding before specimen collection.
2. If initial screening is positive, a repeat test is performed and further diagnostic evaluation is required to verify the diagnosis.
3. Rescreening of infants should be done by 14 days of age if the initial screening was done before 48 hours of age.
4. If phenylketonuria is diagnosed, prepare to implement the following:
   - **a.** Restrict phenylalanine intake; high-protein foods (meats and dairy products) and aspartame are avoided because they contain large amounts of phenylalanine.
   - **b.** Monitor physical, neurological, and intellectual development.
   - **c.** Stress the importance of follow-up treatment.
   - **d.** Encourage the parents to express feelings about the diagnosis and the risk of phenylketonuria in future children.
   - **e.** Reinforce educating the parents about use of special preparation formulas and about the foods that contain phenylalanine.
   - **f.** Consult with social care services to assist the parents with financial burdens of specially prepared formulas.

VI. Diabetes Mellitus

A. Description (Fig. 33-1)

1. Type 1 diabetes mellitus is characterized by the destruction of the pancreatic beta cells, which produce insulin. This results in absolute insulin deficiency.
2. Type 2 diabetes mellitus usually arises as a result of insulin resistance, in which the body fails to use insulin properly, in combination with relative (rather than absolute) insulin deficiency.

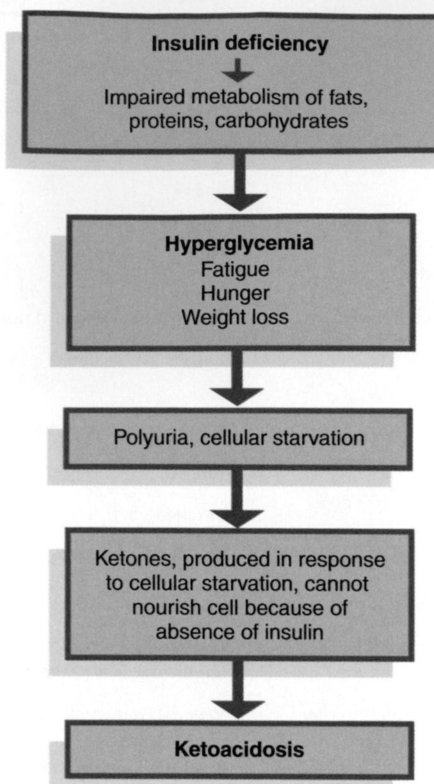

FIGURE 33-1 Insulin deficiency leading to ketoacidosis. (From McKinney E, James S, Murray S, Ashwill J: *Maternal-child nursing*, ed 4, St. Louis, 2013, Saunders.)

3. Insulin deficiency requires the use of exogenous insulin to promote appropriate glucose use and prevent complications related to elevated blood glucose levels, such as hyperglycemia, diabetic ketoacidosis, and death.
4. Diagnosis is based on the presence of classic symptoms and an elevated blood glucose level (a normal blood glucose level is between 70 and 100 mg/dL for a nondiabetic person).
5. Children may be admitted directly to the pediatric intensive care unit because of the manifestations of diabetic ketoacidosis, which may be the initial occurrence when they are diagnosed with diabetes mellitus.

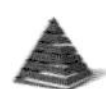

B. Data collection
   1. Polyuria, polydipsia, and polyphagia
   2. Hyperglycemia
   3. Weight loss
   4. Unexplained fatigue or lethargy
   5. Headaches
   6. Occasional enuresis in a previously toilet-trained child
   7. Vaginitis in adolescent girls (caused by *Candida vaginitis,* which thrives in hyperglycemic tissues)
   8. Fruity odor to the breath
   9. Dehydration
   10. Blurred vision
   11. Slow wound healing
   12. Changes in the level of consciousness

C. Long-term effects
   1. Failure to grow at a normal rate
   2. Delayed maturation
   3. Recurrent infections
   4. Neuropathy
   5. Cardiovascular disease
   6. Retinal microvascular disease
   7. Renal microvascular disease

D. Complications
   1. Hypoglycemia
   2. Hyperglycemia
   3. Diabetic ketoacidosis
   4. Coma
   5. Hypokalemia
   6. Hyperkalemia
   7. Microvascular changes
   8. Cardiovascular changes

For a child with diabetes mellitus, plan to initiate a consultation with the diabetic specialist to plan the child's care.

E. Diet
   1. Normal, healthy nutrition is encouraged. The total number of calories is individualized on the basis of the child's age and **growth** expectations.
   2. As prescribed by the HCP, children with diabetes need no special foods or supplements. They need sufficient calories to balance daily expenditure for energy and to satisfy the requirement for growth and development.
   3. Dietary intake should include three well-balanced meals per day, eaten at regular intervals, plus a midafternoon snack and a bedtime snack; a consistent intake of the prescribed protein, fats, and carbohydrates at each meal and snack is needed (concentrated sweets are discouraged; fat is reduced to 30% or less of the total caloric requirement).
   4. Tell the child and the parents that the child should carry a source of glucose (e.g., glucose tablets) with him or her at all times to treat hypoglycemia if it occurs.
   5. Incorporate the diet into the individual child's needs, likes, dislikes, lifestyle, and cultural and socioeconomic patterns.
   6. Allow the child to participate in making food choices to provide a sense of control.

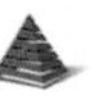

F. Exercise
   1. Instruct the child regarding dietary adjustments to consider when exercising.

2. Extra food needs to be consumed for increased activity (usually 10 to 15 g of carbohydrates for every 30 to 45 minutes of activity).
3. Instruct the child to check the blood glucose level before exercising.
4. Plan an appropriate exercise regimen with the child, and incorporate the child's developmental stage.

G. Insulin
1. Diluted insulin may be required for some infants to provide small enough doses to avoid hypoglycemia. Diluted insulin should be clearly labeled to avoid dosage errors.
2. A laboratory evaluation of the glycosylated hemoglobin level should be performed every 3 months.
3. Illness, infection, and stress increase the need for insulin. Insulin should not be withheld in these situations, because hyperglycemia and ketoacidosis can result.
4. When the child is NPO for a special procedure, verify with the HCP the need to withhold the morning insulin and when food, fluids, and insulin are to be given.
5. Reinforce instructions to the child and parents regarding the administration of the insulin.
6. Reinforce instructions to the child and parents regarding how to recognize the symptoms of hypoglycemia and hyperglycemia.
7. Reinforce instructions to the parents in the administration of glucagon intramuscularly or subcutaneously if the child has a hypoglycemic reaction and is unable to consume items orally (if semiconscious or unconscious).
8. Reinforce instructions to the child and parents to always have a spare bottle of insulin available.
9. Advise the parents to obtain a Medic-Alert bracelet that indicates the type and daily insulin dosage that has been prescribed for the child.
10. See Chapter 46 for information on insulin types, administration sites, and administration procedure.

H. Blood glucose monitoring
1. Results provide information needed to maintain good glycemic control.
2. Blood glucose monitoring is more accurate than urine testing.
3. Requires that the child prick himself or herself several times a day, as prescribed (Box 33-1)
4. Reinforce instructions to the child and parents in the proper procedure for obtaining the blood glucose level.
5. Inform the child and parents that the procedure must be performed precisely to obtain accurate results.
6. Stress the importance of hand washing before and after performing the procedure to prevent infection.

BOX 33-1 Lessening the Pain of Blood Glucose Monitoring

- Hold the finger under warm water for a few seconds before puncture (enhances blood flow to the finger).
- Use the ring finger or thumb to obtain a blood sample because blood flows more easily to these areas; puncture the finger just to the side of the finger pad because there are more blood vessels in this area and fewer nerve endings.
- Press the lancet device lightly against the skin to prevent a deep puncture.
- Use glucose monitors that require very small blood samples for measurement.

Adapted from Perry S, Hockenberry M, Lowdermilk D, Wilson D: *Maternal child nursing care*, ed 4, St. Louis, 2010, Elsevier.

7. Stress the importance of following the manufacturer's instructions for the blood glucose monitoring device.
8. Reinforce instructions to the child and parents to calibrate the monitor as instructed by the manufacturer.
9. Reinforce instructions to the child and parents to check the expiration date on the test strips used for blood glucose monitoring.
10. Reinforce instructions to the child and parents that if the blood glucose results do not seem reasonable, they should reread the instructions, reassess the technique, check the expiration date of the test strips, and perform the procedure again to verify the results.

I. Urine testing
1. Reinforce instructions to the parents and child in the procedure for testing the urine for ketones and glucose.
2. Reinforce instructions to the child that the second voided urine specimen is the most accurate. 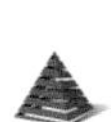
3. The presence of ketones may indicate impending ketoacidosis.

Urine glucose testing is an unreliable method of monitoring the glucose level; however, the urine should be tested for ketones when the child is ill or when the blood glucose level is greater than 200 mg/dL or as specified by the HCP.

J. Hypoglycemia 
1. Description
   a. A blood glucose level less than 70 mg/dL (or as specified by the HCP)
   b. Occurs as a result of too much insulin, not enough food, or excessive activity

c. Signs include headache, nausea, sweating, tremors, lethargy, hunger, confusion, slurred speech, tingling around the mouth, and anxiety.

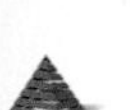

2. Interventions (Boxes 33-2 and 33-3) (see Priority Nursing Actions)

K. Hyperglycemia

PRIORITY NURSING ACTIONS

Actions to Take When a Hospitalized Child with Diabetes Mellitus Experiences Hypoglycemia

1. Check the child's blood glucose level.
2. Give the child ½ cup of fruit juice or other acceptable item.
3. Take the child's vital signs.
4. Retest the blood glucose level.
5. Give the child a small snack of carbohydrate and protein.
6. Document the child's complaints, actions taken, and outcome.

If a child with diabetes mellitus experiences hypoglycemia, the nurse first would check the child's blood glucose level to verify that the child is experiencing hypoglycemia. When this is verified, the nurse gives the child 10 to 15 g of carbohydrates. The nurse retests the blood glucose level in 15 minutes. In the meantime, the nurse checks the child's vital signs. If the child's symptoms of hypoglycemia do not resolve, the nurse gives the child another 10- to 15-g carbohydrate food item. Otherwise, the nurse provides a small snack of carbohydrates and protein if the child's next scheduled meal is more than 1 hour away from the time of the occurrence. After treatment and resolution of the hypoglycemic event, the nurse documents the occurrence, actions taken, and outcome.

Reference(s): Hockenberry, M., & Wilson, D. (2013). *Wong's: Essentials of pediatric nursing* (9th ed., p. 996). St. Louis: Mosby.

BOX 33-2 Interventions for Hypoglycemia

If possible, the nurse should confirm the hypoglycemia with a blood glucose reading.

Administer glucose immediately. The rapid-releasing glucose is followed by a complex carbohydrate and protein, such as a slice of bread or a peanut butter cracker.

Give the child an extra snack if the next meal is not planned for more than 30 minutes or if activity is planned.

If the child becomes unconscious, squeeze cake frosting or glucose paste onto the gums and retest the blood glucose level if the child does not improve in 15 minutes (monitor the child closely); if the reading remains low, administer additional glucose.

If the child remains unconscious, it may be necessary to administer glucagon.

In the hospital setting, prepare for the administration of intravenous dextrose if the child is unable to consume an oral glucose product.

BOX 33-3 Food Items to Treat Hypoglycemia

- ½ cup orange juice or a sugar-sweetened carbonated beverage
- 8 oz milk
- 1 small box of raisins
- 3 or 4 hard candies
- 4 sugar cubes (1 tbsp of sugar)
- 3 or 4 Life Savers
- 1 candy bar
- 1 tsp honey
- 2 or 3 glucose tablets

1. Description: Elevated blood glucose level (>200 mg/dL, or as specified by the HCP)
2. Signs include polydipsia, polyuria, polyphagia, blurred vision, weakness, weight loss, and syncope.

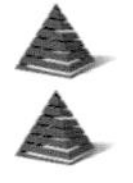

3. Interventions (Box 33-4)
4. Sick-day rules (Box 33-5)

L. Diabetic ketoacidosis (see Fig. 33-1)

1. Description
   a. A complication of diabetes mellitus that develops when a severe insulin deficiency occurs
   b. A life-threatening condition
   c. Hyperglycemia that progresses to metabolic acidosis occurs.
   d. Develops over a period of several hours to days
   e. The blood glucose level is more than 300 mg/dL, and urine and serum ketones are positive.

BOX 33-4 Interventions for Hyperglycemia

Instruct the parents to notify the HCP when the following occur:

- Blood glucose results remain elevated (usually above 200 mg/dL).
- Moderate or high ketonuria is present.
- The child is unable to take food or fluids.
- The child vomits more than once.
- Illness persists.

BOX 33-5 Sick-Day Rules for the Diabetic Child

- Always give insulin, even if the child does not have an appetite, or contact the HCP for specific instructions.
- Test blood glucose levels at least every 4 hours.
- Test for urinary ketones with each voiding.
- Notify the HCP if moderate or large amounts of urinary ketones are present.
- Follow the child's usual meal plan.
- Encourage liquids to aid in clearing ketones.
- Encourage rest, especially if urinary ketones are present.
- Notify the HCP if vomiting, fruity odor to the breath, deep rapid respirations, decreasing level of consciousness, or persistent hyperglycemia occurs.

Adapted from Hockenberry M, Wilson D: *Nursing care of infants and children*, ed 9, St. Louis, 2011, Mosby.

Manifestations of diabetic ketoacidosis include signs of hyperglycemia, Kussmaul's respirations, acetone (fruity) breath odor, increasing lethargy, and decreasing level of consciousness.

2. Interventions
   a. The goal is to restore the circulating volume and protect against cerebral, coronary, or renal hypoperfusion.
   b. Dehydration is corrected with IV infusions of 0.9% or 0.45% saline, as prescribed.
   c. Hyperglycemia is corrected with IV regular insulin administration, as prescribed.
   d. Monitor the vital signs, urine output, and mental status closely.
   e. Correct acidosis and electrolyte imbalances as prescribed.
   f. Administer oxygen, as prescribed.
   g. Monitor the blood glucose level frequently.
   h. Monitor potassium level closely because when the child receives insulin to lower the blood glucose level, the serum potassium level will change; if the potassium level decreases, potassium replacement may be required.
   i. The child should be voiding adequately before administering potassium; if the child does not have an adequate output, hyperkalemia may result.
   j. Monitor the child closely for signs of fluid overload.
   k. Intravenously administered dextrose is added as prescribed when the blood glucose reaches an appropriate level.
   l. The cause of the hyperglycemia is treated.

VII. Cleft Lip and Cleft Palate

A. Description
   1. A congenital anomaly that occurs as a result of the failure of soft tissue or a bony structure to fuse during embryonic development
   2. Involves abnormal openings in the lip or palate that may occur unilaterally or bilaterally and that are readily apparent at birth
   3. Causes include **hereditary** and environmental factors—exposure to radiation or rubella virus, chromosome abnormalities, and teratogenic factors.
   4. Closure of cleft lip defect precedes that of the cleft palate and is usually performed by age 3 to 6 months.
   5. Cleft palate repair is performed sometime between 6 and 24 months of age to allow for the palatal changes that take place with normal growth; a cleft palate is closed as early as possible to facilitate speech development.
   6. The child with cleft palate is at risk for developing frequent otitis media; this can result in hearing loss.
   7. A multidisciplinary team approach is taken to address the many needs of the child; some of these professionals include audiologists, orthodontists, plastic surgeons, and occupational and speech therapists.

B. Data collection (Fig. 33-2)
   1. Cleft lip can range from a slight notch to a complete separation from the floor of the nose.
   2. Cleft palate can include nasal distortion, midline or bilateral cleft, and variable extension from the uvula and the soft and hard palate.

C. Interventions
   1. Check the ability to suck, swallow, handle normal secretions, and breathe without distress.
   2. Monitor the fluid and calorie intake daily, and monitor the weight.
   3. Modify feeding techniques; plan to use specialized feeding techniques, obturators, and special nipples and feeders.
   4. Hold the child in an upright position and direct the formula to the side and back of the mouth to prevent aspiration.
   5. Feed small amounts gradually and burp frequently.
   6. Keep suction equipment and a bulb syringe at the bedside.
   7. Reinforce instructions to the parents about special feeding or suctioning techniques.
   8. Reinforce instructions to the parents about the *ESSR* method of feeding (*e*nlarge the nipple, *s*timulate the sucking reflex, *s*wallow, *r*est to allow the child to finish swallowing what has been placed in the mouth).
   9. Encourage the parents to express their feelings about the disorder.
   10. Encourage parental bonding with the child, including holding and calling the child by name.

D. Postoperative interventions
   1. Cleft lip repair
      a. Provide lip protection; a metal appliance or adhesive strips may be taped securely to the cheeks to prevent trauma to the suture line.
      b. Avoid positioning the child on the side of the repair or in the prone position because these positions can cause rubbing of the surgical site on the mattress (position on the back upright and position to prevent airway obstruction by secretions, blood, or the tongue).
      c. Keep the surgical site clean and dry; after feeding, gently cleanse the suture line of formula or serosanguineous drainage with a solution such as normal saline or as designated by agency procedure.

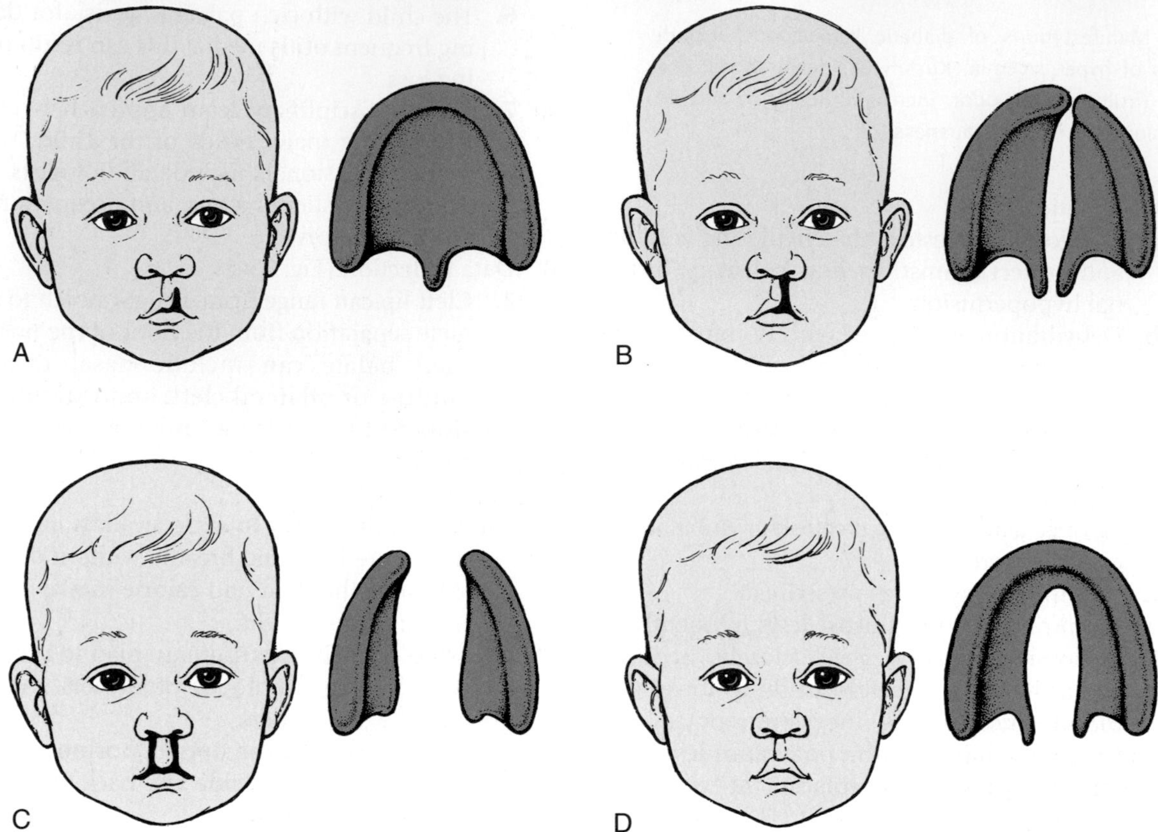

FIGURE 33-2 Variations in clefts of lip and palate at birth. **A,** Notch in vermilion border. **B,** Unilateral cleft lip and palate. **C,** Bilateral cleft lip and palate. **D,** Cleft palate. (From Hockenberry M, Wilson D: *Wong's: Essentials of pediatric nursing*, ed 9, St. Louis, 2013, Mosby.)

- **d.** Apply antibiotic ointment to the site as prescribed.
- **e.** Elbow restraints should be used to prevent the infant from injuring or traumatizing the surgical site.
- **f.** Monitor for signs and symptoms of infection at the surgical site.

2. Cleft palate repair

- **a.** Feedings are resumed by bottle, breast, or cup per surgeon preference; some surgeons prescribe the use of an asepto syringe for feeding or a soft cup such as a Sippy cup.
- **b.** Oral packing may be secured to the palate (usually removed in 2 to 3 days).
- **c.** Do not allow the child to brush his or her teeth.
- **d.** Reinforce instructions to the parents to avoid offering hard food items to the child, such as toast or cookies.

3. Soft elbow or jacket restraints may be used (check agency policies and procedures) to keep the child from touching the repair site; remove restraints at least every 2 hours (or per agency procedure) to check skin integrity and circulation and to allow for exercising the arms.

4. Avoid the use of oral suction or placing objects in the mouth such as a tongue depressor, thermometer, straws, spoons, forks, or pacifiers.
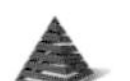
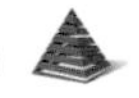

5. Provide analgesics for pain as prescribed.

6. Reinforce instructions to the parents in feeding techniques and in the care of the surgical site.

7. Reinforce instructions to the parents to monitor for signs of infection at the surgical site, such as redness, swelling, or drainage.

8. Encourage the parents to hold the child.

9. Initiate appropriate referrals such as a dental referral and speech therapist referral.

VIII. Esophageal Atresia and Tracheoesophageal Fistula (Fig. 33-3)

A. Description

1. The esophagus terminates before it reaches the stomach, ending in a blind pouch, and/or a fistula is present that forms an unnatural connection with the trachea.

2. The condition causes oral intake to enter the lungs or a large amount of air to enter the stomach. Choking, coughing, and severe abdominal distention can occur.

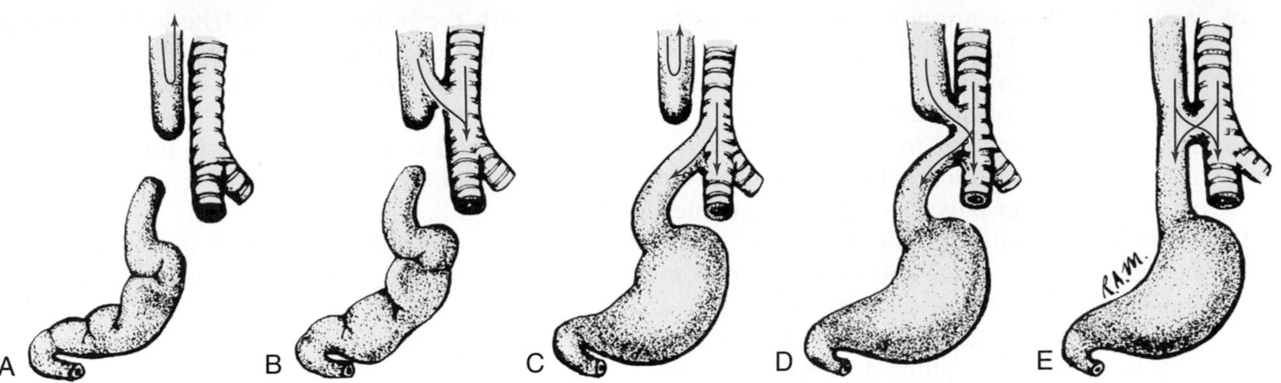

FIGURE 33-3 Congenital atresia of esophagus and tracheoesophageal fistula. **A,** Upper and lower segments of esophagus end in blind sac (occurring in 5% to 8% of such infants). **B,** Upper segment of esophagus ends in atresia and connects to trachea by fistulous tract (occurring rarely). **C,** Upper segment of esophagus ends in blind pouch; lower segment connects with trachea by small fistulous tract (occurring in 80% to 95% of such infants). **D,** Both segments of esophagus connect by fistulous tracts to trachea (occurring in less than 1% of such infants). Infant may aspirate with first feeding. **E,** Esophagus is continuous but connects by fistulous tract to trachea; known as H-type. (From Hockenberry M, Wilson D: *Wong's: Essentials of pediatric nursing,* ed 9, St. Louis, 2013, Mosby.)

3. Aspiration pneumonia and severe respiratory distress will develop, and death will occur without surgical intervention.
4. Treatment includes maintenance of a patent airway, prevention of pneumonia, gastric or blind-pouch decompression, supportive therapy, and surgical repair.

B. Data collection
1. Frothy saliva in the mouth and nose; drooling
2. The "3 C's"—coughing and choking during feedings and unexplained cyanosis
3. **Regurgitation** and vomiting
4. Abdominal distention
5. Increased respiratory distress during and after feeding

C. Preoperative interventions
1. The infant may be placed in a radiant warmer in which humidified oxygen is administered (intubation and mechanical ventilation may be necessary if respiratory distress occurs).
2. Maintain NPO status.
3. Maintain IV fluids, as prescribed.
4. Suction accumulated secretions from the mouth and pharynx.
5. Maintain in a supine upright position (at least 30 degrees upright) to facilitate drainage and prevent aspiration of gastric secretions.
6. The blind pouch is kept empty of secretions by intermittent or continuous suction as prescribed; monitor its patency closely because clogging from mucus can easily occur.
7. If a gastrostomy tube is inserted, it may be left open so that air entering the stomach through the fistula can escape, minimizing the risk of regurgitation of gastric contents into the trachea.
8. Broad-spectrum antibiotics may be prescribed because of the high risk for aspiration pneumonia.

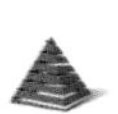

D. Postoperative interventions
1. Monitor vital signs and respiratory status.
2. Assist in maintaining IV fluids, antibiotics, and parenteral nutrition as prescribed.
3. Monitor strict intake and output.
4. Monitor daily weight; monitor for dehydration and possible fluid overload.
5. Monitor for signs of pain.
6. Assist to maintain chest tube patency if present.
7. Inspect the surgical site for signs and symptoms of infection.
8. Monitor for anastomotic leaks as evidenced by purulent drainage from the chest tube, increased temperature, and increased white blood cell count; report these findings to the registered nurse (RN).
9. If a gastrostomy tube is present, it is usually attached to gravity drainage until the infant can tolerate feedings and the anastomosis is healed (usually postoperative day 5 to 7); then feedings are prescribed.
10. Before oral feedings and removal of the chest tube, assist to prepare for an esophagram as prescribed to check the integrity of the esophageal anastomosis.
11. Before feeding, the gastrostomy tube is elevated and secured above the level of the stomach to allow gastric secretions to pass to the duodenum and swallowed air to escape through the open gastrostomy tube.
12. Assist to administer oral feedings with sterile water, followed by frequent small feedings of formula as prescribed.
13. Check the cervical esophagostomy site, if present, for redness, breakdown, or exudate; remove accumulated drainage frequently, and apply protective ointment, barrier dressing, and/or a collection device as prescribed.

14. Assist to provide nonnutritive sucking using a pacifier for infants who remain NPO for extended periods (a pacifier should not be used if the infant is unable to handle secretions).
15. Reinforce instructions to the parents in the techniques of suctioning, gastrostomy tube care and feedings, and skin site care as appropriate.
16. Reinforce instructions to the parents to identify behaviors that indicate the need for suctioning, signs of respiratory distress, and signs of a constricted esophagus (e.g., poor feeding, dysphagia, drooling, coughing during feedings, regurgitated undigested food).

IX. Gastroesophageal Reflux

A. Description

1. Gastroesophageal reflux is backflow of gastric contents into the esophagus as a result of relaxation or incompetence of the lower esophageal or cardiac sphincter.
2. Most infants with gastroesophageal reflux have a mild problem that improves in about 1 year and requires only medical therapy.
3. Gastroesophageal reflux disease (GERD) occurs when gastric contents reflux into the esophagus or oropharynx and produce symptoms.

B. Data collection

1. Passive regurgitation or emesis
2. Poor weight gain
3. Irritability
4. Hematemesis
5. Heartburn (in older children)
6. Anemia from blood loss

C. Interventions

1. Monitor the amount and characteristics of the emesis.
2. Monitor the relationship of the vomiting to the times of feedings and infant activity.
3. Monitor the breath sounds before and after feedings.
4. Monitor for signs of aspiration, such as drooling, coughing, or dyspnea following feeding.
5. Place suction equipment at the bedside.
6. Monitor the I&O.
7. Monitor for signs and symptoms of dehydration.
8. Assist to maintain the IV fluids, as prescribed.

Complications of gastroesophageal reflux disease include esophagitis, esophageal strictures, aspiration of gastric contents, and aspiration pneumonia.

D. Positioning

1. The infant is placed in the supine position during sleep (to reduce the incidence of sudden infant death syndrome) unless the risk of death from aspiration or other serious complications of GERD greatly outweigh the risks associated with the prone position (check the HCP's prescription); otherwise, the prone position is only acceptable while the infant is awake and can be monitored.
2. In children older than 1 year, position with the head of the bed elevated.

E. Diet

1. Provide small, frequent feedings with predigested formula to decrease the amount of regurgitation.
2. Nutrition via nasogastric tube feedings may be prescribed if severe regurgitation and poor growth are present.
3. For infants, formula may be thickened by adding rice cereal to the formula (follow agency procedure); then cross-cut the nipple.
4. Breastfeeding may continue, and the mother may provide more frequent feeding times or express milk for thickening with rice cereal.
5. Burp the infant frequently when feeding and handle the infant minimally after feedings; monitor for coughing during feeding and other signs of aspiration.
6. For toddlers, feed solids first, followed by liquids.
7. Reinforce instructions to the parents to avoid feeding the child fatty foods, chocolate, tomato products, carbonated liquids, fruit juices, citrus products, and spicy foods.
8. Reinforce instructions to the parents that the child should avoid vigorous play after feeding, and avoid feeding just before bedtime.

F. Medications

1. Antacids for symptom relief
2. Proton pump inhibitors and histamine 2 (H_2) antagonists to decrease acid secretion

X. Hypertrophic Pyloric Stenosis (Fig. 33-4)

A. Description

1. Hypertrophy of the circular muscles of the pylorus causes the narrowing of the pyloric canal between the stomach and the duodenum.
2. The stenosis usually develops during the first few weeks of life and causes projectile vomiting, dehydration, metabolic alkalosis, and failure to thrive.

B. Data collection

1. Vomiting that progresses from mild regurgitation to forceful and projectile that usually occurs after a feeding.
2. Vomitus contains gastric contents, such as milk or formula. It may contain mucus, may be blood-tinged, and does not usually contain bile.
3. Hunger and irritability
4. Peristaltic waves visible from left to right across the epigastrium during or immediately after a feeding 
5. Olive-shaped mass in the epigastrium just right of the umbilicus 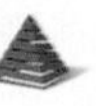

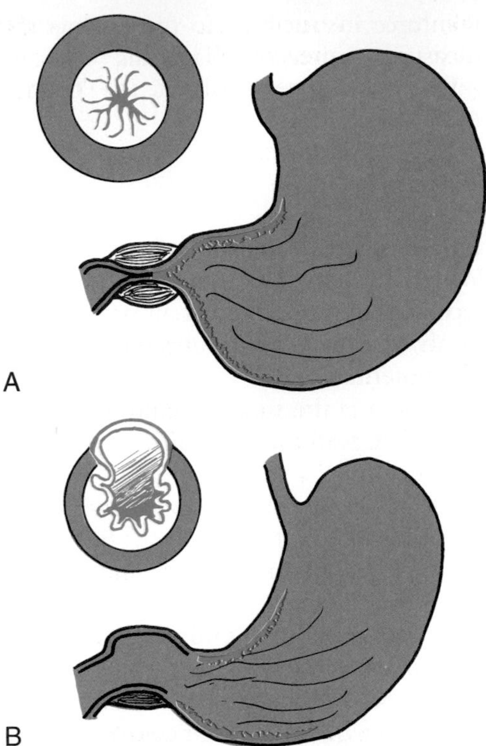

FIGURE 33-4 Hypertrophic pyloric stenosis. **A,** Enlarged muscular tumor nearly obliterates pyloric channel. **B,** Longitudinal surgical division of muscle down to submucosa establishes adequate passageway. (From Hockenberry M, Wilson D: *Wong's: Essentials of pediatric nursing,* ed 9, St. Louis, 2013, Mosby.)

6. Dehydration and malnutrition
7. Electrolyte imbalances
8. Metabolic alkalosis

C. Interventions
1. Monitor strict intake and output.
2. Monitor vomiting episodes and stools.
3. Obtain daily weights.
4. Monitor for signs of dehydration and electrolyte imbalances.
5. Assist to prepare the child and parents for pyloromyotomy, if prescribed.

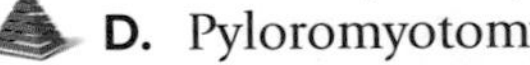

D. Pyloromyotomy
1. Description: An incision through the muscle fibers of the pylorus, which may be performed by laparoscopy
2. Interventions preoperatively
   a. Monitor the hydration status by checking the daily weights, I&O, and urine for specific gravity.
   b. Correct fluid and electrolyte imbalances. IV fluids may be prescribed for rehydration.
   c. Maintain NPO status.
   d. Monitor the number and character of stools.
   e. Maintain the patency of the nasogastric (NG) tube that is placed for stomach decompression.
3. Postoperative interventions
   a. Monitor intake and output.
   b. Begin small, frequent feedings postoperatively as prescribed.
   c. Gradually increase amount and interval between feedings until a full feeding schedule has been reinstated.
   d. Feed the infant slowly, burping frequently, and handle the infant minimally after feedings.
   e. Monitor for abdominal distention.
   f. Monitor the surgical wound and for signs of infection.
   g. Reinforce instructions to the parents about wound care and feeding.

XI. Lactose Intolerance

A. Description: The inability to tolerate lactose as a result of an absence or deficiency of lactase, which is an enzyme found in the secretions of the small intestine that is required for the digestion of lactose

B. Data collection
1. Symptoms occur after the ingestion of milk products.
2. Abdominal distention
3. Crampy, abdominal pain; colic
4. Diarrhea and excessive flatus

C. Interventions
1. Eliminate the offending dairy product or administer an enzyme replacement.
2. Provide information to the parents about enzyme tablets that predigest the lactose in milk or supplement the body's own lactase.
3. Soy-based formula can be substituted for cow's milk formula or human milk.
4. Limit milk consumption to one glass at a time.
5. If milk is consumed, it should be taken when other foods are consumed rather than by itself.
6. Encourage the consumption of hard cheese, cottage cheese, or yogurt (which contains inactive lactase enzyme) rather than milk.
7. Encourage the consumption of small amounts of dairy foods daily to help colonic bacteria adapt to ingested lactose.
8. Reinforce instructions to the parents about the foods that contain lactose, including hidden sources.

A child with lactose intolerance can develop calcium and vitamin D deficiency. Instruct the parents about the importance of providing these supplements.

XII. Celiac Disease

A. Description
1. Celiac disease also is known as gluten enteropathy or celiac sprue.

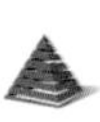

2. Intolerance to gluten, the protein component of wheat, barley, rye, and oats, is characteristic.
3. Celiac disease results in the accumulation of the amino acid glutamine, which is toxic to intestinal mucosal cells.

Pediatric

4. Intestinal villi atrophy occurs, which affects absorption of ingested nutrients.
5. Symptoms of the disorder occur most often between the ages of 1 and 5 years
6. There is usually an interval of 3 to 6 months between the introduction of gluten in the diet and the onset of symptoms.
7. Strict dietary avoidance of gluten minimizes the risk of developing malignant lymphoma of the small intestine and other gastrointestinal malignancies.

B. Data collection
1. Acute or insidious diarrhea. Stools are watery and pale with an offensive odor.
2. Steatorrhea
3. Anorexia
4. Abdominal pain and distention
5. Muscle wasting, particularly in the buttocks and extremities
6. Vomiting
7. Anemia
8. Irritability

C. Celiac crisis (Box 33-6)

D. Interventions
1. Gluten-free diet and the substitution of corn, rice, and millet as grain sources
2. Lifelong elimination of gluten sources such as wheat, rye, oats, and barley
3. Mineral and vitamin supplements, including iron, folic acid, and fat-soluble supplements A, D, E, and K
4. Reinforce teaching the parents about a gluten-free diet and to read food labels carefully for hidden sources of gluten (Box 33-7).
5. Reinforce instructions to the parents regarding measures to prevent celiac crisis.
6. Inform the parents about the Celiac Sprue Association.

BOX 33-6 Celiac Crisis

- Precipitated by infection, fasting, and the ingestion of gluten
- Can lead to electrolyte imbalance, rapid dehydration, and severe acidosis
- Causes profuse, watery diarrhea and vomiting

BOX 33-7 Basics of a Gluten-Free Diet

Foods Allowed

Meat such as beef, pork, and poultry and fish; eggs; milk and dairy products; vegetables; fruits; rice; corn; gluten-free wheat flour; puffed rice; cornflakes; cornmeal; and precooked gluten-free cereals

Foods Prohibited

Commercially prepared ice cream; malted milk; prepared puddings; and grains, including anything made from wheat, rye, oats, or barley, such as breads, rolls, cookies, cakes, crackers, cereal, spaghetti, macaroni noodles, beer, and ale

XIII. Appendicitis

A. Description
1. Inflammation of the appendix
2. When the appendix becomes inflamed or infected, perforation may occur within a matter of hours, leading to peritonitis, sepsis, septic shock, and potential death.
3. Treatment is the surgical removal of the appendix before perforation occurs.

B. Data collection
1. Pain in periumbilical area that descends to the right lower quadrant
2. Abdominal pain that is most intense at McBurney's point
3. Referred pain that indicates the presence of peritoneal irritation
4. Rebound tenderness and abdominal rigidity
5. Elevated white blood cell count
6. Side-lying position with abdominal guarding (legs flexed) to relieve pain
7. Difficulty walking and pain in the right hip
8. Low-grade fever
9. Anorexia, nausea, and vomiting after the pain develops
10. Diarrhea

C. Peritonitis
1. Description: Results from a perforated appendix
2. Data collection
   a. Increased fever
   b. Progressive abdominal distention
   c. Tachycardia and tachypnea
   d. Pallor
   e. Chills
   f. Restlessness and irritability

An indication of a perforated appendix is the sudden relief of pain and then a subsequent increase in pain accompanied by right guarding of the abdomen.

D. Appendectomy
1. Description: Surgical removal of the appendix
2. Preoperative interventions
   a. Maintain NPO status.
   b. IV fluids and electrolytes may be prescribed to prevent dehydration and correct electrolyte imbalances.
   c. Monitor for signs of a ruptured appendix and peritonitis.
   d. Monitor for changes in the level of pain; pain medications may be avoided so as not to mask pain changes associated with perforation.
   e. Antibiotics may be prescribed.

f. Monitor the bowel sounds.
g. Position the child in a right side-lying or low to semi-Fowler's position to promote comfort.
h. Apply ice packs to the abdomen for 20 to 30 minutes every hour, if prescribed.
i. Avoid the application of heat to the abdomen and the administration of laxatives or enemas because of the risk of perforation.

3. Postoperative interventions
   a. Monitor the temperature for signs of infection.
   b. Maintain NPO status until bowel function has returned. Advance the diet gradually, as tolerated and as prescribed, when bowel sounds return.
   c. Monitor the incision for signs of infection, such as redness, swelling, drainage, and pain.
   d. Monitor Penrose drain drainage, which may be inserted if perforation occurred.
   e. Position in a right side-lying or low to semi-Fowler's position with the legs slightly flexed to facilitate drainage.
   f. Change the dressing, as prescribed, and record the type and amount of drainage.
   g. Perform wound irrigations, if prescribed.
   h. Maintain NG tube suction and the patency of the tube, if present.
   i. Administer antibiotics and analgesics, as prescribed.

XIV. Hirschsprung's Disease (Fig. 33-5)

A. Description
1. Congenital anomaly also known as congenital aganglionosis or aganglionic megacolon

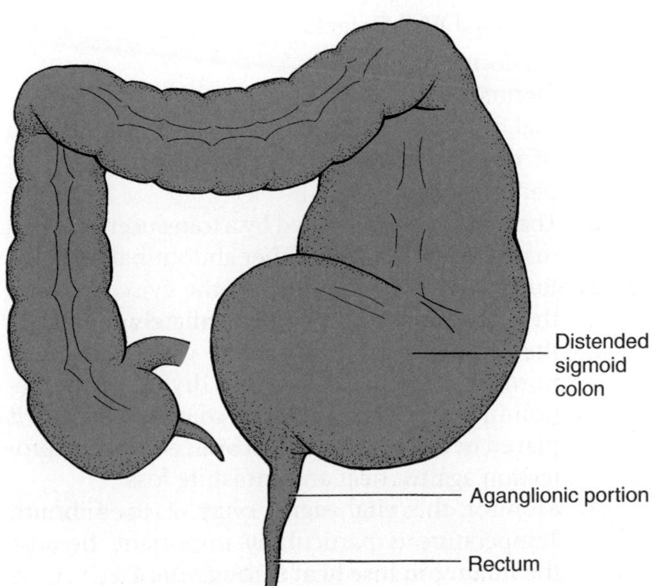

FIGURE 33-5 Hirschsprung's disease. (From Perry S, Hockenberry M, Lowdermilk D, Wilson D: *Maternal-child nursing care*, ed 4, St. Louis, 2010, Mosby.)

2. The disease occurs as the result of an absence of ganglion cells in the rectum and other areas of the affected intestine.
3. The disease results in mechanical obstruction because of inadequate motility in an intestinal segment.
4. The disease may be a familial congenital defect or may be associated with other anomalies, such as Down syndrome and genitourinary abnormalities.
5. A rectal biopsy demonstrates histological evidence of the absence of ganglionic cells.
6. The most serious complication is enterocolitis; signs include fever, severe prostration, gastrointestinal bleeding, and explosive watery diarrhea.
7. Treatment for mild or moderate disease is based on relieving the chronic constipation with stool softeners and rectal irrigations; however, surgery may be required for severe disease.

B. Data collection
1. Newborn infants
   a. Failure to pass meconium stool
   b. Refusal to suck
   c. Abdominal distention
   d. Bile-stained vomitus
2. Children
   a. Failure to gain weight and delayed growth
   b. Abdominal distention
   c. Vomiting
   d. Constipation alternating with diarrhea
   e. Ribbon-like and foul-smelling stools

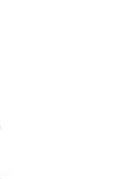

C. Interventions: Medical management
1. Maintain low-fiber, high-calorie, high-protein diet; parenteral nutrition may be necessary in extreme situations.
2. Administer stool softeners as prescribed.
3. Administer daily rectal irrigations with normal saline to promote adequate elimination and prevent obstruction as prescribed.

D. Surgical management: Preoperative interventions
1. Monitor the bowel function and administer bowel preparations, as prescribed.
2. Maintain NPO status.
3. Monitor hydration and fluid and electrolyte status. IV fluids may be prescribed for hydration.
4. Administer antibiotics or colonic irrigations with an antibiotic solution as prescribed to clear the bowel of bacteria.
5. Monitor strict I&O and weight.
6. Measure the abdominal girth.
7. Avoid taking rectal temperatures.
8. Monitor for respiratory distress associated with abdominal distention.

E. Postoperative interventions
1. Monitor vital signs, avoiding taking the temperature rectally.
2. Measure abdominal girth daily and PRN.

Pediatric

3. Check the surgical site for redness, swelling, and drainage.
4. Check the stoma if present for bleeding or skin breakdown (stoma should be red and moist).
5. Check the anal area for the presence of stool, redness, or discharge.
6. Maintain NPO status until bowel sounds return or flatus is passed and as prescribed, usually within 48 to 72 hours
7. Maintain the nasogastric tube to allow intermittent suction until peristalsis returns.
8. Maintain IV fluids until the child tolerates appropriate oral intake, advancing the diet from clear liquids to regular as tolerated and as prescribed.
9. Monitor for dehydration and fluid overload.
10. Monitor strict intake and output.
11. Obtain daily weight.
12. Monitor for pain and provide comfort measures as required and as prescribed.
13. Reinforce instructions to the parents regarding colostomy care and skin care.
14. Reinforce teaching the parents about the appropriate diet and the need for adequate fluid intake.

XV. Intussusception (Fig. 33-6)

A. Description
1. The telescoping of one portion of the bowel into another
2. Results in an obstruction of the passage of intestinal contents

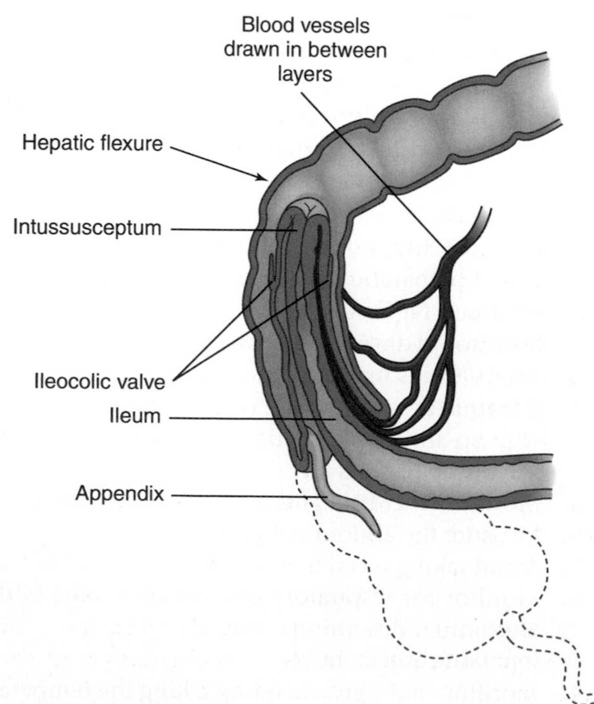

FIGURE 33-6 Ileocolic intussusception. (From Hockenberry M, Wilson D: *Wong's: Essentials of pediatric nursing*, ed 9, St. Louis, 2013, Mosby.)

B. Data collection
1. Colicky abdominal pain that causes the child to scream and draw his or her knees to the abdomen
2. Vomiting of gastric contents
3. Bile-stained fecal emesis
4. Currant jelly-like stools that contain blood and mucus
5. Hypoactive or hyperactive bowel sounds
6. Tender and distended abdomen, possibly with a palpable sausage-shaped mass in the upper right quadrant

C. Interventions
1. Monitor for signs of perforation and shock as evidenced by fever, increased heart rate, changes in level of consciousness or blood pressure, and respiratory distress, and report immediately.
2. Antibiotics, IV fluids, and decompression via nasogastric tube may be prescribed.
3. Monitor for the passage of normal, brown stool, which indicates that the intussusception has reduced itself.
4. Prepare for hydrostatic reduction as prescribed, if no signs of perforation or shock occur (in hydrostatic reduction, air or fluid is used to exert pressure on area involved to lessen, diminish, or rid the intestine of prolapse).
5. Posthydrostatic reduction
   a. Monitor for the return of normal bowel sounds, for the passage of barium, and the characteristics of stool.
   b. Administer clear fluids and advance the diet gradually as prescribed.
6. If surgery is required, postoperative care is similar to that following any abdominal surgery.

XVI. Abdominal Wall Defects

A. Omphalocele

1. Occurs when there is a herniation of the abdominal contents through the umbilical ring (hernia of the umbilical cord), usually with an intact peritoneal sac
2. The protrusion is covered by a translucent sac that may contain bowel or other abdominal organs.
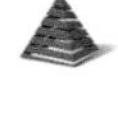
3. Rupture of the sac results in the evisceration of the abdominal contents. Immediately after birth, the sac is covered with sterile gauze soaked in normal saline to prevent the drying of the abdominal contents. A layer of plastic wrap is placed over the gauze to provide additional protection against heat and moisture loss.

4. Monitor the vital signs every 2 to 4 hours. Temperature is particularly important, because the infant can lose heat through the sac.
5. Preoperatively: Maintain NPO status. IV fluids will be prescribed to maintain hydration and electrolyte balance. Monitor for signs of

infection, and handle the infant carefully to prevent the rupture of the sac.
6. Postoperatively: Control pain, prevent infection, maintain fluid and electrolyte balance, and ensure adequate nutrition.

B. Gastroschisis
1. Occurs when the herniation of the intestine is lateral (usually on the right) to the umbilical ring

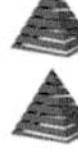

2. There is no membrane covering the exposed bowel.
3. The exposed bowel is loosely covered in saline-soaked pads, and the abdomen is loosely wrapped in a plastic drape. Wrapping around the exposed bowel is contraindicated, because if the exposed bowel expands, the wrapping could cause pressure and necrosis.
4. Preoperatively: Care is similar to that for omphalocele. Surgery is performed within several hours after birth, because there is no membrane covering the sac.
5. Postoperatively: Most infants develop a prolonged ileus and require mechanical ventilation and parenteral nutrition. Otherwise, care is similar to that for omphalocele.

XVII. Umbilical Hernia

A. Description
1. A hernia is a protrusion of the bowel through an abnormal opening in the abdominal wall.
2. In children, a hernia most commonly occurs at the umbilicus and through the inguinal canal.
3. A hydrocele is the presence of abdominal fluid in the scrotal sac.

B. Data collection
1. Umbilical hernia: A soft swelling or protrusion around the umbilicus that is usually reducible with the finger
2. Inguinal hernia
   a. Painless inguinal swelling that is reducible
   b. Swelling may disappear during periods of rest and is most noticeable when the infant cries or coughs.
3. Incarcerated hernia
   a. Occurs when the descended portion of the bowel becomes tightly caught in the hernial sac, compromising blood supply
   b. Represents a medical emergency requiring surgical repair
   c. Data collection findings—irritability, tenderness at site, anorexia, abdominal distention, difficulty defecating
   d. May lead to complete intestinal obstruction and gangrene
4. Noncommunicating hydrocele
   a. Occurs when residual peritoneal fluid is trapped with no communication with the peritoneal cavity
   b. Usually disappears by the age of 1 year
5. Communicating hydrocele
   a. Associated with a hernia that remains open from the scrotum to the abdominal cavity
   b. Data collection findings include a bulge in the inguinal area or the scrotum that increases with crying or straining and that decreases when the child is at rest.

C. Postoperative interventions (hernia)
1. Monitor the vital signs.
2. Monitor for wound infection (redness or drainage).
3. Monitor I&O and hydration status.
4. Advance the diet, as tolerated and as prescribed.
5. Administer analgesics, as prescribed.

D. Postoperative interventions (hydrocele)
1. Provide ice bags and a scrotal support to relieve pain and swelling.
2. Reinforce instructions to the child and parents to avoid tub bathing until the incision heals.
3. Reinforce instructions to the child and parents to avoid strenuous physical activities.

XVIII. Irritable Bowel Syndrome

A. Description
1. Occurs as a result of increased motility, which can lead to spasm and pain
2. Diagnosis is based on the elimination of pathological conditions.
3. Self-limiting, intermittent problem with no definitive treatment
4. Stress and emotional factors may contribute to its occurrence.

B. Data collection
1. Diffuse abdominal pain unrelated to meals or activity
2. Alternating constipation and diarrhea with the presence of undigested food and mucus in the stool

C. Interventions
1. Reassure the parents that the problem is self-limiting and intermittent and that it will resolve.
2. Anticholinergics may be prescribed. (Antidepressants may be needed in severe cases.)
3. Encourage the maintenance of a healthy, well-balanced, moderate-fiber and low-fat diet.
4. Encourage health-promotion activities, such as exercise and school activities.
5. Inform the parents about psychosocial resources, if required.

XIX. Imperforate Anus

A. Description: The incomplete development or absence of the anus in its normal position in the perineum

B. Data collection (Box 33-8)

C. Preoperative interventions

Pediatric

BOX 33-8 Data Collection Findings: Imperforate Anus

- Failure to pass meconium stool
- Absence or stenosis of the anal rectal canal
- Presence of an anal membrane
- External fistula to the perineum

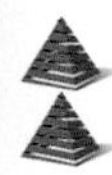

1. Determine the patency of the anus.
2. Monitor for the presence of stool in the urine and vagina. Report this immediately.
3. Assist to administer IV fluids as prescribed.
4. Prepare the child and parents for the surgical procedures, including the potential for colostomy.

D. Postoperative interventions
1. Monitor the skin for signs of infection.
2. The preferred position is a side-lying prone position with the hips elevated or a supine position with the legs suspended at a 90-degree angle to the trunk to reduce edema and pressure on the surgical site.
3. Keep the anal surgical incision clean and dry, and monitor for redness, swelling, or drainage.
4. Maintain NPO status and the nasogastric tube, if one has been placed.
5. Maintain IV fluids until gastrointestinal motility returns as prescribed.
6. Assist to provide colostomy care, if prescribed.
7. A fresh colostomy stoma will be red and edematous, but this should decrease with time.
8. Reinforce instructions to the parents about the procedure to perform anal dilation, if prescribed, to achieve and maintain bowel patency.

XX. Hepatitis

A. This section contains specific information regarding hepatitis as it relates to infants and children. Refer to Chapters 26 and 47 for additional information about hepatitis.

B. Description: An acute or chronic inflammation of the liver that may be caused by a virus, a medication reaction, or another disease process

C. Hepatitis A virus (HAV)
1. Highest incidence occurs among preschool or school-age children who are less than 15 years old.
2. Many affected children are asymptomatic, but mild nausea, vomiting, and diarrhea may occur.
3. Infected children who are asymptomatic can still spread HAV to others.

D. Hepatitis B virus (HBV)
1. Most HBV in children is acquired perinatally.
2. Newborns are at risk if the mother is infected with HBV or was a carrier of HBV during pregnancy.
3. Possible routes of maternal–fetal (infant) transmission include the leakage of the virus across the placenta late in pregnancy or during labor, the ingestion of amniotic fluid or maternal blood, and breastfeeding, especially if the mother has cracked nipples.
4. The severity in the infant varies from no liver disease to fulminant (severe, acute course) or chronic, active disease.
5. In children and adolescents, HBV occurs in specific high-risk groups, including the following:
   a. Children with hemophilia or other disorders who have received multiple blood transfusions
   b. Children or adolescents who are involved in drug abuse
   c. Institutionalized children
   d. Preschool-age children in endemic areas
   e. Children who may be involved with heterosexual activity or sexual activity with homosexual males
6. HBV infection can cause a carrier state and lead to eventual cirrhosis or hepatocellular carcinoma during adulthood.

E. Hepatitis C virus (HCV)
1. Transmission is primarily by the parenteral route.
2. Some children may be asymptomatic, but HCV often becomes a chronic condition, and it can cause cirrhosis and hepatocellular carcinoma.

F. Hepatitis D virus
1. Infection occurs in children already infected with HBV.
2. Acute and chronic forms tend to be more severe than HBV and can lead to cirrhosis.
3. Children with hemophilia are more likely to be infected, as are children who are IV drug users.

G. Hepatitis E virus
1. Uncommon among children
2. Is not a chronic condition, does not cause chronic liver disease, and has no carrier state

H. Data collection (Box 33-9) 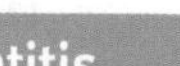

BOX 33-9 Data Collection Findings: Hepatitis

Prodromal or Anicteric Phase

- Lasts 5 to 7 days
- Absence of jaundice
- Anorexia, malaise, lethargy, and easy fatigability
- Fever (especially among adolescents)
- Nausea and vomiting
- Epigastric or right upper quadrant abdominal pain
- Arthralgia and skin rashes (more likely with hepatitis B virus)
- Hepatomegaly

Icteric Phase

- Jaundice, which is best assessed in the sclera, nail beds, and mucous membranes
- Dark urine and pale stools
- Pruritus

I. Diagnostic evaluation: See Chapter 11 for the laboratory studies that are used to diagnose hepatitis.

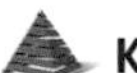

J. Prevention
1. Immunoglobulin provides **passive immunity** and may be effective for preexposure prophylaxis to prevent HAV infection.
2. Hepatitis B immunoglobulin provides passive immunity and may be effective in preventing infection following a one-time exposure (should be given immediately after exposure), such as an accidental needle puncture or other contact of contaminated material with mucous membranes; should also be given to newborns whose mothers are HBsAg-positive.
3. Hepatitis A and hepatitis B vaccines (see Chapter 39 for information on immunizations)

Proper hand washing and standard precautions can prevent the spread of viral hepatitis.

K. Interventions
1. Strict hand washing is required
2. Hospitalization is required in the event of coagulopathy or fulminant hepatitis.
3. Standard precautions and enteric precautions are followed during hospitalization; provide enteric precautions for at least 1 week after the onset of jaundice with HAV.
4. A hospitalized child is not usually isolated in a separate room unless he or she is fecally incontinent and items are likely to become contaminated with feces.
5. Children are discouraged from sharing toys.
6. Reinforce instructions to the child and parents regarding good hand-washing techniques.
7. Reinforce instructions to the parents to thoroughly disinfect diaper-changing surfaces using ¼ cup of bleach in 1 gallon of water.
8. Maintain comfort and provide adequate rest and sleep.
9. Provide a low-fat, balanced diet.
10. Inform the parents that because HAV is not infectious 1 week after the onset of jaundice, the child may return to school at that time if he or she feels well enough.
11. Inform the parents that jaundice may get worse before it resolves.
12. Caution the parents about administering any medications to the child. (Remember that the liver is unable to detoxify and excrete medications.)
13. Reinforce instructions to the parents regarding the signs that indicate the worsening of the child's condition, such as changes in the neurological status, bleeding, and fluid retention.

XXI. Ingestion of Poisons (see Priority Nursing Actions)

PRIORITY NURSING ACTIONS

Actions to Take in the Emergency Department in the Event of a Poisoning

1. Assess the child.
2. Terminate exposure to the poison.
3. Identify the poison.
4. Take measures to prevent absorption of the poison.
5. Document the occurrence, data collection findings, poison ingested, treatment measures, and the child's response.

In the event of a poisoning, the nurse treats the child first, not the poison. Circulation, airway, and breathing and vital signs are assessed. Cardiopulmonary resuscitation is initiated immediately if necessary. Exposure to the poison is terminated next, such as emptying the mouth of pills or other materials or flushing the skin or other body area. The poison is identified next by questioning the parents or witnesses of the event to determine the appropriate treatment. The nurse assists to administer the antidote or takes other measures as prescribed by the HCP, such as administering activated charcoal. The nurse documents the occurrence, data collection findings, poison ingested, treatment measures, and the child's response.

Reference(s): Hockenberry, M., & Wilson, D. (2013). *Wong's: Essentials of pediatric nursing* (9th ed., p. 437). St. Louis: Mosby.

A. Lead poisoning
1. Description: Excessive accumulation of lead in the blood
2. Causes

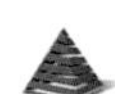

a. The pathway for exposure may be food, air, or water.
b. Dust and soil contaminated with lead may be a source of exposure.
c. Lead enters the child's body through ingestion or inhalation or through placental transmission to an unborn child when the mother is exposed; the most common route is hand to mouth from contaminated objects, such as loose paint chips, pottery, or ceramic ware coupled with the inhalation of lead dust in the environment.
d. When lead enters the body, it affects the erythrocytes, bones, teeth, organs, and tissues, including the brain and nervous system. The most serious consequences are the effects on the central nervous system.
3. Universal screening

a. Recommended in high-risk areas at the age of 1 to 2 years. Children at high risk should be screened earlier.
b. Any child between the ages of 3 and 6 years who has not been screened should be tested.

TABLE 33-2 Blood Lead Level Test Results and Intervention

Level (mcg/dL)	Intervention
Less than 10	Reassess or rescreen in 1 year or sooner if exposure status changes.
10 to 14	Provide family lead education, follow-up testing, and social service referral for home assessment if necessary.
15 to 19	Provide family lead education, follow-up testing, and social service referral if necessary; on follow-up testing, initiate actions for blood lead level of 20 to 44 mcg/dL.
20 to 44	Provide coordination of care, clinical management, including treatment, environmental investigation, and lead-hazard control
45 to 69	Provide coordination of care and clinical management within 48 hours, including treatment, environmental investigation, and lead hazard control (the child must not remain in a lead-hazardous environment if resolution is necessary).
70 or greater	Medical treatment is provided immediately, including coordination of care, clinical management, environmental investigation, and lead-hazard control.

Adapted from Perry S, Hockenberry M, Lowdermilk D, Wilson D: *Maternal child nursing care*, ed 4, St. Louis, 2010, Elsevier.

4. Targeted screening
   a. Acceptable in low-risk areas
   b. At the age of 1 to 2 years (or a child between the ages of 3 and 6 years who has not been screened) may be targeted for screening if determined to be at risk.

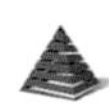

5. Blood lead level test: Used for screening and diagnosis (Table 33-2)

6. Erythrocyte protoporphyrin test
   a. An indicator of anemia
   b. Normal value for a child is 35 mcg/100 mL of whole blood or less

7. Chelation therapy
   a. Removes lead from the circulating blood and from some organs and tissues
   b. Does not counteract any effects of the lead
   c. Medications include calcium disodium edetate ($CaNa_2EDTA$), and succimer (Chemet), an oral preparation; British anti-Lewisite (BAL, dimercaprol) is used in conjunction with EDTA.
   d. British anti-Lewisite (BAL, dimercaprol) is administered by the intravenous route or via deep intramuscular route and is contraindicated in children with an allergy to peanuts because the medication is prepared in a peanut oil solution; it is also contraindicated in children with a glucose 6-phosphate dehydrogenase (G6PD) deficiency and should not be given with iron.
   e. The function of the renal, hepatic, and hematological systems must be monitored closely.
   f. Adequate urinary output is ensured before administering the medication, and it is important to monitor the output and pH of the urine closely during and after therapy.
   g. Provide adequate hydration and monitor kidney function for nephrotoxicity when the medication is given because the medication is excreted via the kidneys.
   h. Follow-up of lead levels needs to be done to monitor progress.
   i. Reinforce instructions to the parents about safety from lead hazards, medication administration, and the need for follow-up.
   j. Confirm that the child will be discharged to a home without lead hazards.

B. Acetaminophen (Tylenol) poisoning

1. Description
   a. The seriousness of the ingestion is determined by the amount ingested and the length of time before intervention.
   b. A toxic dose is 150 mg/kg or higher in children.

2. Data collection
   a. First 2 to 4 hours: Malaise, nausea, vomiting, sweating, pallor, and weakness
   b. Latent period: 24 to 36 hours; child improves.
   c. Hepatic involvement: May last up to 7 days and be permanent; right upper quadrant pain, jaundice, confusion, stupor, elevated liver enzymes and bilirubin levels, and prolonged prothrombin time

3. Interventions
   a. Administer the antidote: *N*-acetylcysteine.
   b. Antidote is diluted in juice or soda because of its offensive odor.
   c. Loading dose is followed by maintenance doses.
   d. In the unconscious child, prepare to administer gastric lavage with activated charcoal to decrease the absorption of acetaminophen.
   e. If using activated charcoal with lavage, do not also use *N*-acetylcysteine because activated charcoal will inactivate the antidote.

C. Acetylsalicylic acid (aspirin) poisoning

1. Description
   a. May be caused by acute or chronic ingestion
   b. Acute: Severe toxicity occurs with 300 to 500 mg/kg.
   c. Chronic: More than 100 mg/kg/day for 2 days or more; can be more serious than acute ingestion

2. Data collection
   a. Gastrointestinal effects: Nausea, vomiting, and thirst from dehydration
   b. Central nervous system effects: Hyperpnea, confusion, tinnitus, seizures, coma, respiratory failure, and circulatory collapse
   c. Renal effects: Oliguria
   d. Hematopoietic effects: Bleeding tendencies
   e. Metabolic effects: Diaphoresis, fever, hyponatremia, hypokalemia, dehydration, and hypoglycemia
3. Interventions
   a. Prepare to administer activated charcoal to decrease the absorption of salicylate.
   b. Emesis or cathartic measures may be prescribed.
   c. Assist to administer IV fluids; sodium bicarbonate may be prescribed to correct metabolic acidosis.
   d. Other interventions may include external cooling, anticonvulsants, vitamin K (if bleeding), and oxygen.
   e. Prepare the child for dialysis as prescribed if the child is unresponsive to the therapy.

D. Corrosives
1. Description
   a. Items that can cause poisoning include household cleaners, detergents, bleach, paint or paint thinners, or batteries.
   b. Liquid corrosives can cause more damage to the victim than other types of corrosives, such as granular.
2. Data collection
   a. Severe burning in the mouth, throat, or stomach
   b. Edema of the mucous membranes, lips, tongue, and pharynx
   c. Vomiting
   d. Drooling and inability to clear secretions
3. Interventions
   a. Dilute corrosive with water or milk as prescribed (usually no more than 4 oz).
   b. Inducing vomiting is contraindicated because vomiting redamages the mucous membranes.
   c. Neutralization of the ingested corrosive is not done because it can cause a reaction producing heat and burns.

Educate parents to call the poison control center immediately in the event of poisoning. The parents need to be instructed to post the poison control center telephone number near each phone in the house.

XXII. Intestinal Parasites

A. Description: Common infections in children are giardiasis and pinworms.
1. Giardiasis is caused by protozoa, and it is prevalent among children in crowded environments, such as classrooms and day-care centers.
2. Pinworms (enterobiasis) are universally present in temperate climate zones and easily transmitted in crowded environments.

B. Data collection
1. Giardiasis
   a. Diarrhea and vomiting
   b. Anorexia
   c. Failure to thrive
   d. Abdominal cramps with intermittent loose stools and constipation
   e. Steatorrhea
   f. Stool specimens from three or more collections are used for diagnosis
2. Pinworms
   a. Intense perianal itching
   b. Irritability and restlessness
   c. Poor sleeping
   d. Bed-wetting

C. Interventions
1. Giardiasis
   a. Medications that may be prescribed include metronidazole (Flagyl), tinidazole (Tindamax), nitazoxanide (Alinia), or albendazole (Albenza).
   b. Performance of meticulous hand washing by caregivers
   c. Reinforce education to the family and caregivers regarding sanitary practices.
2. Pinworms 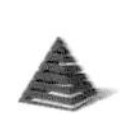
   a. Perform a visual inspection of the anus with a flashlight 2 to 3 hours after sleep.
   b. The tape test is the most common diagnostic test.
   c. Reinforce educating the family and caregivers regarding the tape test. A loop of transparent tape is placed firmly against the child's perianal area; it is removed in the morning and placed in a glass jar or plastic bag and transported to the primary care provider for analysis. 
   d. Medications that may be prescribed include ebendazole (Vermox), pyrantel pamoate (Pin-Rid, Antiminth), and albendazole (Albenza); these medications are not used in children under the age of 2 years.
   e. The medication regimen may be repeated in 2 weeks to prevent reinfection
   f. All members of the family are treated for the infection.
   g. Reinforce teaching the family and caregivers about the importance of meticulous hand washing and about washing all clothes and bed linens in hot water.

CRITICAL THINKING What Should You Do?

Answer: If a child suddenly vomits, the nurse must maintain a patent airway. The child should be positioned upright or on the side to prevent aspiration. Suctioning equipment should be obtained and kept at the bedside. The nurse should check the character and amount of the vomitus. The force of the vomiting should be assessed because projectile vomiting may indicate pyloric stenosis or increased intracranial pressure. The nurse should also monitor intake and output and for signs of dehydration.

Reference(s): McKinney, E., James, S., Murray, S., Nelson, K. & Ashwill, J. (2013). *Maternal-child nursing* (4th ed., pp. 1004–1005). St. Louis: Elsevier.

PRACTICE QUESTIONS

311. The nurse reviews the record of a 3-week-old infant and notes that the health care provider has documented a diagnosis of suspected Hirschsprung's disease. The nurse understands that which manifestation led the mother to seek health care for the infant?

1. Diarrhea
2. Projectile vomiting
3. The regurgitation of feedings
4. Foul-smelling, ribbon-like stools

312. The nurse is caring for a child with a diagnosis of intussusception. Which manifestation should the nurse expect to note in this child?

1. Watery diarrhea
2. Ribbon-like stools
3. Profuse projectile vomiting
4. Blood and mucus in the stools

313. A child with a diagnosis of a hernia has been scheduled for a surgical repair in 2 weeks. The nurse reinforces instructions to the parents about the signs of possible hernial strangulation. The nurse tells the parents that which manifestation requires health care provider (HCP) notification by the parents?

1. Fever
2. Diarrhea
3. Vomiting
4. Constipation

314. The nurse reinforces home-care instructions to the parents of a child with hepatitis regarding the care of the child and the prevention of the transmission of the virus. Which statement by a parent indicates a **need for further teaching?**

1. "Frequent hand washing is important."
2. "I need to provide a well-balanced, high-fat diet to my child."
3. "I need to clean contaminated household surfaces with bleach."
4. "Diapers should not be changed near any surfaces that are used to prepare food."

❖**315.** The nurse is assigned to care for a child who is scheduled for an appendectomy. Which prescriptions does the nurse anticipate to be prescribed? **Select all that apply.**

- ❑ 1. Administer a Fleet enema.
- ❑ 2. Initiate an intravenous line.
- ❑ 3. Maintain nothing-by-mouth status.
- ❑ 4. Administer intravenous antibiotics.
- ❑ 5. Administer preoperative medications.
- ❑ 6. Place a heating pad on the abdomen to decrease pain.

316. A school-age child with type 1 diabetes mellitus has soccer practice three afternoons a week. The nurse reinforces instructions regarding how to prevent hypoglycemia during practice. Which should the nurse tell the child?

1. Drink a half a cup of orange juice before soccer practice.
2. Eat twice the amount that is normally eaten at lunchtime.
3. Take half of the amount of prescribed insulin on practice days.
4. Take the prescribed insulin at noontime rather than in the morning.

317. A mother of a 6-year-old child with type 1 diabetes mellitus calls the clinic nurse and tells the nurse that the child has been sick. The mother reports that she checked the child's urine and it showed positive ketones. Which should the nurse instruct the mother to do?

1. Hold the next dose of insulin.
2. Come to the clinic immediately.
3. Encourage the child to drink liquids.
4. Administer an additional dose of regular insulin.

318. The nurse is caring for an 18-month-old child who has been vomiting. The appropriate position to place the child during naps and sleep time is which?

1. A supine position
2. A side-lying position
3. Prone, with the head elevated
4. Prone, with the face turned to the side

319. The nurse is monitoring for signs of dehydration in a 1-year-old child who has been hospitalized for diarrhea and prepares to take the

child's temperature. Which method of temperature measurement should be avoided?
1. Rectal
2. Axillary
3. Electronic
4. Tympanic

320. An infant returns to the nursing unit after the surgical repair of a cleft lip located on the right side of the lip. The **best** position to place this infant at this time is which?
1. A flat position
2. A prone position
3. On his or her left side
4. On his or her right side

321. The nurse reviews the record of an infant who is seen in the clinic. The nurse notes that a diagnosis of esophageal atresia with tracheoesophageal fistula (TEF) is suspected. The nurse expects to note which **most likely** manifestation of this condition in the medical record?
1. Incessant crying
2. Coughing at nighttime
3. Choking with feedings
4. Severe projectile vomiting

322. The nurse is reviewing the record of a child with a diagnosis of pyloric stenosis. Which data should the nurse expect to note as having been documented in the child's record?
1. Watery diarrhea
2. Projectile vomiting
3. Increased urine output
4. Vomiting large amounts of bile

323. The nurse reinforces instructions to the mother about dietary measures for a 5-year-old child with lactose intolerance. The nurse should tell the mother that which supplement will be required as a result of the need to avoid lactose in the diet?
1. Fats
2. Zinc
3. Calcium
4. Thiamine

324. The nurse reinforces home-care instructions to the parents of a child with celiac disease. Which food item should the nurse advise the parents to include in the child's diet?
1. Rice
2. Oatmeal
3. Rye toast
4. Wheat bread

325. The nursing instructor asks a nursing student about phenylketonuria (PKU). Which statement made by the student indicates an understanding of this disorder?
1. "PKU is an autosomal-dominant disorder."
2. "PKU primarily affects the gastrointestinal system."
3. "Treatment of PKU includes the dietary restriction of tyramine."
4. "All 50 states require routine screening of all newborns for PKU."

ANSWERS

311. 4

Rationale: Chronic constipation that begins during the first month of life and that results in foul-smelling, ribbon-like or pellet-like stools is a clinical manifestation of Hirschsprung's disease. The delayed passage or absence of meconium stool during the neonatal period is a characteristic sign. Bowel obstruction (especially during the neonatal period), abdominal pain and distention, and failure to thrive are also signs and symptoms. This disorder results in a decrease in passage of stool, so diarrhea would not be a presenting manifestation. Hirschsprung's disease affects the colon, so regurgitation and vomiting most often associated with esophageal and stomach pathology would not be presenting manifestations.

Test-Taking Strategy: Knowledge regarding the manifestations associated with the subject, Hirschsprung's disease, is required to answer this question. Think about the pathophysiology associated with this disorder and recall that foul-smelling, ribbon-like or pellet-like stools are manifestations of this disorder. **Review:** Hirschsprung's disease.

Level of Cognitive Ability: Understanding
Client Needs: Physiological Integrity
Integrated Process: Nursing Process/Data Collection
Content Area: Child Health: Gastrointestinal
Priority Concepts: Elimination, Nutrition
Reference(s): Hockenberry, Wilson (2013), p. 780.

312. 4

Rationale: The child with intussusception classically presents with severe abdominal pain that is crampy and intermittent and that causes the child to draw in his or her knees to the chest. Vomiting may be present, but it is not projectile. Bright red blood and mucus are passed through the rectum and commonly described as currant jelly-like stools. Ribbon-like stools are not a manifestation of this disorder.

Test-Taking Strategy: Knowledge related to the manifestations associated with the subject, intussusception, is required to answer this question. Recalling that a classic manifestation is currant jelly-like stools will assist in directing you to the correct option. **Review: intussusception.**

Level of Cognitive Ability: Understanding
Client Needs: Physiological Integrity

Integrated Process: Nursing Process/Data Collection
Content Area: Child Health: Gastrointestinal
Priority Concepts: Acid-Base Balance, Elimination
Reference(s): Hockenberry, Wilson (2013), pp. 809–810.

313. 3
Rationale: The parents of a child with a hernia need to be instructed about the signs of strangulation. These signs include vomiting, pain, and an irreducible mass. The parents should be instructed to contact the HCP immediately if strangulation is suspected. Fever, diarrhea, and constipation are not associated with strangulation of a hernia.
Test-Taking Strategy: Focus on the subject, a hernia and the need to notify the health care provider. Use the definition of the word *strangulation* to help answer this question; this will assist you with eliminating options 1 and 2. From the remaining options, thinking about the signs of strangulation will assist you with answering the question. **Review: hernias.**
Level of Cognitive Ability: Applying
Client Needs: Physiological Integrity
Integrated Process: Teaching and Learning
Content Area: Child Health: Gastrointestinal
Priority Concepts: Client Education, Pain
Reference(s): Hockenberry, Wilson (2013), pp. 806–807.

314. 2
Rationale: The child with hepatitis should consume a well-balanced, low-fat diet to allow the liver to rest. Options 1, 3, and 4 are components of the home-care instructions to the family of a child with hepatitis.
Test-Taking Strategy: Note the strategic words, *need for further teaching*. These words indicate a negative event query and ask you to select an option that is an incorrect statement. Options 1, 3, and 4 can be eliminated by remembering the basic principles related to standard precautions. **Review: hepatitis.**
Level of Cognitive Ability: Evaluating
Client Needs: Safe and Effective Care Environment
Integrated Process: Teaching and Learning
Content Area: Child Health: Gastrointestinal
Priority Concepts: Client Education, Nutrition
Reference(s): McKinney et al (2013), p. 1110.

❖315. 2, 3, 4, 5
Rationale: During the preoperative period, enemas or laxatives should not be administered. In addition, heat should not be applied to the abdomen. Any of these interventions can cause the rupture of the appendix and resultant peritonitis. Intravenous fluids would be started, and the child should receive nothing by mouth while awaiting surgery. Antibiotics are usually administered because of the risk of perforation. Preoperative medications are administered as prescribed.
Test-Taking Strategy: Consider the anatomical location of the subject, appendicitis, and think about the concern of rupture of the appendix for clients with this disorder. This will assist you with determining the correct interventions. **Review: appendicitis.**
Level of Cognitive Ability: Analyzing
Client Needs: Physiological Integrity
Integrated Process: Nursing Process/Planning
Content Area: Child Health: Gastrointestinal
Priority Concepts: Inflammation, Safety
Reference(s): Hockenberry, Wilson (2013), p. 786; McKinney et al (2013), p. 1090.

316. 1
Rationale: An extra snack of 10 g to 15 g of carbohydrates eaten before activities and for every 30 to 45 minutes of activity will prevent hypoglycemia. A half cup of orange juice will provide the needed carbohydrates. The child or parents should not be instructed to adjust the amount or time of insulin administration, and meal amounts should not be doubled.
Test-Taking Strategy: Focus on the subject, preventing hypoglycemia. Options 3 and 4 can be eliminated first using general medication guidelines, because insulin dosages and times should not be adjusted. From the remaining options, recalling the signs/symptoms and treatment associated with hypoglycemia will direct you to the correct option. **Review: diabetes mellitus.**
Level of Cognitive Ability: Applying
Client Needs: Health Promotion and Maintenance
Integrated Process: Teaching and Learning
Content Area: Child Health: Metabolic/Endocrine
Priority Concepts: Glucose Regulation, Nutrition
Reference(s): Hockenberry, Wilson (2013), pp. 996, 1000.

317. 3
Rationale: When the child is sick, the mother should test for urinary ketones with each voiding. If ketones are present, liquids are essential to help with clearing them. The child should be encouraged to drink liquids. It is not necessary to bring the child to the clinic immediately, and insulin doses should not be adjusted or changed.
Test-Taking Strategy: Focus on the subject, sick-day rules for the child with diabetes mellitus. Eliminate options 1 and 4 first, because insulin doses should not be adjusted or changed. From the remaining options, note the words *positive ketones*. This finding does not require immediate health care provider referral. **Review: diabetes mellitus.**
Level of Cognitive Ability: Applying
Client Needs: Physiological Integrity
Integrated Process: Nursing Process/Implementation
Content Area: Child Health: Metabolic/Endocrine
Priority Concepts: Elimination, Glucose Regulation
Reference(s): McKinney et al (2013), p. 1405.

318. 2
Rationale: The vomiting child should be placed in an upright or side-lying position to prevent aspiration. Options 1, 3, and 4 will place the child at risk for aspiration if vomiting occurs.
Test-Taking Strategy: Eliminate options 3 and 4 first, because they are comparable or alike. In addition, these positions would place the child at risk for aspiration if vomiting occurred. Visualize the remaining two positions. Option 1 is also inappropriate and would cause aspiration. **Review: vomiting.**
Level of Cognitive Ability: Applying
Client Needs: Safe and Effective Care Environment
Integrated Process: Nursing Process/Implementation
Content Area: Child Health: Gastrointestinal
Priority Concepts: Clinical Judgment, Safety
Reference(s): McKinney et al (2013), pp. 1004–1005.

319. 1
Rationale: Rectal temperature measurements should be avoided if diarrhea is present. The use of a rectal thermometer can stimulate peristalsis and cause more diarrhea. Axillary or tympanic measurements of temperature would be acceptable. Most measurements are performed via electronic devices.

Test-Taking Strategy: Focus on the subject, the method of temperature measurement that should be avoided. Note that the child has diarrhea. Eliminate option 3 first because most methods of temperature measurement are performed with the use of an electronic device. Next, note the diagnosis stated in the question; this should direct you to the correct option. **Review:** diarrhea.
Level of Cognitive Ability: Applying
Client Needs: Physiological Integrity
Integrated Process: Nursing Process/Implementation
Content Area: Child Health: Gastrointestinal
Priority Concepts: Clinical Judgment, Safety
Reference(s): Hockenberry, Wilson (2013), p. 777.

320. 3
Rationale: After the repair of a cleft lip, the infant should be positioned on the side opposite to the repair to prevent contact of the suture lines with the bed linens. In this case, it is best to place the infant on the left side. Additionally, the flat or prone position can result in aspiration if the infant vomits.
Test-Taking Strategy: Note the strategic word, *best.* Consider the anatomical location of the surgical site, *right side,* and think about the risk of aspiration and the risk of disruption of the surgical site. You should be easily directed to the correct option with the use of these concepts. **Review:** cleft lip.
Level of Cognitive Ability: Applying
Client Needs: Physiological Integrity
Integrated Process: Nursing Process/Implementation
Content Area: Child Health: Gastrointestinal
Priority Concepts: Clinical Judgment, Safety
Reference(s): McKinney et al (2013), p. 1073.

321. 3
Rationale: Any child who exhibits the "3 C's"—coughing and choking during feedings and unexplained cyanosis—should be suspected of having TEF. Options 1, 2, and 4 are not specifically associated with TEF.
Test-Taking Strategy: Note the strategic words, *most likely.* Focus on the subject, signs and symptoms of TEF, and think about the pathophysiology associated with this condition. Recalling the "3 C's" associated with TEF will direct you to the correct option. **Review:** esophageal atresia with tracheoesophageal fistula.
Level of Cognitive Ability: Analyzing
Client Needs: Physiological Integrity
Integrated Process: Nursing Process/Data Collection
Content Area: Child Health: Gastrointestinal
Priority Concepts: Clinical Judgment, Gas Exchange
Reference(s): McKinney et al (2013), pp. 1074–1075.

322. 2
Rationale: Signs and symptoms of pyloric stenosis include projectile, nonbilious vomiting; irritability; hunger and crying; constipation; and signs of dehydration, including a decrease in urine output.
Test-Taking Strategy: Focus on the subject, signs/symptoms of pyloric stenosis. Considering the anatomical location of this disorder and the definition of the word *stenosis* will assist you with eliminating the incorrect options. **Review:** pyloric stenosis.
Level of Cognitive Ability: Analyzing
Client Needs: Physiological Integrity
Integrated Process: Nursing Process/Data Collection
Content Area: Child Health: Gastrointestinal
Priority Concepts: Acid-Base Balance, Clinical Judgment
Reference(s): McKinney et al (2013), p. 1095.

323. 3
Rationale: Lactose intolerance is the inability to tolerate lactose, which is the sugar that is found in dairy products. Removing milk from the diet can provide relief from symptoms. Additional dietary changes may be required to provide adequate sources of calcium and, if the child is an infant, protein and calories.
Test-Taking Strategy: Focus on the subject, adequate nutrition for the child with lactose intolerance. Knowledge that lactose is the sugar that is found in dairy products will easily direct you to the correct option because dairy products are a major source of calcium. **Review:** lactose intolerance.
Level of Cognitive Ability: Applying
Client Needs: Physiological Integrity
Integrated Process: Nursing Process/Implementation
Content Area: Child Health: Gastrointestinal
Priority Concepts: Elimination, Nutrition
Reference(s): Hockenberry, Wilson (2013), p. 527.

324. 1
Rationale: Dietary management is the mainstay of treatment for celiac disease. All wheat, rye, barley, and oats should be eliminated from the diet and replaced with corn and rice. Vitamin supplements, especially fat-soluble vitamins and folate, may be required during the early period of treatment to correct deficiencies. These restrictions are likely to be lifelong, although small amounts of grains may be tolerated after the gastrointestinal ulcerations have healed.
Test-Taking Strategy: Focus on the subject, dietary management for the child with celiac disease. Think about the pathophysiology of this disease. Recalling that corn and rice are substitute food replacements among clients with this disease will direct you to the correct option. **Review:** celiac disease.
Level of Cognitive Ability: Applying
Client Needs: Health Promotion and Maintenance
Integrated Process: Teaching and Learning
Content Area: Child Health: Gastrointestinal
Priority Concepts: Client Education, Nutrition
Reference(s): Hockenberry, Wilson (2013), p. 815.

325. 4
Rationale: PKU is an autosomal-recessive disorder. Treatment includes the dietary restriction of phenylalanine intake (not tyramine intake). PKU is a genetic disorder that results in central nervous system (CNS) damage from toxic levels of phenylalanine in the blood.
Test-Taking Strategy: Focus on the subject, an understanding of phenylketonuria (PKU). Recalling that PKU is a recessive disorder will assist you with eliminating option 1. Reading option 3 carefully will direct you to eliminate it because tyramine is restricted among clients taking monoamine oxidase inhibitors rather than among those with PKU. Recalling that PKU affects the CNS will direct you to the correct option. **Review:** phenylketonuria.
Level of Cognitive Ability: Understanding
Client Needs: Physiological Integrity
Integrated Process: Teaching and Learning
Content Area: Child Health: Metabolic/Endocrine
Priority Concepts: Communication, Health Promotion
Reference(s): McKinney et al (2013), pp. 733, 1380–1381.

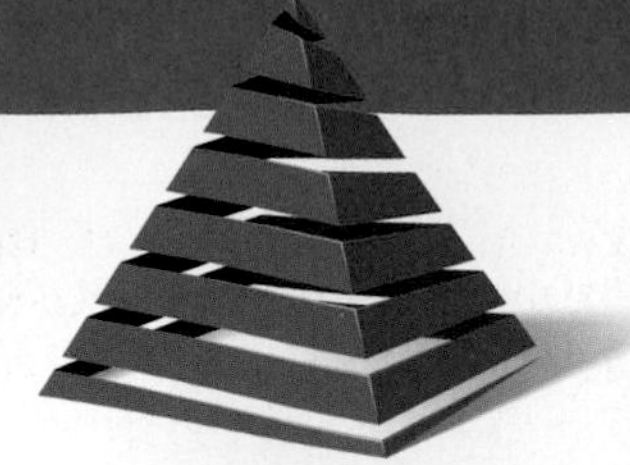

CHAPTER 34

Eye, Ear, Throat, and Respiratory Disorders

CRITICAL THINKING What Should You Do?

A child with pneumonia complains of pain in the pleural area on the affected side. What should the nurse do?

Answer located on p. 420.

I. Strabismus

A. Description
1. Called "squint" or "cross-eye"
2. A condition in which the eyes are not aligned as a result of a lack of coordination of the extraocular muscles
3. Most often results from a muscle imbalance or the paralysis of the extraocular muscles, but it may also result from a congenital defect.
4. Amblyopia (reduced visual acuity) may occur if not treated early because the brain receives two messages as a result of the nonparallel visual axes.
5. Permanent loss of vision can occur if not treated early.
6. This condition is considered a normal finding in a young infant, but it should not be present after about age 4 months.
7. Treatment of the condition depends on the cause.

B. Data collection
1. Crossed eyes
2. Squinting; tilts the head or closes one eye to see
3. Headaches
4. Diplopia; photophobia

C. Interventions
1. Corrective lenses to improve eye alignment
2. Instruct the parents regarding patching (occlusion therapy) of the "good" eye to strengthen the weak eye.
3. Prepare for surgery to realign the weak muscles as prescribed if nonsurgical interventions are unsuccessful; this is usually performed before the age of 2 years.
4. Reinforce instructions to the parents about the need for follow-up visits.

II. Conjunctivitis

A. Description
1. Inflammation of the conjunctiva; frequently known as pinkeye
2. May be caused by allergy, infection, or trauma
3. Bacterial or viral conjunctivitis is extremely contagious.

B. Data collection
1. Itching, burning, or scratchy eyelids
2. Redness of the conjunctiva and sclera
3. Edema
4. Redness

Chlamydial conjunctivitis is rare among older children; if diagnosed in a child who is not sexually active, he or she should be assessed for possible sexual abuse.

C. Interventions
1. Reinforce instructions in infection control measures such as good hand washing and not sharing towels and washcloths.
2. Administer antibiotic or antiviral eyedrops or ointment, as prescribed, if infection is present (severe infection may require therapy with systemic antibiotics).
3. Administer antihistamines, as prescribed, if an allergy is present.
4. Reinforce instructions to the child and parents in the administration of the prescribed medications.
5. Reinforce instructions to the parents that the child should be kept home from school or day care until antibiotics and/or antibiotic eyedrops have been administered for 24 hours.
6. Reinforce instructions to the child and parents in the use of cool compresses to lessen irritation and in the wearing of dark glasses for photophobia.
7. Reinforce instructions to the child to avoid rubbing the eye to prevent injury.
8. Reinforce instructions to the child who is wearing contact lenses to discontinue wearing them until treatment is complete. New lenses need to

be obtained to eliminate the chance of reinfection that can occur from the use of the old lenses.

9. Reinforce instructions to the adolescent that the eye makeup currently being used should be discarded and replaced with new makeup to prevent reinfection.

III. Otitis Media

A. Description
   1. Otitis media is an inflammatory disorder usually caused by an infection of the middle ear occurring as a result of a blocked eustachian tube, which prevents normal drainage; can be acute or chronic.
   2. Otitis media is a common complication of an acute respiratory infection (most commonly from respiratory syncytial virus or influenza).
   3. Infants and children have eustachian tubes that are shorter, wider, and straighter, which makes them more prone to otitis media.

B. Prevention
   1. Feed infants in upright position to prevent reflux.
   2. Maintain routine immunizations.
   3. Encourage breastfeeding for at least the first 6 months of age.
   4. Avoid exposure to tobacco smoke and allergens.

C. Data collection
   1. Fever
   2. Acute onset of ear pain
   3. Crying, irritability, lethargy
   4. Loss of appetite
   5. Rolling of head from side to side
   6. Pulling on or rubbing the ear
   7. Purulent ear drainage may be present
   8. Red, opaque, bulging, immobile tympanic membrane on otoscopic exam
   9. Signs of hearing loss (indicative of chronic otitis media)

D. Interventions
   1. Encourage fluid intake (may be difficult if the child is in pain).
   2. Reinforce instructions to the child to avoid chewing as much as possible during the acute period because chewing increases pain.
   3. Provide local heat or cold as prescribed to relieve discomfort and have the child lie with the affected ear down.
   4. Reinforce instructions to the parents in the appropriate procedure to clean drainage from the external ear canal with sterile swabs or gauze; frequent cleansing and the application of moisture barriers may be prescribed to prevent ear excoriation from the drainage.
   5. Reinforce instructions to the parents in the administration of analgesics or antipyretics such as acetaminophen (Tylenol) or ibuprofen (Motrin IB) as prescribed to decrease fever and pain.
   6. Reinforce instructions to the parents in the administration of antibiotics if prescribed, emphasizing that the prescribed period of administration is necessary to eliminate infective organisms.
   7. In healthy infants over 6 months and children, careful use of antibiotics is recommended because of concerns about drug-resistant *Streptococcus pneumoniae;* usually, waiting up to 72 hours for spontaneous resolution is a safe and appropriate management of acute otitis media.
   8. Reinforce instructions to the parents that screening for hearing loss may be necessary.
   9. Reinforce instructions to the parents about the procedure for administering ear medications such as topical pain relief drops if prescribed.

To administer ear medications in a child younger than age 3, pull the ear lobe down and back. In a child older than 3 years, pull the pinna up and back.

E. Myringotomy
   1. Description
      a. A surgical incision into the tympanic membrane to provide drainage of the purulent middle ear fluid; may be done by a laser-assisted procedure
      b. Insertion of tympanoplasty tubes into the middle ear may be done to allow continued drainage and to equalize pressure and allow ventilation of the middle ear.
   2. Postoperative interventions
      a. Reinforce instructions to the parents and child to keep the ears dry.
      b. The child should wear earplugs while bathing, shampooing, and swimming (diving and submerging under water are not allowed).
      c. Parents can administer an analgesic such as acetaminophen (Tylenol) or ibuprofen (Motrin IB) as prescribed to relieve discomfort following insertion of tympanoplasty tubes.
      d. Parents should be taught that the child should not blow his or her nose for 7 to 10 days after surgery.
      e. Reinforce instructions to the parents that if the tubes fall out, it is not an emergency, but the health care provider (HCP) should be notified; inform the parents of the appearance of the tubes (tiny, white, spool-shaped tubes).

IV. Tonsillitis and Adenoiditis

A. Description
   1. *Tonsillitis* refers to inflammation and infection of the tonsils, which is lymphoid tissue located in the pharynx.
   2. *Adenoiditis* refers to inflammation and infection of the adenoids (pharyngeal tonsils), located on the posterior wall of the nasopharynx.

Pediatric

3. Tonsillectomy (surgical removal of the tonsils) and adenoidectomy (surgical removal of the adenoids) may be necessary.

B. Data collection
1. Persistent or recurrent sore throat
2. Enlarged bright red tonsils that may be covered with white exudate
3. Difficulty swallowing
4. Mouth breathing and an unpleasant mouth odor
5. Fever
6. Cough
7. Enlarged adenoids may cause a nasal quality of speech, mouth breathing, hearing difficulty, snoring, or obstructive sleep apnea.

C. Interventions preoperatively
1. Monitor for signs of active infection.
2. Monitor bleeding and clotting studies, because the throat is very vascular.
3. Prepare the child for a sore throat postoperatively, and inform the child that he or she will need to drink liquids.
4. Check for any loose teeth to decrease the risk of aspiration during surgery.

D. Interventions postoperatively
1. Position the child prone or side-lying to facilitate drainage.
2. Have suction equipment available, but do not suction unless there is an airway obstruction.
3. Monitor for signs of bleeding (frequent swallowing may indicate bleeding). If bleeding occurs, turn the child to the side and notify the registered nurse immediately.
4. Discourage coughing, clearing of the throat, or nose blowing to prevent bleeding.
5. Provide an ice collar or analgesics (rectally or intravenously) for discomfort, as prescribed.
6. Administer antiemetics, as prescribed, to prevent vomiting.
7. Provide clear, cool, noncitrus, and noncarbonated fluids (crushed ice, ice pops).

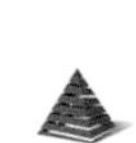

8. Avoid red, purple, or brown liquids, which will simulate the appearance of blood if the child vomits.

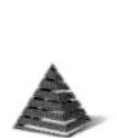

9. Avoid milk products such as milk, ice cream, and pudding initially, because they will coat the throat, causing the child to clear the throat.
10. Soft foods may be prescribed 1 to 2 days postoperatively.
11. Do not give the child any straws, forks, or sharp objects that can be put into the mouth.
12. Mouth odor, slight ear pain, and a low-grade fever may occur for a few days postoperatively, but the parents should be instructed to notify the HCP if bleeding, a persistent earache, or fever occurs.
13. Reinforce instructions to the parents to keep the child away from crowds until healing has occurred; usually the child is able to resume normal activities after 1 to 2 weeks postoperatively.

V. Epistaxis (Nosebleeds)

A. Description
1. The nose, especially the septum, is a highly vascular structure, and bleeding usually results from direct trauma, foreign bodies, nose picking, and mucosal inflammation.
2. Recurrent epistaxis and severe bleeding may indicate underlying disease.

B. Interventions
1. See Priority Nursing Actions.
2. If bleeding cannot be controlled, packing or cauterization of the bleeding vessel may be prescribed.

VI. Epiglottitis

A. Description
1. A bacterial form of croup

PRIORITY NURSING ACTIONS!

Actions to Take if a Child Has a Nosebleed

1. Remain calm and keep the child calm and quiet.
2. Have the child sit up and lean forward (not lying down).
3. Apply continuous pressure to the nose with the thumb and forefinger for at least 10 minutes.
4. Insert cotton or wadded tissue into each nostril, and apply ice or a cold cloth to the bridge of the nose if bleeding persists.

If a nosebleed occurs in a child, it is important for the nurse to remain calm; otherwise, the child becomes agitated and it is difficult to get the child to cooperate with the necessary interventions. The child should be assisted to a sitting up and leaning forward position to prevent aspiration of blood. The child should not be placed in a lying-down position because of the risk of aspiration. Nosebleeds usually originate in the anterior part of the nasal septum and can be controlled by applying pressure to the soft lower portion of the nose with the thumb and forefinger for at least 10 minutes. If bleeding persists, cotton or wadded tissue should be placed into each nostril, and ice or a cold cloth should be applied to the bridge of the nose. In addition, if bleeding does persist, the HCP needs to be notified, and the nose may require packing by the HCP. After the nosebleed has been stopped, petroleum or a water-soluble jelly may be inserted into each nostril to prevent crusting of old blood and to lessen the likelihood of the child picking at the crusted lesions and restarting the bleeding. Repeated bleeding episodes that last longer than 30 minutes may be an indication of the need for evaluation of a bleeding disorder.

Reference(s): Hockenberry, M., & Wilson, D. (2013). *Wong's: Essentials of pediatric nursing* (9th ed., p. 888). St. Louis: Mosby.

2. An inflammation of the epiglottis occurs, which may be caused by *Haemophilus influenzae* type B or *Streptococcus pneumonia*; children immunized with *H influenza* type b (Hib **vaccine**) are at less risk for epiglottitis.
3. Occurs most frequently among children who are 2 to 8 years of age, but can occur from infancy to adulthood
4. Onset is abrupt; occurs most often in the winter.
5. Considered an emergency situation because it can progress rapidly to severe respiratory distress

B. Data collection
1. High fever
2. Sore, red, and inflamed throat (large, cherry red, edematous epiglottis) and pain on swallowing (Fig. 34-1)
3. Absence of spontaneous cough
4. Dysphonia (muffled voice), dysphagia, dyspnea, and drooling
5. Agitation
6. Muffled voice
7. Retractions and the child struggles to breathe (Fig. 34-2)
8. Inspiratory **stridor** aggravated by the supine position
9. Tachycardia
10. Tachypnea progressing to more severe respiratory distress (hypoxia, hypercapnia, respiratory acidosis, decreased level of consciousness)
11. Tripod positioning: while supporting the body with the hands, the child leans forward, thrusts the chin forward, and opens the mouth in an attempt to widen the airway.

C. Interventions
1. Maintain a patent airway.
2. Monitor respiratory status and breath sounds, noting **nasal flaring**, the use of accessory muscles, retractions, and the presence of stridor.
3. Do not measure the temperature by the oral route.
4. Monitor pulse oximetry.

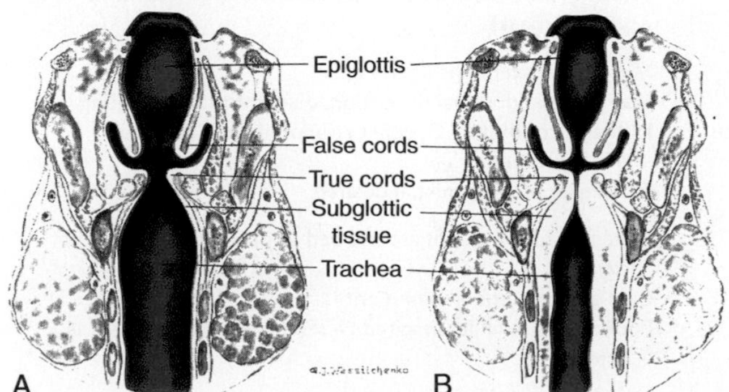

FIGURE 34-1 **A,** Normal larynx. **B,** Obstruction and narrowing resulting from edema of croup. (From Hockenberry M, & Wilson D: *Wong's: Nursing care of infants and children*, ed 9, St. Louis, 2013, Mosby.)

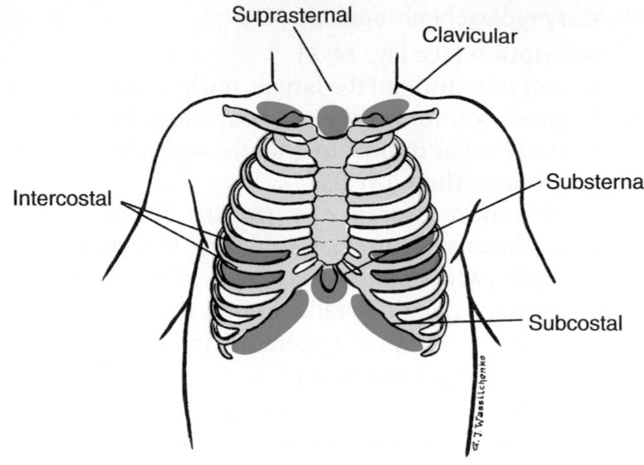

FIGURE 34-2 Location of retractions. (From Hockenberry M, & Wilson D: *Wong's: Nursing care of infants and children*, ed 9, St. Louis, 2013, Mosby.)

5. Prepare the child for lateral neck films to confirm the diagnosis (accompany the child to the radiology department).
6. Maintain an NPO status.
7. Do not leave the child unattended.
8. Avoid placing the child in a supine position because this position will further affect the respiratory status.
9. Do not restrain the child or take any other measure that may agitate the child.
10. Assist to administer intravenous (IV) fluids as prescribed; insertion of an IV may need to be delayed until an adequate airway is established because this procedure may agitate the child.
11. Intravenous antibiotics may be prescribed; these are usually followed by oral antibiotics.
12. Administer analgesics and antipyretics (acetaminophen [Tylenol] or ibuprofen [Motrin]) to reduce fever and throat pain as prescribed.
13. Administer corticosteroids to decrease inflammation and reduce throat edema as prescribed.
14. Medications that promote mucosal vasoconstriction and reduce edema may be prescribed.
15. Provide cool-mist oxygen therapy as prescribed; high humidification cools the airway and decreases swelling.
16. Have resuscitation equipment available, and prepare for endotracheal intubation or tracheotomy for severe respiratory distress.
17. Ensure that the child is up to date with the immunization schedule, including *Haemophilus influenzae* type b (Hib) conjugate vaccine. (See Chapter 39 for information on immunizations.)

⚠ If epiglottitis is suspected, no attempts should be made to visualize the posterior pharynx, obtain a throat culture, or take an oral temperature. Otherwise, spasm of the epiglottis can occur, leading to complete airway occlusion.

Pediatric

VII. Laryngotracheobronchitis (Croup)

A. Description (see Fig. 34-2)
   1. Inflammation of the larynx, trachea, and bronchi
   2. Most common type of croup; may be viral or bacterial and most frequently occurs in children younger than 5 years
   3. Common causative organisms include para-influenzae viruses, respiratory syncytial virus (RSV), *Mycoplasma pneumoniae,* and influenza
   4. Characterized by gradual onset that may be preceded by an upper respiratory infection

B. Data collection (Box 34-1)

C. Interventions
   1. Maintain a patent airway.
   2. Monitor the respiratory status, and check for nasal flaring, sternal **retraction**, and inspiratory stridor.
   3. Monitor for adequate respiratory exchange; monitor for pallor or **cyanosis**.
   4. Elevate the head of the bed and provide rest.
   5. Provide humidified oxygen via a cool-mist tent for the hospitalized child (Table 34-1).
   6. Reinforce instructions to the parents to use a cool-air vaporizer or humidifier at home. Other measures include having the child breathe in the cool night air or the air from an open freezer and taking the child to a cool basement or garage.
   7. Provide and encourage fluid intake. IV fluids may be prescribed to maintain hydration status if the child is unable to take oral fluids.
   8. Administer analgesics as prescribed to reduce fever.

BOX 34-1 Progression of Symptoms in Laryngotracheobronchitis

Stage I
- Low-grade fever
- Hoarseness
- Seal bark and brassy cough (croup cough)
- Inspiratory stridor
- Fear
- Irritability and restlessness

Stage II
- Continuous respiratory stridor
- Retractions
- Use of accessory muscles
- Crackles and wheezing
- Labored respirations

Stage III
- Continued restlessness
- Anxiety
- Pallor
- Diaphoresis
- Tachypnea
- Signs of anoxia and hypercapnia

Stage IV
- Intermittent cyanosis that progresses to permanent cyanosis
- Apneic episodes that progress to cessation of breathing

Modified from Perry S, Hockenberry M, Lowdermilk D, Wilson D: *Maternal-child nursing care*, ed 4, St. Louis, 2010, Mosby.

TABLE 34-1 Advantages and Disadvantages of Various Oxygen-Delivery Systems

Systems	Advantages	Disadvantages
Oxygen mask	Various sizes available Delivers higher O_2 concentration than cannula Able to provide a predictable concentration of oxygen if Venturi mask is used, whether child breathes through nose or mouth	Skin irritation Fear of suffocation Accumulation of moisture on face Possibility of aspiration of vomitus Difficulty with controlling O_2 concentrations (except with Venturi mask)
Nasal cannula	Provides low to moderate O_2 concentration (22%-40%) Child is able to eat and talk while receiving O_2 Possibility of more complete observation of child because nose and mouth remain unobstructed	Must have patent nasal passages May cause abdominal distention, discomfort, or vomiting Difficulty controlling O_2 concentration if child breathes through mouth Inability to provide mist, if desired
Oxygen tent	Provides lower O_2 concentrations (FIO_2 up to 0.3-0.5) Child is able to receive desired inspired O_2 concentrations, even while eating	Necessity for proper fit around bed to prevent the leakage of oxygen Cool and wet tent environment Poor access to child; inspired O_2 levels fall when the tent is entered
Oxygen hood	Provides high O_2 concentrations (FIO_2 up to 1.00) Free access to child's chest for assessment	High-humidity environment Need to remove child for feeding and care

FIO_2, Fraction of inspired oxygen; *O_2*, oxygen.
Data from Hockenberry M, Wilson D: *Wong's: Nursing care of infants and children*, ed 9, St. Louis, 2013, Mosby.

9. Reinforce teaching the parents to avoid administering cough syrups and cold medicines, which may dry and thicken secretions.
10. Assist to administer corticosteroids, if prescribed, for their anti-inflammatory effects.
11. Assist to administer nebulized epinephrine (racemic epinephrine), as prescribed, for children with severe disease experiencing stridor at rest, retractions, or difficulty breathing.
12. Assist to administer antibiotics, as prescribed, noting that they are not indicated unless a bacterial infection is present.
13. Medications that reduce the work of breathing, reduce airway turbulence, and help to relieve airway obstruction may be prescribed.
14. Have resuscitation equipment available.
15. Provide appropriate reassurance and education to the parents or caregivers.

Isolation precautions should be implemented for a hospitalized child with an upper respiratory infection until the cause of the infection is known.

VIII. Bronchitis

A. Description
   1. Inflammation of the trachea and bronchi; may be referred to as *tracheobronchitis*
   2. Usually occurs in association with an upper respiratory infection
   3. Is usually a mild disorder; causative agent is most often viral

B. Data collection
   1. Fever
   2. Dry, hacking, and nonproductive cough that is worse at night and becomes productive in 2 to 3 days

C. Interventions
   1. Treat the symptoms as necessary.
   2. Monitor for respiratory distress.
   3. Provide cool, humidified air to the child.
   4. Encourage increased fluid intake; child may drink beverages that he or she likes as long as the respiratory status is stable.
   5. Administer antipyretics for fever as prescribed.
   6. Medication may be prescribed to promote rest.

IX. Bronchiolitis and Respiratory Syncytial Virus (RSV)

A. Description
   1. An inflammation of the bronchioles that causes a thick production of mucus, which occludes the bronchiole tubes and the small bronchi.
   2. Respiratory syncytial virus is an acute viral infection and a common cause of bronchiolitis (other organisms that cause bronchiolitis include adenoviruses, parainfluenza viruses, and human metapneumovirus).

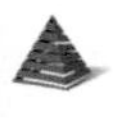

   3. RSV, although not airborne, is highly communicable and is usually transferred by direct contact with respiratory secretions.
   4. Occurs primarily in the winter and spring
   5. Rarer in children older than 2 years, with a peak incidence at approximately 6 months of age
   6. At-risk children include those older than 1 year of age who have a chronic or disabling condition.
   7. Identification of the virus is done via testing of nasal or nasopharyngeal secretions.
   8. Prevention measures include encouraging breastfeeding, avoiding tobacco smoke exposure, using good hand-washing techniques, and administering palivizumab (Synagis), a monoclonal antibody, to high-risk infants; palivizumab is administered via intramuscular injection monthly for a 5-month period (usually from November to March).

B. Data collection (Box 34-2)

C. Interventions
   1. For the child with bronchiolitis, interventions are aimed at treating symptoms and include airway maintenance, cool humidified air and oxygen, adequate fluid intake, and medications.
   2. For the hospitalized child with RSV, isolate the child in a single room or place in a room with another child with RSV.
   3. Ensure that nurses caring for the child with RSV do not care for other high-risk children.
   4. Use contact and standard precautions during care; using good hand-washing techniques and wearing gloves and gowns are necessary.
   5. Monitor airway status and maintain a patent airway.

BOX 34-2 Data Collection: Respiratory Syncytial Virus

Initial Manifestations
- Rhinorrhea
- Eye or ear drainage
- Pharyngitis
- Coughing
- Sneezing
- Wheezing
- Intermittent fever

Manifestations as the Disease Progresses
- Increased coughing and wheezing
- Signs of air hunger
- Tachypnea and retractions
- Periods of cyanosis

Manifestations in Severe Illness
- Tachypnea greater than 70 breaths per minute
- Decreased breath sounds and inadequate air exchange
- Listlessness
- Apneic episodes

Modified from Perry S, Hockenberry M, Lowdermilk D, Wilson D: *Maternal-child nursing care*, ed 4, St. Louis, 2010, Mosby.

6. For most effective airway maintenance, position the child at a 30- to 40-degree angle with the neck slightly extended to maintain an open airway and decrease pressure on the diaphragm.
7. Provide cool, humidified oxygen as prescribed.
8. Monitor pulse oximetry levels.
9. Encourage fluids; fluids administered intravenously may be necessary until the acute stage has passed.
10. Periodic suctioning may be necessary if nasal secretions are copious; use of a bulb syringe for suctioning may be effective and should be done before feeding to promote comfort and adequate intake.
11. Assist to administer ribavirin (Virazole), an antiviral medication, if prescribed.

Cough suppressants are administered with caution because they can interfere with the clearance of respiratory secretions.

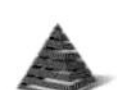

X. Pneumonia

A. Description
1. Inflammation of the pulmonary parenchyma and/or alveoli caused by a virus, mycoplasmal agents, bacteria, or aspiration of foreign substances
2. The causative agent usually is introduced into the lungs through inhalation or from the bloodstream.
3. Viral pneumonia occurs more frequently than bacterial pneumonia, is seen in children of all ages, and often is associated with a viral upper respiratory infection.
4. Primary atypical pneumonia, usually caused by *Mycoplasma pneumoniae* or *Chlamydia pneumoniae,* occurs most often in the fall and winter months and is more common in crowded living conditions; most often seen in children between the ages of 5 and 12 years.
5. Bacterial pneumonia is often a serious infection requiring hospitalization when pleural effusion or empyema accompanies the disease; hospitalization is also necessary for children with staphylococcal pneumonia (*Streptococcus pneumoniae* is a common cause).
6. Aspiration pneumonia occurs when food, secretions, liquids, or other materials enter the lung and cause inflammation and a chemical pneumonitis. Classic symptoms include an increasing cough or fever with foul-smelling sputum, deteriorating results on chest x-rays, and other signs of airway involvement.
7. Prevention of viral and bacterial pneumonia includes immunization of infants and children with pneumococcal vaccine. (See Chapter 39 for information on immunizations.)

B. Viral pneumonia
1. Data collection
   a. Mild fever, slight cough, and malaise to high fever, severe cough, and prostration
   b. Nonproductive or productive cough of small amounts of whitish sputum
   c. Wheezes or fine **crackles**
2. Interventions
   a. Treatment is symptomatic.
   b. Administer oxygen with cool humidified air as prescribed.
   c. Increase fluid intake.
   d. Administer antipyretics for fever as prescribed.
   e. Administer chest physiotherapy and postural drainage as prescribed.

C. Primary atypical pneumonia
1. Data collection
   a. Fever, chills, anorexia, headache, malaise, and muscle pain
   b. Rhinitis, sore throat, and dry, hacking cough
   c. Cough is nonproductive initially and then produces seromucoid sputum, which becomes mucopurulent or blood streaked.
2. Interventions: Symptomatic

D. Bacterial pneumonia
1. Data collection
   a. Infant: Irritability, lethargy, poor feeding, abrupt fever (may be accompanied by seizures), and respiratory distress (air hunger, tachypnea, and circumoral cyanosis)
   b. Older child: Headache, chills, abdominal pain, chest pain, and meningeal symptoms (meningism)
   c. Hacking, nonproductive cough
   d. Diminished breath sounds or scattered crackles
   e. With consolidation, decreased breath sounds are more pronounced.
   f. As the infection resolves, the cough becomes productive and the child expectorates purulent sputum; coarse crackles and wheezing are noted.
2. Interventions
   a. Antibiotic therapy is initiated as soon as the diagnosis is suspected; in the hospitalized infant or child, intravenous antibiotics are usually prescribed.
   b. Administer oxygen for respiratory distress as prescribed and monitor oxygen saturation via pulse oximetry.
   c. Place the child in a cool mist tent as prescribed; cool humidification moistens the airways and assists in temperature reduction.
   d. Suction mucus from the infant using a bulb syringe to maintain a patent airway if the infant is unable to handle secretions.
   e. Administer chest physiotherapy and postural drainage every 4 hours as prescribed.

f. Promote bed rest to conserve energy.
g. Encourage the child to lie on the affected side (if pneumonia is unilateral) to splint the chest and reduce the discomfort caused by pleural rubbing.
h. Encourage fluid intake (administer cautiously to prevent aspiration); intravenously administered fluids may be necessary.
i. Administer antipyretics for fever and bronchodilators as prescribed.
j. Monitor temperature frequently because of the risk for febrile seizures.
k. Institute isolation precautions with pneumococcal or staphylococcal pneumonia (according to agency policy).
l. Cough suppressant may be prescribed before rest times and meals if the cough is disturbing.
m. Continuous closed-chest drainage may be instituted if purulent fluid is present (usually noted in *Staphylococcus* infections).
n. Fluid accumulation in the pleural cavity may be removed by thoracentesis; thoracentesis also provides a means for obtaining fluid for culture and for instilling antibiotics directly into the pleural cavity.

! Children with a respiratory disorder should be monitored for weight loss and for signs of dehydration. Signs of dehydration include a sunken fontanel (infants), nonelastic skin turgor, decreased and concentrated urinary output, dry mucous membranes, and decreased tear production.

XI. Asthma

A. Description
1. Asthma is a chronic inflammatory disease of the airways (see Chapter 49 for additional information about this disorder).
2. Asthma is classified on the basis of disease severity; management includes medications, environmental control of allergens, and child/family education.
3. The allergic reaction in the airways caused by the precipitant can result in an immediate reaction with obstruction occurring, and it can result in a late bronchial obstructive reaction several hours after the initial exposure to the precipitant.
4. Mast cell release of histamine leads to a bronchoconstrictive process, bronchospasm, and obstruction.
5. Diagnosis is made on the basis of the child's symptoms, history and physical exam, chest radiograph, and laboratory tests (Box 34-3).
6. Precipitants triggering an asthma attack (Box 34-4)

BOX 34-3 Laboratory Tests to Assist in Diagnosing Asthma

Pulmonary function tests (PFTs): Spirometry testing assesses the presence and degree of disease and can determine the response to treatment.
Peak expiratory flow rate (PEFR) measurement: Measures the maximum flow of air that can be forcefully exhaled in 1 second; the child uses a peak expiratory flow meter (PEFM) to determine a "personal best value" that can be used for comparison at other times, such as during and after an asthma attack.
Bronchoprovocation testing: Testing done to identify inhaled allergens; the mucous membranes are directly exposed to the suspected allergen in increasing amounts.
Skin testing: Done to identify specific allergens.
Exercise challenges: Exercise is used to identify the occurrence of exercise-induced bronchospasm.
Radioallergosorbent test (RAST): A blood test used to identify a specific allergen.
Chest radiograph: May show hyperexpansion of the airways.

Note: Some tests place the child at risk for an asthma attack; therefore, testing should be done under close supervision.

BOX 34-4 Precipitants Triggering an Asthma Attack

Allergens
- *Outdoor:* Trees, shrubs, weeds, grasses, molds, pollen, air pollution, spores
- *Indoor:* Dust, dust mites, mold, cockroach antigen

Irritants:
- Tobacco smoke, wood smoke, odors, sprays

Exposure to occupational irritants
Exercise
Cold air
Changes in weather or temperature
Environmental change:
- Moving to a new home, starting a new school

Colds and infections
Animals:
- Cats, dogs, rodents, horses

Medications:
- Aspirin, nonsteroidal anti-inflammatory drugs, antibiotics, β-blockers

Strong emotions:
- Fear, anger, laughing, crying

Conditions:
- Gastroesophageal reflux disease, tracheoesophageal fistula

Food additives:
- Sulfite preservatives

Foods:
- Nuts, milk, and other dairy products

Endocrine factors:
- Menses, pregnancy, thyroid disease

Data from Perry S, Hockenberry M, Lowdermilk D, Wilson D: *Maternal-child nursing care*, ed 4, St. Louis, 2010, Mosby.

Pediatric

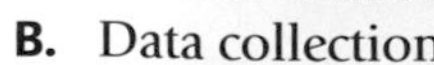

7. Status asthmaticus is an acute asthma attack, and the child displays respiratory distress despite vigorous treatment measures; this is a medical emergency that can result in respiratory failure and death if not treated.

B. Data collection

1. Child has episodes of dyspnea, **wheezing**, breathlessness, chest tightness, and cough, particularly at night and/or in the early morning.
2. Acute asthma attacks
   - **a.** Episodes of progressively worsening shortness of breath, cough, wheezing, chest tightness, decreases in expiratory airflow secondary to bronchospasm, mucosal edema, and mucus plugging; air is trapped behind occluded or narrow airways, and hypoxemia can occur.
   - **b.** The attack begins with irritability, restlessness, headache, feeling tired, and/or chest tightness; just before the attack, the child may present with itching localized at the front of the neck or over the upper part of the back.
   - **c.** Respiratory symptoms include a hacking, irritable, nonproductive cough caused by bronchial edema.
   - **d.** Accumulated secretions stimulate the cough; the cough becomes rattling, and there is production of frothy, clear, gelatinous sputum.
   - **e.** The child experiences retractions.
   - **f.** Hyperresonance on percussion of the chest is noted.
   - **g.** Breath sounds are coarse and loud, with crackles, coarse rhonchi, and inspiratory and expiratory wheezing; expiration is prolonged.
   - **h.** Child may be pale or flushed, and the lips may have a deep, dark red color that may progress to cyanosis (also observed in the nail beds and skin, especially around the mouth).
   - **i.** Restlessness, apprehension, and diaphoresis occur.
   - **j.** Child speaks in short, broken phrases.

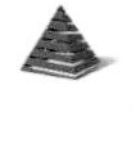

   - **k.** Younger children assume the tripod sitting position; older children sit upright, with the shoulders in a hunched-over position, the hands on the bed or a chair, and the arms braced to facilitate the use of the accessory muscles of breathing (child refuses to lie down).
   - **l.** Exercise-induced attack: A cough, shortness of breath, chest pain or tightness, wheezing, and endurance problems occur during exercise.

   - **m.** Severe spasm or obstruction: Breath sounds and wheezing cannot be heard (silent chest), and the cough is ineffective (represents a lack of air movement).
   - **n.** Ventilatory failure and asphyxia: Shortness of breath, with air movement in the chest restricted to the point of absent breath sounds is noted; this is accompanied by a sudden rise in the respiratory rate.

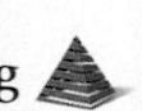

C. Interventions: Acute episode (see Priority Nursing Actions)

PRIORITY NURSING ACTIONS!

Actions to Take in the Event of an Acute Asthma Attack

1. Check airway patency and respiratory status.
2. Assist to administer humidified oxygen by nasal cannula or face mask.
3. Assist to administer quick-relief (rescue) medications.
4. Assist to initiate an intravenous (IV) line.
5. Prepare the child for a chest radiograph if prescribed.
6. Prepare to obtain a blood sample for determining arterial blood gas levels if prescribed.

In the event of an acute asthma attack, several interventions are necessary. First, the nurse checks airway status to ensure airway patency. If the airway is not patent, emergency interventions such as endotracheal intubation may be necessary. The nurse also quickly assesses the child's respiratory status. If the airway is patent, the nurse administers oxygen by nasal cannula or mask as prescribed. Quick-relief (rescue) medications are administered as prescribed to treat the symptoms. An IV line is initiated so that IV medications can be administered if prescribed.

The nurse prepares the child for a chest x-ray to assess airway status and to assist in ruling out a respiratory infection. Blood samples are obtained, and an arterial blood gas may be obtained. When the laboratory results are obtained, the nurse assists to administer medications as prescribed to correct dehydration, acidosis, or electrolyte imbalances. During the episode and during treatment, the nurse stays with the child and continuously monitors respiratory status, pulse oximetry, and color. The nurse also needs to be alert to decreased wheezing or a silent chest, which may signal the inability to move air.

Reference(s): McKinney, E., James, S., Murray, S., Nelson, K. & Ashwill, J. (2013). *Maternal-child nursing* (4th ed., pp. 1181–1182). St. Louis: Elsevier.

D. Medications

1. Quick-relief (rescue medications): Used to treat symptoms and exacerbations (Box 34-5)
2. Long-term control (preventer medications): Used to achieve and maintain control of inflammation (Box 34-6)
3. Nebulizer, metered-dose inhaler (MDI): May be used to administer medications; if the child has difficulty using the MDI, medication can be administered by nebulization (medication is mixed with saline and then nebulized with compressed air by a machine).

BOX 34-5 Quick-Relief (Rescue) Medications

Short-acting β_2-agonists (for bronchodilation)
Anticholinergics (for the relief of acute bronchospasm)
Systemic corticosteroids (for their anti-inflammatory action to treat reversible airflow obstruction)

BOX 34-6 Long-Term Control (Preventer) Medications

Corticosteroids (for anti-inflammatory action)
Antiallergic medications (to prevent an adverse response on exposure to an allergen)
Nonsteroidal anti-inflammatory drugs (for anti-inflammatory action)
Long-acting β_2 agonists (for long-acting bronchodilation)
Leukotriene modifiers (to prevent bronchospasm and inflammatory cell infiltration)
Monoclonal antibody (blocks the binding of IgE to mast cells to inhibit inflammation)

4. If the MDI is used to administer a corticosteroid, a spacer should be used to prevent yeast infections in the child's mouth.
5. The child's **growth** patterns need to be monitored when corticosteroids are prescribed.

E. Chest physiotherapy
1. Includes breathing exercises and physical training.
2. Chest physiotherapy will strengthen the respiratory musculature and produce more efficient breathing patterns.
3. Chest physiotherapy is not recommended during an acute exacerbation.

F. Allergen control
1. Testing may be done to identify allergens.
2. Reinforce teaching the child and parents about measures to prevent and reduce exposure to allergens (see Box 34-4).

G. Home-care measures
1. Reinforce instructions to the family in measures to eliminate environmental allergens.
2. Avoid extremes of environmental temperature; in cold temperatures, instruct the child to breathe through the nose, not the mouth, and to cover the nose and mouth with a scarf.
3. Avoid exposure to individuals with a respiratory infection.
4. Reinforce instructions to the child and family in how to recognize early symptoms of an asthma attack.
5. Reinforce instructions to the child and family in how to administer medications as prescribed.
6. Reinforce instructions to the child and family in how to use a nebulizer, MDI, or peak expiratory flowmeter.
7. Reinforce instructions to the child and family about the importance of home monitoring of the peak expiratory flow rate; a decrease in the expiratory flow rate may indicate impending infection or exacerbation.
8. Reinforce instructions to the child in the cleaning of devices used for inhaled medications (yeast infections can occur with the use of aerosolized corticosteroids).
9. Encourage adequate rest, sleep, and a well-balanced diet.
10. Reinforce instructions to the child in the importance of adequate fluid intake to liquefy secretions.
11. Assist in developing an exercise program.
12. Reinforce instructions to the child in the procedure for respiratory treatments and exercises as prescribed.
13. Encourage the child to cough effectively.
14. Encourage the parents to keep immunizations up to date; annual influenza vaccinations are recommended for children 6 months of age and older.
15. Inform other HCP and school personnel of the asthma condition.
16. Allow the child to take control of self-care measures based on age appropriateness.

XII. Cystic Fibrosis (Fig. 34-3)

A. Description
1. A chronic multisystem disorder and autosomal-recessive trait disorder that is characterized by exocrine gland dysfunction
2. The mucus produced by the exocrine glands is abnormally thick and copious, which causes the obstruction of the small passageways of the affected organs, particularly in the respiratory, gastrointestinal, and reproductive systems.
3. Common symptoms are associated with pancreatic enzyme deficiency and pancreatic fibrosis caused by duct blockage, progressive chronic lung disease as a result of infection, and sweat gland dysfunction, resulting in increased sodium and chloride sweat concentrations.
4. An increase in sodium and chloride in sweat and saliva forms the basis for one diagnostic test, the sweat chloride test (Box 34-7).
5. Cystic fibrosis (CF) is a progressive and incurable disorder, and respiratory failure is a common cause of death; organ transplantations may be an option to increase survival rates.

B. Respiratory system
1. Symptoms are produced by the stagnation of mucus in the airway, which leads to bacterial colonization and the destruction of lung tissue.
2. Emphysema and atelectasis occur as the airways become increasingly obstructed.

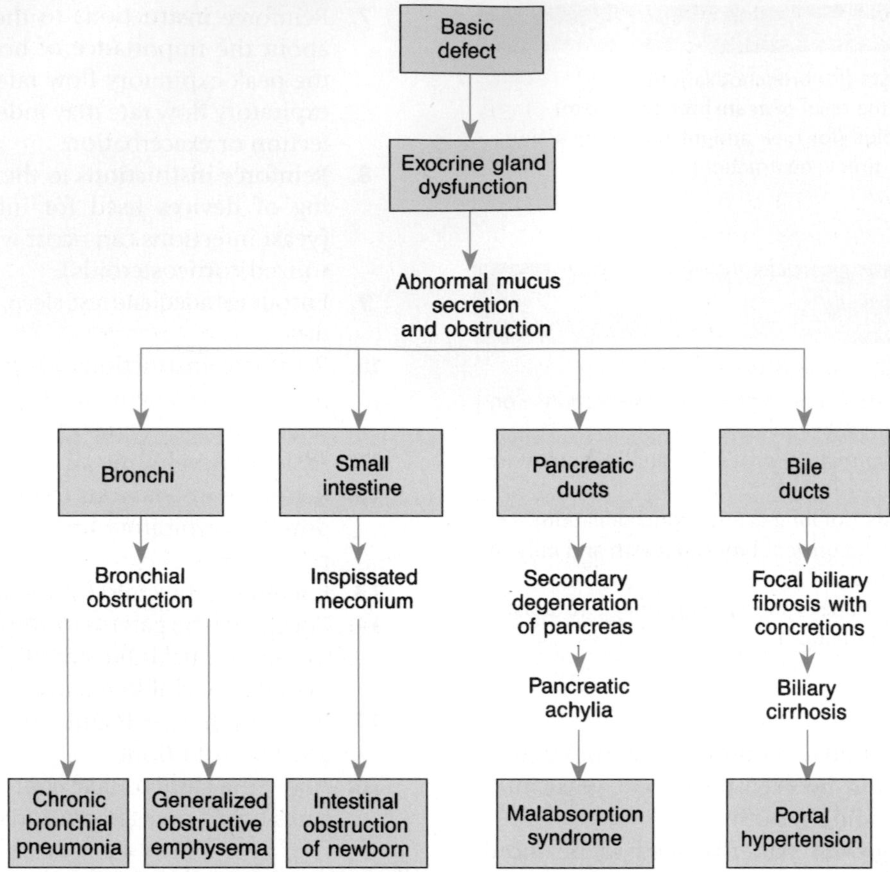

FIGURE 34-3 Various effects of exocrine gland dysfunction in cystic fibrosis. (From Hockenberry M, & Wilson D: *Wong's: Nursing care of infants and children*, ed 9, St. Louis, 2013, Mosby.)

BOX 34-7 Quantitative Sweat Chloride Test

- The production of sweat is stimulated (pilocarpine iontophoresis), the sweat is collected, and the sweat electrolytes are measured (75 mg of sweat is needed).
- Normally, the sweat chloride concentration is lower than 40 mEq/L.
- A chloride concentration higher than 60 mEq/L is a positive test result (higher than 40 mEq/L is diagnostic in infants younger than 3 months of age).
- Chloride concentrations between 40 to 60 mEq/L are highly suggestive of cystic fibrosis and require a repeat test.

3. Chronic hypoxemia causes the contraction and hypertrophy of the muscle fibers in the pulmonary arteries and arterioles, thus leading to pulmonary hypertension and eventual cor pulmonale.
4. Pneumothorax from ruptured bullae and hemoptysis from the erosion of the bronchial wall occur as the disease progresses.
5. Other respiratory symptoms
   - **a.** Wheezing and cough
   - **b.** Dyspnea
   - **c.** Cyanosis
   - **d.** Clubbing of the fingers and toes (Fig. 34-4)
   - **e.** Barrel chest
   - **f.** Repeated episodes of bronchitis and pneumonia

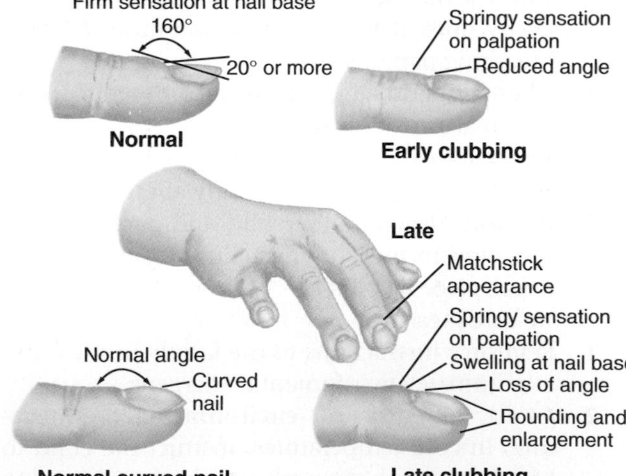

FIGURE 34-4 Clubbing of fingers. (From Hockenberry M, & Wilson D: *Wong's: Nursing care of infants and children*, ed 9, St. Louis, 2013, Mosby.)

C. Gastrointestinal system

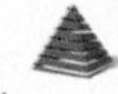

1. Meconium ileus in the newborn is the earliest manifestation.
2. Intestinal obstruction (distal intestinal obstructive syndrome) caused by thick intestinal

secretions. Signs include pain, abdominal distention, nausea, and vomiting.

3. Steatorrhea (frothy, foul-smelling stools)
4. Deficiency of the fat-soluble vitamins A, D, E, and K, which causes easy bruising, bleeding, and anemia
5. Malnutrition and failure to thrive. Hypoalbuminemia from the diminished absorption of protein occurs, which results in generalized edema.
6. Rectal prolapse can result from the large, bulky stools and increased intraabdominal pressure.
7. Pancreatic fibrosis can occur and places the child at risk for diabetes mellitus.

D. Integumentary system

1. Abnormally high concentrations of sodium and chloride in the sweat
2. Parents report that the infant tastes "salty" when kissed.
3. Dehydration and electrolyte imbalances, especially during hyperthermic conditions

E. Reproductive system

1. Can delay **puberty** in females
2. Fertility can be inhibited by highly viscous cervical secretions, which act as a plug and block sperm entry.
3. Males are usually sterile (but not impotent) as a result of the blockage of the vas deferens by abnormal secretions or the failure of the normal development of duct structures.

F. Diagnostic tests

1. Quantitative sweat chloride test is positive (see Box 34-7).
2. Newborn screening may be done in some states and may consist of immunoreactive trypsinogen analysis and direct DNA analysis for mutant genes.
3. Chest x-ray reveals atelectasis and obstructive emphysema.
4. Pulmonary function tests provide evidence of abnormal small airway function.
5. Stool fat and/or enzyme analysis: A 72-hour stool sample is collected to check the fat and/or enzyme (trypsin) content, or both (food intake is recorded during the collection).

G. Interventions: Respiratory system

1. Goals of treatment include preventing and treating pulmonary infection by improving aeration, removing secretions, and administering antibiotic medications.
2. Monitor respiratory status, including lung sounds and the presence and characteristics of a cough.
3. Chest physiotherapy (via percussion and postural drainage) on awakening and in the evening (more frequently during pulmonary infection) may be prescribed to be done every day to maintain pulmonary hygiene; it should not be performed before or immediately after a meal.
4. A Flutter Mucus Clearance Device (a small, handheld plastic pipe with a stainless-steel ball on the inside) facilitates the removal of mucus and may be prescribed; store away from small children because if the device separates, the steel ball poses a choking hazard.
5. Handheld percussors or a special vest device that provides high-frequency chest wall oscillation may be prescribed to help loosen secretions.
6. A positive expiratory pressure mask may be prescribed; use of this mask forces secretions to the upper airway for expectoration.
7. The child should be taught the forced expiratory technique (huffing) to mobilize secretions for expectoration.
8. Bronchodilator medication by aerosol may be prescribed, and the medication opens the bronchi for easier expectoration (administered before the chest physiotherapy when the child has reactive airway disease or is wheezing); medications that decrease the viscosity of mucus may also be prescribed.
9. A physical exercise program with the aim of stimulating mucus expectoration and establishing an effective breathing pattern should be instituted.
10. Aerosolized antibiotics may be prescribed, or intravenous antibiotics may be prescribed and administered at home through a central venous access device.
11. Oxygen may be prescribed during acute episodes; monitor closely for oxygen narcosis (signs include nausea and vomiting, malaise, fatigue, numbness and tingling of extremities, substernal distress) because the child with cystic fibrosis may have chronic carbon dioxide retention.
12. Lung transplantation may be an option.

H. Interventions: Gastrointestinal system 

1. The child with cystic fibrosis requires a high-calorie, high-protein, and well-balanced diet to meet energy and growth needs; multivitamins and vitamins A, D, E, and K are also administered.
2. Monitor weight and for failure to thrive.
3. Monitor stool patterns and for signs of intestinal obstruction.
4. The goal of treatment for pancreatic insufficiency is to replace pancreatic enzymes; pancreatic enzymes are administered within 30 minutes of eating and administered with all meals and all snacks (not given if the child is NPO).
5. The amount of pancreatic enzymes administered depends on the HCP's preference and usually is adjusted to achieve normal growth and a

decrease in the number of stools to two or three daily (additional enzymes are needed if the child is consuming high-fat foods).

6. Enteric-coated pancreatic enzymes should not be crushed or chewed; capsules can be taken apart and the contents can be sprinkled on a small amount of food for administration.
7. Monitor for constipation, intestinal obstruction, and rectal prolapse.
8. Monitor for signs of gastroesophageal reflux; place the infant in an upright position after eating, and teach the child to sit upright after eating.

I. Additional interventions
1. Monitor blood glucose levels and for signs of diabetes mellitus.
2. Ensure adequate salt intake and fluids that provide an adequate supply of electrolytes during extremely hot weather and when the child has a fever.
3. Monitor bone growth in the child.
4. Monitor for signs of retinopathy or nephropathy.
5. Provide emotional support to the parents, particularly when the child is diagnosed; parents will be fearful and uncertain about the disorder and the care involved.
6. Provide support to the child as he or she transitions through the stages of growth.
7. Reinforce teaching to the child and parents about the care involved and encourage independence in the child to care for self, as it is age-appropriate.

J. Home care
1. Home care involves educating the parents and the child about all of the aspects of care for the disorder.
2. Inform the parents and child about the signs of complications and actions to take, and the importance of follow-up care is critical.
3. Reinforce instructions to the parents to be sure that the child receives the recommended immunizations on schedule; in addition, annual influenza vaccinations are recommended for children 6 months of age and older.
4. Inform the child and parents about the Cystic Fibrosis Foundation.

An alteration in respiratory status can create a frightening experience for both the child and parents. A calm and reassuring nursing approach will assist in reducing fear.

XIII. Sudden Infant Death Syndrome (SIDS)

A. Description
1. SIDS refers to the unexpected death of an apparently healthy infant younger than 1 year for whom an investigation of the death and a thorough autopsy fails to demonstrate an adequate cause of death.
2. Several theories are proposed as to the cause, but the exact cause is unknown.
3. Most frequently occurs during winter months
4. Death usually occurs during sleep periods, but not necessarily at night.
5. Most frequently affects infants from 2 months to 3 months of age
6. Incidence is higher in males.
7. Incidence is higher in Native Americans, African Americans, and Hispanics, and in lower socioeconomic groups.
8. Incidence has been found to be lower in breastfed infants and infants sleeping with a pacifier.
9. High-risk conditions for SIDS
   a. Prone position
   b. Use of soft bedding or sleeping in a noninfant bed such as a sofa
   c. Overheating (thermal stress)
   d. Co-sleeping
   e. Mother who is cigarette smoking or partakes in substance **abuse** during pregnancy
   f. Exposure to tobacco smoke after birth.

B. Data collection
1. Child is apneic, blue, and lifeless.
2. Frothy blood-tinged fluid is in the nose and mouth.
3. Child may be found in any position, but typically is found in a disheveled bed, with blankets over the head, and huddled in a corner.
4. Child may appear to have been clutching bedding.
5. Diaper may be wet and full of stool.

C. Prevention and interventions
1. Infants should be placed in the supine position for sleep.
2. Mother needs to be taught about the risk factors: cigarette smoking and substance abuse during pregnancy; use of soft bedding; sleeping in a noninfant bed such as a sofa; overheating (thermal stress); co-sleeping; exposure to tobacco smoke after birth; stuffed animals or other toys should be removed from the crib while the infant is sleeping.
3. Reinforce teaching to the parents about monitoring for positional plagiocephaly caused by the supine sleeping position; signs include flattened posterior occiput and development of a bald spot in the posterior occiput area.
4. To assist in preventing positional plagiocephaly, teach the parents to alter head position during sleep, avoid excessive time in infant seats and bouncers, and place the infant in a prone position while awake (monitor the infant when in the prone position).
5. If SIDS occurs, the parents need a great deal of support as they grieve and mourn, especially because the event was sudden, unexpected, and unexplained.

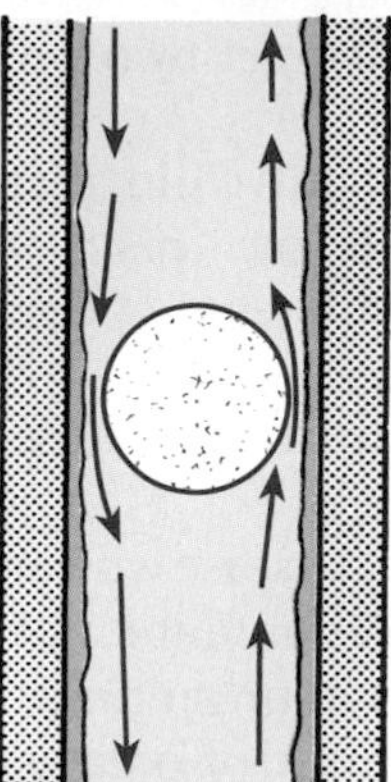

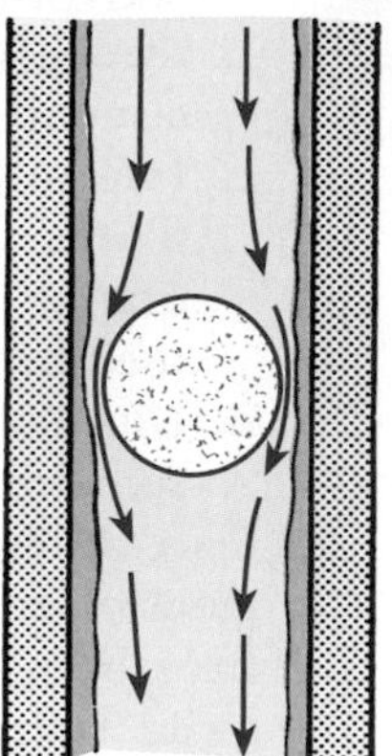

Obstruction allows passage of air in both directions

SECOND-DEGREE OBSTRUCTION
Inhalation
Expiration
Air able to move past the obstruction in one direction only. Air passages enlarge during inspiration and diminish during expiration.
COMPLETE OBSTRUCTION
Air unable to move in either direction. FB and edematous mucosa obliterate passage.

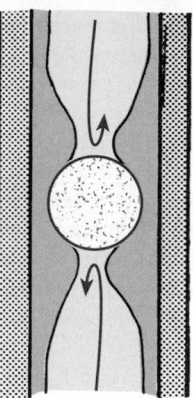

FIGURE 34-5 Manifestations of airway obstruction by foreign body (FB). (From Hockenberry M, & Wilson D: *Wong's: Nursing care of infants and children*, ed 9, St. Louis, 2013, Mosby.)

XIV. Foreign-Body Aspiration

A. Description (Fig. 34-5)

1. Swallowing and aspirating a foreign body (or bodies) into the air passages
2. Most inhaled foreign bodies lodge in the mainstem or lobar bronchus.
3. The most common offending foods are round in shape and include hot dogs, candy, peanuts, popcorn, and grapes.

B. Data collection

1. Initially, choking, gagging, coughing, and retractions are general findings.
2. If the condition worsens, cyanosis may occur.
3. Laryngotracheal obstruction leads to dyspnea, stridor, cough, and hoarseness.
4. Bronchial obstruction produces paroxysmal cough, wheezing, asymmetrical breath sounds, and dyspnea.
5. If any obstruction progresses, unconsciousness and asphyxiation may occur.
6. Partial obstructions may occur without symptoms.
7. The distressed child cannot speak, becomes cyanotic, and collapses.

C. Interventions

1. Emergency care (see Chapter 16)
2. Nonemergency management entails removal by endoscopy.
   - **a.** Postprocedure, the child receives high-humidity air.
   - **b.** Observe for signs and symptoms of airway edema.
3. Prevention
   - **a.** Keep any small object out of reach of small children.
   - **b.** Avoid giving small children small, round, food items.
4. Parent, day care provider, babysitter education
   - **a.** Reinforce teaching about the hazards of aspiration.
   - **b.** Discuss potential situations in which small items may be aspirated.
   - **c.** Reinforce teaching about the symptoms of aspiration.
   - **d.** Reinforce teaching about how to perform emergency care measures.

XV. Tuberculosis

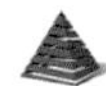

A. Description (see Chapter 49)

1. A contagious disease caused by *Mycobacterium tuberculosis,* which is an acid-fast bacillus
2. Multidrug-resistant strains of *M. tuberculosis* occur as a result of client or family noncompliance with therapeutic regimens.
3. The route of transmission of *M. tuberculosis* is via the inhalation of droplets from an individual with active tuberculosis (TB).

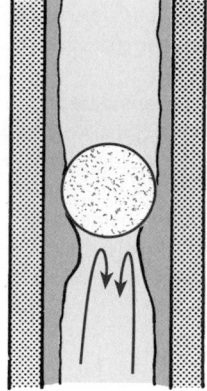

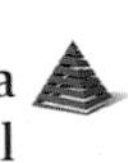

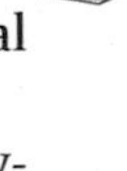

4. There is an increased incidence in urban low-income areas, nonwhite racial or ethnic groups, and first-generation immigrants from endemic countries.
5. Most children are infected by a family member or another individual with whom they have frequent contact (e.g., a babysitter).

B. Data collection

1. May be asymptomatic or develop symptoms such as malaise, fever, cough, weight loss, anorexia, and lymphadenopathy

Pediatric

BOX 34-8 Tuberculin Skin Test Interpretation

Induration that measures 15 mm or more is considered to be a positive reaction in children 4 years old or older who do not have any risk factors.

Induration that measures 10 mm or more is considered to be a positive reaction in children younger than 4 years old and in those with chronic illness or who are at high risk for exposure to tuberculosis.

Induration that measures 5 mm or more is considered to be positive for those in the highest-risk groups, such as children with immunosuppressive conditions or human immunodeficiency virus infection.

2. Specific symptoms related to the site of infection, such as the lungs, brain, bone, may be present.
3. With increased time, asymmetrical expansion of the lungs, decreased breath sounds, crackles, and dullness to percussion develop.

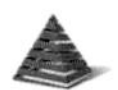
C. Tuberculin skin test (TST) (Box 34-8)
1. Will produce a positive reaction 2 to 10 weeks after the initial infection
2. Determines whether the child has been infected and has developed a sensitivity to the protein of the tubercle bacillus. A positive reaction does not confirm the presence of active disease (exposure versus presence).
3. After the child reacts positively, he or she will always react positively. A positive reaction in a previously negative child indicates that the child has been infected since the last test.

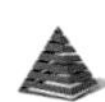
4. Tuberculosis testing should not be done at the same time as measles immunization (viral interference from the measles vaccine may cause a false-negative result).

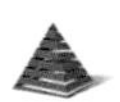
D. Sputum culture
1. A definitive diagnosis is made by demonstrating the presence of mycobacteria in a culture.
2. Chest x-rays are supplemental to sputum cultures and are not definitive alone.
3. Because an infant or young child often swallows sputum rather than expectorates it, gastric washings (aspiration of lavaged contents from the fasting stomach) may be done to obtain a specimen; the specimen is obtained in the early morning before breakfast.

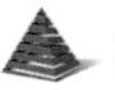
E. Interventions
1. Medications
   a. A 9-month course of isoniazid may be prescribed to prevent a latent infection from progressing to clinically active TB and to prevent initial infection in children in high-risk situations; a 12-month course may be prescribed for the child infected with human immunodeficiency virus.
   b. Recommendation for the child with clinically active tuberculosis may include combination administration of isoniazid, rifampin (Rifadin), and pyrazinamide daily for 2 months, and then isoniazid and rifampin twice weekly for 4 months.
   c. Inform the parents and child that bodily fluids, including urine, may turn an orange-red color with some tuberculosis medications.
   d. Direct observed therapy may be necessary for some children.
2. Place children with active disease who are contagious on respiratory isolation until medications have been initiated, sputum cultures demonstrate a diminished number of organisms, and cough is improving; this includes use of a personally fitted air-purifying N95 or N100 respirator (mask) by the nurse caring for the child.
3. Stress the importance of adequate rest and adequate diet.
4. Reinforce instructions to the child and family about measures to prevent the transmission of tuberculosis.
5. Case finding and follow-up with known contacts is critical to decrease the number of cases of individuals with active TB.

CRITICAL THINKING What Should You Do?

Answer: For the child with pneumonia, to reduce the discomfort in the pleural area, the nurse should encourage the child to lie on the affected side (if pneumonia is unilateral) to splint the chest. This position reduces the discomfort associated with pleural rubbing. The health care provider's prescription for positioning is always followed. In addition, a mild analgesic may be administered if it is prescribed.

Reference(s): McKinney, E., James, S., Murray, S., Nelson, K. & Ashwill, J. (2013). *Maternal-child nursing* (4th ed., p. 1169). St. Louis: Elsevier.

PRACTICE QUESTIONS

❖ **326.** The nurse is preparing for the admission of an infant with a diagnosis of bronchiolitis caused by the respiratory syncytial virus (RSV). Which interventions should be included in the plan of care? **Select all that apply.**

- ❑ **1.** Place the infant in a private room.
- ❑ **2.** Place the infant in a room near the nurses' station.
- ❑ **3.** Ensure that the infant's head is in a flexed position.
- ❑ **4.** Wear a mask at all times when in contact with the infant.

❑ 5. Place the child in a tent that delivers warm, humidified air.
❑ 6. Position the infant side-lying, with the head lower than the chest.

327. After a tonsillectomy, the child begins to vomit bright red blood. Which is the **initial** nursing action?
1. Turn the child to the side.
2. Notify the registered nurse (RN).
3. Administer the prescribed antiemetic.
4. Maintain nothing-by-mouth (NPO) status.

328. After a tonsillectomy, which fluid or food item would be appropriate to offer to the child?
1. Yellow Jell-O
2. Cold ginger ale
3. Vanilla pudding
4. Cherry Popsicle

329. The nurse reinforces instructions to the mother of a child with croup about the measures to take if an acute spasmodic episode occurs. Which statement by the mother indicates the **need for further teaching**?
1. "I will place a steam vaporizer in my child's room."
2. "I will take my child out into the humid night air."
3. "I will place a cool-mist humidifier in my child's room."
4. "I will place my child in a closed bathroom and allow my child to inhale steam from the running water."

330. The nurse reinforces instructions to the mother of a child who has been hospitalized with croup. Which statement made by the mother would indicate the **need for further teaching**?
1. "I will give my child cough syrup if a cough develops."
2. "During an attack, I will take my child to a cool location."
3. "I can give acetaminophen (Tylenol) if my child develops a fever."
4. "I will be sure that my child drinks at least three to four glasses of fluids every day."

331. The nurse is working in the emergency department and is caring for a child who has been diagnosed with epiglottitis. Which is an indication that the child may be experiencing airway obstruction?
1. Nasal flaring and bradycardia
2. A low-grade fever and complaints of a sore throat
3. The child thrusts the chin forward and opens the mouth
4. The child leans backward, supporting himself or herself with the hands and arms

332. The nurse is caring for a hospitalized infant with bronchiolitis. Diagnostic tests have confirmed respiratory syncytial virus (RSV). On the basis of this finding, which should be the appropriate nursing action?
1. Initiate strict enteric precautions.
2. Wear a mask when caring for the child.
3. Plan to move the infant to a room with another child with RSV.
4. Leave the infant in the present room, because RSV is not contagious.

333. The nurse is instructing the mother of a child with cystic fibrosis (CF) about the appropriate dietary measures. Which meal **best** illustrates the **most appropriate** diet for a client with cystic fibrosis?
1. Veggie salad and a caramel apple
2. Strawberry jelly sandwich and pretzels
3. Plate of nachos and cheese and a cupcake
4. Chicken tenders and a baked potato with butter

334. The nurse reviews the results of a tuberculin skin test performed on a 3-year-old child. The results indicate an area of induration that measures 10 mm. How should the nurse interpret this result?
1. Positive
2. Negative
3. Inconclusive
4. Definitive, requiring a repeat test

335. Isoniazid (INH) is prescribed for a 2-year-old child with a positive tuberculin skin test. The mother of the child asks the nurse how long the child will need to take the medication. Which time frame is the appropriate response to the mother?
1. 6 months
2. 9 months
3. 15 months
4. 18 months

336. The day care nurse is observing a 2-year-old child and suspects that the child may have strabismus. Which observation may be indicative of this condition?
1. The child has difficulty hearing.
2. The child does not respond when spoken to.
3. The child consistently tilts his or her head to see.
4. The child consistently turns his or her head to see.

337. The nurse has provided instructions to the mother of a child who has been diagnosed with bacterial conjunctivitis. Which statement by the mother would indicate the **need for further teaching**?
1. "I need to wash my hands frequently."
2. "I need to clean the eye, as prescribed."
3. "It is okay to share towels and washcloths."
4. "I need to give the eyedrops, as prescribed."

338. The nurse is assigned to care for a child after a myringotomy with the insertion of tympanostomy tubes. The nurse notes a small amount of reddish drainage from the child's ear after the surgery. On the basis of this finding, which action should the nurse take?
1. Document the findings.
2. Notify the registered nurse immediately.
3. Change the ear tubes so that they do not become blocked.
4. Check the ear drainage for the presence of cerebrospinal fluid.

339. The nurse assists to prepare a teaching plan regarding the administration of eardrops for the parents of a 2-year-old child. Which should be included in the plan?
1. Wear gloves when administering the eardrops.
2. Pull the ear up and back before instilling the eardrops.
3. Pull the earlobe down and back before instilling the eardrops.
4. Hold the child in a sitting position when administering the eardrops.

340. The nurse should place the child who had a tonsillectomy in which position?
1. Supine position
2. Side-lying position
3. High Fowler's position
4. Trendelenburg's position

ANSWERS

❖ **326. 1, 2**

Rationale: The infant with RSV should be isolated in a private room or in a room with another child with RSV. The infant should be placed in a room near the nurses' station for close observation. The infant should be positioned with the head and chest at a 30- to 40-degree angle and the neck slightly extended to maintain an open airway and to decrease pressure on the diaphragm. Cool, humidified oxygen is delivered to relieve dyspnea, hypoxemia, and insensible water loss from tachypnea. Contact precautions (wearing gloves and a gown) reduce the nosocomial transmission of RSV.
Test-Taking Strategy: Focus on the subject, care of the child with RSV. Recalling the mode of transmission of RSV will assist you with determining that the infant needs to be placed in a private room or in a room with another child with RSV and that contact precautions need to be maintained. Recalling the reasons to maintain a patent airway (edema and the accumulation of mucus obstruct the bronchioles) will assist you with determining that the infant needs to be observed closely, that the infant's head should be elevated, and that the infant should receive cool, humidified oxygen. **Review: respiratory syncytial virus.**
Level of Cognitive Ability: Analyzing
Client Needs: Physiological Integrity
Integrated Process: Nursing Process/Planning
Content Area: Child Health: Throat/Respiratory
Priority Concepts: Gas Exchange, Infection
Reference(s): Hockenberry, Wilson (2013), p. 725; McKinney et al (2013), p. 1167.

327. 1

Rationale: After a tonsillectomy, if bleeding occurs, the child is turned to the side, and the RN or HCP is notified. An NPO status would be maintained, and an antiemetic may be prescribed; however, the initial nursing action would be to turn the child to the side.
Test-Taking Strategy: Note the strategic word, *initial.* Although all of the options may be appropriate to maintain physiological integrity, the initial action is to turn the child to the side. **Review: tonsillectomy.**
Level of Cognitive Ability: Applying
Client Needs: Physiological Integrity
Integrated Process: Nursing Process/Implementation
Content Area: Child Health: Throat/Respiratory
Priority Concepts: Gas Exchange, Safety
Reference(s): McKinney et al (2013), p. 1158.

328. 1

Rationale: After a tonsillectomy, clear, cool liquids should be administered. Citrus, carbonated, and extremely hot or cold liquids need to be avoided because they may irritate the throat. Milk and milk products (pudding) are avoided because they coat the throat and cause the child to clear the throat, thus increasing the risk of bleeding. Red liquids need to be avoided because they give the appearance of blood if the child vomits.
Test-Taking Strategy: Focus on the subject, care of the child following tonsillectomy. Remember that avoiding foods and fluids that may irritate the throat or cause bleeding is the concern; this will assist you with eliminating options 2 and 3. The word *cherry* in option 4 should be the clue that this is not an appropriate food item. **Review: tonsillectomy.**
Level of Cognitive Ability: Applying
Client Needs: Physiological Integrity
Integrated Process: Nursing Process/Implementation
Content Area: Child Health: Throat/Respiratory
Priority Concepts: Gas Exchange, Nutrition
Reference(s): Hockenberry, Wilson (2013), p. 716.

329. 1

Rationale: Steam from warm running water in a closed bathroom and cool mist from a bedside humidifier are effective for reducing mucosal edema. Cool-mist humidifiers are recommended as compared with steam vaporizers, which present a danger of scalding burns. Taking the child out into the humid night air may also relieve mucosal swelling. Remember, however, that a cold mist may precipitate bronchospasm.
Test-Taking Strategy: Note the strategic words, *need for further teaching.* These words indicate a negative event query and the need to select the incorrect statement. Recall the goals of

reducing mucosal edema and providing a safe environment. Note the word *steam* in option 1. Option 1 would provide an unsafe environment for the child. **Review:** acute spasmodic croup.
Level of Cognitive Ability: Evaluating
Client Needs: Safe and Effective Care Environment
Integrated Process: Teaching and Learning
Content Area: Child Health: Throat/Respiratory
Priority Concepts: Client Education, Gas Exchange
Reference(s): McKinney et al (2013), pp. 1160–1161.

330. 1
Rationale: Cough syrups and cold medicines are not to be given because they may dry and thicken secretions. During a croup attack, the child can be taken to a cool basement or garage. Acetaminophen is used if a fever develops. Adequate hydration of 500 to 1000 mL of fluids daily is important for thinning secretions.
Test-Taking Strategy: Note the **strategic words**, *the need for further teaching*. These words indicate a **negative event query** and ask you to select an option that is an incorrect statement. Knowledge of the pathophysiology related to croup will assist you with eliminating options 3 and 4 first. Recalling that taking the child to a cool location during an attack is appropriate will direct you to the correct option from the remaining options. **Review:** croup.
Level of Cognitive Ability: Evaluating
Client Needs: Physiological Integrity
Integrated Process: Teaching and Learning
Content Area: Child Health: Throat/Respiratory
Priority Concepts: Client Education, Gas Exchange
Reference(s): McKinney et al (2013), p. 1162.

331. 3
Rationale: Clinical manifestations that are suggestive of airway obstruction include tripod positioning (leaning forward supported by the hands and arms with the chin thrust out and the mouth open), nasal flaring, tachycardia, a high fever, and a sore throat.
Test-Taking Strategy: Focus on the **subject**, signs/symptoms of airway obstruction. Eliminate option 1 first because tachycardia rather than bradycardia will occur in a child who is experiencing respiratory distress. Eliminate option 2 next, knowing that a high fever occurs with epiglottitis. From the remaining options, visualize the descriptions given in each, and determine which position would best assist a child who is experiencing respiratory distress. **Review:** epiglottitis.
Level of Cognitive Ability: Analyzing
Client Needs: Physiological Integrity
Integrated Process: Nursing Process/Data Collection
Content Area: Child Health: Throat/Respiratory
Priority Concepts: Gas Exchange, Perfusion
Reference(s): McKinney et al (2013), p. 1162.

332. 3
Rationale: RSV is a highly communicable disorder, but it is not transmitted via the airborne route. It is usually transferred by the hands, and meticulous hand washing is necessary to decrease the spread of organisms. The infant with RSV is isolated in a single room or placed in a room with another child with RSV. Enteric precautions are not necessary; however, the nurse should wear a gown when the soiling of clothing may occur.
Test-Taking Strategy: Focus on the **subject**, transmission of RSV. Knowledge regarding the transmission of RSV will direct you to option 3. Remember that RSV is usually transferred by the hands and that meticulous hand washing is necessary to decrease the spread of organisms. **Review:** respiratory syncytial virus.
Level of Cognitive Ability: Applying
Client Needs: Safe and Effective Care Environment
Integrated Process: Nursing Process/Implementation
Content Area: Child Health: Throat/Respiratory
Priority Concepts: Gas Exchange, Infection
Reference(s): Hockenberry, Wilson (2013), p. 725.

333. 4
Rationale: Children with CF are managed with a high-calorie, high-protein diet. Pancreatic enzyme replacement therapy is undertaken, and fat-soluble vitamin supplements are administered. Fats are not restricted unless steatorrhea cannot be controlled by increased levels of pancreatic enzymes. Chicken tenders and a baked potato with butter provide a high-calorie and high-protein meal that includes fat.
Test-Taking Strategy: Focus on the **subject**, dietary measures for a child with cystic fibrosis. Note the **strategic words**, *best* and *most appropriate*. Eliminate options 1, 2, and 3 because they are not high in protein or calories. From the remaining options, recalling the appropriate diet for the child with CF will direct you to the correct option. **Review:** cystic fibrosis.
Level of Cognitive Ability: Applying
Client Needs: Physiological Integrity
Integrated Process: Teaching and Learning
Content Area: Child Health: Throat/Respiratory
Priority Concepts: Gas Exchange, Nutrition
Reference(s): McKinney et al (2013), p. 1190.

334. 1
Rationale: An induration that measures 10 mm or more is considered to be a positive result for children who are younger than 4 years old and for those with chronic illness or with a high risk for environmental exposure to tuberculosis. A reaction of 5 mm or more is considered to be a positive result for those in the highest-risk groups.
Test-Taking Strategy: Focus on the **subject**, interpreting a tuberculin skin test result. Use your knowledge regarding a positive tuberculin skin test in children to answer this question. Option 4 can be easily eliminated first. Note the child's age in the question to determine the correct option from the remaining three options. **Review:** tuberculin skin test.
Level of Cognitive Ability: Analyzing
Client Needs: Physiological Integrity
Integrated Process: Nursing Process/Data Collection
Content Area: Child Health: Throat/Respiratory
Priority Concepts: Gas Exchange, Infection
Reference(s): McKinney et al (2013), pp. 1147, 1192.

335. 2
Rationale: Isoniazid is given to prevent tuberculosis (TB) infection from progressing to active disease. A chest x-ray film is obtained before the initiation of preventive therapy. In infants and children, the recommended duration of isoniazid therapy is 9 months. For children with human immunodeficiency virus infection, a minimum of 12 months is recommended.

Test-Taking Strategy: Focus on the subject, treatment with INH. Knowledge regarding treatment with INH in a 2-year-old child is required to answer this question. Remember that in infants and children, the recommended duration of isoniazid therapy is 9 months. **Review: tuberculosis.**
Level of Cognitive Ability: Applying
Client Needs: Physiological Integrity
Integrated Process: Nursing Process/Implementation
Content Area: Pharmacology: Respiratory Medications
Priority Concepts: Gas Exchange, Infection
Reference(s): Hockenberry, Wilson (2013), p. 731.

336. 3
Rationale: The nurse may suspect strabismus in a child when the child complains of frequent headaches, squints, or tilts the head to see. Options 1, 2, and 4 are not indicative of this condition.
Test-Taking Strategy: Focus on the subject, manifestations of strabismus. Begin by eliminating options 1 and 2 because they are comparable or alike and refer to hearing. From the remaining options, recalling the signs of strabismus will direct you to the correct option. **Review: strabismus.**
Level of Cognitive Ability: Understanding
Client Needs: Physiological Integrity
Integrated Process: Nursing Process/Data Collection
Content Area: Child Health: Eye/Ear
Priority Concepts: Clinical Judgment, Sensory Perception
Reference(s): McKinney et al (2013), pp. 1504–1505.

337. 3
Rationale: Bacterial conjunctivitis is highly contagious, and infection control measures should be taught; these include frequent hand washing and not sharing towels and washcloths. Options 1, 2, and 4 are correct measures.
Test-Taking Strategy: Note the strategic words, *need for further teaching*. These words indicate a negative event query and ask you to select an option that is an incorrect statement. Recalling that bacterial conjunctivitis is highly contagious will direct you to the correct option. **Review: bacterial conjunctivitis.**
Level of Cognitive Ability: Evaluating
Client Needs: Safe and Effective Care Environment
Integrated Process: Teaching and Learning
Content Area: Child Health: Eye/Ear
Priority Concepts: Client Education, Infection
Reference(s): Hockenberry, Wilson (2013), p. 432.

338. 1
Rationale: After a myringotomy with the insertion of tympanostomy tubes, the child is monitored for ear drainage. A small amount of reddish drainage is normal during the first few days after surgery. However, any heavy bleeding or bleeding that occurs after 3 days should be reported. The nurse would document the findings. Options 2, 3, and 4 are not necessary.
Test-Taking Strategy: Note the subject, a small amount of reddish drainage. Considering both the anatomical location of the surgery and the subject of the question will direct you to the correct option. **Review: myringotomy with the insertion of tympanostomy tubes.**
Level of Cognitive Ability: Applying
Client Needs: Physiological Integrity
Integrated Process: Nursing Process/Implementation
Content Area: Child Health: Eye/Ear
Priority Concepts: Clinical Judgment, Safety
Reference(s): McKinney et al (2013), pp. 1152–1153.

339. 3
Rationale: When administering eardrops to a child who is younger than 3 years old, the ear should be pulled down and back. For children who are older than 3 years old, the ear is pulled up and back. Gloves do not need to be worn by the parents, but hand washing needs to be performed before and after the procedure. The child should be in a side-lying position with the affected ear facing upward to facilitate the flow of medication down the ear canal by gravity.
Test-Taking Strategy: Focus on the subject, administering eardrops to a 2-year-old child. Visualizing this procedure will assist you with eliminating options 1 and 4 first. From the remaining options, recalling the anatomy of the 2-year-old's ear canal will direct you to the correct option. **Review:** administration of eardrops.
Level of Cognitive Ability: Applying
Client Needs: Physiological Integrity
Integrated Process: Teaching and Learning
Content Area: Child Health: Eye/Ear
Priority Concepts: Client Education, Safety
Reference(s): Perry, Potter, Ostendorf (2014), pp. 514–515.

340. 2
Rationale: The child should be placed in a semiprone or side-lying position after tonsillectomy to facilitate drainage. Options 1, 3, and 4 will not achieve this goal.
Test-Taking Strategy: Focus on the subject, care following a tonsillectomy. Visualize each of the positions described in the options. Keeping in mind that the goal is to facilitate drainage will direct you to the correct option. **Review: tonsillectomy.**
Level of Cognitive Ability: Applying
Client Needs: Physiological Integrity
Integrated Process: Nursing Process/Implementation
Content Area: Child Health: Throat/Respiratory
Priority Concepts: Gas Exchange, Safety
Reference(s): Hockenberry, Wilson (2013), p. 716.

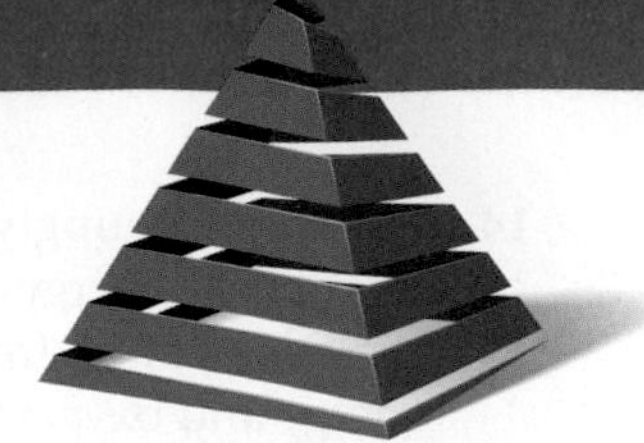

CHAPTER 35

Cardiovascular Disorders

CRITICAL THINKING What Should You Do?

A child diagnosed with a congenital heart defect suddenly develops difficulty breathing. What should the nurse do?

Answer located on p. 432.

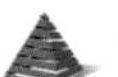

I. Heart Failure (HF)

A. Description

1. The inability of the heart to pump a sufficient amount of blood to meet the metabolic and oxygen needs of the body
2. In infants and children, inadequate cardiac output is most commonly caused by congenital heart defects (**shunt**, obstruction, or a combination of both) that produce an excessive volume or pressure load on the myocardium.
3. In infants and children, a combination of both left- and right-sided heart failure is usually present (Box 35-1).
4. The goals of treatment are to improve cardiac function, remove accumulated fluid and sodium, decrease cardiac demands, improve tissue oxygenation, and decrease oxygen consumption.

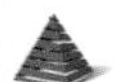

B. Data collection of early signs

1. Tachycardia, especially during rest and slight exertion
2. Tachypnea
3. Profuse scalp diaphoresis, especially in infants
4. Fatigue and irritability
5. Sudden weight gain related to excess fluid retention
6. Respiratory distress

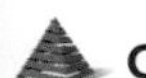

C. Interventions

1. Monitor for early signs of HF.
2. Monitor for respiratory distress (count respirations for 1 minute).
3. Monitor apical pulse (count apical pulse for 1 minute) and monitor for abnormal rhythms.
4. Monitor temperature for hyperthermia and for other signs of infection, particularly respiratory infection.
5. Monitor strict intake and output; weigh diapers as appropriate for most accurate output.
6. Monitor daily weight to check for fluid retention; a weight gain of 0.5 kg (1 lb) in 1 day is caused by the accumulation of fluid.
7. Monitor for facial or peripheral dependent edema, listen to lung sounds, and report abnormal findings indicating excessive fluid in the body.
8. Elevate the head of the bed in a semi-Fowler's position.
9. Maintain a neutral thermal environment to prevent cold stress in infants.
10. Provide rest and decrease environmental stimuli.
11. Administer cool humidified oxygen as prescribed, using an oxygen hood for young infants and a nasal cannula or face mask for older infants and children.
12. Organize nursing activities to allow for uninterrupted sleep.
13. Maintain adequate nutritional status.

BOX 35-1 Signs and Symptoms of Heart Failure

Left-Sided Failure

- Crackles and wheezes
- Cough
- Dyspnea
- Grunting (infants)
- Head bobbing (infants)
- Nasal flaring
- Orthopnea
- Periods of cyanosis
- Retractions
- Tachypnea

Right-Sided Failure

- Ascites
- Hepatosplenomegaly
- Jugular vein distention
- Oliguria
- Peripheral edema, especially dependent edema and periorbital edema
- Weight gain

14. Feed when hungry and soon after awakening, conserving energy and oxygen supply.
15. Provide small, frequent feedings, conserving energy and oxygen supply.
16. Administer sedation as prescribed during the acute stage to promote rest.
17. Administer digoxin (Lanoxin) as prescribed.
    a. Check apical heart rate for 1 minute before administration.
    b. Withhold digoxin if the apical pulse is less than 90 to 110 beats/min in infants and young children and less than 70 beats/min in older children, as prescribed.
    c. Be aware that infants rarely receive more than 1 mL (50 mcg or 0.05 mg) of digoxin in one dose.
18. Monitor digoxin levels and for signs of digoxin toxicity, including anorexia, poor feeding, vomiting, bradycardia, and abnormal heart rhythms; report any signs to the registered nurse immediately.
    a. Normal digoxin level is 0.5 to 2.0 mg/dL.
    b. Digoxin toxicity occurs when level is above 2.0 mg/dL.
19. Administer angiotensin-converting enzyme inhibitors as prescribed.
    a. Monitor for hypotension, kidney dysfunction, and cough when angiotensin-converting enzyme inhibitors are administered.
    b. The blood pressure; serum protein, albumin, blood urea nitrogen, and creatinine levels; white blood cell count; urine output; urinary specific gravity; and urinary protein level are monitored.
20. Administer diuretics such as furosemide (Lasix) as prescribed.
    a. Monitor for signs and symptoms of hypokalemia (serum potassium level less than 3.5 mEq/L), including muscle weakness and cramping and confusion (child), irritability, restlessness, and inverted T wave or prominent U waves on the electrocardiogram (ECG).
    b. If signs and symptoms of hypokalemia are present and the child is also being administered digoxin, then monitor closely for digoxin toxicity because hypokalemia potentiates digoxin toxicity.
21. Administer potassium supplements and provide dietary sources of potassium as prescribed.

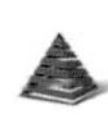

    a. Supplemental potassium is prescribed if the need is indicated by low serum potassium levels and if adequate kidney function is evident; supplemental potassium is usually necessary when administering a potassium-losing diuretic such as furosemide (Lasix).
    b. Encourage foods that the child will eat that are high in potassium, as appropriate, such as bananas, baked potato skins, and peanut butter.
22. Monitor serum electrolyte levels, particularly the potassium level (normal level is 3.5 to 5.0 mEq/L).
23. Limit fluid intake as prescribed in the acute stage.
24. Monitor for signs and symptoms of dehydration, including sunken fontanel (infant), nonelastic skin turgor, dry mucous membranes, decreased tear production, decreased urine output, and concentrated urine.
25. Monitor sodium levels as prescribed.
    a. Normal level is 135 to 145 mEq/L.
    b. Many infant formulas have slightly more sodium than breast milk.
26. Reinforce instructions to the parents regarding the description of the diagnosis and administration of medications (Box 35-2).
27. Reinforce instructions to the parents in cardiopulmonary resuscitation (CPR); see Chapter 16 for information on CPR.

The parents should be provided with a medication guide for any medication prescribed for the infant or child. In addition, the nurse needs to review the instructions in the guide and provide an opportunity for the parents to demonstrate medication administration procedures.

BOX 35-2 Home Care Instructions for Administering Digoxin (Lanoxin)

Administer the medication as prescribed.
Use an accurate measuring device as provided by the pharmacist.
Administer the medication 1 hour before or 2 hours after feedings.
Use a calendar to mark off the dose that has been administered.
Do not mix the medication with food or fluid.
If a dose is missed and more than 4 hours have elapsed, withhold the dose, and give the next dose at the scheduled time. If less than 4 hours have elapsed, administer the missed dose.
If the child vomits, do not administer a second dose (follow health care provider's [HCP's] prescription).
If more than two consecutive doses have been missed, notify the HCP. Do not increase or double the dose to make up for missed doses.
If the child has teeth, give him or her water after the medication. If possible, brush the child's teeth to prevent tooth decay from the sweetened liquid.
Monitor for signs of toxicity such as poor feeding or vomiting.
If the child becomes ill, notify the HCP.
Keep the medication in a locked cabinet.
Call the poison control center immediately if accidental overdose occurs.

II. Defects with Increased Pulmonary Blood Flow

A. Description
   1. Intracardiac communication along the septum or an abnormal connection between the great arteries allows blood to flow from the high-pressure left side of the heart to the low-pressure right side of the heart.
   2. The infant typically demonstrates signs and symptoms of HF.

B. Atrial septal defect (ASD)
   1. An abnormal opening between the atria that causes an increased flow of oxygenated blood into the right side of the heart
   2. Right atrial and ventricular enlargement occurs.
   3. Infant may be asymptomatic or may develop HF.
   4. Signs and symptoms of decreased cardiac output may be present (Box 35-3).
   5. Nonsurgical treatment: May be closed with the use of devices during a cardiac catheterization.
   6. Management: Open repair with cardiopulmonary bypass is usually performed before the child reaches school age.

C. Atrioventricular canal defect
   1. Results from incomplete fusion of the endocardial cushions
   2. Most common cardiac defect in children with Down syndrome
   3. A characteristic murmur is present.
   4. The infant usually has mild to moderate HF. **Cyanosis** increases with crying.
   5. Signs and symptoms of decreased cardiac output may be present.
   6. Management: Can include either pulmonary artery banding for infants with severe symptoms (palliative) or complete repair via cardiopulmonary bypass

D. Patent ductus arteriosus (PDA)
   1. Failure of the fetal ductus arteriosus (shunt that connects the aorta and the pulmonary artery) to close within the first weeks of life
   2. A characteristic machine-like murmur is present. The infant may be asymptomatic or he or she may show signs of HF.
   3. A widened pulse pressure and bounding pulses are present.

BOX 35-3 Signs and Symptoms of Decreased Cardiac Output

- Decreased peripheral pulses
- Exercise intolerance
- Feeding difficulties
- Hypotension
- Irritability, restlessness, and lethargy
- Oliguria
- Pale, cool extremities
- Tachycardia

   4. Signs and symptoms of decreased cardiac output may be present.
   5. Management
      a. Indomethacin (prostaglandin inhibitor) may be administered to close a patent ductus in premature infants and some newborns.
      b. The defect may be closed during cardiac catheterization or may require surgical management.

E. Ventricular septal defect (VSD)
   1. An abnormal opening between the right and left ventricles.
   2. Many VSDs close spontaneously during the first year of life in children who have small or moderate defects.
   3. A characteristic murmur is present; HF is common.
   4. Signs and symptoms of HF and of decreased cardiac output may be present.
   5. Management
      a. Device closure during cardiac catheterization may be possible.
      b. Open repair with cardiopulmonary bypass may be done.

III. Obstructive Defects

A. Description
   1. Blood exiting the heart meets an area of anatomic narrowing (**stenosis**), thus causing obstruction of the blood flow.
   2. The location of narrowing is usually near the valve of the obstructive defect.
   3. Infants and children exhibit signs of HF.
   4. Children with mild obstruction may be asymptomatic.

B. Aortic stenosis
   1. Aortic stenosis is a narrowing or stricture of the aortic valve, causing resistance to blood flow from the left ventricle into the aorta, resulting in decreased cardiac output, left ventricular hypertrophy, and pulmonary vascular congestion.
   2. Valvular stenosis is the most common type and usually is caused by malformed cusps, resulting in a bicuspid rather than a tricuspid valve, or fusion of the cusps.
   3. A characteristic murmur is present.
   4. Infants with severe defects demonstrate signs of decreased cardiac output.
   5. Children show signs of exercise intolerance, chest pain, and dizziness when standing for long periods of time.
   6. Management
      a. Dilation of the narrowed valve may be done during cardiac catheterization.
      b. Surgical aortic valvotomy (palliative) may be done; a valve replacement may be required at a second procedure.

C. Coarctation of the aorta

1. Coarctation of the aorta is localized narrowing near the insertion of the ductus arteriosus.
2. Signs of HF may occur in infants.
3. Signs and symptoms of decreased cardiac output may be present.
4. Children may experience headaches, dizziness, fainting, and epistaxis resulting from hypertension.
5. Management of the defect may be done via balloon angioplasty in children; restenosis can occur. Surgical intervention may be necessary.

With coarctation of the aorta, the blood pressure is higher in the upper extremities than the lower extremities. In addition, bounding pulses in the arms, weak or absent femoral pulses, and cool lower extremities may be present.

D. Pulmonary stenosis

1. Narrowing at the entrance to the pulmonary artery
2. Resistance to blood flow causes right ventricular hypertrophy and decreased pulmonary blood flow. The right ventricle may be hypoplastic.
3. Pulmonary **atresia** is the extreme form of pulmonary stenosis in that there is total fusion of the commissures and no blood flows to the lungs.
4. A characteristic murmur is present.
5. May be asymptomatic
6. Newborns with severe narrowing will be cyanotic.
7. If pulmonary stenosis is severe, HF occurs.
8. Signs and symptoms of decreased cardiac output may occur.
9. Management: Dilation of the narrowed valve may be done during cardiac catheterization. Surgical intervention may be necessary.

IV. Defects with Decreased Pulmonary Blood Flow

A. Description

1. Obstructed pulmonary blood flow and an anatomic defect (ASD or VSD) between the right and left sides of the heart
2. Pressure in the right side of the heart increases as a result of obstructed blood flow, exceeding pressure in the left side, which allows desaturated blood to shunt right to left, causing desaturation in the left side of the heart and in the systemic circulation.
3. Typically, hypoxemia and cyanosis appear.

B. Tetralogy of Fallot

1. Includes four defects: ventricular septal defect, pulmonary stenosis, overriding aorta, and right ventricular hypertrophy
2. If pulmonary vascular resistance is higher than systemic resistance, the shunt is from right to left. If systemic resistance is higher than pulmonary resistance, the shunt is from left to right.
3. Infants
   a. May be acutely cyanotic at birth or may have mild cyanosis that progresses over the first year of life as the pulmonic stenosis worsens
   b. A characteristic murmur is present.
   c. Acute episodes of cyanosis and hypoxia (hypercyanotic spells), called blue spells or tet spells, occur when the infant's oxygen requirements exceed the blood supply (usually during crying, feeding, or defecating). 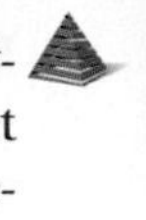
4. Children: With increasing cyanosis, squatting, clubbing of the fingers, and poor **growth** may occur.
   a. Squatting is a compensatory mechanism to facilitate increased return of blood flow to the heart for oxygenation.
   b. Clubbing (an abnormal enlargement in the distal phalanges seen in the fingers)
5. Surgical management: Palliative shunt
   a. The shunt increases pulmonary blood flow and increases oxygen saturation in infants who cannot undergo primary repair.
   b. The shunt provides blood flow to the pulmonary arteries from the left or right subclavian artery.
6. Surgical management: Complete repair, if necessary, usually is performed in the first year of life.

C. Tricuspid atresia

1. Failure of the tricuspid valve to develop
2. There is no communication from the right atrium to the right ventricle.
3. Blood flows through an ASD or a patent foramen ovale to the left side of the heart and through a VSD to the right ventricle and out to the lungs.
4. Often associated with pulmonic stenosis and the transposition of the great arteries.
5. A complete mixing of unoxygenated and oxygenated blood in the left side of the heart occurs, which results in systemic desaturation, pulmonary obstruction, and decreased pulmonary blood flow.
6. Cyanosis, tachycardia, fatigability with feeding, and dyspnea are seen in the newborn. 
7. Older children exhibit signs of chronic hypoxemia and clubbing.
8. Management: If the ASD is small, the defect may be closed during cardiac catheterization; otherwise, surgery is needed.

Clubbing is symptomatic of chronic hypoxia. Peripheral circulation is diminished and oxygenation of vital organs and tissues is compromised.

V. Mixed Defects

A. Description
1. Fully saturated systemic blood flow mixes with the desaturated blood flow, which causes a desaturation of the systemic blood flow.
2. Pulmonary congestion occurs, and cardiac output decreases.
3. Signs of HF are present; symptoms depend on the degree of desaturation.

B. Hypoplastic left heart syndrome
1. The underdevelopment of the left side of the heart that results in a hypoplastic left ventricle and aortic atresia
2. Mild cyanosis and signs of HF occur until the ductus arteriosus closes. Progressive deterioration with cyanosis and decreased cardiac output then occur, which lead to cardiovascular collapse.
3. This is fatal during the first few months of life without intervention.
4. Surgical treatment is necessary.

C. Transposition of the great arteries or transposition of the great vessels
1. The pulmonary artery leaves the left ventricle, and the aorta exits from the right ventricle.
2. No communication exists between the systemic and pulmonary circulations.
3. Infants with minimal communication are severely cyanotic and depressed at birth.
4. Infants with large septal defects or a patent ductus arteriosus may be less severely cyanotic but may have symptoms of HF.
5. Cardiomegaly is evident a few weeks after birth.
6. Surgery is usually required.

D. Total anomalous pulmonary venous connection
1. Failure of the pulmonary veins to join the left atrium
2. Results in mixed blood being returned to the right atrium and shunted from the right to the left through an ASD
3. The right side of the heart hypertrophies, whereas the left side of the heart may remain small.
4. Signs and symptoms of HF develop.
5. Cyanosis worsens with pulmonary vein obstruction. After obstruction occurs, the infant's condition deteriorates rapidly.
6. Surgical treatment is necessary.

E. Truncus arteriosus
1. The failure of normal septation and the division of the embryonic bulbar trunk into the pulmonary artery and the aorta, which results in a single vessel that overrides both ventricles
2. Blood from both ventricles mixes in the common great artery, thus causing desaturation and hypoxemia.

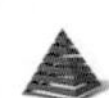

3. A characteristic murmur is present.
4. The infant exhibits moderate to severe HF, variable cyanosis, poor growth, and activity intolerance.
5. Surgical treatment is necessary.

VI. Interventions: Cardiovascular Defects

A. Monitor for signs of a defect in the infant or child (see previous descriptions of defects).

B. Monitor the vital signs closely.

C. Monitor the respiratory status for the presence of **nasal flaring** and the use of accessory muscles. The registered nurse is notified immediately if any changes occur.

D. Breath sounds are auscultated for **crackles,** wheezes, or rhonchi.

E. If respiratory effort is increased, place the child in reverse Trendelenburg's position (elevate the head and upper body) to decrease the work of breathing.

F. Administer humidified oxygen, as prescribed.

G. Endotracheal tube and ventilator care may be necessary.

H. Monitor for hypercyanotic spells and intervene immediately if they occur (see Priority Nursing Actions).

PRIORITY NURSING ACTIONS!

Actions to Take if a Hypercyanotic Spell Occurs in an Infant

1. Place the infant in a knee-chest position.
2. Prepare to administer 100% oxygen.
3. Assist to administer morphine sulfate.
4. Assist to administer fluids intravenously.
5. Document occurrence, actions taken, and the infant's response.

Hypercyanotic spells are also known as tet spells or blue spells and occur in infants or children with certain types of heart defects. The infant or child becomes acutely cyanotic and hyperpneic because of the sudden infundibular spasm. These spells may occur as a result of stressful procedures or from feeding, crying, or defecation. If a spell occurs, the nurse needs to provide a calm and comforting approach, while immediately placing the infant in the knee-chest position. This assists breathing and increases oxygenation to body tissues. Oxygen is administered by face mask or blow-by. Morphine sulfate is administered as prescribed subcutaneously or through an existing intravenous line (morphine sulfate helps reduce the infundibular spasm). Intravenous fluids are administered to replace fluids and to keep the infant well hydrated and the hematocrit and blood viscosity within acceptable limits. Depending on the infant's response, a repeated dose of morphine sulfate may be prescribed. Finally, the nurse documents the occurrence, actions taken, and the infant's response.

Reference(s): Hockenberry, M., & Wilson, D. (2013). *Wong's: Essentials of pediatric nursing* (9th ed., p. 842). St. Louis: Mosby.

I. Monitor for signs of HF, such as fluid retention in the hands, feet, chest, and around the eyes.
J. Monitor the peripheral pulses.
K. Monitor the I&O, and notify the registered nurse immediately if a decrease in urine output occurs (weigh diapers as necessary).
L. Obtain daily weight.
M. Provide adequate nutrition (high-calorie requirements), as prescribed.
N. Assist to administer medications, as prescribed.
O. Plan interventions to allow maximal rest for the child; keep the child as stress-free as possible.
P. Prepare the child and parents for cardiac catheterization, if appropriate.

VII. Cardiac Catheterization

A. Description (see Chapter 51)
   1. An invasive diagnostic procedure used to determine cardiac defects
   2. Provides information about the oxygenation saturation of the blood in the great vessels and heart chambers
   3. May be diagnostic, interventional, or electrophysiological in purpose
   4. Risks include hemorrhage from the entry site, clot formation and subsequent blockage distally, and transient dysrhythmias.

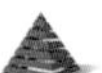

B. Preprocedure interventions
   1. Check the accurate height and weight, because this assists with the selection of the correct catheter size.
   2. Obtain a history of the presence of allergic reactions to iodine.
   3. Check for symptoms of infection, including diaper rash.
   4. Check and mark bilateral pulses (e.g., dorsalis pedis, posterior tibial).
   5. Check the baseline oxygen saturation.
   6. Familiarize the parents and child with hospital procedures and equipment.
   7. Reinforce educating the parents and older child about the procedure.
   8. Allow the parents and child to verbalize their feelings and concerns regarding the procedure and the disorder.

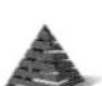

C. Postprocedure interventions
   1. Monitor findings on the cardiac monitor and the oxygen saturation for up to 4 hours after the procedure.
   2. Check the pulses below the catheter site for equality and symmetry.
   3. Check the temperature and color of the affected extremity, and report coolness immediately, which may indicate arterial obstruction.
   4. Monitor the vital signs frequently, per the HCP's prescriptions.
   5. Check the pressure dressing for intactness and signs of hemorrhage.
   6. Check the bedsheets under the extremity for blood, which may indicate bleeding from the entry site.
   7. If bleeding is present, apply continuous direct pressure above the entry site, and report it immediately.
   8. Immobilize the affected extremity for at least 4 to 6 hours for a venous entry site and for 6 to 8 hours for an arterial entry site, as prescribed.
   9. Hydrate the child via the oral route, the intravenous route, or both, as prescribed.
   10. Administer acetaminophen (Tylenol) or ibuprofen (Motrin) for pain or discomfort, as prescribed.
   11. Prepare the parents and child, if appropriate, for surgery.

D. Discharge teaching for the child and parents
   1. Remove the dressing on the day after the procedure and cover it with a bandage for 2 to 3 days.
   2. Keep the site clean and dry.
   3. Have the child avoid tub baths for 2 to 3 days.
   4. Observe for redness, edema, drainage, bleeding, and fever, and report any of these signs immediately.
   5. Avoid strenuous activity, if applicable (the child may return to school, if appropriate).
   6. Provide a diet as tolerated.
   7. Administer acetaminophen (Tylenol) or ibuprofen (Motrin) for pain, discomfort, or fever.
   8. Stress the importance of keeping follow-up appointments with the health care provider.

VIII. Cardiac Surgery

A. Postoperative interventions
   1. Monitor the vital signs and oxygen saturation, per protocol.
   2. Monitor for signs of sepsis, such as fever, chills, diaphoresis, lethargy, and altered levels of consciousness. Notify the registered nurse immediately if any signs occur.
   3. Maintain aseptic technique.
   4. Assist with monitoring lines, tubes, or catheters that are in place. Assist to remove them promptly, as prescribed, when they are no longer needed to prevent infection.
   5. Monitor for signs of discomfort, such as irritability or restlessness, and any changes in heart rate, respiratory rate, and blood pressure.
   6. Assist to administer pain medications, as prescribed, and note their effectiveness.
   7. Assist to administer antibiotics and antipyretics, as prescribed.
   8. Encourage rest and sleep periods.
   9. Facilitate parent–child contact as soon as possible.

B. Postoperative home care (Box 35-4)

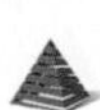

BOX 35-4 Home Care After Cardiac Surgery (Based upon Health Care Provider's Prescription)

- Omit play outside for several weeks.
- Avoid activities in which the child could fall and injure self, such as bike riding, for 2 to 4 weeks.
- Avoid crowds for 2 weeks after discharge.
- Follow a no-added-salt diet if prescribed.
- Do not add any new foods to the infant's diet (if an allergy exists to the new food, the manifestations may be interpreted as a postoperative complication).
- Do not place creams, lotions, or powders on the incision until completely healed.
- The child may return to school usually the third week after discharge, starting with half-days.
- The child should not participate in physical education for 2 months.
- Reinforce instructions to the parents to discipline the child normally.
- Reinforce instructions to the parents about the importance of the 2-week follow-up.
- Avoid immunizations, invasive procedures, and dental visits for 2 months; following this time period, the immunization schedule and dental visits need to be resumed.
- Advise the parents regarding the importance of a dental visit every 6 months after age 3 years and to inform the dentist of the cardiac problem so that antibiotics can be prescribed if necessary.
- Reinforce instructions to the parents to call the health care provider if coughing, tachypnea, cyanosis, vomiting, diarrhea, anorexia, pain, or fever occur, or any swelling, redness, or drainage occurs at the site of the incision.

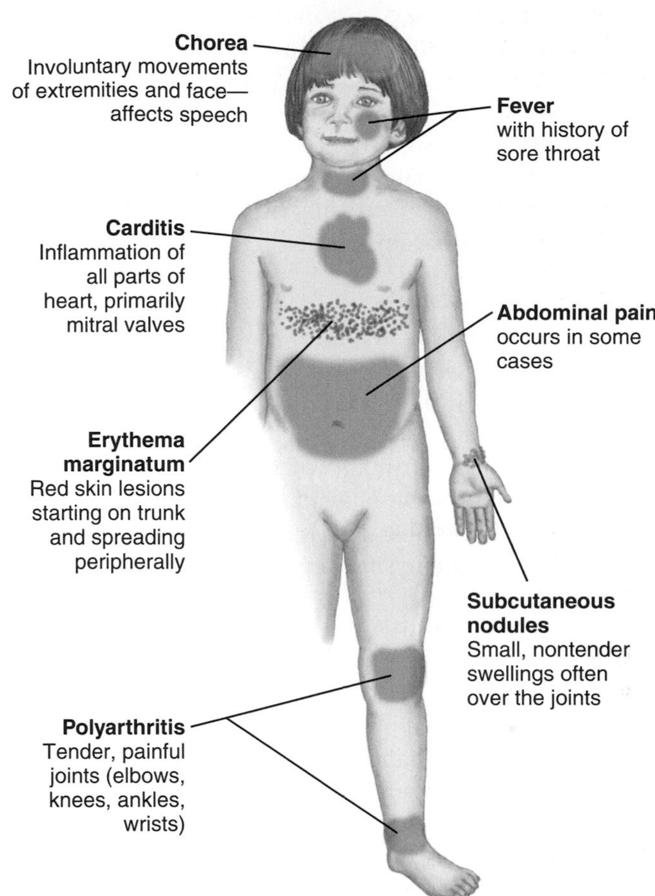

FIGURE 35-1 Clinical manifestations of rheumatic fever. (From McKinney E, James S, Murray S, Ashwill J: *Maternal-child nursing*, ed 4, Philadelphia, 2013, Saunders.)

IX. Rheumatic Fever

A. Description
   1. An inflammatory autoimmune disease that affects the connective tissues of the heart, joints, skin (subcutaneous tissues), blood vessels, and central nervous system.
   2. The most serious complication is rheumatic heart disease, which affects the cardiac valves
   3. Presents 2 to 6 weeks after an untreated or partially treated group A β-hemolytic streptococcal infection of the upper respiratory tract
   4. Jones criteria are used to determine the diagnosis.

B. Data collection (Fig. 35-1)
   1. Low-grade fever that spikes in the late afternoon
   2. Elevated antistreptolysin O titer
   3. Elevated erythrocyte sedimentation rate
   4. Elevated C-reactive protein
   5. Aschoff's bodies (lesions) in the heart, blood vessels, brain, and serous surfaces of the joints and pleurae
   6. A macular erythematous rash, primarily on the trunk and extremities

Data collection of a child with suspected rheumatic fever includes inquiring about a recent sore throat because rheumatic fever manifests 2 to 6 weeks after an untreated or partially treated group A β-hemolytic streptococcal infection of the upper respiratory tract.

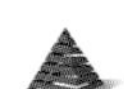

C. Interventions
   1. Monitor the vital signs.
   2. Control joint pain and inflammation with massage and alternating hot and cold applications, as prescribed.
   3. Provide bed rest during the acute febrile phase.
   4. Limit physical exercise in the child with carditis.
   5. Assist to administer antibiotics, as prescribed.
   6. Assist to administer salicylates and anti-inflammatory agents, as prescribed. (These medications should not be instituted before the diagnosis is confirmed, because they mask polyarthritis.)

7. Initiate seizure precautions if the child is experiencing chorea.
8. Reinforce instructions to the parents about the importance of follow-up and the need for antibiotic prophylaxis for dental work, infection, and invasive procedures.
9. Inform the parents to ask the school nurse to notify them if anyone in school develops a streptococcal throat infection.

X. Kawasaki Disease

A. Description
1. Also called mucocutaneous lymph node syndrome. It is an acute systemic inflammatory illness.
2. The cause is unknown but may be associated with an infection by an organism or toxin.

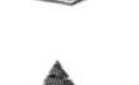

3. Cardiac involvement is the most serious complication. Aneurysms can develop.

B. Data collection
1. Acute stage
   a. Fever
   b. Conjunctival hyperemia
   c. Red throat
   d. Swollen hands, rash, and enlargement of the cervical lymph nodes
2. Subacute stage
   a. Cracking lips and fissures
   b. Desquamation of the skin on the tips of the fingers and toes
   c. Joint pain
   d. Cardiac manifestations
   e. Thrombocytosis
3. Convalescent stage: Child appears normal but signs of inflammation may be present.

C. Interventions
1. Monitor temperature frequently.
2. Check heart sounds and the heart rate and rhythm.
3. Check extremities for edema, redness, and desquamation.
4. Examine eyes for conjunctivitis.
5. Monitor mucous membranes for inflammation.
6. Monitor strict intake and output.
7. Administer soft foods and liquids that are neither too hot nor too cold.
8. Weigh the child daily.
9. Provide passive range-of-motion exercises to facilitate joint movement.
10. Administer acetylsalicylic acid (aspirin) as prescribed for its antipyretic and antiplatelet effects (additional anticoagulation may be necessary if aneurysms are present).
11. Intravenous immunoglobulin (IVIG) may be prescribed to reduce the duration of the fever and the incidence of coronary artery lesions and aneurysms; IVIG is a blood product, so blood precautions when administering it are warranted.
12. Reinforce parent education (Box 35-5).

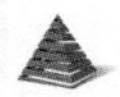

BOX 35-5 Parent Education for Kawasaki Disease

- Follow-up care is essential to recovery.
- The signs and symptoms of Kawasaki disease include the following:
- Irritability that may last for up to 2 months after the onset of symptoms.
- Peeling of the hands and feet.
- Pain in the joints that may persist for several weeks.
- Stiffness in the morning, after naps, and in cold temperatures.
- Record the temperature (because fever is expected) until child has been afebrile for several days.
- Notify the health care provider if the temperature is 101°F or higher.
- Salicylates such as acetylsalicylic acid (aspirin) may be prescribed.
- Signs of aspirin toxicity include tinnitus, headache, vertigo, bruising; do not administer aspirin or aspirin-containing products if child has been exposed to chickenpox or the flu.
- Signs and symptoms of bleeding include epistaxis (nosebleeds), hemoptysis (coughing up blood), hematemesis (vomiting up blood), hematuria (blood in urine), melena (blood in stool), and bruises on body.
- Signs and symptoms of cardiac complications include chest pain or tightness (older children), cool and pale extremities, abdominal pain, nausea and vomiting, irritability, restlessness, and uncontrollable crying.
- Child should avoid contact sports, if age appropriate, if taking aspirin or anticoagulants.
- Avoid administration of measles, mumps, and rubella (MMR) or varicella vaccine to the child for 11 months after intravenous immunoglobulin therapy, if appropriate.
- Contact the health care provider if any signs of complication such as aspirin toxicity, bleeding, or cardiac problems occur.

CRITICAL THINKING What Should You Do?

Answer: The nurse should monitor respiratory status closely in a child who has a congenital heart defect. If respiratory effort is increased, the nurse should place the child in a reverse Trendelenburg's position, elevating the head and upper body, to decrease the work of breathing. In addition, the child should sleep with the head elevated on several pillows and should remain in a semi- or high Fowler's position during waking hours.

Reference(s): Hockenberry, M., & Wilson, D. (2013). *Wong's: Essentials of pediatric nursing* (9th ed., p. 837). St. Louis: Mosby.

PRACTICE QUESTIONS

341. The nurse reviews the record of a child who was just seen by a health care provider (HCP). The HCP has documented a diagnosis of suspected aortic stenosis. Which specific sign/symptom of aortic stenosis should the nurse anticipate?
1. Pallor
2. Hyperactivity
3. Exercise intolerance
4. Gastrointestinal disturbances

342. The nurse has reinforced home care instructions to the mother of a child who is being discharged after cardiac surgery. Which statement by the mother indicates the **need for further teaching**?
1. "A balance of rest and exercise is important."
2. "I can apply lotion or powder to the incision if it is itchy."
3. "Activities during which the child could fall need to be avoided for 2 to 4 weeks."
4. "Large crowds of people need to be avoided for at least 2 weeks after this surgery."

343. The nurse is told that a child with rheumatic fever (RF) will be arriving to the nursing unit for admission. Which question should the nurse ask the family to elicit information specific to the development of RF?
1. "Has the child complained of back pain?"
2. "Has the child complained of headaches?"
3. "Has the child had any nausea or vomiting?"
4. "Did the child have a sore throat or a fever within the past 2 months?"

344. Acetylsalicylic acid (aspirin) is prescribed for a child with rheumatic fever (RF). The nurse should question this prescription if the child had documented evidence of which condition?
1. Arthralgia
2. Joint pain
3. Facial edema
4. A viral infection

345. The nurse assists with admitting a child with a diagnosis of acute-stage Kawasaki disease. When obtaining the child's medical history, which manifestation is likely to be noted?
1. Cracked lips
2. A normal appearance
3. Conjunctival hyperemia
4. Desquamation of the skin

346. The nurse caring for an infant with congenital heart disease is monitoring the infant closely for signs of heart failure (HF). The nurse should observe for which **early** sign of HF?
1. Pallor
2. Cough
3. Tachycardia
4. Slow and shallow breathing

❖ **347.** The nurse is caring for an infant with a diagnosis of tetralogy of Fallot. The infant suddenly becomes cyanotic and the oxygen saturation reading drops to 60%. Which interventions should the nurse perform? **Select all that apply.**
- ❑ 1. Call a code blue.
- ❑ 2. Notify the registered nurse.
- ❑ 3. Place the infant in a prone position.
- ❑ 4. Prepare to administer morphine sulfate.
- ❑ 5. Prepare to administer intravenous fluids.
- ❑ 6. Prepare to administer 100% oxygen by face mask.

348. The nurse is monitoring the daily weight of an infant with heart failure (HF). Which finding alerts the nurse to suspect fluid accumulation and thus the need to notify the registered nurse?
1. Bradypnea
2. Diaphoresis
3. Decreased blood pressure (BP)
4. A weight gain of 1 lb in 1 day

349. The nurse provides home care instructions to the parents of a child with heart failure regarding the procedure for the administration of digoxin (Lanoxin). Which statement by a parent indicates the **need for further teaching**?
1. "I will not mix the medication with food."
2. "If more than one dose is missed, I will call the health care provider."
3. "I will take my child's pulse before administering the medication."
4. "If my child vomits after medication administration, I will repeat the dose."

350. A health care provider has prescribed oxygen as needed for a 10-month-old infant with heart failure (HF). In which situation should the nurse administer the oxygen to the child?
1. When the child is sleeping
2. When changing the child's diapers
3. When the mother is holding the child
4. When drawing blood for electrolyte levels

ANSWERS

341. 3

Rationale: The child with aortic stenosis shows signs of exercise intolerance, chest pain, and dizziness when standing for long periods. Pallor may be noted, but it is not specific to this type of disorder alone. Options 2 and 4 are not related to this disorder.

Test-Taking Strategy: Focus on the subject, a specific sign/symptom of aortic stenosis. Options 2 and 4 can be eliminated first because they are not associated with a cardiac disorder. From the remaining choices, noting the word *specifically* in the question will direct you to the correct option. **Review: aortic stenosis.**

Level of Cognitive Ability: Analyzing
Client Needs: Physiological Integrity
Integrated Process: Nursing Process/Data Collection
Content Area: Child Health: Cardiovascular
Priority Concepts: Gas Exchange, Perfusion
Reference(s): McKinney et al (2013), p. 1216.

342. 2

Rationale: The mother should be instructed that lotions and powders should not be applied to the incision site because these items can affect the skin integrity and the healing process. Options 1, 3, and 4 are accurate instructions regarding home care after cardiac surgery.

Test-Taking Strategy: Note the strategic words, *need for further teaching*. These words indicate a negative event query and ask you to select an option that is an incorrect statement. Using the general principles related to postoperative incisional site care will direct you to the correct option. **Review:** cardiac surgery.

Level of Cognitive Ability: Evaluating
Client Needs: Physiological Integrity
Integrated Process: Teaching and Learning
Content Area: Child Health: Cardiovascular
Priority Concepts: Client Education, Tissue Integrity
Reference(s): McKinney et al (2013), p. 1224.

343. 4

Rationale: Rheumatic fever (RF) characteristically presents 2 to 6 weeks after an untreated or partially treated group A β-hemolytic streptococcal infection of the upper respiratory tract. Initially, the nurse determines if the child has had a sore throat or an unexplained fever within the past 2 months. Options 1, 2, and 3 are unrelated to RF.

Test-Taking Strategy: Focus on the subject, the etiology associated with RF. Note the similarity between rheumatic "fever" in the question and the word *fever* in the correct option. Review: rheumatic fever.

Level of Cognitive Ability: Analyzing
Client Needs: Physiological Integrity
Integrated Process: Nursing Process/Data Collection
Content Area: Child Health: Cardiovascular
Priority Concepts: Infection, Inflammation
Reference(s): Hockenberry, Wilson (2013), p. 849.

344. 4

Rationale: Anti-inflammatory agents, including aspirin, may be prescribed by the health care provider for the child with RF. Aspirin should not be given to a child who has chickenpox or other viral infections such as influenza because of the risk of Reye's syndrome. Options 1 and 2 are clinical manifestations of RF. Facial edema may be associated with the development of a cardiac complication.

Test-Taking Strategy: Options 1 and 2 can be eliminated first because they are comparable or alike. Recalling that facial edema may indicate a cardiac complication will assist you with eliminating this option. **Review: aspirin.**

Level of Cognitive Ability: Applying
Client Needs: Safe and Effective Care Environment
Integrated Process: Nursing Process/Implementation
Content Area: Child Health: Cardiovascular
Priority Concepts: Infection, Inflammation
Reference(s): Hockenberry, Wilson (2013), p. 849.

345. 3

Rationale: During the acute stage of Kawasaki disease, the child presents with fever, conjunctival hyperemia, a red throat, swollen hands, a rash, and enlargement of the cervical lymph nodes. During the subacute stage, cracking lips and fissures, desquamation of the skin on the tips of the fingers and toes, joint pain, cardiac manifestations, and thrombocytosis occur. During the convalescent stage, the child appears normal, but signs of inflammation may be present.

Test-Taking Strategy: Focus on the subject, acute stage of Kawasaki disease. It is necessary to know the manifestations that occur in each stage to answer correctly. **Review: Kawasaki disease.**

Level of Cognitive Ability: Analyzing
Client Needs: Physiological Integrity
Integrated Process: Nursing Process/Data Collection
Content Area: Child Health: Cardiovascular
Priority Concepts: Infection, Perfusion
Reference(s): McKinney et al (2013), pp. 1232–1233.

346. 3

Rationale: The early signs of HF include tachycardia, tachypnea, profuse scalp sweating, fatigue, irritability, sudden weight gain, and respiratory distress. A cough may occur with HF as a result of mucosal swelling and irritation, but it is not an early sign. Pallor may be noted in the infant with HF, but it is also not an early sign.

Test-Taking Strategy: Note the strategic word, *early*. Think about the physiology and the effects on the heart when fluid overload occurs. These concepts will assist with directing you to the correct option. **Review: heart failure.**

Level of Cognitive Ability: Analyzing
Client Needs: Physiological Integrity
Integrated Process: Nursing Process/Data Collection
Content Area: Child Health: Cardiovascular
Priority Concepts: Gas Exchange, Perfusion
Reference(s): Hockenberry, Wilson (2013), pp. 835, 838.

❖ 347. 2, 4, 5, 6

Rationale: The child who is cyanotic with oxygen saturations dropping to 60% is having a hypercyanotic episode. Hypercyanotic episodes often occur among infants with tetralogy of Fallot, and they may occur among infants whose heart defect includes the obstruction of pulmonary blood flow and communication between the ventricles.

If a hypercyanotic episode occurs, the infant is placed in a knee-chest position immediately. The registered nurse is notified, who will then contact the health care provider. The knee-chest position improves systemic arterial oxygen saturation by decreasing venous return so that smaller amounts of highly saturated blood reach the heart. Toddlers and children squat to get into this position and relieve chronic hypoxia. There is no reason to call a code blue unless respirations cease. Additional interventions include administering 100% oxygen by face mask, morphine sulfate, and intravenous fluids, as prescribed.

Test-Taking Strategy: Focus on the **subject**, the infant's diagnosis and the data in the question. Noting that the infant is cyanotic and has an oxygen saturation of 60% will assist in selecting the correct interventions. **Review: hypercyanotic episode.**

Level of Cognitive Ability: Analyzing
Client Needs: Physiological Integrity
Integrated Process: Nursing Process/Implementation
Content Area: Critical Care: Emergency Situations
Priority Concepts: Gas Exchange, Perfusion
Reference(s): Hockenberry, Wilson (2013), p. 842.

348. 4

Rationale: A weight gain of 0.5 kg (1 lb) in 1 day is a result of the accumulation of fluid. The nurse should monitor the urine output, monitor for evidence of facial or peripheral edema, check the lung sounds, and report the weight gain. Tachypnea and an increased BP would occur with fluid accumulation. Diaphoresis is a sign of HF, but it is not specific to fluid accumulation, and it usually occurs with exertional activities.

Test-Taking Strategy: Focus on the **subject**, fluid accumulation. Note the relationship between fluid accumulation in the question and weight gain in the correct option. **Review: heart failure.**

Level of Cognitive Ability: Analyzing
Client Needs: Physiological Integrity
Integrated Process: Nursing Process/Data Collection
Content Area: Child Health: Cardiovascular
Priority Concepts: Gas Exchange, Perfusion
Reference(s): McKinney et al (2013), p. 1204.

349. 4

Rationale: The parents need to be instructed that if the child vomits after the digoxin is administered, they are not to repeat the dose. Options 1, 2, and 3 are accurate instructions regarding the administration of this medication. Additionally, the parents should be instructed that if a dose is missed and it is not noticed until 4 hours later, the dose should not be administered.

Test-Taking Strategy: Note the **strategic words**, *need for further teaching.* These words indicate a **negative event query** and ask you to select an option that is an incorrect statement. Principles related to the administration of medication to children will assist you with eliminating option 1. General knowledge regarding digoxin administration will assist you with eliminating option 3. From the remaining options, select option 4 over option 2 because if the child vomits, it would be difficult to determine whether the medication was absorbed by the body. **Review: digoxin.**

Level of Cognitive Ability: Evaluating
Client Needs: Physiological Integrity
Integrated Process: Teaching and Learning
Content Area: Child Health: Cardiovascular
Priority Concepts: Client Education, Safety
Reference(s): McKinney et al (2013), p. 1207.

350. 4

Rationale: Oxygen administration may be prescribed for the infant with HF for stressful periods, especially during bouts of crying or invasive procedures. Drawing blood is an invasive procedure that would likely cause the child to cry.

Test-Taking Strategy: Focus on the **subject**, care of the infant with heart failure. Read the options and recall the situations that would place stress and an increased workload on the heart. This concept should direct you to the correct option. **Review: heart failure.**

Level of Cognitive Ability: Applying
Client Needs: Physiological Integrity
Integrated Process: Nursing Process/Implementation
Content Area: Child Health: Cardiovascular
Priority Concepts: Gas Exchange, Perfusion
Reference(s): Hockenberry, Wilson (2013), p. 838.

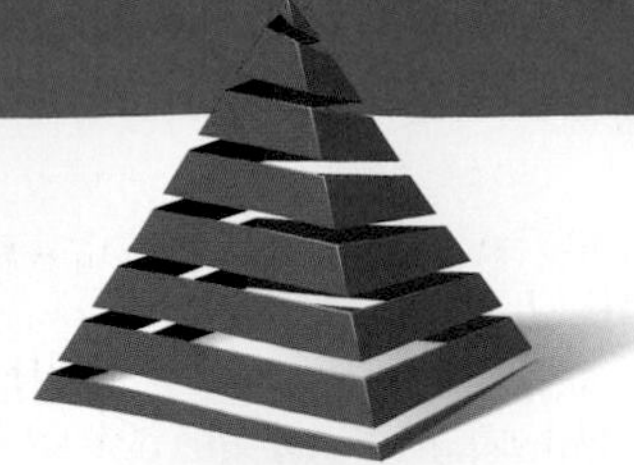

CHAPTER 36

Renal and Urinary Disorders

CRITICAL THINKING What Should You Do?

The nurse notes that there has been no urinary output for 1 hour in an infant who underwent surgical repair of hypospadias. What should the nurse do?

Answer located on p. 440.

I. Glomerulonephritis

A. Description
1. Glomerulonephritis is a term that refers to a group of kidney disorders characterized by inflammatory injuries in the glomerulus, most of which are caused by an immunological reaction.
2. Results in proliferative and inflammatory changes within the glomerular structure
3. Destruction, inflammation, and sclerosis of the glomeruli of both kidneys occur.
4. Inflammation of the glomeruli results from an antigen–antibody reaction produced by an infection elsewhere in the body.
5. Loss of kidney function develops.

B. Causes
1. Immunological diseases
2. Autoimmune diseases

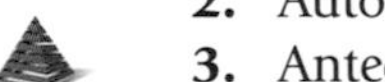

3. Antecedent group A β-hemolytic streptococcal infection of the pharynx or skin
4. History of pharyngitis or tonsillitis 2 to 3 weeks before the onset of symptoms

C. Types
1. Acute: Occurs 2 to 3 weeks after a streptococcal infection
2. Chronic: May occur after the acute phase or slowly over time

D. Complications
1. Kidney failure
2. Hypertensive encephalopathy
3. Pulmonary edema
4. Heart failure

E. Data collection
1. Periorbital and facial edema that is more prominent in the morning
2. Anorexia
3. Decreased urinary output
4. Cloudy, smoky, brown-colored urine (hematuria)
5. Pallor, irritability, and lethargy
6. In the older child, headaches, abdominal or flank pain, and dysuria
7. Hypertension
8. Proteinuria that produces a persistent and excessive foam in the urine
9. Azotemia
10. Increased blood urea nitrogen and creatinine levels
11. Increased antistreptolysin O titer (used to diagnose disorders caused by streptococcal infections)

F. Interventions
1. Monitor the vital signs, daily weight, intake and output (I&O), and characteristics of the urine.
2. Limit activity; provide safety measures.
3. Diet restrictions of sodium depend on the stage and severity of the disease, especially the extent of the edema; in addition, potassium may be restricted during periods of oliguria.
4. Monitor for complications (i.e., kidney failure, hypertensive encephalopathy, seizures, pulmonary edema, and heart failure).
5. Assist to administer diuretics (if significant edema and fluid overload are present), antihypertensives (for hypertension), and antibiotics (to the child with evidence of persistent streptococcal infections), as prescribed.
6. Initiate seizure precautions and assist to administer anticonvulsants, as prescribed, for seizures associated with hypertensive encephalopathy.
7. Reinforce instructions to the parents to report signs of bloody urine, headache, or edema.
8. Reinforce instructions to the parents that the child needs to obtain appropriate and adequate treatment for infections, specifically for sore throats, upper respiratory infections, and skin infections.

Measuring the daily weight and monitoring for weight changes are the most useful and effective methods for determining fluid balance.

Pediatric

II. Nephrotic Syndrome

A. Description

1. A kidney disorder characterized by massive proteinuria, hypoalbuminemia (hypoproteinemia), and edema (Fig. 36-1)
2. The primary objectives of therapeutic management are to reduce the excretion of urinary protein and to maintain protein-free urine.

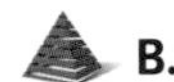

B. Data collection (Box 36-1)

The classic manifestations of nephrotic syndrome are massive proteinuria, hypoalbuminemia, and edema.

C. Interventions

1. Monitor the vital signs, I&O, and daily weights.
2. Monitor the urine for specific gravity and protein.
3. Monitor for edema.
4. Nutrition: A regular diet without added salt is prescribed if the child is in remission. Sodium is restricted during periods of massive edema (fluids may also be restricted).
5. Corticosteroid therapy: Prescribed as soon as the diagnosis has been determined. Monitor the child closely for signs of infection (see Chapter 46).
6. Immunosuppressant therapy may be prescribed to reduce the relapse rate and to induce long-term remission. This may be administered in conjunction with the corticosteroid.
7. Diuretics may be prescribed to reduce edema.
8. Plasma expanders such as salt-poor human albumin may be prescribed for the severely edematous child.
9. Reinforce instructions to the parents about testing the urine for protein, medication administration, the side and adverse effects of the medications, and the general care of the child. 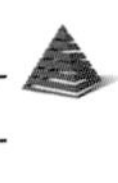
10. Reinforce instructions to the parents regarding the signs of infection and the need to avoid contact with other children who may be infectious. 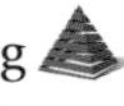

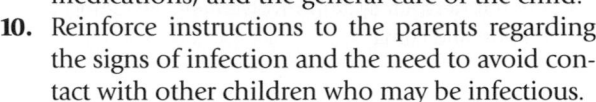

BOX 36-1 Findings in Nephrotic Syndrome

- The child gains weight.
- Periorbital and facial edema are most prominent in the morning.
- Leg, ankle, labial, or scrotal edema occur.
- Urine output decreases, and the urine is dark and frothy.
- Ascites (fluid in the abdominal cavity) is present.
- Blood pressure is normal or slightly decreased.
- Lethargy, anorexia, and pallor occur.
- Massive proteinuria is seen.
- Decreased serum protein (hypoproteinemia) and elevated serum lipid levels occur.

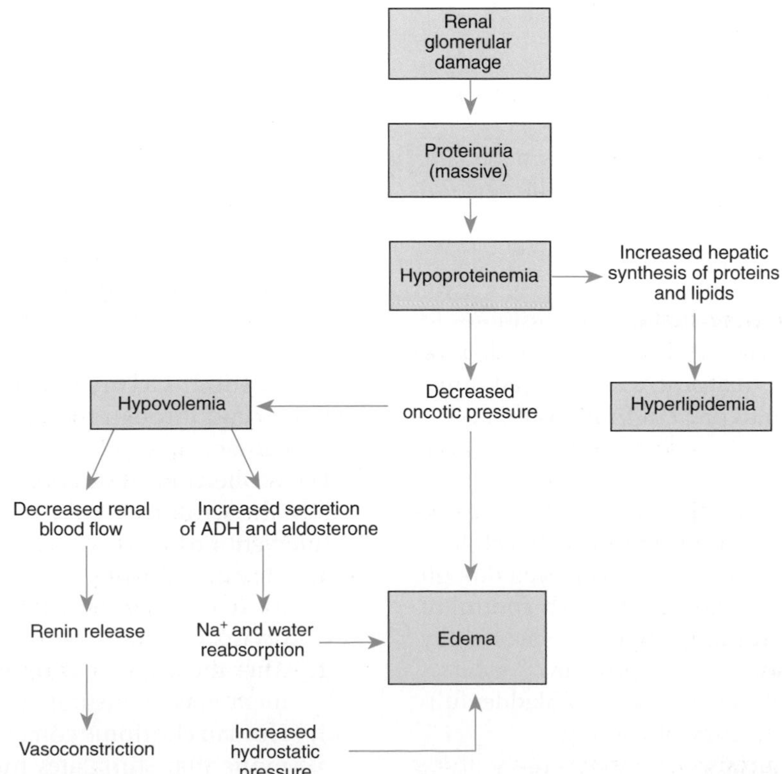

FIGURE 36-1 Sequence of events in the nephrotic syndrome. *ADH*, antidiuretic hormone. (From Perry S, Hockenberry M, Lowdermilk D, Wilson D: *Maternal-child nursing care*, ed 4, St. Louis, 2010, Mosby.)

Pediatric

BOX 36-2 Manifestations of Hemolytic-Uremic Syndrome

- Vomiting
- Irritability
- Lethargy
- Marked pallor
- Hemorrhagic manifestations, such as bruising, petechiae, jaundice, and bloody diarrhea
- Oliguria or anuria
- Central nervous system involvement, including seizures, stupor, and coma

III. Hemolytic-Uremic Syndrome

A. Description
   1. Thought to be associated with bacterial toxins, chemicals, and viruses that cause acute kidney injury in children
   2. Occurs primarily among infants and small children between the ages of 6 months and 5 years
   3. Clinical features include acquired hemolytic anemia, thrombocytopenia, kidney injury, and central nervous system symptoms.

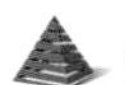

B. Data collection
   1. Triad of anemia, thrombocytopenia, and renal failure is diagnostic (Box 36-2).
   2. Proteinuria, hematuria, and the presence of urinary casts
   3. Blood urea nitrogen and serum creatinine levels are elevated. Hemoglobin and hematocrit levels are decreased.

C. Interventions
   1. Hemodialysis or peritoneal dialysis may be prescribed if the child is anuric.
   2. Strict monitoring of fluid balance is necessary. Fluid restrictions may be prescribed if the child is anuric.
   3. Institute measures to prevent infection.
   4. Provide adequate nutrition.
   5. Other treatments may include medications to treat manifestations or the administration of blood products to treat severe anemia (administered with caution to prevent fluid overload).

IV. Enuresis

A. Description
   1. Enuresis refers to a condition in which a child is unable to control bladder function, even though the child has reached an age at which control of voiding is expected or the child has successfully completed a bladder control program.
   2. By age 5, most children are aware of bladder fullness and are able to control voiding.

B. Primary nocturnal enuresis
   1. Primary nocturnal enuresis is bed-wetting in a child who has never been dry for extended periods.
   2. The condition is common in children, and most children eventually outgrow bed-wetting without therapeutic intervention.
   3. The child is unable to sense a full bladder and does not awaken to void.
   4. The child may have delayed maturation of the central nervous system.
   5. The child should be evaluated for any pathological causes before the diagnosis of primary nocturnal enuresis is made.

C. Secondary or acquired enuresis
   1. The onset of wetting occurs after a period of established urinary continence.
   2. Secondary enuresis may occur during nighttime sleep (nocturnal), only during the waking hours (diurnal), or during daytime and nighttime.
   3. The child may complain of dysuria, urgency, or frequency.
   4. The child should be assessed for urinary tract infections.

D. Assessment: History of bed-wetting with no extended period of dryness in a child older than age 5 years

E. Interventions
   1. A urinalysis and urine culture may be prescribed to rule out infection or an existing disorder.
   2. Assist the family with identifying a treatment plan that best fits the needs of the child.
   3. Limit fluid intake at night, and encourage the child to void just before going to bed.
   4. Involve the child in caring for the wet sheets and changing the bed to assist the child to take ownership of the problem.
   5. Provide reward systems as appropriate for the child.
   6. Incorporate behavioral conditioning techniques.
   7. Medications may be prescribed (such as tricyclic antidepressants, antidiuretics, and antispasmodics) to treat enuresis.
   8. Encourage follow-up to determine the effectiveness of the treatment.

V. Cryptorchidism

A. Description: Occurs when one or both testes fail to descend through the inguinal canal and into the scrotal sac

B. Data collection: Testes not palpable or easily guided into the scrotum

C. Interventions
   1. Monitor during the first 12 months of life to determine whether spontaneous descent occurs.
   2. After the age of 1 year, medical or surgical treatment may be instituted.
   3. Human chorionic gonadotropin, a pituitary hormone that stimulates the production of testosterone, may be prescribed.
   4. Surgical correction, if needed, is performed by orchiopexy before the child's second birthday

(preferably between 1 and 2 years of age) if the testes do not descend spontaneously.

5. Monitor for bleeding and infection postoperatively.
6. Reinforce instructions to the parents regarding postoperative home care measures, including preventing infection, pain control, and activity restrictions.
7. Provide an opportunity for parental counseling if the parents are concerned about the future fertility of the child.

VI. Epispadias and Hypospadias (Fig. 36-2)

A. Description: Congenital defects that involve the abnormal placement of the urethral orifice of the penis; these anatomical defects can lead to the easy entry of bacteria into the urine.

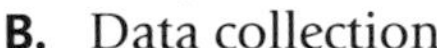

B. Data collection
   1. Epispadias: Urethral orifice is located on the dorsal surface of the penis; often occurs with exstrophy of the bladder
   2. Hypospadias: Urethral orifice is located below the glans penis, along the ventral surface.

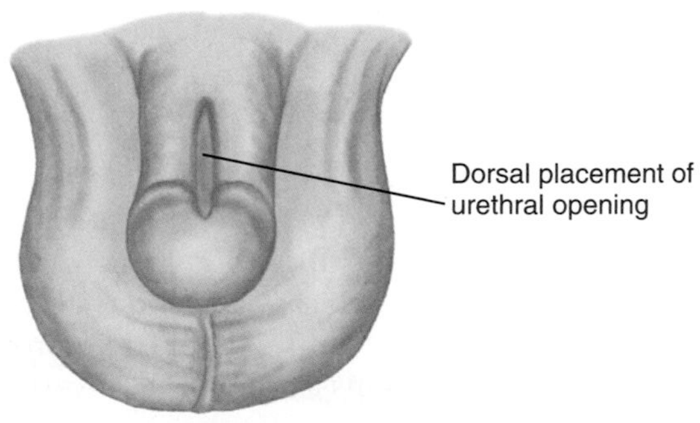

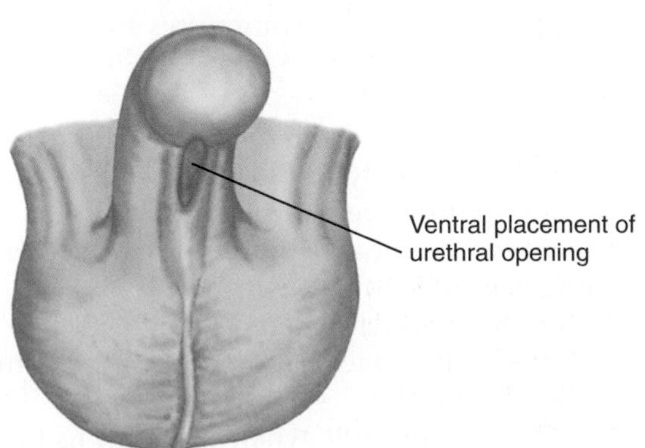

FIGURE 36-2 Epispadias and hypospadias are genital anomalies in which the urethral opening is above or below its normal location on the glans of the penis. (From James S, Ashwill J: *Nursing care of children: Principles and practice*, ed 4, St. Louis, 2012, Saunders.)

C. Surgical interventions: Performed before the age of toilet training, preferably between 16 and 18 months of age

> ⚠ Circumcision is not performed on a newborn with epispadias or hypospadias because the foreskin may be used in surgical reconstruction of the defect.

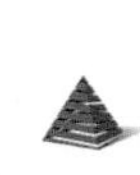

D. Postoperative interventions
   1. The child will have a pressure dressing and may have some type of urinary diversion or a urinary stent (used to maintain the patency of the urethral opening) while the healing of the meatus occurs.
   2. Monitor the vital signs.
   3. Encourage fluid intake to maintain adequate urine output and to maintain the patency of the stent.
   4. Monitor the I&O and the urine for cloudiness or a foul odor.
   5. Notify the registered nurse if there is no urinary drainage for 1 hour, because this may indicate kinks in the system or obstruction by sediment.
   6. Assist to provide pain medication or medication to relieve bladder spasms (anticholinergic), as prescribed.
   7. Assist to administer antibiotics, as prescribed.
   8. Reinforce instructions to the parents regarding the care of the urinary diversion or stent, if present.
   9. Reinforce instructions to the parents to avoid giving the child a tub bath until the stent, if present, is removed.
   10. Reinforce instructions to the parents about fluid intake, medication administration, the signs and symptoms of infection, and the need for health care provider follow-up for dressing removal approximately 4 days after surgery.

VII. Bladder Exstrophy

A. Description
   1. A congenital anomaly characterized by the extrusion of the urinary bladder to the outside of the body through a defect in the lower abdominal wall
   2. Cause is unknown.
   3. Treatment requires surgical management and occurs in a series of staged reconstructions.
   4. Initial surgery for the closure of the abdominal defect is normally planned within the first few days of life.
   5. Goals of subsequent surgeries are to reconstruct the bladder and genitalia and enable the child to achieve urinary continence.

B. Data collection
   1. Exposed bladder mucosa
   2. Widened symphysis pubis
   3. Defects of the external genitalia

C. Interventions
1. Monitor the urinary output.
2. Monitor for signs of urinary tract or wound infection.
3. Maintain the integrity of the exposed bladder mucosa.
4. Prevent the bladder tissue from drying while allowing for the drainage of urine until surgical closure is performed; immediately after birth, as prescribed, the exposed bladder is covered with a sterile, nonadherent dressing to protect it until closure can be performed.
5. Laboratory values and urinalysis are monitored to assess for kidney function.
6. Assist to administer antibiotics, as prescribed.
7. Provide emotional support to the parents, and encourage the verbalization of their fears and concerns.

Applying petroleum jelly to the bladder mucosa is avoided because it tends to dry out, adhere to the bladder mucosa, and damage the delicate tissues when the dressing is removed.

CRITICAL THINKING What Should You Do?

Answer: Following surgical repair for hypospadias, the urinary output is monitored closely. The nurse should notify the registered nurse (RN) if there is no urinary output for 1 hour because this may indicate kinks in the urinary diversion or stent placed during the surgical procedure or an obstruction caused by sediment. The RN will perform an assessment and contact the health care provider if necessary.

Reference(s): Hockenberry, M., & Wilson, D. (2013). *Wong's: Essentials of pediatric nursing* (9th ed., p. 912). St. Louis: Mosby.

McKinney, E., James, S., Murray, S., Nelson, K. & Ashwill, J. (2013). *Maternal-child nursing* (4th ed., pp. 1127–1128). St. Louis: Elsevier.

PRACTICE QUESTIONS

351. The nurse is assigned to care for a child who is suspected of having glomerulonephritis. The nurse reviews the child's record and notes that which finding is associated with the diagnosis of glomerulonephritis?
1. Hypotension
2. Red-brown urine
3. Low urinary specific gravity
4. A low blood urea nitrogen (BUN) level

❖ **352.** A child is admitted to the hospital with a probable diagnosis of nephrotic syndrome. Which findings should the nurse expect to observe? **Select all that apply.**
- ☐ 1. Pallor
- ☐ 2. Edema
- ☐ 3. Anorexia
- ☐ 4. Proteinuria
- ☐ 5. Weight loss
- ☐ 6. Decreased serum lipids

353. The nurse is planning care for a child with hemolytic-uremic syndrome (HUS). The child has been anuric and will be receiving peritoneal dialysis treatment. The nurse should plan to include which intervention in the care of the child?
1. Restriction of fluids, as prescribed
2. Administration of analgesics, as prescribed
3. Monitoring the arteriovenous (AV) fistula
4. Encouraging the intake of foods that are high in potassium

354. The nurse is assisting with gathering admission assessment data on a 2-year-old child who has been diagnosed with nephrotic syndrome. The nurse collects data knowing that which is a common characteristic associated with nephrotic syndrome?
1. Hypotension
2. Generalized edema
3. Increased urinary output
4. Frank, bright red blood in the urine

355. The child with cryptorchidism is being discharged after orchiopexy, which was performed on an outpatient basis. The nurse should reinforce instructions to the parents about which **priority** care measure?
1. Measuring intake and output
2. Administering anticholinergics
3. Preventing infection at the surgical site
4. Applying cold, wet compresses to the surgical site

356. The nurse is reinforcing discharge instructions to the mother of a 2-year-old child who has had an orchiopexy to correct cryptorchidism. Which statement by the mother indicates that **further teaching is needed**?
1. "I'll check his temperature."
2. "I'll give him medication so he'll be comfortable."
3. "I'll let him decide when to return to his play activities."
4. "I'll check his voiding to be sure there are no problems."

357. The nurse collects a urine specimen preoperatively from a child with epispadias who is scheduled for surgical repair. The nurse reviews the child's record for the laboratory results of the urine test and would **most likely** expect to note which finding?
1. Hematuria
2. Bacteriuria
3. Glucosuria
4. Proteinuria

358. An 18-month-old child is being discharged after surgical repair of hypospadias. Which postoperative nursing care measure should the nurse stress to the parents as they prepare to take this child home?
1. Leave diapers off to allow the site to heal.
2. Avoid tub baths until the stent has been removed.
3. Encourage toilet training to ensure that the flow of urine is normal.
4. Restrict the fluid intake to reduce urinary output for the first few days.

359. The parents of a newborn have been told that their child was born with bladder exstrophy, and the parents ask the nurse about this condition. Which response should the nurse give to the parents about bladder exstrophy?
1. "It is a hereditary disorder that occurs in every other generation."
2. "It is caused by the use of medications taken by the mother during pregnancy."
3. "It is a condition in which the urinary bladder is abnormally located in the pelvic cavity."
4. "It is an extrusion of the urinary bladder to the outside of the body through a defect in the lower abdominal wall."

360. The nurse is reviewing the health record of a child who has been recently diagnosed with glomerulonephritis. Which finding noted in the child's record is associated with the diagnosis of glomerulonephritis?
1. The child fell off a bike and onto the handlebars.
2. The child has had nausea and vomiting for the last 24 hours.
3. The child had urticaria and itching for 1 week before diagnosis.
4. The child had a streptococcal throat infection 2 weeks before diagnosis.

ANSWERS

351. 2

Rationale: Gross hematuria resulting in dark, smoky, cola-colored or red-brown urine is a classic symptom of glomerulonephritis, and hypertension is also common. A mid- to high urinary specific gravity is associated with glomerulonephritis. BUN levels may be elevated.

Test-Taking Strategy: Focus on the subject, the manifestations of glomerulonephritis. Eliminate options 1 and 3 first because hypertension and a high specific gravity are likely to occur with this kidney disorder. Recalling that BUN levels elevate in clients with this condition will assist with directing you to the correct option. **Review: glomerulonephritis.**

Level of Cognitive Ability: Analyzing

Client Needs: Physiological Integrity

Integrated Process: Nursing Process/Data Collection

Content Area: Child Health: Renal and Urinary

Priority Concepts: Elimination, Inflammation

Reference(s): Hockenberry, Wilson (2013), p. 915.

❖ **352. 1, 2, 3, 4**

Rationale: Nephrotic syndrome is a kidney disorder that is characterized by massive proteinuria, hypoalbuminemia, edema, elevated serum lipids, anorexia, and pallor. The urine volume is decreased, and the urine is dark and frothy in appearance. The child with this condition gains weight.

Test-Taking Strategy: Note the child's diagnosis and think about the subject, nephrotic syndrome and its associated characteristics, to answer the question. Remember it is characterized by massive proteinuria, hypoalbuminemia, edema, elevated serum lipids, anorexia, and pallor. **Review: nephrotic syndrome.**

Level of Cognitive Ability: Analyzing

Client Needs: Physiological Integrity

Integrated Process: Nursing Process/Data Collection

Content Area: Child Health: Renal and Urinary

Priority Concepts: Elimination, Inflammation

Reference(s): Hockenberry, Wilson (2013), p. 914; McKinney et al (2013), p. 1132.

353. 1

Rationale: HUS is thought to be associated with bacterial toxins, chemicals, and viruses that cause acute renal failure in children. Clinical features of the disease include acquired hemolytic anemia, thrombocytopenia, renal injury, and central nervous system symptoms. A child with HUS who is undergoing peritoneal dialysis for the treatment of anuria will be on fluid restrictions. Pain is not associated with HUS, and potassium would be restricted rather than encouraged if the child was anuric. Peritoneal dialysis does not require an AV fistula (only hemodialysis does).

Test-Taking Strategy: Focus on the subject, hemolytic-uremic syndrome, and recall your knowledge of the care of a client with this diagnosis. Also focus on the data in the question. Noting the word *peritoneal* will assist you with eliminating option 3. From the remaining options, remember that because the child is anuric, fluids will be restricted. **Review: hemolytic-uremic syndrome.**

Level of Cognitive Ability: Analyzing

Client Needs: Physiological Integrity

Integrated Process: Nursing Process/Planning

Content Area: Child Health: Renal and Urinary
Priority Concepts: Fluid and Electrolyte Balance, Inflammation
Reference: McKinney et al (2013), pp. 1136–1137.

354. 2
Rationale: Nephrotic syndrome is defined as massive proteinuria, hypoalbuminemia, and edema. The urine is dark, foamy, and frothy, but microscopic hematuria may be present. Frank, bright red blood in the urine does not occur. Urine output is decreased, and the blood pressure is normal or slightly decreased.
Test-Taking Strategy: Focus on the subject, the characteristics of nephrotic syndrome. Eliminate option 3 first because urine output is likely to be decreased in a client with a renal disorder. From the remaining options, associate edema with nephrotic syndrome, because this will be helpful to you if you encounter a similar question. **Review:** **nephrotic syndrome.**
Level of Cognitive Ability: Applying
Client Needs: Physiological Integrity
Integrated Process: Nursing Process/Data Collection
Content Area: Child Health: Renal and Urinary
Priority Concepts: Elimination, Fluid and Electrolyte Balance
Reference(s): Hockenberry, Wilson (2013), p. 914.

355. 3
Rationale: The most common complications associated with orchiopexy are bleeding and infection. The parents are instructed in postoperative home care measures, including the prevention of infection, pain control, and activity restrictions. The measurement of intake and output is not required. Anticholinergics are prescribed for the relief of bladder spasms; they are not necessary after orchiopexy. Cold, wet compresses are not prescribed. The moisture from a wet compress presents a potential for infection.
Test-Taking Strategy: Note the strategic word, *priority.* Use Maslow's Hierarchy of Needs theory to answer the question. Of the options presented, the potential for infection is the physiological priority. **Review:** home care instructions after **orchiopexy.**
Level of Cognitive Ability: Applying
Client Needs: Physiological Integrity
Integrated Process: Teaching and Learning
Content Area: Child Health: Renal and Urinary
Priority Concepts: Elimination, Infection
Reference(s): Hockenberry, Wilson (2013), pp. 911–912.

356. 3
Rationale: All vigorous activities should be restricted for 2 weeks after surgery to promote healing and prevent injury. This will prevent dislodging of the suture, which is internal. Normally, 2-year-old children will want to be very active. Therefore, allowing the child to decide when to return to his play activities may prevent healing and cause injury. The parents should be taught to monitor the child's temperature; provide analgesics, as needed; and monitor the urine output.
Test-Taking Strategy: Note the strategic words, *further teaching is needed.* These words indicate a negative event query and ask you to select an option that is an incorrect statement. Option 1 is an important action for recognizing signs of infection. Option 2 is appropriate for keeping pain to a minimum. Option 4 monitors the voiding pattern, which is also important after this type of surgery. **Review:** discharge instructions after the surgical correction of **cryptorchidism.**
Level of Cognitive Ability: Evaluating
Client Needs: Physiological Integrity
Integrated Process: Teaching and Learning
Content Area: Child Health: Renal and Urinary
Priority Concepts: Client Education, Infection
Reference(s): Hockenberry, Wilson (2013), p. 912.

357. 2
Rationale: Epispadias is a congenital defect that involves the abnormal placement of the urethral orifice of the penis. In clients with this condition, the urethral opening is located anywhere on the dorsum of the penis. This anatomical characteristic leads to the easy access of bacterial entry into the urine. Options 1, 3, and 4 are not characteristically noted with this condition.
Test-Taking Strategy: Note the strategic words, *most likely.* Use your knowledge regarding the anatomical characteristics of epispadias to answer the question. Options 1, 3, and 4 do not relate to the potential for infection, which can be present with this condition. **Review:** **epispadias.**
Level of Cognitive Ability: Analyzing
Client Needs: Physiological Integrity
Integrated Process: Nursing Process/Data Collection
Content Area: Child Health: Renal and Urinary
Priority Concepts: Elimination, Infection
Reference(s): McKinney et al (2013), p. 1127.

358. 2
Rationale: After hypospadias repair, the parents are instructed to avoid giving the child a tub bath until the stent has been removed to prevent infection. Diapers are placed on the child to prevent the contamination of the surgical site. Toilet training should not be an issue during this stressful period. Fluids should be encouraged to maintain hydration.
Test-Taking Strategy: Focus on the subject, home care instructions following surgical repair of hypospadias. Option 3 is eliminated first because toilet training should not be initiated during times of stress, such as after surgery. Eliminate option 1 because this action can cause the contamination of the surgical site. Option 4 is inappropriate because fluids should be encouraged rather than restricted. **Review:** surgical repair of **hypospadias.**
Level of Cognitive Ability: Applying
Client Needs: Physiological Integrity
Integrated Process: Teaching and Learning
Content Area: Child Health: Renal and Urinary
Priority Concepts: Client Education, Infection
Reference(s): Hockenberry, Wilson (2013), p. 911.

359. 4
Rationale: Bladder exstrophy is a congenital anomaly that is characterized by the extrusion of the urinary bladder to the outside of the body through a defect in the lower abdominal wall. The cause is unknown, and there is a higher incidence among males. Options 1, 2, and 3 are not characteristics of this disorder.
Test-Taking Strategy: Focus on the subject, the characteristics of bladder exstrophy. If you are unfamiliar with this condition,

note the relationship of the word *exstrophy* in the name of the disorder to the word *extrusion* in the correct option; this should remind you that this condition is located *external* to the body. **Review: bladder exstrophy.**
Level of Cognitive Ability: Applying
Client Needs: Physiological Integrity
Integrated Process: Nursing Process/Implementation
Content Area: Child Health: Renal and Urinary
Priority Concepts: Elimination, Infection
Reference(s): Hockenberry, Wilson (2013), p. 912; McKinney et al (2013), p. 1129.

360. 4
Rationale: Group A β-hemolytic streptococcal infection is a cause of glomerulonephritis. The child often becomes ill with streptococcal infection of the upper respiratory tract and then develops symptoms of acute poststreptococcal glomerulonephritis after an interval of 1 to 2 weeks. The data presented in options 1, 2, and 3 are unrelated to a diagnosis of glomerulonephritis.
Test-Taking Strategy: Focus on the **subject,** the etiology associated with glomerulonephritis. Option 1 relates to a kidney injury. Options 2 and 3 are not related to the diagnosis of glomerulonephritis. **Review:** causes of **glomerulonephritis**.
Level of Cognitive Ability: Understanding
Client Needs: Physiological Integrity
Integrated Process: Nursing Process/Data Collection
Content Area: Child Health: Renal and Urinary
Priority Concepts: Elimination, Infection
Reference(s): Hockenberry, Wilson (2013), p. 915.

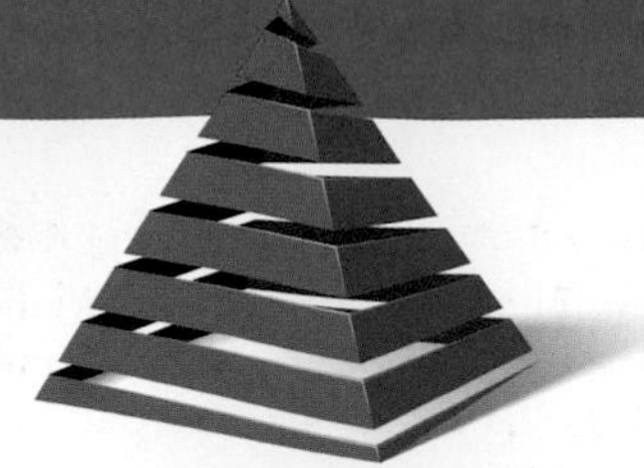

CHAPTER 37

Neurological, Cognitive, and Psychosocial Disorders

CRITICAL THINKING What Should You Do?

The nurse notes signs of increased intracranial pressure (ICP) in a child who has undergone insertion of a ventriculoperitoneal shunt for the treatment of hydrocephalus. What should the nurse do?

Answer located on p. 451.

I. Cerebral Palsy

A. Description

1. A disorder characterized by impaired movement and posture resulting from an abnormality in the extrapyramidal or pyramidal motor system.
2. The most common clinical type is spastic cerebral palsy, which represents an upper motor neuron type of muscle weakness.
3. Less common types of cerebral palsy are athetoid, ataxic, and mixed.

B. Data collection

1. Extreme irritability and crying
2. Feeding difficulties
3. Abnormal motor performance
4. Alterations of muscle tone; stiff and rigid arms or legs
5. Delayed developmental milestones
6. Persistence of primitive infantile reflexes (e.g., Moro, tonic neck) after 6 months (most primitive reflexes disappear by 3 to 4 months of age)
7. Abnormal posturing (e.g., opisthotonic [exaggerated arching of the back]) (Fig. 37-1)
8. Seizures may occur.

C. Interventions

1. The goals of management are early recognition and intervention to maximize the child's abilities.
2. A multidisciplinary team approach is implemented to meet the many needs of the child.
3. Therapeutic management includes physical therapy, occupational therapy, speech therapy, education, and recreation.
4. Determine the child's developmental level and intelligence.
5. Encourage early intervention, and participation in school programs is encouraged.
6. Prepare for using mobilizing devices to help prevent or reduce deformities.
7. Encourage communication and interaction with the child on his or her **developmental age** rather than his or her **chronological age** level.
8. Provide a safe environment by removing sharp objects, using a protective helmet if the child falls frequently, and implementing seizure precautions, if necessary.
9. Provide safe, appropriate toys for the child's age and developmental level.
10. Position the child upright after meals.
11. Medications may be prescribed to relieve muscle spasms, which cause intense pain; antiseizure medications may also be prescribed.
12. Provide the parents with information about the disorder and treatment plan; encourage support groups for parents.

II. Head Injury

A. Description

1. Head injury is the pathological result of any mechanical force to the skull, scalp, meninges, or brain.
   a. Open head injury occurs when there is a fracture of the skull or a penetration of the skull by an object.
   b. Closed head injury is the result of blunt trauma. It is more serious because of the chance of increased intracranial pressure (ICP) in a "closed" vault. This type of injury can also be caused by shaken baby syndrome.
2. Manifestations depend on the type of injury and the subsequent amount of increased ICP.

B. Data collection: Increased ICP

⚠ The child's level of consciousness provides the earliest indication of an improvement or deterioration of the neurological condition.

1. Early signs
   a. Slight change in vital signs

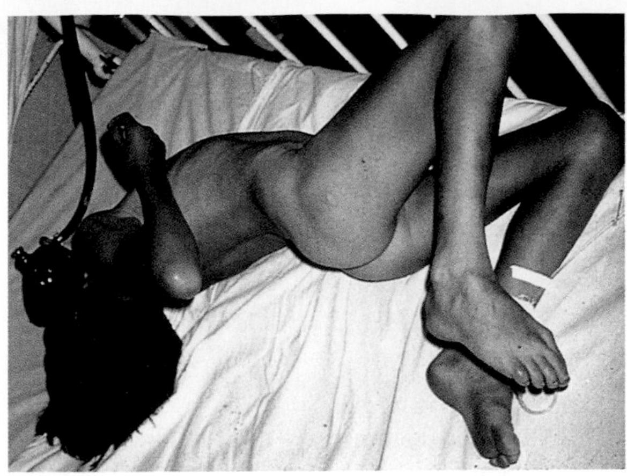

FIGURE 37-1 Abnormal posturing: Opisthotonos. (From Farrar WE: *Atlas of infections of the nervous system*, London, 1993, Mosby-Wolfe.)

b. Slight change in level of consciousness
c. Infant: Irritability, high-pitched cry, bulging fontanel, increased head circumference, dilated scalp veins, Macewen sign (cracked-pot sound on percussion of the head), setting-sun sign (sclera visible above the iris)
d. Child: Headache, nausea, vomiting, visual disturbances (diplopia), seizures

2. Late signs
   a. Decrease in level of consciousness
   b. Bradycardia
   c. Decreased motor and sensory responses
   d. Alteration in pupil size and reactivity
   e. Decorticate (flexion) posturing: Adduction of the arms at the shoulders; arms are flexed on the chest with the wrists flexed and the hands fisted, and the lower extremities are extended and adducted; seen with severe dysfunction of the cerebral cortex (Fig. 37-2).

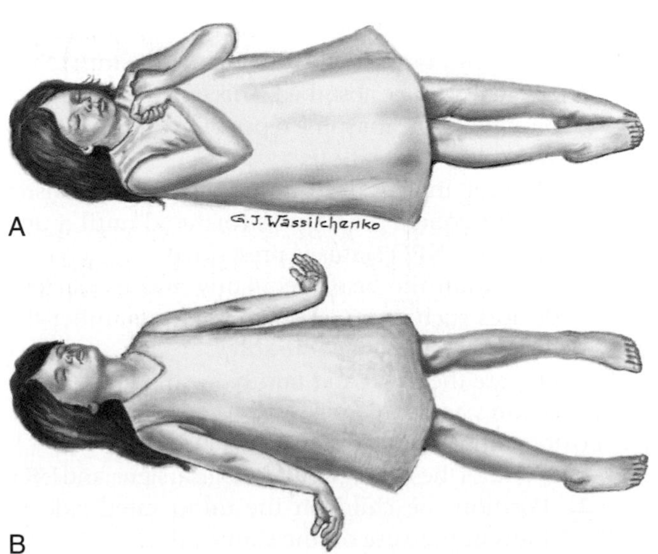

FIGURE 37-2 **A**, Decorticate (flexion) posturing. **B**, Decerebrate (extension) posturing. (From Hockenberry M, Wilson D: *Wong's: Nursing care of infants and children*, ed 9, St. Louis, 2011, Mosby.)

   f. Decerebrate (extension) posturing: Rigid extension and pronation of the arms and the legs; a sign of dysfunction at the level of the midbrain (see Fig. 37-2).
   g. Cheyne-Stokes respirations
   h. Coma

C. Interventions

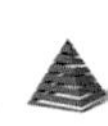

Immobilize the neck and spine after a head injury if a cervical or other spinal injury is suspected. When a spinal cord injury is ruled out, elevate the head of the bed 15 to 30 degrees, if not contraindicated and as prescribed, to facilitate venous drainage.

1. Monitor the airway and administer oxygen as prescribed.
2. Check injuries. (Refer to Chapter 57 for information on spinal cord injuries.)
3. Position the child so that the head is maintained midline to avoid jugular vein compression, which can increase ICP.
4. Monitor vital signs and neurological function. (Monitor level of consciousness closely.)
5. Keep stimuli to a minimum; attempt to minimize crying in the infant.
6. Sedating medications are withheld during the acute phase of the injury so that changes in levels of consciousness can be assessed.
7. Initiate seizure precautions (Box 37-1).
8. Monitor for decreased responsiveness to pain (a significant sign of altered level of consciousness).
9. Maintain an NPO status or provide clear liquids, if prescribed, until it is determined that vomiting will not occur.
10. Assist to monitor prescribed intravenous fluids carefully to avoid increasing any cerebral edema and to minimize the possibility of overhydration.
11. Monitor for a fluid or electrolyte alteration (could indicate injury to the hypothalamus or posterior pituitary).
12. Check wounds and dressings for the presence of drainage and monitor for nose or ear drainage, which could indicate leakage of cerebrospinal

BOX 37-1 Seizure Precautions

Raise the side rails when the child is sleeping or resting.
Pad the side rails and other hard objects.
Place a waterproof mattress or pad on the bed or crib.
Instruct the child to wear or carry medical identification.
Instruct the child regarding precautions to take during potentially hazardous activities.
Instruct the child to swim with a companion.
Instruct the child to use a protective helmet and padding during bicycle riding, skateboarding, and inline skating.
Alert caregivers to the need for any special precautions.

fluid (CSF); if this is noted, notify the registered nurse (RN) immediately.

13. Assist to administer tepid sponge baths or place on a hypothermia blanket as prescribed if hyperthermia occurs.
14. Avoid suctioning through the nares because of the possibility of the catheter entering the brain through a fracture, which places the child at high risk for a secondary infection.
15. As prescribed, assist to administer medications such as acetaminophen (Tylenol) for headache, anticonvulsants for seizures, and antibiotics if a laceration is present; prepare to administer prophylactic tetanus toxoid.
16. A corticosteroid or osmotic diuretic may be prescribed to reduce cerebral edema.
17. Monitor for signs of brainstem involvement (Box 37-2).
18. Monitor for signs of epidural hematoma: Asymmetrical pupils (one dilated, nonreactive pupil) may indicate a neurosurgical emergency that requires evacuation of the hematoma; Notify the RN immediately if this is noted.

Drainage from the nose or ear needs to be tested for the presence of glucose. Drainage that is positive for glucose (as tested with reagent strips) indicates leakage of CSF. The registered nurse and health care provider (HCP) must be notified immediately if the drainage tests positive for glucose.

III. Hydrocephalus

A. Description
   1. An imbalance of CSF absorption and production caused by malformations, tumors, hemorrhage, infections, or trauma
   2. Results in head enlargement and increased ICP

B. Types (Box 37-3)

C. Data collection
   1. Infant
      a. Increased head circumference
      b. Thin, widely separated bones of the head that produce a cracked-pot sound (Macewen's sign) on percussion
      c. Anterior fontanel that is tense, bulging, and nonpulsating; sutures will separate prior to fontanel bulging.
      d. Dilated scalp veins

BOX 37-2 Signs of Brainstem Involvement

- Deep, rapid, or intermittent and gasping respirations
- Wide fluctuations or noticeable slowing of the pulse
- Widening pulse pressure or extreme fluctuations in blood pressure
- Sluggish, dilated, or unequal pupils

Notify the registered nurse or HCP immediately if these signs develop!

BOX 37-3 Types of Hydrocephalus

Communicating

Hydrocephalus occurs as a result of impaired absorption within the subarachnoid space.

Interference of the cerebrospinal fluid in the ventricular system does not occur.

Noncommunicating

The obstruction of cerebrospinal fluid flow in the ventricular system occurs.

      e. Frontal bossing
      f. "Setting sun" eyes
   2. Child
      a. Behavior changes (e.g., irritability, lethargy)
      b. Headache on awakening
      c. Nausea and vomiting
      d. Ataxia
      e. Nystagmus
   3. Late signs: A high, shrill cry and seizures

D. Surgical interventions
   1. The goal of surgical treatment is to prevent further CSF accumulation by bypassing the blockage and draining the fluid from the ventricles to a location where it may be reabsorbed.
   2. In a ventriculoperitoneal **shunt**, the CSF drains into the peritoneal cavity from the lateral ventricle (Fig. 37-3).
   3. In a ventriculoatrial shunt, the CSF drains into the right atrium of the heart from the lateral ventricle, bypassing the obstruction. This is used for older children and those with pathological conditions of the abdomen.
   4. Shunt revision may be necessary as the child grows.
   5. An alternative to shunt placement is endoscopic third ventriculostomy, in which a small opening in the floor of the third ventricle is made that allows CSF to bypass the fourth ventricle and return to the circulation to be absorbed. This treatment may not be appropriate for some types of hydrocephalus.

E. Preoperative interventions
   1. Monitor intake and output (I&O). Administer small frequent feedings as tolerated until a preoperative NPO status is prescribed.
   2. Reposition the head frequently and use special devices such as an egg crate mattress under the head to prevent pressure sores.
   3. Prepare the child and family for diagnostic procedures and surgery.

F. Postoperative interventions
   1. Monitor the vital signs, neurological signs, and I&O.
   2. Position the child on the unoperated side to prevent pressure on the shunt valve.
   3. Keep the child flat, as prescribed, to avoid the rapid reduction of intracranial fluid.
   4. Observe for increased ICP. If increased ICP occurs, elevate the head of the bed to 15 to 30 degrees to 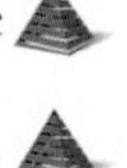

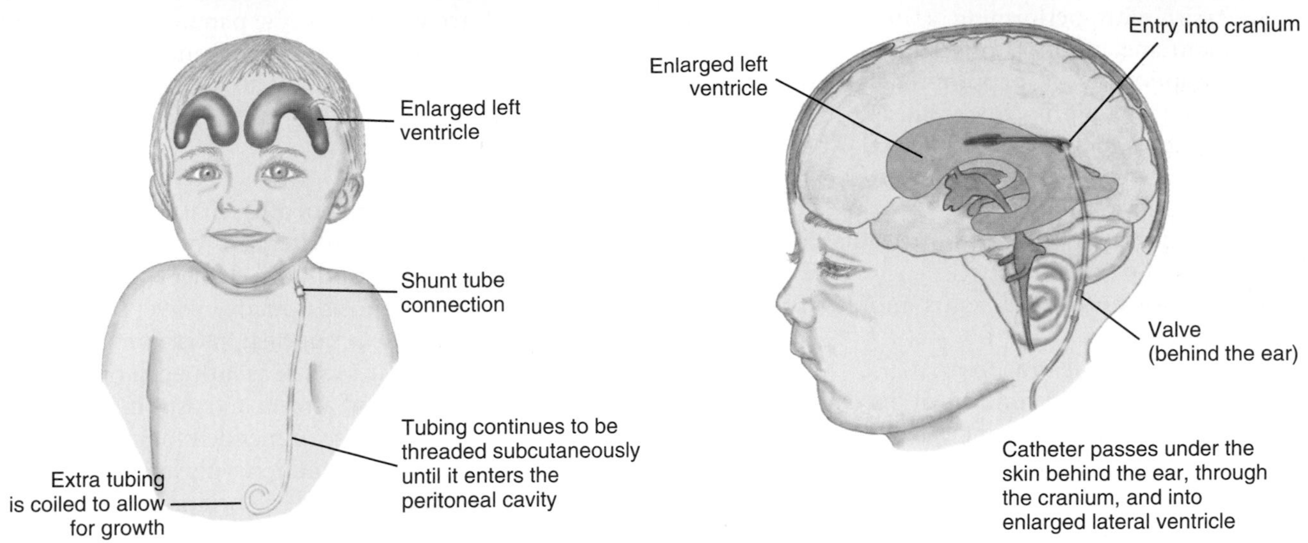

FIGURE 37-3 Ventriculoperitoneal shunt. (From McKinney E, James S, Murray S, Ashwill J: *Maternal-child nursing*, ed 4, St. Louis, 2013, Saunders.)

enhance gravity flow through the shunt and report the observations to the registered nurse.

5. Monitor for signs of infection. Check dressings for drainage.
6. Measure the head circumference.
7. Provide comfort measures. Assist to administer medications, as prescribed.
8. Reinforce instructions to the parents regarding how to recognize shunt infection or malfunction.
9. In an infant, irritability, a high shrill cry, lethargy, and feeding poorly may indicate shunt malfunction or infection.
10. In a toddler, headache and a lack of appetite are the earliest common signs of shunt malfunction.
11. In older children, the most valuable indicator of shunt malfunction is an alteration in the child's level of consciousness.

A high shrill cry in an infant can be a sign of increased ICP.

IV. Meningitis

A. Description
1. Meningitis is an infectious process of the central nervous system that is caused by bacteria and viruses that may be acquired as a primary disease or as a result of complications of neurosurgery, trauma, infection of the sinuses or ears, or systemic infections.
2. The diagnosis of bacterial meningitis is made by testing CSF obtained by lumbar puncture. The fluid of a child with meningitis is cloudy with increased pressure, increased white blood cell count, elevated protein, and decreased glucose levels.
3. Bacterial meningitis can be caused by a variety of organisms, most commonly *Haemophilus influenza* type B, *Streptococcus pneumoniae*, or *Neisseria meningitides*; meningococcal meningitis occurs in epidemic form and can be transmitted by droplets from nasopharyngeal secretions.
4. Viral meningitis is associated with viruses such as mumps, paramyxovirus, herpesvirus, and enterovirus.

B. Data collection
1. Signs and symptoms vary, depending on the type, the age of the child, and the duration of the preceding illness.
2. Fever, chills, and headache
3. Vomiting and diarrhea
4. Poor feeding or anorexia
5. Nuchal rigidity
6. Poor or high-shrill cry
7. Altered level of consciousness (e.g., lethargy, irritability)
8. Bulging anterior fontanel in the infant
9. Positive Kernig's sign (the inability to extend the leg when the thigh is flexed anteriorly at the hip) and Brudzinski's sign (neck flexion causes adduction and flexion movements of the lower extremities) in children and adolescents
10. Muscle or joint pain (meningococcal infection and *Haemophilus influenzae* infection)
11. Petechial or purpuric rashes (meningococcal infection)
12. Ear that chronically drains (pneumococcal meningitis)

C. Interventions
1. Provide respiratory isolation precautions and maintain them for at least 24 hours after antibiotics are initiated.
2. Assist to administer antibiotics and antipyretics as prescribed. (Antibiotics are administered as soon as they are prescribed after lumbar puncture.) Antiseizure medications may also be prescribed.

3. Assist with performing a neurological assessment and monitor for seizures. Monitor for the complication of inappropriate antidiuretic hormone secretion, which causes fluid retention (cerebral edema) and dilutional hyponatremia.
4. Monitor for changes in the level of consciousness and irritability.
5. Monitor for a purpuric or petechial rash and for signs of thromboemboli.
6. Monitor nutritional status; monitor intake and output.
7. Monitor for hearing loss.
8. Determine close contacts of the child with meningitis because the contacts will need prophylactic treatment.
9. Pneumococcal conjugate **vaccine** is recommended for all children beginning at age 2 months to protect against meningitis; streptococcal pneumococci can cause many bacterial infections, including meningitis (see Chapter 39 for information on vaccines).

V. Submersion Injury

A. Description
1. Survival of at least 24 hours after submersion in a fluid medium
2. Hypoxia and asphyxiation are the primary problems because they result in extensive cell damage. Cerebral cells sustain irreversible damage after 4 to 6 minutes of submersion.
3. Additional problems include aspiration and hypothermia.
4. The outcome is predicted based on the length of submersion in non-icy water. The outcome may be good if submersion was for less than 5 minutes and the child exhibits neurological responsiveness, reactive pupils, and a normal cardiac rhythm.
5. A child who was submerged for more than 10 minutes and does not respond to cardiopulmonary life support measures within 25 minutes has an extremely poor prognosis (severe neurological impairment or death).

B. Interventions
1. Provide ventilatory and circulatory support; if child has had a severe cerebral insult, endotracheal intubation and mechanical ventilation may be required.
2. Monitor respiratory status because respiratory compromise and cerebral edema may occur 24 hours after the incident.
3. Monitor for aspiration pneumonia.
4. Monitor neurological status closely; if spontaneous purposeful movement and normal brainstem function is not apparent 24 hours after the event, the child most likely suffered severe neurological deficits.
5. Reinforce teaching to the parents to provide adequate supervision of infants and small children around water to prevent accidents.

VI. Reye's Syndrome

A. Description
1. An acute encephalopathy that follows a viral illness. It is characterized pathologically by cerebral edema and fatty changes in the liver; a definitive diagnosis is made by liver biopsy.
2. The exact cause is not clear; most commonly follows a viral illness such as influenza or varicella.
3. Administration of aspirin and aspirin-containing salicylates is not recommended for children with a febrile illness or children with varicella or influenza because of its association with Reye's syndrome.
4. Acetaminophen (Tylenol) or ibuprofen (Motrin IB) is usually prescribed for pediatric clients.
5. Early diagnosis and aggressive treatment is important; the goal of treatment is to maintain effective cerebral perfusion and control increasing ICP.

B. Data collection
1. History of systemic viral illness 4 to 7 days before the onset of symptoms
2. Malaise
3. Nausea and vomiting
4. Signs of altered hepatic function such as lethargy
5. Progressive neurological deterioration

C. Interventions
1. Provide rest and decrease stimulation in the environment.
2. Monitor neurological status.
3. Monitor for altered level of consciousness and signs of increased ICP.
4. Monitor for signs of altered hepatic function and the results of liver function studies.
5. Monitor intake and output.
6. Monitor for signs of bleeding and signs of impaired coagulation, such as a prolonged bleeding time.

VII. Seizure Disorders

A. Description (see Chapter 57 for additional information on seizures)
1. Excessive and unorganized neuronal discharges in the brain that activate associated motor and sensory organs.
2. Classified as generalized, partial, or unclassified, depending on the area of the brain involved.
3. Types of generalized seizures include tonic-clonic, absence, myoclonic, and atonic.
4. Partial seizures arise from a specific area in the brain and cause limited symptoms; types include simple partial and complex partial.

BOX 37-4 Emergency Treatment for Seizures

Ensure airway patency.
Have suction equipment and oxygen available.
Time the seizure episode.
If the child is standing or sitting, ease the child down to the floor and place him or her in a side-lying position.
Place a pillow or folded blanket under the child's head. If no bedding is available, place your own hands under the child's head, or place the child's head in your own lap.
Loosen restrictive clothing.
Remove eyeglasses from the child, if present.
Clear the area of any hazards or hard objects.
Allow the seizure to proceed and end without interference.
If vomiting occurs, turn the child to one side as a unit.
Do not restrain the child, place anything in the child's mouth, or give any food or liquids to the child.
Prepare to assist to administer medications, as prescribed.
Remain with the child until he or she fully recovers.
Observe for incontinence, which may have occurred during the seizure.
Document the occurrence.

B. Data collection
1. Obtain information from the parents about the time of onset, precipitating events, and behavior before and after the seizure.
2. Determine the child's history related to seizures.
3. Ask the child about the presence of an aura (a warning sign of impending seizure).
4. Monitor for apnea and **cyanosis**.
5. Postseizure: The child is disoriented and sleepy.

C. Seizure precautions (see Box 37-1)

D. Interventions (Box 37-4)

E. Anticonvulsant medications (see Chapter 58 for information about medications)

Never place anything, including an airway device or padded tongue blade, into the mouth of a child experiencing a seizure.

VIII. Neural Tube Defects

A. Description
1. Central nervous system defect that results from the failure of the neural tube to close during embryonic development
2. Associated deficits may include sensorimotor disturbance, dislocated hips, talipes equinovarus (clubfoot), and hydrocephalus.
3. Defect closure is performed immediately after birth.

B. Types
1. Spina bifida occulta
   a. Posterior vertebral arches fail to close in the lumbosacral area.
   b. The spinal cord remains intact and usually is not visible.
   c. Meninges are not exposed on the skin surface.
   d. Neurological deficits are not usually present.
2. Spina bifida cystica
   a. Protrusion of the spinal cord or its meninges, or both, occurs.
   b. The defect results in the incomplete closure of the vertebral and neural tubes, which results in a saclike protrusion in the lumbar or sacral area with varying degrees of nervous tissue involvement.
   c. The defect can include meningocele, myelomeningocele, lipomeningocele, and lipomeningomyelocele.
3. Meningocele
   a. The protrusion involves meninges and a saclike cyst that contains CSF in the midline of the back, usually in the lumbosacral area.
   b. The spinal cord is not involved.
   c. Neurological deficits are usually not present.
4. Myelomeningocele
   a. Protrusion of the meninges, CSF, nerve roots, and a portion of the spinal cord occurs.
   b. The sac (defect) is covered by a thin membrane that is prone to leakage or rupture.
   c. Neurological deficits are evident.

C. Data collection
1. Depends on the spinal cord involvement
2. Visible spinal defect
3. Flaccid paralysis of the legs
4. Altered bladder and bowel function
5. Hip and joint deformities
6. Hydrocephalus

D. Interventions
1. Evaluate the sac and measure the lesion.
2. Assist with performing a neurological assessment.
3. Monitor for increased ICP, which may indicate developing hydrocephalus.
4. Measure the head circumference. Check the anterior fontanel for fullness.
5. Protect the sac as prescribed. Cover with a sterile, moist (normal saline), nonadherent dressing to maintain the moisture of the sac and its contents.
6. Change the dressing that covers the sac on a regular schedule, as prescribed, or whenever it becomes soiled to reduce the risk of infection. Diapering may be contraindicated until the defect has been repaired.
7. Use aseptic technique to prevent infection.
8. Check the sac for redness, clear or purulent drainage, abrasions, irritation, and signs of infection.
9. Early signs of infection include elevated axillary temperature, irritability, lethargy, and nuchal rigidity.
10. Place the child in a prone position to minimize tension on the sac and the risk of trauma; the head is turned to one side for feeding. 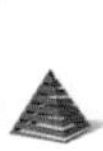

11. Check for physical impairments such as hip and joint deformities.
12. Assist to prepare the child and family for surgery.
13. Assist to administer antibiotics preoperatively and postoperatively, as prescribed, to prevent infection.
14. Reinforce teaching to the parents and eventually the child about long-term home care.
    a. Positioning, feeding, skin care, and range-of-motion exercises
    b. Instituting a bladder elimination program and performing clean intermittent catheterization technique
    c. Administering antispasmodics (these act on the smooth muscle of the bladder) as prescribed to increase bladder capacity and improve continence
    d. Implementing a bowel program as appropriate and as needed, including a high-fiber diet, increased fluids, suppositories
    e. The child is at high risk for allergy to latex and rubber products because of the frequent exposure to latex during implementation of care measures.

IX. Attention Deficit Hyperactivity Disorder

A. Description
1. A behavior disorder that is characterized by inappropriate degrees of inattention, overactivity, and impulsivity
2. Childhood problems include lowered intellectual development, some minor physical abnormalities, sleep disturbances, behavioral or emotional disorders, and difficulty with social relationships.
3. Early diagnosis is important to prevent impaired emotional and psychological development.
4. Diagnosis is established on the basis of self-reports, parent and teacher reports, and the use of assessment tools.

B. Data collection
1. Fidgets with hands or feet or squirms in a seat
2. Easily distracted by external or internal stimuli
3. Difficulty with following through on instructions
4. Poor attention span
5. Shifts from one uncompleted activity to another
6. Talks excessively
7. Interrupts or intrudes on others
8. Engages in physically dangerous activities without considering the possible consequences

C. Interventions
1. Provide parents with information about the disorder and treatment plan; encourage support groups for the parents.
2. Treatment includes behavioral therapy, medication, maintaining a consistent environment, and appropriate classroom placement.
3. Behavioral therapy focuses on preventing undesirable behavior.
4. Maintaining a consistent home and classroom environment and providing environmental and physical safety measures are important.
5. Promote self-esteem.
6. Stimulant medications may be prescribed; possible side/adverse effects include appetite suppression and weight loss, nervousness, tics, insomnia, and increased blood pressure.
7. Reinforce instructions to the child and parents regarding medication administration and the need for regular follow-up.

X. Autism Spectrum Disorders

A. Description
1. Autism spectrum disorders (ASDs) are complex neurodevelopmental disorders of unknown etiology composed of qualitative alterations in social interaction and verbal impairment with repetitive, restricted, and stereotype behavioral patterns.
2. Autism spectrum disorder impairments range from mild to severe; types include autism, Asperger syndrome, Rett syndrome.
3. Symptoms are usually noted by the parents by 3 years of age.
4. The cause of the disorder is not specifically known; however, it has been linked to a wide range of antepartum, intrapartum, and postpartum conditions and exposure to hazardous chemicals. Genetic predisposition is also linked to the disorder.

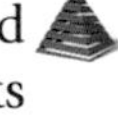

5. The disorder is accompanied by intellectual and social behavioral deficits, and the child exhibits peculiar and bizarre characteristics with social interactions, communication, and behaviors.

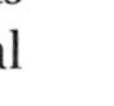

6. Despite their relatively moderate to severe disability, some children with autism (known as savants) excel in particular areas, such as art, music, memory, mathematics, or perceptual skills such as puzzle building.
7. Diagnosis is established on the basis of symptoms and with the use of several screening tools.

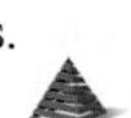

B. Data collection
1. Social
    a. Abnormal lack of comfort-seeking behaviors
    b. Abnormal or lack of social play
    c. Impairment in peer relationships
    d. Lack of awareness of the existence or feelings of others
    e. Abnormal or lack of imitation of others
2. Communication
    a. Lack of, impaired, or abnormal speech such as producing a monotone voice or echolalia
    b. Abnormal nonverbal communication (does not use gestures to communicate)
    c. Lack of imaginative play

3. Behavior
   a. Persistent preoccupation or attachment to objects; range of interests restricted
   b. Self-injurious behaviors
   c. Must maintain routine; any environmental change produces marked distress.
   d. Produces repetitive body movements such as rocking or head banging

C. Interventions
1. Determine the child's routines, habits, and preferences, and maintain consistency as much as possible.
2. Determine the specific ways in which the child communicates and use these methods.
3. Avoid placing demands on the child.
4. Implement safety precautions, as necessary, for self-injurious behaviors such as head banging.
5. Assist to initiate referrals to special programs, as required.
6. Provide support to the parents.

Ensuring a safe environment for a child with autism is a priority.

XI. Intellectual Disability (Mental Retardation)

A. Description
1. In intellectual disability, a child manifests subaverage intellectual functioning along with deficits in adaptive skills.
2. Down syndrome is a congenital condition that results in moderate to severe retardation and has been linked to an extra group G chromosome, chromosome 21 (trisomy 21).

B. Data Collection
1. Deficits in cognitive skills and level of adaptive functioning
2. Delays in fine and gross motor skills
3. Speech delays
4. Decreased spontaneous activity
5. Nonresponsiveness
6. Irritability
7. Poor eye contact during feeding

C. Interventions
1. Medical strategies are focused on correcting structural deformities and treating associated behaviors.
2. Assist to implement community and educational services, using a multidisciplinary approach.
3. Promote care skills as much as possible.
4. Assist with communication and socialization skills.
5. Facilitate appropriate playtimes.
6. Initiate safety precautions as necessary.
7. Assist the family with decisions regarding care.
8. Provide information regarding support services and community agencies.

CRITICAL THINKING What Should You Do?

Answer: Following insertion of a ventriculoperitoneal shunt for the treatment of hydrocephalus, the nurse should monitor the child for signs of increased ICP. In the child, early signs include a change of level of consciousness, headache, nausea, vomiting, visual disturbances (diplopia), and seizures. Normally, the surgeon prescribes that the child be kept flat to avoid rapid reduction of intracranial fluid. If increased ICP occurs, the nurse should elevate the head of the bed to 15 to 30 degrees to enhance gravity flow through the shunt. The nurse should also notify the registered nurse (RN) immediately. The RN will assess the child and contact the surgeon immediately.

Reference(s): Hockenberry, M., & Wilson, D. (2013). *Wong's: Essentials of pediatric nursing* (9th ed., pp. 969–970). St. Louis: Mosby.

McKinney, E., James, S., Murray, S., Nelson, K. & Ashwill, J. (2013). *Maternal-child nursing* (4th ed., pp. 1418–1419). St. Louis: Elsevier.

PRACTICE QUESTIONS

361. The nurse is collecting data about a child who has been admitted to the hospital with a diagnosis of seizures. Which action would **best** assist in determining the causes of the seizure?
1. Testing the child's urine for specific gravity
2. Asking the child what happens during a seizure
3. Obtaining a family history of psychiatric illness
4. Obtaining a history regarding factors that may occur before the seizure activity

362. A child has a basilar skull fracture. Which health care provider's prescription should the nurse question?
1. Restrict fluid intake.
2. Insert an indwelling urinary catheter.
3. Keep an intravenous (IV) line patent.
4. Suction via the nasotracheal route as needed.

363. Which laboratory result would verify the diagnosis of bacterial meningitis?
1. Clear cerebrospinal fluid with high protein and low glucose levels
2. Cloudy cerebrospinal fluid with low protein and low glucose levels
3. Cloudy cerebrospinal fluid with high protein and low glucose levels
4. Decreased pressure and cloudy cerebrospinal fluid with a high protein level

Pediatric

364. A child has been diagnosed with meningococcal meningitis. Which precautionary technique is appropriate to prevent transmission of the disease?

1. Enteric precautions
2. Neutropenic precautions
3. No precautions are required as long as antibiotics have been started.
4. Isolation precautions for at least 24 hours after the initiation of antibiotics

❖ **365.** The nurse is assisting to develop a plan of care for a child who is at risk for seizures. Which interventions apply if the child has a seizure? **Select all that apply.**

- ❑ 1. Time the seizure.
- ❑ 2. Restrain the child.
- ❑ 3. Stay with the child.
- ❑ 4. Place the child in a prone position.
- ❑ 5. Move furniture away from the child.
- ❑ 6. Insert a padded tongue blade into the child's mouth.

366. The parents of a child recently diagnosed with cerebral palsy ask the nurse about the disorder. The nurse bases the response on the understanding that cerebral palsy is which type of condition?

1. An infectious disease of the central nervous system
2. An inflammation of the brain as a result of a viral illness
3. A congenital condition that results in moderate to severe retardation
4. A chronic disability characterized by impaired muscle movement and posture

367. The nurse is assisting with data collection from an infant who has been diagnosed with hydrocephalus. If the infant's level of consciousness diminishes, which is a **priority** intervention?

1. Taking the apical pulse
2. Taking the blood pressure
3. Testing the urine for protein
4. Palpating the anterior fontanel

368. The nurse is reviewing the record of a child with increased intracranial pressure and notes that the child has exhibited signs of decerebrate posturing. On data collection of the child, the nurse expects to note which characteristic of this type of posturing?

1. Flaccid paralysis of all extremities
2. Adduction of the arms at the shoulders
3. Rigid extension and pronation of the arms and legs
4. Abnormal flexion of the upper extremities and extension and adduction of the lower extremities

369. A child is diagnosed with Reye's syndrome. The nurse assists to develop a nursing care plan for the child and should include which intervention in the plan?

1. Assessing hearing loss
2. Monitoring urine output
3. Changing body position every 2 hours
4. Providing a quiet atmosphere with dimmed lighting

370. Which represents a **primary** characteristic of an autism spectrum disorder?

1. Normal social play
2. Consistent imitation of others' actions
3. Lack of social interaction and awareness
4. Normal verbal and nonverbal communication

ANSWERS

361. 4

Rationale: Fever and infections increase the body's metabolic rate. This can cause seizure activity among children who are less than 5 years old. Dehydration and electrolyte imbalance can also contribute to the occurrence of a seizure. Falls can cause head injuries, which would increase intracranial pressure or cerebral edema. Some medications could cause seizures. Specific gravity would not be a reliable test because it varies, depending on the existing condition. Psychiatric illness has no impact on seizure occurrence or cause. Children do not remember what happened during the seizure itself.

Test-Taking Strategy: Note the strategic word, *best*. Also, focus on the subject, the cause of the seizure activity. Note the relationship between the subject and the correct option. **Review:** seizures.

Level of Cognitive Ability: Analyzing

Client Needs: Physiological Integrity

Integrated Process: Nursing Process/Data Collection

Content Area: Child Health: Neurological

Priority Concepts: Clinical Judgment, Intracranial Regulation

Reference(s): Hockenberry, Wilson (2013), pp. 956–957.

362. 4

Rationale: Nasotracheal suctioning is contraindicated in a child with a basilar skull fracture. Because of the location of the injury, the suction catheter may be introduced into the brain. Fluids are restricted to prevent fluid overload. The child may require a urinary catheter for the accurate monitoring of intake and output. An IV line is maintained to administer fluids or medications, if necessary.

Test-Taking Strategy: Focus on the subject, the prescription that the nurse should question. Note that options 1, 2, and 3 are comparable or alike in that they all address the subject of fluid intake or output. **Review: basilar skull fracture.**

Level of Cognitive Ability: Analyzing

Client Needs: Safe and Effective Care Environment

Integrated Process: Nursing Process/Implementation
Content Area: Child Health: Neurological
Priority Concepts: Intracranial Regulation, Safety
Reference(s): Hockenberry, Wilson (2013), p. 944.

363. 3

Rationale: A diagnosis of meningitis is made by testing the cerebrospinal fluid (CSF) obtained by lumbar puncture. In the case of bacterial meningitis, findings usually include increased pressure, cloudy cerebrospinal fluid, a high protein level, and a low glucose level.
Test-Taking Strategy: Focus on the subject, verifying the diagnosis of meningitis. Eliminate options 1 and 4 first because clear CSF and decreased pressure are not likely to be found if an infectious process such as meningitis is suspected. From this point, recalling that a high protein level indicates a possible diagnosis of meningitis will direct you to the correct option. **Review: meningitis.**
Level of Cognitive Ability: Analyzing
Client Needs: Physiological Integrity
Integrated Process: Nursing Process/Data Collection
Content Area: Fundamental Skills: Laboratory Values
Priority Concepts: Cellular Regulation, Infection
Reference(s): McKinney et al (2013), p. 1414.

364. 4

Rationale: Meningococcal meningitis is transmitted primarily by droplet infection. Isolation is begun and maintained for at least 24 hours after antibiotics are given. Options 1, 2, and 3 are incorrect.
Test-Taking Strategy: Focus on the subject, preventing the transmission of meningococcal meningitis. Eliminate options 1 and 2 first. Both enteric and neutropenic precautions are unrelated to the mode of transmission of meningococcal meningitis. Recalling that it takes approximately 24 hours for antibiotics to reach a therapeutic blood level will assist with directing you to the correct option from the remaining options. **Review: meningococcal meningitis.**
Level of Cognitive Ability: Applying
Client Needs: Safe and Effective Care Environment
Integrated Process: Nursing Process/Planning
Content Area: Fundamental Skills: Infection Control
Priority Concepts: Infection, Safety
Reference(s): McKinney et al (2013), pp. 1439–1440.

❖ 365. 1, 3, 5

Rationale: During a seizure, the child is placed on his or her side in a lateral position. This type of positioning will prevent aspiration because saliva will drain out of the corner of the child's mouth. The child is not restrained because this could cause injury. The nurse would loosen clothing around the child's neck and ensure a patent airway. Nothing is placed into the child's mouth during a seizure because this action may cause injury to the child's mouth, gums, or teeth. The nurse would stay with the child to reduce the risk of injury and allow for the observation and timing of the seizure.
Test-Taking Strategy: Focus on the subject, care during a seizure. Visualize this clinical situation. Recalling that airway patency and safety are the priorities will assist you with determining the appropriate interventions. **Review:** interventions **for seizures.**
Level of Cognitive Ability: Analyzing
Client Needs: Physiological Integrity
Integrated Process: Nursing Process/Planning
Content Area: Child Health: Neurological
Priority Concepts: Intracranial Regulation, Safety
Reference(s): Hockenberry, Wilson (2013), p. 965.

366. 4

Rationale: Cerebral palsy is a chronic disability characterized by impaired movement and posture resulting from an abnormality in the extrapyramidal or pyramidal motor system. Meningitis is an infectious process of the central nervous system. Encephalitis is an inflammation of the brain that occurs as a result of viral illness or central nervous system infection. Down syndrome is an example of a congenital condition that results in moderate to severe retardation.
Test-Taking Strategy: Eliminate options 1 and 2 first, noting that they are comparable or alike. Next, note the relationship between the words *palsy* in the question and *impaired muscle movement* in the correct option. **Review: cerebral palsy.**
Level of Cognitive Ability: Applying
Client Needs: Physiological Integrity
Integrated Process: Teaching and Learning
Content Area: Child Health: Neurological
Priority Concepts: Intracranial Regulation; Mobility
Reference(s): Hockenberry, Wilson (2013), pp. 1092–1093.

367. 4

Rationale: A full or bulging anterior fontanel indicates an increase in cerebrospinal fluid collection in the cerebral ventricle. Apical pulse and blood pressure changes and proteinuria are not specifically associated with increasing cerebrospinal fluid in the brain tissue in an infant.
Test-Taking Strategy: Note the strategic word, *priority.* Use the principles associated with excessive fluid buildup in the cranial cavity, and note that the question addresses an infant. Additionally, correlate *hydrocephalus* in the question with *anterior fontanel* in the correct option. **Review: hydrocephalus.**
Level of Cognitive Ability: Analyzing
Client Needs: Physiological Integrity
Integrated Process: Nursing Process/Data Collection
Content Area: Child Health: Neurological
Priority Concepts: Development, Intracranial Regulation
Reference(s): Hockenberry, Wilson (2013), p. 968.

368. 3

Rationale: Decerebrate (extension) posturing is characterized by the rigid extension and pronation of the arms and legs. Option 1 is incorrect. Options 2 and 4 describe decorticate (flexion) posturing.
Test-Taking Strategy: Focus on the subject, characteristics of decerebrate (extension) posturing. Recalling the clinical manifestations associated with decerebrate posturing will direct you to the correct option. Remember that decerebrate posturing is characterized by the rigid extension and pronation of the arms and legs. **Review:** characteristics of **decorticate** and **decerebrate posturing.**
Level of Cognitive Ability: Analyzing
Client Needs: Physiological Integrity
Integrated Process: Nursing Process/Data Collection
Content Area: Child Health: Neurological

Priority Concepts: Clinical Judgment, Intracranial Regulation
Reference(s): Hockenberry, Wilson (2013), pp. 931–932.

369. 4

Rationale: Reye's syndrome is an acute encephalopathy that follows a viral illness and is characterized pathologically by cerebral edema and fatty changes in the liver. A definitive diagnosis is made by liver biopsy. In Reye's syndrome, supportive care is directed toward monitoring and managing cerebral edema. Decreasing stimuli in the environment by providing a quiet environment with dimmed lighting would decrease the stress on the cerebral tissue and neuron responses. Hearing loss and urine output are not affected. Changing the body position every 2 hours would not affect the cerebral edema directly. The child should be positioned with the head elevated to decrease the progression of the cerebral edema and promote drainage of cerebrospinal fluid.
Test-Taking Strategy: Focus on the subject, nursing care for the child with Reye's syndrome. Think about the pathophysiology associated with Reye's syndrome. Recalling that cerebral edema is a concern for a child with Reye's syndrome will direct you to the correct option. **Review:** care of the child with Reye's syndrome.
Level of Cognitive Ability: Applying
Client Needs: Physiological Integrity
Integrated Process: Nursing Process/Planning
Content Area: Child Health: Neurological
Priority Concepts: Clinical Judgment; Intracranial Regulation
Reference(s): Hockenberry, Wilson (2013), p. 956.

370. 3

Rationale: A primary characteristic of an autism spectrum disorder is a lack of social interaction and awareness. Social behaviors include a lack of or an abnormal imitation of others' actions and a lack of or abnormal social play. Additional characteristics include a lack of or impaired verbal communication and markedly abnormal nonverbal communication.
Test-Taking Strategy: Note the strategic word, *primary*. Focus on the subject, a primary characteristic of an autism spectrum disorder. Think about the characteristics of this disorder. Eliminate options 1 and 4 first because they address normal behaviors. From the remaining options, recalling that the child lacks social interaction and awareness will direct you to the correct option. **Review: autism spectrum disorders.**
Level of Cognitive Ability: Understanding
Client Needs: Psychosocial Integrity
Integrated Process: Nursing Process/Data Collection
Content Area: Child Health: Neurological
Priority Concepts: Functional Ability, Sensory Perception
Reference(s): McKinney et al (2013), pp. 590–591.

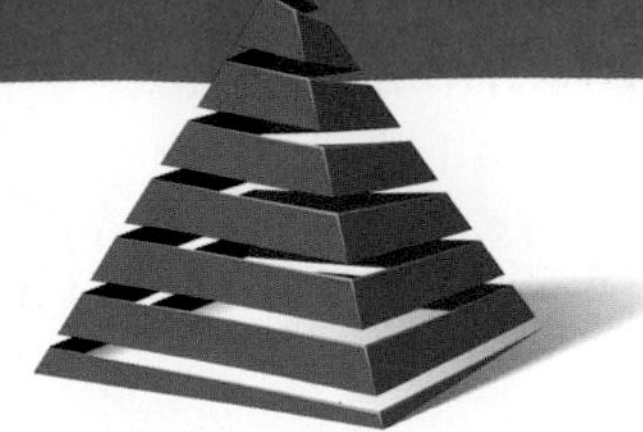

CHAPTER 38

Musculoskeletal Disorders

Pediatric

CRITICAL THINKING What Should You Do?

The nurse is assessing an infant with clubfoot who is in a cast. The nurse notes that the tissue distal to the cast is pale and edematous and the infant shows signs of pain with passive movement. What should the nurse do?
Answer located on p. 460.

I. Developmental Dysplasia of the Hip

A. Description
1. Refers to disorders related to abnormal development of the hip that may develop during fetal life, infancy, or childhood; in these disorders, the head of the femur is seated improperly in the acetabulum or hip socket of the pelvis.
2. Degrees of developmental dysplasia of the hip (see Box 38-1)

B. Data collection (Fig. 38-1)
1. Neonates: Laxity of the ligaments around the hip.
2. Infants beyond the newborn period
   a. Shortening of the limb on the affected side (Galeazzi sign, Allis's sign)
   b. Restricted abduction of the hip on the affected side when the child is placed supine with the knees and hips flexed (limited range of motion in the affected hip)
   c. Unequal gluteal folds when the infant is prone and the legs are extended against the examining table
   d. Positive Ortolani's test: The Ortolani's maneuver is a test to assess for hip instability. In the Ortolani maneuver, the examiner abducts the thigh and applies gentle pressure forward over the greater trochanter. A "clicking" sensation indicates a dislocated femoral head moving into the acetabulum.
   e. Positive Barlow's test: The examiner adducts the hips and applies gentle pressure down and back with the thumbs. In hip dysplasia, the examiner can feel the femoral head move out of the acetabulum.
3. Older infant and child
   a. Affected leg is shorter than the other.
   b. The head of the femur can be felt to move up and down in the buttock when the extended thigh is pushed first toward the child's head and then pulled distally.
   c. Positive Trendelenburg's sign: The child stands on one foot and then the other foot, holding onto a support and bearing weight on the affected hip; the pelvis tilts downward on the normal side instead of upward, as it would with normal stability.
   d. Greater trochanter is prominent.
   e. Marked lordosis or waddling gait is noted in bilateral dislocations.

C. Interventions
1. Birth to 6 months of age: Splinting of the hips with a Pavlik harness to maintain flexion, abduction, and external rotation; worn continuously until the hip is stable, in about 3 to 6 months (Fig. 38-2).
2. Age 6 to 18 months: Gradual reduction by traction followed by closed reduction or open reduction (if necessary) under general anesthesia. The child is then placed in a hip spica cast for 2 to 4 months until the hip is stable, and then a flexion-abduction brace is applied for approximately 3 months.

BOX 38-1 Degrees of Developmental Dysplasia of the Hip

Acetabular Dysplasia (Preluxation)
- Mildest form
- Neither subluxation nor dislocation
- Delay in acetabular development occurs
- Femoral head remains in the acetabulum

Subluxation
- Incomplete dislocation of the hip
- Femoral head remains in the acetabulum
- Stretched capsule and ligamentum teres causes head of the femur to be partially displaced

Dislocation
- Femoral head loses contact with acetabulum and is displaced posteriorly and superiorly over the fibrocartilaginous rim
- Ligamentum teres—elongated and taut

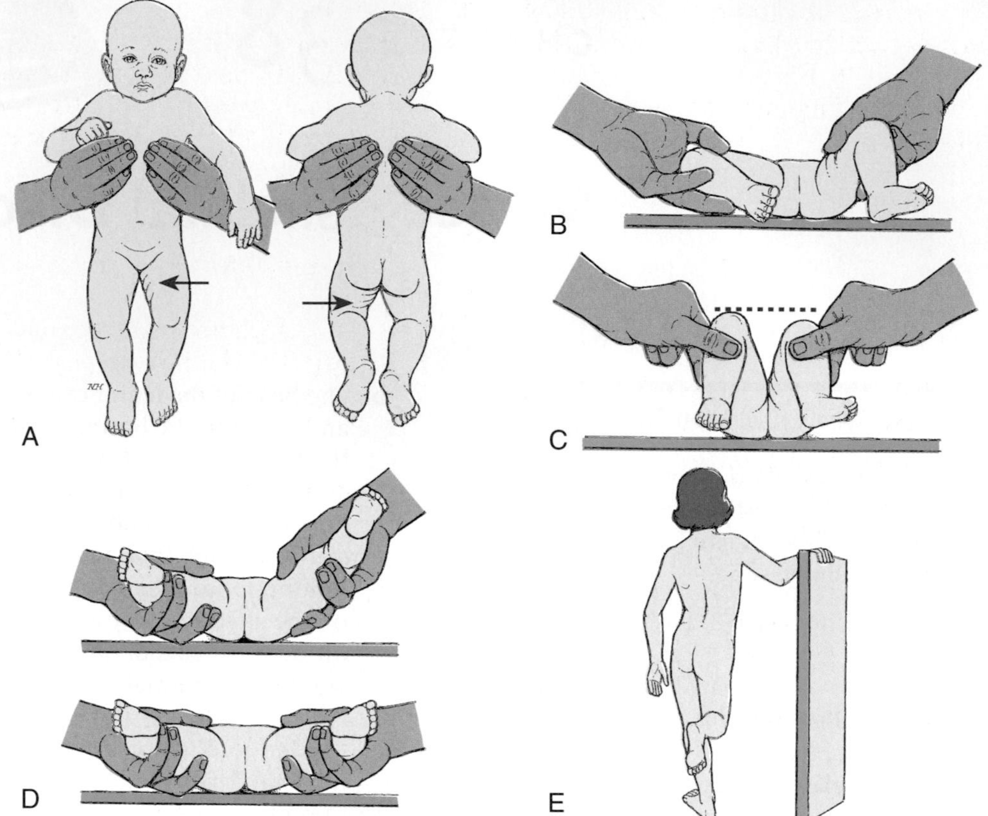

FIGURE 38-1 Signs of developmental dysplasia of the hip. **A,** Asymmetry of gluteal and thigh folds. **B,** Limited hip abduction, as seen in flexion. **C,** Apparent shortening of the femur, as indicated by the level of the knees in flexion. **D,** Ortolani click (if infant is under 4 weeks of age). **E,** Positive Trendelenburg's sign of gait (if child is weight bearing). (From Hockenberry M, Wilson D: *Wong's: Essentials of pediatric nursing,* ed 9, St. Louis, 2013, Mosby.)

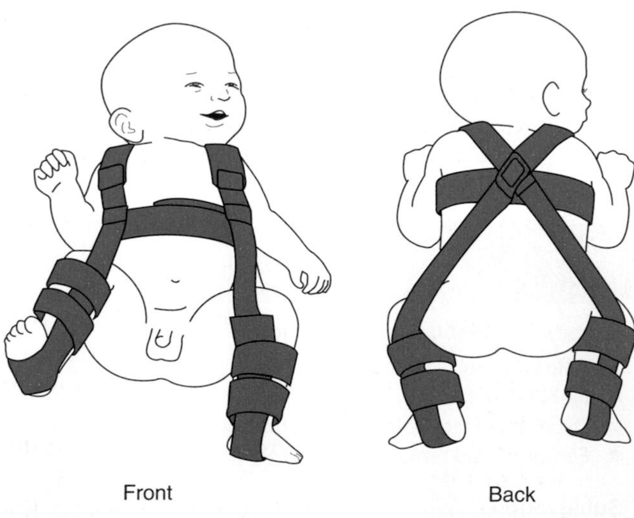

FIGURE 38-2 Child in Pavlik harness. (From Ball JW: *Mosby's: Pediatric patient teaching guides,* St. Louis, 1998, Mosby.)

3. Older child: Operative reduction and reconstruction may be required.
4. Reinforce instructions to the parents regarding the proper care of a Pavlik harness, spica cast, or abduction brace.

II. Congenital Clubfoot

A. Description
   1. Complex deformity of the ankle and foot that includes forefoot adduction, midfoot supination, hindfoot varus, and ankle equinus. The defect may be unilateral or bilateral.
   2. The goal of treatment is to achieve a painless plantigrade (able to walk on the sole of the foot with the heel on the ground) and stable foot.
   3. Long-term interval follow-up is required until the child reaches skeletal maturity.

B. Data collection: Deformities are described on the basis of the position of the ankle and foot.
   1. Talipes varus: An inversion or bending inward
   2. Talipes valgus: An eversion or bending outward
   3. Talipes equinus: Plantar flexion in which the toes are lower than the heel
   4. Talipes calcaneus: Dorsiflexion in which the toes are higher than the heel

C. Interventions
   1. Treatment begins as soon after birth as possible.
   2. Manipulation and casting are performed weekly for about 8 to 12 weeks because of the rapid **growth** of early infancy; a splint is then applied if casting and manipulation are successful.

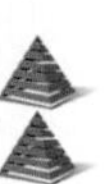

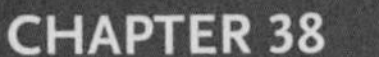

3. Surgical intervention may be necessary if normal alignment is not achieved by about 6 to 12 weeks of age.
4. Monitor for pain and monitor the neurovascular status of the toes.

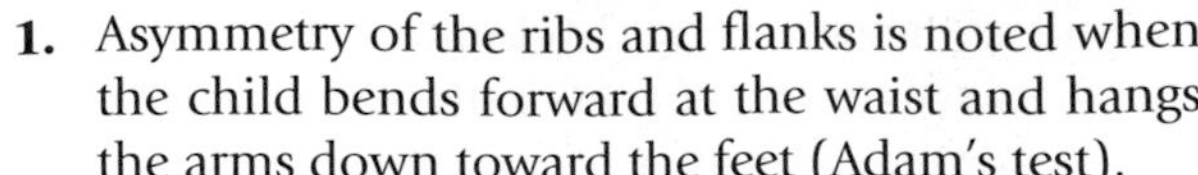

Contact the registered nurse or health care provider immediately if signs of neurovascular impairment are noted in a child with a cast or brace.

III. Idiopathic Scoliosis

A. Description
1. A three-dimensional spinal deformity that usually involves lateral curvature, spinal rotation that results in rib asymmetry, and hypokyphosis of the thorax (Fig. 38-3).
2. Usually diagnosed during the preadolescent growth spurt. Screenings are important at times when growth spurts occur.
3. Surgical (spinal fusion, which may be done by thoracoscopic surgery, placement of an instrumentation system, or use of metallic staples placed into vertebral bodies) and nonsurgical (bracing) interventions are used; the type of treatment depends on the location and degree of the curvatures, the age of the child, the amount of growth that is yet anticipated, and any underlying disease processes.
4. Long-term monitoring is essential to detect any progression of the curve.

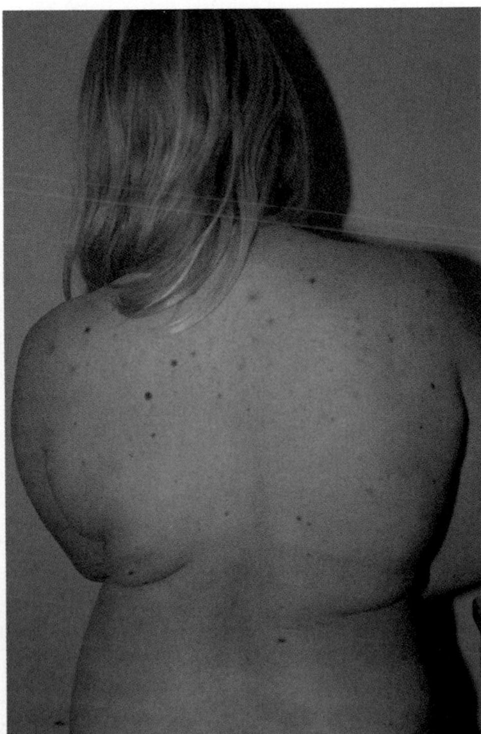

FIGURE 38-3 Scoliosis in a standing erect posture. (From Lemmi FO, Lemmi CAE: *Physical assessment findings CD-ROM*, Philadelphia, 2000, Saunders.)

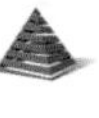

B. Data collection
1. Asymmetry of the ribs and flanks is noted when the child bends forward at the waist and hangs the arms down toward the feet (Adam's test).
2. Hip height, rib positioning, and shoulder height are asymmetrical. (This can be noted when standing behind the undressed child.) A leg-length discrepancy is also apparent.
3. Radiographs are performed to confirm the diagnosis.

C. Interventions
1. Monitor the progression of the curvatures.
2. Prepare the child and parents for the use of a brace, if prescribed.
3. Prepare the child and parents for surgery (spinal fusion and the placement of internal instrumentation systems), if prescribed.

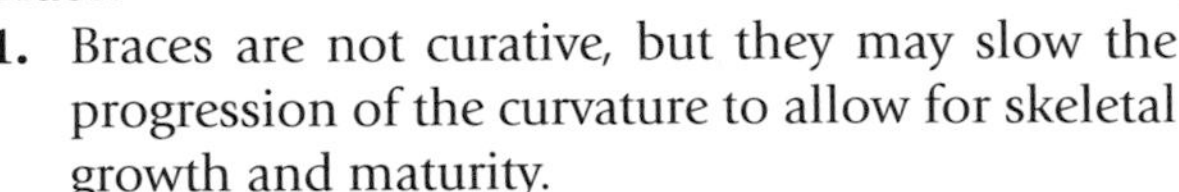

The potential for altered role performance, body image disturbance, fear, anger, and isolation exists for a child with a disabling condition and a condition that requires wearing a body brace.

D. Braces
1. Braces are not curative, but they may slow the progression of the curvature to allow for skeletal growth and maturity.
2. Braces usually are prescribed to be worn from 16 to 23 hours a day.
3. Inspect the skin for signs of redness or breakdown.
4. Keep the skin clean and dry, and avoid lotions and powders because these cake and lead to skin breakdown.
5. Advise the child to wear soft, nonirritating clothing under the brace.
6. Reinforce instructions to the child and parents in the prescribed exercises, which help to maintain and strengthen the spinal and abdominal muscles during treatment.
7. Encourage verbalization about body image and other psychosocial issues.

E. Postoperative interventions
1. Maintain proper alignment. Avoid twisting movements.
2. Logroll the child when turning him or her to maintain alignment.
3. Monitor the neurovascular status of the extremities.
4. Encourage coughing, deep breathing, and the use of incentive spirometry.
5. Check for pain and assist to administer analgesics, as prescribed.
6. Monitor for incontinence.
7. Monitor for signs and symptoms of infection.
8. Monitor for superior mesenteric artery syndrome, which is caused by mechanical changes in the position of the child's abdominal contents during surgery, and notify the registered

nurse immediately if it occurs. Symptoms include emesis and abdominal distention similar to that which occurs with intestinal obstruction or paralytic ileus.

9. Reinforce instructions to the child and parents regarding activity restrictions.
10. Reinforce instructions to the child how to log-roll from a side-lying position to a sitting position, and assist the child with ambulation.
11. Be alert to signs of a body image problem.

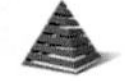

IV. Juvenile Idiopathic Arthritis

A. Description
1. An autoimmune, inflammatory disease affecting the joints and other tissues, such as articular cartilage, that occurs most often in girls.
2. Treatment is supportive (there is no cure) and directed toward preserving joint function, controlling inflammation, minimizing deformity, and reducing the impact that the disease may have on the development of the child.
3. Treatment includes medications, physical and occupational therapies, and child and family education.
4. Surgical intervention may be implemented if the child has problems with joint contractures and unequal growth of extremities.

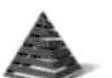

B. Data collection (Box 38-2)
1. There are no definitive tests to diagnose the condition.
2. Certain laboratory tests (e.g., an elevated erythrocyte sedimentation rate, the presence of leukocytosis) may support evidence of the disease.
3. Radiographs may show soft tissue swelling and joint space widening as a result of increased synovial fluid in the joint.

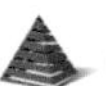

C. Interventions
1. Facilitate social and emotional development.
2. Reinforce instructions to the parents and child in the administration of medications. Medications may be given alone or in combination and are prescribed in a steplike fashion that is dependent on the disease's response to each level (see Chapter 60 for medications).
3. Assist the child with range-of-motion exercises. Instruct the child and parents with regard to prescribed exercises.

BOX 38-2 Data Collection: Juvenile Idiopathic Arthritis

Stiffness, swelling, and limited motion occur in the affected joints.
The affected joints are warm to the touch, tender, and painful.
Joint stiffness is present on arising in the morning and after inactivity.
Uveitis (the inflammation of structures in the uveal tract) can occur and cause blindness.

4. Encourage the normal performance of activities of daily living.
5. Reinforce instructions to the parents and child in the use of hot and cold packs, splinting, and positioning the affected joint in a neutral position during painful episodes.
6. Encourage and support prescribed physical and occupational therapy.
7. Reinforce instructions to the child and parents in the importance of preventive eye care and the reporting of visual disturbances.
8. Assess the child's and family's perceptions regarding the chronic illness. Plan to discuss the nature of a chronic illness and the grief associated with the new recognition of life alterations that result from the chronic progression of the disorder.

V. Marfan Syndrome

A. Description
1. A disorder of connective tissue that affects the skeletal system, cardiovascular system, eyes, and skin

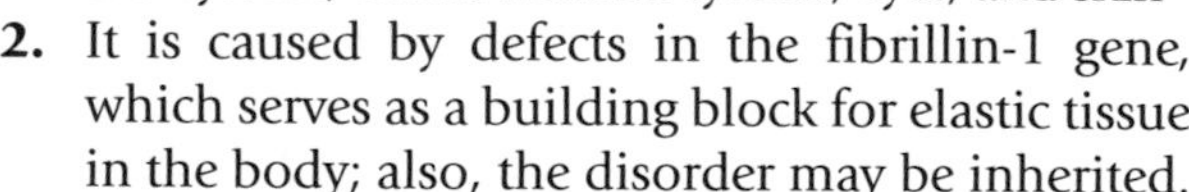

2. It is caused by defects in the fibrillin-1 gene, which serves as a building block for elastic tissue in the body; also, the disorder may be inherited.
3. There is no cure for the disorder.

B. Data collection
1. Tall and thin body structure; slender fingers, long arms and legs, curvature of the spine
2. Presence of visual problems
3. Presence of cardiac problems

C. Interventions
1. Monitor for vision problems and obtain visual exams on a regular schedule.
2. Monitor for curvature of the spine, especially during adolescence.
3. Cardiac medications may be prescribed to slow the heart rate, which will decrease stress on the aorta.
4. Reinforce instructions to the parents that the child should avoid participating in competitive athletics and contact sports to avoid injuring the heart.
5. Reinforce instructions to the parents to inform the dentist of the condition; antibiotics should be taken before dental procedures to prevent endocarditis.
6. Surgical replacement of the aortic root and valve may be necessary.

VI. Fractures (see also Chapter 59)

A. Description
1. A break in the continuity of the bone as a result of trauma, twisting, or bone decalcification

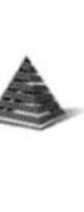

2. Fractures in children usually occur as a result of increased mobility and inadequate or immature motor and cognitive skills; they may result from trauma or bone diseases such as congenital bone disease or bone tumors.

Fractures in infancy are generally rare and warrant further investigation to rule out the possibility of child abuse and recognize bone structure defects.

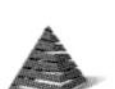

B. Data collection
 1. Pain or tenderness over the involved area
 2. Obvious deformity
 3. Edema
 4. Ecchymosis
 5. Muscle spasm
 6. Loss of function
 7. Crepitation

C. Initial care of a fracture (see Priority Nursing Actions)

PRIORITY NURSING ACTIONS!

Actions to Take if a Child Sustains an Extremity Fracture

1. Check the extent of the injury and immobilize the affected extremity.
2. If a compound fracture exists, cover the wound with a sterile dressing. (Apply a clean dressing if a sterile dressing is unavailable.)
3. Elevate the injured extremity.
4. Apply cold packs to the injured area.
5. Continue to monitor neurovascular status.
6. Transport to the nearest emergency department.

If a child sustains a fracture, the extent of the injury is immediately assessed using the five "Ps"—pain and point of tenderness, pulses distal to fracture site, pallor, paresthesia (sensation) distal to the fracture site, and paralysis (movement distal to fracture site). The extremity is immobilized to prevent movement and further injury to soft tissues. If an open wound is present, it is covered to reduce the risk of infection. The extremity is elevated to reduce swelling, and cold packs are applied to assist in reducing the swelling and to reduce the pain. The neurovascular status is monitored closely, and the child is transported to the nearest emergency facility.

Reference(s): Hockenberry, M., & Wilson, D. (2013). *Wong's: Essentials of pediatric nursing* (9th ed., p. 1059). St. Louis: Mosby.

D. Interventions
 1. Reduction
  a. Restoring the bone to proper alignment
  b. Closed reduction: Accomplished by the manual alignment of the fragments, followed by immobilization
  c. Open reduction: Requires the surgical insertion of internal fixation devices (e.g., rods, wires, pins) that help maintain alignment while healing occurs
 2. Retention: The application of traction or a cast to maintain alignment until healing occurs

E. Traction (see Chapter 59)
 1. Russell's skin traction
  a. Used to stabilize a fractured femur before surgery
  b. Similar to Buck's traction but provides a double pull using a knee sling that pulls at the knee and foot
 2. Balanced suspension
  a. Used with skin or skeletal traction to approximate fractures of the femur, tibia, or fibula
  b. Traction is produced by a counterforce other than the child.
  c. Provide pin care if pins are used with the skeletal traction.
 3. 90-degree–90-degree traction
  a. The lower leg is supported by a boot cast or a calf sling.
  b. A skeletal Steinmann pin or Kirschner wire is placed in the distal fragment of the femur, allowing a 90-degree angle at both the hip and the knee.

 4. Interventions
  a. Maintain the correct amount of weight, as prescribed.
  b. Ensure that the weights hang freely. They must not be resting on the floor or bed.
  c. Check all ropes for fraying and all knots for tightness; be sure that the ropes are appropriately tracking in the grooves of the pulley wheels.

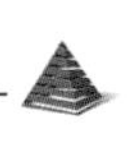

  d. Monitor the neurovascular status of the involved extremity.
  e. Protect the skin from breakdown.

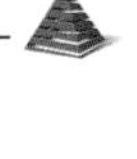

  f. Monitor for signs and symptoms of complications of immobilization, such as constipation, skin breakdown, lung congestion, renal complications, and disuse syndrome of unaffected extremities.
  g. Monitor for sensory deprivation. Provide therapeutic and diversional play.

F. Casts
 1. Description
  a. Made of plaster or fiberglass to provide for the immobilization of bones and joints after a fracture or injury
  b. Fractures of the hip or the knee may require a spica cast.
 2. Interventions
  a. Examine the cast for pressure areas.
  b. Ensure that no rough casting material remains in contact with the skin; assist with petaling the cast edges with waterproof adhesive tape as necessary to ensure a smooth cast edge.
  c. If a hip spica cast is placed, the cast edges around the perineum and buttocks may need to be taped with waterproof tape.

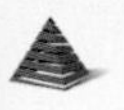

d. Monitor the extremity for circulatory impairment, such as more pain than that expected for the type of injury, edema, rubor, pallor, numbness and tingling, coolness, decreased sensation or mobility, or diminished pulse.

e. Notify the registered nurse immediately if circulatory impairment occurs.

f. Prepare to assist with bivalving or cutting the cast if circulatory impairment occurs; prepare for emergency fasciotomy if cast removal does not improve the neurocirculatory compromise.

g. Reinforce instructions to the family and child not to stick objects down the cast.

h. Reinforce teaching the family and the child to keep the cast clean and dry.

i. Reinforce instructions to the family and the child in isometric exercises to prevent muscle atrophy.

CRITICAL THINKING What Should You Do?

Answer: Compartment syndrome is a condition in which pressure increases in a confined anatomical space, leading to decreased blood flow, ischemia, and dysfunction of these tissues. This complication can occur with casts. Signs of this complication include unrelieved or increased pain in the limb; pale, dusky, or edematous tissue distal to the involved area; pain with passive movement; loss of sensation (paresthesia); and pulselessness (a late sign). The nurse should notify the registered nurse (RN) immediately. The RN will assess the child and then contact the health care provider (HCP) immediately because of the risk of tissue ischemia and necrosis if neurovascular impairment is noted.

Reference(s): Hockenberry, M., & Wilson, D. (2013). *Wong's: Essentials of pediatric nursing* (9th ed., p. 1059). St. Louis: Mosby.

PRACTICE QUESTIONS

371. The nurse is reinforcing instructions to the parents of a child with scoliosis regarding the use of a brace. Which statement by a parent indicates the **need for further teaching**?
1. "I need to have my child wear a soft fabric under the brace."
2. "I will apply lotion under the brace to prevent skin breakdown."
3. "I need to encourage my child to perform the prescribed exercises."
4. "I need to avoid applying powder under the brace, because it will cake."

372. The mother of a child with juvenile idiopathic arthritis calls the nurse because the child is experiencing a painful exacerbation of the disease. The mother asks the nurse if the child should perform range-of-motion (ROM) exercises at this time. The nurse should make which response to the mother?
1. "Avoid all exercise during painful periods."
2. "The ROM exercises must be performed every day."
3. "Have the child perform simple isometric exercises during this time."
4. "Administer additional pain medication before performing the ROM exercises."

373. A 4-year-old child sustains a fall at home and is brought to the emergency department by the mother. After an x-ray, it is determined that the child has a fractured arm, and a plaster cast is applied. The nurse reinforces instructions to the mother regarding cast care for the child. Which statement by the mother indicates the **need for further teaching**?
1. "The cast may feel warm as it dries."
2. "I can use lotion or powder around the cast edges to relieve itching."
3. "A small amount of white shoe polish can touch up a soiled white cast."
4. "If the cast becomes wet, a blow-dryer set on the cool setting may be used to dry it."

374. The nurse is preparing to perform a neurovascular check for tissue perfusion in the child with an arm cast. Which is the **priority** when performing this procedure?
1. Taking the temperature
2. Taking the blood pressure
3. Checking the apical heart rate
4. Checking the peripheral pulse in the affected arm

❖ **375.** The nurse, reinforcing home care instructions, prepares a list for the parents of a child who has a plaster cast applied to the left forearm. Which instructions should be included on the list? **Select all that apply.**
- ❑ 1. Use the fingertips to lift the cast while it is drying.
- ❑ 2. Keep small toys and sharp objects away from the cast.
- ❑ 3. Use a padded ruler or another padded object to scratch the skin under the cast if it itches.
- ❑ 4. Place a heating pad on the lower end of the cast and over the fingers if the fingers feel cold.
- ❑ 5. Contact the health care provider (HCP) if the child complains of numbness or tingling in the extremity.
- ❑ 6. Elevate the extremity on pillows for the first 24 to 48 hours after casting to prevent swelling.

376. The nurse is assisting a health care provider (HCP) during the examination of an infant with hip dysplasia. The HCP performs the Ortolani maneuver.

Which **best** describes the reason for performing the Ortolani maneuver?
1. Determining the extent of range of motion
2. Checking for asymmetry on the affected side
3. Pushing the unstable femoral head out of the acetabulum
4. Reducing the dislocated femoral head back into the acetabulum

377. The nurse provides information to the mother of a 2-week-old infant who was diagnosed with clubfoot at the time of birth. Which statement by the mother indicates the **need for further teaching** regarding this disorder?
1. "Treatment needs to be started as soon as possible."
2. "I realize my child will require follow-up care until full grown."
3. "I need to bring my child back to the clinic in 1 month for a new cast."
4. "I need to come to the clinic every week with my child for the casting."

378. The nurse is assigned to care for a child after a spinal fusion for the treatment of scoliosis. The child complains of abdominal discomfort and begins to have episodes of vomiting. On data collection, the nurse notes abdominal distention. Which action should the nurse take?
1. Administer an antiemetic.
2. Increase the intravenous fluids.
3. Notify the registered nurse (RN).
4. Place the child in a side-lying Sims' position.

379. The nurse is assigned to care for a child who is in skeletal traction. The nurse needs to avoid which action when caring for the child?
1. Keeping the weights hanging freely
2. Ensuring that the ropes are in the pulleys
3. Placing the bed linens on the traction ropes
4. Ensuring that the weights are out of the child's reach

380. The nurse is performing a neurovascular check on a hospitalized child who had a cast applied to the lower leg. The child complains of tingling in the toes distal to the fracture site. Which action should the nurse take?
1. Elevate the extremity.
2. Document the findings.
3. Notify the registered nurse.
4. Ambulate the child with crutches.

ANSWERS

371. 2

Rationale: The use of either lotions or powders should be avoided because they can become sticky or cake under the brace, thus causing irritation. Options 1, 3, and 4 are appropriate statements regarding the care of a child with a brace.

Test-Taking Strategy: Note the strategic words, *need for further teaching.* These words indicate a negative event query and ask you to select an option that is an incorrect statement. Recalling that lotions and powders need to be avoided will direct you to the correct option. **Review: instructions for a child in a brace.**

Level of Cognitive Ability: Evaluating
Client Needs: Physiological Integrity
Integrated Process: Teaching and Learning
Content Area: Child Health: Musculoskeletal
Priority Concepts: Mobility, Tissue Integrity
Reference(s): McKinney et al (2013), p. 1355; Perry, Potter, Ostendorf (2014), p. 271.

372. 3

Rationale: During painful episodes, hot or cold packs, splinting, and positioning the affected joint in a neutral position help to reduce the pain. Although resting the extremity is appropriate, it is important to begin simple isometric or tensing exercises as soon as the child is able. These exercises do not involve joint movement.

Test-Taking Strategy: Use general medication guidelines to assist in eliminating option 4. Additional medication would not be given. Eliminate options 1 and 2 because of the closed-ended words, *all* and *must,* in these options. **Review:** pain management and care during exacerbations of **juvenile idiopathic arthritis.**

Level of Cognitive Ability: Applying
Client Needs: Physiological Integrity
Integrated Process: Nursing Process/Implementation
Content Area: Child Health: Musculoskeletal
Priority Concepts: Inflammation, Pain
Reference(s): McKinney et al (2013), p. 1370.

373. 2

Rationale: The mother needs to be instructed not to use lotion or powders on the skin around the cast edges or inside the cast because they can become sticky or caked and cause skin irritation. Options 1, 3, and 4 are appropriate instructions.

Test-Taking Strategy: Note the strategic words, *need for further teaching.* These words indicate a negative event query and ask you to select an option that is an incorrect statement. Recalling the principles related to routine cast care and the concern of skin breakdown should direct you to the correct option. **Review:** cast care.

Level of Cognitive Ability: Evaluating
Client Needs: Physiological Integrity
Integrated Process: Teaching and Learning

Content Area: Child Health: Musculoskeletal
Priority Concepts: Client Education, Tissue Integrity
Reference(s): McKinney et al (2013), p. 1346.

374. 4
Rationale: The neurovascular check for tissue perfusion is performed on the toes or fingers distal to an injury or cast and includes checking peripheral pulse, color, capillary refill time, warmth, motion, and sensation. Options 1, 2, and 3 may be components of care, but they are not the priority in this situation.
Test-Taking Strategy: Note the **strategic word**, *priority*. Option 4 is the only option that addresses a neurovascular check. Review: **neurovascular check** and **tissue perfusion**.
Level of Cognitive Ability: Applying
Client Needs: Physiological Integrity
Integrated Process: Nursing Process/Data Collection
Content Area: Child Health: Musculoskeletal
Priority Concepts: Perfusion, Tissue Integrity
Reference(s): McKinney et al (2013), p. 1343.

❖375. 2, 5, 6
Rationale: While the cast is drying, the palms of the hands are used to lift the cast. If the fingertips are used, indentations in the cast could occur and cause constant pressure on the underlying skin. Small toys and sharp objects are kept away from the cast, and no objects (including padded objects) are placed inside of the cast because of the risk of altered skin integrity. A heating pad is not applied to the cast or fingers. Cold fingers could indicate neurovascular impairment, and the HCP should be notified. The extremity is elevated to prevent swelling, and the HCP is notified immediately if any signs of neurovascular impairment develop.
Test-Taking Strategy: Focus on the **subject**, cast care instructions. Think about the complications associated with a cast and the safety principles related to the care of a child with a cast. This will assist you with answering the question. **Review: cast care.**
Level of Cognitive Ability: Analyzing
Client Needs: Physiological Integrity
Integrated Process: Teaching and Learning
Content Area: Child Health: Musculoskeletal
Priority Concepts: Safety, Tissue Integrity
Reference(s): Hockenberry, Wilson (2013), p. 1061.

376. 4
Rationale: With the Ortolani maneuver, the examiner reduces the dislocated femoral head back into the acetabulum. A positive Ortolani maneuver is a palpable clunk as the femoral head moves over the acetabular ring. Options 1 and 2 are data collection techniques for the identification of the clinical manifestations of hip dysplasia, but they do not describe the Ortolani maneuver. When performing the Barlow maneuver, the examiner pushes the unstable femoral head out of the acetabulum.
Test-Taking Strategy: Focus on the **subject**, the reason for performing the Ortolani maneuver. Also note the **strategic word**, *best*. Eliminate options 1 and 2 first, because they are **comparable or alike** and are data collection techniques. From the remaining options, it is necessary to know the action/purpose of the Ortolani maneuver. **Review: developmental dysplasia of the hip.**
Level of Cognitive Ability: Understanding
Client Needs: Physiological Integrity
Integrated Process: Nursing Process/Data Collection
Content Area: Child Health: Musculoskeletal
Priority Concepts: Mobility, Safety
Reference(s): Hockenberry, Wilson (2013), p. 1069.

377. 3
Rationale: The treatment for clubfoot is started as soon as possible after birth. Serial manipulation and casting are performed at least weekly. If sufficient correction is not achieved within 3 to 6 months, surgery is usually indicated. Because clubfoot can recur, all children with the condition require long-term interval follow-up until they reach skeletal maturity to ensure an optimal outcome.
Test-Taking Strategy: Focus on the **subject**, the treatment plan for clubfoot. Note the **strategic words**, *need for further teaching*. These words indicate a **negative event query** and the need to select the incorrect statement. This will assist you with eliminating options 1 and 2. Recalling that serial manipulations and casting are required weekly will direct you to the correct option. **Review: clubfoot.**
Level of Cognitive Ability: Evaluating
Client Needs: Physiological Integrity
Integrated Process: Teaching and Learning
Content Area: Child Health: Musculoskeletal
Priority Concepts: Client Education, Mobility
Reference(s): McKinney et al (2013), pp. 1365–1367.

378. 3
Rationale: A complication after the surgical treatment of scoliosis is superior mesenteric artery syndrome. This disorder is caused by mechanical changes in the position of the child's abdominal contents that result from the lengthening of the child's body. It results in a syndrome of emesis and abdominal distention that is similar to that which occurs with intestinal obstruction or paralytic ileus. Postoperative vomiting among children with body casts or among those who have undergone spinal fusion warrants attention because of the possibility of superior mesenteric artery syndrome. Therefore, the remaining options are incorrect.
Test-Taking Strategy: Focus on the **subject**, the complications of spinal fusion. Eliminate option 2 first because it should not be implemented without a prescription. Eliminate option 4 next because this child requires logrolling, and the Sims' position may cause injury after surgery. From the remaining options, note the signs and symptoms in the question. These should alert you that the registered nurse needs to be notified, who will then contact the health care provider. **Review: scoliosis.**
Level of Cognitive Ability: Analyzing
Client Needs: Physiological Integrity
Integrated Process: Nursing Process/Implementation
Content Area: Child Health: Musculoskeletal
Priority Concepts: Clinical Judgment, Safety
Reference(s): Hockenberry, Wilson (2013), pp. 1078–1079.

379. 3
Rationale: Bed linens should not be placed on the traction ropes because of the risk of disrupting the traction apparatus. Options 1, 2, and 4 are appropriate measures when caring for a child who is in skeletal traction.

Test-Taking Strategy: Focus on the subject, the action that the nurse avoids. This tells you that you need to select an option that is an incorrect intervention. Use knowledge regarding the care of the child in traction to direct you to the correct option. Review: child in traction.
Level of Cognitive Ability: Applying
Client Needs: Safe and Effective Care Environment
Integrated Process: Nursing Process/Implementation
Content Area: Child Health: Musculoskeletal
Priority Concepts: Mobility, Safety
Reference(s): Hockenberry, Wilson (2013), p. 1065.

380. 3
Rationale: Reduced sensation to touch or complaints of numbness or tingling at a site distal to the fracture may indicate poor tissue perfusion. This finding should be reported to the registered nurse or health care provider. Options 1, 2, and 4 are inappropriate and would delay the required and immediate interventions.
Test-Taking Strategy: Focus on the subject, the action that the nurse should take. Note the data in the question and recall the signs of circulatory compromise. Noting the child's complaint will assist with directing you to the correct option. **Review:** casts.
Level of Cognitive Ability: Applying
Client Needs: Physiological Integrity
Integrated Process: Nursing Process/Implementation
Content Area: Child Health: Musculoskeletal
Priority Concepts: Perfusion, Tissue Integrity
Reference(s): Hockenberry, Wilson (2013), p. 1060.

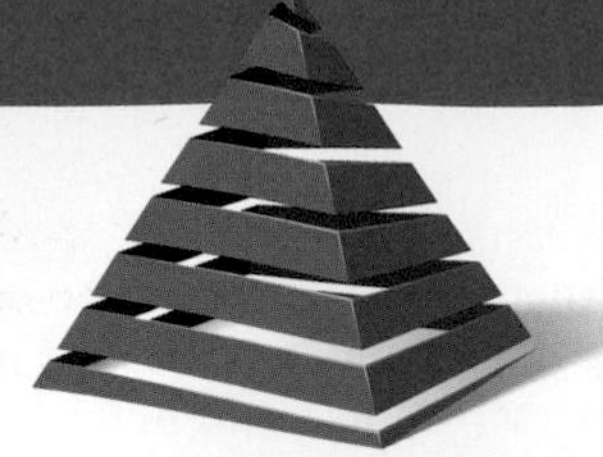

Pediatric

CHAPTER 39

Communicable Diseases and Acquired Immunodeficiency Syndrome

CRITICAL THINKING What Should You Do?

The nurse notes that a 1-year-old infant with human immunodeficiency virus (HIV) has a temperature of 101.2°F axillary. What should the nurse do?
Answer located on p. 472.

I. Rubeola (Measles)

A. Description
1. Agent: Paramyxovirus virus
2. Incubation period: 10 to 20 days
3. Communicable period: From 4 days before to 5 days after the rash appears; mainly during the **prodromal** stage (this pertains to early symptoms that may mark the onset of disease)
4. Source: Respiratory tract secretions, blood, or urine of an infected person
5. Transmission: Airborne particles, direct contact with infectious droplets, or transplacental transmission

B. Data collection
1. Fever
2. Malaise
3. The "three Cs": Coryza, cough, and conjunctivitis
4. Rash appears as red, erythematous maculopapular eruption starting on the face and spreading downward to the feet; blanches easily with pressure and gradually turns a brownish color (lasts 6 to 7 days); may have desquamation.
5. Koplik spots: Small, red spots with a bluish-white center and a red base. They are located on the buccal mucosa and last for approximately 3 days.

C. Interventions
1. Use airborne droplet precautions if the child is hospitalized.
2. Restrict the child to quiet activities and bed rest.
3. Use a cool-mist vaporizer for cough and coryza.
4. Dim the lights if photophobia is present.
5. Administer antipyretics for fever, as prescribed.

II. Roseola (Exanthema Subitum)

A. Description
1. Agent: Human herpesvirus type 6
2. Incubation period: 5 to 15 days
3. Communicable period: Unknown, but thought to extend from the febrile stage to the time that the rash first appears
4. Source and transmission: Unknown

B. Data collection
1. Sudden high fever (greater than 102°F) of 3 to 5 days' duration in a child who appears well, followed by a rash (rose-pink macules that blanch with pressure)
2. The rash appears several hours to 2 days after the fever subsides and lasts 1 to 2 days.

C. Interventions: Supportive

III. Rubella (German Measles)

A. Description
1. Agent: Rubella virus
2. Incubation period: 14 to 21 days
3. Communicable period: 7 days before to about 5 days after the rash appears
4. Source: Nasopharyngeal secretions. The virus is also present in the blood, stool, and urine.
5. Transmission
   a. Airborne or direct contact with infectious droplets
   b. Indirectly via articles that have been freshly contaminated with nasopharyngeal secretions, feces, or urine
   c. Transplacental

B. Data collection
1. Low-grade fever
2. Malaise
3. Pinkish-red maculopapular rash that begins on the face and spreads to the entire body within 1 to 3 days
4. Petechiae red, pinpoint spots may occur on the soft palate.

C. Interventions
1. Use airborne droplet precautions if the child is hospitalized; provide supportive treatment.
2. Isolate the infected child from pregnant women.

IV. Mumps

A. Description

1. Agent: Paramyxovirus
2. Incubation period: 14 to 21 days
3. Communicable period: Immediately before and after parotid gland swelling begins
4. Source: The saliva of an infected person and possibly the urine
5. Transmission: Direct contact or droplet spread from an infected person

B. Data collection

1. Fever
2. Headache and malaise
3. Anorexia
4. Jaw or ear pain aggravated by chewing, followed by parotid glandular swelling
5. Orchitis may occur.
6. Aseptic meningitis may occur.

C. Interventions

1. Institute airborne droplet precautions.
2. Provide bed rest until the parotid gland swelling subsides.
3. Avoid foods that require chewing.
4. Apply hot or cold compresses to the neck, as prescribed.
5. Apply warmth and local support with snug-fitting underpants to relieve orchitis.
6. Monitor closely for signs of aseptic meningitis, a complication of mumps (see Chapter 37 for information on meningitis).

V. Chickenpox (Varicella)

A. Description

1. Agent: Varicella zoster virus
2. Incubation period: 13 to 17 days
3. Communicable period: 1 to 2 days before the onset of the rash to 6 days after the first crop of vesicles, when crusts have formed
4. Source: Respiratory tract secretions of an infected person; skin lesions
5. Transmission: Direct contact, droplet (airborne) spread, and contaminated objects

B. Data collection

1. Slight fever, malaise, and anorexia are followed by a macular rash that first appears on the trunk and scalp and then moves to the face and extremities
2. Lesions become pustules, begin to dry, and develop a crust.
3. Lesions may appear on the mucous membranes of the mouth, the genital area, and the rectal area.

C. Interventions

1. In the hospital setting, ensure strict isolation (i.e., contact and droplet precautions).
2. In the home setting, isolate the infected child until the vesicles have dried.
3. The antiviral agent acyclovir (Zovirax) may be used to treat varicella infections in susceptible immunocompromised persons to decrease the number of lesions; shorten the duration of fever; and decrease itching, lethargy, and anorexia.
4. The use of VCZ immune globulin (VariZIG) or intravenous immune globulin (IVIG) is recommended for children who are immunocompromised, who have no previous history of varicella, and who are likely to contract the disease and have complications as a result.
5. Provide supportive care.

Isolate high-risk children, such as children who have immunosuppressive disorders, from a child with a communicable disease.

VI. Pertussis (Whooping Cough)

A. Description

1. Agent: Bordetella pertussis
2. Incubation period: 5 to 21 days (usually 10 days)
3. Communicable period: Greatest during the catarrhal stage (i.e., when discharge from respiratory secretions occurs)
4. Source: Discharge from the respiratory tract of the infected person
5. Transmission: Direct contact or droplet spread from the infected person; indirect contact with freshly contaminated articles

B. Data collection

1. Symptoms of respiratory infection followed by increased severity of cough with a loud whooping inspiration
2. May experience **cyanosis**, respiratory distress, and tongue protrusion
3. Listlessness, irritability, and anorexia

C. Interventions

1. Isolate the child during the catarrhal stage. If the child is hospitalized, institute droplet precautions.
2. Antimicrobial therapy may be prescribed.
3. Reduce environmental factors that cause coughing spasms, such as dust, smoke, and sudden changes in temperature. 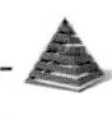
4. Ensure adequate hydration and nutrition.
5. Provide suction and humidified oxygen, if needed.
6. Monitor the cardiopulmonary status (via a monitor as prescribed) and pulse oximetry.
7. Infants do not receive maternal immunity to pertussis.

VII. Diphtheria

A. Description

1. Agent: Corynebacterium diphtheriae
2. Incubation period: 2 to 5 days
3. Communicable period: Variable; until virulent bacilli are no longer present (three negative cultures of discharge from the nose, nasopharynx,

skin, and other lesions); usually 2 weeks but can be as long as 4 weeks
4. Source: Discharge from the mucous membrane of the nose, nasopharynx, skin, and other lesions of the infected person
5. Transmission: Direct contact with an infected person, carrier, or contaminated articles

B. Data collection
1. Low-grade fever, malaise, and sore throat
2. Foul-smelling and mucopurulent nasal discharge
3. Dense pseudomembrane formation in the throat that may interfere with eating, drinking, and breathing
4. Lymphadenitis, neck edema, and "bull neck"

C. Interventions
1. Ensure strict isolation for the hospitalized child.
2. Assist to administer diphtheria antitoxin, as prescribed (after a skin or conjunctival test to rule out sensitivity to horse serum).
3. Provide bed rest.
4. Assist to administer antibiotics, as prescribed.
5. Provide suction and humidified oxygen, as needed.
6. Provide tracheostomy care if a tracheostomy is necessary.

VIII. Poliomyelitis

A. Description
1. Agent: Enteroviruses
2. Incubation period: 7 to 14 days
3. Communicable period: Unknown. The virus is present in the throat and feces shortly after infection and persists for about 1 week in the throat and 4 to 6 weeks in the feces.
4. Source: The oropharyngeal secretions and feces of an infected person
5. Transmission: Direct contact with an infected person; fecal-oral and oropharyngeal routes

B. Data collection
1. Fever, malaise, anorexia, nausea, headache, and sore throat
2. Abdominal pain followed by soreness and stiffness of the trunk, neck, and limbs that may progress to central nervous system paralysis

C. Interventions
1. Enteric precautions
2. Supportive treatment
3. Bed rest
4. Monitoring for signs of respiratory paralysis
5. Physical therapy

IX. Scarlet Fever

A. Description
1. Agent: Group A β-hemolytic streptococci
2. Incubation period: 1 to 7 days
3. Communicable period: During the incubation period and clinical illness; during the first 2 weeks of the carrier stage, although this stage may persist for months
4. Source: Nasopharyngeal secretions of an infected person or carriers
5. Transmission: Direct contact with an infected person or droplet spread; indirectly by contact with contaminated articles or the ingestion of contaminated milk or other foods

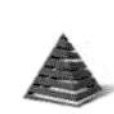
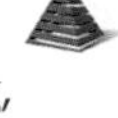

B. Data collection
1. Abrupt high fever, flushed cheeks, vomiting, headache, enlarged lymph nodes in the neck, malaise, and abdominal pain
2. A red, fine, sandpaper-like rash develops in the axilla, groin, and neck and spreads to cover the entire body, except the face
3. The rash blanches with pressure (Schultz-Charlton reaction), except in areas of deep creases and folds of the joints (Pastia's sign).
4. Desquamation, a sheet-like sloughing of the skin of the palms and soles, appears by week 1 to week 3.
5. The tongue is initially coated with a white, furry covering with red projecting papillae (white strawberry tongue). By the third to fifth day, the white coat sloughs off, leaving a red, swollen tongue (red strawberry tongue).
6. Tonsils are reddened, edematous, and covered with exudate.
7. Pharynx is edematous and beefy red.

C. Interventions
1. Institute respiratory precautions until 24 hours after the initiation of antibiotic therapy.
2. Provide supportive therapy.
3. Provide bed rest.
4. Encourage fluid intake.

X. Erythema Infectiosum (Fifth Disease)

A. Description
1. Agent: Human parvovirus B19
2. Incubation period: 4 to 14 days; may be as long as 20 days
3. Communicable period: Uncertain, but before the onset of symptoms in most children
4. Source: Infected person
5. Transmission: Unknown; possibly respiratory secretions and blood

B. Data collection
1. Before rash, asymptomatic or mild fever, malaise, headache, and runny nose
2. Stages of the rash
   a. Erythema of the face (slapped-cheek appearance) develops, chiefly on the cheeks, and disappears by 1 to 4 days.
   b. About 1 day after the rash appears on the face, maculopapular red spots appear and are symmetrically distributed on the extremities. The rash progresses from the proximal to distal surfaces and may last a week or more.

c. The rash subsides but may reappear if the skin is irritated or traumatized by factors such as the sun, heat, cold, exercise, or friction.

C. Interventions
1. The child is not usually hospitalized.
2. Pregnant women should avoid the infected individual.
3. Provide supportive care.
4. Assist to administer antipyretics, analgesics, and anti-inflammatory medications, as prescribed.

XI. Infectious Mononucleosis

A. Description
1. Agent: Epstein-Barr virus
2. Incubation period: 4 to 6 weeks
3. Communicable period: Unknown
4. Source: Oral secretions
5. Transmission: Direct intimate contact

B. Data collection
1. Fever, sore throat, malaise, headache, fatigue, nausea, abdominal pain, and enlarged, red tonsils
2. Lymphadenopathy and hepatosplenomegaly
3. A discrete macular rash that is most prominent over the trunk may occur.

C. Interventions
1. Provide supportive care.
2. Monitor for signs of splenic rupture.

Teach the parents of a child with mononucleosis to monitor for signs of splenic rupture, which include abdominal pain, left upper quadrant pain, and left shoulder pain.

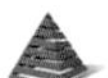

XII. Rocky Mountain Spotted Fever

A. Description
1. Agent: Rickettsia rickettsii
2. Incubation period: 2 to 14 days
3. Source: Tick from a mammal source, most often from wild rodents and dogs
4. Transmission: The bite of an infected tick

B. Data collection
1. Fever, malaise, anorexia, vomiting, headache, and myalgia
2. A maculopapular or petechial rash primarily on the extremities (ankles and wrists) but that may spread to other areas; characteristically on the palms and soles

C. Interventions
1. Provide vigorous supportive care.
2. Assist to administer antibiotics, as prescribed.
3. Reinforce teaching to the child and parents about protection from tick bites (Box 39-1).

BOX 39-1 Protection from Tick Bites

Wear long-sleeved shirts, long pants tucked into long socks (socks should be pulled up over the pant legs), and a hat when walking in tick-infested areas.
Wear light-colored clothing to make ticks more visible if they get onto the child.
Check children for the presence of ticks after they have been in high-risk or tick-infested areas.
Follow paths rather than walking in tall grass and shrub areas because these are the places where most ticks are found.
Apply insect repellents containing diethyltoluamide (DEET) and permethrin before possible exposure to areas where ticks are found (use with caution in infants and small children).
Keep yards at home trimmed and free of accumulating leaves and other brush.
Apply tick repellent to dogs.
Save the tick for later identification if it is removed from the child's body.

XIII. Community-Associated Methicillin-Resistant *Staphylococcus aureus* (CA-MRSA)

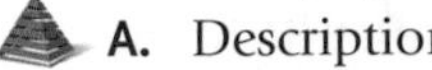

A. Description
1. *Staphylococcus aureus* is a bacterium that is normally located on the skin or in the nose of healthy people. When present without symptoms, it is called *colonization*, and when symptoms are present, it is called an *infection*.
2. MRSA is a strain of *S. aureus* that is resistant to methicillin and most often occurs in people who were hospitalized or treated at a health care facility (hospital-acquired MRSA).
3. CA-MRSA is a MRSA infection that occurs in a healthy person who has not been hospitalized or had a medical procedure done within the past year.
4. Persons at risk for community-associated MRSA include athletes, prisoners, day care attendees, military recruits, persons who abuse intravenous drugs, persons living in crowded settings, persons with poor hygiene practices, persons who use contaminated items, persons who get tattoos, and persons with a compromised immune system.
5. Community-associated MRSA is spread through person-to-person contact, contact with contaminated items, or infection of a preexisting cut or wound that is not protected by a dressing.
6. The bacteria can enter the bloodstream through the cut or wound and cause sepsis, cellulitis, endocarditis, osteomyelitis, septic arthritis, toxic shock syndrome, pneumonia, organ failure, and death.

B. Prevention measures

1. Hand washing and practicing good personal hygiene
2. Avoiding sharing of personal items
3. Regular cleaning of shared equipment such as athletic equipment, whirlpools, or saunas
4. Cleaning a cut or wound thoroughly

C. Data collection
1. Appearance of a skin infection: Red, swollen area, warmth around the area, drainage of pus, pain at the site, fever
2. Symptoms of a more serious infection: Chest pain, cough, fatigue, chills, fever, malaise, headache, muscle aches, shortness of breath, rash

D. Interventions
1. Check skin lesions.
2. Prepare to drain an infected skin site and culture the wound and wound drainage.
3. Prepare to obtain blood cultures, sputum cultures, and urine cultures.
4. Prepare to administer antibiotics as prescribed.
5. Reinforce educating the parent and family about the causes and modes of transmission, signs and symptoms, and importance of treatment prescribed.

XIV. Influenza

A. Description
1. Various strains of influenza can occur.
2. It is a viral infection that affects the respiratory system and is highly contagious.
3. Children, pregnant women, persons with preexisting health conditions, and persons with a compromised immune system are at high risk for developing complications.
4. It is caused by contact with an infected person or by touching something such as a toy or tissue that the infected person has touched.

B. Prevention
1. Flu **vaccine**
2. Wash the child's hands frequently and teach hand-washing techniques.
3. Avoid children who are ill.
4. Keep the child home from school or away from others until the child has been fever-free (without the use of antipyretics) for at least 24 hours.
5. For additional information, refer to Centers for Disease Control and Prevention (CDC) website: http://www.cdc.gov/vaccines/schedules/index.html.

The signs and symptoms of flu usually last a week. If they last longer, the presence of complications should be suspected.

C. Data collection
1. Fever that occurs suddenly and is high
2. Headache, body aches, fatigue, chills, cough, congestion, sore throat, loss of appetite, vomiting, diarrhea

D. Interventions
1. Antiviral medications if prescribed, fluids, rest, pain relievers such as acetaminophen (Tylenol) or ibuprofen (Motrin)
2. Reinforce family and child teaching about prevention measures.

XV. Immunizations

A. Guidelines (see Priority Nursing Actions)

PRIORITY NURSING ACTIONS!

Actions to Take When Administering a Parenteral Vaccine

1. Verify the prescription for the vaccine.
2. Obtain an immunization history from the parents and assess for allergies.
3. Provide information to the parents about the vaccine.
4. Obtain parental consent.
5. Check the lot number and expiration date and prepare the injection.
6. Select the appropriate site for administration.
7. Administer the vaccine.
8. Document the administration and site of administration and lot number and expiration date of the vaccine.
9. Provide a vaccination record to the parents.

The nurse should first verify the prescription and then obtain an immunization history from the parents to ensure that the immunizations are up to date. The nurse should also question the parents about the presence of any allergies in the child because some vaccines contain components to which the child may be allergic. The nurse next provides information to the parents about the vaccine and obtains consent. The expiration date and the lot number (located on the medication vial) of the vaccine should be checked before preparing the vaccine for administration. When the vaccine is prepared, the nurse prepares the child for the procedure, selects an appropriate site, and administers the vaccine. The nurse documents that the vaccination has been administered and provides an updated immunization record to the parents.

Reference(s): Hockenberry, M., & Wilson, D. (2013). *Wong's: Essentials of pediatric nursing* (9th ed., p. 341). St. Louis: Mosby.
McKinney, E., James, S., Murray, S., Nelson, K. & Ashwill, J. (2013). *Maternal-child nursing* (4th ed., p. 85). St. Louis: Elsevier.

1. In the United States, the recommended age for beginning primary immunizations of infants is at birth.
2. Children who began primary immunizations at the recommended age but failed to receive all of the required doses do not need to begin the series again. Rather, they need to receive only the missed doses.
3. If there is a suspicion that the parent will not  bring the child to the pediatrician or health care clinic for follow-up immunizations according to the optimal immunization schedule, any of the recommended vaccines can be administered simultaneously.

B. General contraindications and precautions

1. A vaccine is contraindicated if the child experienced an anaphylactic reaction to a previously administered vaccine or a component in the vaccine.
2. Live virus vaccines generally are not administered to individuals with severely deficient immune systems, those with a severe sensitivity to gelatin, or pregnant women.
3. A vaccine is administered with caution to an individual with a moderate or severe acute illness, with or without fever.

C. Guidelines for administration (Box 39-2)

⚠ Children born prematurely should receive the full dose of each vaccine at the appropriate chronological age.

BOX 39-2 Guidelines for the Administration of Vaccines

Follow the manufacturer's recommendations for the route of administration, storage, and the reconstitution of the vaccine.

If refrigeration is necessary, store the vaccine on a center shelf and not on the door. Frequent temperature changes from opening the refrigerator door can alter the potency of the vaccine.

A vaccine information statement needs to be given to the parents or the individual, and informed consent for administration needs to be obtained.

Check the expiration date on the vaccine bottle.

Parenteral vaccines are given in separate syringes at different injection sites.

Vaccines that are administered intramuscularly are given in the vastus lateralis muscle (best site) or the ventrogluteal muscle. The deltoid can be used for children 36 months and older; the dorsogluteal site (the buttocks) is avoided.

Vaccines that are administered subcutaneously are given into the fatty areas in the lateral upper arms and the anterior thighs.

Adequate needle length and gauge are as follows: intramuscular, 1 inch, 23 to 25 gauge; subcutaneous, 5/8 inch, 25 gauge (needle length may vary, depending on the child's size).

Mild side effects may include fever, soreness, swelling, or redness at the injection site.

A topical anesthetic may be applied to the injection site before the injection.

For painful or red injection sites, advise the parent to apply cool compresses for the first 24 hours and to then use warm or cool compresses as long as needed.

An age-appropriate dose of acetaminophen (Tylenol) or ibuprofen (Motrin), per health care provider's preference, may be administered every 4 to 6 hours for vaccine-associated discomfort.

Maintain an immunization record: document the day, month, and year of administration; the manufacturer and lot number of vaccine; the name, address, and title of the person who administered the vaccine; and the site and route of administration.

A vaccine adverse event report needs to be filed and the health department needs to be notified if an adverse reaction to an immunization occurs.

D. Recommended immunization schedules: For the most up-to-date information about schedules and specific information for each type of vaccine, refer to Centers for Disease Control and Prevention (CDC) website: http://www.cdc.gov/vaccines/schedules/index.html.

XVI. Reactions to a Vaccine

A. Local reactions

1. Tenderness, erythema, and swelling at the injection site
2. Low-grade fever
3. Behavioral changes, such as drowsiness, unusual crying, and eating less

B. Minimizing local reactions

1. Select a needle of adequate length to deposit the vaccine deep into the muscle or subcutaneous mass.
2. Inject the vaccine into the appropriate, recommended site.

C. Anaphylactic reactions

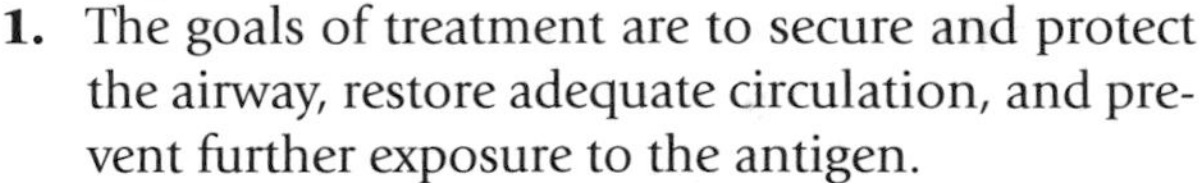

1. The goals of treatment are to secure and protect the airway, restore adequate circulation, and prevent further exposure to the antigen.
2. For a mild reaction with no evidence of respiratory distress or cardiovascular compromise, a subcutaneous injection of an antihistamine such as diphenhydramine (Benadryl), and epinephrine (Adrenalin) may be prescribed.
3. For moderate or severe distress, establish an airway; provide cardiopulmonary resuscitation to the child if necessary; elevate the head; epinephrine, fluids, and vasopressors may be prescribed; monitor the vital signs and the urine output.

XVII. Acquired Immunodeficiency Syndrome (AIDS)

A. Description

1. AIDS is a disorder caused by human immunodeficiency virus (HIV) and characterized by generalized dysfunction of the immune system (Fig. 39-1).
2. HIV virus infects the $CD4^+$ T cells; a gradual decrease in the $CD4^+$ T cell count occurs, and this results in a progressive immune deficiency; the risk for opportunistic infections is present.
3. HIV is transmitted through blood, semen, vaginal secretions, and breast milk; the incubation period is months to years.
4. Horizontal transmission occurs through intimate sexual contact or parenteral exposure to blood or body fluids that contain blood.
5. Vertical (perinatal) transmission occurs through transmission from an HIV-infected pregnant woman to her fetus. (See Chapter 26 for additional information on HIV.)

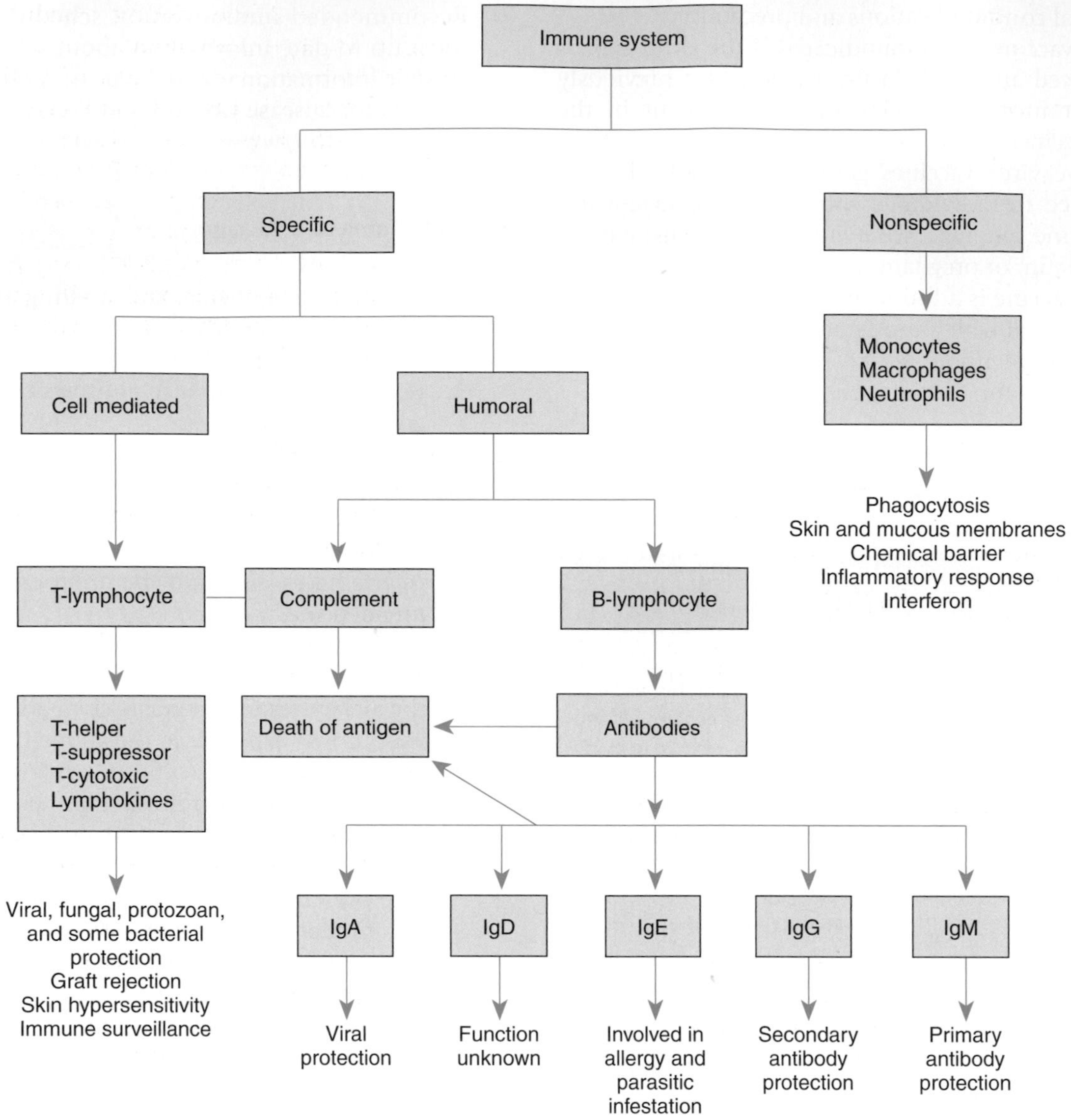

Immune system
Specific
Nonspecific
Cell mediated
Humoral
Monocytes
Macrophages
Neutrophils
Phagocytosis
Skin and mucous membranes
Chemical barrier
Inflammatory response
Interferon
T-lymphocyte
Complement
B-lymphocyte
T-helper
T-suppressor
T-cytotoxic
Lymphokines
Death of antigen
Antibodies
Viral, fungal, protozoan, and some bacterial protection
Graft rejection
Skin hypersensitivity
Immune surveillance
IgA
IgD
IgE
IgG
IgM
Viral protection
Function unknown
Involved in allergy and parasitic infestation
Secondary antibody protection
Primary antibody protection

FIGURE 39-1 Components of the immune system. (From Hockenberry M, Wilson D: *Wong's: Nursing care of infants and children,* ed 9, St. Louis, 2013, Mosby.)

6. The most common opportunistic infection that occurs in children infected with HIV is *Pneumocystis jiroveci* pneumonia; most frequently occurs between the ages of 3 and 6 months.

The infant or child infected with HIV is at risk for developing an opportunistic infection that can be life-threatening. Monitor the infant or child closely for signs of infection, and report these signs immediately if they occur.

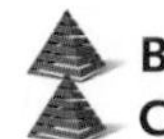

B. Data collection (Boxes 39-3 and 39-4)

C. Diagnostic tests: Before testing, counseling should be provided to parents; issues that should be addressed include the causes of HIV, reasons for testing, implications of positive test results,

BOX 39-3 Common Data Collection Findings in Children with HIV Infection

Chronic cough
Chronic or recurrent diarrhea
Developmental delay or regression of developmental milestones
Failure to thrive
Hepatosplenomegaly
Lymphadenopathy
Malaise and fatigue
Night sweats
Oral candidiasis
Parotitis
Weight loss

Adapted from Perry S, Hockenberry M, Lowdermilk D, Wilson D: *Maternal-child nursing care,* ed 4, St. Louis, 2010, Mosby.

BOX 39-4 Common AIDS-Defining Conditions in Children

Candidal esophagitis
Cryptosporidiosis
Cytomegalovirus disease
Herpes simplex disease
HIV encephalopathy
Lymphoid interstitial pneumonitis
Mycobacterium avium-intracellulare infection
Pneumocystis jiroveci pneumonia
Pulmonary candidiasis
Recurrent bacterial infections
Wasting syndrome

From Perry S, Hockenberry M, Lowdermilk D, Wilson D: *Maternal-child nursing care*, ed 4, St. Louis, 2010, Elsevier.

confidentiality issues, and beneficial effects of early intervention (Table 39-1).

D. Care of the child with HIV infection or AIDS

1. Multidisciplinary health care approach is taken; primary goals are to decelerate the replication of the virus, prevent opportunistic infections, provide nutritional support, treat symptoms, and treat opportunistic infections.
2. Prophylaxis (*P. jiroveci* pneumonia and other opportunistic infections)
   - **a.** Provide prophylaxis as prescribed against *P. jiroveci* pneumonia and other opportunistic infections, particularly during the first year of life of an infant born to an HIV-infected mother.
   - **b.** After 1 year of age, the need for prophylaxis is determined on the basis of the presence and severity of immunosuppression or a history of *P. jiroveci* pneumonia.
   - **c.** Continuing prophylaxis is based on the child's HIV status, history of opportunistic infections, and CD4+ counts.
3. Antiretroviral medications (refer to Chapter 62)
   - **a.** The goal of antiretroviral medications is to suppress viral replication to slow the decline in the number of CD4+ cells, preserve immune function, reduce the incidence and severity of opportunistic infections, and delay disease progression.
   - **b.** The medications affect different stages of the HIV life cycle to prevent reproduction of new virus particles.
   - **c.** Combination therapy may be prescribed and includes the use of more than one antiretroviral medication.

Before administering an antiretroviral medication, ensure that the medication is safe for pediatric administration. Also check the contraindications for use and the adverse effects.

4. Immunizations: Symptomatic HIV or severe immunosuppression
   - **a.** Only the inactivated influenza vaccine that is given intramuscularly should be used (influenza vaccine should be given yearly).
   - **b.** Measles vaccine should not be given; immunoglobulin may be prescribed after measles exposure.
   - **c.** Only the inactivated polio vaccine that is given intramuscularly should be used.

TABLE 39-1 Diagnostic Tests for HIV

Test	Age-Appropriate Use	Test Determines	Special Considerations
Enzyme-linked immunosorbent assay (ELISA)	18 mo or older	Response of antibodies to HIV virus	If used and found to be positive in infants younger than 18 mo, indicates only that the mother is infected because maternal antibodies are transmitted transplacentally; another diagnostic test is used.
Western blot	18 mo or older	Presence of HIV antibodies	Same as above
Polymerase chain reaction (PCR)	Younger than 18 mo	Presence of proviral DNA	Very accurate for diagnosing infants 1-4 mo of age
p24 antigen	Younger than 18 mo	HIV antigen specific	Very accurate for diagnosing infants 1-4 mo of age
CD4+ lymphocyte count, T-lymphocyte count	Infant up to 13 yr	Immune system status related specifically to suppression	Age adjustment is essential because normal counts are relatively high in infants and steadily decline until 6 yr of age. Severe suppression in all age groups is <15% total lymphocytes (less than 750 cells/L in an infant younger than 12 mo, less than 500 cells/L in a child 1-5 yr, less than 200 cells/L in a child 6-12 yr).

Branson BM, Handsfield HH, Lampe MA, et al.; *Centers for Disease Control and Prevention: Revised recommendations for HIV testing of adults, adolescents, and pregnant women in health-care settings.* MMWR Recomm Rep 2006;55(RR14):1–17. Available from: http://www.cdc.gov/mmwr/preview/mmwrhtml/rr5514a1.htm

d. Rotavirus vaccine should not be given.
e. Varicella zoster virus vaccine should not be given; varicella zoster immunoglobulin may be prescribed after chickenpox exposure.
f. Tetanus immune globulin may be prescribed for tetanus-prone wounds.

! Immunizations against common childhood illnesses are recommended for all children exposed to or infected with HIV.

5. Caregiver instructions
   a. Encourage routine good hygiene and frequent hand washing.
   b. Monitor for fever, malaise, fatigue, weight loss, vomiting, diarrhea, altered activity level, and oral lesions. Notify the health care provider if these occur.
   c. Monitor for signs and symptoms of opportunistic infections, such as pneumonia.
   d. Administer antiretroviral medications and other medications, as prescribed. Emphasize the importance of strict adherence to the treatment regimen.
   e. The child needs to be restricted from having contact with persons who have infections or other contagious or potentially contagious illnesses.
   f. Keep immunizations up to date.
   g. Keep the child home when he or she is sick.
   h. Avoid direct unprotected contact with the child's body fluids.
   i. Monitor the child's weight.
   j. Provide a high-calorie, high-protein diet (appetite stimulants may be prescribed).
   k. Do not share eating utensils with the child.
   l. Wash all eating utensils in the dishwasher.
   m. Cover any of the child's unused food and formula and refrigerate (discard unused refrigerated formula and food after 24 hours).
   n. Do not allow the child to eat fresh fruits or vegetables or raw meat or fish (neutropenic diet if immunosuppressed).
   o. Avoid sharing objects that may become contaminated with blood, such as toothbrushes.
   p. Wear gloves when caring for the child, especially when in contact with body fluids and changing diapers.
   q. Change diapers frequently and away from food areas.
   r. Fold soiled disposable diapers inward, close with tabs, and dispose in a tightly covered plastic-lined container.
   s. Dispose of trash daily.
   t. Clean up any of the child's body fluid spills with bleach solution (10:1 ratio of water to bleach).

E. Teaching points for an adolescent infected with HIV
   1. High-risk behaviors and the importance of avoiding high-risk behaviors
   2. Methods of transmission of HIV
   3. The importance of abstinence from sexual contact, such as intercourse
   4. The importance of using safe condoms if intercourse is planned
   5. Resources available for support and other issues

CRITICAL THINKING What Should You Do?

Answer: An infant or child infected with HIV is at risk for developing a life-threatening opportunistic infection. The nurse should monitor the infant or child closely for signs of infection and report these signs immediately if they occur. The normal axillary temperature for a 1-year-old infant is 97° to 99°F. A temperature of 101.2°F axillary may be indicative of the presence of an opportunistic infection and needs to be reported immediately to the registered nurse who will contact the health care provider (HCP).

Reference(s): McKinney, E., James, S., Murray, S., Nelson, K. & Ashwill, J. (2013). *Maternal-child nursing* (4th ed., pp. 727–728). St. Louis: Elsevier.

PRACTICE QUESTIONS

381. A child with rubeola (measles) is being admitted to the hospital. When preparing for the admission of the child, which precautions should be implemented?
1. Enteric
2. Contact
3. Protective
4. Respiratory

382. The nurse reinforces instructions regarding respiratory precautions to the mother of a child with mumps. The mother asks the nurse about the length of time required for the respiratory precautions. The nurse should base the response on which information about mumps?
1. Respiratory isolation is not necessary.
2. Mumps is not transmitted by the respiratory system.
3. Respiratory precautions are indicated during the period of communicability.
4. Respiratory precautions are indicated for 18 days after the onset of parotid swelling.

383. A 6-month-old infant receives a diphtheria, tetanus, and acellular pertussis (DTap) immunization at the well-baby clinic. The mother returns home and calls the clinic to report that the infant

has developed swelling and redness at the site of injection. Which instruction by the nurse is appropriate?
1. Monitor the infant for a fever.
2. Bring the infant back to the clinic.
3. Apply an ice pack to the injection site.
4. Leave the injection site alone, because this always occurs.

384. A child is diagnosed with scarlet fever. The nurse collects data regarding the child. Which is characteristic of scarlet fever?
1. Pastia's sign
2. Abdominal pain and flaccid paralysis
3. Dense pseudoformation membrane in the throat
4. Foul-smelling and mucopurulent nasal drainage

385. A child is diagnosed with infectious mononucleosis. The nurse reinforces home care instructions to the parents about the care of the child. Which instruction should the nurse provide to the parents?
1. Maintain the child on bed rest for 2 weeks.
2. Maintain respiratory precautions for 1 week.
3. Notify the health care provider (HCP) if the child develops a fever.
4. Notify the HCP if the child develops abdominal or left shoulder pain.

386. The health care provider prescribes laboratory studies for an infant of a woman positive for human immunodeficiency virus (HIV) to determine the presence of HIV antigen in the infant. The nurse anticipates that which laboratory study will be prescribed for the infant?
1. Chest x-ray
2. Western blot
3. $CD4^+$ cell count
4. p24 antigen assay

387. A nursing student is assigned to help administer immunizations to children in a clinic. The nursing instructor asks the student about the contraindications to receiving an immunization. Immunization is contraindicated in the presence of which condition?
1. A cold
2. Otitis media
3. Mild diarrhea
4. A severe febrile illness

388. A mother with human immunodeficiency virus (HIV) infection brings her 10-month-old infant to the clinic for a routine checkup. A health care provider has documented that the infant is asymptomatic for HIV infection. After the checkup, the mother tells the nurse that she is so pleased that the infant will not get HIV. Which response by the nurse is appropriate?
1. "I am also so pleased that everything has turned out fine."
2. "Since symptoms have not developed, it is unlikely that the infant will develop HIV infection."
3. "Everything looks great, but be sure that you return with your infant next month for the scheduled visit."
4. "Most children infected with HIV develop symptoms within the first 9 months of life, and some become symptomatic at some point before the age of 3 years."

❖ **389.** Which home care instructions should the nurse plan to reinforce to the mother of a child with acquired immunodeficiency syndrome (AIDS)? **Select all that apply.**

❑ 1. Frequent hand washing is important.
❑ 2. The child should avoid exposure to other illnesses.
❑ 3. The child's immunization schedule will need revision.
❑ 4. Kissing the child on the mouth will never transmit the virus.
❑ 5. Clean up body fluid spills with bleach solution (10:1 ratio of water to bleach).
❑ 6. Fever, malaise, fatigue, weight loss, vomiting, and diarrhea are expected to occur and do not require special intervention.

390. A child is scheduled to receive a measles, mumps, and rubella (MMR) vaccine. The nurse, preparing to administer the vaccine, reviews the child's record. Which finding should make the nurse question the health care provider's prescription?
1. Recent recovery from a cold
2. A history of frequent respiratory infections
3. A history of an anaphylactic reaction to neomycin
4. A local reaction at the site of a previous MMR vaccine injection

ANSWERS

381. 4

Rationale: Rubeola is transmitted via airborne particles or direct contact with infectious droplets. Respiratory precautions are required, and a mask is worn by those who come in contact with the child. Gowns and gloves are not indicated. Articles that are contaminated should be bagged and labeled. Options 1, 2, and 3 are not indicated for rubeola.

Test-Taking Strategy: Focus on the subject, precautions needed for a child with rubeola. Recalling that rubeola is transmitted via the airborne route will direct you to the correct option. **Review: rubeola.**

Level of Cognitive Ability: Applying
Client Needs: Safe and Effective Care Environment
Integrated Process: Nursing Process/Implementation
Content Area: Child Health: Infectious and Communicable Diseases
Priority Concepts: Infection, Safety
Reference(s): Hockenberry, Wilson (2013), p. 427.

382. 3

Rationale: Mumps is transmitted via direct contact or droplets spread from an infected person and possibly by contact with urine. Respiratory precautions are indicated during the period of communicability. Options 1, 2, and 4 are incorrect.

Test-Taking Strategy: Options 1 and 2 can be eliminated first, because they are comparable or alike. From the remaining options, select option 3, because it is the umbrella option, and it addresses communicability. In addition, the time frame indicated in option 4 seems rather lengthy. **Review: mumps.**

Level of Cognitive Ability: Applying
Client Needs: Safe and Effective Care Environment
Integrated Process: Teaching and Learning
Content Area: Child Health: Infectious and Communicable Diseases
Priority Concepts: Infection, Safety
Reference(s): Hockenberry, Wilson (2013), p. 426.

383. 3

Rationale: Occasionally tenderness, redness, or swelling may occur at the site of the injection. This can be relieved with cool packs for the first 24 hours and followed by warm or cool compresses if the inflammation persists. It is not necessary to bring the infant back to the clinic. Option 1 may be an appropriate intervention, but it is not specific to the subject of the question.

Test-Taking Strategy: Option 4 can be eliminated first because of the closed-ended word, *always.* Eliminate option 1 next because it does not relate specifically to the subject of the question, swelling and redness at the injection site. Next, eliminate option 2 as an unnecessary intervention. **Review: immunizations.**

Level of Cognitive Ability: Applying
Client Needs: Physiological Integrity
Integrated Process: Nursing Process/Implementation
Content Area: Child Health: Infectious and Communicable Diseases
Priority Concepts: Immunity, Tissue Integrity
Reference(s): McKinney et al (2013), p. 85.

384. 1

Rationale: Pastia's sign is a rash seen among children with scarlet fever that will blanch with pressure, except in areas of deep creases and in the folds of joints. The tongue is initially coated with a white furry covering with red projecting papillae (white strawberry tongue). By the fourth to fifth day, the white strawberry tongue sloughs off and leaves a red, swollen tongue (strawberry tongue). The pharynx is edematous and beefy red in color. Option 2 is associated with poliomyelitis. Options 3 and 4 are characteristics of diphtheria.

Test-Taking Strategy: Focus on the subject, the characteristic associated with scarlet fever. Remember that Pastia's sign describes the rash noted with scarlet fever. **Review: scarlet fever.**

Level of Cognitive Ability: Analyzing
Client Needs: Physiological Integrity
Integrated Process: Nursing Process/Data Collection
Content Area: Child Health: Infectious and Communicable Diseases
Priority Concepts: Infection, Tissue Integrity
Reference(s): McKinney et al (2013), p. 1025.

385. 4

Rationale: The parents need to be instructed to notify the HCP if abdominal pain (especially in the left upper quadrant) or left shoulder pain occurs, because this may indicate splenic rupture. Children with enlarged spleens are also instructed to avoid contact sports until the splenomegaly resolves. Bed rest is not necessary, and children usually self-limit their activity. Respiratory precautions are not required, although transmission can occur via direct intimate contact or contact with infected blood. Fever is treated with acetaminophen (Tylenol).

Test-Taking Strategy: Focus on the subject, home care instructions for infectious mononucleosis. Use knowledge regarding the organs that are affected in clients with infectious mononucleosis. Options 1 and 2 can be eliminated first because they are unnecessary interventions for this disease. From the remaining options, knowledge that splenic rupture is a concern will direct you to the correct option. **Review: infectious mononucleosis.**

Level of Cognitive Ability: Applying
Client Needs: Physiological Integrity
Integrated Process: Teaching and Learning
Content Area: Child Health: Infectious and Communicable Diseases
Priority Concepts: Infection, Pain
Reference(s): Hockenberry, Wilson (2013), p. 720.

386. 4

Rationale: The detection of HIV in infants is confirmed by a p24 antigen assay, virus culture of HIV, or polymerase chain reaction. A chest x-ray evaluates the presence of other manifestations of HIV infection, such as pneumonia. A Western blot test confirms the presence of HIV antibodies. The $CD4^+$ cell count indicates how well the immune system is working.

Test-Taking Strategy: Note the subject of the question, the test for HIV for an infant. Recalling the laboratory tests used to determine the presence of HIV infection is needed to answer this question. Remember that the detection of HIV in infants is confirmed by a p24 antigen assay, virus culture of HIV, or polymerase chain reaction. **Review:** laboratory tests used to detect **human immunodeficiency virus.**

Level of Cognitive Ability: Understanding

Client Needs: Physiological Integrity
Integrated Process: Nursing Process/Data Collection
Content Area: Child Health: Immune
Priority Concepts: Immunity, Infection
Reference(s): McKinney et al (2013), p. 1046; Pagana, Pagana (2013), pp. 529–533.

387. 4
Rationale: A severe febrile illness is a reason to delay immunization but only until the child has recovered from the acute stage of the illness. Minor illnesses such as a cold, otitis media, or mild diarrhea are not contraindications to immunization.
Test-Taking Strategy: Focus on the subject, a contraindication to receiving an immunization. Noting the word *severe* in option 4 will direct you to this option. **Review: contraindications to immunizations.**
Level of Cognitive Ability: Understanding
Client Needs: Physiological Integrity
Integrated Process: Teaching and Learning
Content Area: Child Health: Infectious and Communicable Diseases
Priority Concepts: Immunity, Safety
Reference(s): Hockenberry, Wilson (2013), pp. 340–341; McKinney et al (2013), pp. 84–85.

388. 4
Rationale: Most children who are infected with HIV develop symptoms within the first 9 months of life. The remainder of these infected children become symptomatic sometime before the age of 3 years. Children, with their immature immune systems, have a much shorter incubation period than adults. Options 1, 2, and 3 are incorrect responses.
Test-Taking Strategy: Eliminate options 1, 2, and 3 because they are comparable or alike in content. Option 4 is the only option that provides specific and accurate data regarding HIV infection in the infant. **Review: human immunodeficiency virus infection.**
Level of Cognitive Ability: Applying
Client Needs: Psychosocial Integrity
Integrated Process: Nursing Process/Implementation
Content Area: Child Health: Immune
Priority Concepts: Immunity, Infection
Reference(s): McKinney et al (2013), p. 1046.

❖ **389.** 1, 2, 5
Rationale: AIDS is a disorder that is caused by the human immunodeficiency virus (HIV) and is characterized by a generalized dysfunction of the immune system. Both cellular and humoral immunity are compromised. The horizontal transmission of HIV occurs through intimate sexual contact or parenteral exposure to blood or body fluids that contain visible blood. Vertical (perinatal) transmission occurs when an HIV-infected pregnant woman passes the infection to her infant. Home care instructions include the following: frequent hand washing; monitoring for fever, malaise, fatigue, weight loss, vomiting, diarrhea, altered activity level, and oral lesions and notifying the health care provider if these occur; monitoring for signs and symptoms of opportunistic infections; administering antiretroviral medications, as prescribed; avoiding exposure to other illnesses; keeping immunizations up to date; avoiding kissing the child on the mouth; monitoring the weight and providing a high-calorie, high-protein diet; washing eating utensils in the dishwasher; and avoiding the sharing of eating utensils. Gloves are worn for care, especially when in contact with body fluids or changing diapers. Diapers are changed frequently and away from food areas, and soiled disposable diapers are folded inward, closed with their tabs, and disposed of in a tightly covered plastic-lined container. Any body fluid spills are cleaned with a bleach solution made up of a 10:1 ratio of water to bleach.
Test-Taking Strategy: Focus on the subject, home care of the child with AIDS. Recalling that this disorder is characterized by a generalized dysfunction of the immune system and recalling the modes of transmission will assist you with selecting the home care instructions. **Review: human immunodeficiency virus and acquired immunodeficiency syndrome.**
Level of Cognitive Ability: Analyzing
Client Needs: Safe and Effective Care Environment
Integrated Process: Teaching and Learning
Content Area: Child Health: Immune
Priority Concepts: Client Education, Infection
Reference(s): McKinney et al (2013), pp. 1053–1054.

390. 3
Rationale: The MMR vaccine contains minute amounts of neomycin. A history of an anaphylactic reaction to neomycin is considered a contraindication to the MMR vaccine. The general contraindication to all immunizations is a severe febrile illness. The presence of a minor illness such as the common cold is not a contraindication. In addition, a history of frequent respiratory infections is not a contraindication to receiving a vaccine. A local reaction to an immunization is treated with cool packs for the first 24 hours after injection, and this is followed by warm or cool compresses if the inflammation persists.
Test-Taking Strategy: Focus on the subject, the health care provider's prescription that should be questioned. Recalling that a general contraindication to all immunizations is a severe febrile illness will assist you with eliminating options 1 and 2. From the remaining options, note that option 4 identifies a local reaction. This will direct you to the correct option, which is a systemic reaction and a potentially life-threatening condition. **Review: immunizations.**
Level of Cognitive Ability: Analyzing
Client Needs: Physiological Integrity
Integrated Process: Nursing Process/Implementation
Content Area: Child Health: Infectious and Communicable Diseases
Priority Concepts: Immunity, Safety
Reference(s): McKinney et al (2013), p. 85.

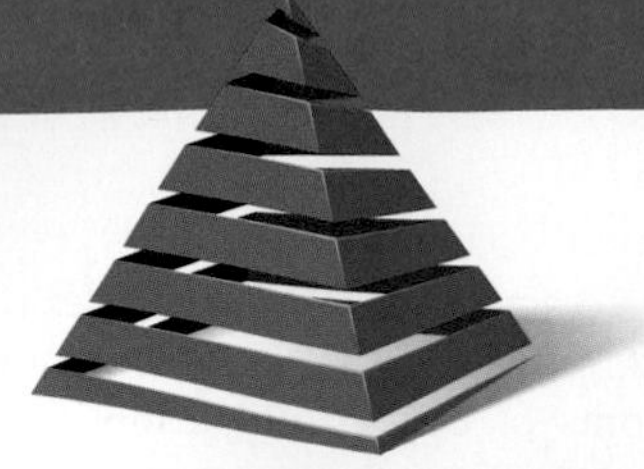

CHAPTER 40

Pediatric Medication Administration and Calculations

CRITICAL THINKING What Should You Do?

The nurse is preparing to administer a medication that has an unpleasant taste to an infant. What should the nurse do to minimize this unpleasant effect?

Answer located on p. 480.

I. Medications and the Pediatric Client

A. Pediatric clients are smaller than adult clients, and their medications have to be adapted to their sizes and ages.

B. Neonates and premature infants have immature body systems.

C. The absorption, distribution, metabolism, and excretion of medications differ substantially, and the pediatric client will react more quickly to medication than will an adult client; also, their renal and hepatic function needs to be checked before medications are administered (Fig. 40-1).

D. Medication reactions are not as predictable in pediatric clients as they are in adult clients.

II. Oral Medications

A. Most oral pediatric medications are in liquid or suspension form because children usually cannot swallow a tablet.

B. Solutions may be measured by using an oral plastic syringe or other acceptable measurement or administration device; the device used depends on the **developmental age** of the child.

C. Medications in suspension settle to the bottom of the bottle between uses, so thorough mixing is required before the pouring of the medication.

D. Suspensions must be administered immediately after measurement to prevent settling and thus the administration of an incomplete dose.

E. Administer oral medications with the child sitting in an upright position with the head elevated to prevent aspiration if the child cries or resists.

F. Place the small child sideways on the adult's lap; the child's closest arm should be placed under the adult's arm and behind the adult's back; cradle the child's head, hold his or her hand, and administer the medication slowly with a plastic spoon, small plastic cup, or a syringe.

G. If a tablet or capsule has been administered, check the child's mouth to ensure that it has been swallowed; if swallowing is a problem, some tablets can be crushed and given in small amounts of puréed food or flavored syrup (enteric-coated tablets, timed-release tablets, and capsules should not be crushed).

H. Follow generally accepted medication administration guidelines for children (Box 40-1).

⚠ Newborns and infants have an immature liver and immature kidneys, so metabolism and elimination of medications are delayed.

III. Parenteral Medications

A. Subcutaneous and intramuscularly administered medications

1. Medications usually given via the subcutaneous route are insulin and some immunizations.
2. Any site with sufficient subcutaneous tissue may be used for subcutaneous injections; common sites include the central third of the lateral aspect of the upper arm, the abdomen, and the center third of the anterior thigh.
3. 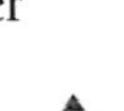 The safe use of all injection sites is based on normal muscle development and the size of the child; the preferred site for intramuscular injections in infants is the vastus lateralis, but agency policies and procedures need to be followed (Table 40-1 and Fig. 40-2).
4. For pediatric clients, the usual needle length is ½ to 1 inch, and the usual needle gauge is 22 to 25; needle length also can be estimated by grasping the muscle between the thumb and forefinger, and half the resulting distance would be the needle length.
5. 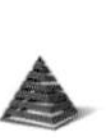 Pediatric dosages for subcutaneous and intramuscular administration are calculated to the nearest hundredth and measured with the use of a tuberculin syringe; always follow agency guidelines.

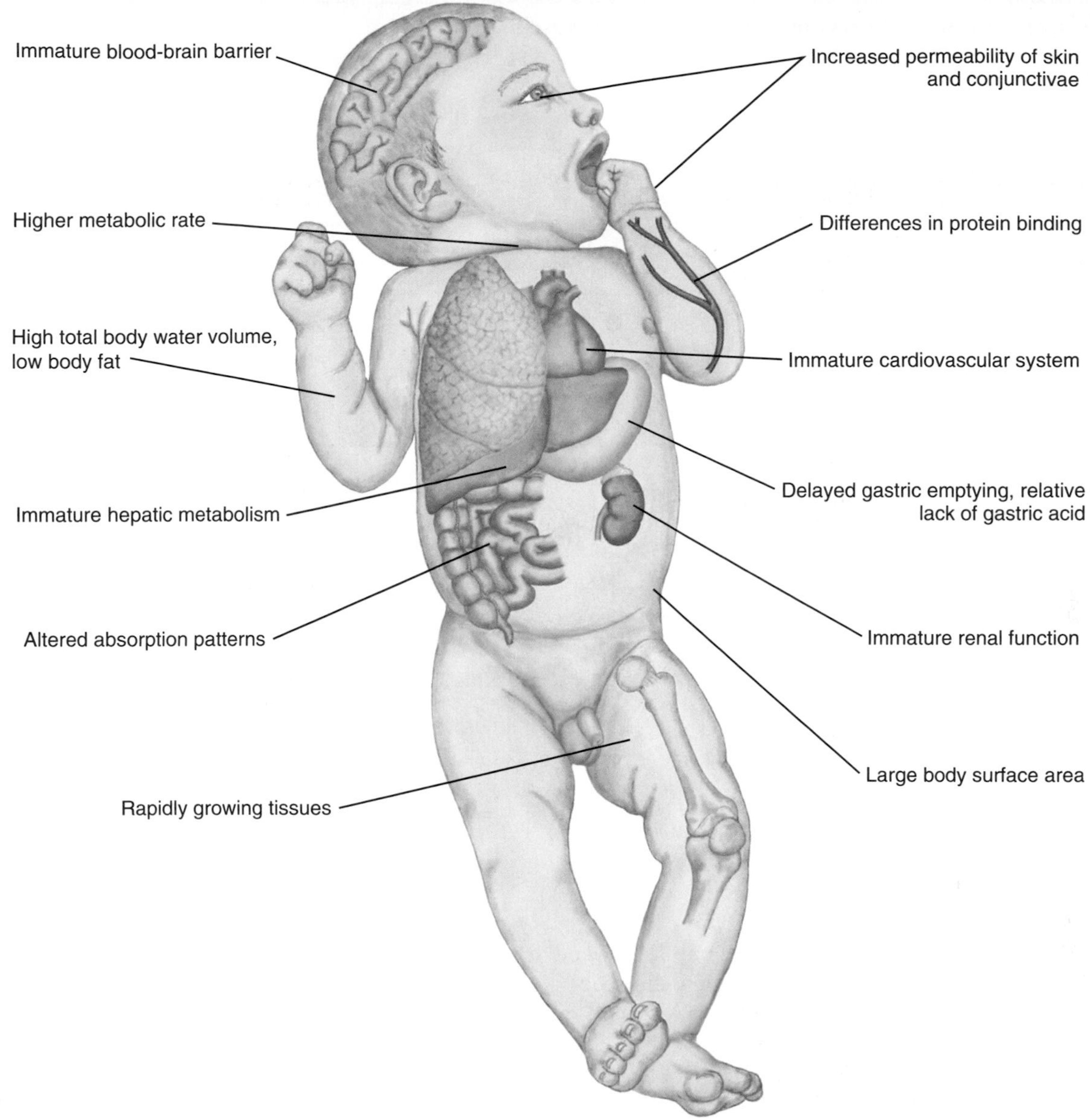

FIGURE 40-1 Some factors that affect drug disposition in children. (From Price D, Gwin J: *Pediatric nursing*, ed 11, St. Louis, 2012, Saunders.)

BOX 40-1 Medication Administration Guidelines for Children

- Two identifiers are required before medication administration, such as name, medical record number, and birth date.
- Obtain information from the parents about successful methods for administering medications to their children.
- Ask the parents about any known allergies.
- To avoid aspiration, liquid forms of medication are safer to swallow than other forms.
- Straws often help older children swallow pills.
- Avoid putting medications in foods, such as milk, cereal, or baby food, because it may cause an unpleasant taste to the food and the child may refuse to accept that same food in the future. In addition, the child may not consume the entire serving and will not receive the required medication dosage.
- If the taste of the medication is unpleasant, have the child drink the medication through a straw.
- Offer juice, a soft drink, or a frozen juice bar after the child swallows a medication.
- Always read the pharmacological indications for administration. Some items such as fruit syrups can be acidic and should not be used with medications that react negatively in an acid medium.
- Record the most successful method of administering medications and pertinent nursing prescriptions on the child's care plan for other nursing staff to follow; this notation also saves the child frustration, fear, and anxiety.

Data from Potter P, Perry A, Stockert P, Hall A: *Fundamentals of nursing*, ed 8, St. Louis, 2013, Mosby; and Perry S, Hockenberry M, Lowdermilk D, Wilson D: *Maternal-child nursing care*, ed 4, St. Louis, 2010, Mosby.

TABLE 40-1 Intramuscular Injections: Amount of mL by Muscle Group

Muscle	Neonate	Infants 1 to 12 months	Toddlers 1 to 2 years	Preschool to child 3 to 12 years	Adolescent 12 to 18 years
Vastus lateralis	0.5	0.5 to 1	0.5 to 2	2	2
Rectus femoris	Not safe	Not safe	0.5 to 1	2	2
Ventrogluteal	Not safe	Not safe	Not safe	0.5 to 3	2 to 3
Deltoid	Not safe	Not safe	0.5 to 1	0.5 to 1	1 to 1.5

Modified from Kee J, Marshall S: *Clinical calculations: With applications to general and specialty areas*, ed 7, St. Louis, 2013, Saunders.

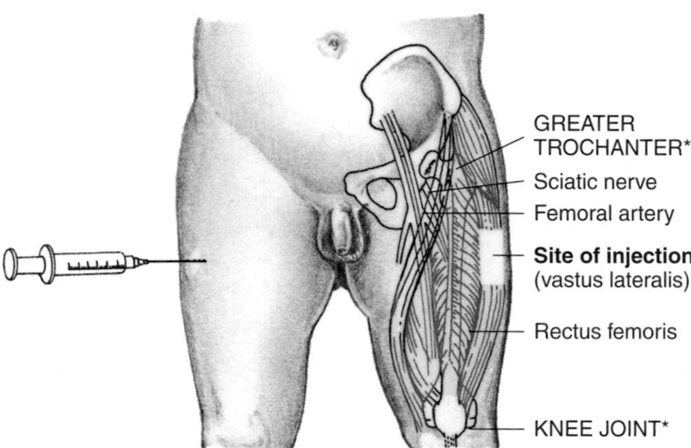

FIGURE 40-2 Intramuscular injection site—vastus lateralis. Landmarks are indicated by asterisks. (From Hockenberry M, Wilson D: *Wong's: Essentials of pediatric nursing*, ed 9, St. Louis, 2012, Mosby.)

6. Place a plain or decorated adhesive bandage over the puncture site to help the child view the experience in a somewhat pleasant way.

B. Monitoring intravenous (IV) medications
   1. When an infant or a child is receiving an IV medication, the IV site needs to be monitored closely for signs of infiltration and inflammation immediately before, during, and after the completion of the administration of each medication.
   2. Signs of infiltration or inflammation need to be reported.

The 24-hour fluid intake must be monitored closely, and all IV fluid amounts, including the amount of flush volume, need to be documented accurately to prevent overhydration. For children, the maximum amount of IV fluid administered in a 24-hour period varies and is usually based on body weight and other factors. Check the health care provider's prescription and agency guidelines for the procedures for the administration of IV fluids and medications.

IV. Calculation of Medication Dosage by Body Weight

A. Conversion of body weight (Box 40-2)

B. Calculating daily dosages
   1. Abbreviations (Box 40-3)

BOX 40-2 Conversion of Body Weight

Measurements

1 lb = 16 oz
1 kg = 2.2 lb

Pounds to Kilograms

2.2 lbs = 1 kg
To convert pounds to kilograms, divide by 2.2.
Kilograms are expressed to the nearest tenth.

Kilograms to Pounds

1 kg = 2.2 lbs
To convert kilograms to pounds, multiply by 2.2.
Pounds are expressed to the nearest tenth.

BOX 40-3 Common Measurement Abbreviations

Abbreviation	Meaning
BSA	body surface area
g	gram(s)
gr	grain(s)
kg	kilogram(s)
lb	pound(s)
m^2	square meters
mcg	microgram(s)
mg	milligram(s)
mL	milliliter(s)
SA	surface area

   2. Dosages are expressed in terms of milligrams per kilogram per day, milligrams per pound per day, or milligrams per kilogram per dose.
   3. The total daily dosage is usually administered in divided (more than one) doses per day.
   4. Express the child's body weight in kilograms or pounds to correlate with the dosage specifications.
   5. Calculate the total daily dosage.
   6. Divide the total daily dosage by the number of doses to be administered in 1 day.

V. Calculation of Body Surface Area

A. The body surface area (BSA) is determined by comparing body weight and height with averages or norms on a graph called a *nomogram.*

B. Not all children are the same size at the same age; therefore, the nomogram chart is used to determine the BSA of the child.

C. Look at the nomogram chart (Fig. 40-3); note that the height is on the left-hand side of the chart, and the weight is on the right-hand side.

D. Place a ruler across the chart.

E. Line up the left side of the ruler on the height and the right side of the ruler on the weight; read the BSA at the point where the straight edge of the ruler intersects the surface area (SA) column.

F. The estimated SA is given in square meters (m^2).

G. Box 40-4 shows an example.

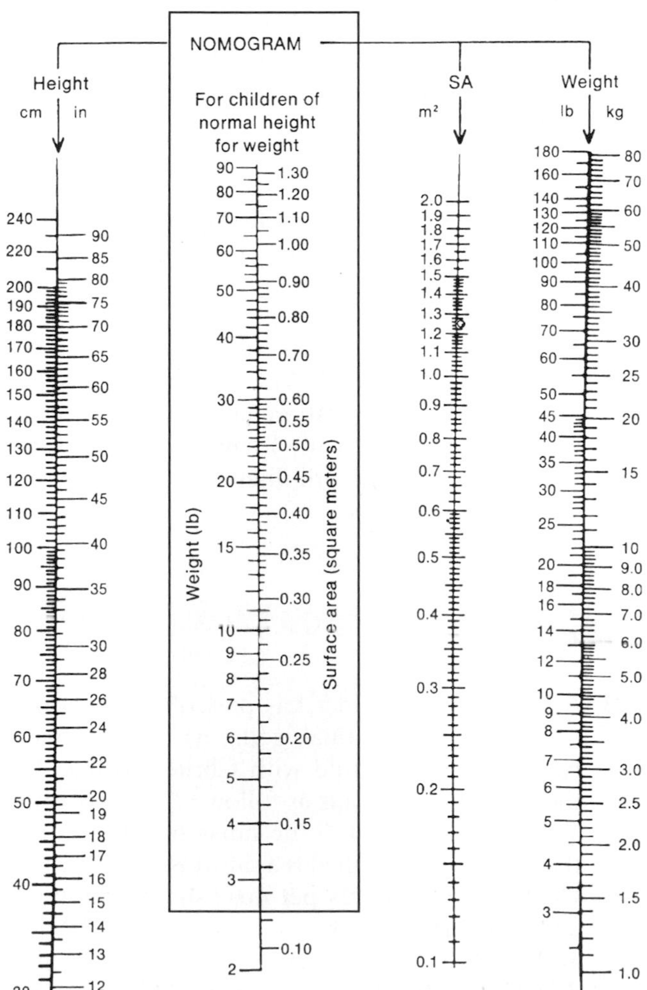

FIGURE 40-3 West nomogram for estimation of surface areas in infants and children. First, find height; next, find weight; finally, draw a straight line connecting the height and weight. The body surface area (in square meters [m^2]) is indicated where a straight line connecting the height and weight intersects the surface area (SA) column or, if the child is approximately of normal proportion, from weight alone (*beige area*). (From Hockenberry M, Wilson D: *Wong's: Essentials of pediatric nursing,* ed 7, St. Louis, 2005, Mosby.)

BOX 40-4 How to Use the Nomogram

Example: Use the nomogram to estimate the body surface area (BSA) of a child whose height is 58 inches and whose weight is 12 kg.

1. Look at Figure 40-3 and note that the height is on the left-hand side of the chart and the weight is on the right-hand side of the chart.
2. Place a ruler on the chart, and line up the left side of the ruler on the height and the right side of the ruler on the weight. Read the BSA at the point where the straight edge of the ruler intersects the surface area (SA) column.
3. The estimated SA is given in square meters (m^2).

Answer: This child's BSA is 0.66 m^2.

VI. Calculations Based on Body Surface Area

A. When dosage recommendations for children are in milligrams, micrograms, or units per square meter, calculating the dosage is simple multiplication (Box 40-5).

B. When dosages are specified only for adults, a formula is used to calculate the child's dosage (Box 40-6).

VII. Developmental Considerations for Administering Medications

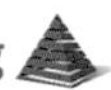

A. When administering medications to children, developmental age must be taken into consideration to ensure safe and effective administration.

BOX 40-5 Calculating Medication Dosage

Example: The dosage recommendation is 4 mg/m^2. The child has a body surface area of 1.1 m^2. What is the dosage to be administered?

Answer: $1.1 \times 4\text{ mg} = 4.4\text{ mg}$

BOX 40-6 Calculating a Child's Dosage from the Adult Dosage

When dosages are specified only for adults, a formula is used to calculate a child's dosage from the adult dosage. The adult dosage is based on a standardized body surface area of 1.73 m^2.

Example: A health care provider has prescribed an antibiotic for a child. The average adult dose is 250 mg. The child has a body surface area (BSA) of 0.41 m^2. What is the dose for the child?

Formula:

$$\frac{\text{BSA of child }(m^2)}{1.73\ m^2} \times \text{Adult dose} = \text{Child's dose}$$

$$\frac{0.41}{1.73} \times 250\text{ mg} = 59.24\text{ mg}$$

Answer: This child's dose is 59.24 mg.

B. General interventions
   1. Always be prepared for the procedure with all necessary equipment and assistance.
   2. For the hospitalized child, ask the parent or child or both if the parent should or should not remain for the procedure.
   3. Determine appropriate preadministration and postadministration comfort measures.
   4. Try to make the event as pleasant as is possible.

C. Box 40-7 lists developmental considerations when giving medications.

BOX 40-7 Developmental Considerations for Administering Medications

Infants

- Perform the procedure quickly, allowing the infant to swallow; then offer comfort measures, such as holding, rocking, and cuddling.
- Allow self-comforting measures, such as the use of a pacifier.

Toddlers

- Offer a brief, concrete explanation of the procedure, and then perform it.
- Accept aggressive behavior, within reasonable limits, as a healthy response, and provide outlets for the toddler.
- Provide comfort measures immediately after the procedure, such as touch, holding, cuddling, and providing a favorite toy.

Preschoolers

- Offer a brief, concrete explanation of the procedure and then perform it.
- Accept aggressive behavior, within reasonable limits, as a healthy response, and provide outlets for the child.
- Provide comfort measures after the procedure, such as touch, holding, or providing a favorite toy.

School-Age Children

- Explain the procedure, allowing for some control over the body and situation.
- Explore feelings and concepts through therapeutic play, drawings of own body and self in the hospital, and the use of books and realistic hospital equipment.
- Set appropriate behavior limits, such as it is all right to cry or scream but not to bite.
- Provide activities for releasing aggression and anger.
- Use the opportunity to teach about how medication helps the disorder.

Adolescents

- Explain the procedure, allowing for some control over the body and situation.
- Explore concepts of self, hospitalization, and illness, and correct any misconceptions.
- Encourage self-expression, individuality, and self-care needs.
- Encourage participation in the procedure.

Data from McKenry L, Salerno E: *Mosby's: Pharmacology in nursing*, St. Louis, 2003, Mosby.

CRITICAL THINKING What Should You Do?

Answer: When administering a medication with an unpleasant taste to an infant, the nurse should draw the required dose into a syringe without the needle and place the syringe into the side and toward the back of the infant's mouth; the medication should be administered slowly, allowing the infant to swallow.

Reference(s): Hockenberry, M., & Wilson, D. (2013). *Wong's: Essentials of pediatric nursing* (9th ed., pp. 666–667). St. Louis: Mosby.

PRACTICE QUESTIONS

391. Morphine sulfate, 2.5 mg, is prescribed for a child. The safe pediatric dose is 0.05 to 0.1 mg/kg/dose. The child weighs 50 kg. Which statement most accurately describes the prescribed dosage for this child?
1. The dose is too low.
2. The dose is too high.
3. The dose is within the safe dosage range.
4. There is not enough information to determine the safe dosage range.

392. A health care provider's prescription reads as follows: "Ampicillin, 125 mg intramuscular every 6 hours." The medication label reads, "1 gram when reconstituted with 7.4 mL of bacteriostatic water." How many milliliters should the nurse draw up for one dose?
1. 0.54 mL
2. 0.92 mL
3. 1.1 mL
4. 7.4 mL

393. A health care provider has prescribed phenobarbital sodium (luminal sodium), 25 mg orally twice daily, for a child with febrile seizures. The medication label reads as follows: "Phenobarbital sodium, 20 mg/5 mL." The nurse has determined that the dose prescribed is a safe dose for the child. How many milliliters per dose should the nurse administer to the child?
1. 2 mL
2. 4.5 mL
3. 6.25 mL
4. 7 mL

394. Sulfisoxazole (Gantrisin), 1 g orally four times daily, is prescribed for an adolescent with a urinary tract infection. The medication label reads, "500-mg tablets." The nurse has determined that

the prescribed dose is safe. How many tablets per dose should the nurse administer to the adolescent?
1. 0.5
2. 1
3. 2
4. 3

❖ **395.** Atropine sulfate, 0.2 mg given intramuscularly, is prescribed for a child. The medication label reads as follows: "0.4 mg/mL." The nurse has determined that the prescribed dose is safe. How many milliliters should the nurse administer to the child? **Fill in the blank.**

Answer: ______ mL

ANSWERS

391. 3
Rationale: Use the formula for calculating a safe dosage range.
Dosage parameters:

$$0.05 \text{ mg/kg/dose} \times 50 \text{ kg} = 2.5 \text{ mg/dose}$$

$$0.1 \text{ mg/kg/dose} \times 50 \text{ kg} = 5 \text{ mg/dose}$$

The dose is within the safe dosage range.
Test-Taking Strategy: Focus on the **subject**, the safe dosage range of the medication. Calculate the dosage parameters with the use of the safe dosage range identified in the question and the child's weight in kilograms. Verify the answer with the use of a calculator. **Review: pediatric medication calculations.**
Level of Cognitive Ability: Applying
Client Needs: Physiological Integrity
Integrated Process: Nursing Process/Planning
Content Area: Fundamental Skills: Medication/IV Calculations
Priority Concepts: Clinical Judgment, Safety
Reference(s): McKinney et al (2013), p. 952.

392. 2
Rationale: Convert grams to milligrams. With the metric system, to convert larger to smaller, multiply by 1000 or move the decimal three places to the right. Then, use the medication calculation formula:

$$1 \text{ g} = 1000 \text{ mg}$$

Formula:

$$\frac{\text{Desired}}{\text{Available}} \times \text{Volume} = \frac{125 \text{ mg}}{1000 \text{ mg}} \times 7.4 \text{ mL} = 0.925 \text{ mL/dose}$$

Test-Taking Strategy: Focus on the **subject**, milliliters per dose. First, convert grams to milligrams. Next, use the formula to determine the correct dosage, knowing that 1000 mg = 7.4 mL. Verify the answer with the use of a calculator. **Review: pediatric medication calculations.**
Level of Cognitive Ability: Applying
Client Needs: Physiological Integrity
Integrated Process: Nursing Process/Implementation
Content Area: Fundamental Skills: Medication/IV Calculations
Priority Concepts: Clinical Judgment, Safety
Reference(s): Potter et al (2013), pp. 573–574.

393. 3
Rationale: Use the medication calculation formula.
Formula:

$$\frac{\text{Desired}}{\text{Available}} \times \text{Volume} = \frac{25 \text{ mg}}{20 \text{ mg}} \times 5 \text{ mL} = 6.25 \text{ mL/dose}$$

Test-Taking Strategy: Focus on the **subject**, milliliters per dose. Use the formula to determine the correct dosage, and use a calculator to verify the answer. **Review: pediatric medication calculations.**
Level of Cognitive Ability: Applying
Client Needs: Physiological Integrity
Integrated Process: Nursing Process/Implementation
Content Area: Fundamental Skills: Medication/IV Calculations
Priority Concepts: Clinical Judgment, Safety
Reference(s): McKinney et al (2013), p. 952.

394. 3
Rationale: Change grams to milligrams, knowing that 1000 mg = 1 g. When converting from grams to milligrams (larger to smaller), move the decimal point three places to the right; thus, 1.0 g = 1000 mg. Then, use the medication calculation formula.
Formula:

$$\frac{\text{Desired}}{\text{Available}} \times \text{Tablet} = \frac{1000 \text{ mg}}{500 \text{ mg}} \times 1 \text{ tablet} = 2 \text{ tablets}$$

Test-Taking Strategy: Focus on the **subject**, tablets per dose. Change grams to milligrams first. Then, use the formula to determine the correct dosage. Remember to verify the answer with the use of a calculator. **Review: pediatric medication calculations.**
Level of Cognitive Ability: Applying
Client Needs: Physiological Integrity
Integrated Process: Nursing Process/Implementation
Content Area: Fundamental Skills: Medication/IV Calculations
Priority Concepts: Clinical Judgment, Safety
Reference(s): Potter et al (2013), pp. 573–574.

❖ **395. 0.5 mL**
Rationale: Use the formula for calculating medication dosage.
Formula:

$$\frac{\text{Desired}}{\text{Available}} \times \text{Volume} = \frac{0.2 \text{ mg}}{0.4 \text{ mg}} \times 1 \text{ mL} = 0.5 \text{ mL/dose}$$

Test-Taking Strategy: Focus on the **subject**, milliliters to be administered. Use the formula to determine the correct dose, and use a calculator to verify your answer. **Review: pediatric medication calculations.**
Level of Cognitive Ability: Applying
Client Needs: Physiological Integrity
Integrated Process: Nursing Process/Implementation
Content Area: Fundamental Skills: Medication/IV Calculations
Priority Concepts: Clinical Judgment, Safety
Reference(s): McKinney et al (2013), p. 952.

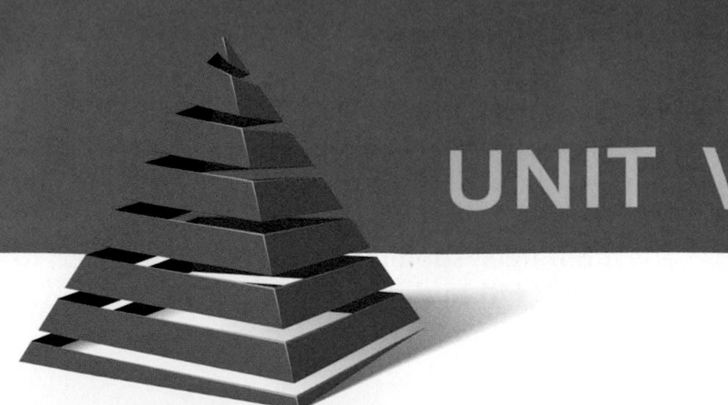

UNIT VIII

The Adult Client with an Integumentary Disorder

PYRAMID TERMS

burns Cell destruction of the layers of the skin caused by heat, friction, electricity, radiation, or chemicals.

carbon monoxide poisoning Carbon monoxide is a colorless odorless and tasteless gas that has an affinity for hemoglobin that is 200 times greater than that of oxygen. Poisoning occurs from the inhalation of carbon monoxide. Oxygen molecules are displaced and carbon monoxide reversibly binds to hemoglobin to form carboxyhemoglobin. Tissue hypoxia results.

deep full-thickness burn Injury extends beyond the skin into underlying fascia and tissues and muscle bone and tendons are damaged.

deep partial-thickness burn Injury extends deep into the dermis.

full-thickness burn Involves injury and destruction of the epidermis and the dermis.

herpes zoster (shingles) An acute viral infection of the nerve structure caused by the varicella zoster virus. Herpes zoster is contagious to individuals who have never had chickenpox and have not been vaccinated against the disease.

pressure ulcer Area of tissue damage that occurs as a result of skin and underlying soft tissue compression from pressure between a surface and a bony prominence.

skin cancer A malignant lesion of the skin that may or may not metastasize.

smoke inhalation injury Respiratory injury that occurs due to inhalation of products or combustion during a fire.

superficial partial-thickness burn Involves injury that extends into the dermis.

superficial-thickness burn Involves injury that extends into the epidermis.

Pyramid to Success

The Pyramid to Success focuses on the concept that the integumentary system provides the first line of defense against infections. Focus is on the protective measures necessary to prevent infection, including infection with methicillin-resistant *Staphylococcus aureas* (MRSA). Pyramid points address the risk factors related to the development of integumentary disorders and the preventive measures related to skin cancer. Also described are the emergency measures related to a client with a burn, fluid resuscitation, monitoring for complications, and skin grafting. Psychosocial issues relate to the body-image disturbances that can occur as the result of an integumentary disorder.

Client Needs

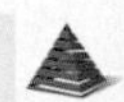

Safe and Effective Care Environment

Assisting the registered nurse (RN) with making referrals to appropriate health care providers
Consulting with the RN and other members of the health care team regarding treatments
Ensuring that informed consent for treatments and procedures has been obtained
Establishing priorities of care
Handling hazardous and infectious materials
Instituting standard and other precautions
Maintaining confidentiality related to the disorder
Practicing asepsis techniques and preventing infection

Health Promotion and Maintenance

Implementing disease prevention measures
Performing data collection regarding the integumentary system
Promoting health screening and health promotion programs to prevent skin disorders
Reinforcing instructions to the client regarding prevention measures and care for an integumentary disorder

Psychosocial Integrity

Addressing end-of-life issues
Discussing unexpected body-image changes
Identifying coping mechanisms
Identifying situational role changes
Using support systems

Physiological Integrity

Assisting the RN with providing emergency care
Monitoring for alterations in body systems
Monitoring for infection
Providing adequate nutrition for healing
Providing basic care and comfort
Monitoring for the expected effects of treatments
Monitoring for fluid and electrolyte imbalances and other complications
Monitoring laboratory values

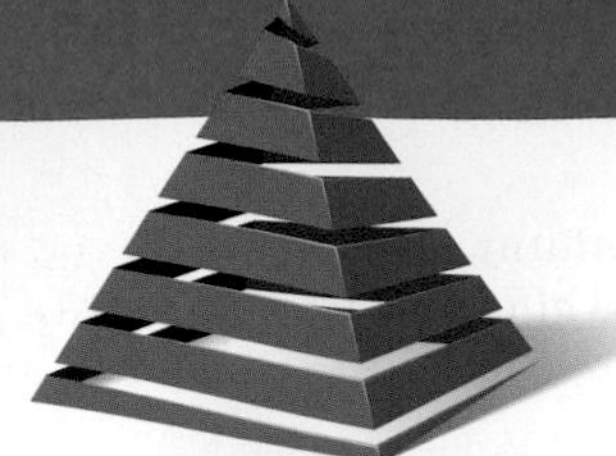

CHAPTER 41

Integumentary System

CRITICAL THINKING What Should You Do?

A burn client undergoes autograft to the lower right leg. What should the nurse do when caring for the graft site?

Answer located on p. 500.

I. Anatomy and Physiology

- **A.** The skin is the largest sensory organ of the body, with a surface area of 15 to 20 square feet and a weight of about 9 lb.
- **B.** Functions
  - **1.** Acts as the first line of defense against infections
  - **2.** Protects underlying tissues and organs from injury
  - **3.** Receives stimuli from the external environment; detects touch, pressure, pain, and temperature stimuli and relays that information to the nervous system
  - **4.** Maintains the normal body temperature
  - **5.** Excretes salts, water, and organic wastes
  - **6.** Protects the body from excessive water loss
  - **7.** Synthesizes vitamin D_3, which converts to calcitriol, for normal calcium metabolism.
  - **8.** Stores nutrients
- **C.** Layers
  - **1.** Epidermis
  - **2.** Dermis
  - **3.** Hypodermis (subcutaneous fat)
- **D.** Epidermal appendages
  - **1.** Nails
  - **2.** Hair
  - **3.** Glands
    - **a.** Sebaceous
    - **b.** Sweat
- **E.** Normal bacterial flora
  - **1.** Types of normal bacterial flora include the following:
    - **a.** Gram-positive and gram-negative staphylococci
    - **b.** *Pseudomonas sp.*
    - **c.** *Streptococcus sp.*
  - **2.** Organisms are shed with normal exfoliation.
  - **3.** A pH of 4.2 to 5.6 halts the growth of bacteria.

II. Risk Factors for Integumentary Disorders

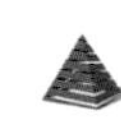

- **A.** Exposure to chemical and environmental pollutants
- **B.** Exposure to radiation
- **C.** Race and age
- **D.** Exposure to the sun or use of indoor tanning
- **E.** Lack of personal hygiene habits
- **F.** Use of harsh soaps or other harsh products
- **G.** Some medications, such as long-term glucocorticoid use or herbal preparations
- **H.** Nutritional deficiencies
- **I.** Moderate to severe emotional stress
- **J.** Infection, with injured areas as the potential entry points for infection
- **K.** Repeated injury or irritation
- **L.** Genetic predisposition
- **M.** Systemic illnesses

III. Psychosocial Impact

- **A.** Change in body image, decreased general well-being, and decreased self-esteem
- **B.** Social isolation and fear of rejection (because of embarrassment about changes in skin appearance)
- **C.** Restrictions in physical activity
- **D.** Pain
- **E.** Disruption or loss of employment
- **F.** Cost of medications, hospitalizations, and follow-up care including dressing supplies

IV. Phases of Wound Healing

- **A.** Phases
  - **1.** Inflammatory: Begins at the time of injury and lasts 3 to 5 days; manifestations include local edema, pain, redness, and warmth.
  - **2.** Fibroblastic: Begins the fourth day after injury and lasts 2 to 4 weeks; scar tissue forms and granulation tissue forms in the tissue bed.
  - **3.** Maturation: Begins as early as 3 weeks after the injury and may last for 1 year; scar tissue becomes thinner and is firm and inelastic on palpation.
- **B.** Healing by intention
  - **1.** First intention: Wound edges are approximated and held in place (i.e., with sutures) until healing occurs; wound is easily closed and dead space is eliminated.

BOX 41-1 Types of Drainage from Wounds

Serous
- Clear or straw-colored
- Occurs as a normal part of the healing process

Serosanguineous
- Pink-colored due to the presence of a small amount of blood cells mixed with serous drainage
- Occurs as a normal part of the healing process

Sanguineous
- Red drainage from trauma to a blood vessel
- May occur with wound cleansing or other trauma to the wound bed
- Sanguineous drainage is uncommon in wounds

Hemorrhaging
- Frank blood from a leaking blood vessel
- May require emergency treatment to control bleeding
- Hemorrhage is an abnormal wound exudate

Purulent
- Yellow, gray, or green drainage due to infection in the wound

2. Second intention: This type of healing occurs with injuries or wounds that have tissue loss and require gradual filling in of the dead space with connective tissue.
3. Third intention: This type of healing involves delayed primary closure and occurs with wounds that are intentionally left open for several days for irrigation or removal of debris and exudates; once debris has been removed and inflammation resolves, the wound is closed by first intention.

C. Types of wound drainage: Refer to Box 41-1.

V. Diagnostic Tests

A. Skin biopsy
1. Description
   a. Skin biopsy is the collection of a small piece of skin tissue for histopathologic study.
   b. Methods include punch, excisional, and shave.
2. Preprocedure interventions
   a. Verify informed consent has been obtained.
   b. Cleanse site as prescribed.
3. Postprocedure interventions
   a. Place specimen in the appropriate container and send to pathology laboratory for analysis.
   b. Use surgically aseptic technique for biopsy site dressings.
   c. Monitor the biopsy site for bleeding and infection.
   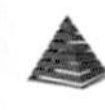
   d. Reinforce instructions to the client to keep the dressing dry and in place for at least 8 hours and to then clean the area daily and use antibiotic ointment, as prescribed.
   e. Reinforce instructions to the client to report signs of excessive drainage or redness or other signs of infection.

B. Skin/wound cultures
1. A small skin culture sample is obtained with the use of a sterile applicator and the appropriate type of culture tube (e.g. bacterial or viral). Methods include scraping, punch biopsy, and collecting fluid.
2. Postprocedure intervention
   a. Viral culture is immediately placed on ice.
   b. Sample is sent to the laboratory to identify an existing organism.
3. Preprocedure intervention: Obtain skin culture samples before instituting antibiotic therapy.

Obtain skin culture samples or any other type of culture specimens before instituting antibiotic therapy.

C. Wood's light examination
1. Description: Skin is viewed under ultraviolet light through a special glass (Wood's glass) to identify superficial infections of the skin.
2. Preprocedure intervention: Darken the room before the examination.
3. Postprocedure intervention: Assist the client during adjustment to light after being in a darkened room.

D. Diascopy
1. Technique allows clearer inspection of lesions by eliminating the erythema caused by increased blood flow to the area.
2. A glass slide is pressed over the lesion, causing blanching and revealing the lesion more clearly.

E. Data collection of the skin (see Chapter 23)

VI. *Candida albicans*

A. Description
1. A superficial fungal infection of the skin and mucous membranes
2. Is also known as a yeast infection or thrush when it occurs in the mouth.
3. Risk factors include immunosuppression such as in clients with acquired immunodeficiency syndrome; cancer clients receiving chemotherapy; clients undergoing long-term antibiotic therapy; clients with diabetes mellitus; and clients with obesity.
4. Common areas of occurrence include the mucous membranes of the mouth, perineum, vagina, axilla, and under the breasts.

B. Data collection
1. Skin: red and irritated appearance that itches and stings
2. Mucous membranes of the mouth: red and whitish patches

C. Interventions
1. Reinforce instructions to the client to keep skinfold areas clean and dry.
2. For the hospitalized client, inspect skinfold areas frequently, turn and reposition the client frequently, and keep the skin and bed linens clean and dry.
3. Provide frequent mouth care as prescribed and avoid irritating products.
4. Provide food and fluids that are tepid in temperature and nonirritating to mucous membranes.
5. Antifungal medications may be prescribed.

VII. Herpes Zoster (Shingles)

A. Description
1. With a history of chickenpox, shingles is caused by the reactivation of the varicella-zoster virus; shingles can occur during any immunocompromised state in a client with a history of chickenpox.
2. The dormant virus is located in the dorsal nerve root ganglia of the sensory cranial and spinal nerves.
3. Herpes zoster eruptions occur in a segmental distribution on the skin area along the infected nerve and show up after several days of discomfort in the area.
4. Diagnosis is determined by visual examination, and a Tzanck smear and viral culture that identify the organism.
5. Postherpetic neuralgia (severe pain) can remain after the lesions resolve.
6. It is contagious to individuals who never had chickenpox and have not been vaccinated against the disease.
7. Herpes simplex virus is another type of virus; Type 1 infection causes a cold sore (usually on the lip), and Type 2 causes genital herpes (both types are contagious).

B. Data collection
1. Unilaterally clustered skin vesicles along peripheral sensory nerves on the trunk, thorax, or face
2. Fever, malaise
3. Burning and pain
4. Pruritus
5. Paresthesia

C. Interventions
1. Isolate the client because exudate from the lesions contains the virus (maintain standard and other precautions as appropriate, such as contact precautions).
2. Assess for signs and symptoms of infection, including skin infections and eye infections; skin necrosis can also occur.
3. Assess neurovascular status and seventh cranial nerve function; Bell's palsy is a complication.
4. Use an air mattress and bed cradle on the client's bed if hospitalized, and keep the environment cool; warmth and touch aggravate the pain.
5. Prevent the client from scratching and rubbing the affected area.
6. Reinforce instructions to the client to wear lightweight, loose cotton clothing and to avoid wool and synthetic clothing.
7. Reinforce teaching the client about the prescribed therapies; astringent compresses may be prescribed to relieve irritation and pain and to promote crust formation and healing.
8. Reinforce teaching the client about measures to keep the skin clean to prevent infection.
9. Reinforce teaching the client about topical treatment or antiviral medications if prescribed.
10. A vaccination for shingles is recommended for adults 60 years of age and older to reduce the risk of occurrence and the long-term pain associated with shingles.
11. Antiviral medications may be prescribed; refer to Chapter 62 for information on antiviral medications.

VIII. Methicillin-Resistant *Staphylococcus aureas* (MRSA)

A. Description
1. Skin or wound becomes infected with methicillin-resistant *Staphylococcus aureus.*
2. MRSA is also referred to as a health care–associated infection. See Chapters 14 and 39 for additional types of health care–associated infections.
3. Infection can range from mild to severe and can present as folliculitis or furuncles.
4. Folliculitis is a superficial infection of the follicle caused by *Staphylococcus* and presents as a raised and red rash and pustules; furuncles are also caused by *Staphylococcus* and occur deep in the follicle and present as large raised bumps that may or may not have a pustule and are very painful.
5. If MRSA infects the blood, sepsis, organ damage, and death can occur.

MRSA is contagious and is spread to others by direct contact with infected skin or infected articles; for the client with MRSA, the infection can also be spread to other parts of the body.

B. Data collection: A culture and sensitivity of the skin or wound confirms the presence of MRSA and leads to the choice of appropriate antibiotic therapy.

C. Interventions
1. Maintain standard precautions and contact precautions as appropriate to prevent spread of infection to others.
2. Monitor the client closely for signs of further infection, which may result in systemic illness or organ damage.
3. Administer antibiotic therapy as prescribed.

4. For additional information on MRSA, refer to Chapters 14 and 39.

IX. Erysipelas and Cellulitis

A. Description
   1. Erysipelas is an acute, superficial, rapidly spreading inflammation of the dermis and lymphatics caused by group A *Streptococcus*, which enters the tissue via an abrasion, bite, trauma, or wound.
   2. Cellulitis is an infection of the dermis and underlying hypodermis; the causative organism is usually group A *Streptococcus* or *Staphylococcus aureas*.

B. Data collection
   1. Pain and tenderness
   2. Erythemia and warmth
   3. Edema
   4. Fever

C. Interventions
   1. Promote rest of the affected area.
   2. Apply warm compresses as prescribed to promote circulation and to decrease discomfort, erythema, and edema.
   3. Apply antibacterial dressings, ointments, or gels as prescribed.
   4. Administer antibiotics as prescribed for an infection; obtain a culture of the area before initiating the antibiotics.

X. Poison Ivy, Poison Oak, and Poison Sumac

A. Description: A dermatitis that develops from contact with urushiol from poison ivy, oak, or sumac plants

B. Data collection
   1. Papulovesicular lesions
   2. Severe pruritis

C. Interventions
   1. Cleanse the skin of the plant oils immediately.
   2. Apply cool, wet compresses to relieve the itching.
   3. Apply topical products to relieve the itching and discomfort.
   4. Topical or oral glucocorticoids may be prescribed for severe reactions.

XI. Bites and Stings

A. Spider bites
   1. Almost all types of spider bites are venomous, and most are not harmful, but bites or stings from brown recluse spiders, black widow spiders, tarantulas, scorpions, bees, and wasps can produce toxic reactions in humans.
   2. Brown recluse spider
      a. Can cause a skin lesion, a necrotic wound, or systemic effects from the toxin (loxoscelism)
      b. Application of ice to decrease enzyme activity of the venom and limit tissue necrosis should be done immediately and intermittently for up to 4 days after the bite.
      c. Topical antiseptics and antibiotics may be necessary if the site becomes infected.
   3. Black widow spider
      a. Causes a small red papule
      b. Venom causes neurotoxicity.
      c. Ice is applied immediately to inhibit the action of the neurotoxin.
      d. Systemic toxicity can occur and the victim may require supportive therapy in the hospital.
   4. Tarantulas
      a. Bite causes swelling, redness, numbness, lymph inflammation, and pain at the bite site.
      b. The tarantula launches its barbed hairs, which penetrate the skin and eyes of the victim, producing a severe inflammatory reaction.
      c. Tarantula hairs are removed as soon as possible using sticky tape to pull hairs from the skin, and the skin is thoroughly irrigated; saline irrigations are done for eye exposure.
      d. The involved extremity is elevated and immobilized to reduce the pain and swelling.
      e. Antihistamines and topical or systemic corticosteroids may be prescribed; tetanus prophylaxis is necessary.

B. Scorpion stings
   1. Scorpions inject venom into the victim through a stinging apparatus on their tail.
   2. Most stings cause local pain, inflammation, and mild systemic reactions that are treated with analgesics, wound care, and supportive treatment.
   3. The bark scorpion can inflict a severe and fatal systemic response, and the venom is neurotoxic; the victim is taken to the emergency department immediately (an antivenom is administered for bark scorpion bites).

C. Bees and wasps
   1. Usually cause a wheal and flare reaction
   2. Emergency care involves quick removal of the stinger and application of an ice pack.
   3. The stinger is removed by gently scraping or brushing it off with the edge of a needle or similar object; tweezers are not used because of the risk of pinching the venom sac.
   4. If the victim is allergic to the venom of a bee or wasp, a severe allergic response can occur (hives, pruritus, swelling of the lips and tongue) that can progress to life-threatening anaphylaxis; immediate emergency care is required.
   5. Individuals who are allergic should carry an EpiPen (epinephrine autoinjector) for self-administration of intramuscular epinephrine if a bee or wasp sting occurs.

D. Snake bites
   1. Some snakes are venomous and can cause a serious systemic reaction in the victim.

2. The victim should be immediately moved to a safe area away from the snake and should rest to decrease venom circulation; the extremity is immobilized and kept below the level of the heart.
3. Constricting clothing and jewelry are removed before swelling occurs.
4. The victim is kept warm and is not allowed to consume beverages such as alcohol or those that contain caffeine because they may speed absorption of the venom.
5. If transport to the emergency room is not done immediately, a constricting band may be applied proximal to the wound to slow the venom circulation; monitor the circulation frequently and loosen the band if edema occurs.
6. The wound is not incised or sucked to remove the venom; ice is not applied to the wound.
7. Emergency care in a hospital is required as soon as possible; an antivenom may be administered along with supportive care.

For spider bites, scorpion bites, or other stings or bites, the Poison Control Center should be contacted as soon as possible to determine the best initial management.

XII. Frostbite

A. Description
   1. Frostbite is damage to tissues and blood vessels as a result of prolonged exposure to cold.
   2. Fingers, toes, face, nose, and ears often are affected.

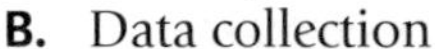

B. Data collection
   1. First-degree: Involves white plaque surrounded by a ring of hyperemia and edema
   2. Second-degree: Large, clear fluid-filled blisters with partial thickness skin necrosis
   3. Third-degree: Involves the formation of small hemorrhagic blisters, usually followed by eschar formation involving the hypodermis, requiring débridement
   4. Fourth-degree: No blisters or edema noted; full thickness necrosis with visible tissue loss extending into muscle and bone, which may result in gangrene. Amputation may be required.

C. Interventions
   1. Rewarm the affected part rapidly and continuously with a warm water bath or towels at 104° to 107.6°F (40° to 42°C) to thaw the frozen part.
   2. Handle the affected area gently, and immobilize.
   3. Avoid the use of dry heat, and never rub or massage the part, which may result in further tissue damage.
   4. The rewarming process may be painful; analgesics may be necessary.
   5. Avoid compression of the injured tissues, and apply only loose and nonadherent sterile dressings.
   6. Monitor for signs of compartment syndrome.
   7. Tetanus prophylaxis is necessary, and topical and systemic antibiotics may be prescribed.
   8. Débridement of necrotic tissue may be necessary; amputation may be necessary if gangrene develops.

XIII. Actinic Keratoses

A. Actinic keratoses is caused by chronic exposure to the sun and appear as rough, scaly, red or brown lesions and are usually found on the face, scalp, arms, and back of the hands.

B. Lesions can progress to squamous cell carcinoma.

C. Treatment includes medications and therapies such as excision, cryotherapy, curettage, and laser therapy. (See Chapter 42 for information on medications.)

XIV. Skin Cancer

A. Description
   1. Skin cancer is a malignant lesion of the skin, which may or may not metastasize.
   2. Overexposure to the sun is a primary cause; other causes and conditions that place the individual at risk include chronic skin damage from repeated injury and irritation, genetic predisposition, ionizing radiation, light-skinned race, age greater than 60 years, an outdoor occupation, and exposure to chemical carcinogens.
   3. Diagnosis is confirmed by a skin biopsy.

B. Types
   1. Basal cell: Basal cell cancer arises from the basal cells contained in the epidermis; metastasis is rare, but underlying tissue destruction can progress to organ tissue.
   2. Squamous cell: Squamous cell cancer is a tumor of the epidermal keratinocytes and can infiltrate surrounding structures and metastasize to lymph nodes.
   3. Melanoma: Melanoma may occur any place on the body, especially where birthmarks or new moles are apparent; it is highly metastatic to the brain, lungs, bone, and liver, with survival depending on early diagnosis and treatment.

C. Data collection (Box 41-2)
   1. Change in color, size, or shape of preexisting lesion
   2. Pruritus
   3. Local soreness

The client needs to be informed about the risks associated with overexposure to the sun and taught about the importance of performing monthly self-skin assessments.

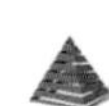

D. Interventions
   1. Reinforce instructions to the client regarding the risk factors and preventive measures.

BOX 41-2 Appearance of Skin Cancer Lesions

Basal Cell Carcinoma

- Waxy border
- Papule, with a red, central crater
- Rarely metastasizes

Squamous Cell Carcinoma

- Oozing, bleeding, crusting lesion
- Potentially metastatic
- Larger tumors associated with higher risk for metastasis

Melanoma

- Irregular, circular, bordered lesion with hues of tan, black, or blue
- Rapid infiltration into tissue
- Rapid metastasis

2. Reinforce instructions to the client to perform monthly self-skin assessments and to monitor for lesions that do not heal or that change characteristics.
3. Reinforce instructions to the client to have moles or lesions removed that are subject to chronic irritation.
4. Reinforce instructions to the client to avoid contact with chemical irritants.
5. Reinforce instructions to the client to wear layered clothing and use sunscreen lotions with an appropriate skin protection factor when outdoors.
6. Reinforce instructions to the client to avoid sun exposure between 10 AM and 4 PM.
7. Management may include surgical or nonsurgical interventions; if medication is prescribed, provide instructions about its use.
8. Assist with surgical management, which may include cryosurgery, curettage and electrodessication, or surgical excision of the lesion.

XV. Psoriasis

A. Description

1. Psoriasis is a chronic, noninfectious skin inflammation involving keratin synthesis that results in psoriatic patches; however, a break in skin integrity can lead to an infection in the affected area.
2. Various forms exist, with psoriasis vulgaris being the most common.
3. Possible causes of the disorder include stress, trauma, infection, hormonal changes, obesity, an autoimmune reaction, and climate changes; a genetic predisposition may also be a cause.
4. The disorder also may be exacerbated by the use of certain medications.
5. Koebner phenomenon is the development of psoriatic lesions at a site of injury, such as a scratched or sunburned area.
6. In some individuals with psoriasis, arthritis develops that leads to joint changes similar to those seen in rheumatoid arthritis.
7. The goal of therapy is to reduce cell proliferation and inflammation, and the type of therapy prescribed depends on the extent of the disease and the client's response to treatment.

B. Data collection

1. Pruritus
2. Shedding, silvery, white scales on a raised, reddened, round plaque that usually affects the scalp, knees, elbows, extensor surfaces of arms and legs, and sacral regions 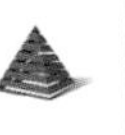
3. A yellow discoloration, pitting, and thickening of the nails is noted, if they are affected
4. Joint inflammation with psoriatic arthritis

C. Pharmacological therapy: Refer to Chapter 42 for medications used to treat psoriasis.

D. Interventions and client education

1. Provide emotional support to the client with altered body image and decreased self-esteem.
2. Reinforce instructions to the client in the use of prescribed therapies and to avoid over-the-counter medications.
3. Reinforce instructions to the client not to scratch the affected areas and to keep the skin lubricated as prescribed to minimize itching.
4. Monitor for and reinforce instructions to the client to recognize the signs and symptoms of secondary skin problems, such as infection and to report these signs.
5. Reinforce instructions to the client to wear light cotton clothing over affected areas.
6. Assist the client to identify ways to reduce stress if stress is a predisposing factor.

XVI. Acne Vulgaris

A. Description

1. Acne is a chronic skin disorder that usually begins in puberty and is more common in males; lesions develop on the face, neck, chest, shoulders, and back.
2. Acne requires active treatment for control until it resolves.
3. The types of lesions include comedones (open and closed), pustules, papules, and nodules.
4. The exact cause is unknown but may include androgenic influence on sebaceous glands, increased sebum production, and proliferation of *Propionibacterium acnes* (the enzymes that reduce lipids to irritating fatty acids).
5. Exacerbations coincide with the menstrual cycle because of hormonal activity; oily skin and a genetic predisposition may be contributing factors.

B. Data collection
   1. Closed comedones are whiteheads and noninflamed lesions that develop as follicles and enlarge, with the retention of horny cells.
   2. Open comedones are blackheads that result from continuing accumulation of horny cells and sebum, which dilates the follicles.
   3. Pustules and papules result as the inflammatory process progresses.
   4. Nodules result from total disintegration of a comedone and subsequent collapse of the follicle.
   5. Deep scarring can result from nodules.

C. Interventions
   1. Reinforce instructions to the client in prescribed skin-cleansing methods, with emphasis on not scrubbing the face and using only the prescribed topical agents.
   2. Reinforce instructions to the client in the administration of topical or oral medications as prescribed.
   3. Reinforce instructions to the client not to squeeze, prick, or pick at lesions.
   4. Reinforce instructions to the client to use products labeled noncomedogenic and cosmetics that are water-based and to avoid contact with excessively oil-based products.
   5. Reinforce instructions to the client on the importance of follow-up treatment.
   6. Refer to Chapter 42 for information on the medications used to treat acne.

XVII. Stevens-Johnson Syndrome

A. A drug-induced skin reaction that occurs through an immunological response

B. Similar to toxic epidermal necrolysis (TEN), another drug-induced skin reaction that results in diffuse erythema and large blister formation

C. May be mild or severe and cause vesicles, erosions, and crusts on the skin; if severe, systemic reactions occur that involve the respiratory system, renal system, and eyes, resulting in blindness.

D. Most commonly occurs in clients with cancer who are receiving chemotherapy or immunotherapy

E. Treatment includes immediate discontinuation of the medication causing the syndrome; antibiotics, corticosteroids, and supportive therapy may be necessary.

XVIII. Pressure Ulcer

A. Description
   1. A pressure ulcer is an impairment of skin integrity.
   2. A pressure ulcer can occur anywhere on the body; tissue damage results when the skin and underlying tissue are compressed between a bony prominence and an external surface for an extended period of time.
   3. The tissue compression restricts blood flow to the skin, and this can result in tissue ischemia, inflammation, and necrosis; once a pressure ulcer forms, it is difficult to heal.
   4. Prevention of skin breakdown in any part of the body is a major role for the nurse.

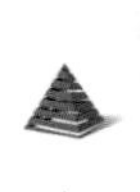

B. Risk factors
   1. Skin pressure
   2. Skin shearing and friction
   3. Immobility
   4. Malnutrition
   5. Incontinence
   6. Decreased sensory perception

C. Data collection and staging (Table 41-1)

D. Interventions

> Avoid direct massage to a reddened skin area because massage can damage the capillary beds and cause tissue necrosis.

   1. Identify clients at risk for developing a pressure ulcer.
   2. Institute measures to prevent pressure ulcers such as appropriate positioning, using pressure relief devices, ensuring adequate nutrition, and developing a plan for skin cleansing and care.
   3. Check the skin frequently and monitor for an alteration in skin integrity.
   4. Keep the client's skin dry and the sheets wrinkle-free; if the client is incontinent, check the client frequently and change pads or any items placed under the client immediately after they are soiled.
   5. Use creams and lotions to lubricate the skin and a barrier protection ointment for the incontinent client.
   6. Turn and reposition the immobile client every 2 hours or more frequently if necessary; provide active and passive range of motion exercises at least every 8 hours.
   7. If a pressure ulcer is present, record the location and size of the wound (length, width, depth), monitor and record the type and amount of exudates (a culture of the exudate may be prescribed), and check for undermining and tunneling.
   8. Serosanguineous exudate (blood-tinged amber fluid) is expected for the first 48 hours; purulent exudates indicate colonization of the wound with bacteria.
   9. Use agency protocols for skin assessment and management of a wound.
   10. Treatment may include wound dressings and débridement procedures; skin grafting may be necessary (Tables 41-2 and 41-3).

TABLE 41-1 Stages of Pressure Ulcers

Stage I

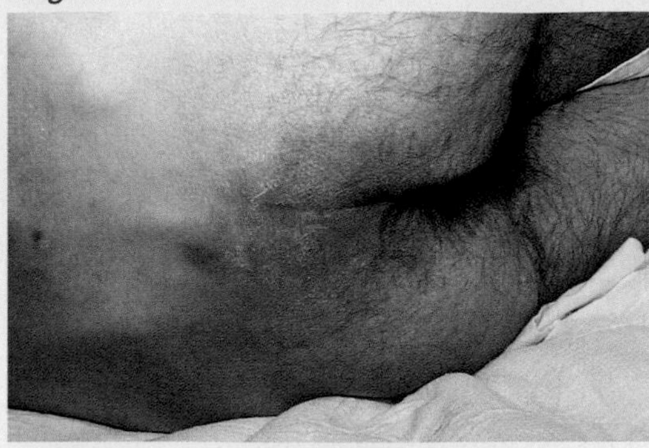

Skin is intact
Area is red and does not blanch with external pressure
Area may be painful, firm, soft, warmer or cooler compared with adjacent tissue

Stage II

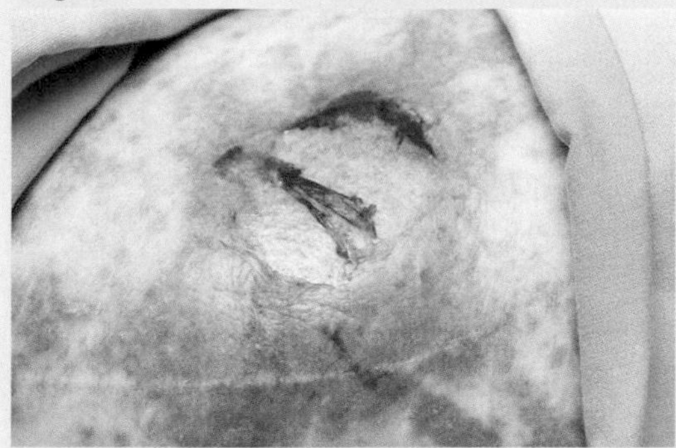

Skin is not intact
Partial-thickness skin loss of the dermis occurs
Presents as a shallow open ulcer with a red-pink wound bed or as intact or open/ruptured serum-filled blister

Stage III

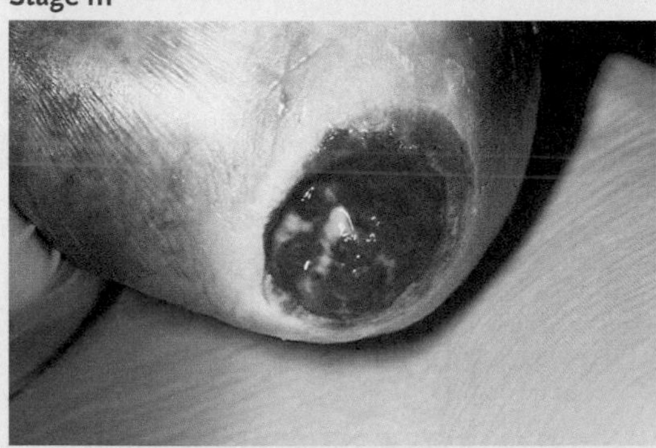

Full-thickness skin loss extends into the dermis and subcutaneous tissues, and slough may be present
Subcutaneous tissue may be visible
Undermining and tunneling may or may not be present

Stage IV

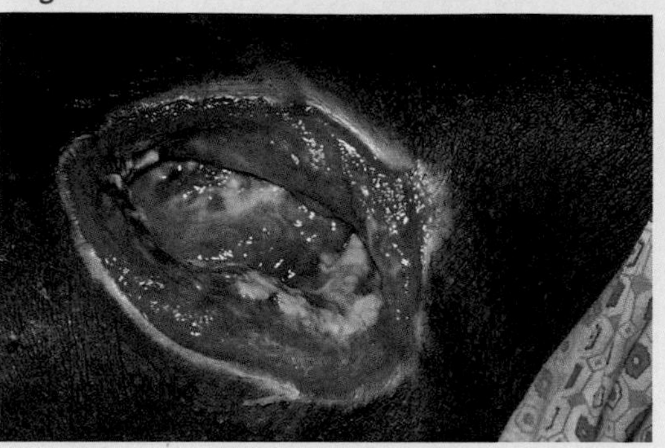

Full-thickness skin loss is present with exposed bone, tendon, or muscle
Slough or eschar may be present
Undermining and tunneling may develop

Suspected Deep-Tissue Injury

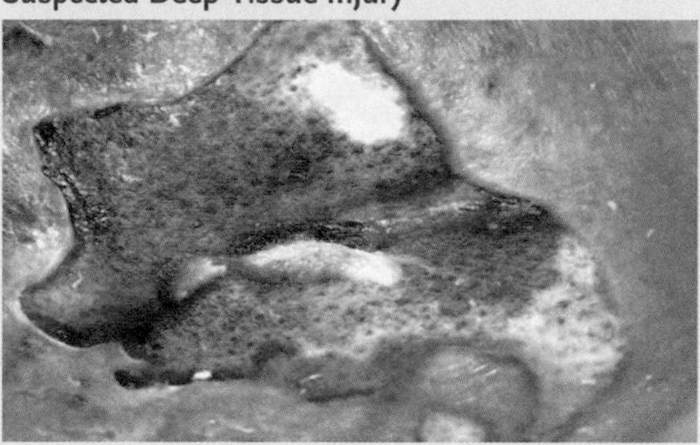

Ischemic subcutaneous tissue injury under intact skin
Appears purple or maroon colored
May be painful, firm, or boggy

Unstageable

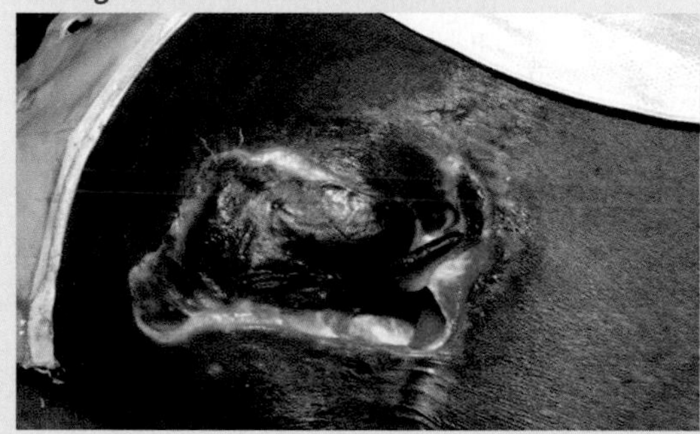

Full-thickness tissue loss in which the wound bed is covered by slough and/or eschar
The true depth, and therefore stage, of the wound cannot be determined until the slough and/or eschar is removed to visualize the wound bed

Adapted from and figures from Ignatavicius D, Workman ML: *Medical-surgical nursing: Patient-centered collaborative care,* ed 7, Philadelphia, 2013, Saunders.

TABLE 41-2 Types of Dressings and Mechanism of Action

Dressing Type	Mechanism of Action
Wet-to-damp saline-moistened gauze	Mechanically removes necrotic debris
Continuous wet gauze	Wound is continually bathed with a prescribed solution; promotes dilution of exudates and softens dry eschar
Topical enzyme preparations	Provides proteolytic action on thick and adherent eschar; this causes breakdown of the denatured protein and more rapid separation of necrotic tissue
Moisture-retentive dressing	Spontaneous separation of necrotic tissue is promoted by autolysis

Data from Ignatavicius D, Workman ML: *Medical-surgical nursing: Patient-centered collaborative care,* ed 7, Philadelphia, 2013, Saunders.

TABLE 41-3 Types of Dressing Materials

Type	Indications, Uses, Considerations	Frequency of Dressing Changes
Alginate	Provides hemostasis, débridement, absorption, and protection Can be used as packing for deep wounds and for infected wounds Requires a secondary dressing for securing	When dressing is saturated (every 3 to 5 days) or more frequently
Biological	Provides protection and débridement after eschar removal May be used for dormant and nonhealing wounds that do not respond to other topical therapies May be used for burns or before pigskin and cadaver skin grafts Conforms to uneven wound surfaces; reduces pain Requires a secondary dressing for securing	Topical growth factors: Changed daily Skin substitutes: The need for dressing change varies
Cotton gauze	Continuous dry dressing provides absorption and protection Continuous wet dressing provides protection, a means for the delivery of topical treatment, and débridement Wet to damp dressing provides atraumatic mechanical débridement May be painful on removal	Clean base: every 12 to 24 hr Necrotic base: every 4 to 6 hr
Foam	Provides absorption, protection, insulation, and débridement Conforms to uneven wound surfaces Requires a secondary dressing for securing	When dressing is saturated or more frequently
Hydrocolloidal	Provides absorption, protection, and débridement Is waterproof and is painless on removal	Clean base: On leakage of exudates Necrotic base: Every 24 hr
Hydrogel	Provides absorption, protection, and débridement Conducive to use with topical agents Conforms to uneven wound surfaces but allows only partial wound visualization Requires a secondary dressing for securing Can promote the growth of *Pseudomonas* and other microorganisms	Clean base: every 24 hr Necrotic base: every 6 to 8 hr
Adhesive transparent film	Provides protection for partial-thickness lesions, débridement, and serves as a secondary (cover) dressing Provides good wound visualization Is waterproof and reduces pain Use is limited to superficial lesions Is nonabsorbent, adheres to normal and healing tissue Dressing may be difficult to apply	Clean base: On leakage of exudates Necrotic base: every 24 hr

From Ignatavicius D, Workman ML: *Medical-surgical nursing: Patient-centered collaborative care,* ed 7, Philadelphia, 2013, Saunders.

11. Other treatments may include electrical stimulation to the wound area (increases blood vessel growth and stimulates granulation), vacuum-assisted wound closure (removes infectious material from the wound and promotes granulation), hyperbaric oxygen therapy (administration of oxygen under high pressure raises tissue oxygen concentration), and the use of topical growth factors (biologically active substances that stimulate cell growth).

XIX. Burn Injuries (See Priority Nursing Actions)

A. Description: Cell destruction of the layers of the skin caused by heat, friction, electricity, radiation, or chemicals

B. Burn size
1. Small burns: The response of the body to injury is localized to the injured area.
2. Large or extensive burns
   a. Major or extensive burns consist of 25% or more of the total body surface area for an adult and 10% or more of the total body surface area for a child.
   b. The response of the body to the injury is systemic.
   c. The burn affects all the major systems of the body.

C. Estimating the extent of injury (Fig. 41-1)

D. Burn depth
1. **Superficial-thickness burn**
   a. Involves injury to the epidermis; the blood supply to the dermis is still intact.
   b. Mild to severe erythema (pink to red) is present, but no blisters.
   c. The skin blanches with pressure.

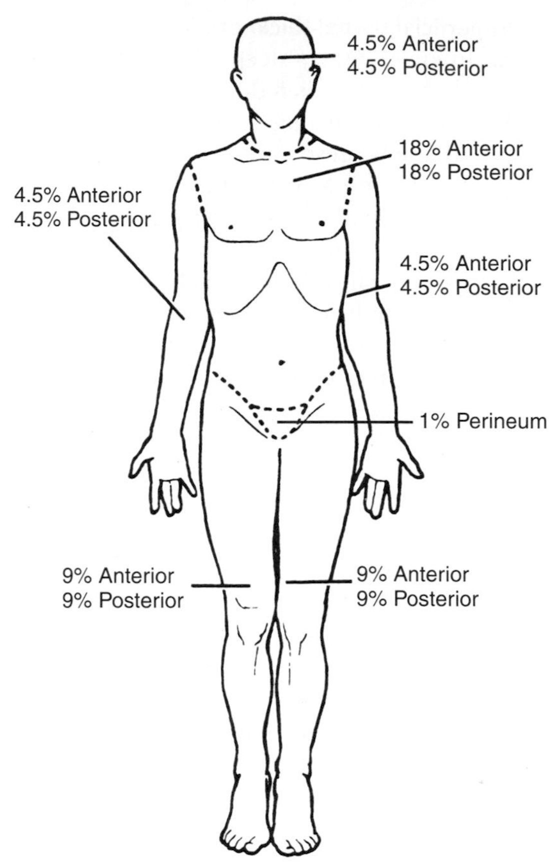

FIGURE 41-1 The rule of nines for estimating burn percentage. (Ignatavicius D, Workman ML: *Medical-surgical nursing: Patient-centered collaborative care*, ed 7, Philadelphia, 2013, Saunders.)

   d. Burn is painful, with tingling sensation, and the pain is eased by cooling.
   e. Discomfort lasts about 48 hours; healing occurs in about 3 to 6 days.
   f. No scarring occurs, and skin grafts are not required.

PRIORITY NURSING ACTIONS!

Actions to Take in the Emergency Department for a Client with a Burn Injury

1. Assess for airway patency.
2. Administer oxygen as prescribed.
3. Obtain vital signs.
4. Assist to initiate an intravenous (IV) line and begin fluid replacement as prescribed.
5. Elevate the extremities if no fractures are obvious.
6. Keep the client warm and place the client on NPO status.

The primary goal for a burn injury is to maintain a patent airway, administer IV fluids to prevent hypovolemic shock, and preserve vital organ functioning. Therefore, the priority action is to assess for airway patency and to maintain a patent airway. The nurse then prepares to administer oxygen. The type of oxygen delivery system is prescribed by the health care provider. Oxygen is necessary to perfuse tissues and organs. Vital signs should be assessed so that a baseline is obtained, which is needed for comparison of subsequent vital signs once fluid resuscitation is initiated. The nurse then assists to initiate an IV line and begins fluid replacement as prescribed. The extremities are elevated (if no obvious fractures are present) to assist in preventing shock. The client is kept warm (using sterile linens) and is placed on NPO status because of the altered gastrointestinal function that occurs as a result of the burn injury. A Foley catheter may be inserted so that the response to the fluid resuscitation can be carefully monitored. Once these actions are taken, the nurse assists to perform a complete assessment, stays with the client, and monitors the client closely. In addition, tetanus toxoid may be prescribed for prophylaxis.

Reference(s): deWit, D. & Kumagai, C. (2013). *Medical-surgical nursing: Concepts & practice.* (2nd ed., pp. 983–984). St. Louis: Saunders.

2. **Superficial partial-thickness burn**
   a. Involves injury deeper into the dermis; the blood supply is reduced
   b. Large blisters may cover an extensive area.
   c. Edema is present.
   d. Mottled pink to red base and a broken epidermis, with a wet, shiny, and weeping surface is characteristic.
   e. Burn is painful and sensitive to cold air.
   f. Heals in 10 to 21 days with no scarring, but some minor pigment changes may occur.
   g. Grafts may be used if the healing process is prolonged.
3. **Deep partial-thickness burn**
   a. Extends deeper into the skin dermis
   b. Blister formation usually does not occur because the dead tissue layer is thick and sticks to underlying viable dermis.
   c. Wound surface is red and dry with white areas in deeper parts.
   d. May or may not blanch, and edema is moderate.
   e. Can convert to a full-thickness burn when tissue damage increases with infection, hypoxia, or ischemia.
   f. Generally heals in 3 to 6 weeks, but scar formation results, and skin grafting may be necessary.
4. **Full-thickness burn**
   a. Involves injury and destruction of the epidermis and the dermis; the wound will not heal by reepithelialization and grafting may be required.
   b. Appears as a dry, hard, leathery eschar (burn crust or dead tissue must slough off or be removed from the wound before healing can occur).
   c. Appears waxy white, deep red, yellow, brown, or black.
   d. Injured surface appears dry.
   e. Edema is present under the eschar.
   f. Sensation is reduced or absent because of nerve ending destruction.
   g. Healing may take weeks to months and depends on establishing an adequate blood supply.
   h. Scarring and wound contractures are likely to develop.
5. **Deep full-thickness burn**
   a. Injury extends beyond the skin into underlying fascia and tissues, and muscle, bone, and tendons are damaged.
   b. Injured area appears black, and sensation is completely absent.
   c. Eschar is hard and inelastic.
   d. Healing takes months, and grafts are required.

E. Age and general health
1. Mortality rates are higher for children younger than 4 years old, particularly for children from birth to 1 year of age, and for clients older than 65 years.
2. Debilitating disorders, such as cardiac, respiratory, endocrine, and renal disorders, negatively influence the client's response to injury and treatment.
3. Mortality rate is higher when the client has a preexisting disorder at the time of the burn injury.

F. Burn location
1. Burns of the head, neck, and chest are associated with pulmonary complications.
2. Burns of the face are associated with corneal abrasion.
3. Burns of the ear are associated with auricular chondritis.
4. Hands and joints require intensive therapy to prevent disability.
5. The perineal area is prone to autocontamination by urine and feces.
6. Circumferential burns of the extremities can produce a tourniquet-like effect and lead to vascular compromise (compartment syndrome).
7. Circumferential thorax burns lead to inadequate chest wall expansion and pulmonary insufficiency.

XX. Inhalation Injuries

A. Smoke inhalation injury
1. Description: Respiratory injury that occurs when the victim inhales products of combustion during a fire

 Airway is a priority concern in an inhalation injury.

2. Data collection
   a. Facial burns
   b. Erythema
   c. Swelling of the oropharynx and nasopharynx
   d. Singed nasal hairs
   e. Flaring nostrils
   f. Stridor, wheezing, and dyspnea
   g. Hoarse voice
   h. Sooty (carbonaceous) sputum and cough
   i. Tachycardia
   j. Agitation and anxiety

B. Carbon monoxide poisoning 
1. Description
   a. Carbon monoxide is a colorless, odorless, and tasteless gas that has an affinity for hemoglobin 200 times greater than that of oxygen.
   b. Oxygen molecules are displaced, and carbon monoxide reversibly binds to hemoglobin to form carboxyhemoglobin.
   c. Tissue hypoxia occurs.
2. Data collection (Table 41-4)

TABLE 41-4 Carbon Monoxide Poisoning

Blood Level (%)	Clinical Manifestations
1-10	Normal level
11-20 (mild poisoning)	Headache Flushing Decreased visual acuity Decreased cerebral functioning Slight breathlessness
21-40 (moderate poisoning)	Headache Nausea and vomiting Drowsiness Tinnitus and vertigo Confusion and stupor Pale to reddish-purple skin Decreased blood pressure Increased and irregular heart rate
41-60 (severe poisoning)	Coma Seizures
61-80 (fatal poisoning)	Death

Modified from Ignatavicius D, Workman ML: *Medical-surgical nursing: Patient-centered collaborative care*, ed 7, Philadelphia, 2013, Saunders.

C. Direct thermal heat injury
  1. Description
    a. Thermal heat injury can occur to the lower airways by the inhalation of steam or explosive gases or the aspiration of scalding liquids.
    b. Injury can occur to the upper airways, which appear erythematous and edematous, with mucosal blisters and ulcerations.
    c. Mucosal edema can lead to upper airway obstruction, especially during the first 24 to 48 hours.
    d. All clients with head or neck burns should be monitored closely for the development of airway obstruction and are considered immediately for endotracheal intubation if obstruction occurs.
  2. Data collection
    a. Erythema and edema of the upper airways
    b. Mucosal blisters and ulcerations

XXI. Pathophysiology of Burns

A. Following a burn, vasoactive substances are released from the injured tissue, and these substances cause an increase in the capillary permeability, allowing the plasma to seep into the surrounding tissues.

B. The direct injury to the vessels increases capillary permeability (capillary permeability decreases 18 to 26 hours after the burn, but it does not normalize until 2 to 3 weeks after the injury).

C. Extensive burns result in generalized body edema and a decrease in circulating intravascular blood volume.

D. The fluid losses result in a decrease in organ perfusion.

E. The heart rate increases, cardiac output decreases, and the blood pressure drops.

F. Initially, hyponatremia and hyperkalemia occur.

G. The hematocrit level increases as a result of plasma loss; this initial increase falls to below normal on the third to fourth day after the burn as a result of red blood cell damage and loss at the time of injury.

H. Initially, the body shunts blood from the kidneys, causing oliguria; then the body begins to reabsorb fluid, and diuresis of the excess fluid occurs over the next days to weeks.

I. Blood flow to the gastrointestinal tract is diminished, which leads to intestinal ileus and gastrointestinal dysfunction.

J. Immune system function is depressed, which results in immunosuppression and thus increases the risk of infection and sepsis.

K. Pulmonary hypertension can develop, resulting in a decrease in the arterial oxygen tension level and a decrease in lung compliance.

L. Evaporative fluid losses through the burn wound are greater than normal, and the losses continue until complete wound closure occurs.

M. If the intravascular space is not replenished with intravenously administered fluids, hypovolemic shock and ultimately death occur.

XXII. Management of the Burn Injury

A. Resuscitation/emergent phase (Table 41-5)
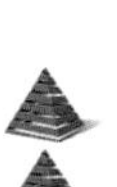
  1. Prehospital care
    a. Begins at the scene of the accident and ends when emergency care is obtained
    b. Remove the victim from the source of the burn.
    c. Check the ABCs—airway, breathing, and circulation.
    d. Check for associated trauma, including inhalation injury.
    e. Conserve body heat.
    f. Cover burns with sterile or clean cloths.
    g. Remove constrictive jewelry and clothing.
    h. Insert intravenous (IV) access.
    i. Transport to the emergency department.
  2. Emergency department care is a continuation of the care administered at the scene of the injury.
  3. Major burns
    a. Evaluate the degree and extent of the burn, and treat life-threatening conditions.
    b. Ensure a patent airway, and administer 100% oxygen as prescribed.
    c. Monitor for respiratory distress, and determine the need for intubation.
    d. Check the oropharynx for blisters and erythema.

TABLE 41-5 Phases of Management of the Burn Injury

Phase	Goal
Resuscitation/Emergent Phase Begins at the time of injury Ends with the restoration of normal capillary permeability Duration usually 48 to 72 hr Includes prehospital care and emergency department care	The primary goal is to maintain the patient's airway, administer intravenous fluids to prevent hypovolemic shock, and preserve vital organ functioning
Resuscitative Phase Begins with the initiation of fluids Ends when capillary integrity returns to near-normal levels and large fluid shifts have decreased Amount of fluid administered is based on client's weight and extent of injury (Most fluid replacement formulas are calculated from the time of injury and not from the time of arrival at the hospital)	The goal is to prevent shock by maintaining adequate circulating blood volume and maintaining vital organ perfusion
Acute Phase Begins when the client is hemodynamically stable, capillary permeability is restored, and diuresis has begun Usually begins 48 to 72 hr after time of injury Focus on infection control, wound care, wound closure, nutritional support, pain management, physical therapy	The emphasis during this phase is placed on restorative therapy, and the phase continues until wound closure is achieved
Rehabilitative Phase Overlaps acute phase of care Extends beyond hospitalization	The goals of this phase are designed so that the client can gain independence and achieve maximal function

e. Monitor arterial blood gases and carboxyhemoglobin level.
f. For an inhalation injury, administer 100% oxygen via a tight-fitting nonrebreather face mask, as prescribed until the carboxyhemoglobin level falls below 15%.
g. Initiate peripheral IV access to nonburned skin proximal to any extremity burn, or prepare for the insertion of a central venous line as prescribed.
h. Monitor for hypovolemia, and prepare to administer fluids intravenously to maintain the fluid balance.
i. Monitor the vital signs closely.
j. Insert a Foley catheter as prescribed, and maintain urine output at 30 to 50 mL per hour.
k. Maintain NPO status.
l. Insert a nasogastric tube as prescribed to remove gastric secretions and prevent aspiration.
m. Administer tetanus prophylaxis as prescribed.
n. Administer pain medication, as prescribed, via the IV route.
o. Prepare the client for an escharotomy or fasciotomy as prescribed.

5. Minor burns
   a. Administer pain medication as prescribed.
   b. Instruct the client regarding the use of oral analgesics as prescribed.
   c. Administer tetanus prophylaxis as prescribed. 
   d. Administer wound care as prescribed, which may include cleansing, débriding loose tissue, removing any damaging agents, followed by the application of topical antimicrobial cream and a sterile dressing.
   e. Reinforce instructions to the client regarding follow-up care, including active range-of-motion exercises and wound care treatments.

B. Resuscitative phase (see Table 41-5) 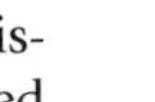
1. Fluid resuscitation
   a. The amount of fluid administered depends on how much IV fluid per hour is required to maintain a urinary output of 30 to 50 mL/hour.
   b. Successful fluid resuscitation is evaluated by stable vital signs, an adequate urine output, palpable peripheral pulses, and intact level of consciousness and thought processes.

c. IV fluid replacement may be titrated (adjusted) on the basis of urinary output plus serum electrolyte levels to meet the perfusion needs of the client with burns.
d. If the hemoglobin and hematocrit levels decrease or if the urinary output exceeds 50 mL/hour, the rate of IV fluid administration may be decreased.

⚠ Urinary output is the most reliable and most sensitive noninvasive assessment parameter for cardiac output and tissue perfusion.

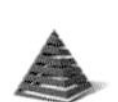

2. Interventions
   a. Monitor for tracheal or laryngeal edema and administer respiratory treatments as prescribed.
   b. Monitor the pulse oximetry and prepare for arterial blood gas and carboxyhemoglobin levels if inhalation injury is suspected.
   c. Elevate the head of the bed to 30 degrees or more for burns of the face and head.
   d. Initiate electrocardiographic monitoring.
   e. Monitor the temperature, and check for infection.
   f. Initiate protective isolation techniques; maintain strict hand washing; use sterile sheets and linens when caring for the client; and use gloves, cap, masks, shoe covers, scrub clothes, and plastic aprons.
   g. Clip body hair around wound margins.
   h. Monitor daily weights, expecting a weight gain of 15 to 20 lbs during the first 72 hours.
   i. Monitor gastric output and pH levels and for gastric discomfort and bleeding, indicating a stress ulcer.
   j. Administer antacids, H_2-receptor antagonists, and antiulcer medications such as prescribed to prevent a stress ulcer.
   k. Auscultate the bowel sounds for ileus and monitor for abdominal distention and gastrointestinal dysfunction.
   l. Monitor stools for occult blood.
   m. Obtain a urine specimen for myoglobin and hemoglobin levels.
   n. Monitor IV fluids and hourly intake and output to determine the adequacy of fluid replacement therapy; notify the HCP if urine output is less than 30 or greater than 50 mL/hour.
   o. Elevate circumferential burns of the extremities on pillows above the level of the heart to reduce dependent edema if no obvious fractures are present; diuretics increase the risk of hypovolemia and are generally avoided as a means of decreasing edema.
   p. Monitor pulses and capillary refill of the affected extremities, and check the perfusion of the distal extremity with a circumferential burn.
   q. Prepare for chest and other radiographs to rule out fractures or associated trauma.
   r. Keep the room temperature warm.
   s. Place the client on an air-fluidized bed or other special mattress and use a bed cradle to keep the sheets off the client's skin.
4. Pain management

⚠ Avoid the intramuscular or subcutaneous medication routes for medication administration because absorption through the soft tissue is unreliable when hypovolemia and large fluid shifts occur.

5. Nutrition
   a. Proper nutrition is essential to promote wound healing and prevent infection.
   b. The basal metabolic rate is 40 to 100 times higher than normal with a burn injury.
   c. Maintain NPO status until bowel sounds are heard, and then advance to clear liquids, as prescribed.
   d. Nutrition may be provided via enteral tube feedings or parenteral nutrition through a central line.
   e. Provide a diet high in protein, carbohydrates, fats, and vitamins.
   f. Monitor calorie intake.
6. Escharotomy
   a. A lengthwise incision is made through the burn eschar to relieve constriction and pressure and to improve circulation.
   b. Escharotomy is performed for circulatory compromise caused by circumferential burns.
   c. Escharotomy is performed at the bedside without anesthesia because nerve endings have been destroyed by the burn injury.
   d. Escharotomy can be performed on the thorax to improve ventilation.
   e. Following escharotomy, check pulses, color, movement, and sensation of affected extremity, and control any bleeding with pressure.
   f. Pack the incision gently with fine-mesh gauze as prescribed after escharotomy.
   g. Apply topical antimicrobial agents to the area as prescribed.
7. Fasciotomy
   a. An incision is made that extends through the subcutaneous tissue and fascia.
   b. The procedure is performed if adequate tissue perfusion does not return following an escharotomy.
   c. Fasciotomy is performed in the operating room with the client under general anesthesia.

d. After the procedure, check the pulses, color, movement, and sensation of the affected extremity, and control any bleeding with pressure.
e. Apply topical antimicrobial agents and dressings to the area, as prescribed.

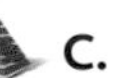
C. Acute phase (see Table 41-5)
1. Continue with protective isolation techniques.
2. Provide wound care as prescribed and prepare for wound closure.
3. Provide pain management.
4. Provide adequate nutrition as prescribed.
5. Prepare the client for rehabilitation.

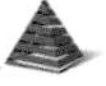
D. Wound care (Table 41-6)
1. Description: The cleansing, débridement, and dressing of the burn wounds
2. Hydrotherapy
a. Wounds are cleansed by immersion, showering, or spraying.
b. Hydrotherapy occurs for 30 minutes or less to prevent increased sodium loss through the burn wound, heat loss, pain, and stress.
c. Client should be medicated before the procedure.
d. Hydrotherapy is generally not used for clients who are hemodynamically unstable or those with new skin grafts.
e. Care is taken to minimize bleeding and to maintain body temperature during the procedure.
f. If hydrotherapy is not used, wounds are washed and rinsed while the client is in bed before the application of antimicrobial agents.
3. Débridement (Box 41-3)
a. Débridement is the removal of eschar or necrotic tissue to prevent bacterial proliferation under the eschar and to promote wound healing.
b. Débridement may be mechanical, enzymatic, or surgical.
c. Deep partial- or **full-thickness burns**: Wound is cleansed and débrided, and topical antimicrobial agents are applied once or twice daily.

E. Wound closure
1. Description
a. Wound closure prevents infection and loss of fluid.
b. Closure promotes healing.
c. Closure prevents contractures.

TABLE 41-6 Open Method versus Closed Method of Wound Care

Method	Advantages	Disadvantages
Open		
Antimicrobial cream is applied as prescribed, and wound is left open to the air without a dressing	Visualization of the wound	Increased chance of hypothermia from exposure
	Easier mobility and joint range of motion	
	Simplicity in wound care	
Closed		
Gauze dressings are carefully wrapped from the distal to the proximal area of the extremity to ensure that circulation is not compromised	Decreases evaporative fluid and heat loss	Mobility limitations
No two burn surfaces should be allowed to touch; touching can promote webbing of digits, contractures, and poor cosmetic outcome	Aids in débridement	Prevents effective range-of-motion exercises
Dressings are changed usually every 8 to 12 hr		Wound assessment limited

BOX 41-3 Débridement

Mechanical
- Performed during hydrotherapy; involves use of washcloths or sponges to cleanse and débride eschar and the use of scissors and forceps to lift and trim away loose eschar
- May include wet-to-dry or wet-to-wet dressing changes
- Painful procedure; may cause bleeding

Enzymatic
- Application of topical enzyme agents directly to the wound; the agent digests collagen necrotic tissue

Surgical
- Excision of eschar or necrotic tissue via a surgical procedure in the operating room

Tangential Technique
- Very thin layers of the necrotic burn surface are excised until bleeding occurs (bleeding indicates that a healthy dermis or subcutaneous fat has been reached).

Fascial Technique
- The burn wound is excised to the level of superficial fascia; this technique is usually reserved for very deep and extensive burns.

BOX 41-4 Wound Coverings

Biological

Amniotic Membranes

- Amniotic membranes from human placentas are used to adhere to the wound.
- This is effective as a dressing until epithelial cell regrowth occurs.
- Frequent changes are required, because amnion does not develop a blood supply, and it disintegrates in about 48 hours.

Allograft or Homograft (Human Tissue)

- Donated human cadaver skin is provided through a skin bank.
- Monitor for wound exudate and signs of infection.
- Rejection can occur within 24 hours.
- The risk of transmitting a blood-borne infection exists with the use of this covering.

Xenograft or Heterograft (Animal Tissue)

- Pigskin is harvested after slaughter and preserved for storage.
- Monitor for infection and wound adherence.
- Rejection can occur within 24 to 72 hours.
- This tissue is placed over granulation tissue and replaced every 2 to 5 days until the wound heals naturally or until closure with an autograft is complete.

Cultured Skin

- Cultured skin is grown in a laboratory from a small specimen of epidermal cells from an unburned portion of the client's body.
- Cell sheets are grafted onto the client to generate a permanent skin surface.
- Cell sheets are not durable; care must be taken when applying them to ensure adherence and prevent sloughing.

Autograft

- Skin is taken from a remote, unburned area of the client's own body and transplanted to cover the burn wound.
- The graft is placed either on a clean granulated bed or over a surgically excised area of the burn.
- Autograft provides for permanent skin coverage.

Nonbiological

Artificial Skin

- Artificial skin consists of two layers: a Silastic epidermis and a porous dermis made from bovine hide collagen and shark cartilage.
- After application, fibroblasts move into the collagen part of the artificial skin and create a structure that is similar to that of normal dermis.
- The artificial dermis then dissolves and is replaced with normal blood vessels and connective tissue called neodermis.
- The neodermis supports a standard autograft that is placed over it when the Silastic layer is removed.

Biosynthetic

- This type of covering is made of a combination of biosynthetic and synthetic materials.
- It is placed in contact with the wound surface, and it forms an adherent bond until epithelialization has occurred.
- Its porous substance allows exudate to pass through it.
- Monitor for wound exudate and signs of infection.

Synthetic

- Synthetic coverings are applied directly to the surface of a clean or surgically prepared wound, and they remain in place until they fall off or are removed.
- The covering is transparent or translucent; therefore, the wound can be inspected without removing the dressing.
- Pain at the wound site is reduced because the covering prevents the contact of the wound with air.

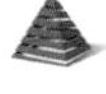

d. Wound closure is performed on day 5 to 21 following the injury, depending on the extent of the burn.

2. Wound coverings (Box 41-4)

3. Autografting (see Box 41-4)

a. Autografting provides permanent wound coverage.

b. Autografting is the surgical removal of a thin layer of the client's own unburned skin, which is then applied to the excised burn wound.

c. Autografting is performed in the operating room with the client under anesthesia.

d. Monitor for bleeding after the graft because bleeding beneath an autograft can prevent adherence.

e. If prescribed, small amounts of blood or serum can be removed by gently rolling the fluid from the center of the graft to the periphery with a sterile gauze pad, where it can be absorbed.

f. For large accumulations of blood, the HCP will aspirate the blood with the use of a small-gauge needle and syringe.

g. Autografts are immobilized after surgery for 3 to 7 days to allow time for the graft to adhere and attach to the wound bed.

h. Position the client for the immobilization and elevation of the graft site to prevent the movement and shearing of the graft.

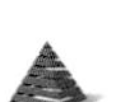
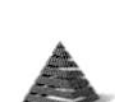

4. Care of the graft site

a. Elevate and immobilize the graft site.

b. Keep the site free from pressure.

c. Avoid weight-bearing.

d. When the graft takes, if prescribed, roll a cotton-tipped applicator over the graft to remove exudate, because exudate can lead to infection and prevent graft adherence.

e. Monitor for foul-smelling drainage, increased temperature, increased white blood cell count, hematoma formation, and fluid accumulation.

f. Reinforce instructions to the client to avoid using fabric softeners and harsh detergents in the laundry.
g. Reinforce instructions to the client to lubricate the healing skin with prescribed agents.
h. Reinforce instructions to the client to protect the affected area from sunlight.
i. Reinforce instructions to the client to use splints and support garments as prescribed.

5. Care of the donor site
   a. Method of care varies, depending on the HCP's preference.
   b. A nonadherent gauze dressing may be applied at the time of surgery to maintain pressure and to stop any oozing; always check surgeon's preference.
   c. The HCP may prescribe site treatment with gauze impregnated with petrolatum or with a biosynthetic dressing.
   d. Keep the donor site clean, dry, and free from pressure.
   e. Prevent the client from scratching the donor site.
   f. Apply lubricating lotions to soften the area and to reduce the itching after the donor site is healed.
   g. Donor site can be reused after healing has occurred (heals spontaneously within 7 to 14 days with proper care).

F. Physical therapy
1. An individualized program of splinting, positioning, exercises, ambulation, and activities of daily living is implemented early during the acute phase of recovery to maximize the functional and cosmetic outcomes.
2. Perform range-of-motion exercises as prescribed to reduce edema and to maintain strength and joint function.
3. Ambulate the client as prescribed to maintain the strength of the lower extremities.
4. Apply splints as prescribed to maintain proper joint position and prevent contractures.
   a. Static splints immobilize the joint and are applied for periods of immobilization, during sleeping, and for clients who cannot maintain proper positioning.
   b. Dynamic splints exercise the affected joint.
   c. Avoid pressure to skin areas when applying splints, which could lead to further tissue and nerve damage.
5. Scarring is controlled by elastic wraps and bandages that apply continuous pressure to the healing skin during the period of time when the skin is vulnerable to shearing.
6. Anti-burn scar support garments are usually worn 23 hours a day until the burn scar tissue has matured, which takes 18 months to 2 years.

G. Rehabilitative phase (see Table 41-5)
1. Description
   a. Rehabilitation is the final phase of burn care.
2. Goals
   a. Promote wound healing.
   b. Minimize deformities.
   c. Increase strength and function.
   d. Provide emotional support.

CRITICAL THINKING What Should You Do?

Answer: The nurse should elevate and immobilize the graft site, keep the site free from pressure, and not allow the client to bear weight on the extremity. When the graft takes, if prescribed, the nurse should roll a cotton-tipped applicator over the graft to remove exudate, because exudate can lead to infection and prevent graft adherence. The nurse should monitor for signs of infection such as foul-smelling drainage, increased temperature, and increased white blood cell count; and monitor for hematoma formation, or fluid accumulation.

Reference(s): Ignatavicius, D., & Workman, M. (2013). *Medical-surgical nursing: Patient-centered collaborative care.* (7th ed., p. 534). St. Louis: Saunders.

PRACTICE QUESTIONS

❖**396.** An adult client was burned as a result of an explosion. The burn initially affected the client's entire face (the anterior half of the head) and the upper half of the anterior torso, and there were circumferential burns to the lower half of both of the arms. The client's clothes caught on fire, and the client ran, which caused subsequent burn injuries of the posterior surface of the head and the upper half of the posterior torso. According to the rule of nines, what is the extent of this client's burn injury? **Fill in the blank.**

Answer: _____%

397. The nurse, employed in a long-term care facility, is planning the clinical assignments for the day. The nurse knows not to assign which staff member to the client with a diagnosis of herpes zoster?
1. A staff member who has never had roseola
2. A staff member who has never had mumps
3. An unlicensed assistive personnel who has never had chickenpox
4. An unlicensed assistive personnel who has never had German measles

398. A client returns to the clinic for follow-up treatment after a skin biopsy of a suspicious lesion that was performed 1 week ago. The biopsy report indicates that the lesion is a melanoma. The nurse

understands that which describes a characteristic of this type of a lesion?
1. Metastasis is rare.
2. It is encapsulated.
3. It is highly metastatic.
4. It is characterized by local invasion.

399. The nurse is reviewing the health care record of a client with a lesion that has been diagnosed as malignant melanoma. The nurse should expect which characteristic of this type of lesion to be documented in the client's record?
1. An irregularly shaped lesion
2. A small papule with a dry, rough scale
3. A firm nodular lesion topped with a crust
4. A pearly papule with a central crater and a waxy border

400. The nurse reinforces instructions to a group of clients regarding measures that will assist with the prevention of skin cancer. Which statement by a client indicates the **need for further teaching**?
1. "I need to wear sunscreen when participating in outdoor activities."
2. "I need to avoid sun exposure before 10:00 AM and after 4:00 PM."
3. "I need to wear a hat, opaque clothing, and sunglasses when in the sun."
4. "I need to examine my body monthly for any lesions that may be suspicious."

401. A client arrives at the emergency department and has experienced frostbite to the right hand. Which should the nurse expect to find when inspecting the client's hand?
1. A pink, edematous hand
2. Fiery red skin with edema in the nail beds
3. Black fingertips surrounded by an erythematous rash
4. A white color of the skin, which is insensitive to touch

402. The evening nurse reviews the nursing documentation in the client's chart and notes that the day nurse has documented that the client has a stage 2 pressure ulcer in the sacral area. Which should the nurse expect to find when checking the client's sacral area?
1. Intact skin
2. The presence of tunneling
3. A deep, crater-like appearance
4. Partial-thickness skin loss of the epidermis

403. The nurse inspects the skin of a client who is suspected of having psoriasis. Which finding should the nurse note if this disorder is present?
1. Oily skin
2. Silvery-white scaly lesions
3. Patchy hair loss and round, red macules with scales
4. The presence of wheal patches scattered about the trunk

404. The nurse is told that an assigned client is suspected of having *methicillin-resistant Staphylococcus aureus* (MRSA). Which precautions should the nurse institute during the care of the client?
1. Wear gloves only.
2. Wear a mask and gloves.
3. Wear a gown and gloves.
4. Avoid touching the client's clothes.

405. The client arrives at the emergency department after a burn injury that occurred in the basement at home, and an inhalation injury is suspected. Which should the nurse anticipate as being prescribed for the client?
1. Oxygen via nasal cannula at 10 L
2. Oxygen via nasal cannula at 15 L
3. 100% oxygen via an aerosol mask
4. 100% oxygen via a tight-fitting, nonrebreather face mask

406. The nurse is caring for a client who has just been admitted to the nursing unit after receiving flame burns to the face and chest. The nurse notes a hoarse cough, and the client is expectorating sputum with black flecks. The client suddenly becomes restless, and his color is becoming dusky. The nurse should interpret this data as indicating which?
1. The client is hypotensive.
2. Pain is present from the burn injury.
3. The burn has probably caused laryngeal edema, which has occluded the airway.
4. The client is afraid and is having a panic attack as a result of the unfamiliar surroundings.

407. Which should be the anticipated therapeutic outcome of an escharotomy procedure performed for a circumferential arm burn?
1. The return of distal pulses
2. Decreasing edema formation
3. Brisk bleeding from the injury site
4. The formation of granulation tissue

408. The nurse is caring for a client with circumferential burns of both legs. Which leg position is appropriate for this type of a burn?
1. A dependent position
2. Elevation of the knees
3. Flat, without elevation
4. Elevation above the level of the heart

409. The nurse is assisting with caring for a client who is receiving intravenous fluids and who has sustained full-thickness burn injuries of the back and legs. The nurse understands that which would provide the **most** reliable indicator for determining the adequacy of the fluid resuscitation?

1. Vital signs
2. Urine output
3. Mental status
4. Peripheral pulses

410. The nurse is assigned to care for a client with herpes zoster. Which characteristics should the nurse expect to note when checking the lesions of this infection?

1. Clustered skin vesicles
2. A generalized body rash
3. Small blue-white spots with red bases
4. A fiery red edematous rash on the cheeks

ANSWERS

❖ **396. 36%**

Rationale: According to the rule of nines, with the initial burn, the anterior half of the head equals 4.5%, the upper half of the anterior torso equals 9%, and the lower halves of both arms equal 9%. The subsequent burn included the posterior half of the head, which equals 4.5%, and the upper half of the posterior torso, which equals 9%. This totals 36%.

Test-Taking Strategy: Focus on the subject, the rule of nines. Knowledge of this rule is necessary in order to answer this question. According to the rule, the entire head equals 9%, each arm equals 9% (both arms, 18%), the anterior and posterior torsos each equal 18% (entire torso, 36%), each leg equals 18% (both legs, 36%), and the perineum equals 1%. Remember the following: 9% (head) + 18% (arms) + 36% (torsos) + 36% (legs) + 1% (perineum) = 100%. **Review:** the **rule of nines.**

Level of Cognitive Ability: Analyzing
Client Needs: Physiological Integrity
Integrated Process: Nursing Process/Data Collection
Content Area: Adult Health: Integumentary
Priority Concepts: Clinical Judgment, Tissue Integrity
Reference(s): deWit, Kumagai (2013), p. 982.

397. 3

Rationale: Herpes zoster is caused by a reactivation of the varicella zoster virus, which is the causative virus of chickenpox. Individuals who have not been exposed to the varicella zoster virus are susceptible to chickenpox. Options 1, 2, and 4 are not associated with the herpes zoster virus.

Test-Taking Strategy: Note the subject, safe assignment-making. Recalling that herpes zoster is caused by a reactivation of the varicella zoster virus will assist you with answering the question. **Review:** the relationship between **herpes zoster** and **chickenpox.**

Level of Cognitive Ability: Applying
Client Needs: Safe and Effective Care Environment
Integrated Process: Nursing Process/Planning
Content Area: Fundamental Skills: Infection Control
Priority Concepts: Immunity, Infection
Reference(s): Linton (2012), p. 1193.

398. 3

Rationale: Melanomas are pigmented malignant lesions that originate in the melanin-producing cells of the epidermis. This skin cancer is highly metastatic, and a person's survival depends on early diagnosis and treatment. Basal cell carcinomas arise in the basal cell layer of the epidermis. Early malignant basal cell lesions often go unnoticed, and although metastasis is rare, underlying tissue destruction can progress to include vital structures. Squamous cell carcinomas are malignant neoplasms of the epidermis. They are characterized by local invasion and the potential for metastasis.

Test-Taking Strategy: Focus on the subject, a melanoma, and use knowledge regarding the various types of skin cancers. Recalling that melanomas are highly metastatic will direct you to the correct option. **Review:** the characteristics of **skin cancers.**

Level of Cognitive Ability: Understanding
Client Needs: Physiological Integrity
Integrated Process: Nursing Process/Data Collection
Content Area: Adult Health: Integumentary
Priority Concepts: Cellular Regulation, Tissue Integrity
Reference(s): Linton (2012), p. 1196.

399. 1

Rationale: A melanoma is an irregularly shaped pigmented papule or plaque with a red, white, or blue color. Basal cell carcinoma appears as a pearly papule with a central crater and a rolled, waxy border. Squamous cell carcinoma is a firm nodular lesion that is topped with a crust or a central area of ulceration. Actinic keratosis, which is a premalignant lesion, appears as a small macule or papule with a dry, rough, adherent yellow or brown scale.

Test-Taking Strategy: Focus on the subject, malignant melanoma. Remembering that irregularly shaped lesions are a cause for concern will assist you with answering the question. **Review:** the characteristics of **malignant skin lesions.**

Level of Cognitive Ability: Analyzing
Client Needs: Physiological Integrity
Integrated Process: Nursing Process/Data Collection
Content Area: Adult Health: Integumentary
Priority Concepts: Cellular Regulation, Tissue Integrity
Reference(s): Linton (2012), p. 1196.

400. 2

Rationale: The client should be instructed to avoid sun exposure between the hours of approximately 10:00 AM and 4:00 PM. Sunscreen, a hat, opaque clothing, and sunglasses should be worn for outdoor activities. The client should be instructed to examine the body monthly for the appearance of any possible cancerous or precancerous lesions.

Test-Taking Strategy: Note the strategic words, *need for further teaching.* These words indicate a negative event query and ask you to select an option that is an incorrect statement. A careful reading of the question will direct you to the correct option. **Review:** client teaching for the prevention of **skin cancer.**

Level of Cognitive Ability: Evaluating
Client Needs: Health Promotion and Maintenance

Integrated Process: Teaching and Learning
Content Area: Adult Health: Integumentary
Priority Concepts: Client Education, Tissue Integrity
Reference(s): deWit, Kumagai (2013), p. 152; Ignatavicius, Workman (2013), p. 503; Lewis et al (2014), pp. 427–428, 431.

401. 4
Rationale: The findings related to frostbite include a white or blue skin color and skin that is hard, cold, and insensitive to touch. As thawing occurs, so does flushing of the skin, the development of blisters or blebs, or tissue edema. Gangrene can develop in 9 to 15 days.
Test-Taking Strategy: Focus on the subject, diagnosis of frostbite. The words, *insensitive to touch,* should assist with directing you to the correct option. **Review:** the characteristics associated with **frostbite.**
Level of Cognitive Ability: Analyzing
Client Needs: Physiological Integrity
Integrated Process: Nursing Process/Data Collection
Content Area: Adult Health: Integumentary
Priority Concepts: Sensory Perception, Tissue Integrity
Reference(s): deWit, Kumagai (2013), pp. 1027–1028.

402. 4
Rationale: With a stage 2 pressure ulcer, the skin is not intact. There is partial-thickness skin loss of the epidermis or dermis. The ulcer is superficial, and it may look like an abrasion, blister, or shallow crater. The skin is intact with a stage 1 pressure ulcer. A deep, crater-like appearance occurs during stage 3, and tunneling develops during stage 4.
Test-Taking Strategy: Focus on the subject, findings associated with a stage 2 pressure ulcer. Use your knowledge of the characteristics associated with each stage of pressure ulcers. Remember, with a stage 2 pressure ulcer, the skin is not intact. **Review:** the characteristics associated with each stage of **pressure ulcers**.
Level of Cognitive Ability: Analyzing
Client Needs: Physiological Integrity
Integrated Process: Nursing Process/Data Collection
Content Area: Adult Health: Integumentary
Priority Concepts: Cellular Regulation, Tissue Integrity
Reference(s): Linton (2012), pp. 339–340.

403. 2
Rationale: Psoriatic patches are covered with silvery white scales. There is no patchy hair loss or round, red macules with scales. The skin is dry and there is no presence of wheal patches scattered about the trunk.
Test-Taking Strategy: Focus on the subject, psoriasis. Recall that psoriasis is associated with the presence of silvery white scaly patches. This will direct you to the correct option. **Review:** signs/symptoms associated with **psoriasis**.
Level of Cognitive Ability: Understanding
Client Needs: Physiological Integrity
Integrated Process: Nursing Process/Data Collection
Content Area: Adult Health: Integumentary
Priority Concepts: Clinical Judgment, Tissue Integrity
Reference(s): deWit, Kumagai (2013), p. 969.

404. 3
Rationale: The Centers for Disease Control and Prevention recommends the wearing of gowns and gloves when in close contact with a person who has *methicillin-resistant Staphylococcus aureus* (MRSA). Masks are not necessary. Transmission via clothing and other inanimate objects is uncommon. *Methicillin-resistant Staphylococcus aureus* (MRSA) is contagious and is spread to others by direct contact with infected skin or infected articles.
Test-Taking Strategy: Focus on the subject, precautions for a client with *methicillin-resistant Staphylococcus aureus* (MRSA). Consider the mode of transmission of *methicillin-resistant Staphylococcus aureus* (MRSA). Because *methicillin-resistant Staphylococcus aureus* (MRSA) is transmitted by direct skin contact, eliminate options 1, 2, and 4. **Review:** standard precautions and the transmission mode of **methicillin-resistant Staphylococcus aureus (MRSA)**.
Level of Cognitive Ability: Applying
Client Needs: Safe and Effective Care Environment
Integrated Process: Nursing Process/Implementation
Content Area: Fundamental Skills: Infection Control
Priority Concepts: Infection, Safety
Reference(s): deWit, Kumagai (2013), pp. 967, 974.

405. 4
Rationale: If an inhalation injury is suspected, the administration of 100% oxygen via a tight-fitting, nonrebreather face mask is prescribed until the carboxyhemoglobin level falls below 15%. With inhalation injuries, the oropharynx is inspected for evidence of erythema, blisters, or ulcerations. The need for endotracheal intubation is also determined. Options 1, 2, and 3 are incorrect.
Test-Taking Strategy: Focus on the subject, inhalation injury. Recalling that 100% oxygen is required after an inhalation injury will assist you with eliminating options 1 and 2. From the remaining options, recall that a tight-fitting nonrebreather mask is preferred so that the client will not rebreathe exhaled air. **Review:** care of the client after an **inhalation injury**.
Level of Cognitive Ability: Analyzing
Client Needs: Physiological Integrity
Integrated Process: Nursing Process/Planning
Content Area: Critical Care: Emergency Situations
Priority Concepts: Gas Exchange, Tissue Integrity
Reference(s): Lewis et al (2014), p. 456.

406. 3
Rationale: The client exhibits several warning signs of an inhalation injury: a history of a flame burn to the face, hoarseness, cough, carbonaceous sputum, singed facial hair, facial edema, and color change. Additionally, one of the cardinal signs of hypoxia is restlessness.
Test-Taking Strategy: Use the ABCs—airway, breathing, and circulation—to answer the question. The only option that addresses the airway is option 3. **Review:** the signs and symptoms associated with **burns** of the face and **laryngeal edema**.
Level of Cognitive Ability: Analyzing
Client Needs: Physiological Integrity
Integrated Process: Nursing Process/Data Collection
Content Area: Critical Care: Emergency Situations
Priority Concepts: Gas Exchange, Tissue Integrity
Reference(s): Lewis et al (2014), p. 456.

407. 1
Rationale: Escharotomies are performed to alleviate the compartment syndrome that can occur when edema forms under

nondistensible eschar in a circumferential burn. Escharotomies are performed through avascular eschar to subcutaneous fat. Although bleeding may occur from the site, it is considered a complication rather than an anticipated therapeutic outcome. The formation of granulation tissue is not the intent of an escharotomy, and escharotomy will not affect the formation of edema.
Test-Taking Strategy: Note the subject, a therapeutic outcome. Use the ABCs—airway, breathing, and circulation—to answer the question. The only option that addresses circulation is the correct option. **Review:** the purpose of an escharotomy.
Level of Cognitive Ability: Evaluating
Client Needs: Physiological Integrity
Integrated Process: Nursing Process/Evaluation
Content Area: Adult Health: Integumentary
Priority Concepts: Perfusion, Tissue Integrity
Reference(s): deWit, Kumagai (2013), p. 986.

408. 4
Rationale: Circumferential burns of the extremities may compromise circulation. Elevating injured extremities above the level of the heart and performing active exercise help to reduce dependent edema formation. Options 1, 2, and 3 are incorrect.
Test-Taking Strategy: Focus on the subject, circumferential burns. Remember that when an injury such as a burn occurs, edema occurs. Option 4 addresses a position that will reduce edema. **Review:** the care of the client with a **circumferential burn injury.**
Level of Cognitive Ability: Applying
Client Needs: Physiological Integrity
Integrated Process: Nursing Process/Implementation
Content Area: Adult Health: Integumentary
Priority Concepts: Perfusion, Tissue Integrity
Reference(s): Lewis et al (2014), p. 455.

409. 2
Rationale: Successful or adequate fluid resuscitation in the adult is signaled by stable vital signs, adequate urine output, palpable peripheral pulses, and a clear sensorium. The most reliable indicator for determining the adequacy of fluid resuscitation is the urine output. For an adult, the hourly urine volume should be 30 to 50 mL.
Test-Taking Strategy: Note the subject, fluid resuscitation. Also note the strategic word, *most.* Note the relationship between urine output and the subject of administering fluids. **Review:** the care of the burn client during **fluid resuscitation.**
Level of Cognitive Ability: Evaluating
Client Needs: Physiological Integrity
Integrated Process: Nursing Process/Evaluation
Content Area: Critical Care: Emergency Situations
Priority Concepts: Fluid and Electrolyte Balance, Tissue Integrity
Reference(s): deWit, Kumagai (2013), p. 985.

410. 1
Rationale: The primary lesion of herpes zoster is a vesicle. The classic presentation is grouped vesicles on an erythematous base along a dermatome. Because they follow nerve pathways, the lesions do not cross the body's midline. Options 2, 3, and 4 are incorrect descriptions.
Test-Taking Strategy: Note the subject, characteristics of herpes zoster. Remembering that these lesions occur as grouped vesicles along a nerve pathway will assist you with answering the question. **Review:** the characteristics of **herpes zoster lesions.**
Level of Cognitive Ability: Understanding
Client Needs: Physiological Integrity
Integrated Process: Nursing Process/Data Collection
Content Area: Adult Health: Integumentary
Priority Concepts: Infection, Tissue Integrity
Reference(s): deWit, Kumagai (2013), pp. 971–972; Linton (2012), pp. 1192–1193.

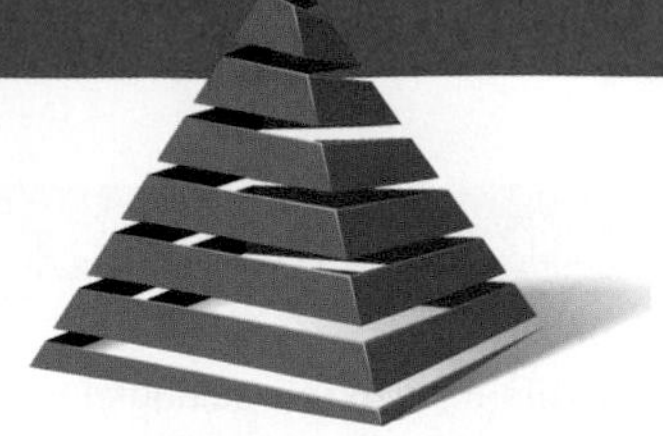

CHAPTER 42

Integumentary Medications

CRITICAL THINKING What Should You Do?

A topical glucocorticoid is prescribed for a hospitalized client to treat an inflammatory skin condition on the neck. What should the nurse do when administering the medication?
Answer located on p.511.

I. Poison Ivy Treatment (Box 42-1 and Fig. 42-1)

A. Treatment of lesions includes calamine lotion and other products that soothe lesions, Burow's solution compresses (Aluminum acetate), and/or Aveeno baths to relieve discomfort.

B. Topical corticosteroids are effective to prevent or relieve inflammation, especially when used before blisters form.

C. Oral corticosteroids may be prescribed for severe reactions, and a sedative such as diphenhydramine (Benadryl) may be prescribed.

II. Medications to Treat Atopic Dermatitis (Box 42-2)

A. Description
  1. A chronic inflammatory skin disease that is also known as eczema and is characterized by dry and scaly skin
  2. May be treated with moisturizer and topical glucocorticoids; systemic immunosuppressants may also be prescribed if topical treatment is ineffective.
  3. Systemic immunosuppressants may include methotrexate, cyclosporine (Sandimmune), or azathioprine (Imuran), and oral glucocorticoids.

B. Topical immunosuppressants
  1. Include tacrolimus (Protopic) and Pimecrolimus 1% cream (Elidel)
  2. Side effects include redness, burning, and itching; causes sensitization of the skin to sunlight.
  3. Tacrolimus (Protopic) increases the risk of varicella zoster infection in children.
  4. Tacrolimus (Protopic) may cause **skin cancer** and lymphoma.

C. Other medications
  1. Topical tricyclic antidepressants such as doxepin, which is available as a Zonalon cream, may be prescribed; side effects include burning or stinging at the application site, drowsiness, dizziness, dry mouth, blurred vision, and changes in taste.
  2. Coal tar may be prescribed: Side/adverse effects include increased risk of skin cancer and skin irritation. (See section on psoriasis for more information on coal tar.)

III. Topical Glucocorticoids

A. Description
  1. Anti-inflammatory, antipruritic, and vasoconstrictive actions
  2. Preparations vary in potency and depend on the concentration and type of preparation and method of application (occlusive dressings enhance absorption, increasing the effects).
  3. Systemic effects are more likely to occur with prolonged therapy and when extensive skin surfaces are treated.

⚠ Topical glucocorticoids can be absorbed into the systemic circulation; absorption is greater in permeable skin areas (scalp, axilla, face and neck, eyelids, perineum) and less in areas where permeability is poor (palms, soles, back).

B. Contraindications
  1. Clients demonstrating previous sensitivity to corticosteroids
  2. Clients with current systemic fungal, viral, or bacterial infections
  3. Clients with current complications related to glucocorticoid therapy

C. Local side/adverse effects
  1. Burning, dryness, irritation, itching
  2. Skin atrophy
  3. Thinning of the skin, striae, purpura, telangiectasia
  4. Acneiform eruptions
  5. Hypopigmentation
  6. Overgrowth of bacteria, fungi, and viruses

D. Systemic adverse effects
  1. Growth retardation in children
  2. Adrenal suppression
  3. Cushing's syndrome
  4. Striae, skin atrophy
  5. Ocular effects (glaucoma and cataracts)

BOX 42-1 Poison Ivy Treatment Products

Bentoquatam—for preventive use (Ivy Block)
Calamine lotion (Caladryl lotion)
Hydrocortisone (Ivy Soothe, Ivy Stat)
Isopropanol; cetyl alcohol (Ivy Cleanse)
Zinc acetate; isopropanol (Ivy Dry)
Zinc acetate; isopropanol; benzyl alcohol (Ivy Super Dry)

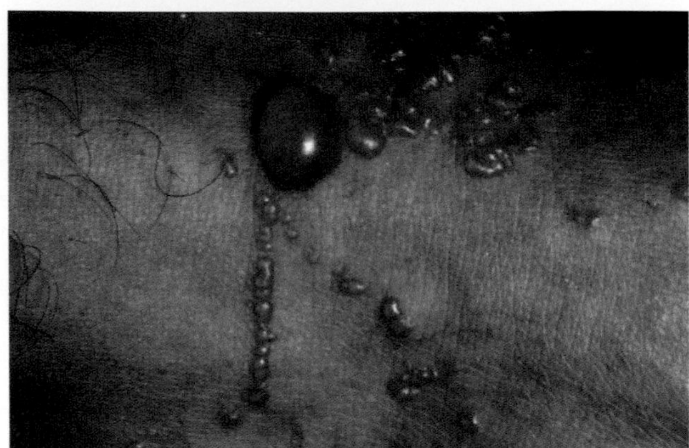

FIGURE 42-1 Poison ivy. Note "streaked" blisters surrounding one large blister. (From Habif TP: *Clinical dermatology: a color guide to diagnosis and therapy*, ed 4, St. Louis, 2004, Mosby.)

BOX 42-2 Medications to Treat Atopic Dermatitis

Systemic Immunosuppressants
Methotrexate
Cyclosporine (Sandimmune)
Azathioprine (Imuran)
Oral glucocorticoids

Topical Immunosuppressants
Tacrolimus (Protopic)
Pimecrolimus 1% cream (Elidel)

Others
Doxepin (Zonalon)
Coal tar

E. Interventions
1. Monitoring plasma cortisol levels may be prescribed if prolonged therapy is necessary.
2. Wash the area just before application to increase medication penetration.
3. Apply sparingly in a thin film, rubbing gently.
4. Avoid the use of a dry occlusive dressing unless specifically prescribed by the health care provider (HCP).
5. Reinforce instructions to the client to report signs of adverse effects to the HCP.

BOX 42-3 Medications to Treat Actinic Keratoses

Aminolevulinic acid (Levulan Kerastick)
Diclofenac sodium 3% gel (Solaraze)
Fluorouracil (Carac, Efudex, Fluoroplex)
Imiquimod 5% cream (Aldara)

⚠ In the adult, intact skin is generally impermeable to most topical medications. However, medications should not be applied to denuded areas unless prescribed because undesired absorption can occur.

IV. Medications to Treat Actinic Keratosis (Box 42-3)

A. Description
1. Actinic keratoses are caused by chronic exposure to the sun and appear as rough, scaly, red or brown lesions and are usually found on the face, scalp, arms, and back of the hands.
2. Lesions can progress to squamous cell carcinoma.
3. Treatment includes medications and therapies such as excision, cryotherapy, curettage, and laser therapy.

B. Medications include fluorouracil (Carac, Efudex, Fluoroplex), diclofenac sodium (Solaraze; Voltaren gel), imiquimod 5% cream (Aldara; Zyclara), and aminolevulinic acid (Levulan Kerastick).
1. Fluorouracil (Carac, Efudex, Fluoroplex)
   a. A topical medication that affects DNA and RNA synthesis and causes a sequence of responses that results in healing; results are usually seen in 2 to 6 weeks, but it may take 1 to 2 months longer for complete healing.
   b. Side effects include itching, burning, inflammation, rash, and increased sensitivity to sunlight.
2. Diclofenac sodium (Solaraze; Voltaren gel)
   a. A nonsteroidal anti-inflammatory topical drug, which may take 3 months to be effective
   b. Side effects include dry skin, itching, redness, and rash.
3. Imiquimod 5% cream (Aldara; Zyclara)
   a. In addition to treating actinic keratoses, this topical medication has been used to treat venereal warts; it may take up to 4 months to be effective.
   b. Side effects include redness, skin swelling, itching, burning, sores, blisters, scabbing, and crusting of the skin.
4. Aminolevulinic acid (Levulan Kerastick)
   a. A topical medication used in conjunction with blue light photoactivation; the medication is applied, and 14 to 18 hours later, the medication is activated by exposing the lesions to the blue light.
   b. Can cause burning, stinging, redness, and swelling of the skin. Treated areas need to be protected from sunlight and bright indoor lights.

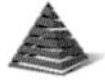

V. Sunscreens

A. Ultraviolet (UV) light can damage the skin and can cause premalignant actinic keratoses and some types of skin cancer.

B. Sunscreens prevent the penetration of UV light and protect the skin.

C. Organic (chemical) sunscreen absorbs UV light; inorganic (physical) sunscreen reflects and scatters UV light.

D. A sunscreen that protects against both UVB and UVA rays and one that has a sun protection factor (SPF) of at least 15 should be used.

E. Sunscreens are most effective when applied at least 30 minutes before exposure to the sun (sunscreens containing para-aminobenzoic acid [PABA] or padimate O require application 2 hours before sun exposure).

F. Sunscreen should be reapplied every 2 to 3 hours and after swimming or sweating; otherwise, the duration of protection is reduced.

G. Products containing PABA need to be avoided by individuals who are allergic to benzocaine, sulfonamides, or thiazides.

H. Sunscreens can cause contact dermatitis and photosensitivity reactions.

> ⚠ The client should be informed that UV light is greatest between the hours of 10:00 AM and 4:00 PM, and sunglasses, protective clothing, and a hat should be worn to reduce the risk of skin damage from the sun.

VI. Medications to Treat Psoriasis (Box 42-4)

A. Description
1. Psoriasis is a chronic inflammatory disorder that has varying degrees of severity.
2. Treatment is based on the severity of symptoms and aims to suppress the proliferation of keratinocytes or the activity of inflammatory cells.

B. Topical medications
1. Glucocorticoids
   - **a.** Used for mild psoriasis
   - **b.** Should not be applied to the face, groin, axilla, or genitalia because the medication is readily absorbable, making the skin vulnerable to glucocorticoid-induced atrophy
2. Anthralin (Dritho-Crème, Zithranol)
   - **a.** Can cause local irritation and skin redness.
   - **b.** Is applied to lesions at bedtime and allowed to remain on the skin overnight
   - **c.** Client should be informed that the medication can stain clothing, skin, and hair.
3. Tazarotene (Tazorac; Avage)
   - **a.** Is a vitamin A derivative
   - **b.** Local reactions include itching, burning, stinging, dry skin, and redness; other, less common effects include rash, desquamation, contact dermatitis, inflammation, fissuring, and bleeding.
   - **c.** Sensitization to sunlight can occur, and the client should be instructed to use sunscreen and wear protective clothing.
   - **d.** Medication is usually applied once daily in the evening to dry skin.
4. Calcipotriene (Dovonex; Calcitrene)
   - **a.** Is an analogue of vitamin D
   - **b.** May take up to 1 to 3 weeks to produce a desired effect
   - **c.** Can cause local irritation; high-dose applications may cause hypercalcemia.
5. Coal tar (Exorex, Alphosyl HC cream)
   - **a.** Suppresses DNA synthesis, miotic activity, and cell proliferation
   - **b.** Has an unpleasant odor and may cause irritation, burning, and stinging; can also stain the skin and hair
6. Keratolytics
   - **a.** Soften scales and loosen the horny layer of the skin, resulting in minimal peeling to extensive desquamation
   - **b.** Salicylic acid: Can be absorbed systemically 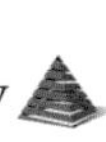 and can cause salicylism, which is characterized by dizziness and tinnitus, hyperpnea, and psychologic disturbances. Salicylic acid is not applied to large surface areas or open wounds because of the risk of systemic effects.

BOX 42-4 Medications and Treatments for Psoriasis

Topical Medications
Anthralin (Dritho-Crème, Zithranol)
Calcipotriene (Dovonex)
Coal tar
Glucocorticoids
Keratolytics (topical salicylic acid; sulfur)
Tazarotene (Tazorac)
Others

Systemic Medications
Acitretin (Soriatane)
Cyclosporine (Neoral)
Methotrexate

Systemic Biologic Medications
Alefacept (Amevive)
Ustekinumab (Stelara)
Adalimumab (Humira)
Infliximab (Remicade)
Etanercept (Enbrel)

Phototherapy
Coal tar and ultraviolet B irradiation
Photochemotherapy (PUVA [psoralen and ultraviolet A] therapy)

c. Sulfur: Promotes peeling and drying and is used to treat acne, dandruff, seborrheic dermatitis, and psoriasis; may be used if there is a concern for using a corticosteroid or a risk of coal tar toxicity

C. Systemic medications
1. Methotrexate
a. Used for moderate to severe psoriasis and reduces proliferation of epidermal cells
b. Can be toxic; causes gastrointestinal effects such as diarrhea and ulcerative stomatitis and bone marrow depression leading to blood dyscrasias
c. Can be hepatotoxic, and hepatic function should be monitored during therapy
2. Acitretin (Soriatane)
a. Inhibits keratinization, proliferation, and differentiation of cells; has anti-inflammatory and immunomodulatory actions; used for severe psoriasis and is reserved for use in those who have not responded to safer medications
b. Is embryotoxic and teratogenic; medication is contraindicated during pregnancy; pregnancy must be ruled out, and two reliable forms of contraception need to be implemented before the medication is started. (Contraception needs to be implemented at least 1 month before treatment starts and continued for at least 3 years after treatment is discontinued.)
c. If pregnancy occurs during treatment with the medication, the medication is discontinued immediately and possible termination of the pregnancy is discussed.
d. Dermatological effects include hair loss, skin peeling, dry skin, rash, pruritus, and nail disorders. Other effects include rhinitis from mucous membrane irritation, inflammation of the lips, dry mouth, dry eyes, nosebleed, gingivitis, stomatitis, bone and joint pain, and spinal disorders.
e. Can be hepatotoxic; can elevate triglyceride levels and reduce levels of high-density lipoprotein cholesterol
f. Medication should be taken with meals to facilitate absorption; alcohol must be avoided.
g. This derivative of vitamin A can cause vitamin A toxicity if taken concurrently with vitamin A supplements.
h. Should not be taken concurrently with tetracycline because it can cause increased intracranial pressure.
3. Cyclosporine (Neoral; Gengraf)
a. An immunosuppressant that inhibits proliferation of B and T cells
b. Can be toxic and can cause kidney damage
c. Is used for severe psoriasis and is reserved for use in those who have not responded to safer medications
d. Systemic agent of choice for pregnant women with severe psoriasis

D. Systemic biologic medications
1. Alefacept (Amevive), Adalimumab (Humira), Infliximab (Remicade), Etanercept (Enbrel)
a. These medications reduce the number and activity of memory CD4$^+$T lymphocytes; therefore, the medication is contraindicated in clients with human immunodeficiency virus infection.
b. CD4$^+$T cell counts should be monitored before each dose and discontinued if the count falls below 250 cells/mL.
c. Risk of cancer is increased, and the medication should not be administered to a client with a history of malignancy; medication should be discontinued if cancer develops.
d. Can cause chills, cough, pruritus, myalgia, inflammation and pain at the intramuscular injection site
2. Ustekinumab (Stelara)
a. A human monoclonal antibody
b. Can decrease the activity of the immune system and increase the risk for certain types of cancer
c. Side/adverse effects of the medication include upper respiratory infections, headache, and tiredness.
d. Contraindicated in clients who have a history of cancer; also contraindicated in clients with infection or posterior leukoencephalopathy syndrome (rare condition that affects the brain and can cause death)
e. The client should not receive any live virus vaccines because the viruses used in some types of vaccines can cause infection in those with a weakened immune system; in addition, the HCP needs to be informed if anyone in the household needs a vaccine.
f. The client should not receive the bacilli Calmette-Guerin (BCG) vaccine during the 1 year before or 1 year after taking the medication.
g. The client should inform the HCP if he or she is receiving phototherapy, has any other medical condition, is pregnant or plans to become pregnant, or is breastfeeding or plans to breastfeed.

E. Phototherapy
1. Coal tar and ultraviolet B irradiation: Treatment involves the application of coal tar for 8 to 10 hours; coal tar is washed off, and the area is exposed to shortwave UV radiation (ultraviolet B, or UVB).

2. Photochemotherapy (PUVA [psoralen and ultraviolet A] therapy)
   a. Combines the use of longwave radiation (ultraviolet A, or UVA) with oral methoxsalen (Oxsoralen Ultra) (photosensitive medication)
   b. Can cause pruritus, nausea, erythema; may accelerate the aging process of the skin and may increase the risk of skin cancer

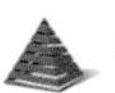

VII. Acne Products (Box 42-5 and Fig. 42-2)

A. Description
1. Acne lesions that are mild may be treated with nonpharmacological measures such as gentle cleansing two or three times daily (oil-based moisturizing products need to be avoided), dermabrasion, or comedo extraction.
2. Mild acne is usually treated pharmacologically with topical agents (antimicrobials and retinoids).
3. Moderate acne is usually treated with oral antibiotics and comedolytics.
4. Severe acne is usually treated with isotretinoin (Amnesteem or Clavaris).
5. Hormonal medications such as oral contraceptives and spironolactone (Aldactone) may be prescribed to treat acne in female clients.
6. Combination therapy may be prescribed to treat the acne.

BOX 42-5 Acne Products

Topical Antibiotics

Benzoyl peroxide
Clindamycin (Cleocin) and erythromycin (Erythroderma)
Dapsone (Aczone)
Fixed dose combinations: clindamycin/benzoyl peroxide (BenzaClin) and erythromycin/benzoyl peroxide (Benzamycin)
Others

Topical Retinoids

Tretinoin (Retin-A)
Adapalene (Differin)
Tazarotene (Tazorac)
Azelaic acid (Azelex)

Oral Medications

Doxycycline (Vibramycin)
Minocycline (Dynacin, Minocin, Solodyn)
Tetracycline (Sumycin)
Erythromycin (Ery-Tab)
Isotretinoin (Amnesteem, Clavaris)

Hormonal Medications

Oral contraceptives
Spironolactone (Aldactone)

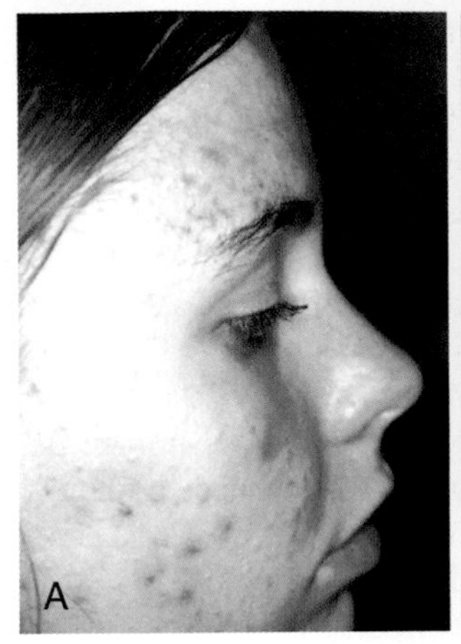

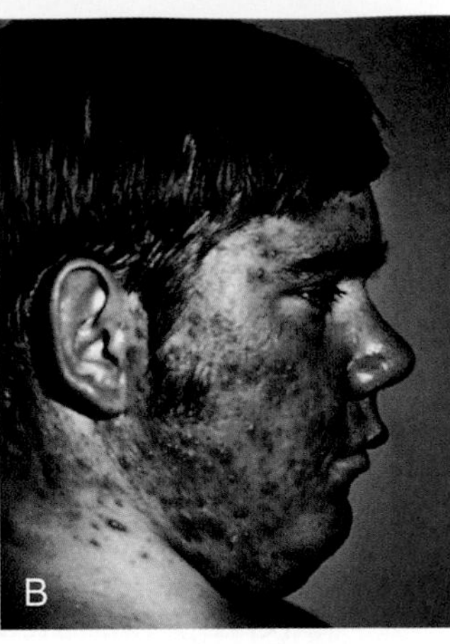

FIGURE 42-2 Acne vulgaris. **A,** Comedones with a few inflammatory pustules. **B,** Papulopustular acne. (From Weston WL, Lane AT: *Color textbook of pediatric dermatology*, ed 4, St. Louis, 2007, Mosby.)

7. Actions of the medications may include suppressing the growth of *Propionibacterium acnes,* reducing inflammation, promoting keratolysis, unplugging existing comedones and preventing their development, and normalizing hyperproliferation of epithelial cells within the hair follicles; some medications cause thinning of the skin, which facilitates penetration of other medications.
8. For topical applications: The site should be washed and allowed to completely dry before application. Hands should be washed after application.
9. All topical products are kept away from the eyes, inside the nose, lips, mucous membranes, hair, and inflamed or denuded skin.

B. Topical antibiotic products
1. Benzoyl peroxide
   a. Can produce drying and peeling
   b. Severe local irritation (burning, blistering, scaling, swelling) may require reducing the frequency of applications.
   c. Some products may contain sulfites. Monitor for allergic reactions.
2. Clindamycin (Cleocin) and erythromycin (Erythroderma)
   a. Both products may be prescribed for use to prevent emergence of resistance.
   b. Combination therapy with benzoyl peroxide can be prescribed to prevent emergence of resistance. Fixed-dose combinations include clindamycin/benzoyl peroxide (BenzaClin) and erythromycin/benzoyl peroxide (Benzamycin).
3. Dapsone (Aczone): Side effects include oiliness, peeling, dryness, and erythema of the skin.

C. Topical retinoids
1. Tretinoin
   a. A derivative of vitamin A (vitamin A supplements should be discontinued during therapy)

b. In addition to treating acne, it may be prescribed to reduce fine wrinkles, skin roughness, mottled hyperpigmentation such as those that occur with age spots (tretinoin [Renova, Retin A as a topical cream]).
c. Can cause localized side effects such as blistering, peeling, crusting, burning, and swelling of the skin
d. The use of abrasive products and keratolytic products should be discontinued before using tretinoin because they can cause localized side effects.
e. Sensitizes the skin to ultraviolet light (UVL); the client needs to be instructed to apply sunscreen with a sun protection factor (SPF) of 15 or greater and to wear protective clothing when outdoors because the medication increases susceptibility to sunburn.

2. Adapalene (Differin): Similar to tretinoin and sensitizes the skin to UVL; side effects include burning and itching after application, redness, dryness, and scaling of the skin.
3. Tazarotene (Tazorac)
   a. Is a derivative of vitamin A (vitamin A supplements should be discontinued during therapy)
   b. In addition to acne, it is used to treat wrinkles and psoriasis.
   c. Can cause itching, burning, and dry skin and sensitizes the skin to UVL
4. Azelaic acid (Azelex) can cause burning, itching, stinging, and redness of the skin; it can also cause hypopigmentation of the skin in clients with a dark complexion.

D. Oral antibiotics
1. Includes doxycycline (Vibramycin); minocycline (Dynacin, Minocin, Solodyn); tetracycline (Sumycin); and erythromycin (Ery-Tab)
2. Improvement develops slowly with the use of oral antibiotics and may take 3 to 6 months for some improvement to be noted; following control of symptoms, the client is usually switched to a topical antibiotic.

E. Isotretinoin (Amnesteem or Clavaris)
1. Derivative of vitamin A (vitamin A supplements should be discontinued during therapy); in addition, the use of tetracyclines can increase the risk of adverse effects and should be discontinued before use of isotretinoin.
2. Used to treat severe cystic acne; reserved for persons who have not responded to other therapies, including systemic antibiotics
3. Side/adverse effects include nosebleeds; inflammation of the lips or eyes; dryness or itching of the skin, nose, or mouth; pain, tenderness, or stiffness in the joints, bones, or muscles; and back pain.
4. Less common side/adverse effects include skin rash, hair loss, peeling of the skin, headache, and reduction in night vision.
5. Causes sensitization of the skin to UVL
6. The medication elevates triglyceride levels, which should be monitored before and during therapy; alcohol consumption needs to be eliminated during therapy because alcohol could potentiate elevation of serum triglyceride levels.
7. May cause depression in some clients; if depression occurs, the medication should be discontinued.

⚠ Isotretinoin (Amnesteem or Clavaris) is highly teratogenic and can cause fetal abnormalities. If prescribed, the client needs to follow strict rules of the iPLEDGE Program. It must not be used if the client is pregnant.

F. iPLEDGE Program
1. A risk management program that ensures that no woman starting isotretinoin is pregnant or no woman taking this medication becomes pregnant
2. Access to the medication is controlled through a central automated system.
3. Strict rules must be followed by the client, HCP prescribing the medication, pharmacist dispensing the medication, and wholesaler of the medication to ensure safety and that no woman is pregnant on initiation of therapy or becomes pregnant while taking the medication.
4. Website on the iPLEDGE Program from the U.S. Food and Drug Administration: http://www.fda.gov/Drugs/DrugSafety/PostmarketDrugSafetyInformationforPatientsandProviders/ucm094307.htm

G. Hormonal medications
1. Hormonal medications such as oral contraceptives and spironolactone (Aldactone) may be prescribed to treat acne in female clients.
2. These medications decrease androgen activity, resulting in decreased production of sebum (substance that combines with keratin to create a plug within a pore).
3. Spironolactone is teratogenic; therefore, contraception during its use is necessary.
4. The adverse effects of spironolactone include breast tenderness, menstrual irregularities, and hyperkalemia.

VIII. Burn Products (Box 42-6)

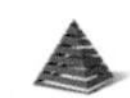

A. Mafenide acetate (Sulfamylon)
1. Water-soluble cream that is bacteriostatic for gram-negative and gram-positive organisms
2. Used to treat **burns** to reduce the bacteria present in avascular tissues

BOX 42-6 Burn Products

Mafenide acetate (Sulfamylon)
Silver sulfadiazine (Silvadene)

3. Diffuses through the devascularized areas of the skin and may precipitate metabolic acidosis (usually compensated for by hyperventilation)
4. Apply 1/16 inch film directly to the burn.
5. Side effects can include local pain and rash.
6. Systemic effects include bone marrow depression, hemolytic anemia, and metabolic acidosis.
7. Keep burn covered with mafenide acetate at all times.
8. Notify the registered nurse, who will then notify the HCP if hyperventilation occurs; if acidosis develops, mafenide acetate is washed off the skin and is usually discontinued for 1 to 2 days.

B. Silver sulfadiazine (Silvadene, Thermazene, SSD Cream)
1. Has broad spectrum of activity against gram-negative bacteria, gram-positive bacteria, and yeast
2. Released slowly from the cream, which is selectively toxic to bacteria
3. Used primarily to prevent sepsis in clients with burns
4. Not a carbonic anhydrase inhibitor; therefore, does not cause acidosis
5. Apply 1/16 inch film (keep burn covered at all times with silver sulfadiazine).
6. Side effects include rash and itching.
7. Systemic effects include leukopenia and interstitial nephritis.
8. Monitor complete blood cell count, particularly the white blood cells, frequently. If leukopenia develops, the registered nurse and HCP are notified (and the medication is usually discontinued).

CRITICAL THINKING What Should You Do?

Answer: Topical glucocorticoids can be absorbed into the systemic circulation; absorption is greater in permeable skin areas (scalp, axilla, face and neck, eyelids, perineum). The nurse should wash the area just before application and apply sparingly in a thin film, rubbing the area gently. The nurse should also monitor the client for signs of systemic absorption.

Reference(s): deWit, D. & Kumagai, C. (2013). *Medical-surgical nursing: Concepts & practice.* (2nd ed., p. 963). St. Louis: Saunders.

Lehne, R. (2013). *Pharmacology for nursing care* (8th ed., p. 1336). St. Louis: Saunders.

PRACTICE QUESTIONS

411. Salicylic acid is prescribed for a client with a diagnosis of psoriasis. The nurse monitors the client knowing that which would indicate the presence of systemic toxicity from this medication?
1. Tinnitus
2. Diarrhea
3. Constipation
4. Decreased respirations

412. The camp nurse asks the children preparing to swim in the lake if they have applied sunscreen. The nurse reminds the children that chemical sunscreens are **most effective** when applied at which time?
1. Immediately before swimming
2. 15 minutes before exposure to the sun
3. Immediately before exposure to the sun
4. At least 30 minutes before exposure to the sun

413. Mafenide acetate (Sulfamylon) is prescribed for the client with a burn injury. When applying the medication, the client complains of local discomfort and burning. Which is the **most appropriate** nursing action?
1. Notifying the registered nurse
2. Discontinuing the medication
3. Informing the client that this is normal
4. Applying a thinner film than prescribed to the burn site

414. The burn client is receiving treatments of topical mafenide acetate (Sulfamylon) to the site of injury. The nurse monitors the client knowing that which indicates a systemic effect has occurred?
1. Hyperventilation
2. Elevated blood pressure
3. Local pain at the burn site
4. Local rash at the burn site

415. Isotretinoin (Amnesteem, Clavaris) is prescribed for a client with severe acne. Before the administration of this medication, the nurse anticipates that which laboratory test will be prescribed?
1. Platelet count
2. Triglyceride level
3. Complete blood count
4. White blood cell count

❖ **416.** The health education nurse reinforces instructions to a group of clients regarding measures that will assist in preventing skin cancer. Which instructions should the nurse reinforce to the clients? **Select all that apply.**
- ❑ 1. Sunscreen should be applied every 8 hours.
- ❑ 2. Use sunscreen when participating in outdoor activities.
- ❑ 3. Wear a hat, opaque clothing, and sunglasses when in the sun.

❑ **4.** Avoid sun exposure in the late afternoon and early evening hours.
❑ **5.** Examine your body monthly for any lesions that may be suspicious.

417. The nurse is applying a topical corticosteroid to a client with eczema. The nurse should monitor for the potential for increased systemic absorption of the medication if the medication is being applied to which body area?
1. Back
2. Axilla
3. Soles of the feet
4. Palms of the hands

418. The clinic nurse is collecting data on a client being admitted. The nurse notes that the client is taking azelaic acid (Azelex). Because of the medication prescription the nurse should suspect that the client is being treated for which condition?
1. Acne
2. Eczema
3. Hair loss
4. Herpes simplex

419. The health care provider has prescribed silver sulfadiazine (Silvadene) for the client with a partial-thickness burn that has cultured positive for gram-negative bacteria. The nurse is reinforcing information to the client about the medication. Which statement made by the client indicates a lack of understanding about the treatments?
1. "The medication is an antibacterial."
2. "The medication will help heal the burn."
3. "The medication will permanently stain my skin."
4. "The medication should be applied directly to the wound."

420. A client with severe acne is seen in the clinic, and the health care provider (HCP) prescribes isotretinoin (Amnesteem, Clavaris). The nurse reviews the client's medication record and should contact the HCP if the client is taking which medication?
1. Vitamin A
2. Digoxin (Lanoxin)
3. Furosemide (Lasix)
4. Phenytoin (Dilantin)

ANSWERS

411. 1
Rationale: Salicylic acid is absorbed readily through the skin, and systemic toxicity (salicylism) can result. Symptoms include tinnitus, dizziness, hyperpnea, and psychological disturbances. Constipation and diarrhea are not associated with salicylism.
Test-Taking Strategy: Focus on the subject, toxicity from use of salicylic acid. Noting the name of the medication will assist in directing you to the correct option if you can recall the toxic effects that occur with acetylsalicylic acid (aspirin). **Review:** the toxic effects of **salicylic acid.**
Level of Cognitive Ability: Analyzing
Client Needs: Physiological Integrity
Integrated Process: Nursing Process/Data Collection
Content Area: Pharmacology: Integumentary Medications
Priority Concepts: Safety, Tissue Integrity
Reference(s): Lehne (2013), p. 1329.

412. 4
Rationale: Sunscreens are most effective when applied at least 30 minutes before exposure to the sun so that they can penetrate the skin. All sunscreens should be reapplied after swimming or sweating.
Test-Taking Strategy: Knowledge that sunscreens need to penetrate the skin will assist in eliminating options 2 and 3. Noting the strategic words, *most effective,* will assist in directing you to option 4. **Review:** protective skin measures and the use of **sunscreen.**
Level of Cognitive Ability: Applying
Client Needs: Physiological Integrity
Integrated Process: Teaching and Learning
Content Area: Pharmacology: Integumentary Medications
Priority Concepts: Client Education, Tissue Integrity
Reference(s): Lehne (2013), p. 1336.

413. 3
Rationale: Mafenide acetate is bacteriostatic for gram-negative and gram-positive organisms and is used to treat burns to reduce bacteria present in avascular tissues. The client should be informed that the medication will cause local discomfort and burning and that this is a normal reaction; therefore, options 1, 2, and 4 are incorrect.
Test-Taking Strategy: Note the strategic words, *most appropriate.* Focus on the subject, client complaint of burning and discomfort. Eliminate options 2 and 4 because these options are comparable or alike and are not within the scope of nursing practice to alter or discontinue a medication therapy. Recalling that this is a normal expected occurrence will direct you to the correct option. **Review:** the effects of **mafenide acetate (Sulfamylon).**
Level of Cognitive Ability: Applying
Client Needs: Physiological Integrity
Integrated Process: Nursing Process/Implementation
Content Area: Pharmacology: Integumentary Medications
Priority Concepts: Pain, Tissue Integrity
Reference(s): Lehne (2013), p. 1106.

414. 1
Rationale: Mafenide acetate is a carbonic anhydrase inhibitor and can suppress renal excretion of acid, thereby causing acidosis. Clients receiving this treatment should be monitored for signs of an acid-base imbalance (hyperventilation). If this occurs, the medication should be discontinued for 1 to 2 days. Options 3 and 4 describe local rather than systemic effects. An elevated blood pressure may be expected from the pain that occurs with a burn injury.
Test-Taking Strategy: Note the subject, a systemic effect. Options 3 and 4 can be eliminated because these are local rather than systemic effects. From the remaining options, recall that the client in pain would likely have an el

pressure. This should direct you to the correct option. **Review:** the systemic effects of **mafenide acetate (Sulfamylon)**.
Level of Cognitive Ability: Analyzing
Client Needs: Physiological Integrity
Integrated Process: Nursing Process/Data Collection
Content Area: Pharmacology: Integumentary Medications
Priority Concepts: Acid-Base Balance, Tissue Integrity
Reference(s): Lehne (2013), p. 1106.

415. 2
Rationale: Isotretinoin can elevate triglyceride levels. Blood triglyceride levels should be measured before treatment and periodically thereafter until the effect on the triglycerides has been evaluated. Options 1, 3, and 4 do not need to be monitored specifically during this treatment.
Test-Taking Strategy: Focus on the subject, laboratory tests associated with isotretinoin. Eliminate options 3 and 4 first because they are comparable or alike and a complete blood count also will measure the white blood cell count. From the remaining options, recall that the medication can affect triglyceride levels in the client. **Review: isotretinoin (Amnesteem, Clavaris).**
Level of Cognitive Ability: Analyzing
Client Needs: Physiological Integrity
Integrated Process: Nursing Process/Data Collection
Content Area: Pharmacology: Integumentary Medications
Priority Concepts: Safety, Tissue Integrity
Reference(s): Hodgson, Kizior (2014), p. 630.

❖ **416. 2, 3, 5**
Rationale: The client should be instructed to avoid sun exposure between the hours of 10:00 AM and 4:00 PM. Sunscreen, a hat, opaque clothing, and sunglasses should be worn for outdoor activities. The client should be instructed to examine the body monthly for the appearance of any possible cancerous or any precancerous lesions. Sunscreen should be reapplied every 2 to 3 hours and after swimming or sweating; otherwise, the duration of protection is reduced.
Test-Taking Strategy: Focus on the subject, measures to prevent skin cancer. Reading each option carefully and thinking about the causes of cancer will direct you to the correct options. **Review:** client teaching points for the prevention of **skin cancer.**
Level of Cognitive Ability: Applying
Client Needs: Health Promotion and Maintenance
Integrated Process: Teaching and Learning
Content Area: Adult Health: Oncology
Priority Concepts: Client Education, Health Promotion
Reference(s): Ignatavicius, Workman (2013), p. 472; Lehne (2013), pp. 1335–1336.

417. 2
Rationale: Topical corticosteroids can be absorbed into the systemic circulation. Absorption is higher from regions where the skin is especially permeable (scalp, axilla, face, eyelids, neck, perineum, genitalia) and lower from regions in which permeability is poor (back, palms, soles).
Test-Taking Strategy: Focus on the subject, areas of high permeability and the potential for increased systemic absorption. Eliminate options 3 and 4 because these body areas are comparable or alike in terms of skin substance. From the remaining options, think about permeability of the skin area. This should direct you to the correct option. **Review:** the principles related to the administration of **topical corticosteroids.**
Level of Cognitive Ability: Analyzing
Client Needs: Physiological Integrity
Integrated Process: Nursing Process/Data Collection
Content Area: Pharmacology: Integumentary Medications
Priority Concepts: Health Promotion, Tissue Integrity
Reference(s): Ignatavicius, Workman (2013), p. 497; Lehne (2013), p. 1336.

418. 1
Rationale: Azelaic acid is a topical medication used to treat mild to moderate acne. The acid appears to work by suppressing the growth of *Propionibacterium acnes* and decreasing the proliferation of keratinocytes. Options 2, 3, and 4 are incorrect.
Test-Taking Strategy: Focus on the subject, the use of azelaic acid. Knowledge on the use of this medication is required to answer this question. This will direct you to the correct option. **Review: azelaic acid (Azelex).**
Level of Cognitive Ability: Analyzing
Client Needs: Physiological Integrity
Integrated Process: Nursing Process/Data Collection
Content Area: Pharmacology: Integumentary Medications
Priority Concepts: Health Promotion, Tissue Integrity
Reference(s): Lehne (2013), p. 1332.

419. 3
Rationale: Silver sulfadiazine (Silvadene) is an antibacterial that has a broad spectrum of activity against gram-negative bacteria, gram-positive bacteria, and yeast. It is applied directly to the wound to assist in healing. It does not stain the skin.
Test-Taking Strategy: Focus on the subject, silver sufadiazine (Silvadene) and note the words, *lack of understanding*. These words ask you to select an option that is an incorrect statement. Recall the characteristics of this medication. Noting the words *permanently stain* in option 3 will direct you to this option. **Review: silver sulfadiazine (Silvadene).**
Level of Cognitive Ability: Evaluating
Client Needs: Physiological Integrity
Integrated Process: Teaching and Learning
Content Area: Pharmacology: Integumentary Medications
Priority Concepts: Client Education, Tissue Integrity
Reference(s): Lilley et al (2014), p. 905.

420. 1
Rationale: Isotretinoin is a metabolite of vitamin A and can produce generalized intensification of isotretinoin toxicity. Because of the potential for increased toxicity, vitamin A supplements should be discontinued before isotretinoin therapy. Options 2, 3, and 4 are not contraindicated with the use of isotretinoin.
Test-Taking Strategy: Focus on the subject, medications that are contraindicated with isotretinoin. Recalling that isotretinoin is a metabolite of vitamin A will direct you to the correct option. **Review:** the contraindications associated with the use of **isotretinoin (Amnesteem, Clavaris).**
Level of Cognitive Ability: Analyzing
Client Needs: Physiological Integrity
Integrated Process: Nursing Process/Implementation
Content Area: Pharmacology: Integumentary Medications
Priority Concepts: Safety, Tissue Integrity
Reference(s): Hodgson, Kizior (2014), p. 630.

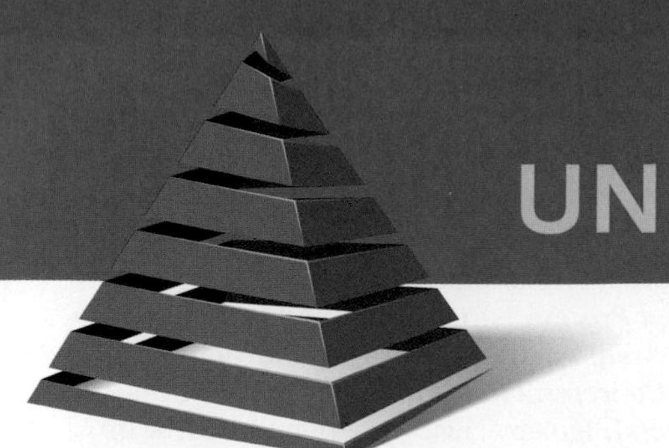

UNIT IX

Hematological and Oncological Disorders of the Adult Client

PYRAMID TERMS

adenocarcinoma A tumor that arises from glandular tissues.

cancer A neoplastic disorder that can involve all body organs. Cells lose their normal growth-controlling mechanism, and the growth of cells is uncontrolled.

carcinogen A physical, chemical, or biological stressor that causes neoplastic changes in normal cells.

carcinoma A new growth or malignant tumor that originates from the epithelial cells, the skin, the gastrointestinal tract, the lungs, the uterus, the breast, or other organs.

carcinoma in situ A premalignant lesion with all of the histological characteristics of a malignancy except invasion.

leukemia Neoplasm involving abnormal overproduction of leukocytes, usually at an immature stage, in the bone marrow.

lymphoma Neoplasm that originates from lymphoid tissue.

malignant Term for growths that are not encapsulated but grow and metastasize. These growths are cancerous lesions that have the characteristics of disorderly, uncontrolled, and chaotic proliferations of cells.

metastasis The transfer of disease from one organ or part to another not directly connected with it. Secondary malignant lesions, originating from the primary tumor, are located in anatomically distant places.

myeloma A malignant proliferation of plasma cells within the bone.

nadir The period of time during which an antineoplastic medication has its most profound effects on the bone marrow.

staging A method of classfiying malignancies on the basis of the presence and extent of the tumor within the body.

tumor marker Specific bodily substances that seem to indicate tumor progression or regression.

Pyramid to Success

The pyramid points focus on the treatment modalities related to an oncological disorder (e.g., pain management, internal and external radiation, chemotherapy). In preparation for the NCLEX®, focus on the following oncological disorders: skin cancer; leukemia; breast cancer; testicular cancer; stomach, bowel, and pancreatic cancers; bladder cancer; prostate cancer; and lung cancer. Particular attention is given to the nursing care related to these disorders and treatment modalities, client adaptation, and the impact of the treatment or the disorder. Also, focus on the complications related to chemotherapy and the nursing measures required to monitor for these complications and preventing life-threatening conditions, such as infection and bleeding.

Client Needs

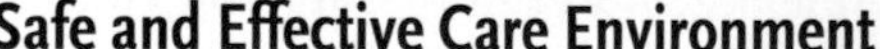

Safe and Effective Care Environment

Discussing oncology-related consultations and referrals
Ensuring advocacy and client autonomy related to the client's decisions
Ensuring that advance directives are in the client's medical record
Ensuring ethical practices
Ensuring informed consent for treatments and procedures has been obtained
Establishing priorities
Handling hazardous and infectious materials related to radiation and chemotherapy safely
Implementing protective, standard, and other precautions
Maintaining medical and surgical asepsis and preventing infection
Providing confidentiality regarding diagnosis
Upholding client's rights

Health Promotion and Maintenance

Discussing expected body image changes related to chemotherapy and treatments
Providing client and family instructions regarding home care

Providing instructions regarding monthly breast or testicular self-examinations
Reinforcing teaching about health promotion programs regarding risks for cancer
Reinforcing teaching about health screening measures for cancer
Respecting client's lifestyle choices

Psychosocial Integrity

Assisting the client and family with coping with alterations in body image
Determining the client's ability to cope, adapt, and/or problem solve during illness or stressful events
Discussing end-of-life and grief and loss issues related to death and the dying process
Mobilizing the appropriate support and resource systems
Promoting a positive environment to maintain an optimal quality of life
Respecting religious and cultural preferences

Physiological Integrity

Assisting the registered nurse (RN) with administering blood and blood products
Assisting the RN with caring for central venous access devices
Assisting the RN with caring for the client who is receiving chemotherapy
Caring for the client who is receiving radiation therapy
Managing pain
Monitoring diagnostic tests and laboratory values, such as white blood cell and platelet counts
Monitoring for expected and unexpected responses to radiation and chemotherapy
Protecting the client from the life-threatening adverse effects of treatments
Providing basic care and comfort
Providing nutrition

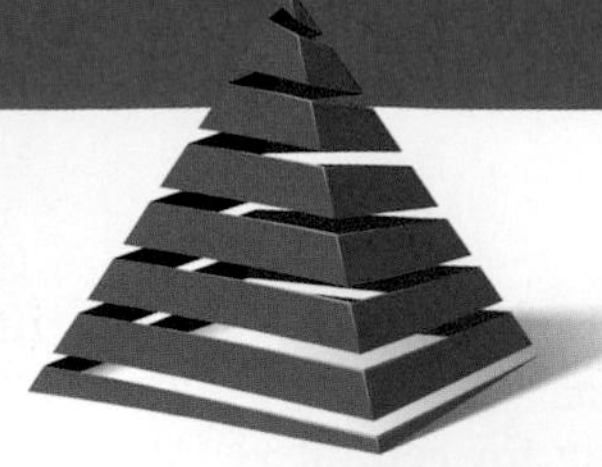

CHAPTER 43

Hematological and Oncological Disorders

CRITICAL THINKING What Should You Do?

The laboratory reports that a client with leukemia has a platelet count of 19,000 cells/mm³. What should the nurse do?
Answer located on p. 539.

I. Cancer

A. Description

1. A neoplastic disorder that can involve any body organ with manifestations that vary according to the body system affected and type of tumor cells
2. Cells lose their normal growth-controlling mechanism, and the growth of cells is uncontrolled.
3. **Cancer** produces serious health problems such as impaired immune and hematopoietic (blood-producing) function; altered gastrointestinal (GI) tract structure and function; motor and sensory deficits; and decreased respiratory function.

B. Metastasis (Box 43-1)

1. Cancer cells move from their original location to other sites.
2. Routes of metastasis
   a. Local seeding: Distribution of shed cancer cells occurs in the local area of the primary tumor.
   b. Blood-borne metastasis: Tumor cells enter the blood; this is the most common cause of cancer spread.
   c. Lymphatic spread: Primary sites rich in lymphatics are more susceptible to early metastatic spread.

C. Cancer classification

1. Solid tumors: Associated with the organs from which they develop, such as breast cancer or lung cancer
2. Hematologic cancers: Originate from blood cell-forming tissues, such as the leukemias, lymphomas, and multiple **myeloma**

D. Grading and **staging**

1. Grading and staging are methods used to describe the tumor.
2. These methods describe the extent of the tumor, the extent to which malignancy has increased in size, the involvement of regional nodes, and metastatic development.
3. Grading classifies the cellular aspects of the cancer.
4. Staging classifies the clinical aspects of the cancer and degree of metastasis at diagnosis.

E. Factors that influence cancer development

1. Environmental factors
   a. Chemical **carcinogens**: Factors include industrial chemicals, drugs, and tobacco.
   b. Physical carcinogens: Factors include ionizing radiation (diagnostic and therapeutic x-rays) and ultraviolet radiation (sun, tanning beds, and germicidal lights), chronic irritation, and tissue trauma.
   c. Viral carcinogens: Viruses capable of causing cancer are known as oncoviruses (e.g., Epstein-Barr virus, hepatitis B virus, human papillomavirus).
   d. *Helicobacter pylori* infection is associated with an increased risk of gastric cancer.
2. Obesity and dietary factors including preservatives, contaminants, additives, and nitrates.

BOX 43-1 Common Sites of Metastasis

Bladder Cancer
Lung
Bone
Liver
Pelvic, retroperitoneal structures

Brain Tumors
Central nervous system

Breast Cancer
Bone
Lung
Brain
Liver

Colorectal Cancer
Liver

Lung Cancer
Brain
Liver

Prostate Cancer
Bone
Spine
Lung
Liver
Kidneys

Testicular Cancer
Lung
Bone
Liver
Adrenal glands
Retroperitoneal lymph nodes

3. Genetic predisposition: Factors include an inherited predisposition to specific cancers, inherited conditions associated with cancer, familial clustering, and chromosomal aberrations.
4. Age: Advancing age is a significant risk factor for the development of cancer.
5. Immune function: The incidence of cancer is higher in immunosuppressed individuals, such as those with acquired immunodeficiency syndrome and organ transplant recipients who are taking immunosuppressive medications.

F. Prevention: Avoidance of known or potential carcinogens and avoidance or modification of the factors associated with the development of cancer cells

G. Early detection (Boxes 43-2 and 43-3)
1. Mammography
2. Papanicolaou (Pap) test
3. Rectal exams and stools for occult blood
4. Sigmoidoscopy, Colonoscopy
5. Breast self-examination and clinical breast examination
6. Testicular self-examination
7. Skin inspection

BOX 43-2 Warning Signs of Cancer

- Any sore that does not heal
- Change in bowel or bladder habits
- Indigestion
- Nagging cough or hoarseness
- Obvious change in wart or mole
- Thickening or lump in breast or elsewhere
- Unusual bleeding or discharge

From WebMD: Understanding Cancer–Symptoms. Retrieved from http://www.webmd.com/cancer/understanding-cancer-symptoms.

BOX 43-3 Diagnostic Tests

- Biopsy
- Bone marrow examination (particularly if a hematolymphoid malignancy is suspected)
- Chest x-ray
- Complete blood count (CBC)
- Computed tomography (CT) scan
- Cytology studies (Papanicolaou smear)
- Liver function studies
- Magnetic resonance imaging (MRI)
- Evaluation of serum tumor markers (e.g., carcinoembryonic antigen and alpha-fetoprotein)
- Proctoscopic examination (including guaiac test for occult blood)
- Radiographic studies (mammography)
- Radioisotope scanning (liver, brain, bone, lung)
- Tumor markers

II. Diagnostic Tests

A. Diagnostic tests to be performed depend on the suspected primary or metastatic sites of the **cancer** (see Box 43-3).

B. Biopsy
1. Description
   a. Definitive means of diagnosing cancer; provides histologic proof of malignancy
   b. Involves the surgical incision of a small piece of tissue for microscopic examination
2. Types
   a. Needle: Aspiration of cells
   b. Incisional: Wedge of suspected tissue is removed from a larger mass
   c. Excisional: Complete removal of the entire lesion
   d. Staging: Multiple needle or incisional biopsies in tissues in which metastasis is suspected or likely (see Box 43-1)
3. Tissue examination
   a. After excision, a frozen section or a permanent paraffin section is obtained to examine the specimen.
   b. The advantage of the frozen section is the speed with which the section can be prepared and the preliminary diagnosis made; only minutes are required for this test.
   c. A permanent paraffin section takes about 24 hours; however, it provides clearer details than the frozen section.
4. Interventions
   a. The procedure is usually performed in an outpatient surgical setting.
   b. Prepare the client for the diagnostic procedure in accordance with the health care provider's (HCP's) instructions, and provide postprocedure instructions.
   c. Ensure that informed consent has been obtained.

III. Pain Control

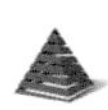

Assess the client's pain; pain is what the client describes or says it is. Do not under medicate the cancer client who is in pain.

A. Causes of pain
1. Bone destruction
2. Obstruction of an organ
3. Compression of peripheral nerves
4. Infiltration and distention of tissue
5. Inflammation and necrosis
6. Psychological factors, such as fear or anxiety

B. Interventions 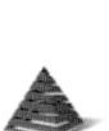
1. Collaborate with other members of the health care team to develop a pain management program.

2. Oral preparations are administered if possible and if they provide adequate relief of pain; the transdermal route may also be prescribed.
3. Mild or moderate pain may be treated with salicylates, acetaminophen (Tylenol), and nonsteroidal anti-inflammatory drugs (NSAIDs).
4. Severe pain is treated with opioids, such as codeine sulfate, morphine sulfate, methadone, and hydromorphone hydrochloride (Dilaudid). Neuropathic pain is treated with a variety of anticonvulsants and antidepressants, as well as opioids.
5. Subcutaneous injections and continuous intravenous (IV) infusions of opioids provide rapid pain control; equianalgesic comparison charts are used when switching routes of administration of opioids.
6. Monitor vital signs and for side/adverse effects of medications; notify the registered nurse (RN) if side/adverse effects occur.
7. Monitor for effectiveness of medications.
8. Provide nonpharmacological techniques of pain control, such as distraction, relaxation, guided imagery, biofeedback, massage, and heat/cold application. Holistic care, such as aromatherapy, may also be beneficial.

IV. Surgery

A. Description: Used to diagnose, stage, and treat cancer

B. Prophylactic surgery
1. Performed in clients with an existing premalignant condition or a known family history that strongly predisposes the person to the development of cancer
2. An attempt is made to remove the tissue or organ at risk and thus prevent the development of cancer.

C. Ablation therapy: Tumor is destroyed (burned) via radio-frequency, microwave therapy, or other type of therapy.

D. NanoKnife: System uses electrical currents to destroy the tumor tissue.

E. Curative surgery: All gross and microscopic tumor is either removed or destroyed.

F. Control (cytoreductive or debulking) surgery
1. A debulking procedure that consists of removing part of the tumor
2. It decreases the number of cancer cells and increases the chance that other therapies will be successful.

G. Palliative surgery
1. Performed to improve the quality of life during the survival time
2. Performed to reduce pain, relieve airway obstruction, relieve obstructions in the gastrointestinal (GI) and urinary tracts, relieve pressure on the brain or spinal cord, prevent hemorrhage, remove infected or ulcerated tumors, or drain abscesses

H. Reconstructive or rehabilitative surgery: Performed to improve the quality of life by restoring maximal function and appearance (e.g., breast reconstruction after mastectomy)

I. Adverse effects of surgery
1. Loss or loss of function of a specific body part
2. Reduced function as a result of organ loss
3. Scarring or disfigurement
4. Grieving about an altered body image or an imposed change in lifestyle
5. Risk for surgical complications, including infection

V. Chemotherapy

A. Description
1. Kills or inhibits the reproduction of neoplastic cells; also attacks and kills normal cells
2. Effects are systemic because chemotherapy is usually administered systemically.
3. Normal cells most profoundly affected include those of the skin, the hair, the lining of the GI tract, the spermatocytes, and the hematopoietic cells.
4. Usually several medications are used in combination (combination therapy) to increase the therapeutic response.
5. Combination chemotherapy is planned by the health care provider (HCP) so that medications with overlapping toxicities and nadirs (the time during which bone marrow activity and white blood cell counts are at their lowest) are not administered at or near the same time; this will minimize immunosuppression.
6. 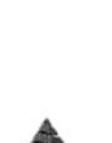 Common side/adverse effects include fatigue, alopecia, nausea and vomiting, mucositis, skin changes, and myelosuppression (neutropenia, anemia, and thrombocytopenia).
7. See Chapter 44 for information about the care of the client who is receiving chemotherapy.

VI. Radiation Therapy (see Priority Nursing Actions)

A. Description
1. Radiation therapy destroys cancer cells with minimal exposure of normal cells to the damaging effects of radiation; the cells that are damaged die or become unable to divide.
2. Radiation therapy is effective on tissues directly within the path of the radiation beam.
3. Side/adverse effects include local skin changes and irritation, alopecia (hair loss), fatigue (most common side effect of radiation), and altered taste sensation; the effects vary according to the site of treatment.
4. External-beam radiation (also called teletherapy) and brachytherapy are the types of radiation therapy that are most commonly used to treat cancer.

BOX 43-4 Client Education Guide: Radiation Therapy for Cancer

Wash the irradiated area gently each day with either water alone or with a mild soap and water.
Use the hand rather than a washcloth to wash the area.
Rinse the soap thoroughly from the skin.
Take care not to remove the markings that indicate exactly where the beam of radiation is to be focused.
Dry the irradiated area with patting motions rather than rubbing motions; use a clean, soft towel or cloth.
Use no powders, ointments, lotions, or creams on the skin at the radiation site unless they are prescribed by the radiologist.
Wear soft clothing over the skin at the radiation site.
Avoid wearing belts, buckles, straps, or any type of clothing that binds or rubs the skin at the radiation site.
Avoid exposure of the irradiated area to the sun.
Avoid heat exposure.

From Ignatavicius D, Workman, M: *Medical-surgical nursing: Patient-centered collaborative care*, ed 7, St. Louis, 2013, Saunders.

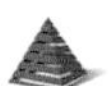

B. External-beam radiation: The radiation source is external to the client.
   1. Instruct the client regarding skin care (Box 43-4).
   2. The client does not emit radiation and does not pose a hazard to anyone else.

C. Brachytherapy: The radiation source is within the client.
   1. The radiation source comes into direct, continuous contact with tumor tissues for a specific time.
   2. For a period of time, the client emits radiation and can pose a hazard to others.
   3. Brachytherapy includes a sealed or unsealed source of radiation.
   4. Unsealed radiation source
      a. Administration is via the oral or IV route or by instillation into the body cavities.
      b. The source is not confined completely to one body area; it enters body fluids and eventually is eliminated via various excreta, which are radioactive and harmful to others; most of the source is eliminated from the body within 48 hours, at which time neither the client nor the excreta are radioactive or harmful.
   5. Sealed radiation source (Box 43-5)
      a. A sealed temporary or permanent radiation source (solid implant) is implanted within the tumor target tissues.
      b. The client emits radiation while the implant is in place, but the excreta are not radioactive.
   6. Removal of sealed radiation sources
      a. The client is no longer radioactive.
      b. Inform the client that cancer is not contagious.
      c. Inform the female client that she may resume sexual intercourse after 7 to 10 days (as prescribed) if the implant was cervical or vaginal.
      d. Provide a douche, if prescribed, if the implant was placed in the cervix.

BOX 43-5 Care of the Client with a Sealed Radiation Implant

Place the client in a private room with a private bath.
Place a caution sign on the client's door.
Organize nursing tasks to minimize exposure to the radiation source.
Nursing assignments to a client with a radiation implant should be rotated.
Limit exposure time to 30 minutes per care provider per 8-hour shift.
Wear a dosimeter film badge to measure radiation exposure.
Wear a lead shield to reduce the transmission of radiation.
The nurse should never care for more than one client with a radiation implant at one time.
Do not allow a pregnant nurse to care for the client.
Do not allow children who are younger than 16 years old or pregnant women to visit the client.
Limit visitors to 30 minutes per day; visitors should be at least 6 feet from the source.
Save the bed linens and dressings until the source is removed, and then dispose of the linens and dressings in the usual manner.
Other equipment can be removed from the room at any time.

PRIORITY NURSING ACTIONS!

Actions to Take If a Sealed Radiation Implant Becomes Dislodged

1. Encourage the client to lie still.
2. Use a long-handled forceps to retrieve the radioactive source.
3. Deposit the radioactive source in a lead container.
4. Contact the RN and radiation oncologist.
5. Document the occurrence and the actions taken.

The client with a sealed radiation implant can emit radiation. Therefore, the nurse and any other person who is in contact with the client needs to take special precautions to protect himself or herself from radiation exposure. In the event that a radiation source becomes dislodged, the nurse would first encourage the client to lie still until the radioactive source has been placed in a safe closed container. The nurse would never touch the dislodged radiation source with his or her hands and would use a long-handled forceps to place the source in the lead container that should be kept in the client's room. The nurse contacts the RN, who will contact the radiation oncologist, and then documents the occurrence and the actions taken. In the event that the radiation source cannot be located, the nurse ensures that no linens or other articles in the client's room are disposed of, prohibits visitors, and notifies the radiation oncologist.

Reference(s): deWit, D. & Kumagai, C. (2013). *Medical-surgical nursing: Concepts & practice.* (2nd ed., p. 161). St. Louis: Saunders.
Linton, A. (2012). *Introduction to medical-surgical nursing* (5th ed., p. 402). St. Louis: Saunders.

e. Administer a ready-to-use saline enema, as prescribed.
f. Advise the client who had a cervical or vaginal implant to notify the HCP if nausea, vomiting, diarrhea, frequent urination, vaginal or rectal bleeding, hematuria, foul-smelling vaginal discharge, abdominal pain or distention, or a fever occurs.

VII. Bone Marrow Transplantation

A. Description
1. Bone marrow transplantation (BMT) and peripheral blood stem cell transplantation (PBSCT) are procedures that replace stem cells that have been destroyed by high doses of chemotherapy and/or radiation therapy.
2. BMT and PBSCT are most commonly used in the treatment of leukemia and lymphoma, but are also used to treat other cancers, such as neuroblastoma and multiple myeloma.
3. The goal of treatment is to rid the client of all leukemic or other malignant cells through treatment with high doses of chemotherapy and whole-body irradiation.
4. Because these treatments are damaging to bone marrow cells, without the replacement of blood-forming stem cell function through transplantation, the client would die of infection or hemorrhage.

B. Transplantation: Stem cells are administered through the client's central line in a manner similar to that of a blood transfusion.

C. Posttransplantation period

> ⚠ During the posttransplantation period, the client remains without any natural immunity until the donor stem cells begin to proliferate and engraftment occurs.

1. The client remains without any natural immunity until the donor marrow begins to proliferate and engraftment occurs.
2. Infection, bleeding, or neutropenia and severe thrombocytopenia are major concerns until engraftment occurs; engraftment involves movement of the transfused cells to marrow-forming sites of the recipient's bones and the white blood cell, erythrocyte, and platelet counts begin to rise.

D. Complications: Major complications include failure to engraft, graft-versus-host disease, and veno-occlusive disease.

VIII. Skin Cancer (See Chapter 41)

IX. Leukemia (Box 43-6)

A. Description
1. Leukemias are a group of hematological malignancies involving abnormal overproduction of leukocytes, usually at an immature stage, in the bone marrow.

BOX 43-6 Classification of Leukemia

Acute Lymphocytic Leukemia
- Mostly lymphoblasts present in the bone marrow
- Age of onset is usually younger than 15 years

Acute Myelogenous Leukemia
- Mostly myeloblasts present in the bone marrow
- Age of onset is usually between 15 and 39 years

Chronic Myelogenous Leukemia
- Mostly granulocytes present in the bone marrow
- Age of onset is usually in the fourth decade

Chronic Lymphocytic Leukemia
- Mostly lymphocytes present in the bone marrow
- Age of onset is usually older than 50 years

2. The two major types of leukemia are lymphocytic (involving abnormal cells from the lymphoid pathway) and myelocytic or myelogenous (involving abnormal cells from the myeloid pathways).
3. Leukemia may be acute, with a sudden onset, or chronic, with a slow onset and persistent symptoms over a period of years.
4. Leukemia affects the bone marrow, causing anemia, leukopenia, the production of immature cells, thrombocytopenia, and a decline in immunity.
5. The cause is unknown and appears to involve genetically damaged cells, leading to the transformation of cells from a normal state to a malignant state.
6. Risk factors include genetic, viral, immunological, and environmental factors and exposure to radiation, chemicals, and medications, such as previous chemotherapy.

B. Data collection 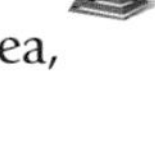
1. Anorexia, fatigue, weakness, pallor, dyspnea, weight loss
2. Anemia
3. Overt bleeding (nosebleeds, gum bleeding, rectal bleeding, hematuria, increased menstrual flow) and occult bleeding (e.g., as detected in a fecal occult blood test)
4. Ecchymoses, petechiae (burst blood vessels under the skin)
5. Prolonged bleeding after minor abrasions or lacerations
6. Elevated temperature
7. Enlarged lymph nodes, spleen, and liver
8. Normal, elevated, or reduced white blood cell (WBC) count 
9. Decreased hemoglobin and hematocrit levels

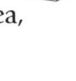

10. Decreased platelet count

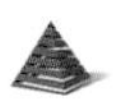

11. Positive bone marrow biopsy identifying leukemic blast-phase cells

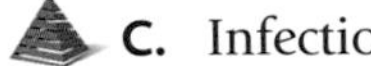

C. Infection

Infection is a major cause of death in the immunosuppressed client.

1. Can occur through autocontamination or cross-contamination. The white blood cell (WBC) count may be extremely low during the period of greatest bone marrow depression, known as the **nadir**.
2. Common sites of infection are the skin, the respiratory tract, and the gastrointestinal tract.
3. Initiate protective isolation procedures.
4. Ensure frequent and thorough hand washing by the client, family, and health care providers.
5. Staff and visitors with known infections or exposure to communicable diseases should avoid contact with the client until risk of infectious spread has passed.
6. Use strict aseptic technique for all procedures.
7. Keep supplies for the client separate from supplies for other clients; keep frequently used equipment in the room for the client's use only.
8. Limit the number of caregivers that enter the client's room to reduce the risk of cross-infection.
9. Maintain the client in a private room with the door closed.
10. Place the client in a room with a high-efficiency particulate air filtration system or a laminar airflow system that moves particles away from the client, if possible.
11. Reduce exposure to environmental organisms by eliminating raw fruits and vegetables (low-bacteria diet) from the diet, eliminating fresh flowers and live plants, and not leaving standing water in the client's room.
12. Be sure that the client's room is cleaned daily.
13. Assist the client with daily bathing with the use of an antimicrobial soap.
14. Assist the client with performing oral hygiene frequently.
15. Initiate a bowel program to prevent constipation and rectal trauma.
16. Avoid invasive procedures, such as injections, insertion of rectal thermometers, enemas, urinary catheterization.
17. Change wound dressings daily, and inspect the wounds for redness, swelling, or drainage.
18. Monitor the urine for cloudiness and other signs of infection.
19. Monitor the skin and oral mucous membranes for signs of infection (Box 43-7).

BOX 43-7 Mouth Care for the Client with Mucositis

Inspect the mouth daily.
Offer complete mouth care before and after every meal and at bedtime.
Brush the teeth and tongue with a soft-bristled toothbrush or sponges.
Provide mouth rinses every 12 hours with the prescribed solution.
Administer topical anesthetic agents to mouth sores, as prescribed.
Avoid the use of alcohol- or glycerin-based mouthwashes or swabs because they are irritating to the mucosa.
Offer soft foods that are cool to warm in temperature rather than foods that are hard or spicy.

20. Encourage the client to cough and deep breathe; check breath sounds.
21. Monitor temperature, pulse, respirations, blood pressure, and for pain.
22. Monitor the white blood cell and neutrophil counts.
23. The health care provider is notified if signs of infection are present; prepare to obtain specimens for the culture of open lesions, urine, and sputum. A chest x-ray may be prescribed.
24. Antibiotic, antifungal, and antiviral medication may be prescribed.
25. Reinforce home care instructions.
    a. To avoid crowds and those with infections
    b. To maintain a low-bacteria diet and to avoid drinking water that has been standing for longer than 15 minutes
    c. To avoid activities that expose him or her to infection, such as changing a pet's litter box, working with houseplants, or gardening
    d. That neither they nor their household contacts should receive immunization with a live virus such as measles, mumps, rubella, polio, varicella, shingles, and some influenza vaccines)

During the period of greatest bone marrow suppression (the nadir), the platelet count and the white blood cell count may be extremely low.

D. Bleeding

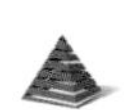

1. The client is at risk for bleeding when the platelet count falls below 50,000 cells/mm^3; spontaneous bleeding frequently occurs when the platelet count is lower than 20,000 cells/mm^3.
2. Clients with platelet counts less than 20,000/mm^3 may need a platelet transfusion.
3. For clients with anemia and fatigue, packed red blood cells may be prescribed.

4. Monitor the laboratory values, as appropriate.
5. Examine the client for signs and symptoms of bleeding; examine all body fluids and excrement for the presence of blood.
6. Handle the client gently; use caution when obtaining blood pressure measurements to prevent skin injury.
7. Monitor for signs of internal hemorrhage (e.g., pain, rapid and weak pulse, increased abdominal girth, and abdomen guarding).
8. Provide soft foods that are cool to warm to avoid oral mucosa damage.
9. Avoid injections, if possible, to prevent trauma to the skin and bleeding; apply firm and gentle pressure to a needle-stick site for at least 5 minutes, or longer if needed.
10. Pad the side rails and sharp corners of the bed and furniture.
11. Avoid rectal suppositories, enemas, and thermometers.
12. If the female client is menstruating, count the number of pads or tampons used.
13. Reinforce instructions to the client to use a soft toothbrush and to avoid dental floss.
14. Reinforce instructions to the client to use only an electric razor for shaving.
15. Reinforce instructions to the client to avoid blowing the nose.
16. Reinforce instructions to the client to avoid constrictive or tight clothing or shoes.
17. Discourage the client from engaging in activities that involve the use of sharp objects.
18. Reinforce instructions to the client to avoid using nonsteroidal anti-inflammatory drugs and products that contain aspirin.

E. Fatigue and nutrition

1. Assist the client with selecting a well-balanced diet.
2. Provide small, frequent meals (high calorie, high protein, high carbohydrate) that require little chewing to reduce energy expenditure at mealtimes.
3. Assist the client with self-care and mobility activities.
4. Allow for adequate rest periods during care.
5. Do not perform activities unless they are essential; assist the client in scheduling important or pleasurable activities during periods of highest energy.
6. Blood products may be prescribed for anemia.

F. Additional interventions

1. Chemotherapy
2. Administer antibiotic, antibacterial, antiviral, and antifungal medications as prescribed.
3. Administer colony-stimulating factors as prescribed.
4. Blood replacements may be prescribed.
5. Maintain infection and bleeding precautions.
6. Bone marrow transplantation may be indicated.
7. Reinforce instructions to the client about appropriate home care measures.
8. Provide psychosocial support and support services for home care.

X. Lymphoma: Hodgkin's Disease

A. Description

1. Lymphomas, classified as Hodgkin's and non-Hodgkin's, depending on the cell type, are characterized by abnormal proliferation of lymphocytes.
2. Hodgkin's disease is a malignancy of the lymph nodes that originates in a single lymph node or a chain of nodes.
3. Metastasis occurs to other, adjacent lymph structures and eventually invades nonlymphoid tissue.
4. Usually involves the lymph nodes, tonsils, spleen, and bone marrow; it is characterized by the presence of Reed-Sternberg cells in the nodes.
5. Possible causes include viral infections; clients treated with combination chemotherapy for Hodgkin's disease have a greater risk of developing acute leukemia and non-Hodgkin's lymphoma, among other secondary malignancies.
6. Prognosis is dependent on the stage of the disease.

B. Data collection

1. Fever
2. Malaise, fatigue, and weakness
3. Night sweats
4. Loss of appetite and significant weight loss
5. Anemia and thrombocytopenia
6. Enlarged lymph nodes, spleen, and liver
7. Positive biopsy of lymph nodes, with cervical nodes most often affected first
8. Presence of Reed-Sternberg cells in nodes 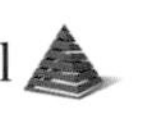
9. Positive computed tomography scan of the liver and spleen

C. Interventions

1. For earlier stages (stages I and II), without mediastinal node involvement, the treatment of choice is extensive external radiation of the involved lymph node regions.
2. With more extensive disease, radiation along with multiagent chemotherapy is used.
3. Monitor for side/adverse effects related to chemotherapy or radiation.
4. Monitor for signs of infection and bleeding.
5. Maintain infection and bleeding precautions.
6. Discuss the possibility of sterility with the client who is receiving radiation; inform the male client of options such as sperm banks.

XI. Multiple Myeloma

A. Description
1. A **malignant** proliferation of plasma cells and tumors within the bone
2. An excessive number of abnormal plasma cells invade the bone marrow, develop into tumors, and ultimately destroy the bone; invasion of the lymph nodes, spleen, and liver occurs.
3. The abnormal plasma cells produce an abnormal antibody (myeloma protein or the Bence-Jones protein) that is found in the blood and urine.
4. Causes the decreased production of immunoglobulin and antibodies and increased levels of uric acid and calcium, which can lead to kidney failure
5. The disease typically develops slowly and the cause is unknown.

B. Data collection
1. Bone (skeletal) pain, especially in the pelvis, spine, and ribs
2. Weakness and fatigue
3. Recurrent infections
4. Anemia
5. Urinalysis shows Bence-Jones proteinuria and elevated total serum protein level
6. Osteoporosis (bone loss and the development of pathological fractures)
7. Thrombocytopenia and leukopenia
8. Elevated calcium and uric acid levels
9. Kidney failure
10. Spinal cord compression and paraplegia
11. Bone marrow aspiration shows an abnormal number of immature plasma cells.

The client with multiple myeloma is at risk for pathological fractures. Therefore, provide skeletal support during moving, turning, and ambulating, and provide a hazard-free environment.

C. Interventions
1. Administer chemotherapy, as prescribed.
2. Provide supportive care to control symptoms and prevent complications, especially bleeding, bone fractures, kidney failure, and infections.
3. Maintain neutropenic and bleeding precautions, as necessary.
4. Encourage the consumption of at least 2L of fluid per day to offset potential problems associated with hypercalcemia, hyperuricemia, and proteinuria.
5. Monitor for signs of kidney failure.
6. Encourage ambulation to prevent renal problems and slow down bone resorption; provide skeletal support during moving, turning, and ambulating to prevent pathological fractures; provide a hazard-free environment.
7. IV fluids and diuretics may be prescribed to increase the renal excretion of calcium.
8. Blood transfusions may be prescribed for anemia.
9. Administer analgesics, as prescribed, to control pain.
10. Administer antibiotics, as prescribed, for infection.
11. Bisphosphonate medications may be prescribed to slow bone damage and reduce pain and risk of fractures.
12. Prepare the client for local radiation therapy, if prescribed.
13. Reinforce instructions to the client regarding home care measures and the signs and symptoms of infection.

XII. Testicular Cancer

A. Description
1. Testicular cancer arises from germinal epithelium from the sperm-producing germ cells or from nongerminal epithelium from other structures in the testicles.
2. Testicular cancer most often occurs between the ages of 15 and 40 years.
3. The cause of testicular cancer is unknown, but a history of undescended testicle (cryptorchidism) and genetic predisposition have been associated with testicular tumor development.
4. Metastasis occurs to the lung, liver, bone, and adrenal glands via the blood, and to the retroperitoneal lymph nodes via lymphatic channels.

B. Early detection: Perform monthly testicular self-examination (Fig. 43-1). 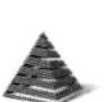

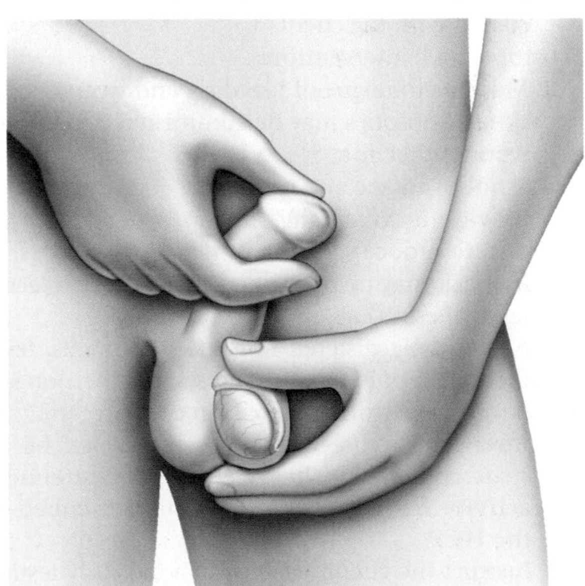

FIGURE 43-1 Testicular self-examination and client instructions. **1.** The best time to perform this examination is right after a shower when your scrotal skin is moist and relaxed, thus making the testicles easy to feel. **2.** Gently lift each testicle. Each one should feel like an egg; it should be firm but not hard, and smooth with no lumps. **3.** Using both hands, place your middle fingers on the underside of each testicle and your thumbs on top. **4.** Gently roll each testicle between the thumb and fingers to feel for any lumps, swellings, or masses. **5.** If you notice any changes from one month to the next, notify your health care provider. (From Harkreader H, Hogan MA: *Fundamentals of nursing: Caring and clinical judgment*, ed 3, Philadelphia, 2007, Saunders.)

1. Performing testicular self-examination: Perform monthly; a day of the month is selected and the examination is performed on the same day each month.
2. Client instructions (see Fig. 43-1)

C. Data Collection
1. Painless testicular swelling occurs.
2. "Dragging" or "pulling" sensation is experienced in the scrotum.
3. Palpable lymphadenopathy, abdominal masses, and gynecomastia may indicate metastasis.
4. Late signs include back or bone pain and respiratory symptoms.

D. Interventions
1. Chemotherapy may be prescribed.
2. Prepare the client for radiation therapy as prescribed.
3. Prepare the client for unilateral orchiectomy, if prescribed, for diagnosis and primary surgical management or radical orchiectomy (surgical removal of the affected testis, spermatic cord, and regional lymph nodes).
4. Prepare the client for retroperitoneal lymph node dissection, if prescribed, to stage the disease and reduce tumor volume so that chemotherapy and radiation therapy are more effective.
5. Reproduction, sexuality, and fertility information and options will be discussed with the client.
6. Reproductive options such as sperm storage, donor insemination, and adoption will be discussed with the client.

E. Postoperative interventions
1. Monitor for signs of bleeding and wound infection; antibiotics may be administered to prevent wound infection.
2. Monitor intake and output.
3. Provide and explain pain management methods; to reduce swelling in the first 48 hours, an ice pack may be prescribed (wrap in a protective layer of cloth).
4. Notify the registered nurse (RN) if chills, fever, increasing pain or tenderness at the incision site, or drainage from the incision occurs.
5. After the orchiectomy, the client will be instructed to avoid heavy lifting and strenuous activity for the length of time prescribed by the HCP.
6. Instruct the client to perform a monthly testicular self-examination on the remaining testicle (see Fig. 43-1).
7. Inform the client that sutures will be removed approximately 7 to 10 days after surgery.

XIII. Cervical Cancer

A. Description
1. Preinvasive cancer is limited to the cervix and is often asymptomatic.
2. Invasive cancer is in the cervix and other pelvic structures.
3. Metastasis is usually confined to the pelvis, but distant metastasis occurs through lymphatic spread.
4. Premalignant changes are described on a continuum from dysplasia, which is the earliest premalignancy change, to **carcinoma in situ**, which is the most advanced premalignant change.

B. Risk factors
1. Human papillomavirus (HPV) infection (vaccination against HPV is effective to avoid HPV infection, and thus cervical cancer)
2. Cigarette smoking, both active and passive
3. Reproductive behavior, including early first intercourse (before age 17), multiple sex partners, or male partners with multiple sex partners.
4. Screening via regular gynecological examinations and Papanicolaou smear (Pap test), with treatment of precancerous abnormalities, decreases the incidence and mortality of cervical cancer. 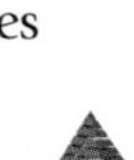

C. Data collection 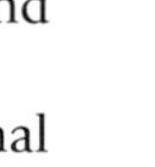
1. Painless vaginal bleeding, postmenstrually and postcoitally (after sexual intercourse)
2. Foul-smelling or serosanguineous vaginal discharge
3. Pelvic, lower back, leg, or groin pain
4. Anorexia and weight loss
5. Leakage of urine and feces from the vagina
6. Dysuria (painful urination)
7. Hematuria
8. Cytological changes on Pap test

D. Interventions (Box 43-8)

E. Cryosurgery
1. Involves freezing of the tissues by a probe with subsequent necrosis
2. No anesthesia is required, although cramping may occur during the procedure.
3. A heavy, watery discharge will occur for several weeks after the procedure.
4. Reinforce instructions to the client to avoid intercourse and the use of tampons while the discharge is present.

BOX 43-8 Treatment for Cervical Cancer

Nonsurgical
- Chemotherapy
- Cryosurgery
- External radiation
- Internal radiation implants (intracavitary)
- Laser therapy

Surgical
- Conization
- Hysterectomy
- Pelvic exenteration

F. Laser therapy
   1. Used when all boundaries of the lesion are visible during colposcopic examination
   2. Energy from the beam is absorbed by fluid in the tissues, which causes them to vaporize.
   3. Minimal bleeding is associated with the procedure.
   4. Slight vaginal discharge is expected after the procedure; healing occurs in 6 to 12 weeks.

G. Conization
   1. A cone-shaped area of the cervix is removed.
   2. Conization allows the woman to retain reproductive capacity.
   3. Long-term follow-up care is needed, because new lesions can develop.
   4. The risks of the procedure include hemorrhage, uterine perforation, incompetent cervix, cervical stenosis, and preterm labor in future pregnancies.

H. Hysterectomy
   1. Description
      a. For microinvasive cancer if childbearing is not desired
      b. A vaginal approach is most commonly performed.
      c. A radical hysterectomy and bilateral lymph node dissection may be performed for cancer that has spread beyond the cervix but not to the pelvic wall.
   2. Postoperative interventions
      a. Monitor the vital signs and respiratory status.
      b. Assist with coughing and deep-breathing exercises and the use of an incentive spirometer.
      c. Assist with range-of-motion (ROM) exercises and provide early ambulation.
      d. Apply antiembolism stockings, as prescribed.
      e. Monitor intake and output (I&O), indwelling bladder catheter drainage, and hydration status.
      f. Monitor bowel sounds.
      g. Monitor the incision site for signs of infection.
      h. Administer pain medication, as prescribed.
      i. Reinforce postoperative instructions to avoid tub baths, sitting for long periods, and stair climbing for 1 month; avoid strenuous activity or lifting anything weighing more than 10 to 20 pounds; consume foods that aid in healing, including protein, fruits, and vegetables; avoid sexual intercourse for 3 to 6 weeks, as prescribed; and about the signs/symptoms associated with complications.

Monitor vaginal bleeding following hysterectomy. More than one saturated pad per hour may indicate excessive bleeding; report this occurrence to the RN.

I. Pelvic exenteration (Box 43-9)
   1. Description
      a. Pelvic exenteration, the removal of all pelvic contents, including bowel, vagina, and bladder, is a radical surgical procedure performed for recurrent cancer if no evidence of tumor outside the pelvis and no lymph node involvement exist.
      b. When the bladder is removed, an ileal conduit will be created and located on the right side of the abdomen to divert urine.
      c. A colostomy may need to be created and will be located on the left side of the abdomen for the passage of feces.
   2. Postoperative interventions
      a. Nursing care measures are similar to postoperative care after hysterectomy.
      b. Administer prophylactic heparin as prescribed.
      c. Administer perineal irrigations and sitz baths, as prescribed.
      d. Inform the client that the perineal opening, if present, may drain for several months.
      e. Reinforce instructions regarding the care of the ileal conduit and colostomy, if present.
      f. Consult with the RN about the need for sexual counseling; vaginal intercourse is not possible after anterior and total pelvic exenteration.

BOX 43-9 Types of Pelvic Exenteration

Anterior

Removal of the uterus, ovaries, fallopian tubes, vagina, bladder, urethra, and pelvic lymph nodes

Posterior

Removal of the uterus, ovaries, fallopian tubes, descending colon, rectum, and anal canal

Total

Combination of anterior and posterior

XIV. Ovarian Cancer

A. Description
   1. Ovarian cancer grows rapidly, spreads quickly, and is often bilateral.
   2. Metastasis occurs by direct spread to the organs in the pelvis, by distal spread through lymphatic drainage, or by peritoneal seeding.
   3. In its early stages, ovarian cancer is often asymptomatic; because most women are diagnosed in advanced stages, ovarian cancer has a higher mortality rate than any other cancer of the female reproductive system, particularly among white women between 55 and 65 years of age of North American or European descent.
   4. An exploratory laparotomy is performed to diagnose and stage the tumor.

B. Data collection 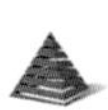
   1. Abdominal discomfort or swelling
   2. GI disturbances
   3. Dysfunctional vaginal bleeding

4. Abdominal mass
5. Elevated **tumor marker** (i.e., CA-125)

C. Interventions
1. External radiation is used if the tumor has invaded other organs.
2. Chemotherapy is used postoperatively for all stages of ovarian cancer.
3. Intraperitoneal chemotherapy, which involves the instillation of chemotherapy into the abdominal cavity, may be prescribed.
4. Total abdominal hysterectomy and bilateral salpingo-oophorectomy may be necessary.

XV. Endometrial (Uterine) Cancer

A. Description
1. A slow-growing tumor arising from the endometrial mucosa of the uterus, associated with the menopausal years
2. Metastasis occurs through the lymphatic system to the ovaries and pelvis and via the blood to the lungs, liver, and bone, or intraabdominally to the peritoneal cavity.

B. Risk factors
1. Use of estrogen replacement therapy (ERT)
2. Nulliparity
3. Polycystic ovary disease
4. Increased age
5. Late menopause
6. Family history of uterine cancer or hereditary nonpolyposis colorectal cancer
7. Obesity
8. Hypertension
9. Diabetes mellitus

C. Data collection
1. Abnormal bleeding, especially in postmenopausal women
2. Vaginal discharge
3. Low back, pelvic, or abdominal pain (pain occurs late in the disease process)
4. Enlarged uterus (in advanced stages)

D. Nonsurgical interventions
1. External radiation or internal radiation (intracavitary radiation), used alone or in combination with surgery, depending on the stage of cancer
2. Chemotherapy to treat advanced or recurrent disease
3. Progesterone therapy with medication for estrogen-dependent tumors may be prescribed.
4. Antiestrogen medication may also be prescribed.

E. Surgical interventions: Total abdominal hysterectomy and bilateral salpingo-oophorectomy

XVI. Breast Cancer

A. Description
1. Classified as invasive when it penetrates the tissue that surrounds the mammary duct and grows in an irregular pattern
2. Metastasis occurs via lymph nodes.
3. Common sites of metastasis are the bones and lungs; can also metastasize to the brain and liver.
4. Diagnosis is made by breast biopsy through a needle aspiration or by the surgical removal of the tumor with a microscopic examination for malignant cells.

B. Risk factors
1. Age
2. Family history of breast cancer
3. Early menarche and late menopause
4. Previous cancer of the breast, uterus, or ovaries
5. Nulliparity, late first birth
6. Obesity
7. High-dose radiation exposure of the chest

C. Data collection
1. Mass felt during breast self-examination (BSE) (usually felt in the upper outer quadrant, beneath the nipple, or in axilla)
2. Presence of the lesion on mammography
3. A fixed, irregular nonencapsulated mass; typically painless except in the late stages
4. Asymmetry, with the affected breast being higher
5. Nipple retraction or elevation
6. Bloody or clear nipple discharge
7. Skin dimpling, retraction, or ulceration
8. Skin edema or peau d'orange skin, which may indicate lymphatic involvement (blocked skin drainage causes skin edema and an "orange peel" appearance)
9. Axillary lymphadenopathy
10. Lymphedema of the affected arm
11. Symptoms of bone or lung metastasis in late stage

D. Early Detection: Monthly BSE
1. Perform 7 to 10 days after menses
2. Postmenopausal clients or clients who have had a hysterectomy should select a specific day of the month and perform a BSE monthly on that day.

E. Reinforce client instructions (Fig. 43-2)

F. Nonsurgical interventions
1. Chemotherapy
2. Radiation therapy
3. Hormonal manipulation via the use of medication in postmenopausal women or other medications for estrogen receptor-positive tumors

G. Surgical interventions: Surgical breast procedures with possible breast reconstruction (Box 43-10)

H. Postoperative interventions
1. Monitor the vital signs.
2. Position the client in a semi-Fowler's position; turn her from the back to the unaffected side, with the affected arm elevated above the level of the heart to promote drainage and prevent lymphedema.
3. Encourage coughing and deep breathing.

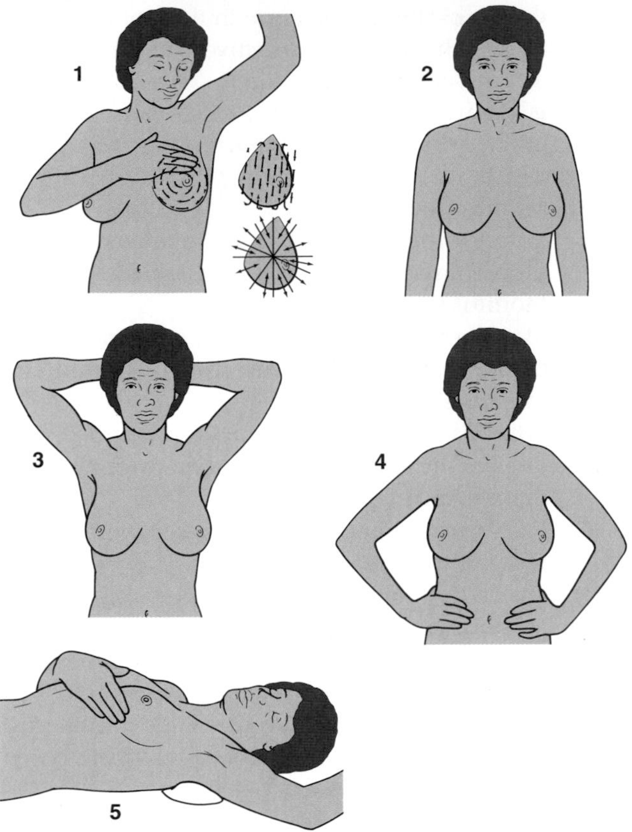

FIGURE 43-2 Breast self-examination and client instructions. 1. While in the shower or bath, when the skin is slippery with soap and water, examine your breasts. Use the pads of your second, third, and fourth fingers to firmly press every part of the breast. Use your right hand to examine your left breast and your left hand to examine your right breast. Using the pads of the fingers on your left hand, examine the entire breast with the use of small circular motions in a spiral or in an up-and-down motion so that the entire breast area is examined. Repeat the procedure using your right hand to examine your left breast. Repeat the pattern of palpation under the arm. Check for any lump, hard knot, or thickening of the tissue. 2. Look at your breasts in a mirror. Stand with your arms at your side. 3. Raise your arms overhead and check for any changes in the shape of your breasts, any dimpling of the skin, or any changes in the nipple. 4. Place your hands on your hips and press down firmly, tightening the pectoral muscles. Observe for asymmetry or changes, keeping in mind that your breasts probably do not match exactly. 5. While lying down, feel your breasts as described in step 1. When examining your right breast, place a folded towel under your right shoulder, and put your right hand behind your head. Repeat the procedure when examining your left breast. Mark on your calendar that you have completed your breast self-examination; note any changes or unique characteristics that you want to discuss with your health care provider. (From Lewis S, Dirksen S, Heitkemper M, Bucher L, Camera I: *Medical-surgical nursing: Assessment and management of clinical problems*, ed 8, St. Louis, 2011, Mosby.)

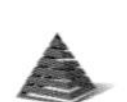

4. If a bulb suction drain is in place, maintain suction, and record the amount of drainage and the drainage characteristics.
5. Monitor the operative site for infection, swelling, or the presence of fluid collection under the skin flaps.
6. Monitor the incision site for constriction from the dressings, impaired sensation, or color changes of the skin.

BOX 43-10 Surgical Breast Procedures

Lumpectomy

The tumor is excised and removed.
Lymph node dissection may also be performed.

Simple Mastectomy

Breast tissue and the nipple are removed.
The lymph nodes are left intact.

Modified Radical Mastectomy

Breast tissue, the nipple, and the lymph nodes are removed.
The muscles are left intact.

7. If breast reconstruction was performed, the client will return from surgery with a surgical support garment and the temporary prosthesis in place.
8. Provide the use of a pressure sleeve, as prescribed, if edema is severe.
9. Maintain fluid and electrolyte balance; administer diuretics and provide a low-salt diet, as prescribed, for severe lymphedema.
10. Consult with the RN and the physical therapist regarding the appropriate exercise program.
11. Reinforce instructions regarding home care measures (Box 43-11).

BOX 43-11 Client Instructions following Mastectomy

- Avoid overuse of the arm during the first few months.
- To prevent lymphedema, keep the affected arm elevated; consultation with lymphedema specialist may be prescribed.
- Provide incision care with an emollient as prescribed to soften and prevent wound contracture.
- Encourage use of Reach to Recovery volunteers.
- Encourage the client to perform breast self-examination on the remaining breast.
- Protect the affected hand and arm.
- Avoid strong sunlight on the affected arm.
- Do not let the affected arm hang dependent.
- Do not carry a pocketbook or anything heavy over the affected arm.
- Avoid trauma, cuts, bruises, or burns to the affected side.
- Avoid wearing constricting clothing or jewelry on the affected side.
- Wear gloves when gardening.
- Use thick oven mitts when cooking.
- Use a thimble when sewing.
- Apply hand cream several times daily.
- Use cream cuticle remover.
- Call the HCP if signs of inflammation occur in the affected arm.
- Wear a Medic-Alert bracelet stating which arm is lymphedematous.

⚠ No IVs, no injections, no blood pressure measurements, and no venipunctures should be done on the arm on the side of the mastectomy. The arm on the side of the mastectomy is protected, and any intervention that could traumatize the affected arm is avoided.

XVII. Esophageal Cancer

A. Description

1. Esophageal cancer is a malignancy found in the esophageal mucosa, formed by squamous cell **carcinoma** (SCC) or **adenocarcinoma**.
2. The cause is unknown, but major risk factors include cigarette smoking, alcohol consumption, and chronic reflux.
3. Complications include dysphagia, painful swallowing, loss of appetite, and malaise.
4. The goal of treatment is to inhibit tumor growth and maintain nutrition.

B. Data Collection

1. Dysphagia
2. Odynophagia
3. Epigastric pain or sternal pain

C. Interventions

1. Monitor nutritional status, including daily weight, intake and output, and calories consumed.
2. Inform the client about diet changes that make eating easier.
3. Surgical interventions may be prescribed.

XVIII. Gastric Cancer

A. Description

1. Gastric cancer is a malignant growth of the mucosal cells in the inner lining of the stomach, with invasion to the muscle and beyond in advanced disease.
2. No single causative agent has been identified, but it is believed that *Helicobacter pylori* infection and a diet of smoked, highly salted, processed, or spiced foods have carcinogenic effects; other risk factors include smoking, alcohol and nitrate ingestion, and a history of gastric ulcers.
3. Complications include gastrointestinal hemorrhage, obstruction, metastasis, and dumping syndrome.
4. The goals of treatment are to remove the tumor and to provide a nutritional program.

B. Data collection

1. Early
   - **a.** Indigestion
   - **b.** Abdominal discomfort
   - **c.** Full feeling
   - **d.** Epigastric, back, or retrosternal pain
2. Late
   - **a.** Weakness and fatigue
   - **b.** Anorexia and weight loss
   - **c.** Nausea and vomiting
   - **d.** A sensation of pressure in the stomach
   - **e.** Dysphagia and obstructive symptoms
   - **f.** Iron deficiency anemia
   - **g.** Ascites
   - **h.** Palpable epigastric mass

C. Interventions

1. Monitor the vital signs.
2. Monitor the hemoglobin and hematocrit levels; blood transfusions may be prescribed.
3. Monitor the weight daily.
4. Monitor the nutritional status; encourage small, bland, easily digestible meals with vitamin and mineral supplements.
5. Administer pain medication, as prescribed.
6. Prepare the client for chemotherapy or radiation therapy, as prescribed.
7. Prepare the client for surgical resection of the tumor, as prescribed (Box 43-12).

D. Postoperative interventions

1. Monitor vital signs.
2. Place in Fowler's position for comfort.
3. Administer analgesics, antiemetics, as prescribed.
4. Monitor intake and output; fluids and electrolyte replacement by IV will be prescribed; parenteral nutrition may also be necessary.
5. Maintain NPO status as prescribed for 1 to 3 days until peristalsis returns; monitor bowel sounds.
6. Monitor nasogastric suction.
7. The nasogastric tube is not irrigated or removed (follow agency procedures); assist the HCP with irrigation or removal. 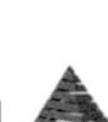
8. Advance the diet from NPO to sips of clear water to six small bland meals a day, as prescribed.
9. Monitor for complications such as hemorrhage, dumping syndrome, diarrhea, hypoglycemia, and vitamin B12 deficiency.

BOX 43-12 Surgical Interventions for Gastric Cancer

Subtotal Gastrectomy

Gastroduodenostomy

- Also called Billroth I
- Partial gastrectomy; the remaining segment is anastomosed to the duodenum

Gastrojejunostomy

- Also called Billroth II
- Partial gastrectomy; the remaining segment is anastomosed to the jejunum

Total Gastrectomy

- Also called esophagojejunostomy
- Removal of the stomach, with the attachment of the esophagus to the jejunum or the duodenum

XIX. Pancreatic Cancer

A. Description

1. Most pancreatic tumors are highly malignant, rapidly growing adenocarcinomas that originate from the epithelium of the ductal system.
2. Pancreatic cancer is associated with increased age, a history of diabetes mellitus, alcohol use, a history of previous pancreatitis, smoking, the ingestion of a high-fat diet, and exposure to environmental chemicals.

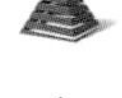

3. Symptoms usually do not occur until the tumor is large; therefore, the prognosis is poor.

B. Data collection

1. Nausea and vomiting
2. Jaundice
3. Unexplained weight loss
4. Clay-colored stools
5. Glucose intolerance
6. Abdominal pain

C. Interventions

1. Radiation
2. Chemotherapy
3. Whipple procedure, which involves a pancreaticoduodenectomy with the removal of the distal third of the stomach, a pancreaticojejunostomy, a gastrojejunostomy, and a choledochojejunostomy (Fig. 43-3)
4. Postoperative care measures are similar to those for the care of a client with pancreatitis and for a client after gastric surgery; monitor the blood glucose levels for transient hyperglycemia or hypoglycemia resulting from the surgical manipulation of the pancreas.

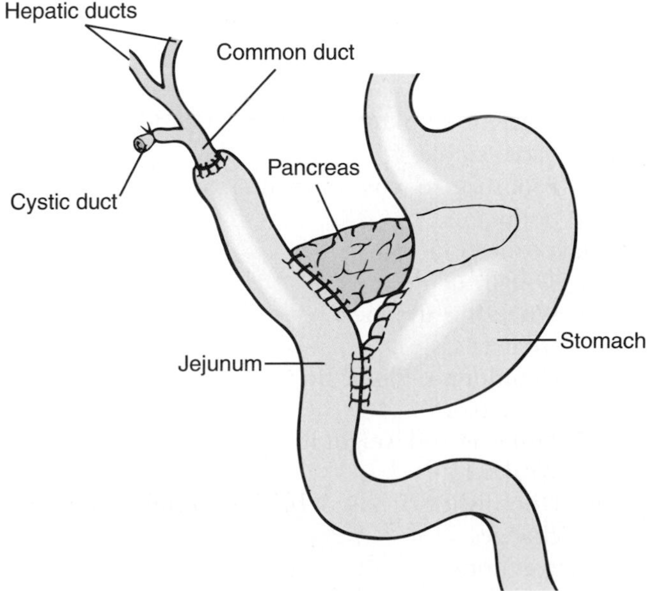

FIGURE 43-3 Whipple procedure or radical pancreaticoduodenectomy. (From Lewis S, Dirksen S, Heitkemper M, Bucher L, Camera I: *Medical-surgical nursing: Assessment and management of clinical problems*, ed 8, St. Louis, 2011, Mosby.)

XX. Intestinal Tumors

A. Description

1. Malignant lesions that develop in the cells lining the bowel wall or that develop as polyps in the colon or rectum
2. Metastasis occurs via the circulatory or lymphatic system or by direct extension to other areas in the colon or other organs.
3. Complications include bowel perforation with peritonitis, abscess and/or fistula formation, hemorrhage, and complete intestinal obstruction.

B. Risk factors for colorectal cancer

1. Age older than 50 years
2. Familial polyposis, family history of colorectal cancer
3. Previous colorectal polyps, history of colorectal cancer
4. History of chronic inflammatory bowel disease
5. History of ovarian or breast cancer

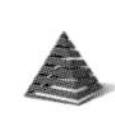

C. Data collection

1. Blood in the stool
2. Anorexia, vomiting, and weight loss
3. Anemia
4. Abnormal stools
   a. Ascending colon tumor: Diarrhea
   b. Descending colon tumor: Constipation, some diarrhea, or flat, ribbon-like stool caused by partial obstruction
   c. Rectal tumor: Alternating constipation and diarrhea
5. Guarding or abdominal distention, abdominal mass (late sign)
6. Cachexia (late sign)
7. Masses noted on barium enema, colonoscopy, CT scan, sigmoidoscopy

D. Interventions

1. Monitor for signs of complications, which include bowel perforation with peritonitis, abscess and/or fistula formation (fever associated with pain), hemorrhage (signs of shock), and complete intestinal obstruction.
2. Monitor for signs of bowel perforation, which include low blood pressure, rapid and weak pulse, distended abdomen, and elevated temperature.

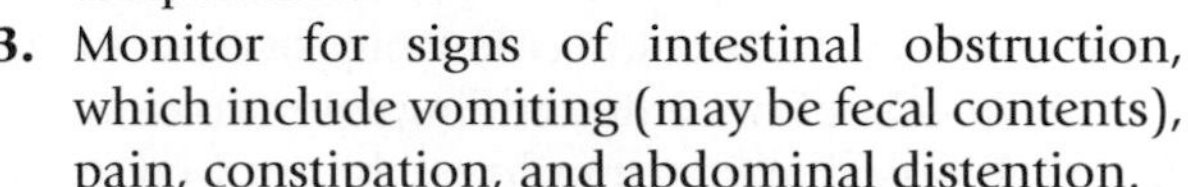

3. Monitor for signs of intestinal obstruction, which include vomiting (may be fecal contents), pain, constipation, and abdominal distention.
4. Note that an early sign of intestinal obstruction is increased peristaltic activity, which produces an increase in bowel sounds; as the obstruction progresses, hypoactive sounds are heard.
5. Prepare for radiation preoperatively if prescribed to facilitate surgical resection and postoperatively to decrease the risk of recurrence or to reduce pain, hemorrhage, bowel obstruction, or metastasis.

E. Nonsurgical interventions
   1. Preoperative radiation for local control and postoperative radiation for palliation may be prescribed.
   2. Postoperative chemotherapy to control symptoms and the spread of disease

F. Surgical interventions: Bowel, local lymph node resection, and creation of a colostomy or ileostomy

G. Colostomy, ileostomy
   1. Preoperative interventions
      a. Consultation with the enterostomal therapist may be necessary to assist with identifying the optimal placement of the ostomy.
      b. Instruct the client in prescribed preoperative diet; bowel preparation (laxatives and enemas) may be prescribed.
      c. Intestinal antiseptics and antibiotics may be prescribed (per surgeon's preference) to decrease the bacterial content of the colon and to reduce the risk of infection from the surgical procedure.
   2. Postoperative: Colostomy
      a. If a pouch system is not in place, apply a petroleum jelly gauze over the stoma to keep it moist, and keep it covered by a dry sterile dressing; place a pouch system on the stoma as soon as possible.
      b. Monitor the pouch system for proper fit and signs of leakage; empty the pouch when one third full.
      c. Monitor the stoma for size, unusual bleeding, and necrotic tissue.
      d. Note that the normal stoma color is red or pink, which indicates high vascularity.
      e. Note that a pale pink stoma indicates low hemoglobin and hematocrit levels and that a purple-black stoma indicates compromised circulation that requires RN and HCP notification.
      f. Monitor the functioning of the colostomy.
      g. Expect that stool will be liquid postoperatively but that it will become more solid, depending on the area of the colostomy.
      h. Expect liquid stool from an ascending colon colostomy, loose to semiformed stool from a transverse colon colostomy, or close to normal stool from a descending colon colostomy.
      i. Fecal matter should not be allowed to remain on the skin.
      j. Administer analgesics and antibiotics, as prescribed.
      k. Irrigate the perineal wound, if present and if prescribed, and monitor for signs of infection.
      l. Inform the client to avoid foods that cause excessive gas formation and odor.
      m. Reinforce instructions about stoma care and irrigations, as prescribed.
      n. Inform the client that normal activities may be resumed when approved by the HCP.
      o. Discuss with the RN about the need for the client to seek counseling or support services as needed for altered body image issues.
   3. Postoperative: Ileostomy
      a. A healthy stoma is red
      b. Postoperative drainage will be dark green and progress to yellow as the client begins to eat.
      c. Stool is liquid.
      d. The risk for dehydration and electrolyte imbalance exists.

⚠ Monitor stoma color. A dark blue, purple, or black stoma indicates compromised circulation, requiring RN and HCP notification.

XXI. Lung Cancer

A. Description
   1. Lung cancer is a malignant tumor of the bronchi and peripheral lung tissue.
   2. The lungs are a common target for metastasis from other organs.
   3. Bronchogenic cancer (tumors originate in the epithelium of the bronchus) spreads through direct extension and lymphatic dissemination.
   4. Classified according to histological cell type; types include small cell lung cancer (SCLC) and non-small cell lung cancer (NSCLC); epidermal (squamous cell), adenocarcinoma, and large cell anaplastic carcinoma are classified as NSCLC because of their similar responses to treatment.
   5. Diagnosis is made by a chest x-ray, CT scan, or magnetic resonance imaging (MRI), which will show a lesion or mass, and by bronchoscopy and sputum studies, which will demonstrate a positive cytological study for cancer cells.

B. Causes 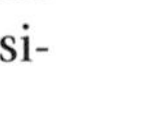
   1. Cigarette smoking; also exposure to "passive" tobacco smoke
   2. Exposure to environmental and occupational pollutants

C. Data collection 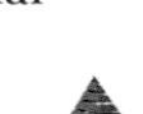
   1. Cough
   2. Wheezing, dyspnea
   3. Hoarseness
   4. Hemoptysis, blood-tinged or purulent sputum
   5. Chest pain
   6. Anorexia and weight loss
   7. Weakness
   8. Diminished or absent breath sounds, respiratory changes

D. Interventions
   1. Monitor the vital signs.
   2. Monitor the breathing patterns and breath sounds and for signs of respiratory impairment; monitor for hemoptysis.

3. Monitor for tracheal deviation.
4. Administer analgesics, as prescribed, for pain management.
5. Place the client in Fowler's position for ease of breathing.
6. Administer oxygen, as prescribed, and humidification to moisten and loosen secretions.
7. Monitor the pulse oximetry.
8. Provide respiratory treatments, as prescribed.
9. Administer bronchodilators and corticosteroids, as prescribed, to decrease bronchospasm, inflammation, and edema.
10. Provide a high-calorie, high-protein, high-vitamin diet.
11. Provide activity (as tolerated), rest periods, and active and passive ROM exercises.

E. Nonsurgical interventions
1. Radiation therapy for localized intrathoracic lung cancers and for the palliation of hemoptysis, obstructions, dysphagia, superior vena cava syndrome, and pain
2. Chemotherapy may be prescribed for the treatment of nonresectable tumors or as adjuvant therapy.

F. Surgical interventions
1. Laser therapy: To relieve endobronchial obstruction
2. Ablation therapy: To destroy the tumor
3. Thoracentesis and pleurodesis: To remove pleural fluid and relieve hypoxia
4. Thoracotomy (opening into the thoracic cavity) with pneumonectomy: Surgical removal of a lung
5. Thoracotomy with lobectomy: Surgical removal of one lobe of the lung for tumors that are confined to a single lobe
6. Thoracotomy with segmental resection: Surgical removal of a lobe segment

G. Preoperative interventions
1. Explain the potential postoperative need for chest tubes.
2. Note that closed-chest drainage is not usually used for a pneumonectomy and that the serum fluid that accumulates in the empty thoracic cavity eventually consolidates, thus preventing shifts of the mediastinum, heart, and remaining lung.

H. Postoperative interventions
1. Monitor the vital signs.
2. Monitor the cardiac and respiratory statuses; monitor lung sounds.
3. Monitor the chest tube drainage system, which will drain air and/or blood that accumulates in the pleural space; monitor for excess bleeding. (See Chapter 19 for care of the client with a chest tube.)
4. Monitor the chest tube insertion site for crepitus (subcutaneous air) and drainage.
5. Administer oxygen, as prescribed.
6. Check prescriptions regarding client positioning; complete lateral turning must be avoided.
7. Monitor the pulse oximetry.
8. Provide activity, as tolerated and prescribed.
9. Encourage active ROM exercises of the operative shoulder, as prescribed.

Airway is the priority for a client with lung or laryngeal cancer.

XXII. Laryngeal Cancer

A. Description
1. Laryngeal cancer is a malignant tumor of the larynx.
2. Laryngeal cancer presents as malignant ulcerations with underlying infiltration and is spread by local extension to adjacent structures in the throat and neck and by the lymphatic system.
3. Diagnosis is made by laryngoscopy and biopsy showing a positive cytological study for cancer cells.
4. Laryngoscopy allows for evaluation of the throat and biopsy of tissues; chest radiography, CT, and MRI are used for staging.

B. Risk factors
1. Cigarette smoking
2. Heavy alcohol use and the combined use of tobacco and alcohol
3. Exposure to environmental pollutants (e.g., asbestos, wood dust)
4. Exposure to radiation

C. Data collection
1. Persistent hoarseness and sore throat
2. Painless neck mass
3. The feeling of a lump in the throat
4. Burning sensation in the throat
5. Dysphagia
6. Change in voice quality
7. Dyspnea
8. Weakness and weight loss
9. Hemoptysis
10. Foul breath odor

D. Interventions
1. Place the client in Fowler's position to promote optimal air exchange. 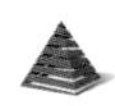
2. Monitor the respiratory status.
3. Monitor for signs of food and fluid aspiration. 
4. Administer oxygen, as prescribed.
5. Provide respiratory treatments, as prescribed.
6. Provide activity, as tolerated.
7. Provide a high-calorie, high-protein diet.
8. Prepare to provide nutritional support via parenteral nutrition or nasogastric, gastrostomy, or jejunostomy tube, as prescribed.
9. Administer analgesics for pain, as prescribed.

E. Nonsurgical interventions
1. Radiation therapy if the cancer is limited to a small area in one vocal cord
2. Chemotherapy, which may be performed in combination with radiation and surgery

F. Surgical interventions
   1. The goal is to remove the cancer while preserving as much normal function as possible.
   2. Depend on the tumor size and the amount of tissue to be resected
   3. Types of resection include cordal stripping, cordectomy, partial laryngectomy, and total laryngectomy.
   4. A tracheostomy is performed with a total laryngectomy; this airway opening is always permanent and is referred to as a laryngectomy stoma.

G. Preoperative interventions
   1. Discuss self-care of the airway, alternative methods of communication, suctioning, pain-control methods, the critical care environment, and nutritional support.
   2. Encourage the client to express feelings about changes in body image and the loss of the voice.
   3. Describe the rehabilitation program and provide information about the tracheostomy and suctioning.

H. Postoperative interventions
   1. Monitor the vital signs.
   2. Monitor the respiratory status and airway patency, and provide frequent suctioning to remove bloody secretions.
   3. Place the client in high Fowler's position.
   4. Maintain mechanical ventilator support or a tracheostomy collar with humidification, as prescribed.
   5. Monitor the pulse oximetry.
   6. Maintain surgical drains in the neck area, if present.
   7. Observe for hemorrhage and edema in the neck.
   8. Monitor IV fluids or parenteral nutrition, if prescribed, until nutrition is administered via nasogastric, gastrostomy, or jejunostomy tube.
   9. Provide oral hygiene.
   10. Monitor the gag and cough reflexes and the ability to swallow.
   11. Increase activity, as tolerated.
   12. Monitor the color, amount, and consistency of the sputum.
   13. Provide stoma and laryngectomy care (Box 43-13).
   14. Provide consultation with a speech and language pathologist, as prescribed.
   15. Reinforce the method of communication that is established preoperatively.
   16. Prepare the client for rehabilitation and speech therapy (Box 43-14).

BOX 43-13 Stoma Care After Laryngectomy

- Protect the neck from injury.
- Provide instructions in how to clean the incision and provide stoma care.
- Provide instructions to wear a stoma guard and/or loose-fitting, high-collared clothing to cover the stoma and for shielding and preventing debris from entering the stoma.
- Avoid swimming, showering, and using aerosol sprays.
- Reinforce teaching the client clean suctioning technique.
- Advise the client to increase humidity in the home.
- Increase fluid intake as prescribed.
- Avoid exposure to persons with infections.
- Demonstrate how to perform range-of-motion exercises for the arms, shoulders, and neck as prescribed.
- Advise the client to wear a Medic-Alert bracelet.

BOX 43-14 Speech Rehabilitation After Laryngectomy

Esophageal Speech
- Client produces esophageal speech by "burping" the air that is swallowed.
- Voice produced is monotone; it cannot be raised or lowered, and it carries no pitch.
- Client must have adequate hearing because he or she uses the mouth to shape words as they are heard.

Mechanical Devices
- One device, the *electrolarynx*, is placed against the side of the neck; the air inside the neck and pharynx is vibrated, and the client articulates.
- Another device consists of a plastic tube that is placed inside the client's mouth and vibrates on articulation.

Tracheoesophageal Fistula
- A fistula is surgically created between the trachea and the esophagus, with the eventual placement of a prosthesis that is used to produce speech.
- Prosthesis provides the client with a means to divert the air from the lungs through the trachea, into the esophagus, and out of the mouth.
- Speech is produced by lip and tongue movements.

XXIII. Prostate Cancer

A. Description
   1. Prostate cancer, a slow-growing malignancy of the prostate gland, is a common cancer in American men; most prostate tumors are adenocarcinomas arising from androgen-dependent epithelial cells.
   2. The risk increases in men with each decade after the age of 50 years.
   3. Prostate cancer can spread via direct invasion of surrounding tissues or by metastasis, through the bloodstream and lymphatics, to the bony pelvis and spine.
   4. Bone metastasis is a concern, as is spread to the lungs, liver, and kidneys. 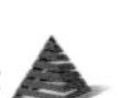
   5. The cause of prostate cancer is unclear, but advancing age, heavy metal exposure, smoking, and history of sexually transmitted infection are contributing factors.

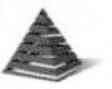
B. Data collection
1. Asymptomatic during the early stages
2. Hard, pea-sized nodule palpated on rectal examination
3. Gross, painless hematuria
4. Late symptoms include weight loss, urinary obstruction, and pain radiating from the lumbosacral area down the leg.
5. Prostate-specific antigen level is elevated in various noncancerous conditions and therefore should not be used as a screening test without a digital rectal exam; it is routinely used to monitor response to therapy.
6. Diagnosis is made through biopsy of the prostate.

C. Nonsurgical interventions
1. Prepare the client for hormone manipulation therapy, as prescribed.
2. Luteinizing hormone may be prescribed to slow the rate of growth of the tumor.
3. Pain medication, radiation therapy, corticosteroids, and bisphosphonates may be prescribed for palliation of advanced prostate cancer.
4. Prepare the client for external beam radiation or brachytherapy, which may be prescribed alone or with surgery, preoperatively or postoperatively, to reduce the lesion and limit metastasis.
5. Prepare the client for the administration of chemotherapy in cases of hormone-resistant tumors.

D. Surgical interventions
1. Prepare the client for orchiectomy (palliative), if prescribed, which will limit the production of testosterone.
2. Prepare the client for prostatectomy, if prescribed.
3. The radical prostatectomy can be performed via a retropubic, perineal, or suprapubic approach.
4. Cryosurgical ablation is a minimally invasive procedure that may be an alternative to radical prostatectomy; liquid nitrogen freezes the gland, and the dead cells are absorbed by the body.

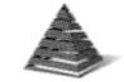
E. Transurethral resection of the prostate (TURP) may be performed for palliation in prostate cancer clients.
1. The procedure involves insertion of a scope into the urethra to excise prostatic tissue.
2. Monitor for hemorrhage; bleeding is common following TURP.
3. Postoperative continuous bladder irrigation (CBI) may be prescribed, which prevents catheter obstruction. (Box 43-15).
4. Monitor for signs of transurethral resection syndrome, which include signs of cerebral edema and increased intracranial pressure, such as increased blood pressure, bradycardia, confusion, disorientation, muscle twitching, visual disturbances, and nausea and vomiting; notify the RN immediately.

BOX 43-15 Continuous Bladder Irrigation

Description

A three-way (lumen) irrigation is used to decrease bleeding and to keep the bladder free from clots. One lumen is for inflating the balloon (30 mL), one is for instillation (inflow), and one lumen is for outflow.

Interventions

Maintain traction on the catheter, if applied, to prevent bleeding by pulling the catheter taut and taping it to the abdomen or thigh.

Instruct the client to keep the leg straight if traction is applied to the catheter and it is taped to the thigh.

Catheter traction is not released without a HCP's prescription; it is usually released after any bright red drainage has diminished.

Use only sterile bladder irrigation solution or prescribed solution to prevent water intoxication.

Run the solution at a rate, as prescribed, to keep the urine pink. Run the solution rapidly if bright red drainage or clots are present; monitor output closely. Run the solution at about 40 drops (gtt)/minute when the bright red drainage clears.

If the urinary catheter becomes obstructed, notify the RN; turn off the continuous bladder irrigation, and assist to irrigate the catheter with 30 to 50 mL of normal saline, if prescribed; notify the HCP if the obstruction does not resolve.

Discontinue continuous bladder irrigation and indwelling urinary catheter as prescribed, usually 24 to 48 hours after surgery.

Monitor for continence and urinary retention when the catheter is removed; inform the client that some burning, frequency, and dribbling may occur after catheter removal.

Inform the client that he should be voiding 150 to 200 mL of clear yellow urine every 3 to 4 hours by 3 days after surgery.

Inform the client that he may pass small clots and tissue debris for several days.

Instruct the client as prescribed to avoid heavy lifting, stressful exercise, driving, the Valsalva's maneuver, and sexual intercourse for 2 to 6 weeks to prevent strain.

Instruct the client to call the HCP if bleeding occurs or if there is a decrease in the urinary stream.

Encourage the client to drink 2400 to 3000 mL of fluid each day, preferably before 8:00 PM to prevent nocturia.

Instruct the client to avoid alcohol, caffeinated beverages, and spicy foods to prevent the overstimulation of the bladder.

Reinforce instructions to the client that if the urine becomes bloody, he should rest and increase the fluid intake; if the bleeding does not subside, he should notify the HCP.

5. Antispasmodics may be prescribed for bladder spasm.
6. Inform the client to monitor and report dribbling or incontinence postoperatively and teach perineal exercises.
7. Sterility is possible following the surgical procedure.

F. Suprapubic prostatectomy
1. Suprapubic prostatectomy is removal of the prostate gland by an abdominal incision with a bladder incision.

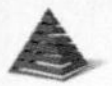

2. The client will have an abdominal dressing that may drain copious amounts of urine, and the abdominal dressing will need to be changed frequently.
3. Severe hemorrhage is possible, and monitoring for blood loss is an important nursing intervention.
4. Antispasmodics may be prescribed for bladder spasms.
5. Continuous bladder irrigation (CBI) is prescribed and carried out to keep the urine pink (see Box 43-15).
6. Sterility occurs with this procedure.

G. Retropubic prostatectomy
1. Retropubic prostatectomy is removal of the prostate gland by a low abdominal incision without opening the bladder.
2. Less bleeding occurs with this procedure compared with the suprapubic procedure, and the client experiences fewer bladder spasms.
3. Abdominal drainage is minimal.
4. CBI may be used (see Box 43-15).
5. Sterility occurs with this procedure.

H. Perineal prostatectomy
1. The prostate gland is removed through an incision made between the scrotum and anus.
2. Minimal bleeding occurs with this procedure.
3. The client needs to be monitored closely for infection because the risk of infection is increased with this type of prostatectomy.
4. Urinary incontinence is common.
5. The procedure causes sterility.
6. Reinforce teaching to the client on how to perform perineal exercises.

I. Postoperative interventions
1. Monitor vital signs.
2. Monitor urinary output and urine for hemorrhage or clots.
3. Increase fluids to 2400 to 3000 mL/day, unless contraindicated.
4. Monitor for arterial bleeding as evidenced by bright red urine with numerous clots; if it occurs, increase CBI and notify the RN immediately (see Box 43-15).
5. Monitor for venous bleeding as evidenced by burgundy-colored urine output; if it occurs, notify the RN; the surgeon may apply traction on the catheter.
6. Monitor hemoglobin and hematocrit levels.
7. Expect red to light pink urine for 24 hours, turning to amber in 3 days.
8. Ambulate the client as early as possible and as soon as urine begins to clear in color.
9. Inform the client that a continuous feeling of an urge to void is normal.
10. Reinforce instructions to the client to avoid attempts to void around the catheter because this will cause bladder spasms.
11. Administer antibiotics, analgesics, stool softeners, and antispasmodics as prescribed.
12. Monitor the three-way indwelling urinary catheter, which usually has a 30- to 45-mL retention balloon.
13. Maintain CBI with sterile bladder irrigation solution as prescribed to keep the catheter free of obstruction and keep the urine pink in color (see Box 43-15).

Following TURP, monitor for transurethral resection syndrome or severe hyponatremia (water intoxication) caused by the excessive absorption of bladder irrigation during surgery (altered mental status, bradycardia, increased blood pressure, and confusion).

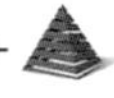

J. Postoperative interventions: Suprapubic prostatectomy
1. Monitor suprapubic and indwelling urinary catheter drainage.
2. Monitor CBI if prescribed.
3. Note that the indwelling urinary catheter will be removed 2 to 4 days postoperatively if the client has a suprapubic catheter.
4. If prescribed, clamp the suprapubic catheter after the indwelling urinary catheter is removed, and instruct the client to attempt to void; after the client has voided, assess the residual urine in the bladder by unclamping the suprapubic catheter and measuring the output.
5. Prepare for removal of the suprapubic catheter when the client consistently empties the bladder and residual urine is 75 mL or less.
6. Monitor the suprapubic incision dressing, which may become saturated with urine, until the incision heals; dressing may need to be changed frequently.

K. Postoperative interventions: Retropubic prostatectomy
1. Note that because the bladder is not entered, there is no urinary drainage on the abdominal dressing; if urinary or purulent drainage is noted on the dressing, notify the RN.
2. Monitor for fever and increased pain, which may indicate an infection.

L. Postoperative interventions: Perineal prostatectomy
1. Note that the client will have an incision, which may or may not have a drain.
2. Avoid the use of rectal thermometers, rectal tubes, and enemas because they may cause trauma and bleeding.

XXIV. Bladder Cancer

A. Description
1. Papillomatous growths in the bladder urothelium that undergo malignant changes and that may infiltrate the bladder wall

2. Predisposing factors include cigarette smoking, exposure to industrial chemicals, and exposure to radiation.
3. Common sites of metastasis include the liver, bones, and lungs.
4. As the tumor progresses, it can extend into the rectum, vagina, other pelvic soft tissues, and retroperitoneal structures.

B. Data collection
1. Gross, painless hematuria
2. Frequency, urgency, and dysuria
3. Clot-induced obstruction
4. Bladder wash specimens and biopsy confirm the diagnosis.

C. Radiation
1. Radiation therapy is indicated for advanced disease that cannot be eradicated by surgery; palliative radiation may be used to relieve pain and bowel obstruction and control potential hemorrhage and leg edema caused by venous or lymphatic obstruction.
2. Intracavitary radiation may be prescribed, which protects adjacent tissue.
3. External beam radiation combined with chemotherapy or surgery may be prescribed to improve survival.
4. Complications of radiation
   - **a.** Abacterial cystitis
   - **b.** Proctitis
   - **c.** Fistula formation
   - **d.** Ileitis or colitis
   - **e.** Bladder ulceration and hemorrhage

D. Chemotherapy
1. Intravesical instillation
   - **a.** An alkylating chemotherapeutic agent is instilled into the bladder.
   - **b.** This method provides a concentrated topical treatment with little systemic absorption.
   - **c.** The medication is injected into a urethral catheter and retained for 2 hours.
   - **d.** Following instillation, the client's position is rotated every 15 to 30 minutes, starting in the supine position, to avoid lying on a full bladder.
   - **e.** After 2 hours, the client voids in a sitting position and is instructed to increase fluids to flush the bladder.

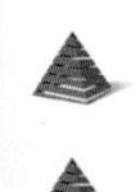

   - **f.** Treat the urine as a biohazard, and send it to the radioisotope laboratory for monitoring.
   - **g.** For 6 hours after intravesical chemotherapy, disinfect the toilet with household bleach after the client has voided.
2. Systemic chemotherapy: Used to treat inoperable or late tumors
3. Complications of chemotherapy
   - **a.** Bladder irritation
   - **b.** Hemorrhagic cystitis

E. Surgical interventions
1. Transurethral resection of the bladder tumor
   - **a.** Local resection and fulguration (destruction of tissue by electrical current through electrodes placed in direct contact with the tissue)
   - **b.** Performed for very early tumors for cure or for inoperable tumors for palliation
2. Partial cystectomy
   - **a.** The removal of up to half of the bladder
   - **b.** Performed for early stage tumors and for clients who cannot tolerate a radical cystectomy
   - **c.** During the initial postoperative period, the bladder capacity is markedly reduced to about 60 mL; however, as the bladder tissue expands, the capacity increases to 200 to 400 mL.
   - **d.** Maintenance of a continuous output of urine after surgery is critical to prevent bladder distention and stress on the suture line.
   - **e.** A urethral catheter and a suprapubic catheter may be in place, and the suprapubic catheter may be left in place for 2 weeks until healing occurs.
3. Cystectomy and urinary diversion (Fig. 43-4)
   - **a.** Various surgical procedures performed to create alternative pathways for urine collection and excretion
   - **b.** Urinary diversion may be performed with or without cystectomy (bladder removal).
   - **c.** The surgery may be performed in two stages if the tumor is extensive, with the creation of the urinary diversion first and the cystectomy several weeks later.
   - **d.** If a radical cystectomy is performed, lower-extremity lymphedema may occur as a result of lymph node dissection, and male impotence may occur.
4. Ileal conduit
   - **a.** Also called ureteroileostomy or Bricker's procedure
   - **b.** Ureters are implanted into a segment of the ileum, with the formation of an abdominal stoma.
   - **c.** The urine flows into the conduit and is continually propelled out through the stoma by peristalsis.
   - **d.** The client is required to wear an appliance over the stoma to collect the urine (Box 43-16).
   - **e.** Complications include obstruction, pyelonephritis, leakage at the anastomosis site, stenosis, hydronephrosis, calculi, skin irritation and ulceration, and stomal defects.
5. Kock pouch
   - **a.** A continent internal ileal reservoir created from a segment of the ileum and the ascending colon

Ureterostomies divert urine directly to the skin surface through a ureteral skin opening (stoma). After ureterostomy, the patient must wear a pouch.

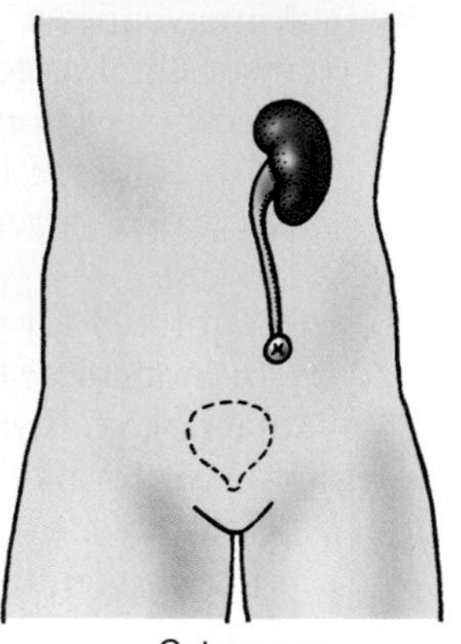

Cutaneous ureterostomy

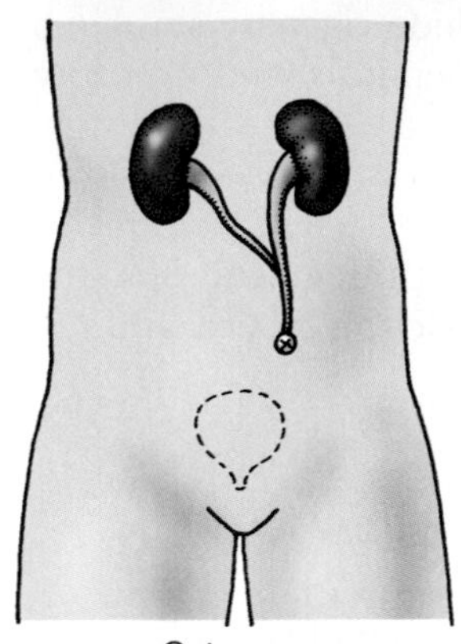

Cutaneous ureteroureterostomy

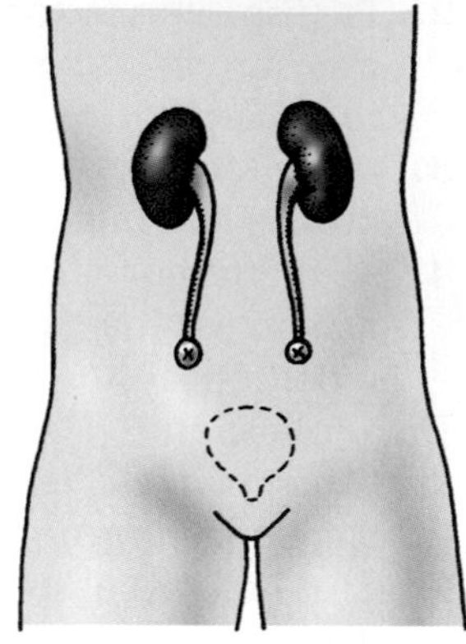

Bilateral cutaneous ureterostomy

Conduits collect urine in a portion of the intestine, which is then opened onto the skin surface as a stoma. After the creation of a conduit, the patient must wear a pouch.

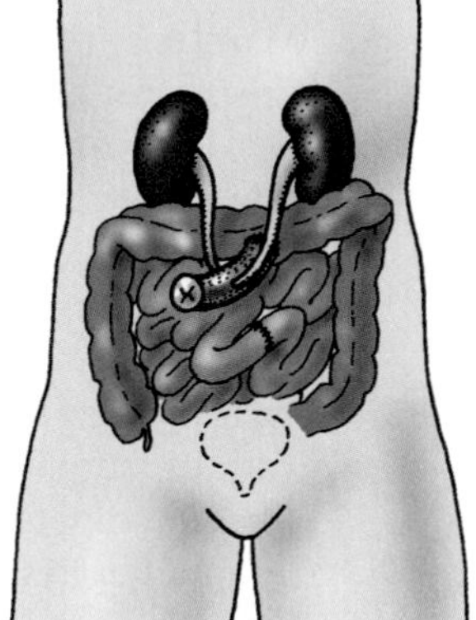

Ileal (Bricker's) conduit

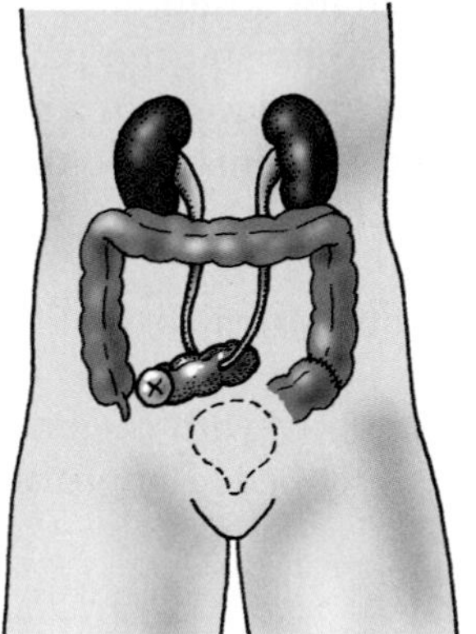

Colon conduit

Ileal reservoirs divert urine into a surgically created pouch, or pocket, that functions as a bladder. The stoma is continent, and the patient removes urine by regular self-catheterization.

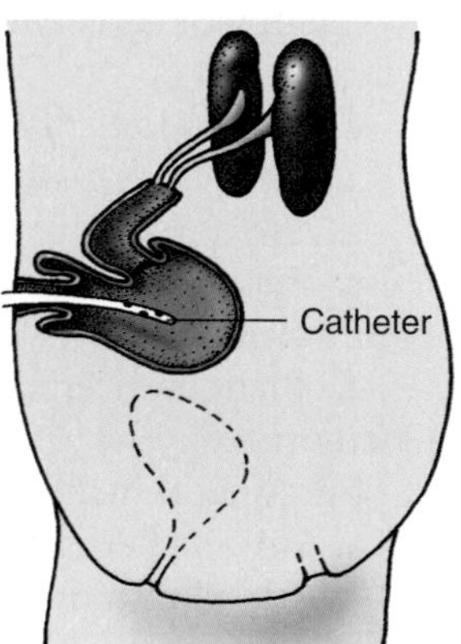

Continent internal ileal reservoir (Kock's pouch)

Sigmoidostomies divert urine to the large intestine, so no stoma is required. The patient excretes urine with bowel movements, and bowel incontinence may result.

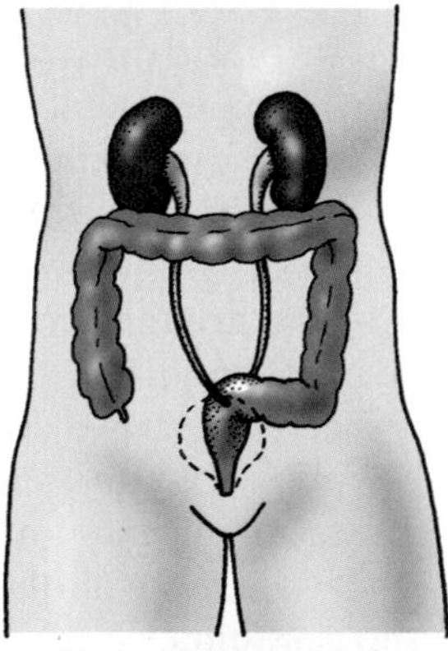

Ureterosigmoidostomy

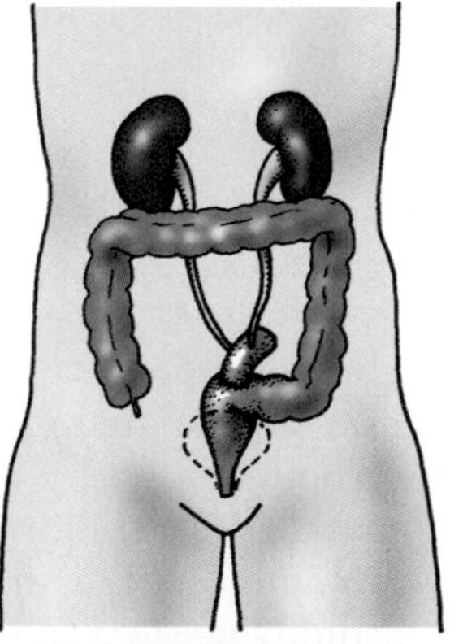

Ureteroiliosigmoidostomy

FIGURE 43-4 Urinary diversion procedures used in the treatment of bladder cancer. (From Ignatavicius D, Workman ML: *Medical-surgical nursing: Patient-centered collaborative care,* ed 7, Philadelphia, 2013, Saunders.)

b. The ureters are implanted into the side of the reservoir, and a special nipple valve is constructed to attach the reservoir to the skin.

c. Postoperatively, the client will have an indwelling urinary catheter in place to drain urine continuously until the pouch has healed.

d. The catheter is irrigated gently with normal saline to prevent obstruction caused by mucus or clots.

e. After the removal of the catheter, the client is instructed in how to self-catheterize and to drain the reservoir at 4- to 6-hour intervals.

6. Indiana pouch

a. A continent reservoir is created from the ascending colon and the terminal ileum, thus making a pouch larger than the Kock pouch (additional continent reservoirs include the Mainz and Florida pouch systems).

BOX 43-16 Urinary Stoma Care

Instruct the client in how to change the appliance.
Encourage self-care; teach the client to use a mirror.
The pouch may be drained by a bedside bag or leg bag, especially at night.
Empty the urinary collection bag when it is one third full to prevent pulling of the appliance and leakage.
Check the appliance seal if perspiring occurs.
Leave the urinary pouch in place as long as it is not leaking
To control odor, the client should drink adequate fluids, wash the appliance thoroughly with soap and lukewarm water, and soak the collection pouch in dilute white vinegar for 20 to 30 minutes; a special deodorant tablet can also be placed into the pouch while it is being worn.
Instruct the client who takes baths to keep the level of the water below the stoma and to avoid oily soaps.
If the client plans to shower, instruct the client to direct the flow of water away from the stoma.

   b. Postoperatively, care is similar as with the Kock pouch.
7. Creation of a neobladder
   a. Similar to the creation of an internal reservoir but different because instead of emptying through an abdominal stoma, it empties through a pelvic outlet into the urethra.
   b. The client empties the neobladder by relaxing the external sphincter and creating abdominal pressure or by intermittent self-catheterization.
8. Percutaneous nephrostomy or pyelostomy
   a. Used when the cancer is inoperable to prevent or treat obstruction
   b. Involves a percutaneous or surgical insertion of a nephrostomy tube into the kidney for drainage
   c. Nursing interventions involve stabilizing the tube to prevent dislodgment and monitoring output.
9. Ureterostomy
   a. May be performed as a palliative procedure if the ureters are obstructed by the tumor
   b. The ureters are attached to the surface of the abdomen, where the urine flows directly into a drainage appliance without a conduit.
   c. Potential problems include infection, skin irritation, and the obstruction of urinary flow as a result of strictures at the opening.
10. Vesicostomy
   a. The bladder is sutured to the abdomen, and a stoma is created in the bladder wall.
   b. The bladder empties through the stoma.

F. Preoperative interventions
1. Reinforce instructions about preoperative, operative, and postoperative management, including diet, medications, nasogastric tube placement, IV lines, NPO status, pain control, coughing and deep breathing, leg exercises, and postoperative activity.
2. Assist the RN to demonstrate appliance application and use for those clients who will have a stoma.
3. Assist the surgeon and the enterostomal nurse with selecting an appropriate skin site for the creation of the abdominal stoma.
4. Encourage the client to talk about his or her feelings related to the stoma creation.

G. Postoperative interventions

! Monitor urinary output closely following bladder surgery. Assist the RN to irrigate the ureteral catheter (if present and if prescribed) gently to prevent obstruction. Follow the HCP's prescriptions and agency policy regarding irrigation.

1. Monitor vital signs.
2. Monitor incision site.
3. Check the stoma (it should be red and moist) every hour for the first 24 hours.
4. Monitor for edema in the stoma, which may be present during the immediate postoperative period.
5. If the stoma appears dark and dusky, notify the RN and the HCP immediately, because this indicates necrosis.

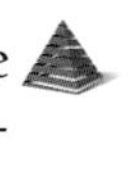

6. Monitor for the prolapse or retraction of the stoma; notify the RN.
7. Monitor for the return of bowel function; monitor for peristalsis, which will return in 3 to 4 days.

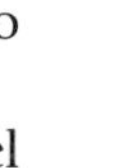

8. Maintain NPO status, as prescribed, until bowel sounds return.
9. Monitor for continuous urine flow (30 to 60 mL/hour).
10. The RN is notified if the urine output is less than 30 mL/hour or if there is no urine output for more than 15 minutes.

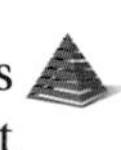

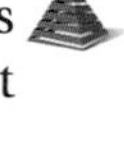

11. Ureteral stents or catheters may be in place for 2 to 3 weeks or until healing occurs; maintain stability of catheters to prevent dislodgment.
12. Monitor for hematuria.
13. Monitor for signs of peritonitis.
14. Monitor for bladder distention after a partial cystectomy.
15. Monitor for shock, hemorrhage, thrombophlebitis, and lower-extremity lymphedema after a radical cystectomy.

Adult—Oncological

16. Monitor the urinary drainage pouch for leaks, and check the skin integrity.
17. Monitor the pH of the urine (do not place the dipstick into the stoma), because highly alkaline or acidic urine can cause skin irritation and facilitate crystal formation.
18. Reinforce instructions to the client regarding the potential for urinary tract infection or the development of calculi.
19. Reinforce instructions to the client to check the skin for irritation and to monitor the urinary drainage pouch for any leakage.
20. Encourage the client to express feelings about changes in body image and sexual function, as well as embarrassment.

XXV. Oncological Emergencies

A. Sepsis and disseminated intravascular coagulation (DIC)
   1. Description: The client with cancer is at increased risk for infection, particularly gram-negative organisms, in the bloodstream (sepsis or septicemia) and DIC, a life-threatening problem frequently associated with sepsis.
   2. Interventions
      a. Prevent the complication through early identification of clients at high risk for sepsis and DIC.
      b. Maintain strict aseptic technique with the immunocompromised client, and monitor closely for infection.
      c. IV antibiotics may be prescribed.
      d. Anticoagulants may be prescribed during the early phase of DIC.
      e. Cryoprecipitated clotting factors may be prescribed when DIC progresses and hemorrhage is the primary problem.

Notify the RN and HCP immediately if signs of an oncological emergency occur.

B. Syndrome of inappropriate antidiuretic hormone
   1. Description
      a. Tumors can produce, secrete, or stimulate substances that mimic antidiuretic hormone.
      b. Mild symptoms include weakness, muscle cramps, loss of appetite, and fatigue; serum sodium levels range from 115 to 120 mEq/L.
      c. More serious signs and symptoms relate to water intoxication and include weight gain, personality changes, confusion, and extreme muscle weakness.
      d. As the serum sodium level approaches 110 mEq/L, seizures, coma, and eventually death will occur unless the condition is rapidly treated.
   2. Interventions
      a. Initiate fluid restriction and increased sodium intake, as prescribed.
      b. As prescribed, assist with the administration of an antagonist to antidiuretic hormone.
      c. Monitor the serum sodium levels.

C. Spinal cord compression
   1. Description
      a. Occurs when a tumor directly enters the spinal cord or when the vertebral column collapses as a result of tumor entry
      b. Causes back pain, usually before neurological deficits occur
      c. Neurological deficits relate to the spinal level of compression and include numbness and tingling; the loss of urethral, vaginal, and rectal sensation; and muscle weakness.
   2. Interventions
      a. Early recognition: Monitor for back pain and neurological deficits.
      b. Prepare the client for immediate radiation and/or chemotherapy to reduce the size of the tumor and relieve compression.
      c. Surgery may need to be performed to remove the tumor and relieve the pressure on the spinal cord.
      d. Reinforce instructions to the client regarding the use of neck or back braces, if prescribed.
      e. High doses of corticosteroids may be given to reduce the edema around the spinal cord.

D. Hypercalcemia
   1. Description
      a. A late manifestation of extensive malignancy that occurs most often in clients with bone metastasis, when the bone releases calcium into the bloodstream
      b. Decreased physical mobility contributes to or worsens hypercalcemia.
      c. Early signs include fatigue, anorexia, nausea, vomiting, constipation, confusion, and polyuria.
      d. More serious signs and symptoms include severe muscle weakness, diminished deep tendon reflexes, paralytic ileus, dehydration, and electrocardiography changes.
   2. Interventions
      a. Monitor the serum calcium level and for cardiac changes.
      b. Oral or parenteral (normal saline) fluids may be prescribed.
      c. Medications to lower the calcium level may be prescribed.
      d. Prepare the client for dialysis if the condition becomes life threatening or is accompanied by kidney impairment.

E. Superior vena cava (SVC) syndrome
  1. Description
    a. Occurs when the SVC is compressed or obstructed by tumor growth (commonly associated with lung cancer and lymphoma)
    b. Signs and symptoms result from the blockage of blood flow in the venous system of the head, neck, and upper trunk.
    c. Early signs and symptoms generally occur in the morning and include edema of the face (especially around the eyes) and tightness of the shirt or blouse collar (Stokes' sign).
    d. As the condition worsens, edema in the arms and hands, dyspnea, erythema of the upper body, and epistaxis (nosebleed) occur.
    e. Life-threatening signs and symptoms include hemorrhage, cyanosis, mental status changes, decreased cardiac output, and hypotension.
  2. Interventions
    a. Monitor for early signs and symptoms of SVC syndrome.
    b. Prepare the client for radiation therapy to the mediastinal area and possible surgery to insert a metal stent in the vena cava.

F. Tumor lysis syndrome (TLS)
  1. Description
    a. Occurs when large quantities of tumor cells are destroyed rapidly and intracellular components such as potassium and uric acid are released into the bloodstream faster than the body can eliminate them.
    b. Tumor lysis syndrome can indicate that cancer treatment is destroying tumor cells; however, if left untreated, it can cause severe tissue damage and death.
    c. Hyperkalemia, hyperphosphatemia with resultant hypocalcemia, and hyperuricemia occur; hyperuricemia can lead to acute kidney injury.
  2. Interventions
    a. Encourage oral hydration; IV hydration may be prescribed for the client experiencing nausea; monitor renal function.
    b. Diuretics may be prescribed to increase the urine flow through the kidneys.
    c. Medications that increase the excretion of purines, such as allopurinol (Zyloprim) may be prescribed.
    d. The IV infusion of glucose and insulin may be prescribed to treat hyperkalemia.
    e. Prepare the client for dialysis if hyperkalemia and hyperuricemia persist despite treatment.

CRITICAL THINKING What Should You Do?

Answer: The normal platelet count is 150,000 to 450,000 cells/mm^3. If the count is low, the client should be placed on bleeding precautions. The registered nurse and health care provider need to be notified of the laboratory result. The nurse should examine the client for signs of bleeding, including checking all body fluids and excrement, and monitor for signs of internal hemorrhage (e.g., pain; rapid and weak pulse, drop in blood pressure, and other signs of shock; increased abdominal girth; and abdomen guarding). The nurse should handle the client gently and use caution when taking blood pressure to prevent skin injury. Other interventions include soft foods that are cool to warm to avoid oral mucosa damage; avoiding injections to prevent trauma to the skin and bleeding; applying firm and gentle pressure to a needlestick site for at least 5 minutes, or longer if needed; padding corners of the bed and furniture; and avoiding rectal suppositories, enemas, and thermometers. The client should use a soft toothbrush and avoid dental floss, use only an electric razor for shaving, and avoid blowing the nose.

Reference(s): deWit, D. & Kumagai, C. (2013). *Medical-surgical nursing: Concepts & practice.* (2nd ed., pp. 359–360). St. Louis: Saunders.

Ignatavicius, D., & Workman, M. (2013). *Medical-surgical nursing: Patient-centered collaborative care.* (7th ed., p. 669). St. Louis: Saunders.

PRACTICE QUESTIONS

421. The nurse is assisting with developing a plan of care for the client with multiple myeloma. Which is a **priority** nursing intervention for this client?
  1. Encouraging fluids
  2. Providing frequent oral care
  3. Coughing and deep breathing
  4. Monitoring the red blood cell count

422. The nurse is assisting with conducting a health-promotion program to community members regarding testicular cancer. The nurse determines that **further teaching is needed** if a community member states that which is a sign/symptom of testicular cancer?
  1. Alopecia
  2. Back pain
  3. Painless testicular swelling
  4. A heavy sensation in the scrotum

423. The nurse is reviewing the laboratory results of a client with leukemia who has received a regimen of chemotherapy. Which laboratory finding would provide information about the massive cell destruction that occurs with the chemotherapy?

1. Anemia
2. Decreased platelets
3. Increased uric acid level
4. Decreased leukocyte count

424. The client is receiving external radiation to the neck for cancer of the larynx. The nurse monitors the client knowing that which is the **most likely** side/adverse effect of the external radiation?
1. Dyspnea
2. Diarrhea
3. Sore throat
4. Constipation

425. The nurse is reinforcing instructions to a client receiving external radiation therapy. The nurse determines that the client **needs further teaching** if the client states an intention to take which action?
1. Eat a high-protein diet.
2. Avoid exposure to sunlight.
3. Wash the skin with a mild soap and pat it dry.
4. Apply pressure on the radiated area to prevent bleeding.

426. The nurse is caring for a client with an internal radiation implant. The nurse should observe which principle?
1. Pregnant women are not allowed into the client's room.
2. Limit the time with the client to 1 hour per 8-hour shift.
3. Remove the dosimeter badge when entering the client's room.
4. Individuals less than 16 years old are allowed in the room if they stay 6 feet away from the client.

427. The nurse provides skin care instructions to the client who is receiving external radiation therapy. Which statement by the client indicates the **need for further teaching**?
1. "I will handle the area gently."
2. "I will wear loose-fitting clothing."
3. "I will avoid the use of deodorants."
4. "I will limit sun exposure to 1 hour daily."

428. The client is hospitalized for the insertion of an internal cervical radiation implant. While giving care, the nurse finds the radiation implant in the bed. Which is the **immediate** nursing action?
1. Call the health care provider (HCP).
2. Reinsert the implant into the vagina.
3. Pick up the implant with gloved hands and flush it down the toilet.
4. Pick up the implant with long-handled forceps and place into a lead container.

429. The nurse is assisting with developing a plan of care for a client who is experiencing hematological toxicity as a result of chemotherapy. The nurse should suggest including which in the plan of care?
1. Restricting all visitors
2. Restricting fluid intake
3. Restricting fresh fruits and vegetables in the diet
4. Inserting an indwelling urinary catheter to prevent skin breakdown

❖ **430.** The client with carcinoma of the lung develops the syndrome of inappropriate antidiuretic hormone (SIADH) as a complication of the cancer. The nurse anticipates that which may be prescribed to treat this complication? **Select all that apply.**
- ❑ 1. Radiation
- ❑ 2. Chemotherapy
- ❑ 3. Increased fluid intake
- ❑ 4. Serum sodium blood levels
- ❑ 5. Decreased oral sodium intake
- ❑ 6. Medication that is antagonistic to antidiuretic hormone (ADH)

431. The client is admitted to the hospital with a diagnosis of suspected Hodgkin's disease. Which finding should the nurse **most likely** expect to find documented in the client's record?
1. Fatigue
2. Weakness
3. Weight gain
4. Enlarged lymph nodes

432. When reviewing the health care record of a client with ovarian cancer, the nurse recognizes which sign/symptom as being a typical manifestation of the disease?
1. Diarrhea
2. Hypermenorrhea
3. Abnormal bleeding
4. Abdominal distention

433. The nurse is caring for a client after a mastectomy. Which finding would indicate that the client is experiencing a complication related to the surgery?
1. Mild pain at the incisional site
2. Arm edema on the operative side
3. Sanguineous drainage in the drainage tube
4. Complaints of decreased sensation near the operative site

434. The nurse is reinforcing discharge instructions to a client with cancer of the prostate after a prostatectomy. The nurse should reinforce which discharge instruction?
1. Avoid driving a car for 1 week.
2. Restrict fluid intake to prevent incontinence.

3. Avoid lifting objects heavier than 20 pounds for at least 6 weeks.
4. Notify the health care provider if small blood clots are noticed during urination.

435. The nurse is reviewing the laboratory results of a client who is receiving chemotherapy and notes that the platelet count is 10,000 cells/mm^3. On the basis of this laboratory value, the nurse should collect which data as a **priority**?
1. Temperature
2. Lung sounds
3. Status of skin turgor
4. Level of consciousness

ANSWERS

421. 1

Rationale: Hypercalcemia secondary to bone destruction is a priority concern in the client with multiple myeloma. The nurse should encourage fluids in adequate amounts to maintain an output of 1.5 to 2 L/day. Clients require about 3 L of fluid per day. The fluid is needed not only to dilute the calcium but also to prevent protein from precipitating in the renal tubules. Options 2, 3, and 4 may be components of the plan of care, but they are not the priorities for this client.

Test-Taking Strategy: Note the strategic word, *priority*. Think about the pathophysiology associated with multiple myeloma. Recalling that hypercalcemia is a concern and that encouraging fluids is specific to the care of a client with this disorder will direct you to the correct option. **Review: multiple myeloma.**

Level of Cognitive Ability: Applying

Client Needs: Physiological Integrity

Integrated Process: Nursing Process/Implementation

Content Area: Adult Health: Oncology

Priority Concepts: Cellular Regulation, Fluid and Electrolyte Balance

Reference(s): deWit, Kumagai (2013), p. 360.

422. 1

Rationale: Alopecia is not a sign/symptom of testicular cancer. However, it may occur as a result of radiation or chemotherapy. Options 2, 3, and 4 are findings in clients with testicular cancer. Back pain may indicate metastasis to the retroperitoneal lymph nodes.

Test-Taking Strategy: Note the strategic words, *further teaching is needed*. These words indicate a negative event query and ask you to select an option that is incorrect. Also focus on the subject, sign/symptom of testicular cancer. Remember that alopecia occurs as a result of chemotherapy rather than of the disease. **Review: testicular cancer.**

Level of Cognitive Ability: Evaluating

Client Needs: Health Promotion and Maintenance

Integrated Process: Teaching and Learning

Content Area: Adult Health: Oncology

Priority Concepts: Client Education, Health Promotion

Reference(s): deWit, Kumagai (2013), p. 933.

423. 3

Rationale: Hyperuricemia is especially common after treatment for leukemias and lymphomas, because the therapy results in massive cell destruction, resulting in the release of uric acid. Although options 1, 2, and 4 may also be noted, an increased uric acid level is specifically related to cell destruction.

Test-Taking Strategy: Focus on the subject, the effects associated with massive cell destruction. Read each option carefully, thinking about the physiology of the cell. Recalling the cell response to destruction will assist with directing you to the correct option. **Review: hyperuricemia.**

Level of Cognitive Ability: Understanding

Client Needs: Physiological Integrity

Integrated Process: Nursing Process/Data Collection

Content Area: Adult Health: Oncology

Priority Concepts: Cellular Regulation, Clinical Judgment

References(s): deWit, Kumagai (2013), pp. 169, 359.

424. 3

Rationale: In general, only the area in the treatment field is affected by the radiation. Skin reactions, fatigue, nausea, and anorexia may occur with radiation to any site, whereas other side/adverse effects occur only when specific areas are involved in treatment. A client who is receiving radiation to the larynx is most likely to experience a sore throat. Options 2 and 4 may occur with radiation to the gastrointestinal (GI) tract. Dyspnea may occur with lung involvement.

Test-Taking Strategy: Note the strategic words, *most likely*. Eliminate options 2 and 4 first because they are comparable or alike, and both are GI related. Consider the anatomical location of the radiation therapy to direct you to the correct option. **Review: radiation therapy.**

Level of Cognitive Ability: Applying

Client Needs: Physiological Integrity

Integrated Process: Nursing Process/Data Collection

Content Area: Adult Health: Oncology

Priority Concepts: Cellular Regulation, Clinical Judgment

Reference(s): deWit, Kumagai (2013), pp. 162, 283; Lewis et al (2014), pp. 515–516.

425. 4

Rationale: The client should avoid pressure on the radiated area and should wear loose-fitting clothing to prevent a disruption in the skin integrity. The remaining options are accurate instructions regarding radiation therapy. Protein assists in the healing process. Options 2 and 3 will assist in preventing skin disruption.

Test-Taking Strategy: Note the strategic words, *needs further teaching*. These words indicate a negative event query and ask you to select an option that is an incorrect statement. The word *pressure* in option 4 should be an indication that this is an inappropriate measure. **Review: radiation therapy and skin care.**

Level of Cognitive Ability: Evaluating

Client Needs: Physiological Integrity

Integrated Process: Teaching and Learning

Content Area: Adult Health: Oncology

Priority Concepts: Client Education, Tissue Integrity

Reference(s): Ignatavicius, Workman (2013), p. 413.

426. 1

Rationale: The time that the nurse spends in the room of a client with an internal radiation implant is 30 minutes per 8-hour shift. The dosimeter badge must be worn when in the client's room. Children less than 16 years old and pregnant women are not allowed in the client's room. These guidelines protect individuals from radiation exposure.
Test-Taking Strategy: Focus on the subject, principles to observe for the client with an internal radiation implant. Option 3 can be eliminated first because the purpose of the dosimeter badge is to measure radiation exposure. Knowledge of the time frame related to exposure to the client will assist you with eliminating option 2. From the remaining options, select option 1 because of the possible risks associated with exposure to the mother and fetus. **Review: radiation and internal radiation implant.**
Level of Cognitive Ability: Applying
Client Needs: Safe and Effective Care Environment
Integrated Process: Nursing Process/Implementation
Content Area: Adult Health/Oncology
Priority Concepts: Cellular Regulation, Safety
Reference(s): deWit, Kumagai (2013), p. 161.

427. 4

Rationale: The client needs to be instructed to avoid exposure to the sun because of the risk of burns, resulting in altered tissue integrity. Options 1, 2, and 3 are accurate measures for the care of a client who is receiving external radiation therapy.
Test-Taking Strategy: Note the strategic words, *need for further teaching.* These words indicate a negative event query and ask you to select an option that is an incorrect statement. Eliminate option 1 because of the word *gently* and option 2 because of the word *loose.* From the remaining options, recalling that sun exposure is to be avoided will assist you with answering the question. **Review: external radiation skin care.**
Level of Cognitive Ability: Evaluating
Client Needs: Physiological Integrity
Integrated Process: Teaching and Learning
Content Area: Adult Health: Oncology
Priority Concepts: Cellular Regulation, Tissue Integrity
Reference(s): Ignatavicius, Workman (2013), p. 413.

428. 4

Rationale: A lead container and long-handled forceps should be kept in the client's room at all times during internal radiation therapy. If the implant becomes dislodged, the nurse should pick up the implant with long-handled forceps and place it into the lead container. Options 2 and 3 are inaccurate interventions. It is not within the realm of nursing responsibilities to insert a radiation implant. Option 3 exposes the nurse and possibly others to the radiation. Although the HCP needs to be notified, this is not the immediate action.
Test-Taking Strategy: Note the strategic word, *immediate,* which indicates a priority nursing action. Option 2 is not an appropriate nursing action. Eliminate option 3 next because the implant would not be discarded, and this action exposes the nurse to the radiation. Although the HCP would be notified, the immediate action is option 4. **Review: internal cervical radiation safety.**
Level of Cognitive Ability: Applying
Client Needs: Safe and Effective Care Environment
Integrated Process: Nursing Process/Implementation
Content Area: Adult Health: Oncology
Priority Concepts: Cellular Regulation, Safety
Reference(s): deWit, Kumagai (2013), p. 161.

429. 3

Rationale: In a client who is experiencing hematological toxicity, a low-bacteria diet is implemented. This includes avoiding fresh fruits and vegetables and performing a thorough cooking of all foods. Not all visitors are restricted, but the client is protected from people with known infections. Fluids should be encouraged. Invasive measures such as an indwelling urinary catheter should be avoided to prevent infections.
Test-Taking Strategy: Note the subject, hematological toxicity and care of the immunocompromised client. Eliminate option 1 because of the word *all.* Next, eliminate option 2; it is not reasonable to restrict fluids for a client who is receiving chemotherapy because he or she is already at risk for fluid and electrolyte imbalances. Eliminate option 4 because of the risk of infection that exists with this measure. **Review: hematological toxicity.**
Level of Cognitive Ability: Applying
Client Needs: Safe and Effective Care Environment
Integrated Process: Nursing Process/Planning
Content Area: Adult Health: Oncology
Priority Concepts: Cellular Regulation, Safety
Reference(s): deWit, Kumagai (2013), p. 168.

❖ **430. 1, 2, 4, 6**

Rationale: Cancer is a common cause of SIADH. In clients with SIADH, excessive amounts of water are reabsorbed by the kidney and put into the systemic circulation. The increased water causes hyponatremia (decreased serum sodium levels) and some degree of fluid retention. SIADH is managed by treating the condition and its cause, and treatment usually includes fluid restriction, increased sodium intake, and a medication with a mechanism of action that is antagonistic to ADH. Sodium levels are monitored closely because hypernatremia can suddenly develop as a result of treatment. The immediate institution of appropriate cancer therapy (usually either radiation or chemotherapy) can cause tumor regression so that ADH synthesis and release processes return to normal.
Test-Taking Strategy: Focus on the subject, the client's diagnosis, and recall that in clients with SIADH, excessive amounts of water are reabsorbed by the kidney and put into the systemic circulation. Option 3 is inappropriate for clients with increased circulating volume. Option 5 is not a correct intervention for SIADH. **Review: Syndrome of inappropriate antidiuretic hormone (SIADH).**
Level of Cognitive Ability: Analyzing
Client Needs: Physiological Integrity
Integrated Process: Nursing Process/Planning
Content Area: Adult Health: Oncology
Priority Concepts: Cellular Regulation, Clinical Judgment
Reference(s): Ignatavicius, Workman (2013), p. 431.

431. 4

Rationale: Hodgkin's disease is a chronic, progressive neoplastic disorder of the lymphoid tissue that is characterized by the painless enlargement of the lymph nodes with progression to extralymphatic sites, such as the spleen and liver. Weight loss is more likely to be noted than weight gain. Fatigue and weakness may occur, but they are not significantly related to the disease.

Test-Taking Strategy: Note the strategic words, *most likely.* Option 3 can be eliminated because weight loss is more likely to occur. Options 1 and 2 are comparable or alike and rather vague symptoms that can occur with many disorders. Recall that Hodgkin's disease specifically affects the lymph nodes. Review: Hodgkin's disease.
Level of Cognitive Ability: Understanding
Client Needs: Physiological Integrity
Integrated Process: Nursing Process/Data Collection
Content Area: Adult Health: Oncology
Priority Concepts: Cellular Regulation, Clinical Judgment
Reference(s): deWit, Kumagai (2013), p. 251.

432. 4
Rationale: Signs and symptoms of ovarian cancer include abdominal distention, urinary frequency and urgency, and abdominal pain, caused by pressure from the growing tumor, resulting in urinary or bowel obstruction, and constipation. Abnormal bleeding is associated with uterine cancer and often results in hypermenorrhea.
Test-Taking Strategy: Eliminate options 2 and 3 first because they are comparable or alike. From the remaining options, think about the anatomical location of the ovaries. Review: ovarian cancer.
Level of Cognitive Ability: Understanding
Client Needs: Physiological Integrity
Integrated Process: Nursing Process/Data Collection
Content Area: Adult Health: Oncology
Priority Concepts: Cellular Regulation, Clinical Judgment
Reference(s): deWit, Kumagai (2013), p. 908.

433. 2
Rationale: Arm edema on the operative side (lymphedema) is a complication after mastectomy that can occur immediately, months, or even years after surgery. Options 1, 3, and 4 are expected occurrences after mastectomy and are not indicative of a complication.
Test-Taking Strategy: Note the subject, a complication of a mastectomy, and consider the normal and expected occurrences after a mastectomy. Option 2 is not an expected outcome. Review: mastectomy.
Level of Cognitive Ability: Analyzing
Client Needs: Physiological Integrity
Integrated Process: Nursing Process/Data Collection
Content Area: Adult Health: Oncology
Priority Concepts: Cellular Regulation, Clinical Judgment
Reference(s): deWit, Kumagai (2013), pp. 253, 913–915.

434. 3
Rationale: Option 3 is an accurate discharge instruction after prostatectomy. Driving a car and sitting for long periods of time are restricted for at least 3 weeks. A daily fluid intake of 2 to 2.5 L/day should be maintained to limit clot formation and prevent infection. Small pieces of tissue or blood clots can be passed during urination for up to 2 weeks after surgery.
Test-Taking Strategy: Focus on the subject, postprostatectomy discharge instructions. Recall that small blood clots are expected after this type of surgery, so option 4 can be eliminated. Option 2 can be eliminated because it is an incorrect and harmful intervention. Eliminate option 1 because 1 week is a short time period. Review: prostatectomy.
Level of Cognitive Ability: Applying
Client Needs: Physiological Integrity
Integrated Process: Teaching and Learning
Content Area: Adult Health: Oncology
Priority Concepts: Cellular Regulation, Client Education
Reference(s): deWit, Kumagai (2013), p. 935.

435. 4
Rationale: A high risk of hemorrhage exists when the platelet count drops below 20,000/mm^3. Fatal central nervous system hemorrhage or massive gastrointestinal hemorrhage can occur when the platelet count is less than 10,000 cells/mm^3. The client should be monitored for changes in the level of consciousness, which may be an early indication of an intracranial hemorrhage. Option 2 is a priority when the white blood cell count is low and the client is at risk for an infection. Although options 1 and 3 are important, they are not the priority in this situation.
Test-Taking Strategy: Note the strategic word, *priority.* Recall the normal platelet count and determine that a low count places the client at risk for bleeding, which is a higher priority than options 1, 2, and 3. Review: platelet count.
Level of Cognitive Ability: Analyzing
Client Needs: Physiological Integrity
Integrated Process: Nursing Process/Implementation
Content Area: Adult Health: Oncology
Priority Concepts: Cellular Regulation, Clotting
Reference(s): deWit, Kumagai (2013), p. 168; Lewis et al (2014), pp. 265, 661; Linton (2012), pp. 636–637.

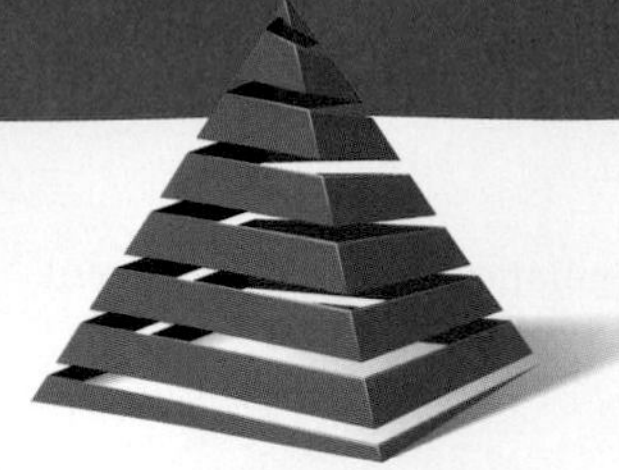

CHAPTER 44

Antineoplastic Medications

CRITICAL THINKING What Should You Do?

The nurse notes that a client who needs to receive a scheduled antineoplastic medication has a neutrophil count of 1000 cells/mm³. What should the nurse do?

Answer located on p. 550.

I. Antineoplastic Medications

A. Description
1. Antineoplastic medications kill or inhibit the reproduction of neoplastic cells.
2. Antineoplastic medications are used to cure, increase survival time, and decrease life-threatening complications.
3. The effect of antineoplastic medications may not be limited to neoplastic cells; normal cells also are affected by the medication.
4. Cell cycle phase-specific medications affect cells only during a certain phase of the reproductive cycle (Fig. 44-1).
5. Cell cycle phase-nonspecific medications affect cells in any phase of the reproductive cycle (see Fig. 44-1).
6. Usually, several medications are used in combination to increase the therapeutic response.
7. Antineoplastic medications may be combined with other treatments, such as surgery and radiation.
8. Although the intravenous (IV) route is most common for administration, antineoplastic medication may be given by the oral, intraarterial, isolated limb perfusion, or intracavitary route; dosing is usually based on the client's body surface area and type of **cancer**.
9. Chemotherapy dosing is usually based on total body surface area (BSA), to ensure that the client receives optimal doses of chemotherapy medications.

⚠ Side and adverse effects from chemotherapy result from the effects of the antineoplastic medication on normal cells.

B. Side/adverse effects 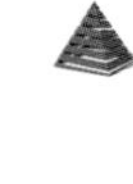
1. Mucositis
2. Alopecia
3. Anorexia, nausea, and vomiting
4. Diarrhea
5. Anemia
6. Low white blood cell count (neutropenia)
7. Thrombocytopenia
8. Infertility, sexual alterations

C. General interventions
1. Physiological integrity
   a. Complete blood count (CBC), white blood cell count, platelet count, uric acid level, and electrolytes are monitored.
   b. Bleeding precautions are initiated if thrombocytopenia occurs. 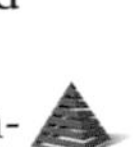
   c. When the platelet count is less than 50,000 cells/mm³, minor trauma can lead to episodes of prolonged bleeding; when less than 20,000 cells/mm³, spontaneous and uncontrollable bleeding can occur. The RN and health care provider is notified, and bleeding precautions are initiated.
   d. Monitor for petechiae, ecchymosis, bleeding of the gums, and nosebleeds because the decreased platelet count can precipitate bleeding tendencies.
   e. Intramuscular injections and venipunctures are avoided as much as possible to prevent bleeding.
   f. Neutropenic precautions are initiated if the white blood cell (WBC) count decreases; if the WBC count is low, the RN and health care provider is notified and bleeding precautions are initiated.
   g. Monitor for fever, sore throat, unusual bleeding, and signs and symptoms of infection.
   h. The client is informed that loss of appetite also may be the result of taste changes or a bitter taste in the mouth from the medications.
   i. Monitor for nausea and vomiting, and provide a high-calorie diet with protein supplements.
   j. Antiemetics are administered several hours before chemotherapy and for 12 to 48 hours after, as prescribed, because antineoplastic medications stimulate the vomiting center in the brain.

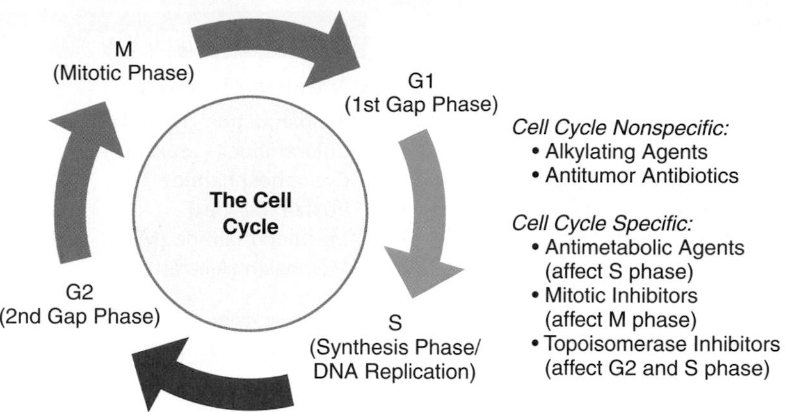

FIGURE 44-1 The cell cycle. *G1*, The cell is preparing for division; *S* (synthesis phase, DNA replication), the cell doubles its DNA content through DNA synthesis; *G2*, the cell produces proteins to be used in cell division and in normal physiological function after cell division is complete; and *M* (mitotic phase), the single cell splits apart into two cells.

k. Encourage hydration; IV fluids will be administered before and during therapy.
l. Promote a fluid intake of at least 2000 mL/day to maintain adequate kidney function.

Antineoplastic medication causes the rapid destruction of cells, resulting in the release of uric acid. Allopurinol (Zyloprim) may be prescribed to lower the serum uric acid level.

2. Safe and effective care environment
a. IV chemotherapy is prepared in an air-vented space (biohazard cabinet area); in most health care agencies, it is prepared in the pharmacy.
b. Gloves, gown, eye protectors, and mask are worn when handling IV medications.
c. Nurses who are pregnant should avoid chemotherapy preparation or the administration of chemotherapy.
d. IV equipment is discarded in designated (biohazard) containers.
e. Antineoplastic medication is administered precisely as prescribed to maximize antineoplastic effects while allowing normal cells to recover.
f. IV administration can cause phlebitis because these medications may irritate the veins; the site needs to be monitored closely.
g. Monitor for extravasation (leakage of medication into surrounding skin and subcutaneous tissue, which causes tissue necrosis), and notify the registered nurse if this occurs; heat or ice is applied, depending on the medication, and an antidote may be injected into the site.

3. Psychosocial integrity
a. The client is instructed about the possibility of hair loss and that varying degrees of hair loss may occur after the first or second treatment.
b. Discuss the purchase of a wig before treatment starts.
c. The client is informed that new hair growth will occur several months after the final treatment.
d. The client is instructed about the need for contraception because these medications have teratogenic effects.
e. The potential effect of infertility is discussed, which may be irreversible.
f. Encourage pretreatment counseling.

4. Health promotion and maintenance
a. The client is instructed that if diarrhea is a problem to avoid spicy foods and high-fiber foods and foods that are hot in temperature, which increase peristalsis.
b. The client is instructed to inspect the oral mucosa frequently for erythema and ulcers, rinse the mouth after meals, and perform good oral hygiene.
c. The client is instructed to use mouth rinses as prescribed for mouth sores if necessary.
d. The client is instructed in the use of antifungal agents for mouth sores, if prescribed, for the development of a fungal infection.
e. The client is instructed to avoid crowds and persons with infections and to report signs of infection such as a low-grade fever, chills, or sore throat.
f. Individuals with colds or infections are instructed to wear a mask when visiting or to avoid visiting the client.
g. The client is instructed to use a soft toothbrush and electric razor to minimize the risk of bleeding.
h. The client is instructed to avoid aspirin-containing products to minimize the risk of bleeding.
i. The client is instructed to consult the health care provider (HCP) before receiving vaccinations (live vaccines should not be administered).

D. Anaphylactic reactions
  1. Precautions
    a. Obtain an allergy history.
    b. A test dose is administered when prescribed by the HCP.
    c. Stay with the client during the administration of medication.
    d. Monitor vital signs.
    e. Have emergency equipment and medications readily available.
    f. An IV line is initiated for the administration of emergency medications if needed.
  2. Signs/symptoms of an anaphylactic reaction
    a. Dyspnea
    b. Chest tightness or pain
    c. Pruritis or urticaria
    d. Tachycardia
    e. Dizziness
    f. Anxiety or agitation
    g. Flushed appearance
    h. Hypotension
    i. Decreased sensorium
    j. Cyanosis

PRIORITY NURSING ACTIONS!

Actions Taken if an Anaphylactic Reaction Occurs from Medication

1. Respiratory status is assessed.
2. The medication is stopped.
3. The HCP is contacted by the RN; the Rapid Response Team is also contacted if necessary.
4. Oxygen is administered.
5. The IV access is maintained with normal saline.
6. The client's feet and legs are raised, if not contraindicated.
7. Prescribed emergency medications are administered.
8. Vital signs are monitored.
9. The event, actions taken, and the client's response are documented.

If anaphylaxis occurs from a medication, the nurse immediately assesses the client's respiratory status. The medication is also immediately stopped. If the client's airway needs to be established or stabilized, the Rapid Response Team is called. Additionally, the RN and HCP are contacted. The IV line is not removed because IV access is needed to administer emergency medications such as diphenhydramine (Benadryl) or epinephrine. The client is positioned appropriately. The legs and feet are elevated. The head of the bed is elevated to improve ventilation; elevate the head of the bed 10 degrees if hypotension is present and 45 degrees or higher if the blood pressure is normal. The nurse stays with the client and monitors the client's status, including the vital signs. The nurse also follows the instructions of the RN. The nurse documents the event, actions taken, and the client's response.

Reference(s): Lewis, S., Dirksen, S., Heitkemper, M., & Bucher, L. (2014). *Medical-surgical nursing: Assessment and management of clinical problems* (9th ed., p. 214). St. Louis: Mosby.

BOX 44-1 Alkylating Medications

Nitrogen Mustards
Bendamustine (Treanda)
Chlorambucil (Leukeran)
Cyclophosphamide
Ifosfamide (Ifex)
Mechlorethamine (Mustargen)
Melphalan (Alkeran)

Nitrosoureas
Carmustine (BiCNU, Gliadel)
Lomustine (CeeNu)
Streptozocin (Zanosar)

Alkylating-Like Medications
Altretamine (Hexalen)
Busulfan (Myleran, Busulfex)
Carboplatin
Cisplatin
Dacarbazine
Oxaliplatin (Eloxatin)
Temozolomide (Temodar)
Thiotepa

  3. Interventions for an anaphylactic reaction (see Priority Nursing Actions)

II. Alkylating Medications (Box 44-1)

A. Description
  1. Breaks the DNA helix, thereby interfering with DNA replication
  2. Cell cycle phase-nonspecific medications

B. Side/adverse effects
  1. Anorexia, nausea, and vomiting may occur.
  2. Stomatitis may occur.
  3. Rash may occur.
  4. Client may feel IV site pain during IV administration.
  5. Busulfan (Myleran, Busulfex) may cause hyperuricemia.
  6. Chlorambucil (Leukeran) and mechlorethamine (Mustargen) may cause gonadal suppression and hyperuricemia.
  7. Cisplatin, a platinum compound, may cause ototoxicity, tinnitus, hypokalemia, hypocalcemia, hypomagnesemia, and nephrotoxicity. 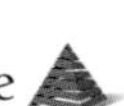
  8. Cyclophosphamide (Neosar) may cause alopecia, gonadal suppression, hemorrhagic cystitis, and hematuria. 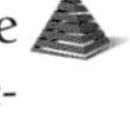

C. Interventions: Refer to Section I.C. Antineoplastic Medications—General Interventions.
  1. Monitor results of pulmonary function tests.
  2. Monitor results of chest radiography and kidney and liver function studies.
  3. When cisplatin is administered, the client is monitored for dizziness, tinnitus, hearing loss, incoordination, and numbness or tingling of extremities.

4. Mesna (Mesnex) may be administered with ifosfamide to reduce the potential of ifosfamide-induced cystitis.
5. Reinforce instructions to the client that cyclophosphamide, when prescribed orally, is administered without food.
6. Reinforce instructions to the client to follow a diet low in purines to alkalinize the urine and lower uric acid blood levels.
7. Reinforce instructions to the client in how to avoid infection.
8. Reinforce instructions to the client to report signs of infection or bleeding.
9. Reinforce instructions to the client about good oral hygiene and use of a soft toothbrush.

⚠ Cyclophosphamide and ifosfamide (Ifex) are medications that can cause hemorrhagic cystitis. The client is encouraged to drink increased fluids (2 to 3 L per day) during therapy, unless contraindicated.

III. Antitumor Antibiotic Medications (Box 44-2)

A. Description
1. Interfere with DNA and RNA synthesis
2. Cell cycle phase-nonspecific medications

B. Side/adverse effects
1. Nausea and vomiting
2. Fever
3. Bone marrow depression
4. Rash
5. Alopecia
6. Stomatitis
7. Gonadal suppression
8. Hyperuricemia
9. Vesication (blistering of tissue at IV site)
10. Daunorubicin may cause heart failure and dysrhythmias.
11. Doxorubicin (Doxil) and idarubicin (Idamycin) may cause cardiotoxicity, cardiomyopathy, and electrocardiographic changes; dexrazoxane (Zinecard) may be administered with doxorubicin to reduce cardiomyopathy.
12. Pulmonary toxicity can occur with bleomycin.

C. Interventions: Refer to Section I.C. Antineoplastic Medications—General Interventions.

BOX 44-2 Antitumor Antibiotic Medications

Bleomycin sulfate
Dactinomycin (Cosmegen)
Daunorubicin (DaunoXome)
Doxorubicin (Doxil)
Epirubicin (Ellence)
Idarubicin (Idamycin)
Mitomycin (Mutamycin)
Mitoxantrone (Novantrone)
Valrubicin (Valstar)

1. Monitor results of pulmonary function tests.
2. Monitor for electrocardiographic changes.
3. Monitor for adventitious lung sounds.
4. Monitor for signs/symptoms of heart failure, including dyspnea, crackle-like sounds, peripheral edema, and weight gain.
5. Monitor for results of chest radiography and kidney and liver function studies.
6. Monitor for myocardial toxicity, dyspnea, dysrhythmias, hypotension, and weight gain when daunorubicin, doxorubicin, or idarubicin are administered.
7. Monitor pulmonary status when bleomycin is administered. 

IV. Antimetabolite Medications (Box 44-3)

A. Description
1. Antimetabolite medications halt the synthesis of cell protein; their presence impairs cell division.
2. Antimetabolite medications are cell cycle phase-specific and affect the S phase.

B. Side/adverse effects
1. Anorexia, nausea, and vomiting
2. Diarrhea
3. Alopecia
4. Stomatitis
5. Depression of bone marrow
6. Cytarabine (Cytosar-U, DepoCyt, Tarabine PFS) may cause alopecia, stomatitis, hyperuricemia, and hepatotoxicity.
7. Fluorouracil (Adrucil) may cause alopecia, stomatitis, diarrhea, phototoxicity reactions, and cerebellar dysfunction. 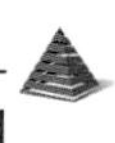
8. Mercaptopurine (Purinethol) may cause hyperuricemia and hepatotoxicity.
9. Methotrexate (Rheumatrex, Trexall) may cause alopecia, stomatitis, hyperuricemia, photosensitivity, hepatotoxicity, and hematological, gastrointestinal, and skin toxicity. 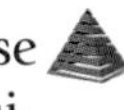

BOX 44-3 Antimetabolite Medications

Capecitabine
Cladribine (Leustatin)
Clofarabine (Clolar)
Cytarabine (DepoCyt)
Floxuridine (FUDR)
Fludarabine (Fludara)
Fluorouracil (Adrucil)
Gemcitabine (Gemzar)
Hydroxyurea (Hydrea, Droxia)
Mercaptopurine (Purinethol)
Methotrexate (Rheumatrex, Trexall)
Nelarabine (Arranon)
Pemetrexed (Alimta)
Pentostatin (Nipent)
Pralatrexate (Folotyn)
Thioguanine (Tabloid)

C. Interventions: Refer to Section I.C. Antineoplastic Medications—General Interventions.
   1. Monitor kidney function studies.
   2. Monitor for cerebellar dysfunction.
   3. Monitor for photosensitivity.
   4. When fluorouracil is administered, monitor for signs of cerebellar dysfunction, such as dizziness, weakness, and ataxia, and monitor for stomatitis and diarrhea, which may necessitate medication discontinuation.
   5. When fluorouracil or methotrexate is administered, the client is instructed to use sunscreen and wear protective clothing to prevent photosensitivity reactions.

When methotrexate is administered in large doses, leucovorin (folinic acid or citrovorum factor) may be administered as prescribed to prevent toxicity. This is known as leucovorin rescue.

V. Mitotic Inhibitor Medications (Vinca Alkaloids) (Box 44-4)

A. Description
   1. Mitotic inhibitors prevent mitosis (i.e., cell division) causing cell death.
   2. Mitotic inhibitors are cell cycle phase-specific and act on the M phase.

B. Side/adverse effects
   1. Leukopenia
   2. Neurotoxicity with vincristine (Vincasar) manifested as numbness and tingling in the fingers and toes, constipation, paralytic ileus.
   3. Ptosis
   4. Hoarseness
   5. Motor instability
   6. Anorexia, nausea, and vomiting
   7. Peripheral neuropathy
   8. Alopecia
   9. Stomatitis
   10. Hyperuricemia
   11. Phlebitis at IV site

C. Interventions: Refer to Section I.C. Antineoplastic Medications—General Interventions.
   1. Monitor for hoarseness.
   2. Monitor eyes for ptosis.
   3. Monitor motor stability and initiate safety precautions as necessary.
   4. Monitor for neurotoxicity with vincristine sulfate manifested as numbness and tingling in the fingers and toes. 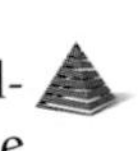
   5. Monitor for constipation and paralytic ileus.

BOX 44-4 Mitotic Inhibitors

Vinca Alkaloids
Vinblastine sulfate
Vincristine sulfate
Vinorelbine (Navelbine)

Taxanes
Docetaxel (Docefrez, Taxotere)
Paclitaxel (Onxol)

VI. Topoisomerase Inhibitors (Box 44-5)

A. Description
   1. Block an enzyme needed for DNA synthesis and cell division.
   2. Cell cycle phase-specific; act on the G2 and S phases

B. Side/adverse effects
   1. Leukopenia, thrombocytopenia, anemia
   2. Anorexia, nausea, and vomiting
   3. Diarrhea
   4. Alopecia
   5. Orthostatic hypotension
   6. Hypersensitivity reaction

C. Interventions: Refer to Section I.C. Antineoplastic Medications—General Interventions.

VII. Hormonal Medications and Enzymes (Box 44-6)

A. Description
   1. Suppress the immune system and block normal hormones in hormone-sensitive tumors
   2. Change the hormonal balance and slow the growth rates of certain tumors

B. Side/adverse effects
   1. Anorexia, nausea, and vomiting
   2. Leukopenia
   3. Impaired pancreatic function with asparaginase (Elspar)
   4. Sex characteristic alterations
      a. Masculinizing effect in women: Chest and facial hair, menses stops.
      b. Feminine manifestations in men: Gynecomastia
   5. Breast swelling
   6. Hot flashes
   7. Weight gain
   8. Hemorrhagic cystitis, hypouricemia, and hyperlipidemia, with mitotane (Lysodren)
   9. Hypertension
   10. Thromboembolic disorders
   11. Edema
   12. Electrolyte imbalances

BOX 44-5 Topoisomerase Inhibitors

Etoposide (Toposar)
Irinotecan (Camptosar)
Teniposide (Vumon)
Topotecan (Hycamtin)

BOX 44-6 Hormonal Medications and Enzymes

Estrogens
Estramustine (Emcyt)
Ethinyl estradiol (Estinyl)

Antiestrogens
Anastrozole (Arimidex)
Exemestane (Aromasin)
Fulvestrant (Faslodex)
Letrozole (Femara)
Raloxifene (Evista)
Tamoxifen citrate (Nolvadex)
Toremifene (Fareston)

Antiandrogens
Bicalutamide (Casodex)
Flutamide
Goserelin acetate (Zoladex)
Nilutamide (Nilandron)
Triptorelin (Trelstar)

Progestins
Medroxyprogesterone (Depo-Provera)
Megestrol acetate (Megace)

Other Hormonal Antagonists and Enzymes
Asparaginase (Elspar)
Leuprolide acetate (Lupron)
Mitotane (Lysodren)

13. Tamoxifen may cause edema, hypercalcemia, and elevated cholesterol and triglyceride levels.
14. Tamoxifen decreases the effects of estrogen.

C. Interventions: Refer to Section I.C. Antineoplastic Medications—General Interventions.
1. Check medications that the client is currently taking.
2. Monitor serum calcium levels with androgens.
3. Monitor for signs of alterations in sexual characteristics.
4. Monitor pancreatic function with asparaginase.
5. Monitor uric acid and cholesterol levels.
6. Monitor for signs of hemorrhagic cystitis.

VIII. Immunomodulator Agents: Biological Response Modifiers (Box 44-7)

A. Description
1. Immunomodulators stimulate the immune system to recognize cancer cells and take action to eliminate or destroy them.
2. Interleukins help various immune system cells recognize and destroy abnormal body cells.
3. Interferons slow down tumor cell division, stimulate proliferation, and cause cancer cells to differentiate into nonproliferative forms.

B. Colony-stimulating factors induce more rapid bone marrow recovery after suppression by chemotherapy (Box 44-8).

BOX 44-7 Immunomodulator Agents

Aldesleukin (Proleukin, interleukin-2)
Interferon alfa-2a
Interferon alfa-2b
Interferon alfa-n3 (Alferon N)
Recombinant interferon alfa-2a (Intron A)
Recombinant interferon alfa-2b (Roferon-A)

Common Monoclonal Antibodies
Alemtuzumab (Campath)
Gemtuzumab ozogamicin (Mylotarg)
Ibritumomab (Zevalin)
Infliximab (Remicade)
Rituximab (Rituxan)
Trastuzumab (Herceptin)

BOX 44-8 Colony-Stimulating Factors

Granulocyte-Macrophage Colony-Stimulating Factor
Sargramostim (Leukine)

Granulocyte Colony-Stimulating Factor
Filgrastim (Neupogen)
Pegfilgrastim (Neulasta)

Erythropoietin
Epoetin alfa (Epogen)
Darbepoetin alfa (Aranesp)

Thrombopoietic Growth Factor
Oprelvekin (Interleukin-11)
Eltrombopag (Promacta)

IX. Other Antineoplastic Medications (Box 44-9)

A. Altretamine (Hexalen): Cytotoxic agent used to treat ovarian cancer

B. Denileukin diftitox (Ontak): Recombinant DNA-derived medication used to treat cutaneous T-cell **lymphoma**

C. Gemcitabine (Gemzar): Used to treat non-small cell lung cancer and **adenocarcinoma** of the pancreas and metastatic breast cancer, and lung cancer (in combination with paclitaxel [Abraxane, Taxol, Onxol]).

D. Irinotecan (Camptosar): Used to treat colorectal or rectal cancer

E. Paclitaxel: Used to treat ovarian or metastatic breast cancer

F. Pegaspargase (Oncaspar): Used in combination chemotherapies for acute lymphoblastic **leukemia** in clients unable to take asparaginase (Elspar)

G. Topotecan (Hycamtin): Indicated for the treatment of relapsed or refractory metastatic ovarian cancer after other therapies have failed

BOX 44-9 Other Antineoplastic Medications

Asparaginase (Elspar)
Arsenic trioxide (Trisenox)
Bexarotene (Targretin)
Bortezomib (Velcade)
Imatinib (Gleevec)
Temozolomide (Temodar)

H. Trastuzumab (Herceptin): Used in combination chemotherapy to treat breast cancer
I. Bexarotene (Targretin): Use to treat advanced stage cutaneous T-cell lymphoma

CRITICAL THINKING What Should You Do?

Answer: If the nurse notes that a client's neutrophil count is low, the nurse would immediately notify the registered nurse (RN). The RN should withhold the medication if the neutrophil count is less than 1800 cells/mm³. The health care provider (HCP) is notified for further prescriptions, and neutropenic precautions are initiated to protect the client from infection.

Reference(s): deWit, D. & Kumagai, C. (2013). *Medical-surgical nursing: Concepts & practice.* (2nd ed., pp. 168–169). St. Louis: Saunders.
Lehne, R. (2013). *Pharmacology for nursing care* (8th ed., p. 1190). St. Louis: Saunders.

PRACTICE QUESTIONS

436. The nurse is caring for a client who is receiving an intravenous (IV) infusion of an antineoplastic medication. During the infusion, the client complains of pain at the insertion site. During an inspection of the site, the nurse notes redness and swelling. The nurse should take which appropriate action?
1. Notify the registered nurse.
2. Administer pain medication to reduce the discomfort.
3. Apply ice and maintain the infusion rate, as prescribed.
4. Elevate the extremity of the IV site, and slow the infusion.

437. The client with squamous cell carcinoma of the larynx is receiving bleomycin intravenously. The nurse caring for the client anticipates that which diagnostic study will be prescribed?
1. Echocardiography
2. Electrocardiography
3. Cervical radiography
4. Pulmonary function studies

438. The client with acute myelocytic leukemia is being treated with busulfan (Myleran). Which laboratory value should the nurse specifically monitor during treatment with this medication?
1. Clotting time
2. Uric acid level
3. Potassium level
4. Blood glucose level

❖ **439.** The nurse is assisting with caring for a client with cancer who is receiving cisplatin. Which adverse effects are associated with this medication? **Select all that apply.**
❑ **1.** Tinnitus
❑ **2.** Ototoxicity
❑ **3.** Hyperkalemia
❑ **4.** Hypercalcemia
❑ **5.** Nephrotoxicity
❑ **6.** Hypomagnesemia

440. The licensed practical nurse (LPN) is assisting the registered nurse (RN) to create a teaching plan for the client receiving an antineoplastic medication. The LPN expects which information to be included?
1. Take aspirin (acetylsalicylic acid) as needed for headache.
2. Drink beverages containing alcohol in moderate amounts each evening.
3. Consult with health care providers (HCPs) before receiving immunizations.
4. It is not necessary to consult HCPs before receiving a flu vaccine at the local health fair.

441. The client with ovarian cancer is being treated with vincristine (Vincasar). The nurse monitors the client, knowing that which adverse effect is specific to this medication?
1. Diarrhea
2. Hair loss
3. Chest pain
4. Extremity numbness

442. The nurse is reviewing the history and physical examination of a client who will be receiving asparaginase (Elspar), an antineoplastic agent. The nurse consults with the registered nurse regarding the administration of the medication if which is documented in the client's history?
1. Pancreatitis
2. Diabetes mellitus
3. Myocardial infarction
4. Chronic obstructive pulmonary disease

443. Tamoxifen (Soltamox) is prescribed for the client with metastatic breast carcinoma. The nurse understands that which is the **primary** action of this medication?

1. Increase DNA and RNA synthesis.
2. Promote the biosynthesis of nucleic acids.
3. Increase estrogen concentration and estrogen response.
4. Compete with estradiol for binding to estrogen in tissues containing high concentrations of receptors.

444. The client with metastatic breast cancer is receiving tamoxifen (Soltamox). The nurse specifically monitors which laboratory value while the client is taking this medication?
1. Glucose level
2. Calcium level
3. Potassium level
4. Prothrombin time

445. The client with small cell lung cancer is being treated with etoposide (Toposar). The nurse assisting in caring for the client during its administration should understand that which side/adverse effect is specifically associated with this medication?
1. Alopecia
2. Chest pain
3. Pulmonary fibrosis
4. Orthostatic hypotension

ANSWERS

436. 1

Rationale: When antineoplastic medications are administered via IV, great care must be taken to prevent the medication from escaping into the tissues surrounding the injection site because pain, tissue damage, and necrosis can result. The nurse monitors for signs of extravasation, such as redness or swelling at the insertion site. If extravasation occurs, the registered nurse needs to be notified; he or she will then contact the health care provider.
Test-Taking Strategy: Focus on the subject, chemotherapy and extravasation. Note the given information about the insertion site. Think about the definition of extravasation; this will assist to eliminate options 2, 3, and 4 as inappropriate nursing actions. **Review: chemotherapy, extravasation.**
Level of Cognitive Ability: Applying
Client Needs: Physiological Integrity
Integrated Process: Nursing Process/Implementation
Content Area: Pharmacology: Oncology Medications
Priority Concepts: Cellular Regulation, Tissue Integrity
Reference(s): deWit, Kumagai (2013), p. 54.

437. 4

Rationale: Bleomycin is an antineoplastic medication that can cause interstitial pneumonitis, which can progress to pulmonary fibrosis. Pulmonary function studies along with hematological, hepatic, and renal function tests need to be monitored. The nurse needs to monitor lung sounds for dyspnea and adventitious sounds, which could indicate pulmonary toxicity. The medication needs to be discontinued immediately if pulmonary toxicity occurs. Options 1, 2, and 3 are unrelated to the specific use of this medication.
Test-Taking Strategy: Focus on the subject, considerations when administering the medication bleomycin. Eliminate options 1 and 2 first because they are cardiac-related and are therefore comparable or alike. From the remaining options, use the ABCs—airway, breathing, and circulation—to direct you to the correct option. **Review: bleomycin.**
Level of Cognitive Ability: Analyzing
Client Needs: Physiological Integrity
Integrated Process: Nursing Process/Planning
Content Area: Pharmacology: Oncology Medications
Priority Concepts: Cellular Regulation, Gas Exchange
Reference(s): Hodgson, Kizior (2014), pp. 139–141.

438. 2

Rationale: Busulfan (Myleran) can cause an increase in the uric acid level. Hyperuricemia can produce uric acid nephropathy, renal stones, and acute kidney injury. Options 1, 3, and 4 are not specifically related to this medication.
Test-Taking Strategy: Focus on the subject, the laboratory value to monitor for busulfan. It is necessary to know the adverse effects associated with this medication. Recalling that busulfan increases the uric acid level will direct you to the correct option. **Review: busulfan.**
Level of Cognitive Ability: Analyzing
Client Needs: Physiological Integrity
Integrated Process: Nursing Process/Data Collection
Content Area: Pharmacology: Oncology Medications
Priority Concepts: Cellular Regulation, Safety
Reference(s): Hodgson, Kizior (2014), p. 163.

❖ **439. 1, 2, 5, 6**

Rationale: Cisplatin is an alkylating medication. Alkylating medications are cell cycle phase-nonspecific medications that affect the synthesis of DNA by causing the cross-linking of DNA to inhibit cell reproduction. Cisplatin may cause ototoxicity, tinnitus, hypokalemia, hypocalcemia, hypomagnesemia, and nephrotoxicity. Amifostine (Ethyol) may be administered before cisplatin to reduce the potential for renal toxicity.
Test-Taking Strategy: Note the subject, the adverse effects of cisplatin. Recall that most antineoplastic medications affect the bone marrow and the hematological system. This concept will assist you with determining that *hypo-* rather than *hyper-* conditions would occur. In addition, recall that this medication affects the ears (ototoxicity and tinnitus) and the kidneys (nephrotoxicity). **Review: cisplatin.**
Level of Cognitive Ability: Analyzing
Client Needs: Physiological Integrity
Integrated Process: Nursing Process/Data Collection
Content Area: Pharmacology: Oncology Medications
Priority Concepts: Cellular Regulation, Clinical Judgment
Reference(s): Hodgson, Kizior (2014), p. 250.

440. *Answer:* 3

Rationale: Because antineoplastic medications lower the immune response of the body, clients must be informed not to receive immunizations without a HCP's approval. Clients also need to avoid contact with individuals who have recently

received a live virus vaccine. Clients need to avoid aspirin and aspirin-containing products to minimize the risk of bleeding, and they need to avoid alcohol to minimize the risk of toxicity and side effects.
Test-Taking Strategy: Focus on the subject, a plan of care for the client receiving an antineoplastic medication. Recalling that antineoplastic medications lower the immune response of the body will direct you to the correct option. **Review: antineoplastic medications.**
Level of Cognitive Ability: Applying
Client Needs: Physiological Integrity
Integrated Process: Nursing Process: Planning
Content Area: Pharmacology: Oncology Medications
Priority Concepts: Cellular Regulation, Immunity
Reference(s): Lilley et al (2014), p. 800.

441. 4
Rationale: An adverse effect specific to vincristine is peripheral neuropathy. Peripheral neuropathy can be manifested as numbness and tingling in the fingers and toes. Depression of the Achilles tendon reflex may be the first clinical sign indicating peripheral neuropathy. Constipation, rather than diarrhea, is most likely to occur with this medication, although diarrhea may occur occasionally. Hair loss occurs with nearly all the antineoplastic medications. Chest pain is unrelated to this medication.
Test-Taking Strategy: Focus on the subject, an adverse effect of vincristine. Eliminate options 1 and 2 first because these effects are associated with many of the antineoplastic agents. Note that the question asks for the adverse effect specific to this medication. Correlate peripheral neuropathy with vincristine. **Review: vincristine.**
Level of Cognitive Ability: Analyzing
Client Needs: Physiological Integrity
Integrated Process: Nursing Process/Data Collection
Content Area: Pharmacology: Oncology Medications
Priority Concepts: Cellular Regulation, Clinical Judgment
Reference(s): Lehne (2013), pp. 1283–1284.

442. 1
Rationale: Asparaginase (Elspar) is contraindicated if hypersensitivity exists, in pancreatitis, or if the client has a history of pancreatitis. The medication impairs pancreatic function, and pancreatic function tests should be performed before therapy begins and when a week or more has elapsed between administration of the doses. The client needs to be monitored for signs of pancreatitis, which include nausea, vomiting, and abdominal pain. The conditions noted in options 2, 3, and 4 are not contraindicated with this medication.
Test-Taking Strategy: Focus on the subject, a contraindication for asparaginase. It is necessary to know the contraindications associated with this medication. Recalling that this medication affects pancreatic function will direct you to the correct option. **Review: asparaginase (Elspar).**
Level of Cognitive Ability: Analyzing
Client Needs: Physiological Integrity
Integrated Process: Nursing Process/Data Collection
Content Area: Pharmacology: Oncology Medications
Priority Concepts: Cellular Regulation, Clinical Judgment
Reference(s): Hodgson, Kizior (2014), pp. 81–83; Lehne (2013), p. 1286.

443. 4
Rationale: Tamoxifen (Soltamox) is an antineoplastic medication that competes with estradiol for binding to estrogen in tissues containing high concentrations of receptors. Tamoxifen reduces DNA synthesis and estrogen response.
Test-Taking Strategy: Note the strategic word, *primary*, and focus on the subject, the action of tamoxifen. Eliminate options 1 and 2 first because they are comparable or alike. Nucleic acids include DNA and RNA. Eliminate option 3 because it is unlikely that treatment of metastatic breast carcinoma would focus on increasing estrogen concentration and estrogen response. **Review: tamoxifen.**
Level of Cognitive Ability: Understanding
Client Needs: Physiological Integrity
Integrated Process: Nursing Process/Implementation
Content Area: Pharmacology: Oncology Medications
Priority Concepts: Cellular Regulation, Clinical Judgment
Reference(s): Hodgson, Kizior (2014), pp. 1122–1123; Lehne (2013), p. 771.

444. 2
Rationale: Tamoxifen may increase calcium, cholesterol, and triglyceride levels. Before the initiation of therapy, a complete blood count, platelet count, and serum calcium levels should be assessed. These blood levels, along with cholesterol and triglyceride levels, should be monitored periodically during therapy. The nurse should assess for hypercalcemia while the client is taking this medication. Signs of hypercalcemia include increased urine volume, excessive thirst, nausea, vomiting, constipation, hypotonicity of muscles, and deep bone and flank pain.
Test-Taking Strategy: Focus on the subject, the laboratory value to monitor for tamoxifen. It is necessary to know the adverse effects associated with this medication. Recalling that this medication causes hypercalcemia will direct you to the correct option. **Review: tamoxifen.**
Level of Cognitive Ability: Analyzing
Client Needs: Physiological Integrity
Integrated Process: Nursing Process/Data Collection
Content Area: Pharmacology: Oncology Medications
Priority Concepts: Cellular Regulation, Clinical Judgment
Reference(s): Skidmore-Roth (2014), p. 1129.

445. 4
Rationale: A side effect specific to etoposide (Toposar) is orthostatic hypotension. The client's blood pressure is monitored during the infusion. Hair loss occurs with nearly all the antineoplastic medications. Chest pain and pulmonary fibrosis are unrelated to this medication.
Test-Taking Strategy: Focus on the subject, a side/adverse effect of etoposide. Eliminate option 1 first because this side effect is associated with many of the antineoplastic agents. Eliminate options 2 and 3 next because they are unrelated to etoposide. Note that the question asks for the side/adverse effect specific to this medication. Correlate hypotension with etoposide. **Review: etoposide.**
Level of Cognitive Ability: Analyzing
Client Needs: Physiological Integrity
Integrated Process: Nursing Process/Data Collection
Content Area: Pharmacology: Oncology Medications
Priority Concepts: Cellular Regulation, Clinical Judgment
Reference(s): Lehne (2013), p. 1286.

UNIT X

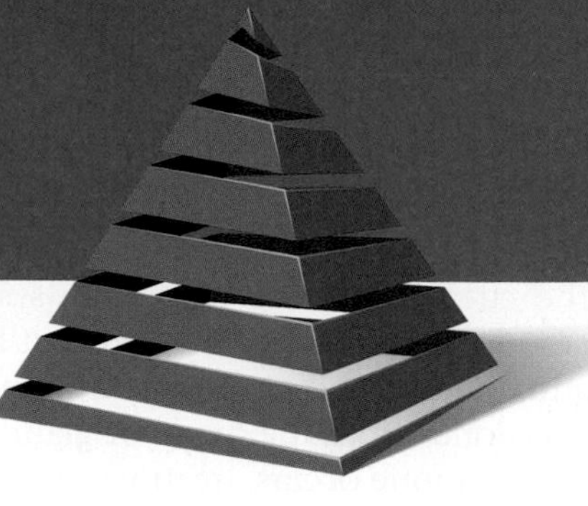

The Adult Client with an Endocrine Disorder

PYRAMID TERMS

addisonian crisis A life-threatening disorder caused by adrenal hormone insufficiency. Crisis is precipitated by infection, trauma, stress, or surgery. Death can occur from shock, vascular collapse, or hyperkalemia.

Addison's disease The hyposecretion of adrenal cortex hormones (glucocorticoids and mineralocorticoids) from the adrenal gland that results in a deficiency of the corticosteroid hormones. The condition is fatal if left untreated.

adrenalectomy The surgical removal of an adrenal gland. Lifelong replacement of glucocorticoids and mineralocorticoids is necessary with a bilateral adrenalectomy. Temporary replacement may be necessary for up to 2 years for a unilateral adrenalectomy.

Chvostek's sign A sign of hypocalcemia. A spasm of the facial muscles elicited by tapping the facial nerve just anterior to the ear.

Cushing's disease A metabolic disorder characterized by abnormally increased secretion (endogenous) of cortisol, caused by increased amounts of adrenoorticotropic hormone (ACTH) secreted by the pituitary gland.

Cushing's syndrome A metabolic disorder resulting from the chronic and excessive production of cortisol by the adrenal cortex or by the administration of glucocorticoids in large doses for several weeks or longer (exogenous or iatrogenic).

dawn phenomenon A nocturnal release of growth hormone, which may cause blood glucose level elevations before breakfast in the client with diabetes mellitus. Treatment includes administering an evening dose of intermediate-acting insulin at 10:00 PM.

diabetes insipidus The hyposecretion of antidiuretic hormone from the posterior pituitary gland, resulting in failure of the tubular reabsorption of water in the kidneys and diuresis.

diabetes mellitus A chronic disorder of glucose intolerance and impaired carbohydrate, protein, and lipid metabolism caused by a deficiency of insulin or resistance to the action of insulin. A deficiency of effective insulin results in hyperglycemia.

diabetic ketoacidosis A life-threatening complication of diabetes mellitus that develops when a severe insulin deficiency occurs. Hyperglycemia progresses to ketoacidosis over a period of several hours to several days. Acidosis occurs in clients with type 1 diabetes mellitus, persons with undiagnosed diabetes, and persons who stop prescribed treatment for diabetes.

hyperglycemia Elevated blood glucose as a result of too little insulin or the inability of the body to use insulin properly.

Hyperosmolar hyperglycemic syndrome (HHS) Extreme hyperglycemia without acidosis. A complication of type 2 diabetes mellitus, which may result in dehydration or vascular collapse. Onset is usually slow, taking from hours to days.

hyperthyroidism A condition that occurs as a result of excessive thyroid hormone secretion.

hypoglycemia Low blood glucose level that results from too much insulin, not enough food, or excess activity.

hypothyroidism A hypothyroid state resulting from a hyposecretion of thyroid hormone.

myxedema coma A rare but serious disorder that results from the persistently low thyroid production. Coma can be precipitated by acute illness, rapid withdrawal of thyroid medication, anesthesia and surgery, hypothermia, and the use of sedatives and opioid analgesics.

Somogyi phenomenon A rebound phenomenon that occurs in clients with type 1 diabetes mellitus. Normal or elevated blood glucose levels are present at bedtime; hypoglycemia occurs at about 2:00 to 3:00 AM. Counterregulatory hormones, produced to prevent further hypoglycemia, result in hyperglycemia (evident in the prebreakfast blood glucose level). Treatment includes decreasing the evening (predinner or bedtime) dose of intermediate-acting insulin or increasing the bedtime snack.

thyroidectomy Surgical removal of the thyroid gland to treat persistent hyperthyroidism or thyroid tumors.

thyroid storm An acute, potentially fatal exacerbation of hyperthyroidism that may result from manipulation of the thyroid gland during surgery, severe infection, or stress.

Trousseau's sign A sign of hypocalcemia. Carpal spasm can be elicited by compressing the brachial artery with a blood pressure cuff for 3 minutes.

Pyramid to Success

The endocrine system is made up of organs or glands that secrete hormones and release them directly into the circulation. The endocrine system can be understood easily if you remember that basically one of two situations can occur: hypersecretion or hyposecretion of hormones from the organ or gland. When an excess of the hormone occurs, treatment is aimed at blocking the hormone release through medication or surgery. When a deficit of the hormone exists, treatment is aimed at replacement therapy. Pyramid Points focus on diabetes mellitus, including its prevention, the prevention and treatment of complications, insulin therapy, hypoglycemic and hyperglycemic reactions, and diabetic ketoacidosis; Addison's disease and addisonian crisis; Cushing's disease or Cushing's syndrome; thyroid disorders and thyroid storm; and care of the client after thyroidectomy or adrenalectomy.

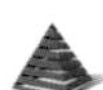

Client Needs

Safe and Effective Care Environment

Acting as a client advocate
Collaborating with the registered nurse (RN), multidisciplinary team, and appropriate care providers regarding treatment
Ensuring informed consent for treatments and procedures has been obtained
Establishing priorities of care based on the endocrine disorder
Handling hazardous and infectious materials
Maintaining confidentiality related to the disorder
Preventing accidents and client injury
Using medical and surgical asepsis to prevent infection

Health Promotion and Maintenance

Discussing expected body image changes
Identifying lifestyle choices related to treatment
Performing data collection techniques related to the endocrine system
Preventing disease
Providing health screening
Reinforcing teaching about self-care measures

Psychosocial Integrity

Discussing grief and loss issues related to complications of the disorder
Discussing situational role changes related to the disorder
Discussing unexpected body image changes
Identifying coping mechanisms
Monitoring for sensory and perceptual alterations as a result of the disorder
Using support systems

Physiological Integrity

Assisting the RN in providing emergency care to the client
Monitoring for alterations in body systems as a result of the disorder
Monitoring for complications from surgical procedures and health alterations
Monitoring for complications of diagnostic tests, treatments, and procedures
Monitoring for expected outcomes and effects of pharmacological therapy
Monitoring for fluid and electrolyte imbalances that can occur
Monitoring for unexpected responses to therapies
Monitoring laboratory values
Preparing the client for diagnostic tests
Providing nonpharmacological comfort interventions
Providing nutrition and oral hydration measures

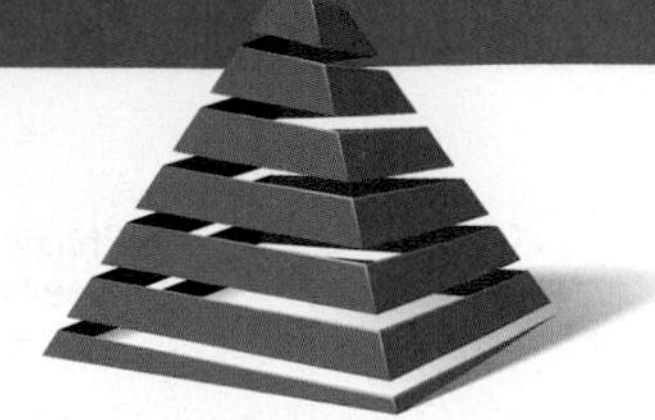

CHAPTER 45

Endocrine System

CRITICAL THINKING What Should You Do?

The nurse suspects that a client with pheochromocytoma is developing hypertensive crisis. What should the nurse do?

Answer located on p. 572.

BOX 45-1 Risk Factors for Endocrine Disorders

- Age
- Heredity
- Congenital factors
- Trauma
- Environmental factors
- Consequence of surgery or other disorders

I. Anatomy and Physiology of the Endocrine Glands

A. Functions
 1. Maintenance and regulation of vital functions
 2. Response to stress and injury
 3. Growth and development
 4. Energy metabolism
 5. Reproduction
 6. Fluid, electrolyte, and acid-base balance

B. Risk factors for endocrine disorders (Box 45-1)

C. Hypothalamus
 1. Portion of the diencephalon of the brain, forming the floor and part of the lateral wall of the third ventricle
 2. Activates, controls, and integrates the peripheral autonomic nervous system, endocrine processes, and many somatic functions, such as body temperature, sleep, and appetite

D. Pituitary gland (Fig. 45-1)

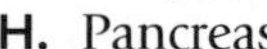

 1. The master gland; located at the base of the brain
 2. Influenced by the hypothalamus; directly affects the function of the other endocrine glands
 3. Promotes the growth of body tissue, influences water absorption by the kidney, and controls sexual development and function

E. Adrenal gland
 1. One adrenal gland is on top of each kidney.
 2. Regulates sodium and electrolyte balance; affects carbohydrate, fat, and protein metabolism; influences the development of sexual characteristics; and sustains the "fight-or-flight" response
 3. Adrenal cortex
  a. The cortex is the outer shell of the adrenal gland.
  b. The cortex synthesizes glucocorticoids and mineralocorticoids and secretes small amounts of sex hormones (androgens, estrogens).
 4. Adrenal medulla
  a. The medulla is the inner core of the adrenal gland.
  b. The medulla works as part of the sympathetic nervous system and produces epinephrine and norepinephrine.

F. Thyroid gland
 1. Located in the anterior part of the neck
 2. Controls the rate of body metabolism and growth and produces thyroxine (T_4), triiodothyronine (T_3), and thyrocalcitonin

G. Parathyroid glands
 1. Located on the thyroid gland
 2. Control calcium and phosphorus metabolism; produce parathyroid hormone 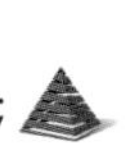

H. Pancreas
 1. Located posteriorly to the stomach
 2. Influences carbohydrate metabolism, indirectly influences fat and protein metabolism, and produces insulin and glucagon

I. Ovaries and testes
 1. The ovaries are located in the pelvic cavity and produce estrogen and progesterone.
 2. The testes are located in the scrotum, control the development of the secondary sex characteristics, and produce testosterone.

J. Negative feedback loop
 1. Regulates hormone secretion by the hypothalamus and pituitary gland
 2. Increased amounts of target gland hormones in the bloodstream decrease secretion of the same hormone and other hormones that stimulate its release.

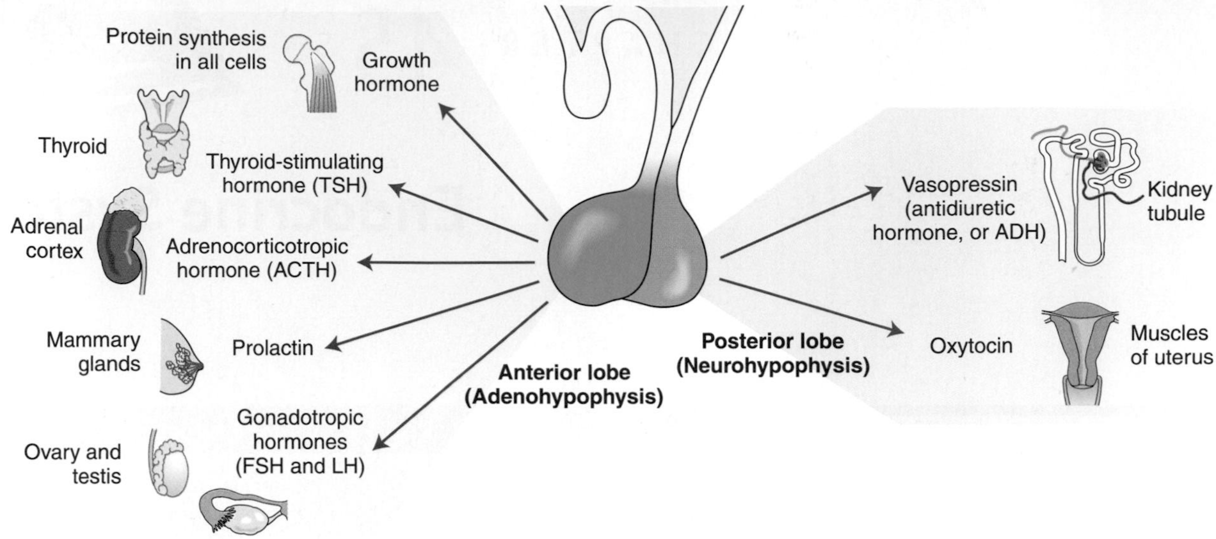

FIGURE 45-1 Pituitary hormones. *FSH*, Follicle-stimulating hormone; *LH*, luteinizing hormone. (From Lilley L, Harrington S, Snyder J: *Pharmacology and the nursing process*, ed 5, St. Louis, 2008, Mosby.)

II. Diagnostic Tests

A. Stimulation and suppression tests

1. Stimulation testing
   a. In the client with suspected underactivity of an endocrine gland, a stimulus may be provided to determine whether the gland is capable of normal hormone production.
   b. Measured amounts of selected hormones or substances are administered to stimulate the target gland to produce its hormone.
   c. Hormone levels produced by the target gland are measured.
   d. Failure of the hormone level to increase with stimulation indicates hypofunction.
2. Suppression tests
   a. Suppression tests are used when hormone levels are high or in the upper range of normal.
   b. Agents that normally induce a suppressed response are administered to determine whether normal negative feedback is intact.
   c. Failure of hormone production to be suppressed during standardized testing indicates hyperfunction.

B. Radioactive iodine uptake

1. This thyroid function test measures the absorption of an iodine isotope to determine how the thyroid gland is functioning.
2. A small dose of radioactive iodine is given by mouth or intravenously; the amount of radioactivity is measured in 2 to 4 hours and again at 24 hours.
3. Normal values are 3% to 10% at 2 to 4 hours and 5% to 30% at 24 hours.
4. Elevated values indicate **hyperthyroidism**, decreased iodine intake, or increased iodine excretion.
5. Decreased values indicate a low T_4 level, the use of antithyroid medications, thyroiditis, myxedema, or **hypothyroidism**.
6. The test is contraindicated during pregnancy.

C. T_3 and T_4 resin uptake test

1. Blood tests are used to diagnose thyroid disorders.
2. T_3 and T_4 regulate thyroid-stimulating hormone.
3. Normal values (normal findings vary among laboratory settings)
   a. T_3: 80 to 230 ng/dL
   b. T_4: 5 to 12 mcg/dL
   c. Thyroxine, free (FT_4): 0.8 to 2.4 ng/dL
4. The T_3 level is elevated in hyperthyroidism, decreases with the aging process, and may be decreased in hypothyroidism.
5. The T_4 level is elevated in hyperthyroidism and decreased in hypothyroidism.

D. Thyroid-stimulating hormone

1. Blood test is used to differentiate the diagnosis of primary hypothyroidism.
2. Normal value is 0.2 to 5.4 microunits/mL (normal findings vary among laboratory settings).
3. Elevated values indicate primary hypothyroidism.
4. Decreased values indicate hyperthyroidism or secondary hypothyroidism.

E. Thyroid scan

1. A thyroid scan is performed to identify nodules or growths in the thyroid gland.
2. A radioisotope of iodine or technetium is administered before scanning the thyroid gland.
3. Reassure the client that the level of radioactive medication is not dangerous to self or others.
4. Determine whether the client has received radiographic contrast agents within the past 3 months, because these may invalidate the scan.

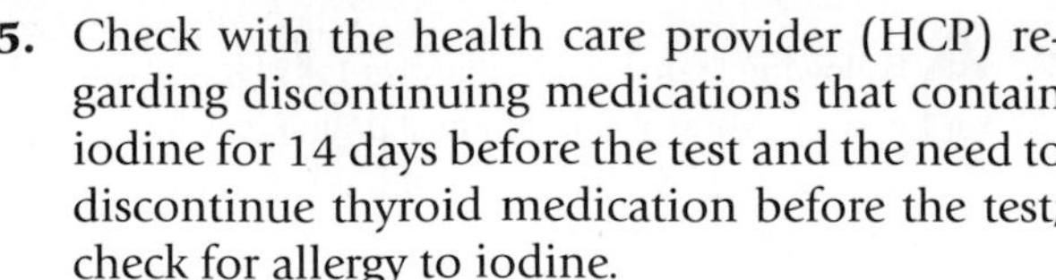

5. Check with the health care provider (HCP) regarding discontinuing medications that contain iodine for 14 days before the test and the need to discontinue thyroid medication before the test; check for allergy to iodine.
6. Reinforce instructions to the client to maintain NPO status after midnight on the day before the test; if iodine is used, the client will fast for an additional 45 minutes after the ingestion of the oral isotope, and the scan will be performed in 24 hours.
7. If technetium is used, it is administered by the IV route 30 minutes before the scan.
8. The test is contraindicated during pregnancy and in those with an iodine allergy.

F. Needle aspiration of thyroid tissue
   1. Aspiration of thyroid tissue is done for cytological examination.
   2. No client preparation is necessary.
   3. Light pressure is applied to the aspiration site after the procedure.

G. Glucose tolerance test
   1. The glucose tolerance test aids in the diagnosis of **diabetes mellitus**.
   2. A 2-hour postload glucose level (2 hours after the injection or ingestion of glucose) greater than 200 mg/dL confirms the diagnosis of diabetes mellitus.
   3. Client preparation (Box 45-2)
   4. Many factors can alter the results, and therefore it is not always a reliable test.

H. Glycosylated hemoglobin
   1. Description
      a. Glycosylated hemoglobin is blood glucose bound to hemoglobin.
      b. Glycosylated hemoglobin A (HbA_{1c}) is a reflection of how well the blood glucose levels have been controlled for the prior 3 to 4 months.

Hyperglycemia in a client with diabetes mellitus is usually the cause of an increase in the HbA_{1c} value.

BOX 45-2 Client Preparation: Glucose Tolerance Test

Eat a diet with at least 150 g of carbohydrates for 3 days before the test.
Avoid alcohol, coffee, and smoking for 36 hours before testing.
Fast for 10 to 12 hours before the test.
Avoid strenuous exercise for 8 hours before and after the test.
Withhold morning insulin or oral hypoglycemic medication (client with diabetes mellitus).
A sample is drawn for determination of the fasting blood glucose level, and then the client will be given a high-glucose drink.
Blood samples will be drawn at 30-minute intervals for a minimum of 2 hours.

   2. Values
      a. Values are expressed as a percentage of the total hemoglobin.
      b. The goal for clients with diabetes mellitus is 7% or lower.
      c. For clients without diabetes mellitus, the normal range is 4.5% to 6%.
   3. Nursing consideration: Fasting is not required.

III. Pituitary Gland Disorders

A. Hypopituitarism
   1. Description: Hyposecretion of one or more of the pituitary hormones caused by tumors, trauma, encephalitis, autoimmunity, or stroke
   2. Hormones most often affected are growth hormone (GH) and the gonadotropins (luteinizing hormone, follicle-stimulating hormone), but thyroid-stimulating hormone (TSH), adrenocorticotropic hormone (ACTH), or antidiuretic hormone (ADH) may be involved.
   3. Data collection
      a. Mild to moderate obesity (GH, TSH)
      b. Reduced cardiac output (GH, ADH)
      c. Infertility and sexual dysfunction (gonadotropins, ACTH)
      d. Fatigue, low blood pressure (TSH, ADH, ACTH, GH)
      e. Tumors of the pituitary also may cause headaches and visual defects (pituitary is located near the optic nerve).
   4. Interventions
      a. Provide emotional support to the client and family.
      b. Encourage the client and family to express feelings related to disturbed body image or sexual dysfunction.
      c. Client may need hormone replacement for specific deficient hormones.
      d. Client education is needed regarding the signs and symptoms of both hypofunction and hyperfunction related to insufficient or excess hormone replacement.

B. Hyperpituitarism
   1. Description
      a. Hypersecretion of growth hormone by the anterior pituitary gland in an adult; caused primarily by pituitary tumors.
      b. Leads to conditions such as acromegaly and **Cushing's disease**
   2. Data collection 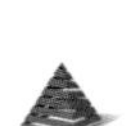
      a. Large hands and feet
      b. Thickening and protrusion of the jaw
      c. Arthritic changes and joint pain
      d. Visual disturbances
      e. Diaphoresis
      f. Oily, rough skin

g. Organomegaly
h. Hypertension
i. Dysphagia
j. Deepening of the voice

3. Interventions
   a. Provide emotional support to the client and family, and encourage the client and family to express feelings related to disturbed body image.
   b. Provide frequent skin care.
   c. Provide pharmacological and nonpharmacological interventions for joint pain.
   d. Prepare the client for radiation of the pituitary gland if prescribed.
   e. Prepare the client for hypophysectomy if planned.

C. Hypophysectomy (pituitary adenectomy, transsphenoidal pituitary surgery)
1. Description
   a. The removal of the pituitary tumor via craniotomy or via transsphenoidal (endoscopic transnasal) approach (the latter approach is preferred because it is associated with fewer complications).
   b. Complications for craniotomy include increased intracranial pressure, bleeding, meningitis, and hypopituitarism.
   c. Complications for the transsphenoidal surgery include cerebrospinal fluid leak, infection, and hypopituitarism.
2. Postoperative interventions
   a. Initiate postoperative care similar to craniotomy care.
   b. Monitor the vital signs, neurological status, and level of consciousness.
   c. Elevate the head of the bed.
   d. Monitor for increased intracranial pressure.
   e. Monitor for bleeding.

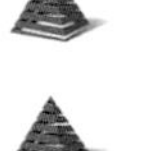

   f. Reinforce instructions to the client to avoid sneezing, coughing, and blowing the nose.
   g. Monitor for signs of temporary diabetes insipidus or syndrome of inappropriate ADH resulting from ADH disturbances.
   h. Monitor the intake and output and avoid water intoxication.
   i. Administer glucocorticoids and other hormone replacements as prescribed.
   j. Administer antibiotics, analgesics, and antipyretics as prescribed.
   k. Reinforce instructions to the client regarding the administration of prescribed medications.
   l. Administer oral mouth rinse as prescribed.
   m. As prescribed, reinforce instructions to the client to brush teeth gently with an ultrasoft toothbrush for at least 2 weeks following surgery (http://www.cc.nih.gov/ccc/patient_education/pepubs/transsphenoidal.pdf).

Following transsphenoidal hypophysectomy, monitor for any postnasal drip or nasal drainage, which might indicate leakage of cerebrospinal fluid (CSF) (check the nasal drainage for glucose; if the drainage is positive for glucose, it is likely CSF).

D. Diabetes insipidus
1. Description
   a. Hyposecretion of ADH caused by stroke or trauma, or may be idiopathic
   b. The kidney tubules fail to reabsorb water.
2. Data collection
   a. Excretion of large amounts of dilute urine
   b. Polydipsia
   c. Dehydration (decreased skin turgor and dry mucous membranes)
   d. Inability to concentrate urine
   e. A low urinary specific gravity, 1.006 or lower
   f. Fatigue
   g. Muscle pain and weakness
   h. Headache
   i. Postural hypotension that may progress to vascular collapse without rehydration
   j. Tachycardia
3. Interventions
   a. Monitor vital signs and neurological and cardiovascular status.
   b. Provide a safe environment, particularly for the client with postural hypotension.

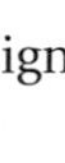

   c. Monitor the electrolyte values and for signs of dehydration.
   d. Maintain client intake of adequate fluids.
   e. Monitor intake and output, weight, serum osmolality, and specific gravity of urine.
   f. Reinforce instructions to the client to avoid foods or liquids that produce diuresis.
   g. Vasopressin tannate (Pitressin) or desmopressin acetate (DDAVP, Stimate) may be prescribed; these are used when the ADH deficiency is severe or chronic.
   h. Reinforce instructions to the client regarding the administration of medications as prescribed; DDAVP may be administered by injection, intranasally, or orally.
   i. Reinforce instructions to the client to wear a Medic-Alert bracelet.

E. Syndrome of inappropriate antidiuretic hormone secretion (SIADH)
1. Description
   a. Excess ADH is released, but not in response to the body's need for it.
   b. Causes include trauma, stroke, malignancies (often in the lungs or pancreas), medications, and stress.
   c. The syndrome results in water intoxication and hyponatremia.

2. Data collection
   a. Signs of fluid volume overload
   b. Changes in the level of consciousness and mental status changes
   c. Weight gain
   d. Hypertension
   e. Tachycardia
   f. Anorexia, nausea, and vomiting
   g. Hyponatremia
3. Interventions
   a. Monitor the vital signs and cardiac and neurological status.
   b. Provide a safe environment, particularly for the client with changes in the level of consciousness or mental status.
   c. Monitor intake and output and obtain weight daily.
   d. Monitor fluid and electrolyte balance.
   e. Monitor the serum and urine osmolality.
   f. Restrict fluid intake as prescribed.
   g. Administer diuretics and IV fluids (usually normal saline or hypertonic saline); monitor IV fluids carefully because of the risk for fluid volume overload. (IV solutions containing water are contraindicated because of the risk of water intoxication).
   h. Medications that inhibit ADH-induced water reabsorption and produce water diuresis may be prescribed.

IV. Adrenal Gland Disorders

A. Addison's disease
1. Description
   a. Hyposecretion of adrenal cortex hormones (glucocorticoids and mineralocorticoids)
   b. Can be primary or secondary.
   c. The condition is fatal if left untreated.
2. Data collection (Table 45-1)
3. Interventions
   a. Monitor vital signs, particularly blood pressure, weight, and intake and output.
   b. Monitor white blood cell (WBC) count; blood glucose; and potassium, sodium, and calcium levels.
   c. Administer glucocorticoid or mineralocorticoid medications as prescribed.

   d. Observe for addisonian crisis caused by stress, infection, trauma, or surgery.

4. Client education
   a. Avoid individuals with infections.
   b. Diet: High protein and carbohydrate intake; normal sodium intake
   c. Avoid strenuous exercise and stressful situations.
   d. Need for lifelong glucocorticoid therapy
   e. Avoid over-the-counter medications.
   f. Wear a Medic-Alert bracelet.

TABLE 45-1 Data Collection: Addison's Disease and Cushing's Disease (Cushing's Syndrome)

Addison's Disease	Cushing's Disease and Syndrome
Lethargy, fatigue, and muscle weakness	Generalized muscle wasting and weakness
Gastrointestinal disturbances	Moon face, buffalo hump
Weight loss	Truncal obesity with thin extremities, supraclavicular fat pads; weight gain
Menstrual changes in women; impotence in men	Hirsutism (masculine characteristics in females)
Hypoglycemia, hyponatremia	Hyperglycemia, hypernatremia
Hyperkalemia, hypercalcemia	Hypokalemia, hypocalcemia
Postural hypotension	Hypertension
Hyperpigmentation of the skin (bronzed) with primary disease	Fragile skin that easily bruises; reddish-purple striae on the abdomen and upper thighs

BOX 45-3 Addisonian Crisis

- A life-threatening disorder caused by acute adrenal insufficiency
- Precipitated by stress, infection, trauma, surgery, or abrupt withdrawal of exogenous corticosteroid use
- Can cause hyponatremia, hyperkalemia, hypoglycemia, and shock

   g. Signs and symptoms of complications such as underreplacement and overreplacement of hormones

B. Addisonian crisis
1. Description (Box 45-3)
2. Data collection 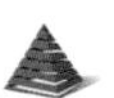
   a. Severe headache
   b. Severe abdominal, leg, and lower back pain
   c. Generalized weakness
   d. Irritability and confusion
   e. Severe hypotension
   f. Shock
3. Interventions
   a. Prepare to assist the RN to administer glucocorticoids intravenously as prescribed; hydrocortisone sodium succinate (Solu-Cortef) usually is prescribed initially.
   b. Following resolution of the crisis, administer glucocorticoids and mineralocorticoids orally as prescribed.
   c. Monitor the vital signs, particularly blood pressure.
   d. Monitor the neurological status, noting irritability and confusion.

e. Monitor intake and output.
f. Monitor the laboratory values, particularly the sodium, potassium, and blood glucose levels.
g. Monitor IV fluids as prescribed to restore electrolyte balance.
h. Protect the client from infection.
i. Maintain bed rest and provide a quiet environment.

Addison's disease is characterized by the hyposecretion of adrenal cortex hormones (glucocorticoids and mineralocorticoids), whereas Cushing's disease is characterized by a hypersecretion of glucocorticoids.

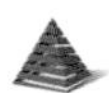

C. **Cushing's disease** and **Cushing's syndrome** (hypercortisolism)
1. Description
a. Characterized by a hypersecretion of glucocorticoids from the adrenal cortex
b. Cushing's disease is a metabolic disorder characterized by the abnormally increased secretion (endogenous) of cortisol, caused by increased amounts of ACTH secreted by the pituitary gland.
c. Cushing's syndrome is a metabolic disorder that results from the chronic and excessive production of cortisol by the adrenal cortex or from the administration of glucocorticoids in large doses for several weeks or longer (exogenous or iatrogenic).

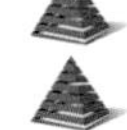

2. Data collection (Table 45-1)
3. Interventions
a. Monitor vital signs, particularly blood pressure.
b. Monitor intake and output, and weight.
c. Monitor laboratory values, particularly the white blood cell count, and serum glucose, sodium, potassium, and calcium levels.
d. Provide meticulous skin care.
e. Allow the client to discuss feelings related to body appearance.
f. Administer chemotherapeutic agents as prescribed for inoperable adrenal tumors.
g. Prepare the client for radiation as prescribed if the condition results from a pituitary adenoma.
h. Prepare the client for the removal of pituitary tumor (hypophysectomy, transsphenoidal adenectomy) if the condition results from the increased pituitary secretion of ACTH.
i. Prepare the client for adrenalectomy if the condition results from an adrenal ademona; glucocorticoid replacement may be required following adrenalectomy.

D. Primary hyperaldosteronism (Conn's syndrome)
1. Description
a. A hypersecretion of mineralocorticoids (aldosterone) from the adrenal cortex of the adrenal gland
b. Most commonly caused by an adenoma
2. Data collection
a. Symptoms related to hypokalemia, hypernatremia, and hypertension
b. Headache, fatigue, muscle weakness, and nocturia
c. Polydipsia and polyuria
d. Paresthesias
e. Visual changes
f. Low urine specific gravity and increased urinary aldosterone level
g. Elevated serum aldosterone levels
3. Interventions
a. Monitor the vital signs, particularly blood pressure.
b. Monitor for signs of hypokalemia and hypernatremia.
c. Monitor intake and output and urine for specific gravity.
d. Spironolactone (Aldactone) may be prescribed to promote fluid balance and to control hypertension; this is a potassium-retaining diuretic and an aldosterone antagonist, and the clients need to be monitored for hyperkalemia, particularly in the presence of impaired renal function or excessive potassium intake.
e. Administer potassium supplements as prescribed.
f. Prepare the client for adrenalectomy.
g. Maintain sodium restriction, if prescribed, preoperatively.
h. Administer glucocorticoids preoperatively as prescribed to prevent adrenal hypofunction.
i. Monitor the client for adrenal insufficiency postoperatively.
j. Reinforce instructions to the client regarding the need for glucocorticoid therapy after adrenalectomy.
k. Reinforce instructions to the client about the need to wear a Medic-Alert bracelet.

E. Pheochromocytoma
1. Description
a. Catecholamine-producing tumor that is usually found in the adrenal medulla, but extra-adrenal locations include the chest, bladder, abdomen, and brain; typically a benign tumor but can be malignant.
b. Excessive amounts of epinephrine and norepinephrine are secreted.
c. Diagnostic tests include a 24-hour urine collection for vanillylmandelic acid (VMA) (a product of catecholamine metabolism), metanephrine, and catecholamines, all of

which are elevated in the presence of pheochromocytoma; the normal range of urinary catecholamines is up to 14 mcg/100 mL of urine, with higher levels occurring in pheochromocytoma.
d. Surgical removal of the adrenal gland is the primary treatment.
e. Symptomatic treatment is initiated if surgical removal is not possible.
f. The complications associated with pheochromocytoma include hypertensive crisis, including hypertensive retinopathy and nephropathy, cardiac enlargement and dysrhythmias, heart failure, myocardial infarction, increased platelet aggregation, and stroke.
g. Death can occur from shock, stroke, renal failure, dysrhythmias, or dissecting aortic aneurysm.

2. Data collection
   a. Paroxysmal or sustained hypertension
   b. Severe headaches
   c. Palpitations
   d. Flushing and profuse diaphoresis
   e. Pain in the chest or abdomen with nausea and vomiting
   f. Heat intolerance
   g. Weight loss
   h. Tremors
   i. **Hyperglycemia**
3. Interventions
   a. Monitor vital signs, particularly the blood pressure and heart rate.
   b. Monitor for hypertensive crisis; monitor for complications that can occur with hypertensive crisis, such as stroke, cardiac dysrhythmias, myocardial infarction.
   c. Reinforce instructions to the client not to smoke, drink caffeine-containing beverages, or change position suddenly.
   d. Prepare to administer a β-adrenergic blocking agent as prescribed to control hypertension.
   e. Monitor serum glucose level.
   f. Promote rest and a nonstressful environment.
   g. Provide a diet high in calories, vitamins, and minerals.
   h. Prepare the client for adrenalectomy.

For the client with pheochromocytoma, avoid stimuli that can precipitate a hypertensive crisis, such as increased abdominal pressure and vigorous abdominal palpation.

F. Adrenalectomy
1. Description (Box 45-4)
2. Preoperative interventions
   a. Monitor electrolyte levels and correct electrolyte imbalances.

BOX 45-4 Adrenalectomy

Surgical removal of an adrenal gland
Lifelong glucocorticoid and mineralocorticoid replacement is necessary with bilateral adrenalectomy.
Temporary glucocorticoid replacement, usually up to 2 years, is necessary after a unilateral adrenalectomy.
Catecholamine levels drop as a result of surgery, which can result in cardiovascular collapse, hypotension, and shock, and the client needs to be monitored closely.
Hemorrhage also can occur because of the high vascularity of the adrenal glands.

   b. Monitor for dysrhythmias.
   c. Monitor for hyperglycemia.
   d. Protect the client from infections.
   e. Administer glucocorticoids as prescribed.
3. Postoperative interventions
   a. Monitor vital signs.
   b. Monitor intake and output; if the urinary output is less than 30 mL/hour, notify the RN because this may indicate kidney failure and impending shock.
   c. Monitor weight daily.
   d. Monitor electrolyte and serum glucose levels.
   e. Monitor for signs of hemorrhage and shock, particularly during the first 24 to 48 hours.
   f. Monitor for manifestations of adrenal insufficiency (see Table 45-1).
   g. Check the dressing for drainage.
   h. Monitor for paralytic ileus. IV fluids will be prescribed to maintain blood volume.
   i. Administer glucocorticoids and mineralocorticoids as prescribed.
   j. Administer pain medication as prescribed.
   k. Provide pulmonary interventions to prevent atelectasis (coughing, deep breathing, incentive spirometry, splinting of incision).
   l. Reinforce instructions to the client regarding the importance of hormone replacement therapy following surgery.
   m. Reinforce instructions to the client regarding the signs and symptoms of complications such as underreplacement and overreplacement of hormones.
   n. Reinforce instructions to the client regarding the need to wear a Medic-Alert bracelet.

V. Thyroid Gland Disorders
A. Hypothyroidism
1. Description
   a. Hypothyroid state resulting from the hyposecretion of the thyroid hormones T_3 and T_4
   b. Characterized by a decreased rate of body metabolism
2. Data collection (Table 45-2) 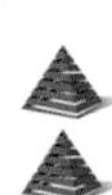
3. Interventions

a. Monitor vital signs, including heart rate and rhythm.
b. Administer thyroid replacement; levothyroxine sodium (Synthroid) is most commonly prescribed.
c. Reinforce instructions to the client about thyroid replacement therapy and about the clinical manifestations of both hypothyroidism and hyperthyroidism related to underreplacement or overreplacement of the hormone.
d. Reinforce instructions to the client to consume a low-calorie, low-cholesterol, and low-saturated fat diet.
e. Monitor the client for constipation; provide roughage and fluids to prevent constipation.
f. Provide a warm environment for the client.
g. Avoid sedatives and opioid analgesics because of increased sensitivity to these medications.
h. Monitor for overdose of thyroid medications, characterized by tachycardia, chest pain, restlessness, nervousness, and insomnia.

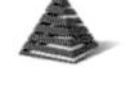

i. Reinforce instructions to the client to immediately report episodes of chest pain or other signs of overdose.

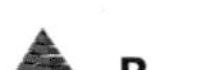

B. Myxedema coma

1. Description (Box 45-5)
2. Data collection
    a. Hypotension
    b. Bradycardia
    c. Hypothermia
    d. Hyponatremia
    e. **Hypoglycemia**
    f. Generalized edema
    g. Respiratory failure
    h. Coma
3. Interventions
    a. Maintain a patent airway.
    b. Institute aspiration precautions.
    c. Monitor IV fluids (normal or hypertonic saline) as prescribed.
    d. Assist RN to administer levothyroxine sodium (Synthroid) intravenously as prescribed.
    e. Assist RN to administer glucose intravenously as prescribed.
    f. Administer corticosteroids as prescribed.
    g. Monitor the client's temperature hourly.
    h. Monitor blood pressure frequently.
    i. Keep the client warm.

BOX 45-5 Myxedema Coma

This rare but serious disorder results from persistently low thyroid production.

Coma can be precipitated by acute illness, rapid withdrawal of thyroid medication, anesthesia and surgery, hypothermia, or the use of sedatives and opioid analgesics.

j. Monitor for changes in mental status.
k. Monitor electrolyte and glucose levels.

C. Hyperthyroidism

1. Description
    a. Hyperthyroid state resulting from the hypersecretion of thyroid hormones T_3 and T_4
    b. Characterized by an increased rate of body metabolism
    c. A common cause is Graves' disease, also known as toxic diffuse goiter.
    d. Clinical manifestations are referred to as *thyrotoxicosis*.
2. Data collection (Table 45-2)
3. Interventions
    a. Provide adequate rest.
    b. Administer sedatives as prescribed.
    c. Provide a cool and quiet environment.
    d. Obtain weight daily.
    e. Provide a high-calorie diet.
    f. Avoid the administration of stimulants.
    g. Administer antithyroid medications (propylthiouracil, PTU) that block thyroid synthesis as prescribed.
    h. Administer iodine preparations that inhibit the release of thyroid hormone as prescribed.

TABLE 45-2 Data Collection: Hypothyroidism and Hyperthyroidism

Hypothyroidism	Hyperthyroidism
Lethargy and fatigue	Personality changes such as irritability, agitation, and mood swings
Weakness, muscle aches, paresthesias	Nervousness and fine tremors of the hands
Intolerance to cold	Heat intolerance
Weight gain	Weight loss
Dry skin and hair and loss of body hair	Smooth, soft skin and hair
Bradycardia	Palpitations, cardiac dysrhythmias, such as tachycardia or atrial fibrillation
Constipation	Diarrhea
Generalized puffiness and edema around the eyes and face (myxedema)	Protruding eyeballs (exophthalmos) may be present
Forgetfulness and loss of memory	Diaphoresis
Menstrual disturbances	Hypertension
Cardiac enlargement, tendency to develop heart failure	Enlarged thyroid gland (goiter)
Goiter may or may not be present	

i. Administer propranolol (Inderal) for tachycardia as prescribed.
j. Prepare the client for radioactive iodine therapy as prescribed to destroy thyroid cells.
k. Prepare the client for thyroidectomy if prescribed.

D. Thyroid storm
1. Description (Box 45-6)
2. Data collection
   a. Elevated temperature (fever)
   b. Tachycardia
   c. Systolic hypertension
   d. Nausea, vomiting, and diarrhea
   e. Agitation, tremors, anxiety
   f. Irritability, agitation, restlessness, confusion, and seizures as the condition progresses
   g. Delirium and coma
3. Interventions
   a. Maintain a patent airway and adequate ventilation.
   b. Administer antithyroid medications, sodium iodide solution, propranolol, and glucocorticoids as prescribed.
   c. Monitor vital signs.
   d. Monitor continually for cardiac dysrhythmias.
   e. Administer nonsalicylate antipyretics as prescribed (salicylates increase free thyroid hormone levels).
   f. Use a cooling blanket to decrease the client's temperature as prescribed.

E. Thyroidectomy
1. Description
   a. Removal of the thyroid gland
   b. Performed when persistent hyperthyroidism exists
2. Preoperative interventions
   a. Obtain vital signs and weight.
   b. Monitor electrolyte levels.
   c. Monitor for hyperglycemia.
   d. Reinforce instructions to the client in how to perform coughing and deep-breathing exercises and how to support the neck during the postoperative period when coughing and moving.
   e. Assist to administer medications as prescribed to prevent the occurrence of thyroid storm.

BOX 45-6 Thyroid Storm

This acute and life-threatening condition occurs in a client with uncontrollable hyperthyroidism.

It can be caused by manipulation of the thyroid gland during surgery and the release of thyroid hormone into the bloodstream; it also can occur from severe infection and stress.

Antithyroid medications, β-blockers, glucocorticoids, and iodides may be administered to the client before thyroid surgery to prevent its occurrence.

3. Postoperative interventions 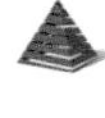
   a. Monitor for respiratory distress.
   b. Have a tracheotomy set, oxygen, and suction at the bedside.
   c. Limit client talking, and determine the level of hoarseness.
   d. Monitor for laryngeal nerve damage as evidenced by respiratory obstruction, dysphonia, high-pitched voice, stridor, dysphagia, and restlessness.
   e. Monitor for signs of hypocalcemia and tetany, which can be the result of trauma to the parathyroid gland (Box 45-7).
   f. Assist RN to administer calcium gluconate as prescribed for tetany.
   g. Monitor for thyroid storm.

⚠ Following thyroidectomy, maintain the client in a semi-Fowler's position. Monitor the surgical site for edema and for signs of bleeding and check the dressing anteriorly and at the back of the neck.

VI. Parathyroid Gland Disorders

A. Hypoparathyroidism
1. Description
   a. Condition caused by hyposecretion of parathyroid hormone by the parathyroid gland
   b. Can occur following thyroidectomy because of removal of parathyroid tissue
2. Data collection
   a. Hypocalcemia and hyperphosphatemia
   b. Numbness and tingling in the face
   c. Muscle cramps and cramps in the abdomen or in the extremities
   d. Positive **Trousseau's sign** or **Chvostek's sign**
   e. Signs of overt tetany, such as bronchospasm, laryngospasm, carpopedal spasm, dysphagia, photophobia, cardiac dysrhythmias, and seizures
   f. Hypotension
   g. Anxiety, irritability, depression
3. Interventions
   a. Monitor vital signs.
   b. Monitor for signs of hypocalcemia and tetany.

BOX 45-7 Signs of Tetany

- Cardiac dysrhythmias
- Carpopedal spasm
- Dysphagia
- Muscle and abdominal cramps
- Numbness and tingling of the face and extremities
- Positive Chvostek's sign
- Positive Trousseau's sign
- Visual disturbances (photophobia)
- Wheezing and dyspnea (bronchospasm, laryngospasm)
- Seizures

c. Initiate seizure precautions.
d. Place a tracheotomy set, oxygen, and suction at the bedside.
e. Assist RN to administer IV calcium gluconate for hypocalcemia.
f. Provide a high-calcium, low-phosphorus diet.
g. Reinforce instructions to the client regarding the administration of calcium supplements as prescribed.
h. Reinforce instructions to the client regarding the administration of vitamin D supplements as prescribed; vitamin D enhances the absorption of calcium from the gastrointestinal tract.
i. Reinforce instructions to the client regarding the administration of phosphate binders as prescribed to promote the excretion of phosphate through the gastrointestinal tract.
j. Reinforce instructions to the client to wear a Medic-Alert bracelet.

B. Hyperparathyroidism
1. Description: Condition caused by the hypersecretion of parathyroid hormone by the parathyroid gland
2. Data collection
a. Hypercalcemia and hypophosphatemia
b. Fatigue and muscle weakness
c. Skeletal pain and tenderness
d. Bone deformities that result in pathological fractures
e. Anorexia, nausea, vomiting, epigastric pain
f. Weight loss
g. Constipation
h. Hypertension
i. Cardiac dysrhythmias
j. Renal stones

3. Interventions
a. Monitor vital signs, particularly the blood pressure.
b. Monitor for cardiac dysrhythmias.
c. Monitor intake and output and for signs of renal stones.
d. Monitor for skeletal pain; move the client slowly and carefully.
e. Encourage fluid intake.
f. Administer furosemide (Lasix) as prescribed to lower calcium levels.
g. Normal saline may be prescribed intravenously to maintain hydration.
h. Assist to administer phosphates, which interfere with calcium reabsorption, as prescribed.
i. Assist to administer calcitonin (Fortical, Miacalcin) as prescribed to decrease skeletal calcium release and increase renal excretion of calcium.
j. Monitor calcium and phosphorus levels.
k. Prepare the client for parathyroidectomy as prescribed.

For the client with a parathyroid gland disorder, the RN and HCP are notified immediately if hypocalcemia occurs. Monitor for tingling and numbness in the face and extremities and for other signs of hypocalcemia.

C. Parathyroidectomy
1. Description: The removal of one or more of the parathyroid glands
2. Preoperative interventions
a. Monitor electrolytes, calcium, phosphate, and magnesium levels.
b. Ensure that calcium levels are decreased to near-normal values.
c. Inform the client that talking may be painful for the first day or two after surgery.
3. Postoperative interventions
a. Monitor for respiratory distress.
b. Place a tracheotomy set, oxygen, and suction at the bedside.
c. Monitor vital signs.
d. Position the client in a semi-Fowler's position.
e. Check the neck dressing for bleeding.
f. Monitor for hypocalcemic crisis as evidenced by tingling and twitching in the extremities and face.
g. Monitor for positive Trousseau's sign or Chvostek's sign, which signals the potential for tetany.
h. Monitor for changes in voice pattern and hoarseness.
i. Monitor for laryngeal nerve damage.
j. Reinforce instructions to the client regarding the administration of calcium and vitamin D supplements as prescribed.

VII. Disorders of the Pancreas

A. Diabetes mellitus
1. Description
a. Chronic disorder of impaired carbohydrate, protein, and lipid metabolism caused by a deficiency of insulin
b. An absolute or relative deficiency of insulin results in hyperglycemia.
c. Type 1 diabetes mellitus is a nearly absolute deficiency of insulin; if insulin is not given, fats are metabolized for energy, which results in ketonemia (acidosis).
d. Type 2 diabetes mellitus is a relative lack of insulin or resistance to the action of insulin; usually, insulin is sufficient to stabilize fat and protein metabolism but not carbohydrate metabolism.
e. Metabolic syndrome is also known as syndrome X, and the individual has coexisting risk factors for developing type 2 diabetes mellitus; these risk factors include abdominal obesity, hyperglycemia, hypertension,

high triglyceride level, and a lowered HDL (high-density lipoprotein) cholesterol level.

f. Diabetes mellitus can lead to chronic health problems and early death as a result of complications that occur in the large and small blood vessels in tissues and organs.

g. Macrovascular complications include coronary artery disease, cardiomyopathy, hypertension, cerebrovascular disease, and peripheral vascular disease. (Refer to Chapter 51 for information on cardiovascular disorders.)

h. Microvascular complications include retinopathy, nephropathy, and neuropathy.

i. Infection is also a concern because of reduced healing ability.

j. Male erectile dysfunction can also occur as a result of the disease.

Obesity is a major risk factor for diabetes mellitus.

2. Data collection
   a. Polyuria, polydipsia, and polyphagia (more common with type 1 diabetes mellitus)
   b. Hyperglycemia
   c. Weight loss (common with type 1 diabetes mellitus, rare with type 2 diabetes mellitus)
   d. Blurred vision
   e. Slow wound healing
   f. Vaginal infections
   g. Weakness and paresthesias
   h. Signs of inadequate circulation to the feet
   i. Signs of accelerated atherosclerosis (renal, cerebral, cardiac, peripheral)
3. Diet
   a. The diabetic client's diet should take into account weight, medication, activity level, and other health problems.
   b. Day-to-day consistency in timing and amount of food intake helps control the blood glucose level.
   c. As prescribed by the HCP, the client may be advised to follow the recommendations of the American Diabetic Association diet or U.S. dietary guidelines (MyPlate: http://www.choosemyplate.gov/) issued by the U.S. Departments of Agriculture and Health and Human Services.
   d. Carbohydrate counting may be a simpler approach for some clients; it focuses on the total grams of carbohydrates eaten per meal. The client may be more compliant with carbohydrate counting, resulting in better glycemic control; it is usually necessary for clients using intense insulin therapy.
   e. Incorporate the diet into individual client needs, lifestyle, and cultural and socioeconomic patterns.
4. Exercise 
   a. Exercise lowers the blood glucose level, encourages weight loss, reduces cardiovascular risks, improves circulation and muscle tone, decreases total cholesterol and triglyceride levels, and decreases insulin resistance and glucose intolerance.
   b. Reinforce instructions to the client regarding dietary adjustments when exercising; dietary adjustments are individualized.
   c. If the client requires extra food during exercise to prevent hypoglycemia, it need not be deducted from the regular meal plan.
   d. If the blood glucose level is greater than 250 mg/dL and urinary ketones (type 1 diabetes mellitus) are present, the client is instructed not to exercise until the blood glucose is closer to normal and urinary ketones are absent.

Instruct the client with diabetes mellitus to monitor the blood glucose level before, during, and after exercising.

5. Oral hypoglycemic medications: Oral medications are prescribed for clients with type 2 diabetes mellitus when diet and weight control therapy have failed to maintain satisfactory blood glucose levels (see Chapter 46).

To prevent a serious reaction, inform the client taking a sulfonylurea to avoid consuming alcohol.

6. Insulin
   a. Insulin is used to treat types 1 and 2 diabetes mellitus when diet, weight-control therapy, and oral hypoglycemic agents have failed to maintain satisfactory blood glucose levels.
   b. Illness, infection, and stress increase blood glucose levels and the need for insulin; insulin should not be withheld during illness, infection, or stress because hyperglycemia and diabetic ketoacidosis can result.
   c. The peak action time of insulin is important because of the possibility of hypoglycemic reactions occurring during that time.

Only short-duration insulin (lispro, aspart, glulisine, and regular insulin) can be administered intravenously.

B. Complications of insulin therapy
1. Local allergic reactions
   a. Redness, swelling, tenderness, and induration or a wheal at the site of injection may occur 1 to 2 hours after administration.
   b. Reactions usually occur during the early stages of insulin therapy.
   c. Reinforce instructions to the client to cleanse the skin with alcohol before injection.

2. Insulin lipodystrophy
   a. Lipoatrophy is a loss of subcutaneous fat, and it appears as a slight dimpling or a more serious pitting of the subcutaneous fat; the use of human insulin helps to prevent this complication.
   b. Lipohypertrophy is the development of fibrous fatty masses at the injection site and is caused by the repeated use of an injection site.
   c. Reinforce instructions to the client to avoid injecting insulin into affected sites.
   d. Reinforce instructions to the client about the importance of rotating insulin injection sites.
3. Insulin resistance
   a. The client receiving insulin develops immune antibodies that bind the insulin, thereby decreasing the insulin available for use in the body.
   b. Treatment consists of administering a purer insulin preparation.
   c. *Insulin resistance* is also the term used for the lack of tissue sensitivity to the insulin from the body, which results in hyperglycemia.
4. **Dawn phenomenon**
   a. Dawn phenomenon results from reduced tissue sensitivity to insulin and usually develops between 5:00 AM and 8:00 AM (prebreakfast hyperglycemia occurs); it may be caused by the nocturnal release of growth hormone.
   b. Treatment includes administering an evening dose (or increasing the amount of a current dose) of intermediate-acting insulin at about 10:00 PM.
5. **Somogyi phenomenon**
   a. Normal or elevated blood glucose levels are present at bedtime; hypoglycemia occurs at about 2:00 to 3:00 AM, which causes an increase in the production of counterregulatory hormones.
   b. By 7:00 AM, in response to the counterregulatory hormones, the blood glucose rebounds significantly to the hyperglycemic range.
   c. Treatment includes decreasing the evening (predinner or bedtime) dose of intermediate-acting insulin or increasing the bedtime snack.

C. Insulin administration
1. Subcutaneous injections and mixing insulin (see Chapter 46)
2. Insulin pumps
   a. Continuous subcutaneous insulin infusion is administered by an externally worn device that contains a syringe attached to a long, thin, narrow-lumen tube with a needle or Teflon catheter attached to the end.
   b. The client inserts the needle or Teflon catheter into the subcutaneous tissue (usually on the abdomen) and secures it with tape or a transparent dressing; the pump is worn on a belt or in a pocket; the needle or Teflon catheter is changed at least every 2 to 3 days.
   c. A continuous basal rate of insulin infuses; in addition, on the basis of the blood glucose level, the anticipated food intake, and the activity level, the client delivers a bolus of insulin before each meal.
   d. Both rapid-acting and regular short-acting insulin (buffered to prevent the precipitation of insulin crystals within the catheter) are appropriate for use in these pumps.
5. Insulin pump and skin sensor
   a. A skin sensor device that monitors the client's blood continuously; the information is transmitted to the pump, determines the need for insulin, and then the insulin is injected.
   b. The pump holds up to a 3-day supply of insulin and can be easily disconnected for activities such as bathing.
4. Pancreas transplants
   a. The goal of pancreatic transplantation is to halt or reverse the complications of diabetes mellitus.
   b. Transplants are performed on a limited number of clients (in general, those clients who are undergoing kidney transplantation simultaneously).
   c. Immunosuppressive therapy is prescribed to prevent and treat rejection.

D. Self-monitoring of blood glucose level
1. Self-monitoring provides the client with the current blood glucose level and information to maintain good glycemic control.
2. Monitoring requires a finger prick to obtain a drop of blood for testing.
3. Alternative site testing (obtaining blood from the forearm, upper arm, abdomen, thigh, or calf) is now available, using specific measurement devices.
4. Tests must be used with caution among clients with diabetic neuropathy.
5. Client instructions (Box 45-8)

E. Urine testing
1. Urine testing for glucose is not a reliable indicator of blood glucose and is not used for monitoring purposes.
2. Reinforce instructions to the client regarding the procedure for testing urine ketones.
3. The presence of ketones may indicate impending ketoacidosis.
4. Urine ketone testing should be performed during illness and whenever the client with type 1 diabetes mellitus has persistently elevated blood glucose levels (higher than 240 mg/dL or as prescribed for two consecutive testing periods).

BOX 45-8 Client Instructions: Monitoring of Blood Glucose Level

Use the proper procedure to obtain the sample for determining the blood glucose level.
Perform the procedure precisely to obtain accurate results.
Follow the manufacturer's instructions for the glucometer.
Wash hands before and after performing the procedure to prevent infection.
Calibrate the monitor as instructed by the manufacturer.
Check the expiration date on the test strips.
If the blood glucose level results do not seem reasonable, reread the instructions, reassess technique, check the expiration date of the test strips, and perform the procedure again to verify results.

VIII. Acute Complications of Diabetes Mellitus

A. Hypoglycemia (see Priority Nursing Actions)
   1. Description
      a. Hypoglycemia occurs when the blood glucose level falls below 70 mg/dL or when the blood glucose drops rapidly from an elevated level.

PRIORITY NURSING ACTIONS!

Actions to Take if the Client Experiences a Hypoglycemic Reaction

1. Check the client's blood glucose level.
2. Give the client a 10- to 15-g carbohydrate item, such as ½ cup of fruit juice, to drink (if client is not responsive or is unable to swallow, assist the RN in preparation of an IV injection of 25 to 50 mL of 50% dextrose in water).
3. Take the client's vital signs.
4. Retest the blood glucose level.
5. Give the client a small snack of carbohydrate and protein.
6. Document the client's complaints, actions taken, and outcome.

If the client experiences symptoms of a hypoglycemic reaction such as hunger, irritability, shakiness, or weakness, the nurse first checks the client's blood glucose level to verify that he or she is experiencing hypoglycemia. Once this is verified, the nurse gives the client 10 to 15 g of carbohydrates. The nurse assists the RN in preparation of an IV injection of 25 to 50 mL of 50% dextrose in water if client is not responsive or able to swallow. The nurse retests the blood glucose level in 15 minutes. In the meantime, the nurse checks the client's vital signs. The nurse gives the client another 10- to 15-g carbohydrate food item if the client's symptoms do not resolve. Otherwise, the nurse provides a small snack of carbohydrates and protein if the client's next scheduled meal is more than an hour away from the time of the occurrence. Following treatment and resolution of the hypoglycemic event, the nurse would document the occurrence, actions taken, and outcome.

Reference(s): deWit, D. & Kumagai, C. (2013). *Medical-surgical nursing: Concepts & practice.* (2nd ed., p. 874). St. Louis: Saunders.

      b. Hypoglycemia is caused by too much insulin or oral hypoglycemic agents, too little food, or excessive activity.
      c. The client needs to be instructed to always carry some form of fast-acting simple carbohydrate with him or her.
      d. If the client has a hypoglycemic reaction and does not have any of the recommended emergency foods available, any available food should be eaten; high-fat foods slow the absorption of glucose, and the hypoglycemic symptoms may not resolve quickly.
   2. Data collection (Box 45-9)
      a. Mild hypoglycemia: The client remains fully awake but displays adrenergic symptoms; the blood glucose level is usually lower than 60 mg/dL.
      b. Moderate hypoglycemia: The client displays symptoms of worsening hypoglycemia; the blood glucose level is usually less than 40 mg/dL.
      c. Severe hypoglycemia: Client displays severe neuroglycopenic symptoms; the blood glucose level is usually lower than 20 mg/dL.
   3. Interventions: Mild hypoglycemia
      a. Give 10 to 15 g of a fast-acting simple carbohydrate (Box 45-10).
      b. Retest the blood glucose level in 15 minutes and repeat the treatment if symptoms do not resolve.

BOX 45-9 Assessment of Hypoglycemia

Mild
- Hunger
- Nervousness
- Palpitations
- Sweating
- Tachycardia
- Tremor

Moderate
- Confusion
- Double vision
- Drowsiness
- Emotional changes
- Headache
- Impaired coordination
- Inability to concentrate
- Irrational or combative behavior
- Light-headedness
- Numbness of the lips and tongue
- Slurred speech

Severe
- Difficulty arousing
- Disoriented behavior
- Loss of consciousness
- Seizures

BOX 45-10 Simple Carbohydrates to Treat Hypoglycemia

- Commercially prepared glucose tablets
- 6 to 10 Life Savers or hard candy
- 4 tsp of sugar
- 4 sugar cubes
- 1 Tbsp of honey or syrup
- ½ cup of fruit juice or regular (nondiet) soft drink
- 8 oz low-fat milk
- 6 saltine crackers
- 3 graham crackers

c. Once symptoms resolve, a snack that contains protein and carbohydrates, such as low-fat milk or cheese and crackers, is recommended unless the client plans to eat a regular meal within 60 minutes.

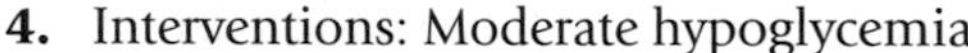

4. Interventions: Moderate hypoglycemia
   a. Administer 15 to 30 g of a fast-acting simple carbohydrate.
   b. Administer additional food such as low-fat milk or cheese and crackers after 10 to 15 minutes.

5. Interventions: Severe hypoglycemia
   a. If a client is unconscious and cannot swallow, an injection of glucagon is administered subcutaneously or intramuscularly.
   b. Administer a second dose in 10 minutes if the client remains unconscious.
   c. A small meal is given to the client when the client awakens as long as the client is not nauseated.
   d. The HCP is notified if a severe hypoglycemic reaction occurs.
   e. In the hospital or emergency department, the client may be treated with an IV injection of 25 to 50 mL of 50% dextrose in water.
   f. Family members need to be instructed regarding the administration of glucagon.

⚠ Do not attempt to administer oral food or fluids to the client experiencing a severe hypoglycemic reaction who is semiconscious or unconscious and is unable to swallow. This client is at risk for aspiration. For this client, an injection of glucagon is administered subcutaneously or intramuscularly. In the hospital or emergency department, the client may be treated with an IV injection of 25 to 50 mL of 50% dextrose in water.

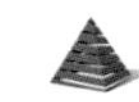

B. **Diabetic ketoacidosis** (DKA)
1. Description (Fig. 45-2)
   a. Diabetic ketoacidosis is a life-threatening complication of type 1 diabetes mellitus that develops when a severe insulin deficiency occurs.

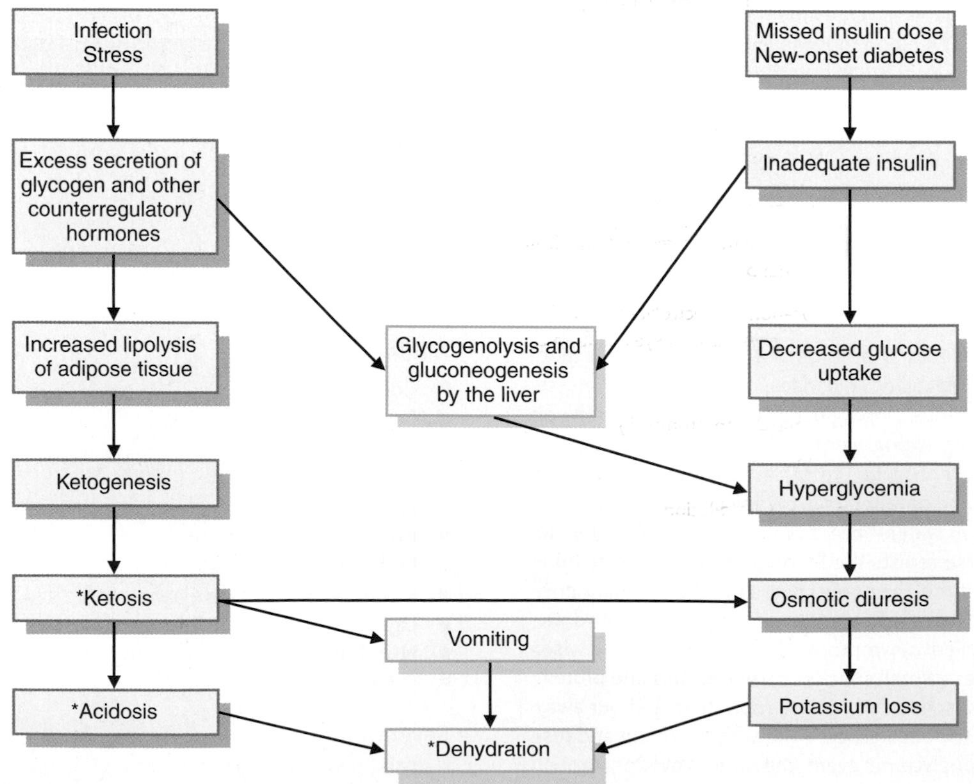

FIGURE 45-2 Pathophysiology of diabetic ketoacidosis (DKA). (From Black J, Hawks J: *Medical-surgical nursing: Clinical management for positive outcomes*, ed 8, St. Louis, 2009, Saunders.)

b. The main clinical manifestations include hyperglycemia, dehydration, electrolyte imbalance, and acidosis.
2. Data collection (Table 45-3)
3. Interventions
a. Restore circulating blood volume and protect against cerebral, coronary, and renal hypoperfusion
b. Dehydration will be treated with rapid IV infusions of 0.9% or 0.45% normal saline (NS), as prescribed; dextrose is added to IV fluids (D_5NS or 5% dextrose in 0.45% saline) when the blood glucose level reaches 250 to 300 mg/dL.
c. Hyperglycemia will be treated with regular insulin administered intravenously as prescribed.
d. Correct electrolyte imbalances (potassium level may be elevated as a result of dehydration and acidosis).
e. Monitor potassium level closely because when the client receives treatment for the dehydration and acidosis, the serum potassium will decrease, and potassium replacement may be required.
4. Insulin IV administration by the RN
a. Short-duration insulin only is used.
b. An IV bolus dose of insulin (usually 5 to 10 units) may be prescribed before a continuous infusion is begun.
c. The insulin solution is flushed through the entire IV infusion set, and the first 50 to 100 mL of solution is discarded before connecting and administering it to the client (insulin molecules adhere to the plastic of IV infusion sets).
d. The insulin infusion is always placed on an IV infusion controller.
e. Insulin is infused continuously until subcutaneous administration resumes to prevent a rebound of the blood glucose level.
f. Monitor vital signs.
g. Monitor urinary output and for signs of fluid overload.
h. Monitor potassium and glucose levels and for signs of increased intracranial pressure.
i. The potassium level will fall rapidly within the first hour of treatment as the dehydration and the acidosis are treated.

TABLE 45-3 Differences between Diabetic Ketoacidosis and Hyperosmolar Hyperglycemic Syndrome

	Diabetic Ketoacidosis (DKA)	Hyperosmolar Hyperglycemic Syndrome (HHS)
Onset	Sudden	Gradual
Precipitating factors	Infection	Infection
	Other stressors	Other stressors
	Inadequate insulin dose	Poor fluid intake
Manifestations	Ketosis: Kussmaul's respiration, "fruity" breath, nausea, abdominal pain	Altered central nervous system function with neurologic symptoms
	Dehydration or electrolyte loss: Polyuria, polydipsia, weight loss, dry skin, sunken eyes, soft eyeballs, lethargy, coma	Dehydration or electrolyte loss: Same as for DKA
Laboratory Findings		
Serum glucose	>300 mg/dL (16.7 mmol/L)	>800 mg/dL (44.5 mmol/L)
Osmolarity	Variable	>350 mOsm/L
Serum ketones	Positive at 1:2 dilution	Negative
Serum pH	<7.35	>7.4
Serum HCO_3	<15 mEq/L	>20 mEq/L
Serum Na	Low, normal, or high	Normal or low
Serum K	Normal; elevated with acidosis, low following dehydration	Normal or low
BUN	>20 mg/dL; elevated because of dehydration	Elevated
Creatinine	>1.5 mg/dL; elevated because of dehydration	Elevated
Urine ketones	Positive	Negative

BUN, blood urea nitrogen; *HCO_3*, bicarbonate.
From Ignatavicius D, Workman M: *Medical-surgical nursing: Patient-centered collaborative care*, ed 7, St. Louis, 2013, Saunders.

BOX 45-11 Client Education: Guidelines During Illness

Take insulin or oral antidiabetic medications as prescribed.
Determine the blood glucose level, and test the urine for ketones every 3 to 4 hours.
If the usual meal plan cannot be followed, substitute soft foods six to eight times a day.
If vomiting, diarrhea, or fever occurs, consume liquids every 30 to 60 minutes to prevent dehydration and to provide calories.
Notify the health care provider if vomiting, diarrhea, or fever persists; if blood glucose levels are higher than 250 to 300 mg/dL; when ketonuria is present for more than 24 hours; when unable to take food or fluids for a period of 4 hours; or when illness persists for more than 2 days.

j. Potassium is administered intravenously in a diluted solution as prescribed when the potassium reaches a normal level to prevent hypokalemia; ensure adequate renal function before administering potassium.

5. Reinforcement of client education (Box 45-11)

Monitor the client being treated for DKA closely for signs of increased intracranial pressure. If the blood glucose level falls too far or too fast before the brain has time to equilibrate, water is pulled from the blood to the cerebrospinal fluid and the brain, causing cerebral edema and increased intracranial pressure.

C. Hyperosmolar hyperglycemic syndrome (HHS)

1. Description
- **a.** Extreme hyperglycemia occurs without ketosis and acidosis.
- **b.** The syndrome occurs most often among individuals with type 2 diabetes mellitus.
- **c.** The major difference between HHS and DKA is that ketosis and acidosis do not occur with HHS; enough insulin is present with HHS to prevent the breakdown of fats for energy, thus preventing ketosis.

2. Data collection (see Table 45-3)

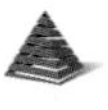

3. Interventions
- **a.** Treatment is similar to that for DKA.
- **b.** Treatment includes fluid replacement, the correction of electrolyte imbalances, and insulin administration.
- **c.** Fluid replacement in the older client must be done very carefully secondary to the potential for heart failure.
- **d.** Insulin plays a less critical role in the treatment of HHS than it does for the treatment of DKA because ketosis and acidosis do not occur; rehydration alone may decrease glucose levels.

IX. Chronic Complications of Diabetes Mellitus

A. Diabetic retinopathy

1. Description
- **a.** Chronic and progressive impairment of the retinal circulation that eventually causes hemorrhage
- **b.** Permanent vision changes and blindness can occur.
- **c.** The client has difficulty with carrying out the daily tasks of blood glucose testing and insulin injections.

2. Data collection
- **a.** A change in vision is caused by the rupture of small microaneurysms in retinal blood vessels.
- **b.** Blurred vision results from macular edema.
- **c.** Sudden loss of vision results from retinal detachment.
- **d.** Cataracts result from lens opacity.

3. Interventions
- **a.** Maintain safety.
- **b.** Early prevention via the control of hypertension and blood glucose levels
- **c.** Photocoagulation (laser therapy) may be done to remove hemorrhagic tissue to decrease scarring and prevent the progression of the disease process.
- **d.** Vitrectomy may be done to remove vitreous hemorrhages and thus decrease tension on the retina, preventing detachment.
- **e.** Cataract removal with a lens implantation improves vision.

B. Diabetic nephropathy

1. Description: Progressive decrease in kidney function

2. Data collection
- **a.** Microalbuminuria
- **b.** Thirst
- **c.** Fatigue
- **d.** Anemia
- **e.** Weight loss
- **f.** Signs of malnutrition
- **g.** Frequent urinary tract infections
- **h.** Signs of a neurogenic bladder

3. Interventions
- **a.** Early prevention measures include the control of hypertension and blood glucose levels.
- **b.** Monitor vital signs.
- **c.** Monitor intake and output.
- **d.** Monitor the blood urea nitrogen, creatinine, and urine albumin levels.
- **e.** Restrict dietary protein, sodium, and potassium intake as prescribed.
- **f.** Avoid nephrotoxic medications.
- **g.** Prepare the client for dialysis procedures if planned.

h. Prepare the client for kidney transplant if planned.
i. Prepare the client for pancreas transplant if planned.

C. Diabetic neuropathy
1. Description
a. A general deterioration of the nervous system throughout the body.
b. Complications include the development of nonhealing ulcers of the feet, gastric paresis, and erectile dysfunction.
2. Classifications
a. Focal neuropathy or mononeuropathy: Involves a single nerve or a group of nerves, most frequently cranial nerves III (oculomotor) and VI (abducens), and results in diplopia
b. Sensory or peripheral neuropathy: Affects the distal portion of the nerves, most frequently in the lower extremities
c. Autonomic neuropathy: Symptoms vary according to the organ system involved.
d. Cardiovascular: Cardiac denervation syndrome (heart rate does not respond to changes in oxygenation needs) and orthostatic hypotension occur.
e. Pupillary: Pupil does not dilate in response to decreased light.
f. Gastric: Decreased gastric emptying (gastroparesis)
g. Urinary: Neurogenic bladder
h. Skin: Decreased sweating
i. Adrenal: Hypoglycemic unawareness
j. Reproductive: Impotence (male) and painful intercourse (female)
3. Data collection: Findings depend on the classification.
a. Paresthesias
b. Decreased or absent reflexes
c. Decreased sensation to vibration or light touch
d. Pain, aching, and burning in the lower extremities
e. Poor peripheral pulses
f. Skin breakdown and signs of infection
g. Weakness or loss of sensation in cranial nerves III (oculomotor), IV (trochlear), V (trigeminal), and VI (abducens)
h. Dizziness and postural hypotension
i. Nausea and vomiting
j. Diarrhea or constipation
k. Incontinence
l. Dyspareunia
m. Impotence
n. Hypoglycemic unawareness
4. Interventions
a. Early prevention measures include the control of hypertension and blood glucose levels.

BOX 45-12 Preventive Foot Care Instructions

Provide meticulous skin care and proper foot care.
Inspect feet daily and monitor feet for redness, swelling, or break in skin integrity.
Notify the health care provider if redness or a break in the skin occurs.
Avoid thermal injuries from hot water, heating pads, and baths.
Wash feet with warm (not hot) water and dry thoroughly (avoid foot soaks).
Avoid treating corns, blisters, or ingrown toenails.
Do not cross legs or wear tight garments that may constrict blood flow.
Apply moisturizing lotion to the feet, but not between the toes.
Prevent moisture from accumulating between the toes.
Wear loose socks and well-fitting (not tight) shoes; do not go barefoot.
Wear clean cotton socks to keep the feet warm, and change the socks daily.
Avoid wearing the same pair of shoes 2 days in a row.
Avoid wearing open-toed shoes or shoes with a strap that goes between the toes.
Check shoes for cracks or tears in the lining and for foreign objects before putting them on.
Break in new shoes gradually.
Cut toenails straight across, and smooth nails with an emery board.
Avoid smoking.

b. Careful foot care is required to prevent trauma (Box 45-12).
c. Administer medications as prescribed for pain relief.
d. Initiate bladder-training programs.
e. Reinforce instructions to the client regarding the use of estrogen-containing lubricants for women with dyspareunia.
f. Prepare the male client with impotence for penile injections or other possible treatment options as prescribed.
g. Prepare for surgical decompression of compression lesions related to the cranial nerves as prescribed.

X. Care of the Diabetic Client Undergoing Surgery

A. Preoperative care
1. Check with the HCP regarding withholding oral hypoglycemic medications or insulin.
2. Some long-acting oral antidiabetic medications are discontinued 24 to 48 hours before surgery.
3. Metformin (Glucophage) may need to be discontinued 48 hours before surgery and may not be restarted until renal function is normal postoperatively.
4. All other oral antidiabetic medications are usually withheld the day of surgery.
5. Insulin dose may be adjusted or withheld if IV insulin administration during surgery is planned.

6. Monitor the blood glucose level.
7. Assist to administer prescribed IV fluids.

B. Intraoperative care
1. Monitor blood glucose levels frequently.
2. As prescribed, the operating room nurse will administer IV short- or rapid-acting insulin as prescribed to maintain blood glucose level lower than 200 mg/dL.

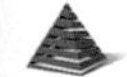

C. Postoperative care
1. Assist the RN to administer IV glucose and regular insulin infusions as prescribed until the client can tolerate oral feedings.
2. Administer supplemental short-acting insulin as prescribed based on blood glucose results.
3. Monitor blood glucose levels frequently if the client is receiving parenteral nutrition.
4. When the client is tolerating food, ensure that the client receives an adequate amount of carbohydrates daily to prevent hypoglycemia.
5. Client is at higher risk for cardiovascular and renal complications postoperatively.
6. Client is also at risk for impaired wound healing.

CRITICAL THINKING What Should You Do?

Answer: Hypertensive crisis can occur as a complication of pheochromocytoma. This can result in stroke, cardiac dysrhythmias, or myocardial infarction. Manifestations include severe headache, extremely high blood pressure (BP), dizziness, blurred vision, shortness of breath, epistaxis (nosebleed), and severe anxiety. If the nurse suspects a hypertensive crisis, the nurse should place the client in a semi-Fowler's position and notify the registered nurse immediately. The health care provider should also be notified immediately, and, as prescribed, the nurse should prepare to administer oxygen, assist the RN to start an intravenous (IV) infusion of 0.9% normal saline (NS) solution and infuse it slowly to prevent fluid overload (which would increase blood pressure), assist the RN to administer intravenous medications to lower the BP, monitor the blood pressure frequently, and monitor for complications.

Reference(s): deWit, D. & Kumagai, C. (2013). *Medical-surgical nursing: Concepts & practice.* (2nd ed., p. 847). St. Louis: Saunders.

Ignatavicius, D., & Workman, M. (2013). *Medical-surgical nursing: Patient-centered collaborative care.* (7th ed., p. 784). St. Louis: Saunders.

PRACTICE QUESTIONS

446. The nurse is caring for a client after a thyroidectomy and notes that calcium gluconate is prescribed for the client. The nurse determines that this medication has been prescribed for which reason?
1. Treat thyroid storm.
2. Prevent cardiac irritability.
3. Treat hypocalcemic tetany.
4. Stimulate the release of parathyroid hormone.

447. The nurse is collecting data regarding a client after a thyroidectomy and notes that the client has developed hoarseness and a weak voice. Which nursing action is appropriate?
1. Check for signs of bleeding.
2. Administer calcium gluconate.
3. Notify the registered nurse immediately.
4. Reassure the client that this is usually a temporary condition.

448. A client is admitted to the emergency department, and a diagnosis of myxedema coma is made. Which action should the nurse prepare to carry out **initially**?
1. Warm the client.
2. Maintain a patent airway.
3. Monitor intravenous fluids.
4. Administer thyroid hormone.

449. The nurse is assisting with preparing a teaching plan for the client with diabetes mellitus regarding proper foot care. Which instruction should be included in the plan of care?
1. Soak the feet in hot water.
2. Avoid using soap to wash the feet.
3. Apply a moisturizing lotion to dry feet, but not between the toes.
4. Always have a podiatrist cut your toenails; never cut them yourself.

450. The nurse provides dietary instructions to a client with diabetes mellitus regarding the prescribed diabetic diet. Which statement made by the client indicates the **need for further teaching**?
1. "I'll eat a balanced meal plan."
2. "I need to drink diet soft drinks."
3. "I need to buy special dietetic foods."
4. "I will snack on fruit instead of cake."

451. A client who has been newly diagnosed with diabetes mellitus has been stabilized with daily insulin injections. Which teaching information should the nurse reinforce upon discharge?
1. Keep insulin vials refrigerated at all times.
2. Rotate the insulin injection sites systematically.
3. Increase the amount of insulin before unusual exercise.
4. Monitor the urine acetone level to determine the insulin dosage.

452. The nurse reinforces teaching with a client with diabetes mellitus regarding differentiating between hypoglycemia and ketoacidosis. The client demonstrates an understanding of the

teaching by stating that glucose will be taken if which symptom develops?
1. Polyuria
2. Shakiness
3. Blurred vision
4. Fruity breath odor

453. When the nurse is reinforcing instructions to a client who has been newly diagnosed with type 1 diabetes mellitus, which statement by the client would indicate that teaching has been **effective**?
1. "I will stop taking my insulin if I'm too sick to eat."
2. "I will decrease my insulin dose during times of illness."
3. "I will adjust my insulin dose according to the level of glucose in my urine."
4. "I will notify my health care provider if my blood glucose level is consistently greater than 250 mg/dL."

454. The nurse is monitoring a client who has been newly diagnosed with diabetes mellitus for signs of complications. Which statement made by the client would indicate hyperglycemia and thus warrant health care provider notification?
1. "I am urinating a lot."
2. "My pulse is really slow."
3. "I am sweating for no reason."
4. "My blood pressure is really high."

455. The nurse is reinforcing instructions with a client with diabetes mellitus who is recovering from diabetic ketoacidosis (DKA) regarding measures to prevent a recurrence. Which instruction is important for the nurse to emphasize?
1. Eat six small meals daily.
2. Test the urine ketone levels.
3. Monitor blood glucose levels frequently.
4. Receive appropriate follow-up health care.

456. The nurse is reinforcing discharge teaching with a client who has Cushing's syndrome. Which statement by the client indicates that the instructions related to dietary management were understood?
1. "I can eat foods that contain potassium."
2. "I will need to limit the amount of protein in my diet."
3. "I am fortunate that I can eat all the salty foods I enjoy."
4. "I am fortunate that I do not need to follow any special diet."

❖ **457.** The nurse educator is asking the nursing student to recall the signs/symptoms of hypothyroidism. The nurse educator determines that the student understands this disorder if which are included in the student's response? **Select all that apply.**
- ❑ 1. Dry skin
- ❑ 2. Irritability
- ❑ 3. Palpitations
- ❑ 4. Weight loss
- ❑ 5. Constipation
- ❑ 6. Cold intolerance

458. The nurse is caring for a postoperative parathyroidectomy client. Which would require the nurse's **immediate** attention?
1. Incisional pain
2. Laryngeal stridor
3. Difficulty voiding
4. Abdominal cramps

459. The nurse notes that a client with type 1 diabetes mellitus has lipodystrophy on both upper thighs. Which further information should the nurse obtain from the client during data collection?
1. Plan for injection rotation
2. Consistency of aspiration
3. Preparation of the injection site
4. Angle at which the medication is administered

460. A client with type 1 diabetes mellitus calls the nurse to report recurrent episodes of hypoglycemia. Which statement by the client indicates a correct understanding of Humulin N insulin and exercise?
1. "I should not exercise after lunch."
2. "I should not exercise after breakfast."
3. "I should not exercise in the late evening."
4. "I should not exercise in the late afternoon."

Adult—Endocrine

ANSWERS

446. 3

Rationale: Hypocalcemia can develop after thyroidectomy if the parathyroid glands are accidentally removed or injured during surgery. Manifestations develop 1 to 7 days after surgery. If the client develops numbness and tingling around the mouth, fingertips, or toes, or muscle spasms or twitching, the health care provider is notified immediately. Calcium gluconate should be accessible for the client who underwent thyroidectomy.

Test-Taking Strategy: Focus on the subject, the intended effect of calcium gluconate. Noting the name of the medication (calcium gluconate) should easily direct you to the correct option. Calcium is given if hypocalcemic tetany occurs. **Review: calcium gluconate.**

Level of Cognitive Ability: Analyzing
Client Needs: Physiological Integrity
Integrated Process: Nursing Process/Planning
Content Area: Pharmacology: Endocrine Medications
Priority Concepts: Clinical Judgment, Fluid and Electrolyte Balance

Reference(s): deWit, Kumagai (2013), p. 843; Linton (2012), pp. 1033, 1041.

447. 4

Rationale: Weakness and hoarseness of the voice can occur as a result of trauma of the laryngeal nerve. If this develops, the client should be reassured that the problem will subside in a few days. Unnecessary talking should be discouraged. It is not necessary to notify the registered nurse immediately. These signs do not indicate bleeding or the need to administer calcium gluconate.

Test-Taking Strategy: Focus on the subject, postoperative expectations in the client who underwent thyroidectomy. The options of checking for bleeding and administering calcium gluconate can easily be eliminated because they are unrelated to the signs presented in the question. From the remaining options, recall that these signs indicate a temporary condition. Review: expected findings after **thyroidectomy**.

Level of Cognitive Ability: Applying

Client Needs: Physiological Integrity

Integrated Process: Nursing Process/Implementation

Content Area: Adult Health: Endocrine

Priority Concepts: Caregiving, Clinical Judgment

Reference(s): Ignatavicius, Workman (2013), p. 1399.

448. 2

Rationale: The initial nursing action would be to maintain a patent airway. Oxygen would be administered, followed by fluid replacement. The nurse would also keep the client warm, monitor intravenous fluids, and administer thyroid hormones.

Test-Taking Strategy: Note the strategic word, *initially.* All of the options are appropriate interventions, but the use of the ABCs—airway, breathing, and circulation—will direct you to the correct option. **Review:** the care of the client with **myxedema coma.**

Level of Cognitive Ability: Analyzing

Client Needs: Physiological Integrity

Integrated Process: Nursing Process/Implementation

Content Area: Critical Care: Emergency Situations

Priority Concepts: Gas Exchange, Safety

Reference(s): deWit, Kumagai (2013), p. 845. Hammond, Zimmermann (2013), p. 310.

449. 3

Rationale: The client should use a moisturizing lotion on his or her feet, but should avoid applying the lotion between the toes. The client should also be instructed not to soak the feet and to avoid hot water to prevent burns. The client may cut the toenails straight across and even with the toe itself, but he or she should consult a podiatrist if the toenails are thick or hard to cut or if his or her vision is poor. The client should be instructed to wash the feet daily with a mild soap.

Test-Taking Strategy: Focus on the subject, foot care for the diabetic client. Eliminate the option regarding *hot water* because hot water can cause injury to the client. Eliminate the option stating to *always have a podiatrist cut your toenails* because the word *always* is a closed-ended word. From the remaining options, recalling the concern related to skin infection will assist you with eliminating the option regarding using soap. **Review: diabetic foot care instructions.**

Level of Cognitive Ability: Applying

Client Needs: Health Promotion and Maintenance

Integrated Process: Nursing Process/Planning

Content Area: Adult Health: Endocrine

Priority Concepts: Client Education, Infection

Reference(s): Linton (2012), p. 1052.

450. 3

Rationale: It is important to emphasize to the client and family that they are not eating a diabetic diet but rather following a balanced meal plan. Adherence to nutrition principles is an important component of diabetic management, and an individualized meal plan should be developed for the client. It is not necessary for the client to purchase special dietetic foods.

Test-Taking Strategy: Note the strategic words, *need for further teaching.* This is a negative event query, which indicates the need to select the incorrect option as the answer. Basic principles related to the diabetic diet will direct you to the correct option. **Review: diabetic diet.**

Level of Cognitive Ability: Evaluating

Client Needs: Physiological Integrity

Integrated Process: Teaching and Learning

Content Area: Adult Health: Endocrine

Priority Concepts: Client Education, Nutrition

Reference(s): deWit, Kumagai (2013), p. 860; Linton (2012), pp. 1056–1057.

451. 2

Rationale: Insulin dosages should not be adjusted or increased before unusual exercise. If acetone is found in the urine, it may possibly indicate the need for additional insulin. To minimize the discomfort associated with insulin injections, the insulin should be administered at room temperature. Injection sites should be systematically rotated from one area to another. The client should be instructed to give injections in one area, about 1 inch apart, until the whole area has been used and then to change to another site. This prevents dramatic changes in daily insulin absorption.

Test-Taking Strategy: Focus on the subject, reinforcement of teaching for a client newly diagnosed with diabetes mellitus. Eliminate the option stating to keep insulin vials *refrigerated at all times* first because of the closed-ended word, *all.* Knowledge regarding insulin administration and the significance of acetone in the urine will assist you with eliminating options of increasing insulin and monitoring urine acetone levels. **Review: insulin management.**

Level of Cognitive Ability: Applying

Client Needs: Physiological Integrity

Integrated Process: Teaching and Learning

Content Area: Adult Health: Endocrine

Priority Concepts: Client Education, Glucose Regulation

Reference(s): deWit, Kumagai (2013), p. 864; Linton (2012), p. 1061.

452. 2

Rationale: Shakiness is a sign of hypoglycemia, and it would indicate the need for food or glucose. Fruity breath odor, blurred vision, and polyuria are signs of hyperglycemia.

Test-Taking Strategy: Knowledge regarding the signs and symptoms of hypoglycemia and hyperglycemia is required to answer this question. Remember that shakiness is a sign of hypoglycemia. The other options are comparable or alike

options and are related to hyperglycemia. **Review:** signs and symptoms of **hypoglycemia** and **hyperglycemia**.
Level of Cognitive Ability: Evaluating
Client Needs: Physiological Integrity
Integrated Process: Nursing Process/Evaluation
Content Area: Adult Health: Endocrine
Priority Concepts: Client Education, Glucose Regulation
Reference(s): deWit, Kumagai (2013), p. 851, 879.

453. 4
Rationale: During illness, the client should monitor the blood glucose level, and he or she should notify the health care provider (HCP) if the level is greater than 250 mg/dL. Insulin should never be stopped. In fact, insulin may need to be increased during times of illness. Doses should not be adjusted without the HCP's advice.
Test-Taking Strategy: Note the strategic word, *effective.* Note that options regarding stopping or decreasing insulin doses and adjusting insulin dosage are comparable or alike; therefore, eliminate these options. Recall that serum blood glucose levels should be monitored rather than urine glucose levels because of unreliability issues associated with urine glucose levels. **Review: diabetic management.**
Level of Cognitive Ability: Evaluating
Client Needs: Physiological Integrity
Integrated Process: Nursing Process/Evaluation
Content Area: Adult Health: Endocrine
Priority Concepts: Client Education, Glucose Regulation
Reference(s): deWit, Kumagai (2013), pp. 827–828; Linton (2012), pp. 1064–1065.

454. 1
Rationale: The classic symptoms of hyperglycemia include polydipsia, polyuria, and polyphagia. Options 2, 3, and 4 are not signs of hyperglycemia.
Test-Taking Strategy: Focus on the subject, signs of hyperglycemia. Remember the 3 Ps—polyuria, polydipsia, and polyphagia. **Review: signs of hyperglycemia.**
Level of Cognitive Ability: Evaluating
Client Needs: Physiological Integrity
Integrated Process: Nursing Process/Evaluation
Content Area: Adult Health: Endocrine
Priority Concepts: Clinical Judgment, Glucose Regulation
Reference(s): deWit, Kumagai (2013), p. 859; Linton (2012), p. 1048.

455. 3
Rationale: Client education after DKA should emphasize the need for home glucose monitoring four to five times per day. It is also important to instruct the client to notify the health care provider when illness occurs. The presence of urinary ketones indicates that DKA has already occurred. The client should eat well-balanced meals with snacks, as prescribed.
Test-Taking Strategy: Focus on the subject, preventing diabetic ketoacidosis. Recall that the treatment of diabetic ketoacidosis focuses on the maintenance of an appropriate blood glucose level. Eating six small meals daily is not an accurate component of diabetic care. Receiving follow-up care will not prevent DKA. Testing the urine ketone levels does not prevent diabetic ketoacidosis but helps to confirm the diagnosis. **Review: diabetic ketoacidosis.**
Level of Cognitive Ability: Applying
Client Needs: Health Promotion and Maintenance
Integrated Process: Teaching and Learning
Content Area: Adult Health: Endocrine
Priority Concepts: Glucose Regulation, Health Promotion
Reference(s): deWit, Kumagai (2013), p. 873.

456. 1
Rationale: A diet that is low in calories, carbohydrates, and sodium but ample in protein and potassium content is encouraged for a client with Cushing's syndrome. Such a diet promotes weight loss, the reduction of edema and hypertension, the control of hypokalemia, and the rebuilding of wasted tissue.
Test-Taking Strategy: Focus on the subject, that instructions related to dietary management were understood. Eliminate the option of not needing to follow a special diet because it indicates that no dietary change is necessary. Eliminate the option of limiting protein next because protein is usually only limited with renal disorders. Excess sodium is not healthy in general, so eliminate that option. **Review:** dietary measures associated with **Cushing's syndrome.**
Level of Cognitive Ability: Evaluating
Client Needs: Physiological Integrity
Integrated Process: Nursing Process/Evaluation
Content Area: Adult Health: Endocrine
Priority Concepts: Client Education, Nutrition
Reference(s): Ignatavicius, Workman (2013), pp. 1387, 1391.

❖457. 1, 5, 6
Rationale: Signs of hypothyroidism include dry skin, hair, and loss of body hair; constipation; cold intolerance; lethargy and fatigue; weakness; muscle aches; paresthesias; weight gain; bradycardia; generalized puffiness and edema around the eyes and face; forgetfulness; menstrual disturbances; cardiac enlargement; and goiter. Irritability, palpitations, and weight loss are signs of hyperthyroidism.
Test-Taking Strategy: Focus on the subject, hypothyroidism. Note the relationship between *hypo-* in *hypothyroidism* and the correct answers, and recall that everything slows down with hypothyroidism. **Review:** signs of **hypothyroidism.**
Level of Cognitive Ability: Evaluating
Client Needs: Physiological Integrity
Integrated Process: Nursing Process: Evaluation
Content Area: Adult Health: Endocrine
Priority Concepts: Clinical Judgment, Thermoregulation
Reference(s): deWit, Kumagai (2013), pp. 844–845.

458. 2
Rationale: During the postoperative period, the nurse carefully observes the client for signs of hemorrhage, which causes swelling and the compression of adjacent tissue. Laryngeal stridor is a harsh, high-pitched sound heard on inspiration and expiration that is caused by the compression of the trachea and that leads to respiratory distress. It is an acute emergency situation that requires immediate attention to avoid the complete obstruction of the airway.
Test-Taking Strategy: Note the strategic word, *immediate.* Focus on the concept of ABCs—airway, breathing, and circulation—and consider the anatomical location of the surgical procedure. The options of incisional pain, difficulty voiding, and abdominal cramps are common postoperative

problems that are not life-threatening. Laryngeal stridor addresses the airway and requires immediate attention. **Review:** care of the client after **parathyroidectomy**.
Level of Cognitive Ability: Analyzing
Client Needs: Physiological Integrity
Integrated Process: Nursing Process/Data Collection
Content Area: Adult Health: Endocrine
Priority Concepts: Gas Exchange, Inflammation
Reference(s): Ignatavicius, Workman (2013), p. 1399.

459. 1
Rationale: Lipodystrophy (i.e., the hypertrophy of subcutaneous tissue at the injection site) occurs in some diabetic clients when the same injection sites are used for prolonged periods of time. Thus clients are instructed to adhere to a rotating injection site plan to avoid tissue changes. Preparation of the site, aspiration, and the angle of insulin administration do not produce tissue damage.
Test-Taking Strategy: Focus on the **subject**, lipodystrophy. Remember that lipodystrophy is the hypertrophy of subcutaneous tissue at the injection site. **Review: insulin therapy.**
Level of Cognitive Ability: Applying
Client Needs: Physiological Integrity
Integrated Process: Nursing Process/Data Collection
Content Area: Adult Health: Endocrine
Priority Concepts: Glucose Regulation, Tissue Integrity
Reference(s): deWit, Kumagai (2013), p. 864; Linton (2012), p. 1061.

460. 4
Rationale: A hypoglycemic reaction may occur in response to increased exercise. Clients should avoid exercise during the peak time of insulin. Humulin N insulin peaks at 12 to 14 hours; therefore, late-afternoon exercise would occur during the peak of the medication.
Test-Taking Strategy: Note the **subject**, the most likely time of a hypoglycemic reaction. Recalling the peak time of Humulin N insulin will direct you to the option of late-afternoon exercise. **Review:** measures to prevent **hypoglycemia**.
Level of Cognitive Ability: Evaluating
Client Needs: Physiological Integrity
Integrated Process: Nursing Process/Evaluation
Content Area: Adult Health: Endocrine
Priority Concepts: Glucose Regulation, Health Promotion
Reference(s): deWit, Kumagai (2013), pp. 861–862; Linton (2012), pp. 1057–1058.

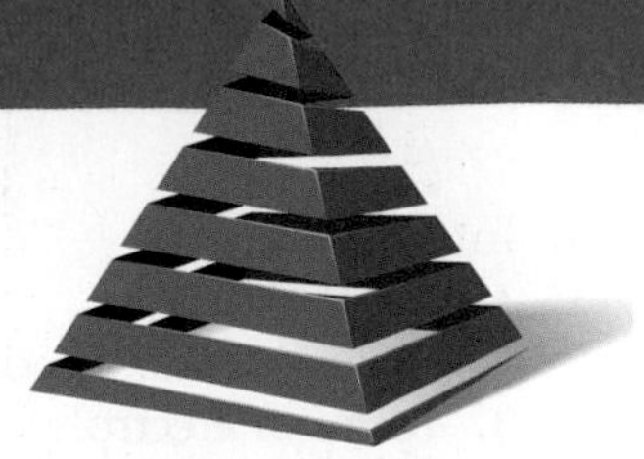

CHAPTER 46

Endocrine Medications

CRITICAL THINKING What Should You Do?

The nurse is reviewing the medical record of a client scheduled for a computerized tomography (CT) scan with an intravenous iodine contrast dye and notes that the client has diabetes mellitus and is taking metformin (Glucophage). What should the nurse do?

Answer located on p. 587.

I. Pituitary Medications

A. Description
   1. The anterior pituitary gland secretes growth hormone (GH), thyroid-stimulating hormone (TSH), adrenocorticotropic hormone (ACTH), prolactin, melanocyte-stimulating hormone (MSH), and gonadotropins (follicle-stimulating hormone [FSH] and luteinizing hormone [LH]).
   2. The posterior pituitary gland secretes antidiuretic hormone (vasopressin) and oxytocin.

B. Growth hormones and related medications (Box 46-1)
   1. Uses
      a. Growth hormones are used to treat pediatric or adult growth hormone deficiency.
      b. Growth hormone receptor antagonists are used to treat acromegaly.
      c. Growth hormone releasing factor is used to evaluate anterior pituitary function.
   2. Side/adverse effects
      a. May vary depending on the medication
      b. Development of antibodies to growth hormone
      c. Headache, muscle pain, weakness, vertigo
      d. Diarrhea, nausea, abdominal discomfort
      e. Mild **hyperglycemia**
      f. Hypertension
      g. Weight gain
      h. Allergic reaction (rash, swelling), pain at injection site
      i. Elevated aspartate aminotransferase (AST) and alanine aminotransferase (ALT)

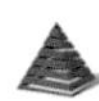

   3. Interventions
      a. Check the child's physical growth and compare growth with standards.
      b. Recommend annual bone age determinations for children receiving growth hormones.
      c. Monitor vital signs, blood glucose levels, AST and ALT levels, and thyroid function tests.
      d. Reinforce teaching to the client and family about the clinical manifestations of hyperglycemia and about other side/adverse effects of therapy and the importance of follow-up regarding periodic blood tests.

II. Antidiuretic Hormones

A. Desmopressin acetate (DDVAP, Stimate, Minirin); vasopressin (Pitressin)

B. Description
   1. Antidiuretic hormones enhance reabsorption of water in the kidneys, promoting an antidiuretic effect and regulating fluid balance.
   2. Antidiuretic hormones are used in **diabetes insipidus**.

C. Side/adverse effects
   1. Flushing
   2. Headache
   3. Nausea and abdominal cramps
   4. Water intoxication
   5. Hypertension with water intoxication
   6. Nasal congestion with nasal administration

BOX 46-1 Growth Hormones and Related Medications

Growth Hormones

Somatropin (Humatrope)
Mecasermin (Increlex)

Growth Hormone Receptor Antagonists

Octreotide acetate (Sandostatin)
Pegvisomant (Somavert)

Growth Hormone Releasing Factor

Tesamorelin (Egrifta)

D. Interventions
1. Monitor weight.
2. Monitor intake and output and urine osmolality.
3. Monitor electrolyte levels.
4. Monitor for signs of dehydration, indicating the need to increase the dosage.
5. Monitor for signs of water intoxication (drowsiness, listlessness, shortness of breath, and headache), indicating need to decrease dosage.
6. Monitor blood pressure.
7. Reinforce instructions to the client in how to use the intranasal medication.
8. Reinforce instructions to the client to weigh himself or herself daily to identify weight gain.
9. Reinforce instructions to the client to report signs of water intoxication or symptoms of headache or shortness of breath.

III. Thyroid Hormones (Box 46-2)

A. Description
1. Thyroid hormones control the metabolic rate of tissues and accelerate heat production and oxygen consumption.
2. Thyroid hormones are used to replace the thyroid hormone deficit in conditions such as **hypothyroidism** and **myxedema coma**.
3. Thyroid hormones enhance the action of oral anticoagulants, sympathomimetics, and antidepressants and decrease the action of insulin, oral hypoglycemics, and digitalis preparations; the action of thyroid hormones is decreased by phenytoin (Dilantin) and carbamazepine (Tegretol).

4. Thyroid hormones should be given at least 4 hours apart from multivitamins, aluminum hydroxide and magnesium hydroxide, simethicone, calcium carbonate, bile acid sequestrants, iron, and sucralfate (Carafate) because these medications decrease the absorption of thyroid replacements.

B. Side/adverse effects
1. Nausea and decreased appetite
2. Abdominal cramps and diarrhea
3. Weight loss
4. Nervousness and tremors
5. Insomnia
6. Sweating
7. Heat intolerance (mild, side effect; extreme, adverse effect)
8. Tachycardia, dysrhythmias, palpitations, chest pain
9. Hypertension
10. Headache
11. Toxicity: **Hyperthyroidism**

C. Interventions
1. The client is assessed for a history of medications currently being taken.
2. Monitor vital signs.
3. Monitor weight.
4. Monitor triiodothyronine, thyroxine, and thyroid-stimulating hormone levels.
5. Reinforce instructions to the client to take the medication at the same time each day, in the morning without food.
6. Reinforce instructions to the client in how to monitor the pulse rate.
7. Reinforce instructions to the client to avoid foods that can inhibit thyroid secretion, such as strawberries, peaches, pears, cabbage, turnips, spinach, kale, Brussels sprouts, cauliflower, radishes, and peas.
8. The client is advised to avoid over-the-counter medications.
9. Reinforce instructions to the client to wear a Medic-Alert bracelet.

The client taking a thyroid hormone is instructed to report symptoms of hyperthyroidism, such as tachycardia, chest pain, palpitations, and excessive sweating. These indicate signs of toxicity.

IV. Antithyroid Medications (Box 46-3)

A. Description
1. Antithyroid medications inhibit the synthesis of thyroid hormone.
2. Antithyroid medications are used for hyperthyroidism, or Graves' disease.

B. Side/adverse effects
1. Nausea and vomiting
2. Diarrhea
3. Drowsiness, headache, fever
4. Hypersensitivity with skin rash

BOX 46-2 Thyroid Hormones

Levothyroxine sodium (Synthroid, Levothroid, Levoxyl, Unithroid)
Liothyronine sodium (Cytomel, Triostat)
Liotrix (Thyrolar)
Thyroid (Armour Thyroid, Nature-Thyroid, Thyroid USP, Westhroid)

BOX 46-3 Antithyroid Medications

Methimazole (Tapazole)
Propylthiouracil
Strong iodine solution (Lugol's solution)
Potassium iodide (SSKI)
Iodide-131 (Iodotope)

5. Agranulocytosis with leukopenia and thrombocytopenia
6. Alopecia and hyperpigmentation
7. Toxicity: Hypothyroidism
8. Iodism: Characterized by vomiting, abdominal pain, metallic or brassy taste in the mouth, rash, and sore gums and salivary glands

C. Interventions
1. Monitor vital signs.
2. Monitor triiodothyronine, thyroxine, and thyroid-stimulating hormone levels.
3. Monitor weight.
4. Reinforce instructions to the client to take medication with meals to avoid gastrointestinal upset.
5. Reinforce instructions to the client in how to monitor the pulse rate.
6. Reinforce instructions to the client of side/adverse effects and when to notify the health care provider (HCP).
7. Reinforce instructions to the client in the signs of hypothyroidism.
8. Reinforce instructions to the client regarding the importance of medication compliance and that abruptly stopping the medication could cause **thyroid storm**.
9. Reinforce instructions to the client to monitor for signs and symptoms of thyroid storm (fever, flushed skin, confusion and behavioral changes, tachycardia, dysrhythmias, and signs of heart failure).
10. Reinforce instructions to the client to monitor for signs of iodism.

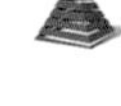

11. Reinforce instructions to the client to consult the HCP before eating iodized salt and iodine-rich foods.

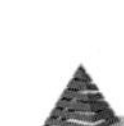

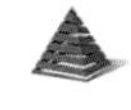

12. Reinforce instructions to the client to avoid acetylsalicylic acid (aspirin) and medications containing iodine.

Propylthiouracil causes agranulocytosis. Therefore, the client is advised to contact the HCP if a fever or sore throat develops.

V. Parathyroid Medications (Box 46-4)

A. Description
1. Parathyroid hormone regulates serum calcium levels.
2. Low serum levels of calcium stimulate parathyroid hormone release.
3. Hyperparathyroidism results in a high serum calcium level and bone demineralization; medication is used to lower the serum calcium level.
4. Hypoparathyroidism results in a low serum calcium level, which increases neuromuscular excitability; treatment includes calcium and vitamin D supplements.

BOX 46-4 Medications to Treat Calcium Disorders

Oral Calcium Supplements
Calcium acetate (PhosLo)
Calcium carbonate (Rolaids, Tums, others)
Calcium chloride
Calcium citrate (Citracal)
Calcium glubionate (Calcionate)
Calcium gluconate (Cal-Glu)
Calcium lactate (Cak-lac)
Tribasic calcium phosphate (Posture)

Vitamin D Supplements
Cholecalciferol (Vitamin D_3)
Ergocalciferol (Vitamin D_2)

Bisphosphonates and Calcium Regulators
Alendronate sodium (Fosamax)
Calcitonin salmon (Fortical, Miacalcin)
Etidronate disodium (Didronel)
Ibandronate (Boniva)
Pamidronate disodium
Risedronate sodium (Actonel)
Tiludronate disodium (Skelid)
Zoledronate (Reclast, Zometa)
Zoledronate (Zometa)

Medications to Treat Hypercalcemia
Cinacalcet hydrochloride (Sensipar)
Doxercalciferol (Hectorol)
Gallium nitrate (Ganite)
Paricalcitol (Zemplar)

5. Calcium salts administered with digoxin (Lanoxin) increase the risk of digoxin toxicity.
6. Oral calcium salts reduce the absorption of tetracycline hydrochloride.

B. Interventions
1. Monitor electrolyte and calcium levels.
2. Monitor for signs and symptoms of hypocalcemia and hypercalcemia.
3. Monitor for symptoms of tetany in the client with hypocalcemia.

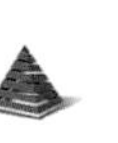

4. Monitor for renal calculi in the client with hypercalcemia.
5. Reinforce instructions to the client in the signs and symptoms of hypercalcemia and hypocalcemia.
6. Reinforce instructions to the client to check over-the-counter medication labels for the possibility of calcium content.
7. Reinforce instructions to the client receiving oral calcium supplements to maintain an adequate intake of vitamin D because vitamin D enhances absorption of calcium.

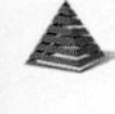

8. Reinforce instructions to the client receiving calcium regulators such as alendronate sodium (Fosamax) to swallow the tablet whole with water at least 30 minutes before breakfast and not to lie down for at least 30 minutes.
9. Reinforce instructions to the client using nasal spray of calcitonin (Miacalcin) to alternate nares.
10. Reinforce instructions to the client using antihypercalcemic agents to avoid foods rich in calcium such as green, leafy vegetables; dairy products; shellfish; and soy.
11. Reinforce instructions to the client not to take other medications within 1 hour of taking a calcium salt.
12. Reinforce instructions to the client to increase fluid and fiber in the diet to prevent constipation associated with calcium supplements.

VI. Corticosteroids (Mineralocorticoids)

A. Fludrocortisone acetate (Florinef)

B. Description
1. Mineralocorticoids are steroid hormones that enhance the reabsorption of sodium and chloride and promote the excretion of potassium and hydrogen from the renal tubules, thereby helping maintain fluid and electrolyte balance.
2. Mineralocorticoids are used for replacement therapy in primary and secondary adrenal insufficiency in **Addison's disease**.

C. Side effects/adverse effects
1. Sodium and water retention (hypernatremia and edema), hypertension
2. Hypokalemia
3. Hypocalcemia
4. Osteoporosis, compression fractures
5. Weight gain
6. Heart failure

D. Interventions
1. Monitor vital signs.
2. Monitor intake and output, weight, and for edema.
3. Monitor electrolyte and calcium levels.
4. The client is instructed to take medication with food or milk.
5. The client is instructed to consume a high-potassium diet.
6. The client is instructed to report illness, such as severe diarrhea, vomiting, and fever.
7. The client is instructed to notify the HCP if low blood pressure, weakness, cramping, palpitations, or changes in mental status occur.
8. The client is instructed to wear a Medic-Alert bracelet.

The client taking a corticosteroid is instructed not to stop the medication abruptly because this could result in adrenal insufficiency.

BOX 46-5 Corticosteroids: Glucocorticoids

Betamethasone
Cortisone acetate
Dexamethasone
Hydrocortisone
Methylprednisolone
Prednisolone
Prednisone
Triamcinolone

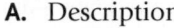

VII. Corticosteroids (Glucocorticoids) (Box 46-5)

A. Description
1. Glucocorticoids affect glucose, protein, and bone metabolism; alter the normal immune response and suppress inflammation; and produce anti-inflammatory, antiallergic, and antistress effects.
2. Glucocorticoids may be used as a replacement for adrenocortical insufficiency.

B. Side/adverse effects
1. Hyperglycemia
2. Hypokalemia
3. Hypocalcemia, osteoporosis
4. Sodium and fluid retention
5. Weight gain
6. Mood swings
7. Moon face, buffalo hump, truncal obesity
8. Increased susceptibility to infection and masking of the signs and symptoms of infection
9. Cataracts
10. Hirsutism, acne, fragile skin, bruising
11. Growth retardation in children
12. Gastrointestinal (GI) irritation, peptic ulcer, pancreatitis
13. Seizures, psychosis

C. Contraindications and cautions
1. Contraindicated in clients with hypersensitivity, psychosis, and fungal infections
2. Should be used with caution in clients with **diabetes mellitus**

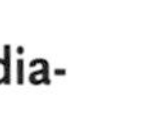

3. Used with extreme caution in clients with infections because they mask the signs and symptoms of an infection
4. Increase the potency of medications taken concurrently, such as aspirin, and nonsteroidal anti-inflammatory drugs, thus increasing the risk of gastrointestinal bleeding and ulceration.
5. Use of potassium-wasting diuretics increases potassium loss, resulting in hypokalemia.
6. Dexamethasone decreases the effects of orally administered anticoagulants and antidiabetic agents.
7. Barbiturates, phenytoin (Dilantin), and rifampin (Rifadin) decrease the effect of prednisone.

D. Interventions
1. Monitor vital signs.
2. Monitor serum electrolyte and blood glucose levels.

3. Monitor for hypokalemia and hyperglycemia.
4. Monitor intake and output, weight, and for edema.
5. Monitor for hypertension.
6. Check medical history for glaucoma, cataracts, peptic ulcer, mental health disorders, or diabetes mellitus.
7. Monitor the older client for signs and symptoms of increased osteoporosis.
8. Check for changes in muscle strength.
9. Prepare a schedule for the client with information on short-term tapered doses.
10. The client is instructed that it is best to take medication in the early morning with food or milk.
11. The client is advised to eat foods high in potassium.
12. The client is instructed to avoid individuals with respiratory infections.
13. The client is instructed to inform all HCPs of the medication regimen.
14. The client is instructed to report signs and symptoms of a medication overdose or **Cushing's syndrome**, including a moon face, puffy eyelids, edema in the feet, increased bruising, dizziness, bleeding, and menstrual irregularities.
15. Note that the client may need additional doses during periods of stress, such as surgery.
16. The client is instructed not to stop the medication abruptly because abrupt withdrawal can result in severe adrenal insufficiency.
17. The client is advised to consult with the HCP before receiving vaccinations.
18. The client is advised to wear a Medic-Alert bracelet.

VIII. Androgens (Box 46-6)

A. Description
1. Used to replace deficient hormones or to treat hormone-sensitive disorders
2. Can cause bleeding if the client is taking oral anticoagulants (increase the effect of anticoagulants)
3. Can cause decreased serum glucose concentration, thereby reducing insulin requirements in the client with diabetes mellitus
4. Hepatotoxic medications are avoided with the use of androgens because of the risk of additive damage to the liver.
5. Androgens usually are avoided in men with known prostate or breast carcinoma because androgens often stimulate growth of these tumors.

B. Side/adverse effects
1. Masculine secondary sexual characteristics (body hair growth, lowered voice, muscle growth)
2. Bladder irritation and urinary tract infections
3. Breast tenderness
4. Gynecomastia
5. Priapism
6. Menstrual irregularities
7. Virilism
8. Sodium and water retention with edema
9. Nausea, vomiting, or diarrhea
10. Acne
11. Changes in libido
12. Hepatotoxicity, jaundice
13. Hypercalcemia

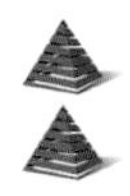

C. Interventions
1. Monitor vital signs.
2. Monitor for edema, weight gain, skin changes
3. Check mental status and neurological function.
4. Check for signs of liver dysfunction, including right upper quadrant abdominal pain, malaise, fever, jaundice, and pruritus.
5. Check for the development of secondary sexual characteristics.
6. The client is instructed to take medication with meals or a snack.
7. The client is instructed to notify the HCP if priapism develops.
8. The client is instructed to notify the HCP if fluid retention occurs.
9. Women are instructed to use a nonhormonal contraceptive while on therapy.
10. For women, monitor for menstrual irregularities and decreased breast size.

BOX 46-6 Androgens

Fluoxymesterone
Methyltestosterone (Testred)
Testosterone preparations:
- Testosterone, pellets (Testopel)
- Testosterone, transdermal (Androderm, AndroGel)
- Testosterone cypionate (Depo-Testosterone)
- Testosterone enanthate (Delatestryl)
- Testosterone (Striant)

IX. Estrogens and Progestins

A. Description
1. Estrogens are steroids that stimulate female reproductive tissue.
2. Progestins are steroids that specifically stimulate the uterine lining.
3. Estrogen and progestin preparations may be used to stimulate the endogenous hormones to restore hormonal balance, to treat hormone-sensitive tumors (suppress tumor growth), or for contraception (Boxes 46-7 and 46-8).

BOX 46-7 Estrogens

Esterified estrogens (Menest)
Estradiol (Estrace, Climara)
Estrogens, conjugated (Premarin, Cenestin, Enjuvia)
Ethinyl estradiol (Estinyl)

BOX 46-8 Progestins

Estradiol/drospirenone (Angelic)
Estradiol/norgestimate (Prefest)
Estradiol/norethindrone (Femhrt, Junel, Loestrin)
Estradiol/etonogestrel (NuvaRing)
Medroxyprogesterone acetate (Depo-Provera, Provera)
Medroxyprogesterone and conjugated estrogens (Premphase, Prempro)
Megestrol acetate (Megace)
Norethindrone acetate (Aygestin)
Norgestrel (Ovrette)
Progesterone (Prometrium)

B. Contraindications and cautions
1. Estrogens
   a. Estrogens are contraindicated in clients with breast cancer, endometrial hyperplasia, endometrial cancer, history of thromboembolism, known or suspected pregnancy, or lactation.
   b. Use estrogens with caution in clients with hypertension, gallbladder disease, or liver or kidney dysfunction.
   c. Estrogens increase the risk of toxicity when used with hepatotoxic medications.
   d. Barbiturates, phenytoin (Dilantin), and rifampin (Rifadin) decrease the effectiveness of estrogen.
2. Progestins are contraindicated in clients with thromboembolic disorders and should be avoided in clients with breast tumors or hepatic disease.

C. Side/adverse effects
1. Breast tenderness, menstrual changes
2. Nausea, vomiting, and diarrhea
3. Malaise, depression, excessive irritability
4. Weight gain
5. Edema and fluid retention
6. Atherosclerosis
7. Hypertension, stroke, myocardial infarction
8. Thromboembolism (estrogen)
9. Migraine headaches and vomiting (estrogen)

D. Interventions
1. Monitor vital signs.
2. Monitor for hypertension.
3. Check for edema and weight gain.
4. The client is advised not to smoke.
5. The client is advised to undergo routine breast and pelvic examinations.

X. Contraceptives

A. Description
1. These medications contain a combination of estrogen and a progestin or a progestin alone.
2. Estrogen-progestin combinations suppress ovulation and change the cervical mucus, making it difficult for sperm to enter.
3. Medications that contain only progestins are less effective than the combined medications.
4. Contraceptives usually are taken for 21 consecutive days and stopped for 7 days. The administration cycle is then repeated.

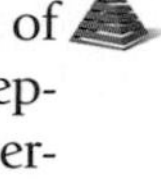

5. Contraceptives provide reversible prevention of pregnancy.
6. Contraceptives are useful in controlling irregular or excessive menstrual cycles.
7. Risk factors associated with the development of complications related to the use of contraceptives include smoking, obesity, and hypertension.

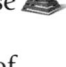

8. Contraceptives are contraindicated in women with hypertension, thromboembolic disease, cerebrovascular or coronary artery disease, estrogen-dependent cancers, and pregnancy.
9. Contraceptives should be avoided with the use of hepatotoxic medications.
10. Contraceptives interfere with the activity of bromocriptine mesylate (Parlodel) and anticoagulants and increase the toxicity of tricyclic antidepressants.
11. Contraceptives may alter blood glucose levels.

12. Antibiotics may decrease the absorption and effectiveness of oral contraceptives.

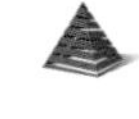

B. Side/adverse effects
1. Breakthrough bleeding
2. Excessive cervical mucus formation
3. Breast tenderness
4. Hypertension
5. Nausea, vomiting

C. Interventions
1. Monitor vital signs and weight.
2. Reinforce instructions to the client in the administration of the medication. (It may take up to 1 week for full contraceptive effect to occur when the medication is begun; the client should be instructed to use a barrier method during this time.)
3. Reinforce instructions to the client with diabetes mellitus to monitor blood glucose levels carefully.
4. The client is instructed to report signs of thromboembolic complications.
5. The client is instructed to notify the HCP if vaginal bleeding or menstrual irregularities occur or if pregnancy is suspected.
6. The client is instructed to use an alternate method of birth control when taking antibiotics because these may decrease absorption of the oral contraceptive.
7. The client is instructed to perform breast self-examination monthly and about the importance of annual physical examinations.
8. Contraceptive patches
   a. Designed to be worn for 3 weeks and removed for a 1-week period

b. Applied on clean, dry, intact skin on the buttocks, abdomen, upper outer arm, or upper torso
c. The client is instructed to peel away half of backing on patch, apply the sticky surface to the skin, remove the other half of the backing, and then press down on the patch with the palm for 10 seconds.
d. The client is instructed to change the patch weekly, using a new location for each patch.
e. If the patch falls off and remains off for less than 24 hours (such as when the client is sleeping or is unaware that it has fallen off), it can be reapplied if still sticky, or it can be replaced with a new patch.
f. If the patch is off for more than 24 hours, a new 4-week cycle must be started immediately.

9. Vaginal ring
    a. Inserted into the vagina by the client, left in place for 3 weeks, and removed for 1 week
    b. The medication is absorbed through mucous membranes of the vagina.
    c. Removed rings should be wrapped in a foil pouch and discarded, not flushed down the toilet.
10. Implants and depo injections provide long-acting forms of birth control, from 3 months to 5 years in duration.

If the client decides to discontinue the contraceptive to become pregnant, recommend that the client use an alternative form of birth control for 2 months after discontinuation to ensure more complete excretion of hormonal agents before conception.

XI. Fertility Medications (Box 46-9)

A. Description
1. Fertility medications act to stimulate follicle development and ovulation in functioning ovaries and are combined with human chorionic gonadotropin to maintain the follicles once ovulation has occurred.
2. Fertility medications are contraindicated in the presence of primary ovarian dysfunction, thyroid or adrenal dysfunction, ovarian cysts, pregnancy, or idiopathic uterine bleeding.

BOX 46-9 Fertility Medications

Chorionic gonadotropin (Novarel, Pregnyl)
Clomiphene citrate (Clomid, Serophene)
Follitropin alfa (Gonal-f)
Follitropin beta (Follistim AQ)
Menotropins (Repronex, Menopur)
Urofollitropin alfa (Bravelle)
Lutropin alfa (Luveris)

3. Fertility medications should be used with caution in clients with thromboembolic or respiratory disease.

B. Side/adverse effects
1. Risk of multiple births and birth defects
2. Ovarian overstimulation (abdominal pain, distention, ascites, pleural effusion)
3. Headache, irritability
4. Fluid retention and bloating
5. Nausea, vomiting
6. Uterine bleeding
7. Ovarian enlargement
8. Gynecomastia
9. Rash
10. Orthostatic hypotension
11. Febrile reactions

C. Interventions
1. The client is instructed regarding administration of the medication.
2. A calendar of treatment days and instructions on when intercourse should occur are provided to increase therapeutic effectiveness of the medication.
3. Information about the risks and hazards of multiple births is provided.
4. The client is instructed to notify the HCP if signs of ovarian overstimulation occur.
5. The client is instructed about the need for regular follow-up for evaluation.

XII. Medications for Erectile Dysfunction

A. Description
1. Alprostadil (Caverject, Edex, Muse) is a prostaglandin that relaxes smooth muscle and promotes blood flow when injected directly into the corpus cavernosum.
2. Sildenafil (Viagra), tadalafil (Cialis), and vardenafil (Levitra) cause smooth muscle relaxation and allow blood flow into the corpus cavernosum.

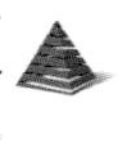
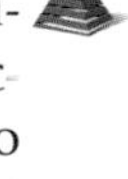
3. Erectile dysfunction medications are contraindicated in the presence of any anatomical obstruction or condition that might predispose to priapism and in clients with penile implants.
4. Caution should be used in clients with bleeding disorders.
5. Sildenafil, tadalafil, and vardenafil are used cautiously in clients with coronary artery disease, active peptic ulcer disease, bleeding disorders, or retinitis pigmentosa.
6. Sildenafil, tadalafil, and vardenafil cannot be administered to clients taking nitrates, nitroprusside, or β-blockers (risk of severe hypotension).

B. Side/adverse effects
1. Alprostadil: Pain at the injection site, infection, priapism, fibrosis, rash
2. Sildenafil, tadalafil, and vardenafil: Headache, flushing, dyspepsia, urinary tract infection,

diarrhea, hypotension, dizziness, rash, neuralgia, insomnia

3. Blurred vision and changes in color vision

C. Interventions

1. A thorough assessment of health and medication history is performed.
2. The client is instructed regarding administration of the medication. Alprostadil is injected intracavernously. Sildenafil, tadalafil, and vardenafil are taken orally.
3. The client is informed of side/adverse effects necessitating the need to notify the HCP.

XIII. Medications for Diabetes Mellitus

A. Insulin and oral hypoglycemic medications

1. Description
   a. Insulin increases glucose transport into cells and promotes conversion of glucose to glycogen, decreasing serum glucose levels.
   b. Oral hypoglycemic agents stimulate the pancreas to produce more insulin, increase the sensitivity of peripheral receptors to insulin, decrease hepatic glucose output, or delay intestinal absorption of glucose, thus decreasing serum glucose levels.
2. Contraindications and concerns
   a. Insulin is contraindicated in clients with hypersensitivity.
   b. Oral hypoglycemic agents are contraindicated in type 1 diabetes mellitus.

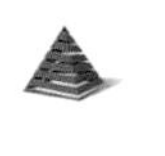

   c. β-Adrenergic blocking agents may mask signs and symptoms of **hypoglycemia** associated with hypoglycemic medications.
   d. Anticoagulants, chloramphenicol (Chloromycetin), salicylates, propranolol (Inderal), monoamine oxidase inhibitors, pentamidine (Pentam 300, Nebupent), and sulfonamides may cause hypoglycemia.

   e. Corticosteroids, sympathomimetics, thiazide diuretics, phenytoin (Dilantin), thyroid preparations, oral contraceptives, and estrogen compounds may cause hyperglycemia.

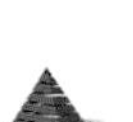

   f. Side/adverse effects of the sulfonylureas include gastrointestinal symptoms and dermatological reactions; hypoglycemia can occur when an excessive dose is administered or when meals are omitted or delayed, food intake is decreased, or activity is increased.

⚠ Sulfonylureas can cause a disulfiram (Antabuse) type of reaction when alcohol is ingested.

B. Oral hypoglycemic medications

1. Prescribed for clients with type 2 diabetes mellitus
2. Sulfonylureas (Box 46-10)
   a. Sulfonylureas may be classified as first- or second-generation sulfonylureas.

BOX 46-10 Sulfonylureas and Nonsulfonylureas

Sulfonylureas
Chlorpropamide
Glimepiride (Amaryl)
Glipizide (Glucotrol)
Glyburide (DiaBeta, Micronase)
Tolazamide (Tolinase)
Tolbutamide

Biguanide
Metformin (Glucophage)

Alpha Glucosidase Inhibitors
Acarbose (Precose)
Miglitol (Glyset)

Thiazolidinediones
Pioglitazone (Actos)
Rosiglitazone (Avandia)

Meglitinides
Nateglinide (Starlix)
Repaglinide (Prandin)

Gliptins
Alogliptin (Nesina)
Alogliptin and pioglitazone (Oseni)
Linagliptin (Tradjenta)
Saxagliptin (Onglyza)
Sitagliptin (Januvia)
Metformin and alogliptin (Kazano)
Metformin and linagliptin (Jentadueto)
Metformin and saxagliptin (Kombiglyze XR)
Metformin and sitagliptin (Janumet)

   b. Sulfonylureas stimulate the beta cells to produce more insulin.
3. Biguanides (see Box 46-10)
   a. May be used alone or in combination with a sulfonylurea
   b. Suppresses hepatic production of glucose and increases insulin sensitivity
   c. Side/adverse effects: Diarrhea (most common), lactic acidosis (most serious)
4. Alpha-glucosidase inhibitors (see Box 46-10)
   a. Delay absorption of ingested carbohydrates (sucrose and complex carbohydrates), resulting in smaller increase in blood glucose level after meals
   b. Do not increase insulin production
   c. Can be given alone or in combination with sulfonylureas
   d. Will not cause hypoglycemia when given alone
   e. Given with first bite of meal
5. Thiazolidinediones (see Box 46-10)
   a. Insulin-sensitizing agents that lower blood glucose by decreasing hepatic glucose production

and improving target cell response to insulin
b. May cause liver toxicity
6. Meglitinides (see Box 46-10)
a. Stimulate pancreatic insulin secretion
b. Quicker and shorter duration of action; therefore, less chance of hypoglycemia because blood glucose-lowering effect wears off quickly
c. Very fast onset of action allows client to take the medication with meals and skip a dose when a meal is skipped.
7. Interventions
a. The client's knowledge of diabetes mellitus and the use of oral antidiabetic agents are assessed.
b. A medication history regarding the medications that the client is taking currently is obtained.
c. Monitor vital signs and blood glucose levels.
d. Reinforce instructions to the client to recognize the signs and symptoms of hypoglycemia and hyperglycemia.
e. Reinforce instructions to the client to avoid over-the-counter medications unless prescribed by the HCP.
f. Reinforce instructions to the client not to ingest alcohol with sulfonylureas.
g. Reinforce instructions to the client that insulin may be needed during stress, surgery, or infection.
h. Reinforce instructions to the client in the necessity of compliance with prescribed medication.
i. Reinforce instructions to the client in how to take each specific medication, such as with the first bite of the meal for meglitinides and alpha-glucosidase inhibitors.
j. Reinforce instructions to the client to wear a Medic-Alert bracelet.

Metformin (Glucophage) may need to be withheld temporarily before and for 48 hours after any radiologic study that involves the administration of intravenous contrast dye because of the risk of contrast-induced nephropathy and lactic acidosis. The HCP needs to be consulted for specific prescriptions.

C. Insulin
1. Insulin primarily acts in the liver, muscle, and adipose tissue by attaching to receptors on cellular membranes and facilitating the passage of glucose, potassium, and magnesium.
2. Insulin is prescribed for clients with type 1 diabetes mellitus and type 2 diabetes mellitus in clients whose blood glucose level is not controlled with oral hypoglycemic agents.
3. The onset, peak, and duration of action depend on the insulin type (Table 46-1).
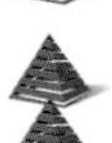
4. Storing of insulin (Box 46-11)
5. Insulin injection sites
a. The main areas for injections are the abdomen, arms (posterior surface), thighs (anterior surface), and hips (Fig. 46-1).
b. Insulin injected into the abdomen may absorb more evenly and rapidly than at other sites.
c. Systematic rotation within one anatomical area is recommended to prevent lipodystrophy; client should be instructed not to use the same site more than once in a 2- to 3-week period.
d. Injections should be 1½ inches apart within the anatomical area.
e. Heat, massage, and exercise of the injected area can increase absorption rates and may result in hypoglycemia.
f. Injection into scar tissue may delay absorption of insulin.
6. Administering insulin

Insulin glargine (Lantus) and insulin detemir (Levemir) cannot be mixed with any other types of insulin.

a. To prevent dosage errors, be certain that there is a match between the insulin concentration noted on the vial and the calibration of units on the insulin syringe. The usual concentration of insulin is U 100 (100 units/mL).
b. Most insulin syringes have a 27- to 29-gauge needle that is about ½ inch long.
c. Before use, swirl the insulin vial gently or rotate between palms to ensure that the insulin and ingredients are mixed well; otherwise, an inaccurate dose will be drawn; vigorously shaking the bottle will cause bubbles to form.
d. Premixed insulins (NPH and regular insulin; insulin aspart protamine and insulin aspart) are available as 70/30 (most commonly used), and premixed insulin lispro protamine and insulin lispro 75/25 and 50/50 are also available.

e. Inject air into the insulin bottle. (A vacuum makes it difficult to draw up the insulin.)
f. When mixing insulins, draw up the shortest-acting insulin first (Fig. 46-2).
g. Short-acting (i.e., regular, lispro, aspart, and glulisine) insulin may be mixed with NPH.
h. Lispro insulin may be mixed with Humulin N.
i. Insulin aspart protamine (Novolog Mix 70/30) may be mixed with NPH insulin only.
j. A mixed dose of insulin is administered within 5 to 15 minutes of preparation; after
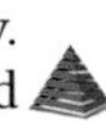

TABLE 46-1 Time Activity of Pharmacological Insulin*

Preparation	Brand	Onset (hr)	Peak (hr)	Duration (hr)
Rapid-Acting Insulin				
Insulin aspart	NovoLog	0.25	1–3	3–5
Insulin glulisine	Apidra	0.3	0.5–1.5	3–4
Human lispro injection	Humalog	0.25	0.5–1.5	5
Short-Acting Insulin				
Regular human insulin injection	Humulin R	0.5	2–4	5–7
	Novolin R	0.5	2.5–5	8
	ReliOn R			
Humulin R (concentrated U-500)	Humulin R (U-500)	1.5	4–12	24
Intermediate-Acting Insulin				
Isophane insulin NPH injection	Humulin N	1.5	4–12	16–24+
	Novolin N	1.5	4–12	16–24+
	ReliOn N			
Insulin detemir injection	Levemir	1	6–8	5.7–24
70% human insulin isophane suspension/30% human insulin injection	Humulin 70/30	0.5	2–12	24
	Novolin 70/30			
	ReliOn 70/30			
50% human insulin isophane suspension/50% human insulin injection	Humulin 50/50	0.5	3–5	24
70% insulin aspart protamine suspension/30% insulin aspart injection	NovoLog Mix 70/30	0.25	1–4	24
75% insulin lispro protamine suspension/25% insulin lispro injection	Humalog Mix 75/25	0.25	1–2	24
Long-Acting Insulin				
Insulin glargine injection	Lantus	2–4	None	24

*Time activity may be dose related.
From Ignatavicius D, Workman M: *Medical-surgical nursing: Patient-centered collaborative care*, ed 7, St. Louis, 2013, Saunders.

this time, the short-acting insulin binds with the NPH insulin and its action is reduced.

k. Aspiration after insertion of the needle is generally not recommended with self-injection of insulin.

l. Insulin is administered at a 45- to 90-degree angle in clients with normal subcutaneous mass and at a 45- to 60-degree angle in thin persons or those with a decreased amount of subcutaneous mass.

BOX 46-11 Storing Insulin

- Avoid exposing insulin to extremes in temperature.
- Insulin should not be frozen or kept in direct sunlight or a hot car.
- Before injection, insulin should be at room temperature.
- If a vial of insulin will be used up in 1 month, it may be kept at room temperature; otherwise, the vial should be refrigerated.

Rapid- and short-acting insulins are the only types of insulin that can be administered intravenously.

D. Exenatide (Byetta)

1. A synthetic hormone classified as an incretin mimetic that is administered subcutaneously
2. Used for clients with type 2 diabetes mellitus (not recommended for clients taking insulin, nor should clients be taken off of insulin and given exenatide)
3. Restores first-phase insulin response (first 10 minutes after food ingestion), lowers the production of glucagon after meals, slows gastric emptying (which limits the rise in the blood

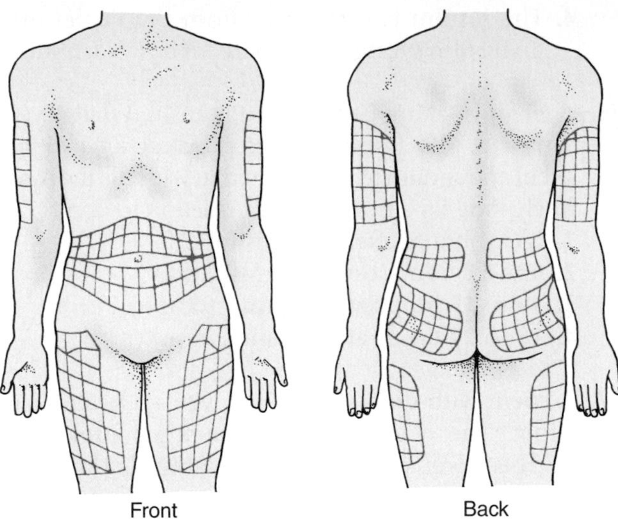

FIGURE 46-1 Common insulin injection sites. (From Ignatavicius D, Workman M: *Medical-surgical nursing: Patient-centered collaborative care*, ed 7, St. Louis, 2013, Saunders.)

1 Wash hands.
2 Gently rotate NPH insulin bottle.
3 Wipe off tops of insulin vials with alcohol sponge.
4 Draw back amount of air into the syringe that equals total dose.
5 Inject air equal to NPH dose into NPH vial. Remove syringe from vial.
6 Inject air equal to regular dose into regular vial.

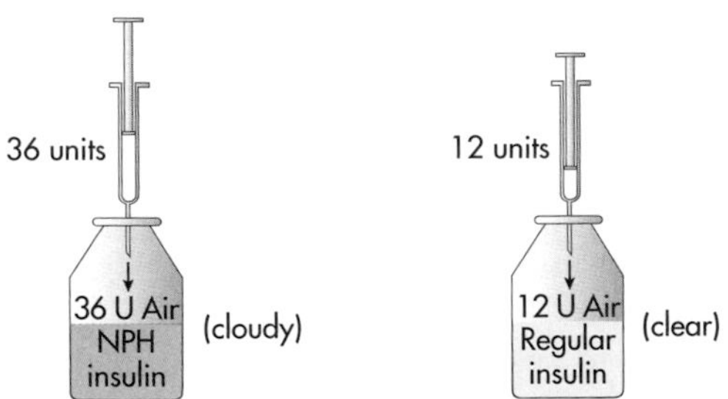

7 Invert regular insulin bottle and withdraw regular insulin dose.
8 Without adding more air to NPH vial, carefully withdraw NPH dose and add to regular insulin already in syringe.

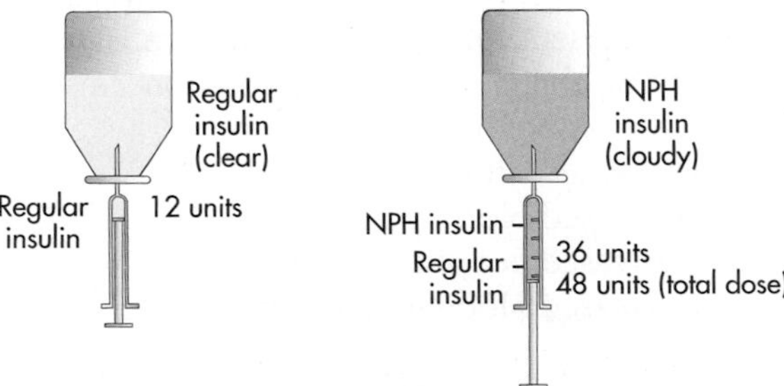

FIGURE 46-2 Steps for mixing insulins. (From Lewis S, Heitkemper M, Dirksen S: *Medical-surgical nursing: Assessment and management of clinical problems*, ed 8, St. Louis, 2011, Mosby.)

glucose level after a meal), reduces fasting and postprandial blood glucose levels, and reduces caloric intake, resulting in weight loss

4. Packaged in premeasured doses (pen) that require refrigeration (cannot be frozen)
5. Administered as a subcutaneous injection in the thigh, abdomen, or upper arm within 60 minutes before morning and evening meals; not taken after meals; if a dose is missed, the treatment regimen is resumed as prescribed with the next scheduled dose.
6. Can cause mild to moderate nausea that abates with use

E. Glucagon (also available as GlucaGen)
1. Hormone secreted by the alpha cells of the islets of Langerhans in the pancreas
2. Increases blood glucose level by stimulating glycogenolysis in the liver
3. Can be administered subcutaneously, intramuscularly, or intravenously
4. Used to treat insulin-induced hypoglycemia when the client is semiconscious or unconscious and is unable to ingest liquids
5. The blood glucose level begins to increase within 5 to 20 minutes after administration.
6. The family is instructed in the procedure for administration.
7. See Chapter 45 for additional information regarding interventions for severe hypoglycemia.

CRITICAL THINKING What Should You Do?

Answer: The nurse needs to notify the registered nurse that the client is taking metformin. The client will need to temporarily discontinue the metformin a day or two before the CT scan and for 48 hours after the scan. Intravenous contrast that contains iodine poses a risk for contrast-induced nephropathy and lactic acidosis. The serum creatinine level is checked prior to giving intravenous contrast, and it may also be checked before allowing the client to resume the medication. Health care provider prescriptions and agency procedures are followed regarding timelines for discontinuing the medication.

Reference(s): deWit, D. & Kumagai, C. (2013). *Medical-surgical nursing: Concepts & practice.* (2nd ed., pp. 459, 862–863). St. Louis: Saunders.

PRACTICE QUESTIONS

461. The nurse is reinforcing teaching for a client regarding how to mix regular insulin and NPH insulin in the same syringe. Which action performed by the client indicates the **need for further teaching**?
1. Withdraws the NPH insulin first
2. Withdraws the regular insulin first
3. Injects air into NPH insulin vial first
4. Injects an amount of air equal to the desired dose of insulin into the vial

462. The home care nurse visits a client recently diagnosed with diabetes mellitus who is taking Humulin NPH insulin daily. The client asks the nurse how to store the unopened vials of insulin. The nurse should provide which information?

1. Freeze the insulin.
2. Refrigerate the insulin.
3. Store the insulin in a dark, dry place.
4. Keep the insulin at room temperature.

❖ **463.** The home care nurse is visiting a client who was recently diagnosed with type 2 diabetes mellitus. The client is prescribed repaglinide (Prandin) and metformin (Glucophage) and asks the nurse to explain these medications. The nurse should reinforce which instructions to the client? **Select all that apply.**

❑ 1. Diarrhea can occur secondary to the metformin.
❑ 2. The repaglinide is not taken if a meal is skipped.
❑ 3. The repaglinide is taken 30 minutes before eating.
❑ 4. Candy or another simple sugar is carried and used to treat mild hypoglycemia episodes.
❑ 5. Metformin increases hepatic glucose production to prevent hypoglycemia associated with repaglinide.
❑ 6. Muscle pain is an expected side effect of metformin and may be treated with acetaminophen (Tylenol).

❖ **464.** The nurse is monitoring a client receiving levothyroxine sodium (Synthroid) for hypothyroidism. Which findings indicate the presence of a side effect associated with this medication? **Select all that apply.**

❑ 1. Insomnia
❑ 2. Weight loss
❑ 3. Bradycardia
❑ 4. Constipation
❑ 5. Mild heat intolerance

465. The health care provider (HCP) prescribes exenatide (Byetta) for a client with type 1 diabetes mellitus who takes insulin. The nurse knows that which is the **most appropriate** intervention?

1. The medication is administered within 60 minutes before the morning and evening meal.
2. The medication is withheld and the HCP is called to question the prescription for the client.
3. The client is monitored for gastrointestinal side effects after administration of the medication.
4. The insulin is withdrawn from the Penlet into an insulin syringe to prepare for administration.

466. A client is taking Humulin NPH insulin daily every morning. The nurse reinforces instructions to the client and should tell the client that which is the **most likely** time for a hypoglycemic reaction to occur?

1. 2 to 4 hours after administration
2. 4 to 12 hours after administration
3. 16 to 18 hours after administration
4. 18 to 24 hours after administration

467. A client with diabetes mellitus visits a health care clinic. The client's diabetes mellitus previously had been well controlled with glyburide (DiaBeta) daily, but recently the fasting blood glucose level has been 180 to 200 mg/dL. Which medication, added to the client's regimen, may have contributed to the hyperglycemia?

1. Prednisone
2. Phenelzine (Nardil)
3. Atenolol (Tenormin)
4. Allopurinol (Zyloprim)

468. The community health nurse visits a client at home who has been prescribed prednisone 5 mg orally daily. The nurse reinforces teaching for the client about the medication. Which statement made by the client indicates a **need for further teaching**?

1. "I can take aspirin or my antihistamine if I need it."
2. "I need to take the medication every day at the same time."
3. "I need to avoid coffee, tea, cola, and chocolate in my diet."
4. "If I gain more than 5 pounds a week, I will call my doctor."

469. Desmopressin acetate (DDAVP) is prescribed for the treatment of diabetes insipidus. The nurse monitors the client after medication administration for which therapeutic response?

1. Decreased urinary output
2. Decreased blood pressure
3. Decreased peripheral edema
4. Decreased blood glucose level

470. Glimepiride (Amaryl) is prescribed for a client with diabetes mellitus. The nurse reinforces instructions for the client and tells the client to avoid which while taking this medication?

1. Alcohol
2. Organ meats
3. Whole-grain cereals
4. Carbonated beverages

ANSWERS

461. 1

Rationale: When preparing a mixture of regular insulin with another insulin preparation, the regular insulin is drawn into the syringe first. This sequence will avoid contaminating the vial of regular insulin with insulin of another type. Options 2, 3, and 4 identify the correct actions for preparing NPH and regular insulin.
Test-Taking Strategy: Note the strategic words, *need for further teaching*. These words indicate a negative event query and ask you to select an option that is an incorrect action. Remember *RN*—draw up the ***R***egular insulin before the ***N***PH insulin. **Review:** **mixing insulins**.
Level of Cognitive Ability: Evaluating
Client Needs: Physiological Integrity
Integrated Process: Teaching and Learning
Content Area: Pharmacology: Endocrine Medications
Priority Concepts: Client Education, Glucose Regulation
Reference(s): deWit, Kumagai (2013), p. 864; Lilley et al (2014), pp. 516, 528.

462. 2

Rationale: Insulin in unopened vials should be stored under refrigeration until needed. Vials should not be frozen because freezing affects the chemical composition of the insulin. When stored unopened under refrigeration, insulin can be used up to the expiration date on the vial. Freezing insulin, storing insulin in a dark, dry place and keeping the insulin at room temperature are all incorrect actions.
Test-Taking Strategy: Focus on the subject, how to store unopened vials of insulin. Remembering that insulin should not be frozen will assist in eliminating this option. The options for storing insulin at room temperature or in a dark, dry place are comparable or alike and should be eliminated. **Review:** client teaching points related to **storing insulin**.
Level of Cognitive Ability: Applying
Client Needs: Physiological Integrity
Integrated Process: Teaching and Learning
Content Area: Pharmacology: Endocrine Medications
Priority Concepts: Client Education, Glucose Regulation
Reference(s): Lilley et al (2014), pp. 527–528.

❖ **463. 1, 2, 3, 4**

Rationale: Repaglinide is a rapid-acting oral hypoglycemic agent that stimulates pancreatic insulin secretion that should be taken before meals and that should be withheld if the client does not eat. Hypoglycemia is a side effect of repaglinide, and the client should always be prepared by carrying a simple sugar with her or him at all times. Metformin is an oral hypoglycemic given in combination with repaglinide and works by decreasing hepatic glucose production. A common side effect of metformin is diarrhea. Muscle pain may occur as an adverse effect from metformin but it might signify a more serious condition that warrants health care provider notification, not the use of acetaminophen.
Test-Taking Strategy: Focus on the subject, client teaching points related to repaglinide and metformin. Also focus on the data in the question and the client's diagnosis to assist in answering the question. Recalling the actions and effects of these medications will assist in answering correctly. **Review:** **repaglinide and metformin**.
Level of Cognitive Ability: Analyzing
Client Needs: Physiological Integrity
Integrated Process: Nursing Process/Implementation
Content Area: Pharmacology: Endocrine Medications
Priority Concepts: Client Education, Glucose Regulation
Reference(s): Lehne (2013), pp. 735, 737.

❖ **464. 1, 2, 5**

Rationale: Insomnia, weight loss, and mild heat intolerance are side effects of levothyroxine sodium. Bradycardia and constipation are not side effects associated with this medication, but rather are associated with hypothyroidism, which is the disorder that this medication is prescribed to treat.
Test-Taking Strategy: Focus on the subject, side effects of levothyroxine. Thinking about the pathophysiology of hypothyroidism and the action of the medication will assist you in determining that insomnia, weight loss, and mild heat intolerance are side effects of thyroid hormones. **Review:** **levothyroxine sodium (Synthroid)**.
Level of Cognitive Ability: Analyzing
Client Needs: Physiological Integrity
Integrated Process: Nursing Process/Data Collection
Content Area: Pharmacology: Endocrine Medications
Priority Concepts: Clinical Judgment, Safety
Reference(s): Lehne (2013), pp. 747–748.

465. 2

Rationale: Exenatide (Byetta) is an incretin mimetic used for type 2 diabetes mellitus only. It is not recommended for clients taking insulin. Hence, the nurse should hold the medication and question the HCP regarding this prescription. Although options 1 and 3 are correct statements about the medication, in this situation the medication should not be administered. The medication is packaged in prefilled pens ready for injection without the need for drawing it up into another syringe.
Test-Taking Strategy: Focus on the subject, type 1 diabetes and exenatide, and note the strategic words, *most appropriate*. Eliminate the option regarding drawing up the medication because the medication is packaged in prefilled pens ready for injection without the need for drawing it up into another syringe. From the remaining options, focus on the data in the question. Although the other options are appropriate when administering this medication, this client should not receive the medication. **Review:** type 1 diabetes and **exanatide**.
Level of Cognitive Ability: Applying
Client Needs: Physiological Integrity
Integrated Process: Nursing Process/Planning
Content Area: Pharmacology: Endocrine Medications
Priority Concepts: Glucose Regulation, Health Promotion
Reference(s): Lehne (2013), p. 728.

466. 2

Rationale: Humulin NPH is an intermediate-acting insulin. The onset of action is 1.5 hours, it peaks in 4 to 12 hours, and its duration of action is 24 hours. Hypoglycemic reactions most likely occur during peak time.
Test-Taking Strategy: Note the strategic words, *most likely*, and focus on the subject, peak time of NPH insulin. Use knowledge regarding the onset, peak, and duration of action for NPH insulin. Remember that NPH peaks in 4 to 12 hours. **Review:** the characteristics of **NPH insulin**.

Level of Cognitive Ability: Applying
Client Needs: Physiological Integrity
Integrated Process: Teaching and Learning
Content Area: Pharmacology: Endocrine Medications
Priority Concepts: Client Education, Glucose Regulation
Reference(s): Hodgson, Kizior (2014), p. 613; Lehne (2013), p. 712.

467. 1
Rationale: Prednisone may decrease the effect of oral hypoglycemics, insulin, diuretics, and potassium supplements. Option 2, a monoamine oxidase inhibitor, and option 3, a β-blocker, have their own intrinsic hypoglycemic activity. Option 4 decreases urinary excretion of sulfonylurea agents, causing increased levels of the oral agents, which can lead to hypoglycemia.
Test-Taking Strategy: Focus on the **subject**, medications that cause an increase in the blood glucose level. Recalling that prednisone decreases the effects of oral hypoglycemics will direct you to the correct option. **Review:** medication interactions with **oral hypoglycemic medications.**
Level of Cognitive Ability: Analyzing
Client Needs: Physiological Integrity
Integrated Process: Nursing Process/Data Collection
Content Area: Pharmacology: Endocrine Medications
Priority Concepts: Clinical Judgment, Glucose Regulation
Reference(s): Hodgson, Kizior (2014), pp. 977–978.

468. 1
Rationale: Aspirin and other over-the-counter medications should not be taken unless the client consults with the health care provider (HCP). The client needs to take the medication at the same time every day and should be instructed not to stop the medication. A slight weight gain as a result of an improved appetite is expected, but after the dosage is stabilized, a weight gain of 5 lb or more weekly should be reported to the HCP. Caffeine-containing foods and fluids need to be avoided because they may contribute to steroid-ulcer development.
Test-Taking Strategy: Note the **strategic words**, *need for further teaching.* This indicates a **negative event query** and a need to select the incorrect statement as the answer. Remember that a client should not take other medications, especially over-the-counter medications, without first consulting with his or her HCP. **Review:** teaching points for the client taking **prednisone.**
Level of Cognitive Ability: Evaluating
Client Needs: Physiological Integrity
Integrated Process: Teaching and Learning
Content Area: Pharmacology: Endocrine Medications
Priority Concepts: Client Education, Safety
Reference(s): Lehne (2013), pp. 917–918.

469. 1
Rationale: Desmopressin promotes renal conservation of water. The hormone carries out this action by acting on the collecting ducts of the kidney to increase their permeability to water, which results in increased water reabsorption. The therapeutic effect of this medication would be manifested by a decreased urine output. Options 2, 3, and 4 are unrelated to the effects of this medication.
Test-Taking Strategy: Note the **subject**, therapeutic response of DDAVP. Focus on the diagnosis in the question to assist in answering the question. Recalling the signs and symptoms related to the loss of large volumes of urine in this disorder will help direct you to the option describing decreased urine output. **Review:** **diabetes insipidus** and the action of **desmopressin.**
Level of Cognitive Ability: Evaluating
Client Needs: Physiological Integrity
Integrated Process: Nursing Process/Evaluation
Content Area: Pharmacology: Endocrine Medications
Priority Concepts: Clinical Judgment, Safety
Reference(s): Lehne (2013), pp. 758–759.

470. 1
Rationale: When alcohol is combined with glimepiride (Amaryl), a disulfiram-like reaction may occur. This syndrome includes flushing, palpitations, and nausea. Alcohol can also potentiate the hypoglycemic effects of the medication. Clients need to be instructed to avoid alcohol consumption while taking this medication. The items in options 2, 3, and 4 do not need to be avoided.
Test-Taking Strategy: Focus on the **subject**, the substance to avoid. Eliminate organ meats, whole-grain cereals, and carbonated beverages because these food items are allowed in a diabetic diet. Remembering that alcohol can affect the action of many medications will assist in directing you to the correct option. **Review:** interactions with **glimepiride.**
Level of Cognitive Ability: Applying
Client Needs: Physiological Integrity
Integrated Process: Teaching and Learning
Content Area: Pharmacology: Endocrine Medications
Priority Concepts: Client Education, Glucose Regulation
Reference(s): Hodgson, Kizior (2014), p. 542.

UNIT XI

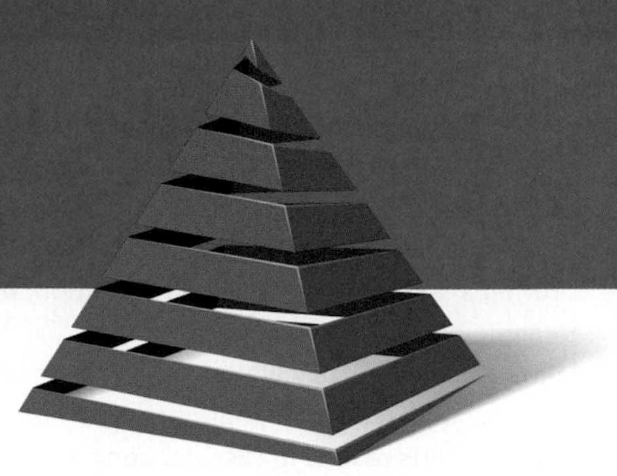

The Adult Client with a Gastrointestinal Disorder

PYRAMID TERMS

ascites The accumulation of fluid within the peritoneal cavity that results from venous congestion of the hepatic capillaries, which leads to plasma leaking directly from the liver surface and portal vein.

asterixis A coarse tremor characterized by rapid, nonrhythmic extensions and flexions in the wrist and fingers; also termed liver flap.

Billroth I Partial gastrectomy, with the remaining segment being anastomosed to the duodenum; also termed gastroduodenostomy.

Billroth II Partial gastrectomy, with the remaining segment being anastomosed to the jejunum; also termed gastrojejunosotomy.

cholecystectomy Removal of the gallbladder.

cholecystitis An inflammation of the gallbladder that may occur as an acute or chronic process. Acute inflammation is associated with gallstones (cholelithiasis). Chronic cholecystitis results when inefficient bile emptying and gallbladder muscle wall disease cause a fibrotic and contracted gallbladder.

choledocholithotomy Incision into the common bile duct to remove a gallstone.

cirrhosis A chronic progressive disease of the liver characterized by diffuse degeneration and destruction of hepatocytes. Repeated destruction of hepatic cells causes the formation of scar tissue.

Crohn's disease An inflammatory disease that can occur anywhere in the gastrointestinal tract but most often affects the terminal ileum; leads to thickening and scarring, a narrowed lumen, fistulas, ulcerations, and abscesses. The disease is characterized by remissions and exacerbations.

Cullen's sign Bluish discoloration of the abdomen and periumbilical area seen in acute hemorrhagic pancreatitis.

diverticulitis Inflammation of one or more diverticula from penetration of fecal matter through the thin-walled diverticula, resulting in local abscess formation. A perforated diverticulum can progress to intraabdominal perforation with generalized peritonitis.

diverticulosis Outpouchings or herniations of the intestinal mucosa that can occur in any part of the intestine but are most common in the sigmoid colon.

dumping syndrome Rapid emptying of the gastric contents into the small intestine, which occurs following gastric resection.

esophageal varices Dilated and tortuous veins in the submucosa of the esophagus caused by portal hypertension, often associated with liver cirrhosis; at high risk for rupture if portal circulation pressure rises.

fetor hepaticus The fruity, musty breath odor associated with severe chronic liver disease.

gastrectomy Removal of the stomach with attachment of the esophagus to the jejunum or duodenum; also termed esophagojejunostomy or esophagoduodenostomy.

gastric resection Removal of the lower half of the stomach, usually including a vagotomy; also termed antrectomy.

hepatitis Inflammation of the liver caused by a virus, bacteria, or exposure to medications or hepatotoxins.

hiatal hernia A portion of the stomach that herniates through the diaphragm and into the thorax. Herniation results from weakening of the muscles of the diaphragm and is aggravated by factors that increase abdominal pressure, such as pregnancy, ascites, obesity, tumors, heavy lifting; also termed esophageal or diaphragmatic hernia.

melena Black, tarry stools as a result of bleeding in the upper gastrointestinal tract.

Murphy's sign A sign of gallbladder disease consisting of pain on taking a deep breath when the examiner's fingers are on the approximate location of the gallbladder.

pancreatitis An acute or chronic inflammation of the pancreas, with associated escape of pancreatic enzymes into surrounding tissue. Acute pancreatitis can occur suddenly as one attack or can be recurrent with resolution. Chronic pancreatitis is a continual inflammation and destruction of the pancreas, with scar tissue replacing pancreatic tissue.

peristalsis Wavelike rhythmic contractions that propel material through the gastrointestinal tract.

portal hypertension A persistent increase in pressure within the portal vein that develops as a result of obstruction to flow.

pyloroplasty Enlarging the pylorus to prevent or decrease pyloric obstruction, thereby enhancing gastric emptying.

Turner's sign A gray-blue discoloration of the flanks seen in acute hemorrhagic pancreatitis.

ulcerative colitis Ulcerative and inflammatory disease of the bowel that results in poor absorption of nutrients. Acute ulcerative colitis results in vascular congestion, hemorrhage, edema, and ulceration of the bowel mucosa. Chronic ulcerative colitis causes muscular hypertrophy, fat deposits, and fibrous tissue with bowel thickening, shortening, and narrowing.

vagotomy Surgical division of the vagus nerve to eliminate the vagal impulses that stimulate hydrochloric acid secretion in the stomach.

Pyramid to Success

Pyramid points focus on diagnostic tests and nursing care related to the various gastric or intestinal tubes, gastric surgery, cirrhosis, hepatitis, pancreatitis, and colostomy care. Focus on preprocedure and postprocedure care of the client undergoing a gastrointestinal diagnostic test. Remember that an informed consent is required for any invasive procedure. Focus on diet restrictions before and after the diagnostic test, and remember that the gag reflex or bowel sounds must return before allowing a client to consume food or fluids. Pyramid points also include reinforcing instructions to the client and family regarding the prevention of gastrointestinal disorders and the complications associated with the disorder. Focus on reinforcing client and family teaching about diet and nutrition specific to the disorder, tube and wound care, preventing the transmission of infection such as with hepatitis, and care of a colostomy or ileostomy. Remember that body image disturbances can occur in clients with a gastrointestinal disorder. Specific focus relates to the client with a diversion, such as an ileostomy or colostomy; the social isolation issues that can occur; and effective coping strategies.

Client Needs

Safe and Effective Care Environment

Assisting the registered nurse (RN) in obtaining referrals for home care and community services

Consulting with the RN and other health care professionals regarding the client's nutritional status

Ensuring that confidentiality issues related to the gastrointestinal disorder are maintained

Ensuring that informed consent for treatments and surgical procedures has been obtained

Establishing priorities of care

Handling infectious drainage and secretions safely

Maintaining standard precautions and other precautions as appropriate

Preventing disease transmission

Health Promotion and Maintenance

Performing data collection techniques of the gastrointestinal system

Preventing disease related to the gastrointestinal system

Providing health screening and health promotion programs related to gastrointestinal disorders

Reinforcing teaching related to colostomy or ileostomy care

Reinforcing teaching related to prescribed dietary and other treatment measures

Reinforcing teaching related to preventing the transmission of disease

Psychosocial Integrity

Asking about coping mechanisms

Considering end-of-life and grief and loss issues

Identifying available support systems

Monitoring for expected body image changes

Physiological Integrity

Administering medications as prescribed specific to the gastrointestinal disorder

Assisting with personal hygiene

Monitoring elimination patterns

Monitoring for complications related to tests, procedures, and surgical interventions

Monitoring for fluid and electrolyte imbalances

Monitoring for signs and symptoms of infectious diseases of the gastrointestinal tract

Monitoring laboratory values related to gastrointestinal disorders

Monitoring parenterally administered fluids, including parenteral nutrition

Providing adequate nutrition and oral hydration

Providing care for gastrointestinal tubes

Providing nonpharmacological and pharmacological comfort measures

Providing preprocedure and postprocedure care for diagnostic tests related to the gastrointestinal system

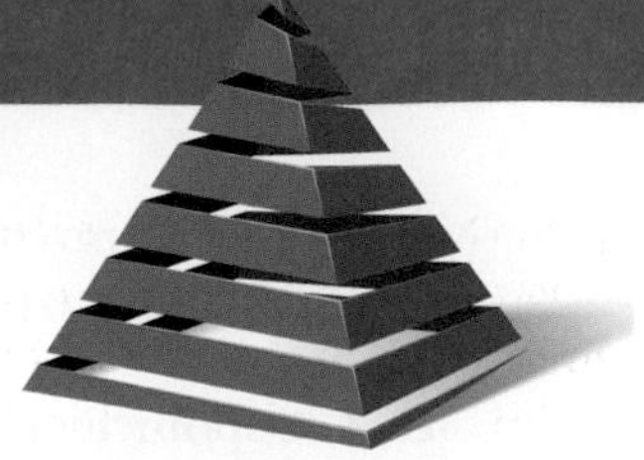

CHAPTER 47

Gastrointestinal System

CRITICAL THINKING What Should You Do?

The nurse is preparing a client for a liver biopsy. On review of the client's laboratory results, the nurse notes that the client's bleeding time is 10 minutes and the prothrombin time is 35 seconds. What should the nurse do?

Answer located on p. 612.

BOX 47-1 Risk Factors Associated with the Gastrointestinal (GI) System

Allergic reactions to food or medications
Cardiac, respiratory, and endocrine disorders that may lead to slowed gastrointestinal (GI) movement or constipation
Chronic alcohol use
Chronic high stress levels
Chronic laxative use
Chronic use of aspirin or nonsteroidal anti-inflammatory drugs
Diabetes mellitus, which may predispose to oral candidal infections or other GI disorders
Family history of GI disorders
Long-term GI conditions, such as ulcerative colitis, that may predispose to colorectal cancer
Neurological disorders that can impair movement, particularly with chewing and swallowing
Previous abdominal surgery or trauma, which may lead to adhesions
Tobacco use

I. Anatomy and Physiology

A. Functions of the gastrointestinal system
1. Process food substances
2. Absorb the products of digestion into the blood
3. Excrete unabsorbed materials
4. Provide an environment for microorganisms to synthesize nutrients, such as vitamin K
5. For risk factors associated with the gastrointestinal system, see Box 47-1.

B. Mouth
1. Contains the lips, cheeks, palate, tongue, teeth, salivary glands, muscles, and maxillary bones
2. Saliva contains the amylase enzyme (ptyalin) that aids in digestion.

C. Esophagus
1. A collapsible muscular tube about 10 inches long
2. Carries food from the pharynx to the stomach

D. Stomach
1. Contains the cardia, fundus, the body, and the pylorus
2. Mucous glands are located in the mucosa and prevent autodigestion by providing an alkaline protective covering.
3. The lower esophageal (cardiac) sphincter prevents reflux of gastric contents into the esophagus.
4. The pyloric sphincter regulates the rate of stomach emptying into the small intestine.
5. Hydrochloric acid kills microorganisms, breaks food into small particles, and provides a chemical environment that facilitates gastric enzyme activation.
6. Pepsin is the chief coenzyme of gastric juice, which converts proteins into proteoses and peptones.
7. Intrinsic factor is necessary for the absorption of vitamin B_{12}.
8. Gastrin controls gastric acidity.

E. Liver
1. The largest gland in the body, weighing 3 to 4 lb
2. Contains Kupffer's cells, which remove bacteria in the portal venous blood
3. Removes excess glucose and amino acids from the portal blood
4. Synthesizes glucose, amino acids, and fats
5. Aids in the digestion of fats, carbohydrates, and proteins
6. Stores and filters blood (200 to 400 mL of blood stored)
7. Stores vitamins A, D, and B and iron
8. The liver secretes bile to emulsify fats (500 to 1000 mL of bile/day)
9. Hepatic ducts
   a. Deliver bile to the gallbladder via the cystic duct and to the duodenum via the common bile duct

   b. The common bile duct opens into the duodenum with the pancreatic duct at the ampulla of Vater.
   c. The sphincter prevents the reflux of intestinal contents into the common bile duct and pancreatic duct.

F. Gallbladder
   1. Stores and concentrates bile and contracts to force bile into the duodenum during the digestion of fats
   2. The cystic duct joins the hepatic duct to form the common bile duct.
   3. The sphincter of Oddi is located at the entrance to the duodenum.
   4. The presence of fatty materials in the duodenum stimulates the liberation of cholecystokinin, which causes contraction of the gallbladder and relaxation of the sphincter of Oddi.

G. Pancreas
   1. Exocrine gland
      a. Secretes sodium bicarbonate to neutralize the acidity of the stomach contents that enter the duodenum
      b. Pancreatic juices contain enzymes for digesting carbohydrates, fats, and proteins.
   2. Endocrine gland
      a. Secretes glucagon to raise blood glucose levels and secretes somatostatin to exert a hypoglycemic effect
      b. The islets of Langerhans secrete insulin.
      c. Insulin is secreted into the bloodstream and is important for carbohydrate metabolism.

H. Pancreatic intestinal juice enzymes
   1. Amylase digests starch to maltose.
   2. Maltase reduces maltose to monosaccharide glucose.
   3. Lactase splits lactose into galactose and glucose.
   4. Sucrase reduces sucrose to fructose and glucose.
   5. Nucleases split nucleic acids to nucleotides.
   6. Enterokinase activates trypsinogen to trypsin.

I. Small intestine
   1. The duodenum contains the openings of the bile and pancreatic ducts.
   2. The jejunum is about 8 feet long.
   3. The ileum is about 12 feet long.
   4. The small intestine terminates in the cecum.

J. Large intestine
   1. Is about 5 feet long
   2. Absorbs water and eliminates wastes
   3. Intestinal bacteria play a vital role in the synthesis of some B vitamins and vitamin K.
   4. Colon: includes the ascending, transverse, descending, and sigmoid colons and rectum
   5. The ileocecal valve prevents contents of the large intestine from entering the ileum.
   6. The internal and external anal sphincters control the anal canal.

BOX 47-2 Common Gastrointestinal System Diagnostic Studies

- Capsule endoscopy
- Endoscopic retrograde cholangiopancreatography (ERCP)
- Endoscopic ultrasound
- Fiberoptic colonoscopy
- Laparoscopy: Liver and pancreas laboratory studies
- Liver biopsy
- Paracentesis
- Percutaneous transhepatic cholangiography
- Stool specimens
- Upper gastrointestinal endoscopy or esophagogastroduodenoscopy
- Upper gastrointestinal tract study (barium swallow)
- Videofluoroscopic swallowing study

Note: Informed consent is obtained for a diagnostic study that is invasive.

K. Peritoneum: lines the abdominal cavity and forms the mesentery that supports the intestines and blood supply

II. Diagnostic Procedures (Box 47-2)

A. Upper gastrointestinal tract study (barium swallow)
   1. Description: Examination of the upper gastrointestinal tract under fluoroscopy after the client drinks barium sulfate
   2. Preprocedure: NPO after midnight before the day of the test
   3. Postprocedure
      a. A laxative may be prescribed.
      b. The client is instructed to increase oral fluid intake to help pass the barium.
      c. Monitor stools for the passage of barium (stools will appear chalky white) because barium can cause a bowel obstruction.

B. Capsule endoscopy 
   1. A procedure that uses a small wireless camera shaped like a medication capsule that the client swallows; the test will detect bleeding or changes in the lining of the small intestine.
   2. The camera travels through the entire digestive tract and sends pictures to a small box that the client wears like a belt; the small box saves the pictures, which are then transferred to a computer for viewing once the test is complete.
   3. The client visits the HCP office in the morning and swallows the capsule, the recording belt is applied by the office staff, and then the client returns at the end of the day so that pictures can be transferred to the computer.
   4. Preprocedure, a bowel preparation will be prescribed; the client will need to maintain a clear liquid diet the evening before the exam; additionally, NPO status is maintained for 3 hours before and after swallowing the capsule (time

for NPO status is prescribed by the health care provider but is usually 2 to 3 hours).

C. Upper gastrointestinal endoscopy
1. Description
a. Is also known as esophagogastroduodenoscopy
b. Following sedation, an endoscope is passed down the esophagus to view the gastric wall, sphincters, and duodenum; tissue specimens can be obtained.
2. Preprocedure
a. The client must be NPO for 6 to 12 hours before the test.
b. A local anesthetic (spray or gargle) may be administered along with medication that provides conscious sedation and relieves anxiety, such as midazolam (Versed), just before the scope is inserted.
c. Medication may be administered to reduce secretions, and medication may be administered to relax smooth muscle.
d. Client is positioned on the left side to facilitate saliva drainage and provide easy access of the endoscope.
e. Airway patency is monitored during the test, and pulse oximetry is used to monitor oxygen saturation; emergency equipment should be readily available.
3. Postprocedure
a. Client must be NPO until the gag reflex returns (1 to 2 hours).
b. Monitor for signs of perforation (pain, bleeding, unusual difficulty in swallowing, elevated temperature).
c. Maintain bed rest for the sedated client until alert.
d. Lozenges, saline gargles, or oral analgesics can relieve a minor sore throat (not given to the client until the gag reflex returns).

D. Fiberoptic colonoscopy
1. Description
a. Colonoscopy is a fiberoptic endoscopy study in which the lining of the large intestine is visually examined; biopsies and polypectomies can be performed.
b. Cardiac and respiratory functions are monitored continuously during the test.
c. Colonoscopy is performed with the client lying on the left side with the knees drawn up to the chest; the position may be changed during the test to facilitate passing of the scope.
2. Preprocedure
a. Adequate cleansing of the colon is necessary, as prescribed by the health care provider (HCP).
b. A clear liquid diet is started on the day before the test.
c. Consult with the HCP regarding medications that must be withheld before the test.
d. The client is NPO after midnight on the day before the test.
e. A mild sedative is administered intravenously.
f. Medication may be administered to relax smooth muscle.

The client receiving enemas or colon cleansing agents is at risk for fluid and electrolyte imbalances.

3. Postprocedure
a. Provide bed rest until alert.
b. Monitor for signs of bowel perforation and peritonitis.
c. The client is instructed to report any bleeding to the HCP.

Signs of bowel perforation and peritonitis include restlessness, guarding of the abdomen, progressive abdominal distension and abdominal pain, increased temperature and chills, tachycardia and tachypnea, and pallor.

E. Laparoscopy is performed with a fiberoptic laparoscope that allows direct visualization of organs and structures within the abdomen; biopsies may be obtained.

F. Endoscopic retrograde cholangiopancreatography (ERCP)
1. Description
a. Examination of the hepatobiliary system is performed via a flexible endoscope inserted into the esophagus to the descending duodenum; multiple positions are required during the procedure to pass the endoscope.
b. If medication is administered before the procedure, the client is monitored closely for signs of respiratory and central nervous system depression, hypotension, oversedation, and vomiting.
2. Preprocedure
a. Client is NPO for several hours before the procedure.
b. Sedation is administered before the procedure.
3. Postprocedure
a. Monitor the vital signs.
b. Monitor for the return of the gag reflex.
c. Monitor for signs of perforation or peritonitis.

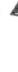

Following endoscopic procedures, monitor for the return of a gag reflex before giving the client any oral substance. If the gag reflex has not returned, the client could aspirate.

G. Endoscopic ultrasonography
1. Description: Provides images of the gastrointestinal (GI) wall and digestive organs

2. Preprocedure and postprocedure: Care is similar to that implemented for endoscopy. Following endoscopic procedures, monitor for the return of the gag reflex before giving the client any oral substance. If the gag reflex has not returned, the client could aspirate.

H. Percutaneous transhepatic cholangiography
1. Description
   a. The examination involves the injection of dye directly into the biliary tree.
   b. The hepatic ducts within the liver, the entire length of the common bile duct, the cystic duct, and the gallbladder are outlined clearly.
2. Preprocedure
   a. Client is NPO, usually from midnight preprocedure.
   b. Sedating medication is administered.
3. Postprocedure
   a. Monitor vital signs.
   b. Monitor for signs of bleeding, peritonitis, and septicemia; report the presence of pain immediately.
   c. Administer antibiotics as prescribed to reduce the risk of sepsis.

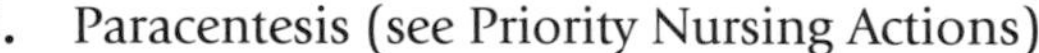

I. Paracentesis (see Priority Nursing Actions)

The rapid removal of fluid from the abdominal cavity during paracentesis leads to decreased abdominal pressure, which can cause vasodilation and resultant shock.

J. Liver biopsy
1. Description: A needle is inserted through the abdominal wall to the liver to obtain a tissue sample for biopsy and microscopic examination.
2. Preprocedure
   a. Check results of coagulation tests (prothrombin time, partial thromboplastin time, platelet count).
   b. Administer a sedative as prescribed.
   c. Note that the client is placed in the supine or left lateral position during the procedure to expose the right side of the upper abdomen.

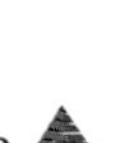

3. Postprocedure
   a. Monitor vital signs.
   b. Check biopsy site for bleeding.
   c. Monitor for peritonitis,
   d. Maintain bed rest for time frame as prescribed, usually 2 hours.
   e. The client is instructed to avoid heavy lifting and strenuous exercise for 1 week.

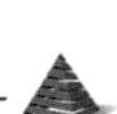

PRIORITY NURSING ACTIONS!

Actions to Take in Caring for a Client with a Paracentesis

1. Ensure that the client understands the procedure and that informed consent has been obtained.
2. Obtain vital signs, including weight.
3. Have the client void.
4. Position the client upright.
5. Assist the HCP. Monitor the vital signs and provide comfort and support during the procedure.
6. Apply a dressing to the site of puncture.
7. Weigh the client, and maintain the client on bed rest.
8. Measure the amount of fluid removed.
9. Label and send the fluid for laboratory analysis.
10. Document the event, client's response, and appearance and amount of fluid removed.

Paracentesis is the transabdominal removal of fluid from the peritoneal cavity. The nurse first ensures that the client understands the procedure and that informed consent has been obtained because the procedure is invasive. The nurse next obtains preprocedure vital signs, including measuring abdominal girth and weight so that a baseline is obtained. Weight is taken before and after the procedure to provide an indication of the effectiveness of the procedure in fluid removal. The nurse assists the client to void before the start of the procedure to empty the bladder and to move the bladder out of the way of the paracentesis needle. The client is positioned upright on the edge of the bed, with the back supported and the feet resting on a stool or in a Fowler's position in bed. The nurse assists the HCP, monitors vital signs per protocol, and provides comfort and support to the client during the procedure. Once the procedure is complete the nurse applies a dressing to the site of puncture and monitors for leakage or bleeding. The client is placed in a position of comfort, bed rest is maintained as prescribed, and vital signs are monitored to assess for complications. The fluid removed from the client is measured, labeled and sent to the laboratory for analysis. Weight and abdominal girth are measured postprocedure for comparison to preprocedure values. The nurse should also monitor for hypovolemia, electrolyte loss, mental status changes, or encephalopathy. Since bladder trauma can occur, the nurse monitors for hematuria. The nurse documents the event, the client's response, the appearance and amount of fluid removed, and any additional pertinent data. The nurse also reports any signs of complications to the RN immediately.

Reference(s): deWit, Kumagai (2013), pp. 51, 702–703. St. Louis: Saunders.

Ignatavicius, D. & Workman, M. (2013). *Medical-surgical nursing: Patient-centered collaborative care.* (7th ed., p. 1300). St. Louis: Saunders.

Following a liver biopsy, place the client on the right side with a pillow (or agency-approved pressure item such as a sandbag) under the costal margin to decrease the risk of hemorrhage; the client is instructed to avoid coughing and straining.

K. Stool specimens
1. Testing of stool specimens includes inspecting the specimen for consistency and color and testing for occult blood.
2. Tests for fecal urobilinogen, fat, nitrogen, parasites, pathogens, food substances, and other substances may be performed; these tests require that the specimen be sent to the laboratory.
3. Random specimens are sent promptly to the laboratory.
4. Quantitative 24- to 72-hour collections must be kept refrigerated until they are taken to the laboratory.
5. Some specimens require that a certain diet be followed or that certain medications be withheld; check agency guidelines regarding specific procedures.

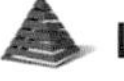

L. Liver and pancreas laboratory studies (refer to Chapter 11).
1. Alkaline phosphatase is released with liver damage or biliary obstruction.
2. Prothrombin time is prolonged with liver damage.
3. The serum ammonia level assesses the ability of the liver to deaminate protein by-products.
4. Liver enzymes (transaminase studies) are elevated with liver damage.
5. An increase in cholesterol indicates **pancreatitis** or biliary obstruction.
6. An increase in bilirubin level indicates liver damage or biliary obstruction.
7. Increased values for amylase and lipase levels indicate pancreatitis.

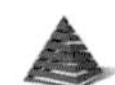

III. Data Collection (See Chapter 23)

IV. Gastrointestinal Tubes (Refer to Chapter 19)

V. Gastroesophageal Reflux Disease

A. Description
1. Gastroesophageal reflux is the backflow of gastric and duodenal contents into the esophagus.
2. The reflux is caused by an incompetent lower esophageal sphincter, pyloric stenosis, or a motility disorder.

B. Data collection
1. Epigastric pain; heartburn
2. Dyspepsia
3. Nausea; regurgitation
4. Pain and difficulty with swallowing
5. Hypersalivation

C. Interventions
1. The client is instructed to avoid factors that decrease lower esophageal sphincter pressure or cause esophageal irritation such as peppermint, chocolate, coffee, fried or fatty foods, carbonated beverages, alcoholic beverages, and cigarette smoking.
2. The client is instructed to eat a low-fat, high-fiber diet and to avoid eating and drinking 2 hours before bedtime and wearing tight clothes; also, elevate the head of the bed on 6- to 8-inch blocks.
3. Avoid the use of anticholinergics, which delay stomach emptying; also nonsteroidal anti-inflammatory medications and other medications that contain acetylsalicylic acid need to be avoided.
4. Reinforce instructions regarding prescribed medications, such as antacids, histamine 2 (H_2)-receptor antagonists, or proton pump inhibitors.
5. Reinforce instructions regarding the administration of prokinetic medications, if prescribed, which accelerate gastric emptying.
6. Surgery may be required in extreme cases when medical management is unsuccessful; this involves fundoplication (wrapping a portion of the gastric fundus around the sphincter area of the esophagus); surgery may be performed by laparoscopy.

VI. Gastritis

A. Description
1. Inflammation of the stomach or gastric mucosa
2. Acute gastritis is caused by the ingestion of food contaminated with disease-causing microorganisms or food that is irritating or too highly seasoned, the overuse of aspirin or other nonsteroidal anti-inflammatory drugs (NSAIDs), excessive alcohol intake, bile reflux, or radiation therapy.
3. Chronic gastritis is caused by benign or malignant ulcers or by the bacteria *H. pylori*, and it may be caused by autoimmune diseases, dietary factors, medications, alcohol, smoking, or reflux.

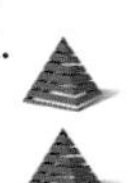

B. Data collection (Box 47-3)

C. Interventions
1. Acute gastritis: Food and fluids may be withheld until symptoms subside; afterward, ice chips can be given, followed by clear liquids, and then solid food.
2. Monitor for signs of hemorrhagic gastritis such as hematemesis, tachycardia, and hypotension, and notify the HCP if these signs occur.
3. Reinforce instructions to avoid irritating foods, fluids, and other substances such as spicy and highly seasoned foods, caffeine, alcohol, and nicotine.
4. Reinforce instructions on the use of prescribed medications, such as antibiotics and antacids.

BOX 47-3 Data Collection: Acute and Chronic Gastritis

Acute

Abdominal discomfort
Anorexia, nausea, and vomiting
Headache
Hiccuping
Reflux

Chronic

Anorexia, nausea, and vomiting
Belching
Heartburn after eating
Sour taste in the mouth
Vitamin B_{12} deficiency

BOX 47-4 Data Collection: Gastric and Duodenal Ulcers

Gastric

Gnawing, sharp pain in or to the left of the midepigastric region occurs 30 to 60 minutes after a meal (food ingestion accentuates the pain).
Hematemesis is more common than melena.

Duodenal

Burning pain in the midepigastric area 1½ to 3 hours after a meal and during the night (often awakens the client).
Melena is more common than hematemesis.
Pain is often relieved by the ingestion of food.

5. Provide the client with information about the importance of vitamin B_{12} injections if a deficiency is present.

VII. Peptic Ulcer Disease

A. Description
1. A peptic ulcer is an ulceration in the mucosal wall of the stomach, pylorus, duodenum, or esophagus in portions accessible to gastric secretions; erosion may extend through the muscle.
2. The ulcer may be referred to as *gastric, duodenal,* or *esophageal,* depending on its location.
3. The most common peptic ulcers are gastric ulcers and duodenal ulcers.

B. Gastric ulcers
1. Description
   a. A gastric ulcer involves ulceration of the mucosal lining that extends to the submucosal layer of the stomach.
   b. Predisposing factors include stress, smoking, the use of corticosteroids, NSAIDs, alcohol, history of gastritis, family history of gastric ulcers, or infection with *H. pylori.*
   c. Complications include hemorrhage, perforation, and pyloric obstruction.

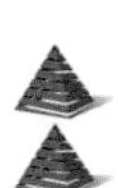

2. Data collection (Box 47-4)
3. Interventions
   a. Monitor vital signs and for signs of bleeding.
   b. Administer small, frequent, bland feedings during the active phase.
   c. Administer H_2-receptor antagonists or proton pump inhibitors as prescribed to decrease the secretion of gastric acid.
   d. Administer antacids as prescribed to neutralize gastric secretions.
   e. Administer anticholinergics as prescribed to reduce gastric motility.
   f. Administer mucosal barrier protectants as prescribed 1 hour before each meal.
   g. Administer prostaglandins as prescribed for their protective and antisecretory actions.
4. Client education
   a. Avoid consuming alcohol and substances that contain caffeine or chocolate.
   b. Avoid smoking.
   c. Avoid aspirin or NSAIDs.
   d. Obtain adequate rest and reduce stress.
5. Interventions during active bleeding
   a. Monitor vital signs closely.
   b. Monitor for signs of dehydration, hypovolemic shock, sepsis, and respiratory insufficiency.
   c. Maintain NPO status and assist to administer intravenous (IV) fluid replacement as prescribed; monitor intake and output.
   d. Monitor hemoglobin and hematocrit.
   e. Assist to administer blood transfusions as prescribed.
   f. Prepare to assist with administering medications as prescribed to induce vasoconstriction and reduce bleeding.
6. Surgical interventions
   a. Total **gastrectomy**: Removal of the stomach with attachment of the esophagus to the jejunum or duodenum; also called esophagojejunostomy or esophagoduodenostomy
   b. **Vagotomy**: Surgical division of the vagus nerve to eliminate the vagal impulses that stimulate hydrochloric acid secretion in the stomach
   c. **Gastric resection**: Removal of the lower half of the stomach and usually includes a vagotomy; also called antrectomy
   d. **Billroth I**: Partial gastrectomy, with the remaining segment anastomosed to the duodenum; also called *gastroduodenostomy*
   e. **Billroth II**: Partial gastrectomy, with the remaining segment anastomosed to the jejunum; also called *gastrojejunostomy*
   f. **Pyloroplasty**: Enlargement of the pylorus to prevent or decrease pyloric obstruction, thereby enhancing gastric emptying

7. Postoperative interventions
   a. Monitor vital signs.
   b. Place in a Fowler's position for comfort and to promote drainage.
   c. Assist to administer fluids and electrolyte replacements intravenously as prescribed; monitor intake and output.
   d. Check bowel sounds.
   e. Monitor nasogastric suction as prescribed.
   f. Maintain NPO status as prescribed for 1 to 3 days until **peristalsis** returns.
   g. Progress the diet from NPO to sips of clear water to six small bland meals a day, as prescribed when the bowel sounds return.
   h. Monitor for postoperative complications of hemorrhage, **dumping syndrome**, diarrhea, hypoglycemia, and vitamin B_{12} deficiency.

Following gastric surgery, do not irrigate or remove the nasogastric (NG) tube unless specifically prescribed because of the risk for disruption of the gastric sutures. Monitor closely to ensure proper functioning of the NG tube to prevent strain on the anastomosis site. Contact the HCP if the tube is not functioning properly.

C. Duodenal ulcers
1. Description
   a. A duodenal ulcer is a break in the mucosa of the duodenum.
   b. Risk factors and causes include infection with *H. pylori*; alcohol intake; smoking; stress; caffeine; and the use of aspirin, corticosteroids, and NSAIDs.
   c. Complications include bleeding, perforation, gastric outlet obstruction, and intractable disease.

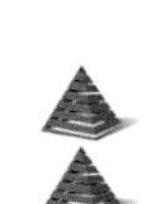
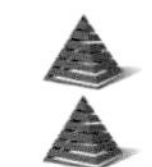

2. Data collection (see Box 47-4)
3. Interventions
   a. Monitor vital signs.
   b. Instruct the client about a bland diet, with small frequent meals.
   c. Provide for adequate rest.
   d. Encourage the cessation of smoking.
   e. Reinforce instructions to avoid alcohol intake, caffeine, the use of aspirin, corticosteroids, and NSAIDs.
   f. Administer medications to treat *H. pylori* and antacids to neutralize acid secretions as prescribed.
   g. Administer H_2-receptor antagonists or proton pump inhibitors as prescribed to block the secretion of acid.
4. Surgical interventions: Surgery is performed only if the ulcer is unresponsive to medications or if hemorrhage, obstruction, or perforation occurs.

D. Dumping syndrome
1. Description: The rapid emptying of the gastric contents into the small intestine that occurs following gastric resection

BOX 47-5 Client Education: Preventing Dumping Syndrome

Avoid sugar, salt, and milk.
Eat a high-protein, high-fat, low-carbohydrate diet.
Eat small meals, and avoid consuming fluids with meals.
Lie down after meals.
Take antispasmodic medications as prescribed to delay gastric emptying.

2. Data collection
   a. Symptoms occurring 30 minutes after eating
   b. Nausea and vomiting
   c. Feelings of abdominal fullness and abdominal cramping
   d. Diarrhea
   e. Palpitations and tachycardia
   f. Perspiration
   g. Weakness and dizziness
   h. Borborygmi (loud gurgles indicating hyperperistalsis)
3. Client education (Box 47-5)

VIII. Vitamin B_{12} Deficiency

A. Description
1. Vitamin B_{12} deficiency results from an inadequate intake of vitamin B_{12} or a lack of absorption of ingested vitamin B_{12} from the intestinal tract.
2. Pernicious anemia results from a deficiency of intrinsic factor, necessary for intestinal absorption of vitamin B_{12}; gastric disease or surgery can result in a lack of intrinsic factor.

B. Data collection
1. Severe pallor
2. Fatigue
3. Weight loss
4. Smooth, beefy red tongue
5. Slight jaundice
6. Paresthesias of the hands and feet
7. Disturbances with gait and balance

C. Interventions
1. Increase dietary intake of foods rich in vitamin B_{12} if the anemia is the result of a dietary deficiency (refer to Chapter 12).
2. Administer vitamin B_{12} injections initially as prescribed weekly and then monthly for maintenance (lifelong) if the anemia is the result of a deficiency of the intrinsic factor or disease or surgery of the ileum.

IX. Bariatric Surgery

A. Description
1. Surgical reduction of gastric capacity that may be performed on a client with morbid obesity to produce long-term weight loss
2. Surgery may be performed by laparoscopy; the decision is based on the client's weight, body

build, history of abdominal surgery, and current medical disorders.

3. Obese clients are at increased postoperative risk for pulmonary and thromboembolic complications and death.
4. Surgery can prevent the complications of obesity, such as diabetes mellitus, hypertension and other cardiovascular disorders, or sleep apnea.
5. The client needs to agree to modify his or her lifestyle, lose weight and keep the weight off, and obtain support from available community resources (Box 47-6).
6. Various procedures are available; the type performed depends on the HCP and the client's choice (Fig. 47-1).

BOX 47-6 Community Resources After Bariatric Surgery

American Obesity Association
American Society of Bariatric Surgery
Overeaters Anonymous

B. Postoperative interventions
1. Care is similar to that for the client undergoing abdominal surgery.
2. Dietary measures are prescribed per surgeon's preference.
3. Usually clear liquids are introduced slowly once bowel sounds have returned and the client passes flatus; then protein shakes (1 to 2 ounces as tolerated) or other liquids may be introduced, with diet progression as prescribed.

C. Client teaching points (Box 47-7)

X. Gastric Cancer (see Chapter 43)

XI. Hiatal Hernia

A. Description
1. A hiatal hernia is also known as esophageal or diaphragmatic hernia.
2. A portion of the stomach herniates through the diaphragm and into the thorax.
3. Herniation results from weakening of the muscles of the diaphragm and is aggravated by factors that increase abdominal pressure such as pregnancy, **ascites**, obesity, tumors, and heavy lifting.

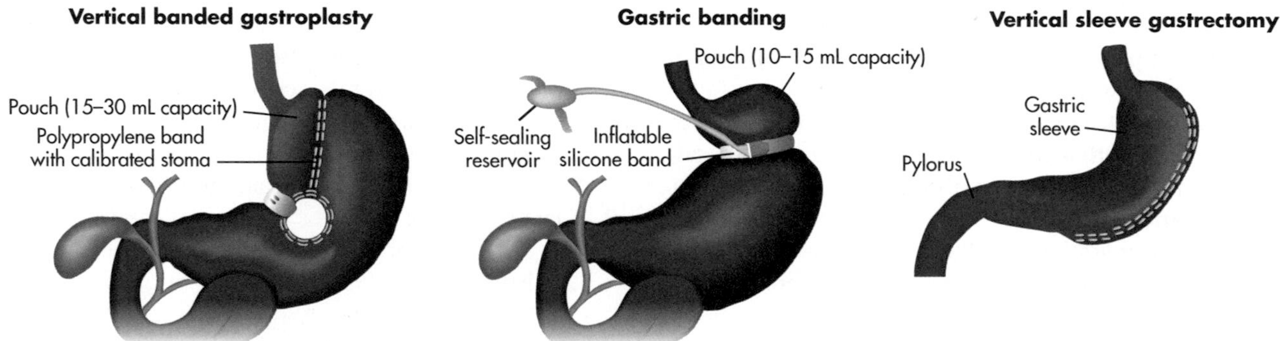

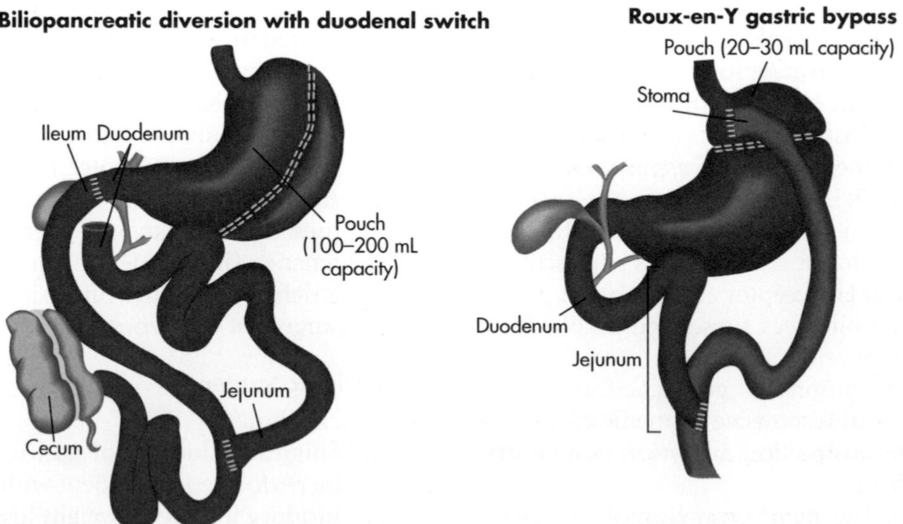

FIGURE 47-1 Bariatric surgical procedures. (From Lewis S, Dirksen S, Heitkemper M, Bucher L, Camera I: *Medical-surgical nursing: Assessment and management of clinical problems*, ed 8, St. Louis, 2011, Mosby.)

BOX 47-7 Client Education Following Bariatric Surgery

Avoid alcohol, high-protein foods, and foods high in sugar and fat.
Eat slowly and chew food well.
Progress food types and amounts as prescribed.
Take nutritional supplements as prescribed, which may include calcium, iron, multivitamins, and vitamin B_{12}.
Monitor and report signs and symptoms of complications, such as dehydration and gastric leak (persistent abdominal pain and nausea and vomiting).

4. Complications include ulceration, hemorrhage, regurgitation, aspiration of stomach contents, strangulation, and incarceration of the stomach in the chest with possible necrosis, peritonitis, and mediastinitis.

B. Data collection
1. Heartburn
2. Regurgitation or vomiting
3. Dysphagia
4. Feeling of fullness

C. Interventions
1. Medical and surgical management are similar to those for gastroesophageal reflux disease.
2. Provide small, frequent meals and limit the amount of liquids taken with meals.
3. The client is advised not to recline for 1 hour after eating.
4. Anticholinergics are avoided, which delay stomach emptying.

XII. Cholecystitis

A. Description
1. Inflammation of the gallbladder that may occur as an acute or chronic process
2. Acute inflammation is associated with gallstones (cholelithiasis).
3. Chronic cholecystitis results when inefficient bile emptying and gallbladder muscle wall disease cause a fibrotic and contracted gallbladder.
4. Acalculous cholecystitis occurs in the absence of gallstones and is caused by bacterial invasion via the lymphatic or vascular systems.

B. Data collection
1. Nausea and vomiting
2. Indigestion
3. Belching
4. Flatulence
5. Epigastric pain that radiates to the scapula 2 to 4 hours after eating fatty foods and may persist for 4 to 6 hours
6. Pain localized in right upper quadrant
7. Guarding, rigidity, and rebound tenderness
8. Mass palpated in the right upper quadrant
9. **Murphy's sign** (cannot take a deep breath when the examiner's fingers are passed below the hepatic margin because of pain)
10. Elevated temperature
11. Tachycardia
12. Signs of dehydration

C. Biliary obstruction

1. Jaundice
2. Dark orange and foamy urine
3. Steatorrhea and clay-colored feces
4. Pruritus

D. Interventions
1. Maintain NPO status during nausea and vomiting episodes.
2. Maintain nasogastric decompression as prescribed for severe vomiting.
3. Administer antiemetics as prescribed for nausea and vomiting.
4. Administer analgesics as prescribed to relieve pain and reduce spasm.
5. Administer antispasmodics (anticholinergics) as prescribed to relax smooth muscle.
6. Reinforce instructions with chronic **cholecystitis** to eat small, low-fat meals.
7. Reinforce instructions to avoid gas-forming foods.
8. Prepare the client for nonsurgical and surgical procedures as prescribed.

E. Surgical interventions
1. **Cholecystectomy** is the removal of the gallbladder.
2. **Choledocholithotomy** requires incision into the common bile duct to remove the stone.
3. Surgical procedures may be performed by laparoscopy.

F. Postoperative interventions
1. Monitor for respiratory complications caused by pain at the incisional site.
2. Encourage coughing and deep breathing.
3. Encourage early ambulation.
4. Reinforce instructions about splinting the abdomen to prevent discomfort during coughing.
5. Administer antiemetics as prescribed for nausea and vomiting.
6. Administer analgesics as prescribed for pain relief.
7. Maintain NPO status and nasogastric tube suction as prescribed.
8. Advance diet from clear liquids to solids when prescribed and as tolerated by the client.
9. Maintain and monitor drainage from the T-tube, if present (Box 47-8).

XIII. Cirrhosis (Box 47-9)

A. Description
1. A chronic, progressive disease of the liver characterized by diffuse degeneration and destruction of hepatocytes

BOX 47-8 Care of a T-Tube

Purpose and Description

A T-tube is placed after surgical exploration of the common bile duct. The tube preserves the patency of the duct and ensures drainage of bile until edema resolves and bile is effectively draining into the duodenum. A gravity drainage bag is attached to the T-tube to collect the drainage.

Interventions

Place the client in a semi-Fowler's position to facilitate drainage.
Monitor the amount, color, consistency, and odor of the drainage.
Report sudden increases in bile output to the HCP.
Monitor for inflammation and protect the skin from irritation.
Keep the drainage system below the level of the gallbladder.
Monitor for foul odor and purulent drainage, and report its presence to the HCP.
Avoid irrigation, aspiration, or clamping of the T-tube without a HCP's prescription.
As prescribed, clamp the tube before a meal and observe for abdominal discomfort and distention, nausea, chills, or fever; unclamp the tube if nausea or vomiting occurs.

BOX 47-9 Types of Cirrhosis

Laënnec's Cirrhosis

Cirrhosis is alcohol induced, nutritional, or portal.
Cellular necrosis causes eventual widespread scar tissue, with fibrotic infiltration of the liver.

Postnecrotic Cirrhosis

Cirrhosis occurs after massive liver necrosis.
Cirrhosis results as a complication of hepatitis or exposure to hepatotoxins.
Scar tissue causes destruction of liver lobules and entire lobes.

Biliary Cirrhosis

Cirrhosis develops from chronic biliary obstruction, bile stasis, and inflammation, resulting in severe obstructive jaundice.

Cardiac Cirrhosis

Cirrhosis is associated with severe, right-sided heart failure and results in an enlarged, edematous, congested liver.
The liver becomes anoxic, resulting in liver cell necrosis and fibrosis.

2. Repeated destruction of hepatic cells causes the formation of scar tissue.

B. Complications
1. **Portal hypertension**: A persistent increase in pressure in the portal vein that develops as a result of obstruction to flow
2. **Ascites**
   a. Accumulation of fluid within the peritoneal cavity that results from venous congestion of the hepatic capillaries
   b. Capillary congestion leads to plasma leaking directly from the liver surface and portal vein.
3. Bleeding **esophageal varices**: Fragile, thin-walled, distended esophageal veins that become irritated and rupture
4. Coagulation defects
   a. Decreased synthesis of bile fats in the liver prevents the absorption of fat-soluble vitamins.
   b. Without vitamin K and clotting factors II, VII, IX, and X, the client is prone to bleeding.
5. Jaundice: Occurs because the liver is unable to metabolize bilirubin and the edema, fibrosis, and scarring of the hepatic bile ducts interfere with normal bile and bilirubin secretion
6. Portal systemic encephalopathy: End-stage hepatic failure characterized by altered level of consciousness, neurological symptoms, impaired thinking, and neuromuscular disturbances; caused by failure of the diseased liver to detoxify neurotoxic agents such as ammonia
7. Hepatorenal syndrome
   a. Progressive renal failure associated with hepatic failure
   b. Characterized by a sudden decrease in urinary output, elevated blood urea nitrogen and creatinine levels, decreased urine sodium excretion, and increased urine osmolarity

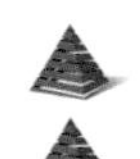

C. Data collection (Fig. 47-2)

D. Interventions
1. Elevate the head of the bed to minimize shortness of breath.
2. If ascites and edema are absent and the client does not exhibit signs of impending coma, a high-protein diet supplemented with vitamins is prescribed.
3. Provide supplemental vitamins (B complex; vitamins A, C, and K, folic acid, and thiamine) as prescribed.
4. Restrict sodium intake and fluid intake as prescribed.
5. Initiate enteral feedings or assist with parenteral nutrition as prescribed.
6. Administer diuretics as prescribed to treat ascites.
7. Monitor intake and output and electrolyte balance.
8. Weigh the client and measure abdominal girth daily.
9. Monitor level of consciousness; monitor for a precoma state (tremors, delirium).
10. Monitor for **asterixis**, a coarse tremor characterized by rapid, nonrhythmic extension and flexions in the wrist and fingers.

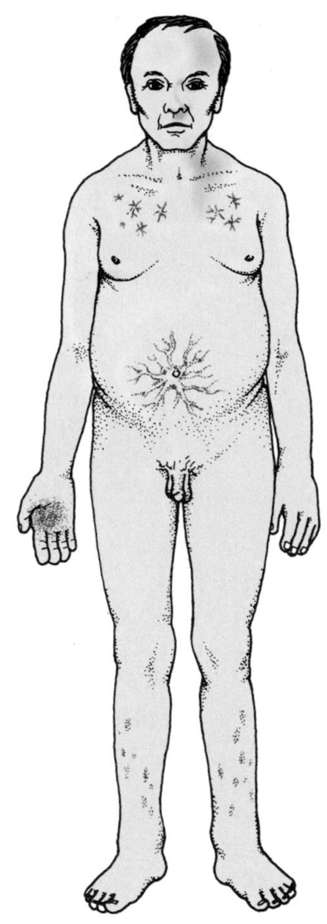

NEUROLOGIC FINDINGS
Asterixis
Paresthesias of feet
Peripheral nerve degeneration
Portal-systemic encephalopathy
Reversal of sleep-wake pattern
Sensory disturbances
GASTROINTESTINAL (GI) FINDINGS
Abdominal pain
Anorexia
Ascites
Clay-colored stools
Diarrhea
Esophageal varices
Fetor hepaticus
Gallstones
Gastritis
Gastrointestinal bleeding
Hemorrhoidal varices
Hepatomegaly
Hiatal hernia
Hypersplenism
Malnutrition
Nausea
Small nodular liver
Vomiting
RENAL FINDINGS
Hepatorenal syndrome
Increased urine bilirubin
ENDOCRINE FINDINGS
Increased aldosterone
Increased antidiuretic hormone
Increased circulating estrogens
Increased glucocorticoids
Gynecomastia
IMMUNE SYSTEM DISTURBANCES
Increased susceptibility to infection
Leukopenia
CARDIOVASCULAR FINDINGS
Cardiac dysrhythmias
Development of collateral circulation
Fatigue
Hyperkinetic circulation
Peripheral edema
Portal hypertension
Spider angiomas
PULMONARY FINDINGS
Dyspnea
Hydrothorax
Hyperventilation
Hypoxemia
HEMATOLOGIC FINDINGS
Anemia
Disseminated intravascular coagulation
Impaired coagulation
Splenomegaly
Thrombocytopenia
DERMATOLOGIC FINDINGS
Axillary and pubic hair changes
Caput medusae
Ecchymosis
Increased skin pigmentation
Jaundice
Palmar erythema
Pruritus
Spider angiomas
FLUID AND ELECTROLYTE DISTURBANCES
Ascites
Decreased effective blood volume
Dilutional hyponatremia or hypernatremia
Hypocalcemia
Hypokalemia
Peripheral edema
Water retention

FIGURE 47-2 Clinical picture of a client with liver dysfunction. Manifestations vary according to the progression of the disease. (From Ignatavicius D, Workman ML: *Medical-surgical nursing: Patient-centered collaborative care*, ed 7, Philadelphia, 2013, Saunders.)

11. Monitor for **fetor hepaticus**—the fruity, musty breath odor of severe chronic liver disease.
12. Assist to maintain gastric intubation to monitor bleeding or esophagogastric balloon tamponade to control bleeding varices if prescribed.
13. Assist to administer blood products as prescribed.
14. Monitor coagulation laboratory results; vitamin K may be prescribed.
15. Administer antacids as prescribed.
16. Administer lactulose (Constulose, Enulose, Generlac) as prescribed, which decreases the pH of the bowel, decreases production of ammonia by bacteria in the bowel, and facilitates the excretion of ammonia.
17. Administer antibiotics as prescribed to inhibit protein synthesis in bacteria and decrease the production of ammonia.
18. Avoid medications such as opioids, sedatives, and barbiturates and any hepatotoxic medications or substances.
19. Reinforce instructions about the importance of abstinence of alcohol intake.
20. Prepare the client for paracentesis to remove abdominal fluid.
21. Prepare the client for surgical shunting procedures if prescribed to divert fluid from ascites into the venous system.

XIV. Esophageal Varices

A. Description
   1. Dilated and tortuous veins in the submucosa of the esophagus
   2. Caused by portal hypertension, are often associated with liver cirrhosis, and are at high risk for rupture if portal circulation pressure rises

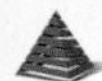

3. Bleeding varices are an emergency.
4. The goal of treatment is to control bleeding, prevent complications, and prevent the reoccurrence of bleeding.

B. Data collection
1. Hematemesis
2. **Melena**
3. Ascites
4. Jaundice
5. Hepatomegaly and splenomegaly
6. Dilated abdominal veins
7. Signs of shock

Rupture and resultant hemorrhage of the esophageal varices are a primary concern because it presents a life-threatening situation.

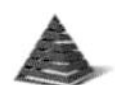

C. Interventions
1. Monitor vital signs.
2. Elevate the head of the bed.
3. Monitor for orthostatic hypotension.
4. Assist to monitor lung sounds and for the presence of respiratory distress.
5. Administer oxygen as prescribed to prevent tissue hypoxia.
6. Monitor level of consciousness.
7. Maintain NPO status.
8. Intravenous fluids may be prescribed to restore fluid volume and electrolyte imbalances; monitor intake and output.
9. Monitor hemoglobin and hematocrit and coagulation factors.
10. Assist to administer blood transfusions or clotting factors as prescribed.
11. A nasogastric tube or a balloon tamponade may be inserted if prescribed; balloon tamponade is not used frequently because it is very uncomfortable for the client and its use is associated with complications.
12. Prepare to assist with administering medications to induce vasoconstriction and reduce bleeding.
13. Reinforce instructions to avoid activities that will initiate vasovagal responses.
14. Prepare the client for endoscopic procedures or surgical procedures as prescribed.

D. Endoscopic injection (sclerotherapy)
1. The procedure involves the injection of a sclerosing agent into and around bleeding varices.
2. Complications include chest pain, pleural effusion, aspiration pneumonia, esophageal stricture, and perforation of the esophagus.

E. Endoscopic variceal ligation
1. The procedure involves ligation of the varices with an elastic rubber band.
2. Sloughing, followed by superficial ulceration, occurs in the area of ligation within 3 to 7 days.

F. Shunting procedures
1. Description: Shunt blood away from the esophageal varices
2. Portacaval shunt involves anastomosis of the portal vein to the inferior vena cava, diverting blood from the portal system to the systemic circulation
3. Distal splenorenal shunt
   a. The shunt involves anastomosis of the splenic vein to the left renal vein.
   b. The spleen conducts blood from the high-pressure varices to the low-pressure renal vein.
4. Mesocaval shunting involves a side anastomosis of the superior mesenteric vein to the proximal end of the inferior vena cava.
5. Transjugular intrahepatic portosystemic shunt (TIPS)
   a. The nonsurgical procedure uses the normal vascular anatomy of the liver to create a shunt with the use of a metallic stent.
   b. The shunt is between the portal and systemic venous system in the liver and is aimed at relieving portal hypertension.

XV. Hepatitis

A. Description
1. Inflammation of the liver caused by a virus, bacteria, or exposure to medications or hepatotoxins
2. The goals of treatment include resting the inflamed liver to reduce metabolic demands and increasing the blood supply, thus promoting cellular regeneration and preventing complications.

B. Types of viral hepatitis
1. Hepatitis A virus (HAV)
2. Hepatitis B virus (HBV)
3. Hepatitis C virus (HCV)
4. Hepatitis D virus (HDV)
5. Hepatitis E virus (HEV)

C. Stages of viral hepatitis (Box 47-10)

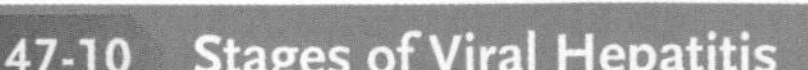

BOX 47-10 Stages of Viral Hepatitis

Preicteric Stage

The first stage of hepatitis, preceding the appearance of jaundice; includes flu-like symptoms

Icteric Stage

The second stage of hepatitis; includes the appearance of jaundice and associated symptoms such as elevated bilirubin levels, dark or tea-colored urine, and clay-colored stools

Posticteric Stage

The convalescent stage of hepatitis, in which the jaundice decreases and the color of the urine and stool returns to normal

D. Data collection
  1. Preicteric stage
    a. Flu-like symptoms—malaise, fatigue
    b. Anorexia, nausea, vomiting, diarrhea
    c. Pain—headache, muscle aches, polyarthritis
    d. Serum bilirubin and enzyme levels are elevated.
  2. Icteric stage
    a. Jaundice
    b. Pruritus
    c. Dark or tea-colored urine
    d. Clay-colored stools
    e. Decrease in preicteric-phase symptoms
  3. Posticteric stage
    a. Increased energy levels
    b. Subsiding of pain
    c. Minimal to absent gastrointestinal symptoms
    d. Serum bilirubin and enzyme levels return to normal.

E. Laboratory findings: Elevated liver enzyme levels (alkaline phosphatase, alanine aminotransferase [ALT], aspartate aminotransferase [AST]); elevated ammonia level; elevated bilirubin level

XVI. Hepatitis A

A. Description
  1. Formerly known as *infectious hepatitis*
  2. Commonly seen during the fall and early winter

B. Individuals at increased risk
  1. Commonly seen in young children
  2. Individuals in institutionalized settings
  3. Health care personnel

C. Transmission
  1. Fecal-oral route
  2. Person-to-person contact
  3. Parenteral
  4. Contaminated fruits, vegetables, or uncooked shellfish
  5. Contaminated water or milk
  6. Poorly washed utensils

D. Incubation and infectious period
  1. Incubation period is 2 to 6 weeks.
  2. Infectious period is 2 to 3 weeks before and 1 week after development of jaundice.

E. Testing
  1. Infection is established by the presence of HAV antibodies (anti-HAV) in the blood.
  2. Immunoglobulin M (IgM) and G (IgG) are normally present in the blood, and increased levels indicate infection and inflammation.
  3. Ongoing inflammation of the liver is evidenced by the presence of elevated IgM antibodies, which persist in the blood for 4 to 6 weeks.
  4. Previous infection is indicated by the presence of elevated IgG antibodies.

F. Complication: Fulminant (severe acute and often fatal) hepatitis

G. Prevention
  1. Strict hand washing
  2. Stool and needle precautions
  3. Treatment of municipal water supplies
  4. Serological screening of food handlers
  5. Hepatitis A vaccine (HAVRIX, VAQTA)
  6. Immune globulin: For individuals exposed to HAV who have never received the hepatitis A vaccine; administer immune globulin during the period of incubation and within 2 weeks of exposure.
  7. Immune globulin and hepatitis A vaccine are recommended for household members and sexual contacts of individuals with hepatitis A.
  8. Preexposure prophylaxis with immunoglobulin is recommended to individuals traveling to countries with poor or uncertain sanitation conditions.

Strict and frequent hand washing is key to preventing the spread of all types of hepatitis.

XVII. Hepatitis B

A. Description
  1. Hepatitis B is nonseasonal.
  2. All age groups are affected.

B. Individuals at increased risk
  1. IV drug users
  2. Clients undergoing long-term hemodialysis
  3. Health care personnel

C. Transmission

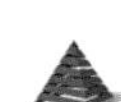
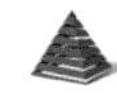

  1. Blood or body fluid contact
  2. Infected blood products
  3. Infected saliva or semen
  4. Contaminated needles
  5. Sexual contact
  6. Parenteral
  7. Perinatal period
  8. Blood or body fluids contact at birth

D. Incubation period: 6 to 24 weeks

E. Testing
  1. Infection is established by the presence of hepatitis B antigen-antibody systems in the blood.
  2. Presence of hepatitis B surface antigen (HBsAg) is the serological marker establishing the diagnosis of hepatitis B.
  3. The client is considered infectious if these antigens are present in the blood.
  4. If the serological marker (HBsAg) is present after 6 months, it indicates a carrier state or chronic hepatitis.
  5. Normally the serological marker (HBsAg) level declines and disappears after the acute hepatitis B episode.
  6. The presence of antibodies to HBsAg (anti-HBs) indicates recovery and immunity to hepatitis B.

7. Hepatitis B early antigen (HBeAg) is detected in the blood about 1 week after the appearance of HBsAg, and its presence determines the infective state of the client.

F. Complications
1. Fulminant hepatitis
2. Chronic liver disease
3. Cirrhosis
4. Primary hepatocellular carcinoma

G. Prevention
1. Strict hand washing
2. Screening blood donors
3. Testing of all pregnant women
4. Needle precautions
5. Avoiding intimate sexual contact if test for hepatitis B surface antigen (HBsAg) is positive.
6. Hepatitis B vaccine: Engerix-B (adult), Recombivax HB (pediatric); there is also an adult vaccine that protects against hepatitis A and B known as Twinrix.
7. Hepatitis B immune globulin is for individuals exposed to HBV through sexual contact or through the percutaneous or transmucosal routes, who have never had hepatitis B and have never received hepatitis B vaccine.

XVIII. Hepatitis C

A. Description
1. Hepatitis C virus infection occurs year-round.
2. Infection can occur in any age group.
3. Infection with HCV is common among drug abusers and is the major cause of posttransfusion hepatitis.
4. Risk factors are similar to those for HBV because hepatitis C is also transmitted parenterally.

B. Individuals at increased risk
1. Parenteral drug users
2. Clients receiving frequent transfusions
3. Health care personnel

C. Transmission: Same as for HBV, primarily through blood

D. Incubation period: 5 to 10 weeks

E. Testing: Anti-HCV is the antibody to HCV and is measured to detect chronic states of hepatitis C.

F. Complications
1. Chronic liver disease
2. Cirrhosis
3. Primary hepatocellular carcinoma

G. Prevention
1. Strict hand washing
2. Needle precautions
3. Screening of blood donors

XIX. Hepatitis D

A. Description
1. Hepatitis D is common in the Mediterranean and Middle Eastern areas.
2. Hepatitis D occurs with hepatitis B and may cause infection only in the presence of active HBV infection.
3. Coinfection with the delta-agent (HDV) intensifies the acute symptoms of hepatitis B.
4. Transmission and risk of infection are the same as for HBV, via contact with blood and blood products.
5. Prevention of HBV infection with vaccine also prevents HDV infection, because HDV depends on HBV for replication.

B. High-risk individuals
1. Drug users
2. Clients receiving hemodialysis
3. Clients receiving frequent blood transfusions

C. Transmission: Same as for HBV

D. Incubation period: 7 to 8 weeks

E. Testing: Serological HDV determination is made by detection of the hepatitis D antigen (HDAg) early in the course of the infection and by detection of anti-HDV antibody in the later disease stages.

F. Complications
1. Chronic liver disease
2. Fulminant hepatitis

G. Prevention: Because hepatitis D must coexist with hepatitis B, the precautions that help prevent hepatitis B are also useful in preventing delta hepatitis.

XX. Hepatitis E

A. Description
1. Hepatitis E is a waterborne virus.
2. Hepatitis E is prevalent in areas where sewage disposal is inadequate or communal bathing in contaminated rivers is practiced.
3. The risk of infection is the same as for HAV.
4. Infection with HEV presents as a mild disease except in infected women in the third trimester of pregnancy, in whom the mortality rate is high.

B. Individuals with increased risk
1. Travelers to countries that have a high incidence of hepatitis E such as India, Burma (Myanmar), Afghanistan, Algeria, and Mexico
2. Eating or drinking of food or water contaminated with the virus

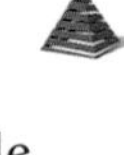

C. Transmission: Same as for HAV

D. Incubation period: 2 to 9 weeks

E. Testing: Specific serological tests for HEV include detection of IgM and IgG antibodies to hepatitis E (anti-HEV).

F. Complications
1. High mortality rate in pregnant women
2. Fetal demise

G. Prevention
1. Strict hand washing
2. Treatment of water supplies and sanitation measures

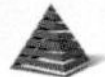

XXI. Client and Family Home Care Instructions for Hepatitis (Box 47-11)

XXII. Pancreatitis

A. Description

1. Acute or chronic inflammation of the pancreas, with associated escape of pancreatic enzymes into surrounding tissue
2. Acute pancreatitis occurs suddenly as one attack or can be recurrent, with resolutions.
3. Chronic pancreatitis is a continual inflammation and destruction of the pancreas, with scar tissue replacing pancreatic tissue.
4. Precipitating factors include trauma, the use of alcohol, biliary tract disease, viral or bacterial disease, hyperlipidemia, hypercalcemia, cholelithiasis, hyperparathyroidism, ischemic vascular disease, and peptic ulcer disease.

B. Acute pancreatitis

1. Data collection
   a. Abdominal pain, including a sudden onset at the midepigastric or left upper quadrant location with radiation to the back
   b. Pain aggravated by a fatty meal, alcohol, or by lying in a recumbent position
   c. Abdominal tenderness and guarding
   d. Nausea and vomiting
   e. Weight loss
   f. Absent or decreased bowel sounds
   g. Elevated white blood cell count, glucose, bilirubin, alkaline phosphatase, and urinary amylase
   h. Elevated serum lipase and amylase
   i. **Cullen's sign**
   j. Turner's sign

Cullen's sign is the discoloration of the abdomen and periumbilical area. Turner's sign is the bluish discoloration of the flanks. Both signs are indicative of pancreatitis.

2. Interventions
   a. Maintain NPO status and assist to maintain hydration with IV fluids as prescribed.
   b. Assist to administer parenteral nutrition for severe nutritional depletion.
   c. Administer supplemental preparations and vitamins and minerals to increase caloric intake if prescribed.
   d. Maintain nasogastric tube to decrease gastric distention and suppress pancreatic secretion.
   e. Administer opiates as prescribed for pain.
   f. Administer antacids as prescribed to neutralize gastric secretions.
   g. Administer H_2-receptor antagonists or proton pump inhibitors as prescribed to decrease hydrochloric acid production and prevent activation of pancreatic enzymes.
   h. Administer anticholinergics as prescribed to decrease vagal stimulation, decrease gastrointestinal motility, and inhibit pancreatic enzyme secretion.
   i. Reinforce instructions on the importance of avoiding alcohol.
   j. Reinforce instructions on the importance of follow-up visits with the HCP.
   k. Reinforce instructions to notify the HCP if acute abdominal pain, jaundice, clay-colored stools, or dark urine develops. 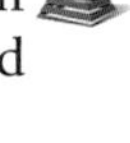

C. Chronic pancreatitis

1. Data collection 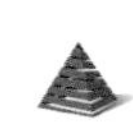
   a. Abdominal pain and tenderness
   b. Left upper quadrant mass
   c. Steatorrhea and foul-smelling stools that may increase in volume as pancreatic insufficiency increases
   d. Weight loss
   e. Muscle wasting
   f. Jaundice
   g. Signs and symptoms of diabetes mellitus
2. Interventions
   a. The client is instructed on the prescribed dietary measures (fat and protein intake may be limited).
   b. The client is instructed to avoid heavy meals.
   c. The client is instructed about the importance of avoiding alcohol.

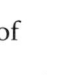

BOX 47-11 Home Care Instructions for the Client with Hepatitis

Hand washing must be strict and frequent.
Do not share bathrooms unless the client strictly adheres to personal hygiene measures.
Individual washcloths, towels, drinking and eating utensils, toothbrushes, and razors must be labeled and identified.
The client must not prepare food for other family members.
The client should avoid alcohol and over-the-counter medications, particularly acetaminophen (Tylenol) and sedatives, because these medications are hepatotoxic.
The client should increase activity gradually to prevent fatigue.
The client should consume small, frequent, high-carbohydrate, low-fat foods.
The client is not to donate blood.
The client may maintain normal contact with persons as long as proper personal hygiene is maintained.
Close personal contact such as kissing should be discouraged until hepatitis B surface antigen test results are negative.
The client is to avoid sexual activity until hepatitis B surface antigen results are negative.
The client needs to carry a Medic-Alert card noting the date of hepatitis onset.
The client needs to inform other health professionals, such as medical or dental personnel, of the onset of hepatitis.
The client needs to keep follow-up appointments with the HCP.

d. Provide supplemental preparations and vitamins and minerals to increase caloric intake.
e. Administer pancreatic enzymes as prescribed to aid in the digestion and absorption of fat and protein.
f. Administer insulin or oral hypoglycemic medications as prescribed to control diabetes mellitus, if present.
g. Reinforce instructions on the use of pancreatic enzyme medications.
h. Reinforce instructions to the client on the treatment plan for glucose management.
i. Reinforce instructions to notify the HCP if increased steatorrhea occurs, abdominal distention or cramping, or skin breakdown develops.
j. Reinforce instructions in the importance of follow-up visits.

XXIII. Pancreatic Tumors, Intestinal Tumors, and Bowel Obstruction (Refer to Chapter 43)

XXIV. Ulcerative Colitis

A. Description
1. An ulcerative and inflammatory disease of the bowel that results in poor absorption of nutrients
2. Commonly begins in the rectum and spreads upward toward the cecum
3. The colon becomes edematous and may develop bleeding lesions and ulcers; the ulcers may lead to perforation.
4. Scar tissue develops and causes loss of elasticity and loss of the ability to absorb nutrients.
5. Colitis is characterized by various periods of remissions and exacerbations.
6. Acute ulcerative colitis results in vascular congestion, hemorrhage, edema, and ulceration of the bowel mucosa.
7. Chronic ulcerative colitis causes muscular hypertrophy, fat deposits, and fibrous tissue, with bowel thickening, shortening, and narrowing.

B. Data collection
1. Anorexia
2. Weight loss
3. Malaise
4. Abdominal tenderness and cramping
5. Severe diarrhea that may contain blood and mucus

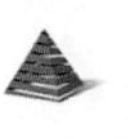

6. Malnutrition, dehydration, electrolyte imbalances
7. Anemia
8. Vitamin K deficiency

C. Interventions
1. Acute phase: Maintain NPO status and assist to administer fluids and electrolytes intravenously or via parenteral nutrition as prescribed.
2. Restrict the client's activity to reduce intestinal activity.
3. Monitor bowel sounds and for abdominal tenderness and cramping.
4. Monitor stools, noting color, consistency, and the presence or absence of blood.
5. Monitor for bowel perforation, peritonitis, and hemorrhage.
6. Following the acute phase, the diet progresses from clear liquids to low-fiber diet as tolerated.
7. Reinforce instructions about diet; usually a low-fiber, high-protein diet with vitamins and iron supplements is prescribed.
8. Reinforce instructions to avoid gas-forming foods, milk products, and foods such as whole-wheat grains, nuts, raw fruits and vegetables, pepper, alcohol, and caffeine-containing products.
9. Reinforce instructions to avoid smoking.
10. Administer medications as prescribed, which may include a combination of medications such as salicylate compounds, corticosteroids, immunosuppressants, and antidiarrheals.

D. Surgical interventions: Performed in extreme cases if medical management is unsuccessful
1. Total proctocolectomy with permanent ileostomy
   a. The procedure is curative and involves the removal of the entire colon (colon, rectum, and anus with anal closure).
   b. The end of the terminal ileum forms the stoma, which is located in the right lower quadrant.
2. Kock ileostomy (continent ileostomy) (Fig. 47-3)
   a. The Kock ileostomy is an intraabdominal pouch that stores the feces and is constructed from the terminal ileum.
   b. The pouch is connected to the stoma with a nipple-like valve constructed from a portion of the ileum. The stoma is flush with the skin.
   c. A catheter is used to empty the pouch, and a small dressing or adhesive bandage is worn over the stoma between emptyings.
3. Ileoanal reservoir (Fig. 47-4)
   a. Creation of an ileoanal reservoir is a two-stage procedure that involves the excision of the rectal mucosa, an abdominal colectomy, construction of a reservoir to the anal canal, and a temporary loop ileostomy.
   b. The ileostomy is closed 3 to 4 months after the capacity of the reservoir is increased and has had time to heal.
4. Ileoanal anastomosis (ileorectostomy)
   a. Does not require an ileostomy
   b. A 12- to 15-cm rectal stump is left after the colon is removed, and the small intestine is inserted into this rectal sleeve and anastomosed.
   c. Ileorectostomy requires a large, compliant rectum.

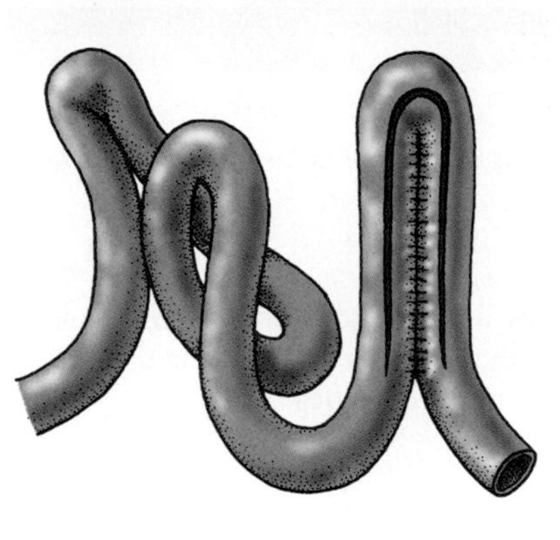
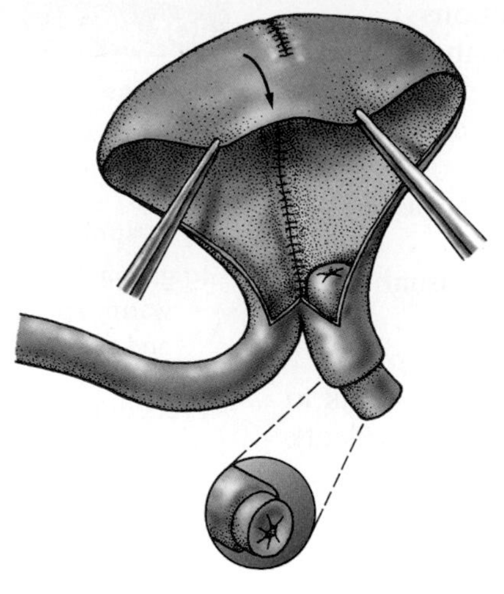
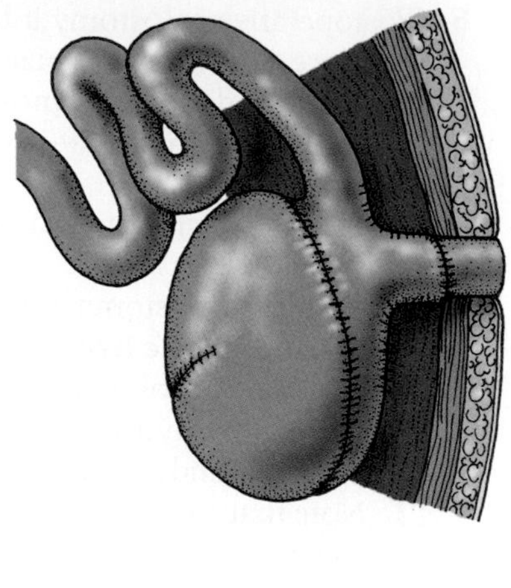

1. A reservoir, in which the patient will retain stool until draining it, is constructed from a loop of ileum folded and sutured together, then cut.

2. A portion of the ileum is intussuscepted to form a nipple valve, and the upper part of the stitched and cut ileum is pulled down and sutured to form a pouch.

3. The nipple valve, which shuts tight against pressure from a filled pouch, is pulled through the stoma and sutured flush with the abdomen.

FIGURE 47-3 Creation of a Kock (continent) ileostomy. (From Ignatavicius D, Workman ML: *Medical-surgical nursing: Patient-centered collaborative care,* ed 7, Philadelphia, 2013, Saunders.)

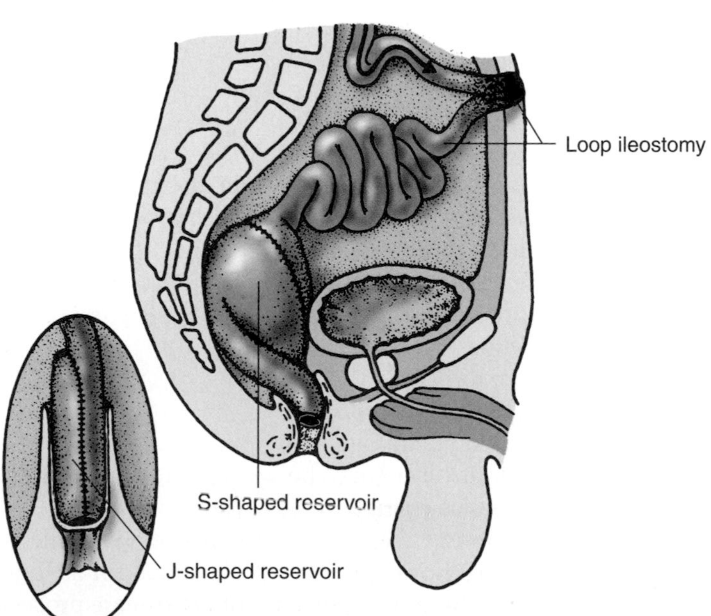

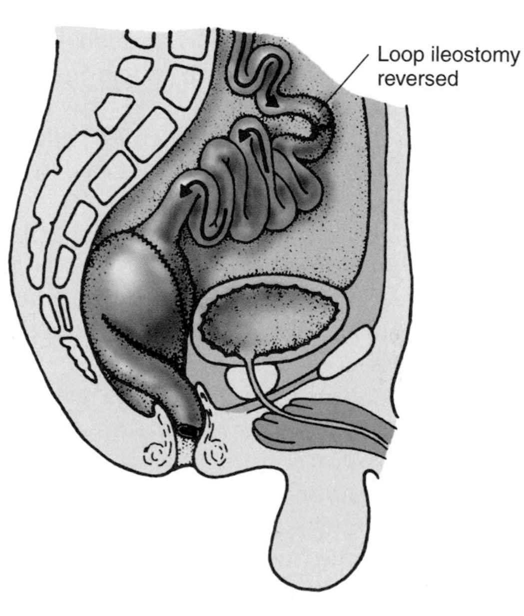

Stage 1.
After removal of the colon, a temporary loop ileostomy is created and an ileoanal reservoir is formed. The reservoir is created in an S-shaped reservoir (using three loops of ileum) or a J-shaped reservoir (suturing a portion of ileum to the rectal cuff, with an upward loop).

Stage 2.
After the reservoir has had time to heal—usually several months—the temporary loop ileostomy is reversed, and stool is allowed to drain into the reservoir.

FIGURE 47-4 Creation of an ileoanal reservoir. (From Ignatavicius D, Workman ML: *Medical-surgical nursing: Patient-centered collaborative care,* ed 7, Philadelphia, 2013, Saunders.)

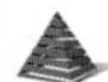

5. Preoperative colostomy and ileostomy interventions
   a. Consult with an enterostomal therapist to assist in identifying optimal placement of the ostomy.
   b. Reinforce instructions to eat a low-fiber diet for 1 to 2 days before surgery as prescribed.
   c. Administer intestinal antiseptics and antibiotics if prescribed to cleanse the bowel and to decrease the bacterial content of the colon.
   d. Administer laxatives and enemas as prescribed.

6. Postoperative colostomy interventions
    a. Place petrolatum gauze over the stoma as prescribed to keep it moist, followed by a dry, sterile dressing if a pouch (external) system is not in place.
    b. Place a pouch system on the stoma as soon as possible.
    c. Monitor the stoma for size, unusual bleeding, or necrotic tissue.
    d. Monitor for color changes in the stoma.
    e. Note that the normal stoma color is pink to bright red and shiny, indicating high vascularity.
    f. Note that a pale pink stoma indicates low hemoglobin and hematocrit levels, and a purple-black stoma indicates compromised circulation, requiring HCP notification.
    g. Monitor the functioning of the colostomy and check for bowel sounds.
    h. Expect that stool is liquid in the immediate postoperative period but becomes more solid, depending on the area of the colostomy: ascending colon—liquid; transverse colon—loose to semiformed; and descending colon—close to normal.
    i. Monitor the pouch system for proper fit and signs of leakage.
    j. Empty the pouch when it is one third full.
    k. Fecal matter should not be allowed to remain on the skin.
    l. Administer analgesics and antibiotics as prescribed.
    m. Assist to irrigate the perineal wound (if present) as prescribed, and monitor for signs of infection.
    n. Reinforce instructions to avoid foods that cause excess gas formation and odor.
    o. Reinforce instructions about stoma care and irrigations as prescribed (Box 47-12).
    p. Reinforce instructions that normal activities may be resumed when approved by the HCP.

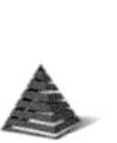
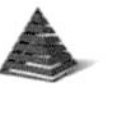

7. Postoperative ileostomy interventions
    a. Note that normal stool is liquid.
    b. Monitor for dehydration and electrolyte imbalance.

A stoma that is purple-black in color indicates compromised circulation, requiring immediate HCP notification.

XXV. Crohn's Disease

A. Description
1. An inflammatory disease that can occur anywhere in the gastrointestinal tract, but most often affects the terminal ileum and leads to thickening and scarring, a narrowed lumen, fistulas, ulcerations, and abscesses
2. Characterized by remissions and exacerbations

BOX 47-12 Colostomy Irrigation

Purpose

An enema is given through the stoma to stimulate bowel emptying.

Description

Irrigation is performed by instilling 500 to 1000 mL of lukewarm tap water through the stoma and allowing the water and stool to drain into a collection bag.

Procedure

If ambulatory, position the client sitting on the toilet.
If on bed rest, position the client on his or her side.
Hang the irrigation bag so that the bottom of the bag is at the level of the client's shoulder or slightly higher.
Insert the irrigation tube carefully without force.
Begin the flow of irrigation.
Clamp the tubing if cramping occurs; release the tubing as cramping subsides.
Avoid frequent irrigations, which can lead to loss of fluids and electrolytes.
Perform irrigation at about the same time each day.
Perform irrigation preferably 1 hour after a meal.
To enhance effectiveness of the irrigation, massage the abdomen gently.

B. Data collection
1. Fever
2. Cramp-like and colicky pain after meals
3. Diarrhea (semisolid), which may contain mucus and pus
4. Abdominal distention
5. Anorexia, nausea, and vomiting
6. Weight loss
7. Anemia
8. Dehydration
9. Electrolyte imbalances
10. Malnutrition (may be worse than that seen in **ulcerative colitis**)

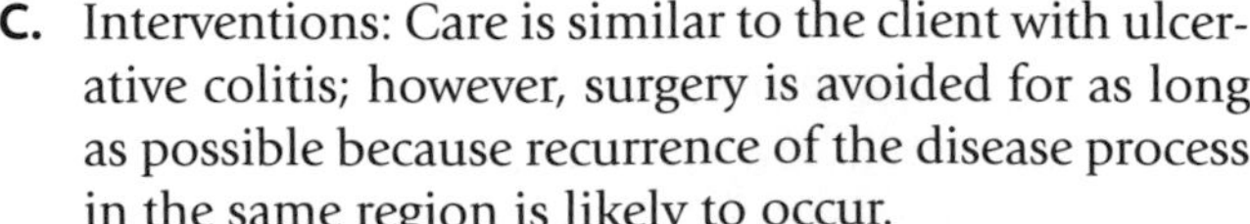
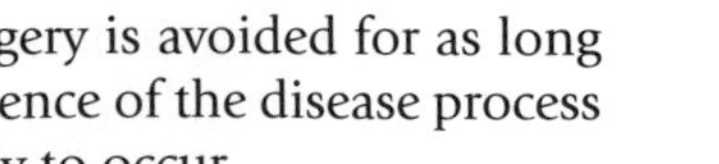
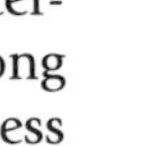

C. Interventions: Care is similar to the client with ulcerative colitis; however, surgery is avoided for as long as possible because recurrence of the disease process in the same region is likely to occur.

XXVI. Appendicitis

A. Description
1. Inflammation of the appendix
2. When the appendix becomes inflamed or infected, rupture may occur within a matter of hours, leading to peritonitis and sepsis.

B. Data collection
1. Pain in the periumbilical area that descends to the right lower quadrant

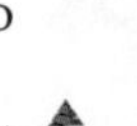
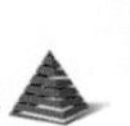

2. Abdominal pain that is most intense at McBurney's point
3. Rebound tenderness and abdominal rigidity
4. Low-grade fever

5. Elevated white blood cell count
6. Anorexia, nausea, and vomiting
7. Client in side-lying position, with abdominal guarding and legs flexed
8. Constipation or diarrhea

C. Peritonitis: Inflammation of the peritoneum

D. Appendectomy: surgical removal of the appendix
1. Preoperative interventions
   a. Maintain NPO status.
   b. Assist to administer fluids intravenously to prevent dehydration.
   c. Monitor for changes in level of pain.
   d. Monitor for signs of ruptured appendix and peritonitis.
   e. Position the client right side–lying or low to semi-Fowler's position to promote comfort.
   f. Monitor bowel sounds.
   g. Apply ice packs to the abdomen for 20 to 30 minutes every hour as prescribed.
   h. Assist to administer antibiotics as prescribed.
   i. Avoid laxatives or enemas.

Avoid the application of heat to the abdomen of a client with appendicitis. Heat can cause rupture of the appendix leading to peritonitis, a life-threatening condition.

2. Postoperative interventions
   a. Monitor temperature for signs of infection.
   b. Monitor incision for signs of infection such as redness, swelling, and pain.
   c. Maintain NPO status until bowel function has returned.
   d. Advance diet gradually as tolerated and as prescribed, when bowel sounds return.
   e. If rupture of the appendix occurred, expect a drain to be inserted, or the incision may be left open to heal from the inside out.
   f. Expect that drainage from the drain may be profuse for the first 12 hours.
   g. Position the client in a right side–lying or low to semi-Fowler's position, with legs flexed, to facilitate drainage.
   h. Change the dressing as prescribed and record the type and amount of drainage.
   i. Perform wound irrigations if prescribed.
   j. Maintain nasogastric suction and patency of the nasogastric tube if present.
   k. Assist to administer antibiotics and analgesics as prescribed.

XXVII. Diverticulosis and Diverticulitis

A. Description
1. Diverticulosis
   a. Diverticulosis is an outpouching or herniation of the intestinal mucosa.
   b. The disorder can occur in any part of the intestine but is most common in the sigmoid colon.
2. Diverticulitis
   a. Diverticulitis is the inflammation of one or more diverticula that occurs from penetration of fecal matter through the thin-walled diverticula and can result in local abscess formation and perforation.
   b. A perforated diverticulum can progress to intraabdominal perforation with generalized peritonitis.

B. Data collection
1. Left lower quadrant abdominal pain that increases with coughing, straining, or lifting
2. Elevated temperature
3. Nausea and vomiting
4. Flatulence
5. Cramp-like pain
6. Abdominal distention and tenderness
7. Palpable, tender rectal mass may be present.
8. Blood in the stools

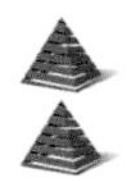

C. Interventions
1. Provide bed rest during the acute phase.
2. Maintain NPO status or provide clear liquids during the acute phase as prescribed.
3. Introduce a fiber-containing diet gradually, when the inflammation has resolved.
4. Administer antibiotics, analgesics, and anticholinergics to reduce bowel spasms as prescribed.
5. Reinforce instructions to refrain from lifting, straining, coughing, or bending to avoid increased intraabdominal pressure.

6. Monitor for perforation, hemorrhage, fistulas, and abscesses.
7. Reinforce instructions to increase fluid intake to 2500 to 3000 mL daily, unless contraindicated.
8. Reinforce instructions to eat soft high-fiber foods, such as whole grains; the client should avoid high-fiber foods when inflammation occurs because these foods will irritate the mucosa further.
9. Reinforce instructions to avoid gas-forming foods or foods containing indigestible roughage, seeds, or nuts because these food substances become trapped in diverticula and cause inflammation.
10. Reinforce instructions to consume a small amount of bran daily and to take bulk-forming laxatives as prescribed to increase stool mass.

D. Surgical interventions
1. Colon resection with primary anastomosis may be an option.
2. Temporary or permanent colostomy may be required for increased bowel inflammation.

XXVIII. Hemorrhoids

A. Description
1. Dilated varicose veins of the anal canal

2. May be internal, external, or prolapsed
3. Internal hemorrhoids lie above the anal sphincter and cannot be seen on inspection of the perianal area.
4. External hemorrhoids lie below the anal sphincter and can be seen on inspection.
5. Prolapsed hemorrhoids can become thrombosed or inflamed.
6. Hemorrhoids are caused by portal hypertension, straining, irritation, or increased venous or abdominal pressure.

B. Data collection
1. Bright red bleeding with defecation
2. Rectal pain
3. Rectal itching

C. Interventions
1. Apply cold packs to the anal/rectal area followed by sitz baths as prescribed.
2. Apply witch hazel soaks and topical anesthetics as prescribed.
3. Encourage a high-fiber diet and fluids to promote bowel movements without straining.
4. Administer stool softeners as prescribed.

D. Surgical interventions: May include ultrasound, sclerotherapy, circular stapling, or simple resection of the hemorrhoids (hemorrhoidectomy)

E. Postoperative interventions after hemorrhoidectomy
1. Assist the client to a prone or side-lying position to prevent bleeding.
2. Maintain ice packs over the dressing as prescribed until the packing is removed by the HCP.
3. Monitor for urinary retention.
4. Administer stool softeners as prescribed.
5. Reinforce instructions to increase fluids and high-fiber foods.
6. Reinforce instructions to limit sitting to short periods of time.
7. Reinforce instructions in the use of sitz baths three to four times a day as prescribed.

CRITICAL THINKING What Should You Do?

Answer: Bleeding is a primary concern for a liver biopsy because of the high vascularity of the liver. Therefore, a preprocedure data collection procedure is to check the client's status related to the risk for bleeding. The normal bleeding time ranges from 1 to 6 minutes, depending on the testing method used, and the normal prothrombin time ranges from 9.5 to 11.8 seconds. Since the client's bleeding time and prothrombin times are prolonged, the client is at risk for bleeding. Therefore, the nurse should immediately notify the registered nurse and the health care provider of these abnormal laboratory values.

Reference(s): deWit, D. & Kumagai, C. (2013). *Medical-surgical nursing: Concepts & practice.* (2nd ed., pp. 628–630). St. Louis: Saunders.

PRACTICE QUESTIONS

471. The nurse is reinforcing teaching to a client about an upcoming colonoscopy procedure. The nurse should include in the instructions that the client will be placed in which position for the procedure?
1. Left Sims' position
2. Lithotomy position
3. Knee-chest position
4. Right Sims' position

472. The nurse is preparing to perform an abdominal examination. The **initial** step should be which?
1. Palpation
2. Inspection
3. Percussion
4. Auscultation

473. The nurse reinforces postoperative liver biopsy procedures to a client. Which should the nurse tell the client?
1. Avoid alcohol for 8 hours.
2. Remain NPO for 24 hours.
3. Lie on the right side for 2 hours.
4. Save all stools to be checked for blood.

474. The nurse is caring for a client with a diagnosis of chronic gastritis. The nurse anticipates that the client is at risk for which vitamin deficiency?
1. Vitamin A
2. Vitamin C
3. Vitamin E
4. Vitamin B_{12}

475. The nurse is caring for a client after a Billroth II (gastrojejunostomy) procedure. On review of the postoperative prescriptions, which should the nurse clarify?
1. Leg exercises
2. Early ambulation
3. Irrigating the nasogastric (NG) tube
4. Coughing and deep-breathing exercises

476. The nurse is reinforcing discharge instructions to a client after a gastrectomy. Which measure should the nurse include in client teaching to help prevent dumping syndrome?
1. Ambulate after a meal.
2. Eat high-carbohydrate foods.
3. Limit the fluids taken with meals.
4. Sit in a high Fowler's position during meals.

477. The nurse is monitoring a client for the **early** signs and symptoms of dumping syndrome. Which indicates this occurrence?
1. Sweating and pallor
2. Dry skin and stomach pain
3. Bradycardia and indigestion
4. Double vision and chest pain

478. The nurse is reviewing the record of a client with Crohn's disease. Which stool characteristic should the nurse expect to see documented in the record?
1. Diarrhea
2. Constipation
3. Bloody stools
4. Stool constantly oozing from the rectum

479. A client with ascites is scheduled for a paracentesis. The nurse is assisting the health care provider in performing the procedure. Which position should the nurse assist the client into for this procedure?
1. Flat
2. Upright
3. Left side–lying
4. Right side–lying

❖ **480.** The nurse is reviewing the prescriptions of a client admitted to the hospital with a diagnosis of acute pancreatitis. Which interventions should the nurse expect to note? **Select all that apply.**
❑ 1. Administer antacids, as prescribed.
❑ 2. Encourage small, frequent, high-calorie feedings.
❑ 3. Encourage coughing and deep breathing.
❑ 4. Administer anticholinergics, as prescribed.
❑ 5. Maintain the client in a supine and flat position.

481. It has been determined that a client with hepatitis has contracted the infection from contaminated food. Which type of hepatitis is this client **most likely** experiencing?
1. Hepatitis A
2. Hepatitis B
3. Hepatitis C
4. Hepatitis D

482. The nurse is reviewing the health care provider's prescriptions written for a client admitted with acute pancreatitis. Which health care provider prescription should the nurse verify if noted in the client's chart?
1. NPO status
2. An anticholinergic medication
3. Position the client supine and flat
4. Prepare to insert a nasogastric tube

483. A client with hiatal hernia chronically experiences heartburn after meals. Which should the nurse teach the client to avoid?
1. Lying recumbent after meals
2. Eating small, frequent, bland meals
3. Raising the head of the bed on 6-inch blocks
4. Taking histamine receptor antagonist medication, as prescribed

484. The nurse is monitoring for stoma prolapse in a client with a colostomy. Which stoma observation should indicate that a prolapse has occurred?
1. Dark and bluish
2. Sunken and hidden
3. Narrowed and flattened
4. Protruding and swollen

485. An ultrasound of the gallbladder is scheduled for the client with a suspected diagnosis of cholecystitis. Which should the nurse explain to the client about this test?
1. The test is uncomfortable.
2. The test requires that the client be NPO.
3. The test requires the client to lie still for short intervals.
4. The test is preceded by the administration of oral tablets.

ANSWERS

471. 1

Rationale: The client is placed in the left Sims' position for the procedure. This position takes the best advantage of the client's anatomy for ease in introducing the colonoscope. The other options are incorrect.
Test-Taking Strategy: Focus on the subject, position for a colonoscopy. Use concepts related to gastrointestinal anatomy to answer this question. The position would be the same as that used for giving the client an enema while lying down. When answering factual questions such as these, remember the guiding principles and attempt to visualize the procedure to help you select the correct option. **Review:** positions for a colonoscopy.
Level of Cognitive Ability: Applying
Client Needs: Physiological Integrity
Integrated Process: Nursing Process/Implementation
Content Area: Fundamental Skills: Diagnostic Tests
Priority Concepts: Client Education, Elimination
Reference(s): deWit, Kumagai (2013), p. 628; Chernecky, Berger (2013), p. 358.

472. 2

Rationale: The appropriate technique for abdominal examination is inspection, auscultation, percussion, and palpation. Auscultation is performed after inspection and before percussion and palpation to ensure that the motility of the bowel and bowel sounds are not altered. The sequence of maneuvers is inspect, auscultate, percuss, and palpate.
Test-Taking Strategy: Focus on the subject, abdominal examination. Note the strategic word, *initial.* Visualize the procedure. Remember that inspection is first, and the sequence for abdominal examination is different from the

usual systematic approach. **Review:** techniques for **abdominal assessment.**
Level of Cognitive Ability: Applying
Client Needs: Health Promotion and Maintenance
Integrated Process: Nursing Process/Data Collection
Content Area: Developmental Stages: Health Assessment/Physical Exam
Priority Concepts: Clinical Judgment, Health Promotion
Reference(s): deWit, Kumagai (2013), pp. 20, 22; Jarvis (2012), pp. 115–116.

473. 3
Rationale: To splint the puncture site, the client is kept on the right side for a minimum of 2 hours. It is not necessary to remain NPO for 24 hours. Permission regarding the consumption of alcohol should be obtained from the health care provider. It is not necessary to save all stools.
Test-Taking Strategy: Focus on the **subject**, a liver biopsy. Recalling the anatomical location of this procedure will direct you to the correct option. **Review:** postprocedure instructions after a **liver biopsy.**
Level of Cognitive Ability: Applying
Client Needs: Physiological Integrity
Integrated Process: Nursing Process/Implementation
Content Area: Fundamental Skills: Diagnostic Tests
Priority Concepts: Client Education, Clinical Judgment
Reference(s): Pagana, Pagana (2013), p. 604.

474. 4
Rationale: Deterioration and atrophy of the lining of the stomach lead to the loss of function of the parietal cells. When the acid secretion decreases, the source of the intrinsic factor is lost, which results in the inability to absorb vitamin B_{12}. This leads to the development of pernicious anemia. Options 1, 2, and 3 are incorrect.
Test-Taking Strategy: Focus on the **subject**, vitamin deficiency with chronic gastritis. Knowledge regarding the pathophysiology related to the lining of the stomach is required to answer this question. **Review: vitamin B_{12} deficiency** and its relationship to gastric disorders.
Level of Cognitive Ability: Understanding
Client Needs: Physiological Integrity
Integrated Process: Nursing Process/Data Collection
Content Area: Adult Health: Gastrointestinal
Priority Concepts: Clinical Judgment, Nutrition
Reference(s): Cooper, Gosnell (2015), pp. 1417–1418, 1500.

475. 3
Rationale: In a Billroth II resection, the proximal remnant of the stomach is anastomosed to the proximal jejunum. Patency of the NG tube is critical for preventing the retention of gastric secretions. The nurse, however, should never irrigate or reposition the gastric tube after gastric surgery unless specifically prescribed by the health care provider. In this situation, the nurse should clarify the prescription. Options 1, 2, and 4 are appropriate postoperative interventions.
Test-Taking Strategy: Focus on the **subject**, care of the client who underwent a Billroth II procedure. Eliminate the incorrect options because they are **comparable or alike** and are general postoperative measures. Also, consider the anatomical location of the surgical procedure to assist in directing you to the correct option. **Review:** postoperative measures for a **Billroth II procedure.**
Level of Cognitive Ability: Analyzing
Client Needs: Safe and Effective Care Environment
Integrated Process: Nursing Process/Implementation
Content Area: Adult Health: Gastrointestinal
Priority Concepts: Clinical Judgment, Safety
Reference(s): deWit, Kumagai (2013), p. 656; Cooper, Gosnell (2015), p. 1426.

476. 3
Rationale: The client should be instructed to decrease the amount of fluid taken at meals. The client should also be instructed to avoid high-carbohydrate foods, including fluids such as fruit nectars; assume a low-Fowler's position during meals; lie down for 30 minutes after eating to delay gastric emptying; and take antispasmodics as prescribed.
Test-Taking Strategy: Focus on the **subject**, dumping syndrome. Eliminate options 1 and 4 first because these measures are **comparable or alike** and will promote gastric emptying. From the remaining options, select option 3 because this measure will delay gastric emptying. **Review:** client teaching points for **dumping syndrome.**
Level of Cognitive Ability: Applying
Client Needs: Physiological Integrity
Integrated Process: Teaching and Learning
Content Area: Adult Health: Gastrointestinal
Priority Concepts: Client Education, Nutrition
Reference(s): deWit, Kumagai (2013), p. 657.

477. 1
Rationale: Early manifestations occur 5 to 30 minutes after eating. Symptoms include vertigo, tachycardia, syncope, sweating, pallor, palpitations, and the desire to lie down.
Test-Taking Strategy: Focus on the **subject**, dumping syndrome. Note the **strategic word**, *early*. Knowledge regarding the early signs and symptoms associated with dumping syndrome is required to answer this question. Remember, sweating and pallor occur and are early signs of dumping syndrome. **Review:** signs and symptoms of **dumping syndrome.**
Level of Cognitive Ability: Analyzing
Client Needs: Physiological Integrity
Integrated Process: Nursing Process/Data Collection
Content Area: Adult Health: Gastrointestinal
Priority Concepts: Elimination, Nutrition
Reference(s): deWit, Kumagai (2013), p. 657.

478. 1
Rationale: Crohn's disease is characterized by nonbloody diarrhea of usually not more than four or five stools daily. Over time, the diarrhea episodes increase in frequency, duration, and severity. Options 2, 3, and 4 are not characteristics of Crohn's disease.
Test-Taking Strategy: Focus on the **subject**, Crohn's disease. Recalling the pathophysiology related to Crohn's disease will direct you to the correct option. **Review: Crohn's disease.**
Level of Cognitive Ability: Understanding
Client Needs: Physiological Integrity
Integrated Process: Nursing Process/Data Collection
Content Area: Adult Health: Gastrointestinal
Priority Concepts: Elimination, Inflammation

Reference(s): deWit, Kumagai (2013), p. 671; Cooper, Gosnell (2015), pp. 1437–1438.

479. 2

Rationale: An upright position allows the intestine to float posteriorly and helps prevent intestinal laceration during catheter insertion. Options 1, 3, and 4 are incorrect positions.
Test-Taking Strategy: Focus on the subject, position for a paracentesis. Visualize this procedure in selecting the correct option. Knowing that fluid will be aspirated from the abdominal cavity will assist in directing you to the correct option. **Review:** the procedure for a **paracentesis**.
Level of Cognitive Ability: Applying
Client Needs: Physiological Integrity
Integrated Process: Nursing Process/Implementation
Content Area: Fundamental Skills: Diagnostic Tests
Priority Concepts: Clinical Judgment, Safety
Reference(s): Cooper, Gosnell (2015), p. 380; Pagana, Pagana (2013), p. 692.

❖**480. 1, 3, 4**

Rationale: The client with acute pancreatitis is normally placed on an NPO status to rest the pancreas and suppress gastrointestinal (GI) secretions. Because abdominal pain is a prominent symptom of pancreatitis, pain medication will be prescribed. Some clients experience lessened pain by assuming positions that flex the trunk and draw the knees up to the chest. A side-lying position with the head elevated 45 degrees decreases tension on the abdomen and may also help ease the pain. The client is susceptible to respiratory infections because the retroperitoneal fluid raises the diaphragm, which causes the client to take shallow, guarded abdominal breaths. Therefore, measures such as turning, coughing, and deep breathing are instituted. Antacids and anticholinergics may be prescribed to suppress GI secretions.
Test-Taking Strategy: Focus on the subject, interventions associated with acute pancreatitis. Remember the pathophysiology associated with pancreatitis and note the word *acute* in the question. This will assist in selecting the correct interventions. **Review:** treatment measures for **acute pancreatitis**.
Level of Cognitive Ability: Analyzing
Client Needs: Physiological Integrity
Integrated Process: Nursing Process/Planning
Content Area: Adult Health: Gastrointestinal
Priority Concepts: Clinical Judgment, Pain
Reference(s): deWit, Kumagai (2013), pp. 708–709.

481. 1

Rationale: Hepatitis A is transmitted by the fecal-oral route via contaminated food or infected food handlers. Hepatitis B, C, and D are most commonly transmitted via infected blood or body fluids.
Test-Taking Strategy: Focus on the subject, transmission of hepatitis, and note the strategic words, *most likely.* Knowledge regarding the modes of transmission of the various types of hepatitis is required to answer this question. Remember, hepatitis A is transmitted by the fecal-oral route via contaminated food or infected food handlers. **Review:** the modes of **transmission of hepatitis**.
Level of Cognitive Ability: Understanding
Client Needs: Physiological Integrity
Integrated Process: Nursing Process/Data Collection
Content Area: Adult Health: Gastrointestinal
Priority Concepts: Clinical Judgment, Infection
Reference(s): deWit, Kumagai (2013), pp. 694–695; Cooper, Gosnell (2015), p. 1472.

482. 3

Rationale: The pain associated with acute pancreatitis is aggravated when the client lies in a supine and flat position. Therefore, the nurse would verify this prescription. Options 1, 2, and 4 are appropriate interventions for the client with acute pancreatitis.
Test-Taking Strategy: Focus on the subject, contraindications in care for the client with acute pancreatitis. Recalling the treatment measures for acute pancreatitis and the contraindications in the care of the client will direct you to the correct option. **Review:** measures for **acute pancreatitis**.
Level of Cognitive Ability: Analyzing
Client Needs: Safe and Effective Care Environment
Integrated Process: Nursing Process/Implementation
Content Area: Adult Health: Gastrointestinal
Priority Concepts: Clinical Judgment, Pain
Reference(s): deWit, Kumagai (2013), p. 709; Cooper, Gosnell (2015), pp. 1481–1485.

483. 1

Rationale: Hiatal hernia is caused by a protrusion of a portion of the stomach above the diaphragm, where the esophagus usually is positioned. The client generally experiences pain caused by reflux resulting from ingestion of irritating foods, lying flat following meals or at night, and consuming large or fatty meals. Relief is obtained by eating small, frequent, and bland meals; histamine antagonists and antacids; and elevation of the thorax after meals and during sleep.
Test-Taking Strategy: Focus on the subject, the action to "avoid." This tells you that the correct answer will be the option that represents an aggravating factor for hiatal hernia discomfort. Visualize each option and think about the anatomical location of a hiatal hernia to direct you to the correct option. **Review:** the teaching points for a **hiatal hernia**.
Level of Cognitive Ability: Applying
Client Needs: Physiological Integrity
Integrated Process: Teaching and Learning
Content Area: Adult Health: Gastrointestinal
Priority Concepts: Client Education, Health Promotion
Reference(s): deWit, Kumagai (2013), p. 646; Cooper, Gosnell (2015), pp. 1444–1445.

484. 4

Rationale: A prolapsed stoma is one in which bowel protrudes through the stoma, with an elongated and swollen appearance. A stoma retraction is characterized by sinking of the stoma. Ischemia of the stoma would be associated with dusky or bluish color. A stoma with a narrowed opening, either at the level of the skin or fascia, is said to be stenosed.
Test-Taking Strategy: Focusing on the subject, the characteristics of stoma prolapse. Thinking about the definition of *prolapse* will direct you to the correct option. **Review:** the different complications that can occur with an **ostomy**.

Level of Cognitive Ability: Analyzing
Client Needs: Physiological Integrity
Integrated Process: Nursing Process/Data Collection
Content Area: Adult Health: Gastrointestinal
Priority Concepts: Clinical Judgment, Tissue Integrity
Reference(s): deWit, Kumagai (2013), p. 683; Linton (2012), p. 432; Cooper, Gosnell (2015), pp. 689–690, 692.

485. 3

Rationale: Ultrasound of the gallbladder is a noninvasive procedure and is frequently used for emergency diagnosis of acute cholecystitis. The client may need to lie still during the procedure for short intervals of time while visualization of the gallbladder is done. The client may or may not need to be NPO (per health care provider preference), but may be instructed to avoid carbonated beverages for 48 hours before the test to help decrease intestinal gas. It is a painless test and does not require the administration of oral tablets as preparation.
Test-Taking Strategy: Focus on the **subject**, an ultrasound of the gallbladder. Visualizing this procedure will direct you to the correct option. **Review:** the procedure for an **ultrasound.**
Level of Cognitive Ability: Applying
Client Needs: Physiological Integrity
Integrated Process: Nursing Process/Implementation
Content Area: Fundamental Skills: Diagnostic Tests
Priority Concepts: Client Education, Clinical Judgment
Reference(s): Chernecky, Berger (2013), p. 553; Cooper, Gosnell (2015), pp. 382–383; Pagana, Pagana (2013), p. 3.

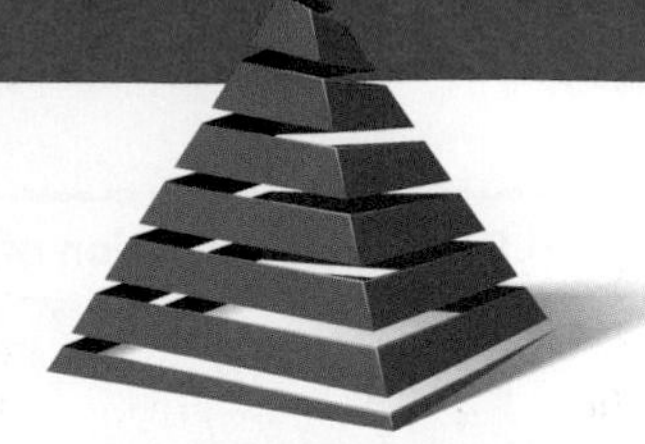

CHAPTER 48

Gastrointestinal Medications

Adult—Gastrointestinal

CRITICAL THINKING What Should You Do?

The nurse checks the ammonia level of a client with hepatic dysfunction who is receiving lactulose (Constulose) and notes that the level is 40 mcg/dL. What should the nurse do?

Answer located on p. 622.

I. Antacids (Table 48-1 and Fig. 48-1)

A. React with gastric acid to produce neutral salts or salts of low acidity
B. Inactivate pepsin and enhance mucosal protection but do not coat the ulcer crater
C. These medications are used for peptic ulcer disease and gastroesophageal reflux disease.
D. These medications should be taken on a regular schedule; some are prescribed to be taken 1 and 3 hours after each meal and at bedtime.
E. To provide maximum benefit, treatment should elevate the gastric pH above 5.
F. Antacid tablets should be chewed thoroughly and followed with a glass of water or milk.
G. Liquid preparations should be shaken before dispensing.

To prevent interactions with other medications and the interference with the action of other medications, allow 1 hour between antacid administration and the administration of other medications.

II. Gastric Protectants

A. Misoprostol (Cytotec)
   1. An antisecretory medication that enhances mucosal defenses
   2. Suppresses secretion of gastric acid and maintains submucosal blood flow by promoting vasodilation
   3. Used to prevent gastric ulcers caused by nonsteroidal anti-inflammatory medications and aspirin
   4. Administered with meals
   5. Causes diarrhea and abdominal pain
   6. Contraindicated for use in pregnancy

B. Sucralfate (Carafate)
   1. Creates a protective barrier against acid and pepsin 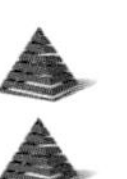
   2. Administered orally; should be taken on an empty stomach
   3. May cause constipation
   4. May impede absorption of warfarin sodium (Coumadin), phenytoin (Dilantin), theophylline, digoxin (Lanoxin), and some antibiotics; should be administered at least 2 hours apart from these medications

III. Muscarinic Antagonist

A. Description: Suppresses acid secretion by blocking muscarinic cholinergic receptors
B. Medication: Pirenzepine (Gastrozepine)

IV. Histamine (H_2)-Receptor Antagonists

A. Description
   1. Suppress secretion of gastric acid
   2. Alleviate symptoms of heartburn and assist in preventing complications of peptic ulcer disease
   3. Prevent stress ulcers and reduce the recurrence of all ulcers
   4. Promote healing in gastroesophageal reflux disease
   5. Are contraindicated in hypersensitive clients
   6. Should be used with caution in clients with impaired renal or hepatic function

B. Cimetidine (Tagamet) 
   1. Can be administered orally, intramuscularly, or intravenously
   2. Food reduces the rate of absorption; if taken with meals, absorption will be slowed.
   3. Intravenous administration can cause hypotension and dysrhythmias.
   4. Antacids can decrease the absorption of oral cimetidine.
   5. Cimetidine and antacids should be administered at least 1 hour apart from each other.
   6. Cimetidine passes the blood-brain barrier, and central nervous system side/adverse effects can

TABLE 48-1 Classification of Antacids and Considerations

Classification	Considerations
Aluminum compounds	Aluminum hydroxide is used to treat hyperphosphatemia; therefore, it can cause hypophosphatemia. Aluminum hydroxide can reduce the effects of tetracyclines, warfarin sodium (Coumadin), and digoxin (Lanoxin) and can reduce phosphate absorption and thereby cause hypophosphatemia. Contain significant amounts of sodium; should be used with caution in clients with hypertension and heart failure. The most common side effect is constipation.
Magnesium compounds	Magnesium hydroxide is also a saline laxative, and the most prominent side effect is diarrhea; it is usually administered in combination with aluminum hydroxide, an antacid that assists in preventing diarrhea. Magnesium compounds are contraindicated in clients with intestinal obstruction, appendicitis, or undiagnosed abdominal pain. In clients with renal impairment, magnesium can accumulate to high levels, causing signs of toxicity.
Calcium compounds	Calcium carbonate can cause acid rebound. Calcium compounds are rapid-acting and release carbon dioxide in the stomach, causing belching and flatulence. A common side effect is constipation. Milk-alkali syndrome (headache, urinary frequency, anorexia, nausea/vomiting, fatigue) can occur (the client should avoid milk products and vitamin D supplements).
Sodium bicarbonate	Has a rapid onset, liberates carbon dioxide, increases intraabdominal pressure, and promotes flatulence. Should be used with caution in clients with hypertension and heart failure. Can cause systemic alkalosis in clients with renal impairment. Sodium bicarbonate is useful for treating acidosis and elevating urinary pH to promote excretion of acidic medications after overdose.

occur; it may cause mental confusion, agitation, psychosis, depression, anxiety, and disorientation.

7. Dosage should be reduced in clients with renal impairment.
8. If cimetidine is administered with warfarin sodium (Coumadin), phenytoin (Dilantin), theophylline, or lidocaine, the dosages of these medications should be reduced.

C. Ranitidine (Zantac)

1. Can be administered orally, intramuscularly, or intravenously
2. Side effects are uncommon, and it does not penetrate the blood-brain barrier, as does cimetidine.
3. Ranitidine is not affected by food.

D. Famotidine (Pepcid) and nizatidine (Axid)

1. Famotidine and nizatidine are similar to ranitidine and cimetidine.
2. These medications do not need to be administered with food.

V. Proton Pump Inhibitors (Box 48-1)

A. Suppress gastric acid secretion

B. Used to treat active ulcer disease, erosive esophagitis, and pathological hypersecretory conditions

C. Contraindicated in hypersensitivity

D. Common side effects include headache, diarrhea, abdominal pain, and nausea.

VI. Medication Regimens to Treat *Helicobacter pylori* Infections (Box 48-2)

A. An antibacterial agent alone is not effective for eradicating *Helicobacter pylori* because the bacterium readily becomes resistant to the agent.

B. Triple or quadruple therapy with a variety of medication combinations is used (if triple therapy fails, quadruple therapy is recommended).

VII. Prokinetic Agent

A. Medication: Metoclopramide (Reglan)

B. Stimulates motility of the upper gastrointestinal tract and increases the rate of gastric emptying without stimulating gastric, biliary, or pancreatic secretions

C. Used to treat gastroesophageal reflux and paralytic ileus

D. May cause restlessness, drowsiness, extrapyramidal reactions, dizziness, insomnia, and headache

E. Usually administered 30 minutes before meals and at bedtime 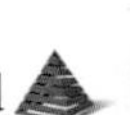

F. Contraindicated in clients with sensitivity and in clients with mechanical obstruction, perforation, or gastrointestinal hemorrhage

G. Can precipitate hypertensive crisis in clients with pheochromocytoma 

H. Safety in pregnancy has not been established.

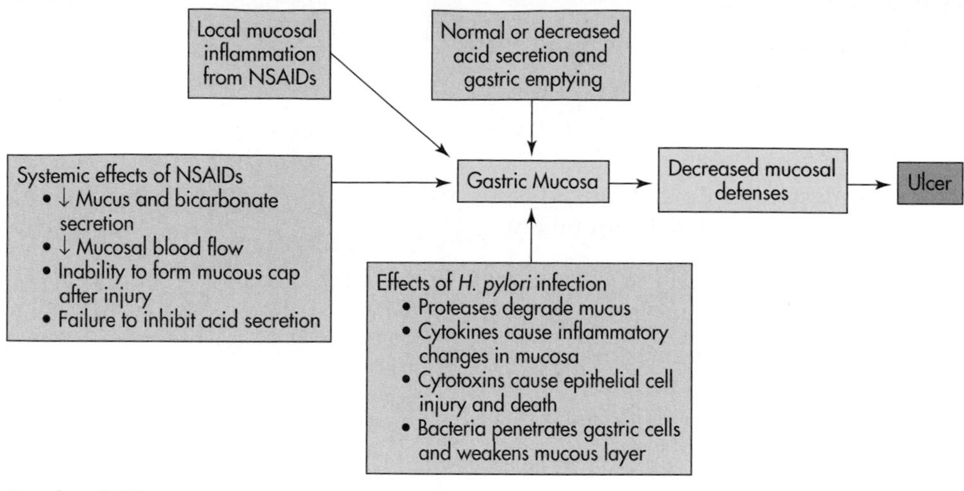

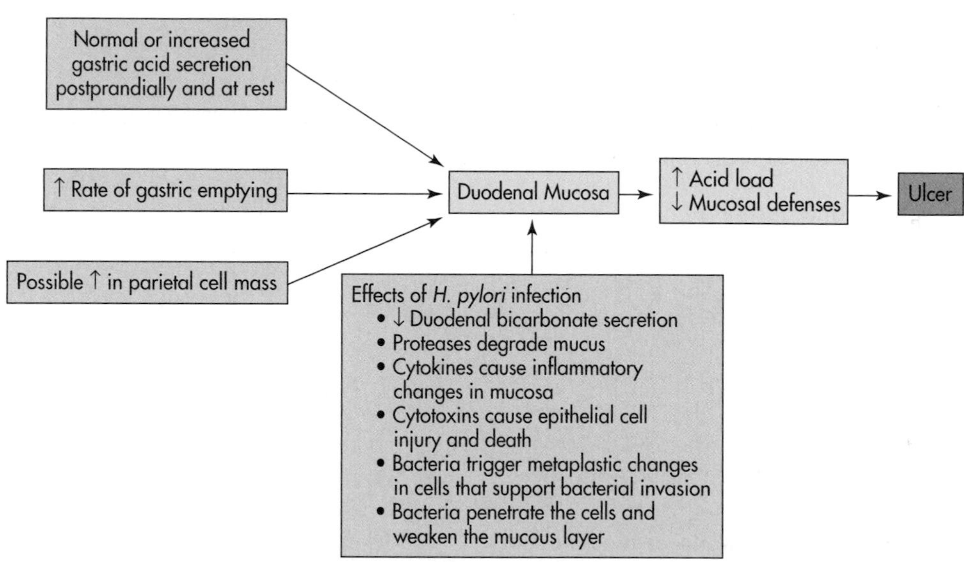

FIGURE 48-1 Pathophysiological components of peptic ulcer. *H. pylori, Helicobacter pylori; NSAIDs,* nonsteroidal anti-inflammatory drugs. (From Monahan F, Sands J, Neighbors M, Marek J, Green C: *Phipps' medical-surgical nursing: Health and illness perspectives,* ed 8, St. Louis, 2007, Mosby.)

BOX 48-1 Proton Pump Inhibitors

Esomeprazole (Nexium)
Lansoprazole (Prevacid)
Omeprazole (Prilosec)
Pantoprazole (Protonix)
Rabeprazole (AcipHex)

I. Metoclopramide (Reglan) can cause parkinsonian reactions; if this occurs, the medication will be discontinued by the health care provider.
J. Anticholinergics and opioid analgesics antagonize the effects of metoclopramide.
K. Alcohol, sedatives, cyclosporine (Sandimmune), and tranquilizers produce an additive effect.

BOX 48-2 Medication Regimens for Treating *Helicobacter pylori* Infections

Triple Therapy

Esomeprazole (Nexium), amoxicillin (Amoxil), clarithromycin (Biaxin)

Quadruple Therapies

Esomeprazole (Nexium) or Ranitidine (Zantac), metronidazole (Flagyl), tetracycline, bismuth subsalicylate

Note: Additional medications may be prescribed for each level of therapy.

VIII. Bile Acid Sequestrants (Box 48-3)

A. Act by absorbing and combining with intestinal bile salts, which then are secreted in the feces, preventing intestinal reabsorption

BOX 48-3 Bile Acid Sequestrants

Colesevelam (WelChol)
Cholestyramine (Questran, Prevalite)
Colestipol (Colestid)

B. Used to treat hypercholesterolemia in adults, biliary obstruction, and pruritis associated with biliary disease

C. With powdered forms, taste and palatability are often reasons for noncompliance and can be improved by the use of flavored products or mixing the medication with various juices.

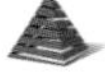

D. Side effects include nausea, bloating, and constipation. Fecal impaction and intestinal obstruction can result (adverse effects).

E. Stool softeners and other sources of fiber can be used to abate the gastrointestinal side effects.

⚠ Bile acid sequestrants should be used cautiously in clients with suspected bowel obstruction or severe constipation because they can worsen these conditions.

IX. Treating Hepatic Encephalopathy

A. Medication: Lactulose (Constulose, Enulose, Generlac)

B. Used in the prevention and treatment of portal systemic encephalopathy, including hepatic precoma and coma; also used in the treatment of chronic constipation

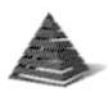

C. Promotes increased **peristalsis** and bowel evacuation, expelling ammonia from the colon and thus lowering the ammonia level

D. Improves protein tolerance in clients with advanced hepatic **cirrhosis**

E. Administered orally in the form of a syrup or rectally

X. Pancreatic Enzyme Replacements

A. Pancreatin, pancrelipase (Pancrease MT, Lipram, Pancrecarb MS, Creon)

B. Used to supplement or replace pancreatic enzymes and thus improve nutritional status and reduce the amount of fatty stools (a deficiency of pancreatic enzymes can compromise digestion, especially the digestion of fats)

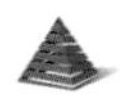

C. Should be taken with every meal and snack.

D. Side effects include abdominal cramps or pain, nausea, and diarrhea.

E. Products that contain calcium carbonate or magnesium hydroxide interfere with the action of these medications.

XI. Treatment for Inflammatory Bowel Disease (Box 48-4)

A. Inflammatory bowel disease has two forms, including **Crohn's disease** and **ulcerative colitis**.

BOX 48-4 Medications to Treat Inflammatory Bowel Disease

Antimicrobial

Metronidazole (Flagyl)
Ciprofloxacin (Cipro)
Rifaximin (Xifaxan)
Clarithromycin (Biaxin)

5-Aminosalicylates

Balsalazide (Colazal)
Mesalamine (Rowasa Asacol, Pentasa, Canasa)
Olsalazine (Dipentum)
Sulfasalazine (Azulfidine)

Corticosteroids

Budesonide (Entocort-EC)
Prednisone

Immunosuppressants

Azathioprine (Imuran)
Cyclosporine (Sandimmune)
Mercaptopurine (Purinethol)

Immunomodulators

Adalimumab (Humira)
Certolizumab (Cimzia)
Infliximab (Remicade)
Natalizumab (Tysabri)

B. Antimicrobials: May be prescribed to prevent or treat secondary infection (see Chapter 62 for information on antimicrobials)

C. 5-Aminosalicylates (5-ASAs [Asacol, Rowasa]): Decrease gastrointestinal inflammation; adverse effects include nausea, rash, arthralgia, and hematological disorders.

D. Corticosteroids: Act as an anti-inflammatory to decrease gastrointestinal inflammation (see Chapter 46 for information on glucocorticoids and corticosteroids)

E. Immunosuppressants: Suppress the immune system; can cause **pancreatitis** and neutropenia secondary to bone marrow depression, and their use is reserved for those who have not responded to other traditional therapies (see Chapter 62 for information on immunosuppressants)

F. Immunomodulators: Monoclonal antibodies that modulate the immune response to induce and maintain remission

XII. Treatment for Irritable Bowel Syndrome (IBS)

A. Irritable bowel syndrome is a gastrointestinal disorder that is characterized by crampy abdominal pain accompanied by diarrhea, constipation, or both.

B. Symptomatic relief is sometimes provided with the use of antispasmodics that relax the smooth muscle of the gastrointestinal tract, bulk-forming medications, antidiarrheals, and antidepressants.

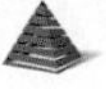

C. Alosetron (Lotronex)
   1. Used for severe IBS
   2. Can cause severe adverse effects such as constipation, impaction, bowel obstruction, perforation of the bowel, and ischemic colitis
   3. A strict risk management procedure must be followed by both the prescriber of the medication and the client, which includes several guidelines that must be followed, including monitoring for serious adverse effects, reporting them, and immediate discontinuation of the medication if they arise.

D. Lubiprostone (Amitiza)
   1. Increases intestinal motility and increases the passage of stool, thereby reducing abdominal pain
   2. Side effects include nausea, headache, diarrhea, flatulence; adverse effects include urinary tract infection and upper respiratory tract infection.

E. Linaclotide (Linzess)
   1. Used to treat irritable bowel syndrome with constipation (IBS-C) and chronic idiopathic constipation (CIC)
   2. Contraindicated in intestinal obstruction; not administered to children, and it is not known if it is harmful to the fetus during pregnancy or to the baby during breastfeeding
   3. If severe diarrhea, severe abdominal pain, or red or black stools occur, the health care provider should be notified.
   4. The daily dose should be taken 30 minutes before the first meal of the day.

XIII. Antiemetics (Box 48-5)

A. Medications used to control vomiting and motion sickness

B. The choice of the antiemetic is determined by the cause of the nausea and vomiting.

C. Monitor vital signs and intake and output.

D. Limit odors in the client's room when the client is nauseated or vomiting.

E. Limit oral intake to clear liquids when the client is nauseated or vomiting.

Antiemetics can cause drowsiness; therefore, a priority intervention is to protect the client from injury.

XIV. Laxatives (Box 48-6)

A. Bulk-forming
   1. Description
      a. Absorb water into the feces and increase bulk to produce large and soft stools
      b. Contraindicated in bowel obstruction
      c. Dependency can occur with chronic use.
   2. Side effects include gastrointestinal disturbances; dehydration and electrolyte imbalances are adverse effects.

B. Stimulants: Stimulate motility of large intestine

C. Surfactants
   1. Inhibit absorption of water so fecal mass remains large and soft
   2. Used to avoid straining

BOX 48-5 Commonly Administered Antiemetics

Serotonin Antagonists
Dolasetron (Anzemet)
Granisetron (Kytril, Granisol)
Ondansetron (Zofran)
Palonosetron (Aloxi)

Glucocorticoids
Dexamethasone (Decadron)
Methylprednisolone (Solu-Medrol)

Substance P/Neurokinin-1 Antagonists
Aprepitant (Emend)
Fosaprepitant (Emend)

Benzodiazepines
Lorazepam (Ativan)
Diazepam (Valium)
Midazolam (Versed)

Dopamine Antagonists
Phenothiazines
Chlorpromazine (Thorazine) DISC
Perphenazine (Trilafon)
Prochlorperazine (Compazine)
Promethazine (Phenergan)

Butyrophenones
Haloperidol (Haldol)
Droperidol (Inapsine)

Others
Metoclopramide (Reglan)
Domperidone (Motilium)

Cannabinoids
Dronabinol (Marinol)
Nabilone (Cesamet)

Anticholinergics
Scopolamine transdermal (Transderm Scop)

Antihistamines
Cyclizine (Marezine)
Dimenhydrinate (Dramamine)
Diphenhydramine (Benadryl)
Hydroxyzine (Vistaril, Atarax)
Meclizine hydrochloride (Bonine, Antivert)

Modified from Lehne R: *Pharmacology for nursing care*, ed 8. Philadelphia, 2013, Saunders.

BOX 48-6 Laxatives

Bulk-Forming
Methylcellulose (Citrucel)
Polycarbophil (FiberCon)
Psyllium (Metamucil, others)

Stimulants
Bisacodyl (Correctol, Dulcolax, Feen-a-Mint, Fleet laxative, others)
Senna (Senokot Ex-Lax, others), Cascara sagrada

Surfactant
Docusate sodium (Colace, others)

Osmotics
Magnesium hydroxide (Milk of Magnesia)
Magnesium citrate (Citrate of magnesia)
Sodium phosphates (Fleet enema, Fleet Phospho-Soda)
Polyethylene glycol and electrolytes (GoLYTELY)

Lubricant
Mineral oil

D. Osmotics: Attract water into the large intestine to produce bulk and stimulate peristalsis
E. Lubricants
   1. Act to soften the feces, ease the strain of passing stool, and lessen irritation to hemorrhoids
   2. Mineral oil: Interferes with absorption of the fat-soluble vitamins A, D, E, and K and can cause lipid pneumonia if accidentally aspirated

The client receiving a laxative needs to increase fluid intake to prevent dehydration.

XV. Medications to Control Diarrhea (Box 48-7)

A. Goals: Identify and treat the underlying cause, treat dehydration, replace fluids and electrolytes, relieve abdominal discomfort and cramping, and reduce the passage of stool
B. Opioids
   1. Opioids are effective antidiarrheal medications and decrease intestinal motility and peristalsis.

BOX 48-7 Medications to Control Diarrhea

Opioids and Related Medications
Difenoxin with atropine sulfate (Motofen)
Diphenoxylate with atropine sulfate (Lomotil)
Loperamide (Imodium)
Paregoric (camphorated tincture of opium)
Tincture of opium

Other Antidiarrheals
Bismuth subsalicylate (Pepto-Bismol, Kaopectate, Kapectolin)

   2. When poisons, infections, or bacterial toxins are the cause of the diarrhea, opioids worsen the condition by delaying the elimination of toxins. 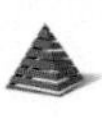
   3. Tincture of opium has an unpleasant taste and can be diluted with 15 to 30 mL of water for administration.

CRITICAL THINKING What Should You Do?

Answer: Lactulose is used in the prevention and treatment of portal systemic encephalopathy, including hepatic precoma and coma. It promotes increased peristalsis and bowel evacuation, expelling ammonia from the colon and thus lowering the ammonia level. The normal ammonia level is 10 to 80 mcg/dL. If the level is 40 mcg/dL, then the nurse determines that the medication is effective in lowering the ammonia level. The nurse should report the level to the registered nurse.

Reference(s): deWit, D. & Kumagai, C. (2013). *Medical-surgical nursing: Concepts & practice.* (2nd ed., pp. 630, 696). St. Louis: Saunders.

PRACTICE QUESTIONS

486. A client with Crohn's disease is scheduled to receive an infusion of infliximab (Remicade). The nurse assisting in caring for the client should take which action to monitor the **effectiveness** of treatment?
1. Monitoring the leukocyte count for 2 days after the infusion
2. Checking the frequency and consistency of bowel movements
3. Checking serum liver enzyme levels before and after the infusion
4. Carrying out a Hematest on gastric fluids after the infusion is completed

487. The client has a PRN prescription for loperamide hydrochloride (Imodium). The nurse understands that this medication is used for which condition?
1. Constipation
2. Abdominal pain
3. An episode of diarrhea
4. Hematest-positive nasogastric tube drainage

488. The client has a PRN prescription for ondansetron (Zofran). For which condition should this medication be administered to the postoperative client?
1. Paralytic ileus
2. Incisional pain
3. Urinary retention
4. Nausea and vomiting

489. The client has begun medication therapy with pancrelipase (Pancrease MT). The nurse evaluates that

the medication is having the optimal intended benefit if which effect is observed?
1. Weight loss
2. Relief of heartburn
3. Reduction of steatorrhea
4. Absence of abdominal pain

490. An older client recently has been taking cimetidine (Tagamet). The nurse should monitor the client for which **most** frequent central nervous system side effect of this medication?
1. Tremors
2. Dizziness
3. Confusion
4. Hallucinations

❖ **491.** A histamine (H_2)-receptor antagonist will be prescribed for a client. The nurse understands that which medications are H_2-receptor antagonists? **Select all that apply.**
❑ 1. Nizatidine (Axid)
❑ 2. Ranitidine (Zantac)
❑ 3. Famotidine (Pepcid)
❑ 4. Cimetidine (Tagamet)
❑ 5. Esomeprazole (Nexium)
❑ 6. Lansoprazole (Prevacid)

492. The client who frequently uses nonsteroidal anti-inflammatory drugs (NSAIDs) has been taking misoprostol (Cytotec). The nurse determines that the medication is having the intended therapeutic effect if which is noted?
1. Resolved diarrhea
2. Relief of epigastric pain
3. Decreased platelet count
4. Decreased white blood cell count

493. The client has been taking omeprazole (Prilosec) for 4 weeks. The nurse evaluates that the client is receiving an optimal intended effect of the medication if the client reports the absence of which symptom?
1. Diarrhea
2. Heartburn
3. Flatulence
4. Constipation

494. A client with a peptic ulcer is diagnosed with a *Helicobacter pylori* infection. The nurse is reinforcing teaching for the client about the medications prescribed, including clarithromycin (Biaxin), esomeprazole (Nexium), and amoxicillin (Amoxil). Which statement by the client indicates the **best** understanding of the medication regimen?
1. "My ulcer will heal because these medications will kill the bacteria."
2. "These medications are only taken when I have pain from my ulcer."
3. "The medications will kill the bacteria and stop the acid production."
4. "These medications will coat the ulcer and decrease the acid production in my stomach."

495. The client with a gastric ulcer has a prescription for sucralfate (Carafate) 1 g by mouth four times daily. The nurse should schedule the medication for which times?
1. With meals and at bedtime
2. Every 6 hours around the clock
3. One hour after meals and at bedtime
4. One hour before meals and at bedtime

ANSWERS

486. 2
Rationale: The principal manifestations of Crohn's disease are diarrhea and abdominal pain. Infliximab (Remicade) is an immunomodulator that reduces the degree of inflammation in the colon, thereby reducing the diarrhea. Options 1, 3, and 4 are unrelated to this medication.
Test-Taking Strategy: Focus on the **subject**, Crohn's disease and nursing implications associated with infliximab, and note the **strategic word**, *effectiveness*. Eliminate option 1 because gastric bleeding is not a characteristic of Crohn's disease. Monitoring the leukocyte count and liver enzyme levels is appropriate when infliximab (Remicade) is given but not to evaluate the effectiveness of treatment, eliminating options 3 and 4. **Review:** the signs and symptoms of **Crohn's disease** and **infliximab (Remicade)**.
Level of Cognitive Ability: Evaluating
Client Needs: Physiological Integrity
Integrated Process: Nursing Process/Evaluation
Content Area: Pharmacology: Gastrointestinal Medications
Priority Concepts: Elimination, Inflammation
Reference(s): Hodgson, Kizior (2015), p. 622.

487. 3
Rationale: Loperamide is an antidiarrheal agent. It is used to manage acute and also chronic diarrhea in conditions such as inflammatory bowel disease. Loperamide also can be used to reduce the volume of drainage from an ileostomy. It is not used for the conditions in options 1, 2, and 4.
Test-Taking Strategy: Focus on the **subject**, the intended use of loperamide. Recalling that this medication is an antidiarrheal agent will direct you to option 3. **Review:** the action of **loperamide**.
Level of Cognitive Ability: Understanding
Client Needs: Physiological Integrity
Integrated Process: Nursing Process/Planning
Content Area: Pharmacology: Gastrointestinal Medications
Priority Concepts: Elimination, Inflammation
Reference(s): Hodgson, Kizior (2015), pp. 715–716.

488. 4

Rationale: Ondansetron is an antiemetic used to treat postoperative nausea and vomiting, as well as nausea and vomiting associated with chemotherapy. The other options are incorrect.

Test-Taking Strategy: Focus on the **subject**, the intended effect of ondansetron. Recalling that this medication is an antiemetic will direct you to the correct option. **Review:** the action of **ondansetron**.

Level of Cognitive Ability: Applying

Client Needs: Physiological Integrity

Integrated Process: Nursing Process/Implementation

Content Area: Pharmacology: Gastrointestinal Medications

Priority Concepts: Clinical Judgment, Elimination

Reference(s): Hodgson, Kizior (2015), pp. 889–890.

489. 3

Rationale: Pancrelipase (Pancrease MT) is a pancreatic enzyme used in clients with pancreatitis as a digestive aid. The medication should reduce the amount of fatty stools (steatorrhea). Another intended effect could be improved nutritional status. It is not used to treat abdominal pain or heartburn. Its use could result in weight gain but should not result in weight loss if it is aiding in digestion.

Test-Taking Strategy: Focus on the **subject**, optimal intended effect of the medication as well as the name of the medication. Use knowledge of physiology of the pancreas to assist in directing you to the correct option. **Review: pancrelipase.**

Level of Cognitive Ability: Evaluating

Client Needs: Physiological Integrity

Integrated Process: Nursing Process/Evaluation

Content Area: Pharmacology: Gastrointestinal Medications

Priority Concepts: Elimination, Nutrition

Reference(s): Hodgson, Kizior (2015), pp. 919–920.

490. 3

Rationale: Cimetidine is a histamine 2 (H_2)-receptor antagonist. Older clients are especially susceptible to the central nervous system side effects of cimetidine. The most frequent of these is confusion. Less common central nervous system side effects include headache, dizziness, drowsiness, and hallucinations.

Test-Taking Strategy: Note the **strategic word**, *most*. Use knowledge of the older client and medication effects to direct you to the correct option. **Review:** the side effects of **cimetidine**.

Level of Cognitive Ability: Analyzing

Client Needs: Physiological Integrity

Integrated Process: Nursing Process/Data Collection

Content Area: Pharmacology: Gastrointestinal Medications

Priority Concepts: Clinical Judgment, Cognitive Function

Reference(s): Lehne (2013), pp. 998–999.

❖ **491. 1, 2, 3, 4**

Rationale: H_2-receptor antagonists suppress secretion of gastric acid, alleviate symptoms of heartburn, and assist in preventing complications of peptic ulcer disease. These medications also suppress gastric acid secretions and are used in active ulcer disease, erosive esophagitis, and pathological hypersecretory conditions. The other medications listed are proton pump inhibitors.

Test-Taking Strategy: Focus on the **subject**, H_2-receptor antagonists. Recalling that these medication names end with *-dine* will assist in answering this question. Also, recall that proton pump inhibitor medication names end with *-zole*. **Review:** **H_2-receptor antagonists.**

Level of Cognitive Ability: Understanding

Client Needs: Physiological Integrity

Integrated Process: Nursing Process/Implementation

Content Area: Pharmacology: Gastrointestinal Medications

Priority Concepts: Clinical Judgment, Tissue Integrity

Reference(s): Lehne (2013), pp. 998–999.

492. 2

Rationale: The client who frequently uses nonsteroidal anti-inflammatory drugs (NSAIDs) is prone to gastric mucosal injury. Misoprostol is a gastric protectant and is given specifically to prevent this occurrence. Diarrhea can be a side effect of the medication, but it is not an intended effect. Options 3 and 4 are incorrect.

Test-Taking Strategy: Note the **subject**, intended therapeutic effect of this medication. This tells you that the medication is being given to prevent the occurrence of specific symptoms. Recalling that NSAIDs can cause gastric mucosal injury will direct you to the correct option. **Review: misoprostol** and the side effects of **NSAIDs.**

Level of Cognitive Ability: Evaluating

Client Needs: Physiological Integrity

Integrated Process: Nursing Process/Evaluation

Content Area: Pharmacology: Gastrointestinal Medications

Priority Concepts: Clinical Judgment, Tissue Integrity

Reference(s): Hodgson, Kizior (2015), pp. 800–801.

493. 2

Rationale: Omeprazole is a proton pump inhibitor classified as an antiulcer agent. The intended effect of the medication is relief of pain from gastric irritation, often called "heartburn" by clients. Omeprazole is not used to treat the conditions identified in options 1, 3, and 4.

Test-Taking Strategy: Focus on the **subject**, the intended effect of omeprazole. Recalling that this medication is a proton pump inhibitor will direct you to the correct option. **Review:** the action of **omeprazole**.

Level of Cognitive Ability: Analyzing

Client Needs: Physiological Integrity

Integrated Process: Nursing Process/Evaluation

Content Area: Pharmacology: Gastrointestinal Medications

Priority Concepts: Pain, Tissue Integrity

Reference(s): Hodgson, Kizior (2015), pp. 888–889.

494. 3

Rationale: Triple therapy for *Helicobacter pylori* infection usually includes two antibacterial drugs and a proton pump inhibitor. Clarithromycin and amoxicillin are antibacterials. Esomeprazole is a proton pump inhibitor. These medications will kill the bacteria and decrease acid production.

Test-Taking Strategy: Note the **strategic word**, *best*, and focus on the **subject**, the name of the medications and their actions. Eliminate option 1 because the medications do more than kill the bacteria. These medications are taken not only when there is pain but continually until pain is gone, usually for 1 to 2 weeks. This will eliminate option 2. These medications do not coat the ulcer, eliminating option 4. **Review:** the medication regimens for treatment of ***H. pylori*** and their actions.

Level of Cognitive Ability: Evaluating
Client Needs: Physiological Integrity
Integrated Process: Nursing Process/Evaluation
Content Area: Pharmacology: Gastrointestinal Medications
Priority Concepts: Client Education, Tissue Integrity
Reference(s): deWit, Kumagai (2013), pp. 650, 652; Lilley et al (2014), pp. 817–818.

495. 4

Rationale: Sucralfate is a gastric protectant. The medication should be scheduled for administration 1 hour before meals and at bedtime. The medication is timed to allow it to form a protective coating over the ulcer before food intake stimulates gastric acid production and mechanical irritation. The other options are incorrect.

Test-Taking Strategy: Note the **subject**, scheduling of sucralfate. Focusing on the client's diagnosis and thinking about the pathophysiology associated with a gastric ulcer will assist in directing you to the correct option. **Review:** the administration of sucralfate.

Level of Cognitive Ability: Applying
Client Needs: Physiological Integrity
Integrated Process: Nursing Process/Implementation
Content Area: Pharmacology: Gastrointestinal Medications
Priority Concepts: Inflammation, Tissue Integrity
Reference(s): Hodgson, Kizior (2015), pp. 1131–1132.

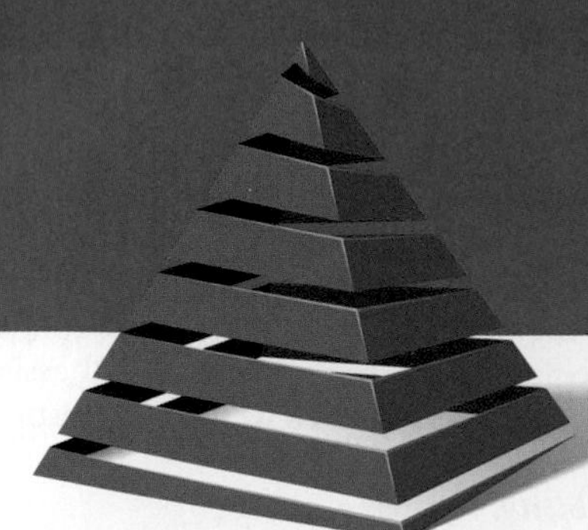

UNIT XII

The Adult Client with a Respiratory Disorder

PYRAMID TERMS

asthma A chronic inflammatory disorder of the airways marked by airway hyperresponsiveness. Asthma causes recurrent episodes of wheezing, breathlessness, chest tightness, and coughing associated with airflow obstruction that is often reversible with treatment.

bacille Calmette-Guérin vaccine A vaccine containing attenuated tubercle bacilli that may be given to persons in foreign countries or to those traveling to foreign countries to produce increased resistance to tuberculosis.

chronic obstructive pulmonary disease A disease state characterized by pulmonary airflow obstruction that is usually progressive, not fully reversible, and sometimes accompanied by airway hyperreactivity. Airflow obstruction may be caused by chronic bronchitis and/or emphysema. In chronic hypercapnia the stimulus to breathe is a low PO_2 instead of an increased PCO_2.

emphysema Abnormal permanent enlargement of air spaces distal to the terminal bronchioles, with destruction of alveolar walls without obvious fibrosis.

mechanical ventilation The use of a ventilator to move room air or oxygen-enriched air into and out of the lungs mechanically to maintain proper levels of oxygen and carbon dioxide in the blood. Types of ventilators include negative-pressure and positive-pressure ventilators. Various ventilator modes are adjusted to the client's individual needs.

multidrug-resistant strain A multidrug-resistant strain of tuberculosis (MDR-TB) can occur as a result of improper or noncompliant use of treatment programs and the development of mutations in the tubercle bacilli.

pneumothorax The accumulation of atmospheric air in the pleural space caused by a rupture in the visceral or parietal pleura. The loss of negative intrapleural pressure results in collapse of the lung. Diagnosis of pneumothorax is made by chest radiography.

suctioning A sterile procedure involving the removal of respiratory secretions that accumulate in the tracheobronchial airway when the client is unable to expectorate secretions; performed to maintain a patent airway.

tuberculin skin test (TST) The standard determinant of infection with tuberculosis. The TST is performed by injecting 0.1 mL of tuberculin purified protein derivative (PPD) intradermally in the forearm. The skin test reaction is read between 48 and 72 hours later. The reaction is measured in millimeters of the induration (raised, hardened area).

tuberculosis A highly communicable disease caused by *Mycobacterium tuberculosis*, an acid-fast rod bacterium. Tuberculosis is transmitted by the airborne route via droplet infection.

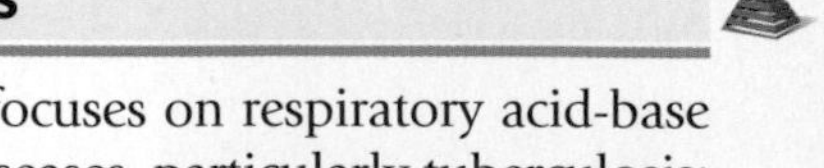

Pyramid to Success

The Pyramid to Success focuses on respiratory acid-base imbalances; infectious diseases, particularly tuberculosis; and respiratory care in relation to oxygen delivery systems and mechanical ventilation. Pyramid Points focus on the client with pneumonia, chronic obstructive pulmonary disease, pneumothorax, influenza, and tuberculosis. The Pyramid to Success includes the care of the client with tuberculosis, especially regarding the importance of the medication regimen, providing adequate nutrition and adequate rest to promote the healing process, and prevention of progression of the disease. Focus on assisting the client to cope with the social isolation issues that exist during the period of illness and on teaching the client and family the critical measures of screening, of preventing respiratory disease, and the transmission of infectious airborne disease.

Client Needs

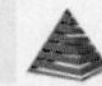

Safe and Effective Care Environment

Collaborating with the registered nurse (RN) and multidisciplinary team in the management of the respiratory disorder

Discussing consultations and referrals with the RN related to the respiratory disorder
Ensuring that informed consent related to diagnostic and surgical procedures has been obtained
Establishing priorities
Handling infectious materials such as sputum or body fluids safely
Maintaining asepsis when caring for wounds or tracheostomy sites and during mechanical ventilation or suctioning
Maintaining confidentiality related to the respiratory disorder
Maintaining respiratory precautions, standard precautions, and other precautions

Health Promotion and Maintenance

Informing the client about health promotion programs
Performing data collection techniques related to the respiratory system
Preventing respiratory disorders and infectious diseases
Providing health screening related to risks for respiratory disorders
Reinforcing instructions about adequate fluid and nutritional intake, about breathing exercises and respiratory therapy and care, about medication administration, about the need for follow-up care, and about the prevention of transmission of infection

Psychosocial Integrity

Considering religious, cultural, and spiritual influences when providing care
Discussing body image changes related to a tracheostomy if performed
Discussing end-of-life and grief and loss issues
Discussing situational role changes
Identifying coping mechanisms
Identifying support systems and community resources

Physiological Integrity

Administering medications
Assisting in caring for the client on mechanical ventilation
Caring for the client receiving respiratory care and supplemental oxygen
Managing respiratory illnesses
Monitoring for acid-base imbalances
Monitoring for alterations in body systems
Monitoring for infectious diseases
Providing nutrition and oral hygiene
Providing personal hygiene and promoting comfort, rest, and sleep

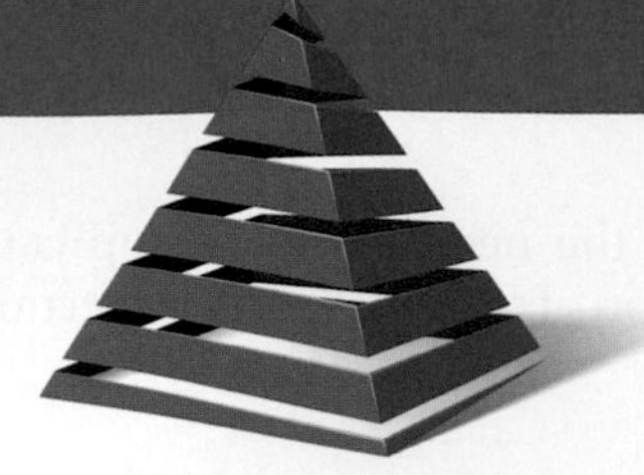

CHAPTER 49

Respiratory System

CRITICAL THINKING What Should You Do?

A victim of a gunshot wound to the chest sustained a penetrating injury. The emergency medical response team applied a nonporous dressing over the victim's sucking chest wound at the site of the accident. On arrival at the emergency department, the victim is cyanotic, and the nurse notes subcutaneous emphysema (crepitus) and tracheal deviation away from the affected side. What should the nurse do?

Answer located on p. 646.

I. Anatomy and Physiology

A. Primary functions of the respiratory system
- **1.** Provides oxygen for metabolism in the tissues
- **2.** Removes carbon dioxide, the waste product of metabolism

B. Secondary functions of the respiratory system
- **1.** Facilitates sense of smell
- **2.** Produces speech
- **3.** Maintains acid-base balance
- **4.** Maintains body water levels
- **5.** Maintains heat balance

C. Upper respiratory tract
- **1.** Nose: Humidifies, warms, and filters inspired air
- **2.** Sinuses: Air-filled cavities within the hollow bones that surround the nasal passages and provide resonance during speech
- **3.** Pharynx
  - **a.** Passageway for the respiratory and digestive tracts located behind the oral and nasal cavities
  - **b.** Is divided into the nasopharynx, oropharynx, and laryngopharynx
- **4.** Larynx
  - **a.** Located just below the pharynx at the root of the tongue; commonly called the *voice box*
  - **b.** Contains two pairs of vocal cords: the false and true cords
  - **c.** The opening between the true vocal cords is the glottis.
  - **d.** The glottis plays an important role in coughing, which is the most fundamental defense mechanism of the lungs.
- **5.** Epiglottis
  - **a.** Leaf-shaped elastic flap structure at the top of the larynx
  - **b.** Prevents food from entering the tracheobronchial tree by closing over the glottis during swallowing

D. Lower respiratory tract
- **1.** Trachea: Located in front of the esophagus; branches into the right and left mainstem bronchi at the carina
- **2.** Mainstem bronchi
  - **a.** Begins at the carina
  - **b.** The right bronchus is slightly wider, shorter, and more vertical than the left bronchus.
  - **c.** The mainstem bronchi divide into secondary or lobar bronchi that enter each of the five lobes of the lung.
  - **d.** The bronchi are lined with cilia, which propel mucus up and away from the lower airway to the trachea, where it can be expectorated or swallowed.
- **3.** Bronchioles
  - **a.** Branch from the secondary bronchi and subdivide into the small terminal and respiratory bronchioles
  - **b.** The bronchioles contain no cartilage and depend on the elastic recoil of the lung for patency.
  - **c.** The terminal bronchioles contain no cilia and do not participate in gas exchange.
- **4.** Alveolar ducts and alveoli
  - **a.** *Acinus* (plural, *acini*) is a term used to indicate all structures distal to the terminal bronchiole.
  - **b.** Alveolar ducts branch from the respiratory bronchioles.
  - **c.** Alveolar sacs, which arise from the ducts, contain clusters of alveoli, which are the basic units of gas exchange.
  - **d.** Type II alveolar cells in the walls of the alveoli secrete surfactant, a phospholipid protein that reduces the surface tension in the alveoli; without surfactant, the alveoli would collapse.
- **5.** Lungs
  - **a.** Located in the pleural cavity in the thorax
  - **b.** Extend from just above the clavicles to the diaphragm, the major muscle of inspiration

c. The right lung, which is larger than the left, is divided into three lobes: upper, middle, and lower lobes.
d. The left lung, which is narrower than the right lung to accommodate the heart, is divided into two lobes.
e. The respiratory structures are innervated by the phrenic nerve, the vagus nerve, and the thoracic nerves.
f. The parietal pleura lines the inside of the thoracic cavity, including the upper surface of the diaphragm.
g. The visceral pleura covers the pulmonary surfaces.
h. A thin fluid layer, which is produced by the cells lining the pleura, lubricates the visceral pleura and the parietal pleura, allowing them to glide smoothly and painlessly during respiration.
i. Blood flows throughout the lungs via the pulmonary circulation system.

6. Accessory muscles of respiration include the scalene muscles, which elevate the first two ribs; the sternocleidomastoid muscles, which raise the sternum; and the trapezius and pectoralis muscles, which fix the shoulders.
7. The respiratory process
   a. The diaphragm descends into the abdominal cavity during inspiration, causing negative pressure in the lungs.
   b. The negative pressure draws air from the area of greater pressure, the atmosphere, into the area of lesser pressure, the lungs.
   c. In the lungs, air passes through the terminal bronchioles into the alveoli to oxygenate the body tissues.
   d. At the end of inspiration, the diaphragm and intercostal muscles relax and the lungs recoil.
   e. As the lungs recoil, pressure within the lungs becomes greater than atmospheric pressure, causing the air, which now contains the cellular waste products of carbon dioxide and water, to move from the alveoli in the lungs to the atmosphere.
   f. Effective gas exchange depends on distribution of gas (ventilation) and blood (perfusion) in all portions of the lungs.

II. Diagnostic Tests

A. Risk factors for respiratory disorders (Box 49-1)

B. Chest x-ray film (radiograph)
1. Description: Provides information regarding the anatomical location and appearance of the lungs
2. Preprocedure
   a. Remove all jewelry and other metal objects from the chest area.
   b. Determine the client's ability to inhale and hold breath.

BOX 49-1 Risk Factors for Respiratory Disorders

Allergies
Chest injury
Crowded living conditions
Exposure to chemicals and environmental pollutants
Family history of infectious disease
Frequent respiratory illnesses
Geographic residence and travel to foreign countries
Smoking
Surgery
Use of chewing tobacco
Viral syndromes

3. Postprocedure: Help the client get dressed.

Question women regarding pregnancy or the possibility of pregnancy before performing radiography studies.

C. Sputum specimen: Specimen is obtained by expectoration or tracheal **suctioning** to assist in the identification of organisms or abnormal cells (see Priority Nursing Actions for suctioning procedure).
1. Preprocedure
   a. Determine the specific purpose of specimen collection and check with institutional policy for appropriate method for collection of the specimen.
   b. Obtain an early-morning sterile specimen by suctioning or expectoration after a respiratory treatment if a treatment is prescribed.
   c. Instruct the client to rinse the mouth with water before collection.
   d. Instruct the client to take several deep breaths and then cough deeply to obtain sputum (15 mL is needed).
   e. Always collect the specimen before the client begins antibiotic therapy. 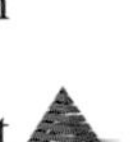
2. Postprocedure
   a. If a culture of sputum is prescribed, transport the specimen to the laboratory immediately.
   b. Assist the client with mouth care.

Ensure informed consent has been obtained for any procedure that is invasive.

D. Laryngoscopy and bronchoscopy
1. Description: Direct visual examination of the larynx, trachea, and bronchi with a fiberoptic bronchoscope
2. Preprocedure
   a. Maintain NPO status for the client from midnight before the procedure.
   b. Obtain vital signs.
   c. Check the results of coagulation studies.
   d. Remove dentures and eyeglasses.

PRIORITY NURSING ACTIONS!

Actions to Take to Perform Respiratory Suctioning

1. Explain the procedure to the client.
2. Assist the client to an upright position.
3. Perform hand hygiene and don protective garb.
4. Prepare suctioning equipment and turn on the suction.
5. Hyperoxygenate the client.
6. Insert the catheter without suction applied.
7. Once inserted, apply suction intermittently while rotating and withdrawing the catheter.
8. Hyperoxygenate the client.
9. Listen to breath sounds.
10. Document the procedure, client response, and effectiveness.

After the nurse has collected data on the client, the nurse explains the procedure. The client is assisted to a sitting upright position such as semi-Fowler's, with the head hyperextended (unless contraindicated). The nurse next performs hand hygiene (hand hygiene is also performed before positioning the client) and applies appropriate protective garb, using aseptic technique. The nurse prepares the needed suctioning equipment, turns on the suction device, and sets it to the appropriate pressure. The nurse hyperoxygenates the client with a resuscitation bag, increasing the oxygen flow rate, or asking the client to take deep breaths. The nurse next lubricates the catheter with sterile water or water-soluble lubricant (per agency procedure), inserts the catheter without the application of suction, and then applies intermittent suction for up to 10 seconds while rotating and withdrawing the catheter. After suctioning, the nurse hyperoxygenates the client again and encourages the client to take deep breaths if possible. During the procedure the nurse monitors the client for toleration of the procedure and the presence of complications. Finally, the nurse listens to breath sounds to assist in determining effectiveness and documents the procedure, the client's response, and effectiveness.

Reference(s): deWit, D. & Kumagai, C. (2013). *Medical-surgical nursing: Concepts & practice.* (2nd ed., p. 272). St. Louis: Saunders.

- **e.** Prepare suction equipment.
- **f.** Ensure that the client has an intravenous (IV) access, and assist to administer medication for sedation as prescribed.
- **g.** Have emergency resuscitation equipment readily available.

3. Postprocedure
- **a.** Monitor vital signs.
- **b.** Maintain the client in the semi-Fowler's position.
- **c.** Check for the return of the gag reflex.

- **d.** Maintain NPO status until the gag reflex returns.
- **e.** Have an emesis basin readily available for the client to expectorate sputum.
- **f.** Monitor for bloody sputum.
- **g.** Monitor respiratory status, particularly if sedation has been administered.
- **h.** Monitor for complications, such as bronchospasm or bronchial perforation, indicated by facial or neck crepitus, dysrhythmias, hemorrhage, hypoxemia, and pneumothorax.

- **i.** Notify the RN and health care provider (HCP) if fever, difficulty in breathing, or other signs of complications occur following the procedure.

E. Endobronchial ultrasound (EBUS)

1. Tissue samples are obtained from central lung masses and lymph nodes, using a bronchoscope with the help of ultrasound guidance.

2. A minimally invasive procedure performed on an outpatient basis

3. Tissue samples are used for diagnosing and staging lung cancer, detecting infections, and identifying inflammatory diseases that affect the lungs, such as sarcoidosis.

4. Postprocedure, the client is monitored for signs of bleeding and respiratory distress.

F. Pulmonary angiography

1. Description
- **a.** An invasive fluoroscopic procedure in which a catheter is inserted through the antecubital or femoral vein into the pulmonary artery or one of its branches
- **b.** Involves an injection of iodine or radiopaque or contrast material

2. Preprocedure
- **a.** Check for allergies to iodine, seafood, or other radiopaque dyes.
- **b.** Maintain NPO status of the client for 8 hours before the procedure.
- **c.** Monitor vital signs.
- **d.** Check the results of coagulation studies.
- **e.** Ensure an intravenous access is established.
- **f.** Assist to administer sedation as prescribed.
- **g.** Reinforce instructions about the need to lie still during the procedure.
- **h.** Tell the client that he or she may feel an urge to cough, flushing, nausea, or a salty taste following injection of the dye.
- **i.** Have emergency resuscitation equipment available.

3. Postprocedure
- **a.** Monitor vital signs.
- **b.** Avoid taking blood pressures for 24 hours in the extremity used for the injection.
- **c.** Monitor peripheral neurovascular status of the affected extremity.

d. Check insertion site for bleeding.
e. Monitor for delayed reaction to the dye.

G. Thoracentesis
1. Description: Removal of fluid or air from the pleural space via transthoracic aspiration
2. Preprocedure
a. Obtain vital signs.
b. Prepare the client for ultrasound or chest radiograph, if prescribed, before the procedure.
c. Check results of coagulation studies.
d. Note that the client is positioned sitting upright, with the arms and shoulders supported by a table at the bedside during the procedure.
e. If the client cannot sit up, the client is placed lying in bed toward the unaffected side with the head of the bed elevated.
f. Instruct the client not to cough, breathe deeply, or move during the procedure.
3. Postprocedure
a. Monitor vital signs.
b. Monitor respiratory status.
c. Apply a pressure dressing, and check the puncture site for bleeding and crepitus.
d. Monitor for signs of pneumothorax, air embolism, and pulmonary edema; notify the RN and HCP if signs of complications occur.

H. Pulmonary function test
1. Description: Tests used to evaluate lung mechanics, gas exchange, and acid-base disturbance through spirometric measurements, lung volumes, and arterial blood gas levels.
2. Preprocedure
a. Determine whether an analgesic that may depress the respiratory function is being administered.
b. Consult with the HCP regarding withholding bronchodilators before testing.
c. The client is instructed to void before the procedure and to wear loose clothing.
d. Remove dentures.
e. Reinforce instructions to the client to refrain from smoking or eating a heavy meal for 4 to 6 hours before the test.
3. Postprocedure: Client may resume a normal diet and any bronchodilators and respiratory treatments that were withheld before the procedure.

I. Lung biopsy
1. Description
a. A transbronchial biopsy and a transbronchial needle aspiration may be performed to obtain tissue for analysis by culture or cytological examination.
b. An open lung biopsy is performed in the operating room.
2. Preprocedure
a. Maintain NPO status of the client before the procedure.
b. Inform the client that a local anesthetic will be used for a needle biopsy, but a sensation of pressure during needle insertion and aspiration may be felt.
c. Administer analgesics and sedatives as prescribed.
3. Postprocedure 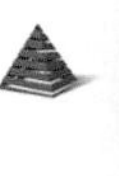
a. Monitor vital signs.
b. Apply a dressing to the biopsy site and monitor for drainage or bleeding.
c. Monitor for signs of respiratory distress, and notify the RN and HCP if they occur.
d. Monitor for signs of pneumothorax and air emboli, and notify the RN and HCP if they occur.
e. Prepare the client for chest radiography if prescribed.

J. Ventilation-perfusion lung scan
1. Description
a. The perfusion scan evaluates blood flow to the lungs.
b. The ventilation scan determines the patency of the pulmonary airways and detects abnormalities in ventilation.
c. A radionuclide may be injected for the procedure.
2. Preprocedure
a. Check the client for allergies to dye, iodine, or seafood.
b. Remove jewelry around the chest area.
c. Review breathing methods that may be required during testing.
d. Ensure intravenous access has been established.
e. Assist to administer sedation if prescribed.
f. Have emergency resuscitation equipment available.
3. Postprocedure
a. Monitor the client for reaction to the radionuclide.
b. Inform the client that the radionuclide clears from the body in about 8 hours.

K. Skin tests: A skin test is an intradermal injection to help diagnose various infectious diseases (Box 49-2).

L. Arterial blood gases (ABGs)
1. Description: Measurement of the dissolved oxygen and carbon dioxide in the arterial blood helps indicate the acid-base state and how well the oxygen is being carried to the body.
2. Preprocedure and postprocedure care, and analysis of results: Refer to Chapter 10.

Avoid suctioning the client before drawing an ABG sample because the suctioning procedure will deplete the client's oxygen, resulting in inaccurate ABG results.

BOX 49-2 Skin Test Procedure

1. Determine hypersensitivity or previous reactions to skin tests.
2. Use a skin site that is free of excessive body hair, dermatitis, and blemishes.
3. Apply the injection at the upper one third of the inner surface of the left arm.
4. Circle and mark the injection test site.
5. Document the date, time, and test site.
6. Advise the client not to scratch the test site in order to prevent infection and possible abscess formation.
7. Instruct the client to avoid washing the test site.
8. Interpret the reaction at the injection site between 24 to 72 hours after administration of the test antigen, depending on the test.
9. Check the test site for the amount of induration (hard swelling) in millimeters and for the presence of erythema and vesiculation (small blister-like elevations).

M. Pulse oximetry
   1. Description
      a. Pulse oximetry is a noninvasive test that registers the oxygen saturation (SaO_2) of the client's hemoglobin.
      b. The capillary SaO_2 is recorded as a percentage.
      c. The normal value is 96% to 100%.
      d. After a hypoxic client uses up the readily available oxygen (measured as the arterial oxygen pressure [PaO_2] on ABG testing), the reserve oxygen—that oxygen attached to the hemoglobin (SaO_2)—is drawn on to provide oxygen to the tissues.
      e. A pulse oximeter reading can alert the nurse to hypoxemia before clinical signs occur.

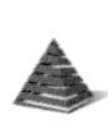

   2. Procedure
      a. A sensor is placed on the client's finger, toe, nose, earlobe, or forehead to measure SaO_2, which is then displayed on a monitor.
      b. Maintain the transducer at heart level.
      c. Do not select an extremity with an impediment to blood flow.

! A pulse oximetry reading lower than 91% necessitates HCP notification; if the reading is lower than 85%, oxygenation to body tissues is compromised, and a reading lower than 70% is life-threatening. Agency procedures and health care provider prescriptions are followed regarding actions to take for specific readings.

III. Respiratory Treatments

A. Breathing retraining (Box 49-3)

B. Chest physiotherapy (CPT)
   1. Description: Percussion, vibration, and postural drainage techniques performed over the thorax to loosen secretions in the affected area of the lungs and move them into more central airways

BOX 49-3 Client Education: Breathing Retraining and Huff Coughing

Breathing Retraining

Includes exercises to decrease the use of the accessory muscles of breathing to decrease fatigue, and to promote CO_2 elimination

The main types of exercises include pursed lip breathing and diaphragmatic breathing.

The client should inhale slowly through the nose.

The client should place the hand over the abdomen while inhaling; the abdomen should expand with inhalation and contract during exhalation.

The client should exhale three times longer than inhalation by blowing through pursed lips.

Huff Coughing

An effective coughing technique that conserves energy, reduces fatigue, and facilitates mobilization of secretions

The client should perform three or four deep breaths using pursed lip and diaphragmatic breathing. Leaning slightly forward, the client should cough three or four times during exhalation.

The client may need to splint the thorax or abdomen to achieve a maximum cough.

   2. Interventions (Box 49-4)
   3. Contraindications
      a. Unstable vital signs
      b. Increased intracranial pressure
      c. Bronchospasm

BOX 49-4 Chest Physiotherapy (CPT) Procedure

CPT is performed in the morning on rising, 1 hour before meals, or 2 to 3 hours after meals.

CPT is stopped if pain occurs.

If the client is receiving a tube feeding, the feeding is stopped and the residual is aspirated before beginning CPT.

A bronchodilator (if prescribed) may be administered 15 minutes before the procedure.

A layer of material (gown or pajamas) is placed between the hands or percussion device and the client's skin.

The client is positioned for postural drainage based on data collection.

The area is percussed for 1 to 2 minutes.

The same area is vibrated while the client exhales four or five deep breaths.

The client is monitored for respiratory tolerance to the procedure.

The procedure is stopped if cyanosis or exhaustion occurs.

The client's position is maintained for 5 to 20 minutes after the procedure.

All necessary positions are repeated until the client no longer expectorates mucus.

Sputum is disposed of properly.

Mouth care is provided after the procedure.

d. History of pathological fractures
e. Rib fractures
f. Chest incisions

C. Incentive spirometry (Box 49-5)

BOX 49-5 Client Instructions for Incentive Spirometry

1. Instruct the client to assume a sitting or upright position.
2. Instruct the client to place the mouth tightly around the mouthpiece of the device.
3. Instruct the client to inhale slowly to raise and maintain the flow rate indicator between the 600 and 900 marks.
4. Instruct the client to hold the breath for 5 seconds and then to exhale through pursed lips.
5. Instruct the client to repeat this process 10 times every hour.

IV. Oxygen

A. Supplemental oxygen delivery systems (Table 49-1)

1. Nasal cannula for low flow: Used for the client with chronic airflow limitation and for long-term oxygen use
2. Nasal high-flow (NHF) respiratory therapy: Used for hypoxemic clients in mild to moderate respiratory depression (Box 49-6)
3. Simple face mask: Used for short-term oxygen therapy or to deliver oxygen in an emergency (Fig. 49-1)
4. Venturi mask: Used for clients at risk for or experiencing acute respiratory failure (Fig. 49-2)
5. Partial rebreather mask: Useful when the oxygen concentration needs to be raised; not usually prescribed for a client with **chronic obstructive pulmonary disease** (COPD) (Fig. 49-3)

TABLE 49-1 Supplemental Oxygen Delivery Systems

Device	Oxygen Delivered	Nursing Considerations
Nasal cannula (nasal prongs)	1–6 L/min for oxygen concentration (FiO_2) of 24% (at 1 L/min) to 44% (at 6 L/min)	Easily tolerated Can dislodge easily. Doesn't get in the way of eating or talking Effective oxygen concentration can be delivered to nose and mouth breathers Ensure that prongs are in the nares, with openings facing the client Check the nasal mucosa for irritation from drying effect of higher flow rates Check skin integrity as tubing can irritate skin Add humidification as prescribed and check water levels
Simple face mask (Fig. 49-1)	5–8 L/min oxygen flow for FiO_2 of 40%–60% Minimum flow of 5 L/min needed to flush CO_2 from mask	Interferes with eating and talking Can be warm and confining Ensure that mask fits securely over nose and mouth Remove saliva and mucus from the mask Provide skin care to area covered by mask Provide emotional support to decrease anxiety in the client who feels claustrophobic Monitor for risk of aspiration from inability of client to clear mouth—that is, if vomiting occurs
Venturi mask (Ventimask) (Fig. 49-2)	4–10 L/min oxygen flow for FiO_2 of 24%–55% Delivers exact desired selected concentrations of O_2	Keep the air entrapment port for the adapter open and uncovered to ensure adequate oxygen delivery Keep mask snug on the face and ensure tubing is free of kinks because the FiO_2 is altered if kinking occurs or if the mask fits poorly Check the nasal mucosa for irritation; humidity or aerosol can be added to the system as needed
Partial rebreather mask (mask with reservoir bag) (Fig. 49-3)	6–15 L/min oxygen flow for FiO_2 of 70%–90%	The client rebreathes one third of the exhaled tidal volume, which is high in oxygen, thus providing a high FiO_2 Adjust flow rate to keep the reservoir bag two thirds full during inspiration Keep mask snug on face Make sure the reservoir bag does not twist or kink Deflation of the bag results in decreased oxygen delivered and rebreathing of exhaled air

Continued

TABLE 49-1 Supplemental Oxygen Delivery Systems—cont'd

Device	Oxygen Delivered	Nursing Considerations
Nonrebreather mask (Fig. 49-4)	FiO_2 of 60%–100% at a rate of flow that maintains the bag two thirds full	Adjust flow rate to keep the reservoir bag inflated. Keep mask snug on the face Remove mucus and saliva from the mask Provide emotional support to decrease anxiety in the client who feels claustrophobic Ensure that the valves and flaps are intact and functional during each breath (valves should open during expiration and close during inhalation) Make sure the reservoir bag does not twist or kink or that the oxygen source does not disconnect; otherwise, the client will suffocate
Tracheostomy collar and T-bar or T-piece (face tent; face shield)	The tracheostomy collar can be used to deliver the desired amount of oxygen to a client with a tracheostomy A special adaptor (T-bar or T-piece) can be used to deliver any desired FiO_2 to client with tracheostomy, laryngectomy, or endotracheal tube The face tent provides 8–12 L/min, and the FiO_2 varies due to environmental loss	Change the delivery system to a nasal cannula during mealtime if indicated for the client with a face shield Ensure that aerosol mist escapes from the vents of the delivery system during inspiration and expiration Empty condensation from the tubing to prevent the client from being lavaged with water and to promote an adequate oxygen flow rate (remove and clean the tubing at least every 4 hr) Keep the exhalation port in the T-piece open and uncovered (if the port is occluded, the client can suffocate) Position the T-piece so that it does not pull on the tracheostomy or endotracheal tube and cause erosion of the skin at the tracheostomy insertion site

FiO_2, Fraction of inspired oxygen.

BOX 49-6 Nasal High-Flow (NHF) Respiratory Therapy

- Comfortably delivers high flows of heated and humidified oxygen through a wide-bore nasal cannula and humidification system
- Can deliver nasal flow rates up to 50 to 60 L/minute to deliver humidified high-flow oxygen therapy

6. Nonrebreather mask: Most frequently used for the client with a deteriorating respiratory status who might require intubation (Fig. 49-4)
7. Tracheostomy collar and T-bar or T-piece: Tracheostomy collar is used to deliver high humidity and the desired oxygen to the client with a tracheostomy; the T-bar or T-piece is used to deliver the desired FiO_2 to the client with a tracheostomy, laryngectomy, or endotracheal tube.
8. Face tent: Used instead of a tight-fitting mask for the client who has facial trauma or burns.

B. Continuous positive airway pressure (CPAP) and bilevel positive airway pressure (BiPAP)

1. CPAP: A machine that provides continuous positive airway pressure in which a constant flow of air is provided via a face mask; used to treat obstructive sleep apnea, a chronic disorder in which one repeatedly stops breathing during the night with events that last 10 seconds or longer, and may occur numerous times during the night.

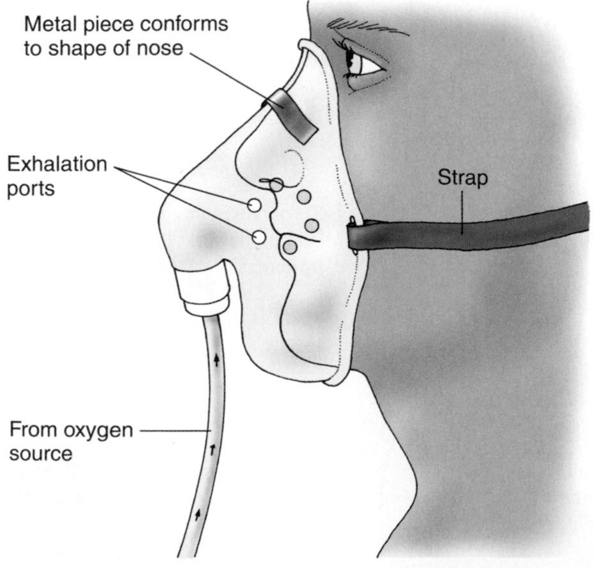

FIGURE 49-1 A simple face mask used to deliver oxygen. (From Ignatavicius D, Workman M: *Medical-surgical nursing: Patient-centered collaborative care*, ed 7, St. Louis, 2013, Saunders.)

2. BiPAP: Similar to a CPAP, except the BiPAP offers two pressure flows in which the machine is able to alternate between, allowing the client to breathe out against a slightly lower pressure; used to treat central sleep apnea, a condition similar to obstructive sleep apnea, in which the effort to breathe stops, but there is no clear obstruction of the airway.

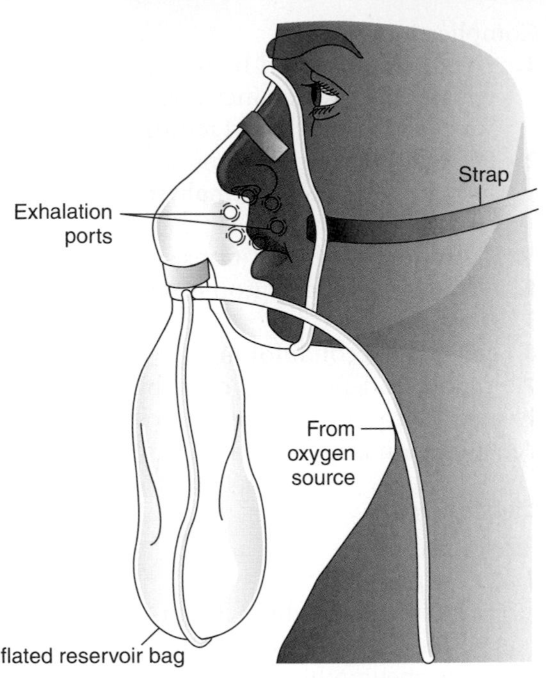

FIGURE 49-2 A Venturi mask for precise oxygen delivery. (From Ignatavicius D, Workman M: *Medical-surgical nursing: Patient-centered collaborative care*, ed 7, St. Louis, 2013, Saunders.)

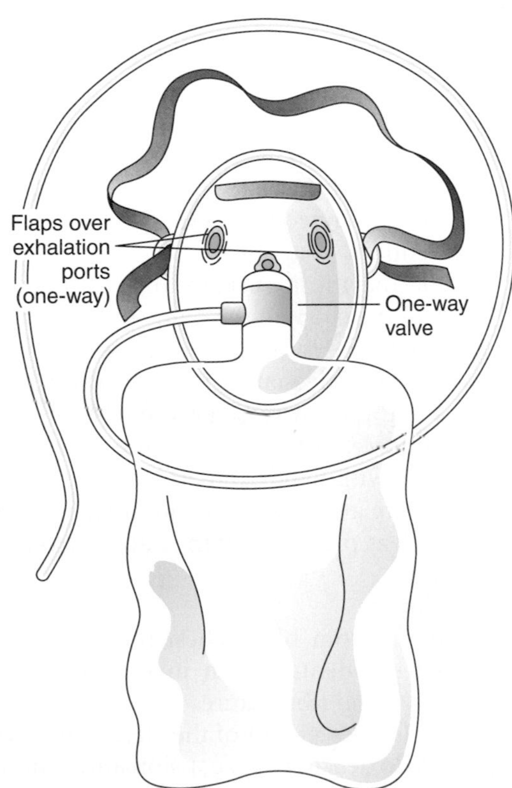

FIGURE 49-3 A partial rebreather mask. (From Ignatavicius D, Workman M: *Medical-surgical nursing: Patient-centered collaborative care*, ed 7, St. Louis, 2013, Saunders.)

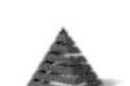

C. General interventions
1. Check color and vital signs before and during treatment.
2. Place an *Oxygen in Use* sign at the client's bedside.
3. Check for the presence of chronic lung problems before administering oxygen.

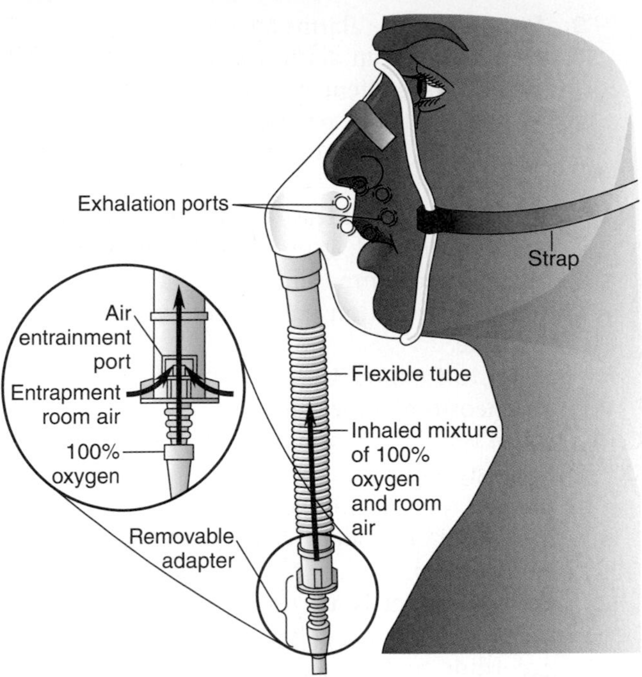

FIGURE 49-4 A non-rebreather mask. (From Ignatavicius D, Workman M: *Medical-surgical nursing: Patient-centered collaborative care*, ed 7, St. Louis, 2013, Saunders.)

4. Humidify the oxygen if indicated.
5. For specific interventions for each supplemental oxygen delivery system, see Table 49-1.

⚠ A client who is hypoxemic and has chronic hypercapnia requires low levels of oxygen delivery at 1 to 2 L/min because a low arterial oxygen level is the client's primary drive for breathing.

V. Mechanical Ventilation

A. Description: Used to overcome the client's inability to ventilate or oxygenate adequately.

⚠ For a client receiving mechanical ventilation, always check the client first and then check the ventilator.

B. Interventions 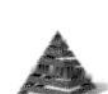
1. Check vital signs, lung sounds, respiratory status, and breathing patterns (the client will never breathe at a rate lower than the rate set on the ventilator).
2. Monitor skin color, particularly in the lips and nail beds.
3. Monitor the chest for bilateral expansion.
4. Obtain pulse oximetry readings.
5. Monitor ABG results.
6. Determine the need for suctioning and observe the type, color, and amount of secretions.
7. Check ventilator settings.
8. Check the level of water in the humidifier and the temperature of the humidification system because extremes in temperature can damage the mucosa in the airway.

9. Ensure that the alarms are set.
10. If a cause for an alarm cannot be determined, ventilate the client manually with a resuscitation bag until the problem is corrected.
11. Empty the ventilator tubing when moisture collects.
12. Turn the client at least every 2 hours or get the client out of bed, as prescribed, to prevent complications of immobility.
13. Have resuscitation equipment available at the bedside.
14. Refer to Chapter 19 for endotracheal tube and tracheostomy tube care.

C. Causes of ventilator alarms (Box 49-7)

D. Alarm safety and alarm fatigue
1. It is the responsibility of the nurse to be alert to the sound of an alarm because this signals a client problem.
2. The nurse needs to respond promptly to an alarm and immediately check the client.
3. According to The Joint Commission (TJC), the most common contributing factor related to alarm-related sentinel events is alarm fatigue.
4. Alarm fatigue results when the numerous alarms and the resulting noise tend to desensitize the nursing staff and cause them to ignore alarms or even disable them.
5. Some recommendations of TJC include establish alarm safety as a facility policy, identify default alarm settings, identify the most important alarms to manage, establish policies and procedures for managing alarms, and staff education.
6. For additional information access: http://www.pwrnewmedia.com/2013/joint_commission/medical_alarm_safety/downloads/SEA_50_alarms.pdf
http://www.jointcommission.org/assets/1/6/Field_Review_NPSG_Alarms_20130109.pdf

Never set ventilator alarm controls to the off position.

BOX 49-7 Causes of Ventilator Alarms

High-Pressure Alarm

Increased secretions are in the airway.
Wheezing or bronchospasm is causing decreased airway size.
The endotracheal tube is displaced.
The endotracheal tube is obstructed as a result of water or a kink in the tubing.
The client coughs, gags, or bites on the oral endotracheal tube.
The client is anxious or fights the ventilator.

Low-Pressure Alarm

Disconnection or leak in the ventilator or in the client's airway cuff occurs.
The client stops spontaneous breathing.

E. Complications
1. Hypotension caused by the application of positive pressure, which increases intrathoracic pressure and inhibits blood return to the heart
2. Respiratory complications such as pneumothorax or subcutaneous **emphysema** as a result of positive pressure
3. Gastrointestinal alterations such as stress ulcers
4. Malnutrition if nutrition is not maintained
5. Infections
6. Muscular deconditioning
7. Ventilator dependence or inability to wean

F. Weaning: Process of going from ventilator dependence to spontaneous breathing

VI. Chest Injuries

A. Rib fracture
1. Description
   a. Results from direct blunt chest trauma and causes a potential for intrathoracic injury, such as pneumothorax or pulmonary contusion
   b. Pain with movement and chest splinting result in impaired ventilation and inadequate clearance of secretions.
2. Data collection
   a. Pain at the injury site that increases with inspiration
   b. Tenderness at the site
   c. Shallow respirations
   d. Client splints chest
   e. Fractures noted on chest x-ray
3. Interventions
   a. Note that the ribs usually unite spontaneously.
   b. Place the client in the high Fowler's position.
   c. Administer pain medication as prescribed to maintain adequate ventilatory status.
   d. Monitor for increased respiratory distress.
   e. Reinforce instructions to the client to self-splint with hands and arms. 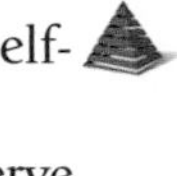
   f. Prepare the client for an intercostal nerve block as prescribed if the pain is severe.

B. Flail chest
1. Description
   a. Occurs from blunt chest trauma associated with accidents, which may result in hemothorax and rib fractures
   b. The loose segment of the chest wall becomes paradoxical to the expansion and contraction of the rest of the chest wall.  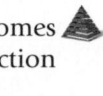
2. Data collection
   a. Paradoxical respirations (inward movement of a segment of the thorax during inspiration with outward movement during expiration)
   b. Severe pain in the chest
   c. Dyspnea
   d. Cyanosis
   e. Tachycardia

f. Hypotension
g. Tachypnea, shallow respirations
h. Diminished breath sounds
3. Interventions
a. Maintain the client in a Fowler's position.
b. Administer humidified oxygen as prescribed.
c. Monitor for increased respiratory distress.
d. Encourage coughing and deep breathing.
e. Administer pain medication as prescribed.
f. Maintain bed rest and limit activity to reduce oxygen demands.
g. Prepare for intubation with **mechanical ventilation** for severe flail chest associated with respiratory failure and shock.

C. Pulmonary contusion
1. Description
a. Characterized by interstitial hemorrhage associated with intraalveolar hemorrhage, resulting in decreased pulmonary compliance
b. The major complication is acute respiratory distress syndrome.
2. Data collection
a. Dyspnea
b. Hypoxemia
c. Increased bronchial secretions
d. Hemoptysis
e. Restlessness
f. Decreased breath sounds
g. Crackles and wheezes
3. Interventions
a. Maintain a patent airway and adequate ventilation.
b. Place the client in a Fowler's position.
c. Administer oxygen as prescribed.
d. Monitor for increased respiratory distress.
e. Maintain bed rest and limit activity to reduce oxygen demands.
f. Prepare for mechanical ventilation if required.

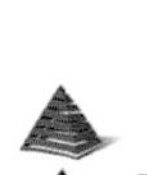
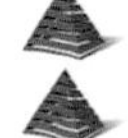
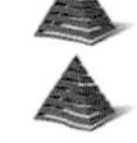

D. **Pneumothorax** (Fig. 49-5)
1. Description
a. Accumulation of atmospheric air in the pleural space, which results in a rise in intrathoracic pressure and reduced vital capacity
b. The loss of negative intrapleural pressure results in collapse of the lung.
c. A spontaneous pneumothorax occurs with the rupture of a pulmonary bleb.
d. An open pneumothorax occurs when an opening through the chest wall allows the entrance of positive atmospheric air pressure into the pleural space.
e. A tension pneumothorax occurs from a blunt chest injury or from mechanical ventilation when a buildup of positive pressure occurs in the pleural space.
f. Diagnosis of pneumothorax is made by chest x-ray.

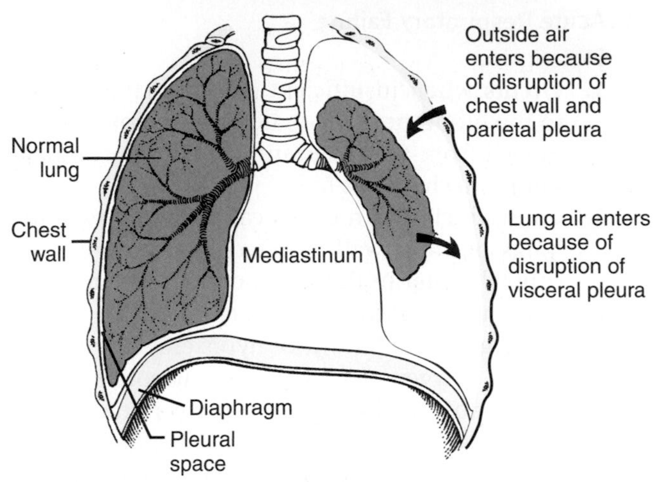

FIGURE 49-5 Pneumothorax. Air in the pleural space causes the lungs to collapse around the hilus and may push the mediastinal contents (heart and great vessels) toward the other lung. (From McCance K, Huether S: *Pathophysiology: The biologic basis for disease in adults and children*, ed 6, St. Louis, 2010, Mosby.)

BOX 49-8 Data Collection Findings: Pneumothorax

Absent breath sounds on affected side
Cyanosis
Decreased chest expansion unilaterally
Dyspnea
Hypotension
Sharp chest pain
Subcutaneous emphysema as evidenced by crepitus on palpation
Sucking sound with open chest wound
Tachycardia
Tachypnea
Tracheal deviation to the unaffected side with tension pneumothorax

2. Data collection (Box 49-8)
3. Interventions
a. Apply a nonporous dressing over an open chest wound.
b. Administer oxygen as prescribed.
c. Place the client in the Fowler's position.
d. Prepare for chest tube placement, which will remain in place until the lung has expanded fully.
e. Monitor the chest tube drainage system.
f. Monitor for subcutaneous emphysema.
g. Refer to Chapter 19 for information on caring for a client with chest tubes.

! Clients with a respiratory disorder should be positioned with the head of the bed elevated.

VII. Acute Respiratory Failure

A. Description
1. Occurs when insufficient oxygen is transported to the blood or inadequate carbon dioxide is removed from the lungs and the client's compensatory mechanisms fail
2. Causes include a mechanical abnormality of the lungs or chest wall, a defect in the respiratory control center in the brain, or an impairment in the function of the respiratory muscles.
3. In oxygenation failure, or hypoxemic respiratory failure, oxygen may reach the alveoli but cannot be absorbed or used properly, resulting in a PaO_2 less than 60 mm Hg, arterial oxygen saturation (SaO_2) lower than 90%, or partial pressure of arterial carbon dioxide ($PaCO_2$) greater than 50 mm Hg occurring with acidemia.
4. Many clients experience both hypoxemic and hypercapnic respiratory failure, and retained carbon dioxide in the alveoli displaces oxygen, contributing to the hypoxemia.
5. Manifestations of respiratory failure are related to the extent and rapidity of change in PaO_2 and $PaCO_2$.

B. Data collection
1. Dyspnea
2. Headache
3. Restlessness
4. Confusion
5. Decreased level of consciousness
6. Tachycardia
7. Hypertension
8. Dysrhythmias
9. Alterations in respirations and breath sounds

C. Interventions
1. Identify and treat the cause of the respiratory failure
2. Administer oxygen to maintain the PaO_2 level greater than 60 to 70 mm Hg.
3. Place the client in a Fowler's position.
4. Encourage deep breathing.
5. Assist to administer bronchodilators as prescribed.
6. Prepare the client for mechanical ventilation if supplemental oxygen cannot maintain acceptable PaO_2 and $PaCO_2$ levels.

VIII. Acute Respiratory Distress Syndrome

A. Description
1. A form of acute respiratory failure that occurs as a complication of some other condition; it is caused by a diffuse lung injury and leads to extravascular lung fluid.
2. The major site of injury is the alveolar capillary membrane.
3. The interstitial edema causes compression and obliteration of the terminal airways and leads to reduced lung volume and compliance.
4. The ABG levels identify respiratory acidosis and hypoxemia that do not respond to an increased percentage of oxygen.
5. The chest x-ray shows bilateral interstitial and alveolar infiltrates; interstitial edema may not show until there is a 30% increase in fluid content.
6. Some of the causes include sepsis, fluid overload, shock, trauma, neurological injuries, burns, disseminated intravascular coagulation, drug ingestion, aspiration, and the inhalation of toxic substances.

B. Data collection
1. Tachypnea
2. Dyspnea
3. Decreased breath sounds
4. Deteriorating ABG levels
5. Hypoxemia despite high concentrations of delivered oxygen
6. Decreased pulmonary compliance
7. Pulmonary infiltrates

C. Interventions
1. Identify and treat the cause of the acute respiratory distress syndrome.
2. Administer oxygen as prescribed.
3. Place the client in a Fowler's position.
4. Restrict fluid intake as prescribed.
5. Provide respiratory treatments as prescribed.
6. Administer diuretics, anticoagulants, or corticosteroids as prescribed.
7. Prepare the client for intubation and mechanical ventilation.

IX. Asthma

A. Refer to Chapter 34 for information on asthma.

X. Chronic Obstructive Pulmonary Disease

A. Description
1. Is also known as chronic obstructive lung disease and chronic airflow limitation
2. Chronic obstructive pulmonary disease is a disease state characterized by airflow obstruction caused by emphysema or chronic bronchitis.
3. Progressive airflow limitation occurs, associated with an abnormal inflammatory response of the lungs that is not completely reversible.
4. Chronic obstructive pulmonary disease leads to pulmonary insufficiency, pulmonary hypertension, and cor pulmonale.

B. Data collection
1. Cough
2. Exertional dyspnea
3. Wheezing and crackles
4. Sputum production
5. Weight loss
6. Barrel chest (emphysema) (Fig. 49-6) 
7. Use of accessory muscles for breathing 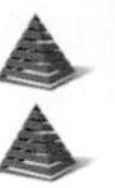
8. Prolonged expiration
9. Orthopnea

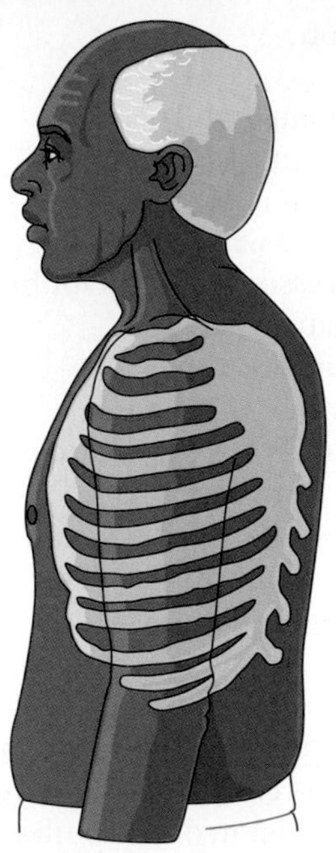

FIGURE 49-6 Typical barrel chest in a client with chronic obstructive pulmonary disease. (From Ignatavicius D, Workman M: *Medical-surgical nursing: Critical thinking for collaborative care*, ed 7, St. Louis, 2013, Saunders.)

10. Dysrhythmias
11. Congestion and hyperinflation on chest x-ray film (Fig. 49-7)
12. ABG levels that indicate respiratory acidosis and hypoxemia
13. Pulmonary function tests that demonstrate decreased vital capacity

C. Interventions
1. Monitor vital signs.
2. Administer a low concentration of oxygen (1 to 2 L/minute) as prescribed; the stimulus to breathe is a low arterial PO_2 instead of an increased PCO_2.
3. Monitor pulse oximetry.
4. Provide respiratory treatments and CPT.
5. Instruct the client in diaphragmatic or abdominal breathing techniques and pursed lip breathing techniques, which increase airway pressure and keep air passages open, promoting maximal carbon dioxide expiration.
6. Record the color, amount, and consistency of sputum.
7. Suction fluids from the client's lungs, if necessary, to clear the airway and prevent infection.
8. Monitor weight.
9. Encourage small, frequent meals to maintain nutrition and prevent dyspnea.
10. Provide a high-calorie, high-protein diet with supplements.
11. Encourage fluid intake up to 3000 mL/day to keep secretions thin, unless contraindicated.
12. Place the client in a Fowler's position and leaning forward to aid in breathing.
13. Allow activity as tolerated.
14. Administer bronchodilators as prescribed, and instruct the client in the use of oral and inhalant medications.
15. Administer corticosteroids as prescribed for exacerbation.
16. Administer mucolytics as prescribed to thin secretions.
17. Administer antibiotics for infection if prescribed.

D. Client education (Box 49-9).

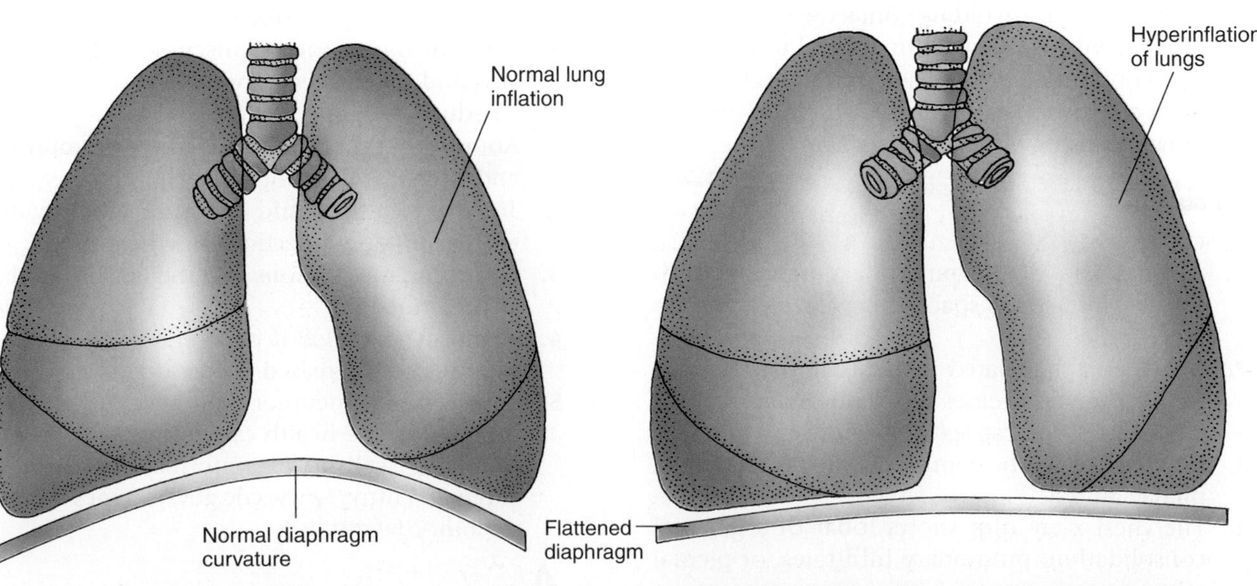

FIGURE 49-7 Diaphragm shape and lung inflation in the normal client and in the client with chronic obstructive pulmonary disease. (From Ignatavicius D, Workman M: *Medical-surgical nursing: Patient-centered collaborative care*, ed 7, St. Louis, 2013, Saunders.)

BOX 49-9 Client Education: Chronic Obstructive Pulmonary Disease

Adhere to activity limitations, alternating rest periods with activity.
Avoid gas-producing foods, spicy foods, and extremely hot or cold foods.
Avoid exposure to individuals with infections, and avoid crowds.
Avoid extremes in temperature.
Avoid fireplaces, pets, feather pillows, and other environmental allergens.
Avoid powerful odors.
Meet nutritional requirements.
Receive immunizations as recommended.
Recognize the signs and symptoms of respiratory infection and hypoxia.
Eliminate smoking and avoid environments with secondary smoke exposure.
Use medications and inhalers as prescribed.
Use oxygen therapy as prescribed.
Use pursed lip and diaphragmatic or abdominal breathing.
When dusting, use a wet cloth.

XI. Severe Acute Respiratory Syndrome (SARS)

A. Respiratory illness caused by the coronavirus, called *SARS-associated coronavirus*
B. The syndrome begins with a fever, an overall feeling of discomfort, body aches, and mild respiratory symptoms.
C. After 2 to 7 days, the client may develop a dry cough and dyspnea.
D. Infection is spread by close person-to-person contact by direct contact with infectious material (respiratory secretions from infected persons or contact with objects contaminated with infectious droplets).
E. Prevention includes avoiding contact with those suspected of having SARS, avoiding travel to countries where an outbreak of SARS exists, avoiding close contact with crowds in areas where SARS exists, and frequent hand washing if in an area where SARS exists.

XII. Pneumonia

A. Description
   1. An infection of the pulmonary tissue, including the interstitial spaces, the alveoli, and the bronchioles
   2. The edema associated with inflammation stiffens the lung, decreases lung compliance and vital capacity, and causes hypoxemia.
   3. Pneumonia can be community acquired or hospital acquired.
   4. The chest x-ray film shows lobar or segmental consolidation, pulmonary infiltrates, or pleural effusions.

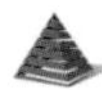
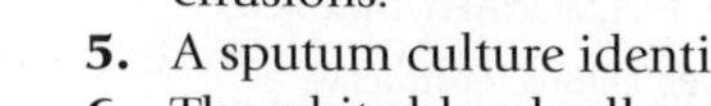

   5. A sputum culture identifies the organism.
   6. The white blood cell count and erythrocyte sedimentation rate are elevated.

B. Data collection
   1. Chills
   2. Elevated temperature
   3. Pleuritic pain
   4. Tachypnea
   5. Rhonchi and wheezes
   6. Use of accessory muscles for breathing
   7. Mental status changes
   8. Sputum production
C. Interventions
   1. Administer oxygen as prescribed.
   2. Monitor respiratory status.
   3. Monitor for labored respirations, cyanosis, and cold and clammy skin.
   4. Encourage coughing and deep breathing and use of the incentive spirometer.
   5. Place the client in the semi-Fowler's position to facilitate breathing and lung expansion.
   6. Change the client's position frequently and ambulate as tolerated to mobilize secretions.
   7. Provide CPT.
   8. Perform nasotracheal suctioning if the client is unable to clear secretions.
   9. Monitor pulse oximetry.
   10. Monitor and record color, consistency, and amount of sputum.
   11. Provide a high-calorie, high-protein diet with small, frequent meals.
   12. Encourage fluids up to 3 L/day to thin secretions, unless contraindicated.
   13. Provide a balance of rest and activity, increasing activity gradually.
   14. Administer antibiotics as prescribed.
   15. Administer antipyretics, bronchodilators, cough suppressants, mucolytic agents, and expectorants as prescribed.
   16. Prevent the spread of infection by hand washing and the proper disposal of secretions.
D. Client education
   1. About the importance of rest, proper nutrition, and adequate fluid intake
   2. To avoid chilling and exposure to individuals with respiratory infections or viruses
   3. Regarding medications and the use of inhalants as prescribed
   4. To notify the HCP if chills, fever, dyspnea, hemoptysis, or increased fatigue occurs
   5. To receive a pneumococcal vaccine as recommended by the health care provider, refer to the following website for information about this vaccine: http://www.cdc.gov/vaccines/vpd-vac/pneumo/default.htm

Teach clients that using proper hand-washing techniques, disposing respiratory secretions properly, and receiving vaccines as appropriate will assist in preventing the spread of infection.

XIII. Influenza

A. Description

1. Also known as the seasonal flu; highly contagious acute viral respiratory infection
2. May be caused by several viruses usually known as A, B, and C
3. Yearly vaccination is recommended to prevent the disease, especially for those who are older than 50 years of age, individuals with chronic illness or who are immunocompromised, those living in institutions, and health care personnel providing direct care to clients (the vaccination is contraindicated in individuals with egg allergies).
4. Additional prevention measures include avoiding those who have developed influenza, frequent and proper hand washing, and cleaning and disinfecting surfaces that have become contaminated with secretions.
5. Avian influenza A (H5N1)
   - **a.** Affects birds; does not usually affect humans; however, human cases have been reported in some countries.
   - **b.** An H5N1 vaccine has been developed for use if a pandemic virus were to emerge.
   - **c.** Reported symptoms are similar to those that are associated with influenza A, B, and C.
   - **d.** Prevention measures include thoroughly cooking poultry products, avoiding contact with wild animals, frequent and proper hand washing, and cleaning and disinfecting surfaces that have become contaminated with secretions.
6. Swine (H1N1) influenza
   - **a.** A strain of flu that consists of genetic materials from swine, avian, and human influenza viruses
   - **b.** Signs and symptoms are similar to those that present with seasonal flu; in addition, vomiting and diarrhea commonly occur.
   - **c.** Prevention measures and treatment are the same as for the seasonal flu.
   - **d.** Refer to Chapter 39 for additional information on influenza and Chapter 50 for information on H1N1 vaccines.

B. Data collection

1. Acute onset of fever and muscle aches
2. Headache
3. Fatigue, weakness, and anorexia
4. Sore throat, cough, and rhinorrhea

C. Interventions

1. Encourage rest.
2. Encourage fluids to prevent pulmonary complications (unless contraindicated).
3. Monitor lung sounds.
4. Provide supportive therapy such as antipyretics or antitussives as indicated.
5. Administer antiviral medications as prescribed for current strain of influenza (refer to Chapter 50).

XIV. Legionnaire's Disease

A. Description

1. Acute bacterial infection caused by *Legionella pneumophila*
2. Sources of the organism include contaminated air conditioner cooling tower water and warm stagnant water supplies, including water vaporizers, water sonicators, whirlpool spas, and showers.
3. Person-to-person contact does not occur, and the risk for infection is increased by the presence of other conditions.

B. Data collection: Influenza-like symptoms with a high fever, chills, muscle aches, and headache that may progress to dry cough, pleurisy, and sometimes diarrhea.

C. Interventions: Treatment is supportive, and antibiotics may be prescribed.

XV. Pleural Effusion

A. Description

1. Pleural effusion is the collection of fluid in the pleural space.
2. Any condition that interferes with secretion or drainage of fluid in the pleural space will lead to pleural effusion.

B. Data collection

1. Pleuritic pain that is sharp and increases with inspiration
2. Progressive dyspnea with decreased movement of the chest wall on the affected side

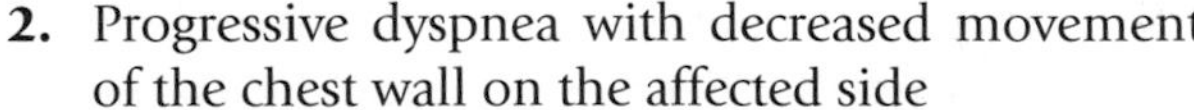

3. Dry, nonproductive cough caused by bronchial irritation or mediastinal shift
4. Tachycardia
5. Elevated temperature
6. Decreased breath sounds over affected area
7. Chest x-ray film that shows pleural effusion and a mediastinal shift away from the fluid if the effusion is greater than 250 mL

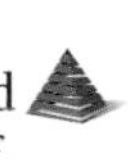

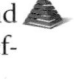

C. Interventions

1. Identify and treat the underlying cause.
2. Monitor breath sounds.
3. Place the client in a Fowler's position.
4. Encourage coughing and deep breathing.
5. Prepare the client for thoracentesis.
6. If pleural effusion is recurrent, prepare the client for pleurectomy or pleurodesis as prescribed.

D. Pleurectomy

1. Consists of surgically stripping the parietal pleura away from the visceral pleura
2. This produces an intense inflammatory reaction that promotes adhesion formation between the two layers during healing.

E. Pleurodesis
   1. Involves the instillation of a sclerosing substance into the pleural space via a thoracotomy tube
   2. The substance creates an inflammatory response that scleroses tissues together.

XVI. Empyema

A. Description
   1. Collection of pus within the pleural cavity
   2. The fluid is thick, opaque, and foul smelling.
   3. The most common cause is pulmonary infection and lung abscess caused by thoracic surgery or chest trauma, in which bacteria are introduced directly into the pleural space.
   4. Treatment focuses on treating the infection, emptying the empyema cavity, reexpanding the lung, and controlling the infection.

B. Data collection
   1. Recent febrile illness or trauma
   2. Chest pain
   3. Cough
   4. Dyspnea
   5. Anorexia and weight loss
   6. Malaise
   7. Elevated temperature and chills
   8. Night sweats
   9. Pleural exudate on chest x-ray

C. Interventions
   1. Monitor breath sounds.
   2. Place the client in a semi-Fowler's or high Fowler's position.
   3. Encourage coughing and deep breathing.
   4. Administer antibiotics as prescribed.
   5. Instruct the client to splint the chest as necessary.
   6. Assist with thoracentesis or chest tube insertion to promote drainage and lung expansion.
   7. If marked pleural thickening occurs, prepare the client for decortication, if prescribed; this is a surgical procedure that involves removal of the restrictive mass of fibrin and inflammatory cells.

XVII. Pleurisy

A. Description
   1. Inflammation of the visceral and parietal membranes; may be caused by pulmonary infarction or pneumonia
   2. The visceral and parietal membranes rub together during respiration and cause pain.
   3. Pleurisy usually occurs on one side of the chest, usually in the lower lateral portions in the chest wall.

B. Data collection
   1. Knifelike pain that is aggravated on deep breathing and coughing
   2. Apprehension
   3. Dyspnea
   4. Pleural friction rub heard on auscultation

C. Interventions
   1. Identify and treat the cause.
   2. Monitor lung sounds.
   3. Administer analgesics as prescribed.
   4. Apply hot or cold applications as prescribed.
   5. Encourage coughing and deep breathing.
   6. The client is instructed to lie on the affected side to splint the chest.

XVIII. Pulmonary Embolism

A. Description
   1. Occurs when a thrombus forms (most commonly in a deep vein), detaches, travels to the right side of the heart, and then lodges in a branch of the pulmonary artery
   2. Clients prone to pulmonary embolism are those at risk for deep vein thrombosis, including those with prolonged immobilization, surgery, obesity, pregnancy, heart failure, advanced age, or a history of thromboembolism.
   3. Fat emboli can occur as a complication after a fracture of a long bone and can cause pulmonary emboli.
   4. Treatment is aimed at prevention through risk factor recognition and elimination.
   5. If the suspicion for pulmonary embolism is low, a d-Dimer blood test may be prescribed, which measures one of the breakdown products of a blood clot. If normal, then the likelihood of a pulmonary embolism is very low (D-dimer values 250 ng/mL [0.50 mcg/mL fibrinogen equivalent units] or less are normal).

B. Data collection (Box 49-10) 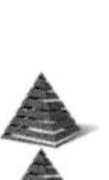

C. Interventions (see Priority Nursing Actions)

BOX 49-10 Data Collection Findings: Pulmonary Embolism

Apprehension and restlessness
Blood-tinged sputum
Chest pain
Cough
Crackles and wheezes on auscultation
Cyanosis
Distended neck veins
Dyspnea accompanied by anginal and pleuritic pain, exacerbated by inspiration
Feeling of impending doom
Hypotension
Petechiae over the chest and axilla
Shallow respirations
Tachypnea and tachycardia

PRIORITY NURSING ACTIONS!

Actions to Take If a Pulmonary Embolism Is Suspected

1. Notify the Rapid Response Team.
2. Reassure the client and elevate the head of the bed.
3. Prepare to administer oxygen.
4. Obtain vital signs and check lung sounds.
5. Prepare to obtain an arterial blood gas.
6. Prepare for the administration of heparin therapy or other therapies.
7. Document the event, interventions taken, and the client's response to treatment.

Signs and symptoms of a pulmonary embolism include the sudden onset of dyspnea, apprehension and restlessness, a feeling of impending doom, cough, hemoptysis, tachypnea, crackles, petechiae over the chest and axillae, and a decreased arterial oxygen saturation. If suspected, the nurse immediately notifies the RN and Rapid Response Team. The nurse stays with the client, reassures the client, and elevates the head of the bed. The health care provider is also notified. The nurse prepares to administer oxygen and obtains the vital signs and checks lung sounds. The nurse continues to monitor the client closely, prepares the client for tests prescribed to confirm the diagnosis, and prepares to assist to obtain an arterial blood gas. When prescribed, the client is prepared for the administration of heparin therapy or other therapies such as embolectomy or placement of a vena cava filter if necessary. Finally, the nurse documents the event, interventions taken, and the client's response to treatment.

Reference(s): deWit, D. & Kumagai, C. (2013). *Medical-surgical nursing: Concepts & practice.* (2nd ed., p. 312). St. Louis: Saunders.

XIX. Lung Cancer and Laryngeal Cancer (See Chapter 43)

XX. Carbon Monoxide Poisoning (See Chapter 41)

XXI. Histoplasmosis

A. Description
   1. Pulmonary fungal infection caused by spores of *Histoplasma capsulatum*
   2. Transmission occurs by the inhalation of spores, which are commonly found in contaminated soil.
   3. Spores are also usually found in bird droppings.

B. Data collection
   1. Similar to pneumonia
   2. Positive skin test for histoplasmosis
   3. Positive agglutination test
   4. Splenomegaly, hepatomegaly

C. Interventions
   1. Administer oxygen as prescribed.
   2. Monitor breath sounds.
   3. Assist to administer antiemetics, antihistamines, antipyretics, and corticosteroids as prescribed.
   4. Assist to administer fungicidal medications as prescribed.
   5. Encourage coughing and deep breathing.
   6. Place the client in a semi-Fowler's position.
   7. Monitor vital signs.
   8. Monitor for nephrotoxicity from fungicidal medications.
   9. As appropriate, the client is educated about the importance of spraying the floor area with water before sweeping barn and chicken coops.

XXII. Sarcoidosis

A. Description
   1. Presence of epithelioid cell tubercles in the lung
   2. The cause is unknown, but a high titer of Epstein-Barr virus may be noted.
   3. Viral incidence is highest in African Americans and young adults.

B. Data collection
   1. Night sweats
   2. Fever
   3. Weight loss
   4. Cough
   5. Skin nodules
   6. Polyarthritis
   7. Kveim test: Sarcoid node antigen is injected intradermally and causes a local nodular lesion in about 1 month. 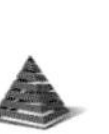

C. Interventions
   1. Administer corticosteroids to control symptoms.
   2. Monitor temperature.
   3. Increase fluid intake.
   4. Provide frequent periods of rest.
   5. Encourage small, nutritious meals.

XXIII. Occupational Lung Disease

A. Description
   1. Caused by exposure to environmental or occupational fumes, dust, vapors, gases, bacterial or fungal antigens, and allergens; can result in acute reversible effects or chronic lung disease
   2. Common disease classifications include occupational **asthma**, pneumoconiosis (silicosis or coal miner's [black lung] disease), diffuse interstitial fibrosis (asbestosis, talcosis, berylliosis), or extrinsic allergic alveolitis (farmer's lung, bird fancier's lung, or machine operator's lung).

B. Data collection: Signs/Symptoms depend on the type of disease and are respiratory symptoms.

C. Interventions

1. Prevention through the use of respiratory protective devices
2. Treatment is based on the symptoms experienced by the client.

XXIV. **Tuberculosis**

A. Description

1. Highly communicable disease caused by *Mycobacterium tuberculosis*
2. *M. tuberculosis* is a nonmotile, nonsporulating, acid-fast rod that secretes niacin; when the bacillus reaches a susceptible site, it multiplies freely.
3. Because *M. tuberculosis* is an aerobic bacterium, it primarily affects the pulmonary system, especially the upper lobes where the oxygen content is highest, but it also can affect other areas of the body, such as the brain, intestines, peritoneum, kidney, joints, and liver.
4. An exudative response causes a nonspecific pneumonitis and the development of granulomas in the lung tissue.
5. Tuberculosis has an insidious onset, and many clients are not aware of symptoms until the disease is well advanced.
6. Improper or noncompliant use of treatment programs may cause the development of mutations in the tubercle bacilli, resulting in a **multidrug-resistant strain** of tuberculosis (MDR-TB).
7. The goal of treatment is to prevent transmission, control symptoms, and prevent progression of the disease.

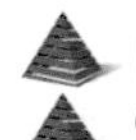

B. Risk factors (Box 49-11)

C. Transmission

1. Via the airborne route by droplet infection.
2. When an infected individual coughs, laughs, sneezes, or sings, droplet nuclei containing tuberculosis bacteria enter the air and may be inhaled by others.
3. Identification of those in close contact with the infected individual is important so they can be tested and treated as necessary.
4. When contacts have been identified, these persons are assessed with a tuberculin skin test and chest x-rays to determine infection with tuberculosis.
5. After the infected individual has received tuberculosis medication for 2 to 3 weeks, the risk of transmission is reduced greatly.

BOX 49-11 Risk Factors for Tuberculosis

Children younger than 5 years of age

Drinking of unpasteurized milk if the cow is infected with bovine tuberculosis

Homeless individuals or those from a lower socioeconomic group, minority groups, or immigrant group

Individuals in constant, frequent contact with an untreated or undiagnosed individual

Individuals living in crowded areas, such as long-term care facilities, prisons, and mental health facilities

Older clients

Individuals with malnutrition, an infection, or an immune dysfunction or human immunodeficiency virus infection; or immunosuppressed as a result of medication therapy

Individuals who abuse alcohol or are intravenous drug users

D. Disease progression

1. Droplets enter the lungs, and the bacteria form a tubercle lesion.
2. The defense systems of the body encapsulate the tubercle, leaving a scar.
3. If encapsulation does not occur, bacteria may enter the lymph system, travel to the lymph nodes, and cause an inflammatory response called *granulomatous inflammation*.
4. Primary lesions form; the primary lesions may become dormant but can be reactivated and become a secondary infection when reexposed to the bacterium.
5. In an active phase, tuberculosis can cause necrosis and cavitation in the lesions, leading to rupture, the spread of necrotic tissue, and damage to various parts of the body.

E. Client history

1. Past exposure to tuberculosis
2. Client's country of origin and travel to foreign countries in which the incidence of tuberculosis is high
3. Recent history of influenza, pneumonia, febrile illness, cough, or foul-smelling sputum production
4. Previous positive tests for tuberculosis; results of the testing
5. Recent **bacille Calmette-Guérin vaccine** (a vaccine containing attenuated tubercle bacilli that may be given to persons in foreign countries or to persons traveling to foreign countries to produce increased resistance to tuberculosis)

An individual who has received a bacilli Calmette-Guérin vaccine will have a positive tuberculin skin test result and should be evaluated for tuberculosis with a chest x-ray.

F. Clinical manifestations

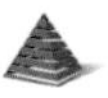

1. May be asymptomatic in primary infection
2. Fatigue
3. Lethargy
4. Anorexia

5. Weight loss
6. Low-grade fever
7. Chills
8. Night sweats
9. Persistent cough and the production of mucoid and mucopurulent sputum, which is occasionally streaked with blood
10. Chest tightness and a dull, aching chest pain that may accompany the cough

G. Chest: Data collection
1. A physical examination of the chest does not provide conclusive evidence of tuberculosis.
2. A chest x-ray film is not definitive, but the presence of multinodular infiltrates with calcification in the upper lobes suggests tuberculosis.
3. If the disease is active, caseation and inflammation may be seen on the chest x-ray.
4. Advanced disease
   a. Dullness with percussion over the involved parenchymal areas, bronchial breath sounds, rhonchi, and crackles indicate advanced disease.
   b. Partial obstruction of a bronchus caused by endobronchial disease or compression by lymph nodes may produce localized wheezing and dyspnea.

H. QuantiFERON-TB Gold test
1. A blood analysis test by an enzyme-linked immunosorbent assay
2. A sensitive and rapid test (results can be available in 24 hours) that assists in diagnosing the client

I. Sputum cultures
1. Sputum specimens are obtained for an acid-fast smear.
2. A sputum culture identifying *Mycobacterium tuberculosis* confirms the diagnosis.
3. After medications are started, sputum samples are obtained again to determine the effectiveness of therapy.
4. Most clients have negative cultures after 3 months of treatment.

J. **Tuberculin skin test (TST)** (Table 49-2)
1. A positive reaction does not mean that active disease is present but indicates previous exposure to tuberculosis or the presence of inactive (dormant) disease.
2. Skin test interpretation depends on two factors: measurement in millimeters of the induration and the person's risk of being infected with TB and progression to disease if infected.
3. Once an individual's skin test is positive, it will be positive in any future tests; a chest x-ray is necessary to rule out active tuberculosis or to detect old healed lesions.

K. The hospitalized client
1. The client with active tuberculosis is placed in an airborne infection isolation (AII) room; the door of the room must be tightly closed.
2. The nurse wears a particulate filter respirator (a special individually fitted mask) when caring for the client and a gown when a possibility exists of contamination of clothing.
3. Thorough hand washing is required before and after caring for the client.
4. If the client needs to leave the room for a test or procedure, the client is required to wear a surgical mask.
5. Respiratory isolation is discontinued when the client is no longer considered infectious.
6. After the infected individual has received tuberculosis medication for 2 to 3 weeks, the risk of transmission is reduced greatly.

L. Client education (Box 49-12)

M. Medications (see Chapter 50)

TABLE 49-2 Classification of the Tuberculin Skin Test Reaction

Induration = 5 mm or Greater Considered Positive in:	Induration = 10 mm or Greater Considered Positive in:	Induration = 15 mm or Greater Considered Positive in:
HIV-infected persons Recent contact of a person with TB disease Persons with fibrotic changes on chest x-ray consistent with prior TB Clients with organ transplants Persons immunosuppressed for other reasons	Recent immigrants from high-prevalence countries Injection drug users Residents and employees in high-risk congregate settings Mycobacteriology laboratory personnel Persons with clinical conditions that place them at high risk Children younger than 4 years of age Infants, children, and adolescents exposed to adults in high-risk categories	Any person, including persons with no known risk factors for TB

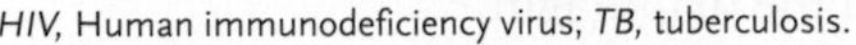

HIV, Human immunodeficiency virus; *TB*, tuberculosis.
From Centers for Disease Control and Prevention. *Tuberculosis (TB) fact sheets*. Available from: http://www.cdc.gov/tb/publications/factsheets/testing/skintesting.htm

BOX 49-12 Client Education: Tuberculosis

Provide the client and family with information about tuberculosis and allay concerns about the contagious aspect of the infection.
Instruct the client to follow the medication regimen exactly as prescribed and always to have a supply of the medication on hand.
Advise the client that the medication regimen is continued over 6 to 12 months, depending on the situation.
Advise the client of the side/adverse effects of the medication and ways of minimizing them to ensure compliance.
Reassure the client that after 2 to 3 weeks of medication therapy, it is unlikely that the client will infect anyone.
Inform the client to resume activities gradually.
Instruct the client about the need for adequate nutrition and a well-balanced diet to promote healing and prevent recurrence of the infection.
Instruct the client to increase intake of foods rich in iron, protein, and vitamin C.
Inform the client and family that respiratory isolation is not necessary because family members have already been exposed.
Instruct the client to cover the mouth and nose when coughing or sneezing and confine used tissues to plastic bags.
Instruct the client and family about thorough hand washing.
Inform the client that a sputum culture is needed every 2 to 4 weeks once medication therapy is initiated.
Inform the client that when the results of three sputum cultures are negative, the client is no longer considered infectious and usually can return to former employment.
Advise the client to avoid excessive exposure to silicone or dust because these substances can cause further lung damage.
Instruct the client regarding the importance of compliance with treatment, follow-up care, and sputum cultures, as prescribed.

CRITICAL THINKING What Should You Do?

Answer:

A tension pneumothorax can occur when there is a buildup of intrathoracic pressure in the pleural space and air cannot escape. One cause is the covering of an open chest wound. Signs include cyanosis, air hunger, violent agitation, tracheal deviation away from the affected side, subcutaneous emphysema, neck vein distension, and hyperresonance to percussion. The nurse should immediately release the chest wound dressing and contact the RN and health care provider. This is a medical emergency requiring possible needle decompression followed by chest tube insertion with a chest drainage system.

Reference(s): deWit, D. & Kumagai, C. (2013). *Medical-surgical nursing: Concepts & practice.* (2nd ed., p. 1025). St. Louis: Saunders.

PRACTICE QUESTIONS

496. The nurse is reinforcing instructions to a hospitalized client with a diagnosis of emphysema about positions that will enhance the effectiveness of breathing during dyspneic episodes. Which position should the nurse instruct the client to assume?

1. Side-lying in bed
2. Sitting in a recliner chair
3. Sitting up in bed at a 90 degree angle
4. Sitting on the side of the bed, leaning on an overbed table

497. The nurse is gathering data on a client with a diagnosis of tuberculosis (TB). The nurse should review the results of which diagnostic test to confirm this diagnosis?

1. Chest x-ray
2. Bronchoscopy
3. Sputum culture
4. Tuberculin skin test

498. Which identifies the route of transmission of tuberculosis (TB)?

1. Hand to mouth
2. The enteric route
3. The airborne route
4. Blood and body fluids

❖ **499.** The nurse is preparing a list of home care instructions for the client who has been hospitalized and treated for tuberculosis. Which instructions should the nurse reinforce? **Select all that apply.**

❑ 1. Activities should be resumed gradually.
❑ 2. Avoid contact with other individuals, except family members, for at least 6 months.
❑ 3. A sputum culture is needed every 2 to 4 weeks once medication therapy is initiated.
❑ 4. Respiratory isolation is not necessary because family members have already been exposed.
❑ 5. Cover the mouth and nose when coughing or sneezing and confine used tissues to plastic bags.
❑ 6. When one sputum culture is negative, the client is no longer considered infectious and can usually return to his or her former employment.

500. The nurse is instructing a client about pursed lip breathing, and the client asks the nurse about its purpose. The nurse should tell the client that the **primary** purpose of pursed lip breathing is which?

1. Promote oxygen intake
2. Strengthen the diaphragm

3. Strengthen the intercostal muscles
4. Promote carbon dioxide elimination

501. The low-pressure alarm sounds on the ventilator. The nurse checks the client and then attempts to determine the cause of the alarm but is unsuccessful. Which **initial** action should the nurse take?
1. Administer oxygen.
2. Ventilate the client manually.
3. Check the client's vital signs.
4. Start cardiopulmonary resuscitation (CPR).

502. The nurse is assigned to care for a client after a left pneumonectomy. Which position is contraindicated for this client?
1. Lateral position
2. Low Fowler's position
3. Semi-Fowler's position
4. Head of the bed elevation at 40 degrees

503. The nurse is caring for a client after pulmonary angiography via catheter insertion into the left groin. The nurse monitors for an allergic reaction to the contrast medium by observing for the presence of which?
1. Hypothermia
2. Respiratory distress
3. Hematoma in the left groin
4. Discomfort in the left groin

504. The nurse is reinforcing discharge instructions to the client with pulmonary sarcoidosis. The nurse knows that the client understands the information if the client verbalizes which **early** sign of exacerbation?
1. Fever
2. Fatigue
3. Weight loss
4. Shortness of breath

505. The nurse is caring for several clients with respiratory disorders. Which client is at **least** risk for developing a tuberculosis infection?
1. An uninsured man who is homeless
2. A woman newly immigrated from Korea
3. A man who is an inspector for the U.S. Postal Service
4. An older woman admitted from a long-term care facility

506. The nurse is reading the results of a tuberculin skin test on a client with no documented health problems. The site has no induration and a 1-mm area of ecchymosis. Which interpretation should the nurse make of these results?
1. Positive
2. Negative
3. Uncertain
4. Borderline

507. The nurse notes that a hospitalized client has experienced a positive reaction to the tuberculin skin test. Which action by the nurse is the **priority**?
1. Report the findings.
2. Document the finding in the client's record.
3. Call the employee health service department.
4. Call the radiology department for a chest x-ray.

508. A client being discharged from the hospital to home with a diagnosis of tuberculosis (TB) is worried about the possibility of infecting family members and others. Which information should reassure the client that contaminating family members and others is not likely?
1. The family does not need therapy, and the client will not be contagious after 1 month of medication therapy.
2. The family does not need therapy, and the client will not be contagious after 6 consecutive weeks of medication therapy.
3. The family will receive prophylactic therapy, and the client will not be contagious after 1 continuous week of medication therapy.
4. The family will receive prophylactic therapy, and the client will not be contagious after 2 to 3 consecutive weeks of medication therapy.

509. The nurse is reinforcing discharge teaching with a client diagnosed with tuberculosis (TB) and has been on medication for 1½ weeks. The nurse knows that the client has understood the information if which statement is made?
1. "I can't shop at the mall for the next 6 months."
2. "I need to continue medication therapy for 2 months."
3. "I can return to work if a sputum culture comes back negative."
4. "I should not be contagious after 2 to 3 weeks of medication therapy."

510. The nurse is caring for a client with emphysema receiving oxygen. The nurse should check the oxygen flow rate to ensure the client does not exceed how many L/min of oxygen?
1. 1
2. 2
3. 6
4. 10

ANSWERS

496. 4

Rationale: Positions that will assist the client with breathing include sitting up and leaning on an overbed table, sitting up and resting with the elbows on the knees, or standing or leaning against the wall. The positions in options 1, 2, and 3 will not enhance the effectiveness of breathing.
Test-Taking Strategy: Focus on the subject, positioning for a client with emphysema. Eliminate option 2 because side-lying will not promote appropriate lung expansion. Next, eliminate options 1 and 3 because they are comparable or alike and will restrict lung expansion. **Review:** the positions that will decrease the work of breathing in a client with **emphysema**.
Level of Cognitive Ability: Applying
Client Needs: Physiological Integrity
Integrated Process: Teaching and Learning
Content Area: Adult Health: Respiratory
Priority Concepts: Gas Exchange, Perfusion
Reference(s): deWit, Kumagai (2013), pp. 263, 303–304; Cooper, Gosnell (2015), pp. 1657–1659.

497. 3

Rationale: A definitive diagnosis of TB is confirmed through culture and isolation of *Mycobacterium tuberculosis*. A presumptive diagnosis is made on the basis of a tuberculin skin test, a sputum smear that is positive for acid-fast bacteria, a chest x-ray, and histologic evidence of granulomatous disease on biopsy.
Test-Taking Strategy: Focus on the subject by noting the word confirm in the question. Confirmation is made by identifying *Mycobacterium tuberculosis*. This will direct you to the correct option. **Review:** the diagnostic procedures related to **tuberculosis**.
Level of Cognitive Ability: Applying
Client Needs: Physiological Integrity
Integrated Process: Nursing Process/Data Collection
Content Area: Adult Health: Respiratory
Priority Concepts: Evidence, Infection
Reference(s): deWit, Kumagai (2013), p. 299; Cooper, Gosnell (2015), pp. 1634–1635.

498. 3

Rationale: Tuberculosis is an infectious disease caused by the bacillus *Mycobacterium tuberculosis* and is spread primarily by the airborne route. Options 1, 2, and 4 are incorrect.
Test-Taking Strategy: Focus on the subject, transmission of TB. Recalling that TB is a respiratory disease will direct you to the correct option. **Review:** the transmission of **tuberculosis**.
Level of Cognitive Ability: Understanding
Client Needs: Safe and Effective Care Environment
Integrated Process: Nursing Process/Planning
Content Area: Fundamental Skills: Infection Control
Priority Concepts: Infection, Safety
Reference(s): deWit, Kumagai (2013), p. 296; Cooper, Gosnell (2015), pp. 1638–1639.

❖ **499. 1, 3, 4, 5**

Rationale: The nurse should provide the client and family with information about tuberculosis and allay concerns about the contagious aspect of the infection. The client is reassured that after 2 to 3 weeks of medication therapy, it is unlikely that the client will infect anyone. The client is also informed that activities should be resumed gradually. The client and family are informed that respiratory isolation is not necessary, because family members have already been exposed. The client is instructed about thorough hand washing and to cover the mouth and nose when coughing or sneezing and confine used tissues to plastic bags. The client is informed that a sputum culture is needed every 2 to 4 weeks once medication therapy is initiated and that when the results of three sputum cultures are negative, the client is no longer considered infectious and can usually return to his or her former employment.
Test-Taking Strategy: Note the subject, home care instructions for the client with TB. Knowledge regarding the pathophysiology, transmission, and treatment of tuberculosis is needed to answer this question. Using this knowledge will assist in directing you to the correct options. **Review:** home care instructions for the client with **tuberculosis**.
Level of Cognitive Ability: Analyzing
Client Needs: Safe and Effective Care Environment
Integrated Process: Teaching and Learning
Content Area: Adult Health: Respiratory
Priority Concepts: Client Education, Infection
Reference(s): Lewis et al (2014), p. 533.

500. 4

Rationale: Pursed lip breathing facilitates maximal expiration for clients with obstructive lung disease and promotes carbon dioxide elimination. This type of breathing allows better expiration by increasing airway pressure, which keeps air passages open during exhalation. Options 1, 2, and 3 are not the purposes of this type of breathing.
Test-Taking Strategy: Focus on the subject, pursed lip breathing, and note the strategic word, *primary*. Visualize the use of this breathing technique to assist in answering correctly. Recalling the respiratory conditions in which this type of breathing is helpful will also assist in directing you to the correct option. **Review:** the purpose of **pursed lip breathing** technique.
Level of Cognitive Ability: Applying
Client Needs: Physiological Integrity
Integrated Process: Teaching and Learning
Content Area: Adult Health: Respiratory
Priority Concepts: Client Education, Gas Exchange
Reference(s): deWit, Kumagai (2013), pp. 321–322; Potter et al (2013), p. 854.

501. 2

Rationale: If an alarm is sounding at any time and the nurse cannot quickly ascertain the problem, the client is disconnected from the ventilator and a manual resuscitation device is used to support respirations until the problem can be corrected. Although oxygen is helpful, it will not provide ventilation to the client. Checking vital signs is not the initial action. There is no reason to begin CPR.
Test-Taking Strategy: Use the concept of ABCs—airway breathing, circulation—and note the strategic word, *initial*. Read the question carefully to note that the subject relates to adequate ventilation of the client. Focusing on this subject will direct you to the correct option. **Review:** care of the client with **mechanical ventilation**.
Level of Cognitive Ability: Applying

Client Needs: Physiological Integrity
Integrated Process: Nursing Process/Implementation
Content Area: Adult Health: Respiratory
Priority Concepts: Clinical Judgment, Gas Exchange
Reference(s): deWit, Kumagai (2013), p. 327.

502. 1
Rationale: Complete lateral positioning is contraindicated for a client following pneumonectomy. Because the mediastinum is no longer held in place on both sides by lung tissue, lateral positioning may cause mediastinal shift and compression of the remaining lung. The head of the bed should be elevated.
Test-Taking Strategy: Focus on the **subject**, the position that is contraindicated. Think about what is involved in this surgical procedure. Eliminate options 2, 3, and 4 because they are **comparable or alike**. **Review:** care of the client after **pneumonectomy**.
Level of Cognitive Ability: Applying
Client Needs: Physiological Integrity
Integrated Process: Nursing Process/Implementation
Content Area: Adult Health: Respiratory
Priority Concepts: Clinical Judgment, Gas Exchange
Reference: deWit, Kumagai (2013), p. 316; Cooper, Gosnell (2015), pp. 1649–1650.

503. 2
Rationale: Signs of allergic reaction to the contrast medium include localized itching and edema, respiratory distress, stridor, and decreased blood pressure. Hypothermia is an unrelated event. Hematoma formation is a complication of the procedure but does not indicate an allergic reaction. Discomfort is expected.
Test-Taking Strategy: Focus on the **subject**, an allergic reaction, and use the **ABCs—airway, breathing, and circulation**. This will direct you to the correct option. **Review:** the signs of an allergic reaction to the **contrast medium**.
Level of Cognitive Ability: Applying
Client Needs: Physiological Integrity
Integrated Process: Nursing Process/Data Collection
Content Area: Adult Health: Respiratory
Priority Concepts: Clinical Judgment, Immunity
Reference(s): Cooper, Gosnell (2015), p. 368.

504. 4
Rationale: Shortness of breath is an early sign of exacerbation of pulmonary sarcoidosis. Others include chest pain, hemoptysis, and pneumothorax. Systemic signs and symptoms that occur later include weakness and fatigue, malaise, fever, and weight loss.
Test-Taking Strategy: Note the **strategic word**, *early*, in the question. Because sarcoidosis is a pulmonary problem, eliminate options 1 and 3 first. Choose option 4 over option 2 because the shortness of breath (and impaired ventilation) appears first and would cause the fatigue as a secondary symptom. **Review:** **sarcoidosis**.
Level of Cognitive Ability: Evaluating
Client Needs: Physiological Integrity
Integrated Process: Nursing Process/Evaluation
Content Area: Adult Health: Respiratory
Priority Concepts: Client Education, Gas Exchange
Reference(s): Cooper, Gosnell (2015), p. 1661.

505. 3
Rationale: People at high risk for acquiring tuberculosis include children younger than 5 years of age; homeless individuals or those from a lower socioeconomic group, minority groups, or immigrant group; individuals in constant, frequent contact with an untreated or undiagnosed individual; individuals living in crowded areas, such as long-term care facilities, prisons, and mental health facilities; older clients; individuals with malnutrition, an infection, or an immune dysfunction or human immunodeficiency virus infection, or individuals who are immunosuppressed as a result of medication therapy; and individuals who abuse alcohol or are intravenous drug users.
Test-Taking Strategy: Note the **strategic word**, *least*. Begin to answer this question by eliminating options 1 and 2, because immigrants and the medically underserved are more frequently affected by this infection. From the remaining options, note that the postal inspector may or may not come in contact with many people, depending on job description. The client from the long-term care facility, however, lives in a group setting, where a large number of people share a common environment 24 hours a day. **Review:** the risks associated with **tuberculosis**.
Level of Cognitive Ability: Analyzing
Client Needs: Health Promotion and Maintenance
Integrated Process: Nursing Process/Data Collection
Content Area: Adult Health: Respiratory
Priority Concepts: Health Promotion, Infection
Reference(s): deWit, Kumagai (2013), p. 298.

506. 2
Rationale: A positive tuberculin skin test reading has an induration measuring 10 mm or more in diameter and indicates exposure to tuberculosis. A small area of ecchymosis is insignificant and is probably related to injection technique. Therefore, the remaining options are incorrect.
Test-Taking Strategy: Focus on the **subject**, tuberculin skin test results. To answer this question accurately, it is necessary to know that induration is necessary for a positive response. Because the client in this question has no induration, the result is negative. **Review: tuberculin skin test** interpretation.
Level of Cognitive Ability: Understanding
Client Needs: Physiological Integrity
Integrated Process: Nursing Process/Data Collection
Content Area: Adult Health: Respiratory
Priority Concepts: Infection, Tissue Integrity
Reference(s): deWit, Kumagai (2013), p. 299.

507. 1
Rationale: The nurse who interprets a tuberculin skin test as positive notifies the health care provider (HCP) immediately. The HCP would prescribe a chest x-ray to determine whether the client has clinically active tuberculosis (TB) or old, healed lesions. A sputum culture would be done to confirm the diagnosis of active TB. The client is placed on TB precautions prophylactically until a final diagnosis is made. The findings are documented in the client's record, but this action is not the highest priority. Calling the employee health service would be of no benefit to the client.
Test-Taking Strategy: Note the **strategic word**, *priority*. Because the nurse may not prescribe diagnostic tests, eliminate option

4 first. Option 3 can be eliminated because calling the employee health service is of no benefit to the client. From the remaining options, notifying the HCP should have a higher priority than the documentation, even though both may be done in the same narrow time period. **Review:** nursing interventions related to **tuberculin skin testing**.
Level of Cognitive Ability: Applying
Client Needs: Safe and Effective Care Environment
Integrated Process: Nursing Process/Implementation
Content Area: Adult Health: Respiratory
Priority Concepts: Infection, Safety
Reference(s): deWit, Kumagai (2013), p. 299.

508. 4
Rationale: Family members or others who have been in close contact with a client diagnosed with TB are placed on prophylactic therapy with isoniazid for 6 to 12 months. The client is usually not contagious after taking medication for 2 to 3 consecutive weeks. However, the client must take the full course of therapy (for 6 months or longer) to prevent reinfection or drug-resistant TB.
Test-Taking Strategy: Focus on the subject, treatment of those exposed to TB and reassuring the client. Recalling that the family requires prophylactic therapy allows you to eliminate options 1 and 2. From the remaining options, it is necessary to know that the client is not contagious after 2 to 3 weeks of therapy. **Review:** the concepts related to the prevention of the spread of **tuberculosis**.
Level of Cognitive Ability: Applying
Client Needs: Psychosocial Integrity
Integrated Process: Caring
Content Area: Adult Health: Respiratory
Priority Concepts: Anxiety, Infection
Reference(s): deWit, Kumagai (2013), p. 301.

509. 4
Rationale: The client is continued on medication therapy for 6 to 12 months, depending on the situation. The client is generally considered to be not contagious after 2 to 3 weeks of medication therapy. The client is instructed to wear a mask if there will be exposure to crowds until the medication is effective in preventing transmission. The client is allowed to return to employment when the results of three sputum cultures are negative.
Test-Taking Strategy: Focus on the subject, client understanding of discharge teaching regarding treatment of TB. Knowing that the medication therapy lasts for at least 6 months helps you eliminate option 2 first. Knowing that three sputum cultures must be negative helps you eliminate option 3 next. From the remaining options, recalling that the client is not contagious after 2 to 3 weeks of therapy helps you choose option 4. **Review:** the infectious period of **tuberculosis**.
Level of Cognitive Ability: Evaluating
Client Needs: Physiological Integrity
Integrated Process: Nursing Process/Evaluation
Content Area: Adult Health: Respiratory
Priority Concepts: Client Education, Infection
Reference(s): Ignatavicius, Workman (2013), pp. 657–658.

510. 2
Rationale: Between 1 and 3 L/min of oxygen by nasal cannula may be required to raise the PaO_2 level to 60 to 80 mm Hg. However, oxygen is used cautiously in the client with emphysema and should not exceed 2 L/min. Because of the long-standing hypercapnia that occurs in this disorder, the respiratory drive is triggered by low oxygen levels rather than by increased carbon dioxide levels, which is the case in a normal respiratory system.
Test-Taking Strategy: Focus on the subject, oxygen administration with emphysema. Recalling the physiology associated with emphysema is required to answer this question. Remember that oxygen is used cautiously in the client with emphysema and should not exceed 2 L/min. **Review:** oxygen administration with **emphysema**.
Level of Cognitive Ability: Applying
Client Needs: Physiological Integrity
Integrated Process: Nursing Process/Data Collection
Content Area: Adult Health: Respiratory
Priority Concepts: Gas Exchange, Safety
Reference(s): deWit, Kumagai (2013), p. 323.

CHAPTER 50

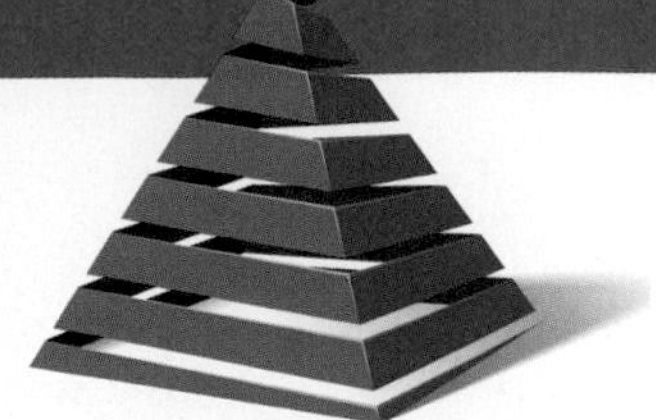

Respiratory Medications

CRITICAL THINKING What Should You Do?

A client who has been taking isoniazid for the past 4 months to treat tuberculosis reports to the nurse that he has been experiencing a lack of appetite and nausea and that his urine is dark in color. What should the nurse do?

Answer located on p. 663.

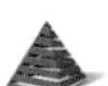

I. Medication Inhalation Devices

A. Metered-dose inhaler (MDI): Uses a chemical propellant to push the medication out of the inhaler (Figs. 50-1 and 50-2)

B. Dry powder inhaler (DPI): Delivers medication without using chemical propellants, but it requires strong and fast inhalation

C. Nebulizer: Delivers fine liquid mists of medication through a tube or a mask that fits over the nose and mouth, using air or oxygen under pressure

D. If two different inhaled medications are prescribed and one of the medications contains a glucocorticoid (corticosteroid), administer the bronchodilator first and the corticosteroid second.

If two different inhaled medications are prescribed, instruct the client to wait 5 minutes following administration of the first before inhaling the second. If a second dose of the same medication is needed, instruct the client to wait 1 to 2 minutes before taking the second dose.

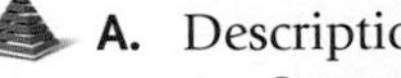

II. Bronchodilators (Box 50-1)

A. Description

1. Sympathomimetic bronchodilators relax the smooth muscle of the bronchi and dilate the airways of the respiratory tree, making air exchange and respiration easier for the client.
2. Methylxanthine bronchodilators stimulate the central nervous system and respiration, dilate coronary and pulmonary vessels, cause diuresis, and relax smooth muscle.
3. Used to treat allergic rhinitis and sinusitis, acute bronchospasm, acute and chronic **asthma**, bronchitis, **chronic obstructive pulmonary disease, emphysema**, and other restrictive airway diseases.
4. Contraindicated in individuals with hypersensitivity, peptic ulcer disease, severe cardiac disease and cardiac dysrhythmias, hyperthyroidism, or uncontrolled seizure disorders

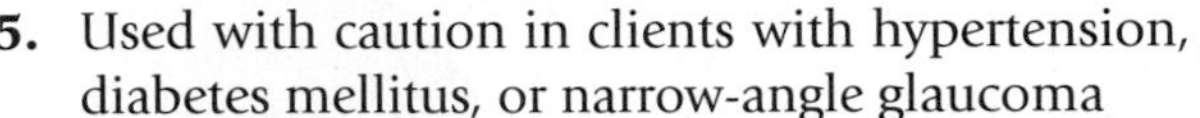

5. Used with caution in clients with hypertension, diabetes mellitus, or narrow-angle glaucoma

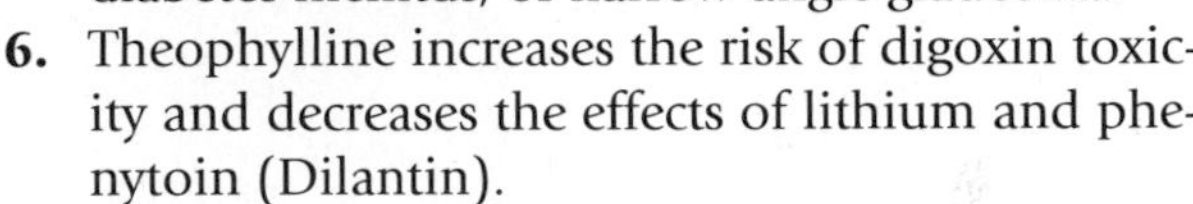

6. Theophylline increases the risk of digoxin toxicity and decreases the effects of lithium and phenytoin (Dilantin).
7. If theophylline and a β_2-adrenergic agonist are administered together, cardiac dysrhythmias may result.
8. β-Blockers, cimetidine (Tagamet), and erythromycin increase the effects of theophylline.
9. Barbiturates and carbamazepine (Tegretol) decrease the effects of theophylline.

B. Side/adverse effects

1. Palpitations and tachycardia
2. Dysrhythmias
3. Restlessness, nervousness, tremors
4. Anorexia, nausea, and vomiting
5. Headaches and dizziness
6. Hyperglycemia
7. Mouth dryness and throat irritation with inhalers
8. Tolerance and paradoxical bronchoconstriction with inhalers

C. Interventions

1. Monitor for restlessness and confusion.
2. Monitor vital signs and lung sounds.
3. Monitor for cardiac dysrhythmias.
4. Check for cough, wheezing, decreased breath sounds, and sputum production.
5. Provide adequate hydration.
6. The medication is administered at regular intervals around the clock to maintain a sustained therapeutic level.
7. Oral medications are administered with or after meals to decrease gastrointestinal irritation.
8. Monitor for a therapeutic serum theophylline level of 10 to 20 mcg/mL.
9. Intravenously administered aminophylline or theophylline preparations should be administered slowly and always via an infusion pump.

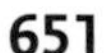

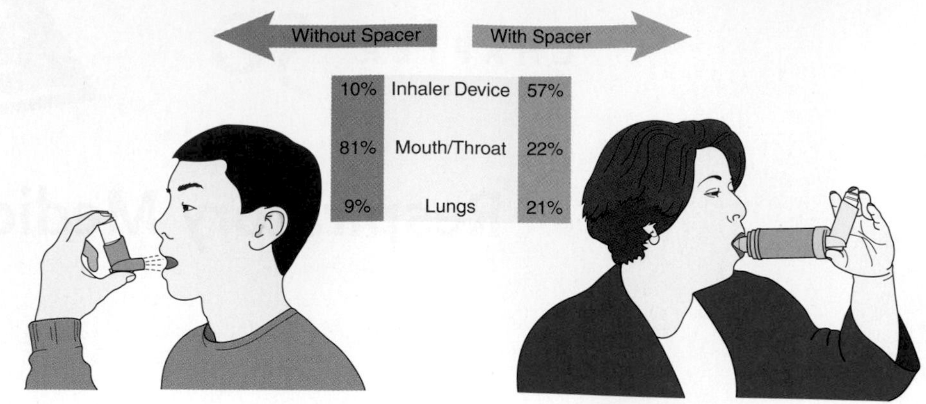

FIGURE 50-1 Distribution of medication with and without a spacer. (From Kee J, Marshall S: *Clinical calculations: With applications to general and specialty areas*, ed 7, St. Louis, 2013, Saunders.)

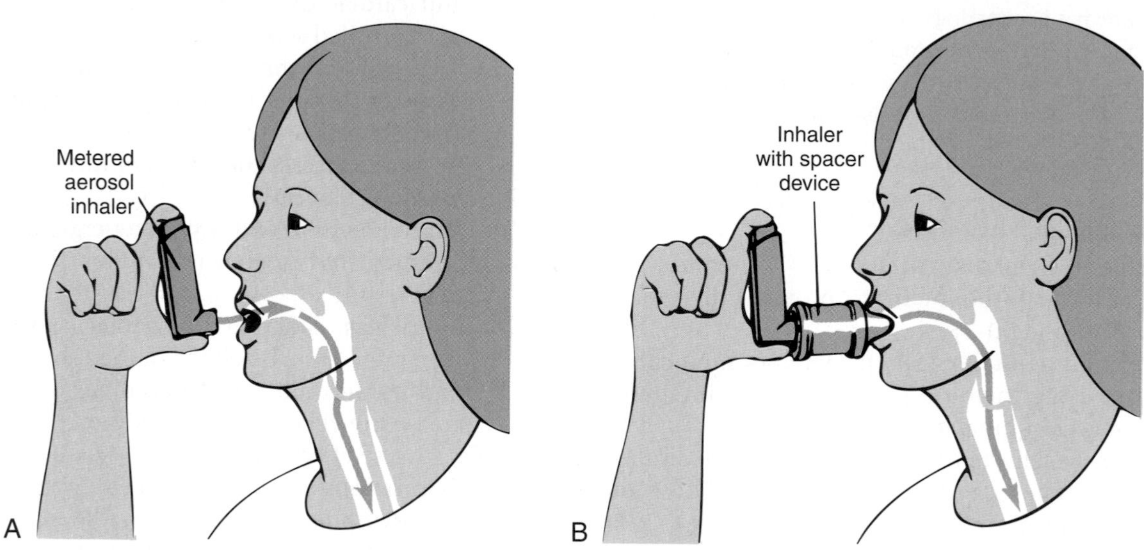

FIGURE 50-2 Inhaled drugs commonly used in asthma treatment include β-adrenergic bronchodilators, cromolyn sodium, and aerosol glucocorticoids. **A,** The metered-dose inhaler should not be put in the mouth but held about two fingerwidths (1½ inches) in front of the mouth. **B,** Alternatively, an inhaler with a spacer device can be used. Clients should breathe deeply once before activating the inhaler and then continue breathing in for about 5 seconds. Clients then should hold their breath for 10 to 15 seconds before breathing out slowly. If a second dose is needed, clients should wait 1 to 2 minutes before taking another dose. (From Clark J, Queener S, Karb V: *Pharmacologic basis of nursing practice*, ed 6, St. Louis, 2000, Mosby.)

10. Client education
- **a.** Not to crush enteric-coated or sustained-release tablets or capsules
- **b.** To avoid caffeine-containing products such as coffee, tea, cola, and chocolate, as well as over-the-counter medications
- **c.** About the side/adverse effects of bronchodilators
- **d.** How to monitor the pulse and to report any abnormalities to the health care provider (HCP)
- **e.** How to use an inhaler, spacer, or nebulizer (see Figs. 50-1 and 50-2) and how to monitor the amount of medication remaining in an inhaler canister
- **f.** The importance of smoking cessation and information regarding support resources
- **g.** To monitor blood glucose levels if diabetes mellitus is a coexisting condition
- **h.** To wear a Medic-Alert bracelet, particularly if the client has asthma

Theophylline toxicity is likely to occur when the serum level is higher than 20 mcg/mL. Early signs of toxicity include restlessness, nervousness, tremors, palpitations, and tachycardia.

III. Anticholinergics (see Box 50-1)

A. Inhaled medications that improve lung function by blocking muscarinic receptors in the bronchi, which results in bronchodilation

B. Effective for treating chronic obstructive pulmonary disease, allergy-induced asthma, and exercise-induced bronchospasm

BOX 50-1 Medications to Treat Restrictive Airway Disorders

Bronchodilators

β_2-Adrenergic Agonists

Inhaled

Albuterol (Proventil HFA, AccuNeb, ProAir HFA, Ventolin HFA)
Arformoterol (Brovana)
Formoterol (Foradil Aerolizer, Perforomist)
Levalbuterol (Xopenex, Xopenex HFA)
Pirbuterol (Maxair Autohaler)
Salmeterol (Serevent Diskus)

Oral

Albuterol (VoSpire, Proventil)
Terbutaline

Methylxanthines

Theophylline, oral (Theo-24, Theochron, Uniphyl, Elixophyllin)

Anticholinergics

Ipratropium, inhaled (Atrovent HFA, Combivent)
Tiotropium, inhaled (Spiriva)

Glucocorticoids (Corticosteroids)

Inhaled

Beclomethasone dipropionate (Qvar, Beclovent)
Budesonide (Pulmicort Turbuhaler, Pulmicort Respules, Pulmicort Flexhaler)
Ciclesonide (Alvescol)
Flunisolide (AeroBid)
Fluticasone propionate (Flovent HFA, Flovent Diskus)
Mometasone furoate (Asmanex Twisthaler)
Triamcinolone acetonide (Azmacort)

Oral

Prednisone
Prednisolone

Leukotriene Modifiers

Montelukast, oral (Singulair)
Zafirlukast, oral (Accolate)
Zileuton, oral (Zyflo, Zyflo CR)

Inhaled Nonsteroidal Antiallergy Agent

Cromolyn sodium, inhaled

Monoclonal Antibody

Omalizumab (Xolair)

Modified from Lehne R: *Pharmacology for nursing care*, ed 7. St. Louis, 2010, Saunders.

C. Side effects include dry mouth and irritation of the pharynx; sucking on sugarless candy will help to relieve symptoms

D. Systemic anticholinergic effects rarely occur but can include increased intraocular pressure, blurred vision, tachycardia, cardiovascular events, urinary retention, and constipation.

⚠ The client with a peanut allergy should not take ipratropium (Atrovent HFA and Combivent) because both products contain soy lecithin, which is in the same plant family as peanuts.

IV. Glucocorticoids (Corticosteroids) (see Box 50-1)

A. Glucocorticoids act as anti-inflammatory agents and reduce edema of the airways; they are used to treat asthma and other inflammatory respiratory conditions.

B. See Chapter 46 for information on glucocorticoids.

V. Leukotriene Modifiers (see Box 50-1)

A. Description
1. Used in the prophylaxis and treatment of chronic bronchial asthma (not used for acute asthma episodes)
2. Inhibit bronchoconstriction caused by specific antigens and reduce airway edema and smooth muscle constriction
3. Contraindicated in clients with hypersensitivity and in breastfeeding mothers
4. Should be used with caution in clients with impaired hepatic function
5. Coadministration of inhaled glucocorticoids increases the risk of upper respiratory infection.

B. Side/adverse effects
1. Headache
2. Nausea and vomiting
3. Dyspepsia
4. Diarrhea
5. Generalized pain, myalgia
6. Fever
7. Dizziness

C. Interventions
1. Monitor vital signs.
2. Check lung sounds for adventitious breath sounds.
3. Monitor liver function laboratory values.
4. Monitor for cyanosis.

D. Client education
1. To take medication 1 hour before or 2 hours after meals
2. To increase fluid intake
3. Not discontinue the medication and to take as prescribed, even during symptom-free periods

VI. Inhaled Nonsteroidal Antiallergy Agent (see Box 50-1)

A. Description
1. Antiasthmatic, antiallergic, and mast cell stabilizers inhibit mast cell release after exposure to antigens.
2. Used to treat allergic rhinitis, bronchial asthma, and exercise-induced bronchospasm
3. It is contraindicated in clients with known hypersensitivity.

4. Orally administered cromolyn sodium is used with caution in clients with impaired hepatic or renal function.

B. Side/adverse effects
1. Cough, sneezing, nasal sting, or bronchospasm after inhalation
2. Unpleasant taste in the mouth

C. Interventions
1. Monitor vital signs.
2. Monitor respirations and check lungs for adventitious sounds.

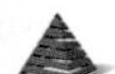

D. Client education
1. To administer oral capsules at least 30 minutes before meals
2. Not to discontinue the medication abruptly because a rebound asthmatic attack can occur; the medication needs to be taken as prescribed.

The client taking inhaled medications is instructed to drink a few sips of water before and after inhalation to prevent a cough and an unpleasant taste in the mouth.

VII. Monoclonal Antibody

A. Description
1. Omalizumab (Xolair) is a recombinant DNA-derived humanized immunoglobulin G (IgG) murine monoclonal antibody that selectively binds to IgE to limit the release of mediators in the allergic response.
2. Used to treat allergy-related asthma; administered subcutaneously every 2 to 4 weeks
3. Dose is titrated on the basis of the serum IgE level and body weight.
4. Contraindicated in those with hypersensitivity to the medication

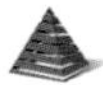

B. Side/adverse effects
1. Injection site reactions
2. Viral infections
3. Upper respiratory infections
4. Sinusitis
5. Headache
6. Pharyngitis
7. Anaphylaxis
8. Malignancies

C. Interventions
1. Monitor respiratory rate, rhythm, and depth and listen to lung sounds.
2. Check for allergies and/or allergic reaction symptoms such as rash or urticaria.
3. Have medications for the treatment of severe hypersensitivity reactions available during initial administration in case anaphylaxis occurs.

D. Client education
1. That respiratory improvement will not be immediate
2. Not stop taking or decrease the currently prescribed asthma medications unless instructed to do so
3. To avoid live virus vaccines for the duration of treatment

BOX 50-2 Antihistamines

Cetirizine (Zyrtec) Chlorpheniramine (Chlor-Trimeton, Chlorphen, Aller-Chlor, others)
Cyproheptadine
Desloratadine (Clarinex)
Dimenhydrinate (Dramamine)
Diphenhydramine (Benadryl)
Fexofenadine (Allegra)
Levocetirizine (Xyzal)
Loratadine (Claritin, Alavert, others)
Olopatadine (Patanase, Patanol)

VIII. Antihistamines (Box 50-2)

A. Description
1. Called *histamine antagonists* or H_1 *blockers*; these medications compete with histamine for receptor sites, thus preventing a histamine response.
2. When the H_1 receptor is stimulated, the extravascular smooth muscles, including those lining the nasal cavity, are constricted.
3. Decrease nasopharyngeal, gastrointestinal, and bronchial secretions by blocking the H_1 receptor
4. Used for the common cold, rhinitis, nausea and vomiting, motion sickness, urticaria, and as a sleep aid
5. Can cause central nervous system (CNS) depression if taken with alcohol, opioids, hypnotics, or barbiturates

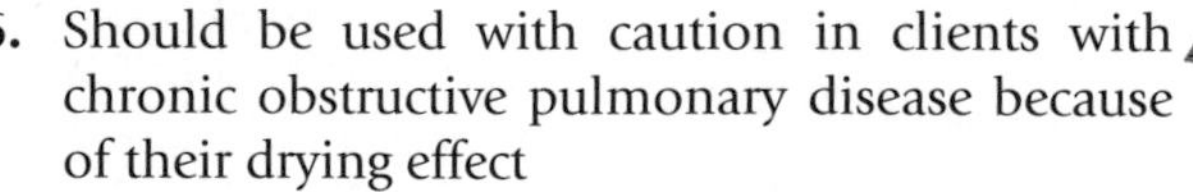

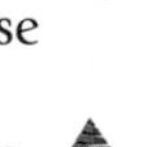

6. Should be used with caution in clients with chronic obstructive pulmonary disease because of their drying effect

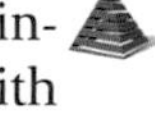

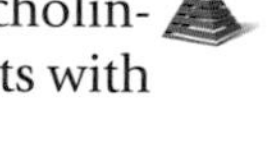

7. Diphenhydramine (Benadryl) has an anticholinergic effect and should be avoided in clients with narrow-angle glaucoma.

B. Side/adverse effects
1. Drowsiness and fatigue
2. Dizziness
3. Urinary retention
4. Blurred vision
5. Wheezing
6. Constipation
7. Dry mouth
8. Gastrointestinal irritation
9. Hypotension
10. Hearing disturbances
11. Photosensitivity
12. Nervousness and irritability
13. Confusion
14. Nightmares

C. Interventions
1. Monitor vital signs.
2. Monitor for signs of urinary dysfunction.
3. Administered with food or milk.

BOX 50-3 Nasal Decongestants

Nonglucocorticoids
Naphazoline (Privine)
Oxymetazoline (Afrin 12-Hour, others)
Phenylephrine hydrochloride (Neo-Synephrine, others)
Pseudoephedrine hydrochloride (Sudafed)
Tetrahydrozoline (Tyzine)
Xylometazoline (Natru-Vent, Otrivin)

Glucocorticoids
Beclomethasone (Beconase AQ, QNASL)
Budesonide (Rhinocort Aqua)
Ciclesonide (Omnaris)
Flunisolide (Nasarel, Nasalide)
Fluticasone furoate (Veramyst)
Fluticasone propionate (Flonase)
Mometasone (Nasonex)
Triamcinolone (Nasacort AQ)

4. Subcutaneous injection is avoided; administered by intramuscular injection in a large muscle if the intramuscular route is prescribed.

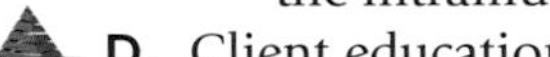

D. Client education
   1. To avoid hazardous activities, alcohol, and other CNS depressants
   2. If the medication is being taken for motion sickness, take it 30 minutes before the event and then before meals and at bedtime during the event as prescribed.
   3. To suck on hard candy or ice chips for dry mouth

IX. Nasal Decongestants (Box 50-3)

A. Description
   1. Include adrenergic, anticholinergic, and corticosteroid medications
   2. Shrink nasal mucosal membranes and reduce fluid secretion
   3. Used for allergic rhinitis, hay fever, and acute coryza (profuse nasal discharge)
   4. Contraindicated or used with extreme caution in clients with hypertension, cardiac disease, hyperthyroidism, or diabetes mellitus

B. Side/adverse effects
   1. Nervousness
   2. Restlessness, insomnia
   3. Hypertension
   4. Hyperglycemia

Nasal decongestants can cause tolerance and rebound nasal congestion (vasodilation) as a result of irritation of the nasal mucosa. Therefore, the client needs to be informed that these medications should not be used for longer than 48 hours.

C. Interventions
   1. The client is assessed for existing medical disorders.
   2. Monitor for cardiac dysrhythmias.
   3. Monitor blood glucose levels.

D. Client education
   1. To avoid consuming caffeine in large amounts because it can increase restlessness and palpitations
   2. About the importance of limiting the use of nasal sprays and drops to prevent rebound nasal congestion

X. Expectorants and Mucolytic Agents

A. Description
   1. Expectorants, like guaifenesin (Humibid, Mucinex, Robitussin), loosen bronchial secretions so they can be eliminated with coughing; they are used for dry nonproductive cough and to stimulate bronchial secretions.
   2. Mucolytic agents thin mucous secretions to help make the cough more productive.
   3. Mucolytic agents with dextromethorphan should not be used by clients with chronic obstructive pulmonary disease because they suppress the cough.
   4. Acetylcysteine (Mucomyst) can increase airway resistance and should not be used in clients with asthma.

B. Side/adverse effects
   1. Gastrointestinal irritation
   2. Skin rash
   3. Oropharyngeal irritation

C. Interventions
   1. Acetylcysteine (Mucomyst), administered by nebulization, and should not be mixed with another medication
   2. If acetylcysteine is administered with a bronchodilator, the bronchodilator should be administered 5 minutes before the acetylcysteine.
   3. Monitor for side effects of acetylcysteine, such as nausea and vomiting, stomatitis, and runny nose.

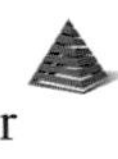

D. Client education
   1. To take the medication with a full glass of water to loosen mucus
   2. To maintain adequate fluid intake
   3. To periodically take some deep breaths and cough

XI. Antitussives (Box 50-4)

A. Description: Act on the cough control center in the medulla to suppress the cough reflex; used for a cough that is nonproductive and irritating

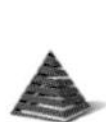

B. Side/adverse effects
   1. Dizziness, drowsiness, sedation
   2. Gastrointestinal irritation, nausea
   3. Dry mouth

BOX 50-4 Antitussives

Opioids

Codeine phosphate, codeine sulfate
Hydrocodone

Nonopioids

Benzonatate (Tessalon)
Dextromethorphan (Mucinex DM, Robitussin DM, others)
Diphenhydramine hydrochloride (Benadryl)

4. Constipation
5. Respiratory depression

C. Interventions
1. The client is encouraged to take adequate fluids with the medication.
2. The client is encouraged to sleep with the head of the bed elevated.
3. Note that drug dependency can occur.

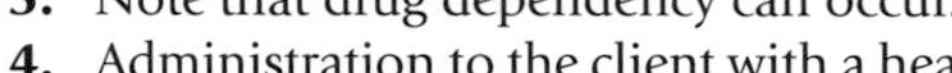

4. Administration to the client with a head injury or a postoperative cranial surgery client is avoided.
5. Administration to the client using opioids, sedative-hypnotics, barbiturates, or antidepressants is avoided because CNS depression can occur.

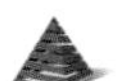

D. Client education
1. If the cough lasts longer than 1 week and a fever or a rash occurs to notify the HCP
2. To avoid hazardous activities
3. To avoid the use of alcohol

XII. Opioid Antagonists (Box 50-5)

A. Description
1. Reverses respiratory depression in opioid overdose
2. Avoid its use for nonopioid respiratory depression.
3. Reoccurrence of respiratory depression can occur if duration of opiate exceeds duration of opioid antagonist.

B. Side/adverse effects
1. Nausea, vomiting
2. Tremors
3. Sweating
4. Increased blood pressure
5. Tachycardia

C. Interventions
1. Monitor vital signs, especially respirations.
2. The registered nurse is responsible for intravenous administration and for titrating the dose administered every 2 to 5 minutes, as prescribed.

BOX 50-5 Opioid Antagonists

Alvimopan (Entereg)
Methylnaltrexone (Relistor)
Naloxone (Narcan)
Naltrexone (Vivitrol)

BOX 50-6 First- and Second-Line Medications for Tuberculosis

First-Line Agents

Ethambutol (Myambutol)
Isoniazid
Pyrazinamide
Rifabutin (Mycobutin)
Rifampin (Rifadin)
Rifapentine (Priftin)

Second-Line Agents

Amikacin (Amikin)
Capreomycin sulfate (Capastat Sulfate)
Ciprofloxacin (Cipro)
Cycloserine (Seromycin)
Ethionamide (Trecator)
Kanamycin (Kantrex)
Levofloxacin (Levaquin)
Moxifloxacin (Avelox)
p-Aminosalicylic acid (Paser)
Streptomycin

3. Have oxygen and resuscitative equipment available during administration.

XIII. Tuberculosis Medications (Box 50-6)

A. Description
1. Offers the most effective method for treating the disease and preventing transmission
2. Treatment of identified lesions depends on whether the individual has active disease or has been exposed to the disease.
3. Treatment is difficult because the bacterium has a waxy substance on the capsule that makes penetration and destruction difficult.

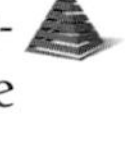

4. The use of a multidrug regimen destroys organisms as quickly as possible and minimizes the emergence of drug-resistant organisms.
5. Active tuberculosis is treated with a combination of medications to which the organism is susceptible.

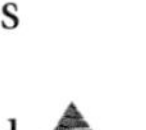
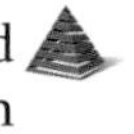

6. Individuals with active tuberculosis are treated for 6 to 9 months; however, clients with human immunodeficiency virus (HIV) infection are treated for a longer period of time.

7. After the infected individual has received medication for 2 to 3 weeks, the risk of transmission is greatly reduced.

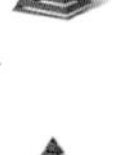

8. Most clients have negative sputum cultures after 3 months of compliance with medication therapy.

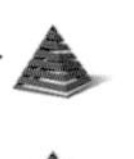
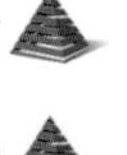

9. Individuals who have been exposed to active tuberculosis are treated with preventive isoniazid for 9 to 12 months.

B. First- or second-line medications
1. First-line medications provide the most effective antituberculosis activity.

2. Second-line medications are used in combination with first-line medications but are more toxic.
3. Current infecting organisms are proving resistant to standard first-line medications; the resistant organisms develop because individuals with the disease fail to complete the course of treatment, so surviving bacteria adapt to the medication and become resistant.
4. Multidrug therapies are instituted because of the resistant organisms.

C. Multidrug-resistant strain of tuberculosis (MDR-TB)
1. Resistance occurs when a client receiving two medications (first-line and second-line medications) discontinues one of the medications.
2. The client briefly experiences some response from the single medication, but then large numbers of resistant organisms begin to grow.
3. The client, infectious again, transmits the drug-resistant organism to other individuals.
4. As this event is repeated, an organism develops that is resistant to many of the first-line tuberculosis medications.

XIV. First-Line Medications for Tuberculosis (see Box 50-6)

A. Isoniazid
1. Description
   a. Bactericidal
   b. Inhibits the synthesis of mycolic acids and acts to kill actively growing organisms in the extracellular environment
   c. Inhibits the growth of dormant organisms in the macrophages and caseating granulomas
   d. Is active only during cell division and is used in combination with other antitubercular medications
2. Contraindications and cautions
   a. Contraindicated in clients with hypersensitivity or with acute liver disease
   b. Use with caution in clients with chronic liver disease, alcoholism, or renal impairment.
   c. Use with caution in clients taking nicotinic acid (niacin).
   d. Use with caution in clients taking hepatotoxic medications because the risk for hepatotoxicity increases.
   e. Alcohol increases the risk of hepatotoxicity.
   f. May increase the risk of toxicity of carbamazepine (Tegretol) and phenytoin (Dilantin)
   g. Isoniazid may decrease ketoconazole (Nizoral) concentrations.
3. Side/adverse effects
   a. Hypersensitivity reactions
   b. Peripheral neuritis
   c. Neurotoxicity
   d. Hepatotoxicity and hepatitis; increased liver function test levels
   e. Pyridoxine (vitamin B_6) deficiency
   f. Irritation at injection site with intramuscular administration
   g. Nausea and vomiting
   h. Dry mouth
   i. Dizziness
   j. Hyperglycemia
   k. Vision changes

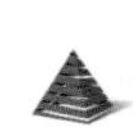

4. Interventions
   a. Monitor for hypersensitivity.
   b. Monitor for hepatic dysfunction.
   c. Monitor for sensitivity to nicotinic acid.
   d. Monitor liver function test results.
   e. Monitor for signs of hepatitis, such as anorexia, nausea, vomiting, weakness, fatigue, dark urine, or jaundice; if these symptoms occur, withhold the medication and notify the registered nurse.
   f. Monitor for tingling, numbness, or burning of the extremities.
   g. Monitor mental status.
   h. Monitor for visual changes, and notify the registered nurse if they occur.
   i. Monitor for dizziness and initiate safety precautions.
   j. Monitor complete blood count (CBC) and blood glucose levels.
   k. Isoniazid is administered 1 hour before or 2 hours after a meal because food may delay absorption.
   l. Isoniazid is administered at least 1 hour before antacids, especially those antacids that contain aluminum.
   m. Pyridoxine is administered as prescribed to reduce the risk of neurotoxicity.

Many tuberculosis medications can cause toxic effects such as hepatotoxicity, nephrotoxicity, neurotoxicity, optic neuritis, or ototoxicity. Teach the client about the signs of toxicity and inform the client that the HCP needs to be notified if any signs arise.

5. Client education
   a. Not to skip doses and to take the medication for the full length of the prescribed therapy
   b. Not to take any other medication without consulting the HCP
   c. About the importance of follow-up HCP visits, vision testing, and laboratory tests
   d. To avoid alcohol
   e. To take medication on an empty stomach with 8 oz of water 1 hour before or 2 hours after meals and to avoid taking antacids with the medication

f. To avoid tyramine-containing foods because they may cause a reaction such as red and itching skin, a pounding heartbeat, lightheadedness, a hot or clammy feeling, or a headache; if this does occur, the client should notify the HCP.
g. To recognize the signs of neurotoxicity, hepatitis, and hepatotoxicity
h. To notify the HCP if signs of neurotoxicity, hepatitis and hepatotoxicity, or visual changes occur.

B. Rifampin (Rifadin)
1. Description
a. Inhibits bacterial RNA synthesis
b. Binds to DNA-dependent RNA polymerase and blocks RNA transcription
c. Used with at least one other antitubercular medication
2. Contraindications and cautions
a. Contraindicated in clients with hypersensitivity
b. Used with caution in clients with hepatic dysfunction or alcoholism
c. Use of alcohol or hepatotoxic medications may increase the risk of hepatotoxicity.
d. Decreases the effects of several medications, including oral anticoagulants, oral hypoglycemics, chloramphenicol (Chloromycetin), digoxin (Lanoxin), disopyramide phosphate (Norpace), mexiletine (Mexitil), quinidine polygalacturonate, fluconazole (Diflucan), methadone hydrochloride (Dolophine), phenytoin (Dilantin), and verapamil hydrochloride (Calan SR)
3. Side/adverse effects
a. Hypersensitivity reaction, including fever, chills, shivering, headache, muscle and bone pain, and dyspnea
b. Heartburn, nausea, vomiting, diarrhea
c. Red-orange–colored body secretions

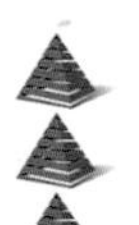

d. Vision changes
e. Hepatotoxicity and hepatitis

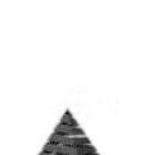

f. Increased uric acid levels
g. Blood dyscrasias
h. Colitis

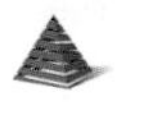

4. Interventions
a. Monitor for hypersensitivity.
b. Monitor CBC, uric acid, and liver function test results.
c. Monitor for signs of hepatitis; if they occur, the medication is withheld and the HCP is notified.
d. Monitor stools for signs of colitis.
e. Monitor mental status.
f. Monitor for visual changes.

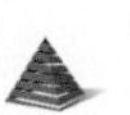

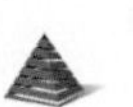

5. Client education
a. Not to skip doses and to take medication for the full length of the prescribed therapy
b. Not to take any other medication without consulting the HCP
c. About the importance of follow-up HCP visits and laboratory tests
d. To avoid alcohol
e. To take medication on an empty stomach with 8 oz of water 1 hour before or 2 hours after meals and to avoid taking antacids with the medication
f. That urine, feces, sweat, and tears will be red-orange and that soft contact lenses can become permanently discolored
g. To notify the HCP if jaundice (yellow eyes or skin) develops or if weakness, fatigue, nausea, vomiting, sore throat, fever, or unusual bleeding occurs

C. Ethambutol (Myambutol)
1. Description
a. Bacteriostatic
b. Interferes with cell metabolism and multiplication by inhibiting one or more metabolites in susceptible organisms
c. Inhibits bacterial RNA synthesis and is active only during cell division
d. Slow-acting and must be used with other bactericidal agents
2. Contraindications and cautions
a. Contraindicated in clients with hypersensitivity or optic neuritis and children younger than 13 years
b. Used with caution in clients with renal dysfunction, gout, ocular defects, diabetic retinopathy, cataracts, or ocular inflammatory conditions
c. Used with caution in clients taking neurotoxic medications because the risk for neurotoxicity increases
3. Side/adverse effects
a. Hypersensitivity reactions
b. Anorexia, nausea, vomiting
c. Dizziness
d. Malaise
e. Mental confusion
f. Joint pain
g. Dermatitis
h. Optic neuritis
i. Peripheral neuritis
j. Thrombocytopenia
k. Increased uric acid levels
l. Anaphylactoid reaction
4. Interventions
a. Monitor the client for hypersensitivity.
b. Monitor results of CBC, uric acid, and renal and liver function tests.
c. Monitor for visual changes such as altered color perception and decreased visual acuity; if changes occur, the medication is withheld and the HCP is notified.

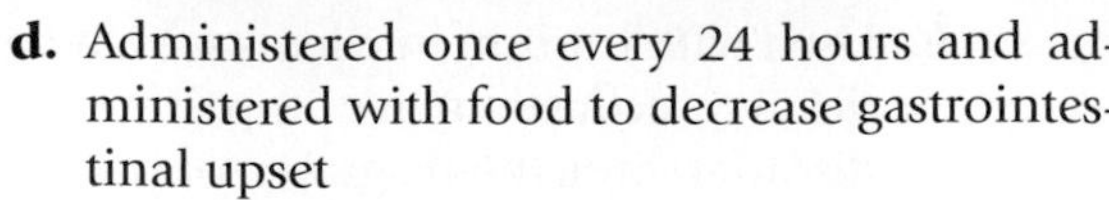

d. Administered once every 24 hours and administered with food to decrease gastrointestinal upset
e. Monitor uric acid concentration and check for painful or swollen joints or signs of gout.
f. Monitor intake and output and for adequate renal function.
g. Monitor mental status.
h. Monitor for dizziness and initiate safety precautions.
i. Monitor for peripheral neuritis (numbness, tingling or burning of the extremities); if it occurs, the HCP is notified.

5. Client education
   a. That nausea, related to the medication, can be prevented by taking the daily dose at bedtime or by taking the prescribed antinausea medications
   b. Not to skip doses and to take the medication for the full length of the prescribed therapy
   c. Not to take any other medication without consulting the HCP
   d. About the importance of follow-up HCP visits, vision testing, and laboratory tests
   e. To notify the HCP immediately if any visual problems occur, or a rash, swelling and pain in the joints, numbness, tingling, or burning in the hands or feet occurs

D. Pyrazinamide
1. Description
   a. The exact mechanism of action of pyrazinamide is unknown.
   b. May be bacteriostatic or bactericidal, depending on its concentration at the infection site and susceptibility of infecting organism
   c. Used with at least one other antitubercular medication after failure or ineffectiveness of the primary medication(s)
2. Contraindications and cautions
   a. Contraindicated in clients with hypersensitivity
   b. Used with caution in clients with diabetes mellitus, renal impairment, or gout, and in children
   c. May decrease the effects of allopurinol (Zyloprim), colchicine (Colcrys), and probenecid
   d. Cross-sensitivity is possible with isoniazid, ethionamide (Trecator), or nicotinic acid
3. Side/adverse effects
   a. Increases liver function tests and uric acid levels
   b. Arthralgia, myalgia
   c. Photosensitivity
   d. Hepatotoxicity
   e. Thrombocytopenia

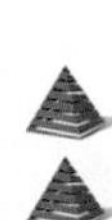

4. Interventions
   a. Monitor for hypersensitivity.
   b. Monitor CBC, liver function test results, and uric acid levels.
   c. Observe for hepatotoxic effects; if they occur, the medication is withheld and the HCP is notified.
   d. Monitor for painful or swollen joints.
   e. Monitor blood glucose level because diabetes mellitus may be difficult to control while client is taking the medication.
5. Client education
   a. To take the medication with food to reduce gastrointestinal distress
   b. To avoid sunlight or ultraviolet light until photosensitivity is determined
   c. To notify the HCP if any side/adverse effects occur
   d. Not to skip doses and to take the medication for the full length of the prescribed therapy
   e. Not to take any other medication without consulting the HCP
   f. About the importance of follow-up HCP visits and laboratory tests

E. Rifabutin (Mycobutin)
1. Description
   a. Inhibits mycobacterial DNA-dependent RNA polymerase and suppresses protein synthesis
   b. Used to prevent disseminated *Mycobacterium avium* complex (MAC) disease in clients with advanced HIV infection
   c. Used to treat active MAC disease and tuberculosis in clients with HIV infection
2. Cautions
   a. Can affect blood levels of some medications, including oral contraceptives and some medications used to treat HIV infection
   b. A nonhormonal method of birth control should be used instead of an oral contraceptive.
3. Side/adverse effects
   a. Rash
   b. Gastrointestinal (GI) disturbances
   c. Neutropenia
   d. Red-orange–colored body secretions
   e. Uveitis
   f. Myositis
   g. Arthralgia
   h. Hepatitis
   i. Chest pain with dyspnea
   j. Flu-like syndrome

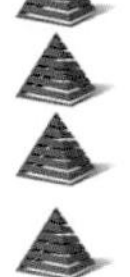

4. Interventions
   a. A medication history is obtained.
   b. Observe for hepatotoxic effects; if they occur, the medication is withheld and the HCP is notified.
   c. Monitor for painful or swollen joints.
   d. Monitor for ocular pain or blurred vision.

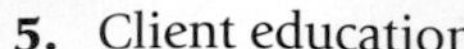

5. Client education
   a. That the medication can be taken without regard to food
   b. To notify the HCP if any side effects occur
   c. Not to skip doses and to take the medication for the full length of the prescribed therapy
   d. Not to take any other medication without consulting the HCP
   e. About the importance of follow-up HCP visits and laboratory tests

F. Rifapentine (Priftin)
1. Description: Used only for pulmonary tuberculosis
2. Cautions: Can affect blood levels of some medications, including oral contraceptives and warfarin (Coumadin), and some medications used to treat HIV infection
3. Side/adverse effects
   a. Red-orange–colored body secretions
   b. Hepatotoxicity
4. Interventions
   a. A medication history is obtained.
   b. Monitor baseline liver function studies and monitor throughout therapy.
   c. Observe for hepatotoxic effects; if they occur, the medication is withheld and the HCP is notified.
5. Client education
   a. That the medication can be taken without regard to food
   b. To avoid sunlight or ultraviolet light until photosensitivity is determined
   c. That red-orange–colored body secretions may occur
   d. Not to skip doses and to take the medication for the full length of the prescribed therapy
   e. Not to take any other medication without consulting the HCP
   f. About the importance of follow-up HCP visits and laboratory tests

⚠ Some tuberculosis medications can cause red-orange–colored body secretions. The client is informed that this is not a harmful effect but that the secretions can stain and permanently discolor items.

XV. Second-Line Medications for Tuberculosis (see Box 50-6)

A. Capreomycin sulfate (Capastat sulfate)
1. Description
   a. Mechanism of action is unknown
   b. Used to treat MDR-TB when significant resistance to other medications is expected
   c. Must be given intramuscularly
2. Contraindications and cautions
   a. The risk of nephrotoxicity, ototoxicity, and neuromuscular blockade is increased with the use of aminoglycosides or loop diuretics.
   b. Used with caution in clients with renal insufficiency, acoustic nerve impairment, hepatic disorder, myasthenia gravis, or parkinsonism
   c. Not administered to clients receiving streptomycin
3. Side/adverse effects
   a. Nephrotoxicity
   b. Ototoxicity
   c. Neuromuscular blockade
4. Interventions
   a. Baseline audiometric testing is performed.
   b. Renal, hepatic, and electrolyte levels are monitored before administration.
   c. Monitor intake and output.
   d. Administered intramuscularly deep into a large muscle mass (reconstituted medication may be stored for 48 hours at room temperature)
   e. Injection sites are rotated.
   f. Observe injection site for redness, excessive bleeding, and inflammation.
5. Client education
   a. Not to perform tasks that require mental alertness
   b. To report any hearing loss, balance disturbances, respiratory difficulty, weakness, or signs of hypersensitivity reactions

B. Antibiotics
1. Description
   a. Aminoglycoside antibiotics (kanamycin; amikacin [Amikin]) or fluoroquinolones (levofloxacin [Levaquin]; moxifloxacin [Avelox]) are given with at least one other antitubercular medication.
   b. Bactericidal because of receptor-binding action interfering with protein synthesis in susceptible microorganisms
   c. Gastrointestinal disturbances are the most common side effect.
   d. Fluoroquinolones are not recommended for use in children.
2. Contraindications and cautions
   a. Contraindicated in clients with hypersensitivity, neuromuscular disorders, or eighth cranial nerve damage
   b. Used with caution in the older client, in neonates because of renal insufficiency and immaturity, and in young infants because it may cause CNS depression
   c. The risk of toxicity increases if taken with other aminoglycosides or nephrotoxicity- or ototoxicity-producing medications.

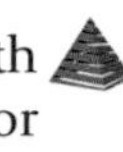

3. Side/adverse effects
   a. Hypersensitivity
   b. Pain and irritation at the injection site
   c. Nephrotoxicity is indicated by increased blood urea nitrogen and serum creatinine levels.

   d. Ototoxicity is indicated by tinnitus, dizziness, ringing or roaring in the ears, and reduced hearing.
   e. Neurotoxicity is indicated by headache, dizziness, lethargy, tremors, and visual disturbances.
   f. Superinfections
4. Interventions
   a. Monitor for hypersensitivity.
   b. Monitor for ototoxic, neurotoxic, and nephrotoxic reactions.
   c. Monitor liver and renal function test results.
   d. Baseline audiometric test is obtained and repeated every 1 to 2 months because the medication impairs the eighth cranial nerve.
   e. Determine acuteness of hearing.
   f. Monitor for visual changes.
   g. Determine hydration status and maintain adequate hydration during therapy.
   h. Monitor intake and output.
   i. Monitor urinalysis results.
   j. Monitor for superinfection.
5. Client education
   a. Not to skip doses and to take the medication for the full length of the prescribed therapy
   b. Not to take any other medication without consulting the HCP
   c. About the importance of follow-up HCP visits and laboratory tests
   d. To notify the HCP if hearing loss, changes in vision, or urinary problems occur

C. Ethionamide (Trecator)
1. Description
   a. Mechanism of action is unknown.
   b. Used to treat MDR-TB when significant resistance to other medications is expected
2. Contraindications and cautions
   a. Contraindicated in clients with hypersensitivity
   b. Used with caution in clients with diabetes mellitus or renal dysfunction
3. Side/adverse effects
   a. Anorexia, nausea, vomiting
   b. Metallic taste in the mouth
   c. Orthostatic hypotension
   d. Jaundice
   e. Mental changes
   f. Peripheral neuritis
   g. Rash
4. Interventions
   a. Monitor liver and renal function test results.
   b. Monitor glucose levels in the client with diabetes mellitus.
   c. Administered as prescribed to reduce the risk of neurotoxicity
5. Client education
   a. To take medication with food or meals to minimize gastrointestinal irritation
   b. To change positions slowly
   c. To report signs of a rash, which can progress to exfoliative dermatitis if the medication is not discontinued
   d. To avoid alcohol
   e. To report signs of jaundice and other side/adverse effects of the medication if they occur

D. Aminosalicylic acid (Paser)
1. Description
   a. Inhibits folic acid metabolism in mycobacteria
   b. Used to treat MDR-TB when significant resistance to other medications is expected
2. Contraindications and cautions
   a. Contraindicated with hypersensitivity to aminosalicylates, salicylates, or compounds containing the *para*-aminophenol group
   b. Aminobenzoates block the absorption of aminosalicylate sodium.
3. Side/adverse effects
   a. Hypersensitivity
   b. Bitter taste in the mouth
   c. Gastrointestinal tract irritation
   d. Exfoliative dermatitis
   e. Blood dyscrasias
   f. Crystalluria
   g. Changes in thyroid function
4. Interventions
   a. Monitor for hypersensitivity.
   b. Offer clear water to rinse the mouth and chewing gum or hard candy to alleviate the bitter taste.
   c. Encourage fluid intake to prevent crystalluria.
   d. Monitor intake and output.

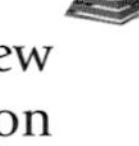

5. Client education
   a. To discard the medication and obtain a new supply if a purplish-brown discoloration occurs

   b. To take the medication with food
   c. That urine may turn red on contact with hypochlorite bleach if bleach was used to clean a toilet
   d. Not to take aspirin or over-the-counter medications without the HCP's approval
   e. To report signs of a blood dyscrasia, such as sore throat or mouth, malaise, fatigue, bruising, or bleeding

E. Cycloserine (Seromycin)
1. Description
   a. Interferes with cell wall biosynthesis
   b. Used to treat MDR-TB when significant resistance to other medications is expected
2. Contraindications and cautions
   a. Use of alcohol or ethionamide increases the risk of seizures
   b. Used with caution in clients with epilepsy, depression, severe anxiety, psychosis, or renal insufficiency, or in clients who use alcohol

3. Side/adverse effects
    a. Hypersensitivity
    b. CNS reactions
    c. Neurotoxicity
    d. Seizures
    e. Heart failure
    f. Headache
    g. Vertigo
    h. Altered level of consciousness
    i. Irritability, nervousness, anxiety
    j. Confusion
    k. Mood changes, depression, suicidal thoughts
4. Interventions
    a. Monitor level of consciousness.
    b. Monitor for changes in mental status and thought processes.
    c. Monitor renal and hepatic function tests.
    d. Monitor serum drug level to avoid the risk of neurotoxicity; the peak concentration, measured 2 hours after dosing, should be 25 to 35 mcg/mL.
5. Client education
    a. To take the medication after meals to prevent gastrointestinal upset
    b. To avoid alcohol
    c. To report signs of a rash or signs of CNS toxicity
    d. To avoid driving or performing tasks that require alertness until the reaction to the medication has been determined
    e. About the need for monitoring serum drug levels weekly, as prescribed

F. Streptomycin
1. Description
    a. An aminoglycoside antibiotic used with at least one other antitubercular medication
    b. Bactericidal because of receptor-binding action that interferes with protein synthesis in susceptible organisms
2. Contraindications and cautions
    a. Contraindicated in clients with hypersensitivity, myasthenia gravis, parkinsonism, or eighth cranial nerve damage
    b. Use with caution in the older client, in neonates because of renal insufficiency and immaturity, and in young infants because the medication may cause CNS depression.
    c. The risk of toxicity increases when streptomycin is taken with other aminoglycosides or nephrotoxicity- or ototoxicity-producing medications.
3. Side/adverse effects (Box 50-7)
4. Interventions
    a. Monitor for hypersensitivity.
    b. Monitor liver and renal function test results.

    c. Monitor for ototoxic, neurotoxic, and nephrotoxic reactions.

BOX 50-7 Side and Adverse Effects of Streptomycin

Nephrotoxicity
Changes in urine output
Decreased appetite
Increased thirst
Nausea, vomiting

Neurotoxicity
Muscle numbness
Seizures
Tingling
Twitching

Vestibular Toxicity
Clumsiness
Dizziness
Unsteadiness

Auditory Toxicity (ototoxicity)
A full feeling in the ears
Ringing in the ears
Loss of hearing

    d. Baseline audiometric testing is performed and repeated every 1 to 2 months because the medication impairs the eighth cranial nerve.
    e. Check hearing acuity.
    f. Monitor for visual changes.
    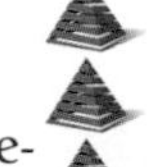
    g. Monitor hydration status and maintain adequate hydration during therapy.
    h. Monitor intake and output.
    i. Monitor urinalysis results.
    j. Monitor for signs of peripheral neuritis.
    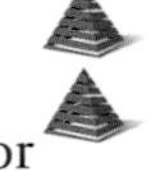
5. Client education
    a. Not to skip doses and to take medication for the full length of the prescribed therapy
    b. Not to take any other medication without consulting the HCP
    c. About the importance of follow-up HCP visits and laboratory tests
    d. To notify the HCP if hearing loss, changes in vision, or urinary problems occur

XVI. Influenza Medications

A. Vaccines
1. Description
    a. Because the strain of influenza virus is different every year, annual vaccination is recommended.
    b. Refer to the Centers for Disease Control and Prevention for current information about the influenza vaccine, vaccines available, and contraindications and cautions at http://www.cdc.gov/flu/protect/vaccine/index.htm.
2. Side/adverse effects
    a. Of the inactivated vaccine: Localized pain and swelling at the injection site, general body aches and pains, malaise, fever
    b. Of the attenuated vaccine (nasal): Runny nose or nasal congestion, cough, headache, and sore throat
3. Interventions
    a. The intramuscular route is recommended for the inactivated vaccine; adults and older

children should be vaccinated in the deltoid muscle.
   b. Monitor for side/adverse effects of the vaccine.
   c. Monitor for hypersensitivity reactions in clients receiving vaccination for the first time.
4. Client education
   a. About the importance of an annual vaccination
   b. That the inactivated vaccine contains non-infectious killed viruses and cannot cause influenza
   c. That any respiratory disease unrelated to influenza can occur after the vaccination
   d. That if the attenuated vaccine is received, the virus may be shed up to 2 days after vaccination
   e. That development of antibodies in adults takes approximately 2 weeks

B. Antiviral medications (Box 50-8)
1. Description
   a. Use during outbreaks of influenza depends on the current strain of influenza.
   b. Diagnosis of influenza should include rapid diagnostic tests because symptoms of infection from other pathogens may cause symptoms similar to those of influenza infection.
   c. May also be administered as prophylaxis against infection but should not replace vaccination
2. Contraindicated in hypersensitive clients.
3. Side/adverse effects
   a. Common side effects include headache, dizziness, fatigue, nausea, and vomiting.
   b. Some side/adverse effects depend on the medication (Table 50-1).
4. Interventions
   a. Administered within 2 days of onset of symptoms and continued for the entire prescription.
   b. Monitor for side/adverse effects of specific medications.
5. Client education
   a. That the medication may not prevent the transmission of influenza to others
   b. About the need to adjust activities if dizziness or fatigue occur
   c. About management of side/adverse effects of various medications
   d. To take medication exactly as prescribed and for the duration of prescription

BOX 50-8 Antiviral Influenza Medications

Amantadine (Symmetrel)
Oseltamivir (Tamiflu)
Rimantadine (Flumadine)
Zanamivir (Relenza)

TABLE 50-1 Side/Adverse Effects of Antiviral Influenza Medications

Antiviral Medications	Side/Adverse Effects
Amantadine (Symmetrel)	Drowsiness, anxiety, psychosis, depression, hallucinations, tremors, confusion, insomnia, orthostatic hypotension, heart failure, blurred vision, constipation, dry mouth, urinary frequency and retention, leukopenia, photosensitivity, dermatitis
Oseltamivir (Tamiflu)	Insomnia, diarrhea, abdominal pain, cough
Rimantadine (Flumadine)	Depression, hallucinations, tremors, seizures, insomnia, poor concentration, asthenia, gait abnormalities, anxiety, confusion, pallor, palpitations, hypotension, edema, tinnitus, eye pain, constipation, dry mouth, anorexia, abdominal pain, diarrhea, dyspepsia, rash
Zanamivir (Relenza)	Ear, nose, and throat infections; diarrhea; nasal symptoms; cough; sinusitis; bronchitis

XVII. Pneumococcal Conjugate Vaccine

A. Pneumococcal conjugate vaccine (PCV, Prevnar) is used for the prevention of invasive pneumococcal disease in infants and children.

B. Pneumococcal polysaccharide vaccine (Pneumovax 23) is used for adults and high-risk children older than 2 years.

C. Side/adverse effects include erythema, swelling, pain and tenderness at the injection site, fever, irritability, drowsiness, and reduced appetite.

D. See Chapter 39 for additional information about vaccines for pneumonia.

CRITICAL THINKING What Should You Do?

Answer: An adverse effect of isoniazid is nonviral hepatitis. Manifestations include anorexia, nausea, vomiting, weakness, fatigue, dark urine, or jaundice. If these symptoms occur, the nurse should withhold the medication and notify the registered nurse. The health care provider is also notified. The nurse should also check the client's liver function test results for elevations, such as alanine aminotransferase (ALT), the normal level being 10 to 40 units/L; aspartate aminotransferase (AST), the normal level being 10 to 30 units/L; and the total bilirubin level, which should be lower than 1.5 mg/dL. If these are elevated, the client could be experiencing nonviral hepatitis.

Reference(s): Lewis, S., Dirksen, S., Heitkemper, M., & Bucher, L. (2014). *Medical-surgical nursing: Assessment and management of clinical problems* (9th ed., pp. 531–532). St. Louis: Mosby.

PRACTICE QUESTIONS

❖ **511.** Rifabutin (Mycobutin) is prescribed for a client with active *Mycobacterium avium* complex (MAC) disease and tuberculosis. The nurse should monitor for which side/adverse effects of the medication? **Select all that apply.**

- ☐ **1.** Signs of hepatitis
- ☐ **2.** Flu-like syndrome
- ☐ **3.** Low neutrophil count
- ☐ **4.** Vitamin B_6 deficiency
- ☐ **5.** Ocular pain or blurred vision
- ☐ **6.** Tingling and numbness of the fingers

512. A client has a prescription to take guaifenesin (Humibid) every 4 hours, as needed. The nurse determines that the client understands the **most effective** use of this medication if the client makes which statement?

1. "I will watch for irritability as a side effect."
2. "I will take the tablet with a full glass of water."
3. "I will take an extra dose if the cough is accompanied by fever."
4. "I will crush the sustained-release tablet if immediate relief is needed."

513. A postoperative client has received a dose of naloxone hydrochloride (Narcan) for respiratory depression shortly after transfer to the nursing unit from the postanesthesia care unit. After administration of the medication, the nurse should check the client for which sign/ symptom?

1. Pupillary changes
2. Scattered lung wheezes
3. Sudden increase in pain
4. Sudden episodes of diarrhea

514. A client has been taking isoniazid for 2 months. The client complains to the nurse about numbness, paresthesias, and tingling in the extremities. The nurse interprets that the client is experiencing which problem?

1. Hypercalcemia
2. Peripheral neuritis
3. Small blood vessel spasm
4. Impaired peripheral circulation

515. A client is to begin a 6-month course of therapy with isoniazid. The nurse should plan to provide which information to the client?

1. Drink alcohol in small amounts only.
2. Report yellow eyes or skin immediately.
3. Increase intake of Swiss or aged cheeses.
4. Avoid vitamin supplements during therapy.

516. A client has been started on long-term therapy with rifampin (Rifadin). Which information about this medication should the nurse provide to the client?

1. Should always be taken with food or antacids
2. Should be double-dosed if one dose is forgotten
3. Causes red-orange discoloration of sweat, tears, urine, and feces
4. May be discontinued independently if symptoms are gone in 3 months

517. The nurse has given a client taking ethambutol (Myambutol) information about the medication. The nurse determines that the client understands the instructions if the client states to report which occurrence **immediately**?

1. Impaired sense of hearing
2. Problems with visual acuity
3. Gastrointestinal (GI) side effects
4. Red-orange discoloration of body secretions

518. Cycloserine (Seromycin) is added to the medication regimen for a client with tuberculosis. Which instruction should the nurse reinforce in the client-teaching plan regarding this medication?

1. To take the medication before meals
2. To return to the clinic weekly for serum drug-level testing
3. It is not necessary to restrict alcohol intake with this medication.
4. It is not necessary to call the health care provider (HCP) if a skin rash occurs.

519. A client with tuberculosis is being started on antituberculosis therapy with isoniazid. Before giving the client the first dose, the nurse ensures that which baseline study has been completed?

1. Electrolyte levels
2. Coagulation times
3. Liver enzyme levels
4. Serum creatinine level

520. A client is receiving acetylcysteine (Mucomyst), 20% solution diluted in 0.9% normal saline by nebulizer. The nurse should have which item available for a possible adverse event after giving this medication?

1. Ambu bag
2. Intubation tray
3. Nasogastric tube
4. Suction equipment

ANSWERS

❖**511. 1, 2, 3, 5**

Rationale: Rifabutin (Mycobutin) may be prescribed for a client with active MAC disease and tuberculosis. It inhibits mycobacterial DNA–dependent RNA polymerase and suppresses protein synthesis. Side effects include rash, gastrointestinal disturbances, neutropenia (low neutrophil count), red-orange body secretions, uveitis (blurred vision and eye pain), myositis, arthralgia, hepatitis, chest pain with dyspnea, and flu-like syndrome. Vitamin B_6 deficiency and numbness and tingling in the extremities are associated with the use of isoniazid. Ethambutol (Myambutol) also causes peripheral neuritis.

Test-Taking Strategy: Focus on the **subject**, side/adverse effects of this medication. Note the name of the medication to assist in answering the question. Recalling that vitamin B_6 deficiency and numbness and tingling in the extremities are associated with the use of isoniazid not rifabutin, will assist in answering. **Review:** the side/adverse effects associated with **rifabutin (Mycobutin)**.

Level of Cognitive Ability: Analyzing

Client Needs: Physiological Integrity

Integrated Process: Nursing Process/Data Collection

Content Area: Pharmacology: Respiratory Medications

Priority Concepts: Infection, Safety

Reference(s): Hodgson, Kizior (2015), pp. 1051–1052; Lehne (2013), p. 1124.

512. 2

Rationale: Guaifenesin (Humibid) is an expectorant. It should be taken with a full glass of water to decrease viscosity of secretions. Sustained-release preparations should not be broken open, crushed, or chewed. The medication may occasionally cause dizziness, headache, or drowsiness as side effects. The client should contact the health care provider if the cough lasts longer than 1 week or is accompanied by fever, rash, sore throat, or persistent headache.

Test-Taking Strategy: Note the **strategic words**, *most effective.* Begin to answer this question by eliminating option 4 first. Sustained-release preparations are not crushed or broken. Option 3 is eliminated next because fever indicates infection, and an "extra dose" of an expectorant is not helpful in treating infection. From the remaining options, recalling that increased fluids help liquefy secretions for more effective coughing will direct you to the correct option. **Review:** the administration of **guaifenesin**.

Level of Cognitive Ability: Evaluating

Client Needs: Physiological Integrity

Integrated Process: Nursing Process/Evaluation

Content Area: Pharmacology: Respiratory Medications

Priority Concepts: Client Education, Gas Exchange

Reference(s): Skidmore-Roth (2014), p. 615.

513. 3

Rationale: Naloxone hydrochloride is an antidote to opioids and may also be given to the postoperative client to treat respiratory depression. When given to the postoperative client for respiratory depression, it may also reverse the effects of analgesics. Therefore, the nurse must check the client for a sudden increase in the level of pain experienced. Options 1, 2, and 4 are not associated with this medication.

Test-Taking Strategy: Focus on the **subject**, the purpose and effect of administering naloxone hydrochloride. Recalling that this medication is an antidote to opioid analgesics will assist in directing you to option 3. Remember that this medication will cause sudden pain in the postoperative client or return of pain in the client who received opioid analgesics. **Review: naloxone hydrochloride**.

Level of Cognitive Ability: Analyzing

Client Needs: Physiological Integrity

Integrated Process: Nursing Process/Data Collection

Content Area: Pharmacology: Respiratory Medications

Priority Concepts: Cellular Regulation, Gas Exchange

Reference(s): Hodgson, Kizior (2015), pp. 825–827.

514. 2

Rationale: A common adverse effect of isoniazid is peripheral neuritis. This is manifested by numbness, tingling, and paresthesias in the extremities. This adverse effect can be minimized by pyridoxine (vitamin B_6) intake. Options 1, 3, and 4 are incorrect.

Test-Taking Strategy: Focus on the **subject**, a problem associated with isoniazid. Options 3 and 4 would not cause the symptoms presented in the question but instead would cause pallor and coolness. From the remaining options, you should know either that peripheral neuritis is an adverse effect of the medication or that the data in the question do not correlate with hypercalcemia. **Review:** the side/adverse effects associated with **isoniazid**.

Level of Cognitive Ability: Analyzing

Client Needs: Physiological Integrity

Integrated Process: Nursing Process/Data Collection

Content Area: Pharmacology: Respiratory Medications

Priority Concepts: Clinical Judgment, Sensory Perception

Reference(s): Hodgson, Kizior (2015), pp. 645–646; Lehne (2013), pp. 1122–1123, 1129.

515. 2

Rationale: Isoniazid is hepatotoxic, and therefore the client is taught to report signs and symptoms of hepatitis immediately (which include yellow skin and sclera). For the same reason, alcohol should be avoided during therapy. The client should avoid intake of Swiss cheese, fish such as tuna, and foods containing tyramine because they may cause a reaction characterized by redness and itching of the skin, flushing, sweating, tachycardia, headache, or light-headedness. The client can avoid developing peripheral neuritis by increasing the intake of pyridoxine (vitamin B_6) during the course of isoniazid therapy.

Test-Taking Strategy: Focus on the **subject**, signs/symptoms to report associated with use of isoniazid. Alcohol intake is avoided when the client is taking a prescribed medication, so option 1 should be eliminated first. Because the client receiving this medication typically is supplemented with vitamin B_6, option 4 is incorrect and is eliminated next. From the remaining options, recalling that the medication is hepatotoxic will direct you to the correct option. **Review:** client teaching for **isoniazid**.

Level of Cognitive Ability: Applying

Client Needs: Physiological Integrity

Integrated Process: Teaching and Learning

Content Area: Pharmacology: Respiratory Medications

Priority Concepts: Client Education, Infection
Reference(s): Lehne (2013), pp. 1122, 1129.

516. 3
Rationale: Rifampin (Rifadin) should be taken exactly as directed. Doses should not be doubled or skipped. The client should not stop therapy until directed to do so by a health care provider. The medication should be administered on an empty stomach unless it causes gastrointestinal upset, and then it may be taken with food. Antacids, if prescribed, should be taken at least 1 hour before the medication. Rifampin causes red-orange discoloration of body secretions and will permanently stain soft contact lenses.
Test-Taking Strategy: Focus on the subject, client teaching associated with rifampin. Use of general medication administration principles will assist in eliminating options 2 and 4. Eliminate option 1 next because of the closed-ended word, *always.* **Review:** client teaching points associated with **rifampin.**
Level of Cognitive Ability: Applying
Client Needs: Physiological Integrity
Integrated Process: Teaching and Learning
Content Area: Pharmacology: Respiratory Medications
Priority Concepts: Client Education, Safety
Reference(s): Hodgson, Kizior (2015), p. 1054.

517. 2
Rationale: Ethambutol (Myambutol) causes optic neuritis, which decreases visual acuity and the ability to discriminate between the colors red and green. This poses a potential safety hazard when a client is driving a motor vehicle. The client is taught to report this symptom immediately. The client is also taught to take the medication with food if GI upset occurs. Impaired hearing results from antitubercular therapy with streptomycin. Red-orange discoloration of secretions occurs with rifampin (Rifadin).
Test-Taking Strategy: Focus on the subject, client understanding of instructions given regarding ethambutol. Also note the strategic word, *immediately.* Option 3 is the least likely symptom to report; rather, it should be managed by taking the medication with food. To select from the other options, it is necessary to know that this medication causes optic neuritis, resulting in difficulty with red-green discrimination. **Review:** client teaching related to **ethambutol (Myambutol).**
Level of Cognitive Ability: Evaluating
Client Needs: Physiological Integrity
Integrated Process: Nursing Process/Evaluation
Content Area: Pharmacology: Respiratory Medications
Priority Concepts: Infection, Sensory Perception
Reference(s): Hodgson, Kizior (2015), p. 458.

518. 2
Rationale: Cycloserine (Seromycin) is an antitubercular medication that requires weekly serum drug level determinations to monitor for the potential of neurotoxicity. Serum drug levels lower than 30 mcg/mL reduce the incidence of neurotoxicity. The medication must be taken after meals to prevent gastrointestinal irritation. The client must be instructed to notify the HCP if a skin rash or signs of central nervous system toxicity are noted. Alcohol must be avoided because it increases the risk of seizure activity.
Test-Taking Strategy: Focus on the subject, client teaching regarding the use of cycloserine. Eliminate options 3 and 4 first, using guidelines related to general medication administration principles. From this point, knowing that the medication level needs to be monitored will assist in selecting the correct option. **Review:** client instructions related to **cycloserine (Seromycin).**
Level of Cognitive Ability: Applying
Client Needs: Physiological Integrity
Integrated Process: Teaching and Learning
Content Area: Pharmacology: Respiratory Medications
Priority Concepts: Client Education, Infection
Reference(s): Lehne (2013), p. 1126.

519. 3
Rationale: Isoniazid therapy can cause an elevation of hepatic enzyme levels and hepatitis. Therefore, liver enzyme levels are monitored when therapy is initiated and during the first 3 months of therapy. They may be monitored longer in the client who is greater than age 50 or abuses alcohol.
Test-Taking Strategy: Focus on the subject, laboratory monitoring associated with isoniazid. In order to answer this question correctly, it is necessary to know that this medication can be toxic to the liver. **Review:** the adverse effects of the various **antituberculosis medications.**
Level of Cognitive Ability: Analyzing
Client Needs: Physiological Integrity
Integrated Process: Nursing Process/Data Collection
Content Area: Pharmacology: Respiratory Medications
Priority Concepts: Clinical Judgment, Infection
Reference(s): Hodgson, Kizior (2015), pp. 645–646.

520. 4
Rationale: Acetylcysteine can be given orally or by nasogastric tube to treat acetaminophen overdose, or it may be given by inhalation for use as a mucolytic. The nurse administering this medication as a mucolytic should have suction equipment available in case the client cannot manage to clear the increased volume of liquefied secretions.
Test-Taking Strategy: Focus on the subject, equipment necessary in the administration of acetylcysteine. To answer this question, it is necessary to know that acetylcysteine may be given for either acetaminophen overdose or as a mucolytic agent. It is also necessary to know that the inhalation route is only used for mucolytic effects. With this in mind, options 1 and 2 are eliminated because the client does not need resuscitation. Option 3 is eliminated as well because a nasogastric tube may be used in the client with acetaminophen overdose but is not necessary when used as a mucolytic. **Review:** the purpose of **acetylcysteine** and the related nursing interventions.
Level of Cognitive Ability: Applying
Client Needs: Physiological Integrity
Integrated Process: Nursing Process/Implementation
Content Area: Pharmacology: Respiratory Medications
Priority Concepts: Clinical Judgment, Gas Exchange
Reference(s): Skidmore-Roth (2014), p. 68.

UNIT XIII

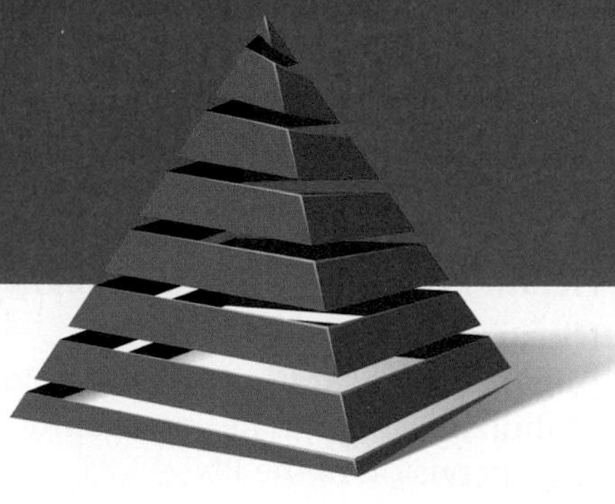

The Adult Client with a Cardiovascular Disorder

PYRAMID TERMS

arterial pressure The pressure of the blood against the arterial walls. Pressure can be measured indirectly by sphygmomanometer or directly by arterial catheter. Readings are expressed as systolic over diastolic. Arterial pressure increases when the cardiac output, peripheral resistance, or blood volume increases.

blood pressure (BP) The force exerted by the blood against the walls of the blood vessels; if the BP falls too low, blood flow to the tissues, heart, brain, and other organs becomes inadequate; if the BP becomes too high, the risk of vessel rupture and damage increases.

cardiac output The total volume of blood pumped through the heart in 1 minute; the normal cardiac output is 4 to 7 L/min; cardiac output = stroke volume × heart rate. Cardiac output equals stroke volume multiplied by heart rate.

collateral circulation Circulation in an area of tissue or in an organ with a number of different pathways for blood flow to the tissue or organ. This is often a result of anastamoses, branches formed between adjacent blood vessels. Collateral circulation can be established in the venous system (between veins) or in the arterial system (between arteries).

contractility Refers to the inherent ability of the myocardium to alter contractile force and velocity; sympathetic stimulation increases myocardial contractility, thus increasing stroke volume; conditions that decrease myocardial contractility reduce stroke volume.

diastole The phase of the cardiac cycle in which the heart relaxes between contractions; it represents the period when the two ventricles are dilated by the blood flowing into them.

diastolic pressure The force of the blood exerted against the artery walls when the heart relaxes or fills.

postural (orthostatic) hypotension A blood pressure decrease of more than 10 to 15 mm Hg of the systolic pressure or a decrease of more than 10 mm Hg of the diastolic pressure and a 10% to 20% increase in heart rate; occurs when the client's blood pressure is not adequately maintained when moving from a lying to a sitting or standing position.

pulse pressure The difference between the systolic and diastolic pressures; normal pulse pressure is 30 to 40 mm Hg.

systole The phase of contraction of the heart, especially of the ventricles, during which blood is forced into the aorta and pulmonary artery.

systolic pressure The maximum pressure of blood exerted against the artery walls when the heart contracts.

venous pressure The force exerted by the blood against the vein walls; normal venous pressures are highest in the extremities (5 to 14 cm H_2O in the arm), and lowest closest to the heart (6 to 8 cm H_2O in the inferior vena cava).

Pyramid to Success

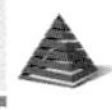

Pyramid points focus on data collection related to cardiovascular risks, health screening and promotion, complications of the various cardiovascular disorders, emergency implementation measures, and reinforcing client education. Focus on the findings in angina, myocardial infarction (MI), heart failure and pulmonary edema, pericarditis, aneurysms, hypertension, and arterial and venous disorders. Focus also on the care of the client following diagnostic treatments and surgical procedures. Note appropriate and therapeutic client positions, particularly with arterial and venous disorders of the extremities. Focus on treatments and medications prescribed for the various cardiovascular disorders and reinforcing client teaching related to prescribed treatment plans. Be familiar with the components related to cardiac rehabilitation.

Client Needs

Safe and Effective Care Environment

Consulting with the registered nurse (RN) and other members of the health care team

Discussing cardiovascular consultations and referrals with the RN

Ensuring that informed consent related to cardiovascular treatments and procedures has been obtained

Establishing priorities

Maintaining asepsis
Maintaining standard and other precautions
Upholding client rights

Health Promotion and Maintenance

Discussing alterations in lifestyle
Implementing cardiovascular data collection techniques
Mobilizing appropriate community resources under the supervision of the RN
Preventing cardiovascular disease
Promoting cardiac rehabilitation under the direction of the RN
Providing health screening and health promotion programs with the RN
Reinforcing teaching related to diet, therapy, exercise, and medications

Psychosocial Integrity

Assisting the client to accept lifestyle changes
Considering religious, spiritual, and cultural influences on health
Discussing grief and loss, and end-of-life issues
Discussing situational role changes
Discussing unexpected body-image changes
Identifying coping mechanisms
Identifying fear, anxiety, and denial
Identifying support systems

Physiological Integrity

Assisting with basic care measures
Discussing activity limitations and promoting rest and sleep
Monitoring for complications related to cardiovascular disorders
Monitoring for therapeutic effects of medications
Monitoring of cardiac enzymes, troponin levels, and other laboratory values related to the cardiovascular system
Providing interventions required in emergencies
Providing nonpharmacological and pharmacological comfort interventions
Responding to medical emergencies

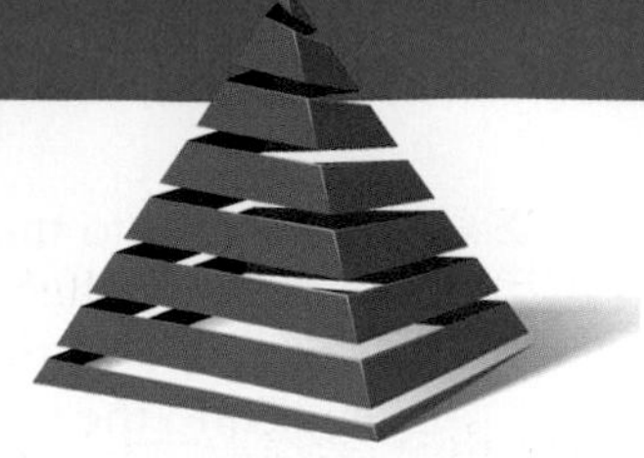

CHAPTER 51

Cardiovascular Disorders

CRITICAL THINKING What Should You Do?

A hospitalized client with a diagnosis of abdominal aortic aneurysm suddenly complains of severe back pain and shortness of breath. What should the nurse do?

Answer located on p. 700.

I. Anatomy and Physiology

A. Heart and heart wall layers
  1. The heart is located in the left side of the mediastinum.
  2. The heart consists of three layers.
    a. The epicardium is the outermost layer of the heart.
    b. The myocardium is the middle layer and actual contracting muscle of the heart.
    c. The endocardium is the innermost layer and lines the inner chambers and heart valves.

B. Pericardial sac
  1. Encases and protects the heart from trauma and infection
  2. Has two layers
    a. The parietal pericardium is the tough, fibrous outer membrane that attaches anteriorly to the lower half of the sternum, posteriorly to the thoracic vertebrae, and inferiorly to the diaphragm.
    b. The visceral pericardium is the thin, inner layer that closely adheres to the heart.
  3. The pericardial space is between the parietal and visceral layers. It holds 5 to 20 mL of pericardial fluid, lubricates the pericardial surfaces, and cushions the heart.

C. There are four heart chambers.
  1. The right atrium receives deoxygenated blood from the body via the superior and inferior vena cava.
  2. The right ventricle receives blood from the right atrium and pumps it to the lungs via the pulmonary artery.
  3. The left atrium receives oxygenated blood from the lungs via four pulmonary veins.
  4. The left ventricle is the largest and most muscular chamber. It receives oxygenated blood from the lungs via the left atrium and pumps blood into the systemic circulation via the aorta.

D. There are four valves in the heart.
  1. There are two atrioventricular (AV) valves—the tricuspid and the mitral—that lie between the atria and ventricles.
    a. The tricuspid valve is located on the right side of the heart.
    b. The bicuspid (mitral) valve is located on the left side of the heart.
    c. The AV valves close at the beginning of ventricular contraction and prevent blood from flowing back into the atria from the ventricles. These valves open when the ventricle relaxes.
  2. There are two semilunar valves: the pulmonic and the aortic.
    a. The pulmonic semilunar valve lies between the right ventricle and the pulmonary artery.
    b. The aortic semilunar valve lies between the left ventricle and the aorta.
    c. The semilunar valves prevent blood from flowing back into the ventricles during relaxation. They open during ventricular contraction and close when the ventricles begin to relax.

E. Sinoatrial (SA) node
  1. The main pacemaker that initiates each heartbeat
  2. Located at the junction of the superior vena cava and the right atrium
  3. The SA node generates electrical impulses at 60 to 100 times per minute and is controlled by the sympathetic and parasympathetic nervous systems.

F. Atrioventricular (AV) node
  1. Located in the lower aspect of the atrial septum
  2. Receives electrical impulses from the SA node
  3. If the SA node fails, the AV node can initiate and sustain a heart rate of 40 to 60 beats/min.

G. The bundle of His
  1. A continuation of the AV node and located at the interventricular septum

2. It branches into the right bundle branch, which extends down the right side of the interventricular septum, and the left bundle branch, which extends into the left ventricle.
3. The right and left bundle branches terminate into Purkinje fibers.

H. Purkinje fibers
1. Purkinje fibers are a diffuse network of conducting strands located beneath the ventricular endocardium.
2. These fibers spread the wave of depolarization through the ventricles.
3. Purkinje fibers can act as the pacemaker with a rate between 20 and 40 beats/min when higher pacemakers (such as the sinoatrial and atrioventricular nodes) fail.

I. Coronary arteries: Supply the capillaries of the myocardium with blood
1. The right main coronary artery supplies the right atrium and ventricle, the inferior portion of the left ventricle, the posterior septal wall, and the sinoatrial and atrioventricular nodes.
2. The left main coronary artery consists of two major branches, the left anterior descending and the circumflex arteries.
3. The left anterior descending artery supplies blood to the anterior wall of the left ventricle, the anterior ventricular septum, and the apex of the left ventricle.
4. The circumflex artery supplies blood to the left atrium and the lateral and posterior surfaces of the left ventricle.

The coronary arteries supply the capillaries of the myocardium with blood. If blockage occurs in these arteries, the client is at risk for myocardial infarction.

J. Heart sounds
1. The first heart sound (S_1) is heard as the AV valves close and is heard loudest at the apex of the heart.
2. The second heart sound (S_2) is heard when the semilunar valves close and is heard loudest at the base of the heart.
3. A third heart sound (S_3) may be heard if ventricular wall compliance is decreased and structures in the ventricular wall vibrate; this can occur in conditions such as heart failure or valvular regurgitation. However, a third heart sound may be normal in individuals younger than 30 years.
4. A fourth heart sound (S_4) may be heard on atrial systole if resistance to ventricular filling is present; this is an abnormal finding, and the causes include cardiac hypertrophy, disease, or injury to the ventricular wall.

K. Heart rate
1. The faster the heart rate, the less time the heart has for filling, and the **cardiac output** decreases.
2. An increase in heart rate increases oxygen consumption.
3. The normal sinus heart rate is 60 to 100 beats/min.
4. Sinus tachycardia is a rate greater than 100 beats/min.
5. Sinus bradycardia is a rate less than 60 beats/min.

L. Autonomic nervous system
1. Stimulation of sympathetic nerve fibers releases the neurotransmitter norepinephrine, producing an increased heart rate, increased conduction speed through the AV node, increased atrial and ventricular **contractility**, and peripheral vasoconstriction. Stimulation occurs when a decrease in pressure is detected.
2. Stimulation of the parasympathetic nerve fibers releases the neurotransmitter acetylcholine, which decreases the heart rate and lessens atrial and ventricular contractility and conductivity. Stimulation occurs when an increase in pressure is detected.

M. Blood pressure (BP) control
1. Baroreceptors, also called pressoreceptors, are located in the walls of the aortic arch and carotid sinuses.
2. Baroreceptors are specialized nerve endings that are affected by changes in the arterial BP.
3. Increases in arterial pressure stimulate baroreceptors, and the heart rate and arterial pressure decrease.
4. Decreases in arterial pressure reduce stimulation of the baroreceptors, and vasoconstriction and an increase in heart rate occur.
5. Stretch receptors, located in the vena cava and the right atrium, respond to pressure changes that affect circulatory blood volume.
6. When the BP decreases as a result of hypovolemia, a sympathetic response occurs, causing an increased heart rate and blood vessel constriction. When the BP increases as a result of hypervolemia, an opposite effect occurs.
7. Antidiuretic hormone (vasopressin) influences BP indirectly by regulating vascular volume.
8. Increases in blood volume result in decreased antidiuretic hormone release, increasing diuresis, and decreasing blood volume and thus decreasing BP.
9. Decreases in blood volume result in increased antidiuretic hormone release. This promotes an increase in blood volume and thus BP.
10. Renin, a potent vasoconstrictor, causes the BP to increase.

11. Renin converts angiotensinogen to angiotensin I. Angiotensin I is then converted to angiotensin II in the lungs.
12. Angiotensin II stimulates the release of aldosterone, which promotes water and sodium retention by the kidneys. This action increases blood volume and BP.

N. The vascular system
1. Arteries are vessels through which the blood passes away from the heart to various parts of the body. They convey highly oxygenated blood from the left side of the heart to the tissues.
2. Arterioles control the blood flow into the capillaries.
3. Capillaries allow the exchange of fluid and nutrients between the blood and the interstitial spaces.
4. Venules receive blood from the capillary bed and move blood into the veins.
5. Veins transport deoxygenated blood from the tissues back to the right heart and then the lungs for oxygenation.
6. Valves help return blood to the heart against the force of gravity.
7. The lymphatics drain the tissues and return the tissue fluid to the blood.

II. Diagnostic Tests and Procedures (Refer to Chapter 11 for further information)

A. Cardiac enzymes
1. CK-MB (creatine kinase, myocardial muscle)
   - **a.** An elevation in value indicates myocardial damage.
   - **b.** An elevation occurs within 4 to 6 hours and peaks 18 to 24 hours following an acute ischemic attack.
   - **c.** Normal value is 0% to 5% of total; total CK is 26 to 174 units/L.
2. Troponin
   - **a.** Troponin is composed of three proteins: troponin C, cardiac troponin I, and cardiac troponin T.
   - **b.** Troponin I especially has a high affinity for myocardial injury; it rises within 3 hours and persists for up to 7 to 10 days.
   - **c.** Normal values are low, with troponin I being lower than 0.6 ng/mL and troponin T normally ranging from 0 to 0.2 ng/mL; thus any rise can indicate myocardial cell damage.
3. Myoglobin
   - **a.** Myoglobin is an oxygen-binding protein found in cardiac and skeletal muscle.
   - **b.** The level rises within 1 hour after cell death, peaks in 4 to 6 hours, and returns to normal within 24 to 36 hours (even faster in some clients).

B. Complete blood count
1. The red blood cell count decreases in rheumatic heart disease and infective endocarditis and increases in conditions characterized by inadequate tissue oxygenation.
2. The white blood cell count increases in infectious and inflammatory diseases of the heart and after MI because large numbers of white blood cells are needed to dispose of the necrotic tissue resulting from the infarction.
3. An elevated hematocrit can result from vascular volume depletion.
4. Decreases in hematocrit and hemoglobin can indicate anemia.

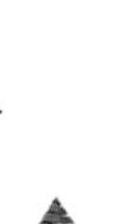

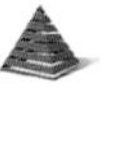

C. Blood coagulation factors: An increase in coagulation factors can occur during and after MI, which places the client at greater risk of thrombophlebitis and extension of clots in the coronary arteries.

D. Serum lipids: Used to assess the risk of developing coronary artery disease
1. The lipid profile measures serum cholesterol, triglyceride, and lipoprotein levels.
2. The lipid profile is used to assess the risk of developing coronary artery disease.
3. The desirable range for serum cholesterol is lower than 200 mg/dL, with low-density lipoprotein cholesterol lower than 130 mg/dL and high-density lipoprotein cholesterol at 30 to 70 mg/dL.
4. Lipoprotein-*a* or *Lp(a)*, a modified form of LDL, increases atherosclerotic plaques and increases clots; value should be less than 30 mg/dL.

E. Homocysteine: Elevated levels may increase the risk of cardiovascular disease; level should be less than 14 mmol/dL.

F. Highly sensitive C-reactive protein (hsCRP): Detects an inflammatory process such as that associated with the development of atherothrombosis; a level less than 1 mg/dL is considered low risk, and a level over 3 mg/dL places the client at risk for heart disease.

G. Microalbuminuria: A small amount of protein in the urine has been a marker for endothelial dysfunction in cardiovascular disease.

H. Electrolytes
1. Potassium
   - **a.** Hypokalemia causes increased cardiac electrical instability, ventricular dysrhythmias, and increased risk of digoxin toxicity.
   - **b.** In hypokalemia, the electrocardiogram would show flattening and inversion of the T wave, the appearance of a U wave, and ST depression.
   - **c.** Hyperkalemia causes asystole and ventricular dysrhythmias.
   - **d.** In hyperkalemia, the electrocardiogram may show tall peaked T waves, widened QRS complexes, prolonged PR intervals, or flat P waves.

2. Sodium
   a. The serum sodium level decreases with the use of diuretics.
   b. The serum sodium level decreases in heart failure, indicating water excess.

I. Calcium
   1. Hypocalcemia can cause ventricular dysrhythmias, prolonged ST and QT interval, and cardiac arrest.
   2. Hypercalcemia can cause a shortened ST segment and widened T wave, AV block, tachycardia or bradycardia, digitalis hypersensitivity, and cardiac arrest.

J. Phosphorus level: Phosphorus levels should be interpreted with calcium levels because the kidneys retain or excrete one electrolyte in an inverse relationship to the other.

K. Magnesium
   1. A low magnesium level can cause ventricular tachycardia (VT) and fibrillation.
   2. Electrocardiographic changes that may be observed with hypomagnesemia include tall T waves and depressed ST segments.
   3. A high magnesium level can cause muscle weakness, hypotension, and bradycardia.
   4. Electrocardiographic changes that may be observed with hypermagnesemia include a prolonged PR interval and widened QRS complex.

Electrolyte and mineral imbalances can cause cardiac electrical instability that can result in life-threatening dysrhythmias.

L. Blood urea nitrogen: The blood urea nitrogen is elevated in heart disorders that adversely affect renal circulation, such as heart failure and cardiogenic shock.

M. Blood glucose: An acute cardiac episode can elevate the blood glucose level.

N. B-type natriuretic peptide (BNP)
   1. BNP is released in response to atrial and ventricular stretch; serves as a marker for heart failure.
   2. BNP levels should be less than 100 pg/mL. The higher the level, the more severe the heart failure.

O. Chest x-ray film
   1. Description
      a. Radiography of the chest is done to determine the size, silhouette, and position of the heart.
      b. Specific pathological changes are difficult to determine via x-ray film, but anatomical changes can be seen.
   2. Interventions
      a. Prepare the client for x-ray film, explaining the purpose and procedure.
      b. Remove jewelry.
      c. Ensure that the client is not pregnant.

P. Electrocardiography
   1. Description: This common noninvasive diagnostic test records the electrical activity of the heart and is useful in detecting cardiac dysrhythmias, detecting location and extent of myocardial infarction, cardiac hypertrophy, and for evaluation of the effectiveness of cardiac medications.
   2. Interventions
      a. Determine the client's ability to lie still. Advise the client to lie still, breathe normally, and refrain from talking during the test.
      b. Reassure the client that an electrical shock will not occur.
      c. Document any cardiac medications the client is taking.

Q. Holter monitoring
   1. Description
      a. In this noninvasive test, the client wears a Holter monitor, and an electrocardiographic tracing is recorded continuously over a period of 24 hours or more while the client performs his activities of daily living.
      b. The Holter monitor identifies dysrhythmias if they occur and evaluates the effectiveness of antidysrhythmics or pacemaker therapy.
   2. Interventions
      a. Reinforce instructions to the client to resume normal daily activities and to maintain a diary documenting activities and any symptoms that may develop for correlation to the electrocardiographic tracing.
      b. Reinforce instructions to the client to avoid tub baths or showers because they will interfere with the electrocardiographic recorder device.

R. Echocardiography
   1. Description
      a. This noninvasive procedure is based on the principles of ultrasound and evaluates structural and functional changes in the heart.
      b. Heart chamber size is measured, ejection fraction is calculated, and flow gradient across the valves is determined.
      c. A transesophageal echocardiography may be done in which the echocardiogram is done through the esophagus; this is an invasive exam and requires pre- and postprocedure preparation, and care is similar to endoscopy procedures.
   2. Interventions: Determine the client's ability to lie still, and advise the client to lie still, breathe normally, and refrain from talking during the test.

S. Exercise electrocardiography testing (stress test)
   1. Description
      a. This noninvasive test studies the heart during activity and detects and evaluates coronary artery disease.

b. Treadmill testing is the most commonly used mode of stress testing.
c. Stress testing may be used with myocardial radionuclide testing (perfusion imaging), at which point the procedure becomes invasive because a radionuclide must be injected.
d. If the client is unable to tolerate exercise, an intravenous (IV) infusion of dipyridamole (Persantine), dobutamine hydrochloride, or adenosine (Adenocard) is given to dilate the coronary arteries and simulate the effect of exercise.
e. An informed consent is required if a radionuclide is to be injected.

2. Preprocedure interventions
a. Obtain an informed consent if required.
b. Provide adequate rest the night before the procedure.
c. Reinforce instructions to the client about oral intake as prescribed (to maintain an NPO status or eat a light meal 1 to 2 hours before the procedure).
d. Reinforce instructions to the client to avoid smoking, alcohol, and caffeine before the procedure.
e. Reinforce instructions to the client to ask the health care provider (HCP) about taking prescribed medication on the day of the procedure. Theophylline products are usually held 12 hours before the test, and calcium channel blockers and β-blockers are usually withheld on the day of the test to allow the heart rate to increase during the stress portion of the test.
f. Reinforce instructions to the client to wear nonconstrictive, comfortable clothing and supportive rubber-soled shoes for the exercise stress test.
g. Reinforce instructions to the client to notify the HCP if any chest pain, dizziness, or shortness of breath occurs during the procedure.

3. Postprocedure interventions: Instruct the client to avoid taking a hot bath or shower for at least 1 to 2 hours.

T. Digital subtraction angiography
1. Description
a. This test combines x-ray techniques and a computerized subtraction technique with fluoroscopy for visualization of the cardiovascular system.
b. A contrast medium (dye) is injected.
2. Preprocedure interventions
a. Check for allergies to seafood, iodine, or radiopaque dyes. If allergic, the client may be premedicated with antihistamines and steroids to prevent a reaction.
b. Obtain informed consent.
3. Postprocedure interventions
a. Monitor vital signs.
b. Monitor injection site for bleeding or discomfort.

U. Myocardial nuclear perfusion imaging (MNPI)
1. Description
a. Nuclear cardiology is the use of radionuclide techniques and scanning in cardiovascular assessment.
b. The most common tests include technetium pyrophosphate scanning, thallium imaging, and multigated cardiac blood pool imaging; can evaluate cardiac motion and calculate the ejection fraction.
2. Preprocedure interventions
a. Obtain informed consent.
b. Inform the client that a small amount of radioisotope will be injected and that the radiation exposure and risks are minimal.
3. Postprocedure interventions
a. Monitor vital signs.
b. Monitor injection site for bleeding or discomfort.
c. Inform the client that fatigue is possible.

V. Magnetic resonance imaging (MRI)
1. Description
a. This is a noninvasive diagnostic test that produces an image of the heart or great vessels through interaction of magnetic fields, radio waves, and atomic nuclei.
b. It provides information on chamber size and thickness, valve and ventricular function, and blood flow through the great vessels and coronary arteries.
2. Preprocedure interventions
a. Evaluate the client for the presence of a pacemaker or other implanted items that present a contraindication to the test.
b. Ensure that the client has removed all metallic objects such as watches, jewelry, clothing with metal fasteners, and metal hair fasteners.
c. Inform the client that he or she may experience claustrophobia while in the scanner.

W. Eletrophysiologic studies: An invasive procedure in which a programmed electrical stimulation of the heart is induced to cause dysrhythmias and conduction defects; assists in finding an accurate diagnosis and aids in determining treatment

X. Electronic-Beam Computer Tomography Scan (EBCT): Determines whether calcifications are present in the arteries; coronary artery calcium (CAC) score is provided (a score higher than 400 requires intensive preventive treatment).

Y. Cardiac catheterization

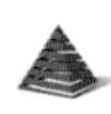

1. Description
a. An invasive test involving insertion of a catheter into the heart and surrounding vessels

b. Obtains information about the structure and performance of the heart chambers and valves and the coronary circulation

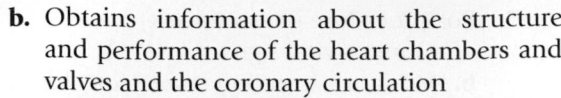

2. Preprocedure interventions
   a. Obtain informed consent.
   b. Monitor for allergies to seafood, iodine, or radiopaque dyes. If allergic, the client may be premedicated with antihistamines and corticosteroids to prevent a reaction.
   c. Withhold solid food for 6 to 8 hours and liquids for 4 hours as prescribed to prevent vomiting and aspiration during the procedure.
   d. Document the client's height and weight because these data will be needed to determine the amount of dye to be administered.
   e. Document baseline vital signs and note the quality and presence of peripheral pulses for postprocedure comparison.
   f. Inform the client that a local anesthetic will be administered before catheter insertion.
   g. Inform the client that he or she may feel fatigued because of the need to lie still and quiet on a hard table for up to 2 hours.
   h. Inform the client that he or she may feel a fluttery feeling as the catheter passes through the heart; a flushed, warm feeling when the dye is injected; a desire to cough; and palpitations caused by heart irritability.
   i. Prepare the insertion site by shaving and cleaning with an antiseptic solution, if prescribed.
   j. Administer preprocedure medications such as sedatives, if prescribed.
   k. Insert an IV line, if prescribed.

If a client taking metformin (Glucophage) is schedule to undergo a procedure requiring the administration of iodine dye, the metformin is withheld 24 to 48 hours (as prescribed) prior because of the risk of lactic acidosis. The medication is not resumed until directed to do so by the HCP (usually 48 hours after the procedure or after renal function studies are done and the results are evaluated).

3. Postprocedure interventions
   a. Monitor vital signs and cardiac rhythm for dysrhythmias at least every 30 minutes for 2 hours initially.
   b. Monitor for chest pain. If dysrhythmias or chest pain occurs, notify the HCP.
   c. Monitor peripheral pulses and the color, warmth, and sensation of the extremity distal to the insertion site at least every 30 minutes for 2 hours initially.
   d. Notify the HCP if the client complains of numbness and tingling; the extremity becomes cool, pale, or cyanotic; or loss of the peripheral pulses occurs.
   e. Monitor the pressure dressing for bleeding or hematoma formation.
   f. Apply a sandbag or compression device to the insertion site to provide additional pressure if prescribed.
   g. Monitor for bleeding. If bleeding occurs, apply manual pressure immediately and notify the HCP.
   h. Monitor for hematoma. If a hematoma develops, notify the HCP.
   i. Keep extremity extended for 4 to 6 hours, as prescribed, keeping the leg straight to prevent arterial occlusion.
   j. Maintain strict bed rest for 6 to 12 hours, as prescribed; however, the client may turn from side to side. Do not elevate the head of the bed more than 15 degrees.
   k. If the antecubital vessel was used, immobilize the arm with an armboard.
   l. Encourage fluid intake, if not contraindicated, to promote renal excretion of the dye and replace fluid loss caused by the osmotic diuretic effect of the dye.
   m. Monitor for nausea, vomiting, rash, or other signs of hypersensitivity to the dye.
   n. Do not resume the administration of metformin (Glucophage) until directed by the HCP (usually 48 hours after catheterization).

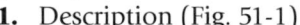

III. Therapeutic Management

A. Percutaneous transluminal coronary angioplasty (PTCA) 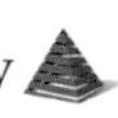

1. Description (Fig. 51-1)
   a. An invasive, nonsurgical technique in which one or more arteries are dilated with a balloon catheter to open the vessel lumen and improve arterial blood flow.
   b. PTCA may be used for clients with an evolving MI alone, or in combination with medications to achieve reperfusion.
   c. The client can experience reocclusion after the procedure; thus the procedure may need to be repeated.
   d. Complications can include arterial dissection or rupture, emobilization of plaque fragments, spasm, and acute MI.
   e. A firm commitment is needed on the part of the client to stop smoking, adhere to dietary restrictions, lose weight, alter exercise patterns, and stop any behaviors that could lead to the progression of artery occlusion.
2. Preprocedure interventions 
   a. Maintain NPO status after midnight.
   b. Obtain informed consent and allergy assessment to iodine, and withhold metformin (as for cardiac catheterization).

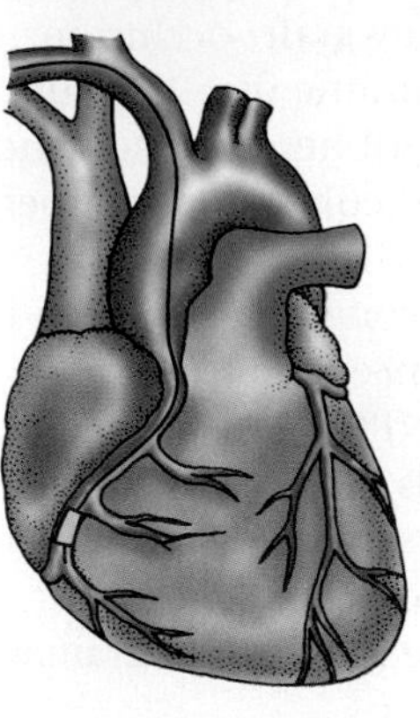

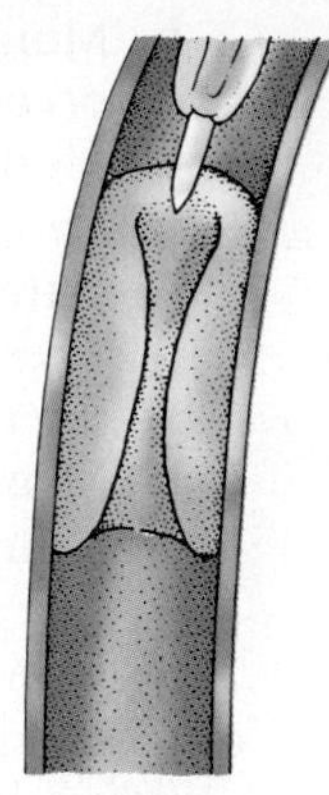

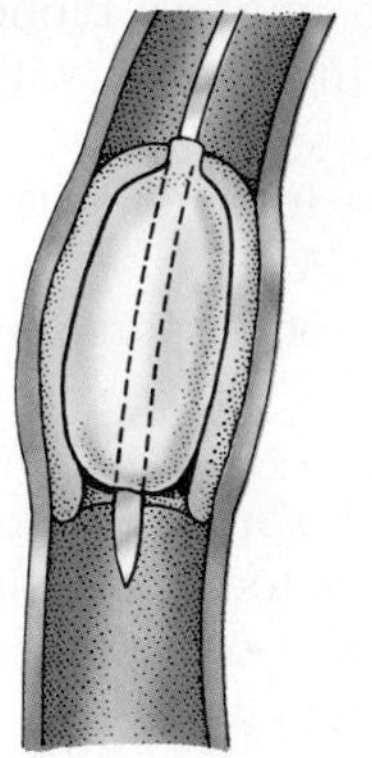

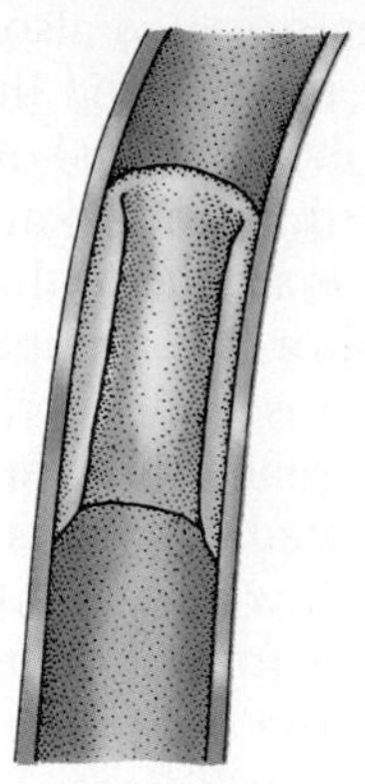

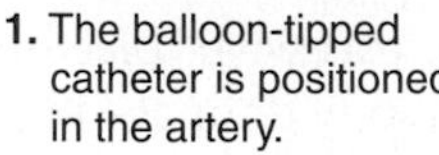

1. The balloon-tipped catheter is positioned in the artery.
2. The uninflated balloon is centered in the obstruction.
3. The balloon is inflated, which flattens plaque against the artery wall.
4. The balloon is removed, and the artery is left unoccluded.

FIGURE 51-1 Percutaneous transluminal coronary angioplasty. (From Ignatavicius D, Workman ML: *Medical-surgical nursing: Patient-centered collaborative care*, ed 7, St. Louis 2013, Saunders.)

c. Prepare the groin area with antiseptic soap and shave per institutional procedure and as prescribed.
d. Monitor baseline vital signs and peripheral pulses.
e. Reinforce instructions to the client that chest pain may occur during balloon inflation and to report it if it does occur.

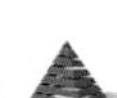

3. Postprocedure interventions
a. Monitor vital signs closely.
b. Check distal pulses in both extremities.
c. Maintain bed rest as prescribed, keeping the limb straight for 6 to 8 hours.
d. Administer anticoagulants such as IV heparin and antiplatelet agents as prescribed to prevent thrombus formation.
e. Intravenous nitroglycerin may be prescribed to prevent coronary artery vasospasm.
f. Encourage fluids if not contraindicated to enhance renal excretion of dye.
g. Reinforce instructions to the client in the administration of nitrates, calcium channel blockers, antiplatelet agents, and anticoagulants as prescribed.
h. Reinforce instructions to the client to take acetylsalicylic acid (aspirin) daily permanently if prescribed.
i. Assist the client with planning lifestyle modifications.

B. Laser-assisted angioplasty
1. Description
a. A laser probe is advanced through a cannula similar to that used for PTCA.
b. Laser-assisted angioplasty is also used for clients with small occlusions in the distal superficial femoral, proximal popliteal, and common iliac arteries, and in the coronary arteries.
c. Heat from the laser vaporizes the plaque to open the occluded artery.
2. Preprocedure and postprocedure interventions
a. Care is similar to that for PTCA.
b. Monitor for complications of coronary dissection, acute occlusion, perforation, embolism, and myocardial infarction.

C. Coronary artery stents 
1. Description
a. Coronary artery stents (usually bare metal or drug-eluting) are used in conjunction with PTCA to provide a supportive scaffold to eliminate the risk of acute coronary vessel closure and improve long-term patency of the vessel.
b. A balloon catheter bearing the stent is inserted into the coronary artery and positioned at the site of occlusion. Balloon inflation deploys the stent.
c. When placed in the coronary artery, the stent reopens the blocked artery.
2. Preprocedure and postprocedure interventions
a. Care is similar to that for PTCA.
b. Acute thrombosis is a major concern following the procedure, and the client is placed on antiplatelet therapy such as clopidogrel (Plavix) and acetylsalicylic acid (aspirin) for several months after the procedure. Length of time of antiplatelet therapy is determined by the type of stent that has been deployed.
c. Monitor for complications of the procedure such as stent migration or occlusion, coronary artery dissection, and bleeding resulting from anticoagulation.

D. Atherectomy
1. Description
a. Atherectomy removes plaque from a coronary artery by the use of a cutting chamber on the inserted catheter or a rotating blade that pulverizes the plaque.

b. Atherectomy is also used to improve blood flow to ischemic limbs in individuals with peripheral arterial disease.
2. Preprocedure and postprocedure interventions
a. Care is similar to that for PTCA.
b. Monitor for complications of perforation, embolus, and reocclusion.

E. Transmyocardial revascularization
1. May be used for clients with widespread atherosclerosis involving vessels that are too small and numerous for replacement or balloon catheterization. The procedure is performed through a small chest incision.
2. Transmyocardial revascularization uses a high-powered laser that creates 20 to 24 channels through the ventricular muscle of the left ventricle, and blood enters these small channels, providing the affected region of the heart with oxygenated blood.
3. The opening on the surface of the heart heals; however, the main channels remain and perfuse the myocardium.

F. Peripheral arterial revascularization
1. Description
a. Performed to increase arterial blood flow to the affected limb
b. Inflow procedures involve bypassing the arterial occlusion above the superficial femoral arteries.
c. Outflow procedures involve bypassing the arterial occlusions at or below the superficial femoral arteries.
d. Graft material is sutured above and below the occlusion to facilitate blood flow around the occlusion.
2. Preoperative interventions
a. Monitor baseline vital signs and peripheral pulses.
b. Insert an IV line and urinary catheter as prescribed.
c. Maintain a central venous catheter and/or arterial line if inserted.

3. Postoperative interventions
a. Monitor vital signs.
b. Monitor the BP and notify the HCP if changes occur.
c. Monitor for hypotension, which may indicate hypovolemia.
d. Monitor for hypertension, which may place stress on the graft and facilitate clot formation.
e. Maintain bed rest for 24 hours as prescribed.
f. Instruct the client to keep the affected extremity straight, limit movement, and avoid bending the knee and hip.
g. Monitor for warmth, redness, and edema, which are often expected outcomes because of increased blood flow.
h. Monitor for graft occlusion, which often occurs within the first 24 hours.
i. Monitor peripheral pulses and for adverse changes in color and temperature of the extremity.
j. Encourage coughing and deep breathing and the use of incentive spirometry.
k. Maintain NPO status, with progression to clear liquids as prescribed.
l. Use strict aseptic technique when in contact with the incision.
m. Monitor the incision for drainage, warmth, or swelling.
n. Monitor for excessive bleeding. (A small amount of bloody drainage is expected.)
o. Monitor the area over the graft for hardness, tenderness, and warmth, which may indicate infection. If this occurs, notify the HCP immediately.
p. Reinforce instructions to the client about proper foot care and measures to prevent ulcer formation.
q. Reinforce instructions to the client to take medications as prescribed.
r. Reinforce instructions to the client on how to care for the incision.
s. Assist the client in modifying lifestyle (such as diet) to prevent further plaque formation.

After arterial vascularization, monitor for a sharp increase in pain because pain is frequently the first indicator of postoperative graft occlusion. If signs of graft occlusion occur, notify the HCP immediately.

G. Coronary artery bypass grafting
1. Description
a. The occluded coronary arteries are bypassed with the client's own **venous** or arterial blood vessels.
b. The saphenous vein, internal mammary artery, or other arteries may be used to bypass lesions in the coronary arteries.
c. Coronary artery bypass grafting is performed when the client does not respond to medical management of coronary artery disease or when vessels are severely occluded.
2. Preoperative interventions
a. Familiarize the client and family with the cardiac surgical critical care unit.
b. Inform the client to expect a sternal incision, possible arm or leg incision(s), one or two chest tubes, a Foley catheter, and several IV fluid catheters.
c. Inform the client that an endotracheal tube will be in place and that he or she will be unable to speak.

   d. Advise the client that he or she will be on mechanical ventilation and to breathe with the ventilator and not fight it.
   e. Reinforce instructions to the client to inform the nurse of any postoperative pain because pain medication will be available.
   f. Reinforce instructions to the client on how to splint the chest incision, cough and deep breathe, use the incentive spirometer, and perform arm and leg exercises.
   g. Encourage the client and family to discuss anxieties and fears related to surgery.
   h. Note that prescribed medications may be discontinued preoperatively (usually diuretics 2 to 3 days before surgery, digoxin 12 hours before surgery, and aspirin and anticoagulants 1 week before surgery).
   i. Administer medications as prescribed, which may include potassium chloride, antihypertensives, antidysrhythmics, and antibiotics.
3. Transfer from the cardiac surgical unit
   a. Monitor vital signs, level of consciousness, and peripheral perfusion. (Alarm safety and alarm fatigue: Refer to Chapter 49.)
   b. Monitor for dysrhythmias.
   c. Auscultate lungs and monitor respiratory status.
   d. Encourage the client to splint the incision, cough and deep breathe, and use the incentive spirometer to raise secretions and prevent atelectasis.
   e. Monitor temperature and white blood cell count, which indicate infection if elevated after 3 to 4 days.
   f. Provide adequate fluids and hydration as prescribed to liquefy secretions.
   g. Monitor suture line and chest tube insertion sites for redness, purulent discharge, and signs of infection.
   h. Monitor sternal suture line for instability, which may indicate an infection.
   i. Guide the client to gradually resume activity.
   j. Monitor the client for tachycardia, **postural (orthostatic) hypotension**, and fatigue before, during, and after activity.
   k. Discontinue activities if the BP drops more than 10 to 20 mm Hg or the pulse increases more than 10 beats/min.
   l. Monitor episodes of pain closely.
   m. See Box 51-1 for home care instructions.

H. Heart transplant
1. A donor heart from an individual with a comparable body weight and ABO compatibility is transplanted into a recipient within 6 hours of procurement.
2. The surgeon removes the diseased heart, leaving the posterior portion of the atria to serve as an anchor for the new heart.

BOX 51-1 Home Care Instructions After Cardiac Surgery

Progressively return to activities at home.
Limit pushing or pulling activities for 6 weeks after discharge.
Maintain incisional care, and record signs of redness, swelling, or drainage.
Sternotomy incision heals in about 6 to 8 weeks.
Avoid crossing legs. Wear elastic hose if prescribed until edema subsides, and elevate surgical limb when sitting in a chair.
Follow prescribed medications as instructed by the HCP.
Follow prescribed dietary measures such as avoiding saturated fat, cholesterol, and salt.
Sexual intercourse can be resumed on the advice of the HCP after exercise tolerance is assessed. If prescribed, if the client can walk one block or climb two flights of stairs without symptoms, he or she can resume sexual activity safely.

3. Because a remnant of the client's atria remains, two unrelated P waves are noted on the electrocardiogram.
4. The transplanted heart is denervated and unresponsive to vagal stimulation. Because the heart is denervated, clients do not experience angina.
5. Symptoms of heart rejection include hypotension, dysrhythmias, weakness, fatigue, and dizziness.
6. Endomyocardial biopsies are performed at regular scheduled intervals and whenever rejection is suspected.
7. The client requires lifetime immunosuppressive therapy.
8. Strict aseptic technique and vigilant hand washing must be maintained when caring for the posttransplant client because of increased risk for infection from immunosuppression.
9. The heart rate approximates 100 beats/min and responds slowly to exercise or stress with regard to increases in heart rate, contractility, and cardiac output.

IV. Cardiac Dysrhythmias

A. Normal sinus rhythm (Fig. 51-2)

1. Rhythm originates from the sinoatrial node.
2. Atrial and ventricular rhythms are regular at 60 to 100 beats/min.

B. Sinus bradycardia

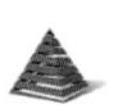

1. Atrial and ventricular rates are regular and are less than 60 beats/min.
2. Note that a low heart rate may be normal for some individuals.
3. Treatment may be necessary if the client is symptomatic (signs of decreased cardiac output).
4. Treatment depends on the cause and may include holding a medication, oxygen, atropine sulfate, or a pacemaker; notify the registered nurse (RN).

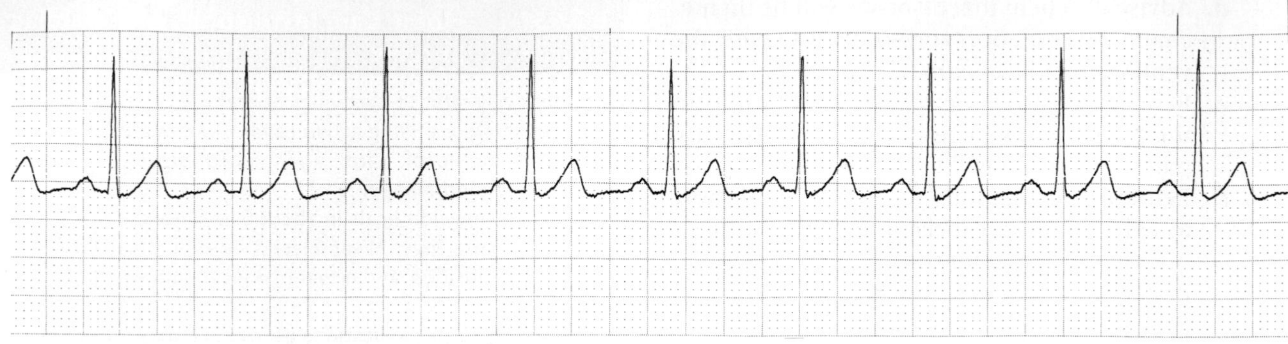

FIGURE 51-2 Normal sinus rhythm. (From Ignatavicius D, Workman ML: *Medical-surgical nursing: Patient-centered collaborative care,* ed 7, St. Louis, 2013, Saunders.)

BOX 51-2 Premature Ventricular Contractions (PVCs)

Bigeminy: PVC every other heartbeat
Trigeminy: PVC every third heartbeat
Quadrigeminy: PVC every fourth heartbeat
Couplet or pair: Two sequential PVCs
Unifocal: Uniform upward or downward deflection, arising from the same ectopic focus
Multifocal: Different shapes, with the impulse generation from different sites
R-on-T phenomenon: PVC falls on the T wave of the preceding beat and may precipitate ventricular fibrillation

C. Sinus tachycardia
   1. Atrial and ventricular rhythms are regular.
   2. Atrial and ventricular rates are 100 to 180 beats/min.
   3. Treatment depends on the cause; notify the registered nurse (RN).

D. Atrial fibrillation
   1. Multiple rapid impulses from many foci depolarize in the atria in a totally disorganized manner at a rate of 350 to 600 times per minute; the atria quiver, which can lead to the formation of thrombi.
   2. Usually no definitive P wave can be observed—only fibrillatory waves before each QRS.
   3. Treatment includes oxygen, anticoagulants, cardiac medications, and possible cardioversion. Notify the RN.

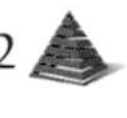

E. Premature ventricular contractions (PVCs) (Box 51-2 and Fig. 51-3)
   1. Early ventricular complexes result from increased irritability of the ventricles.
   2. Treatment depends on the cause, and the RN is notified if PVCs occur.

For the client experiencing PVCs, notify the HCP if the client complains of chest pain or if the PVCs increase in frequency, are multifocal, occur on the T wave (R on T), or occur in runs of ventricular tachycardia.

F. Ventricular tachycardia (VT) (Fig. 51-4)
   1. VT occurs because of a repetitive firing of an irritable ventricular ectopic focus at a rate of 140 to 250 beats/min or more and can lead to cardiac arrest. Notify the RN if VT occurs.
   2. A stable client with sustained VT (with pulse and no signs or symptoms of decreased cardiac output) will be treated with oxygen and antidysrhythmics.
   3. An unstable client with VT (with pulse and signs and symptoms of decreased cardiac output) will be treated with oxygen and antidysrhythmics

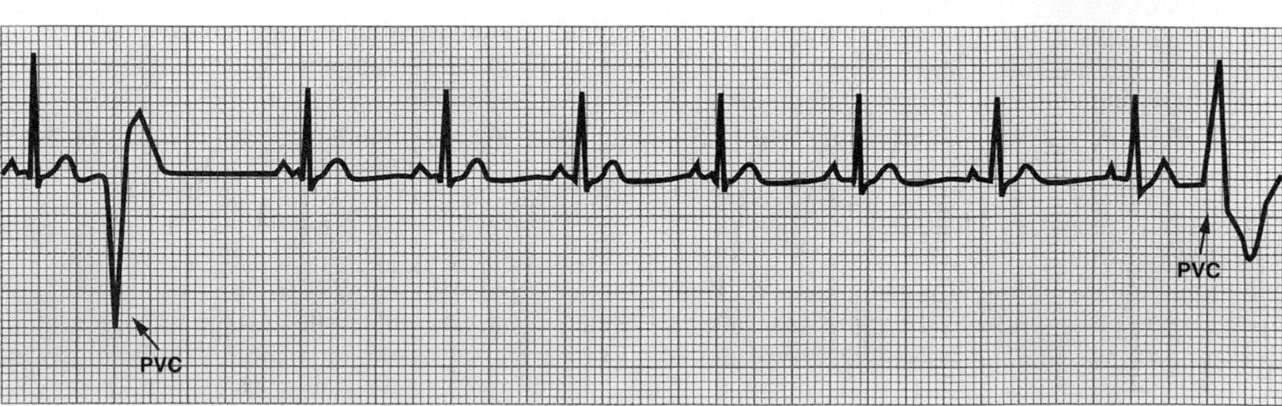

FIGURE 51-3 Normal sinus rhythm with multifocal premature ventricular contractions (one negative and the other positive). (From Ignatavicius D, Workman ML: *Medical-surgical nursing: Patient-centered collaborative care,* ed 7, St. Louis, 2013, Saunders.)

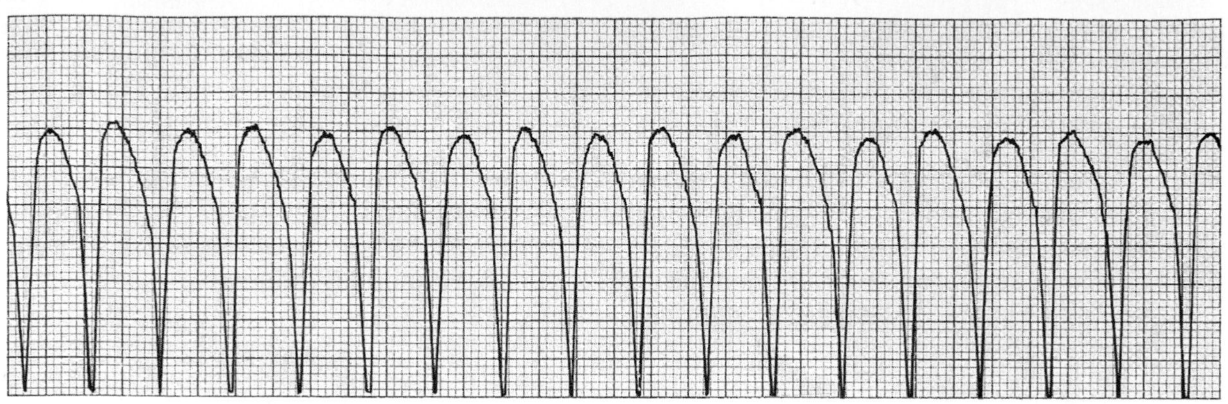

FIGURE 51-4 Ventricular tachycardia. (From Ignatavicius D, Workman ML: *Medical-surgical nursing: Patient-centered collaborative care*, ed 7, St. Louis, 2013, Saunders.)

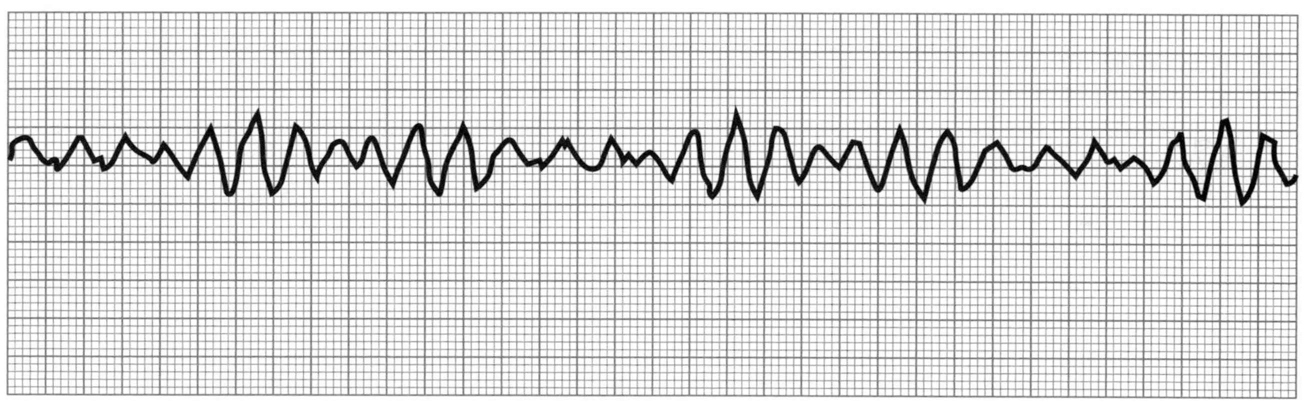

FIGURE 51-5 Ventricular fibrillation. (From Ignatavicius D, Workman ML: *Medical-surgical nursing: Patient-centered collaborative care*, ed 7, St. Louis, 2013, Saunders.)

and possible synchronized cardioversion. The HCP may attempt cough cardiopulmonary resuscitation (CPR) by asking the client to cough hard every 1 to 3 seconds.

4. A pulseless client with VT will be treated with defibrillation and CPR.

G. Ventricular fibrillation (VF) (Fig. 51-5)
   1. Ventricular fibrillation is a chaotic rapid rhythm in which the ventricles quiver and there is no cardiac output.
   2. Client lacks a pulse, BP, respirations, and heart sounds, and VF is fatal if not successfully terminated within 3 to 5 minutes
   3. Treatment includes CPR and immediate defibrillation.

V. Management of Dysrhythmias

A. Vagal maneuvers
   1. Description: Vagal maneuvers induce vagal stimulation of the cardiac conduction system and are used to terminate supraventricular tachydysrhythmias.
   2. Carotid sinus massage
      a. The HCP instructs the client to turn the head away from the side to be massaged.
      b. The HCP massages over one carotid artery for a few seconds to determine if a change in cardiac rhythm occurs.
      c. The client should be on a cardiac monitor, and an electrocardiogram rhythm strip before, during, and after the procedure should be obtained and documented on the chart.
      d. Have a defibrillator and resuscitative equipment available.
      e. Monitor vital signs, cardiac rhythm, and level of consciousness after the procedure.
   3. Valsalva's maneuver
      a. The HCP instructs the client to bear down or induces a gag reflex in the client to stimulate a vagal response.
      b. Monitor the heart rate, rhythm, and BP.
      c. Observe the cardiac monitor for a change in rhythm.
      d. Record an electrocardiographic rhythm strip before, during, and after the procedure.
      e. Provide an emesis basin if the gag reflex is stimulated, and initiate precautions to prevent aspiration.
      f. Have a defibrillator and resuscitative equipment available.

B. Cardioversion

1. Description

a. Cardioversion is synchronized countershock to convert an undesirable rhythm to a stable rhythm.

b. Cardioversion can be an elective procedure performed by the HCP for stable tachydysrhythmias resistant to medical therapies or an emergent procedure for hemodynamically unstable ventricular or supraventricular tachydysrhythmias.

c. A lower amount of energy is used than with defibrillation.

d. Defibrillator is synchronized to the client's R wave to avoid discharging the shock during the vulnerable period (T wave).

e. If the defibrillator were not synchronized, it could discharge on the T wave and cause VF.

2. Preprocedure interventions

a. Obtain an informed consent if it is an elective procedure.

b. Administer sedation as prescribed.

c. If it is an elective procedure, hold digoxin (Lanoxin) 48 hours preprocedure as prescribed to prevent postcardioversion ventricular irritability.

d. If it is an elective procedure for atrial fibrillation or atrial flutter, the client should receive anticoagulant therapy for 4 to 6 weeks preprocedure and a transesophageal echocardiogram (TEE) should be performed to rule out clots in the atria prior to the procedure.

3. During the procedure

a. Ensure that the skin is clean and dry in the area where the electrode paddles/hands off pads will be placed.

b. Stop the oxygen during the procedure to avoid the hazard of fire.

c. Be sure that no one is touching the bed or the client when delivering the countershock.

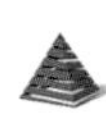
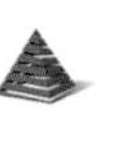

4. Postprocedure interventions

a. Priority data collection includes the ability of the client to maintain airway and breathing.

b. Resume oxygen administration as prescribed.

c. Monitor the vital signs.

d. Monitor the level of consciousness.

e. Monitor the cardiac rhythm.

f. Monitor for indications of successful response such as conversion to sinus rhythm, strong peripheral pulses, an adequate BP, and adequate urine output.

g. Check the skin on the chest for evidence of burns from the edges of the paddles/pads.

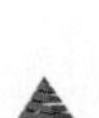

C. Defibrillation

1. Defibrillation is an asynchronous countershock used to terminate pulseless VT or VF.

2. The defibrillator is charged to 120 to 200 joules (biphasic) or 360 joules (monophasic) for one countershock from the defibrillator, and then CPR is immediately resumed and continued for 5 cycles or about 2 minutes.

3. The rhythm is rechecked after 2 minutes, and if VF or pulseless VT continues, the defibrillator is charged to give a second shock, and the life support protocol is continued.

Before defibrillating a client, be sure that the oxygen is shut off to avoid the hazard of fire and be sure that no one is touching the bed or the client.

D. Use of paddle electrodes

1. Apply conductive pads.

2. One paddle is placed at the third intercostal space to the right of the sternum; the other is placed at the fifth intercostal space on the left midaxillary line.

3. Apply firm pressure of at least 25 lb to each of the paddles.

4. Be sure that no one is touching the bed or the client when delivering the countershock.

5. Pads for hands-off biphasic defibrillation may be applied in an anterior-posterior position or apex-posterior position, and placement directly over breast tissue should be avoided.

E. Automatic external defibrillator

1. An automatic external defibrillator is used by laypersons and emergency medical technicians for prehospital cardiac arrest.

2. Place the client on a firm, dry surface.

3. Stop CPR.

4. Ensure that no one is touching the client to avoid motion artifact during rhythm analysis.

5. Place the electrode patches in the correct position on the client's chest.

6. Press the analyzer button to identify the rhythm, which may take 30 seconds. The machine will advise whether a shock is necessary.

7. Shocks are recommended for pulseless VT or VF only.

F. Implantable cardioverter defibrillator (ICD)

1. Description

a. An ICD monitors cardiac rhythm and detects and terminates episodes of VT and VF.

b. The ICD senses VT or VF and delivers 25 to 30 J up to four times if necessary.

c. An ICD is used in clients with episodes of spontaneous sustained VT or VF unrelated to an MI or in clients whose medication therapy has been unsuccessful in controlling life-threatening dysrhythmias.

d. Transvenous electrode leads are placed in the right atrium and ventricle in contact with the endocardium. Leads are used for sensing, pacing, and delivery of cardioversion or defibrillation.

e. The generator is most commonly implanted in the left pectoral region.

2. Reinforce client education
   a. Instruct the client in the basic functions of the ICD.
   b. Know the rate cutoff of the ICD and the number of consecutive shocks that it will deliver.
   c. Wear loose-fitting clothing over the ICD generator site.
   d. Avoid contact sports to prevent trauma to the ICD generator and lead wires.
   e. Report any fever, redness, swelling, or drainage from the insertion site.
   f. Report symptoms of fainting, nausea, weakness, blackouts, and rapid pulse rates to the HCP.
   g. During shock discharge, the client may feel faint or short of breath.
   h. Instruct the client to sit or lie down if he or she feels a shock and to notify the HCP.
   i. Advise the client to maintain a log of the date, time, and activity preceding the shock, the symptoms preceding the shock, and post-shock sensations.
   j. Instruct the client and family in how to access the emergency medical system.
   k. Encourage the family to learn CPR.
   l. Instruct the client to avoid electromagnetic fields directly over the ICD because they can inactivate the device.
   m. Instruct the client to move away from a magnetic field immediately if beeping tones are heard, and notify the HCP.
   n. Keep an ICD identification card in the wallet and obtain and wear a Medic-Alert bracelet.
   o. Inform all HCPs that an ICD has been inserted. Certain diagnostic tests, such as an MRI, and procedures using diathermy or electrocautery interfere with ICD function.
   p. Advise the client of restrictions on activities such as driving and operating dangerous equipment.

VI. Pacemakers

A. Description: a temporary or permanent device that provides electrical stimulation and maintains the heart rate when the client's intrinsic pacemaker fails to provide a perfusing rhythm

B. Settings
   1. A synchronous (demand) pacemaker senses the client's rhythm and paces only if the client's intrinsic rate falls below the set pacemaker rate to stimulate depolarization.
   2. An asynchronous (fixed rate) pacemaker paces at a preset rate regardless of the client's intrinsic rhythm and is used when the client is asystolic or profoundly bradycardic.
   3. Overdrive pacing suppresses the underlying rhythm in tachydysrhythmias so that the sinus node will regain control of the heart.

C. Spikes
   1. When a pacing stimulus is delivered to the heart, a spike (straight vertical line) is seen on the monitor or electrocardiogram strip.
   2. Spikes precede the chamber being paced. A spike preceding a P wave indicates that the atrium is being paced, and a spike preceding the QRS indicates the ventricle is being paced.
   3. An atrial spike followed by a P wave indicates atrial depolarization, and a ventricular spike followed by a QRS represents ventricular depolarization. This is referred to as "capture."
   4. If the electrode is in the atrium, the spike is before the P wave; if the electrode is in the ventricle, the spike is before the QRS complex.

D. Temporary pacemakers
   1. Noninvasive transcutaneous pacing
      a. Noninvasive transcutaneous pacing is used as a temporary emergency measure in the profoundly bradycardic or asystolic client until invasive pacing can be initiated.
      b. Large electrode pads are placed on the client's chest and back and connected to an external pulse generator.
      c. Wash the skin with soap and water before applying electrodes.
      d. It is not necessary to shave the hair or apply alcohol or tinctures to the skin.
      e. Place the posterior electrode between the spine and left scapula, behind the heart, avoiding placement over bone.
      f. Place the anterior electrode between the V_2 and V_5 positions over the heart.
      g. Do not place the anterior electrode over female breast tissue; rather, displace breast tissue and place under the breast.
      h. Do not take the pulse or BP on the left side. The results will not be accurate because of the muscle twitching and electrical current.
      i. Ensure that electrodes are in good contact with the skin.
      j. If loss of "capture" occurs, check the skin contact of the electrodes and increase the current until "capture" is regained.
      k. Evaluate the client for discomfort from cutaneous and muscle stimulation. Administer analgesics as needed.
   2. Invasive transvenous pacing
      a. Pacing lead wire is placed through the antecubital, femoral, jugular, or subclavian vein into the right atrium or right ventricle so that it is in direct contact with the endocardium.
      b. Monitor cardiac rhythm continuously.
      c. Monitor vital signs.

d. Monitor the pacemaker insertion site.
e. Restrict client movement to prevent lead wire displacement.

3. Invasive epicardial pacing: Applied by using a transthoracic approach. The lead wires are threaded loosely on the epicardial surface of the heart after cardiac surgery.
4. Reducing the risk of microshock
   a. Use only inspected and approved equipment.
   b. Insulate the exposed portion of wires with plastic or rubber material (fingers of rubber gloves) when wires are not attached to the pulse generator, and cover with nonconductive tape.
   c. Ground all electrical equipment using a three-pronged plug.
   d. Wear gloves when handling exposed wires.
   e. Keep dressings dry.

E. Permanent pacemakers
1. The pulse generator is internal and surgically implanted in a subcutaneous pocket below the clavicle.
2. The leads are passed transvenously via the cephalic or subclavian vein to the endocardium on the right side of the heart. Postoperatively, limitation of arm movement on the operative side is required to prevent lead wire dislodgement.
3. Permanent pacemakers may be single chambered, in which the lead wire is placed in the chamber to be paced, or dual chambered, with lead wires placed in both the right atrium and ventricle.
4. A permanent pacemaker is programmed when inserted and can be reprogrammed if necessary by noninvasive transmission from an external programmer to the implanted generator.
5. Pacemakers are powered by a lithium battery that has an average life span of 10 years, are nuclear powered with a life span of 20 years or longer, or are designed to be recharged externally.
6. Pacemaker function can be checked in the HCP's office or clinic by a pacemaker interrogator or programmer or from home using telephone transmitter devices.
7. The client may be provided with a device that is placed over the pacemaker battery generator with an attachment to the telephone. The heart rate then can be transmitted to the clinic.
8. Reinforce client teaching as per Box 51-3.

Box 51-3 Pacemakers: Client Education

Instruct the client about the pacemaker, including the programmed rate.
Instruct the client on the signs of battery failure and when to notify the HCP.
Instruct the client to report any fever, redness, swelling, or drainage from the insertion site.
Report signs of dizziness, weakness or fatigue, swelling of the ankles or legs, chest pain, or shortness of breath.
Keep a pacemaker identification card in the wallet, and obtain and wear a Medic-Alert bracelet.
Instruct the client on how to take the pulse, to take the pulse daily, and to maintain a diary of pulse rates.
Wear loose-fitting clothing over the pulse generator site.
Avoid contact sports.
Inform all HCPs that a pacemaker has been inserted.
Instruct the client to inform airport security that he or she has a pacemaker because the pacemaker may set off the security detector.
Instruct the client that most electrical appliances can be used without any interference with the functioning of the pacemaker; however, advise the client not to operate electrical appliances directly over the pacemaker site.
Avoid transmitter towers and antitheft devices in stores.
Instruct the client that if any unusual feelings occur when near any electrical devices to move 5 to 10 feet away and check the pulse.
Instruct the client about the methods of monitoring the function of the device.
Emphasize the importance of follow-up with the HCP.
Use cell phones on the side opposite to the pacemaker.

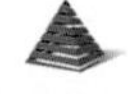

VII. Coronary Artery Disease

A. Description
1. Coronary artery disease is a narrowing or obstruction of one or more coronary arteries as a result of atherosclerosis, an accumulation of lipid-containing plaque in the arteries (Fig. 51-6).
2. The disease causes decreased perfusion of myocardial tissue and inadequate myocardial oxygen supply, leading to hypertension, angina, dysrhythmias, MI, heart failure, and death.
3. **Collateral circulation,** more than one artery supplying a muscle with blood, is normally present in the coronary arteries, especially in older persons.
4. The development of collateral circulation takes time and develops when chronic ischemia occurs to meet the metabolic demands. Therefore, an occlusion of a coronary artery in a younger individual is more likely to be lethal than in an older individual.
5. Symptoms occur when the coronary artery is occluded to the point that inadequate blood supply to the muscle occurs, causing ischemia.
6. Coronary artery narrowing is significant if the lumen diameter of the left main artery is reduced at least 50%, or any major branch is reduced at least 75%.
7. The goal of treatment is to alter the atherosclerotic progression.

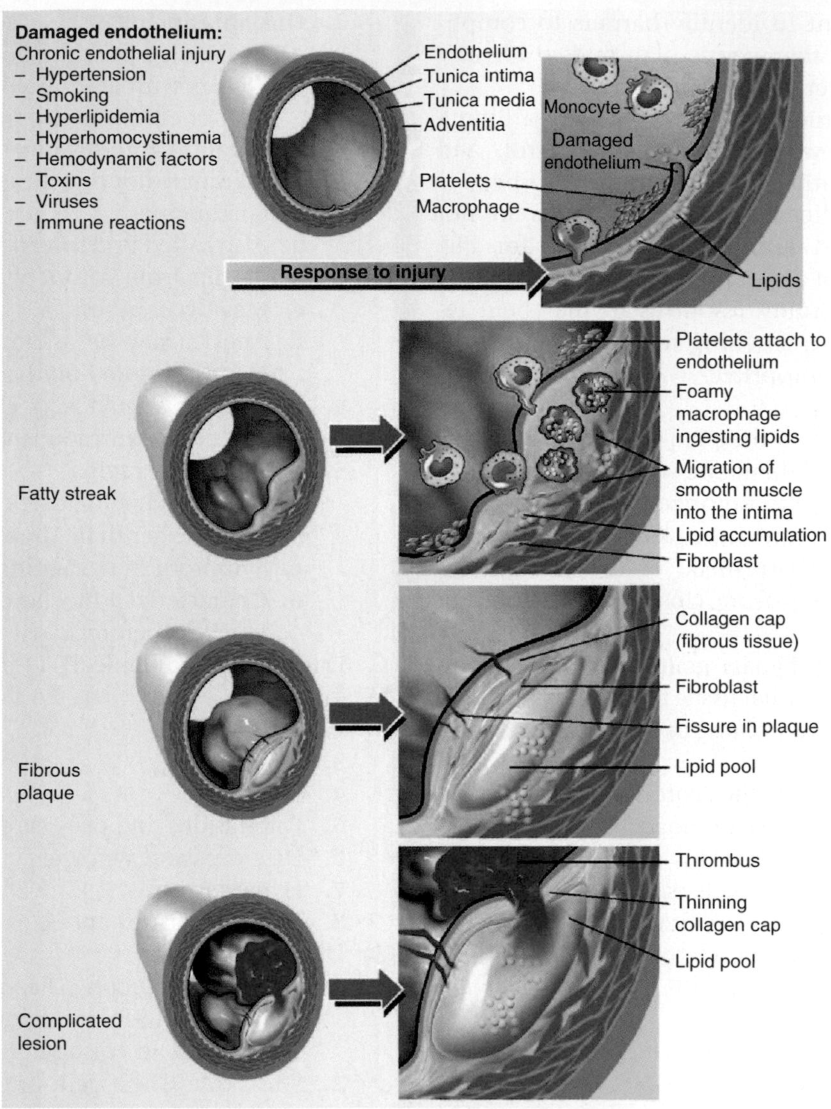

FIGURE 51-6 Cross section of an atherosclerotic coronary artery. (From Ignatavicius D, Workman ML: *Medical-surgical nursing: Patient-centered collaborative care*, ed 7, St. Louis, 2013, Saunders.)

B. Data collection
   1. Possibly normal findings during asymptomatic periods
   2. Chest pain
   3. Palpitations
   4. Dyspnea
   5. Syncope
   6. Cough or hemoptysis
   7. Excessive fatigue

C. Diagnostic studies
   1. Electrocardiography
      a. When blood flow is reduced and ischemia occurs, ST segment depression, T wave inversion, or both are noted. The ST segment returns to normal when the blood flow returns.
      b. With infarction, cell injury results in ST segment elevation, followed by T wave inversion and an abnormal Q wave.
   2. Cardiac catheterization
      a. Cardiac catheterization provides the most definitive source for diagnosis.
      b. Cardiac catheterization shows the presence of atherosclerotic lesions.
   3. Blood lipid levels
      a. Blood lipid levels may be elevated.
      b. Cholesterol-lowering medications may be prescribed to reduce the development of atherosclerotic plaques.

D. Interventions
   1. Reinforce instructions to the client regarding the purpose of diagnostic medical and surgical procedures and the preprocedure and postprocedure expectations.
   2. Assist the client to identify risk factors that can be modified.
   3. Assist the client to set goals to promote lifestyle changes that will reduce the impact of risk factors.

4. Assist the client to identify barriers to compliance with the therapeutic plan and to identify methods to overcome barriers.
5. Reinforce instructions to the client regarding a low-calorie, low-sodium, low-cholesterol, and low-fat diet, with an increase in dietary fiber.
6. Stress to the client that dietary changes are not temporary and must be maintained for life. Teach the client about prescribed medications.
7. Provide community resources to the client regarding exercise, smoking reduction, and stress reduction as appropriate.

E. Surgical procedures
1. PTCA to compress the plaque against the walls of the artery and dilate the vessel
2. Laser angioplasty to vaporize the plaque
3. Atherectomy to remove the plaque from the artery
4. Vascular stent (bare metal or drug-eluting) to prevent the artery from closing and to prevent restenosis
5. Coronary artery bypass graft to improve blood flow to the myocardial tissue that is at risk for ischemia or infarction because of the occluded artery

F. Medications
1. Nitrates to dilate the coronary arteries and decrease preload and afterload
2. Calcium channel blockers to dilate coronary arteries and reduce vasospasm
3. Cholesterol-lowering medications to reduce the development of atherosclerotic plaques
4. β-blockers to reduce the BP in individuals who are hypertensive

VIII. Angina

A. Description
1. Angina is chest pain resulting from myocardial ischemia caused by inadequate myocardial blood and oxygen supply.
2. Angina is caused by an imbalance between oxygen supply and demand.
3. Causes include obstruction of coronary blood flow because of atherosclerosis, coronary artery spasm, and conditions increasing myocardial oxygen consumption.

The goal of treatment for angina is to provide relief of the acute attack, correct the imbalance between myocardial oxygen supply and demand, and prevent the progression of the disease and further attacks to reduce the risk of MI.

B. Patterns of angina
1. Stable angina
   a. Also called exertional angina
   b. Occurs with activities that involve exertion or emotional stress and is relieved with rest or nitroglycerin
   c. Usually has a stable pattern of onset, duration, severity, and relieving factors
2. Unstable angina
   a. Also called preinfarction angina
   b. Occurs with an unpredictable degree of exertion or emotion and increases in occurrence, duration, and severity over time
   c. Pain may not be relieved with nitroglycerin.
3. Variant angina
   a. Also called Prinzmetal's or vasospastic angina
   b. Results from coronary artery spasm
   c. May occur at rest
   d. Attacks may be associated with ST segment elevation noted on the electrocardiogram.
4. Intractable angina is a chronic, incapacitating angina that is unresponsive to interventions.
5. Preinfarction angina
   a. Associated with acute coronary insufficiency
   b. Lasts longer than 15 minutes
   c. Symptom of worsening cardiac ischemia
   d. Characterized by chest pain that occurs days to weeks before an MI

C. Data collection (Table 51-1) 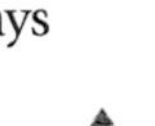
1. Pain
2. Dyspnea
3. Pallor
4. Sweating
5. Palpitations and tachycardia
6. Dizziness and syncope
7. Hypertension
8. Digestive disturbances

D. Diagnostic studies
1. Electrocardiography: Readings are normal during rest, with ST depression and/or T wave inversion during an episode of pain.
2. Stress test: Chest pain or changes in the electrocardiogram or vital signs during testing may indicate ischemia.
3. Cardiac enzymes and troponins: Findings are normal in angina.
4. Cardiac catheterization: Catheterization provides a definitive diagnosis by providing information about the patency of the coronary arteries.

TABLE 51-1 Characteristics of Pain: Angina and Myocardial Infarction

Angina	Myocardial Infarction
Can develop slowly or quickly	Occurs without cause, primarily early in the morning
Usually described as mild or moderate pain	Crushing substernal pain
Substernal, crushing, squeezing pain	May radiate to the jaw, back, and left arm
May radiate to the shoulders, arms, jaw, neck, and back	Lasts 30 minutes or longer
Usually lasts less than 5 minutes; however, can last up to 15–20 minutes	Is unrelieved by rest or nitroglycerin, and relieved only by opioids
Relieved by nitroglycerin or rest	

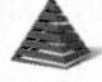

E. Interventions
1. Immediate management includes the following:
   a. Monitoring pain; instituting pain relief measures.
   b. Administering oxygen by nasal cannula as prescribed.
   c. Checking vital signs and providing continuous cardiac monitoring and nitroglycerin as prescribed to dilate the coronary arteries, reduce the oxygen requirements of the myocardium, and relieve the chest pain.
   d. Ensuring bed rest is maintained, placing the client in semi-Fowler's position, and staying with the client.
   e. Obtaining a 12-lead ECG.
   f. Establishing an IV access route.

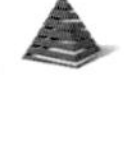

2. Establishing an IV access route.
   a. Reinforce instructions to the client regarding the purpose of diagnostic medical and surgical procedures and the preprocedure and postprocedure expectations.
   b. Assist the client to identify angina-precipitating events.
   c. Reinforce instructions to the client to stop activity and rest if chest pain occurs and to take nitroglycerin as prescribed.
   d. Reinforce instructions to the client to seek medical attention if pain persists.
   e. Reinforce instructions to the client regarding prescribed medications.
   f. Provide diet instructions to the client, stressing that dietary changes are not temporary and must be maintained for life.
   g. Assist the client to identify risk factors that can be modified.
   h. Assist the client to set goals that will promote changes in lifestyle to reduce the impact of risk factors.
   i. Assist the client to identify barriers to compliance with therapeutic plan and to identify methods to overcome barriers.
   j. Provide community resources to the client regarding exercise, smoking reduction, and stress reduction.

F. Surgical procedures: See VII. Coronary Artery Disease.

G. Medications
1. See Section VII, Coronary Artery Disease.
2. Antiplatelet therapy may be prescribed that inhibits platelet aggregation and reduces the risk of developing an acute MI.

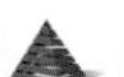

IX. Myocardial Infarction

A. Description
1. Myocardial infarction occurs when myocardial tissue is abruptly and severely deprived of oxygen.
2. Ischemia can lead to necrosis of myocardial tissue if blood flow is not restored.
3. Infarction does not occur instantly but evolves over several hours.
4. Obvious physical changes do not occur in the heart until 6 hours after the infarction, when the infarcted area appears blue and swollen.
5. After 48 hours, the infarct turns gray with yellow streaks developing as neutrophils invade the tissue.
6. By 8 to 10 days after infarction, granulation tissue forms.
7. Over 2 to 3 months, the necrotic area develops into a scar. Scar tissue permanently changes the size and shape of the entire left ventricle.
8. Not all clients experience the classic symptoms of an MI.
9. Women may experience atypical discomfort, shortness of breath, or fatigue and often present with NSTEMI (non-ST-elevation myocardial infarction) or T-wave inversion.
10. An older client may experience shortness of breath, pulmonary edema, dizziness, altered mental status, or dysrhythmia.

B. Location of MI
1. Obstruction of the left anterior descending artery results in anterior or septal MI or both.
2. Obstruction of the circumflex artery results in posterior wall MI or lateral wall MI.
3. Obstruction of the right coronary artery results in inferior wall MI.

C. Risk factors
1. Atherosclerosis
2. Coronary artery disease
3. Elevated cholesterol levels
4. Smoking
5. Hypertension
6. Obesity
7. Physical inactivity
8. Impaired glucose tolerance
9. Stress

D. Diagnostic studies
1. Troponin level
   a. Level rises within 3 hours.
   b. Level remains elevated for up to 7 to 10 days.
2. Total creatine kinase level
   a. Level rises within 6 hours after the onset of chest pain.
   b. Level peaks within 18 hours after damage and death of cardiac tissue.
3. CK-MB isoenzyme
   a. Peak elevation occurs 18 hours after the onset of chest pain.
   b. Level returns to normal 48 to 72 hours later.
4. Myoglobin: Level rises within 2 hours after cell death, with a rapid decline in the level after 7 hours.
5. White blood cell count: An elevated white blood cell count of 10,000 to 20,000 cells/mm^3 appears on the second day after the MI and lasts up to 1 week.

6. Electrocardiogram
   a. Electrocardiogram shows either ST elevation MI (STEMI), T wave inversion, or non-ST elevation MI (NSTEMI); an abnormal Q wave may also be present.
   b. Hours to days after, the MI, ST, and T wave changes will return to normal, but the Q wave usually remains permanently.
7. Diagnostic tests following the acute stage
   a. Exercise tolerance test or stress test may be prescribed to assess for electrocardiographic changes and ischemia and to evaluate for medical therapy or identify clients who may need invasive therapy.
   b. Thallium scans may be prescribed to assess for ischemia or necrotic muscle tissue.
   c. Multigated cardiac blood pool imaging scans may be used to evaluate left ventricular function.
   d. Cardiac catheterization is performed to determine the extent and location of obstructions of the coronary arteries.

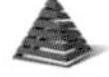

E. Data collection (see Table 51-1)
   1. Pain
   2. Nausea and vomiting
   3. Diaphoresis
   4. Dyspnea
   5. Dysrhythmias
   6. Feelings of fear and anxiety
   7. Pallor, cyanosis, and coolness of extremities

F. Complications of MI (Box 51-4)

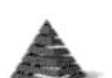

G. Interventions, acute stage

> ⚠ Pain relief increases oxygen supply to the myocardium. Morphine sulfate is administered as a priority in managing pain in the client having an MI.

1. Obtain a description of the chest discomfort.
2. Administer oxygen by nasal cannula as prescribed and institute pain relief measures (morphine, nitroglycerin as prescribed).
3. Monitor vital signs and cardiovascular status and maintain cardiac monitoring.
4. Ensure bed rest and place the client in a semi-Fowler's position to enhance comfort and tissue oxygenation; stay with the client.
5. Assist to establish an IV access route.
6. Obtain a 12-lead ECG.
7. Assist to administer antidysrhythmics as prescribed.
8. Assist to administer thrombolytic therapy, which may be prescribed within the first 6 hours of the coronary event.
9. Monitor for signs of bleeding if the client is receiving thrombolytic therapy.
10. Monitor laboratory values as prescribed.
11. Administer β-blockers as prescribed to slow the heart rate and increase myocardial perfusion while reducing the force of myocardial contraction.
12. Monitor for complications related to the MI.
13. Monitor for cardiac dysrhythmias because tachycardia and PVCs frequently occur in the first few hours after MI.
14. Monitor distal peripheral pulses and skin temperature because poor cardiac output may be identified by cool diaphoretic skin and diminished or absent pulses.
15. Monitor intake and output.
16. Monitor respiratory rate and breath sounds for signs of heart failure, as indicated by the presence of crackles or wheezes or dependent edema.
17. Monitor **blood pressure (BP)** closely after the administration of medications. If the systolic BP is lower than 100 or 25 mm Hg lower than the previous reading, lower the head of the bed and notify the HCP.
18. Provide reassurance to the client and family.

BOX 51-4 Complications of Myocardial Infarction

Dysrhythmias
Heart failure
Pulmonary edema
Cardiogenic shock
Thrombophlebitis
Pericarditis
Mitral valve insufficiency
Postinfarction angina
Ventricular rupture
Dressler's syndrome (a combination of pericarditis, pericardial effusion, and pleural effusion, which can occur several weeks to several months after a myocardial infarction)

H. Interventions following the acute episode
   1. Maintain bed rest for the first 24 to 36 hours as prescribed.
   2. Allow the client to stand to void or use a bedside commode if prescribed.
   3. Provide range-of-motion exercises to prevent thrombus formation and maintain muscle strength.
   4. Progress to dangling legs at the side of the bed or out of bed to the chair for 30 minutes three times a day as prescribed.
   5. Progress to ambulation in the client's room and to the bathroom and then in the hallway three times a day.
   6. Monitor for complications.
   7. Encourage the client to verbalize feelings regarding the MI.

I. Cardiac rehabilitation: Process of actively assisting the client with cardiac disease to achieve and maintain a vital and productive life within the limitations of the heart disease

X. Heart Failure

A. Description
1. Heart failure is the inability of the heart to maintain adequate cardiac output to meet the metabolic needs of the body because of impaired pumping ability.
2. Diminished cardiac output results in inadequate peripheral tissue perfusion.
3. Congestion of the lungs and periphery may occur. The client can develop acute pulmonary edema.

B. Classification
1. Acute heart failure occurs suddenly.
2. Chronic heart failure develops over time; however, a client with chronic heart failure can develop an acute episode.

C. Types of heart failure
1. Right ventricular failure/left ventricular failure
   a. Because the two ventricles of the heart represent two separate pumping systems, it is possible for one to fail alone for a short period.
   b. Most heart failure begins with left ventricular failure and progresses to failure of both ventricles.
   c. Acute pulmonary edema—a medical emergency—results from left ventricular failure.
   d. If pulmonary edema is not treated, death will occur from suffocation because the client literally drowns in his or her own fluids.
2. Forward failure/backward failure
   a. In forward failure, an inadequate output of the affected ventricle causes decreased perfusion to vital organs.
   b. In backward failure, blood backs up behind the affected ventricle, causing increased pressure in the atrium behind the affected ventricle.
3. Low output/high output
   a. In low-output failure, not enough cardiac output is available to meet the demands of the body.
   b. High-output failure occurs when a condition causes the heart to work harder to meet the demands of the body.
4. Systolic failure/diastolic failure
   a. Systolic failure leads to problems with contraction and the ejection of blood.
   b. Diastolic failure leads to problems with the heart relaxing and filling with blood.

D. Compensatory mechanisms
1. Compensatory mechanisms act to restore cardiac output to near-normal levels.
2. Initially these mechanisms increase cardiac output; however, they eventually have a damaging effect on pump action.
3. Compensatory mechanisms contribute to an increase in myocardial oxygen consumption; when this occurs, myocardial reserve is exhausted and clinical manifestations of heart failure develop.

TABLE 51-2 Clinical Manifestations of Right-Sided and Left-Sided Heart Failure

Right-Sided Heart Failure	Left-Sided Heart Failure
Dependent edema (legs and sacrum)	Signs of pulmonary congestion
Jugular venous distention	Dyspnea
Abdominal distention	Tachypnea
Hepatomegaly	Crackles in the lungs
Splenomegaly	Dry, hacking cough
Anorexia and nausea	Paroxysmal nocturnal dyspnea
Weight gain	Increased BP (from fluid volume excess) or decreased BP (from pump failure)
Nocturnal diuresis	
Swelling of the fingers and hands	
Increased BP (from fluid volume excess) or decreased BP (from pump failure)	

4. Compensatory mechanisms include increased heart rate, improved stroke volume, arterial vasoconstriction, sodium and water retention, and myocardial hypertrophy.

Signs of left ventricular failure are evident in the pulmonary system. Signs of right ventricular failure are evident in the systemic circulation.

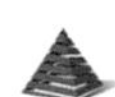

E. Data collection (Table 51-2)
1. Acute pulmonary edema
   a. Severe dyspnea and orthopnea
   b. Pallor
   c. Tachycardia
   d. Expectoration of large amounts of blood-tinged, frothy sputum
   e. Wheezing and crackles on auscultation
   f. Bubbling respirations
   g. Acute anxiety, apprehension, and restlessness
   h. Profuse sweating
   i. Cold, clammy skin
   j. Cyanosis
   k. Nasal flaring
   l. Use of accessory breathing muscles
   m. Tachypnea
   n. Hypocapnia, evidenced by muscle cramps, weakness, dizziness, and paresthesias

F. Immediate management (see Priority Nursing Actions)

G. Following the acute episode
1. Encourage the client to verbalize feelings about the lifestyle changes required as a result of the heart failure.
2. Assist the client to identify precipitating risk factors of heart failure and methods of eliminating these risk factors.
3. Reinforce instructions to the client in the prescribed medication regimen, which may include digoxin (Lanoxin), a diuretic,

PRIORITY NURSING ACTIONS!

Actions to Take If a Client Develops Pulmonary Edema

1. Place the client in a high Fowler's position.
2. Administer oxygen.
3. Check the client quickly, including checking lung sounds.
4. Ensure an intravenous access device is in place.
5. Prepare for the administration of a diuretic and morphine sulfate.
6. Insert a Foley catheter as prescribed.
7. Prepare for intubation and ventilator support, if required.
8. Document the event, actions taken, and the client's response.

Pulmonary edema is a life-threatening event that can result from severe heart failure. In pulmonary edema, the left ventricle fails to eject sufficient blood, and pressure increases in the lungs because of the accumulated blood. The nurse assists the registered nurse in implementing emergency measures. The client is immediately placed in a high Fowler's position, with the legs in a dependent position, to reduce pulmonary congestion and relieve edema. Oxygen is always prescribed, usually in high concentrations by mask or cannula to improve gas exchange and pulmonary function; the goal is to keep the oxygen saturation above 90%. The client is then checked quickly, including checking the lung sounds. Next, it is important to ensure that an IV access device is in place for the administration of a diuretic and morphine sulfate. Furosemide, a rapid-acting diuretic, will eliminate accumulated fluid. Morphine sulfate reduces venous return (preload), decreases anxiety, and also reduces the work of breathing. A Foley catheter is inserted to measure output accurately. The nurse then prepares for intubation and ventilator support, if required. The nurse stays with the client and provides reassurance. Vital signs are monitored and a cardiac monitor is used to monitor the heart rate and for dysrhythmias. The lung sounds are monitored for crackles, decreased breath sounds, and for a response to treatment. A weight measurement will also determine a response to treatment. Other interventions may include the administration of digoxin to increase ventricular contractility and improve cardiac output; bronchodilators for severe bronchospasm or bronchoconstriction; medications to facilitate myocardial contractility and enhance stroke volume; and vasodilators to reduce afterload, increase the capacity of the systemic venous bed, and decrease venous return to the heart. The nurse finally documents the event, the actions taken, and the client's response.

Reference(s): deWit, Kumagai (2013), p. 431. St. Louis: Saunders.

angiotensin-converting enzyme (ACE) inhibitors, low-dose β-blockers, and vasodilators.

4. Advise the client to notify the HCP if side effects occur from the medications.
5. Advise the client to avoid over-the-counter medications.
6. Reinforce instructions to the client to contact the HCP if he or she is unable to take medications because of illness.
7. Reinforce instructions to the client to avoid large amounts of caffeine, found in coffee, tea, cocoa, chocolate, and some carbonated beverages.
8. Reinforce instructions to the client about the prescribed low-sodium, low-fat, and low-cholesterol diet.
9. Provide the client with a list of potassium-rich foods because diuretics can cause hypokalemia (except for potassium-sparing diuretics).
10. Reinforce instructions to the client regarding fluid restriction, if prescribed, advising the client to spread the fluid out during the day and to suck on hard candy to reduce thirst.
11. Reinforce instructions to the client to balance periods of activity and rest.
12. Advise the client to avoid isometric activities, which increase pressure in the heart.
13. Reinforce instructions to the client to monitor daily weight.
14. Reinforce instructions to the client to report signs of fluid retention such as edema or weight gain.

XI. Cardiogenic Shock (see Box 51-5)

XII. Inflammatory Diseases of the Heart

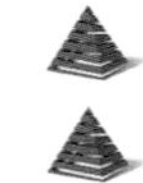

A. Pericarditis

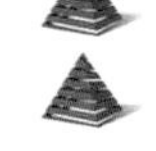

1. Description
   a. Pericarditis is an acute or chronic inflammation of the pericardium.
   b. Chronic pericarditis, a chronic inflammatory thickening of the pericardium, constricts the heart, causing compression.
   c. The pericardial sac becomes inflamed.
   d. Pericarditis can result in loss of pericardial elasticity or an accumulation of fluid within the sac.
   e. Heart failure or cardiac tamponade may result.
2. Data collection
   a. Precordial pain in the anterior chest that radiates to the left side of the neck, shoulder, or back.
   b. Pain is grating and is aggravated by breathing (particularly inspiration), coughing, and swallowing.

Box 51-5 Cardiogenic Shock

Failure of the heart to pump adequately, thereby reducing cardiac output and compromising tissue perfusion

Necrosis of more than 40% of the left ventricle, usually as a result of occlusion of major coronary vessels

Goal of treatment: to maintain tissue oxygenation and perfusion and improve the pumping ability of the heart

c. Pain is worse when in the supine position and may be relieved by leaning forward.
d. Pericardial friction rub (scratchy, high-pitched sound) heard on auscultation and produced by the rubbing of the inflamed pericardial layers
e. Fever and chills
f. Fatigue and malaise
g. Elevated white blood cell count
h. Electrocardiogram changes with acute pericarditis; ST segment elevation with the onset of inflammation; atrial fibrillation is common
i. Signs of right ventricular failure in clients with chronic constrictive pericarditis

3. Interventions
a. Determine the nature of the pain.
b. Position the client in the high Fowler's position, or upright and leaning forward.
c. Administer analgesics, nonsteroidal anti-inflammatory drugs, or corticosteroids for pain as prescribed.
d. Auscultate for a pericardial friction rub.
e. Check results of blood culture to identify causative organism.
f. Administer antibiotics for bacterial infection as prescribed.
g. Administer diuretics and digoxin (Lanoxin) as prescribed to the client with chronic constrictive pericarditis. Surgical incision of the pericardium (pericardiectomy) may be necessary.
h. Monitor for signs of cardiac tamponade, which include pulsus paradoxus, jugular vein distention with clear lung sounds, muffled heart sounds, narrowed **pulse pressure**, tachycardia, and decreased cardiac output.
i. Notify the HCP if signs of cardiac tamponade occur.

B. Myocarditis
1. Description: An acute or chronic inflammation of the myocardium as a result of pericarditis, systemic infection, or allergic response
2. Data collection
a. Fever
b. Pericardial friction rub
c. A gallop rhythm
d. A murmur that sounds like fluid passing an obstruction
e. Pulsus alternans
f. Signs of heart failure
g. Fatigue
h. Dyspnea
i. Tachycardia
j. Chest pain
3. Interventions
a. Assist the client to a position of comfort such as sitting up and leaning forward.
b. Administer analgesics, salicylates, and nonsteroidal anti-inflammatory drugs as prescribed to reduce fever and pain.
c. Administer oxygen as prescribed.
d. Provide adequate rest periods.
e. Limit activities to avoid overexertion and to decrease the workload of the heart.
f. Administer digoxin (Lanoxin) as prescribed, and monitor for signs of digoxin toxicity.
g. Administer antidysrhythmics as prescribed.
h. Administer antibiotics as prescribed to treat the causative organism.
i. Monitor for complications, which can include thrombus, heart failure, or cardiomyopathy.

C. Endocarditis
1. Description
a. Endocarditis is an inflammation of the inner lining of the heart and valves.
b. Occurs primarily in clients who are IV drug abusers, have had valve replacements, or have mitral valve prolapse or other structural defects.
c. Ports of entry for the infecting organism include the oral cavity (especially if the client had a dental procedure in the previous 3 to 6 months), infections (cutaneous, genitourinary, gastrointestinal, and systemic) and surgery or invasive procedures, including IV line placement.
2. Data collection
a. Fever
b. Anorexia
c. Weight loss
d. Fatigue
e. Cardiac murmurs
f. Heart failure
g. Embolic complications from vegetation fragments traveling through the circulation
h. Petechiae
i. Splinter hemorrhages in the nail beds
j. Osler's nodes (reddish tender lesions) on the pads of the fingers, hands, and toes
k. Janeway lesions (nontender hemorrhagic lesions) on the fingers, toes, nose, or ear lobes
l. Splenomegaly
m. Clubbing of the fingers
3. Interventions
a. Provide adequate rest balanced with activity to prevent thrombus formation.
b. Maintain antiembolism stockings.
c. Monitor cardiovascular status.
d. Monitor for signs of heart failure.
e. Monitor for signs of emboli.
f. Monitor for splenic emboli, as evidenced by sudden abdominal pain radiating to the left shoulder, and the presence of rebound abdominal tenderness on palpation.

g. Monitor for renal emboli, as evidenced by flank pain radiating to the groin, hematuria, and pyuria.
h. Monitor for confusion, aphasia, or dysphasia, which may indicate central nervous system emboli.
i. Monitor for pulmonary emboli as evidenced by pleuritic chest pain, dyspnea, and cough.
j. Monitor skin, mucous membranes, and conjunctiva for petechiae.
k. Monitor nail beds for splinter hemorrhages.
l. Monitor for Osler's nodes on the pads of the fingers, hands, and toes.
m. Monitor for Janeway lesions on the fingers, toes, nose, or earlobes.
n. Monitor for clubbing of the fingers.
o. Evaluate blood culture results.
p. Administer antibiotics intravenously as prescribed.
q. Plan and arrange for discharge, providing resources required for the continued administration of antibiotics intravenously.

4. Client education (Box 51-6)

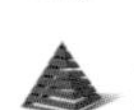

XIII. Cardiac Tamponade (see Box 51-7)

Acute cardiac tamponade can occur when small volumes (20 to 50 mL) of fluid accumulate rapidly in the pericardium.

XIV. Valvular Heart Disease

A. Description
1. Valvular heart disease occurs when the heart valves cannot fully open (stenosis) or close completely (insufficiency or regurgitation).

BOX 51-6 Home Care Instructions for the Client with Infective Endocarditis

Teach the client to maintain aseptic technique during setup and administration of IV antibiotics.
Instruct the client to administer IV antibiotics at scheduled times to maintain the blood level.
Instruct the client to monitor IV catheter sites for signs of infection and report immediately to the HCP.
Instruct the client to record his or her temperature daily for up to 6 weeks and report fever.
Encourage oral hygiene at least twice a day with a soft toothbrush and rinse well with water after brushing.
Client should avoid use of oral irrigation devices and flossing to avoid bacteremia.
Teach the client to thoroughly cleanse any skin lacerations thoroughly and apply an antibiotic ointment as prescribed.
Client should inform all HCPs of a history of endocarditis and request prophylactic antibiotics prior to every invasive procedure, including dental procedures.
Teach the client to observe for signs and symptoms of embolic phenomena and heart failure.

BOX 51-7 Cardiac Tamponade

A pericardial effusion occurs when the space between the parietal and visceral layers of the pericardium fills with fluid.
Pericardial effusion places the client at risk for cardiac tamponade, an accumulation of fluid in the pericardial cavity.
Tamponade restricts ventricular filling, and cardiac output drops. Distant, muffled heart sounds are heard.
Acute tamponade occurs when a small volume (20 to 50 mL) of fluid accumulates quickly in the pericardium.

2. Valvular heart disease prevents efficient blood flow through the heart.

B. Types
1. Mitral stenosis: Valvular tissue thickens and narrows the valve opening, preventing blood flow from the left atrium to left ventricle.
2. Mitral insufficiency/regurgitation: The valve is incompetent, preventing complete valve closure during **systole**.
3. Mitral valve prolapse: Valve leaflets protrude into the left atrium during systole.
4. Aortic stenosis: Valvular tissue thickens and narrows the valve opening, preventing blood flow from the left ventricle into the aorta.
5. Aortic insufficiency: Valve is incompetent, preventing complete valve closure during **diastole**.
6. For aortic disorders see Table 51-3.
7. For tricuspid disorders see Table 51-4.
8. For pulmonary valve disorders see Table 51-5.

C. Repair procedures
1. Balloon valvuloplasty
a. Balloon valvuloplasty is an invasive, nonsurgical procedure.
b. A balloon catheter is passed from the femoral vein through the atrial septum to the mitral valve or through the femoral artery to the aortic valve.
c. The balloon is inflated to enlarge the orifice.

TABLE 51-3 Aortic Valve Disorders

Symptoms	
Aortic Stenosis	**Aortic Insufficiency**
Dyspnea on exertion	Dyspnea
Angina	Angina
Syncope on exertion	Tachycardia
Fatigue	Fatigue
Orthopnea	Orthopnea
Paroxysmal nocturnal dyspnea	Paroxysmal nocturnal dyspnea
Harsh systolic crescendo-decrescendo murmur	Blowing decrescendo diastolic murmur
Interventions	
Refer to section on repair procedures	
Prepare the client for valve replacement as indicated	

TABLE 51-4 Tricuspid Valve Disorders

Symptoms	
Tricuspid Stenosis	**Tricuspid Insufficiency**
Easily fatigued Effort intolerance Complaints of fluttering sensations in the neck (obstructed venous flow) Cyanosis Signs of right ventricular failure including ascites, hepatomegaly, peripheral edema, jugular vein distention with clear lung fields Symptoms of decreased cardiac output Rumbling diastolic murmur	Asymptomatic in mild situations Signs of right ventricular failure including ascites, hepatomegaly, peripheral edema Pleural effusion Systolic murmur heard at the left sternal border, fourth intercostal space
Interventions Refer to section on repair procedures Prepare the client for valve replacement as indicated	

TABLE 51-5 Pulmonary Valve Disorders

Symptoms	
Pulmonary Stenosis	**Pulmonary Insufficiency**
Asymptomatic in a mild condition Dyspnea Fatigue Syncope Signs of right ventricular failure including ascites, hepatomegaly, peripheral edema Systolic thrill heard at left sternal border	Asymptomatic in mild condition Dyspnea Fatigue Syncope Signs of right ventricular failure including ascites, hepatomegaly, peripheral edema Systolic thrill heard at the left sternal border
Interventions Refer to section on repair procedures Prepare the client for pulmonary valve commissurotomy as indicated	Refer to section on repair procedures Prepare the client for valve replacement as indicated

 d. Institute precautions for arterial puncture if appropriate.
 e. Monitor for bleeding from the catheter insertion site.
 f. Monitor for signs of systemic emboli.
 g. Monitor for signs of a regurgitant valve by monitoring cardiac rhythm, heart sounds, and cardiac output.
2. Mitral annuloplasty: Tightening and suturing the malfunctioning valve annulus to eliminate or greatly reduce regurgitation
3. Commissurotomy/valvotomy
 a. The procedure is accomplished with cardiopulmonary bypass during open heart surgery.
 b. The valve is visualized, thrombi are removed from the atria, fused leaflets are incised, and calcium is débrided from the leaflets, thus widening the orifice.

D. Valve replacement procedures
1. Mechanical prosthetic valves: These prosthetic valves are durable.

⚠ Thromboembolism is a problem after valve replacement with a mechanical prosthetic valve, and lifetime anticoagulant therapy is required.

2. Bioprosthetic valves
 a. Biological grafts are xenografts (valves from other species): porcine valves (pig), bovine valves (cow), or homografts (human cadavers).
 b. The risk of clot formation is small; therefore, long-term anticoagulation is not indicated.
3. Preoperative interventions: Consult with the HCP regarding discontinuing anticoagulants 72 hours before surgery.
4. Postoperative interventions 
 a. Monitor closely for signs of bleeding.
 b. Monitor cardiac output and for signs of heart failure.
 c. Administer digoxin (Lanoxin) as prescribed to maintain cardiac output and prevent atrial fibrillation.
 d. Reinforce client teaching (Box 51-8). 

BOX 51-8 Client Instructions After Valve Replacement

Adequate rest is important, and fatigue is common.
Anticoagulant therapy is necessary if a mechanical prosthetic valve was inserted.
Instruct the client concerning hazards related to anticoagulant therapy and to notify the HCP if bleeding or excessive bruising occurs.
Instruct the client concerning the importance of good oral hygiene to reduce the risk of infective endocarditis.
Brush teeth twice daily with a soft toothbrush, followed by oral rinses.
Avoid irrigation devices, electric toothbrushes, and flossing because these activities can cause the gums to bleed, allowing bacteria to enter the mucous membranes and bloodstream.
Monitor incision and report any drainage or redness.
Avoid any dental procedures for 6 months.
Heavy lifting (greater than 10 lb) is to be avoided, and be cautious when in an automobile to prevent injury to the sternal incision.
If a prosthetic valve was inserted, a soft audible clicking sound may be heard.
Instruct the client concerning the importance of prophylactic antibiotics before any invasive procedure and the importance of informing all HCPs of the valvular disease history.
Obtain and wear a Medic-Alert bracelet.

XV. Cardiomyopathy

A. Cardiomyopathy is a subacute or chronic disorder of the heart muscle.

B. Treatment is palliative, not curative, and the client needs to deal with numerous lifestyle changes and a shortened life span.

C. Types, signs and symptoms, and treatment: Refer to Table 51-6.

XVI. Vascular Disorders

A. Venous thrombosis

1. Description

a. Thrombus can be associated with an inflammatory process.

b. When a thrombus develops, inflammation occurs, thickening the vein wall and leading to embolization.

2. Types

a. Thrombophlebitis: A thrombus associated with inflammation

b. Phlebothrombosis: A thrombus without inflammation

c. Phlebitis: Vein inflammation associated with invasive procedures such as IV lines

d. Deep vein thrombophlebitis: More serious than a superficial thrombophlebitis because of the risk for pulmonary embolism

3. Risk factors for thrombus formation

a. Venous stasis from varicose veins, heart failure, and immobility

b. Hypercoagulability disorders

c. Injury to the venous wall from IV injections; administration of vessel irritants (chemotherapy, hypertonic solutions)

TABLE 51-6 Pathophysiology, Signs and Symptoms, and Treatment of Cardiomyopathies

	Hypertrophic Cardiomyopathy		
Dilated Cardiomyopathy	**Nonobstructed**	**Obstructed**	**Restrictive Cardiomyopathy**
Pathophysiology			
Fibrosis of myocardium and endocardium Dilated chambers Mural wall thrombi prevalent	Hypertrophy of the walls Hypertrophied septum Relatively small chamber size	Same as for nonobstructed, except for obstruction of left ventricular outflow tract associated with the hypertrophied septum and mitral valve incompetence	Mimics constrictive pericarditis Fibrosed walls cannot expand or contract Chambers narrowed; emboli common
Signs and Symptoms			
Fatigue and weakness Heart failure (left side) Dysrhythmias or heart block Systemic or pulmonary emboli S$_3$ and S$_4$ gallops Moderate to severe cardiomegaly	Dyspnea Angina Fatigue, syncope, palpitations Mild cardiomegaly S$_4$ gallop Ventricular dysrhythmias Sudden death common Heart failure	Same as for nonobstructed except with mitral regurgitation murmur Atrial fibrillation	Dyspnea and fatigue Heart failure (right-sided) Mild to moderate cardiomegaly S$_3$ and S$_4$ gallops Heart block Emboli
Treatment			
Symptomatic treatment of heart failure Vasodilators Control of dysrhythmias Surgery: heart transplant	For both: Symptomatic treatment β-Blockers Conversion of atrial fibrillation Surgery: ventriculomyotomy or muscle resection with mitral valve replacement Digoxin, nitrates, and other vasodilators contraindicated with the obstructed form		Supportive treatment of symptoms Treatment of hypertension Conversion from dysrhythmias Exercise restrictions Emergency treatment of acute pulmonary edema

From Ignatavicius D, Workman ML: *Medical-surgical nursing: Patient-centered collaborative care*, ed 7, St. Louis, 2013, Saunders.

d. Following surgery, particularly orthopedic and abdominal surgery
e. Pregnancy
f. Ulcerative colitis
g. Use of oral contraceptives
h. Certain malignancies
i. Fractures or other injuries of the pelvis or lower extremities

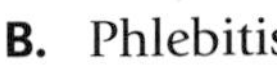

B. Phlebitis
1. Data collection
a. Red, warm area radiating up the vein of an extremity
b. Pain and soreness
c. Swelling
2. Interventions
a. Apply warm, moist soaks as prescribed to dilate the vein and promote circulation (check temperature of soak before applying).
b. Monitor for signs of complications such as tissue necrosis, infection, or pulmonary embolus.

C. Deep vein thrombophlebitis
1. Data collection
a. Calf or groin tenderness or pain with or without swelling
b. Positive Homans' sign may be noted; however, false-positive results are common so this is not a reliable measure.
c. Warm skin that is tender to touch

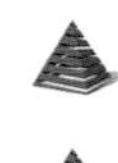

2. Interventions
a. Provide bed rest as prescribed.
b. Elevate the affected extremity above the level of the heart as prescribed.

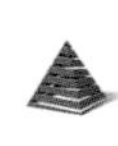

c. Avoid using the knee gatch or a pillow under the knees.
d. Do not massage the extremity.
e. Support stockings may be prescribed (although their use is controversial) to reduce venous stasis and to assist in the venous return of blood to the heart.
f. Administer intermittent or continuous warm, moist compresses as prescribed.
g. Palpate the site gently, monitoring for warmth and edema.
h. Measure and record the circumferences of the thighs and calves.
i. Monitor for shortness of breath and chest pain, which can indicate pulmonary emboli.
j. Administer thrombolytic therapy (tissue plasminogen activator) if prescribed, which must be initiated within 5 days after the onset of symptoms.
k. Administer heparin therapy as prescribed to prevent enlargement of the existing clot and prevent the formation of new clots.
l. Monitor activated partial thromboplastin time during heparin therapy.
m. Administer warfarin (Coumadin) as prescribed following heparin therapy when the symptoms of deep vein thrombophlebitis have resolved.
n. Monitor prothrombin time and international normalized ratio during warfarin (Coumadin) therapy.
o. Monitor for the hazards and side effects associated with anticoagulant therapy.
p. Administer analgesics as prescribed to reduce pain.
q. Administer diuretics as prescribed to reduce lower extremity edema.
r. Reinforce client teaching (Box 51-9).

D. Venous insufficiency
1. Description
a. Venous insufficiency results from prolonged venous hypertension, which stretches the veins and damages the valves.
b. The resultant edema and venous stasis cause venous stasis ulcers, swelling, and cellulitis.
c. Treatment focuses on decreasing edema and promoting venous return from the affected extremity.
d. Treatment for venous stasis ulcers focuses on healing the ulcer and preventing stasis and ulcer recurrence.
2. Data collection
a. Stasis dermatitis or brown discoloration along the ankles and extending up to the calf
b. Edema
c. Ulcer formation: Edges are uneven, ulcer bed is pink, and granulation is present.

BOX 51-9 Instructions for the Client with Deep Vein Thrombophlebitis

Instruct the client concerning the hazards of anticoagulation therapy.
Recognize the signs and symptoms of bleeding.
Avoid prolonged sitting or standing, constrictive clothing, or crossing legs when seated.
Elevate the legs for 10 to 20 minutes every few hours each day.
Plan a progressive walking program.
Inspect the legs for edema, and measure the circumference of the legs.
Wear antiembolism stockings if they are prescribed.
Avoid smoking.
Avoid any medications unless prescribed by the HCP.
Instruct the client concerning the importance of follow-up HCP visits and laboratory studies.
Obtain and wear a Medic-Alert bracelet.

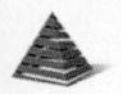

3. Interventions

For venous insufficiency, leg elevation is usually prescribed to assist with the return of the blood to the heart.

   a. Reinforce instructions to the client to avoid prolonged sitting or standing, constrictive clothing, or crossing legs when seated.
   b. Reinforce instructions to the client to elevate the legs for 10 to 20 minutes every few hours each day.
   c. Reinforce instructions to the client to elevate legs above the level of the heart when in bed.
   d. Reinforce instructions to the client in the use of an intermittent sequential pneumatic compression system, if prescribed. Instruct the ambulatory client to apply the compression system twice daily for 1 hour in the morning and evening.
   e. Advise the client with an open ulcer that the compression system is applied over a dressing.

4. Wound care
   a. Provide care to the wound as prescribed by the HCP.
   b. Monitor the client's ability to care for the wound, and initiate home care resources as necessary.
   c. If an Unna boot (a dressing constructed of gauze moistened with zinc oxide) is prescribed, the HCP will change it weekly.
   d. The wound is cleansed with normal saline before application of the Unna boot. Povidone-iodine (Betadine) and hydrogen peroxide are not used because they destroy granulation tissue.
   e. The Unna boot is covered with an elastic wrap that hardens to promote venous return and prevent stasis.
   f. Monitor for signs of arterial occlusion from an Unna boot that may be too tight.
   g. Keep tape off the client's skin.
   h. Occlusive dressings such as polyethylene film or hydrocolloid dressings may be used to cover the ulcer.

5. Medications
   a. Apply topical agents to the wound as prescribed to débride the ulcer, eliminate necrotic tissue, and promote healing.
   b. When applying topical agents, apply an oil-based agent such as petroleum jelly (Vaseline) on surrounding skin, because débriding agents can injure healthy tissue.
   c. Administer antibiotics as prescribed if infection or cellulitis occurs.

E. Varicose veins

1. Description
   a. Distended, protruding veins that appear darkened and tortuous are evident.
   b. Vein walls weaken and dilate, and valves become incompetent.

2. Data collection
   a. Pain in the legs with dull aching after standing
   b. A feeling of fullness in the legs
   c. Ankle edema

3. Trendelenburg's test
   a. Place the client in a supine position with the legs elevated.
   b. When the client sits up, if varicosities are present, veins fill from the proximal end. Veins normally fill from the distal end.

4. Interventions
   a. Assist with Trendelenburg's test.
   b. Reinforce instructions to the client to elevate the legs as much as possible.
   c. Reinforce instructions to the client to avoid constrictive clothing and pressure on the legs.
   d. Prepare the client for sclerotherapy or vein stripping as prescribed.

5. Sclerotherapy
   a. A solution is injected into the vein, followed by the application of a pressure dressing.
   b. An incision and drainage of the trapped blood in the sclerosed vein are performed 14 to 21 days after the injection, followed by the application of a pressure dressing for 12 to 18 hours.

6. Vein stripping
   a. Varicose veins are removed if they are larger than 4 mm in diameter or are in clusters; other treatments are usually tried before vein stripping.
   b. Preoperatively assist the HCP with vein marking.
   c. Evaluate pulses as a baseline for comparison postoperatively.
   d. Maintain elastic (Ace) bandages on the client's legs postoperatively.
   e. Monitor the groin and leg for bleeding through the elastic bandages.
   f. Monitor the extremity for edema, warmth, color, and pulses.
   g. Check for paresthesias, which could include saphenous nerve damage.
   h. Elevate the legs above the level of the heart postoperatively.
   i. Encourage range-of-motion exercises of the legs.
   j. Reinforce instructions to the client to avoid leg dangling or chair sitting.
   k. Reinforce instructions to the client to elevate the legs when sitting.

XVII. Arterial Disorders

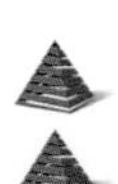

A. Peripheral arterial disease

1. Description
   a. A chronic disorder in which partial or total arterial occlusion deprives the lower extremities of oxygen and nutrients

b. Tissue damage occurs below the level of the arterial occlusion.
c. Atherosclerosis is the most common cause of peripheral arterial disease.

2. Data collection
   a. Intermittent claudication (pain in the muscles resulting from an inadequate blood supply)
   b. Rest pain, characterized by numbness, burning, or aching in the distal portion of the lower extremities, which awakens the client at night and is relieved by placing the extremity in a dependent position
   c. Lower back or buttock discomfort
   d. Loss of hair and dry, scaly skin on the lower extremities
   e. Thickened toenails
   f. Cold and gray-blue skin in the lower extremities
   g. Elevational pallor and dependent rubor in the lower extremities

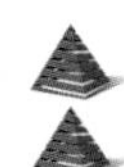

   h. Decreased or absent peripheral pulses
   i. Signs of arterial ulcer formation occurring on or between the toes or on the upper aspect of the foot that are characterized as painful
   j. BP measurements at the thigh, calf, and ankle are lower than the brachial pressure. (Normally BP readings in the thigh and calf are higher than those in the upper extremities.)
3. Interventions

Because swelling in the extremities prevents arterial blood flow, the client with peripheral arterial disease is instructed to elevate the feet at rest but to refrain from elevating them above the level of the heart because extreme elevation slows arterial blood flow to the feet. In severe cases of peripheral arterial disease, clients with edema may sleep with the affected limb hanging from the bed, or they may sit upright (without leg elevation) in a chair for comfort.

   a. Monitor pain.
   b. Monitor the extremities for color, motion and sensation, and pulses.
   c. Obtain BP measurements.
   d. Monitor for signs of ulcer formation or signs of gangrene.
   e. Assist in developing an individualized exercise program, which is initiated gradually and slowly increased.
   f. Encourage prescribed exercise, which will improve arterial flow through the development of collateral circulation.
   g. Reinforce instructions to the client to walk to the point of claudication, stop and rest, and then walk a little farther.
   h. Reinforce instructions to the client with peripheral arterial disease to avoid crossing the legs, which interferes with blood flow.
   i. Reinforce instructions to the client to avoid exposure to cold (causes vasoconstriction) to the extremities and to wear socks or insulated shoes for warmth at all times.
   j. Reinforce instructions to the client never to apply direct heat to the limb, such as with a heating pad or hot water, because the decreased sensitivity in the limb will cause burning.
   k. Reinforce instructions to the client to inspect the skin on the extremities daily and report any signs of skin breakdown.
   l. Reinforce instructions to the client to avoid tobacco and caffeine because of their vasoconstrictive effects.
   m. Reinforce instructions to the client in the use of hemorheologic and antiplatelet medications as prescribed.
   n. Inform the client of the importance of taking all medications prescribed by the HCP.
4. Procedures to improve arterial blood flow
   a. Percutaneous transluminal angioplasty with or without intravascular stent
   b. Laser-assisted angioplasty
   c. Atherectomy
   d. Bypass surgery: Inflow procedures bypass the occlusion above the superficial femoral arteries and include aortoiliac, aortofemoral, and axillofemoral bypasses. Outflow procedures bypass the occlusion at or below the superficial femoral arteries and include femoropopliteal and femorotibial bypasses.

B. Raynaud's disease
1. Description
   a. Raynaud's disease is vasospasm of the arterioles and arteries of the upper and lower extremities.
   b. Vasospasm causes constriction of the cutaneous vessels.
   c. Attacks are intermittent and occur with exposure to cold or stress.
   d. Primarily affects fingers, toes, ears, and cheeks
2. Data collection
   a. Blanching of the extremity, followed by cyanosis during vasoconstriction
   b. Reddened tissue when the vasospasm is relieved
   c. Numbness, tingling, swelling, and a cold temperature at the affected body part
3. Interventions
   a. Monitor pulses.
   b. Administer vasodilators as prescribed.
   c. Reinforce instructions to the client regarding medication therapy.

d. Assist the client to identify and avoid precipitating factors such as cold and stress.
e. Reinforce instructions to the client to avoid smoking.
f. Reinforce instructions to the client to wear warm clothing, socks, and gloves in cold weather.
g. Advise the client to avoid injuries to fingers and hands.

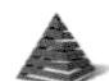
C. Buerger's disease (thromboangiitis obliterans)
1. Description
a. Buerger's disease is an occlusive disease of the median and small arteries and veins.
b. The distal upper and lower limbs are affected most commonly.
2. Data collection
a. Intermittent claudication
b. Ischemic pain occurring in the digits while at rest
c. Aching pain that is more severe at night
d. Cool, numb, or tingling sensation
e. Diminished pulses in the distal extremities
f. Extremities that are cool and red in the dependent position
g. Development of ulcerations in the extremities
3. Interventions
a. Reinforce instructions to the client to stop smoking.
b. Monitor pulses.
c. Reinforce instructions to the client to avoid injury to the upper and lower extremities.
d. Administer vasodilators as prescribed.
e. Reinforce instructions to the client regarding medication therapy.

XVIII. Aortic Aneurysms

A. Description
1. An aortic aneurysm is an abnormal dilation of the arterial wall caused by localized weakness and stretching in the medial layer or wall of the aorta.
2. The aneurysm can be located anywhere along the abdominal aorta.
3. The goal of treatment is to limit the progression of the disease by modifying risk factors, controlling the BP to prevent strain on the aneurysm, recognizing symptoms early, and preventing rupture.

B. Types of aortic aneurysm
1. Fusiform: Diffuse dilation that involves the entire circumference of the arterial segment
2. Saccular: Distinct localized outpouching of the artery wall
3. Dissecting: Created when blood separates the layers of the artery wall, forming a cavity between them
4. False (pseudoaneurysm)
a. Pseudoaneurysm occurs when the clot and connective tissue are outside the arterial wall.
b. Pseudoaneurysm occurs as a result of vessel injury or trauma to all three layers of the arterial wall.

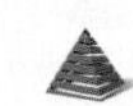
C. Data collection
1. Thoracic aneurysm
a. Pain extending to neck, shoulders, lower back, or abdomen
b. Syncope
c. Dyspnea
d. Increased pulse
e. Cyanosis
f. Weakness
g. Hoarseness/difficulty swallowing because of pressure from the aneurysm
2. Abdominal aneurysm
a. Prominent, pulsating mass in the abdomen, at or above the umbilicus
b. Systolic bruit over the aorta
c. Tenderness on deep palpation
d. Abdominal or lower back pain
3. Rupturing aneurysm
a. Severe abdominal or back pain
b. Lumbar pain radiating to the flank and groin
c. Hypotension
d. Increased pulse rate
e. Signs of shock
f. Hematoma at flank area
4. Diagnostic tests
a. Diagnostic tests are done to confirm the presence, size, and location of the aneurysm.
b. Tests include abdominal ultrasound, computed tomography scan, and arteriography.
5. Interventions
a. Monitor vital signs.
b. Check risk factors for the arterial disease process.
c. Obtain information regarding back or abdominal pain.
d. Question the client regarding the sensation of pulsation in the abdomen.
e. Inspect the skin for the presence of vascular disease or breakdown.
f. Check peripheral circulation, including pulses, temperature, and color.
g. Observe for signs of rupture.
h. Note any tenderness over the abdomen.
i. Monitor for abdominal distention.
6. Nonsurgical interventions
a. Modify the risk factors.
b. Reinforce instructions to the client regarding the procedure for monitoring BP.
c. Reinforce instructions to the client on the importance of regular HCP visits to follow the size of the aneurysm.
d. Reinforce instructions to the client to notify the HCP immediately if any of the following

occur: severe back or abdominal pain or fullness, soreness over the umbilicus, sudden development of discoloration in the extremities, or a persistent elevation of BP.

Instruct the client with an aortic aneurysm to report immediately the occurrence of chest or back pain, shortness of breath, difficulty swallowing, or hoarseness.

D. Pharmacological interventions
 1. Administer antihypertensives to maintain the BP within normal limits and prevent strain on the aneurysm.
 2. Reinforce instructions to the client on the purpose of the medications.
 3. Reinforce instructions to the client about the side effects and schedule of the medications.

E. Abdominal aortic aneurysm resection
 1. Description: Surgical resection or excision of the aneurysm. The excised section is replaced with a graft that is sewn end to end.
 2. Preoperative interventions
  a. Check all peripheral pulses as a baseline for postoperative comparison.
  b. Instruct the client on coughing and deep-breathing exercises.
  c. Administer bowel preparation as prescribed.
 3. Postoperative interventions
  a. Monitor the vital signs.
  b. Monitor peripheral pulses distal to the graft site.
  c. Monitor for signs of graft occlusion, including changes in pulses, cool to cold extremities below the graft, white or blue extremities or flanks, severe pain, or abdominal distention.
  d. Limit elevation of the head of the bed to 45 degrees to prevent flexion of the graft.
  e. Monitor for hypovolemia and kidney failure resulting from significant blood loss during surgery.
  f. Monitor urine output hourly, and notify the HCP if it is less than 30 to 50 mL/hour.
  g. Monitor serum creatinine and blood urea nitrogen daily.
  h. Monitor respiratory status and auscultate breath sounds to identify respiratory complications.
  i. Encourage turning, coughing, and deep breathing, as well as splinting of the incision.
  j. Ambulate as prescribed.
  k. Maintain nasogastric tube to low suction until bowel sounds return.
  l. Monitor bowel sounds and report their return to the HCP.
  m. Monitor for pain and administer medication as prescribed.
  n. Monitor incision site for bleeding or signs of infection.
  o. Prepare the client for discharge by providing instructions regarding pain management, wound care, and activity restrictions.
  p. Reinforce instructions to the client not to lift objects heavier than 15 to 20 lb for 6 to 12 weeks.
  q. Advise the client to avoid activities requiring pushing, pulling, or straining.
  r. Reinforce instructions to the client not to drive a vehicle until approved by the HCP.

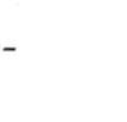

F. Thoracic aneurysm repair
 1. Description
  a. A thoracotomy or median sternotomy approach is used to enter the thoracic cavity.
  b. The aneurysm is exposed and excised, and a graft or prosthesis is sewn onto the aorta.
  c. Total cardiopulmonary bypass is necessary for excision of aneurysms in the ascending aorta.
  d. Partial cardiopulmonary bypass is used for clients with an aneurysm in the descending aorta.
 2. Postoperative interventions
  a. Monitor the vital signs, and neurological and renal status.
  b. Monitor for signs of hemorrhage, such as a drop in BP and increased pulse rate and respirations, and report to the HCP immediately.
  c. Monitor chest tubes for an increase in chest drainage, which may indicate bleeding or separation at the graft site.
  d. Monitor sensation and motion of all extremities and notify the HCP if deficits occur, which can be caused by a lack of blood supply to the spinal cord during surgery.
  e. Monitor respiratory status and auscultate breath sounds to identify respiratory complications.
  f. Encourage turning, coughing, and deep breathing while splinting the incision.
  g. Monitor cardiac status for dysrhythmias.
  h. Monitor for pain and administer medication as prescribed.
  i. Monitor the incision site for bleeding or signs of infection.
  j. Prepare the client for discharge by providing instructions regarding pain management, wound care, and activity restrictions.
  k. Reinforce instructions to the client not to lift objects heavier than 15 to 20 lb for 6 to 12 weeks.
  l. Advise the client to avoid activities requiring pushing, pulling, or straining.
  m. Reinforce instructions to the client not to drive a vehicle until approved by the HCP.

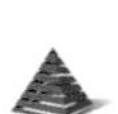

XIX. Embolectomy

A. Description
 1. Embolectomy is removal of an embolus from an artery using a catheter.
 2. A patch graft may be required to close the artery.

B. Preoperative interventions
   1. Obtain a baseline vascular assessment.
   2. Administer anticoagulants as prescribed.
   3. Administer thrombolytics as prescribed.
   4. Place a bed cradle on the bed.
   5. Avoid bumping or jarring the bed.
   6. Maintain the extremity in slightly dependent position.

C. Postoperative interventions
   1. Monitor cardiac, respiratory, and neurological status.
   2. Monitor the affected extremity for color, temperature, and pulse.
   3. Monitor sensory and motor function of the affected extremity.
   4. Monitor for signs and symptoms of new thrombi or emboli.
   5. Administer oxygen as prescribed.
   6. Monitor pulse oximetry.
   7. Monitor for complications caused by reperfusion of the artery, such as spasms and swelling of the skeletal muscles.
   8. Monitor for signs of swollen skeletal muscles such as edema, pain on passive movement, poor capillary refill, numbness, and muscle tenseness.
   9. Maintain bed rest initially, with the client in a semi-Fowler's position.
   10. Place a bed cradle on the bed.
   11. Check incision site for bleeding or hematoma.
   12. Administer anticoagulants as prescribed.
   13. Instruct the client to recognize the signs and symptoms of infection and edema.
   14. Instruct the client to avoid prolonged sitting or crossing the legs when sitting.
   15. Reinforce instructions to the client to elevate the legs when sitting.
   16. Reinforce instructions to the client to ambulate daily.
   17. Reinforce instructions to the client about anticoagulant therapy and the hazards associated with anticoagulants.

XX. Vena Caval Filter and Ligation of Inferior Vena Cava

A. Vena cava filter: Insertion of an intracaval filter (umbrella) that partially occludes the inferior vena cava and traps emboli to prevent pulmonary emboli

B. Ligation: Suturing or placing clips on the inferior vena cava to prevent pulmonary emboli; performed via abdominal laparotomy

C. Preoperative interventions: If the client has been taking an anticoagulant, consult with the HCP regarding discontinuation of the medication to prevent hemorrhage.

D. Postoperative interventions
   1. Maintain a semi-Fowler's position.
   2. Avoid hip flexion.
   3. Refer to postoperative interventions for embolectomy.

XXI. Hypertension

A. Description
   1. For an adult (aged 18 and older), a normal BP is a systolic BP below 120 mm Hg and a diastolic below 80 mm Hg.
   2. An individual classified with prehypertension has a systolic BP between 120 and 139 mm Hg or a **diastolic pressure** between 80 and 89 mm Hg.
   3. Stage 1 hypertension can be classified as a systolic BP between 140 and 159 mm Hg or a diastolic pressure between 90 and 99 mm Hg.
   4. Stage 2 hypertension can be classified as a systolic BP equal to or greater than 160 mm Hg or a diastolic pressure equal to or greater than 100 mm Hg.
   5. Hypertension is a major risk factor for coronary, cerebral, renal, and peripheral vascular disease.
   6. The disease is initially asymptomatic.
   7. The goals of treatment include reduction of the BP and preventing or lessening the extent of organ damage (Table 51-7).
   8. Nonpharmacological approaches, such as lifestyle changes, may be prescribed initially; if the BP cannot be decreased after a reasonable period (1 to 3 months), the client may require pharmacological treatment.

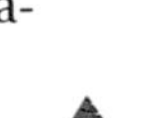
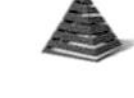

B. Primary or essential hypertension
   1. No known cause
   2. Risk factors
      a. Aging
      b. Family history
      c. African-American race
      d. Obesity
      e. Smoking
      f. Stress
      g. Excessive alcohol
      h. Hyperlipidemia
      i. Increased intake of salt or caffeine

C. Secondary hypertension
   1. Treatment depends on the cause and the organs involved.
   2. Secondary hypertension occurs as a result of other disorders or conditions.
   3. Precipitating disorders or conditions
      a. Cardiovascular disorders

TABLE 51-7 Hypertension

Organ Involvement	Complications
Eyes	Visual changes
Brain	Stroke
Cardiovascular system	Heart failure, hypertensive crisis
Kidneys	Kidney failure

b. Renal disorders
c. Endocrine system disorders
d. Pregnancy
e. Medications (such as estrogens, glucocorticoids, and mineralocorticoids)

D. Data collection
1. May be asymptomatic
2. Headache
3. Visual disturbances
4. Dizziness
5. Chest pain
6. Tinnitus
7. Flushed face
8. Epistaxis

E. Interventions
1. Goals
a. One treatment goal is to reduce the BP.
b. Another treatment goal is to prevent or lessen the extent of organ damage.
2. Question the client regarding the signs and symptoms indicative of hypertension.
3. Obtain the BP two or more times on both arms with the client supine and standing.
4. Compare the BP with prior documentation.
5. Determine family history of hypertension.
6. Identify current medication therapy.
7. Obtain weight.
8. Evaluate dietary patterns and sodium intake.
9. Monitor for visual changes or retinal damage.
10. Monitor for cardiovascular changes such as distended neck veins, increased heart rate, and dysrhythmias.
11. Evaluate chest x-ray film for heart enlargement.
12. Monitor neurological system.
13. Evaluate renal function.
14. Evaluate results of diagnostic and laboratory studies.

F. Nonpharmacological interventions
1. Weight reduction, if necessary, or maintenance of ideal weight
2. Dietary sodium restriction to 2 g daily as prescribed
3. Moderate intake of alcohol and caffeine-containing products
4. Initiation of a regular exercise program
5. Avoidance of smoking
6. Relaxation techniques and biofeedback therapy
7. Elimination of unnecessary medications that may contribute to the hypertension

G. Pharmacological interventions
1. Medication therapy is individualized for each client, and the selection of the medication is based on such factors as client's age, culture, presence of coexisting conditions, severity of hypertension, and client's preferences.
2. See Chapter 52 for medications to treat hypertension.

H. See Box 51-10 for client education reinforcement.

BOX 51-10 Client Education for Hypertension

Describe the importance of compliance with the treatment plan.
Describe the disease process, explaining that symptoms usually do not develop until organs have suffered damage.
Initiate and assist the client in planning a regular exercise program, avoiding heavy weight lifting and isometric exercises.
Emphasize the importance of beginning the exercise program gradually.
Encourage the client to express feelings about daily stress.
Assist the client to identify ways to reduce stress.
Teach relaxation techniques.
Instruct the client on how to incorporate relaxation techniques into the daily living pattern.
Instruct the client and family in the technique for monitoring blood pressure.
Instruct the client to maintain a diary of blood pressure readings.
Emphasize the importance of lifelong medication and the need for follow-up treatment.
Instruct the client and family about the dietary restrictions, which may include sodium, fat, calories, and cholesterol.
Instruct the client on how to shop for and prepare low-sodium meals.
Provide a list of products that contain sodium.
Instruct the client to read labels of products to determine sodium content, focusing on substances listed as sodium, NaCl, or MSG (monosodium glutamate).
Instruct the client to bake, roast, or boil foods. Avoid salt in preparation of foods, and avoid using salt at the table.
Instruct the client that fresh foods are best to consume and to avoid canned foods.
Instruct the client about the actions, side effects, and scheduling of medications.
Advise the client that if uncomfortable side effects occur to contact the HCP and not to stop the medication.
Instruct the client to avoid over-the-counter medications.
Stress the importance of follow-up care.

XXII. Hypertensive Crisis

A. Description
1. A hypertensive crisis is any clinical condition requiring immediate reduction in BP.
2. A hypertensive crisis is an acute and life-threatening condition.
3. The accelerated hypertension requires emergency treatment because target organ damage (brain, heart, kidneys, retina of the eye) can occur quickly.
4. Death can be caused by stroke, kidney failure, or cardiac disease.

B. Data collection
1. An extremely high BP and usually the diastolic pressure is greater than 120 mm Hg
2. Headache
3. Drowsiness and confusion

4. Blurred vision
5. Changes in neurological status
6. Tachycardia and tachypnea
7. Dyspnea
8. Cyanosis
9. Seizures

C. Interventions
1. Maintain a patent airway.
2. IV antihypertensive medications may be prescribed.
3. Monitor vital signs, checking the BP every 5 minutes.
4. Monitor for hypotension during the administration of antihypertensives. Place the client in a supine position if hypotension occurs.
5. Have emergency medications and resuscitation equipment readily available.
6. Maintain bed rest, with the head of the bed elevated at 45 degrees.
7. Monitor IV therapy, monitoring for fluid overload.
8. Monitor I&O.
9. Insert a Foley catheter as prescribed.
10. Monitor urinary output, and if oliguria or anuria occurs, notify the HCP.

CRITICAL THINKING What Should You Do?

Answer: If the client with an abdominal aortic aneurysm suddenly complains of severe back pain and shortness of breath, the nurse should suspect rupture (a surgical emergency) and should immediately contact the health care provider (HCP). The nurse should also obtain information about the back pain, stay with the client while waiting for the arrival of the HCP, monitor vital signs and neurological status, and provide support to the client. Other signs of rupture include severe abdominal pain or fullness, soreness over the umbilicus, and sudden development of discoloration in the extremities.

Reference(s): Ignatavicius, D., & Workman, M. (2013). *Medical-surgical nursing: Patient-centered collaborative care.* (7th ed., pp. 793–794). St. Louis: Saunders.

PRACTICE QUESTIONS

521. A postcardiac surgery client with a blood urea nitrogen (BUN) level of 45 mg/dL and a serum creatinine level of 2.2 mg/dL has a total 2-hour urine output of 25 mL. The nurse understands that the client is at risk for which?
1. Hypovolemia
2. Acute kidney injury
3. Glomerulonephritis
4. Urinary tract infection

522. The nurse is preparing to ambulate a postoperative client after cardiac surgery. The nurse plans to do which to enable the client to **best** tolerate the ambulation?
1. Provide the client with a walker.
2. Remove the telemetry equipment.
3. Encourage the client to cough and deep breathe.
4. Premedicate the client with an analgesic before ambulating.

523. A client is wearing a continuous cardiac monitor, which begins to alarm at the nurse's station. The nurse sees no electrocardiographic complexes on the screen. The nurse should do which **first**?
1. Call a code blue.
2. Call the health care provider.
3. Check the client status and lead placement.
4. Press the recorder button on the ECG console.

❖ **524.** The nurse in a medical unit is caring for a client with heart failure. The client suddenly develops extreme dyspnea, tachycardia, and lung crackles, and the nurse suspects pulmonary edema. The nurse immediately notifies the registered nurse and expects which interventions to be prescribed? **Select all that apply.**
- ❑ 1. Administering oxygen
- ❑ 2. Inserting a Foley catheter
- ❑ 3. Administering furosemide (Lasix)
- ❑ 4. Administering morphine sulfate intravenously
- ❑ 5. Transporting the client to the coronary care unit
- ❑ 6. Placing the client in a low Fowler's side-lying position

525. The nurse is caring for a client on a cardiac monitor who is alone in a room at the end of the hall. The client has a short burst of ventricular tachycardia (VT), followed by ventricular fibrillation (VF). The client suddenly loses consciousness. Which intervention should the nurse do **first**?
1. Go to the nurse's station quickly and call a code.
2. Run to get a defibrillator from an adjacent nursing unit.
3. Call for help and initiate cardiopulmonary resuscitation (CPR).
4. Start oxygen by cannula at 10 L/minute and lower the head of the bed.

526. The nurse is monitoring a client following cardioversion. Which observations should be of **highest priority** to the nurse?
1. Blood pressure
2. Status of airway
3. Oxygen flow rate
4. Level of consciousness

527. To use an external cardiac defibrillator on a client, which action should be performed to check the cardiac rhythm?
1. Holding the defibrillator paddles firmly against the chest
2. Applying the adhesive patch electrodes to the skin and moving away from the client
3. Connecting standard electrocardiographic electrodes to a transtelephonic monitoring device
4. Applying standard electrocardiographic monitoring leads to the client and observing the rhythm

528. The nurse is assisting in caring for the client immediately after insertion of a permanent demand pacemaker via the right subclavian vein. The nurse prevents dislodgement of the pacing catheter by implementing which intervention?
1. Limiting movement and abduction of the left arm
2. Limiting movement and abduction of the right arm
3. Assisting the client to get out of bed and ambulate with a walker
4. Having the physical therapist do active range of motion to the right arm

529. A client diagnosed with thrombophlebitis 1 day ago suddenly complains of chest pain and shortness of breath, and the client is visibly anxious. The nurse understands that a life-threatening complication of this condition is which?
1. Pneumonia
2. Pulmonary edema
3. Pulmonary embolism
4. Myocardial infarction

530. A 24-year-old man seeks medical attention for complaints of claudication in the arch of the foot. The nurse also notes superficial thrombophlebitis of the lower leg. The nurse should check the client for which **next**?
1. Smoking history
2. Recent exposure to allergens
3. History of recent insect bites
4. Familial tendency toward peripheral vascular disease

531. The nurse has reinforced instructions to the client with Raynaud's disease about self-management of the disease process. The nurse determines that the client **needs further teaching** if the client states which?
1. "Smoking cessation is very important."
2. "Moving to a warmer climate should help."
3. "Sources of caffeine should be eliminated from the diet."
4. "Taking nifedipine (Procardia) as prescribed will decrease vessel spasm."

532. A client with myocardial infarction suddenly becomes tachycardic, shows signs of air hunger, and begins coughing frothy, pink-tinged sputum. The nurse listens to breath sounds, expecting to hear which breath sounds bilaterally?
1. Rhonchi
2. Crackles
3. Wheezes
4. Diminished breath sounds

533. The nurse is collecting data on a client with a diagnosis of right-sided heart failure. The nurse should expect to note which specific characteristic of this condition?
1. Dyspnea
2. Hacking cough
3. Dependent edema
4. Crackles on lung auscultation

534. The nurse is checking the neurovascular status of a client who returned to the surgical nursing unit 4 hours ago after undergoing an aortoiliac bypass graft. The affected leg is warm, and the nurse notes redness and edema. The pedal pulse is palpable and unchanged from admission. The nurse interprets that the neurovascular status is which?
1. Moderately impaired, and the surgeon should be called
2. Normal, caused by increased blood flow through the leg
3. Slightly deteriorating, and should be monitored for another hour
4. Adequate from an arterial approach, but venous complications are arising

535. A client with a diagnosis of rapid rate atrial fibrillation asks the nurse why the health care provider is going to perform carotid massage. The nurse responds that this procedure may stimulate which?
1. Vagus nerve to slow the heart rate
2. Vagus nerve to increase the heart rate
3. Diaphragmatic nerve to slow the heart rate
4. Diaphragmatic nerve to increase the heart rate

ANSWERS

521. 2

Rationale: The client who undergoes cardiac surgery is at risk for acute kidney injury from poor perfusion, hemolysis, low cardiac output, or vasopressor medication therapy. Kidney injury is signaled by a decreased urine output and increased BUN and creatinine levels. The client may need medications to increase renal perfusion and could need peritoneal dialysis or hemodialysis.
Test-Taking Strategy: Focus on the subject, postoperative laboratory values. The question provides no evidence of any infection, so eliminate options 3 and 4 first. Noting the laboratory values in the question will assist with eliminating option 1. **Review:** laboratory values and **postcardiac surgery complications**.
Level of Cognitive Ability: Analyzing
Client Needs: Physiological Integrity
Integrated Process: Nursing Process/Data Collection
Content Area: Adult Health: Cardiovascular
Priority Concepts: Fluid and Electrolyte Balance, Perfusion
Reference(s): Lewis et al (2014), pp. 772, 1112; Pagana, Pagana (2013), p. 944.

522. 4

Rationale: The nurse should encourage regular use of pain medication for the first 48 to 72 hours after cardiac surgery, because analgesia will promote rest, decrease myocardial oxygen consumption caused by pain, and allow better participation in activities such as coughing, deep breathing, and ambulation.
Test-Taking Strategy: Focus on the subject, ambulating a client after surgery, and note the strategic word, *best*. The question asks for the *best* action of the nurse to help a client tolerate ambulation. Coughing and deep breathing will not actively help endurance, so eliminate option 3. Eliminate option 2 because removal of telemetry equipment is contraindicated unless prescribed. From the remaining options, noting that the client is postoperative will direct you to option 4. **Review: postoperative nursing care.**
Level of Cognitive Ability: Applying
Client Needs: Physiological Integrity
Integrated Process: Nursing Process/Planning
Content Area: Adult Health: Cardiovascular
Priority Concepts: Clinical Judgment, Pain
Reference(s): deWit, Kumagai (2013), p. 468.

523. 3

Rationale: Sudden loss of electrocardiographic complexes indicates ventricular asystole or possibly electrode displacement. Checking of the client and equipment is the first action by the nurse.
Test-Taking Strategy: Note the strategic word, *first*. Use the steps of the nursing process, and remember that data collection is the first step. Options 1 and 2 are incorrect because they indicate calling for assistance before collecting data. Option 4 may sound reasonable, but the electrocardiographic monitor automatically starts recording when an alarm sounds. Option 3 is the first action because you should always check the client directly before taking any action. **Review:** care of a client on a **cardiac monitor**.
Level of Cognitive Ability: Applying
Client Needs: Physiological Integrity
Integrated Process: Nursing Process/Implementation
Content Area: Adult Health: Cardiovascular
Priority Concepts: Clinical Judgment, Technology and Informatics
Reference(s): Lewis et al (2014), p. 790.

❖524. 1, 2, 3, 4

Rationale: Pulmonary edema is a life-threatening event that can result from severe heart failure. In pulmonary edema the left ventricle fails to eject sufficient blood, and pressure increases in the lungs because of the accumulated blood. Oxygen is always prescribed, and the client is placed in a high Fowler's position to ease the work of breathing. Furosemide, a rapid-acting diuretic, will eliminate accumulated fluid. A Foley catheter is inserted to accurately measure output. Intravenously administered morphine sulfate reduces venous return (preload), decreases anxiety, and reduces the work of breathing. Transporting the client to the coronary care unit is not a priority intervention. In fact, this may not be necessary at all if the client's response to treatment is successful.
Test-Taking Strategy: Focus on the subject, the client's diagnosis. Recalling the pathophysiology associated with pulmonary edema and using the ABCs—airway, breathing, and circulation—will assist in determining the priority interventions. Review: interventions for the client with **pulmonary edema**.
Level of Cognitive Ability: Analyzing
Client Needs: Physiological Integrity
Integrated Process: Nursing Process/Implementation
Content Area: Adult Health: Cardiovascular
Priority Concepts: Clinical Judgment, Gas Exchange
Reference(s): deWit, Kumagai (2013), pp. 314, 431; Cooper, Gosnell (2015), pp. 1571, 1653–1655.

525. 3

Rationale: When ventricular fibrillation occurs, the nurse remains with the client and initiates CPR until a defibrillator is available and attached to the client. Options 1, 2, and 4 are incorrect.
Test-Taking Strategy: Note the strategic word, *first*. Eliminate options 1 and 2 first because you would never leave the client alone. From the remaining options, lowering the head of the bed is appropriate (for resuscitation), but the oxygen by cannula at 10 L/minute is incorrect. Option 3 is the correct choice. Review: care of the client with **ventricular fibrillation**.
Level of Cognitive Ability: Applying
Client Needs: Physiological Integrity
Integrated Process: Nursing Process/Implementation
Content Area: Critical Care: Basic Life Support/Cardiopulmonary Resuscitation
Priority Concepts: Clinical Judgment, Gas Exchange
Reference(s): deWit, Kumagai (2013), p. 440.

526. 2

Rationale: Nursing responsibilities after cardioversion include maintenance of a patent airway, oxygen administration, assessment of vital signs and level of consciousness, and dysrhythmia detection. Airway is the priority.
Test-Taking Strategy: Focus on the strategic words, *highest priority*, and use the ABCs—airway, breathing, and circulation—to answer the question. This will direct you to the correct option. Remember, airway comes first. **Review:** care of the client after **cardioversion**.
Level of Cognitive Ability: Analyzing

Client Needs: Physiological Integrity
Integrated Process: Nursing Process/Data Collection
Content Area: Adult Health: Cardiovascular
Priority Concepts: Gas Exchange, Perfusion
Reference(s): deWit, Kumagai (2013), p. 440.

527. 2

Rationale: The nurse or rescuer puts two large adhesive patch electrodes on the client's chest in the usual defibrillator position. The nurse stops cardiopulmonary resuscitation and orders anyone near the client to move away and not touch the client. The defibrillator then analyzes the rhythm, which may take up to 30 seconds. The machine then indicates if it is necessary to defibrillate. Although automatic external defibrillation can be done transtelephonically, it is done through the use of patch electrodes (not standard electrocardiographic electrodes) that interact via telephone lines to a base station that controls any actual defibrillation. It is not necessary to hold defibrillator paddles against the client's chest with this device.
Test-Taking Strategy: If you are not familiar with this piece of equipment, look first at the word *automatic* in the name. This implies that someone is not as involved in the process as with a conventional defibrillator and thus may help you eliminate option 1. Because standard electrocardiographic monitoring leads are not used (options 3 and 4), you can eliminate these **comparable or alike**, and incorrect, options. Although automatic external defibrillation can be done transtelephonically, it is done through the use of patch electrodes. **Review:** the use of an **external cardiac defibrillator**.
Level of Cognitive Ability: Analyzing
Client Needs: Physiological Integrity
Integrated Process: Nursing Process/Implementation
Content Area: Critical Care: Basic Life Support/Cardiopulmonary Resuscitation
Priority Concepts: Clinical Judgment, Safety
Reference(s): deWit, Kumagai (2013), p. 440.

528. 2

Rationale: In the first several hours after insertion of either a permanent or temporary pacemaker, the most common complication is pacing electrode dislodgment. The nurse helps prevent this complication by limiting the client's activities.
Test-Taking Strategy: Focus on the **subject**, permanent pacemaker insertion. The question tells you that the pacemaker was inserted on the right side. Therefore, to prevent pacing electrode dislodgment, motion must be limited on that side. Options 3 and 4 involve movement of the right arm. Limiting the movement of the left arm (option 1) is of no benefit to the client. Thus option 2 is correct. **Review:** care of the client following **pacemaker insertion**.
Level of Cognitive Ability: Applying
Client Needs: Physiological Integrity
Integrated Process: Nursing Process/Implementation
Content Area: Adult Health: Cardiovascular
Priority Concepts: Caregiving, Safety
Reference(s): deWit, Kumagai (2013), p. 441; Cooper, Gosnell (2015), pp. 1550–1551.

529. 3

Rationale: Pulmonary embolism is a life-threatening complication of deep vein thrombosis and thrombophlebitis. Chest pain is the most common symptom, which is sudden in onset and may be aggravated by breathing. Other signs and symptoms include dyspnea, cough, diaphoresis, and apprehension.
Test-Taking Strategy: This question tests your ability to analyze signs and symptoms of pulmonary embolism in a client at risk. Options 2 and 4 should be eliminated because myocardial infarction and pulmonary edema are cardiac-related problems and are therefore **comparable or alike**. Eliminate option 1 because pneumonia is an infectious process. **Review:** the complications of **thrombophlebitis**.
Level of Cognitive Ability: Analyzing
Client Needs: Physiological Integrity
Integrated Process: Nursing Process/Data Collection
Content Area: Adult Health: Cardiovascular
Priority Concepts: Clotting, Gas Exchange
Reference(s): deWit, Kumagai (2013), pp. 92, 311–312.

530. 1

Rationale: The mixture of arterial and venous manifestations (claudication and phlebitis, respectively) in the young male client suggests thromboangiitis obliterans (Buerger's disease). This is a relatively uncommon disorder, characterized by inflammation and thrombosis of smaller arteries and veins. This disorder is typically found in young men who smoke. The cause is unknown but is suspected to have an autoimmune component.
Test-Taking Strategy: Focus on the **subject**, claudication and phlebitis. You can first eliminate options 2 and 3 because they would most likely cause local skin reactions. Also, note the **strategic word**, *next*. It is often better to assess a modifiable factor before a nonmodifiable one. This will direct you to the correct option. **Review:** the causes of **Buerger's disease**.
Level of Cognitive Ability: Analyzing
Client Needs: Health Promotion and Maintenance
Integrated Process: Nursing Process/Data Collection
Content Area: Adult Health: Cardiovascular
Priority Concepts: Clotting, Gas Exchange
Reference(s): deWit, Kumagai (2013), p. 385; Cooper, Gosnell (2015), pp. 1593–1595.

531. 2

Rationale: Raynaud's disease responds favorably to the elimination of nicotine and caffeine. Medications such as calcium channel blockers may inhibit vessel spasm and prevent symptoms. Avoiding exposure to cold through a variety of means is very important. However, moving to a warmer climate may not necessarily be beneficial because the symptoms could still occur with the use of air conditioning and during periods of cooler weather.
Test-Taking Strategy: Note the **strategic words**, *needs further teaching.* These words indicate a **negative event query** and the need to select the incorrect client statement. All of the options seem reasonable. However, when you analyze each of them, note that relocation is the least favorable of all the options from the viewpoints of practicality and encountering new environmental concerns. **Review:** treatment measures for Reynaud's.
Level of Cognitive Ability: Evaluating
Client Needs: Health Promotion and Maintenance
Integrated Process: Teaching and Learning

Content Area: Adult Health: Cardiovascular
Priority Concepts: Health Promotion, Stress
Reference(s): deWit, Kumagai (2013), p. 414.

532. 2
Rationale: Pulmonary edema is characterized by extreme breathlessness, dyspnea, air hunger, and production of frothy, pink-tinged sputum. Auscultation of the lungs reveals crackles. Wheezes, rhonchi, and diminished breath sounds are not associated with pulmonary edema.
Test-Taking Strategy: Focus on the subject, breath sounds in a client with pulmonary edema. Recall that fluid produces sounds that are called crackles. This will assist in eliminating the incorrect options. **Review:** the signs/symptoms found in **pulmonary edema.**
Level of Cognitive Ability: Analyzing
Client Needs: Physiological Integrity
Integrated Process: Nursing Process/Data Collection
Content Area: Adult Health: Cardiovascular
Priority Concepts: Gas Exchange, Perfusion
Reference(s): deWit, Kumagai (2013), pp. 314, 431.

533. 3
Rationale: Right-sided heart failure is characterized by signs of systemic congestion that occur as a result of right ventricular failure, fluid retention, and pressure buildup in the venous system. Edema develops in the lower legs and ascends to the thighs and abdominal wall. Other characteristics include jugular (neck vein) congestion, enlarged liver and spleen, anorexia and nausea, distended abdomen, swollen hands and fingers, polyuria at night, and weight gain. Left-sided heart failure produces pulmonary signs. These include dyspnea, crackles on lung auscultation, and a hacking cough.
Test-Taking Strategy: Focus on the subject, right-sided heart failure. Eliminate options 1, 2, and 4 because they are comparable or alike and are pulmonary signs. **Review:** the signs of **right- and left-sided heart failure.**
Level of Cognitive Ability: Analyzing
Client Needs: Physiological Integrity
Integrated Process: Nursing Process/Data Collection
Content Area: Adult Health: Cardiovascular
Priority Concepts: Clinical Judgment, Fluid and Electrolyte Balance
Reference(s): deWit, Kumagai (2013), pp. 427–428, 432.

534. 2
Rationale: An expected outcome of surgery is warmth, redness, and edema in the surgical extremity caused by increased blood flow. Options 1, 3, and 4 are incorrect.
Test-Taking Strategy: Focus on the subject, aortoiliac bypass graft. Option 1 can be eliminated because the pedal pulse is unchanged. Venous complications from immobilization caused by surgery would not be apparent within 4 hours, so eliminate option 4 next. To choose between options 2 and 3, think about the effects of sudden reperfusion in an ischemic limb. There would be redness from new blood flow and edema from the sudden change in pressure in the blood vessels. Thus option 2 is correct. **Review:** the expected findings after **aortoiliac bypass graft.**
Level of Cognitive Ability: Analyzing
Client Needs: Physiological Integrity
Integrated Process: Nursing Process/Data Collection
Content Area: Adult Health: Cardiovascular
Priority Concepts: Clinical Judgment, Perfusion
Reference(s): deWit, Kumagai (2013), p. 409.

535. 1
Rationale: Carotid sinus massage is one maneuver used for vagal stimulation to decrease a rapid heart rate and possibly terminate a tachydysrhythmia. The other maneuvers are the Valsalva maneuver of inducing the gag reflex and asking the client to strain or bear down. Medication therapy is often needed as an adjunct to keep the rate down or maintain the normal rhythm.
Test-Taking Strategy: Focus on the subject, carotid massage. Eliminate options 2 and 4 first because these options indicate increasing an already rapid rate. From the remaining options, use knowledge of anatomy and physiology. A rapid-rate dysrhythmia would need to be slowed, which is the function of the vagus nerve. The diaphragmatic nerve affects respiration. **Review:** the functions of the **vagus and diaphragmatic nerves.**
Level of Cognitive Ability: Understanding
Client Needs: Physiological Integrity
Integrated Process: Nursing Process/Implementation
Content Area: Adult Health: Cardiovascular
Priority Concepts: Clinical Judgment, Perfusion
Reference(s): Ignatavicius, Workman (2013), p. 733.

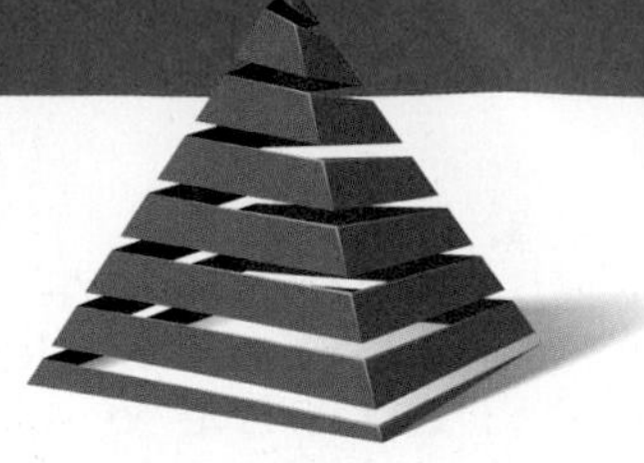

CHAPTER 52

Cardiovascular Medications

CRITICAL THINKING What Should You Do?

The nurse notes that a client taking warfarin sodium (Coumadin) has an international normalized ratio (INR) of 2.8. What should the nurse do?
Answer located on p. 716.

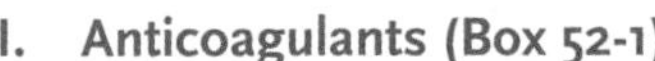

I. Anticoagulants (Box 52-1)

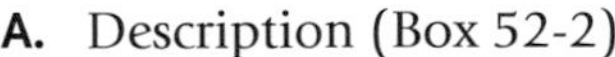

A. Description (Box 52-2)
  1. Anticoagulants prevent the extension and formation of clots by inhibiting factors in the clotting cascade and decreasing blood coagulability.
  2. Anticoagulants are administered when there is evidence or likelihood of clot formation: myocardial infarction, unstable angina, atrial fibrillation, deep vein thrombosis, pulmonary embolism, and the presence of mechanical heart valves.
  3. Anticoagulants are contraindicated with active bleeding (except for disseminated intravascular coagulation), bleeding disorders or blood dyscrasias, ulcers, liver and kidney disease, and hemorrhagic brain injuries.

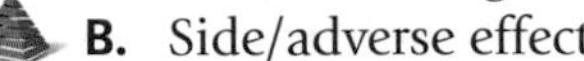

B. Side/adverse effects
  1. Hemorrhage
  2. Hematuria
  3. Epistaxis
  4. Ecchymosis
  5. Bleeding gums
  6. Thrombocytopenia
  7. Hypotension

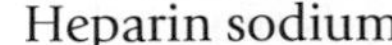

C. Heparin sodium
  1. Description
    a. Heparin prevents thrombin from converting fibrinogen to fibrin.
    b. Heparin prevents thromboembolism.
    c. The therapeutic dose does not dissolve clots but prevents new thrombus formation.

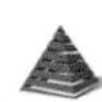

  2. Blood levels
    a. The normal activated partial thromboplastin time (aPTT) is 20 to 36 seconds in most laboratories but may be as high as 40 seconds.
    b. To maintain a therapeutic level of anticoagulation when the client is receiving a continuous infusion of heparin, the aPTT should be 1.5 to 2.5 times the normal value.
    c. Activated partial thromboplastin time therapy should be measured every 4 to 6 hours during initial continuous infusion therapy and then daily.
    d. If the aPTT is too long (longer than 80 seconds), the dosage should be lowered.
    e. If aPTT is too short (less than 60 seconds), the dosage should be increased.

BOX 52-1 Anticoagulants

Oral
Warfarin sodium (Coumadin)
Dabigatran etexilate mesylate (Pradaxa)
Rivaroxaban (Xarelto)

Parenteral
Argatroban
Bivalirudin (Angiomax)
Dalteparin (Fragmin)
Desirudin (Iprivask)
Enoxaparin (Lovenox)
Fondaparinux (Arixtra)
Heparin sodium
Lepirudin (Refludan)
Tinzaparin (Innohep)

BOX 52-2 Substances to Avoid with Anticoagulants

Allopurinol (Zyloprim)
Cimetidine (Tagamet)
Corticosteroids
Gingko and ginseng (herbs)
Green leafy vegetables and foods high in vitamin K
Nonsteroidal anti-inflammatory drugs
Oral hypoglycemic agents
Phenytoin (Dilantin)
Salicylates
Sulfonamides

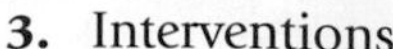

3. Interventions
   a. Monitor aPTT.
   b. Monitor platelet count.
   c. Observe for bleeding gums, bruises, nosebleeds, hematuria, hematemesis, occult blood in the stool, and petechiae.
   d. When heparin is administered subcutaneously, it is injected into the abdomen with a ⅝-inch needle (25 to 28 gauge) at a 90-degree angle; the injection site should not be aspirated or rubbed
   e. Continuous infusions must be delivered through an infusion pump and the infusion pump should be pre-programmed to ensure precise rate of delivery.
   f. Reinforce instructions to the client regarding measures to prevent bleeding.
   g. The antidote to heparin is protamine sulfate.

D. Enoxaparin (Lovenox)—low-molecular-weight heparin
1. Description: Enoxaparin has the same mechanism of action and use as heparin but is not interchangeable. It has a longer half-life than heparin.
2. Interventions
   a. Administered by subcutaneous injection only to the recumbent client in the anterolateral or posterolateral abdominal wall. Do not expel the air bubble from the prefilled syringe or aspirate during injection.
   b. Monitor the same laboratory values as for heparin and observe for bleeding.
   c. The antidote to enoxaparin is protamine sulfate.

E. Warfarin sodium (Coumadin, Jantoven)
1. Description
   a. Warfarin suppresses coagulation by acting as an antagonist of vitamin K by inhibiting four dependent clotting factors (X, IX, VII, and II).
   b. Warfarin prolongs clotting time and is monitored by the prothrombin time (PT) and the international normalized ratio (INR).
   c. It is used for long-term anticoagulation and is used mainly to prevent thromboembolic conditions such as thrombophlebitis, pulmonary embolism, and embolism formation caused by atrial fibrillation, thrombosis, myocardial infarction, or heart valve damage; it is also used in clients who have had a heart valve replaced with a mechanical heart valve.
2. Blood levels
   a. The normal PT is 9.6 to 11.8 seconds.
   b. Warfarin sodium prolongs the PT. The therapeutic range is 1.5 to 2 times the control value.
3. International normalized ratio (INR)
   a. The normal INR is 1.3 to 2.0.
   b. The INR is determined by multiplying the observed PT ratio (the ratio of the client's PT to a control PT) by a correction factor specific to a particular thromboplastin preparation used in the testing.
   c. The treatment goal is to raise the INR to an appropriate value.
   d. An INR of 2 to 3 is appropriate for most clients, although for some clients the target INR is 3 to 4.5, such as for clients with mechanical heart valves.
   e. If the INR is below the recommended range, warfarin sodium should be increased.
   f. If the INR is above the recommended range, warfarin sodium should be reduced.
4. Interventions
   a. Monitor PT and INR.
   b. Observe for bleeding gums, bruises, nosebleeds, hematuria, hematemesis, occult blood in the stool, and petechiae.
   c. Reinforce instructions to the client regarding measures to prevent bleeding.
   d. The antidote for warfarin is phytonadione (vitamin K).

F. Dabigatran etexilate (Pradaxa)
1. Description
   a. Dabigatran etexilate works through direct inhibition of thrombin, preventing the conversion of fibrinogen into fibrin and activation of factor XIII.
   b. Its only approved use is for clot prevention associated with nonvalvular atrial fibrillation.
   c. It is administered in a fixed dose twice daily.
2. Blood levels: No blood testing is required.
3. Interventions: Observe for bleeding gums, bruises, nosebleeds, hematuria, hematemesis, occult blood in the stool, and petechiae.

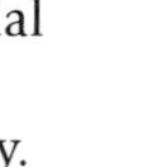

G. Rivaroxaban (Xarelto)
1. Description
   a. Rivaroxaban works through inhibition of factor Xa.
   b. Approved uses include clot prevention associated with nonvalvular atrial fibrillation and after knee and hip replacement
2. Blood levels: No blood testing is required.
3. Interventions
   a. Observe for bleeding gums, bruises, nosebleeds, hematuria, hematemesis, occult blood in the stool, and petechiae.
   b. No antidote is available.

II. Thrombolytic Medications (Box 52-3)

A. Description
1. Thrombolytic medications activate plasminogen. Plasminogen generates plasmin (the enzyme that dissolves clots).

BOX 52-3 Thrombolytic Medications

Alteplase (Activase, tPA)
Reteplase (Retavase)
Tenecteplase (TNKase)

2. Thrombolytic medications are used early in the course of myocardial infarction (within 4 to 6 hours of the onset of the infarct) to restore blood flow, limit myocardial damage, preserve left ventricular function, and prevent death.
3. Thrombolytics are also used in arterial thrombosis, deep vein thrombosis, occluded shunts or catheters, and pulmonary emboli.

B. Contraindications
1. Active internal bleeding
2. History of hemorrhagic brain attack (stroke)
3. Intracranial problems, including trauma
4. Intracranial or intraspinal surgery within the previous 2 months
5. History of thoracic, pelvic, or abdominal surgery in the previous 10 days
6. History of hepatic or renal disease
7. Uncontrolled hypertension
8. Recently required, prolonged cardiopulmonary resuscitation
9. Known allergy to the specific product or any of its preservatives

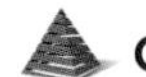
C. Side/adverse effects
1. Bleeding
2. Dysrhythmias
3. Allergic reactions

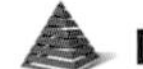
D. Interventions
1. Determine aPTT, PT, fibrinogen level, hematocrit, and platelet count.
2. Monitor the vital signs.
3. Check the pulses.
4. Monitor for bleeding.
5. Monitor all excretions for occult blood.
6. Monitor for neurological changes such as slurred speech, lethargy, confusion, and hemiparesis.
7. Monitor for hypotension and tachycardia.
8. Injections are avoided if possible.
9. Direct pressure is applied over a puncture site for 20 to 30 minutes.
10. The client is handled as little as possible when moving.
11. Reinforce instructions to the client to use an electric razor for shaving and brush teeth gently.
12. The medication is withheld if bleeding develops, and the health care provider (HCP) is notified.
13. Antidote
   a. Aminocaproic acid (Amicar) is the antidote
   b. Used only in acute, life-threatening conditions

⚠ Bleeding is the primary concern for a client taking an anticoagulant, thrombolytic, or antiplatelet medication.

III. Antiplatelet Medications (Box 52-4)

A. Description
1. Antiplatelet medications inhibit the aggregation of platelets in the clotting process, thereby prolonging the bleeding time.
2. Antiplatelet medications may be used with anticoagulants.
3. Used in the prophylaxis of long-term complications after myocardial infarction, coronary revascularization, stents, and brain attacks (stroke).
4. These medications are contraindicated in those with bleeding disorders and known sensitivity.

B. Side/adverse effects
1. Gastrointestinal bleeding
2. Bruising
3. Hematuria
4. Tarry stools

C. Interventions
1. Sensitivity is determined before administration.
2. Monitor vital signs.
3. The client is instructed to take medication with food if gastrointestinal upset occurs.
4. Monitor the bleeding time.
5. Monitor for side/adverse effects related to bleeding.
6. Reinforce instructions to the client in the use of the medication.
7. Reinforce instructions to the client to monitor for side/adverse effects related to bleeding and the measures to prevent bleeding.

IV. Cardiac Glycosides

A. Digoxin (Lanoxin)

B. Description
1. Cardiac glycosides inhibit the sodium-potassium pump, thus increasing intracellular calcium, which causes the heart muscle fibers to contract more efficiently.

BOX 52-4 Antiplatelet Medications

Oral

Aspirin (acetylsalicylic acid, ASA)
Cilostazol (Pletal)
Clopidogrel (Plavix)
Dipyridamole (Persantine)
Dipyridamole; aspirin (Aggrenox)
Ticlopidine (Ticlid)

Parenteral

Abciximab (ReoPro)
Eptifibatide (Integrilin)
Tirofiban (Aggrastat)

2. Cardiac glycosides produce a positive inotropic action, which increases the force of myocardial contractions.
3. Cardiac glycosides produce a negative chronotropic action, which slows the heart rate.
4. Cardiac glycosides produce a negative dromotropic action that slows conduction velocity through the atrioventricular (AV) node.
5. The increase in myocardial **contractility** increases cardiac, peripheral, and kidney function by increasing **cardiac output**, decreasing preload, improving blood flow to the periphery and kidneys, decreasing edema, and increasing fluid excretion. As a result, fluid retention in the lungs and extremities is decreased.
6. Cardiac glycosides are used for heart failure and cardiogenic shock, atrial tachycardia, atrial fibrillation, and atrial flutter; used less frequently for rate control in atrial dysrhythmias (β-blockers and calcium channel blockers are used more often) (Fig. 52-1).
7. These medications are contraindicated in those with ventricular dysrhythmias and second- or third-degree heart block and should be used with caution in clients with renal disease, hypothyroidism, and hypokalemia.

C. Side/adverse effects and toxic effects
1. Anorexia, nausea, vomiting, diarrhea
2. Headache
3. Visual disturbances: Diplopia, blurred vision, yellow-green halos, photophobia
4. Drowsiness
5. Bradycardia
6. Fatigue, weakness

Early signs of digoxin toxicity present as gastrointestinal manifestations (anorexia, nausea, vomiting, diarrhea). Then heart rate abnormalities and visual disturbances appear.

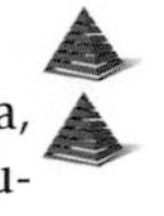

D. Interventions
1. Monitor for toxicity as evidenced by anorexia, nausea, vomiting, visual disturbances, confusion, bradycardia, heart block, premature ventricular contractions, and tachydysrhythmias.
2. Monitor serum digoxin level, electrolyte levels, and renal function test results.
3. The therapeutic digoxin range is 0.5 to 2 ng/mL. Levels greater than 2 ng/mL are toxic.
4. An increased risk of toxicity exists in clients with hypercalcemia, hypokalemia, hypomagnesemia, or hypothyroidism.
5. Monitor the potassium level. If hypokalemia occurs (potassium lower than 3.5 mEq/L), notify the HCP.
6. Reinforce instructions to the client to avoid over-the-counter medications.
7. Monitor the client taking a potassium-wasting diuretic or corticosteroids closely for hypokalemia because the hypokalemia can cause digoxin toxicity.
8. Note that older clients are more sensitive to digoxin toxicity.
9. Advise the client to eat foods high in potassium, such as fresh and dried fruits, fruit juices, vegetables, and potatoes.
10. Monitor the apical pulse for 1 full minute.
11. If the apical pulse rate is lower than 60 beats/min, the medication should be withheld and the HCP notified.
12. Reinforce teaching the client how to measure the pulse.
13. Reinforce teaching the client to notify the HCP if the pulse rate is lower than 60 or higher than 100 beats/min.
14. Reinforce teaching the client the signs and symptoms of toxicity.
15. Antidote: Digoxin immune Fab (Digibind) is used in extreme toxicity.

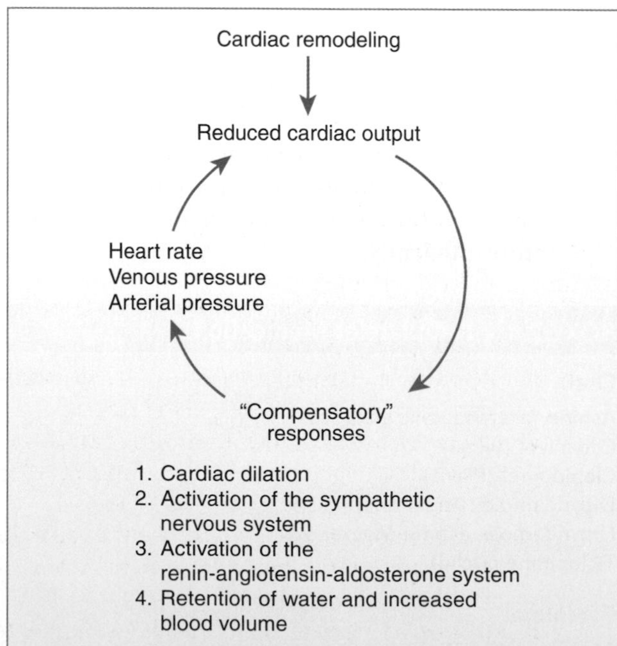

FIGURE 52-1 The vicious cycle of maladaptive compensatory responses to a failing heart. (From Lehne R: *Pharmacology for nursing care*, ed 7, St. Louis, 2010, Saunders.)

V. Antihypertensive Medications

A. Thiazide diuretics (Box 52-5)
1. Description
   a. Thiazide diuretics increase sodium and water excretion by inhibiting sodium reabsorption in the distal tubule of the kidney.
   b. Used for hypertension and peripheral edema
   c. Not effective for immediate diuresis

BOX 52-5 Thiazide and Thiazide-Like Diuretics

Chlorothiazide (Diuril)
Chlorthalidone (Thalitone)
Hydrochlorothiazide
Indapamide
Methyclothiazide
Metolazone (Zaroxolyn)
Polythiazide (Renese)

d. Used in clients with normal renal function (contraindicated in clients with renal failure)
e. Thiazide diuretics should be used with caution in the client taking lithium because lithium toxicity can occur in the client taking digoxin, corticosteroids, or hypoglycemic medications.

2. Side/adverse effects
   a. Hypercalcemia, hyperglycemia, hyperuricemia
   b. Hypokalemia, hyponatremia
   c. Hypovolemia
   d. Hypotension
   e. Headaches
   f. Nausea, vomiting
   g. Constipation
   h. Rashes
   i. Photosensitivity
   j. Blood dyscrasias
3. Interventions
   a. Monitor vital signs.
   b. Monitor the weight.
   c. Monitor the urine output.
   d. Monitor electrolyte, glucose, calcium, blood urea nitrogen (BUN), creatinine, and uric acid levels.
   e. Check peripheral extremities for edema.
   f. Reinforce instructions to the client to take the medication in the morning to avoid nocturia and sleep interruption.
   g. Reinforce instructions to the client in how to record the **blood pressure (BP)**.
   h. Reinforce instructions to the client to eat foods high in potassium.
   i. Reinforce instructions to the client in how to take potassium supplements if prescribed.
   j. Reinforce instructions to the client to take medication with food to avoid gastrointestinal upset.
   k. Reinforce instructions to the client to change positions slowly to prevent orthostatic hypotension.
   l. Reinforce instructions to the client to use sunscreen when in direct sunlight because of increased photosensitivity.
   m. Reinforce instructions to the client with diabetes mellitus to have the blood glucose level checked periodically.

BOX 52-6 Loop Diuretics

Bumetanide
Ethacrynic acid (Edecrin)
Furosemide (Lasix)
Torsemide (Demadex)

B. Loop diuretics (Box 52-6)
1. Description
   a. Loop diuretics inhibit sodium and chloride reabsorption from the loop of Henle and the distal tubule.
   b. Loop diuretics have little effect on the blood glucose level; however, they cause depletion of water and electrolytes, increased uric acid levels, and the excretion of calcium.
   c. Loop diuretics are more potent than thiazide diuretics, causing rapid diuresis and thus decreasing vascular fluid volume, cardiac output, and BP.
   d. Loop diuretics are used for hypertension, pulmonary edema, edema associated with heart failure, hypercalcemia, and renal disease.
   e. Use loop diuretics with caution in the client taking digoxin or lithium and the client on aminoglycosides, anticoagulants, corticosteroids, or amphotericin B.

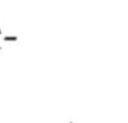
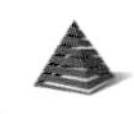

2. Side/adverse effects
   a. Hypokalemia, hyponatremia, hypocalcemia, hypomagnesemia
   b. Thrombocytopenia
   c. Hyperuricemia
   d. Orthostatic hypotension
   e. Skin disturbances
   f. Ototoxicity and deafness
   g. Thiamine deficiency
   h. Dehydration
3. Interventions
   a. Monitor vital signs.
   b. Monitor the weight.
   c. Monitor the urine output.
   d. Monitor electrolyte, calcium, magnesium, BUN, creatinine, and uric acid levels.
   e. Check the peripheral extremities for edema.
   f. Monitor for signs of digoxin or lithium toxicity if the client is on these medications.
   g. Reinforce instructions to the client to take the medication in the morning to avoid nocturia and sleep interruption.
   h. Reinforce instructions to the client in how to record the BP.
   i. Reinforce instructions to the client to eat foods high in potassium.

j. Reinforce instructions to the client in how to take potassium supplements if prescribed.
k. Reinforce instructions to the client to take medication with food to avoid gastrointestinal upset.
l. Reinforce instructions to the client to change positions slowly to prevent orthostatic hypotension.
m. IV furosemide (Lasix) is administered slowly because hearing loss can occur if injected rapidly.

C. Osmotic diuretics
See Chapter 58 for information regarding osmotic diuretics.

D. Potassium-retaining diuretics (Box 52-7)
1. Description
a. Potassium-retaining diuretics act on the distal tubule to promote sodium and water excretion and potassium retention.
b. Used for edema and hypertension, to increase urine output, and to treat fluid retention and overload associated with heart failure, ascites resulting from cirrhosis or nephrotic syndrome, and diuretic-induced hypokalemia.
c. Potassium-retaining diuretics are contraindicated in severe kidney or hepatic disease and severe hyperkalemia.
d. Potassium-retaining diuretics should be used with caution in the client with diabetes mellitus, taking antihypertensives or lithium, taking angiotensin-converting enzyme inhibitors or potassium supplements because hyperkalemia can result.

The primary concern with administering potassium-retaining diuretics is hyperkalemia.

2. Side/adverse effects
a. Hyperkalemia
b. Nausea, vomiting, diarrhea
c. Rash
d. Dizziness, weakness
e. Headache
f. Dry mouth
g. Photosensitivity
h. Anemia
i. Thrombocytopenia

BOX 52-7 Potassium-Retaining Diuretics

Amiloride hydrochloride; hydrochlorothiazide
Eplerenone (Inspra)
Spironolactone (Aldactone)
Spironolactone; hydrochlorothiazide (Aldactazide)
Triamterene (Dyrenium)

3. Interventions
a. Monitor vital signs.
b. Monitor urine output.
c. Monitor for signs and symptoms of hyperkalemia such as nausea, diarrhea, abdominal cramps, tachycardia followed by bradycardia, tall peaked T wave on the electrocardiogram, and oliguria.
d. Monitor for a potassium level greater than 5.1 mEq/L, which indicates hyperkalemia.
e. Reinforce instructions to the client to avoid foods high in potassium.
f. Reinforce instructions to the client to avoid exposure to direct sunlight.
g. Reinforce instructions to the client to monitor for signs of hyperkalemia.
h. Reinforce instructions to the client to avoid salt substitutes because they contain potassium.
i. Reinforce instructions to the client to take with or after meals to decrease gastrointestinal irritation.

VI. Peripherally Acting α-Adrenergic Blockers (Box 52-8)

A. Description
1. These medications decrease sympathetic vasoconstriction by reducing the effects of norepinephrine at peripheral nerve endings, resulting in vasodilation and decreased BP.
2. These medications are used to maintain renal blood flow.
3. These medications are used to treat hypertension.

B. Side/adverse effects
1. Orthostatic hypotension
2. Reflex tachycardia
3. Sodium and water retention
4. Gastrointestinal disturbances
5. Nausea
6. Drowsiness
7. Nasal congestion
8. Edema
9. Weight gain

C. Interventions 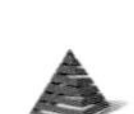
1. Monitor vital signs.
2. Monitor for fluid retention and edema.
3. Reinforce instructions to the client to change positions slowly to prevent orthostatic hypotension.
4. Reinforce instructions to the client in how to monitor the BP.

BOX 52-8 Peripherally Acting α-Adrenergic Blockers

Doxazosin (Cardura)
Prazosin (Minipress)
Terazosin (Hytrin)

BOX 52-9 Centrally Acting Sympatholytics

Clonidine (Catapres)
Guanabenz
Guanfacine (Tenex)
Methyldopa

5. Reinforce instructions to the client to monitor for edema.
6. Reinforce instructions to the client to decrease salt intake.
7. Reinforce instructions to the client to avoid over-the-counter medications.

VII. Centrally Acting Sympatholytics (Adrenergic Blockers) (Box 52-9)

A. Description
   1. Centrally acting sympatholytics stimulate alpha receptors in the central nervous system to inhibit vasoconstriction, thus reducing peripheral resistance.
   2. Used to treat hypertension
   3. Contraindicated in impaired liver function

B. Side/adverse effects
   1. Sodium and water retention
   2. Drowsiness, dizziness
   3. Dry mouth
   4. Bradycardia
   5. Edema
   6. Impotence
   7. Hypotension
   8. Depression

C. Interventions
   1. Monitor vital signs.
   2. Reinforce instructions to the client not to discontinue medication because abrupt withdrawal can cause severe rebound hypertension.
   3. Monitor liver function tests.

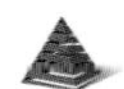

VIII. Angiotensin-Converting Enzyme (ACE) Inhibitors and Angiotensin II Receptor Blockers (ARBs) (Box 52-10)

A. Description
   1. ACE inhibitors prevent peripheral vasoconstriction by blocking conversion of angiotensin I to angiotensin II (AII).
   2. ARBs prevent peripheral vasoconstriction and secretion of aldosterone and block the binding of AII to type 1 AII receptors.
   3. These medications are used to treat hypertension and heart failure. ACE inhibitors are also administered for their cardioprotective effect after myocardial infarction.
   4. Use with potassium supplements and potassium-retaining diuretics is avoided.

BOX 52-10 Angiotensin-Converting Enzyme Inhibitors and Angiotensin Receptor Blockers

Angiotensin-Converting Enzyme Inhibitors
Benazepril (Lotensin)
Captopril (Capoten)
Enalapril (Vasotec)
Lisinopril (Prinivil, Zestril)
Moexipril (Univasc)
Quinapril (Accupril)
Ramipril (Altace)
Trandolapril (Mavik)

Angiotensin II Receptor Blockers
Candesartan (Atacand)
Eprosartan (Teveten)
Irbesartan (Avapro)
Losartan (Cozaar)
Olmesartan (Benicar)
Telmisartan (Micardis)
Valsartan (Diovan)

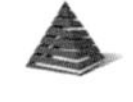

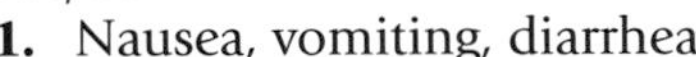

B. Side/adverse effects
   1. Nausea, vomiting, diarrhea
   2. Persistent dry cough (ACE inhibitors only)
   3. Hypotension
   4. Hyperkalemia
   5. Tachycardia
   6. Headache
   7. Dizziness, fatigue
   8. Insomnia
   9. Hypoglycemic reaction in the client with diabetes mellitus
   10. Bruising, petechiae, bleeding
   11. Diminished taste (ACE inhibitors)

A persistent dry cough is a common complaint for those taking an ACE inhibitor. The client is instructed to contact the HCP if this side effect occurs and persists.

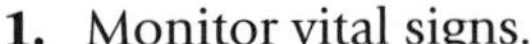

C. Interventions
   1. Monitor vital signs.
   2. Monitor white blood cells, and protein, albumin, BUN, creatinine, and potassium levels.
   3. Monitor for hypoglycemic reactions in the client with diabetes mellitus.
   4. Reinforce instructions to the client to take captopril (Capoten) 20 to 60 minutes before a meal.
   5. Monitor for bruising, petechiae, or bleeding with captopril.
   6. Reinforce instructions to the client not to discontinue medications because rebound hypertension can occur.
   7. Reinforce instructions to the client not to take over-the-counter medications.

8. Reinforce instructions to the client in how to take the BP.
9. Reinforce instructions to the client that if dizziness or any other side/adverse effects occur and persist to notify the HCP.
10. Reinforce instructions to the client that the taste of food may be diminished during the first month of therapy.
11. Reinforce instructions to the client to report the side effect of angioedema immediately to the HCP.

IX. Antianginal Medications (Box 52-11)

A. Nitrates (see Priority Nursing Actions)
 1. Description
  a. Nitrates produce vasodilation.
  b. Nitrates decrease preload and afterload and reduce myocardial oxygen consumption.
  c. Contraindicated in the client with significant hypotension, increased intracranial pressure, severe anemia, and in those taking medication to treat erectile dysfunction (because of the risk for severe hypotension).
  d. Should be used with caution with severe renal or hepatic disease
  e. Abrupt withdrawal of long-acting preparations is avoided to prevent the rebound effect of severe pain from myocardial ischemia.
 2. Side/adverse effects 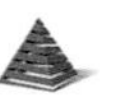
  a. Headache
  b. Orthostatic hypotension
  c. Dizziness, weakness
  d. Faintness
  e. Nausea, vomiting
  f. Flushing or pallor
  g. Confusion
  h. Rash
  i. Dry mouth
  j. Reflex tachycardia
 3. Sublingual medications
  a. Monitor the vital signs.
  b. Offer sips of water before giving because dryness may inhibit medication absorption.
  c. Reinforce instructions to the client to place under the tongue and leave until fully dissolved.
  d. Reinforce instructions to the client not to swallow the medication.
  e. Reinforce instructions to the client to take 1 tablet for pain and to immediately contact emergency medical services if pain is

Box 52-11 Antianginal Medications (Organic Nitrates)

Amyl nitrate inhalant
Isosorbide dinitrate (Isordil, Dilitrate-SR)
Isosorbide mononitrate (Imdur, Monoket)
Nitroglycerin, sublingual (Nitrostat)
Nitroglycerin, translingual (Nitrolingual pumpspray)
Nitroglycerin, transdermal patches (Minitran, Nitro-Dur)
Nitroglycerin ointment
Intravenous nitroglycerin

PRIORITY NURSING ACTIONS!

Actions to Take If a Hospitalized Client with Cardiac Disease Complains of Chest Pain

1. The client is quickly assessed, specifically characteristics of pain, heart rate and rhythm, and blood pressure (BP).
2. A nitroglycerin tablet is administered.
3. The client should not be left alone.
4. The client is reassessed in 5 minutes.
5. Another nitroglycerin tablet is administered if pain is not relieved and the BP is stable.
6. The client is reassessed in 5 minutes.
7. A third nitroglycerin tablet is administered if pain is not relieved and the BP is stable.
8. The client is reassessed in 5 minutes. The HCP is contacted if the third nitroglycerin tablet does not relieve the pain.
9. The event, actions taken, and the client's response to treatment are documented.

The usual guidelines for administering nitroglycerin tablets for chest pain include administering one tablet every 5 minutes PRN for chest pain, for a total dose of three tablets. If the client does not obtain relief after taking a third dose of nitroglycerin, the HCP is notified. Before administering the first dose of nitroglycerin, the nurse quickly assesses the client, specifically the characteristics of the pain, the heart rate and rhythm, and blood pressure (BP). The nurse always stays with the client during the event to provide reassurance and relieve anxiety. Additionally the nurse must be present if a life-threatening situation develops. The nurse assesses the client before administering each subsequent dose of nitroglycerin and pays particular attention to the BP because nitroglycerin causes hypotension. The nurse must lower the head of the bed and contact the HCP before administering another nitroglycerin if hypotension occurs. Agency protocols for this type of event should also be followed. The nurse documents the event, actions taken, and the client's response to treatment.

Reference(s): Lewis, S., Dirksen, S., Heitkemper, M., & Bucher, L. (2014). *Medical-surgical nursing: Assessment and management of clinical problems* (9th ed., p. 750). St. Louis: Mosby.

not relieved; in the hospitalized client, 1 tablet is administered every 5 minutes for a total of three doses and the health care provider is notified immediately if pain is not relieved following the three doses (the blood pressure is checked before each dose administration).

   f. The client is informed that a stinging or burning sensation may indicate that the tablet is fresh.

   g. Reinforce instructions to the client to store medication in a dark, tightly closed bottle.

   h. Reinforce instructions to the client to take acetaminophen (Tylenol) for a headache.

4. Translingual medications (spray)

   a. The client is instructed to direct the spray against the oral mucosa.

   b. The client is instructed to avoid inhaling the spray.

5. Sustained-released medications: The client is instructed to swallow and not chew or crush the medication.

6. Transdermal patch

   a. The client is instructed to apply the patch to a hairless area, using a new patch and different site each day.

   b. As prescribed, the client is instructed to remove the patch after 12 to 14 hours, allowing 10 to 12 "patch-free" hours each day to prevent tolerance.

7. Topical ointments

   a. Reinforce instructions to the client to remove the ointment on the skin from the previous dose.

   b. Reinforce instructions to the client to squeeze a ribbon of ointment of the prescribed length onto the applicator paper.

   c. Reinforce instructions to the client to spread the ointment over a 2.5x3.5-inch area and cover with plastic wrap, using either the chest, back, abdomen, upper arm, or anterior thigh (avoid hairy areas).

   d. Reinforce instructions to the client to rotate sites and avoid touching the ointment when applying.

8. Patches and ointments

   a. Wear gloves when applying.

   b. Do not apply on the chest in the area of defibrillator-cardioverter pads/paddle placement because skin burns can result if the paddles need to be used.

Instruct the client using nitroglycerin tablets to check the expiration date on the medication bottle because expiration may occur within 6 months of obtaining the medication. The tablets will not relieve the chest pain if they have expired.

BOX 52-12 β-Adrenergic Blockers

Nonselective (Block β_1 and β_2)

Carvedilol (Coreg)
Labetalol (Trandate)
Nadolol (Corgard)
Nebivolol (Bystolic)
Penbutolol (Levatol)
Propranolol (Inderal LA)
Sotalol (Betapace)

Cardioselective (Block β_1)

Acebutolol (Sectral)
Atenolol (Tenormin)
Betaxolol
Bisoprolol (Zebeta, Ziac)
Metoprolol (Lopressor, Toprol-XL)

X. β-Adrenergic Blockers (Box 52-12)

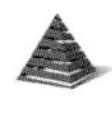

A. Description

1. β-Adrenergic blockers inhibit response to β-adrenergic stimulation, thus decreasing cardiac output.

2. β-Adrenergic blockers block the release of catecholamines, epinephrine, and norepinephrine, thus decreasing the heart rate and BP.

3. β-Adrenergic blockers decrease the workload of the heart and decrease oxygen demands.

4. Used for angina, dysrhythmias, hypertension, migraine headaches, prevention of myocardial infarction, and glaucoma.

5. β-Adrenergic blockers are contraindicated in the client with asthma, bradycardia, heart failure (with exceptions), severe renal or hepatic disease, hyperthyroidism, or brain attack (stroke). Carvedilol, metoprolol, and bisoprolol have been approved for use in heart failure once the client has been stabilized with ACE inhibitor and diuretic therapy.

6. β-Adrenergic blockers should be used with caution in the client with diabetes mellitus because the medication may mask the symptoms of hypoglycemia.

7. β-Adrenergic blockers should be used with caution in the client taking antihypertensive medications.

B. Side/adverse effects

1. Bradycardia
2. Bronchospasm
3. Hypotension
4. Weakness, fatigue
5. Nausea, vomiting
6. Dizziness
7. Hyperglycemia
8. Agranulocytosis
9. Behavioral or psychotic response
10. Depression
11. Nightmares

C. Interventions
1. Monitor the vital signs.
2. Withhold the medication if the pulse or BP is not within the prescribed parameters.
3. Monitor for signs of heart failure or worsening heart failure.
4. Check for respiratory distress and for signs of wheezing and dyspnea.
5. Reinforce instructions to the client to report dizziness, light-headedness, or nasal congestion.
6. Reinforce instructions to the client not to stop the medication because rebound hypertension, rebound tachycardia, or an anginal attack can occur.
7. Reinforce instructions to the client taking insulin that the β-adrenergic blocker can mask early signs of hypoglycemia, such as tachycardia and nervousness.
8. Reinforce instructions to the client taking insulin to monitor the blood glucose level.
9. Reinforce instructions to the client in how to take pulse and BP.
10. Reinforce instructions to the client to change positions slowly to prevent orthostatic hypotension.
11. Reinforce instructions to the client to avoid over-the-counter medications, especially cold medications and nasal decongestants.

XI. Calcium Channel Blockers (Box 52-13)

A. Description
1. Calcium channel blockers decrease cardiac contractility (negative inotropic effect by relaxing smooth muscle) and the workload of the heart, thus decreasing the need for oxygen.
2. Calcium channel blockers promote vasodilation of the coronary and peripheral vessels.
3. Used for angina, dysrhythmias, or hypertension
4. Should be used with caution in the client with heart failure, bradycardia, or atrioventricular block

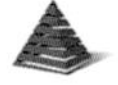
B. Side/adverse effects
1. Bradycardia
2. Hypotension
3. Reflex tachycardia as a result of hypotension
4. Headache
5. Dizziness, light-headedness
6. Fatigue
7. Peripheral edema
8. Constipation
9. Flushing of the skin
10. Changes in liver and kidney function

C. Interventions
1. Monitor vital signs.
2. Monitor for signs of heart failure.
3. Monitor liver enzyme levels.
4. Monitor kidney function tests.
5. Reinforce instructions to the client not to discontinue the medication.
6. Reinforce instructions to the client in how to take a pulse.
7. Reinforce instructions to the client to notify the HCP if dizziness or fainting occurs.
8. Reinforce instructions to the client to not crush or chew sustained-release tablets.

XII. Peripheral Vasodilators (Box 52-14)

A. Description
1. Peripheral vasodilators decrease peripheral resistance by exerting a direct action on the arteries or the arteries and the veins.
2. Peripheral vasodilators increase blood flow to the extremities and are used in peripheral vascular disorders of venous and arterial vessels.
3. Peripheral vasodilators are most effective for disorders resulting from vasospasm (Raynaud's disease).
4. These medications may decrease some symptoms of cerebral vascular insufficiency.

B. Side/adverse effects
1. Light-headedness, dizziness
2. Orthostatic hypotension
3. Tachycardia
4. Palpitations
5. Flushing
6. Gastrointestinal distress

BOX 52-13 Calcium Channel Blockers

Amlodipine (Norvasc)
Clevidipine (Cleviprex)
Diltiazem (Cardizem, Dilacor XR, others)
Felodipine (Plendil)
Nicardipine (Cardene)
Nifedipine (Adalat, Procardia)
Nimodipine
Nisoldipine (Sular)
Verapamil (Calan, Covera-HS, Verelan)

BOX 52-14 Peripheral Vasodilators

α-Adrenergic Blockers
Doxazosin (Cardura)
Prazosin (Minipress)
Terazosin (Hytrin)

Calcium Channel Blockers
Diltiazem (Cardizem, Dilacor XR, others)
Nifedipine (Adalat, Procardia)
Nimodipine
Verapamil (Calan, Covera-HS, Verelan)

Hemorheological
Pentoxifylline (Trental; increases microcirculation and tissue perfusion)

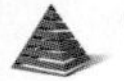

C. Interventions
 1. Monitor the vital signs, especially the BP and heart rate.
 2. Monitor for orthostatic hypotension and tachycardia.
 3. Monitor for signs of inadequate blood flow to the extremities, such as pallor, feeling cold, and pain.
 4. Reinforce instructions to the client that it may take up to 3 months for a desired therapeutic response.
 5. The client is advised not to smoke because smoking increases vasospasm.
 6. Reinforce instructions to the client to avoid aspirin or aspirin-like compounds unless approved by the HCP.
 7. Reinforce instructions to the client to take the medication with meals if gastrointestinal disturbances occur.
 8. Reinforce instructions to the client to avoid alcohol because it may cause a hypotensive reaction.
 9. The client is encouraged to change positions slowly to avoid orthostatic hypotension.

Vasodilators cause orthostatic hypotension. The client is instructed about safety measures when taking these medications, such as the need to rise from a lying to a sitting or standing position slowly.

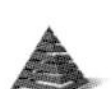

XIII. Antilipemic Medications (Box 52-15)

A. Description
 1. Antilipemic medications reduce serum levels of cholesterol, triglycerides, or low-density lipoprotein.

BOX 52-15 Antilipemic Medications

Bile Acid Sequestrants
Cholestyramine (Questran)
Colesevelam (WelChol)
Colestipol (Colestid)

HMG-CoA Reductase Inhibitors
Atorvastatin (Lipitor)
Fluvastatin (Lescol)
Lovastatin (Mevacor)
Pitavastatin (Livalo)
Pravastatin (Pravachol)
Rosuvastatin (Crestor)
Simvastatin (Zocor)

Other Antilipemic Medications
Ezetimibe (Zetia)
Ezetimibe; simvastatin (Vytorin)
Fenofibrate (Tricor)
Gemfibrozil (Lopid)
Nicotinic acid (Niacin)
Probucol
Sitagliptin; simvastatin (Juvisync)

 2. When cholesterol, triglyceride, and low-density lipoprotein levels are elevated, the client is at increased risk for coronary artery disease.
 3. In many cases, diet alone will not lower blood lipid levels; therefore antilipemic medications will be prescribed.

B. Bile sequestrants
 1. Description
  a. Bind with acids in the intestines, which prevents reabsorption of cholesterol
  b. Should not be used as the only therapy in clients with elevated triglyceride levels because they may raise triglyceride levels.
 2. Side/adverse effects
  a. Constipation
  b. Gastrointestinal disturbances: Heartburn, nausea, belching, bloating
 3. Interventions
  a. Cholestyramine (Questran) comes in a gritty powder that must be mixed thoroughly in juice or water before administration.
  b. Monitor the client for early signs of peptic ulcer such as nausea and abdominal discomfort followed by abdominal pain and distention.
  c. Reinforce instructions to the client that the medication must be taken with and followed by sufficient fluids.

C. HMG-CoA reductase inhibitors
 1. Description
  a. Lovastatin (Mevacor) is highly protein-bound and should not be administered with anticoagulants.
  b. Lovastatin should not be administered with gemfibrozil (Lopid).
  c. Lovastatin is administered with caution to the client taking immunosuppressive medications.

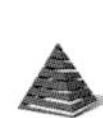

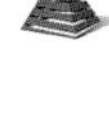

 2. Side/adverse effects
  a. Nausea
  b. Diarrhea or constipation
  c. Abdominal pain or cramps
  d. Flatulence
  e. Dizziness
  f. Headache
  g. Blurred vision
  h. Rash
  i. Pruritus
  j. Elevated liver enzyme levels
  k. Muscle cramps and fatigue
 3. Interventions
  a. Monitor serum liver enzyme levels.
  b. Reinforce instructions to the client to receive an annual eye examination because the medications can cause cataract formation.
  c. If lovastatin is not effective in lowering the lipid level after 3 months, it should be discontinued.

The client who is taking an antilipemic medication is instructed to report any unexplained muscular pain to the HCP immediately.

D. Other antilipemic medications
  1. Description
    a. Gemfibrozil should not be taken with anticoagulants because they compete for protein sites. If the client is taking an anticoagulant, the anticoagulant dose should be reduced during antilipemic therapy and the INR should be monitored closely.
    b. Do not administer gemfibrozil with HMG-CoA reductase inhibitors because it increases the risk for myositis, myalgias, and rhabdomyolysis.
    c. Fish oil supplements have been associated with a decreased risk for cardiovascular heart disease. Plant stanol and sterol esters and Cholestin have been associated with reducing cholesterol levels.

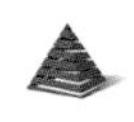

  2. Interventions
    a. Monitor vital signs.
    b. Monitor the liver enzyme levels.
    c. Monitor the serum cholesterol and triglyceride levels.
    d. Reinforce instructions to the client to restrict intake of fats, cholesterol, carbohydrates, and alcohol.
    e. Reinforce instructions to the client to follow an exercise program.
    f. Reinforce instructions to the client that it will take several weeks before the lipid level declines.
    g. Reinforce instructions to the client to have an annual eye examination and report any changes in vision.
    h. Reinforce instructions to the client with diabetes mellitus who is taking gemfibrozil to monitor blood glucose levels regularly.
    i. Reinforce instructions to the client to increase fluid intake.
    j. Note that nicotinic acid has numerous side effects, including gastrointestinal disturbances, flushing of the skin, elevated liver enzyme levels, hyperglycemia, and hyperuricemia.
    k. Reinforce instructions to the client that aspirin or nonsteroidal anti-inflammatory drugs taken 30 minutes before may assist in reducing the side effect of cutaneous flushing from nicotinic acid.
    l. Reinforce instructions to the client to take nicotinic acid with meals to reduce gastrointestinal discomfort.

CRITICAL THINKING What Should You Do?

Answer: The normal INR is 1.3 to 2.0. The treatment goal of warfarin sodium is to raise the INR to an appropriate value. An INR of 2 to 3 is appropriate for most clients, although for some clients the target INR is 3 to 4.5. If the INR is below the recommended range, warfarin sodium should be increased. If the INR is above the recommended range, warfarin sodium should be reduced. If the INR is 2.8, the nurse should plan to administer the same dosage as prescribed.

Reference(s): Lehne, R. (2013). *Pharmacology for nursing care* (8th ed., p. 615). St. Louis: Saunders.

PRACTICE QUESTIONS

536. The nurse reinforces discharge instructions to a postoperative client who is taking warfarin sodium (Coumadin). Which statement made by the client reflects the **need for further teaching**?
1. "I will take my pills every day at the same time."
2. "I will be certain to avoid alcohol consumption."
3. "I have already called my family to pick up a Medic-Alert bracelet."
4. "I will take Ecotrin (enteric-coated aspirin) for my headaches because it is coated."

❖ **537.** A client is receiving digoxin (Lanoxin) daily. The nurse suspects digoxin toxicity after noting which signs and symptoms? **Select all that apply.**
- ☐ 1. Visual disturbances
- ☐ 2. Nausea and vomiting
- ☐ 3. Serum digoxin level of 2.3 ng/mL
- ☐ 4. Serum potassium level of 3.9 mEq/L
- ☐ 5. Apical pulse rate of 63 beats per minute

538. Heparin sodium is prescribed for the client. Which laboratory result indicates that the heparin is prescribed at a therapeutic level?
1. Prothrombin time (PT) of 21 seconds
2. Thrombocyte count of 100,000 cells/mm^3
3. International normalized ratio (INR) of 2.3
4. Activated partial thromboplastin time (aPTT) of 55 seconds

539. The nurse is monitoring a client who is taking propranolol (Inderal LA). Which data collection finding would indicate a potential serious complication associated with propranolol?
1. The development of complaints of insomnia
2. The development of audible expiratory wheezes
3. A baseline blood pressure of 150/80 mm Hg, followed by a blood pressure of 138/72 mm Hg after two doses of the medication

4. A baseline resting heart rate of 88 beats/min, followed by a resting heart rate of 72 beats/min after two doses of the medication

540. Isosorbide mononitrate (Imdur) is prescribed for a client with angina pectoris. The client tells the nurse that the medication is causing a chronic headache. Which action should the nurse suggest to the client?
1. Cut the dose in half.
2. Discontinue the medication.
3. Take the medication with food.
4. Contact the health care provider (HCP).

541. A client is diagnosed with an acute myocardial infarction and is receiving tissue plasminogen activator, alteplase (Activase, tPA). Which action is a **priority** nursing intervention?
1. Monitor for kidney failure.
2. Monitor psychosocial status.
3. Monitor for signs of bleeding.
4. Have heparin sodium available.

❖**542.** A client with coronary artery disease complains of substernal chest pain. After checking the client's heart rate and blood pressure, the nurse administers nitroglycerin, 0.4 mg, sublingually. After 5 minutes, the client states, "My chest still hurts." Which appropriate actions should the nurse take? **Select all that apply.**
- ❑ 1. Call a code blue.
- ❑ 2. Contact the client's family.
- ❑ 3. Assess the client's pain level.
- ❑ 4. Check the client's blood pressure.
- ❑ 5. Administer a second nitroglycerin, 0.4 mg, sublingually.

543. The home health care nurse is visiting a client with elevated triglyceride levels and a serum cholesterol level of 398 mg/dL. The client is taking cholestyramine (Questran). Which statement made by the client indicates the **need for further teaching**?
1. "Constipation and bloating might be a problem."
2. "I'll continue to watch my diet and reduce my fats."
3. "Walking a mile each day will help the whole process."
4. "I'll continue my nicotinic acid from the health food store."

544. A client is on nicotinic acid (niacin) for hyperlipidemia, and the nurse reinforces instructions to the client about the medication. Which statement by the client indicates an understanding of the instructions?
1. "It is not necessary to avoid the use of alcohol."
2. "The medication should be taken with meals to decrease flushing."
3. "Clay-colored stools are a common side effect and should not be of concern."
4. "Ibuprofen (Motrin IB) taken 30 minutes before the nicotinic acid should decrease the flushing."

545. The nurse is planning to administer hydrochlorothiazide to a client. Which are concerns related to the administration of this medication?
1. Hypouricemia, hyperkalemia
2. Increased risk of osteoporosis
3. Hypokalemia, hyperglycemia, sulfa allergy
4. Hyperkalemia, hypoglycemia, penicillin allergy

ANSWERS

536. 4

Rationale: Ecotrin is an aspirin-containing product and should be avoided. Alcohol consumption should be avoided by a client taking warfarin sodium. Taking prescribed medication at the same time each day increases client compliance. The Medic-Alert bracelet provides health care personnel emergency information.
Test-Taking Strategy: Note the strategic words, *need for further teaching.* These words indicate a negative event query and ask you to select an option that is an incorrect statement. Recalling that warfarin (Coumadin) is an anticoagulant and that Ecotrin is an aspirin-containing product will direct you to the correct option. **Review:** client teaching points related to warfarin.
Level of Cognitive Ability: Evaluating
Client Needs: Physiological Integrity
Integrated Process: Teaching and Learning
Content Area: Pharmacology: Cardiovascular Medications
Priority Concepts: Client Education, Pain
Reference(s): Hodgson, Kizior (2015), pp. 89; 1289–1290; Lehne (2013), pp. 659–660.

❖**537. 1, 2, 3**

Rationale: Signs and symptoms of digoxin toxicity include gastrointestinal signs, bradycardia, visual disturbances, and hypokalemia. A therapeutic serum digoxin level ranges from 0.5 to 2 ng/mL. The serum potassium level should be between 3.5 and 5.0 mEq/L. The apical pulse must be 60 or higher beats per minute.
Test-Taking Strategy: Focus on the subject, digoxin toxicity. Knowledge of the signs and symptoms of digoxin toxicity is needed to answer correctly. **Review:** the signs and symptoms of digoxin toxicity.
Level of Cognitive Ability: Analyzing
Client Needs: Physiological Integrity
Integrated Process: Nursing Process/Data Collection
Content Area: Pharmacology: Cardiovascular Medications
Priority Concepts: Clinical Judgment, Safety
Reference(s): deWit, Kumagai (2013), p. 439; Hodgson, Kizior (2015), p. 363.

538. 4

Rationale: The aPTT will assess the therapeutic effect of Heparin sodium. The PT and INR will assess for the therapeutic effect of warfarin sodium (Coumadin). A decreased thrombocyte count can cause bleeding.

Test-Taking Strategy: Note the subject of the question, laboratory values for heparin and Coumadin. Eliminate options 1 and 3 because these laboratory values are related to warfarin sodium (Coumadin therapy). The remaining option 2 is an unrelated test for monitoring therapeutic values of both heparin sodium and warfarin sodium (Coumadin). **Review:** therapeutic laboratory tests and values for **Heparin sodium** and **warfarin sodium (Coumadin)**.

Level of Cognitive Ability: Analyzing
Client Needs: Physiological Integrity
Integrated Process: Nursing Process/Data Collection
Content Area: Pharmacology: Cardiovascular Medications
Priority Concepts: Clotting, Perfusion
Reference(s): Lehne (2013), pp. 658–659.

539. 2

Rationale: Audible expiratory wheezes may indicate a serious adverse reaction: bronchospasm. β-Blockers may induce this reaction, particularly in clients with chronic obstructive pulmonary disease or asthma. Normal decreases in blood pressure and heart rate are expected. Insomnia is a frequent mild side effect and should be monitored.

Test-Taking Strategy: Note the subject, a potential serious complication. Eliminate options 3 and 4 because these are expected effects from the medication. Next, focusing on the subject will direct you to the correct option. **Review:** the adverse effects of **propranolol (Inderal LA)**.

Level of Cognitive Ability: Analyzing
Client Needs: Physiological Integrity
Integrated Process: Nursing Process/Data Collection
Content Area: Pharmacology: Cardiovascular Medications
Priority Concepts: Clotting, Gas Exchange
Reference(s): Hodgson, Kizior (2015), p. 1011; Lehne (2013), pp. 175–176.

540. 3

Rationale: Isosorbide mononitrate is an antianginal medication. Headache is a frequent side effect of isosorbide mononitrate and usually disappears during continued therapy. If a headache occurs during therapy, the client should be instructed to take the medication with food or meals. It is not necessary to contact the HCP unless the headaches persist with therapy. It is not appropriate to instruct the client to discontinue therapy or adjust the dosages.

Test-Taking Strategy: Focus on the subject, isosorbide mononitrate. Eliminate options 1 and 2 first because it is not within the scope of nursing practice to instruct a client to discontinue or adjust dosages. From the remaining options, recalling that the headache can be relieved with the administration of food with the medication will assist in directing you to option 3. Review: **isosorbide mononitrate**.

Level of Cognitive Ability: Applying
Client Needs: Physiological Integrity
Integrated Process: Teaching and Learning
Content Area: Pharmacology: Cardiovascular Medications
Priority Concepts: Client Education, Pain
Reference(s): Hodgson, Kizior (2015), p. 648.

541. 3

Rationale: Tissue plasminogen activator is a thrombolytic. Hemorrhage is a complication of any type of thrombolytic medication. The client is monitored for bleeding. Monitoring for renal failure and monitoring the client's psychosocial status are important but are not the most critical interventions. Heparin is given after thrombolytic therapy, but the question is not asking about follow-up medications.

Test-Taking Strategy: Note the strategic word, *priority*. Think about the action of the medication and remember that bleeding is a priority. **Review:** care of the client on tissue **plasminogen activator**.

Level of Cognitive Ability: Applying
Client Needs: Physiological Integrity
Integrated Process: Nursing Process/Implementation
Content Area: Pharmacology: Cardiovascular Medications
Priority Concepts: Clinical Judgment, Clotting
Reference(s): Lehne (2013), pp. 655, 661.

❖ **542. 3, 4, 5**

Rationale: The usual guideline for administering nitroglycerin tablets for a hospitalized client with chest pain is to administer one tablet every 5 minutes PRN for chest pain, for a total dose of three tablets. The registered nurse is notified immediately if a client complains of chest pain. In this situation, because the client is still complaining of chest pain, the nurse would administer a second nitroglycerin tablet. The nurse would assess the client's pain level and check the client's blood pressure before administering each nitroglycerin dose. There are no data in the question that indicate the need to call a code blue. In addition, it is not necessary to contact the client's family unless the client has requested this.

Test-Taking Strategy: Focus on the data in the question. Use the steps of the nursing process to determine that assessing the client's pain level and checking the client's blood pressure are appropriate actions. Next, recalling the usual guidelines for administering nitroglycerin tablets will assist in determining that an appropriate action is to administer a second nitroglycerin, 0.4 mg, sublingually. **Review:** care of the client with chest pain and the guidelines for the administration of **nitroglycerin**.

Level of Cognitive Ability: Analyzing
Client Needs: Physiological Integrity
Integrated Process: Nursing Process/Implementation
Content Area: Pharmacology: Cardiovascular Medications
Priority Concepts: Clinical Judgment, Pain
Reference(s): Hodgson, Kizior (2015), p. 860.

543. 4

Rationale: Nicotinic acid, even an over-the-counter form, should be avoided because it may lead to liver abnormalities. All lipid-lowering medications also can cause liver abnormalities, so a combination of nicotinic acid and cholestyramine resin is to be avoided. Constipation and bloating are the two most common side effects. Walking and the reduction of fats in the diet are therapeutic measures to reduce cholesterol and triglyceride levels.

Test-Taking Strategy: Note the strategic words, *need for further teaching*. These words indicate a negative event query and ask you to select an option that is an incorrect statement. Remembering that over-the-counter medications should be avoided when a client is taking a prescription medication will

direct you to the correct option. **Review:** client teaching points related to **cholestyramine (Questran)**.
Level of Cognitive Ability: Evaluating
Client Needs: Physiological Integrity
Integrated Process: Teaching and Learning
Content Area: Pharmacology: Cardiovascular Medications
Priority Concepts: Client Education, Nutrition
Reference(s): Lehne (2013), pp. 609, 616.

544. 4
Rationale: Flushing is a side effect of this medication. Aspirin or a nonsteroidal anti-inflammatory drug can be taken 30 minutes before taking the medication to decrease flushing. Alcohol consumption needs to be avoided because it will enhance this side effect. The medication should be taken with meals; this will decrease gastrointestinal upset. Taking the medication with meals has no effect on the flushing. Clay-colored stools are a sign of hepatic dysfunction and should be immediately reported to the health care provider (HCP).
Test-Taking Strategy: Focus on the **subject**, niacin and flushing. Option 1 can be eliminated because alcohol must be abstained from. Option 2 can be eliminated because taking the medication with meals helps decrease the gastrointestinal symptoms. The clay-colored stools in option 3 are a sign of hepatic dysfunction and should be immediately reported to the HCP. **Review:** the client teaching points related to **nicotinic acid (niacin)**.
Level of Cognitive Ability: Evaluating
Client Needs: Physiological Integrity
Integrated Process: Nursing Process/Evaluation
Content Area: Pharmacology: Cardiovascular Medications
Priority Concepts: Client Education, Safety
Reference(s): Lehne (2013), p. 615.

545. 3
Rationale: Thiazide diuretics such as hydrochlorothiazide are sulfa-based medications, and a client with a sulfa allergy is at risk for an allergic reaction. Also, clients are at risk for hypokalemia, hyperglycemia, hypercalcemia, hyperlipidemia, and hyperuricemia.
Test-Taking Strategy: Focus on the **subject**, hydrochlorothiazide. Recalling that thiazide diuretics carry a sulfa ring in their chemical structure will direct you to the correct option. **Review:** the nursing considerations related to administering **hydrochlorothiazide**.
Level of Cognitive Ability: Analyzing
Client Needs: Physiological Integrity
Integrated Process: Nursing Process/Data Collection
Content Area: Pharmacology: Cardiovascular Medications
Priority Concepts: Cellular Regulation, Fluid and Electrolyte Balance
Reference(s): Hodgson, Kizior (2015), pp. 572–574; Lehne (2013), pp. 486–487.

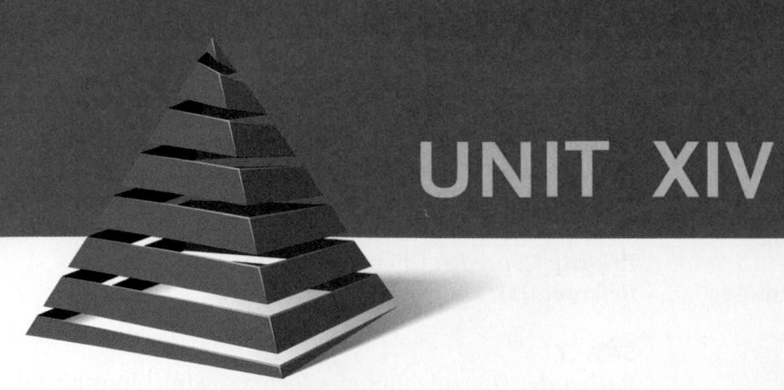

UNIT XIV

The Adult Client with a Renal Disorder

PYRAMID TERMS

acute kidney injury (AKI) The sudden loss of kidney function caused by renal cell damage from ischemia or toxic substances; occurs abruptly and can be reversible; acute kidney injury leads to hypoperfusion, cell death, and decompensation in kidney function; prognosis depends on the cause and the condition of the client; near-normal or normal kidney function may resume gradually.

anuria Urine output of less than 100 mL/day.

arterial steal syndrome A syndrome that can develop following the insertion of an arteriovenous (AV) fistula when too much blood is diverted to the vein and arterial perfusion to the hand is compromised.

azotemia The retention of nitrogenous waste products in the blood.

chronic kidney disease (CKD) The progressive loss and ongoing deterioration in kidney function. It is characterized by a glomerular filtration rate of less than 60 mL/minute for a period of 3 months or longer. It is irreversible and results in uremia or end-stage renal disease. Chronic kidney disease requires dialysis or kidney transplantation to maintain life.

dialysis A blood filtering procedure that is indicated when kidney function deteriorates and the accumulation of water and waste products interferes with life functions. Dialysis is performed via the blood stream (hemodialysis) or through the peritoneal cavity (peritoneal dialysis).

disequilibrium syndrome A rapid change in the composition of the extracellular fluid (ECF) that occurs during hemodialysis; solutes are removed from the blood faster than from the cerebrospinal fluid (CSF) and brain; fluid is pulled into the brain, causing cerebral edema.

kidney failure The loss of kidney function. The types of renal failure include acute kidney injury and chronic kidney disease. The signs and symptoms of kidney disease are caused by the retention of wastes, the retention of fluids, and the inability of the kidneys to regulate electrolytes.

nephrolithiasis The formation of kidney stones, which are formed in the renal parenchyma.

oliguria Urine output of less than 400 mL/day.

urolithiasis The formation of urinary stones or calculi. Urinary calculi are formed in the ureter.

Pyramid to Success

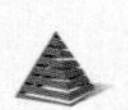

Pyramid points focus on acute kidney injury and chronic kidney disease, dialysis procedures such as hemodialysis and peritoneal dialysis, urinary diversions, and postoperative care following urinary or renal surgery. Focus on the major problems associated with renal failure and the rationale for the prescribed treatment modalities. Be familiar with the complications associated with hemodialysis and peritoneal dialysis, the specific assessment data related to complications, and the expected treatment. Focus on the care of a peritoneal catheter and hemodialysis access devices, the complications associated with these access devices, and the appropriate nursing interventions if a complication is suspected. Review preoperative and postoperative care related to renal transplantation and the assessment data indicating rejection. Be familiar with urinary diversions, care for the client with prostatectomy, and treatment measures for the client with urinary or renal calculi.

Client Needs

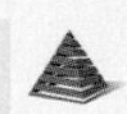

Safe and Effective Care Environment

Consulting with the RN and other members of the health care team

Establishing priorities

Maintaining asepsis related to wound care and dialysis access devices

Maintaining confidentiality related to the kidney disorder

Maintaining standard and other precautions related to care for the client
Ensuring that informed consent related to diagnostic and surgical procedures has been obtained
Preventing injury related to complications associated with the disorder
Upholding client rights

Health Promotion and Maintenance

Discussing expected body image changes
Performing data collection techniques specific to the renal system
Reinforcing client instructions regarding care of a urinary diversion, dialysis access device, and dialysis procedures
Reinforcing client instructions regarding postoperative management
Reinforcing client instructions regarding prescribed treatments related to urinary or renal disorder
Reinforcing client instructions regarding the prevention of the recurrence of a urinary and renal disorder

Psychosocial Integrity

Assisting the client to use appropriate coping mechanisms
Discussing body-image disturbances
Discussing the loss of function of a body part that occurs in clients with a kidney disorder
Identifying appropriate community resources
Identifying grief and loss, and end-of-life issues
Identifying religious and spiritual influences on health
Identifying support systems

Physiological Integrity

Assisting with care related to dialysis access devices
Assisting with care related to hemodialysis and peritoneal dialysis
Assisting with care to the client after prostatectomy
Assisting with providing comfort interventions
Assisting with providing pharmacological therapy
Assisting with providing preoperative and postoperative care related to renal transplantation
Assisting with providing treatment measures for the client with urinary or renal calculi or the client with a urinary diversion
Ensuring elimination measures
Informing the client about diagnostic tests and laboratory results
Monitoring for data indicating rejection of renal transplant
Monitoring for fluid and electrolyte and acid-base disorders
Preventing complications arising as a result of dialysis
Providing adequate rest and sleep
Reinforcing teaching the client about the prescribed nutrition and fluid measures

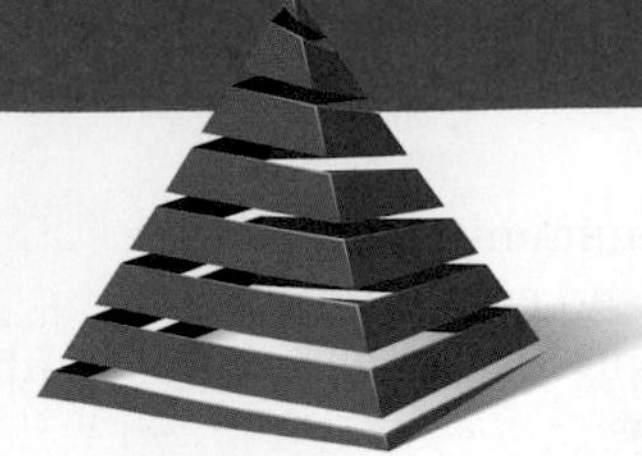

CHAPTER 53

Renal System

CRITICAL THINKING What Should You Do?

On data collection, the nurse notes that a client with glomerulonephritis has developed fine crackles in the lung bases bilaterally. What should the nurse do?
Answer located on p. 749.

I. Anatomy and Physiology

A. Kidney anatomy
  1. Each person has two kidneys; one is attached to the left abdominal wall at the level of the last thoracic and first three lumbar vertebrae and the other is on the right.
  2. The kidneys are enclosed in the renal capsule.
  3. The renal cortex is the outer layer of the renal capsule, which contains blood-filtering mechanisms (glomeruli).
  4. The renal medulla is the inner region, which contains the renal pyramids and renal tubules.
  5. Together the renal cortex, pyramids, and medulla constitute the parenchyma or functional unit of the kidneys.
  6. Nephron
    a. Located within the parenchyma
    b. Composed of glomerulus and tubules
    c. Selectively secretes and reabsorbs ions and filtrates, including fluid, wastes, electrolytes, acids, and bases

⚠ The nephrons are the functional units of the kidney.

  7. Glomerulus
    a. Each nephron contains a tuft of capillaries, which filters large plasma proteins and blood cells
    b. Blood flows into the glomerular capillaries from the afferent arteriole and flows out of the glomerular capillaries into the efferent arteriole.
  8. Bowman's capsule
    a. Thin double-walled capsule that surrounds the glomerulus
    b. Fluid and particles from the blood, such as electrolytes, glucose, amino acids, and metabolic waste (glomerular filtrate), are filtered through the glomerular membrane into a fluid-filled space in Bowman's capsule (Bowman's space) and then enter the proximal convoluted tubule (PCT).
  9. Tubules
    a. The tubules include the PCT, Henle's loop, and the distal convoluted tubule (DCT).
    b. The PCT receives filtrate from the glomerular capsule and reabsorbs water and electrolytes through active and passive transport.
    c. The descending loop of Henle passively reabsorbs water from the filtrate.
    d. The ascending loop of Henle passively reabsorbs sodium and chloride from the filtrate and helps to maintain osmolality.
    e. The DCT actively and passively removes sodium and water.
    f. The filtered fluid is converted to urine in the tubules, and then the urine moves to the pelvis of the kidney.
    g. The urine flows from the pelvis of the kidneys through the ureters and empties into the bladder.

B. Functions of kidneys
  1. Maintain acid-base balance
  2. Excrete end products of body metabolism
  3. Control fluid and electrolyte balance
  4. Excrete bacterial toxins, water-soluble drugs, and drug metabolites
  5. Secrete renin to regulate the blood pressure and erythropoietin to stimulate the bone marrow to produce red blood cells.
  6. Synthesize vitamin D for calcium absorption and regulation of the parathyroid hormones

C. Urine production
  1. As fluid flows through the tubules, water, electrolytes, and solutes are reabsorbed and other solutes such as creatinine, hydrogen ions, and potassium are secreted.
  2. Water and solutes that are not reabsorbed become urine.
  3. The process of selective reabsorption determines the amount of water and solutes to be secreted.

D. Homeostasis of water
1. The antidiuretic hormone (ADH) is primarily responsible for the reabsorption of water by the kidneys.
2. ADH is produced by the hypothalamus and secreted from the posterior lobe of the pituitary gland.
3. Secretion of ADH is stimulated by dehydration or high sodium intake and by a decrease in blood volume.
4. ADH makes the DCTs and collecting duct permeable to water.
5. Water is drawn out of the tubules by osmosis and returns to the blood. Concentrated urine remains in the tubule to be excreted.
6. When ADH is lacking, the client develops diabetes insipidus (DI).
7. Clients with DI produce large amounts of dilute urine; treatment is necessary because the client cannot drink sufficient water to survive.

E. Homeostasis of sodium
1. When the amount of sodium increases, extra water is retained to preserve osmotic pressure.
2. An increase in sodium and water produces an increase in the blood volume and blood pressure (BP).
3. When BP increases, glomerular filtration increases, and extra water and sodium are lost; blood volume is reduced, returning the BP to normal.
4. Reabsorption of sodium in the DCTs is controlled by the renin-angiotensin system.
5. Renin, an enzyme, is released from the nephron when the BP or fluid concentration in the DCT is low.
6. Renin catalyzes the splitting of angiotensin I from angiotensinogen. Angiotensin I converts to angiotensin II as blood flows through the lung.
7. Angiotensin II, a potent vasoconstrictor, stimulates the secretion of aldosterone.
8. Aldosterone stimulates the distal convoluted tubules to reabsorb sodium and secrete potassium.
9. The additional sodium increases water reabsorption and increases blood volume and BP, returning the BP to normal; the stimulus for the secretion of renin then is removed.

F. Homeostasis of potassium
1. Increase in serum potassium level stimulates the secretion of aldosterone.
2. Aldosterone stimulates the distal convoluted tubules to secrete potassium; this action returns the serum potassium concentration to normal.

G. Homeostasis of acidity (pH)
1. Blood pH is controlled by maintaining the concentration of buffer systems.
2. Carbonic acid and sodium bicarbonate form the most important buffers for neutralizing acids in the plasma.
3. The concentration of carbonic acid is controlled by the respiratory system.
4. The concentration of sodium bicarbonate is controlled by the kidneys.
5. Normal arterial pH is 7.35 to 7.45, maintained by keeping the ratio of concentrations of sodium bicarbonate to carbon dioxide constant at 20:1.
6. Strong acids are neutralized by sodium bicarbonate to produce carbonic acid and the sodium salts of the strong acid; this process quickly restores the ratio and thus blood pH.
7. The carbonic acid dissociates into carbon dioxide and water; because the concentration of carbon dioxide is maintained at a constant level by the respiratory system, the excess carbonic acid is rapidly excreted.
8. Sodium combined with the strong acid is actively reabsorbed in the DCTs in exchange for hydrogen or potassium ions. The strong acid is neutralized by ammonia and excreted as ammonia or potassium salts.

H. Adrenal glands (refer to Chapter 45 for information about the adrenal glands)
1. One adrenal gland is on top of each kidney.
2. The adrenal glands influence blood pressure and sodium and water retention

I. Bladder
1. The bladder detrusor muscle, composed of smooth muscle, distends during bladder filling and contracts during bladder emptying.
2. The ureterovesical sphincter prevents reflux of urine from the bladder to the ureter.
3. The total bladder capacity is 1 L; normal adult urine output is 1500 mL/day.

J. Prostate gland
1. The prostate gland surrounds the male urethra.
2. The prostate gland contains a duct that opens into the prostatic portion of the urethra and secretes the alkaline portion of seminal fluid, which protects passing sperm.

K. Risk factors associated with renal disorders (Box 53-1)

II. Diagnostic Tests

A. Refer to Chapter 11 for information regarding normal values for renal function studies.

B. Determination of serum creatinine level
1. Description: A test that measures the amount of creatinine in the serum; creatinine is an end-product of protein and muscle metabolism.
2. Analysis
   a. Creatinine level reflects glomerular filtration rate.

BOX 53-1 Risk Factors Associated with Kidney Disorders

Chemical or environmental toxin exposure
Contact sports
Diabetes mellitus
Family history of renal disease
Frequent urinary tract infections
Heart failure
High-sodium diet
Hypertension
Medications
Trauma
Urolithiasis or nephrolithiasis

b. Kidney disease is the only pathological condition that increases the serum creatinine level.
c. Serum creatinine level increases only when at least 50% of renal function is lost.

C. Determination of blood urea nitrogen (BUN) level
1. Description: A serum test that measures the amount of nitrogenous urea, a by-product of protein metabolism in the liver
2. Analysis
a. BUN levels indicate the extent of renal clearance of urea nitrogenous waste products.
b. An elevation does not always mean kidney disease is present.
c. Some factors that can elevate the BUN include dehydration, poor renal perfusion, intake of a high-protein diet, infection, stress, corticosteroid use, gastrointestinal (GI) bleeding, and factors that cause muscle breakdown.
d. When the BUN and serum creatinine levels increase at the same rate, the ratio of the BUN to creatinine remains constant; elevated serum creatinine and BUN levels suggest renal dysfunction.

D. Glomerular filtration rate (GFR): A blood test that checks how well the kidneys are working by estimating how much blood passes through the glomeruli every minute

E. Urinalysis
1. Description: A urine test for evaluation of the renal system and determination of renal disease
2. Interventions
a. Wash perineal area and use a clean container for collection.
b. Obtain 10 to 15 mL of the first morning voiding.
c. Refrigerated samples may alter the specific gravity.
d. If the client is menstruating, note this on the laboratory requisition form.

F. A 24-hour urine collection
1. Check with the laboratory about specific instructions for the client to follow, such as dietary or medication restrictions.
2. The client is instructed about the urine collection.
3. At the start time, the client is instructed to void and discard the sample.
4. Collect all urine at the prescribed time.
5. Keep the urine specimen on ice or refrigerated and check with the laboratory regarding adding a preservative to the specimen during collection.
6. At the end of the prescribed time, the client is instructed to empty the bladder and add that urine to the collection container.

G. Specific gravity determination
1. Description: A urine test that measures the ability of the kidneys to concentrate urine
2. Interventions
a. Specific gravity can be measured by a multiple-test dipstick method (most common method), refractometer (an instrument used in the laboratory setting), or urinometer (least accurate method).
b. Factors that interfere with an accurate reading include radiopaque contrast agents, glucose, and proteins.
c. Cold specimens may produce a false high reading.
d. Normal value is 1.016 to 1.022 (may vary depending on the laboratory).
e. An increase in specific gravity (more concentrated urine) occurs with insufficient fluid intake, decreased renal perfusion, or increased ADH.
f. A decrease in specific gravity (less concentrated urine) occurs with increased fluid intake or diabetes insipidus; it may also indicate renal disease or the kidneys' inability to concentrate urine.

H. Urine culture and sensitivity testing
1. Description: A urine test that identifies the presence of microorganisms (culture) and determines the specific antibiotics to treat the existing microorganism (sensitivity) appropriately
2. Interventions
a. Clean the perineal area and urinary meatus with a bacteriostatic solution.
b. Collect the midstream sample in a sterile container.
c. Send the collected specimen to the laboratory immediately.
d. Identify any sources of potential contaminants during the collection of the specimen, such as the hands, skin, clothing, hair, or vaginal or rectal secretions.
e. Urine from the client who drank a very large amount of fluids may be too dilute to provide a positive culture.

I. Creatinine clearance test

1. Description

a. The creatinine clearance test evaluates how well the kidneys remove creatinine from the blood.

b. The test includes obtaining a blood sample and timed urine specimens.

c. Blood is drawn at the start of the test and when the urine specimen collection is complete.

d. The urine specimen for the creatinine clearance is usually collected for 24 hours, but shorter periods (8 or 12 hours) could be prescribed.

The creatinine clearance test provides the best estimate of the glomerular filtration rate (GFR); the normal GFR is 125 mL/min.

2. Interventions

a. Encourage fluids before and during the test.

b. Reinforce instructions to the client to avoid caffeinated beverages during testing.

c. Check with the health care provider (HCP) regarding the administration of any prescribed medications during testing.

d. Reinforce instructions to the client about the urine collection.

e. At the start time, ask the client to void (or empty the tubing and drainage bag if the client has an indwelling urinary catheter) and discard the first sample.

f. Collect all urine for the prescribed time.

g. Keep the urine specimen on ice or refrigerated and check with the laboratory regarding adding a preservative to the specimen during collection.

h. At the end of the prescribed time, ask the client to empty the bladder (or empty the tubing and drainage bag if the client has an indwelling urinary catheter catheter) and add that urine to the collection container.

i. Send the labeled urine specimen to the laboratory in a biohazard bag along with the requisition.

j. Document specimen collection, time started and completed, and other pertinent data.

J. Uric acid test

1. Description: A 24-hour urine collection sample is tested to diagnose gout and kidney disease

2. Interventions

a. Encourage fluid intake and a regular diet during testing.

b. Follow the same procedure for urine collection as with the creatinine clearance test.

K. Vanillylmandelic acid (VMA) test

1. Description

a. The test is a 24-hour urine collection to diagnose pheochromocytoma, a tumor of the adrenal gland.

b. The test determines catecholamine levels in the urine.

2. Interventions

a. Check with the laboratory regarding medication restrictions.

b. Reinforce instructions to the client to avoid foods such as caffeine, cocoa, vanilla, cheese, gelatin, licorice, and fruits for at least 2 days before and during urine collection and to check with the HCP regarding the administration of any prescribed medications before or during testing.

c. Reinforce instructions to the client to avoid stress and encourage adequate food and fluid intake during the test.

d. Follow the same procedure for urine collection as with the creatinine clearance test.

L. KUB (kidneys, ureters, and bladder) radiography

1. Description: An x-ray film of the urinary system and adjacent structures used to detect urinary calculi

2. Interventions: No specific preparation is necessary.

M. Bladder ultrasonography (bladder scanning)

1. Bladder ultrasonography is a noninvasive method for measuring the volume of urine in the bladder.

2. Bladder ultrasonography may be performed to evaluate urinary frequency, inability to urinate, or residual urine (the amount of urine remaining in the bladder after voiding).

N. Computed tomography (CT) and magnetic resonance imaging (MRI)

1. Description: These imaging methods provide cross-sectional views of the kidney and urinary tract.

2. Interventions (see Chapter 57)

O. Intravenous urography

1. Description: An x-ray procedure in which an intravenous injection of a radiopaque dye is used to visualize and identify abnormalities in the renal system

2. Preprocedure interventions

a. Ensure an informed consent has been obtained.

b. Check the client for allergies to iodine, seafood, and radiopaque dyes.

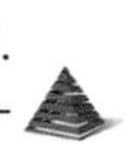

c. Withhold food and fluids after midnight on the night before the test.

d. Administer laxatives if prescribed.

e. Inform the client about possible throat irritation, flushing of the face, warmth, or a salty or metallic taste during the test.

3. Postprocedure interventions

a. Monitor vital signs.

b. Reinforce instructions to the client to drink at least 1 L of fluid unless contraindicated.

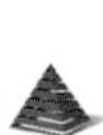

c. Monitor the venipuncture site for bleeding.
d. Monitor urinary output.
e. Monitor for signs of a possible allergic reaction to the dye used during the test, and instruct the client to notify the HCP if any signs of an allergic reaction occur.
f. Contrast dye is potentially damaging to kidneys; the risk is greater in older clients and those experiencing dehydration.

The dye used in a renal angiography may be nephrotoxic; therefore, encourage increased fluids unless contraindicated, and monitor urinary output.

P. Renography (Kidney scan)
1. Description: An intravenous (IV) injection of a radioisotope for visual imaging of renal blood flow, glomerular filtration, tubular function, and excretion
2. Preprocedure interventions
a. Ensure an informed consent has been obtained.
b. Check for allergies.
c. Inform the client that the test requires no dietary or activity restrictions.
d. Assist with administering the radioisotope as necessary.
e. Reinforce instructions to the client to remain motionless during the test.
f. Reinforce instructions to the client that imaging may be repeated at various intervals before the test is complete.
3. Postprocedure interventions
a. Encourage fluid intake unless contraindicated.
b. Monitor the client for signs of delayed allergic reaction such as itching and hives.
c. The radioactivity is eliminated in 24 hours; wear gloves for excretion precautions.
d. Follow standard precautions when caring for incontinent clients and double-bag client linens per agency policy.

Q. Cystoscopy and biopsy of the bladder
1. Description: The bladder mucosa is examined for inflammation, calculi, or tumors by means of a cystoscope; a sample for biopsy may be obtained.
2. Preprocedure interventions
a. Ensure an informed consent has been obtained.
b. If a biopsy is planned, withhold food and fluids after midnight the night before the test.
c. If a cystoscopy alone is planned, no special preparation is necessary, and the procedure may be performed in the HCP's office; postprocedure interventions include increasing fluid intake.
3. Postprocedure interventions following biopsy
a. Monitor the vital signs.
b. Increase fluid intake as prescribed.
c. Monitor intake and output.
d. Encourage deep-breathing exercises to relieve bladder spasms.
e. Administer analgesics as prescribed.
f. Administer sitz baths for back and abdominal pain.
g. Note that leg cramps are common because of the lithotomy position maintained during the procedure.
h. Monitor the urine for color and consistency.
i. Reinforce instructions to the client that burning on urination, pink-tinged or tea-colored urine, and urinary frequency are common after cystoscopy and resolve in a few days.
j. Monitor for bright red urine or clots, and notify the registered nurse (RN) or HCP if a fever (with or without chills) occurs; an increase in white blood cell (WBC) count suggests infection.

R. Renal biopsy
1. Description: Insertion of a needle into the kidney to obtain a sample of tissue for examination; usually done percutaneously
2. Preprocedure interventions
a. Check vital signs.
b. Check baseline coagulation studies. The HCP is notified if abnormal results are noted.
c. Ensure an informed consent has been obtained.
d. Withhold food and fluids 4 to 6 hours before the procedure.
3. Interventions during the procedure: Position the client prone with a pillow under the abdomen and shoulders.
4. Postprocedure interventions
a. Monitor vital signs, especially for hypotension and tachycardia, which could indicate bleeding.

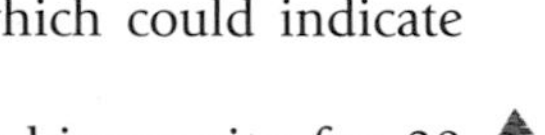

b. Provide pressure to the biopsy site for 30 minutes.
c. Monitor the hemoglobin and hematocrit levels for decreases, which could indicate bleeding.

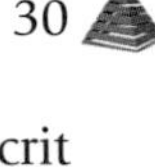
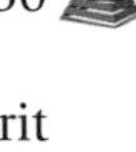

d. Place the client on strict bed rest in the supine position, as prescribed, with a back roll for additional support for 2 to 6 hours after the biopsy.

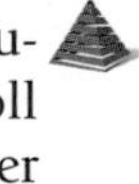
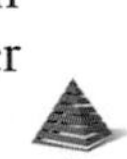

e. Check the biopsy site and under the client for bleeding.
f. Encourage fluid intake of 1500 to 2000 mL as prescribed.
g. Observe the urine for gross and microscopic bleeding.
h. Reinforce instructions to the client to avoid heavy lifting and strenuous activity for 2 weeks.

i. Reinforce instructions to the client to notify the health care provider if either a temperature greater than 100 degrees or hematuria occurs after the first 24 hours postprocedure.

III. Acute Kidney Injury

A. Description

1. **Acute kidney injury (AKI)** is the rapid loss of kidney function from renal cell damage.
2. This occurs abruptly and can be reversible.
3. AKI leads to cell hypoperfusion, cell death, and decompensation of renal function.
4. The prognosis depends on the cause and the condition of the client.
5. Near-normal or normal kidney function may resume gradually.

B. Causes

1. Prerenal: Outside the kidney; caused by intravascular volume depletion, dehydration, decreased cardiac output, decreased peripheral vascular resistance, decreased renovascular blood flow, and prerenal infection or obstruction.
2. Intrarenal: Within the parenchyma of the kidney; caused by tubular necrosis, prolonged prerenal ischemia, intrarenal infection or obstruction, and nephrotoxicity
3. Postrenal: Between the kidney and urethral meatus, such as bladder neck obstruction, bladder cancer, calculi, and postrenal infection

C. Phases of AKI and interventions (Box 53-2)

1. Onset: Begins with precipitating event
2. Oliguric phase
    - **a.** For some clients, **oliguria** does not occur and the urine output is normal; otherwise, the duration of oliguria is 8 to 15 days; the longer the duration, the less chance of recovery.

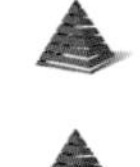

    - **b.** Sudden decrease in urine output. Urine output is less than 400 mL/day.

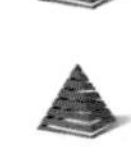

    - **c.** Signs of excess fluid volume: hypertension, edema, pleural and pericardial effusions, dysrhythmias, heart failure (HF), and pulmonary edema
    - **d.** Signs of **uremia**: anorexia, nausea, vomiting, and pruritus
    - **e.** Signs of metabolic acidosis: Kussmaul's respirations
    - **f.** Signs of neurological changes: tingling of extremities, drowsiness progressing to disorientation, and then coma

    - **g.** Signs of pericarditis: friction rub, chest pain with inspiration, and low-grade fever

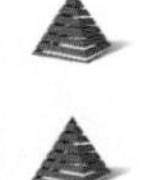

    - **h.** Laboratory analysis (see Box 53-2)
    - **i.** Fluid intake may be restricted. If hypertension is present, daily fluid allowances may be 400 mL to 1000 mL plus the measured urinary output.

BOX 53-2 Acute Kidney Injury: Phases and Laboratory Findings

Onset

Begins with precipitating event

Oliguric Phase

Elevated blood urea nitrogen and serum creatinine
Decreased urine specific gravity (prerenal causes) or normal (intrarenal causes)
Decreased glomerular filtration rate
Hyperkalemia
Normal or decreased serum sodium
Hypervolemia
Hypocalcemia
Hyperphosphatemia

Diuretic Phase

Gradual decline in blood urea nitrogen and serum creatinine, but still elevated
Low creatinine clearance
Hypokalemia
Hyponatremia
Hypovolemia

Recovery Phase (Convalescent)

Increased glomerular filtration rate
Stabilization or continual decline in blood urea nitrogen and serum creatinine levels toward normal
Complete recovery may take 1 to 2 years

    - **j.** Assist to administer medications as prescribed such as diuretics (furosemide [Lasix]) to increase renal blood flow and diuresis.
3. Diuretic phase
    - **a.** Urine output rises slowly, followed by diuresis (4 to 5 L/day).
    - **b.** Excessive urine output indicates that damaged nephrons are recovering their ability to excrete wastes.
    - **c.** Dehydration, hypovolemia, hypotension, and tachycardia can occur.
    - **d.** Level of consciousness improves
    - **e.** Laboratory analysis (see Box 53-2)
    - **f.** IV fluids may be prescribed, which may contain electrolytes to replace losses.
4. Recovery phase (convalescent)
    - **a.** Recovery is a slow process. Complete recovery may take 1 to 2 years.
    - **b.** Urine volume returns to normal.
    - **c.** Memory improves.
    - **d.** Strength increases.
    - **e.** The older adult is less likely than a younger adult to regain full kidney function.
    - **f.** Laboratory analysis (see Box 53-2)
    - **g.** AKI can progress to chronic kidney disease (CKD).

The signs and symptoms of acute kidney injury are primarily caused by the retention of nitrogenous wastes, the retention of fluids, and the inability of the kidneys to regulate electrolytes.

D. Data collection: Obtain objective and subjective data noted in the phases of AKI (see Box 53-2).

E. Other interventions

1. Monitor vital signs, especially for signs of hypertension, tachycardia, tachypnea, and an irregular heart rate.
2. Monitor intake and output (hourly in AKI) and urine color and characteristics.
3. Monitor daily weight (same scale, same clothes, same time of the day), noting that an increase of to 1 lb daily indicates fluid retention.
4. BUN, serum creatinine, and serum electrolyte values are monitored for changes.
5. Acidosis can occur, which may be treated with sodium bicarbonate.
6. Monitor urinalysis for protein level, hematuria, casts, and specific gravity.
7. Monitor for altered level of consciousness caused by uremia.
8. Monitor for signs of infection because the client may not exhibit an elevated temperature or an increased white blood cell count.
9. Monitor the lungs for adventitious sounds and monitor for edema, which can indicate fluid overload.
10. Administer prescribed diet, which is usually a low- to moderate-protein (to decrease the workload on the kidneys) and a high-carbohydrate diet.
11. Restrict potassium and sodium intake as prescribed based on the electrolyte level.
12. Assist to administer medications as prescribed. Be alert to the mechanism for metabolism and excretion of all prescribed medications.
13. Be alert to nephrotoxic medications, which may be prescribed.
14. Be alert to the HCP's adjustment of medication dosages for kidney injury.
15. Assist to prepare the client for dialysis if prescribed. Continuous renal replacement therapy may be used in AKI to treat fluid volume overload or rapidly developing azotemia and metabolic acidosis.
16. Provide emotional support by allowing opportunities for the client to express concerns and fears and encouraging family interactions.
17. Promote consistency in caregivers.
18. Also refer to the Section IV, E in this chapter (Special Problems in Kidney Disease and Interventions).

IV. Chronic Kidney Disease

A. Description

1. Chronic Kidney Disease (CKD) is a slow, progressive, irreversible loss in kidney function with a GFR less than or equal to 60 mL/min for 3 months or longer.
2. Occurs in stages and results in uremia or end-stage kidney disease (Table 53-1)
3. Hypervolemia can occur because of the kidneys' inability to excrete sodium and water, or hypovolemia can occur because of the kidneys' inability to conserve sodium and water.

Chronic kidney disease affects all major body systems and requires dialysis or kidney transplantation to maintain life.

B. Primary causes

1. May follow AKI
2. Diabetes mellitus and other metabolic disorders
3. Hypertension
4. Chronic urinary obstruction
5. Recurrent infections
6. Renal artery occlusion
7. Autoimmune disorders

C. Data collection

1. Monitor body systems for the manifestations of CKD (Box 53-3).
2. Monitor psychological changes, which could include emotional lability, withdrawal, depression, anxiety, suicidal behavior, denial, dependence/independence conflict, and changes in body image.

D. Interventions

1. Same as the interventions for AKI
2. Administer prescribed diet, which is usually a moderate-protein (to decrease the workload on the kidneys) and a high-carbohydrate, low-potassium, and low-phosphorus diet.
3. Provide oral care to prevent stomatitis and reduce discomfort from mouth sores.
4. Provide skin care to prevent pruritus.

TABLE 53-1 Progression of Chronic Kidney Disease

Signs of CKD	Estimated GFR
At risk; normal kidney function (early kidney disease may or may not be present)	>90 mL/min
Mild CKD	60–89 mL/min
Moderate CKD	30–59 mL/min
Severe CKD	15–29 mL/min
ESKD	<15 mL/min

CKD, Chronic kidney disease; *ESKD*, end-stage kidney disease; *GFR*, glomerular filtration rate.

From Ignatavicius D, Workman M: *Medical-surgical nursing: Patient-centered collaborative care*, ed 7, St. Louis, 2013, Saunders.

BOX 53-3 Essential Features of Chronic Kidney Disease

Neurological Signs and Symptoms

- Lethargy and daytime drowsiness
- Inability to concentrate or decreased attention span
- Seizures
- Coma
- Slurred speech
- Asterixis
- Tremors, twitching, or jerky movements
- Myoclonus
- Ataxia (alteration in gait)
- Paresthesias

Cardiovascular Signs and Symptoms

- Cardiomyopathy
- Hypertension
- Peripheral edema
- Heart failure
- Uremic pericarditis
- Pericardial effusion
- Pericardial friction rub
- Cardiac tamponade

Respiratory Signs and Symptoms

- Uremic halitosis
- Tachypnea
- Deep sighing, yawning
- Kussmaul respirations
- Uremic pneumonitis
- Shortness of breath
- Pulmonary edema
- Pleural effusion
- Depressed cough reflex
- Crackles

Hematological Signs and Symptoms

- Anemia
- Abnormal bleeding and bruising

Gastrointestinal Signs and Symptoms

- Anorexia
- Nausea
- Vomiting
- Metallic taste in mouth
- Changes in taste acuity and sensation
- Uremic colitis (diarrhea)
- Constipation
- Uremic gastritis (possible gastrointestinal bleeding)
- Uremic fetor
- Stomatitis
- Diarrhea

Urinary Signs and Symptoms

- Polyuria, nocturia (early)
- Oliguria, anuria (later)
- Proteinuria
- Hematuria
- Diluted, strawlike appearance

Integumentary Signs and Symptoms

- Decreased skin turgor
- Yellow-gray pallor
- Dry skin
- Pruritus
- Ecchymosis
- Purpura
- Soft tissue calcifications
- Uremic frost (late, premorbid)

Musculoskeletal Signs and Symptoms

- Muscle weakness and cramping
- Bone pain
- Pathological fractures
- Renal osteodystrophy

Reproductive Signs and Symptoms

- Decreased fertility
- Infrequent or absent menses
- Decreased libido
- Impotence

From Ignatavicius D, Workman M: *Medical-surgical nursing: Patient-centered collaborative care*, ed 7, St. Louis, 2013, Saunders.

5. Teach the client about fluid and dietary restrictions and the importance of daily weights.
6. Provide support to promote acceptance of the chronic illness and prepare the client for long-term dialysis and transplantation or explain to the client about his or her choice to decline **dialysis** or transplantation.

E. Special problems in kidney disease and interventions
1. Activity intolerance and insomnia
   a. Fatigue results from anemia and the buildup of wastes from the diseased kidneys.
   b. Provide adequate rest periods.
   c. Teach the client to plan activities to avoid fatigue.
   d. Assist to administer mild central nervous system (CNS) depressants as prescribed to promote rest.
2. Anemia
   a. Anemia results from the decreased secretion of erythropoietin by damaged nephrons, resulting in decreased production of red blood cells.
   b. Monitor for decreased hemoglobin and hematocrit levels.
   c. Assist to administer epoetin alfa (Epogen, Procrit) or darbepoetin alfa (Aranesp), or hematopoietics, as prescribed to stimulate the production of red blood cells. 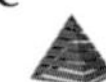

d. Assist to administer folic acid (vitamin B_9) as prescribed.
e. Assist to administer iron orally as prescribed, but not at the same time as phosphate binders.
f. Assist to administer stool softeners as prescribed because of the constipating effects of iron.
g. Note that oral iron is not well absorbed by the gastrointestinal tract in chronic kidney disease and causes nausea and vomiting. Parenteral iron (iron sucrose [Venofer] or sodium ferric gluconate complex [Ferrlecit]) may be used if iron deficiencies persist despite folic acid or oral iron administration.
h. Assist to administer blood transfusions if prescribed. Blood transfusions are prescribed only when necessary (acute blood loss, symptomatic anemia) because they decrease the stimulus to produce red blood cells; note that certain clients (e.g. Jehovah's Witness) may refuse blood and blood products because of their religious beliefs
i. Blood transfusions also cause the development of antibodies against human tissues, which can make matching for organ transplantation difficult.

3. Gastrointestinal bleeding
a. Urea is broken down by the intestinal bacteria to ammonia. Ammonia irritates the gastrointestinal mucosa, causing ulceration and bleeding.
b. Monitor for decreasing hemoglobin and hematocrit levels.
c. Monitor stools for occult blood.
d. Reinforce instructions to the client to use a soft toothbrush.
e. Avoid the administration of acetylsalicylic acid (aspirin) because it is excreted by the kidneys. If administered, aspirin toxicity can occur and prolong the bleeding time.

4. Hyperkalemia
a. Monitor vital signs for hypertension or hypotension and the apical heart rate. An irregular heart rate could indicate dysrhythmias.
b. Monitor the serum potassium level. An elevated serum potassium level can cause tall peaked T waves, flat P waves, a widened QRS complex, and a prolonged PR interval; decreased cardiac output; heart blocks; fibrillation; or asystole (Fig. 53-1).
c. Provide a low-potassium diet, avoiding foods high in potassium. (See Chapter 9 for a listing of foods that are high in potassium.)
d. Assist to administer electrolyte-binding and -excreting medications such as oral or rectal sodium polystyrene sulfonate (Kayexalate) as prescribed to lower the serum potassium level.

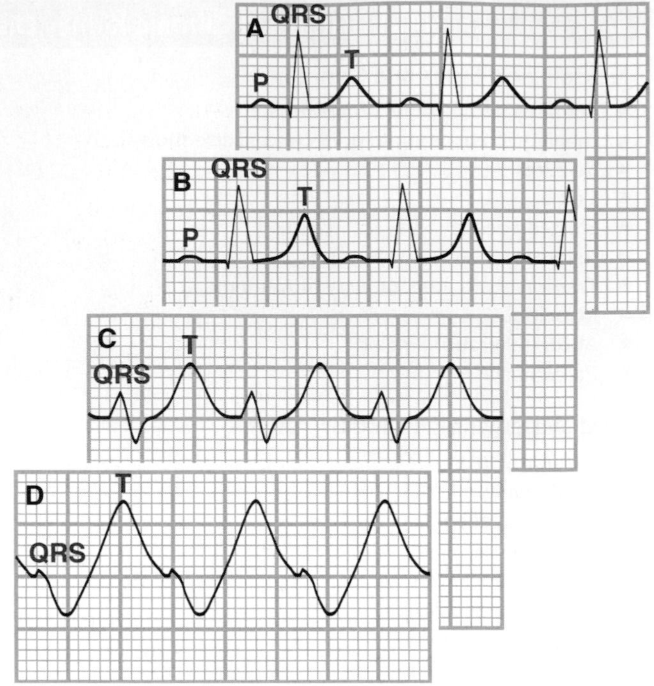

FIGURE 53-1 Cardiac rhythm changes with hyperkalemia. (From Huszar RJ: *Basic dysrhythmias: Interpretation & management*, ed 3, St. Louis, 2007, Mosby.)

e. Assist to administer prescribed medications: 50% dextrose and insulin may be prescribed to shift potassium into the cell. Calcium gluconate IV may be prescribed to reduce myocardial irritability from hyperkalemia, and sodium bicarbonate IV may be prescribed to correct acidosis.
f. Assist to administer prescribed loop diuretics to excrete potassium.
g. Avoid potassium-retaining medications such as spironolactone (Aldactone) and triamterene (Dyrenium), because these medications will increase the potassium level.
h. Assist to prepare the client for peritoneal **dialysis** or hemodialysis as prescribed.

Place the client with kidney disease on continuous cardiac monitoring. The client can develop hyperkalemia and is at risk for dysrhythmias.

5. Hypermagnesemia
a. Results from decreased renal excretion of magnesium.
b. Monitor cardiac manifestations of bradycardia, peripheral vasodilation, and hypotension.

c. Monitor CNS manifestations of decreased nerve impulse transmission such as drowsiness or lethargy.
d. Monitor neuromuscular manifestations such as reduced or absent deep tendon reflexes or weak or absent voluntary skeletal muscle contractions.
e. Assist to administer loop diuretics as prescribed such as furosemide (Lasix).
f. Assist to administer calcium as prescribed for resulting cardiac problems.
g. Avoid medications that contain magnesium such as antacids, laxatives, or enemas.
h. During severe elevations, avoid foods that increase magnesium levels. (See Chapter 9 for a listing of foods that are high in magnesium.)

6. Hyperphosphatemia
a. As the phosphorus level rises, the calcium level drops; this leads to the stimulation of parathyroid hormone, causing bone demineralization.
b. Treatment is aimed at lowering the serum phosphorus levels.
c. Assist to administer phosphate binders as prescribed with meals to lower serum phosphate levels.
d. Avoid the use of aluminum hydroxide preparations to bind phosphates because they are associated with dementia and osteomalacia.
e. Administer stool softeners and laxatives as prescribed because phosphate binders are constipating.
f. Reinforce teaching the client about the need to limit the intake of foods high in phosphorus. (See Chapter 9 for a listing of foods that are high in phosphorus.)

7. Hypertension
a. Caused by failure of the kidneys to maintain BP homeostasis
b. Monitor vital signs for elevated blood pressure.
c. Maintain fluid and sodium restrictions as prescribed.
d. Assist to administer diuretics and antihypertensives as prescribed.
e. Assist to administer propranolol (Inderal)—a β-blocker—as prescribed. Propranolol decreases renin release (renin causes vasoconstriction and subsequent hypertension).

8. Hypervolemia
a. Monitor vital signs for an elevated blood pressure.
b. Monitor intake and output and daily weight for indications of fluid retention.
c. Monitor for periorbital, sacral, and peripheral edema.
d. Monitor the serum electrolyte levels.
e. Monitor for hypertension, and notify the HCP for sustained elevations.
f. Monitor for signs of heart failure and pulmonary edema such as restlessness, heightened anxiety, tachycardia, dyspnea, basilar lung crackles, and blood-tinged sputum. Notify the RN immediately if signs occur. 
g. Maintain fluid restriction.
h. Avoid the administration of large amounts of IV fluids.
i. Assist to administer diuretics such as furosemide (Lasix) as prescribed.
j. Reinforce teaching the client to maintain a low-sodium diet.
k. Reinforce teaching the client to avoid antacids or cold remedies containing sodium bicarbonate.

9. Hypocalcemia
a. Results from the high phosphorus level and the inability of the diseased kidney to activate vitamin D
b. The absence of vitamin D causes poor calcium absorption from the intestinal tract.
c. Monitor the serum calcium level.
d. Administer calcium supplements as prescribed.
e. Administer activated vitamin D as prescribed.
f. See Chapter 9 for a listing of foods that are high in calcium.

10. Hypovolemia
a. Monitor vital signs for hypotension and tachycardia.
b. Monitor for decreasing intake and output and a reduction in the daily weight.
c. Monitor for dehydration.
d. Monitor the electrolyte levels.
e. Assist to administer replacement therapy based on the serum electrolyte level.
f. Assist to administer sodium supplements as prescribed, based on the serum electrolyte value.

11. Infection
a. The client is at risk for infection caused by a suppressed immune system, dialysis access site, and possible malnutrition.
b. Monitor for signs of infection.
c. Avoid urinary catheters when possible; if used, provide catheter care.
d. Provide strict asepsis during urinary catheter insertion and other invasive procedures.
e. Reinforce instructions to the client to avoid fatigue, which decreases body resistance.
f. Reinforce instructions to the client to avoid persons with infections.
g. Assist to administer antibiotics as prescribed, monitoring for nephrotoxic effects.

12. Metabolic acidosis
a. The kidneys are unable to excrete hydrogen ions or manufacture bicarbonate, resulting in acidosis.

b. Assist to administer alkalizers such as sodium bicarbonate as prescribed.
c. Note that clients with CKD adjust to low bicarbonate levels and do not become acutely ill.

13. Muscle cramps
    a. Occur from electrolyte imbalances and the effects of uremia on peripheral nerves
    b. Monitor the serum electrolytes.
    c. Assist to administer electrolyte replacements and medications to control muscle cramps as prescribed.
    d. Administer heat and massage as prescribed.
14. Neurological changes
    a. The buildup of active particles and fluids causes changes in the brain cells and leads to confusion and impairment in decision-making ability.
    b. Peripheral neuropathy results from the effects of uremia on peripheral nerves.
    c. Monitor the level of consciousness and for confusion.
    d. Monitor for restless leg syndrome, which is also common during dialysis treatments.
    e. Reinforce teaching the client to examine areas of decreased sensation for signs of injury.
15. Ocular irritation
    a. Calcium deposits in the conjunctiva cause burning and watering of the eyes.
    b. Assist to administer medications to control the calcium and phosphate levels as prescribed.
    c. Administer lubricating eye drops.
    d. Protect the client from injury.
    e. Provide a safe and hazard-free environment.
    f. Use side rails as needed.
16. Potential for injury
    a. The client is at risk for fractures caused by alterations in the absorption of calcium, excretion of phosphate, and altered vitamin D metabolism.
    b. Provide for a safe environment.
    c. Avoid injury; tissue breakdown causes increased serum potassium levels.
17. Pruritus
    a. To rid the body of excess wastes, urate crystals are excreted through the skin, causing pruritus.
    b. The deposit of urate crystals (uremic frost) occurs in advanced stages of kidney failure.
    c. Monitor for skin breakdown, rash, and uremic frost.
    d. Provide meticulous skin care and oral hygiene.
    e. Avoid the use of soaps.
    f. Assist to administer antihistamines and antipruritics as prescribed to relieve itching.
    g. Reinforce teaching the client to keep the nails trimmed to prevent local infection from scratching.
18. Psychosocial problems
    a. Listen to the client's concerns to determine how the client is handling the situation.
    b. Allow the client time to mourn the loss of kidney function.
    c. With the client's permission, include the family members in discussions of the client's concerns.
    d. Reinforce education about treatment options and support their decision.
    e. Offer information about support groups.
    f. Provide end-of-life care for the client with end-stage kidney disease.

V. Uremic Syndrome

A. Description
1. The accumulation of nitrogenous waste products in the blood caused by the kidneys' inability to filter out these waste products.
2. Uremic syndrome may occur as a result of AKI or CKD.

B. Data collection
1. Oliguria
2. The presence of protein, red blood cells, and casts in the urine
3. Elevated levels of urea, uric acid, potassium, and magnesium in the urine
4. Hypotension or hypertension
5. Alterations in the level of consciousness
6. Electrolyte imbalances
7. Stomatitis
8. Nausea or vomiting
9. Diarrhea or constipation

C. Interventions
1. Monitor vital signs for hypertension, tachycardia, and an irregular heart rate.
2. Monitor serum electrolyte levels.
3. Monitor intake and output and for oliguria.
4. Provide a limited, but high-quality, protein diet as prescribed.
5. Provide a limited sodium, nitrogen, potassium, and phosphate diet as prescribed.
6. Assist the client to cope with body-image disturbances caused by uremic syndrome. 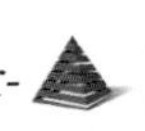

VI. Hemodialysis

A. Description
1. Hemodialysis is the process of cleansing the client's blood.
2. It involves the diffusion of dissolved particles from one fluid compartment into another across a semipermeable membrane. The client's blood flows through one fluid compartment of a dialysis filter, and the dialysate is in another fluid compartment.

B. Functions of hemodialysis
1. Cleanses the blood of accumulated waste products

2. Removes the by-products of protein metabolism such as urea, creatinine, and uric acid from the blood
3. Removes excess body fluids
4. Maintains or restores the buffer system of the body
5. Maintains or restores electrolyte levels in the body

C. Principles of hemodialysis
1. The semipermeable membrane is made of thin, porous cellophane.
2. The pore size of the membrane allows small particles to pass through, such as urea, creatinine, uric acid, and water molecules.
3. Proteins, bacteria, and some blood cells are too large to pass through the membrane.
4. The client's blood flows into the dialyzer. The movement of substances occurs from the blood to the dialysate by the principles of osmosis and diffusion.
5. Diffusion is the movement of particles from an area of greater concentration to one of lower concentration.
6. Osmosis is the movement of fluids across a semipermeable membrane from an area of lower concentration of particles to an area of higher concentration of particles.
7. Ultrafiltration is the movement of fluid across a semipermeable membrane as a result of an artificially created pressure gradient.

D. Dialysate bath
1. A dialysate bath is composed of water and major electrolytes
2. Dialysate need not be sterile because bacteria and viruses are too large to pass through the pores of the semipermeable membrane; however, the dialysate must meet specific standards, and water is treated to ensure a safe water supply.

E. Interventions
1. Monitor vital signs before, during, and after dialysis; the client's temperature may elevate because of slight warming of the blood from the dialysis machine. (Notify the RN, who will notify the HCP, about excessive temperature elevations because this could indicate sepsis; assist to obtain samples for blood culture as prescribed for excessive temperature elevations.)
2. Monitor laboratory values before, during, and after dialysis.
3. Monitor the client for fluid overload before dialysis and fluid volume deficit after dialysis.
4. Weigh the client before and after dialysis to determine fluid loss.
5. Monitor the patency of the blood access device before, during, and after dialysis.
6. Monitor for bleeding. Heparin is added to the dialysis bath to prevent clots from forming within the dialyzer or the blood tubing.
7. Monitor for hypovolemia and shock during dialysis, which can occur from blood loss or excess fluid and electrolyte removal.
8. Provide adequate nutrition. The client may eat before or during dialysis.
9. Identify the client's reactions to the treatment and support coping mechanisms. Encourage independence and involvement in care.

Withhold antihypertensives and other medications that can affect the blood pressure or result in hypotension until after the hemodialysis treatment. Also withhold medications that could be removed by dialysis, such as water-soluble vitamins, certain antibiotics, and digoxin (Lanoxin).

VII. Access for Hemodialysis

A. Subclavian and femoral catheter
1. Description
   a. A subclavian (subclavian vein) or femoral (femoral vein) catheter may be inserted for short-term or temporary use in AKI.
   b. The catheter is used until a fistula or graft matures or develops, which is typically 6 weeks, or may be required when the client's fistula or graft access has failed because of infection or clotting.
2. Interventions
   a. Monitor the insertion site for hematoma, bleeding, catheter dislodgement, and infection.
   b. These catheters should only be used for dialysis treatments.

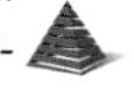
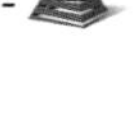
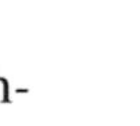
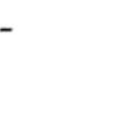

   c. Maintain an occlusive dressing over the catheter insertion site.
3. Subclavian vein catheter
   a. The catheter is usually filled with heparin and capped to maintain patency between dialysis treatments.
   b. The catheter should not be uncapped except for dialysis treatments.
   c. The catheter may be left in place for up to 6 weeks if no complications occur.
4. Femoral vein catheter
   a. Monitor the extremity for circulation, temperature, and pulses.
   b. Prevent pulling or disconnecting of the catheter when giving care.
   c. Because the groin is not a clean site, meticulous perineal care is required.
   d. Use an IV infusion pump or controller with microdrip tubing if a heparin infusion through the catheter to maintain patency is prescribed.

The client with a femoral vein catheter should not sit up more than 45 degrees or lean forward, because the catheter may kink and occlude.

B. External arteriovenous shunt

1. Description

a. Two Silastic cannulas are surgically inserted into an artery and a vein in the forearm or the leg to form an external blood path.

b. The cannulas are connected to form a U shape. Blood flows from the client's artery through the shunt into the vein.

c. A tube leading to the membrane compartment of the dialyzer is connected to the arterial cannula.

d. Blood fills the membrane compartment, passes through the dialyzer, and is returned back to the client through a tube connected to the venous cannula.

e. When dialysis is complete, the cannulas are clamped and reattached, reforming the U shape.

2. Advantages

a. The external arteriovenous shunt can be used immediately after its creation.

b. No venipuncture is necessary for dialysis.

3. Disadvantages

a. Disconnection or dislodgment of the external shunt

b. Risk of hemorrhage, infection, or clotting

c. Potential for skin erosion around the catheter site

4. Interventions

a. Avoid getting the shunt wet.

b. A dressing is wrapped completely around the shunt to keep it dry and intact.

c. Keep cannula clamps at the client's bedside or attached to the arteriovenous dressing for use in the event of accidental disconnection.

d. Reinforce teaching the client that the shunt extremity should not be used for monitoring BP, drawing blood, placing IV lines, or administering injections.

e. Fold back the dressing to expose the shunt tubing and check for signs of hemorrhage, infection, or clotting.

f. Monitor skin integrity around the insertion site.

g. Auscultate for a bruit and palpate for a thrill, although a bruit may not be heard with the shunt.

h. Notify the RN immediately, who will notify the HCP, if signs of clotting, hemorrhage, or infection occur.

5. Signs of clotting

a. Fibrin-white flecks in the tubing

b. Separation of serum and cells

c. Absence of a previously heard bruit; thrill absent on palpation

d. Coolness of the tubing or extremity

e. Tingling sensation at site or in extremity

C. Internal arteriovenous fistula (Fig. 53-2)

1. Description

a. A permanent access of choice for the client with CKD requiring dialysis

b. The fistula is created surgically by anastomosis of a large artery and a large vein in the arm.

c. The flow of arterial blood into the venous system causes the vein to become engorged (matured or developed).

d. Maturity takes about 4 to 6 weeks, depending on the client's ability to do hand-flexing exercises such as "ball squeezing," which will help the fistula mature.

e. The fistula is required to be mature before it can be used because the engorged vein is punctured with a large-bore needle for the dialysis procedure.

f. Subclavian or femoral catheters, **peritoneal dialysis**, or an external arteriovenous shunt can be used for dialysis while the fistula is maturing or developing.

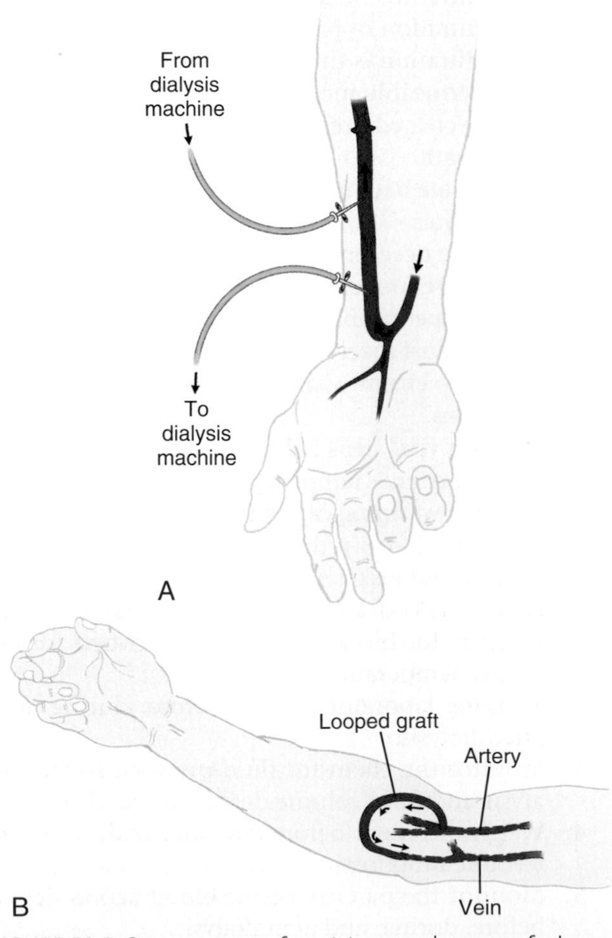

FIGURE 53-2 Common means for gaining vascular access for hemodialysis include **A,** arteriovenous fistula, and **B,** arteriovenous graft. (From Monahan F, Sands J, Neighbors M, et al.: *Phipps' medical-surgical nursing: Health and illness perspectives*, ed 8, St. Louis, 2007, Mosby.)

2. Advantages
   a. Because the fistula is internal, the risks of clotting and bleeding are low.
   b. The fistula can be used indefinitely.
   c. The fistula has a decreased incidence of infection because it is internal and is not exposed.
   d. Once healing has occurred, no external dressing is required.
   e. The fistula allows freedom of movement.
3. Disadvantages
   a. The fistula cannot be used immediately after insertion, so planning ahead for alternate access for dialysis is important.
   b. Needle insertions through the skin and tissues to the fistula are required for dialysis.
   c. Infiltration of the needles during dialysis can occur and cause hematomas.
   d. An aneurysm can form in the fistula.
   e. Heart failure (HF) can occur from the increased blood flow in the venous system.

Arterial steal syndrome can develop in a client with an internal arteriovenous fistula. In this complication, too much blood is diverted to the vein, and arterial perfusion to the hand is compromised.

D. Internal arteriovenous graft (see Fig. 53-2)
1. Description
   a. The internal graft may be used for chronic dialysis clients who do not have adequate blood vessels for the creation of a fistula.
   b. An artificial graft made of Gore-Tex or a bovine (cow) carotid artery is used to create an artificial vein for blood flow.
   c. The procedure involves the anastomosis of an artery to a vein using an artificial graft.
   d. The graft can be used 2 weeks after insertion.
   e. Complications of the graft include clotting, aneurysms, and infection.
2. Advantages
   a. Because the graft is internal, the risks of clotting and bleeding are low.
   b. The graft can be used indefinitely.
   c. The graft has a decreased incidence of infection.
   d. Once healing has occurred, no external dressing is required.
   e. The graft allows freedom of movement.
3. Disadvantages
   a. The graft cannot be used immediately after insertion.
   b. Needle insertions through the skin and tissues to the graft are required for dialysis.
   c. Infiltration of the needles during dialysis can occur and cause hematomas.
   d. An aneurysm can form in the graft; in addition, grafts clot more frequently than arteriovenous fistulas.

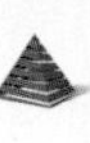

   e. **Arterial steal syndrome** can develop (too much blood is diverted to the vein, and arterial perfusion to the hand is compromised).
   f. Heart failure can occur from the increased blood flow in the venous system.

E. Interventions for an arteriovenous fistula and arteriovenous graft
1. Reinforce teaching the client that the extremity should not be used for monitoring blood pressure, drawing blood, placing IV lines, or administering injections.
2. Reinforce teaching the client with an arteriovenous fistula to perform hand-flexing exercises, if prescribed, such as "ball squeezing" to promote graft maturity.
3. Palpate pulses below the fistula or graft, and monitor for hand swelling as an indication of ischemia.
4. Note the temperature and capillary refill of the extremity.
5. Monitor for clotting.
   a. Complaints of tingling or discomfort in the extremity
   b. Inability to palpate a thrill or auscultate a bruit over the fistula or graft

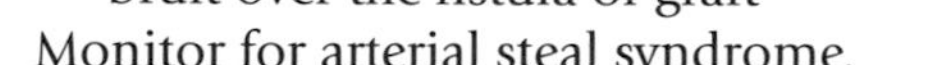

6. Monitor for arterial steal syndrome.
7. Monitor for infection.
8. Monitor lung and heart sounds for signs of HF.
9. Notify the RN immediately, who will notify the HCP, if signs of clotting, infection, or arterial steal syndrome occur.

To ensure patency, palpate for a thrill or auscultate for a bruit over the fistula or graft. Notify the RN and the HCP if a thrill or bruit is absent.

VIII. Complications of Hemodialysis (Box 53-4)

A. Air embolus
1. Description
   a. Introduction of air into the circulatory system
   b. Results in cardiopulmonary complications
2. Data collection
   a. Dyspnea and tachypnea
   b. Chest pain

BOX 53-4 Complications of Hemodialysis

Air embolus
Disequilibrium syndrome
Electrolyte alterations
Encephalopathy
Hemorrhage
Hepatitis
Hypotension
Sepsis
Shock

c. Hypotension
d. Reduced oxygen saturation
e. Cyanosis
f. Anxiety
g. Changes in sensorium

3. Interventions (see Priority Nursing Actions)

B. Disequilibrium syndrome

1. Description
   a. A rapid change in the composition of the extracellular fluid occurs during hemodialysis.
   b. Solutes are removed from the blood faster than from the cerebrospinal fluid and brain; fluid is pulled into the brain, causing cerebral edema.
   c. Occurs more frequently in a new client during the initial onset of hemodialysis.
2. Data collection
   a. Nausea and vomiting
   b. Headache
   c. Hypertension
   d. Restlessness and agitation
   e. Muscle cramps
   f. Confusion
   g. Seizures

PRIORITY NURSING ACTIONS!

Actions to Take If a Client Receiving Hemodialysis Develops an Air Embolism

1. Stop the hemodialysis.
2. Turn the client on the left side, with the head down (Trendelenburg's).
3. Notify the RN and HCP.
4. Administer oxygen.
5. Check the vital signs and pulse oximetry.
6. Document the event, actions taken, and the client's response.

Air embolism occurs when air enters the catheter system and is a complication of hemodialysis. The signs of air embolism include dyspnea, tachypnea, chest pain, hypotension, reduced oxygen saturation, cyanosis, anxiety, and changes in sensorium. Air embolism is a critical situation and if it is suspected, hemodialysis is stopped immediately and the client should be placed in a left side-lying position with the head lower than the feet. This position is used to try to prevent the air from traveling as a bolus to the lungs by trapping it in the right side of the heart. The RN and HCP is notified immediately and oxygen is administered. Vital signs are checked, including the pulse oximetry, and other prescribed interventions are done. The event, actions taken, and the client's response are documented.

Reference(s): Ignatavicius, D., & Workman, M. (2013). *Medical-surgical nursing: Patient-centered collaborative care.* (7th ed., p. 231). St. Louis: Saunders.

3. Interventions
   a. Slow or stop the dialysis.
   b. Notify the RN, who will notify the HCP, if signs of disequilibrium syndrome occur.
   c. Reduce environmental stimuli.
   d. Assist to administer intravenous hypertonic saline solution, albumin, or mannitol (Osmitrol) if prescribed.
   e. The client will be dialyzed for a shorter period at reduced flow rates to prevent its occurrence.

C. Dialysis encephalopathy

1. Description: An aluminum toxicity from dialysate water sources containing aluminum; also can occur from ingestion of aluminum-containing antacids (phosphate binders). This is not a common occurrence.
2. Data collection
   a. Progressive neurological impairment
   b. Mental cloudiness
   c. Speech disturbances
   d. Dementia
   e. Muscle incoordination
   f. Bone pain
   g. Seizures
3. Interventions
   a. Monitor for the signs of dialysis encephalopathy.
   b. Notify the RN, who will contact the HCP, if signs of dialysis encephalopathy occur.
   c. Assist to administer aluminum-chelating agents as prescribed so that aluminum is released and dialyzed from the body.

IX. Peritoneal Dialysis

A. Description

1. The peritoneum acts as the dialyzing membrane (semipermeable membrane) to achieve dialysis.
2. Peritoneal dialysis (PD) works on the principles of osmosis, diffusion, and ultrafiltration; PD occurs via the transfer of fluid and solute from the bloodstream through the peritoneum into the dialysate solution.
3. The peritoneal membrane is large and porous, allowing solutes and fluid to move via osmosis from an area of higher concentration in the body to an area of lower concentration in the dialyzing fluid.
4. The peritoneal cavity is rich in capillaries; therefore, it provides a ready access to the blood supply.

B. Contraindications to peritoneal dialysis

1. Peritonitis
2. Recent abdominal surgery
3. Abdominal adhesions
4. Other gastrointestinal problems such as diverticulosis

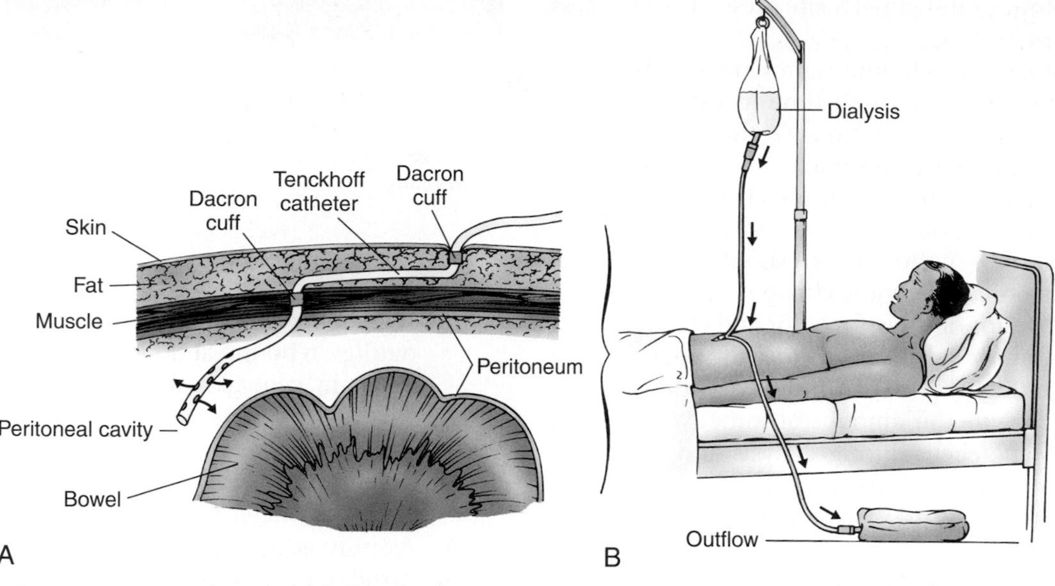

FIGURE 53-3 Manual peritoneal dialysis via an implanted abdominal catheter (Tenckhoff catheter). **A,** Implanted abdominal catheter. **B,** Dialysate inflow and outflow through implanted abdominal catheter. (From Ignatavicius D, Workman M: *Medical-surgical nursing: Patient-centered collaborative care,* ed 6, St. Louis, 2010, Saunders.)

C. Access for peritoneal dialysis (Fig. 53-3)

1. A siliconized rubber catheter such as a Tenckhoff catheter is surgically inserted into the client's peritoneal cavity to allow infusion of dialysis fluid.

2. The preferred insertion site is 3 to 5 cm below the umbilicus. This area is relatively avascular and has less fascial resistance.

3. The catheter is tunneled under the skin, through the fat and muscle tissue, and to the peritoneum. It is stabilized with Dacron cuffs in the muscle and under the skin.

4. Over a period of 1 to 2 weeks after insertion, fibroblasts and blood vessels grow around the cuffs, fixing the catheter in place and providing an extra barrier against dialysate leakage and bacterial invasion.

5. If the client is scheduled for transplant surgery, the peritoneal dialysis catheter may either be removed or left in place if the need for dialysis is suspected posttransplantation.

D. Dialysate solution

1. The dialysate solution is sterile.

2. All dialysis solutions are prescribed by the HCP; the solution contains electrolytes and minerals and has a specific osmolarity, specific glucose concentration, and other medication additives as prescribed.

3. The higher the glucose concentration, the greater the hypertonicity and the amount of fluid removed during a peritoneal dialysis exchange.

4. Increasing the glucose concentration increases the concentration of active particles that cause osmosis, the rate of ultrafiltration, and the amount of fluid removed.

5. If hyperkalemia is not a problem, potassium may be added to each bag of dialysate solution.

6. Heparin is added to the dialysate solution to prevent clotting of the catheter.

7. Prophylactic antibiotics may be added to the dialysate solution to prevent peritonitis.

8. Insulin may be added to the dialysate solution for the client with diabetes mellitus.

E. Peritoneal dialysis infusion

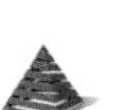

1. Description

a. One infusion (fill), dwell, and drain is considered one exchange.

b. Fill: 1 to 2 L of dialysate as prescribed is infused by gravity into the peritoneal space, which usually takes 10 to 20 minutes.

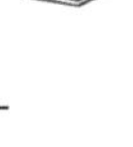

c. Dwell time: The amount of time that the dialysate solution remains in the peritoneal cavity is prescribed by the HCP and can last 20 to 30 minutes to 8 or more hours, depending on the type of dialysis used.

d. Drain (outflow): Fluid drains out of body by gravity into the drainage bag.

2. Interventions before treatment

a. Monitor vital signs.

b. Obtain weight.

c. Have the client void, if possible.

d. Monitor electrolyte and glucose levels.

3. Interventions during treatment

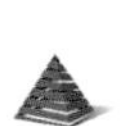

a. Monitor vital signs.

b. Monitor for respiratory distress, pain, or discomfort.

c. Monitor for signs of pulmonary edema.

d. Monitor for hypotension and hypertension.

e. Monitor for malaise, nausea, vomiting.

f. Monitor the catheter site dressing for wetness or bleeding.
g. Monitor dwell time as prescribed by the HCP.
h. Do not allow dwell time to extend beyond the HCP's order because this increases the risk for hyperglycemia.
i. Initiate outflow; turn the client from side to side if the outflow is slow to start.
j. Monitor outflow, which should be a continuous stream after the clamp is opened.
k. Monitor outflow for color and clarity.
l. Monitor intake and output accurately. If outflow is less than inflow, the difference is equal to the amount absorbed or retained by the client during dialysis and should be counted as intake.
m. An outflow greater than inflow should be reported to the HCP, as well as the appearance of frank blood or cloudiness in outflow.
n. The RN is notified if signs of complications occur.

F. Types of peritoneal dialysis
1. Continuous ambulatory peritoneal dialysis (CAPD)
   a. Closely resembles renal function because it is a continuous process
   b. Does not require a machine for the procedure
   c. Promotes client independence
   d. The client performs self-dialysis 24 hours a day, 7 days a week.
   e. Four dialysis cycles are usually administered in a 24-hour period, including an overnight 8-hour dwell time.
   f. Dialysate, 1.5 to 2 L is instilled into the abdomen four times daily and allowed to dwell as prescribed.
   g. After dwell, the bag is placed lower than the insertion site so that fluid drains by gravity flow.
   h. After fluid is drained, the bag is changed, new dialysate is instilled into the abdomen, and the process continues.
   i. Between exchanges, the catheter is clamped.
2. Automated peritoneal dialysis
   a. Automated dialysis requires a peritoneal cycling machine.
   b. Automated dialysis can be done as intermittent peritoneal dialysis, continuous cycling peritoneal dialysis, or nightly peritoneal dialysis.
   c. The exchanges are automated instead of manual.

X. Complications of Peritoneal Dialysis (Box 53-5)

Infection is a concern with peritoneal dialysis. Sites of infection are either at the catheter insertion site or in the peritoneum, which can cause peritonitis.

BOX 53-5 Complications of Peritoneal Dialysis

Abdominal pain
Bladder or bowel perforation
Insufficient outflow
Leakage around the catheter site
Peritonitis

A. Peritonitis
1. Monitor for symptoms of peritonitis: fever, cloudy outflow, rebound abdominal tenderness, abdominal pain, general malaise, nausea, and vomiting.
2. Cloudy or opaque outflow is an early sign of peritonitis.
3. If peritonitis is suspected, obtain a culture of the outflow to determine the infective organism.
4. Assist to administer antibiotics as prescribed.
5. Avoid infections by maintaining meticulous sterile technique when connecting and disconnecting PD solution bags and when caring for the catheter insertion site.
6. Prevent the catheter insertion site dressing from becoming wet during care of the client or the dialysis procedure; change the dressing if wet or soiled.
7. Follow institutional procedure for connecting and disconnecting PD solution bags, which may include scrubbing the connection sites with an antiseptic solution.

B. Abdominal pain
1. Peritoneal irritation during inflow commonly causes pain during the first few exchanges. The pain usually disappears after 1 to 2 weeks of dialysis treatments.
2. Warm the dialysate before administration using a special dialysate warmer pad, because the cold temperature of the dialysate can cause discomfort. 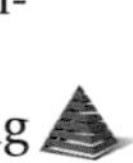

C. Abnormal outflow characteristics are indicative of complications.
1. Bloody outflow after the first few exchanges indicates vascular complications (the outflow should be clear and colorless after the initial exchanges).
2. Brown outflow indicates bowel perforation.
3. Urine-colored outflow indicates bladder perforation.
4. Cloudy outflow indicates peritonitis.

D. Insufficient outflow
1. The main cause of insufficient outflow is a full colon. Encourage a high-fiber diet (because constipation can cause inflow and outflow problems) and administer stool softeners as prescribed.
2. Insufficient outflow may also be caused by catheter migration out of the peritoneal area. If this occurs, an x-ray will be prescribed to evaluate catheter position.

3. Maintain the drainage bag below the client's abdomen.
4. Check for kinks in the tubing.
5. Check for fibrin clots in the tubing, and milk the tubing to dislodge the clot as prescribed.
6. Change the client's outflow position by turning the client to a side-lying position or ambulating the client.

E. Leakage around the catheter site
1. Clear fluid that leaks from the catheter exit site will be noted.
2. It takes 1 to 2 weeks after insertion of the catheter before fibroblasts and blood vessels grow into the catheter cuffs, fixing it in place and providing an extra barrier against dialysate leakage and bacterial invasion.
3. Smaller amounts of dialysate need to be used, and it may take up to 2 weeks for the client to tolerate a full 2-L exchange without leaking around the catheter site.

XI. Continuous Renal Replacement Therapy (CRRT)

A. Description
1. Continuous renal replacement therapy (CRRT) provides continuous ultrafiltration of extracellular fluid and clearance of urinary toxins over a period of 8 to 24 hours; used primarily for clients in AKI or critically ill clients with CKD who cannot tolerate hemodialysis.
2. Water, electrolytes, and other solutes are removed as the client's blood passes through a hemofilter.
3. Because rapid shifts in fluids and electrolytes typically do not occur, hemofiltration is usually well tolerated by critically ill clients.
4. There are five variations of CRRT, some requiring a hemodialysis machine, whereas others rely on the client's blood pressure to power the system.

XII. Kidney Transplantation

A. Description
1. A human kidney from a compatible donor is implanted into a recipient.
2. Kidney transplantation is performed for irreversible kidney failure; specific criteria are established for eligibility for a transplant.
3. The recipient must take immunosuppressive medications for life.

B. Living related donors
1. The most desirable source of kidneys for transplant is living related donors who closely match the client.
2. Donors are screened for ABO blood group, tissue-specific antigen, human leukocyte antigen suitability, mixed lymphocyte culture index (histocompatibility); donors are also screened for the presence of any communicable diseases, and they undergo a complete medical evaluation as well as a nephrology consultation.
3. The donor must be in excellent health with two properly functioning kidneys.
4. The emotional well-being of the donor is determined.
5. Complete understanding of the donation process and outcome by the donor is necessary.

C. Cadaver donors
1. Cadaver donors must meet the criteria of brain death.
2. Cadaver donors usually need to be younger than 70 years.
3. Cadaver donors must have normal renal function, although "marginal" donor organs have been used with the consent of the recipient.
4. No malignant disease outside of the central nervous system can be present.
5. No generalized infection or communicable disease can be present.
6. No renal trauma can be present.
7. The potential donor must be negative for communicable diseases at the time of donation.
8. Once cerebral death has been established for a potential donor, restoration of intravascular volume, weaning from vasopressors, and establishing diuresis are crucial; management of the donor is determined by organ bank personnel.
9. Continuous ventilation, and a normal blood pressure and heart rate are maintained until the kidneys are surgically removed.

D. Preoperative interventions
1. Histocompatibility tests will be done by organ bank personnel.
2. Immunosuppressive medications will be administered to the recipient as prescribed for 2 days before the transplantation, if possible. 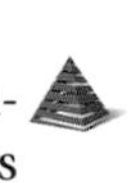
3. Maintain strict aseptic technique for the recipient.
4. Assist to verify that hemodialysis of the recipient was completed 24 hours before transplantation.
5. Ensure that the recipient is free of any infections.
6. Monitor renal function studies.
7. Encourage discussion of feelings of the donor and the recipient.
8. Provide psychological support to the live donor or cadaver donor family and the recipient.

E. Postoperative interventions for the recipient
1. Urine output usually begins immediately if the donor was a living donor. It is usually delayed for a few days or more with a cadaver kidney.
2. Hemodialysis may be performed until adequate kidney function is established.
3. Monitor vital signs, central venous pressure (CVP), and pulse oximetry for signs of complications.

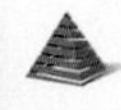

4. Monitor urine output hourly. Immediately report a urine output less than 100 mL/hr.
5. Monitor IV fluids closely; for the first 12 to 24 hours, IV fluid replacement is based on hourly urine output.
6. Assist to administer prescribed diuretics and osmotic agents.
7. Monitor daily weight to evaluate fluid status.
8. Monitor daily laboratory results to evaluate renal function, including hematocrit, BUN, and serum creatinine levels, and monitor urine for blood and specific gravity.
9. Position the client in the semi-Fowler's position to promote gas exchange, turning from the back to the nonoperative side.
10. Monitor indwelling urinary catheter patency. The indwelling urinary catheter remains in the bladder for 3 to 5 days to allow for anastomosis healing.
11. Note that urine is pink and bloody initially but gradually returns to normal within several days to weeks.
12. Notify the RN, who will notify the HCP, if gross hematuria and clots are noted in the urine.
13. Monitor the three-way bladder irrigation, if present, for clots; the RN may irrigate the catheter if a HCP's prescription is present.
14. Assist to remove the indwelling urinary catheter as soon as possible to prevent infection.
15. Maintain aseptic technique and monitor for infection; infection is the primary cause of death in the first year posttransplantation.
16. Monitor for bowel sounds and for the passage of flatus; initiate a specific diet and oral fluids as prescribed when flatus and bowel sounds return (usually fluids, sodium, and potassium are restricted if the client is oliguric).
17. Maintain good oral hygiene, monitoring for stomatitis and bacterial and fungal infections.
18. Encourage coughing and deep-breathing exercises.
19. Assist to administer medications as prescribed, which may include antifungal medications, antibiotics, immunosuppressive agents, and corticosteroids.
20. The client is usually ambulated after 24 hours.

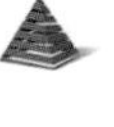

21. Monitor for signs of organ rejection by monitoring laboratory results.
22. Promote live donor and recipient relationship.
23. Monitor both the donor and recipient for depression.
24. Assist to provide the recipient with instructions following the kidney transplantation (Box 53-6).

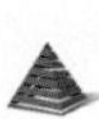
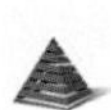

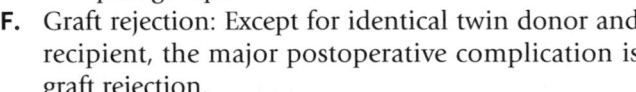

25. Assist the recipient to cope with the body-image disturbances that occur from long-term use of immunosuppressants.

BOX 53-6 Client Instructions After Kidney Transplantation

Avoid prolonged periods of sitting.
Monitor intake and output.
Recognize the signs and symptoms of infection and rejection.
Use medications as prescribed, and maintain immunosuppressive therapy for life.
Avoid contact sports.
Avoid exposure to persons with infections.
Know the signs and symptoms that require the need to contact the RN and HCP.
Ensure follow-up care.

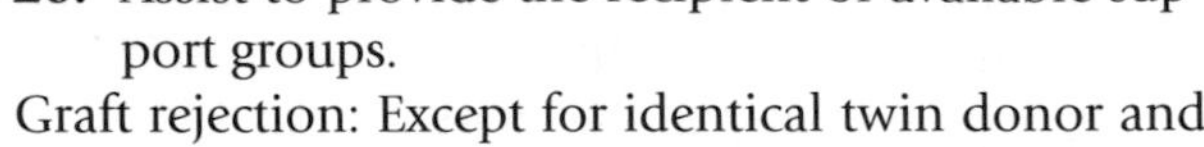

26. Assist to provide the recipient of available support groups.

F. Graft rejection: Except for identical twin donor and recipient, the major postoperative complication is graft rejection.
   1. Data collection (Box 53-7)
   2. Hyperacute rejection
      a. Hyperacute rejection occurs at the time of anastomosis of the organ.
      b. Interventions: Removal of rejected kidney
   3. Acute rejection
      a. Most common type; occurs most frequently within 6 weeks postoperatively but can occur any time posttransplantation
      b. Interventions: Potentially reversible with increased immunosuppression and if treated early; administering high doses of corticosteroids, or monoclonal antibodies if corticosteroids are ineffective.
   4. Chronic rejection
      a. Occurs slowly months to years after transplant and mimics CKD
      b. Interventions: Immunosuppressive medications and retransplantation if necessary

Except for identical twin donors and recipients, the major postoperative complication after renal transplant is graft rejection.

BOX 53-7 Clinical Signs of Renal Transplant (Graft) Rejection

Fever greater than 100° F (37.7° C)
Pain or tenderness over the grafted kidney
A 2- to 3-lb weight gain in 24 hours
Edema
Hypertension
Malaise
Elevated BUN and serum creatinine
Decreased creatinine clearance
Elevated white blood cell count
Rejection indicated by ultrasound or biopsy

XIII. Cystitis/Urinary Tract Infections (UTI)

A. Description

1. Cystitis (urinary tract infection, UTI) is an inflammation of the bladder from an infection, obstruction of the urethra, or other irritants (Box 53-8)
2. The most common causative organisms are *Escherichia coli, Enterobacter, Pseudomonas,* and *Serratia* species.
3. Cystitis is more common in women because women have a shorter urethra than men and the urethra in the woman is located close to the rectum.
4. Sexually active and pregnant women are most vulnerable to cystitis.

B. Data collection

1. Frequency and urgency
2. Burning on urination
3. Voiding in small amounts
4. Inability to void
5. Incomplete emptying of the bladder
6. Lower abdominal discomfort or back discomfort
7. Cloudy, dark, foul-smelling urine
8. Hematuria
9. Bladder spasms
10. Malaise, chills, and fever
11. Nausea and vomiting
12. WBC count greater than 100,000 cells/mm^3 on urinalysis
13. An elevated specific gravity and pH may be noted on urinalysis.

Altered mentation is a sign of a urinary tract infection in older adults; frequency and urgency may not be specific symptoms of UTI because of urinary elimination changes that occur with aging.

C. Interventions

1. Before administering prescribed antibiotics, obtain a urine specimen for culture and sensitivity, if prescribed, to identify bacterial growth.
2. Encourage the client to increase fluids up to 3000 mL/day, especially if the client is taking a sulfonamide. Sulfonamides can form crystals in concentrated urine.
3. Assist to administer prescribed medications, which may include analgesics, antiseptics, antispasmodics, antibiotics, and antimicrobials.
4. Maintain an acid urine pH (5.5). Instruct the client about foods to consume to maintain acidic urine.
5. Provide heat to the abdomen or sitz baths for complaints of discomfort as prescribed.
6. 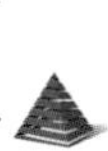 Note that if the client is prescribed an aminoglycoside, a sulfonamide, or nitrofurantoin (Macrodantin), the actions of these medications are decreased by acidic urine.
7. 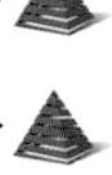 Use sterile technique when inserting a urinary catheter.
8. 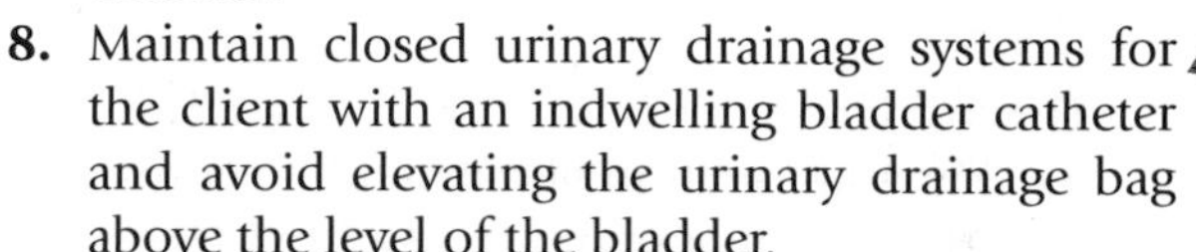 Maintain closed urinary drainage systems for the client with an indwelling bladder catheter and avoid elevating the urinary drainage bag above the level of the bladder.
9. 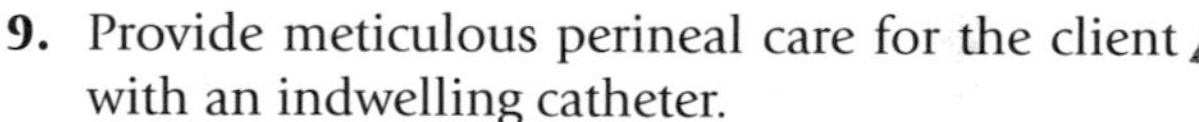 Provide meticulous perineal care for the client with an indwelling catheter.
10. 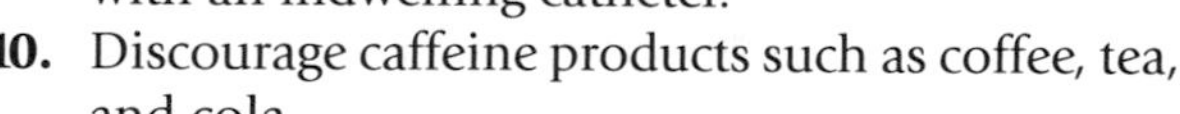 Discourage caffeine products such as coffee, tea, and cola.
11. Reinforce client education
    - **a.** Avoid alcohol.
    - **b.** Take medications as prescribed.
    - **c.** 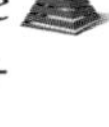 Take antibiotics on schedule and complete the entire course of medications as prescribed, which may be 10 to 14 days.
    - **d.** Repeat the urine culture after treatment.
    - **e.** Prevent recurrence of cystitis (Box 53-9).

XIV. Urosepsis

A. Description

1. Urosepsis is a gram-negative bacteremia originating in the urinary tract.
2. The most common causative organism is *Escherichia coli.*

BOX 53-8 Causes of Cystitis

Allergens or irritants, such as soaps, sprays, bubble bath, and perfumed sanitary napkins
Bladder distention
Calculus
Hormonal changes, influencing alterations in vaginal flora
Indwelling urinary catheters
Invasive urinary tract procedures
Loss of bactericidal properties of prostatic secretions in the male
Microorganisms
Poor-fitting vaginal diaphragms
Sexual intercourse
Synthetic underwear and pantyhose
Urinary stasis
Use of spermicides
Wet bathing suits

BOX 53-9 Teaching for Prevention of Cystitis

Use good perineal care, wiping front to back.
Avoid bubble baths, tub baths, and vaginal deodorants or sprays.
Void every 2 to 3 hours.
Wear cotton pants and avoid wearing tight clothes or pantyhose with slacks.
Avoid sitting in a wet bathing suit for prolonged periods.
If pregnant, void every 2 hours.
If menopausal, use estrogen vaginal creams to restore pH.
Use water-soluble lubricants for intercourse, especially after menopause.
Void and drink a glass of water after intercourse.

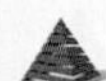

3. In a client who is immunocompromised, the most common cause is infection from an indwelling urinary catheter or an untreated UTI.
4. The major problem is the ability of this bacterium to develop resistant strains.
5. Urosepsis can lead to septic shock if not treated aggressively.

B. Data collection: Fever is the most common and earliest manifestation.

C. Interventions
1. Obtain a urine specimen for urine culture and sensitivity before administering antibiotics.
2. Intravenous antibiotics are administered as prescribed, usually until the client has been afebrile for 3 to 5 days.
3. Assist to administer oral antibiotics as prescribed after the 3- to 5-day afebrile period.

XV. Urethritis

A. Description
1. An inflammation of the urethra commonly associated with sexually transmitted infections and may occur with cystitis.
2. In men, urethritis most often is caused by gonorrhea or chlamydial infection.
3. In women, urethritis is most often caused by feminine hygiene sprays, perfumed toilet paper or sanitary napkins, spermicidal jelly, UTIs, or changes in the vaginal mucosal lining.

B. Data collection
1. Pain or burning on urination
2. Frequency and urgency
3. Nocturia
4. Difficulty voiding
5. Males may have clear to mucopurulent discharge from the penis.
6. Females may have lower abdominal discomfort.

C. Interventions
1. Encourage fluid intake.
2. Assist to prepare the client for testing to determine if a sexually transmitted infection (STI) is present.
3. Assist to administer antibiotics as prescribed.
4. Reinforce instructions to the client in the administration of sitz baths.
5. If stricture occurs, prepare the client for dilation of the urethra and instillation of an antiseptic solution.
6. Reinforce instructions to the female client to avoid the use of perfumed toilet paper or sanitary napkins and feminine hygiene sprays.
7. Reinforce instructions to the client to avoid intercourse until the symptoms subside or treatment of the STI is complete.
8. Reinforce instructions to the client on STIs if this is the cause.
   a. Prevent STIs by the use of latex condoms or abstinence.
   b. All sexual partners during the 30 days before diagnosis with chlamydial infection should be notified, examined, and treated if indicated.
   c. Chlamydial infection often coexists with gonorrhea; diagnostic testing is done for both STIs.
   d. Treatment for STIs includes antibiotics, as prescribed, to treat the causative organism.
   e. The most serious complication of chlamydial infection is sterility.
   f. Follow-up culture may be requested in 4 to 7 days to evaluate the effectiveness of medications.

XVI. Ureteritis

A. Ureteritis
1. Description: An inflammation of the ureter commonly associated with bacterial or viral infections and pyelonephritis
2. Data collection
   a. Dysuria
   b. Frequent urination
   c. Clear to mucopurulent penile discharge in males
3. Interventions
   a. Treatment includes identifying and treating the underlying cause and providing symptomatic relief.
   b. Assist to administer metronidazole (Flagyl) or clotrimazole (Mycelex) as prescribed for treating *Trichomonas* infection.
   c. Assist to administer nystatin (Mycostatin) or fluconazole (Diflucan) as prescribed for treating yeast infections.
   d. Doxycycline (Vibramycin) or azithromycin (Zithromax) may be prescribed for treating chlamydial infections.

XVII. Pyelonephritis

A. Description
1. An inflammation of the renal pelvis and the parenchyma commonly caused by bacterial invasion
2. Acute pyelonephritis often occurs after bacterial contamination of the urethra or an invasive procedure of the urinary tract.
3. Chronic pyelonephritis most commonly occurs after chronic urinary flow obstruction with reflux.
4. *Escherichia coli* is the most common bacterial causative organism.

B. Acute pyelonephritis
1. Acute pyelonephritis occurs as a new infection or recurs as a relapse of a previous infection.
2. It can progress to bacteremia or chronic pyelonephritis.

3. Data collection
   a. Fever and chills
   b. Nausea
   c. Flank pain on the affected side
   d. Costovertebral angle tenderness
   e. Headache
   f. Dysuria
   g. Frequency and urgency
   h. Cloudy, bloody, or foul-smelling urine
   i. Increased white blood cells in the urine

C. Chronic pyelonephritis
   1. A slow, progressive disease usually associated with recurrent acute attacks
   2. Causes contraction of the kidney and dysfunctioning of the nephrons, which are replaced by scar tissue
   3. Causes the ureter to become fibrotic and narrowed by strictures
   4. Can lead to **AKI** or **CKD**
   5. Data collection
      a. Frequently diagnosed incidentally when a client is being evaluated for hypertension
      b. Inability to conserve sodium
      c. Poor urine-concentrating ability
      d. Pyuria
      e. **Azotemia**
      f. Proteinuria

D. Interventions
   1. Monitor the vital signs, especially for elevated temperature.
   2. Encourage fluid intake up to 3000 mL/day to reduce fever and prevent dehydration.
   3. Monitor intake and output (ensure that output is a minimum of 1500 mL/24 hr).
   4. Monitor weight.
   5. Encourage adequate rest.
   6. Instruct the client in a high-calorie, low-protein diet.
   7. Provide warm, moist compresses to the flank area to help relieve pain.
   8. Assist to administer analgesics, antipyretics, antibiotics, urinary antiseptics, and antiemetics as prescribed.
   9. Monitor for signs of kidney failure.
   10. Encourage follow-up urine culture.

XVIII. Glomerulonephritis (See Chapter 36)

XIX. Nephrotic Syndrome (See Chapter 36)

XX. Polycystic Kidney Disease

A. Description
   1. A cystic formation and hypertrophy of the kidneys, which leads to cystic rupture, infection, formation of scar tissue, and damaged nephrons
   2. There is no specific treatment to arrest the progress of the destructive cysts.
   3. The ultimate result of this disease is chronic kidney disease.

B. Types
   1. Infantile polycystic disease: An inherited autosomal recessive trait that results in the death of the infant within a few months after birth
   2. Adult polycystic disease: An autosomal dominant trait that manifests between 30 and 40 years of age and results in chronic kidney disease.

C. Data collection
   1. Often asymptomatic until the ages of 30 to 40 years
   2. Flank, lumbar, or abdominal pain that worsens with activity and is relieved when lying down
   3. Fever and chills
   4. Recurrent urinary tract infections
   5. Hematuria, proteinuria, and pyuria
   6. Calculi
   7. Hypertension
   8. Palpable abdominal masses and enlarged kidneys
   9. Increased abdominal girth

D. Interventions
   1. Monitor for gross hematuria, which indicates cyst rupture.
   2. Increase sodium and water intake because sodium loss rather than retention occurs.
   3. Provide bed rest if ruptured cysts and bleeding occur.
   4. Prepare the client for percutaneous cyst puncture for relief of obstruction or draining an abscess.
   5. Assist to administer antihypertensives as prescribed.
   6. Prevent and/or treat urinary tract infections.
   7. Assist to prepare the client for dialysis or renal transplantation.
   8. Encourage the client to seek genetic counseling.
   9. Provide psychological support to the client and family.
   10. Provide psychosocial support and genetic counseling for family members who may want to donate a kidney.

XXI. Hydronephrosis (Fig. 53-4)

A. Description
   1. The distention of the renal pelvis and calices caused by an obstruction of normal urine flow
   2. The urine becomes trapped proximal to the obstruction.
   3. The causes include calculus, tumors, scar tissue, ureter obstructions, and hypertrophy of the prostate.

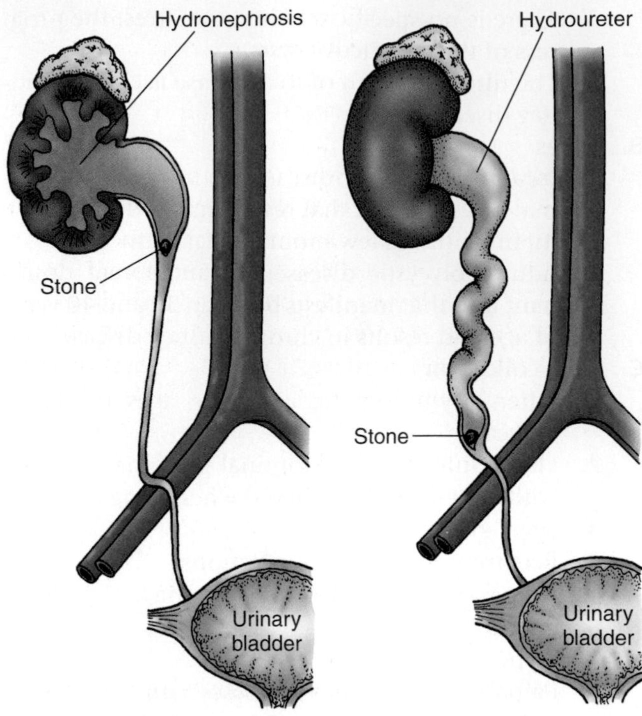

FIGURE 53-4 Hydronephrosis and hydroureter. (From Ignatavicius D, Workman M: *Medical-surgical nursing: Patient-centered collaborative care*, ed 6, St. Louis, 2010, Saunders.)

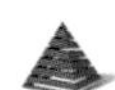

B. Data collection
1. Hypertension
2. Headache
3. Colicky or dull flank pain that radiates to the groin

C. Interventions

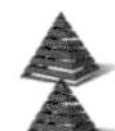

1. Monitor vital signs frequently.
2. Monitor for fluid and electrolyte imbalances, including dehydration after the obstruction is relieved.

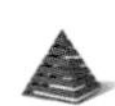

3. Monitor for diuresis, which can lead to fluid depletion.
4. Monitor weight daily.
5. Monitor urine for specific gravity, albumin, and glucose levels.
6. Assist to administer fluid replacement as prescribed.
7. Assist to prepare the client for insertion of a nephrostomy tube or a surgical procedure to relieve the obstruction if prescribed.

XXII. Renal Calculi

A. Description
1. Calculi are stones that can form anywhere in the urinary tract; however, the most frequent site is the kidneys.
2. Problems resulting from calculi are pain, obstruction, tissue trauma, secondary hemorrhage, and infection.
3. The stone can be located through radiography of the kidneys, ureters, and bladder; intravenous pyelography; CT scanning; and renal ultrasonography.
4. A stone analysis will be done after passage to determine the type of stone and assist in determining treatment.
5. **Urolithiasis** refers to the formation of urinary calculi; these form in the ureters.
6. **Nephrolithiasis** refers to the formation of kidney calculi; these form in the renal parenchyma.
7. When a calculus occludes the ureter and blocks the flow of urine, the ureter dilates, producing hydroureter (see Fig. 53-4).
8. If the obstruction is not removed, urinary stasis results in infection, impairment of renal function on the side of the blockage, hydronephrosis (see Fig. 53-4), and irreversible kidney damage.

B. Causes
1. Family history of stone formation
2. Diet high in calcium, vitamin D, protein, oxalate, purines, or alkali
3. Obstruction and urinary stasis
4. Dehydration
5. Use of diuretics, which can cause volume depletion
6. Urinary tract infections and prolonged urinary catheterization
7. Immobilization
8. Hypercalcemia and hyperparathyroidism
9. Elevated uric acid level, such as in gout

C. Data collection
1. Renal colic, which originates in the lumbar region and radiates around the side and down to the testicle in men and to the bladder in women
2. Ureteral colic, which radiates toward the genitalia and thigh
3. Sharp, severe pain of sudden onset

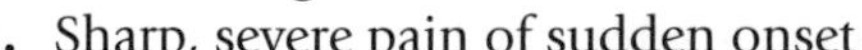

4. Dull, aching pain in the kidney

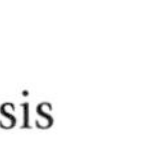

5. Nausea and vomiting, pallor, and diaphoresis during acute pain
6. Urinary frequency with alternating retention
7. Signs of a urinary tract infection
8. Low-grade fever
9. High numbers of red blood cells, white blood cells, and bacteria in the urinalysis report
10. Gross hematuria

D. Interventions
1. Monitor vital signs, especially the temperature, for signs of infection.
2. Monitor intake and output.
3. Monitor for fever, chills, and infection.
4. Monitor for nausea, vomiting, and diarrhea.
5. Encourage fluid intake up to 3000 mL/day, unless contraindicated, to facilitate the passage of the stone and prevent infection; monitor for obstruction.
6. Assist to administer fluids intravenously as prescribed if unable to take fluids orally or in

adequate amounts to increase the flow of urine and facilitate the passage of the stone.

7. Provide heat to the flank area as prescribed (massage therapy should be avoided).
8. Assist to administer analgesics at regularly scheduled intervals as prescribed to relieve pain.
9. Monitor the client's response to pain medication.
10. Assist the client in performing relaxation techniques to assist in relieving pain.
11. Encourage client ambulation if stable to promote the passage of the stone.
12. Turn and reposition the immobilized client to promote the passage of the stone.
13. Reinforce instructions to the client in the diet specific to the stone composition if prescribed.
14. Prepare the client for surgical procedures if prescribed.

For the client with renal calculi, strain all urine for the presence of stones and send the stones to the laboratory for analysis.

XXIII. Treatment Options for Renal Calculi (Fig. 53-5)

A. Cystoscopy
   1. Cystoscopy may be done for stones located in the bladder or lower ureter.
   2. No incision is made.
   3. One or two ureteral catheters are inserted past the stone. The stone may be manipulated and dislodged by the procedure, and the catheters may guide the stones mechanically downward as they are removed.
   4. The catheters are left in place for 24 hours to drain the urine trapped proximal to the stone and to dilate the ureter.
   5. A continuous chemical irrigation may be prescribed to dissolve the stone. 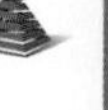

B. Extracorporeal shock wave lithotripsy (ESWL)
   1. A noninvasive mechanical procedure for breaking up stones located in the kidney or upper ureter so that they can pass spontaneously or be removed by other methods
   2. No incision is made and no drains are placed. A stent may be placed to facilitate passing stone fragments.
   3. Fluoroscopy is used to visualize the stone, and ultrasonic waves are delivered to the areas of the stone to disintegrate it.
   4. The stones are passed in the urine within a few days.
   5. Preprocedure: Maintain the client on NPO status for 8 hours before the procedure as prescribed.
   6. Postprocedure
      a. Monitor vital signs, especially for hypotension and tachycardia, which could indicate bleeding.
      b. Monitor intake and output.
      c. Monitor for bleeding.
      d. Monitor for pain and signs of urinary obstruction.
      e. Reinforce instructions to the client that if a ureteral stent is placed to help the stone pass, it is usually removed in 1 to 2 weeks
      f. Reinforce instructions to the client to increase fluid intake to flush out the stone fragments. 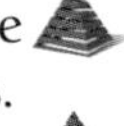
      g. Inform the client that ambulation is important.

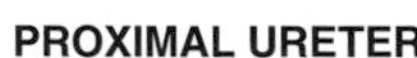

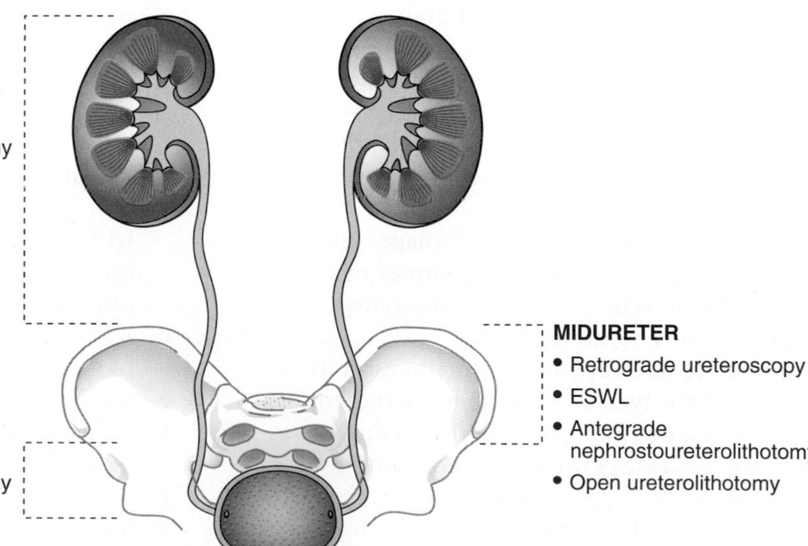

FIGURE 53-5 Treatment options for ureteral stones. *ESWL*, Extracorporeal shockwave lithotripsy. (From Ignatavicius D, Workman M: *Medical-surgical nursing: Patient-centered collaborative care*, ed 6, St. Louis, 2010, Saunders. Adapted from Singal RK, Denstedt JD: Contemporary management of ureteral stones. *Urologic Clinics of North America*, 24(1), 59–70, 1997.)

C. Percutaneous lithotripsy
1. Performed for stones in the bladder, ureter, or kidney
2. An invasive procedure in which a guide is inserted under fluoroscopy near the area of the stone; an ultrasonic wave is aimed at the stone to break it into fragments.
3. Percutaneous lithotripsy may be performed via cystoscopy or nephroscopy.
4. No incision is required for cystoscopy; a small flank incision is needed for nephroscopy.
5. The client may possibly have a indwelling bladder catheter.
6. A nephrostomy tube may be placed to administer chemical irrigations to break up the stone. The nephrostomy tube may remain in place for 1 to 5 days.
7. Encourage the client to drink 3000 to 4000 mL of fluid/day following the procedure as prescribed.
8. Monitor for and instruct the client to monitor for complications of infection, hemorrhage, and extravasation of fluid into the retroperitoneal cavity.

D. Ureterolithotomy
1. An open surgical procedure is performed if lithotripsy is not effective for removal of a stone in the ureter.
2. An incision is made through the lower abdomen or flank and then into the ureter to remove the stone.
3. The client may have a drain, a ureteral stent catheter, and an indwelling bladder catheter.

E. Pyelolithotomy and nephrolithotomy
1. Pyelolithotomy is an incision into the renal pelvis to remove a stone. A large flank incision is required, and the client may have a drain and an indwelling bladder catheter.
2. Nephrolithotomy is an incision into the kidney made to remove a stone. A large flank incision is required, and the client may have a nephrostomy tube and an indwelling bladder catheter.

F. Partial or total nephrectomy
1. Performed for extensive kidney damage, renal infection, severe obstruction from stones or tumors, and the prevention of stone recurrence
2. Postoperative interventions
   a. The plan of care depends on the incision location and the type of drainage tubes present.
   b. Monitor the incision, particularly if a drain is in place, because it will drain large amounts of urine.
   c. Protect the skin from urinary drainage, changing dressings frequently if necessary.
   d. Monitor the nephrostomy tube, which may be attached to a drainage bag, for a continuous flow of urine.
   e. The nephrotomy or bladder catheters are not irrigated unless specifically prescribed; if prescribed, this is done by the RN. 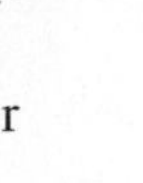
   f. Monitor the indwelling bladder catheter for drainage.
   g. Encourage fluid intake to ensure a urine output of 2500 to 3000 mL/day or more.
   h. Measure intake and output accurately.
   i. If a stone was removed, its composition is determined from laboratory analysis.

XXIV. Kidney Tumors

A. Description
1. Kidney tumors may be benign or malignant, bilateral or unilateral.
2. Common sites of metastasis include bone, lungs, liver, spleen, and the other kidney.
3. The exact cause of renal carcinoma is unknown.

B. Data collection for those with advanced disease
1. Dull flank pain
2. Palpable renal mass
3. Painless gross hematuria

C. Radical nephrectomy
1. Description
   a. The surgical removal of the entire kidney, adjacent adrenal gland, and renal artery and vein
   b. Radiation therapy and possibly chemotherapy may follow radical nephrectomy.
   c. Before surgery, radiation may be used to embolize (occlude) the arteries supplying the kidney to reduce bleeding during nephrectomy.
2. Postoperative interventions
   a. Monitor vital signs for indicators of bleeding (hypotension and tachycardia).
   b. Monitor for abdominal distention, decreases in urinary output, and alterations in level of consciousness as signs indicative of bleeding. Check the bed linens under the client for bleeding.
   c. Monitor for signs of adrenal insufficiency, which include a large urinary output followed by hypotension and subsequent oliguria. 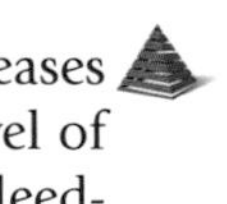
   d. Assist to administer fluids and packed red blood cells intravenously as prescribed.
   e. Monitor intake and output and daily weight.
   f. Monitor for a urinary output of 30 to 50 mL/hour to ensure adequate renal function.
   g. Monitor urine specific gravity.
   h. Maintain the client in a semi-Fowler's position.
   i. Monitor for signs of respiratory complications related to surgery; encourage coughing and deep-breathing exercises.

j. Monitor for passing of flatus and bowel sounds (lack of flatus and bowel sounds can indicate paralytic ileus).
k. If a nephrostomy tube is in place, it is not irrigated (unless specifically prescribed); if prescribed, this is done by the RN.
l. Assist to administer pain medications as prescribed.

XXV. Epididymitis

A. Description
1. An acute or chronic inflammation of the epididymis that occurs as a result of a UTI, sexually transmitted infection (STI), prostatitis, or from long-term use of an indwelling bladder catheter.
2. The infective organism travels upward through the urethra and ejaculatory duct and along the vas deferens to the epididymis.

B. Data collection
1. Scrotal pain
2. Groin pain
3. Swelling in the scrotum and groin
4. Pus and bacteria in the urine
5. Fever and chills
6. Abscess development

C. Interventions
1. Encourage fluid intake.
2. Encourage bed rest with the scrotum elevated to prevent traction on the spermatic cord, facilitate drainage, and relieve pain.
3. Reinforce instructions to the client in the intermittent application of cold compresses to the scrotum.
4. Reinforce instructions to the client in the use of sitz baths.
5. Reinforce instructions to the client in the administration of antibiotics for self and sexual partner if the cause is chlamydial or gonorrheal infection.
6. Reinforce instructions to the client to avoid lifting, straining, and sexual contact until the infection subsides.
7. Reinforce instructions to the client to limit the force of the stream because organisms can be forced into the vas deferens and epididymis from strain or pressure during voiding.
8. Reinforce teaching the client that condom use can help prevent urethritis and epididymitis.
9. Reinforce teaching the client measures to prevent UTI or STI recurrence.

XXVI. Prostatitis

A. Description
1. Inflammation of the prostate gland commonly caused by an infectious agent; may be acute or chronic.
2. The bacterial type occurs as a result of the organism reaching the prostate via the urethra, bladder, bloodstream, or lymphatic channels.
3. The abacterial type usually occurs following a viral illness or a decrease in sexual activity.

B. Data collection
1. Bacterial prostatitis
   a. Client becomes acutely ill
   b. Fever and chills
   c. Frequency and urgency of urination; dysuria
   d. Perineal and low back pain
   e. Urethral discharge
   f. Prostate is tender, indurated, and warm to touch.
   g. Urethral discharge on palpation of prostate
   h. White blood cells found in prostatic secretions
   i. Urine culture is usually positive for gram-negative bacteria, especially after prostate massage.
2. Abacterial prostatitis (most common form of chronic prostatitis)
   a. Backache
   b. Dysuria
   c. Perineal pain
   d. Frequency
   e. Hematuria
   f. Irregularly enlarged, firm, and tender prostate

C. Interventions
1. Encourage adequate fluid intake.
2. Reinforce instructions to the client in the use of sitz baths to promote comfort.
3. Assist to administer antibiotics, analgesics, antispasmodics, and stool softeners as prescribed.
4. Inform the client of activities to drain the prostate, such as intercourse, masturbation, and prostatic massage.
5. Reinforce instructions to the client to avoid spicy foods, coffee, alcohol, prolonged automobile rides, and sexual intercourse during an acute inflammation.

XXVII. Benign Prostatic Hypertrophy or Hyperplasia (BPH)

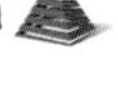

A. Description
1. Benign prostatic hypertrophy (hyperplasia; BPH) is a slow enlargement of the prostate gland, with hypertrophy and hyperplasia of normal tissue.
2. Enlargement compresses the urethra, resulting in partial or complete obstruction.
3. Usually occurs in men older than 50 years

B. Data collection

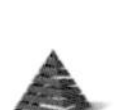

1. Diminished size and force of urinary stream (early sign of BPH)

2. Urinary urgency and frequency
3. Nocturia
4. Inability to start (hesitancy) or continue a urinary stream
5. Feelings of incomplete bladder emptying
6. Postvoid dribbling from overflow incontinence (later sign)
7. Urinary retention and bladder distention
8. Hematuria
9. Urinary stasis
10. Dysuria and bladder pain
11. UTIs

C. Interventions
1. Encourage fluid intake of up to 2000 to 3000 mL/day unless contraindicated.
2. Prepare for urinary catheterization to drain the bladder and prevent distention.

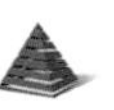

3. Avoid administering medications that cause urinary retention, such as anticholinergics, antihistamines, decongestants, and antidepressants.
4. Assist to administer medications as prescribed to shrink the prostate gland and improve urine flow.
5. Assist to administer medications as prescribed to relax prostatic smooth muscle and improve urine flow.
6. Reinforce instructions to the client to decrease intake of caffeine and artificial sweeteners and limit spicy or acidic foods.
7. Reinforce instructions to the client to follow a timed voiding schedule.
8. Prepare the client for surgery or invasive procedures as prescribed (Box 53-10).

D. Surgical interventions and postoperative care (see Chapter 43)

BOX 53-10 Surgical and Invasive Procedures for Prostatic Hyperplasia

Transurethral resection of the prostate (TURP): Removal of benign prostatic tissue surrounding the urethra with use of a resectoscope introduced through the urethra; there is little risk of impotence and is most commonly used for benign prostatic hypertrophy (BPH)

Transurethral incision of the prostate (TUIP): Removal of prostatic tissue through an incision made in the bladder neck

Transurethral microwave thermotherapy: Application of heat to destroy the hypertrophied tissue

Transurethral needle ablation of the prostate (TUNA): Placement of interstitial radiofrequency needles through the urethra and into the lateral lobes of the prostate, causing heat-induced coagulation necrosis of the prostate for treating BPH

Laser prostatectomy: Ablation of the enlarged prostate using laser instead of radiofrequency waves

Transurethral electrovaporization of the prostate: Placement of a special metal instrument that emits a high-frequency electrical current that cuts and vaporizes excess tissue and seals the remaining tissue to prevent bleeding; especially useful for men on anticoagulants and those at risk for complications

Perineal prostatectomy: Removal of prostatic tissue (may be performed for prostatic cancer) low in the pelvic region through an incision between the scrotum and rectum; impotence and incontinence usually result

Retropubic prostatectomy: Removal of hypertrophied prostatic tissue high in the pelvic region through a low abdominal incision; the bladder is not incised

Suprapubic prostatectomy: Removal of prostatic tissue mass through a low midline incision; an incision into the bladder and urethral mucosa to the anterior aspect of the prostate is made

Urethral stents: Application of stents or coils in the urethra where it is narrowed by the prostate

XXVIII. Bladder Cancer (See Chapter 43)

XXIX. Bladder Trauma

A. Description
1. Occurs following a blunt or penetrating injury to the lower abdomen
2. Blunt trauma causes compression of the abdominal wall and bladder.
3. Penetrating wounds occur as a result of a stabbing, gunshot wound, or other objects piercing the abdominal wall.
4. A fractured pelvis that results in bone fragments puncturing the bladder is a common cause of bladder trauma.

B. Data collection
1. **Anuria**
2. Hematuria
3. Pain below the level of the umbilicus; can radiate to the shoulders
4. Nausea and vomiting

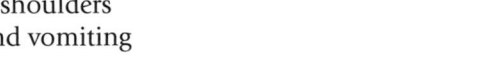

C. Interventions
1. Monitor vital signs.
2. Monitor for hematuria, bleeding, and signs of shock.
3. Promote bed rest.
4. Monitor pain level.
5. If blood is seen at the meatus, avoid urinary catheterization until a retrograde urethrogram can be performed.
6. Assist to prepare the client for insertion of a suprapubic catheter to aid in urinary drainage if prescribed.
7. Assist to prepare the client for surgical repair of the laceration if indicated.

CRITICAL THINKING What Should You Do?

Answer: Glomerulonephritis results in proliferative and inflammatory changes within the glomerular structure. Destruction, inflammation, and sclerosis of the glomeruli of both kidneys occur. Loss of kidney function occurs. With this disorder, the nurse should monitor for complications such as fluid overload, ascites, pulmonary edema, and heart failure. If fine crackles in the lung bases develop bilaterally, the nurse should contact the registered nurse (RN), who will notify the health care provider (HCP) because this could be a sign of one of these complications.

Reference(s): deWit, D. & Kumagai, C. (2013). *Medical-surgical nursing: Concepts & practice.* (2nd ed., pp. 789–790). St. Louis: Saunders.

PRACTICE QUESTIONS

❖ **546.** The nurse is caring for the client with epididymitis. Which treatment modalities should be implemented? **Select all that apply.**

- ❑ **1.** Bed rest
- ❑ **2.** Sitz bath
- ❑ **3.** Antibiotics
- ❑ **4.** Heating pad
- ❑ **5.** Scrotal elevation

547. A client has epididymitis as a complication of a urinary tract infection (UTI). The nurse is giving the client instructions to prevent a recurrence. The nurse determines that the client **needs further teaching** if the client states the intention to do which?

1. Drink increased amounts of fluids
2. Limit the force of the stream during voiding
3. Continue to take antibiotics until all symptoms are gone
4. Use condoms to eliminate risk from chlamydia and gonorrhea

548. The nurse is collecting data from a client who has had benign prostatic hyperplasia (BPH) in the past. To determine if the client is currently experiencing exacerbation of BPH, the nurse should ask the client about the presence of which **early** symptom?

1. Nocturia
2. Urinary retention
3. Urge incontinence
4. Decreased force in the stream of urine

549. A client newly diagnosed with chronic kidney disease has recently begun hemodialysis. Which are signs/symptoms of disequilibrium syndrome?

1. Hypertension, tachycardia, and fever
2. Hypotension, bradycardia, and hypothermia
3. Restlessness, irritability, and generalized weakness
4. Headache, deteriorating level of consciousness, and twitching

550. A client with chronic kidney disease has been on dialysis for 3 years. The client is receiving the usual combination of medications for the disease, including aluminum hydroxide as a phosphate-binding agent. The client now has mental cloudiness, dementia, and complaints of bone pain. Which does this data indicate?

1. Advancing uremia
2. Phosphate overdose
3. Folic acid deficiency
4. Aluminum intoxication

551. A hemodialysis client with a left arm fistula is at risk for arterial steal syndrome. The nurse monitors this client for which signs/symptoms of this disorder?

1. Edema and purpura of the left arm
2. Warmth, redness, and pain in the left hand
3. Aching pain, pallor, and edema of the left arm
4. Pallor, diminished pulse, and pain in the left hand

552. The nurse is reviewing the medical record of a client with a diagnosis of pyelonephritis. Which disorder noted on the client's record should the nurse identify as a risk factor for this disorder?

1. Hypoglycemia
2. Diabetes mellitus
3. Coronary artery disease
4. Orthostatic hypotension

❖ **553.** The nurse is reviewing the client's record and notes that the health care provider has documented that the client has a renal disorder. Which laboratory results would indicate a decrease in renal function? **Select all that apply.**

- ❑ **1.** Elevated serum creatinine level
- ❑ **2.** Elevated thrombocyte cell count
- ❑ **3.** Decreased red blood cell (RBC) count
- ❑ **4.** Decreased white blood cell (WBC) count
- ❑ **5.** Elevated blood urea nitrogen (BUN) level

554. A client is scheduled for intravenous pyelography (IVP). Which **priority** nursing action should the nurse take?

1. Restrict fluids.
2. Administer a sedative.
3. Determine a history of allergies.
4. Administer an oral preparation of radiopaque dye.

555. After a renal biopsy, the client complains of pain at the biopsy site, which radiates to the front of the abdomen. Which would this indicate?
1. Bleeding
2. Infection
3. Renal colic
4. Normal, expected pain

❖ **556.** The nurse monitoring a client receiving peritoneal dialysis notes that the client's outflow is less than the inflow. The nurse should take which actions? **Select all that apply.**
- ❑ 1. Contact the health care provider (HCP).
- ❑ 2. Check the level of the drainage bag.
- ❑ 3. Reposition the client to his or her side.
- ❑ 4. Place the client in good body alignment.
- ❑ 5. Check the peritoneal dialysis system for kinks.
- ❑ 6. Increase the flow rate of the peritoneal dialysis solution.

557. The nurse is collecting data on a newly admitted client with a diagnosis of bladder cancer. Which sign/symptom should be noted **first**?
1. Dysuria
2. Urgency
3. Frequency
4. Hematuria

558. A client with benign prostatic hypertrophy (BPH) undergoes a transurethral resection of the prostate (TURP) and is receiving continuous bladder irrigations postoperatively. Which are the signs/symptoms of transurethral resection (TUR) syndrome?
1. Tachycardia and diarrhea
2. Bradycardia and confusion
3. Increased urinary output and anemia
4. Decreased urinary output and bladder spasms

559. A client with prostatitis resulting from kidney infection has received instructions on management of the condition at home and prevention of recurrence. Which statement indicates that the client understood the instructions?
1. Stop antibiotic therapy when pain subsides.
2. Exercise as much as possible to stimulate circulation.
3. Use warm sitz baths and analgesics to increase comfort.
4. Keep fluid intake to a minimum to decrease the need to void.

560. The nurse is monitoring an older client suspected of having a urinary tract infection (UTI) for signs of the infection. Which sign/symptom should occur **first**?
1. Fever
2. Urgency
3. Confusion
4. Frequency

ANSWERS

❖ **546. 1, 2, 3, 5**

Rationale: Common interventions used in the treatment of epididymitis include bed rest, elevation of the scrotum, ice packs, sitz baths, analgesics, and antibiotics. A heating pad should not be used because direct application of heat could increase blood flow to the area and increase the swelling.

Test-Taking Strategy: Focus on the **subject**, epididymitis. A sitz bath provides heat that is moist and soothing. Knowing that direct heat may increase inflammation in tissue that is already at risk will guide you to eliminate option 4 as the item that could increase swelling. **Review:** care of the client with epididymitis.

Level of Cognitive Ability: Analyzing
Client Needs: Physiological Integrity
Integrated Process: Nursing Process/Implementation
Content Area: Adult Health: Renal and Urinary
Priority Concepts: Inflammation, Tissue Integrity
Reference(s): deWit, Kumagai (2013), p. 932.

547. 3

Rationale: The client who experiences epididymitis from UTI should increase intake of fluids to flush the urinary system. Because organisms can be forced into the vas deferens and epididymis from strain or pressure during voiding, the client should limit the force of the stream. Condom use can help prevent urethritis and epididymitis from sexually transmitted infections. Antibiotics are always taken until the full course of therapy is completed.

Test-Taking Strategy: Note the **strategic words**, *needs further teaching*. These words indicate a **negative event query** and the need to select the incorrect client statement. Because option 1 is consistent with good practices in the prevention of UTI, this option can be eliminated first. From the remaining options, it is necessary to know that the force of stream should be limited to prevent backflow into the epididymis and that condoms are helpful in preventing this disorder from occurring as a complication of a sexually transmitted infection. Remember that antibiotics are not stopped when symptoms subside but must be taken until the full course of therapy is completed. **Review:** care of the client with epididymitis.

Level of Cognitive Ability: Evaluating
Client Needs: Physiological Integrity
Integrated Process: Teaching and Learning
Content Area: Adult Health: Renal and Urinary
Priority Concepts: Infection, Inflammation
Reference(s): deWit, Kumagai (2013), pp. 120, 932.

548. 4

Rationale: Decreased force in the stream of urine is an early sign of BPH. The stream later becomes weak and dribbling. The client may then develop hematuria, frequency, urgency, urge incontinence, and nocturia. If untreated, complete obstruction and urinary retention can occur.

Test-Taking Strategy: Note the strategic word, *early.* Option 2 identifies the most severe symptom and therefore is eliminated first. From the remaining options, focusing on the strategic words and recalling the pathophysiology related to BPH will direct you to the correct option. **Review:** the signs of **benign prostatic hypertrophy**.

Level of Cognitive Ability: Analyzing

Client Needs: Physiological Integrity

Integrated Process: Nursing Process/Data Collection

Content Area: Adult Health: Renal and Urinary

Priority Concepts: Elimination, Fluid and Electrolyte Balance

Reference(s): Cooper, Gosnell (2015), pp. 1701–1702.

549. 4

Rationale: Disequilibrium syndrome is characterized by headache, mental confusion, decreasing level of consciousness, nausea and vomiting, twitching, and possible seizure activity. It is caused by rapid removal of solutes from the body during hemodialysis. At the same time, the blood-brain barrier interferes with the efficient removal of wastes from brain tissue. As a result, water goes into cerebral cells because of the osmotic gradient, causing brain swelling and onset of symptoms. It most often occurs in clients who are new to dialysis and is prevented by dialyzing for shorter times or at reduced blood flow rates.

Test-Taking Strategy: Focus on the subject, disequilibrium syndrome. Noting the relation between the words *disequilibrium syndrome* and the signs in option 4 will direct you to this option. **Review:** signs and symptoms of **disequilibrium syndrome**.

Level of Cognitive Ability: Analyzing

Client Needs: Physiological Integrity

Integrated Process: Nursing Process/Data Collection

Content Area: Adult Health: Renal and Urinary

Priority Concepts: Cognitive Function, Fluid and Electrolyte Balance

Reference(s): Ignatavicius, Workman (2013), p. 1563.

550. 4

Rationale: Aluminum intoxication may occur when there is accumulation of aluminum, an ingredient in many phosphate-binding antacids. It results in mental cloudiness, dementia, and bone pain from infiltration of the bone with aluminum. This condition was formerly known as dialysis dementia. It may be treated with aluminum-chelating agents, which make aluminum available to be dialyzed from the body. It can be prevented by avoiding or limiting the use of phosphate-binding agents that contain aluminum.

Test-Taking Strategy: Focus on the subject, aluminum hydroxide. Note the relation between the medication name in the question and option 4. **Review:** the signs of **aluminum intoxication**.

Level of Cognitive Ability: Analyzing

Client Needs: Physiological Integrity

Integrated Process: Nursing Process/Data Collection

Content Area: Adult Health: Renal and Urinary

Priority Concepts: Elimination, Fluid and Electrolyte Balance

Reference(s): Ignatavicius, Workman (2013), pp. 1556–1557.

551. 4

Rationale: Arterial steal syndrome results from vascular insufficiency after creation of a fistula. The client exhibits pallor and diminished pulse distal to the fistula and complains of pain distal to the fistula, which is caused by tissue ischemia. Warmth, redness, and pain should more likely characterize a problem with infection. Options 2 and 3 are not characteristics of steal syndrome.

Test-Taking Strategy: Focus on the subject, arterial steal syndrome. Recalling that arterial steal syndrome results from vascular insufficiency will direct you to the correct option. **Review:** the signs of **arterial steal syndrome**.

Level of Cognitive Ability: Analyzing

Client Needs: Physiological Integrity

Integrated Process: Nursing Process/Data Collection

Content Area: Adult Health: Renal and Urinary

Priority Concepts: Perfusion, Pain

Reference(s): Ignatavicius, Workman (2013), p. 1562.

552. 2

Rationale: Risk factors associated with pyelonephritis include diabetes mellitus, hypertension, chronic renal calculi, chronic cystitis, structural abnormalities of the urinary tract, presence of urinary stones, and indwelling or frequent urinary catheterization.

Test-Taking Strategy: Focus on the subject, pyelonephritis. Eliminate options 1 and 4 first as least likely being associated as risk factors. From the remaining options, remember that diabetes mellitus can cause renal complications. This will direct you to the correct option. **Review:** the risk factors of **pyelonephritis**.

Level of Cognitive Ability: Analyzing

Client Needs: Health Promotion and Maintenance

Integrated Process: Nursing Process/Data Collection

Content Area: Adult Health: Renal and Urinary

Priority Concepts: Glucose Regulation; Inflammation

Reference(s): Ignatavicius, Workman (2013), p. 1524.

❖ **553. 1, 3, 5**

Rationale: BUN testing is a frequently used laboratory test to determine renal function. The BUN and serum creatinine levels start to rise when the glomerular filtration rate falls below 40% to 60%. A decreased RBC count may be noted if erythropoietic function by the kidney is impaired. An increased WBC is most likely to be noted in renal disease. Thrombocyte cell counts do not indicate decreased renal function.

Test-Taking Strategy: Focus on the subject, laboratory results indicating a decrease in renal function. Eliminate option 2 first because it is unassociated with the renal system. An increased WBC is most likely to be noted in renal disease, so option 4 can be eliminated. Remember that the BUN and creatinine levels are frequently used laboratory tests to determine renal function. **Review:** the **laboratory tests to determine renal function**.

Level of Cognitive Ability: Analyzing

Client Needs: Physiological Integrity

Integrated Process: Nursing Process/Data Collection

Content Area: Adult Health: Renal and Urinary
Priority Concepts: Cellular Regulation, Fluid and Electrolyte Balance
Reference(s): deWit, Kumagai (2013), pp. 767, 770.

554. 3
Rationale: An iodine-based dye may be used during the IVP and can cause allergic reactions such as itching, hives, rash, tight feeling in the throat, shortness of breath, and bronchospasm. Checking for allergies is the priority. Options 1, 2, and 4 are unnecessary.
Test-Taking Strategy: Note the strategic word, *priority*, and use the steps of the nursing process as a guide. Options 1, 2, and 4 address implementation. Option 3 is the only option that addresses data collection. **Review: intravenous pyelography (IVP).**
Level of Cognitive Ability: Applying
Client Needs: Physiological Integrity
Integrated Process: Nursing Process/Implementation
Content Area: Adult Health: Renal and Urinary
Priority Concepts: Clinical Judgment, Safety
Reference(s): deWit, Kumagai (2013), p. 770; Pagana, Pagana (2013), p. 782.

555. 1
Rationale: If pain originates at the biopsy site and begins to radiate to the flank area and around the front of the abdomen, bleeding should be suspected. Hypotension, a decreasing hematocrit, and gross or microscopic hematuria should also indicate bleeding. Signs of infection should not appear immediately after a biopsy. Pain of this nature is not normal. There are no data to support the presence of renal colic.
Test-Taking Strategy: Focusing on the subject, pain at the renal biopsy site, will assist in eliminating options 3 and 4. Recalling that signs of infection may not appear immediately after biopsy will assist in directing you to option 1 from the remaining choices. **Review:** the **complications following renal biopsy.**
Level of Cognitive Ability: Analyzing
Client Needs: Physiological Integrity
Integrated Process: Nursing Process/Data Collection
Content Area: Adult Health: Renal and Urinary
Priority Concepts: Pain, Perfusion
Reference(s): deWit, Kumagai (2013), p. 772.

❖ **556. 2, 3, 4, 5**
Rationale: If outflow drainage is inadequate, the nurse attempts to stimulate outflow by changing the client's position. Turning the client to the other side or making sure that the client is in good body alignment may assist with outflow drainage. The drainage bag needs to be lower than the client's abdomen to enhance gravity drainage. The connecting tubing on the peritoneal dialysis system is also checked for kinks or twisting, and the clamps on the system are checked to ensure that they are open. There is no reason to contact the HCP. Increasing the flow rate is an inappropriate action and is unassociated with the amount of outflow solution.
Test-Taking Strategy: Focus on the subject, peritoneal dialysis outflow and inflow. Use the principles related to gravity flow and preventing obstruction to flow to answer this question. This will assist in determining the correct interventions. **Review:** the nursing interventions related to **insufficient flow of dialysate.**
Level of Cognitive Ability: Analyzing
Client Needs: Physiological Integrity
Integrated Process: Nursing Process/Implementation
Content Area: Adult Health: Renal and Urinary
Priority Concepts: Clinical Judgment, Elimination
Reference(s): Ignatavicius, Workman (2013), p. 1567.

557. 4
Rationale: Gross, painless hematuria is most frequently the first manifestation of bladder cancer. As the disease progresses, the client may experience dysuria, frequency, and urgency.
Test-Taking Strategy: Note the strategic word, *first.* Focus on the subject, a sign/symptom of bladder cancer. Eliminate options 1, 2, and 3, because although they are common signs of bladder cancer, they also are common signs/symptoms of urinary tract infection. **Review:** the specific signs and symptoms associated with **bladder cancer.**
Level of Cognitive Ability: Applying
Client Needs: Physiological Integrity
Integrated Process: Nursing Process/Data Collection
Content Area: Adult Health: Renal and Urinary
Priority Concepts: Clinical Judgment, Elimination
Reference(s): deWit, Kumagai (2013), p. 795.

558. 2
Rationale: TUR syndrome is caused by increased absorption of nonelectrolyte irrigating fluid used during surgery. The client may show signs of cerebral edema and increased intracranial pressure, such as increased blood pressure, bradycardia, confusion, disorientation, muscle twitching, visual disturbances, and nausea and vomiting.
Test-Taking Strategy: Knowledge regarding the subject, TUR syndrome, is required to answer this question. Recalling that increased intracranial pressure is the concern will direct you to option 2. **Review: transurethral resection syndrome.**
Level of Cognitive Ability: Analyzing
Client Needs: Physiological Integrity
Integrated Process: Nursing Process/Data Collection
Content Area: Adult Health: Renal and Urinary
Priority Concepts: Clinical Judgment, Fluid and Electrolyte Balance
Reference(s): Ignatavicius, Workman (2013), p. 1636.

559. 3
Rationale: Treatment of prostatitis includes medication with antibiotics, analgesics, and stool softeners. The client is also taught to rest, increase fluid intake, and use sitz baths for comfort. Antimicrobial therapy is always continued until the prescription is completely finished.
Test-Taking Strategy: Focus on the subject, prostatitis. Eliminate option 1 first because stopping medication therapy before the end of the course is contraindicated. Option 4 is also eliminated because fluid intake should be increased. From the remaining options, it is necessary to understand that sitz baths provide comfort and that rest is helpful in the healing process. Knowledge of either of these concepts will direct you to option 3. **Review:** the **measures to prevent prostatitis.**
Level of Cognitive Ability: Evaluating
Client Needs: Physiological Integrity
Integrated Process: Nursing Process/Evaluation
Content Area: Adult Health: Renal and Urinary

Priority Concepts: Client Education, Inflammation
Reference(s): deWit, Kumagai (2013), p. 933.

560. 3

Rationale: In an older client, the only symptom of a UTI may be something as vague as increasing mental confusion or frequent unexplained falls. Frequency and urgency may commonly occur in an older client, and fever can be associated with a variety of conditions.

Test-Taking Strategy: Note the **strategic word**, *first*. Although all may be signs/symptoms of urinary tract infection, note the client's age in the question to determine which one occurs *first*. Eliminate options 2 and 4 because they may commonly occur in an older client. Eliminate option 1 next because fever can be associated with a variety of conditions. **Review:** the signs and symptoms of **urinary tract infection that occur in the older client.**
Level of Cognitive Ability: Analyzing
Client Needs: Physiological Integrity
Integrated Process: Nursing Process/Data Collection
Content Area: Adult Health: Renal and Urinary
Priority Concepts: Cognitive Function, Infection
Reference(s): deWit, Kumagai (2013), p. 786.

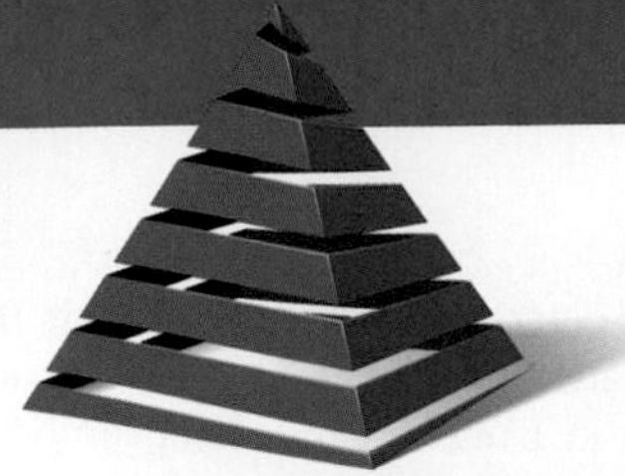

CHAPTER 54

Renal Medications

CRITICAL THINKING What Should You Do?

A client who is taking levofloxacin (Levaquin) complains of dizziness and blurred vision and sensitivity to light. What should the nurse do?

Answer located on p. 759.

I. Urinary Tract Antiseptics

A. Description

1. Urinary tract antiseptics inhibit the growth of bacteria in the urine (Box 54-1).
2. Act as disinfectants within the urinary tract.
3. Used to treat acute cystitis or urinary tract infections (UTIs).
4. Urinary tract antiseptics do not achieve effective antibacterial concentrations in blood or tissues and therefore cannot be used for infections outside the urinary tract.

B. Side/adverse effects and nursing considerations

1. Fosomycin (Monurol)
   - **a.** The medication is available as granules that must be dissolved; instruct the client to mix the contents of a package in about ½ cup of cold water, stir well, and drink all the liquid.
   - **b.** Medications that increase gastrointestinal motility reduce the absorption of fosfomycin.
2. Methenamine (Hiprex, Urex)
   - **a.** Used to treat chronic UTIs, but not recommended for acute infections.
   - **b.** Administer after meals and at bedtime to minimize gastric distress.
   - **c.** Chronic high-dose therapy can cause bladder irritation.
   - **d.** Methenamine can cause crystalluria and should not be used in clients with renal impairment.
   - **e.** Decomposition of the medication generates ammonia; therefore, it should not be used for clients with liver dysfunction.

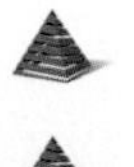

   - **f.** Methenamine requires acidic urine with a pH of 5.5 or lower.

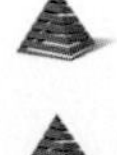

   - **g.** Increasing fluid intake reduces antibacterial effects by diluting the medication and raising urine pH; alkalizing fluids such as milk and citrus juices should be avoided however, cranberry juice is allowed.
   - **h.** Methenamine should not be combined with sulfonamides because of the risk of crystalluria and urinary tract injury.
   - **i.** Clients taking this medication should avoid alkalinizing agents, including over-the-counter (OTC) antacids containing sodium bicarbonate or sodium carbonate.
3. Nitrofurantoin (Furadantin, Macrodantin, Macrobid)
   - **a.** Gastrointestinal effects include anorexia, nausea, vomiting, and diarrhea; administration with milk or meals minimizes gastrointestinal distress.
   - **b.** Pulmonary reactions include dyspnea, chest pain, chills, fever, cough, and alveolar infiltrates. These resolve in 2 to 4 days following cessation of treatment.
   - **c.** Hematological effects include agranulocytosis, leukopenia, thrombocytopenia, and megaloblastic anemia.
   - **d.** Peripheral neuropathy effects include muscle weakness, tingling sensations, and numbness.
   - **e.** Neurological effects include headache, vertigo, drowsiness, and nystagmus.
   - **f.** Allergic reactions include anaphylaxis, hives, rash, and tingling sensations around the mouth.
   - **g.** Nitrofurantoin may impart a harmless brown color to the urine.
   - **h.** Nitrofurantoin is contraindicated in clients with renal impairment.
   - **i.** The client is instructed about the expected side effects, signs warranting notification of the health care provider (HCP), and not to take nitrofurantoin with antacids.

BOX 54-1 Urinary Tract Antiseptics

- Amoxicillin (Amoxil)
- Cefixime (Suprax)
- Fosfomycin (Monurol)
- Methenamine (Hiprex, Urex)
- Nitrofurantoin (Furadantin, Macrodantin, Macrobid)

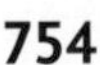

BOX 54-2 Fluoroquinolones

- Ciprofloxacin (Cipro)
- Gemifloxacin (Factive)
- Levofloxacin (Levaquin)
- Moxifloxacin (Avelox)
- Norfloxacin (Noroxin)
- Ofloxacin (Floxin)
- Gatifloxacin (Zymaxid)

BOX 54-3 Sulfonamides

- Sulfadiazine
- Sulfamethoxazole
- Trimethoprim (Trimpex)
- Trimethoprim (TMP)-sulfamethoxazole (SMZ) (Bactrim, Septra)

II. Fluoroquinolones (Box 54-2)

A. Description: Suppress bacterial growth by inhibiting an enzyme necessary for DNA synthesis; active against a broad spectrum of microbes

B. Side/adverse effects and nursing considerations
1. Side effects include dizziness, drowsiness, gastric distress, diarrhea, vaginitis (trovafloxacin), nausea, and vomiting.
2. Adverse effects include psychoses, hallucinations, confusion, tremors, hypersensitivity, and interstitial nephritis.
3. Fluoroquinolones should be used with caution in clients with hepatic, renal, or central nervous system (CNS) disorders.
4. Monitor client for side effects and adverse effects.
5. Enoxacin and norfloxacin (Noroxin) are to be taken on an empty stomach.
6. Ciprofloxacin (Cipro), lomefloxacin (Maxaquin), and ofloxacin (Floxin) may be taken with or without food.
7. Intravenously administered ciprofloxacin and ofloxacin are infused slowly over 60 minutes to minimize discomfort and vein irritation.
8. The client is advised to report dizziness, lightheadedness, visual disturbances, increased light sensitivity, and feelings of depression, because these signs could indicate CNS toxicity.
9. The client is informed of signs of hepatic and renal toxicity and the importance of reporting these signs to the HCP.
10. Avoid ultraviolet light and sun exposure, using protective clothing and sunscreen.

Fluoroquinolones are administered with a full glass of water, and the client is taught that it is necessary to maintain a urine output of at least 1200 to 1500 mL daily to minimize the development of crystalluria.

III. Sulfonamides (Box 54-3)

A. Description: Suppress bacterial growth by inhibiting the synthesis of folic acid; active against a broad spectrum of microbes; used primarily to treat acute urinary tract infections

B. Side/adverse effects and nursing considerations
1. Hypersensitivity reactions include rash, fever, and photosensitivity.
2. Stevens-Johnson syndrome, the most severe hypersensitivity response, produces symptoms that include widespread lesions of the skin and mucous membranes, fever, malaise, and toxemia.
3. Sulfonamides can cause hemolytic anemia, agranulocytosis, leukopenia, and thrombocytopenia. The client is instructed to notify the HCP if sore throat or fever occurs.
4. Sulfonamides are administered with caution in clients with renal impairment.
5. Sulfonamides are contraindicated if hypersensitivity exists to sulfonamides, sulfonylureas, or thiazide or loop diuretics.
6. Sulfonamides are contraindicated in infants younger than 2 months and in pregnant women or mothers who are breastfeeding.
7. Sulfonamides can potentiate the effects of warfarin sodium (Coumadin), phenytoin (Dilantin), and orally administered hypoglycemics such as tolbutamide (Orinase). When combined with sulfonamides, these medications may require a reduction in dosage.
8. Reinforce instructions to the client to take the medication on an empty stomach with a full glass of water.
9. Reinforce instructions to the client to complete the entire course of prescribed medication. 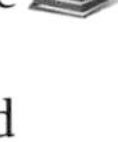
10. Reinforce instructions to the client to avoid prolonged exposure to sunlight, wear protective clothing, and apply a sunscreen to exposed skin.
11. Adults should maintain a daily urine output of 1200 mL by consuming 8 to 10 glasses of water each day to minimize the risk of renal damage from the medication. 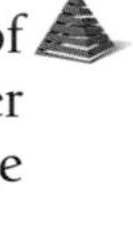
12. The client is informed that some combination medications of sulfonamides can cause the urine to turn dark brown or red.
13. The sulfonamide combination of trimethoprim-sulfamethoxazole (TMP-SMZ; Bactrim, Septra) is more effective than either medication alone because it inhibits the sequential steps in bacterial folic acid synthesis.
14. TMP-SMZ is used cautiously with clients experiencing impaired kidney function, folate deficiency, severe allergy, or bronchial asthma. 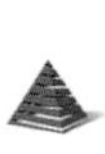

BOX 54-4 Urinary Tract Analgesic

- Pentosan polysulfate sodium (Elmiron)
- Phenazopyridine (Pyridium, Azo-Standard, Pyridiate)

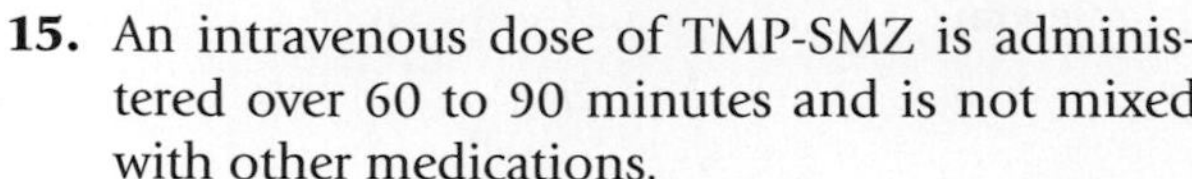

15. An intravenous dose of TMP-SMZ is administered over 60 to 90 minutes and is not mixed with other medications.

Sulfonamides should be withheld if a rash is noted. The client is informed to contact the HCP if a rash appears.

IV. Urinary Tract Analgesic (Box 54-4)

A. Description: A urinary tract analgesic is administered with an antibiotic because the analgesic only treats pain, not the infection.

B. Side/adverse effects
1. Nausea
2. Headache
3. Vertigo

C. Nursing considerations
1. The client is instructed that the urine will turn red or orange and stain clothing.
2. A urinary tract analgesic is contraindicated in clients with renal or hepatic disease.
3. The medication interferes with accurate urine testing for glucose and ketones.

V. Anticholinergics-Antispasmodics (Box 54-5)

A. Description: Used for overactive bladder (urge incontinence)

B. Side/adverse effects
1. Anorexia, nausea, vomiting, and dry mouth
2. Blurred vision
3. Confusion in older clients
4. Constipation
5. Decreased sweating
6. Dizziness
7. Drowsiness
8. Dry eyes
9. Gastric distress
10. Headache
11. Tachycardia
12. Urinary retention

BOX 54-5 Anticholinergics-Antispasmodics

- Darifenacin (Enablex)
- Dicyclomine (Barmine, Bentyl)
- Oxybutynin chloride (Ditropan, Ditropan XL)
- Propantheline (Pro-Banthine, Propanthel)
- Solifenacin (VESIcare)
- Tolterodine (Detrol, Detrol LA)
- Trospium (Sanctura, Sanctura XR)

C. Nursing considerations
1. Extended-release capsules should not be split, chewed, or crushed.
2. Detrol LA should be used cautiously in clients with narrow-angle glaucoma.
3. Oxybutynin is not administered to clients with known hypersensitivity, gastrointestinal or genitourinary obstruction, glaucoma, severe colitis, or myasthenia gravis.
4. Propantheline is not administered to clients with narrow-angle glaucoma, obstructive uropathy, gastrointestinal disease, or ulcerative colitis.
5. Reinforce instructions to the client to avoid hazardous activities because of the side effects of dizziness and drowsiness.
6. Monitor intake and output.
7. Provide gum or hard candy for dry mouth.
8. Monitor for signs of toxicity (CNS stimulation) such as hypotension, hypertension, confusion, tachycardia, flushed or red face, signs of respiratory depression, nervousness, restlessness, hallucinations, and irritability.

VI. Cholinergic

A. Description: Bethanechol chloride (Urecholine) is a cholinergic used to increase bladder tone and function and to treat nonobstructive urinary retention and neurogenic bladder.

B. Side/adverse effects
1. Headache
2. Hypotension
3. Flushing and sweating
4. Increased salivation
5. Abdominal cramps
6. Nausea and vomiting
7. Diarrhea
8. Urinary urgency
9. Bronchoconstriction
10. Transient complete heart block

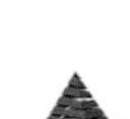

C. Nursing considerations
1. Administered on an empty stomach, 1 hour before or 2 hours after meals to lessen nausea and vomiting
2. Never administered by the intramuscular or intravenous (IV) routes
3. Monitor intake and output.
4. Monitor for increased bladder tone and function.
5. Monitor for cholinergic overdose (excessive salivation, sweating, involuntary urination and defecation, bradycardia, and severe hypotension).
6. Have atropine sulfate (antidote) readily available for IV or subcutaneous administration.

A cholinergic such as bethanechol chloride (Urecholine) is not given to a client who has a urinary stricture or obstruction.

BOX 54-6 Preventing Organ Rejection

Immunosuppressants
- Cyclosporine (Sandimmune, Gengraf, Neoral)
- Sirolimus (Rapamune)
- Tacrolimus (Prograf) Glucocorticoid
- Prednisone

Cytotoxic Medications
- Azathioprine (Imuran)
- Mycophenolate mofetil (CellCept)

Antibodies
- Anti-thymocyte globulin, equine (Atgam)
- Basiliximab (Simulect)
- Daclizumab (Zenapax)

VII. Medications for Preventing Organ Rejection (Box 54-6)

A. Medications include immunosuppressants, corticosteroids, cytotoxic medications, and antibodies.

B. Some medications may be used in combination with one another to produce different actions on the immune system. Combination therapy also allows for administration of the medications in lower doses, reducing the possibility of side/adverse effects.

C. Cyclosporine (Sandimmune, Gengraf, Neoral)

1. Cyclosporine inhibits calcineurin and acts on T lymphocytes to suppress the production of interleukin-2, interferon-γ, and other cytokines.
2. Cyclosporine may be used to prevent rejection of allogeneic kidney, liver, and heart transplants.
3. Prednisone may be administered concurrently.
4. Oral administration of cyclosporine is preferred. Intravenous administration is reserved for clients who cannot take the medication orally.
5. Blood levels of the medication should be measured regularly because of its nephrotoxic effects.
6. The most common adverse effects are nephrotoxicity, infection, hypertension, tremor, and hirsutism.
7. The client is assured that hirsutism is reversible and instructed in the use of a depilatory.
8. Other adverse effects include neurotoxicity, gastrointestinal effects, hyperkalemia, and hyperglycemia.
9. The risk of infection and lymphomas is increased with the use of cyclosporine.
10. Cyclosporine is contraindicated in the presence of hypersensitivity, pregnancy and breastfeeding, recent inoculation with live virus vaccines, and recent contact with an active infection such as chickenpox or herpes zoster.
11. Cyclosporine is embryotoxic, and women of childbearing age should use a mechanical form of contraception and avoid oral contraceptives.
12. The client should be informed about the possibility of renal damage and liver damage and the need for periodic liver function tests and determination of coagulation factors and blood urea nitrogen, serum creatinine, serum potassium, and blood glucose levels.
13. The client should be instructed to monitor for early signs of infection and report these signs immediately.
14. Available in a pill form. If the client is unable to swallow the pill, the client is instructed to dispense the oral liquid medication into a glass container by using a specially calibrated pipette, mix well, and drink immediately; rinse the glass container with diluent and drink it to ensure ingestion of the complete dose; dry the outside of the pipette and return it to its cover for storage.

15. To promote palatability, the client is instructed to mix the liquid medication with milk, chocolate milk, or orange juice just before administration.
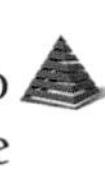
16. Consuming grapefruit juice is prohibited because it raises cyclosporine levels and increases the risk of toxicity.
17. Ketoconazole (Nizoral), erythromycin, and amphotericin B (Abelcet, Amphotec, AmBisome) can elevate cyclosporine levels.
18. Phenytoin (Dilantin), phenobarbital, rifampin (Rifadin), and TMP-SMZ can decrease cyclosporine levels.
19. Renal damage can be intensified by the concurrent use of other nephrotoxic medications.

D. Sirolimus (Rapamune)

1. Sirolimus is used for the prevention of renal transplant rejection by inhibiting the response of helper T lymphocytes and B lymphocytes to cytokinesis.
2. It may be used with cyclosporine or tacrolimus (Prograf) and corticosteroids.
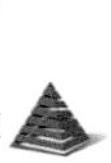
3. Increases the risk of infection, increases the risk of renal injury, increases the risk of lymphocele (a complication of renal transplant surgery), and raises cholesterol and triglyceride levels
4. Side/adverse effects include rash, acne, anemia, thrombocytopenia, joint pain, diarrhea, and hypokalemia.

E. Tacrolimus (Prograf)

1. Tacrolimus inhibits calcineurin and thereby prevents T cells from producing interleukin-2, interferon-γ, and other cytokines.
2. Tacrolimus is more effective than cyclosporine but is more toxic.
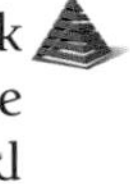
3. Adverse effects are similar to those of cyclosporine and include nephrotoxicity, infection, hypertension, tremor, hirsutism, neurotoxicity, gastrointestinal effects, hyperkalemia, and hyperglycemia.

4. Tacrolimus should be used cautiously in immunosuppressed clients and those with renal, hepatic, or pancreatic impairment.
5. Tacrolimus is contraindicated for clients hypersensitive to cyclosporine.
6. Blood glucose levels are monitored, and prescribed insulin or oral hypoglycemics are administered.

F. Prednisone
1. Prednisone is a glucocorticoid that inhibits accumulation of inflammatory cells at inflammation sites.
2. Hyperglycemia and hypokalemia can occur with prednisone use. Monitor glucose and serum potassium levels.
3. See Chapter 46 for additional information about prednisone.

G. Azathioprine (Imuran)
1. Azathioprine suppresses cell-mediated and humoral immune responses by inhibiting the proliferation of B and T lymphocytes.
2. Not used routinely since the advent of newer medications that prevent transplant rejection
3. Can cause neutropenia and thrombocytopenia from bone marrow suppression
4. Contraindicated in pregnancy; associated with an increased incidence of neoplasms
5. Monitor hematocrit, white blood cell count, platelet count, liver enzyme levels, and coagulation factors.

H. Mycophenolate mofetil (CellCept)
1. Mycophenolate mofetil causes selective inhibition of B- and T-lymphocyte proliferation.
2. May be used with cyclosporine or tacrolimus and glucocorticoids for prophylaxis against organ rejection
3. Adverse effects include diarrhea, severe neutropenia, vomiting, and sepsis.
4. Mycophenolate mofetil is associated with an increased risk of infection and malignancies.
5. Absorption is decreased by the use of magnesium and aluminum antacids and cholestyramine (Questran, Prevalite).
6. It is contraindicated in pregnancy and during breastfeeding.
7. Reinforce instructions to the client to take the medication on an empty stomach and not to open or crush capsules.
8. Reinforce instructions to the client to contact the HCP for unusual bleeding or bruising, sore throat, mouth sores, abdominal pain, or fever.

I. Basiliximab (Simulect) and daclizumab (Zenapax)
1. Basiliximab and daclizumab bind to interleukin-2 receptors on lymphocytes, resulting in diminished cell-mediated immune reactions.
2. Used primarily as an induction agent at the time of transplantation; may be used with other immunosuppressants to prevent acute rejection of transplanted kidneys
3. Administered by the intravenous route
4. Basiliximab (Simulect)
   a. Initial dose is administered within 2 hours before transplantation.
   b. Side/adverse effects are similar to those for daclizumab; in addition, headache, insomnia, dizziness, and tremors can occur.
5. Daclizumab (Zenapax)
   a. The initial dose is administered within 24 hours before transplantation.
   b. Side/adverse effects include chest pain, gastrointestinal distress, edema, shortness of breath, pain in the joints, and slow wound healing.

J. Antithymocyte globulin, equine (Atgam)
1. Antithymocyte globulin, equine, causes a decrease in the number and activity of thymus-derived lymphocytes and is used to suppress organ rejection following renal, liver, bone marrow, and heart transplantation.
2. It is used primarily to treat acute rejection episodes.
3. Before the first infusion, the client should undergo intradermal skin testing to determine hypersensitivity. 
4. Because this product is made using equine and human blood components, it may carry a risk of transmitting infectious agents, such as viruses.
5. Monitor the platelet count and report it if below 100,000 cells/mm^3.
6. Arrange for outpatient referral for repeated infusions after discharge.

VIII. Hematopoietic Growth Factors (Box 54-7) 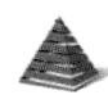

A. Erythropoietic growth factors
1. Stimulate the production of red blood cells
2. Used to treat anemia of **chronic kidney disease**, chemotherapy-induced anemia, anemia caused by zidovudine (AZT), and anemia in clients requiring surgery

BOX 54-7 Hematopoietic Growth Factors

Erythropoietic Growth Factors
- Epoetin alfa (Epogen, Procrit)
- Darbepoetin alfa (Aranesp)
- Peginesatide (Omontys)

Leukopoietic Growth Factors
- Filgrastim (Neupogen)
- Pegfilgrastim (Neulasta)
- Sargramostim (Leukine)

Thrombopoietic Growth Factor
- Oprelvekin (Neumega)

3. Initial effects can be seen within 1 to 2 weeks, and the hematocrit reaches normal levels (30% to 33%) in 2 to 3 months.
4. Side effect: The major side effect is hypertension.
5. Adverse effects can include heart failure, thrombotic effects such as stroke or myocardial infarction, and cardiac arrest.

B. Leukopoietic growth factors
1. Stimulate the production of white blood cells (leukocytes)
2. Used for clients undergoing myelosuppressive chemotherapy or bone marrow transplantation and those with severe chronic neutropenia
3. Can cause bone pain, leukocytosis, and elevation of plasma uric acid, lactate dehydrogenase, and alkaline phosphatase levels. Long-term therapy has caused splenomegaly.

C. Thrombopoietic growth factor
1. Stimulates the production of platelets
2. Used for clients undergoing myelosuppressive chemotherapy to minimize thrombocytopenia and decrease the need for platelet transfusions
3. Adverse effects include fluid retention, cardiac dysrhythmias, conjunctival infection, visual blurring, and papilledema.

CRITICAL THINKING What Should You Do?

Answer: Levofloxacin is a fluoroquinolone that is used to treat urinary tract infections by suppressing bacterial growth. Complaints of dizziness, light-headedness, visual disturbances, increased light sensitivity, and feelings of depression are signs of central nervous system (CNS) toxicity. Therefore, the nurse should withhold the medication and notify the registered nurse, who will contact the health care provider (HCP).

Reference(s): deWit, D. & Kumagai, C. (2013). *Medical-surgical nursing: Concepts & practice.* (2nd ed., p. 786). St. Louis: Saunders.

Lehne, R. (2013). *Pharmacology for nursing care* (8th ed., p. 1053). St. Louis: Saunders.

PRACTICE QUESTIONS

561. The client who has a cold is seen in the emergency department with an inability to void. Because the client has a history of benign prostatic hyperplasia, the nurse determines that the client should be questioned about the use of which medication?
1. Diuretics
2. Antibiotics
3. Antitussives
4. Decongestants

562. A sulfonamide is prescribed for a client with a urinary tract infection. On review of the client's record, the nurse notes that the client is taking warfarin sodium (Coumadin) daily. Which prescription should the nurse anticipate for this client?
1. Discontinuation of warfarin sodium (Coumadin)
2. A decrease in the warfarin sodium (Coumadin) dosage
3. An increase in the warfarin sodium (Coumadin) dosage
4. A decrease in the usual dose of the sulfonamide

❖ **563.** Methenamine (Urex), a urinary antiseptic, is prescribed for the client. The nurse reviews the client's medical record and should contact the health care provider regarding which documented finding to verify the prescription? **Refer to chart.**
1. Renal insufficiency
2. Chest x-ray: normal
3. Blood glucose, 102 mg/dL
4. Folic acid (vitamin B_6) 0.5 mg, orally daily

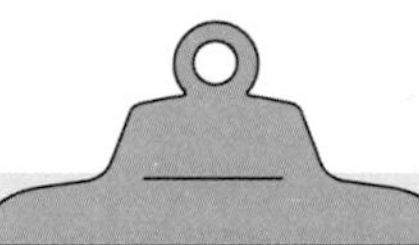

CHART/EXHIBIT

CLIENT'S MEDICAL RECORD

Laboratory Test Result: Blood glucose, 102 mg/dL
Diagnostic Test Result: Chest x-ray: normal
Client's History: Renal Insufficiency
Medication History: Folic acid (vitamin B_6) 0.5 mg, orally daily

564. Trimethoprim-sulfamethoxazole (TMP-SMZ) is prescribed for a client. The nurse should instruct the client to report which symptom if it developed during the course of this medication therapy?
1. Nausea
2. Diarrhea
3. Headache
4. Sore throat

565. Phenazopyridine hydrochloride (Pyridium) is prescribed for a client for symptomatic relief of pain resulting from a lower urinary tract infection. Which should the nurse reinforce to the client?
1. Take the medication at bedtime.
2. Take the medication before meals.
3. Discontinue the medication if a headache occurs.
4. A reddish-orange discoloration of the urine may occur.

566. Bethanechol chloride (Urecholine) is prescribed for a client with urinary retention. Which disorder should be a contraindication to the administration of this medication?
1. Gastric atony
2. Urinary strictures
3. Neurogenic atony
4. Gastroesophageal reflux

567. The nurse who is administering bethanechol chloride (Urecholine) is monitoring for acute toxicity associated with the medication. The nurse should check the client for which sign of toxicity?
1. Dry skin
2. Dry mouth
3. Bradycardia
4. Signs of dehydration

568. Oxybutynin chloride (Ditropan XL) is prescribed for a client with neurogenic bladder. Which sign would indicate a possible toxic effect related to this medication?
1. Pallor
2. Drowsiness
3. Bradycardia
4. Restlessness

569. After kidney transplantation, cyclosporine (Sandimmune) is prescribed for a client. Which laboratory result would indicate an adverse effect from the use of this medication?
1. Decreased creatinine level
2. Decreased hemoglobin level
3. Elevated white blood cell count
4. Elevated blood urea nitrogen level

570. The nurse is reinforcing discharge instructions to a client receiving sulfadiazine. Which should be included in the list of instructions?
1. Restrict fluid intake.
2. Maintain a high fluid intake.
3. If the urine turns dark brown, call the health care provider (HCP) immediately.
4. Decrease the dosage when symptoms are improving to prevent an allergic response.

ANSWERS

561. 4
Rationale: Episodes of urinary retention can be triggered by certain medications such as decongestants, anticholinergics, and antidepressants. Diuretics, antibiotics, and antitussives generally do not trigger urinary retention. Retention also can be precipitated by other factors such as alcoholic beverages, infection, bed rest, and becoming chilled.
Test-Taking Strategy: Focus on the subject, medications that cause urinary retention. The question is asking about medications that could exacerbate or contribute to urinary retention. Diuretics should help voiding; therefore, readily eliminate option 1. Antibiotics should have no effect at all, eliminating option 2. From the remaining options, recalling that medications that contain anticholinergics may cause urinary retention will direct you to option 4. **Review:** medication classifications that can precipitate **urinary retention.**
Level of Cognitive Ability: Analyzing
Client Needs: Physiological Integrity
Integrated Process: Nursing Process/Data Collection
Content Area: Pharmacology: Renal and Urinary Medications
Priority Concepts: Elimination, Infection
Reference(s): deWit, Kumagai (2013), pp. 780, 782.

562. 2
Rationale: Sulfonamides can potentiate the effects of warfarin sodium (Coumadin), phenytoin (Dilantin), and orally administered hypoglycemics such as tolbutamide (Orinase). When an oral anticoagulant is combined with a sulfonamide, a decrease in the anticoagulant dosage may be needed.
Test-Taking Strategy: Focus on the subject, a sulfonamide and interaction with oral anticoagulants. Knowledge about the medication interactions associated with the use of sulfonamides is needed to answer this question. Remember that a sulfonamide can intensify the effects of oral anticoagulants. **Review: sulfonamides.**
Level of Cognitive Ability: Analyzing
Client Needs: Physiological Integrity
Integrated Process: Nursing Process/Planning
Content Area: Pharmacology: Renal and Urinary Medications
Priority Concepts: Clinical Judgment, Safety
Reference(s): deWit, Kumagai (2013), p. 787.

❖**563. 1**
Rationale: Methenamine is a urinary antiseptic. Methenamine can cause crystalluria and should not be used in clients with renal impairment. Therefore, the nurse would verify the prescription if the client had a documented history of renal insufficiency. The laboratory and diagnostic test results are normal findings. Folic acid (vitamin B_6) may be prescribed for a client with renal insufficiency to prevent anemia.
Test-Taking Strategy: Note the subject, caution with the use of methenamine. Focus on the need to contact the health care provider. Eliminate options 2 and 3 because the laboratory and diagnostic test results are normal findings. From the remaining options, note the disorder in the client's history. This directs you to the correct option. **Review:** the contraindications associated with **methenamine.**
Level of Cognitive Ability: Analyzing
Client Needs: Physiological Integrity

Integrated Process: Nursing Process/Data Collection
Content Area: Pharmacology: Renal and Urinary Medications
Priority Concepts: Elimination, Safety
Reference(s): Lehne (2013), p. 1113.

564. 4
Rationale: Clients taking trimethoprim-sulfamethoxazole (TMP-SMZ) should be informed about early signs of blood disorders that can occur from this medication. These include sore throat, fever, and pallor, and the client should be instructed to notify the health care provider (HCP) if these symptoms occur. The other options do not require HCP notification.
Test-Taking Strategy: Focus on the subject, the symptom to be reported. Knowledge that this medication can cause blood dyscrasias will direct you to the correct option. **Review:** side/adverse effects of **trimethoprim-sulfamethoxazole (TMP-SMZ).**
Level of Cognitive Ability: Applying
Client Needs: Physiological Integrity
Integrated Process: Teaching and Learning
Content Area: Pharmacology: Renal and Urinary Medications
Priority Concepts: Client Education, Safety
Reference(s): Hodgson, Kizior (2015), pp. 1238–1239.

565. 4
Rationale: The nurse should instruct the client that a reddish-orange discoloration of urine may occur. The nurse also should instruct the client that this discoloration can stain fabric. The medication should be taken after meals to reduce the possibility of gastrointestinal upset. A headache is an occasional side effect of the medication and does not warrant discontinuation of the medication.
Test-Taking Strategy: Eliminate options 1 and 2 first because they are comparable or alike in that they address time schedules for the administration of the medication. From the remaining options, eliminate option 3 because the nurse would not advise the client to discontinue this medication. **Review:** client instructions regarding **phenazopyridine hydrochloride (Pyridium).**
Level of Cognitive Ability: Applying
Client Needs: Physiological Integrity
Integrated Process: Teaching and Learning
Content Area: Pharmacology: Renal and Urinary Medications
Priority Concepts: Client Education, Pain
Reference(s): Hodgson, Kizior (2015), pp. 949–950.

566. 2
Rationale: Bethanechol chloride (Urecholine) can be harmful to clients with urinary tract obstruction or weakness of the bladder wall. The medication has the ability to contract the bladder and thereby increase pressure within the urinary tract. Elevation of pressure within the urinary tract could rupture the bladder in clients with these conditions.
Test-Taking Strategy: Focus on the subject, a contraindication to bethanechol chloride. Noting that the medication is used for urinary retention may assist in directing you to the correct option. **Review:** the contraindications associated with **bethanechol chloride (Urecholine).**
Level of Cognitive Ability: Analyzing
Client Needs: Physiological Integrity
Integrated Process: Nursing Process/Data Collection
Content Area: Pharmacology: Renal and Urinary Medications
Priority Concepts: Elimination, Safety
Reference(s): Hodgson, Kizior (2015), pp. 135–136; Ignatavicius, Workman (2013), p. 1505.

567. 3
Rationale: Toxicity (overdose) produces manifestations of excessive muscarinic stimulation such as salivation, sweating, involuntary urination and defecation, bradycardia, and severe hypotension. Treatment includes supportive measures and the administration of atropine sulfate subcutaneously or intravenously.
Test-Taking Strategy: Noting the comparable and alike similarity in options 1, 2, and 4 will assist in eliminating these options. **Review:** the signs of toxicity of **bethanechol chloride (Urecholine).**
Level of Cognitive Ability: Analyzing
Client Needs: Physiological Integrity
Integrated Process: Nursing Process/Data Collection
Content Area: Pharmacology: Renal and Urinary Medications
Priority Concepts: Clinical Judgment, Safety
Reference(s): Hodgson, Kizior (2015), pp. 135–136.

568. 4
Rationale: Toxicity (overdose) of this medication produces central nervous system excitation, such as nervousness, restlessness, hallucinations, and irritability. Other signs of toxicity include hypotension or hypertension, confusion, tachycardia, flushed or red face, and signs of respiratory depression. Drowsiness is a frequent side effect of the medication but does not indicate overdose.
Test-Taking Strategy: Focus on the subject, toxicity associated with oxybutynin chloride. Knowledge regarding the signs and symptoms related to toxicity is required to answer this question. Remember that restlessness is a sign of toxicity. **Review:** the signs that indicate toxicity of **oxybutynin chloride (Ditropan XL).**
Level of Cognitive Ability: Analyzing
Client Needs: Physiological Integrity
Integrated Process: Nursing Process/Data Collection
Content Area: Pharmacology: Renal and Urinary Medications
Priority Concepts: Clinical Judgment, Safety
Reference(s): Hodgson, Kizior (2015), pp. 902–903.

569. 4
Rationale: Nephrotoxicity can occur from the use of cyclosporine (Sandimmune). Nephrotoxicity is evaluated by monitoring for elevated blood urea nitrogen and serum creatinine levels. Cyclosporine does not depress the bone marrow.
Test-Taking Strategy: Focus on the subject, indication of an adverse effect of cyclosporine. Eliminate options 2 and 3 first because they are unrelated to renal function. Next, eliminate option 1 because the creatinine level would be elevated, not decreased. Option 4 is the only option that indicates an increased level of a renal function test. **Review:** the adverse effects related to **cyclosporine (Sandimmune).**
Level of Cognitive Ability: Analyzing
Client Needs: Physiological Integrity
Integrated Process: Nursing Process/Data Collection
Content Area: Pharmacology: Renal and Urinary Medications
Priority Concepts: Clinical Judgment, Safety
Reference(s): Hodgson, Kizior (2015), p. 301.

570. 2

Rationale: Each dose of sulfadiazine should be administered with a full glass of water, and the client should maintain a high fluid intake. The medication is more soluble in alkaline urine. The client should not be instructed to taper or discontinue the dose. Some forms of sulfadiazine cause urine to turn dark brown or red. This does not indicate the need to notify the HCP.

Test-Taking Strategy: Focus on the **subject**, client teaching points related to sulfadiazine. Recalling that this medication is used to treat urinary tract infections will direct you to the correct option. **Review:** client instructions regarding **sulfadiazine.**

Level of Cognitive Ability: Applying
Client Needs: Physiological Integrity
Integrated Process: Teaching and Learning
Content Area: Pharmacology: Renal and Urinary Medications
Priority Concepts: Client Education, Elimination
Reference(s): deWit, Kumagai (2013), p. 786.

UNIT XV

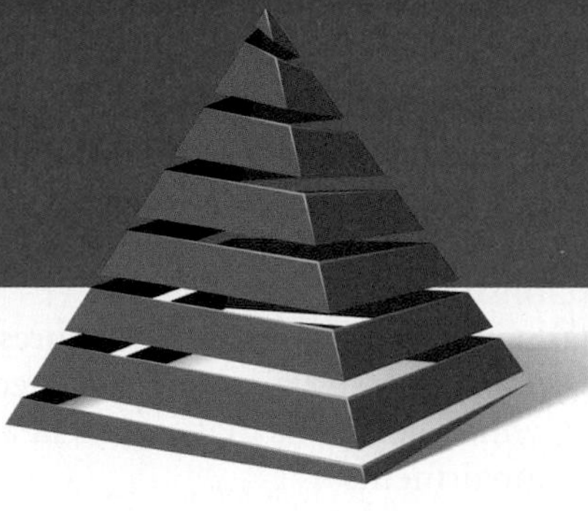

The Adult Client with an Eye or Ear Disorder

PYRAMID TERMS

accommodation Process by which a clear visual image is maintained as the gaze is shifted from a distant to a near point.

astigmatism A condition that results from an uneven curvature of the cornea or lens in which light rays do not focus on a single point on the retina.

cataract An opacity of the lens that distorts the image projected onto the retina and that can progress to blindness.

conductive hearing loss A mechanical dysfunction or blockage of sound waves to the inner ear fibers because of external ear or middle ear disorders; the blockage can be caused by impacted cerumen, foreign bodies, pus, or serum in the middle ear; disorders can often be corrected with no damage to hearing or minimal permanent hearing loss.

cycloplegia The paralysis of the ciliary muscles by medications that block muscarinic receptors; cycloplegia causes blurred vision because the shape of the lens can no longer be adjusted to near vision.

glaucoma Increased intraocular pressure as a result of inadequate drainage of aqueous humor from the canal of Schlemm or overproduction of aqueous humor; the condition damages the optic nerve and can result in blindness.

hyperopia Farsightedness; objects converge to a point behind the retina; vision beyond 20 feet is normal, but near vision is poor; correction is done by a convex lens.

legally blind The best visual acuity with corrective lenses in the better eye of 20/200 or less, or the visual field is no greater than 20 degrees in its widest diameter in the better eye.

macular degeneration A blurred central vision caused by progressive degeneration of the center of the retina; condition may be atrophic or age related, or dry or exudative (wet).

miosis Constriction of the pupil, which occurs primarily by stimulation of the muscarinic receptors of the sphincter muscles. It is seen with the use of pilocarpine drops when treating glaucoma, when using opioids, or when there is brain damage of the pons.

miotics Constricting the pupil; a medication that causes constriction of the pupil.

mydriasis A dilated pupil that occurs because of blockage of the muscarinic receptors of the sphincter muscles or by stimulation of the α-receptors of the dilator muscles. Enlarged pupils occur with stimulation of the sympathetic nervous system, use of dilating drops, acute glaucoma, or past or recent trauma.

mydriatic Dilating the pupil; a medication that dilates the pupil.

myopia Nearsightedness; rays coming from an object are focused in front of the retina; near vision is normal, but distant vision is defective; a biconcave lens is used for correction.

presbycusis Gradual nerve degeneration associated with aging; a common cause of sensorineural hearing loss.

sensorineural hearing loss A pathological process of the inner ear or the sensory fibers that lead to the cerebral cortex; such hearing loss is often permanent, and measures must be taken to reduce further damage or attempt to amplify sound as a means of improving hearing to some degree.

Pyramid to Success

Pyramid points focus on safety and nursing interventions for clients with impairment of sight or hearing and on the nursing care related to disorders such as cataracts, glaucoma, and retinal detachment. Communicating with clients who are visual or hearing impaired is also a priority. Emergency interventions for eye and ear disorders and injuries are a priority point. Pyramid points also focus on client instructions related to medication administration, sensory perceptual alterations and safety issues, and available support systems.

Client Needs

Safe and Effective Care Environment

Assisting with care for the recipient of a tissue (corneal) donation

Consulting with the registered nurse and other members of the health care team
Ensuring that informed consent for invasive procedures has been obtained
Establishing priorities
Maintaining asepsis with procedures and treatments
Maintaining standard and other precautions
Preventing accidents that can occur as a result of sensory impairments
Upholding client rights

Health Promotion and Maintenance

Discussing changes that occur with the aging process
Discussing expected body-image changes and self-care deficits
Implementing measures for the prevention and early detection of health problems and diseases related to the eye and ear
Performing data collection techniques for eye and ear disorders
Reinforcing home care instructions after procedures related to the eye and ear
Reinforcing instructions regarding activity limitations or postoperative activities
Reinforcing instructions regarding the administration of eye and ear medications
Reinforcing the importance of compliance to the prescribed therapy

Psychosocial Integrity

Determining the client's ability to cope with feelings of isolation, fear, or anxiety regarding a possible change in vision and/or hearing status, and loss of independence
Discussing role changes
Identifying family support systems
Informing the client about available community resources
Monitoring for sensory perceptual alterations
Using appropriate communication techniques for impaired vision and hearing

Physiological Integrity

Monitoring for complications related to procedures
Monitoring for expected responses to therapy
Providing care to assistive devices such as glasses, contact lenses, and hearing aids
Taking action in medical emergencies

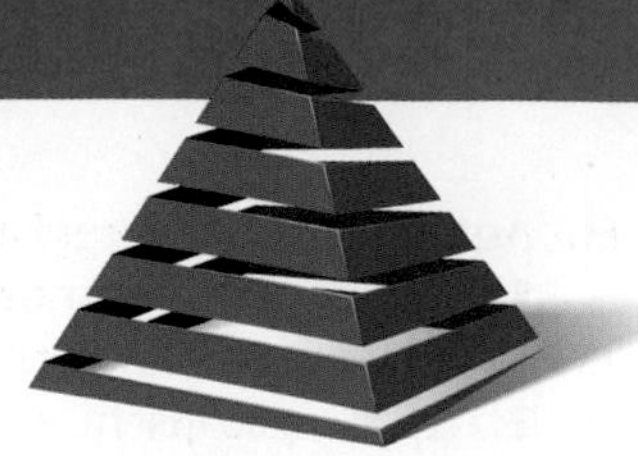

CHAPTER 55

The Eye and the Ear

CRITICAL THINKING What Should You Do?

A client enters the emergency department and tells the nurse that he suddenly felt something hit his eye and has severe eye pain. The nurse notes an entrance wound in the client's affected eye. What should the nurse do?
Answer located on p. 780.

I. Anatomy and Physiology of the Eye

A. The eye
 1. Is 1 inch in diameter and is located in the anterior portion of the orbit
 2. The orbit is the bony structure of the skull that surrounds the eye and offers protection to the eye.

B. Layers of the eye
 1. External layer
  a. The fibrous coat that supports the eye
  b. Contains the sclera, which is an opaque white tissue
  c. Contains the cornea, which is a dense transparent layer
 2. Middle layer
  a. Called the uveal tract
  b. Consists of the choroid, the ciliary body, and the iris
  c. The choroid is the dark brown membrane located between the sclera and the retina that has dark pigmentation to prevent light from reflecting internally.
  d. The choroid lines most of the sclera and is attached to the retina but can detach easily from the sclera.
  e. The choroid contains many blood vessels and supplies nutrients to the retina.
  f. The ciliary body connects the choroid with the iris and secretes aqueous humor that helps give the eye its shape. The muscles of the ciliary body control the thickness of the lens.
  g. The iris is the colored portion of the eye, is located in front of the lens, and has a central circular opening called the pupil. The pupil controls the amount of light admitted into the retina (darkness produces dilation and light produces constriction).
 3. Internal layer
  a. Consists of the retina, a thin, delicate structure in which the fibers of the optic nerve are distributed
  b. The retina is bordered externally by the choroid and sclera and internally by the vitreous.
  c. The retina is the visual receptive layer of the eye in which light waves are changed into nerve impulses and contains blood vessels and photoreceptors called rods and cones.

C. Vitreous body
 1. Contains a gelatinous substance that occupies the vitreous chamber, which is the space between the lens and the retina
 2. The vitreous body transmits light and gives shape to the posterior eye.

D. Vitreous
 1. Gel-like substance that maintains the shape of the eye
 2. Provides additional physical support to the retina

E. Rods and cones
 1. Rods are responsible for peripheral vision and function at reduced levels of illumination.
 2. Cones function at bright levels of illumination and are responsible for color vision and central vision.

F. Optic disk
 1. The optic disk is a creamy pink to white depressed area in the retina.
 2. The optic nerve enters and exits the eyeball at this area.
 3. This area is called the blind spot because it contains only nerve fibers, lacks photoreceptor cells, and is insensitive to light.

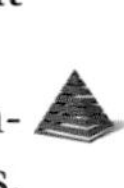

G. Macula lutea
 1. A small, oval, yellowish-pink area located lateral and temporal to the optic disc
 2. The central depressed part of the macula is the fovea centralis, the area of sharpest and keenest vision, where most acute vision occurs.

H. Aqueous humor
1. The aqueous humor is a clear, watery fluid that fills the anterior and posterior chambers of the eye.
2. The aqueous humor is produced by the ciliary processes, and the fluid drains into the canal of Schlemm.
3. The anterior chamber lies between the cornea and the iris.
4. The posterior chamber lies between the iris and the lens.

I. Canal of Schlemm: A passageway that extends completely around the eye that permits fluid to drain out of the eye into the systemic circulation so that a constant intraocular pressure is maintained

J. Lens
1. A transparent convex structure behind the iris and in front of the vitreous body
2. The lens bends rays of light so that the light falls on the retina.
3. The curve of the lens changes to focus on near or distant objects.

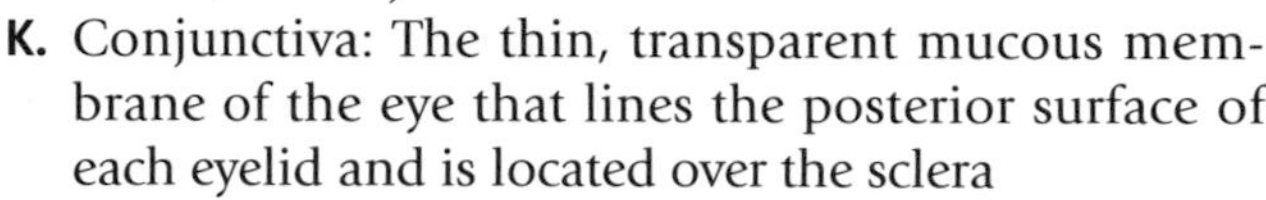

K. Conjunctiva: The thin, transparent mucous membrane of the eye that lines the posterior surface of each eyelid and is located over the sclera

L. Lacrimal gland
1. The lacrimal gland produces tears.
2. Tears are drained through the punctum into the lacrimal duct and sac.

M. Eye muscles
1. Muscles do not work independently but work with the muscle that produces the opposite movement
2. Rectus muscles exert their pull when the eye turns temporally.
3. Oblique muscles exert their pull when the eye turns nasally.

N. Nerves
1. Cranial nerve II: Optic nerve (nerve of sight)
2. Cranial nerve III: Oculomotor
3. Cranial nerve IV: Trochlear
4. Cranial nerve VI: Abducens

O. Blood vessels
1. The ophthalmic artery is the major artery supplying the structures in the eye.
2. The ophthalmic veins drain the blood from the eye.

II. Assessment of Vision (See Chapter 23)

III. Diagnostic Tests for the Eye

A. Fluorescein angiography
1. Description
   a. A detailed imaging and recording of ocular circulation by a series of photographs after the administration of a dye
   b. This test is useful for assessing problems with retinal circulation, such as those that occur in diabetic retinopathy, retinal bleeding, and macular degeneration, or to rule out intraocular tumors.
2. Preprocedure interventions
   a. Check the client for allergies and previous reactions to dyes.
   b. Ensure informed consent has been obtained.
   c. A mydriatic medication, which causes pupil dilation, is instilled into the eye 1 hour before the test.
   d. The dye is injected into a vein of the client's arm.
   e. Inform the client that the dye may cause the skin to appear yellow for several hours after the test and is eliminated gradually through the urine.
   f. The client may experience nausea, vomiting, sneezing, paresthesia of the tongue, or pain at the injection site.
   g. If hives appear, orally or intramuscularly administered antihistamines such as diphenhydramine (Benadryl) are given as prescribed.
3. Postprocedure interventions
   a. Encourage rest.
   b. Encourage fluid intake to assist in eliminating the dye from the client's system.
   c. Remind the client that the yellow skin appearance will disappear.
   d. Inform the client that the urine will appear bright green until the dye is excreted.
   e. Advise the client to avoid direct sunlight for a few hours after the test and to wear sunglasses if staying inside is not possible.
   f. Inform the client that the photophobia will continue until pupil size returns to normal.

B. Computed tomography (CT)
1. Description
   a. The test is performed to examine the eyes, the bony structures around the eye, and the extraocular muscles.
   b. A beam of x-rays scans the skull and orbits of the eye.
   c. A cross-sectional image is formed by the use of a computer.
   d. Contrast material may be used unless eye trauma is suspected.
2. Interventions
   a. No special client preparation or follow-up care is required.
   b. Reinforce instructions to the client that he or she will be positioned in a confined space and will need to keep his or her head still during the procedure.

C. Slit lamp
1. Description
   a. A slit lamp allows examination of the anterior ocular structures under microscopic magnification.

b. The client leans on a chin rest to stabilize the head, while a narrowed beam of light is aimed so it illuminates only a narrow segment of the eye.

2. Interventions

a. Explain the procedure to the client.

b. Advise the client about the brightness of the light and the need to look forward at a point over the examiner's ear.

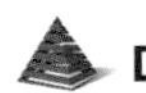

D. Corneal staining

1. Description

a. A topical dye is instilled into the conjunctival sac to outline irregularities of the corneal surface that are not easily visible.

b. The eye is viewed through a blue filter, and a bright green color indicates areas of a nonintact corneal epithelium.

2. Interventions

a. If the client wears contact lenses, the lenses must be removed.

b. Reinforce instructions to the client to blink after the dye has been applied to distribute the dye evenly across the cornea.

E. Tonometry

1. Description: The test is used primarily to assess for an increase of intraocular pressure and potential glaucoma.

2. Noncontact tonometry measurement

a. No direct contact with the client's cornea is needed, and no topical eye anesthetic is needed.

b. A puff of air is directed at the cornea to indent the cornea, which can be unpleasant and may startle the client.

c. It is a less accurate method of measurement as compared with contact tonometry.

3. Contact tonometry measurement

a. Requires a topical anesthetic

b. A flattened cone is brought in contact with the cornea, and the amount of pressure needed to flatten the cornea is measured.

c. The client must be instructed to avoid rubbing the eye after the examination if the eye has been anesthetized because of the potential for scratching the cornea.

Normal intraocular pressure is 10 to 21 mm Hg. Intraocular pressure varies throughout the day and is normally higher in the morning. Always document the time of intraocular measurement.

F. Ultrasound: Procedure is similar to an ultrasound procedure done in other parts of the body and is done to detect lesions or tumors in the eye.

G. Magnetic resonance imaging (MRI): Similar to an MRI done in other parts of the body; refer to Chapter 57 for additional information on MRI.

BOX 55-1 Risk Factors of Eye Disorders

Aging process
Congenital
Diabetes mellitus
Hereditary
Medications
Trauma

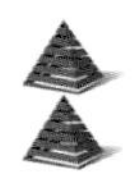

IV. Disorders of the Eye

A. Risk factors related to eye disorders (Box 55-1)

B. Refractive errors

1. Description

a. Refraction is the bending of light rays. Any problem associated with either eye length or refraction can lead to refractive errors.

b. Myopia (nearsightedness): Refractive ability of the eye is too strong for the eye length; images are bent and fall in front of, not on, the retina.

c. Hyperopia (farsightedness): Refractive ability of the eye is too weak; images are focused behind the retina.

d. Presbyopia: Loss of lens elasticity caused by aging; less able to focus the eye for close work, and images fall behind the retina.

e. Astigmatism: Occurs because of the irregular curvature of the cornea; image does not focus on the retina.

2. Data collection

a. Refractive errors are diagnosed through a process called refraction.

b. The client views an eye chart while various lenses of different strengths are systematically placed in front of the eye and is asked whether each lens sharpens or worsens the vision.

3. Nonsurgical interventions: Eyeglasses or contact lenses

4. Surgical interventions

a. Radial keratotomy: Incisions are made through the peripheral cornea to flatten the cornea, which allows the image to be focused closer to the retina; used to treat myopia.

b. Photorefractive keratotomy: A laser beam is used to remove small portions of the corneal surface to reshape the cornea to focus an image properly on the retina; used to treat myopia and astigmatism.

c. Laser in situ keratomileusis (LASIK): The superficial layers of the cornea are lifted as a flap, a laser reshapes the deeper corneal layers, and then the corneal flap is replaced; used to treat hyperopia, myopia, and astigmatism.

d. Corneal ring: The shape of the cornea is changed by placing a flexible ring in the outer edges of the cornea; used to treat myopia.

C. Legally blind

1. Description: The best visual acuity with corrective lenses in the better eye of 20/200 or less or the visual field is no greater than 20 degrees in its widest diameter in the better eye
2. Interventions
   a. When speaking to the client who has limited sight or is blind, the nurse uses a normal tone of voice.
   b. Alert the client when approaching.
   c. Orient the client to the environment.
   d. Use a focal point and provide further orientation to the environment from that focal point.
   e. Allow the client to touch objects in the room.
   f. Use the clock placement of foods on the meal tray to orient the client.
   g. Promote independence as much as possible.
   h. Provide radios, televisions, and clocks that give the time orally, or provide a Braille watch.
   i. When ambulating, allow the client to grasp the nurse's arm at the elbow. The nurse keeps his or her arm close to the body so that the client can detect the direction of movement.
   j. Reinforce instructions to the client to remain one step behind the nurse when ambulating.
   k. Reinforce instructions to the client in the use of the cane used for the blind client, which is differentiated from other canes by its straight shape and white color with red tip.
   l. Reinforce instructions to the client that the cane is held in the dominant hand several inches off the floor.
   m. Reinforce instructions to the client that the cane sweeps the ground where the client's foot will be placed next to determine the presence of obstacles.

D. Cataracts (Fig. 55-1)

1. Description
   a. A cataract is opacity of the lens that distorts the image projected onto the retina and that can progress to blindness.

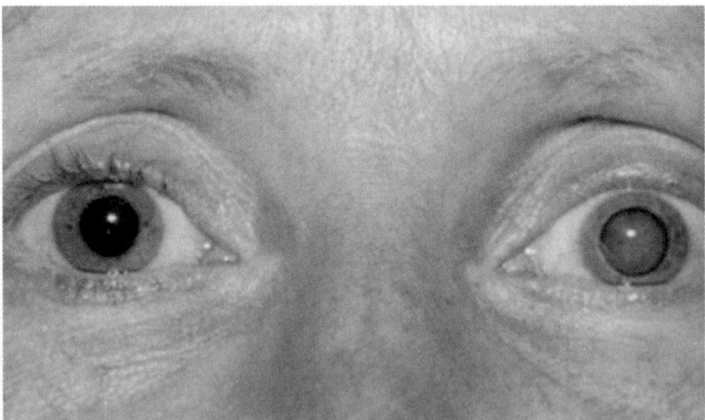

FIGURE 55-1 The cloudy appearance of a lens affected by cataract. (From Patton KT, Thibodeau GA: *Anatomy and physiology*, ed 7, St. Louis, 2010, Mosby.)

   b. Causes include the aging process (senile cataracts), heredity (congenital cataracts), and injury (traumatic cataracts). Cataracts can also result from another eye disease (secondary cataracts).
   c. Causes of secondary cataracts include diabetes mellitus, maternal rubella, severe myopia, ultraviolet light exposure, and medications such as corticosteroids.
   d. Intervention is indicated when visual acuity has been reduced to a level that the client finds to be unacceptable or adversely affects lifestyle.
2. Data collection
   a. Blurred vision and decreased color perception are early signs.
   b. Diplopia, reduced visual acuity, absence of the red reflex, and the presence of a white pupil are late signs.
   c. Pain or eye redness is associated with age-related cataract formation.
   d. Loss of vision is gradual.
3. Interventions
   a. Surgical removal of the lens, one eye at a time, is performed.
   b. With extracapsular extraction, the lens is lifted out without removing the lens capsule. The procedure may be performed by phacoemulsification, in which the lens is broken up by ultrasonic vibrations and is extracted.
   c. With intracapsular extraction, the lens and capsule are removed completely.
   d. A partial iridectomy may be performed with the lens extraction to prevent acute secondary glaucoma.
   e. A lens implantation may be performed at the time of the surgical procedure.
4. Preoperative interventions
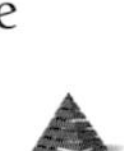
   a. Reinforce instructions to the client regarding the postoperative measures to prevent or decrease intraocular pressure, such as bending over, coughing, straining, and rubbing the eye.
   b. Stress to the client that care after surgery requires instillation of different types of eyedrops several times a day for 2 to 4 weeks.
   c. Administer eye medications preoperatively, including **mydriatics** and **cycloplegics** as prescribed.
5. Postoperative interventions
   a. Elevate the head of the bed 30 to 45 degrees.
   b. Turn the client to the back or nonoperative side.
   c. Provide an eye patch as prescribed. Orient the client to the environment.
   d. Position the client's personal belongings to the nonoperative side.

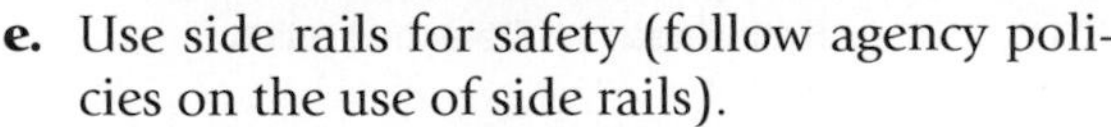

e. Use side rails for safety (follow agency policies on the use of side rails).
f. Assist with ambulation.

6. Client education (Box 55-2)

E. Glaucoma

1. Description
   a. A group of ocular diseases resulting in increased intraocular pressure
   b. Intraocular pressure is the fluid (aqueous humor) pressure within the eye. (Normal intraocular pressure is 10 to 21 mm Hg.)
   c. Increased intraocular pressure results from inadequate drainage of aqueous humor from the canal of Schlemm or overproduction of aqueous humor.
   d. The condition damages the optic nerve and can result in blindness.
   e. The gradual loss of visual fields may go unnoticed because central vision is unaffected.
2. Types
   a. Primary open-angle glaucoma (POAG) results from obstruction to outflow of aqueous humor, is the most common type, is painless, and vision changes are slow; results in "tunnel" vision.
   b. Primary angle-closure glaucoma (PACG) results from blocking the outflow of aqueous humor into the trabecular meshwork; causes include lens or pupil dilation from medications or sympathetic stimulation. Symptoms include blurred vision, halos around lights, and ocular erythemia.

BOX 55-2 Client Education After Cataract Surgery

Avoid eye straining.
Avoid rubbing or placing pressure on the eyes.
Avoid rapid movements, straining, sneezing, coughing, bending, vomiting, or lifting objects of more than 5 lb.
Take measures to prevent constipation.
Follow instructions for dressing changes and prescribed eyedrops and medications.
Wipe excess drainage or tearing with a sterile wet cotton ball from the inner to the outward canthus.
Use an eye shield at bedtime.
If a lens implant is not performed, accommodation is affected and glasses must be worn at all times.
Cataract glasses act as magnifying glasses and replace central vision only.
Because cataract glasses magnify, objects appear closer; therefore, the client needs to accommodate, judge distance, and climb stairs carefully.
Contact lenses provide sharp visual acuity, but dexterity is needed to insert them.
Contact the health care provider (HCP) for any decrease in vision, severe eye pain, or increase in eye discharge.

3. Data collection
   a. Early signs include diminished **accommodation** and increased intraocular pressure.
   b. Primary open-angle glaucoma (POAG): painless, and vision changes are slow; results in "tunnel" vision.
   c. Primary angle-closure glaucoma (PACG): blurred vision, halos around lights, and ocular erythema.
4. Interventions for acute glaucoma

⚠ Acute angle-closure glaucoma is a medical emergency that causes sudden eye pain and possible nausea and vomiting.

   a. Treat acute glaucoma as a medical emergency.
   b. Assist to administer medications as prescribed to lower intraocular pressure.
   c. Prepare the client for peripheral iridectomy, which allows aqueous humor to flow from the posterior to the anterior chamber.
5. Interventions for chronic glaucoma
   a. Reinforce instructions to the client on the importance of medications (**miotics**) to constrict the pupils, carbonic anhydrase inhibitors to decrease the production of aqueous humor, and β-blockers to decrease the production of aqueous humor and intraocular pressure.

   b. Reinforce instructions to the client on the need for lifelong medication use.
   c. Reinforce instructions to the client to wear a Medic-Alert bracelet.
   d. Reinforce instructions to the client to avoid anticholinergic medications.
   e. Reinforce instructions to the client to report eye pain, halos around the eyes, and changes in vision to the HCP.
   f. Reinforce instructions to the client that when maximal medical therapy has failed to halt the progression of visual field loss and optic nerve damage, surgery will be recommended.
   g. Reinforce instructions to the client to contact the health care provider before taking medications, including over-the-counter medications.
   h. Prepare the client for trabeculectomy as prescribed, which allows drainage of aqueous humor into the conjunctival spaces by the creation of an opening.

F. Retinal detachment

1. Description
   a. Detachment or separation of the retina from the epithelium
   b. Retinal detachment occurs when the layers of the retina separate because of the accumulation of fluid between them or when both

retinal layers elevate away from the choroid as a result of a tumor.

c. Partial detachment becomes complete if untreated.

d. When detachment becomes complete, blindness occurs.

2. Data collection
   a. Flashes of light
   b. Floaters or black spots (signs of bleeding)
   c. Increase in blurred vision
   d. Sense of a curtain being drawn over the eye
   e. Loss of a portion of the visual field; painless loss of central or peripheral vision
3. Immediate interventions
   a. Provide bed rest.
   b. Cover both eyes with patches as prescribed to prevent further detachment.
   c. Speak to the client before approaching.
   d. Position the client's head as prescribed.
   e. Protect the client from injury.
   f. Avoid jerky head movements.
   g. Minimize eye stress.
   h. Assist to prepare the client for a surgical procedure as prescribed.
4. Surgical procedures
   a. Draining fluid from the subretinal space so that the retina can return to the normal position
   b. Sealing retinal breaks by cryosurgery, a cold probe applied to the sclera, to stimulate an inflammatory response leading to adhesions
   c. Diathermy, the use of an electrode needle and heat through the sclera, to stimulate an inflammatory response
   d. Laser therapy, to stimulate an inflammatory response and to seal small retinal tears before the detachment occurs
   e. Scleral buckling, to hold the choroid and retina together with a splint until scar tissue forms and closes the tear (Fig. 55-2)
   f. Insertion of gas or silicone oil to promote reattachment. These agents float against the retina to hold it in place until healing occurs.

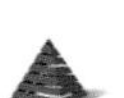

5. Postoperative interventions
   a. Maintain eye patches as prescribed.
   b. Monitor for hemorrhage.
   c. Prevent nausea and vomiting and monitor for restlessness, which can cause hemorrhage.
   d. Monitor for sudden, sharp eye pain (notify the RN and HCP).
   e. Encourage deep breathing, but avoid coughing.
   f. Provide bed rest for 1 to 2 days as prescribed.
   g. Position the client as prescribed. (Positioning depends on the location of the detachment.)

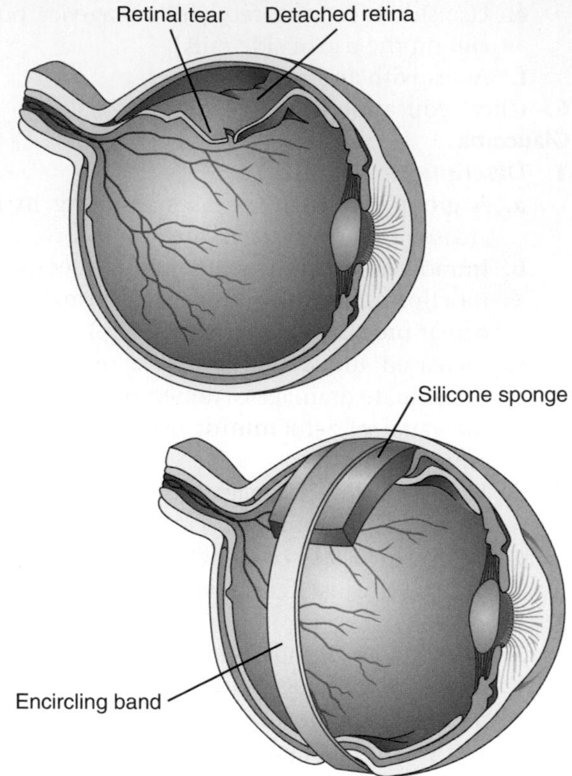

FIGURE 55-2 The scleral buckling procedure for repair of retinal detachment. (From Ignatavicius D, Workman ML: *Medical-surgical nursing: Patient-centered collaborative care*, ed 6, Philadelphia, 2010, Saunders.)

   h. Assist to administer eye medications as prescribed.
   i. Assist the client with activities of daily living.
   j. Avoid sudden head movements or anything that increases intraocular pressure.
   k. Reinforce instructions to the client to limit reading for 3 to 5 weeks.
   l. Reinforce instructions to the client to avoid squinting, straining and constipation, lifting heavy objects, and bending from the waist.
   m. Reinforce instructions to the client to wear dark glasses during the day and an eye patch at night.
   n. Encourage follow-up care because of the danger of recurrence or occurrence in the other eye.

G. Macular degeneration

1. A deterioration of the macula, the area of central vision
2. Can be atrophic (age-related or dry) or exudative (wet)
3. Age-related: Caused by gradual blocking of retinal capillaries, leading to an ischemic and necrotic macula; rods and cones photoreceptors die.
4. Exudative: Serous detachment of pigment epithelium in the macula occurs, and fluid and blood collect under the macula, resulting in scar formation and visual distortion.

5. Interventions are aimed at maximizing the remaining vision.
6. Data collection
   a. A decline in central vision
   b. Blurred vision and distortion
7. Interventions
   a. Initiate strategies to assist in maximizing remaining vision and maintaining independence.
   b. Assist to provide referrals to community organizations.
   c. Laser therapy or photodynamic therapy may be prescribed to seal the leaking blood vessels in or near the macula.

H. Ocular melanoma
1. Most common malignant eye tumor in adults
2. Tumor usually found in the uveal tract and can spread easily because of rich blood supply
3. Data collection
   a. Tumor can be discovered during routine examination.
   b. If macular area is invaded, blurring of vision occurs.
   c. Increased intraocular pressure is present if the canal of Schlemm is invaded.
   d. Change of iris color is noted if the tumor invades the iris.
   e. Ultrasonography may be performed to detect the tumor size and location.
4. Interventions
   a. Enucleation: The entire eyeball is removed surgically, and a ball implant is inserted to provide a base for socket prosthesis.
   b. Radiation via a radioactive plaque that is sutured to the sclera. The radioactive plaque remains in place until the prescribed radiation dose is delivered.

I. Enucleation and exenteration
1. Description
   a. Enucleation is the removal of the entire eyeball.
   b. Exenteration is the removal of the eyeball and surrounding tissues and bone.
   c. The procedures are performed for the removal of ocular tumors.
   d. After the eye is removed, a ball implant is inserted to provide a firm base for socket prosthesis and facilitate the best cosmetic result.
   e. A prosthesis is fitted about 1 month after surgery.
2. Preoperative interventions
   a. Provide emotional support to the client.
   b. Encourage the client to verbalize feelings related to loss.
3. Postoperative interventions
   a. Monitor the vital signs.
   b. Monitor a pressure patch or dressing as prescribed.
   c. Report changes in vital signs or the presence of bright red drainage on the pressure patch or dressing.

J. Hyphema
1. Description
   a. The presence of blood in the anterior chamber that occurs as a result of an injury
   b. The condition usually resolves in 5 to 7 days.

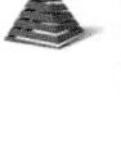

2. Interventions
   a. Encourage rest with the client in the semi-Fowler's position.
   b. Avoid sudden eye movements for 3 to 5 days to decrease the likelihood of bleeding.
   c. Assist to administer cycloplegic eyedrops as prescribed to relax the eye muscles and place the eye at rest.
   d. Reinforce instructions to the client in the use of eye shields or eye patches as prescribed.
   e. Reinforce instructions to the client to restrict reading and limit watching television.

K. Contusions
1. Description
   a. Bleeding into the soft tissue as a result of an injury
   b. A contusion causes a black eye, and the discoloration disappears in about 10 days.
   c. Pain, photophobia, edema, and diplopia may occur.
2. Interventions
   a. Place ice on the eye immediately.
   b. Reinforce instructions to the client to receive a thorough eye examination.

L. Foreign bodies
1. Description: An object such as dust or dirt that enters the eye and causes irritation
2. Interventions
   a. Have the client look upward, expose the lower lid, wet a cotton-tipped applicator with sterile normal saline, and gently twist the swab over the particle, and remove it.
   b. If the particle cannot be seen, have the client look downward, place a cotton applicator horizontally on the outer surface of the upper eye lid, grasp the lashes, and pull the upper lid outward and over the cotton applicator. If the particle is seen, gently twist a swab over it to remove.

M. Penetrating objects
1. Description: An injury that occurs to the eye in which an object penetrates the eye

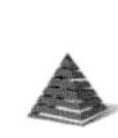

2. Interventions
   a. Never remove the object because it may be holding ocular structures in place. The object must be removed by the HCP.
   b. Cover the object with a cup.
   c. Do not allow the client to bend over or lie flat.
   d. Do not place pressure on the eye.

e. The client must be seen by a HCP immediately.
f. X-rays and computed tomography (CT) scans of the orbit are usually performed.
g. Magnetic resonance imaging (MRI) is contraindicated because of the possibility of metal-containing projectile movement during the procedure.

N. Chemical injury (see Priority Nursing Actions)
1. Description: An eye injury in which a caustic substance enters the eye
2. Interventions

⚠ If a chemical splash to the eye occurs, treatment should begin immediately. Immediately flush the eyes at the scene of the injury with water for at least 15 to 20 minutes.

a. At the scene of the injury, obtain a sample of the chemical involved.
b. At the emergency department, the eye is irrigated with normal saline solution or an ophthalmic irrigation solution for at least 10 minutes or longer as prescribed; the pH is then checked.
c. The solution is directed across the cornea and toward the lateral canthus.

PRIORITY NURSING ACTIONS!

Actions to Take If a Client Sustains a Chemical Eye Injury

1. Irrigate the eye.
2. Check the pH of the eye.
3. Assess visual acuity.
4. Document the event, actions taken, and the client's response.

Emergency care after a chemical splash to the eye includes irrigating the eye immediately with sterile normal saline or ocular irrigating solution. If the injury occurred outside the hospital, the eye is irrigated immediately with tap water and then the client is brought to the emergency department. In the emergency department, the irrigation should be maintained for at least 10 minutes (and at least 1 liter should be used to irrigate). After irrigation, the pH of the eye is checked, and if a pH of 6 to 7 has not returned, the irrigation should be continued. Some HCP's prefer the use of lactated Ringer's solution for irrigation because its pH is 6 to 7.5, which is closer to the pH of tears (7.1) than that of normal saline, which may range from 4.5 to 7. After this emergency treatment, visual acuity is assessed. It is also important for the nurse to find out what chemical splashed into the eye. Finally, the event is documented, as well as the actions taken and the client's response.

Reference(s): deWit, D. & Kumagai, C. (2013). *Medical-surgical nursing: Concepts & practice.* (2nd ed., p. 597). St. Louis: Saunders.
Lewis, S., Dirksen, S., Heitkemper, M., & Bucher, L. (2014). *Medical-surgical nursing: Assessment and management of clinical problems* (9th ed., p. 390). St. Louis: Mosby.

d. Prepare for visual acuity assessment.
e. Apply an antibiotic ointment as prescribed.
f. Cover the eye with a patch as prescribed.

O. Eye (tissue) donation 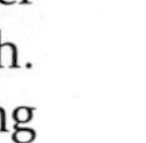
1. Donor eyes
a. Donor eyes are obtained from cadavers.
b. Donor eyes must be enucleated soon after death because of rapid endothelial cell death.
c. Donor eyes must be stored in a preserving solution.
d. Storage, handling, and coordination of donor tissue with surgeons are provided by a network of state eye bank associations.
2. Care to the deceased client as a potential eye donor
a. The option of eye donation is discussed with the HCP and family.
b. Raise the head of the bed 30 degrees.
c. Instill antibiotic eyedrops as prescribed.
d. Close the eyes and place a small ice pack as prescribed to the closed eyes.
3. Preoperative care to the recipient of the cornea 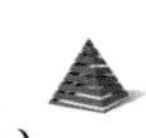
a. Recipient may be told of the tissue (cornea) availability only several hours to 1 day before the surgery.
b. Assist in alleviating client anxiety.
c. Assess the recipient's eye for signs of infection.
d. Report the presence of any redness, watery or purulent drainage, or edema around the recipient's eye to the RN and HCP.
e. Instill antibiotic drops into the recipient's eye as prescribed to reduce the number of microorganisms.
f. Assist to administer fluids and medications intravenously as prescribed.
4. Postoperative care to the recipient
a. The eye is covered with a pressure patch and protective shield that is left in place for 1 day, as prescribed.
b. Do not remove or change the dressing without a HCP's prescription.
c. Monitor vital signs.
d. Monitor level of consciousness.
e. Monitor the eye dressing.
f. Position the client with the head elevated and on the nonoperative side to reduce intraocular pressure.
g. Orient the client frequently.
h. Monitor for complications of bleeding, wound leakage, infection, and tissue rejection.
i. Reinforce instructions to the client on how to apply a patch and eye shield.
j. Reinforce instructions to the client to wear the eye shield at night for 1 month (as prescribed) and whenever around small children or pets.
k. Advise the client not to rub the eye.

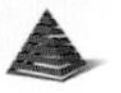

5. Graft rejection
   a. Rejection can occur at any time.
   b. Inform the client of the signs of rejection.
   c. Signs include *r*edness, *s*welling, decreased *v*ision, and *p*ain (RSVP).
   d. The eye is treated with topical corticosteroids.

V. Anatomy and Physiology of the Ear

A. Functions
   1. Hearing
   2. Maintenance of balance

B. External ear (pinna)
   1. The external ear is embedded in the temporal bone bilaterally at the level of the eyes.
   2. The external ear extends from the auricle through the external canal to the tympanic membrane or eardrum.
   3. The external ear includes the mastoid process, which is the bony ridge located over the temporal bone.

C. Middle ear
   1. The middle ear consists of the medial side of the tympanic membrane.
   2. The middle ear contains three bony ossicles.
      a. Malleus
      b. Incus
      c. Stapes
   3. Functions of the middle ear
      a. Conduct sound vibrations from the outer ear to the central hearing apparatus in the inner ear
      b. Protect the inner ear by reducing the amplitude of loud sounds
      c. The eustachian tube allows equalization of air pressure on each side of the tympanic membrane so that the membrane does not rupture.

D. Inner ear
   1. The inner ear contains the semicircular canals, the cochlea, and the distal end of the eighth cranial nerve.
   2. The semicircular canals contain fluid and hair cells connected to sensory nerve fibers of the vestibular portion of the eighth cranial nerve.
   3. The inner ear maintains sense of balance or equilibrium.
   4. The cochlea is the spiral-shaped organ of hearing.
   5. The organ of Corti (within the cochlea) is the receptor and organ of hearing.
   6. Eighth cranial nerve
      a. The cochlear branch of the nerve transmits neuroimpulses from the cochlea to the brain, where they are interpreted as sound.
      b. The vestibular branch maintains balance and equilibrium.

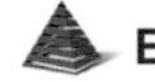

E. Hearing and equilibrium
   1. The external ear conducts sound waves to the middle ear.
   2. The middle ear, also called the tympanic cavity, conducts sound waves to the inner ear.
   3. The middle ear is filled with air, which is kept at atmospheric pressure by the opening of the auditory canal.
   4. The inner ear contains sensory receptors for sound and for equilibrium.
   5. The receptors in the inner ear transmit sound waves and changes in body position to the nerve impulses.

VI. Assessment of the Ear (See Chapter 23)

VII. Diagnostic Tests for the Ear

A. Tomography
   1. Description
      a. Tomography may be performed with or without contrast medium.
      b. Tomography assesses the mastoid, middle ear, and inner ear structures.
      c. Multiple radiographs of the head are obtained.
      d. Tomography is especially helpful in the diagnosis of acoustic tumors.
   2. Interventions
      a. All jewelry is removed.
      b. Lead eye shields are used to cover the cornea to diminish the radiation dose to the eyes.
      c. The client must remain still in a supine position.
      d. No follow-up care is required.

B. Audiometry
   1. Description
      a. Audiometry measures hearing acuity.
      b. Audiometry uses two types: pure tone audiometry and speech audiometry.
      c. Pure tone audiometry is used to identify problems with hearing, speech, music, and other sounds in the environment.
      d. In speech audiometry, the client's ability to hear spoken words is measured.
      e. After testing, audiogram patterns are depicted on a graph to determine the type and level of the hearing loss.
   2. Interventions
      a. Inform the client regarding the procedure.
      b. Reinforce instructions to the client to identify the sounds as they are heard.

C. Electronystagmography (ENG)
   1. Description
      a. The ENG is used to detect disorders of the peripheral vestibular system (the parts of the inner ear that interpret balance and spatial orientation) or the nerves that connect the vestibular system to the brain and the muscles of the eye.
      b. Electrodes are placed at locations above and below the eye to record electrical activity.
      c. By measuring the changes in the electrical field within the eye, ENG can detect

nystagmus (involuntary rapid eye movement) in response to various stimuli.

d. ENG is used to distinguish between normal nystagmus and medication-induced nystagmus or nystagmus caused by a lesion in the central or peripheral vestibular pathway.

e. If nystagmus does not occur on stimulation, a problem may exist within the ear, nerves that supply the ear, or certain parts of the brain.

2. Interventions

a. The client is instructed to remain NPO for 3 hours before testing and to avoid caffeine-containing beverages for 24 to 48 hours before the test.

b. Unnecessary medications are omitted for 24 hours before testing.

c. Instruct the client that this may be a long and tiring procedure.

d. The client should bring prescription eyeglasses to the examination.

e. The client sits and is instructed to gaze at lights, focus on a moving pattern, focus on a moving point, and then close the eyes.

f. While sitting in a chair, the client may be rotated to provide information about vestibular function.

g. In addition, the client's ears are irrigated with cool and warm water, which may cause nausea and vomiting.

h. After the procedure, the client begins taking clear fluids slowly and cautiously because nausea and vomiting may occur.

i. Assistance with ambulation may also be necessary after the procedure.

D. Magnetic resonance imaging (MRI): Refer to Chapter 57 for information on MRI.

VIII. Disorders of the Ear

A. Risk factors related to ear disorders (Box 55-3)

B. **Conductive hearing loss** (Fig. 55-3)

1. Description

a. Conductive hearing loss occurs when sound waves are blocked to the inner ear fibers because of external ear or middle ear disorders.

b. Disorders can often be corrected with no damage to hearing or with minimal permanent hearing loss.

2. Causes

a. Any inflammatory process or obstruction of the external or middle ear

BOX 55-3 Risk Factors of Ear Disorders

Aging process
Infection
Medications
Ototoxicity
Trauma
Tumors

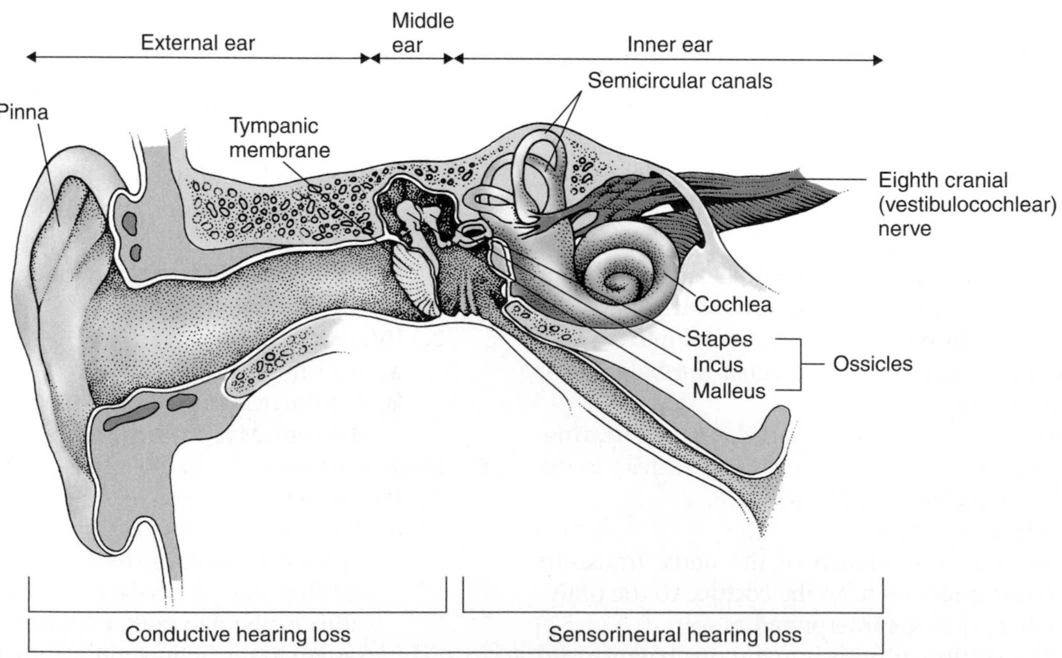

FIGURE 55-3 Anatomy of hearing loss. Hearing loss can be divided into three types: (1) conductive (difficulty in the external or the middle ear); (2) sensorineural (difficulty in the inner ear or acoustic nerve); and (3) mixed conductive-sensorineural (a combination of the two). (From Ignatavicius D, Workman ML: *Medical-surgical nursing: Patient-centered collaborative care*, ed 7, Philadelphia, 2013, Saunders.)

b. Tumors
c. **Otosclerosis**
d. A buildup of scar tissue on the ossicles from previous middle ear surgery

C. **Sensorineural hearing loss** (Fig. 55-3)
1. Description
   a. Sensorineural hearing loss is a pathological process of the inner ear or of the sensory fibers that lead to the cerebral cortex.
   b. Sensorineural hearing loss is often permanent, and measures must be taken to reduce further damage.
2. Causes
   a. Damage to the inner ear structures
   b. Damage to the eighth cranial nerve
   c. Prolonged exposure to loud noise
   d. Medications
   e. Trauma
   f. Inherited disorders
   g. Metabolic and circulatory disorders
   h. Infections
   i. Surgery
   j. Ménière's syndrome
   k. Diabetes mellitus
   l. Myxedema

D. Mixed hearing loss (Fig. 55-3)
1. Mixed hearing loss also is known as conductive-sensorineural hearing loss.
2. Client has sensorineural and conductive hearing loss.

E. Central hearing loss: Involves the inability to interpret sound, including speech, due to a problem in the brain.

F. Signs of hearing loss and facilitating communication (Boxes 55-4 and 55-5)

G. Cochlear implantation
1. Cochlear implants are used for sensorineural hearing loss.
2. A small computer converts sound waves into electrical impulses.
3. Electrodes are placed by the internal ear with a computer device attached to the external ear.
4. Electronic impulses directly stimulate nerve fibers.

BOX 55-4 Signs of Hearing Loss

Frequently asking others to repeat statements
Straining to hear
Turning head or leaning forward to favor one ear
Shouting in conversation
Ringing in the ears
Failing to respond when not looking in the direction of the sound
Answering questions incorrectly
Raising the volume of the television or radio
Avoiding large groups
Better understanding of speech when in small groups
Withdrawing from social interactions

H. Hearing aids
1. Hearing aids are used for the client with conductive hearing loss.

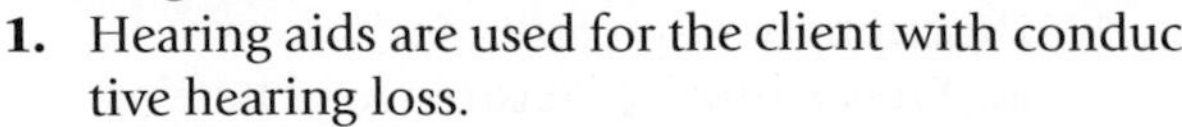

2. Hearing aids have limited value for the client with sensorineural hearing loss, because they only make sounds louder, not clearer.

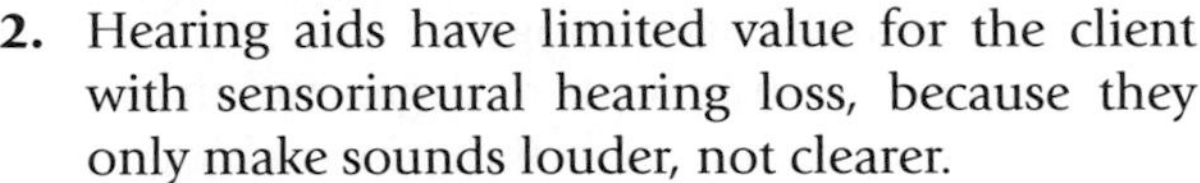

3. A difficulty that exists in the use of hearing aids is the amplification of background noise and voices.
4. Reinforce client education (Box 55-6)

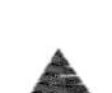

BOX 55-5 Facilitation of Communication

Using written words if the client is able to see, read, and write
Providing plenty of light in the room
Getting the attention of the client before beginning to speak
Facing the client when speaking
Talking in a room without distracting noises
Moving close to the client and speaking slowly and clearly
Keeping hands and other objects away from the mouth when talking to the client
Talking in normal volume and lower pitch, since shouting is not helpful and higher frequencies are less easily heard
Rephrasing sentences and repeating information
Validating with the client the understanding of statements made by asking the client to repeat what was said
Using lip-reading
Encouraging the client to wear glasses when talking to someone to improve vision for lip reading
Using sign language, which combines speech with hand movements that signify letters, words, or phrases
Using telephone amplifiers
Using flashing lights that are activated by ringing of the telephone or doorbell
Using specially trained dogs that help the client to be aware of sound and to alert the client to potential dangers

BOX 55-6 Client Education Regarding a Hearing Aid

Encourage the client to begin using the hearing aid slowly to adjust to the device.
Adjust the volume to the minimal hearing level to prevent feedback squeaking.
Teach the client to concentrate on the sounds that are to be heard and filter out background noise.
Instruct the client to clean the ear mold with mild soap and water.
Avoid excessive wetting of the hearing aid, and try to keep the hearing aid dry.
Clean the ear cannula of the hearing aid with a toothpick or pipe cleaner.
Turn off the hearing aid before removing from the ear to prevent squealing feedback. Remove the battery when not in use.
Keep extra batteries on hand.
Keep the hearing aid in a safe place.
Prevent hair sprays, oils, or other hair and face products from coming in contact with the receiver of the hearing aid.

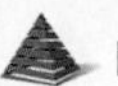

I. Presbycusis

1. Description
   a. Presbycusis is a sensorineural hearing loss associated with aging.
   b. Presbycusis leads to degeneration or atrophy of the ganglion cells in the cochlea and a loss of elasticity of the basilar membranes.
   c. Presbycusis leads to compromise of the vascular supply to the inner ear with changes in several areas of the ear structure.
2. Data collection
   a. Hearing loss is gradual and bilateral.
   b. The client states that he or she has no problem with hearing but cannot understand what the words are.
   c. The client thinks that the speaker is mumbling.

J. External otitis

1. Description
   a. External otitis is an infective inflammatory or allergic response involving the structure of the external auditory canal or the auricles.
   b. An irritating or infective agent comes in contact with the epithelial layer of the external ear.
   c. Contact leads to an allergic response or signs and symptoms of an infection.
   d. The skin becomes red, swollen, and tender to touch on movement.
   e. The extensive swelling of the canal can lead to conductive hearing loss because of obstruction.
   f. External otitis is more common in children, is termed "swimmer's ear," and occurs more often in hot, humid environments.
   g. Prevention includes the elimination of irritating or infecting agents.
2. Data collection
   a. Pain
   b. Itching
   c. Plugged feeling in the ear
   d. Redness and edema
   e. Exudate
   f. Hearing loss
3. Interventions
   a. Apply heat locally for 20 minutes three times a day.
   b. Encourage rest to assist in reducing pain.
   c. Administer antibiotics or corticosteroids as prescribed.
   d. Administer analgesics such as aspirin or acetaminophen (Tylenol) for the pain as prescribed.
   e. Reinforce instructions to the client that the ears should be kept clean and dry.
   f. Reinforce instructions to the client to use earplugs for swimming.
   g. Reinforce instructions to the client that cotton-tipped applicators should not be used to dry ears because their use can lead to trauma to the canal.

BOX 55-7 Client Education After Myringotomy

Avoid strenuous activities.
Avoid rapid head movements, bouncing, or bending.
Avoid straining on bowel movement.
Avoid drinking through a straw.
Avoid traveling by air.
Avoid forceful coughing.
Avoid contact with persons with colds.
Avoid washing hair, showering, or getting the head wet for 1 week as prescribed.
Instruct the client that if he or she needs to blow the nose, to blow one side at a time with the mouth open.
Instruct the client to keep ears dry by keeping a ball of cotton coated with petroleum jelly in the ear and to change the cotton ball daily.
Instruct the client to report excessive ear drainage to the HCP.

   h. Reinforce instructions to the client that irritating agents such as hair products or headphones should be discontinued.

K. Otitis media: See Chapter 34.

1. Myringotomy: See Chapter 34.
2. Reinforce client education (Box 55-7).

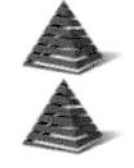

L. Chronic otitis media

1. Description
   a. Chronic otitis media is a chronic infective, inflammatory, or allergic response involving the structure of the middle ear.
   b. Frequent removal of debris from the canal may be required.
   c. Myringoplasty can reconstruct the tympanic membrane and ossicles and improve conductive hearing loss.
   d. Mastoidectomy may be performed if the infection has spread to involve the mastoid bone.

Monitor the client with otitis media closely for response to treatment. Otic and systemic antibiotics may be used to treat the infection, but often the organism is resistant.

2. Preoperative interventions
   a. Administer antibiotic drops as prescribed.
   b. Clean the ear of debris as prescribed. Irrigate the ear with a solution as prescribed to restore the normal pH of the ear.
   c. Reinforce instructions to the client to avoid persons with upper respiratory infections.
   d. Reinforce instructions to the client to obtain adequate rest, eat a balanced diet, and drink adequate fluids.
   e. Reinforce instructions to the client in deep breathing and coughing. Forceful coughing, which increases pressure in the middle ear, is to be avoided postoperatively.

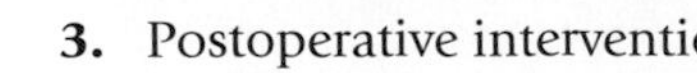

3. Postoperative interventions
    a. Inform the client that initial hearing after surgery is diminished because of the packing in the ear canal and that hearing improvement will occur after the packing is removed.
    b. Keep the dressing clean and dry.
    c. Keep the client flat with the operative ear up for at least 12 hours as prescribed.
    d. Administer antibiotics as prescribed.
    e. Position the client flat with the operative side up.
    f. Restrict the client to bed with bedside commode privileges for 24 hours as prescribed.
    g. Assist the client with getting out of bed to prevent falling or injuries from dizziness.
    h. With reconstruction of the ossicles via a graft, take precautions to prevent dislodging of the graft.

M. Mastoiditis

1. Description
    a. Mastoiditis may be acute or chronic and results from untreated or inadequately treated chronic or acute otitis media.
    b. The pain is not relieved by myringotomy.
2. Data collection
    a. Swelling behind the ear and pain with minimal movement of the head
    b. Cellulitis on the skin or external scalp over the mastoid process
    c. A reddened, dull, thick, immobile tympanic membrane with or without perforation
    d. Tender and enlarged postauricular lymph nodes
    e. Low-grade fever
    f. Malaise
    g. Anorexia
3. Interventions
    a. Prepare the client for surgical removal of infected material.
    b. Monitor for complications.
    c. Simple or modified radical mastoidectomy with tympanoplasty is the most common treatment.
    d. Once infected tissue is removed, the tympanoplasty is performed to reconstruct the ossicles and the tympanic membranes in an attempt to restore normal hearing.
4. Complications
    a. Damage to the abducens and facial cranial nerves
    b. Damage exhibited by inability to look laterally (cranial nerve VI, abducens) and a drooping of the mouth on the affected side (cranial nerve VII, facial)
    c. Meningitis
    d. Brain abscess
    e. Chronic purulent otitis media
    f. Wound infections
    g. Vertigo, if the infection spreads into the labyrinth
5. Postoperative interventions
    a. Monitor for dizziness.
    b. Monitor for signs of meningitis as evidenced by a stiff neck and vomiting.
    c. Prepare for a wound dressing change 24 hours postoperatively.
    d. Monitor the surgical incision for edema, drainage, and redness.

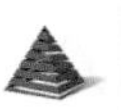

N. Otosclerosis

1. Description
    a. Otosclerosis is a disease of the labyrinthine capsule of the middle ear that results in a bony overgrowth of the tissue surrounding the ossicles.
    b. Otosclerosis causes the development of irregular areas of new bone formation and causes the fixation of the bones.
    c. Stapes fixation leads to a conductive hearing loss.
    d. If the disease involves the inner ear, sensorineural hearing loss is present.
    e. Bilateral involvement is not uncommon, although hearing loss may be worse in one ear.
    f. It is thought to be a hereditary autosomal dominant disorder; is most commonly seen in young women.
    g. Nonsurgical intervention promotes the improvement of hearing through amplification.
    h. Surgical intervention involves removal of the bony growth that is causing the hearing loss.
    i. A partial stapedectomy or complete stapedectomy with prosthesis (fenestration) may be performed surgically.
2. Data collection
    a. Slowly progressing conductive hearing loss
    b. Bilateral hearing loss
    c. A ringing or roaring type of constant tinnitus
    d. Loud sounds heard in the ear when chewing
    e. Pinkish discoloration (Schwartze's sign) of the tympanic membrane, which indicates vascular changes within the ear
    f. Negative Rinne test
    g. Weber test that shows lateralization of sound to the ear with the most conductive hearing loss

O. Fenestration

1. Description
    a. Fenestration is removal of the stapes, with a small hole drilled in the footplate; a prosthesis is connected between the incus and footplate.
    b. Sounds cause the prosthesis to vibrate in the same manner as did the stapes.
    c. Complications include complete hearing loss, prolonged vertigo, infection, or facial nerve damage.

2. Preoperative interventions
   a. Reinforce instructions to the client on measures to prevent middle ear or external ear infections.
   b. Reinforce instructions to the client to avoid excessive nose blowing.
   c. Reinforce instructions to the client not to clean the ear canal with cotton-tipped applicators and to avoid trauma or injury to the ear canal.
3. Postoperative interventions
   a. Inform the client that hearing is initially worse after the surgical procedure because of swelling and that no noticeable improvement in hearing may occur for as long as 6 weeks.
   b. Inform the client that the Gelfoam ear packing interferes with hearing but is used to decrease bleeding.
   c. Assist with ambulating during the first 1 to 2 days after surgery.
   d. Provide side rails when the client is in bed (per agency policy).
   e. Administer antibiotics, antivertiginous, and pain medications as prescribed.
   f. Monitor for facial nerve damage, weakness, changes in tactile sensation, changes in taste sensation, vertigo, nausea, and vomiting.
   g. Reinforce instructions to the client to move the head slowly when changing positions to prevent vertigo.
   h. Reinforce instructions to the client to avoid persons with upper respiratory tract infections.
   i. Reinforce instructions to the client to avoid showering and getting the head and wound wet.
   j. Reinforce instructions to the client to avoid using small objects (cotton-tipped applicators) to clean the external ear canal.
   k. Reinforce instructions to the client to avoid rapid, extreme changes in pressure caused by quick head movements, sneezing, nose blowing, straining, and changes in altitude.
   l. Reinforce instructions to the client to avoid changes in middle ear pressure because they could dislodge the graft or prosthesis.

P. Labyrinthitis
1. Description: Infection of the labyrinth that occurs as a complication of acute or chronic otitis media
2. May result from growth of a cholesteatoma—benign overgrowth of squamous cell epithelium
3. Data collection
   a. Hearing loss that may be permanent on the affected side
   b. Tinnitus
   c. Spontaneous nystagmus to the affected side
   d. Vertigo
   e. Nausea and vomiting
4. Interventions
   a. Monitor for signs of meningitis, the most common complication, as evidenced by headache, stiff neck, and lethargy.
   b. Assist to administer systemic antibiotics as prescribed.
   c. Advise the client to rest in bed in a darkened room.
   d. Assist to administer antiemetics and antivertiginous medications as prescribed.
   e. Reinforce instructions to the client that the vertigo subsides as the inflammation resolves.
   f. Reinforce instructions to the client that balance problems that persist may require gait training through physical therapy.

Q. Ménière's syndrome
1. Description
   a. Ménière's syndrome is also called endolymphatic hydrops and refers to dilation of the endolymphatic system by overproduction or decreased reabsorption of endolymphatic fluid.
   b. The syndrome is characterized by tinnitus, unilateral sensorineural hearing loss, and vertigo.
   c. Symptoms occur in attacks and last for several days, and the client becomes totally incapacitated during the attacks.
   d. Initial hearing loss is reversible, but as the frequency of attacks continues, hearing loss becomes permanent.

A priority nursing intervention in the care of a client with Ménière's syndrome is instituting safety measures.

2. Causes
   a. Any factor that increases endolymphatic secretion in the labyrinth
   b. Viral and bacterial infections
   c. Allergic reactions
   d. Biochemical disturbances
   e. Vascular disturbance producing changes in the microcirculation in the labyrinth
   f. Long-term stress may be a possible contributing factor.

3. Data collection
   a. Feelings of fullness in the ear
   b. Tinnitus, as a continuous low-pitched roar or humming sound, that is present much of the time but worsens just before and during severe attacks
   c. Hearing loss that is worse during an attack
   d. Vertigo, as periods of whirling, that might cause the client to fall to the ground
   e. Vertigo that is so intense that even while lying down, the client holds the bed or ground in an attempt to prevent the whirling

f. Nausea and vomiting
g. Nystagmus
h. Severe headaches

4. Nonsurgical interventions
   a. Prevent injury during vertigo attacks.
   b. Provide bed rest in a quiet environment.
   c. Provide assistance with walking.
   d. Reinforce instructions to the client to move the head slowly to prevent worsening of the vertigo.
   e. Initiate sodium and fluid restrictions as prescribed.
   f. Reinforce instructions to the client to stop smoking.
   g. Reinforce instructions to the client to avoid watching television because the flickering of lights may exacerbate symptoms.
   h. Assist to administer nicotinic acid (niacin) as prescribed for its vasodilatory effect.
   i. Assist to administer antihistamines as prescribed, which will reduce the production of histamine and the inflammation.
   j. Assist to administer antiemetics as prescribed.
   k. Assist to administer tranquilizers and sedatives as prescribed to calm the client and allow him or her to rest and to control vertigo, nausea, and vomiting.
   l. Mild diuretics may be prescribed to decrease endolymph volume.
   m. Inform the client about vestibular rehabilitation as prescribed.
5. Surgical interventions
   a. Surgery is performed when medical therapy is ineffective and the functional level of the client has decreased significantly.
   b. Endolymphatic drainage and insertion of a shunt may be performed early in the course of the disease to assist with the drainage of excess fluids.
   c. A resection of the vestibular nerve or total removal of the labyrinth or a labyrinthectomy may be performed.
6. Postoperative interventions
   a. Monitor packing and dressing on the ear.
   b. Speak to the client on the side of the unaffected ear.
   c. Assist to perform neurological assessments.
   d. Maintain side rails as appropriate per agency policy.
   e. Assist with ambulating.
   f. Encourage the client to use a bedside commode rather than ambulating to the bathroom.
   g. Assist to administer antivertiginous and antiemetic medications as prescribed.

R. Acoustic neuroma
1. Description
   a. Acoustic neuroma is a benign tumor of the vestibular or acoustic nerve.
   b. The tumor may cause damage to hearing and to facial movements and sensations.
   c. Treatment includes surgical removal of the tumor via craniotomy.
   d. Care is taken to preserve the function of the facial nerve.
   e. The tumor rarely recurs after surgical removal.
   f. Postoperative nursing care is similar to postoperative craniotomy care.
2. Data collection
   a. Symptoms usually begin with tinnitus and progress to gradual sensorineural hearing loss.
   b. As the tumor enlarges, damage to adjacent cranial nerves occurs.

S. Trauma
1. Description
   a. The tympanic membrane has a limited stretching ability and gives way under high pressure.
   b. Foreign objects placed in the external canal may exert pressure on the tympanic membrane and cause perforation.
   c. If the object continues through the canal, the bony structure of the stapes, incus, and malleus may be damaged.
   d. A blunt injury to the basal skull and ear can damage the middle ear structures through fractures extending to the middle ear.
   e. Excessive nose blowing and rapid changes of pressure that occur with nonpressurized air flights can increase pressure in the middle ear.
   f. Depending on the damage to the ossicles, hearing loss may or may not return.

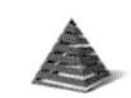

2. Interventions
   a. Tympanic membrane perforations usually heal within 24 hours.
   b. Surgical reconstruction of the ossicles and tympanic membrane through tympanoplasty or myringoplasty may be performed to improve hearing.

T. Cerumen and foreign bodies
1. Description
   a. Cerumen or wax is the most common cause of impacted canals.
   b. Foreign bodies can include vegetables, beads, pencil erasers, insects, or other objects.
2. Data collection
   a. Sensation of fullness in the ear with or without hearing loss
   b. Pain, itching, or bleeding
3. Cerumen
   a. Removal of wax by irrigation may be a slow process.
   b. Irrigation is contraindicated in clients with a history of tympanic membrane perforation or otitis media.

c. If prescribed to soften cerumen, glycerin or mineral oil is placed in the ear at bedtime; hydrogen peroxide may also prescribed.
d. After several days, the ear is irrigated.
e. The maximal amount of solution that should be used for irrigation is 50 to 70 mL.

Inform the client that ear candles should never be used to remove cerumen. Their use can cause burns and a vacuum effect, causing a perforation in the tympanic membrane.

4. Foreign bodies
   a. With a foreign object of vegetable matter, irrigation is used with care because this material expands with hydration.
   b. Insects are killed before removal, unless they can be coaxed out by flashlight or a humming noise.
   c. Mineral oil or diluted alcohol is instilled to suffocate the insect, which then is removed using ear forceps.
   d. A small ear forceps is used to remove the object; care is taken to avoid pushing the object farther into the canal and damaging the tympanic membrane.

CRITICAL THINKING What Should You Do?

Answer: This situation is an emergency. The nurse should immediately accompany the client to a room and notify the registered nurse (RN) and health care provider to assess the client. A penetrating eye wound is a serious injury that can cause loss of sight or require loss of the eye (surgical removal). The object is removed only by an ophthalmologist, because it may be holding eye structures in place. X-rays and computed tomography (CT) scans of the orbit are usually obtained to ensure that the orbit of the eye is intact and to look for fractures that might entrap orbital muscles. Magnetic resonance imaging (MRI) is contraindicated because of the possibility of metal-containing projectile movement during the procedure. Surgery is usually needed to remove the foreign object.

Reference(s): Ignatavicius, D., & Workman, M. (2013). *Medical-surgical nursing: Patient-centered collaborative care.* (7th ed., pp. 1071–1072). St. Louis: Saunders.

PRACTICE QUESTIONS

❖ **571.** The nurse is preparing to reinforce a teaching plan for a client who is undergoing cataract extraction with intraocular implant. Which home care measures should the nurse include in the plan? **Select all that apply.**

- ☐ 1. To avoid activities that require bending over
- ☐ 2. To contact the surgeon if eye scratchiness occurs
- ☐ 3. To place an eye shield on the surgical eye at bedtime
- ☐ 4. That episodes of sudden severe pain in the eye are expected
- ☐ 5. To contact the surgeon if a decrease in visual acuity occurs
- ☐ 6. To take acetaminophen (Tylenol) for minor eye discomfort

572. The nurse is assisting in developing a teaching plan for the client with glaucoma. Which instruction should the nurse suggest to include in the plan of care?
1. Decrease the amount of salt in the diet.
2. Decrease fluid intake to control the intraocular pressure.
3. Avoid reading the newspaper and watching television.
4. Eye medications will need to be administered for the rest of your life.

573. The nurse is assigned to care for a client with a detached retina. Which finding should the nurse expect to be documented in the client's record?
1. Blurred vision
2. Pain in the effected eye
3. A yellow discoloration of the sclera
4. A sense of a curtain falling across the field of vision

574. The nurse is assigned to care for a client with a diagnosis of detached retina. Which finding would indicate that bleeding has occurred as a result of retinal detachment?
1. Total loss of vision
2. A reddened conjunctiva
3. A sudden sharp pain in the eye
4. Complaints of a burst of black spots or floaters

575. A client arrives in the emergency department after an automobile crash. The client's forehead hit the steering wheel, and a hyphema has been diagnosed. Which position should the nurse prepare to position the client?
1. Flat on bed rest
2. On bed rest in a semi-Fowler's position
3. In lateral position on the unaffected side
4. In the lateral position on the affected side

576. A client sustains a contusion of the eyeball after a traumatic injury with a blunt object. The nurse should take which **immediate** action?
1. Notify the health care provider (HCP)
2. Apply ice to the affected eye

3. Irrigate the eye with cool water
4. Accompany the client to the emergency department

577. A client sustains a chemical eye injury from a splash of battery acid. The nurse should prepare the client for which **immediate** measure?
1. Checking visual acuity
2. Covering the eye with a pressure patch
3. Swabbing the eye with antibiotic ointment
4. Irrigating the eye with sterile normal saline

578. The nurse is caring for a client after enucleation and notes the presence of bright red drainage on the dressing. The nurse should take which appropriate action?
1. Document the finding
2. Continue to monitor vital signs
3. Report the finding to the registered nurse (RN)
4. Mark the drainage on the dressing and monitors for any increase in bleeding

579. The nurse is preparing to administer eardrops to an adult client. The nurse administers the eardrops by which technique?
1. Pulling the pinna up and back
2. Pulling the earlobe down and back
3. Tilting the client's head forward and down
4. Instructing the client to stand and lean to one side

580. The nurse is caring for a client who is hearing-impaired and should take which approach to facilitate communication?
1. Speak loudly
2. Speak frequently
3. Speak in a normal tone
4. Speak directly into the impaired ear

581. A client arrives at the emergency department with a foreign body in the left ear that has been determined to be an insect. Which **initial** intervention should the nurse anticipate to be prescribed?
1. Irrigation of the ear
2. Instillation of antibiotic eardrops
3. Instillation of corticosteroid ointment
4. Instillation of mineral oil or diluted alcohol

582. The nurse notes that the health care provider has documented a diagnosis of presbycusis on the client's chart. The nurse understands that this condition is accurately described as which?
1. Tinnitus that occurs with aging
2. Nystagmus that occurs with aging
3. A conductive hearing loss that occurs with aging
4. A sensorineural hearing loss that occurs with aging

583. A client with Ménière's disease is experiencing severe vertigo. The nurse reinforces instructions to the client to do which to assist in controlling the vertigo?
1. Increase sodium in the diet.
2. Lie still and watch television.
3. Avoid sudden head movements.
4. Increase fluid intake to 3000 mL/day.

584. The nurse is assigned to care for a client hospitalized with Ménière's disease. The nurse expects that which would **most likely** be prescribed for the client?
1. Low-fat diet
2. Low-sodium diet
3. Low-cholesterol diet
4. Low-carbohydrate diet

585. A client is diagnosed with glaucoma. Which data gathered by the nurse indicate a risk factor associated with glaucoma?
1. Cardiovascular disease
2. A history of migraine headaches
3. Frequent urinary tract infections
4. Frequent upper respiratory infections

ANSWERS

❖ **571. 1, 3, 5, 6**

Rationale: After eye surgery, some scratchiness and mild eye discomfort may occur in the operative eye and is usually relieved by mild analgesics. If the eye pain becomes severe, the client should notify the surgeon because this may indicate hemorrhage, infection, or increased intraocular pressure. The nurse would also instruct the client to notify the surgeon of purulent drainage, increased redness, or any decrease in visual acuity. The client is instructed to place an eye shield over the operative eye at bedtime to protect the eye from injury during sleep and to avoid activities that increase intraocular pressure such as bending over.

Test-Taking Strategy: Note the subject of the question, cataract extraction with intraocular implant. Recalling that the eye needs to be protected and that a concern is increased intraocular pressure will assist in determining the home care measures to be included in the plan. **Review:** home care measures for cataract surgery.

Level of Cognitive Ability: Applying
Client Needs: Physiological Integrity
Integrated Process: Teaching and Learning
Content Area: Adult Health: Eye
Priority Concepts: Client Education, Sensory Perception
Reference(s): deWit, Kumagai (2013), p. 600.

572. 4

Rationale: The administration of eyedrops is a critical component of the treatment plan for the client with glaucoma.

The client needs to be instructed that medications will need to be taken for the rest of his or her life. Limiting fluids and reducing salt will not decrease intraocular pressure. Option 3 is not necessary.
Test-Taking Strategy: Focus on the subject, glaucoma. Knowing that medications are an integral component of the treatment plan will assist in directing you to the correct option. **Review:** the treatment associated with the care of the client with **glaucoma**.
Level of Cognitive Ability: Applying
Client Needs: Health Promotion and Maintenance
Integrated Process: Teaching and Learning
Content Area: Adult Health: Eye
Priority Concepts: Client Education, Sensory Perception
Reference(s): deWit, Kumagai (2013), p. 605; Lewis et al (2014), p. 401.

573. 4
Rationale: A characteristic clinical manifestation of retinal detachment described by clients is the feeling that a shadow or curtain is falling across the field of vision. There is no pain associated with detachment of the retina. A retinal detachment is an ophthalmic emergency and even more so if visual acuity is still normal. Options 1 and 3 are not specifically associated with a detached retina.
Test-Taking Strategy: Focus on the subject, detached retina. Think about the pathophysiology associated with detached retina. Remember that a characteristic clinical manifestation is the feeling that a shadow or curtain is falling across the field of vision. Retinal detachment can occur suddenly and is an ophthalmic emergency. **Review:** the signs and symptoms associated with a **detached retina**.
Level of Cognitive Ability: Understanding
Client Needs: Physiological Integrity
Integrated Process: Nursing Process/Data Collection
Content Area: Adult Health: Eye
Priority Concepts: Clinical Judgment, Sensory Perception
Reference(s): deWit, Kumagai (2013), p. 606.

574. 4
Rationale: Complaints of a sudden burst of black spots or floaters indicate that bleeding has occurred as a result of the detachment. Options 1, 2, and 3 are not specifically associated with bleeding as a result of detached retina.
Test-Taking Strategy: Focus on the subject, detached retina and bleeding. Hemorrhage is a serious complication associated with retinal detachment. Remember, complaints of a sudden burst of black spots or floaters indicate that bleeding has occurred as a result of the detachment. **Review:** the signs and symptoms associated with the complications of a **detached retina**.
Level of Cognitive Ability: Analyzing
Client Needs: Physiological Integrity
Integrated Process: Nursing Process/Data Collection
Content Area: Adult Health: Eye
Priority Concepts: Perfusion, Sensory Perception
Reference(s): deWit, Kumagai (2013), p. 606.

575. 2
Rationale: A hyphema is the presence of blood in the anterior chamber. It is produced when a force is sufficient to break the integrity of the blood vessels in the eye. It can be caused by direct injury, such as a penetrating injury from a BB pellet, or indirectly, such as from striking the forehead on a steering wheel during an accident. The client is treated by bed rest in a semi-Fowler's position to assist gravity in keeping the hyphema away from the optical center of the cornea.
Test-Taking Strategy: Focus on the subject, hyphema. Think about this type of injury. Eliminate options 1, 3, and 4 because they are comparable or alike. Placing the client flat will produce an increase in pressure at the injured site. **Review:** care of the client with **hyphema**.
Level of Cognitive Ability: Applying
Client Needs: Physiological Integrity
Integrated Process: Nursing Process/Implementation
Content Area: Adult Health: Eye
Priority Concepts: Intracranial Regulation, Sensory Perception
Reference(s): Lewis et al (2014), p. 390.

576. 2
Rationale: Treatment for a contusion begins at the time of injury. Ice is applied immediately. The client should receive a thorough eye examination to rule out the presence of other eye injuries. Eye irrigation is not indicated in a contusion. Options 1 and 4 will delay immediate treatment. After the application of ice, the HCP would be notified.
Test-Taking Strategy: Note the strategic word, *immediate.* Noting that the client sustained a contusion to the eye will direct you to the correct option. **Review:** immediate treatment of an **eye contusion**.
Level of Cognitive Ability: Applying
Client Needs: Physiological Integrity
Integrated Process: Nursing Process/Implementation
Content Area: Adult Health: Eye
Priority Concepts: Inflammation, Sensory Perception
Reference(s): Ignatavicius, Workman (2013), p. 1071; Potter et al (2013), p. 1212.

577. 4
Rationale: Emergency care after a chemical burn to the eye includes irrigating the eye immediately with sterile normal saline or ocular irrigating solution. The irrigation should be maintained for at least 10 minutes. After this emergency treatment, visual acuity is assessed. Options 2 and 3 are not immediate measures.
Test-Taking Strategy: Note the strategic word, *immediate* and focus on the subject, chemical eye injury. Read the question carefully, noting the type of injury to the eye. The question asks about emergency care; therefore, in this type of injury, it is necessary to irrigate the eye first. **Review:** treatment for a **chemical eye injury**.
Level of Cognitive Ability: Applying
Client Needs: Physiological Integrity
Integrated Process: Nursing Process/Implementation
Content Area: Adult Health: Eye
Priority Concepts: Clinical Judgment, Sensory Perception
Reference(s): Hammond, Zimmermann (2013), p. 288; Ignatavicius, Workman (2013), p. 1072.

578. 3
Rationale: If the nurse notes the presence of bright red drainage on the dressing, it must be reported to the registered nurse

because this can indicate hemorrhage. Options 1, 2, and 4 will delay necessary treatment.
Test-Taking Strategy: Note the subject, enucleation. Bright red drainage indicates active bleeding. The registered nurse needs to be notified if this type of drainage occurs. **Review:** postoperative complications associated with an **enucleation**.
Level of Cognitive Ability: Applying
Client Needs: Physiological Integrity
Integrated Process: Nursing Process/Implementation
Content Area: Adult Health: Eye
Priority Concepts: Clinical Judgment, Sensory Perception
Reference(s): deWit, Kumagai (2013), p. 597.

579. 1
Rationale: The nurse tilts the client's head slightly away and pulls the pinna up and back. Asking the client to stand and lean to one side is inappropriate and unsafe.
Test-Taking Strategy: Focus on the subject, administering eardrops. Note that the question addresses an adult client. Use basic knowledge regarding the administration of ear medications in selecting the correct option. In the adult, the pinna is pulled up and back. **Review:** the procedure for administering eardrops to an **adult**.
Level of Cognitive Ability: Applying
Client Needs: Physiological Integrity
Integrated Process: Nursing Process/Implementation
Content Area: Adult Health: Ear
Priority Concepts: Safety, Sensory Perception
Reference(s): deWit, Kumagai (2013), pp. 587–588; Cooper, Gosnell (2015), p. 588.

580. 3
Rationale: It is important to speak in a normal tone to the client with impaired hearing and avoid shouting. The nurse should talk directly to the client while facing the client and should speak clearly. If the client does not seem to understand what is said, the nurse should express it differently. Moving closer to the client and toward the better ear may facilitate communication, but it is important to avoid talking directly into the impaired ear.
Test-Taking Strategy: Focus on the subject, effective communication techniques for the hearing impaired. Knowledge regarding effective communication techniques for the hearing impaired is required to answer this question. Thinking about the effect of each action identified in the options will direct you to the correct option. **Review:** communication with a client with a **hearing impairment**.
Level of Cognitive Ability: Applying
Client Needs: Psychosocial Integrity
Integrated Process: Communication and Documentation
Content Area: Adult Health: Ear
Priority Concepts: Communication, Sensory Perception
Reference(s): deWit, Kumagai (2013), p. 587.

581. 4
Rationale: Insects are killed before removal unless they can be coaxed out by a flashlight or a humming noise. Mineral oil or diluted alcohol is instilled into the ear to suffocate the insect, which is then removed by using ear forceps. When the foreign object is vegetable matter, irrigation is not used because this material expands with hydration and the impaction becomes worse. Options 1, 2, and 3 may be prescribed after the initial treatment if necessary and if inflammation or infection is a concern.
Test-Taking Strategy: Use knowledge regarding care of the client with a foreign body in the ear to answer this question. Note the strategic word, *initial*. Remember, insects are killed before removal with mineral oil or diluted alcohol. **Review:** care for a **foreign body in the ear**.
Level of Cognitive Ability: Applying
Client Needs: Physiological Integrity
Integrated Process: Nursing Process/Planning
Content Area: Adult Health: Ear
Priority Concepts: Clinical Judgment, Safety
Reference(s): Cooper, Gosnell (2015), pp. 1884-1885.

582. 4
Rationale: Presbycusis is a type of hearing loss that occurs with aging. It is a gradual sensorineural loss caused by nerve degeneration in the inner ear or auditory nerve. Options 1, 2, and 3 are not accurate descriptions.
Test-Taking Strategy: Focus on the subject, presbycusis. Knowledge regarding the description of presbycusis is required to answer this question. Remember, presbycusis is a sensorineural hearing loss that occurs with aging. **Review:** **presbycusis**.
Level of Cognitive Ability: Understanding
Client Needs: Physiological Integrity
Integrated Process: Nursing Process/Data Collection
Content Area: Adult Health: Ear
Priority Concepts: Caregiving, Sensory Perception
Reference(s): deWit, Kumagai (2013), pp. 589–590. Cooper, Gosnell (2015), pp. 729; 1890.

583. 3
Rationale: The nurse instructs the client to make slow head movements to prevent worsening of the vertigo. Dietary changes such as salt and fluid restrictions that reduce the amount of endolymphatic fluid are sometimes prescribed. Watching television can increase the vertigo.
Test-Taking Strategy: Identify the subject of the question, *severe vertigo*. Note the relation between severe vertigo and the correct option, avoiding sudden head movements. **Review:** measures that will reduce vertigo in the client with Ménière's disease.
Level of Cognitive Ability: Applying
Client Needs: Physiological Integrity
Integrated Process: Teaching and Learning
Content Area: Adult Health: Ear
Priority Concepts: Client Education, Sensory Perception
Reference(s): deWit, Kumagai (2013), pp. 589–590.

584. 2
Rationale: Dietary changes such as salt and fluid restrictions that reduce the amount of endolymphatic fluid are sometimes prescribed. Options 1, 3, and 4 are not specific dietary prescriptions for this condition.
Test-Taking Strategy: Note the strategic words, *most likely* and focus on the subject, Ménière's disease. Recalling the pathophysiology related to Ménière's disease will direct you to the correct option. **Review:** the pathophysiology related to **Ménière's disease**.
Level of Cognitive Ability: Understanding

Client Needs: Physiological Integrity
Integrated Process: Nursing Process/Planning
Content Area: Adult Health: Ear
Priority Concepts: Nutrition, Sensory Perception
Reference(s): Lewis et al (2014), p. 406.

585. 1

Rationale: Hypertension, cardiovascular disease, diabetes mellitus, and obesity are associated with the development of glaucoma. Smoking, ingestion of caffeine or large amounts of alcohol, illicit drugs, corticosteroids, altered hormone levels, posture, and eye movements may cause varying transient increases in intraocular pressure.

Test-Taking Strategy: Focus on the **subject**, glaucoma. Use knowledge regarding the risk factors associated with glaucoma to answer this question. Remember, cardiovascular disease is associated with the development of glaucoma. **Review:** the risk factors associated with **glaucoma.**
Level of Cognitive Ability: Analyzing
Client Needs: Health Promotion and Maintenance
Integrated Process: Nursing Process/Data Collection
Content Area: Adult Health: Eye
Priority Concepts: Health Promotion, Sensory Perception
Reference(s): deWit, Kumagai (2013), p. 602; Lewis et al (2014), p. 401.

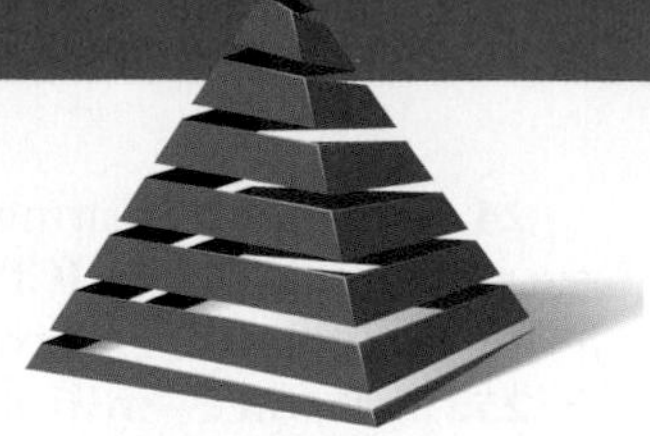

CHAPTER 56

Ophthalmic and Otic Medications

CRITICAL THINKING What Should You Do?

A client who requires the instillation of eyedrops three times daily tells the clinic nurse that he lives alone. He verbalizes concern about the ability to administer the drops because his hands are shaky. What should the nurse do?

Answer located on p. 792.

I. Ophthalmic Medication Administration

A. Guidelines for the use of eye medications

1. Eye medications are usually in the form of drops or ointments.
2. To prevent overflow of medication into the nasal and pharyngeal passages, thus reducing systemic absorption, the client is instructed to apply pressure over the inner canthus next to the nose for 30 to 60 seconds after administration of the medication. The client is instructed to close the eye gently to help distribute the medication.
3. If both an eyedrop and an eye ointment are scheduled to be administered at the same time, the eyedrop is administered first.
4. Hands should be washed and gloves donned before administering eye medications to avoid contaminating the eye or medication dropper or applicator.
5. A separate bottle or tube of medication is used for each client to avoid accidental cross-contamination.
6. The prescribed dose of eye medication is placed in the lower conjunctival sac, never directly onto the cornea.
7. Touching any part of the eye with the dropper or applicator is avoided.
8. Glucocorticoid preparations are administered before other medications.
9. Monitor the pulse of the client receiving an ophthalmic β-blocker. The client is instructed to do the same. If the pulse is less than 50 to 60 beats/min (adult), the next dose of eye medication is withheld and the health care provider (HCP) is notified.
10. Reinforce instructions to the client in how to instill medication correctly, and instillation is supervised until he or she can do it safely.
11. Reinforce instructions to the client to read the medication labels carefully to ensure administration of the correct medication and correct strength.
12. The client is reminded to keep these medications out of the reach of children.
13. Reinforce instructions to the client to avoid driving or operating hazardous equipment if vision is blurred.
14. The client is informed that he or she may be unable to drive home after eye examinations when a medication to dilate the pupil (mydriatic) or to paralyze the ciliary muscle (cycloplegic) is used.
15. If photophobia occurs, the client is instructed to wear sunglasses and avoid bright lights.
16. Reinforce instructions to the client to administer a missed dose of the eye medication as soon as it is remembered, unless the next dose is scheduled to be administered in 1 to 2 hours.
17. The client with **glaucoma** is informed that the disorder cannot be cured, only controlled.
18. Reinforce the importance of using medications to treat glaucoma as prescribed and not to discontinue these medications without consulting the HCP.
19. The client is informed that medications used to treat glaucoma may cause pain and blurred vision, especially when therapy is begun.
20. Reinforce instructions to the client to report the development of any eye irritation.
21. The client using eye gel is instructed to store the gel at room temperature or in the refrigerator, but not to freeze it.
22. Reinforce instructions to the client to discard unused eye gel kept at room temperature as recommended by the HCP and/or the pharmacist.
23. The client is informed that soft contact lenses may absorb certain eye medications and that preservatives in eye medications may discolor the contact lenses.

24. The client wearing contact lenses is advised to question the HCP carefully about special precautions to observe with eye medications.
25. Reinforce instructions to the parents to keep a record of the infant's bowel movements if atropine sulfate eyedrops are being administered.
26. Bowel sounds of the infant or child receiving atropine sulfate eyedrops are auscultated.

⚠ Because the timing of medication administration is critical, eye medications are administered at precise intervals. Instillation is separated by 3 to 5 minutes if two medications must be administered at the same time in the same eye(s).

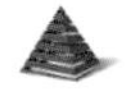

B. Instillation of eye medications
1. Drops
   a. Wash hands.
   b. Put on gloves.
   c. Check the name, strength, and expiration date of the medication.
   d. Instruct the client to tilt the head backward, open the eyes, and look up.
   e. Pull the lower lid down against the cheekbone.
   f. Hold the bottle like a pencil, with the tip downward.
   g. Holding the bottle, gently rest the wrist of the hand on the client's cheek.
   h. Squeeze the bottle gently to allow the drop to fall into the conjunctival sac.
   i. Reinforce instructions to the client to close the eyes gently and not to squeeze the eyes shut.
   j. Wait 3 to 5 minutes before instilling another drop, if more than one drop is prescribed, to promote maximal absorption of the medication.
   k. Do not allow the medication bottle, dropper, or applicator to come in contact with the eyelid or conjunctival sac.
   l. To prevent systemic absorption of the medication, apply gentle pressure with a clean tissue to the client's nasolacrimal duct for 30 to 60 seconds.
2. Ointments
   a. Reinforce instructions to the client to lie down or tilt head backward and look up.
   b. Hold the ointment tube near but not touching the eye or eyelashes.
   c. Squeeze a thin ribbon of ointment along the lining of the lower conjunctival sac from the inner to the outer canthus.
   d. Reinforce instructions to the client to close the eyes gently, rolling the eyeball in all directions (which increases contact area of medication to eye).
   e. Reinforce instructions to the client that vision may be blurred by the ointment.
   f. If possible, apply ointment just before bedtime.

II. Mydriatic-Cycloplegic and Anticholinergic Medications (Box 56-1)

A. Description (Fig. 56-1)
1. **Mydriatics** and cycloplegics dilate the pupils and relax the ciliary muscles (**cycloplegia**).
2. Anticholinergics block responses of the sphincter muscle in the ciliary body, producing **mydriasis** and cycloplegia.
3. These medications are used preoperatively or for eye examinations to produce mydriasis.
4. Mydriatics are contraindicated in cardiac dysrhythmias and cerebral atherosclerosis and should be used with caution in the older client and in those with prostatic hypertrophy, diabetes mellitus, or parkinsonism.

B. Side/adverse effects
1. Tachycardia
2. Photophobia

BOX 56-1 Mydriatic, Cycloplegic, and Anticholinergic Medications

- Atropine (Isopto Atropine)
- Cyclopentolate (AK-Pentolate, Cyclogyl)
- Homatropine (Isopto Homatropine)
- Phenylephrine (AK-Dilate, Mydfrin)
- Scopolamine (Isopto Hyoscine)
- Tropicamide (Mydriacyl, Tropicacyl)

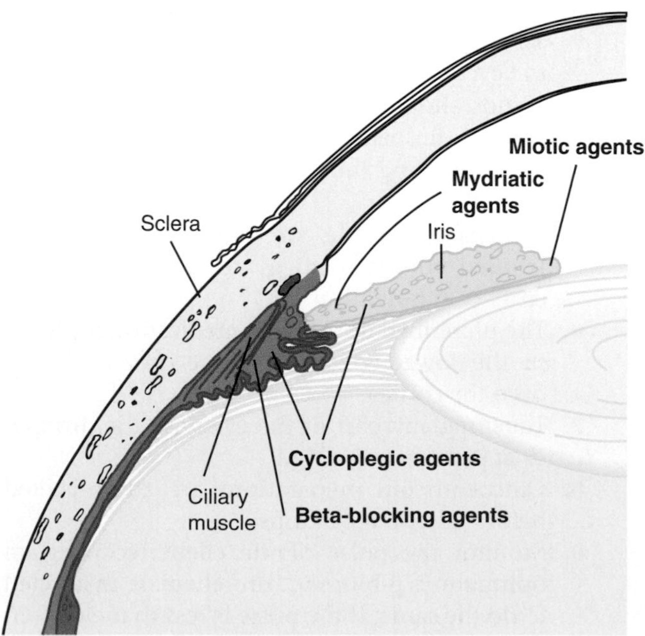

FIGURE 56-1 Sites of action of mydriatic, β-blocking, cycloplegic, and miotic agents. (From Black J, Hawks J: *Medical-surgical nursing: Clinical management for positive outcomes*, ed 8, St. Louis, 2009, Saunders.)

3. Conjunctivitis
4. Dermatitis
5. Elevated blood pressure

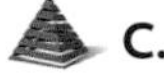

C. Atropine toxicity
1. Dry mouth
2. Blurred vision
3. Photophobia
4. Tachycardia
5. Fever
6. Urinary retention
7. Constipation
8. Headache, brow pain
9. Confusion
10. Hallucinations, delirium
11. Coma
12. Worsening of glaucoma

D. Systemic reactions to anticholinergics
1. Dry mouth and skin
2. Fever
3. Thirst
4. Confusion
5. Hyperactivity

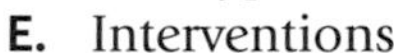

E. Interventions
1. Monitor for allergic response.
2. Determine risk for injury.
3. Check for constipation and urinary retention.
4. Reinforce instructions to the client that a burning sensation may occur on instillation.
5. Reinforce instructions to the client not to drive or perform hazardous activities for 24 hours after instillation of the medication unless otherwise directed by the HCP.
6. Reinforce instructions to the client to wear sunglasses until the effects of the medication wear off.
7. Reinforce instructions to the client to notify the HCP if blurring of vision, loss of sight, difficulty breathing, sweating, or flushing occurs.
8. Reinforce instructions to the client to report eye pain to the HCP.

Mydriatics are contraindicated in clients with glaucoma because of the risk of increased intraocular pressure.

III. Anti-infective Eye Medications (Box 56-2)

A. Description: Anti-infective medications kill or inhibit the growth of bacteria, fungi, and viruses.

B. Side/adverse effects
1. Superinfection
2. Global irritation

C. Interventions
1. Determine risk for injury.
2. Reinforce instructions to the client in how to apply the eye medication. The client is reminded to clean exudates from the eyes before administering drops.
3. The importance of completing the prescribed medication regimen is reinforced.
4. Reinforce instructions to the client to wash the hands thoroughly and frequently.
5. The client is advised that if improvement does not occur to notify the HCP.

BOX 56-2 Anti-infective Eye Medications

Antibacterial
- Chloramphenicol
- Erythromycin (Ilotycin, Romycin)

Aminoglycosides
- Gentamicin sulfate (Garamycin, Genoptic)
- Tobramycin (Tobrex)

Antifungal
- Natamycin (Natacyn)

Antiviral
- Ganciclovir (Zirgan)
- Trifluridine (Viroptic)

Sulfonamide
- Sulfacetamide (Bleph-10)

IV. Anti-inflammatory Eye Medications (Box 56-3)

A. Description

BOX 56-3 Anti-inflammatory Eye Medications

Corticosteroids
- Dexamethasone (Maxidex, others)
- Fluorometholone; sulfacetamide (FML-S eyedrop suspension)
- Loteprednol etabonate (Alrex, Lotemax)
- Prednisolone, gentamicin (PRED FORTE, PRED-G, others)
- Rimexolone (Vexol)

Ophthalmic Immunosuppressant and Anti-inflammatory Agent
- Cyclosporine (Restasis)

Nonsteroidal Anti-inflammatory Agents
- Diclofenac (Voltaren)
- Flurbiprofen sodium (Ocufen)
- Ketorolac tromethamine

Mast Cell Stabilizers
- Azelastine hydrochloride (Optivar)
- Cromolyn sodium (Crolom)
- Epinastine (Elestat)
- Ketotifen fumarate (Zaditor, Alaway)
- Lodoxamide (Alomide)
- Nedocromil sodium (Alocril)
- Olopatadine hydrochloride (Patanol)
- Pemirolast potassium (Alamast)

H_1 Receptor Blocker
- Emedastine difumarate (Emadine)

1. Anti-inflammatory medications control inflammation, thereby reducing vision loss and scarring.
2. Anti-inflammatory medications are used for uveitis, allergic conditions, and inflammation of the conjunctiva, cornea, and lids.

B. Side/adverse effects
1. **Cataracts**
2. Increased intraocular pressure
3. Impaired healing
4. Masking signs and symptoms of infection

C. Interventions
1. Interventions are the same as for anti-infective medications.
2. Note that dexamethasone (Maxidex) should not be used for eye abrasions and wounds.

V. Topical Eye Anesthetics

A. Description
1. Topical anesthetics produce corneal anesthesia.
2. Topical anesthetics are used for anesthesia for eye examinations and surgery or to remove foreign bodies from the eye.
3. Do not use discolored solution and store the bottle tightly closed.
4. Medications: Proparacaine hydrochloride (Ophthetic); tetracaine (Altacaine, TetraVisc)

B. Side/adverse effects
1. Temporary stinging or burning of the eye
2. Temporary loss of corneal reflex

C. Interventions
1. Determine risk for injury.
2. Note that the medications should not be given to the client for home use and are not to be self-administered by the client.
3. The client is instructed not to rub or touch the eye while it is anesthetized.
4. Note that the blink reflex is lost temporarily and that the corneal epithelium must be protected.
5. An eye patch is provided to protect the eye from injury until the corneal reflex returns.

VI. Eye Lubricants (Box 56-4)

A. Description
1. Replace tears or add moisture to the eyes
2. Moisten contact lenses or an artificial eye and protect the eyes during surgery or diagnostic procedures
3. Used for keratitis, during anesthesia, or for a disorder that results in unconsciousness or decreased blinking

BOX 56-4 Eye Lubricants

- Carboxymethylcellulose (Refresh, Theratears)
- Hydroxypropyl methylcellulose (Lacril, Isopto Plain)
- Petroleum-based ointment (Artificial Tears)
- Polyvinyl alcohol (Liquifilm Tears)

B. Side/adverse effects
1. Burning on instillation
2. Discomfort or pain on instillation
3. Allergic reaction

C. Interventions
1. The client is informed that burning may occur on instillation.
2. Be alert to allergic responses to the preservatives in the lubricants.

VII. Medications to Treat Glaucoma (Box 56-5; also see Fig. 56-1)

A. Description
1. These medications reduce intraocular pressure by constricting the pupil and contracting the ciliary muscle, thereby increasing the blood flow to the retina and decreasing retinal damage and loss of vision.
2. These medications open the anterior chamber angle and increase the outflow of aqueous humor.
3. Cholinergic medications reduce intraocular pressure by mimicking the action of acetylcholine.

BOX 56-5 Medications to Treat Glaucoma

Miotics
- Echothiophate
- Pilocarpine hydrochloride (Isopto Carpine)

β-Adrenergic Blocking Eye Medications
- Betaxolol hydrochloride (Betoptic)
- Carteolol hydrochloride (Ocupress)
- Levobunolol hydrochloride (Betagan Liquifilm)
- Metipranolol (OptiPranolol)
- Timolol maleate (Timoptic)

α-Adrenergic Agonists
- Apraclonidine (Iopidine)
- Brimonidine (Alphagan P)

Prostaglandin Analogues
- Latanoprost (Xalatan)
- Tafluprost (Zioptan)
- Travoprost (Travatan)
- Bimatoprost (Lumigan)

Cholinergic Agonists
- Pilocarpine hydrochloride (Isopto Carpine, others)
- Echothiophate iodide (Phospholine Iodide)

Carbonic Anhydrase Inhibitors
- Dorzolamide (Trusopt)
- Brinzolamide (Azopt)

Nonselective Adrenergic Agonist
- Dipivefrin (Propine)

4. Acetylcholine inhibitors reduce intraocular pressure by inhibiting the action of cholinesterase.
5. Some may be used to achieve **miosis** during eye surgery.
6. Contraindicated in clients with **retinal detachment**, adhesions between the iris and lens, or inflammatory diseases.
7. Used with caution in clients with asthma, hypertension, corneal abrasion, hyperthyroidism, coronary vascular disease, urinary tract obstruction, gastrointestinal obstruction, ulcer disease, parkinsonism, and bradycardia.

B. Side effects
1. **Myopia**
2. Headache
3. Eye pain
4. Decreased vision in poor light
5. Local irritation
6. Adverse/Systemic effects
   a. Flushing
   b. Diaphoresis
   c. Gastrointestinal upset and diarrhea
   d. Frequent urination
   e. Increased salivation
   f. Muscle weakness
   g. Respiratory difficulty
7. Toxicity
   a. Vertigo and syncope
   b. Bradycardia
   c. Hypotension
   d. Cardiac dysrhythmias
   e. Tremors
   f. Seizures

C. Interventions
1. Monitor the vital signs.
2. Determine risk for injury.
3. Monitor the client for the degree of diminished vision.
4. Monitor for side/adverse effects and toxic effects.
5. Monitor for postural hypotension, and instruct the client to change positions slowly.
6. Check breath sounds for wheezes and rhonchi because cholinergic medications can cause bronchospasms and increased bronchial secretions.
7. Maintain oral hygiene because of the increase in salivation.
8. Have atropine sulfate available as an antidote for pilocarpine.
9. The client or family is instructed regarding the correct administration of eye medications.
10. Reinforce instructions to the client not to stop the medication suddenly.
11. Reinforce instructions to the client to avoid activities such as driving while vision is impaired.

⚠ The client with glaucoma is instructed to read labels on over-the-counter medications and avoid atropine-like medications because atropine increases intraocular pressure.

VIII. β-Adrenergic Blocker Eye Medications (see Box 56-5)

A. Description (see Fig. 56-1)
1. These medications reduce intraocular pressure by decreasing sympathetic impulses and decreasing aqueous humor production without affecting accommodation or pupil size.
2. These medications are used to treat glaucoma.
3. These medications are contraindicated in the client with asthma or chronic obstructive pulmonary disease because systemic absorption can cause increased airway resistance.
4. These medications are used with caution in the client receiving oral β-blockers.

B. Side/adverse effects
1. Ocular irritation
2. Visual disturbances
3. Bradycardia
4. Hypotension
5. Bronchospasm

C. Interventions
1. Monitor the vital signs, especially blood pressure and pulse, before administering medication.
2. If the pulse is 60 beats/min or less or if the systolic blood pressure is less than 90 mm Hg, the medication is withheld and the RN and HCP is contacted.
3. Monitor for shortness of breath.
4. Determine risk for injury.
5. Monitor intake and output (I&O).
6. The client is instructed to notify the health care provider if shortness of breath occurs.
7. Reinforce instructions to the client not to discontinue the medication abruptly.
8. Reinforce instructions to the client to change positions slowly because of the potential for orthostatic hypotension.
9. Reinforce instructions to the client to avoid hazardous activities.
10. Reinforce instructions to the client to avoid over-the-counter medications without the HCP's approval.
11. Clients with diabetes mellitus using β-adrenergic blockers are instructed to monitor blood glucose levels frequently.

IX. Carbonic Anhydrase Inhibitors (see Box 56-5)

A. Description
1. Carbonic anhydrase inhibitors interfere with the production of carbonic acid, which leads to decreased aqueous humor formation and decreased intraocular pressure.

2. These medications are used for long-term treatment of glaucoma.
3. These medications are contraindicated in the client allergic to sulfonamides.
4. Used with caution for clients with severe renal or liver disease.

B. Side/adverse effects
1. Appetite loss
2. Gastrointestinal upset
3. Paresthesias in the fingers, toes, and face
4. Polyuria
5. Hypokalemia
6. Renal calculi
7. Photosensitivity
8. Lethargy and drowsiness
9. Depression

C. Interventions
1. Monitor the vital signs.
2. Check visual acuity.
3. Determine risk for injury.
4. Monitor intake and output.
5. Monitor weight.
6. Maintain oral hygiene.
7. Monitor for side effects such as lethargy, anorexia, drowsiness, polyuria, nausea, and vomiting.
8. Monitor electrolyte levels for hypokalemia.
9. Fluid intake is increased unless contraindicated.
10. The client is advised to avoid prolonged exposure to sunlight.
11. The use of artificial tears for dry eyes is encouraged.
12. Reinforce instructions to the client not to discontinue the medication abruptly.
13. Reinforce instructions to the client to avoid hazardous activities while vision is impaired.
14. Reinforce instructions to the client not to wear contact lenses during or within 15 minutes of instilling these medications.

X. Ocusert System

A. Description
1. A thin eye wafer (disk) is impregnated with a time-release dose of pilocarpine (Ocusert Pilo-20, Ocusert Pilo-40).
2. The Ocusert system was devised to overcome the frequent application of pilocarpine.
3. It is placed in the upper or lower cul-de-sac of the eye.
4. The pilocarpine is released over 1 week.
5. The disk is replaced every 7 days.
6. Drawbacks of its use include sudden leakage of pilocarpine, migration of the system over the cornea, and unnoticed loss of the system.

B. Interventions
1. Determine the client's ability to insert the medication disk.
2. Store the medication in the refrigerator.
3. Reinforce instructions to the client to discard damaged or contaminated disks.
4. The client is informed that temporary stinging is expected, but to notify the HCP if blurred vision or brow pain occurs.
5. Reinforce instructions to the client to check for the presence of the disk in the conjunctival sac daily at bedtime and on arising.
6. Because vision may change in the first few hours after the eye system is inserted, the client is instructed to replace the disk at bedtime.

XI. Osmotic Medications

A. Mannitol (Osmitrol)

B. Description
1. Lower intraocular pressure.
2. Used in emergency treatment of glaucoma.
3. Used preoperatively and postoperatively to decrease vitreous humor volume.

C. Side/adverse effects
1. Headache
2. Nausea, vomiting, diarrhea, dehydration
3. Disorientation
4. Electrolyte imbalances

D. Interventions
1. Monitor the vital signs.
2. Check visual acuity.
3. Determine risk for injury.
4. Monitor intake and output.
5. Monitor weight.
6. Monitor electrolyte imbalances.
7. Increase fluid intake unless contraindicated.
8. Monitor for changes in level of orientation.

XII. Medications to Treat **Macular Degeneration**

A. Pegaptanib (Macugen), ranizumab (Lucentis), bevacizumab (Avastin), aflibercept (EYLEA)

B. Description
1. Age-related macular degeneration (ARMD) can be either dry ARMD (atrophic ARMD) or wet ARMD (neovascular).
2. Dry is more common; macular photoreceptors undergo gradual breakdown, leading to gradual blurring of central vision.
3. Wet progresses faster, and macular degeneration is caused by growth of new subretinal blood vessels that leads to fluid leakage that lifts the macula and causes permanent injury.
4. Characterized by the presence of drusen (yellow deposits under the retina)

C. Side/adverse effects
1. Endophthalmitis (eye inflammation caused by bacterial, viral, or fungal infection)
2. Blurred vision
3. Cataracts
4. Corneal edema

5. Eye discomfort and discharge
6. Conjunctival hemorrhage
7. Increased intraocular pressure
8. Reduced visual acuity

D. Interventions
1. Reinforce teaching the client about administration of the medications.
2. Reinforce teaching the client about the side effects and the need to notify the HCP.

XIII. Otic Medication Administration

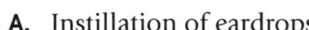

A. Instillation of eardrops
1. In an adult, pull the pinna up and back to straighten the external canal to instill eardrops.
2. Tilt the client's head in the opposite direction of the affected ear and apply the drops into the ear.
3. With the head tilted, gently move the head back and forth five times.
4. Pull the pinna down and back for infants and children younger than 3 years, up and back for older children.

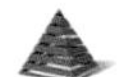

B. Irrigation of the ear
1. Irrigation of the ear needs to be prescribed by the HCP.
2. Ensure direct visualization of the tympanic membrane.
3. Warm irrigating solution to 98°F because solution temperature not close to the client's body temperature will cause ear injury, nausea, and vertigo.
4. Irrigation must be done gently to avoid damage to the eardrum.
5. When irrigating, do not direct irrigation solution directly toward the eardrum.

C. Systemic medications that affect hearing (Box 56-6)

BOX 56-6 Medications That Affect Hearing

Antibiotics
- Amikacin (Amikin)
- Chloramphenicol
- Erythromycin (ERYC, Ery-Tab, PCE Dispertab, Ilotycin)
- Gentamicin (Garamycin, Gentak)
- Streptomycin sulfate
- Tobramycin sulfate (Nebcin)
- Vancomycin (Vancocin)

Diuretics
- Ethacrynic acid (Edecrin)
- Furosemide (Lasix)

Others
- Cisplatin (Platinol)
- Nitrogen mustard (Mustargen)
- Quinine (Qualaquin)
- Quinidine

BOX 56-7 Anti-infective Ear Medications
- Acetic acid; aluminum acetate (Domeboro Otic)
- Amoxicillin (Amoxil)
- Ampicillin
- Cefaclor (Ceclor)
- Chloramphenicol
- Clarithromycin (Biaxin)
- Clindamycin hydrochloride (Cleocin)
- Erythromycin (Ilotycin)
- Gentamicin sulfate otic solution (Garamycin)
- Penicillin V potassium (Veetids)
- Trimethoprim; sulfamethoxazole (Bactrim)

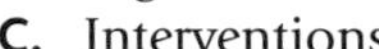

If a perforation of the eardrum is suspected, do not perform ear irrigation.

XIV. Anti-infective Ear Medications (Box 56-7)

A. Description
1. Anti-infective medications kill or inhibit the growth of bacteria and are used for otitis media or otitis externa.
2. Anti-infective medications are contraindicated if a prior hypersensitivity exists.

B. Side/adverse effect: Overgrowth of nonsusceptible organisms 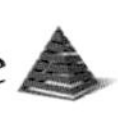

C. Interventions
1. Monitor the vital signs.
2. Check for allergies.
3. Monitor for pain.
4. Monitor for nephrotoxicity.
5. Reinforce instructing the client to report dizziness, fatigue, fever, or sore throat, which may indicate a superimposed infection.
6. Reinforce instructing the client to complete the entire course of the medication.
7. Reinforce instructing the client to keep ear canals dry.

XV. Antihistamines and Decongestants (Box 56-8)

A. Description
1. These medications produce vasoconstriction.
2. These medications stimulate the receptors of the respiratory mucosa.
3. These medications reduce respiratory tissue hyperemia and edema to open obstructed eustachian tubes.
4. These medications are used for acute otitis media.

BOX 56-8 Antihistamines and Decongestants
- Loratadine (Claritin)
- Diphenhydramine (Benadryl)
- Fexofenadine (Allegra)
- Pseudoephedrine (Sudafed)

B. Side/adverse effects
 1. Drowsiness
 2. Blurred vision
 3. Dry mucous membranes

C. Interventions
 1. The client is informed that drowsiness, blurred vision, and a dry mouth may occur.
 2. Reinforce instructing the client to increase fluid intake unless contraindicated and suck on hard candy to alleviate the dry mouth.
 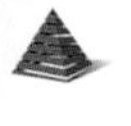
 3. Reinforce instructing the client to avoid hazardous activities if drowsiness occurs.

XVI. Local Anesthetics

A. Description
 1. Local anesthetics block nerve conduction at or near the application site to control pain.
 2. Local anesthetics are used for pain associated with ear infections.

B. Medication: Benzocaine-antipyrine-phenylephrine (Tympagesic)

C. Side/adverse effects
 1. Allergic reaction
 2. Irritation

D. Interventions
 1. Monitor for effectiveness if used for pain relief.
 2. Check for irritation or allergic reaction.

XVII. Ceruminolytic Medications

A. Carbamide peroxide (Debrox)

B. Description
 1. Ceruminolytic medications emulsify and loosen cerumen deposits.
 2. Ceruminolytic medications are used to loosen and remove impacted wax from the ear canal.

C. Side/adverse effects
 1. Irritation
 2. Redness or swelling of the ear canal

D. Interventions
 1. Reinforce instructing the client not to use drops more often than prescribed.
 2. A cotton plug is moistened with medication before insertion.
 3. Keep the container tightly closed and away from moisture.
 4. Touching the ear with the dropper is avoided.
 5. Thirty minutes after instillation, the ear is gently irrigated as prescribed with warm water, using a soft rubber bulb ear syringe.
 6. Irrigation may be done with hydrogen peroxide solution as prescribed to flush cerumen deposits out of the ear canal.
 7. For a chronic cerumen impaction, one or two drops of mineral oil will soften the wax.
 8. Reinforce instructing the client to notify the health care provider if redness, pain, or swelling persists.

CRITICAL THINKING What Should You Do?

Answer: If the client lives alone and has a physical condition that may affect instilling the eyedrops, the clinic nurse should assist to arrange for a home care nurse to assess the client and the home situation. If the client is unable to instill eyedrops independently, a friend, neighbor, or family member can be taught the technique if possible. In addition, adaptive equipment that positions the bottle of eyedrops directly over the eye can be purchased and used by the client who has difficulty instilling eyedrops.

Reference(s): Ignatavicius, D., & Workman, M. (2013). *Medical-surgical nursing: Patient-centered collaborative care.* (7th ed., pp. 1061–1062). St. Louis: Saunders.

PRACTICE QUESTIONS

586. Betaxolol hydrochloride (Betoptic) eyedrops have been prescribed for the client with glaucoma. Which nursing action is **most appropriate** related to monitoring for the side/adverse effects of this medication?
 1. Monitoring temperature
 2. Monitoring blood pressure
 3. Checking peripheral pulses
 4. Checking the blood glucose level

587. The nurse assists to prepare the client for ear irrigation as prescribed by the health care provider. Which action should the nurse plan to take?
 1. Warm the irrigating solution to 98°F.
 2. Position the client with the affected side up after the irrigation.
 3. Direct a slow, steady stream of irrigation solution toward the eardrum.
 4. Assist the client to turn his or her head so that the ear to be irrigated is facing upward.

588. In preparation for cataract surgery, the nurse is to administer cyclopentolate (Cyclogyl) eyedrops. The nurse administers the eyedrops knowing that the purpose of this medication is which?
 1. Produce miosis of the operative eye
 2. Dilate the pupil of the operative eye
 3. Provide lubrication to the operative eye
 4. Constrict the pupil of the operative eye

589. The nurse is providing instructions to a client who will be self-administering eyedrops. To minimize the systemic effects that eyedrops can produce, the client is instructed to perform which?
 1. Eat before instilling the drops.
 2. Swallow several times after instilling the drops.
 3. Blink vigorously to encourage tearing after instilling the drops.

4. Occlude the nasolacrimal duct with a finger over the inner canthus for 30 to 60 seconds after instilling the drops.

590. The client is receiving an eyedrop and an eye ointment to the right eye. Which action should the nurse take?
1. Administer the eyedrop first, followed by the eye ointment.
2. Administer the eye ointment first, followed by the eyedrop.
3. Administer the eyedrop, wait 10 minutes, and administer the eye ointment.
4. Administer the eye ointment, wait 10 minutes, and administer the eyedrop.

591. The nurse is caring for a client with glaucoma. Which medication prescribed for the client should the nurse question?
1. Betaxolol (Betoptic)
2. Pilocarpine (Ocusert Pilo-20)
3. Atropine sulfate (Isopto Atropine)
4. Pilocarpine hydrochloride (Isopto Carpine)

❖ **592.** The nurse is preparing to administer eyedrops. Which interventions should the nurse take to administer the drops? **Select all that apply.**
- ❑ 1. Wash hands.
- ❑ 2. Put on gloves.
- ❑ 3. Place the drop in the conjunctival sac.
- ❑ 4. Pull the lower lid down against the cheekbone.
- ❑ 5. Instruct the client to squeeze the eyes shut after instilling the eyedrop.
- ❑ 6. Instruct the client to tilt the head forward, open the eyes, and look down.

593. A client was just admitted to the hospital to rule out a gastrointestinal (GI) bleed. The client has brought several bottles of medications prescribed by different specialists. During the admission assessment, the client states, "Lately, I have been hearing some roaring sounds in my ears, especially when I am alone." Which medication should the nurse determine to be the cause of the client's complaint?
1. Doxycycline (Vibramycin)
2. Acetylsalicylic acid (aspirin)
3. Atropine sulfate (Isopto Atropine)
4. Diltiazem hydrochloride (Cardizem)

594. Pilocarpine hydrochloride (Isopto Carpine) is prescribed for the client with glaucoma. Which medication should the nurse plan to have available in the event of systemic toxicity?
1. Atropine sulfate
2. Timolol maleate (Timoptic)
3. Metipranolol (OptiPranolol)
4. Carteolol hydrochloride (Ocupress)

595. A miotic medication has been prescribed for the client with glaucoma. The client asks the nurse about the purpose of the medication. The nurse should tell the client which?
1. "The medication will help dilate the eye to prevent an increase in eye pressure."
2. "The medication will relax the muscles of the eyes and prevent blurred vision."
3. "The medication causes the pupil to constrict and will lower the pressure in the eye."
4. "The medication will help block the responses that are sent to the muscles in the eye."

ANSWERS

586. 2

Rationale: Hypotension, dizziness, nausea, diaphoresis, headache, fatigue, constipation, and diarrhea are systemic effects of the medication. Nursing interventions include monitoring the blood pressure for hypotension and assessing the pulse for strength, weakness, irregular rate, and bradycardia. Options 1, 3, and 4 are not specifically associated with this medication.

Test-Taking Strategy: Note the strategic words, *most appropriate*. Use the ABCs—airway, breathing, and circulation—to direct you to the correct option. Although option 3, peripheral pulses, also is related to circulation monitoring, the blood pressure is the umbrella option. **Review:** the side effects of Betaxolol hydrochloride.

Level of Cognitive Ability: Applying
Client Needs: Physiological Integrity
Integrated Process: Nursing Process/Data Collection
Content Area: Adult Health: Eye
Priority Concepts: Perfusion, Sensory Perception
Reference(s): Lehne (2013), pp. 175–176.

587. 1

Rationale: Irrigation solutions that are not close to the client's body temperature can be uncomfortable and may cause injury, nausea, and vertigo. The client is positioned so that the ear to be irrigated is facing downward, because this allows gravity to assist in the removal of the ear wax and solution. After the irrigation, the client is to lie on the affected side to finish draining the irrigating solution. A slow, steady stream of solution should be directed toward the upper wall of the ear canal and not toward the eardrum. Too much force could cause the tympanic membrane to rupture.

Test-Taking Strategy: Focus on the subject, ear irrigations. Read each option carefully and remember that the nurse's concern is to prevent damage to the tympanic membrane. Additionally, remember that the client should be positioned with the

affected side downward to allow drainage of the irrigation solution. **Review:** the procedure for performing **ear irrigations**.
Level of Cognitive Ability: Applying
Client Needs: Physiological Integrity
Integrated Process: Nursing Process/Implementation
Content Area: Adult Health: Ear
Priority Concepts: Safety, Sensory Perception
Reference(s): Cooper, Gosnell (2015), pp. 619–620.

588. 2
Rationale: Cyclopentolate is a rapidly acting mydriatic and cycloplegic medication. Cyclopentolate is effective in 25 to 75 minutes, and accommodation returns in 6 to 24 hours. Cyclopentolate is used for preoperative mydriasis.
Test-Taking Strategy: Options 1 and 4 are **comparable or alike** and are eliminated first. Miosis refers to a constricted pupil. Note that the question identifies a client being prepared for eye surgery. The pupil would need to be dilated for the surgical procedure. **Review:** the action and purpose of cyclopentolate.
Level of Cognitive Ability: Applying
Client Needs: Physiological Integrity
Integrated Process: Nursing Process/Implementation
Content Area: Adult Health: Eye
Priority Concepts: Clinical Judgment, Sensory Perception
Reference(s): Lehne (2013), p. 1322.

589. 4
Rationale: Applying pressure on the nasolacrimal duct prevents systemic absorption of the medication. Options 1, 2, and 3 will not prevent systemic absorption.
Test-Taking Strategy: Focus on the **subject**, administration of eyedrops. Eating and swallowing are **comparable or alike** and are not related to the systemic absorption of an eye medication. Blinking vigorously to produce tearing may result in the loss of the administered medication. **Review:** the procedure for administering eyedrops to prevent **systemic absorption**.
Level of Cognitive Ability: Applying
Client Needs: Physiological Integrity
Integrated Process: Teaching and Learning
Content Area: Adult Health: Eye
Priority Concepts: Client Education, Sensory Perception
Reference(s): Ignatavicius, Workman (2013), pp. 1044, 1062; Perry, Potter, Ostendorf (2014), p. 512.

590. 1
Rationale: When an eyedrop and an eye ointment is scheduled to be administered at the same time, the eyedrop is administered first. Options 2, 3, and 4 are incorrect.
Test-Taking Strategy: Focus on the **subject**, administration of eyedrops and eye ointments. Recalling the guidelines for administering eye medications will direct you to the correct option. **Review:** guidelines for administering **eyedrops and eye ointments**.
Level of Cognitive Ability: Applying
Client Needs: Physiological Integrity
Integrated Process: Nursing Process/Implementation
Content Area: Adult Health: Eye
Priority Concepts: Safety, Sensory Perception
Reference(s): deWit, Kumagai (2013), p. 578.

591. 3
Rationale: Options 1, 2, and 4 are miotic agents used to treat glaucoma. Option 3 is a mydriatic and cycloplegic medication, and its use is contraindicated in clients with glaucoma. Mydriatic medications dilate the pupil and can cause an increase in intraocular pressure in the eye.
Test-Taking Strategy: Focus on the **subject**, glaucoma. Knowledge regarding the classifications of the medications identified in the options will assist in answering the question. Remember that mydriatics dilate, and that these medications are contraindicated in glaucoma. **Review:** the **contraindications related to medications for the client with glaucoma**.
Level of Cognitive Ability: Analyzing
Client Needs: Safe and Effective Care Environment
Integrated Process: Nursing Process/Implementation
Content Area: Adult Health: Eye
Priority Concepts: Safety, Sensory Perception
Reference(s): Hodgson, Kizior (2015), p. 99.

❖**592. 1, 2, 3, 4**
Rationale: To administer eye medications, the nurse would wash hands and put on gloves. The client is instructed to tilt the head backward, open the eyes, and look up. The nurse pulls the lower lid down against the cheekbone and holds the bottle like a pencil, with the tip downward. Holding the bottle, the nurse gently rests the wrist of the hand on the client's cheek and squeezes the bottle gently to allow the drop to fall into the conjunctival sac. The client is instructed to close the eyes gently and not to squeeze the eyes shut to prevent the loss of medication.
Test-Taking Strategy: Focus on the **subject**, administering eyedrops. Use guidelines related to standard precautions and visualize this procedure. This will assist in determining the correct interventions. **Review:** the procedure for administering **eye medications**.
Level of Cognitive Ability: Applying
Client Needs: Physiological Integrity
Integrated Process: Nursing Process/Implementation
Content Area: Adult Health: Eye
Priority Concepts: Safety, Sensory Perception
Reference(s): Ignatavicius, Workman (2013), p. 1050.

593. 2
Rationale: Aspirin is contraindicated for gastrointestinal bleed and is potentially ototoxic. The client should be advised to notify the prescribing health care provider so the medication can be discontinued and/or a substitute that is less toxic to the ear can be taken instead. Options 1, 3, and 4 do not have side effects that are potentially associated with hearing difficulties.
Test-Taking Strategy: Focus on the **subject**, the client's complaint. Review the classifications and/or therapeutic effects, as well as the side/adverse effects, of each medication in the options. Of the medications identified, only aspirin can cause ototoxicity. Additionally, it is contraindicated for GI bleed as well. **Review:** medications that can cause **ototoxicity**.
Level of Cognitive Ability: Analyzing
Client Needs: Physiological Integrity
Integrated Process: Nursing Process/Data Collection

Content Area: Adult Health: Ear
Priority Concepts: Clinical Judgment, Sensory Perception
Reference(s): Hodgson, Kizior (2015), pp. 90–91.

594. 1
Rationale: Systemic absorption of pilocarpine hydrochloride can produce toxicity and includes manifestations of vertigo, bradycardia, tremors, hypotension, and seizures. Atropine sulfate must be available in the event of systemic toxicity. Pindolol, timolol maleate, and carteolol hydrochloride are β-blockers.
Test-Taking Strategy: Note that options 2, 3, and 4 are comparable or alike and are β-blockers. Also remember that atropine sulfate is the antidote for systemic reactions that occur with pilocarpine hydrochloride. **Review: antidotes.**
Level of Cognitive Ability: Applying
Client Needs: Physiological Integrity
Integrated Process: Nursing Process/Implementation
Content Area: Adult Health: Eye
Priority Concepts: Clinical Judgment, Sensory Perception
Reference(s): Lehne (2013), p. 1321.

595. 3
Rationale: Miotics cause pupillary constriction and are used to treat glaucoma. They lower the intraocular pressure, thereby increasing blood flow to the retina and decreasing retinal damage and loss of vision. Miotics cause a contraction of the ciliary muscle and a widening of the trabecular meshwork. Options 1, 2, and 4 are incorrect.
Test-Taking Strategy: Focus on the subject, miotic medication. Note that the client has glaucoma. Recall that prevention of increased intraocular pressure is the goal in the client with glaucoma. Options 1, 2, and 4 describe actions related to mydriatic medications, which primarily dilate the pupils and relax the ciliary muscles. **Review:** the action of a **miotic** medication.
Level of Cognitive Ability: Understanding
Client Needs: Physiological Integrity
Integrated Process: Nursing Process/Implementation
Content Area: Adult Health: Eye
Priority Concepts: Client Education, Sensory Perception
Reference(s): deWit, Kumagai (2013), p. 602.

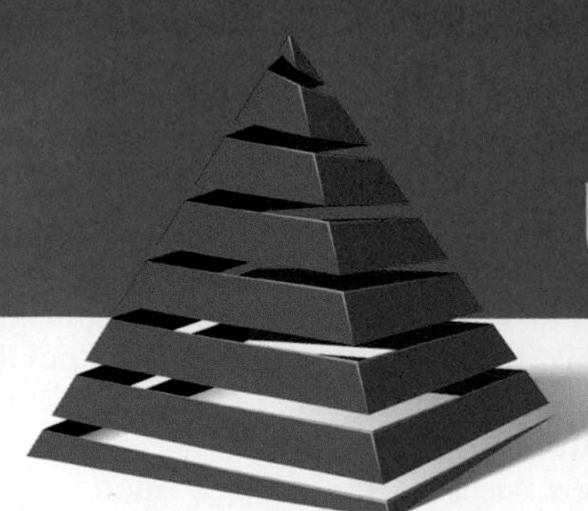

UNIT XVI

The Adult Client with a Neurological Disorder

PYRAMID TERMS

autonomic dysreflexia Syndrome characterized by paroxysmal hypertension, bradycardia, excessive sweating, facial flushing, nasal congestion, pilomotor responses, and headache. The syndrome occurs with spinal lesions above T6 after the period of spinal shock is complete. Triggers include visceral stimulation from a distended bladder or impacted rectum. The syndrome is a neurological emergency and must be treated immediately to prevent a hypertensive stroke. It is also known as *autonomic hyperreflexia*.

Babinski's reflex Dorsiflexion of the big toe with extension; elicited by firmly stroking the lateral aspect of the sole of the foot.

Brudzinski's sign Involuntary flexion of the hip and knee when the neck is passively flexed; indicates meningeal irritation.

decerebrate (extensor) posturing Stiff extension of one or both arms and possibly the legs that indicates a brainstem lesion.

Decorticate (flexor) posturing Flexure of one or both arms on the chest and possibly stiff extension of the legs; indicates a damaged cortex.

edrophonium test Test used to diagnose myasthenia gravis and to differentiate between myasthenic crisis and cholinergic crisis; may also be called the *Tensilon test*.

flaccid posturing No motor response display in any extremity.

hemianopsia Blindness in half of the visual field.

homonymous hemianopsia Loss of half of the field of view on the same side in both eyes.

increased intracranial pressure (ICP) Increased pressure within the skull caused by trauma, hemorrhage, growths or tumors, hydrocephalus, edema, or inflammation. Increased pressure can impede circulation to the brain and absorption of cerebrospinal fluid and can affect nerve cell functioning, leading to brainstem compression and death.

Kernig's sign Loss of the ability of a supine client to straighten the leg completely when it is fully flexed at the knee and hip: indicates meningeal irritation.

neurogenic shock Occurs most commonly in clients with injuries above T6 and usually is experienced soon after the injury. Massive vasodilation occurs, leading to pooling of the blood in blood vessels, tissue hypoperfusion, and impaired cellular metabolism.

nuchal rigidity Stiff neck; flexion of the neck onto the chest causes intense pain.

spinal shock Also known as *spinal shock syndrome*. It is a complete but temporary loss of motor, sensory, reflex, and autonomic function that occurs immediately after injury as the cord's response to the injury. It usually lasts less than 48 hours but can continue for several weeks.

unconscious client A state of depressed cerebral functioning with unresponsiveness to sensory and motor function; causes include head trauma, cerebral toxins, shock, hemorrhage, tumor, and infections.

unilateral neglect An inability to recognize a physical impairment on one side of the body. It occurs most commonly in clients who have had a right cerebral stroke; also known as *neglect syndrome*.

Pyramid to Success

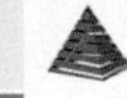

Pyramid points related to neurological disorders focus on safety issues; care of the unconscious client; monitoring for increased intracranial pressure; monitoring level of consciousness; positioning clients; nursing interventions during a seizure, and care of the client with a head injury, brain attack (stroke), spinal cord injury, Parkinson's disease, meningitis, or myasthenia gravis. Focus on the points related to the psychsocial effects as a result of the neurological disorder, such as anxiety, unexpected body image changes, and the appropriate and available support services needed for the client.

Client Needs

Safe and Effective Care Environment

Acting as a client advocate
Assisting to initiate referrals to appropriate services
Collaborating with members of the health care team
Ensuring advance directives are in the client's medical record

Ensuring that informed consent has been obtained for invasive procedures
Establishing priorities
Maintaining asepsis with procedures and treatments
Maintaining confidentiality
Maintaining standard, transmission-based and other precautions
Preventing accidents that can occur as a result of neurological deficits
Upholding client rights

Health Promotion and Maintenance

Assisting the RN in teaching about the importance of prescribed therapy
Discussing expected and unexpected body image changes resulting from neurological deficits
Providing information about local support groups and community resources
Performing neurological data collection techniques
Preventing and detecting health problems associated with neurological deficits
Providing home care instructions regarding care related to the neurological disorder

Psychosocial Integrity

Acknowledging end-of-life issues and grief and loss issues
Considering the cultural, religious, and spiritual influences of the client when planning care
Determining the ability to cope with feelings of isolation and loss of independence
Identifying sensory and perceptual alterations
Identifying support systems and encouraging the use of community resources
Mobilizing coping mechanisms

Physiological Integrity

Assisting to administer pharmacological therapy
Maintaining nutrition
Monitoring for alterations in body systems
Monitoring for complications related to procedures
Monitoring for fluid and electrolyte imbalances
Providing assistive devices for mobility
Providing emergency care
Providing measures to promote comfort
Promoting normal elimination patterns
Promoting self-care measures

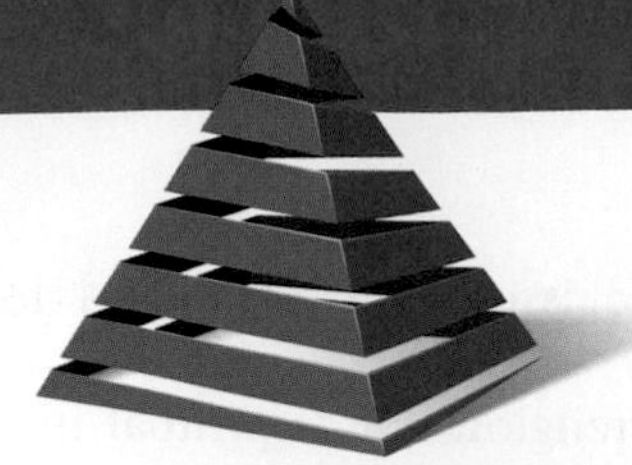

CHAPTER 57

Neurological System

CRITICAL THINKING What Should You Do?

The nurse notes that a client who experienced a stroke is sitting in a chair and is leaning to the left with the arm caught in the side of the chair seat. The nurse suspects unilateral body neglect syndrome. What should the nurse do?

Answer located on p. 821.

I. Anatomy and Physiology of the Brain and Spinal Cord

A. Cerebrum
- **1.** The cerebrum consists of the right and left hemispheres.
- **2.** Each hemisphere receives sensory information from the opposite side of the body and controls the skeletal muscles of the opposite side.
- **3.** The cerebrum governs sensory and motor activity and thought and learning.

B. Cerebral cortex (Box 57-1)
- **1.** The cerebral cortex is the outer gray layer, and it is divided into five lobes.

BOX 57-1 Cerebral Cortex

Frontal Lobe

Broca's area for speech

Motor cortex for voluntary motor function, voluntary eye movement, memory storage, morals, emotions, reasoning and judgment, concentration, and abstraction

Parietal Lobe

Interpretation of taste, pain, touch, temperature, and pressure

Spatial perception

Temporal Lobe

Auditory center

Wernicke's area for sensory and speech

Occipital Lobe

Visual area

Limbic Lobe

Emotional and visceral patterns for survival

Learning and memory

- **2.** It is responsible for the conscious activities of the cerebrum.

C. Basal ganglia: Cell bodies in white matter that help the cerebral cortex in producing smooth voluntary movements

D. Diencephalon
- **1.** Thalamus
  - **a.** Relays sensory impulses to the cortex
  - **b.** Provides a pain gate
  - **c.** Is part of the reticular activating system
- **2.** Hypothalamus
  - **a.** Regulates autonomic responses of the sympathetic and parasympathetic nervous systems
  - **b.** Regulates the stress response, sleep, appetite, body temperature, fluid balance, and emotions
  - **c.** Responsible for the production of hormones secreted by the pituitary gland and the hypothalamus

E. Brainstem
- **1.** Midbrain
  - **a.** Responsible for motor coordination
  - **b.** Contains the visual reflex and auditory relay centers
- **2.** Pons: Contains the respiratory centers and regulates breathing
- **3.** Medulla oblongata
  - **a.** Contains all afferent and efferent tracts and contains cardiac, respiratory, vomiting, and vasomotor centers
  - **b.** Controls heart rate, respiration, blood vessel diameter, sneezing, swallowing, vomiting, and coughing

F. Cerebellum: Coordinates smooth muscle movement, posture, equilibrium, and muscle tone

G. Spinal cord
- **1.** Provides neuron and synapse networks to produce involuntary responses to sensory stimulation
- **2.** Controls body movement and regulates visceral function
- **3.** Carries sensory information to and motor information from the brain
- **4.** Extends from the first cervical to the second lumbar vertebra

5. Protected by the meninges, cerebrospinal fluid (CSF), and adipose tissue
6. Horns
   a. Inner column of gray matter contains two anterior and two posterior horns.
   b. Posterior horns connect with afferent (sensory) nerve fibers.
   c. Anterior horns contain efferent (motor) nerve fibers.
7. Nerve tracts
   a. White matter contains the nerve tract.
   b. Ascending tracts (sensory pathway)
   c. Descending tract (motor pathway)

H. Meninges
1. The dura mater is the tough and fibrous membrane.
2. The arachnoid membrane is the delicate membrane and contains cerebrospinal fluid.
3. The pia mater is a vascular membrane.
4. The subarachnoid space is formed by the arachnoid membrane and the pia mater.

I. Cerebrospinal fluid (CSF)
1. Secreted in the ventricles; circulates in the subarachnoid space and through the ventricles to the subarachnoid space of the meninges, where it is reabsorbed
2. Acts as a protective cushion and aids in the exchange of nutrients and wastes
3. Normal pressure is 50 to 175 mm H_2O.
4. Normal volume is 125 to 150 mL.

J. Ventricles
1. Four ventricles
2. The ventricles communicate between the subarachnoid spaces and produce and circulate CSF.

K. Blood supply
1. Right and left internal carotids
2. Right and left vertebral arteries
3. These arteries supply the brain via an anastomosis at the base of the brain called the circle of Willis.

L. Neurotransmitters
1. Acetylcholine
2. Norepinephrine
3. Dopamine
4. Serotonin
5. Amino acids
6. Polypeptides

M. Neurons
1. The neuron consists of cell body, axons, and dendrites.
2. The cell body contains the nucleus.
3. Neurons carrying impulses to the central nervous system (CNS) are called sensory neurons.
4. Neurons carrying impulses away from the CNS are called motor neurons.
5. Synapse is the chemical transmission of impulses from one neuron to another.

N. Axons and dendrites
1. The axon conducts impulses from the cell body.
2. The dendrites receive stimuli from the body and transmit them to the axon.
3. The neurons are protected and insulated by Schwann cells.
4. The Schwann cell sheath is called the neurolemma.
5. Neurons do not reproduce after the neonatal period.
6. If an axon or dendrite is damaged, it will die and be replaced slowly only if the neurilemma is intact and the cell body has not died.

O. Spinal nerves
1. Human beings have 31 pairs of spinal nerves.
2. Mixed nerve fibers are formed by the joining of the anterior motor and posterior sensory roots.
3. Posterior roots contain afferent (sensory) nerve fibers.
4. Anterior roots contain efferent (motor) nerve fibers.

P. Autonomic nervous system
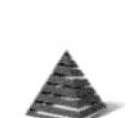
1. Sympathetic (adrenergic) fibers dilate pupils, increase heart rate and rhythm, contract blood vessels, and relax smooth muscles of the bronchi.
2. Parasympathetic (cholinergic) fibers produce the opposite effect.

II. Diagnostic Tests

A. Skull and spinal radiography
1. Description
   a. Radiographs of the skull reveal the size and shape of the skull bones, suture separation in infants, fractures or bony defects, erosion, and calcification.
   b. Spinal radiographs identify fractures, dislocation, compression, curvature, erosion, narrowed spinal cord, and degenerative processes.
2. Preprocedure interventions
   a. Provide nursing support for the confused, combative, or ventilator-dependent client.
   b. Maintain immobilization of the neck if a spinal fracture is suspected.
   c. Remove metal items from body parts.
   d. If the client has thick and heavy hair, this should be documented because it could affect interpretation of the x-ray film.
3. Postprocedure intervention: Maintain immobilization until results are known.

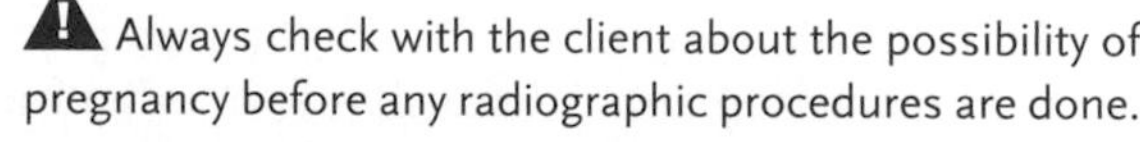

Always check with the client about the possibility of pregnancy before any radiographic procedures are done.

B. Computed tomography (CT) scan of the brain
1. Description
   a. CT is a type of brain scanning that may or may not require injection of a dye.

b. It is used to detect intracranial bleeding, space-occupying lesions, cerebral edema, infarctions, hydrocephalus, cerebral atrophy, and shifts of brain structures.

2. Preprocedure interventions
   a. Ensure an informed consent is obtained if a contrast dye is used.
   b. Check for allergies to iodine, contrast dyes, or shellfish if a dye is used.
   c. Reinforce instructions to the client on the need to lie still and flat during the test.
   d. Reinforce instructions to the client to hold his or her breath when requested.
   e. Assist to initiate an IV line if prescribed.
   f. Remove objects from the head, such as wigs, barrettes, earrings, and hairpins.
   g. Check for claustrophobia.
   h. The client is informed of possible mechanical noises as the scanning occurs.
   i. Inform the client that there may be a hot, flushed sensation and a metallic taste in the mouth when the dye is injected.
   j. Note that some clients may be given the dye even if they report an allergy; they are treated with an antihistamine and corticosteroids before the injection to reduce the severity of a reaction.

Determine the need to withhold metformin (Glucophage) if iodinated contrast dye is used for a diagnostic procedure because of the risk for metformin-induced lactic acidosis.

3. Postprocedure interventions
   a. Provide replacement fluids because diuresis from the dye is expected.
   b. Monitor for an allergic reaction to the dye.
   c. Check dye injection site for bleeding or hematoma, and monitor the extremity for color, warmth, and the presence of distal pulses.

C. Magnetic resonance imaging (MRI)
1. Description
   a. MRI is a noninvasive procedure that identifies types of tissues, tumors, and vascular abnormalities.
   b. It is similar to the CT scan but provides more detailed pictures.
2. Preprocedure interventions
   a. Remove all metal objects from the client.
   b. Determine whether the client has a pacemaker, implanted defibrillator, or other metal implants such as a hip prosthesis or vascular clips because these clients cannot have this test performed.
   c. An intermittent infusion device (saline lock) is attached to all intravenous accesses prior to the procedure (intravenous fluid pumps are not allowed in the MRI room).
   d. Provide precautions for the client who is attached to a pulse oximeter because it can cause a burn during testing if coiled around the body or a body part.
   e. Determine if the client has claustrophobia (unless an open MRI machine is used).
   f. Inform the client of possible mechanical noises as the scanning occurs.
   g. Administer medication as prescribed for the client with claustrophobia.
   h. Determine whether a contrast agent is to be used, and follow the prescription related to the administration of food, fluids, and medications.
   i. Reinforce instructions to the client that he or she will need to remain still during the procedure.

An MRI is contraindicated in a pregnant woman because the increase in amniotic fluid temperature that occurs during the procedure may be harmful to the fetus.

3. Postprocedure interventions
   a. Client may resume normal activities.
   b. Expect diuresis if a contrast agent was used.

D. Lumbar puncture
1. Description
   a. Insert a spinal needle through the L3-L4 interspace into the lumbar subarachnoid space to obtain cerebrospinal fluid (CSF), measure CSF fluid or pressure, or instill air, dye, or medications.
   b. The test is contraindicated in clients with **increased intracranial pressure (ICP)** because the procedure will cause a rapid decrease in pressure within the CSF around the spinal cord, leading to brain herniation.
2. Preprocedure interventions
   a. Ensure that an informed consent has been obtained.
   b. Have the client empty the bladder.
3. Interventions during the procedure
   a. Position the client in a lateral recumbent position, and have the client draw the knees up to the abdomen and the chin onto the chest. (The prone position may be required for radiologically guided punctures.) 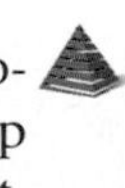
   b. Assist with the collection of specimens. (Label the specimens in sequence.)
   c. Maintain strict asepsis.
4. Postprocedure interventions
   a. Monitor vital signs and neurological signs to check for the presence of leakage of cerebrospinal fluid and also monitor for a headache.
   b. Position the client flat as prescribed. 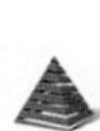

c. Encourage fluids to replace CSF obtained from the specimen collection or from leakage.
d. Monitor intake and output (I&O).

E. Cerebral angiography
1. Description: Injection of a contrast material usually through the femoral artery (or another artery) into the carotid arteries to visualize the cerebral arteries and assess for lesions
2. Preprocedure interventions
a. Ensure that an informed consent has been obtained.
b. Check the client for allergies to iodine and shellfish.
c. Encourage hydration for 2 days before the test.
d. Maintain the client on NPO status 4 to 6 hours before the test as prescribed.
e. A neurological assessment is obtained, which will serve as a baseline for postprocedure assessments.
f. Mark the peripheral pulses.
g. Remove metal items from the hair.
h. Assist to administer premedication as prescribed.
3. Postprocedure interventions
a. Monitor neurological status, vital signs, and neurovascular status of the affected extremity frequently until stable.
b. Monitor for swelling in the neck and for difficulty swallowing, and notify the health care provider (HCP) if these symptoms occur.
c. Maintain bed rest for 12 hours as prescribed.
d. Elevate the head of the bed 15 to 30 degrees only if prescribed.
e. The head of the bed may be kept flat if the femoral artery is used; always follow the health care provider's prescriptions for positioning.
f. Check peripheral pulses.
g. Apply sandbags or another device to immobilize the limb and a pressure dressing to the injection site to decrease bleeding, as prescribed.
h. Place ice on the puncture site, if prescribed.
i. Encourage fluid intake.

F. Electroencephalography
1. Description: A graphic recording of the electrical activity of the superficial layers of the cerebral cortex
2. Preprocedure interventions
a. Wash the client's hair.
b. Inform the client that electrodes are attached to the head and that electricity does not enter the head.
c. Withhold stimulants, such as coffee, tea, and caffeine beverages; antidepressants; tranquilizers; and possibly anticonvulsants for 24 to 48 hours before the test as prescribed.
d. Allow the client to have breakfast if prescribed.
e. Assist to premedicate for sedation, as prescribed.
3. Postprocedure interventions
a. Wash the client's hair.
b. Maintain side rails (per agency policy) and safety precautions if the client was sedated.

G. Caloric testing (oculovestibular reflex)
1. Description: Caloric testing provides information about the function of the vestibular portion of the eighth cranial nerve and aids in the diagnosis of cerebellar and brainstem lesions.
2. Procedure
a. Patency of the external auditory canal is confirmed.
b. The client is positioned supine with the head of the bed elevated 30 degrees.
c. Water that is warmer or cooler than body temperature is infused into the ear.
d. A normal response is the onset of vertigo and nystagmus (involuntary eye movements) within 20 to 30 seconds.
e. Absent or dysconjugate eye movements indicate brainstem damage.

III. Neurological Data Collection (refer to Chapter 23 for information)

A. Risk factors
1. Trauma
2. Hemorrhage
3. Tumors
4. Infection
5. Toxicity
6. Metabolic disorders
7. Hypoxic conditions
8. Hypertension
9. Stress
10. Cigarette smoking
11. Aging process
12. Chemicals, either ingestion or environmental exposure

Level of consciousness is the most sensitive indicator of neurological status.

B. Vital signs: Monitor for blood pressure or pulse changes, which may indicate increased Intracranial pressure (ICP) (rise in blood pressure with widening pulse pressure, slowing of the pulse, elevated temperature, abnormal respirations).

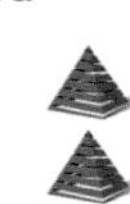

C. Respirations (Box 57-2)
D. Temperature
1. An elevated temperature increases the metabolic rate of the brain.
2. An elevation in temperature may indicate a dysfunction of the hypothalamus or brainstem.
3. A slow rise in temperature may indicate infection.

BOX 57-2 Data Collection: Respirations

Cheyne-Stokes
Rhythmic with periods of apnea
Can indicate a metabolic dysfunction or dysfunction in the cerebral hemisphere or basal ganglia

Neurogenic Hyperventilation
Regular rapid and deep sustained respirations
Indicates a dysfunction in the low midbrain and middle pons

Apneustic
Irregular respirations with pauses at the end of inspiration and expiration
Indicates a dysfunction in the middle or caudal pons

Ataxic
Totally irregular in rhythm and depth
Indicates a dysfunction in the medulla

Cluster
Clusters of breaths with irregularly spaced pauses
Indicates a dysfunction in the medulla and pons

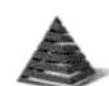

E. Pupils (Fig. 57-1)
1. Unilateral pupil dilation indicates compression of the third cranial nerve.
2. Midposition fixed pupil indicates midbrain injury.
3. Pinpoint fixed pupil indicates pontine damage.
4. See Figure 23-1 for checking extraocular eye movements.

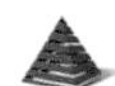

F. Motor function
1. Check muscle tone, including strength and equality.
2. Check for voluntary and involuntary movements and purposeful and nonpurposeful movements.

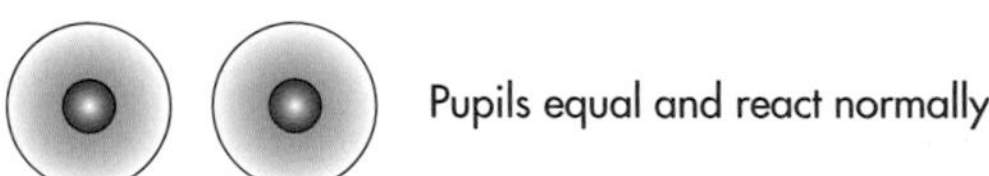

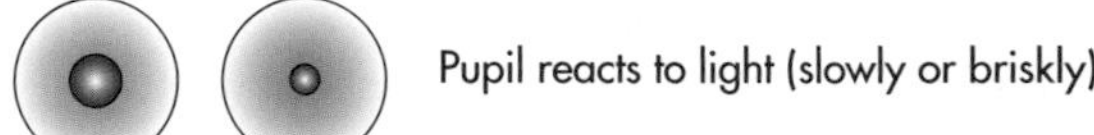
Pupil reacts to light (slowly or briskly)

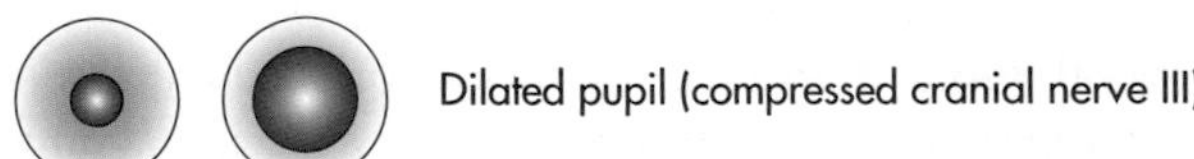
Dilated pupil (compressed cranial nerve III)

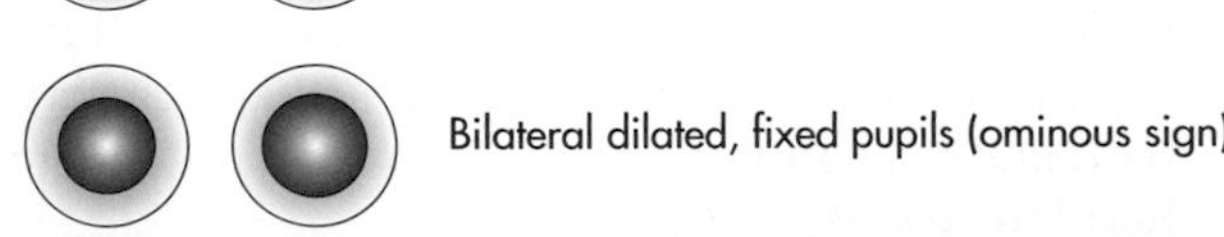

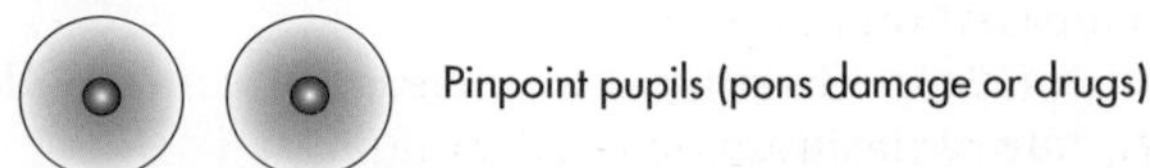

FIGURE 57-1 Pupillary check for size and response. (From Lewis S, Heitkemper M, Dirksen S, O'Brien P, Bucher L: *Medical-surgical nursing: Assessment and management of clinical problems*, ed 7, St. Louis, 2007, Mosby.)

G. Posturing (see Fig. 37-1)
1. Posturing indicates a deterioration of the condition.
2. Flexor (**decorticate posturing**)
   a. The client flexes one or both arms on the chest and may extend the legs stiffly.
   b. Flexor posturing indicates a nonfunctioning cortex.
3. Extensor (decerebrate posturing)
   a. The client stiffly extends one or both arms and possibly the legs.
   b. Extensor posturing indicates a brainstem lesion.
4. **Flaccid posturing**: The client displays no motor response in any extremity.

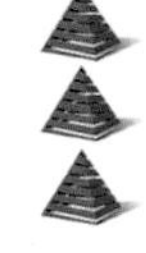

H. Reflexes (Box 57-3)

I. Meningeal irritation (Box 57-4)

J. Autonomic system
1. Sympathetic functions/adrenergic responses
   a. Increased pulse and blood pressure
   b. Dilated pupils
   c. Decreased peristalsis
   d. Increased perspiration
2. Parasympathetic function/cholinergic responses
   a. Decreased pulse and blood pressure
   b. Constricted pupils
   c. Increased salivation
   d. Increased peristalsis
   e. Dilated blood vessels
   f. Bladder contraction

K. Sensory function: touch, pressure, pain

L. **Glasgow Coma Scale** (Box 57-5)
1. The scale is a method of assessing a client's neurological condition.
2. The scoring system is based on a scale of 1 to 15 points.
3. A score lower than 8 indicates that coma is present.

BOX 57-3 Data Collection: Reflexes

Babinski's Reflex
- Dorsiflexion of the big toe, and fanning of the other toes; elicited by firmly stroking the lateral aspect of the sole of the foot
- Is a pathologic or abnormal reflex in anyone older than 2 years and represents the presence of central nervous system (CNS) disease

Corneal Reflex
- Involuntary closure of the eyelids in response to stimulation of the cornea
- Loss of the blink reflex indicates a dysfunction of cranial nerve V

Gag Reflex
- Contraction of pharyngeal muscle, elicited by touching the back of the throat
- Loss of the gag reflex indicates a dysfunction of cranial nerves IX and X

BOX 57-4 Data Collection: Meningeal Irritation

General Findings

Irritability
Nuchal rigidity
Severe, unrelenting headaches
Generalized muscle aches and pains
Nausea and vomiting
Fever and chills
Tachycardia
Photophobia
Nystagmus
Abnormal pupil reaction and eye movement

Brudzinski's Sign

Involuntary flexion of the hip and knee when the neck is passively flexed; indicates meningeal irritation

Kernig's Sign

Loss of the ability of a supine client to straighten the leg completely when it is fully flexed at the knee and hip; indicates meningeal irritation

Motor Response

Hemiparesis, hemiplegia, and decreased muscle tone
Cranial nerve dysfunction, especially cranial nerves III, IV, VI, VII, and VIII

Memory Changes

Short attention span
Personality and behavioral changes

BOX 57-5 Glasgow Coma Scale

Score

- The lowest possible score is 3 points (deep coma or death).
- The highest possible score is 15 points (fully awake).

Motor Response Points

Obeys a simple response = 6
Localizes painful stimuli = 5
Normal flexion (withdrawal) = 4
Abnormal flexion (decorticate posturing) = 3
Extensor response (decerebrate posturing) = 2
No motor response to pain = 1

Verbal Response Points

Oriented = 5
Confused conversation = 4
Inappropriate words = 3
Responds with incomprehensible sounds = 2
No verbal response = 1

Eye-Opening Points

Spontaneous = 4
In response to sound = 3
In response to pain = 2
No response even to painful stimuli = 1

Adapted from Ignatavicius D, Workman M: *Medical-surgical nursing: Patient-centered collaborative care*, ed 6, St. Louis, 2010, Saunders.

IV. The Unconscious Client

A. Description
1. The **unconscious client** is in a state of depressed cerebral functioning with unresponsiveness to stimulation of sensory and motor function.

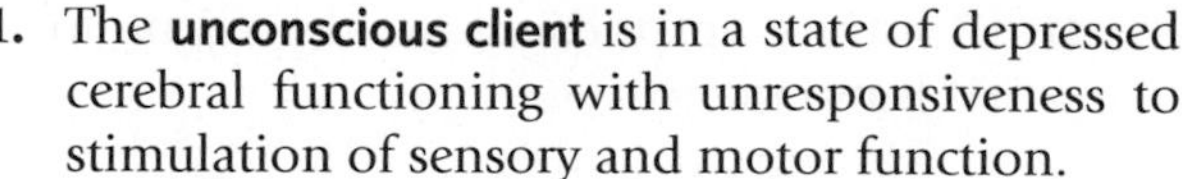

2. Some of the causes include head trauma, cerebral toxins, shock, hemorrhage, tumor, and infection.

B. Data collection
1. Unarousable
2. Primitive or no response to painful stimuli
3. Altered respirations
4. Decreased cranial nerve and reflex activity

C. Interventions (Box 57-6)

V. Increased Intracranial Pressure (ICP)

A. Description
1. Increased ICP may be caused by trauma, hemorrhage, growths or tumors, hydrocephalus, edema, or inflammation.
2. Increased ICP can impede circulation to the brain, hinder the absorption of CSF, affect the functioning of nerve cells, and lead to brainstem compression and death.

B. Data collection
1. Altered level of consciousness (LOC), which is the most sensitive and earliest indication of increasing ICP

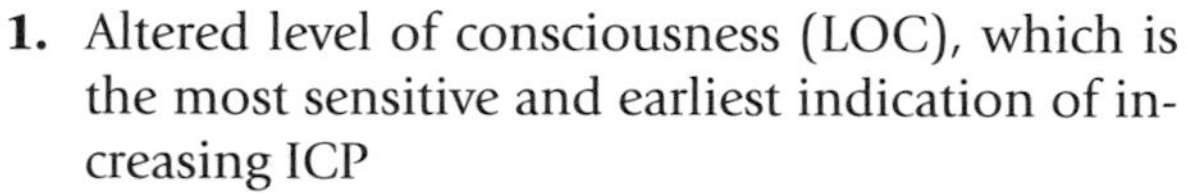

2. Headache

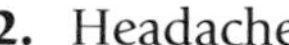

3. Abnormal respirations (see Box 57-2)
4. Rise in blood pressure with widening pulse pressure
5. Slowing of pulse
6. Elevated temperature
7. Vomiting
8. Pupil changes
9. Late signs of increased ICP, including increased systolic blood pressure, widened pulse pressure, and slowed heart rate

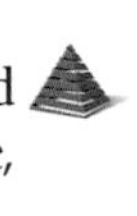

10. Other late signs include changes in motor function from weakness to hemiplegia, a positive **Babinski's reflex**, decorticate or **decerebrate posturing**, and seizures.

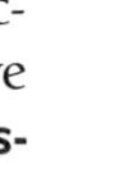

C. Interventions
1. Monitor respiratory status and prevent hypoxia.
2. The administration of morphine sulfate is avoided to prevent the occurrence of hypoxia.
3. Mechanical ventilation is maintained as prescribed; maintaining the $PaCO_2$ at 30 to 35 mm Hg will result in vasoconstriction of the cerebral blood vessels, decreased blood flow, and therefore decreased ICP.
4. Maintain body temperature.
5. Prevent shivering, which can increase ICP.
6. Decrease environmental stimuli.
7. Monitor electrolyte levels and acid–base balance.
8. Monitor intake and output.
9. Limit fluid intake to 1200 mL/day as prescribed.

10. Reinforce instructions to the client to avoid straining activities, such as coughing and sneezing.
11. Reinforce instructions to the client to avoid Valsalva maneuver.

For the client with increased intracranial pressure, the head of the bed is elevated 30 to 40 degrees, the Trendelenburg's position is avoided, and flexion of the neck and hips is prevented.

D. Medications (Box 57-7)
E. Surgical intervention: See Chapter 37 for additional information on ventriculoperitoneal shunt.

VI. Hyperthermia

A. Description
1. A temperature greater than 105°F, which increases the cerebral metabolism and increases the risk of hypoxia

BOX 57-6 Care of the Unconscious Client

Monitor patency of the airway and keep an airway and emergency equipment at the bedside.
Monitor blood pressure, pulse, and heart sounds.
Monitor respiratory and circulatory status.
Maintain a patent airway and ventilation because a high CO_2 level increases intracranial pressure.
Check lung sounds for the accumulation of secretions; suction fluids from the airway as needed.
Monitor neurological status, including level of consciousness, pupillary reactions, and motor and sensory function, using a coma scale.
Place the client in a semi-Fowler's position (avoid Trendelenburg's position).
Change position of the client every 2 hours, avoiding injury when turning.
Use side rails unless contraindicated or according to agency protocol.
Monitor intake and output and daily weight, monitoring for edema and dehydration.
Maintain NPO status until consciousness returns.
Maintain nutrition as prescribed, and monitor fluid and electrolyte balance.
Check the gag and swallow reflex before resuming a diet, and begin the diet with ice chips and fluids when the client becomes alert.
Assist to provide intravenous or enteral feedings as prescribed.
Check bowel sounds.
Monitor elimination patterns.
Monitor for constipation, impaction, and paralytic ileus.
Maintain urinary output to prevent stasis, infection, and calculus formation.
Monitor the status of skin integrity.
Initiate measures to prevent skin breakdown.
Provide frequent mouth care.
Remove dentures and contact lenses.
Check the eyes for the presence of a corneal reflex and irritation, and instill artificial tears or cover the eyes with eye patches.
Monitor drainage from the ears or nose for the presence of cerebrospinal fluid.
Assume that the unconscious client can hear.
Avoid restraints (security devices).
Do not leave the client unattended if unstable.
Initiate seizure precautions if necessary.
Provide range-of-motion exercises to prevent contractures.
Use a footboard or high-top sneakers to prevent foot drop.
Use splints to prevent wrist deformities.
Initiate physical therapy as appropriate.

BOX 57-7 Medications for Intracranial Pressure

Anticonvulsants

Seizures increase metabolic requirements and cerebral blood flow and volume, thus increasing intracranial pressure.
Anticonvulsants may be given prophylactically to prevent seizures.

Antipyretics and Muscle Relaxants

Temperature reduction decreases metabolism, cerebral blood flow, and thus intracranial pressure.
Antipyretics prevent temperature elevations.
Muscle relaxants prevent shivering.

Blood Pressure Medication

Blood pressure medication may be required to maintain cerebral perfusion at a normal level.
Notify the HCP if the blood pressure range is less than 100 or greater than 150 mm Hg systolic.

Corticosteroids

Corticosteroids stabilize the cell membrane and reduce the leakiness in the blood–brain barrier.
Corticosteroids decrease cerebral edema.
A histamine blocker may be administered to counteract the excess gastric secretion that occurs with the corticosteroid.
Clients must be withdrawn slowly from corticosteroid therapy to reduce the risk of adrenal crisis.

Intravenous Fluids

Fluids are administered intravenously via an infusion pump to control the amount administered.
Hypertonic intravenous solutions are usually avoided because of the risk of promoting additional cerebral edema.

Hyperosmotic Agent

A hyperosmotic agent increases intravascular pressure by drawing fluid from the interstitial spaces and from the brain cells.
Monitor kidney function.
Diuresis is expected.

2. The causes include infection, heatstroke, exposure to high environmental temperatures, and dysfunction of the thermoregulatory center.

B. Data collection
1. Temperature greater than 105 °F
2. Shivering
3. Nausea and vomiting

C. Interventions
1. Maintain a patent airway.
2. Initiate seizure precautions.
3. Monitor intake and output (I&O), and monitor the skin and mucous membranes for signs of dehydration.
4. Monitor lung sounds.
5. Monitor for dysrhythmias.
6. Check peripheral pulses for systemic blood flow.
7. Induce normothermia with fluids, cool baths, fans, or a hypothermia blanket.

D. Induction of normothermia
1. Prevent shivering, which will increase ICP and oxygen consumption.
2. Assist to administer medications as prescribed to prevent shivering and to lower body temperature.
3. Monitor neurological status.
4. Monitor for infection and respiratory complications because hypothermia may mask the signs of infection.
5. Monitor for cardiac dysrhythmias.
6. Monitor I&O.
7. Prevent trauma to the skin and tissues.
8. Apply lotion to the skin frequently.
9. Inspect for frostbite if a hypothermia blanket is used.

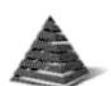

VII. Traumatic Head Injury

A. Description
1. Head injury is trauma to the scalp, skull, or brain, resulting in mild to extensive damage to the brain.
2. Immediate complications include cerebral bleeding, hematomas, increased ICP, infections, and seizures.
3. Changes in personality or behavior, cranial nerve deficits, and any other residual deficits depend on the area of the brain damage and the extent of the damage.

B. Types of head injuries (Box 57-8)
1. Open
a. Scalp lacerations
b. Fractures in the skull
c. Interruption of the dura mater
2. Closed
a. Concussions
b. Contusions
c. Fractures

C. Hematoma
1. Description: Hematoma is a collection of blood in the tissues and can occur as a result of a subarachnoid hemorrhage, subdural hemorrhage, or intracerebral hemorrhage.

BOX 57-8 Types of Head Injuries

Concussion

Concussion is a jarring of the brain within the skull with temporary loss of consciousness.

Contusion

Contusion is a bruising type of injury to the brain tissue.
Contusion may occur along with other neurological injuries, such as with subdural or extradural collections of blood.

Skull Fractures

Linear
Depressed
Compound
Comminuted

Epidural Hematoma

As the most serious type of hematoma, epidural hematoma forms rapidly and results from arterial bleeding.
Epidural hematoma forms between the dura and the skull from a tear in the meningeal artery.
Often associated with temporary loss of consciousness, followed by a lucid period, that rapidly progresses to coma.
Epidural hematoma is a surgical emergency.

Subdural Hematoma

Subdural hematoma forms slowly and results from a venous bleed.
Subdural hematoma occurs under the dura as a result of tears in the veins crossing the subdural space.

Intracerebral Hemorrhage

Intracerebral hemorrhage occurs when a blood vessel within the brain ruptures allowing blood to leak inside the brain.

Subarachnoid Hemorrhage

A subarachnoid hemorrhage is bleeding into the subarachnoid space. It may occur as a result of head trauma or spontaneously, such as from a ruptured cerebral aneurysm.

2. Data collection 
a. Findings depend on the injury.
b. Clinical manifestations usually result from increased ICP.
c. Changing neurological signs in the client
d. Changes in LOC
e. Airway and breathing pattern changes
f. Vital signs changes reflecting increasing ICP
g. Headache, nausea, and vomiting
h. Visual disturbances, pupillary changes, and papilledema
i. **Nuchal rigidity** (not tested until spinal cord injury is ruled out)
j. CSF drainage from the ears or nose
k. Weakness and paralysis
l. Posturing
m. Decreased sensation or absence of feeling
n. Reflex activity changes
o. Seizure activity

CSF can be distinguished from other fluids by the presence of concentric rings (bloody fluid surrounded by a yellow stain) when the fluid is placed on a white sterile background, such as a gauze pad. CSF also tests positive for glucose when tested using a strip test.

3. Interventions
   a. Monitor respiratory status and maintain a patent airway because increased CO_2 levels increase cerebral edema.
   b. Monitor neurological status and vital signs, including temperature.
   c. Monitor for increased ICP.
   d. Maintain head elevation to reduce venous pressure.
   e. Protect the cervical spine, maintain a neutral head position, and prevent neck flexion.
   f. Initiate normothermia measures for increased temperature, and prevent shivering.
   g. Check cranial nerve function, reflexes, and motor and sensory function.
   h. Initiate seizure precautions.
   i. Monitor for pain and restlessness.
   j. Morphine sulfate may be prescribed to decrease agitation and control restlessness caused by pain for the head-injured client on a ventilator; it is administer with caution because it is a respiratory depressant and may increase ICP.
   k. Monitor for drainage from the nose or ears because this fluid may be CSF; notify the registered nurse immediately if this is noted.
   l. Do not attempt to clean the nose, suction, or allow the client to blow his or her nose if drainage occurs.
   m. Do not clean the ear if drainage is noted, but apply a loose, dry sterile dressing.
   n. Reinforce instructions to the client to avoid coughing because this increases ICP.
   o. Prevent complications of immobility.
   p. The client and family are informed about the possible behavior changes that may occur, including those that are expected and those that need to be reported.

D. Craniotomy
1. Description
   a. A surgical procedure that involves an incision through the cranium to remove accumulated blood or a tumor
   b. Complications of the procedure include increased ICP from cerebral edema, hemorrhage, or obstruction of normal flow of CSF.
   c. Additional complications include hematomas, hypovolemic shock, hydrocephalus, respiratory and neurogenic complications, pulmonary edema, and wound infections.
   d. Complications related to fluid and electrolyte imbalances include diabetes insipidus and inappropriate secretion of antidiuretic hormone. 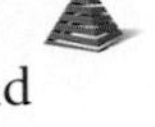
   e. Stereotactic radiosurgery (SRS) may be an alternative to traditional surgery and is usually used to treat tumors and arteriovenous malformations.
2. Preoperative interventions
   a. Explain the procedure to the client and family.
   b. Ensure that an informed consent has been obtained.
   c. Prepare to shave the client's head as prescribed (usually done in the operating room) and cover the head with appropriate covering.
   d. Stabilize the client before surgery.
3. Postoperative interventions (Box 57-9)
4. Postoperative positioning (Box 57-10)

BOX 57-9 Nursing Care After Craniotomy

Monitor vital signs and neurological status every 30 to 60 minutes.
Monitor for increased intracranial pressure.
Monitor for decreased level of consciousness, motor weakness or paralysis, aphasia, visual changes, and personality changes.
Mechanical ventilation and slight hyperventilation is maintained for the first 24 to 48 hours as prescribed to prevent increased intracranial pressure.
Check the HCP's prescriptions regarding client positioning.
Avoid extreme hip or neck flexion, and maintain the head in a midline neutral position.
Provide a quiet environment.
Monitor the head dressing frequently for signs of drainage.
Mark any area of drainage on the dressing at least once each nursing shift for baseline comparison.
Monitor any drains, which may be in place for 24 hours.
Maintain suction on the drain as appropriate; measure drainage every 8 hours, and record the amount and color.
The HCP is notified if drainage is greater than the normal of 30 to 50 mL per shift.
The HCP is notified immediately of excessive amounts of drainage or a saturated head dressing.
Provide basic hygiene.
Record strict measurement of hourly intake and output.
Maintain fluid restriction at 1500 mL/day as prescribed.
Monitor electrolyte values.
Monitor for dysrhythmias, which may occur as a result of fluid and electrolyte imbalance.
Apply ice packs or cool compresses as prescribed. Expect periorbital edema and ecchymosis of one or both eyes, which is not an unusual occurrence.
Provide range-of-motion exercises every 8 hours.
Assist to administer anticonvulsants, antacids, corticosteroids, and antibiotics as prescribed.
Assist to administer analgesics such as codeine sulfate and acetaminophen (Tylenol) as prescribed for pain.

BOX 57-10 Client Positioning After Craniotomy

Positions prescribed after craniotomy vary with the type of surgery and the specific postoperative HCP's prescriptions.
Always check the HCP's prescriptions regarding client positioning.
Incorrect positioning may cause serious and possibly fatal complications.

Removal of a Bone Flap for Decompression

To facilitate brain expansion, the client should be turned from the back to the nonoperative side but not to the side where the operation was performed.

Posterior Fossa Surgery

To protect the operative site from pressure and to minimize tension on the suture line, position the client on the side, with a pillow under the head for support, and not on the back.

Infratentorial Surgery

Infratentorial surgery involves surgery below the tentorium of the brain.
The HCP may prescribe a flat position without head elevation or may prescribe the head of the bed to be elevated at 30 to 45 degrees.
Do not elevate the head of the bed in the acute phase of care after surgery without a HCP's prescription.

Supratentorial Surgery

Supratentorial surgery involves surgery above the tentorium of the brain.
The HCP may prescribe the head of the bed to be elevated at 30 degrees to promote venous outflow through the jugular veins.
Do not lower the head of the bed in the acute phase of care after surgery without a HCP's prescription.

VIII. Spinal Cord Injury

A. Description
1. Trauma to the spinal cord causes partial or complete disruption of the nerve tracts and neurons.
2. The injury can involve contusion, laceration, or compression of the cord.
3. Spinal cord edema develops, and necrosis of the spinal cord can develop as a result of compromised capillary circulation and venous return.
4. Loss of motor function, sensation, reflex activity, and bowel and bladder control may result.
5. The most common causes include motor vehicle accidents, falls, sporting and industrial accidents, and gunshot or stab wounds.

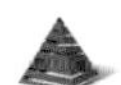

6. Complications related to the injury include respiratory failure, **autonomic dysreflexia**, spinal shock, further cord damage, and death.

B. Most frequently involved vertebrae
1. Cervical: C5, C6, and C7
2. Thoracic: T12
3. Lumbar: L1

C. Transection of the cord
1. Complete transection of the cord. The spinal cord is severed completely, with total loss of sensation, movement, and reflex activity below the level of injury.
2. Partial transection of the cord
   a. The spinal cord is damaged or severed partially.
   b. The symptoms depend on the extent and location of the damage.
   c. If the cord has not suffered irreparable damage, early treatment is needed to prevent partial damage from developing into total and permanent damage.

D. Types of injuries (Fig. 57-2)
1. Central cord syndrome
   a. Central cord syndrome occurs from a lesion in the central portion of the spinal cord.
   b. Loss of motor function is more pronounced in the upper extremities, and varying degrees and patterns of sensation remain intact.
2. Anterior cord syndrome
   a. Anterior cord syndrome is caused by damage to the anterior portion of the gray and white matter of the spinal cord.
   b. Motor function, pain, and temperature sensation are lost below the level of injury; however, the sensations of position, vibration, and touch remain intact.
3. Posterior cord syndrome
   a. Posterior cord syndrome is caused by damage to the posterior portion of the gray and white matter of the spinal cord.
   b. Motor function remains intact, but the client experiences a loss of vibratory sense, crude touch, and position sensation.
4. Brown-Séquard's syndrome
   a. Brown-Séquard's syndrome results from penetrating injuries that cause hemisection of the spinal cord or injuries that affect half of the cord.
   b. Motor function, vibration, proprioception, and deep touch sensations are lost on the same side of the body (ipsilateral) as the lesion or cord damage.
   c. On the opposite side of the body (contralateral) from the lesion or cord damage, the sensations of pain, temperature, and light touch are affected.
5. Conus medullaris syndrome
   a. Conus medullaris syndrome follows damage to the lumbar nerve roots and conus medullaris in the spinal cord.
   b. Client experiences bowel and bladder areflexia and flaccid lower extremities.

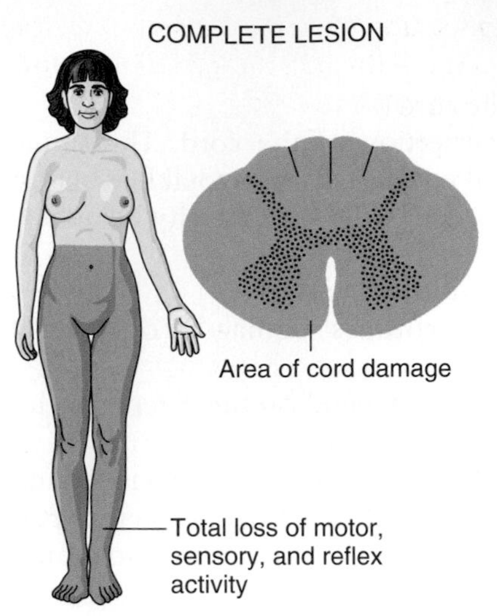

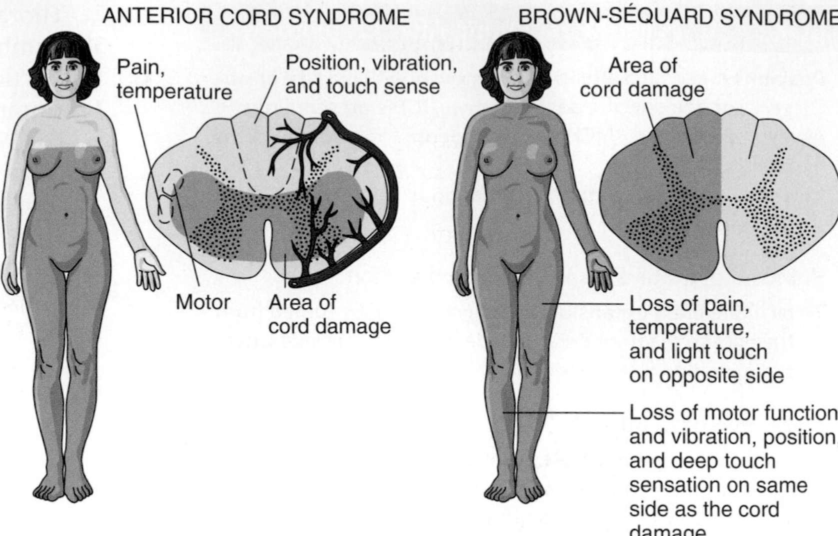

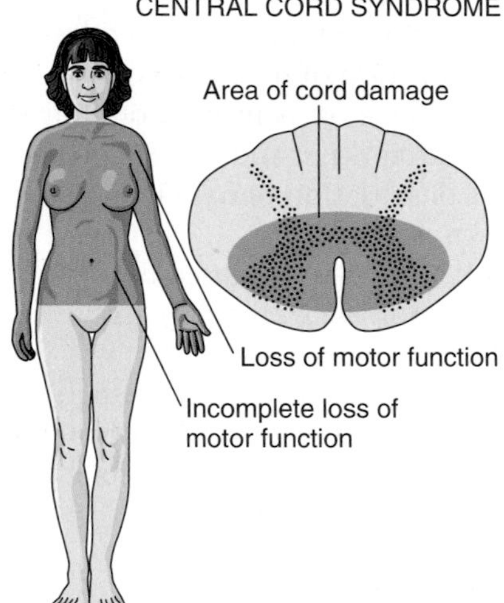

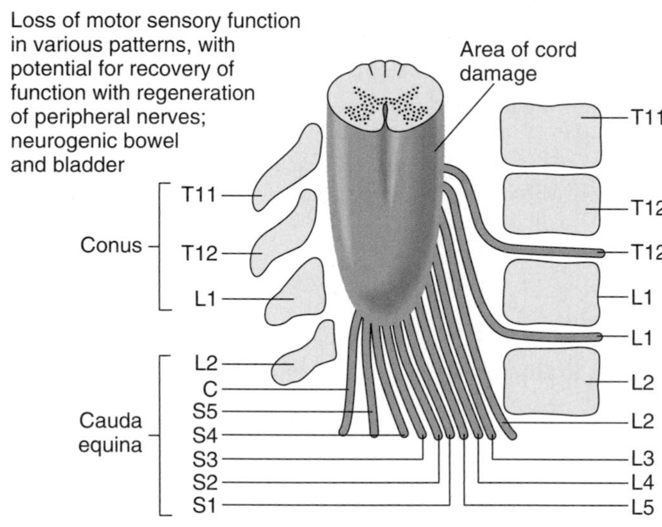

FIGURE 57-2 Common spinal cord syndromes. (From Ignatavicius D, Workman ML: *Medical-surgical nursing: Patient-centered collaborative care*, ed 6, Philadelphia, 2010, Saunders.)

c. If damage is limited to the upper sacral segments of the spinal cord, bulbospongiosus penile (erection) and micturition reflexes will remain.

6. Cauda equina syndrome
   a. Cauda equina syndrome occurs from injury to the lumbosacral nerve roots below the conus medullaris.
   b. The client experiences areflexia of the bowel, bladder, and lower reflexes.

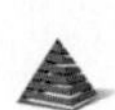

E. Data collection: Spinal cord injuries (Box 57-11)
1. Dependent on the level of the cord injury
2. Level of the spinal cord injury: The lowest spinal cord segment with intact motor and sensory function
3. Respiratory status changes
4. Motor and sensory changes below the level of injury
5. Total sensory loss and motor paralysis below the level of injury
6. Loss of reflexes below the level of injury
7. Loss of bladder and bowel control
8. Urinary retention and bladder distention
9. Presence of sweat, which does not occur on paralyzed areas

BOX 57-11 Effects of Spinal Cord Injury

Tetraplegia (Quadriplegia)

Injury occurring between C1 and C8
Paralysis involving all four extremities

Paraplegia

Injury occurring between T1 and L4
Paralysis involving only the lower extremities

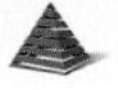

F. Cervical injuries
   1. Injury at C2 to C3 is usually fatal.
   2. C4 is the major innervation to the diaphragm by the phrenic nerve.
   3. Involvement above C4 causes respiratory difficulty and paralysis of all four extremities.
   4. Client may have movement in the shoulder if the injury is at C5 through C8, and may also have decreased respiratory reserve.

G. Thoracic-level injuries
   1. Loss of movement of the chest, trunk, bowel, bladder, and legs may occur, depending on the level of injury.
   2. Leg paralysis (paraplegia) may occur.
   3. Autonomic dysreflexia with lesions or injuries above T6 and in cervical lesions may occur.
   4. Visceral distention from a noxious stimulus such as a distended bladder or impacted rectum may cause reactions such as sweating, bradycardia, hypertension, nasal stuffiness, and goose flesh.

H. Lumbar and sacral level injuries
   1. Loss of movement and sensation of the lower extremities may occur.
   2. S2 and S3 center on micturition; therefore, below this level, the bladder will contract but not empty (neurogenic bladder).
   3. Injury above S2 in males allows them to have an erection, but they are unable to ejaculate because of sympathetic nerve damage.
   4. Injury between S2 and S4 damages the sympathetic and parasympathetic response, preventing erection or ejaculation.

Always suspect spinal cord injury when trauma occurs until this injury is ruled out. Immobilize the client on a spinal backboard with the head in a neutral position to prevent an incomplete injury from becoming complete.

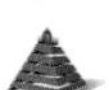

I. Emergency interventions
   1. Emergency management is critical because improper movement can cause further damage and loss of neurological function.
   2. Monitor the respiratory pattern and maintain a patent airway.
   3. Prevent head flexion, rotation, or extension.
   4. During immobilization, maintain traction and alignment on the head by placing hands on either side of the head by the ears.
   5. Maintain an extended position.
   6. Logroll the client.
   7. No part of the body should be twisted or turned, and the client is not allowed to assume a sitting position.
   8. In the emergency department, a client who has sustained a severe cervical fracture should be placed immediately in skeletal traction via skull tongs or halo traction to immobilize the cervical spine and to reduce the fracture and dislocation.

J. Interventions during hospitalization
   1. Respiratory system
      a. Monitor respiratory status because paralysis of the intercostal and abdominal muscles occurs with C4 injuries.
      b. Monitor arterial blood gases and maintain mechanical ventilation if prescribed to prevent respiratory arrest, especially with cervical injuries.
      c. Encourage deep breathing and the use of an incentive spirometer.
      d. Monitor for signs of infection, particularly pneumonia.
   2. Cardiovascular system
      a. Monitor for cardiac dysrhythmias.
      b. Monitor for signs of hemorrhage or bleeding around the fracture site.
      c. Monitor for signs of shock, such as hypotension, tachycardia, and a weak and thready pulse.
      d. Monitor the lower extremities for deep vein thrombosis.
      e. Measure circumferences of the calf and thigh to identify increases in size.
      f. Use sequential compression devices (SCDs) as prescribed.
      g. Remove SCDs daily or as prescribed and check the skin integrity.
      h. Monitor for orthostatic hypotension when repositioning the client.
   3. Neuromuscular system
      a. Monitor neurological status.
      b. Monitor motor and sensory status to determine the level of injury.
      c. Monitor motor ability by testing the client's ability to squeeze hands, spread the fingers, move the toes, and turn the feet.
      d. Check for the absence of sensation, hyposensation, or hypersensation by pinching the skin or pricking it with a pin, starting at the shoulders and working down the extremities.
      e. Monitor for signs of autonomic dysreflexia and spinal shock.
      f. Immobilize the client to promote healing and prevent further injury.
      g. Monitor pain.
      h. Initiate measures to reduce pain.
      i. Assist to administer analgesics as prescribed.
      j. Monitor for complications of immobility.
      k. Prepare the client for decompression laminectomy, spinal fusion, or insertion of instrumentation or rods if prescribed.
      l. Collaborate with the physical therapist and occupational therapist to determine appropriate exercise techniques, check the need for

hand and wrist splints, and develop an appropriate plan to prevent footdrop.

4. Gastrointestinal system
   a. Check abdomen for distention and hemorrhage.
   b. Monitor bowel sounds and assess for paralytic ileus.
   c. Prevent bowel retention.
   d. Initiate a bowel control program as appropriate.
   e. Maintain adequate nutrition and a high-fiber diet.
5. Renal system
   a. Prevent urinary retention.
   b. Initiate a bladder control program as appropriate.
   c. Maintain fluid and electrolyte balance.
   d. Maintain adequate fluid intake of 2000 mL/day.
   e. Monitor for urinary tract infection and calculi.
6. Integumentary system
   a. Check skin integrity.
   b. Turn the client every 2 hours.
7. Psychosocial integrity
   a. Monitor psychosocial status.
   b. Encourage the client to express feelings of anger and depression.
   c. Discuss the sexual concerns of the client.
   d. Promote rehabilitation with self-care, setting realistic goals based on the client's potential functional level.
   e. Encourage contact with appropriate community resources.

K. Spinal shock and neurogenic shock
1. Description
   a. **Spinal shock** is a complete but temporary loss of motor, sensory, reflex, and autonomic function that occurs immediately after injury as the cord's response to the injury. It usually lasts less than 48 hours but can continue for several weeks
   b. **Neurogenic shock** occurs most commonly in clients with injuries above T6 and usually is experienced soon after the injury. Massive vasodilation occurs leading to pooling of the blood in blood vessels, tissue hypoperfusion, and impaired cellular metabolism.

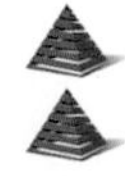

2. Data collection (Box 57-12)
3. Interventions
   a. Monitor for signs of spinal shock following a spinal cord injury.
   b. Monitor for hypotension and bradycardia.
   c. Monitor for reflex activity.
   d. Check bowel sounds.
   e. Monitor for bowel and urinary retention.

BOX 57-12 Neurogenic Shock, Spinal Shock, and Autonomic Dysreflexia

Neurogenic Shock

Hypotension
Bradycardia

Spinal Shock

Flaccid paralysis
Loss of reflex activity below the level of injury
Bradycardia
Hypotension
Paralytic ileus

Autonomic Dysreflexia

Sudden onset of severe, throbbing headache
Severe hypertension and bradycardia
Flushing above the level of the lesion
Pale extremities below the level of injury
Nasal stuffiness
Nausea
Dilated pupils or blurred vision
Sweating
Piloerection (goose bumps)
Restlessness and a feeling of apprehension

   f. Provide supportive measures as prescribed, based on the presence of symptoms.
   g. Monitor for the return of reflexes.

L. Autonomic dysreflexia
1. Description
   a. Autonomic dysreflexia is also known as autonomic hyperreflexia.
   b. Autonomic dysreflexia generally occurs after the period of spinal shock is resolved and occurs with lesions or injuries above T6 and in cervical lesions.
2. Data collection (see Box 57-12)
3. Interventions (see Priority Nursing Actions)

M. Cervical spine traction for cervical injuries
1. Description
   a. Skeletal traction is used to stabilize fractures or dislocations of the cervical or upper thoracic spine.
   b. Two types of equipment used for cervical traction are skull (cervical) tongs and halo traction (halo fixation device).
2. **Skull tongs**
   a. Skull tongs are inserted into the outer aspect of the client's skull, and traction is applied.

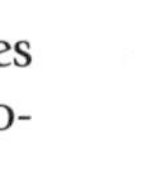

   b. Weights are attached to the tongs, and the client is used as countertraction. The nurse should not add or remove weights.
   c. Monitor the neurological status of the client.
   d. Determine the amount of weight prescribed to be added to the traction.

PRIORITY NURSING ACTIONS!

Actions to Take for a Spinal Cord Injury Client Who Develops Autonomic Dysreflexia

1. Raise the head of the bed.
2. Loosen tight clothing on the client.
3. Check for bladder distention or other noxious stimulus.
4. Assist to administer an antihypertensive medication.
5. Document the occurrence, treatment, and response.

Autonomic dysreflexia is characterized by severe hypertension, bradycardia, severe headache, nasal stuffiness, and flushing. The cause is a noxious stimulus, most often a distended bladder or constipation. Autonomic dysreflexia is a neurological emergency and must be treated promptly to prevent a hypertensive stroke. The registered nurse is notified immediately while emergence measures are implemented. Immediate nursing actions are to sit the client up in bed in a high Fowler's position and remove the noxious stimulus. The nurse would loosen any tight clothing and then check for bladder distention. If the client has a Foley catheter, the nurse would check for kinks in the tubing. The nurse also would check for a fecal impaction and disimpact the client, if necessary. The HCP is contacted. The nurse checks the environment to ensure that it is not too cool or too drafty and also monitors vital signs, particularly the blood pressure, every 15 minutes. Antihypertensive medication may be prescribed by the HCP to minimize cerebral hypertension. Finally, the nurse documents the occurrence, treatment, and client response.

Reference(s): deWit, D. & Kumagai, C. (2013). *Medical-surgical nursing: Concepts & practice.* (2nd ed., pp. 514–515). St. Louis: Saunders.

Lewis, S., Dirksen, S., Heitkemper, M., & Bucher, L. (2014). *Medical-surgical nursing: Assessment and management of clinical problems* (9th ed., p. 1479). St. Louis: Mosby.

e. Ensure that weights hang securely and freely at all times.
f. Ensure that the ropes for the traction remain within the pulley.
g. Maintain body alignment and maintain care of the client on a special bed (such as a Roto-Rest bed, or Stryker, or Foster frame), as prescribed.
h. Turn the client every 2 hours.
i. Check insertion site of the tongs for infection.
j. Provide sterile pin site care as prescribed.

3. **Halo traction**
   a. Halo traction is a static traction device that consists of a headpiece with four pins—two anterior and two posterior—inserted into the client's skull.
   b. The metal halo ring may be attached to a vest (jacket) or cast when the spine is stable, allowing increased client mobility.
   c. Monitor the client's neurological status for changes in movement or decreased strength.
   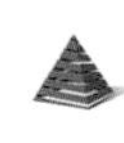
   d. Never move or turn the client by holding or pulling on the halo traction device.
   e. Check tightness of the jacket by ensuring that one finger can be placed under the jacket.
   f. Check skin integrity to ensure that the jacket or cast is not causing pressure.
   g. Provide sterile pin site care as prescribed.

4. Reinforce client education for the halo traction device (Box 57-13)
5. Initiate interventions in support of the client's self-image.
6. Reinforce teaching the client and family pin care, care of the vest, and signs and symptoms of infection to report to his or her health care provider.

BOX 57-13 Client Education for a Halo Fixation Device

Notify the HCP if the halo vest (jacket) or ring bolts loosen.
Use fleece or foam inserts to relieve pressure points.
Keep the vest lining dry.
Clean the pin site daily.
Notify the HCP if redness, swelling, drainage, open areas, pain, tenderness, or a clicking sound occurs from the pin site.
A sponge bath or tub bath is allowed. Showers are prohibited.
Check the skin under the vest daily for breakdown, using a flashlight.
Do not use any products other than shampoo on the hair.
When shampooing the hair, cover the vest with plastic.
When getting out of bed, roll onto the side and push on the mattress with the arms.
Never use the metal frame for turning or lifting.
Use a rolled towel or pillowcase between the back of the neck and the bed or next to the cheek when lying on the side, and raise the head of the bed to increase sleep comfort.
Adapt clothing to fit over the halo device.
Eat foods high in protein and calcium to promote bone healing.
Have the correct-size wrench available at all times for an emergency (tape the wrench to the vest).
If cardiopulmonary resuscitation is required, the anterior portion of the vest will be loosened and the posterior portion will remain in place to provide stability.

N. Interventions for thoracic and lumbar and sacral injuries
   1. Bed rest
   2. Immobilize with a body cast if prescribed.
   3. Monitor for respiratory impairment and paralytic ileus as possible complications of the body cast. 
   4. Use a brace or corset when the client is out of bed.

O. Surgical interventions for thoracic and lumbar/sacral injuries
   1. Decompressive laminectomy
      a. Removal of one or more laminae
      b. Allows for cord expansion from edema; performed if conventional methods fail to prevent neurological deterioration
   2. Spinal fusion
      a. Spinal fusion is used for thoracic spinal injuries.
      b. Bone is grafted between the vertebrae for support and to strengthen the back.
   3. Postoperative interventions
      a. Monitor for respiratory impairment.
      b. Monitor vital signs, motor function, sensation, and circulatory status in the lower extremities.
      c. Encourage breathing exercises.
      d. Monitor for signs of fluid and electrolyte imbalance.
      e. Observe for complications of immobility.
      f. Keep the client in a flat position as prescribed.
      g. Provide cast care if the client is in a full body cast.
      h. Turn and reposition frequently by logrolling side to back to side, using turning sheets and pillows between the legs to maintain alignment.
      i. Assist to administer pain medication as prescribed.
      j. Maintain an NPO status until the client is passing flatus.
      k. Monitor bowel sounds.
      l. Provide the use of a fracture bedpan.
      m. Monitor I&O.
      n. Maintain nutritional status.

P. Medications
   1. Dexamethasone (Decadron)
      a. Used for its anti-inflammatory and edema-reducing effects
      b. May interfere with healing
   2. Dextran: A plasma expander used to increase capillary blood flow within the spinal cord and to prevent or treat hypotension
   3. Baclofen (Lioresal)/Cyclobenzaprine hydrochloride (Flexeril): These medications are used for clients with upper motor neuron injuries to control muscle spasticity.

IX. Cerebral Aneurysm

A. Description
   1. A dilation of the walls of a weakened cerebral artery
   2. Aneurysm can lead to rupture.

B. Data collection
   1. Headache and pain
   2. Irritability
   3. Diplopia
   4. Blurred vision
   5. Tinnitus
   6. Hemiparesis
   7. Nuchal rigidity
   8. Seizures

C. Interventions
   1. Maintain a patent airway (suction only with a HCP's prescription).
   2. Administer oxygen as prescribed.
   3. Monitor vital signs and for hypertension or dysrhythmias.
   4. Avoid taking temperatures via the rectum.
   5. Initiate aneurysm precautions (Box 57-14).

X. Seizures

A. Description
   1. Seizures are an abnormal, sudden, excessive discharge of electrical activity within the brain.
   2. Epilepsy is a disorder characterized by chronic seizure activity and indicates brain or CNS irritation.
   3. Causes include genetic factors, trauma, tumors, circulatory or metabolic disorders, toxicity, and infections.
   4. Status epilepticus involves a rapid succession of epileptic spasms without intervals of consciousness; it is a potential complication that can occur with any type of seizure, and brain damage may result.

BOX 57-14 Aneurysm Precautions

Maintain the client on bed rest in a semi-Fowler's or side-lying position.
Maintain a darkened room (subdued lighting and no direct, bright, artificial lights) without stimulation (a private room is optimal).
Provide a quiet environment (avoid activities or startling noises); telephone in the room is not usually allowed.
Reading, watching television, and listening to music are permitted, provided they do not overstimulate the client.
Limit visitors.
Maintain fluid restrictions.
Provide diet as prescribed; avoid stimulants in the diet.
Prevent any activities that initiate the Valsalva maneuver (straining at stooling, coughing); provide stool softeners to prevent straining.
Administer care gently (e.g., the bath, back rub, range of motion).
Limit invasive procedures.
Maintain normothermia.
Prevent hypertension.
Provide sedation.
Provide pain control.
Assist to administer prophylactic anticonvulsant medications.
Assist to provide deep vein thrombosis (DVT) prophylaxis as prescribed.

B. Types of seizures (Box 57-15)
   1. Generalized seizures
   2. Partial seizures

C. Data collection
   1. Seizure history
   2. Type of seizure
   3. Occurrences before, during, and after the seizure
   4. Prodromal signs, such as mood changes, irritability, and insomnia
   5. Aura: Sensation that warns the client of the impending seizure
   6. Loss of motor activity or bowel and bladder function or loss of consciousness during the seizure
   7. Occurrences during the postictal state, such as headache, loss of consciousness, sleepiness, and impaired speech or thinking

BOX 57-15 Types of Seizures

Generalized Seizures

Tonic-Clonic

Tonic-clonic seizures may begin with an aura.

The tonic phase involves the stiffening or rigidity of the muscles of the arms and legs and usually lasts 10 to 20 seconds, followed by loss of consciousness.

The clonic phase consists of hyperventilation and jerking of the extremities and usually lasts about 30 seconds.

Full recovery from the seizure may take several hours.

Absence

A brief seizure lasts seconds, and the individual may or may not lose consciousness.

No loss or change in muscle tone occurs.

Seizures may occur several times during a day.

The victim appears to be daydreaming.

This type of seizure is more common in children.

Myoclonic

Myoclonic seizures present as a brief generalized jerking or stiffening of extremities.

The victim may fall to the ground from the seizure.

Atonic or Akinetic (Drop Attacks)

An atonic seizure is a sudden momentary loss of muscle tone.

The victim may fall to the ground as a result of the seizure.

Partial Seizures

Simple Partial

The simple partial seizure produces sensory symptoms accompanied by motor symptoms that are localized or confined to a specific area.

The client remains conscious and may report an aura.

Complex Partial

The complex partial seizure is a psychomotor seizure.

The area of the brain most involved is the temporal lobe.

The seizure is characterized by periods of altered behavior of which the client is not aware.

The client loses consciousness for a few seconds.

D. Interventions

⚠ If the client is having a seizure, maintain a patent airway. Do not force the jaws open or place anything in the client's mouth.

   1. Note the time and duration of the seizure.
   2. Monitor behavior at the onset of the seizure. Note if the client experienced an aura, a change in facial expression occurred, or a sound or cry occurred from the client.
   3. If the client is standing, place him or her on the floor and protect the head and body.
   4. Monitor airway, breathing, and circulation.
   5. Administer oxygen.
   6. Prepare to suction secretions from the airway.
   7. Turn the client to the side to allow secretions to drain while maintaining the airway.
   8. Prevent injury during the seizure.
   9. Remain with the client.
   10. Do not restrain the client.
   11. Loosen restrictive clothing.
   12. Note the type, character, and progression of the movements during the seizure.
   13. Monitor for incontinence.
   14. Assist to administer IV medications as prescribed to stop the seizure.
   15. Document the characteristics of the seizure.
   16. Provide privacy, if possible.
   17. Monitor behavior following the seizure, such as the state of consciousness, motor ability, and speech ability.
   18. Reinforce instructions to the client about the importance of lifelong medication and the need for follow-up determination of medication blood levels.
   19. Reinforce instructions to the client to avoid alcohol, excessive stress, fatigue, and strobe lights.
   20. Encourage the client to contact available community resources, such as the Epilepsy Foundation of America.
   21. Encourage the client to wear a Medic-Alert bracelet.

XI. Stroke (Brain Attack)

A. Description
   1. A stroke or brain attack is a sudden focal neurological deficit caused by cerebrovascular disease.
   2. A stroke is a syndrome in which the cerebral circulation is interrupted, causing neurological deficits.
   3. Cerebral anoxia lasting longer than 10 minutes causes cerebral infarction with irreversible change.
   4. Cerebral edema and congestion cause further dysfunction.
   5. Diagnosis is determined by CT scan, electroencephalogram, cerebral arteriography, and MRI.

Adult—Neurological

6. Transient ischemic attack may be a warning sign of an impending stroke
7. The permanent disability cannot be determined until the cerebral edema subsides.
8. The order in which function may return is facial, swallowing, lower limb, speech, and arms.
9. Carotid endarterectomy is a surgical intervention used in stroke management and is targeted at stroke prevention, especially in clients with symptomatic carotid stenosis.
10. The National Institutes of Health through the National Institute of Neurological Disorders and Stroke (NINDS) developed the *Know Stroke. Know the Signs. Act in Time* campaign to help educate the public about the symptoms of stroke and the importance of getting to the hospital quickly (http://stroke.nih.gov/).

A transient ischemic attack (TIA) may be a warning sign of an impending stroke.

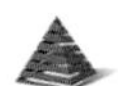
B. Causes
1. Thrombosis
2. Embolism
3. Hemorrhage from rupture of a vessel

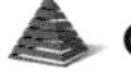
C. Risk factors
1. Atherosclerosis
2. Hypertension
3. Anticoagulation therapy
4. Diabetes mellitus
5. Stress
6. Obesity
7. Oral contraceptives

A critical factor in the early intervention and treatment of stroke is the accurate identification of stroke manifestations and establishing the onset of the manifestations. Stroke screening scales may be used to quickly identify stroke manifestations.

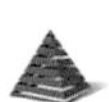
D. Data collection (Boxes 57-16 and 57-17 and Fig. 57-3)
1. Findings depend on the area of the brain affected; stroke scales such as the National Institutes of Health stroke scale may be used by the health care facility for assessment.

BOX 57-16 Neurological Data Collection: Stroke

Changes in level of consciousness
Signs of increasing intracranial pressure
Assessment of cranial nerves V, VII, IX, X, and XII
Cranial nerve V: difficulty with chewing
Cranial nerve VII: facial paralysis or paresis
Cranial nerves IX and X: dysphagia
Cranial nerve IX: absent gag reflex
Cranial nerve XII: impaired tongue movement

BOX 57-17 Data Collection Findings: Stroke

Agnosia
Inability to recognize and use an object correctly

Apraxia
Called *dyspraxia* if the condition is mild
Characterized by loss of ability to execute or carry out skilled movements or gestures, despite having the desire and physical ability to perform them

Hemianopsia
Blindness in half of the visual field

Homonymous Hemianopsia
Loss of half of the field of view on the same side in both eyes.

Neglect Syndrome (Unilateral Neglect)
Client unaware of the existence of his or her paralyzed side

Proprioception Alterations
Altered position sense that places the client at increased risk of injury
Note: With visual problems, the client must turn the head to scan the complete range of vision.

For more information:
U.S. Department of Health and Human Services. National Institute of Health. NIH Publication #10–4872. July 2010. Know Stroke. Know the Signs. Act in Time.
National Institutes of Health. http://stroke.nih.gov/

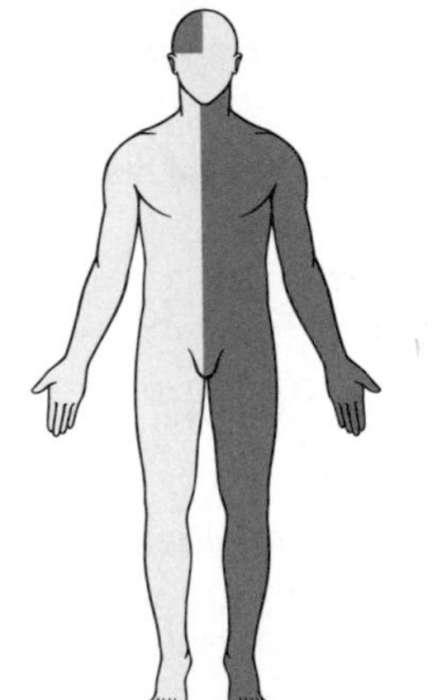

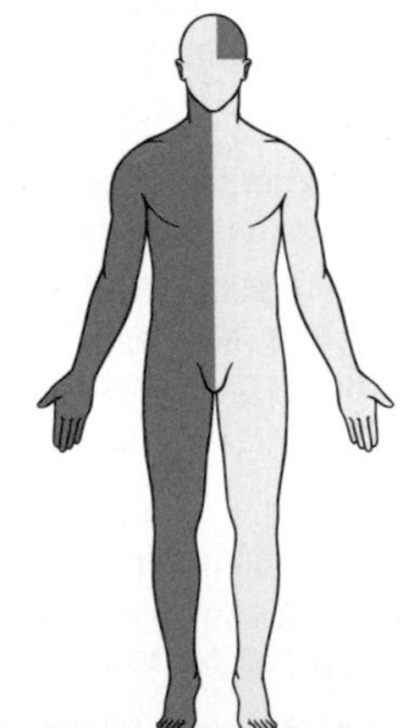

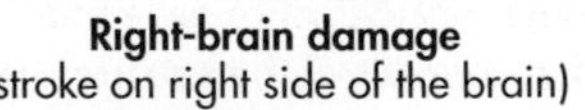

Right-brain damage (stroke on right side of the brain)	**Left-brain damage** (stroke on left side of the brain)
• Paralyzed left side: hemiplegia	• Paralyzed right side: hemiplegia
• Left-sided neglect	• Impaired speech/language aphasias
• Spatial-perceptual deficits	• Impaired right/left discrimination
• Tends to deny or minimize problems	• Slow performance, cautious
• Rapid performance, short attention span	• Aware of deficits: depression, anxiety
• Impulsive, safety problems	• Impaired comprehension related to language, math
• Impaired judgment	
• Impaired time concepts	

FIGURE 57-3 Manifestations of right brain and left brain stroke. (From Lewis S, Dirksen S, Heitkemper M, Bucher L, Camera I: *Medical-surgical nursing: Assessment and management of clinical problems,* ed 8, St. Louis, 2011, Mosby.)

2. Lesions in the cerebral hemisphere result in manifestations on the contralateral side, which is the side of the body opposite the stroke.
3. Airway patency is always a priority.
4. Pulse (may be slow and bounding)
5. Respirations (Cheyne-Stokes)
6. Blood pressure (hypertension)
7. Headache, nausea, and vomiting
8. Facial drooping
9. Nuchal rigidity
10. Visual changes
11. Ataxia
12. Dysarthria
13. Dysphagia
14. Speech changes
15. Decreased sensation to pressure, heat, and cold
16. Bowel and bladder dysfunctions
17. Paralysis

E. Aphasia
1. Expressive
   a. Damage occurs in Broca's area of the frontal brain.
   b. The client understands what is said but is unable to communicate verbally.
2. Receptive
   a. The injury involves Wernicke's area in the temporoparietal area.
   b. The client is unable to understand the spoken and often the written word.
3. Global or mixed: Language dysfunction occurs in expression and reception.
4. Interventions for aphasia
   a. Provide repetitive directions.
   b. Break down tasks to one step at a time.
   c. Repeat names of objects frequently used.
   d. Allow time for the client to communicate.
   e. Use a picture board, communication board, or computerized technology.

F. Interventions during the acute phase of stroke
1. Maintain a patent airway, and administer oxygen as prescribed.
2. Monitor vital signs.
3. Usually a blood pressure of 150/100 mm Hg or as prescribed is maintained to ensure cerebral perfusion.
4. Suction secretions as prescribed, but never suction nasally or for longer than 10 seconds to prevent increasing ICP.
5. Monitor for increasing ICP because the client is at most risk during the first 72 hours following the stroke.
6. Position the client on the side, with the head of the bed elevated 15 to 30 degrees as prescribed.
7. Monitor LOC, pupillary response, motor and sensory response, cranial nerve function, and reflexes.
8. Maintain a quiet environment.
9. Insert a Foley catheter as prescribed.
10. Assist to administer prescribed IV fluids and monitor closely.
11. Maintain fluid and electrolyte balance.
12. Anticoagulants, antiplatelets, diuretics, antihypertensives, and anticonvulsants may prescribed.
13. Establish a form of communication.

G. Interventions in the postacute phase of a stroke
1. Continue with interventions from the acute phase.
2. Position the client 2 hours on the unaffected side and 20 minutes on the affected side.
3. Position the client in the prone position if prescribed, for 30 minutes three times daily.
4. Provide skin, mouth, and eye care.
5. Perform passive range-of-motion exercises to prevent contractures.
6. Place sequential compression devices (SCDs) as prescribed on the client.
7. Measure the thighs and calves for an increase in size.
8. Monitor the gag reflex and ability to swallow. 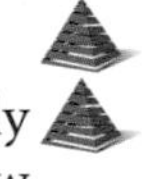
9. As prescribed, provide sips of fluids, and slowly advance the diet to foods that are easy to chew and swallow.
10. As prescribed, provide soft and semisoft foods and flavored, cool or warm, thickened fluids rather than thin liquids because the stroke client is better able to tolerate these types of foods. Speech therapists may do swallow studies to recommend consistency of food and fluids.
11. When the client is eating, position him or her sitting in a chair or sitting up in bed, with the head and neck positioned slightly forward and flexed.
12. Place food in the back of the mouth on the unaffected side to prevent trapping of food in the affected cheek.

H. Interventions in the chronic phase of stroke 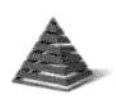
1. Neglect syndrome
   a. The client is unaware of the existence of the paralyzed side (**unilateral neglect**), which places him or her at risk for injury.
   b. Teach the client to touch and use both sides of the body.
2. **Hemianopsia**
   a. The client has blindness in half of the visual field.
   b. **Homonymous hemianopsia** is blindness in the same visual field of both eyes.
   c. Encourage the client to turn the head to scan the complete range of vision; otherwise, he or she does not see half of the visual field.
3. Approach the client from the unaffected side.
4. Place the client's personal objects within the visual field.

5. Provide eye care for visual deficits.
6. Place a patch over the affected eye if the client has diplopia.
7. Increase mobility as tolerated.
8. Encourage fluid intake and a high-fiber diet.
9. Monitor for pain.
10. Administer stool softeners as prescribed.
11. Encourage the client to express his or her feelings.
12. Encourage independence in activities of daily living.
13. Determine the need for assistive devices such as a cane, walker, splints, or braces.
14. Teach transfer technique from bed to chair and chair to bed.
15. Provide gait training.
16. Initiate physical and occupational therapy for assessment and the need for adaptive equipment or other supports for self-care and mobility.
17. Refer the client to a speech and language pathologist as prescribed.
18. Encourage the client and family to contact available community resources.

XII. Multiple Sclerosis

A. Description
1. Multiple sclerosis is a chronic, progressive, noncontagious, degenerative disease of the CNS characterized by demyelinization of the neurons.
2. It usually occurs between the ages of 20 and 40 years and consists of periods of remissions and exacerbations.
3. The causes are unknown, but the disease is thought to be a result of an autoimmune response or viral infection.
4. Precipitating factors include pregnancy, fatigue, stress, infection, and trauma.
5. Electroencephalogram findings are abnormal.
6. A lumbar puncture indicates an increased gamma-globulin level, but the serum globulin level is normal.

B. Data collection
1. Fatigue and weakness
2. Ataxia and vertigo
3. Tremors and spasticity of the lower extremities
4. Paresthesias
5. Blurred vision, diplopia, and transient blindness
6. Nystagmus
7. Dysphasia
8. Decreased perception to pain, touch, and temperature
9. Bladder and bowel disturbances, including urgency, frequency, retention, and incontinence
10. Abnormal reflexes, including hyperreflexia, absent reflexes, and a positive Babinski's reflex
11. Emotional changes such as apathy, euphoria, irritability, and depression
12. Memory changes and confusion

C. Interventions
1. Provide energy conservation measures exacerbation.
2. Protect the client from injury by providing safety measures.
3. Place an eye patch on the eye for diplopia.
4. Monitor for potential complications such as urinary tract infections, calculi, pressure ulcers, respiratory tract infections, and contractures.
5. Promote regular elimination by bladder and bowel training.
6. Encourage independence.
7. Assist the client to establish a regular exercise and rest program.
8. Reinforce instructions to the client to balance moderate activity with rest periods.
9. Assess the need for and provide assistive devices.
10. Initiate physical and speech therapy.
11. Reinforce instructions to the client to avoid fatigue, stress, infection, overheating, and chilling.
12. Reinforce instructions to the client to increase fluid intake and eat a balanced diet, including low-fat, high-fiber foods and foods high in potassium.
13. Reinforce instructions to the client on safety measures related to sensory loss, such as regulating the temperature of bathwater and avoiding heating pads.
14. Reinforce instructions to the client on safety measures related to motor loss, such as avoiding the use of scatter rugs and using assistive devices.
15. Reinforce instructions to the client in the self-administration of prescribed medications.
16. Provide information about the National Multiple Sclerosis Society.

XIII. Myasthenia Gravis

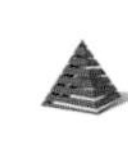

A. Description
1. Myasthenia gravis is a neuromuscular disease that is characterized by considerable weakness and abnormal fatigue of the voluntary muscles.
2. A defect in the transmission of nerve impulses at the myoneural junction occurs.
3. Causes include insufficient secretion of acetylcholine, excessive secretion of cholinesterase, and unresponsiveness of the muscle fibers to acetylcholine.

B. Data collection
1. Weakness and fatigue
2. Difficulty chewing and swallowing 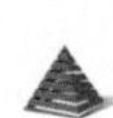
3. Dysphagia
4. Ptosis
5. Diplopia

6. Weak, hoarse voice
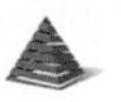
7. Difficulty breathing
8. Diminished breath sounds
9. Respiratory paralysis and failure

C. Interventions
1. Monitor respiratory status and ability to cough and deep breathe adequately.
2. Monitor for respiratory failure.
3. Maintain suctioning and emergency equipment at the bedside.
4. Monitor the vital signs.
5. Monitor speech and swallowing abilities to prevent aspiration.
6. Encourage the client to sit up when eating.
7. Assess muscle status.
8. Reinforce instructions to the client to conserve strength.
9. Plan short activities that coincide with times of maximal muscle strength.
10. Monitor for myasthenic and cholinergic crises.
11. Assist to administer anticholinesterase medications as prescribed.
12. Reinforce instructions to the client to avoid stress, infection, fatigue, and over-the-counter medications.
13. Reinforce instructions to the client to wear a Medic-Alert bracelet.
14. Reinforce instructions to the client about services from the Myasthenia Gravis Foundation.

D. Anticholinesterase medications: Increase levels of acetylcholine at the myoneural junction (see Chapter 58)

E. Myasthenic crisis
1. Description
a. Myasthenic crisis is an acute exacerbation of the disease.
b. The crisis is caused by a rapid, unrecognized progression of the disease; an inadequate amount of medication; infection; fatigue; or stress.
2. Data collection
a. Increased pulse, respirations, and blood pressure
b. Dyspnea, anoxia, and cyanosis
c. Bowel and bladder incontinence
d. Decreased urine output
e. Absent cough and swallow reflex
3. Interventions
a. Monitor for signs of myasthenic crisis.
b. Increase anticholinesterase medication, as prescribed.

F. Cholinergic crisis
1. Description
a. Cholinergic crisis results in depolarization of the motor end plates.
b. The crisis is caused by overmedication with anticholinesterase.
2. Data collection
a. Abdominal cramps
b. Nausea, vomiting, and diarrhea
c. Blurred vision
d. Pallor
e. Facial muscle twitching
f. Hypotension
g. Pupillary miosis
3. Interventions
a. Withhold anticholinesterase medication.
b. Prepare to administer the antidote, atropine sulfate, if prescribed.

G. Edrophonium (Enlon) test

Have atropine sulfate available when performing the edrophonium test.

1. May also be known as the Tensilon test; this test is performed by the neurologist to diagnose myasthenia gravis and to differentiate between myasthenic crisis and cholinergic crisis.
2. The test places the client at risk for ventricular fibrillation and cardiac arrest; the nurse must prepare for this possibility.
3. To diagnose myasthenia gravis
a. An edrophonium injection is administered to the client.
b. Positive for myasthenia gravis: The client shows improvement in muscle strength after the administration of edrophonium.
c. Negative for myasthenia gravis: The client shows no improvement in muscle strength, and strength may even deteriorate after injection of edrophonium.
4. To differentiate crisis
a. Myasthenic crisis: Edrophonium is administered and if strength improves, the client needs more medication.
b. Cholinergic crisis: Edrophonium is administered and if the client's weakness is more severe, then the client is overmedicated. Atropine sulfate, which is the antidote, may be prescribed.

XIV. Parkinson's Disease

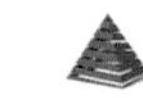

A. Description
1. Parkinson's disease is a degenerative disease caused by the depletion of dopamine, which interferes with the inhibition of excitatory impulses, resulting in a dysfunction of the extrapyramidal system.
2. It is a slow, progressive disease that results in a crippling disability.
3. The debilitation can result in falls, self-care deficits, failure of body systems, and depression.
4. Mental deterioration occurs late in the disease.

B. Data collection
  1. Bradykinesia, abnormal slowness of movement, and sluggishness of physical and mental responses
  2. Akinesia
  3. Monotonous speech
  4. Handwriting that becomes progressively smaller
  5. Tremors in hands and fingers at rest (pill rolling)
  6. Tremors increasing when fatigued and decreasing with purposeful activity or sleep
  7. Rigidity with jerky movements
  8. Restlessness and pacing
  9. Blank facial expression; masklike facies
  10. Drooling
  11. Difficulty swallowing and speaking
  12. Loss of coordination and balance
  13. Shuffling steps, stooped position, and propulsive gait

C. Interventions
  1. Monitor neurological status.
  2. Check ability to swallow and chew.
  3. Provide a high-calorie, high-protein, high-fiber soft diet with small, frequent feedings.
  4. Increase fluid intake to 2000 mL/day.
  5. Monitor for constipation.
  6. Promote independence along with safety measures.
  7. Avoid rushing the client with activities.
  8. Assist with ambulation and provide assistive devices.
  9. Reinforce instructions to the client to rock back and forth to initiate movement.
  10. Reinforce instructions to the client to wear low-heeled shoes.
  11. Encourage the client to lift his or her feet when walking and to avoid prolonged sitting.
  12. Provide a firm mattress, and position the client prone, without a pillow, to facilitate proper posture.
  13. Reinforce instructions for proper posture by teaching the client to hold the hands behind the back to keep the spine and neck erect.
  14. Promote physical therapy and rehabilitation.
  15. Assist to administer antiparkinsonian medications to increase the level of dopamine in the CNS.
  16. Reinforce instructions to the client to avoid foods high in vitamin B_6 because they block the effects of antiparkinsonian medications.
  17. Reinforce instructions to the client to avoid monoamine oxidase inhibitors because they precipitate hypertensive crisis.
  18. See Chapter 58 regarding medication to treat Parkinson's disease.

XV. Trigeminal Neuralgia

A. Description
  1. Trigeminal neuralgia is a sensory disorder of the trigeminal (fifth cranial) nerve.
  2. It results in severe, recurrent, sharp, facial pain along the trigeminal nerve.

B. Data collection
  1. The client has severe pain on the lips, gums, or nose, or across the cheeks.
  2. Situations that stimulate symptoms include cold, washing the face, chewing, or food or fluids of extreme temperatures.

C. Interventions
  1. Reinforce instructions to the client to avoid hot or cold foods and fluids.
  2. Provide small feedings of liquid and soft foods.
  3. Reinforce instructions to the client to chew food on the unaffected side.
  4. Asisst to administer medications as prescribed (see Chapter 58).

D. Surgical interventions
  1. Microvascular decompression: Surgical relocation of the artery that compresses the trigeminal nerve as it enters the pons may relieve pain without compromising facial sensation.
  2. Radiofrequency wave forms: Creates lesions that provide relief from pain without compromising touch or motor function
  3. Rhizotomy: Resection of the root of the nerve to relieve pain
  4. Glycerol injection: Destroys the myelinated fibers of the trigeminal nerve (may take up to 3 weeks for pain relief to occur)

XVI. Bell's Palsy (Facial Paralysis)

A. Description
  1. Bell's palsy is caused by a lower motor neuron lesion of the seventh cranial nerve that may result from infection, trauma, hemorrhage, meningitis, or a tumor.
  2. It results in paralysis of one side of the face.
  3. Recovery usually occurs in a few weeks without residual effects.

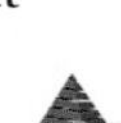

B. Data collection
  1. Flaccid facial muscles
  2. Inability to raise the eyebrows, frown, smile, close the eyelids, or puff out the cheeks
  3. Upward movement of the eye when attempting to close the eyelid
  4. Loss of taste

C. Interventions
  1. Encourage the client to do facial exercises to prevent the loss of muscle tone. (A face sling may be prescribed to prevent stretching of weak muscles.)
  2. Protect the eyes from dryness and prevent injury.

3. Promote frequent oral care.
4. Reinforce instructions to the client to chew on the unaffected side.

XVII. Guillain-Barré Syndrome

A. Description
   1. Guillain-Barré syndrome is an acute infectious neuronitis of the cranial and peripheral nerves.
   2. The immune system overreacts to the infection and destroys the myelin sheath.
   3. The syndrome is usually preceded by a mild upper respiratory infection or gastroenteritis.
   4. Recovery is a slow process and can take years.

⚠ The major concern in Guillain-Barré syndrome is difficulty breathing. Monitor respiratory status closely.

B. Data collection
   1. Paresthesias
   2. Pain and/or hypersensitivity such as with the weight of bed sheets or other items touching the body
   3. Weakness of lower extremities
   4. Gradual progressive weakness of the upper extremities and facial muscles
   5. Possible progression to respiratory failure
   6. Cardiac dysrhythmias
   7. CSF that reveals an elevated protein level
   8. Abnormal electroencephalogram

C. Interventions
   1. Care is directed toward the treatment of symptoms, including pain management.
   2. Monitor respiratory status.
   3. Provide respiratory treatments.
   4. Prepare to initiate respiratory support.
   5. Monitor cardiac status.
   6. Monitor for complications of immobility.
   7. Provide the client and family with support.

XVIII. Amyotrophic Lateral Sclerosis

A. Description
   1. Amyotrophic lateral sclerosis is also known as Lou Gehrig's disease.
   2. It is a progressive degenerative disease involving the motor system.
   3. The sensory and autonomic systems are not involved, and mental status changes do not result from the disease.
   4. The cause of the disease may be related to an excess of glutamate, a chemical responsible for relaying messages between the motor neurons.
   5. As the disease progresses, muscle weakness and atrophy develop until a flaccid tetraplegia develops.
   6. Eventually the respiratory muscles become affected, leading to respiratory compromise, pneumonia, and death.
   7. No cure is known, and the treatment is symptomatic.

B. Data collection
   1. Respiratory difficulty
   2. Fatigue while talking
   3. Muscle weakness and atrophy
   4. Tongue atrophy
   5. Dysphagia
   6. Weakness of the hands and arms
   7. Fasciculations of the face
   8. Nasal quality of speech
   9. Dysarthria

C. Interventions
   1. Care is directed toward the treatment of symptoms.
   2. Monitor the respiratory status and institute measures to prevent aspiration.
   3. Provide respiratory treatments.
   4. Prepare to initiate respiratory support.
   5. Monitor for complications of immobility.
   6. Provide the client and family with support.

XIX. Encephalitis

A. Description
   1. Encephalitis is an inflammation of the brain parenchyma and often the meninges.
   2. It affects the cerebrum, brainstem, and cerebellum.
   3. It is most often caused by a viral agent, although bacteria, fungi, or parasites may also be involved.
   4. Viral encephalitis is almost always preceded by a viral infection.

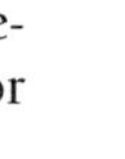

B. Transmission
   1. Arboviruses can be transmitted to human beings through the bite of an infected mosquito or tick.
   2. Echovirus, coxsackievirus, poliovirus, herpes zoster, and viruses that cause mumps and chickenpox are common enteroviruses associated with encephalitis.
   3. Herpes simplex type 1 virus can cause viral encephalitis.
   4. The organism that causes amebic meningoencephalitis can enter the nasal mucosa of persons swimming in warm fresh water, for example, in a pond or lake.

C. Data collection
   1. Presence of cold sores, lesions, or ulcerations of the oral cavity
   2. History of insect bites and swimming in freshwater
   3. Exposure to infectious diseases

4. Travel to areas where the disease is prevalent
5. Fever
6. Nausea and vomiting
7. Nuchal rigidity
8. Changes in LOC and mental status
9. Signs of increased ICP
10. Motor dysfunction and focal neurological deficits

D. Interventions

1. Monitor vital and neurological signs.
2. Check LOC using the Glasgow Coma Scale.
3. Monitor for mental status changes and personality and behavior changes.
4. Monitor for signs of increased ICP.
5. Check for the presence of nuchal rigidity and a positive **Kernig's sign** or **Brudzinski's sign**, indicating meningeal irritation.
6. Assist the client to turn, cough, and deep breathe frequently.
7. Elevate the head of the bed 30 to 45 degrees.
8. Assess for muscle and neurological deficits.
9. Acyclovir (Zovirax) may be prescribed (usually is the medication of choice for herpes encephalitis).
10. Assist to initiate rehabilitation as needed for motor dysfunction or neurological deficits.

XX. West Nile Virus

A. Description

1. West Nile virus is a potentially serious illness that affects the CNS.
2. The virus is contracted primarily by the bite of an infected mosquito. (Mosquitoes become carriers when they feed on infected birds.)
3. Symptoms typically develop between 3 and 14 days after being bitten by the infected mosquito.
4. Neurological effects can be permanent.

B. Data collection

1. Many individuals will not experience any symptoms.
2. Mild symptoms include fever, headache and body aches, nausea, vomiting, swollen glands, or a rash on the chest, stomach, or back.
3. Severe symptoms include a high fever, headache, neck stiffness, stupor, disorientation, tremors, muscle weakness, vision loss, numbness, paralysis, seizures, or coma.

C. Interventions are supportive. There is no specific treatment for the virus.

D. Prevention

1. Use insect repellents containing DEET (diethyltoluamide) when outdoors, and wear long sleeves and long pants and light-colored clothing.
2. Stay indoors at dusk and dawn when mosquitoes are most active.
3. Ensure that mosquito breeding sites are eliminated, such as standing water and water in birdbaths, and keep wading pools empty and on their sides when not in use.

XXI. Meningitis

A. Description

1. Meningitis is inflammation of the arachnoid and pia mater of the brain and spinal cord.
2. It is caused by bacterial and viral organisms, although fungal and protozoan meningitis also occur.
3. Predisposing factors include skull fractures, brain or spinal surgery, sinus or upper respiratory infections, the use of nasal sprays, and individuals with a compromised immune system.
4. CSF is analyzed to determine the diagnosis and the type of meningitis. In meningitis, CSF is cloudy, with increased protein, increased white blood cells, and decreased glucose counts.

B. Transmission: Occurs in areas of high-population density and crowded living areas such as college dormitories and prisons

Transmission of meningitis is by direct contact, including droplet spread.

C. Data collection (see Box 57-4)

1. Mild lethargy; photophobia
2. Deterioration in the level of consciousness
3. Signs of meningeal irritation such as nuchal rigidity and positive Kernig's sign and Brudzinski's sign
4. Red, macular rash with meningococcal meningitis
5. Abdominal and chest pain with viral meningitis

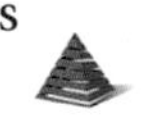

D. Interventions

1. Monitor vital signs and neurological signs.
2. Watch for signs of increasing ICP.
3. Initiate seizure precautions.
4. Monitor for seizure activity.
5. Monitor for signs of meningeal irritation.
6. Assist to perform cranial nerve assessment.
7. Check peripheral vascular status. (Septic emboli may block circulation.)
8. Maintain isolation precautions as necessary with bacterial meningitis.
9. Maintain urine and stool precautions with viral meningitis.
10. Maintain respiratory isolation for the client with pneumococcal meningitis.
11. Elevate the head of the bed 30 degrees, and avoid neck flexion and extreme hip flexion.
12. Prevent stimulation and restrict visitors.
13. Administer analgesics as prescribed.
14. Administer antibiotics as prescribed.

CRITICAL THINKING What Should You Do?

Answer: Unilateral body neglect syndrome is particularly common with strokes in the right cerebral hemisphere. In this syndrome, the client is unaware of his or her left or paralyzed side and neglects that side. If the nurse makes this observation, the nurse should immediately check the client for signs of injury and provide safety to the client. The registered nurse (RN) is also notified. The client with this syndrome often indicates that everything is fine and believes that he or she is sitting up straight in the chair. The client should be taught to use both sides of the body and to attend to the affected side first. If the client is experiencing visual problems, the client is taught to turn the head from side to side to expand the visual field.

Reference(s): Ignatavicius, D., & Workman, M. (2013). *Medical-surgical nursing: Patient-centered collaborative care.* (7th ed., pp. 1011, 1019). St. Louis: Saunders.

PRACTICE QUESTIONS

❖ **596.** A client with a seizure disorder is being admitted to the hospital. Which should the nurse plan to implement for this client? **Select all that apply.**

- ☐ 1. Pad the bed's side rails.
- ☐ 2. Place an airway at the bedside.
- ☐ 3. Place oxygen equipment at the bedside.
- ☐ 4. Place suction equipment at the bedside.
- ☐ 5. Tape a padded tongue blade to the wall at the head of the bed.

597. The client has just undergone computed tomography (CT) scanning with a contrast medium. Which statement by the client demonstrates an understanding of postprocedure care?

1. "I should drink extra fluids for the remainder of the day."
2. "I should not take any medication for at least 4 hours."
3. "I should eat lightly for the remainder of the day."
4. "I should rest quietly for the remainder of the day."

598. The nurse is caring for a client with increased intracranial pressure (ICP). Which change in vital signs would occur if ICP is rising?

1. Increasing temperature, increasing pulse, increasing respirations, decreasing BP
2. Decreasing temperature, decreasing pulse, increasing respirations, decreasing BP
3. Decreasing temperature, increasing pulse, decreasing respirations, increasing BP
4. Increasing temperature, decreasing pulse, decreasing respirations, increasing BP

599. The nurse observes the unlicensed assistive personnel (UAP) positioning the client with increased intracranial pressure (ICP). Which position would require intervention by the nurse?

1. Head midline
2. Head turned to the side
3. Neck in neutral position
4. Head of bed elevated 30 to 45 degrees

600. The client recovering from a head injury is arousable and participating in care. The nurse determines that the client understands measures to prevent elevations in intracranial pressure (ICP) if the nurse observes the client doing which activity?

1. Blowing the nose
2. Isometric exercises
3. Coughing vigorously
4. Exhaling during repositioning

601. The client has clear fluid leaking from the nose after a basilar skull fracture. The nurse determines that this is cerebrospinal fluid (CSF) if the fluid meets which criteria?

1. Is grossly bloody in appearance and has a pH of 6
2. Clumps together on the dressing and has a pH of 7
3. Is clear in appearance and tests negative for glucose
4. Separates into concentric rings and tests positive for glucose

602. The client is admitted to the hospital for observation with a probable minor head injury after an automobile crash. The nurse expects the cervical collar will remain in place until which time?

1. The client is taken for spinal x-rays
2. The family comes to visit after surgery
3. The nurse needs to provide physical care
4. The health care provider reviews the x-ray results

603. The client was seen and treated in the emergency department (ED) for a concussion. Before discharge, the nurse explains the signs/symptoms of a worsening condition. The nurse determines that the family **needs further teaching** if they state they will return to the ED if the client experiences which sign/symptom?

1. Vomiting
2. Minor headache
3. Difficulty speaking
4. Difficulty awakening

604. The nurse is caring for a client who has undergone craniotomy with a supratentorial incision. The nurse should plan to place the client in which position postoperatively?

1. Head of bed flat, head and neck midline
2. Head of bed flat, head turned to the nonoperative side

3. Head of bed elevated 30 to 45 degrees, head and neck midline
4. Head of bed elevated 30 to 45 degrees, head turned to the operative side

605. The client with a cervical spine injury has Crutchfield tongs applied in the emergency department. The nurse should perform which **essential** action when caring for this client?
1. Providing a standard bed frame
2. Removing the weights to reposition the client
3. Removing the weights if the client is uncomfortable
4. Comparing the amount of prescribed weights with the amount in use

606. The nurse has provided discharge instructions to a client with an application of a halo device. The nurse determines that the client **needs further teaching** if which statement is made?
1. "I will use a straw for drinking."
2. "I will drive only during the daytime."
3. "I will use caution because the device alters balance."
4. "I will wash the skin daily under the lamb's-wool liner of the vest."

607. The nurse is caring for the client who has suffered spinal cord injury. The nurse further monitors the client for signs of autonomic dysreflexia and suspects this complication if which sign/symptom is noted?
1. Sudden tachycardia
2. Pallor of the face and neck
3. Severe, throbbing headache
4. Severe and sudden hypotension

608. The client with spinal cord injury is prone to experiencing autonomic dysreflexia. The **least appropriate** measure to minimize the risk of autonomic dysreflexia is which action?
1. Strictly adhering to a bowel retraining program
2. Keeping the linen wrinkle-free under the client
3. Avoiding unnecessary pressure on the lower limbs
4. Limiting bladder catheterization to once every 12 hours

609. The client with spinal cord injury suddenly experiences an episode of autonomic dysreflexia. After checking vital signs, which **immediate** action should the nurse take?
1. Raise the head of the bed and remove the noxious stimulus
2. Lower the head of the bed and remove the noxious stimulus
3. Lower the head of the bed and administer an antihypertensive agent
4. Remove the noxious stimulus and administer an antihypertensive agent

610. The client is having a lumbar puncture (LP) performed. The nurse should place the client in which position for the procedure?
1. Supine, in semi-Fowler's
2. Prone, in slight Trendelenburg's
3. Prone, with a pillow under the abdomen
4. Side-lying, with legs pulled up and chin to the chest

ANSWERS

❖ **596. 1, 2, 3, 4**

Rationale: The nurse should plan seizure precautions for a client with a seizure disorder. The precautions include padded side rails and an airway, and oxygen and suction equipment at the bedside. Attempts to force a padded tongue blade between clenched teeth may result in injury to the teeth and mouth; therefore a padded tongue blade is not placed at the bedside.

Test-Taking Strategy: Focus on the subject, preparation for a client being admitted with a seizure disorder. Consider the items that are needed to keep a client safe if a seizure occurs. Eliminate the padded tongue blade as this item could cause injury if placed in the mouth during a seizure. **Review: seizure precautions.**

Level of Cognitive Ability: Analyzing

Client Needs: Safe and Effective Care Environment

Integrated Process: Nursing Process/Implementation

Content Area: Adult Health: Neurological

Priority Concepts: Clinical Judgment, Safety

Reference(s):deWit, Kumagai (2013), pp. 526–527.

597. 1

Rationale: After CT scanning, the client may resume all usual activities. The client should be encouraged to take in extra fluids to replace those lost with diuresis from the contrast dye. Options 2, 3, and 4 are unnecessary.

Test-Taking Strategy: Eliminate options 3 and 4 because they are comparable or alike. Next, focus the subject, that a contrast medium was given. This will direct you to the correct option. **Review: computed tomography scan.**

Level of Cognitive Ability: Evaluating

Client Needs: Physiological Integrity

Integrated Process: Nursing Process/Evaluation

Content Area: Fundamental Skills: Diagnostic Tests

Priority Concepts: Client Education, Fluid and Electrolyte Balance

Reference(s): Pagana, Pagana (2013), p. 283.

598. 4

Rationale: A change in vital signs may be a late sign of increased ICP. Trends include increasing temperature and blood pressure and decreasing pulse and respirations. Respiratory irregularities may also arise.

Test-Taking Strategy: Think about the pathophysiology of increased ICP. If you remember that blood pressure rises, you are able to eliminate options 1 and 2 as comparable or alike. To select from the remaining options, remember that the temperature rises. **Review: increased ICP.**
Level of Cognitive Ability: Analyzing
Client Needs: Physiological Integrity
Integrated Process: Nursing Process/Data Collection
Content Area: Adult Health: Neurological
Priority Concepts: Gas Exchange, Intracranial Regulation
Reference(s): deWit, Kumagai (2013), pp. 506–507.

599. 2
Rationale: The head of the client with increased ICP should be positioned so that the head is in a neutral, midline position. The nurse should avoid flexing or extending the neck or turning the head side to side. The head of the bed should be raised to 30 to 45 degrees. Use of proper positions promotes venous drainage from the cranium to keep ICP down.
Test-Taking Strategy: Focus on the subject, the need for the nurse to intervene. This indicates a position that interferes with arterial circulation to the brain or with venous drainage from the brain. The only answer that meets one of those criteria is option 2. **Review:** client positioning with **increased intracranial pressure.**
Level of Cognitive Ability: Applying
Client Needs: Physiological Integrity
Integrated Process: Nursing Process/Implementation
Content Area: Adult Health: Neurological
Priority Concepts: Intracranial Regulation, Safety
Reference(s): deWit, Kumagai (2013), pp. 505, 508.

600. 4
Rationale: Activities that increase intrathoracic and intraabdominal pressures cause indirect elevation of the ICP. Some of these activities include isometric exercises, Valsalva maneuver, coughing, sneezing, and blowing the nose. Exhaling during activities such as repositioning or pulling up in bed opens the glottis, which prevents intrathoracic pressure from rising.
Test-Taking Strategy: Focus on the subject, activities that increase intracranial pressure. Evaluate each option in terms of the tension it puts on the body to help you eliminate each of the incorrect options. **Review: increased intracranial pressure.**
Level of Cognitive Ability: Evaluating
Client Needs: Physiological Integrity
Integrated Process: Nursing Process/Evaluation
Content Area: Adult Health: Neurological
Priority Concepts: Client Education, Intracranial Regulation
Reference(s): deWit, Kumagai (2013), pp. 508–509.

601. 4
Rationale: Leakage of CSF from the ears or nose may accompany basilar skull fracture. It can be distinguished from other body fluids because the drainage will separate into bloody and yellow concentric rings on dressing material, which is known as the halo sign. It also tests positive for glucose. Options 1, 2, and 3 are not characteristics of CSF.
Test-Taking Strategy: Focus on the subject, the characteristics of CSF. Recall that CSF contains glucose, whereas other secretions such as mucus do not. Also, remember that CSF separates into rings. **Review: cerebrospinal fluid.**
Level of Cognitive Ability: Analyzing
Client Needs: Physiological Integrity
Integrated Process: Nursing Process/Data Collection
Content Area: Adult Health: Neurological
Priority Concepts: Glucose Regulation, Intracranial Regulation
Reference(s): deWit, Kumagai (2013), p. 502; Lewis et al (2014), p. 1374.

602. 4
Rationale: There is a significant association between cervical spine injury and head injury. For this reason, the nurse leaves any form of spinal immobilization in place until lateral cervical spine x-rays rule out fracture or other damage and the results have been reviewed by the health care provider.
Test-Taking Strategy: Focus on the subject, the client's injury. Remember that the reason for spinal immobilization is to protect the spine from movement, which could cause further damage if the cervical spine were injured. If x-ray results are negative, the health care provider will discontinue the cervical collar. **Review: cervical injury.**
Level of Cognitive Ability: Applying
Client Needs: Physiological Integrity
Integrated Process: Nursing Process/Implementation
Content Area: Adult Health: Neurological
Priority Concepts: Clinical Judgment, Mobility
Reference(s): deWit, Kumagai (2013), p. 511.

603. 2
Rationale: A concussion after head injury is a temporary loss of consciousness (from a few seconds to a few minutes) without evidence of structural damage. After concussion, the family is taught to monitor the client and call the health care provider or return the client to the emergency department if certain signs and symptoms are noted. These include confusion, difficulty awakening or speaking, one-sided weakness, vomiting, or severe headache. Minor headache is expected.
Test-Taking Strategy: Note the strategic words, *needs further teaching.* These words indicate a negative event query and the need to select the incorrect family statement. Noting the word *minor* in option 2 will direct you to this option. **Review: concussions.**
Level of Cognitive Ability: Evaluating
Client Needs: Physiological Integrity
Integrated Process: Teaching and Learning
Content Area: Adult Health: Neurological
Priority Concepts: Client Education, Cognition
Reference(s): Lewis et al (2014), pp. 1369–1370.

604. 3
Rationale: Following supratentorial surgery, the head of the bed is kept at a 30- to 45-degree angle. The head and neck should not be angled either anteriorly or laterally, but rather should be kept in a neutral (midline) position. This will promote venous return through the jugular veins, which will help prevent a rise in intracranial pressure.
Test-Taking Strategy: This question tests knowledge of the subject, differences in positioning the craniotomy client with an infratentorial versus supratentorial incision. If you remember that with *supra-* one should *keep the head up,* and with *infra-* one should *keep the head down,* options 1 and 2 can be eliminated. Knowing how to position the head for optimal

venous drainage helps you select option 3 over option 4. Review: craniotomy.
Level of Cognitive Ability: Applying
Client Needs: Physiological Integrity
Integrated Process: Nursing Process/Planning
Content Area: Adult Health: Neurological
Priority Concepts: Clinical Judgment, Intracranial Regulation
Reference(s): deWit, Kumagai (2013), pp. 502–503.

605. 4
Rationale: Crutchfield tongs are applied after drilling holes in the client's skull under local anesthesia. Weights are attached to the tongs, which exert pulling pressure on the longitudinal axis of the cervical spine. The nurse ensures that weights hang freely and that the amount of weight matches the current prescription. The client with Crutchfield tongs is placed on a Stryker frame or Roto-Rest bed. The nurse does not remove the weights to administer care or change the level of tension or traction based on client comfort level.
Test-Taking Strategy: Note the **strategic word**, *essential.* Recalling the basic principles of traction care and that weights are not removed will direct you to the correct option. **Review: cervical tongs.**
Level of Cognitive Ability: Applying
Client Needs: Physiological Integrity
Integrated Process: Nursing Process/Planning
Content Area: Adult Health: Neurological
Priority Concepts: Mobility, Safety
Reference(s): Lewis et al (2014), p. 1476.

606. 2
Rationale: The client should not drive because the device impairs the range of vision. The halo device alters balance and can cause fatigue because of its weight. The client should cleanse the skin daily under the vest or the device to protect the skin from ulceration and should use powder or lotions sparingly or not at all. The wool liner should be changed if odor becomes a problem. The client should have food cut into small pieces to facilitate chewing and use a straw for drinking. Pin care is done as instructed.
Test-Taking Strategy: Note the **strategic words**, *needs further teaching.* These words indicate a **negative event query** and the need to select the incorrect client statement. Recall that a halo device is used to allow mobility for the client who needs continuous cervical traction; it maintains the head and spine in a neutral position. With this in mind, select option 2 as the correct option. The inability to turn the head without turning the torso would contraindicate driving. **Review: halo device.**
Level of Cognitive Ability: Evaluating
Client Needs: Safe and Effective Care Environment
Integrated Process: Teaching and Learning
Content Area: Adult Health: Neurological
Priority Concepts: Intracranial Regulation, Safety
Reference(s): Lewis et al (2014), p. 1482.

607. 3
Rationale: The client with spinal cord injury above the level of T7 is at risk for autonomic dysreflexia. It is characterized by a severe, throbbing headache, flushing of the face and neck, bradycardia, and sudden severe hypertension. Other signs include nasal stuffiness, blurred vision, nausea, and sweating. It is a life-threatening syndrome triggered by a noxious stimulus below the level of the injury.
Test-Taking Strategy: Focus on the **subject**, autonomic dysreflexia. Remember that it results from the sudden exaggerated response of the sympathetic nervous system to a noxious stimulus. A massive sympathetic nervous system response causes severe hypertension. This would account for the throbbing headache (the correct answer) and cause flushing of the face and neck. Baroreceptors sense the sudden hypertension, causing a reflex bradycardia. Also remember that the pulse and blood pressure changes that occur with autonomic dysreflexia are actually the opposite of what would occur with hypovolemic shock. **Review: autonomic dysreflexia.**
Level of Cognitive Ability: Analyzing
Client Needs: Physiological Integrity
Integrated Process: Nursing Process/Data Collection
Content Area: Adult Health: Neurological
Priority Concepts: Clinical Judgment, Intracranial Regulation
Reference(s): deWit, Kumagai (2013), p. 515.

608. 4
Rationale: The most frequent cause of autonomic dysreflexia is a distended bladder. Straight catheterization should be performed every 4 to 6 hours, and indwelling bladder catheters should be checked frequently for kinks in the tubing. It is not appropriate to catheterize the client every 12 hours. Constipation and fecal impaction are other causes, so maintaining bowel regularity is important. Other causes include stimulation of the skin from tactile, thermal, or painful stimuli. The nurse administers care to minimize risk in these areas.
Test-Taking Strategy: Note the **strategic words**, *least appropriate.* The least appropriate action is the action that should not be taken. Remember that autonomic dysreflexia is caused by noxious stimuli to the bowel, bladder, or skin. With this in mind, you can eliminate the incorrect options because they are the correct thing to do for the client. **Review: autonomic dysreflexia.**
Level of Cognitive Ability: Applying
Client Needs: Physiological Integrity
Integrated Process: Nursing Process/Implementation
Content Area: Adult Health: Neurological
Priority Concepts: Clinical Judgment, Intracranial Regulation
Reference(s): Lewis et al (2014), p. 1479.

609. 1
Rationale: Key nursing actions are to sit the client up in bed, remove the noxious stimulus, and bring the blood pressure under control with antihypertensive medication per protocol. The nurse can also clearly label the client's chart identifying the risk for autonomic dysreflexia. Client and family should be taught to recognize, and later manage, the signs and symptoms of this syndrome.
Test-Taking Strategy: Note the **strategic word**, *immediate.* This indicates that this is the first action you would take. If you know to raise the head of the client's bed first (to try to minimize cerebral hypertension), then this eliminates each of the incorrect options. **Review: autonomic dysreflexia.**
Level of Cognitive Ability: Applying
Client Needs: Physiological Integrity
Integrated Process: Nursing Process/Implementation
Content Area: Adult Health: Neurological

Priority Concepts: Clinical Judgment, Intracranial Regulation
Reference(s): deWit, Kumagai (2013), p. 515.

610. 4

Rationale: The client undergoing a lumbar puncture (LP) is positioned lying on the side, with the knees bent, drawn up to the abdomen, and the chin tucked into the chest. This position helps to open the spaces between the vertebrae.
Test-Taking Strategy: Focus on the subject, positioning for a lumbar puncture (LP). Recall that an LP is the introduction of a needle into the subarachnoid space, so it is reasonable that the position of the client must facilitate this. The correct answer is the only position that flexes the vertebrae for easier needle insertion. **Review: lumbar puncture.**
Level of Cognitive Ability: Applying
Client Needs: Physiological Integrity
Integrated Process: Nursing Process/Implementation
Content Area: Fundamental Skills: Diagnostic Tests
Priority Concepts: Clinical Judgment, Safety
Reference(s): deWit, Kumagai (2013), pp. 481, 489.

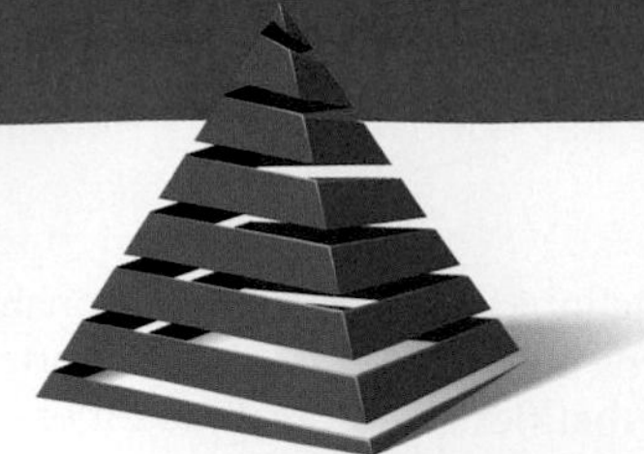

CHAPTER 58

Neurological Medications

CRITICAL THINKING What Should You Do?

A client with a traumatic brain injury experiencing restlessness and agitation due to the pain is receiving morphine sulfate. On data collection the nurse measures the respiratory rate and notes it to be 10 breaths/minute. What should the nurse do?

Answer located on p. 835.

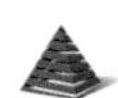

I. Antimyasthenic Medications

A. Description

1. Antimyasthenic medications, also called anticholinesterase medications relieve muscle weakness associated with myasthenia gravis by blocking acetylcholine breakdown at the neuromuscular junction.
2. Antimyasthenic medications are used to treat or diagnose myasthenia gravis or distinguish cholinergic crisis from myasthenic crisis.
3. Neostigmine bromide (Prostigmin), pyridostigmine (Mestinon), and ambenonium chloride (Mytelase) are used to control myasthenic symptoms.
4. Edrophonium chloride (Enlon) is used to diagnose myasthenia gravis and distinguish cholinergic crisis from myasthenic crisis.

B. Medications (Box 58-1)

C. Side/adverse effects: Cholinergic crisis (Box 58-2)

D. Interventions

1. Monitor neuromuscular status, including reflexes, muscle strength, and gait.
2. Monitor the client for signs and symptoms of medication overdose (cholinergic crisis) and underdose (myasthenic crisis).
3. Reinforce instructions to the client to take medications on time to maintain therapeutic blood level, thus preventing weakness, because weakness can impair the client's ability to breathe and swallow.
4. Reinforce instructions to the client to take the medication with a small amount of food to prevent gastrointestinal symptoms.
5. Reinforce instructions to the client to eat 45 to 60 minutes after taking medications to decrease the risk for aspiration.
6. Reinforce instructions to the client to wear a Medic-Alert bracelet.
7. Note that antimyasthenic therapy is lifelong therapy.
8. Evaluate for medication effectiveness, which is based on the improvement of neuromuscular symptoms or strength without cholinergic signs and symptoms.
9. When administering edrophonium chloride, have emergency resuscitation equipment on hand and atropine sulfate available for cholinergic crisis.

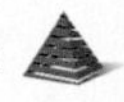

E. Edrophonium (Enlon) test (may be known as the Tensilon test)

1. Edrophonium (Enlon) is injected intravenously.
2. The edrophonium (Enlon) can cause bronchospasm, laryngospasm, hypotension, bradycardia, and cardiac arrest.
3. Atropine sulfate is the antidote for overdose.
4. Diagnosis of myasthenia gravis: Most myasthenic clients show a significant improvement in muscle tone within 30 to 60 seconds after injection, and the muscle improvement lasts 4 to 5 minutes.

BOX 58-1 Antimyasthenic Medications

Ambenonium chloride (Mytelase)
Edrophonium chloride (Enlon, Tensilon)
Neostigmine bromide (Prostigmin)
Pyridostigmine (Mestinon)

BOX 58-2 Signs of Cholinergic Crisis

Abdominal cramps
Nausea, vomiting, and diarrhea
Pupillary miosis
Hypotension and dizziness
Increased bronchial secretions
Increased tearing and salivation
Increased perspiration
Increased bronchial secretions
Bronchospasm, wheezing, and bradycardia

5. The test is used to diagnose cholinergic crisis (overdose with anticholinesterase) or myasthenic crisis (undermedication).
   a. In cholinergic crisis, muscle tone does not improve after the administration of edrophonium, and muscle twitching may be noted around the eyes and face.
   b. An edrophonium injection temporarily worsens the condition when a client is in cholinergic crisis (negative edrophonium test).
   c. An edrophonium injection temporarily improves the condition when the client is in myasthenic crisis (positive test).

II. Antiparkinsonian Medications

A. Description
   1. Antiparkinsonian medications restore the balance of the neurotransmitters acetylcholine and dopamine in the central nervous system (CNS), decreasing the signs and symptoms of Parkinson's disease to maximize the client's functional abilities.
   2. These medications include the dopaminergics, which stimulate the dopamine receptors; the anticholinergics, which block the cholinergic receptors; and the catechol-*O*-methyltransferase inhibitors, which inhibit the metabolism of dopamine in the periphery.

B. Dopaminergic medications
   1. Description
      a. Dopaminergic medications stimulate the dopamine receptors and increase the amount of dopamine available in the CNS or enhance neurotransmission of dopamine.
      b. Dopaminergic medications are contraindicated in clients with cardiac, renal, or psychiatric disorders.

⚠ Levodopa taken with a monoamine oxidase inhibitor antidepressant can cause a hypertensive crisis.

   2. Medications (Box 58-3 and Fig. 58-1)
   3. Side/adverse effects
      a. Dyskinesia
      b. Involuntary body movements
      c. Chest pain
      d. Nausea and vomiting
      e. Urinary retention
      f. Constipation
      g. Sleep disturbances, insomnia, or periods of sedation
      h. Orthostatic hypotension and dizziness
      i. Confusion
      j. Mood changes, especially depression
      k. Hallucinations
      l. Dry mouth

BOX 58-3 Medications to Treat Parkinson's Disease

Medications Affecting the Amount of Dopamine
Amantadine
Apomorphine (Apokyn)
Bromocriptine (Parlodel)
Carbidopa; levodopa (Sinemet)
Levodopa (Larodopa)
Pramipexole (Mirapex)
Ropinirole (Requip)
Selegiline hydrochloride (Eldepryl)

Anticholinergics
Benztropine mesylate (Cogentin)
Biperiden hydrochloride (Akineton)
Trihexyphenidyl hydrochloride

Catechol *O*-Methyltransferase (COMT) Inhibitors
Carbidopa/levodopa/entacapone (Stalevo)
Entacapone (Comtan)
Tolcapone (Tasmar)

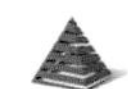

   4. Interventions
      a. Monitor the vital signs.
      b. Determine the risk for injury.
      c. The client is instructed to take the medication with food if nausea or vomiting occurs.
      d. Check for signs and symptoms of parkinsonism, such as rigidity, tremors, akinesia and bradykinesia, a stooped forward posture, shuffling gait, and masked facies.
      e. Monitor for signs of dyskinesia.
      f. The client is instructed to report side/adverse effects and symptoms of dyskinesia.
      g. Monitor the client for improvement in signs and symptoms of parkinsonism without the development of side/adverse effects from the medications.
      h. The client is instructed to change positions slowly to minimize orthostatic hypotension.
      i. Reinforce instructions to the client to not discontinue the medication abruptly.
      j. Reinforce instructions to the client to avoid alcohol.
      k. The client is informed that urine or perspiration may be discolored and that this is harmless but may stain clothing.
      l. The client with diabetes mellitus is advised that glucose testing should not be done by urine testing because the results will not be reliable.
      m. Reinforce instructions to the client taking carbidopa-levodopa (Sinemet) to divide the total daily prescribed protein intake among all meals of the day. High-protein diets interfere with medication availability to the CNS.

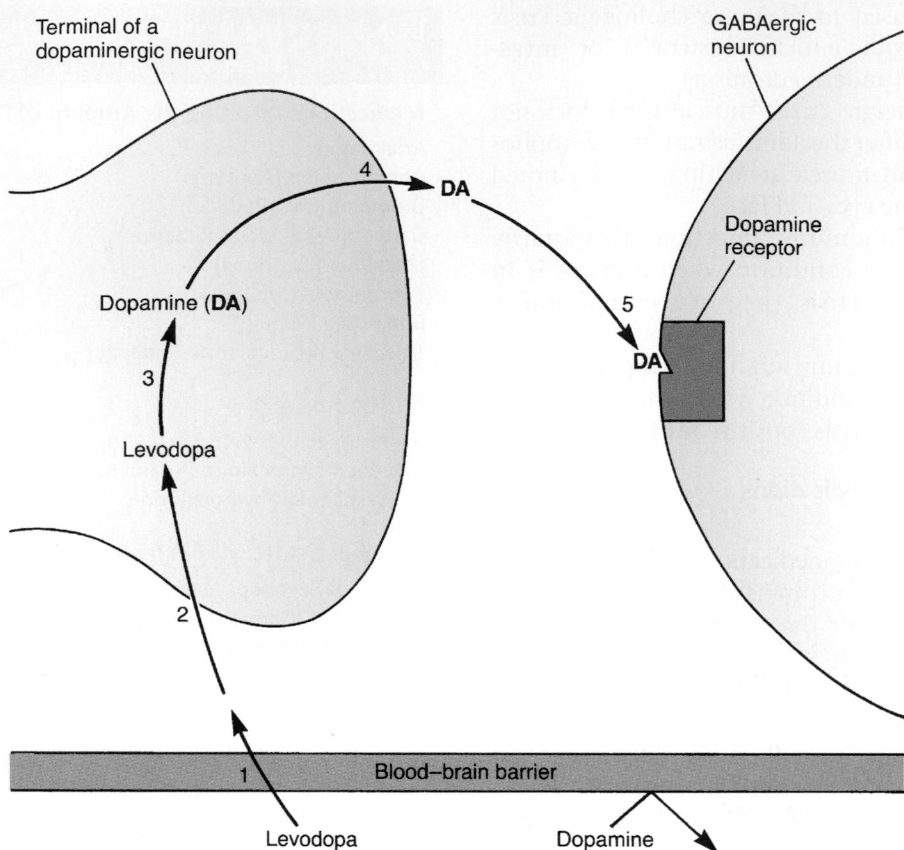

FIGURE 58-1 Steps leading to alteration of central nervous system function by levodopa. To produce its beneficial effects in Parkinson's disease (PD), levodopa must be (1) transported across the blood–brain barrier; (2) taken up by dopaminergic nerve terminals in the striatum; (3) converted into dopamine (DA); (4) released into the synaptic space; and (5) bound to DA receptors on striatal GABAergic neurons, causing them to fire at a slower rate. Note that DA itself is unable to cross the blood–brain barrier and thus cannot be used to treat PD. (From Lehne RA: *Pharmacology for nursing care*, ed 7, St. Louis, 2010, Saunders.)

- **n.** When administering levodopa, the client is instructed to avoid excessive vitamin B_6 intake to prevent medication reactions.

C. Anticholinergic medications

1. Description

- **a.** Anticholinergic medications block the cholinergic receptors in the CNS, thereby suppressing acetylcholine activity.
- **b.** Anticholinergic medications reduce tremors and drooling but have a minimal effect on bradykinesia, rigidity, and balance abnormalities.

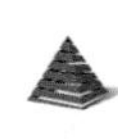
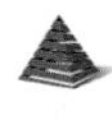

- **c.** Anticholinergic medications are contraindicated in clients with glaucoma.
- **d.** The client with chronic obstructive lung disease can develop dry, thick mucus secretions.

2. Medications (see Box 58-3)

3. Side/adverse effects

- **a.** Blurred vision
- **b.** Dryness of the nose, mouth, throat, and respiratory secretions
- **c.** Increased pulse rate, palpitations, and dysrhythmias
- **d.** Constipation
- **e.** Urinary retention
- **f.** Restlessness, confusion, depression, and hallucinations
- **g.** Photophobia

4. Interventions

- **a.** Monitor the vital signs.
- **b.** Determine the risk for injury.
- **c.** Monitor the client for improvement in signs and symptoms.
- **d.** Check the client's bowel and urinary function, and monitor for urinary retention, constipation, and paralytic ileus.
- **e.** Monitor for involuntary movements.
- **f.** The client is encouraged to avoid alcohol, smoking, caffeine, and aspirin to decrease gastric acidity.
- **g.** Reinforce instructions to the client to consult with the health care provider (HCP) before taking any nonprescription medications.
- **h.** Reinforce instructions to the client to minimize dry mouth by increasing fluid intake and using ice chips, hard candy, or gum.

i. Reinforce instructions to the client to prevent constipation by increasing fluids and fiber in the diet.
j. Reinforce instructions to the client to use sunglasses in direct sunlight because of possible photophobia.
k. Reinforce instructions to the client to have routine eye examinations to assess for intraocular pressure.

If an anticholinergic medication is discontinued abruptly, the signs and symptoms of parkinsonism, such as rigidity, tremors, akinesia and bradykinesia, a stooped forward posture, shuffling gait, and masked facies may be intensified.

III. Anticonvulsant Medications

A. Description
1. Anticonvulsant medications are used to depress abnormal neuronal discharges and prevent the spread of seizures to adjacent neurons.
2. Anticonvulsant medications should be used with caution in clients taking anticoagulants, aspirin, sulfonamides, cimetidine (Tagamet), and antipsychotic drugs.
3. Absorption is decreased with the use of antacids, calcium preparations, and antineoplastic medications.

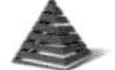

B. Interventions for clients on anticonvulsants
1. Initiate seizure precautions.
2. Monitor urinary output.
3. Monitor liver and renal function tests and medication blood serum levels (Table 58-1).
4. Monitor for signs of medication toxicity, which would include CNS depression, ataxia, nausea, vomiting, drowsiness, dizziness, restlessness, and visual disturbances.
5. If a seizure occurs, monitor seizure activity, including location and duration.

TABLE 58-1 Anticonvulsant Medications

Medication	Therapeutic Serum Range
Amobarbital (Amytal)	1–5 mcg/mL
Carbamazepine (Tegretol)	3–14 mcg/mL
Clonazepam (Klonopin)	20–80 ng/mL
Ethosuximide (Zarontin)	40–100 mcg/mL
Ethotoin (Peganone)	10–50 mcg/mL
Lorazepam (Ativan)	50–240 ng/mL
Mephobarbital (Mebaral)	15–40 mcg/mL
Phenobarbital (Luminal)	15–40 mcg/mL
Phenytoin (Dilantin)	10–20 mcg/mL

BOX 58-4 Client Education: Anticonvulsants

- Take the prescribed medication in the prescribed dose and frequency.
- Take anticonvulsants with food to decrease gastrointestinal irritation, but avoid milk and antacids, which impair absorption.
- If taking liquid medication, shake well before ingesting.
- Do not discontinue the medications.
- Avoid alcohol.
- Avoid over-the-counter medications.
- Wear a Medic-Alert bracelet.
- Use caution when driving or performing activities that require alertness.
- Maintain good oral hygiene, and use a soft toothbrush.
- Maintain preventive dental checkups.
- Maintain follow-up health care visits with periodic blood studies related to determining toxicity.
- Monitor serum glucose levels (diabetes mellitus).
- Urine may be a harmless pink-red or red-brown in color.
- Report symptoms of sore throat, bruising, and nosebleeds, which may indicate a blood dyscrasia.
- Inform the HCP if side/adverse effects occur, such as gingivitis, nystagmus, slurred speech, rash, or dizziness.

6. Protect the client from hazards in the environment during a seizure.

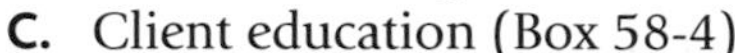
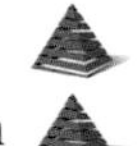

C. Client education (Box 58-4)

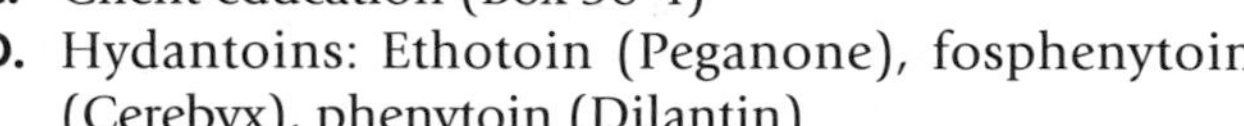

D. Hydantoins: Ethotoin (Peganone), fosphenytoin (Cerebyx), phenytoin (Dilantin)

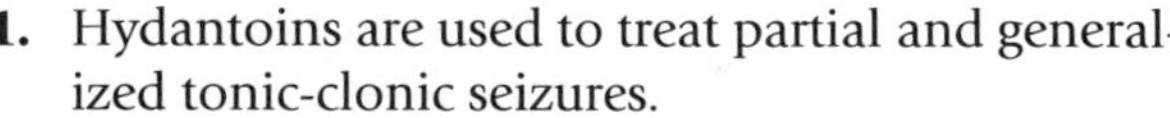

1. Hydantoins are used to treat partial and generalized tonic-clonic seizures.
2. Phenytoin (Dilantin) also is used to treat dysrhythmias.

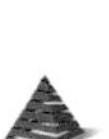
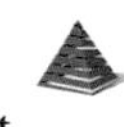

3. Side/adverse effects
a. Gingival hyperplasia (reddened gums that bleed easily)
b. Slurred speech
c. Confusion
d. Sedation and drowsiness
e. Nausea and vomiting
f. Blurred vision and nystagmus
g. Headaches
h. Blood dyscrasias: Decreased platelet count and decreased white blood cell count
i. Elevated blood glucose level
j. Alopecia or hirsutism
k. Skin rash or pruritus
4. Interventions
a. Tube feedings may interfere with the absorption of the enteral form of phenytoin and diminish the effectiveness of the medication; therefore, feedings should be scheduled as far as possible from the time of phenytoin administration.
b. Monitor therapeutic serum levels to assess for toxicity.

c. Monitor for signs of toxicity.
d. Monitor for ataxia (staggering gait).
e. Reinforce instructions to the client to consult with the health care provider before taking other medications to ensure compatibility with anticonvulsants.

⚠ Phenytoin decreases the effectiveness of some birth control pills and can have teratogenic effects if taken during pregnancy.

E. Barbiturates: Amobarbital (Amytal), mephobarbital (Mebaral), phenobarbital (Luminal)
1. Barbiturates are used for tonic-clonic seizures and acute episodes of seizures caused by status epilepticus.
2. Barbiturates also may be used as adjuncts to anesthesia.
3. Side/adverse effects
a. Sedation, ataxia, and dizziness during initial treatment
b. Mood changes
c. Hypotension
d. Respiratory depression
e. Tolerance to the medication

F. Benzodiazepines: Clonazepam (Klonopin), clorazepate (Tranxene), diazepam (Valium), lorazepam (Ativan), alprazolam (Xanax)
1. Benzodiazepines are used to treat absence seizures.
2. Diazepam (Valium), alprazolam (Xanax), and lorazepam (Ativan) are used to treat status epilepticus, anxiety, and skeletal muscle spasms.
3. Clorazepate (Tranxene) is used as adjunctive therapy for partial seizures.
4. Side/adverse effects
a. Sedation, drowsiness, dizziness, blurred vision
b. Bradycardia can occur when administered rapidly by the intravenous route.
c. Medication tolerance and drug dependency
d. Blood dyscrasias: Decreased platelet count and decreased white blood cell count
e. Hepatotoxicity

⚠ Flumazenil (Romazicon) reverses the effects of benzodiazepines. It should not be administered to clients with increased intracranial pressure or status epilepticus who were treated with benzodiazepines because these problems may recur with reversal.

G. Succinimides: Ethosuximide (Zarontin), methsuximide (Celontin)
1. Succinimides are used to treat absence seizures.
2. Side/adverse effects
a. Anorexia, nausea, vomiting
b. Blood dyscrasias

H. Valproates: valproic acid (Depakene, Depacon), divalproex sodium (Depakote ER)
1. Valproates are used to treat tonic-clonic, partial and myoclonic seizures.
2. Side/adverse effects
a. Transient nausea, vomiting, and indigestion
b. Sedation, drowsiness, and dizziness
c. Pancreatitis
d. Blood dyscrasias
e. Hepatotoxicity

I. Iminostilbenes
1. Iminostilbenes are used to treat seizure disorders that have not responded to other anticonvulsants
2. Iminostilbenes are used to treat trigeminal neuralgia.
3. Side/adverse effects
a. Drowsiness
b. Dizziness
c. Nausea and vomiting, dry mouth
d. Constipation or diarrhea
e. Rash
f. Visual abnormalities
g. Blood dyscrasias
h. Headache

J. Other anticonvulsants (Box 58-5)

IV. Central Nervous System Stimulants

A. Description
1. Amphetamines and caffeine stimulate the cerebral cortex of the brain (Box 58-6).
2. Amphetamines have a high potential for abuse.
3. Analeptics and caffeine act on the brainstem and medulla to stimulate respiration.

BOX 58-5 Other Anticonvulsants

Carbamazepine (Tegretol)
Gabapentin (Neurontin)
Lacosamide (Vimpat)
Lamotrigine (Lamictal)
Levetiracetam (Keppra)
Oxcarbazepine (Trileptal)
Pregabalin (Lyrica)
Tiagabine (Gabitril Filmtab tablets)
Topiramate (Topamax)
Zonisamide (Zonegran)
Vigabatrin (Sabril)

Box 58-6 Amphetamines

Amphetamine sulfate
Amphetamine; dextroamphetamine (Adderall)
Atomoxetine (Strattera)
Dexmethylphenidate (Focalin)
Methylphenidate hydrochloride (Ritalin, Concerta)

BOX 58-7 Anorexiants

Benzphetamine hydrochloride (Didrex)
Orlistat (Xenical, Alli)
Phendimetrazine (Bontril, Melfiat-105)
Phentermine hydrochloride (Adipex-P, Ionamin)
Phentermine/topiramate (Qsymia)

4. Anorexiants act on the cerebral cortex and hypothalamus to suppress appetite (Box 58-7).
5. Central nervous system stimulants are used to treat narcolepsy and attention-deficit/hyperactivity disorders.
6. Central nervous system stimulants are used as adjunctive therapy for exogenous obesity.
7. Other central nervous system stimulants: Doxapram (Dopram), theobromine, theophylline (Theo-24)

B. Side/adverse effects
1. Irritability
2. Restlessness
3. Tremors
4. Insomnia
5. Heart palpitations
6. Tachycardia and dysrhythmias
7. Hypertension
8. Dry mouth
9. Anorexia and weight loss
10. Abdominal cramping
11. Diarrhea or constipation
12. Hepatic failure
13. Psychoses
14. Impotence
15. Dependence and tolerance

C. Interventions
1. Monitor the vital signs.
2. Monitor the mental status.
3. Degrees of inattention, impulsivity, hyperactivity, and periods of sleepiness are documented.
4. Check height, weight, and growth if prescribed for a child.
5. Monitor the complete blood count and white blood cell and platelet counts before and during therapy.
6. Monitor for side/adverse effects.
7. Monitor the sleep patterns.
8. Monitor for withdrawal symptoms such as nausea, vomiting, weakness, and headache.
9. Reinforce instructions to the client to take the medication before meals.
10. Reinforce instructions to the client to avoid foods and beverages containing caffeine to prevent additional stimulation.
11. Reinforce instructions to the client to not chew or crush long-acting forms of the medications.
12. Reinforce instructions to the client to read labels on over-the-counter products because many contain caffeine.
13. Reinforce instructions to the client to avoid alcohol.
14. Reinforce instructions to the client not to discontinue the medication abruptly.
15. Reinforce instructions to the client to take the last daily dose of the CNS stimulant at least 6 hours before bedtime to prevent insomnia.
16. Monitor for drug dependence and abuse with amphetamines.
17. If a child is taking a CNS stimulant, instruct the parents to notify the school nurse.
18. Monitor for calming effects of CNS stimulants within 3 to 4 weeks on children with attention-deficit/hyperactivity disorder.
19. Monitor growth in the child on long-term therapy with methylphenidate hydrochloride (Ritalin) or other medication to treat attention-deficit/hyperactivity disorder.

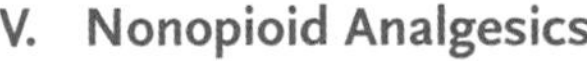

V. Nonopioid Analgesics

A. Nonsteroidal anti-inflammatory drugs (NSAIDs) (Box 58-8)

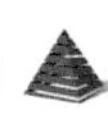

BOX 58-8 Nonopioid Analgesics

Acetaminophen
Acetaminophen (Tylenol)

Aspirin
Aspirin (acetylsalicylic acid) (ASA, Aspergum, Bayer Aspirin, Ecotrin)
Buffered aspirin (acetylsalicylic acid) (Alka-Seltzer, Bufferin, others)

Nonsteroidal Anti-inflammatory Drugs
Fenoprofen (Nalfon)
Ibuprofen (Motrin, Advil)
Naproxen (Anaprox, Aleve, Naprelan, Naprosyn)
Oxaprozin (Daypro)

Cyclooxygenase-2 (COX-2) Inhibitor
Celecoxib (Celebrex)

Other Nonsteroidal Anti-inflammatory Drugs
Diclofenac (Voltaren)
Diflunisal (Dolobid)
Etodolac (Lodine)
Indomethacin (Indocin)
Ketoprofen (Orudis)
Ketorolac (Toradol)
Meclofenamate
Mefenamic acid (Ponstel)
Meloxicam (Mobic)
Piroxicam (Feldene)
Sulindac (Clinoril)

1. Description
   a. NSAIDs are aspirin and aspirin-like medications that inhibit the synthesis of prostaglandins.
   b. The medications act as an analgesic to relieve pain, as an antipyretic to reduce body temperature, and as an anticoagulant to inhibit platelet aggregation.
   c. NSAIDs are used to relieve inflammation and pain and treat rheumatoid arthritis, bursitis, tendinitis, osteoarthritis, and acute gout.
   d. NSAIDs are contraindicated in clients with hypersensitivity or liver or renal disease.
   e. Clients taking anticoagulants should not take aspirin or NSAIDs.
   f. Aspirin and an NSAID should not be taken together because aspirin decreases the blood level and the effectiveness of the NSAID and can increase the risk of bleeding.
   g. NSAIDs can increase the effects of warfarin (Coumadin), sulfonamides, cephalosporins, and phenytoin (Dilantin).
   h. Hypoglycemia can result if ibuprofen (Motrin) is taken with insulin or an oral hypoglycemic medication.
   i. A high risk of toxicity exists if ibuprofen is taken concurrently with calcium channel blockers.

BOX 58-9 Side Effects of Aspirin and Nonsteroidal Anti-inflammatory Drugs

Aspirin

Allergic reactions (anaphylaxis, laryngeal edema)
Bleeding (anemia, hemolysis, increased bleeding time)
Decreased renal function
Dizziness
Drowsiness
Flushing
Gastrointestinal symptoms (distress, heartburn, nausea, vomiting)
Headaches
Tinnitus
Visual changes

Nonsteroidal Anti-inflammatory Drugs

Dysrhythmias
Blood dyscrasias
Cardiovascular thrombotic events
Decreased renal function
Dizziness
Gastric irritation
Hepatotoxicity
Hypotension
Pruritus
Sodium and water retention
Tinnitus

Adolescents and children with flu symptoms, viral illnesses, and varicella should not take aspirin because of the risk of Reye's syndrome.

2. Side/adverse effects (Box 58-9)
3. Interventions
   a. Check client for allergies.
   b. Obtain a medication history on the client.
   c. Check for history of gastric upset or bleeding, or liver or renal disease.
   d. Monitor the client for gastrointestinal upset during medication administration.
   e. Monitor for edema.
   f. Monitor serum salicylate (aspirin) level when the client is taking high doses.
   g. Monitor for signs of bleeding such as tarry stools, bleeding gums, petechiae, ecchymosis, and purpura.
   h. Reinforce instructions to the client to take the medication with water, milk, or food.
   i. An enteric-coated or buffered form of aspirin can be taken to decrease gastric distress.
   j. Reinforce instructions to the client that enteric-coated tablets cannot be crushed or broken.
   k. Clients taking aspirin should sit upright for 20 to 30 minutes after taking the dose.
   l. The client is advised to inform other health care professionals they are taking aspirin. 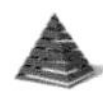
   m. Note that aspirin should be discontinued 3 to 7 days before surgery to reduce the risk of bleeding.
   n. Reinforce instructions to the client to avoid alcoholic beverages.

B. Acetaminophen (Tylenol)  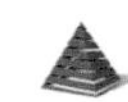 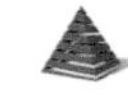 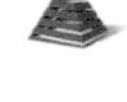 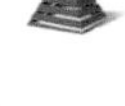      
1. Description
   a. Acetaminophen is used to decrease pain and fever.
   b. Acetaminophen should not be taken if liver dysfunction exists.
2. Side/adverse effects
   a. Anorexia, nausea, vomiting
   b. Rash
   c. Hypoglycemia
   d. Oliguria
   e. Hepatotoxicity
3. Interventions
   a. Monitor the vital signs.
   b. Check the client for a history of liver and renal dysfunction, alcoholism, and malnutrition.
   c. Monitor for hepatic damage, which includes nausea, vomiting, diarrhea, and abdominal pain.
   d. Monitor the liver enzyme test results.

e. Reinforce instructions to the client that self-medication should not be used longer than 10 days for an adult and 5 days for a child.
f. Note that the antidote for acetaminophen is acetylcysteine.
g. Evaluate for the effectiveness of the medication.

Acetaminophen is contraindicated in clients with hepatic or renal disease, alcoholism, and/or hypersensitivity.

VI. Opioid Analgesics

A. Description
1. Opioid analgesics suppress pain impulses but can suppress respiration and coughing by acting on the respiratory and cough center in the medulla of the brainstem.
2. Opioid analgesics can produce euphoria and sedation and cause physical dependence.
3. Opioid analgesics are used for relief of mild, moderate, or severe pain.

B. Medications (Box 58-10)
1. Codeine sulfate
a. Codeine sulfate also is an effective cough suppressant at low doses.
b. Codeine sulfate can cause constipation.
2. Hydromorphone hydrochloride (Dilaudid)
a. Hydromorphone can decrease respiration.
b. Hydromorphone can cause constipation.
3. Meperidine hydrochloride (Demerol)
a. Meperidine can cause hypotension, dizziness, and urinary retention.
b. Meperidine may be used for acute pain and as a preoperative medication.

BOX 58-10 Opioid Analgesics

Acetaminophen/hydrocodone (Lortab)
Buprenorphine hydrochloride (Butrans)
Butorphanol tartrate (Stadol)
Codeine sulfate, codeine phosphate
Fentanyl (Duragesic, Sublimaze)
Hydrocodone (Hycodan)
Hydromorphone hydrochloride (Dilaudid)
Levorphanol tartrate
Meperidine hydrochloride (Demerol)
Methadone hydrochloride (Dolophine, Methadose)
Morphine sulfate (Duramorph, MS Contin, Kadian, Oramorph SR)
Nalbuphine hydrochloride (Nubain)
Oxycodone (Roxicodone, OxyContin)
Oxycodone hydrochloride; acetaminophen (Percocet)
Oxycodone; aspirin (Percodan)
Oxymorphone hydrochloride (Opana)
Remifentanil (Ultiva)
Sufentanil (Sufenta)
Tramadol (Ultram)

c. Meperidine may lead to increased intracranial pressure in clients with head injuries.
d. Meperidine is contraindicated in clients with head injuries and **increased intracranial pressure**, respiratory disorders, hypotension, shock, and severe hepatic and renal disease and in clients taking monoamine oxidase inhibitors.
e. Meperidine should not be taken with alcohol or a sedative-hypnotic because it may increase the CNS depression.
f. Meperidine should be used cautiously in children and adults with a seizure disorder or a history of seizures because it decreases the seizure threshold.
4. Morphine sulfate
a. Morphine can cause respiratory depression, orthostatic hypotension, and constipation.
b. Morphine may cause nausea and vomiting because of increased vestibular sensitivity.
c. Morphine is used for acute pain caused by myocardial infarction or cancer, for dyspnea caused by pulmonary edema, surgery, and as a preoperative medication.
d. Morphine is contraindicated in clients with severe respiratory disorders; head injuries; increased intracranial pressure; severe renal, hepatic, or pulmonary disease; or seizure activity.
e. Morphine is used with caution in clients with shock or blood loss.

Respiratory depression is the priority concern with opioid analgesics.

5. Oxycodone with acetaminophen (Percocet)
a. Percocet can cause constipation.
b. Percocet can cause gastrointestinal upset and should be taken with food.
6. Nalbuphine hydrochloride (Nubain) is preferable for treating the pain of a myocardial infarction because it reduces the oxygen needs of the heart without reducing blood pressure.
7. Methadone hydrochloride (Dolophine)
a. Doses of oral concentrate are diluted with at least 90 mL of water.
b. Dispersible tablets are diluted in at least 120 mL of water, orange juice, or acidic fruit beverage.
c. Methadone is used as a replacement medication for opiate dependence and to facilitate withdrawal.
8. Hydrocodone/homatropine (Hycodan) frequently is used for cough suppression.

C. Interventions for opioid analgesics 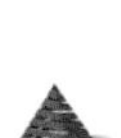
1. Monitor the vital signs.
2. Check the client thoroughly before administering pain medication.

3. Initiate nursing measures such as massage, distraction, deep breathing and relaxation exercises, the application of heat or cold as prescribed, and providing care and comfort before administration of the opioid analgesic.
4. Medications are administered 30 to 60 minutes before painful activities.
5. Monitor respiratory rate, and if the rate is less than 12 breaths/minute in an adult, the medication is withheld unless ventilatory support is being provided.
6. Monitor pulse, and if bradycardia develops, the dose is withheld and the HCP is notified.
7. Monitor the blood pressure for hypotension.
8. Auscultate breath sounds because opioid analgesics suppress the cough reflex.
9. Activities such as turning, deep breathing, and incentive spirometry to prevent atelectasis and pneumonia are encouraged.
10. Monitor the level of consciousness.
11. Initiate safety precautions such as side rails, a night light, and supervised ambulation.
12. Monitor the intake and output (I&O).
13. Monitor for urinary retention.
14. Reinforce instructions to the client to take oral doses with milk or a snack to reduce gastric irritation.
15. Reinforce instructions to the client to avoid alcohol.
16. Reinforce instructions to the client to avoid activities that require alertness.
17. Monitor bowel function for constipation, abdominal distention, and decreased peristalsis.
18. The effectiveness of medication is evaluated.
19. Have the opioid antagonist, oxygen, and resuscitation equipment available.

D. Morphine sulfate and hydromorphone hydrochloride (Dilaudid)
  1. Side/adverse effects
    a. Respiratory depression
    b. Orthostatic hypotension
    c. Urinary retention
    d. Nausea and vomiting
    e. Constipation
    f. Sedation, confusion, and hallucinations
    g. Cough suppression
    h. Reduction in pupillary size
    i. Miosis
  2. Interventions
    a. Have naloxone (Narcan) available for overdose.
    b. Monitor the vital signs and level of consciousness.
    c. Compare the rate and depth of respirations to the baseline.
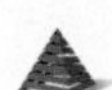
    d. The medication is withheld if the respiratory rate is less than 12 breaths/min (agency policies are followed). Respirations of less than 10 breaths/min can indicate respiratory distress.
    e. Monitor urinary output, which should be at least 30 mL/hr.
    f. Monitor bowel sounds for decreased peristalsis because constipation can occur.
    g. Monitor for pupil changes because pinpoint pupils can indicate morphine overdose.
    h. Reinforce instructions to the client to avoid alcohol or CNS depressants because they can cause respiratory depression.
    i. Reinforce instructions to the client to report dizziness or difficulty breathing.
    j. If taking sustained-release morphine, the client may need short-acting opioid doses for breakthrough pain.
    k. The side/adverse effects of the medication is explained to the client and his or her family.

E. Meperidine hydrochloride (Demerol)
  1. Side/adverse effects
    a. Respiratory depression
    b. Hypotension and dizziness
    c. Tachycardia
    d. Drowsiness and confusion
    e. Constipation
    f. Urinary retention
    g. Nausea and vomiting
    h. Seizures
    i. Tremors
  2. Interventions
    a. Monitor the vital signs.
    b. Monitor for respiratory depression and hypotension.
    c. Have naloxone available for overdose.
    d. Monitor for urinary retention.
    e. Monitor bowel sounds and for constipation.

VII. Opioid Antagonists

A. Opioid antagonists (Box 58-11) are used to treat respiratory depression from opioid overdose.

B. Interventions
  1. Monitor blood pressure, pulse, and respiratory rate every 5 minutes initially, tapering to every 15 minutes, and then every 30 minutes until the client is stable.
  2. Place the client on a cardiac monitor and monitor cardiac rhythm.
  3. Auscultate breath sounds.

BOX 58-11 Opioid Antagonists

Alvimopan (Entereg)
Methylnaltrexone (Relistor)
Naloxone (Narcan)
Naltrexone (Vivitrol)

4. Have resuscitation equipment available.
5. Do not leave the client unattended.
6. Monitor the client closely for several hours because when the effects of the antagonist wear off, the client may again display signs of opioid overdose.

VIII. Osmotic Diuretics

A. Description
1. Osmotic diuretics increase osmotic pressure of the glomerular filtrate, inhibiting reabsorption of water and electrolytes.
2. Osmotic diuretics are used for oliguria and to prevent renal failure, decrease intracranial pressure, and decrease intraocular pressure in clients with narrow-angle glaucoma.
3. Mannitol is used with chemotherapy to induce diuresis.

B. Side/adverse effects
1. Fluid and electrolyte imbalances
2. Pulmonary edema from the rapid shifts of fluid
3. Nausea and vomiting
4. Headache
5. Tachycardia from the rapid fluid loss
6. Hyponatremia and dehydration

C. Interventions
1. Monitor the vital signs.
2. Monitor the weight.
3. Monitor the urine output.
4. Monitor the electrolyte levels.
5. Monitor the lungs and heart sounds for signs of pulmonary edema.
6. Monitor for signs of dehydration.
7. Monitor the neurological status.
8. Monitor for increased intraocular pressure.
9. Check for signs of decreasing intracranial pressure if appropriate.
10. Change the client's position slowly to prevent orthostatic hypotension.

CRITICAL THINKING What Should You Do?

Answer: Morphine sulfate is an opioid analgesic, and an adverse effect is respiratory depression. The nurse needs to monitor the respiratory rate closely, and if the rate is less than 12 breaths/minute in an adult, the nurse needs to withhold the medication unless ventilatory support is being provided and contact the registered nurse and health care provider. The nurse needs to continue to monitor the client closely. Agency policies are always followed regarding the administration of morphine sulfate.

References: Hodgson, Kizior (2015), pp. 812–813; Ignatavicius, Workman (2013), p. 1028.

PRACTICE QUESTIONS

611. The client with myasthenia gravis is suspected of having cholinergic crisis. Which sign/symptom indicates this crisis is taking place?
1. Ataxia
2. Mouth sores
3. Hypothermia
4. Hypertension

❖**612.** The client is receiving meperidine hydrochloride (Demerol) for pain. Which are side/adverse effects of this medication? **Select all that apply.**
- ☐ 1. Diarrhea
- ☐ 2. Tremors
- ☐ 3. Drowsiness
- ☐ 4. Hypotension
- ☐ 5. Urinary frequency
- ☐ 6. Increased respiratory rate

613. The client with myasthenia gravis becomes increasingly weak. The health care provider prepares to identify whether the client is reacting to an overdose of the medication (cholinergic crisis) or increasing severity of the disease (myasthenic crisis). An injection of edrophonium (Enlon) is administered. Which indicates that the client is in cholinergic crisis?
1. No change in the condition
2. Complaints of muscle spasms
3. An improvement of the weakness
4. A temporary worsening of the condition

614. Carbidopa-levodopa (Sinemet) is prescribed for a client with Parkinson's disease, and the nurse monitors the client for adverse effects of the medication. Which sign/symptom indicates the client is experiencing an adverse effect?
1. Pruritus
2. Tachycardia
3. Hypertension
4. Impaired voluntary movements

615. Phenytoin (Dilantin), 100 mg orally three times daily, has been prescribed for a client for seizure control. The nurse reinforces instructions regarding the medication to the client. Which statement by the client indicates an understanding of the instructions?
1. "I will use a soft toothbrush to brush my teeth."
2. "It's all right to break the capsules to make it easier for me to swallow them."
3. "If I forget to take my medication, I can wait until the next dose and eliminate that dose."
4. "If my throat becomes sore, it's a normal effect of the medication and it's nothing to be concerned about."

616. The client is taking phenytoin (Dilantin) for seizure control, and a blood sample for a serum drug level is drawn. Which laboratory finding indicates a therapeutic serum drug result?
1. 5 mcg/mL
2. 15 mcg/mL
3. 25 mcg/mL
4. 30 mcg/mL

617. Ibuprofen (Advil) is prescribed for a client. Which instruction should the nurse give the client about taking this medication?
1. Take with 8 oz of milk.
2. Take in the morning after arising.
3. Take 60 minutes before breakfast.
4. Take at bedtime on an empty stomach.

618. The nurse is caring for a client who is taking phenytoin (Dilantin) for control of seizures. During data collection, the nurse notes that the client is taking birth control pills. Which information should the nurse provide to the client?
1. Pregnancy should be avoided while taking phenytoin (Dilantin).
2. The client may stop taking the phenytoin (Dilantin) if it is causing severe gastrointestinal effects.
3. The potential for decreased effectiveness of the birth control pills exists while taking phenytoin (Dilantin).
4. The increased risk of thrombophlebitis exists while taking phenytoin (Dilantin) and birth control pills together.

619. The client with trigeminal neuralgia is being treated with carbamazepine (Tegretol). Which laboratory result indicates that the client is experiencing an adverse effect of the medication?
1. Sodium level, 140 mEq/L
2. Uric acid level, 5.0 mg/dL
3. White blood cell count, 3000 cells/mm^3
4. Blood urea nitrogen (BUN) level, 15 mg/dL

620. The client with myasthenia gravis is receiving pyridostigmine (Mestinon). The nurse monitors for signs and symptoms of cholinergic crisis caused by overdose of the medication. The nurse checks the medication supply to ensure that which medication is available for administration if a cholinergic crisis occurs?
1. Vitamin K
2. Acetylcysteine
3. Atropine sulfate
4. Protamine sulfate

ANSWERS

611. 4

Rationale: Cholinergic crisis occurs as a result of an overdose of medication. Indications of cholinergic crisis include gastrointestinal disturbances, nausea, vomiting, diarrhea, abdominal cramps, increased salivation and tearing, miosis, hypertension, sweating, and increased bronchial secretions.
Test-Taking Strategy: Note the subject, cholinergic crisis, and recall the signs/symptoms of cholinergic crisis, including hypertension. Note that mouth sores represents a condition that takes time to occur and is not an immediate sign of a crisis. Review: signs and symptoms of cholinergic crisis.
Level of Cognitive Ability: Analyzing
Client Needs: Physiological Integrity
Integrated Process: Nursing Process/Data Collection
Content Area: Pharmacology: Neurological Medications
Priority Concepts: Clinical Judgment, Stress
Reference(s): deWit, Kumagai (2013), p. 564.

❖ **612. 2, 3, 4**

Rationale: Meperidine hydrochloride is an opioid analgesic. Side/adverse effects include respiratory depression, drowsiness, hypotension, constipation, urinary retention, nausea, vomiting, and tremors.
Test-Taking Strategy: Focus on the subject, side/adverse effects of meperidine hydrochloride. Recalling that this medication is an opioid analgesic and recalling the effects of an opioid analgesic will assist in identifying the side/adverse effects. Review: the side/adverse effects of meperidine hydrochloride.
Level of Cognitive Ability: Analyzing
Client Needs: Physiological Integrity
Integrated Process: Nursing Process/Data Collection
Content Area: Pharmacology: Neurological Medications
Priority Concepts: Clinical Judgment, Pain
Reference(s): Hodgson, Kizior (2015), p. 751.

613. 4

Rationale: An edrophonium (Enlon) injection makes the client in cholinergic crisis temporarily worse. This is known as a negative test. An improvement of weakness would occur if the client were experiencing myasthenia gravis. Options 1 and 2 would not occur in either crisis.
Test-Taking Strategy: Focus on the subject, the difference between myasthenic and cholinergic crisis and the Enlon (Tensilon) test. Noting the words, *overdose of the medication (cholinergic crisis)*, will direct you to option 4. It makes sense that administering additional medication will worsen the condition. Review: cholinergic and myasthenic crisis.
Level of Cognitive Ability: Analyzing
Client Needs: Physiological Integrity
Integrated Process: Nursing Process/Data Collection
Content Area: Pharmacology: Neurological Medications
Priority Concepts: Clinical Judgment, Mobility
Reference(s): Lehne (2013), pp. 141–142.

614. 4

Rationale: Dyskinesia and impaired voluntary movement may occur with high levodopa dosages. Nausea, anorexia, dizziness, orthostatic hypotension, bradycardia, and akinesia (the temporary muscle weakness that lasts 1 minute to 1 hour, also known as the "on-off phenomenon") are frequent side effects of the medication.

Test-Taking Strategy: Focus on the subject, signs and symptoms of adverse effects associated with carbidopa and levodopa. Options 2 and 3 are cardiac-related options, so these options can be eliminated first as comparable or alike, and not related to the subject. Note that the question asks for an adverse effect; therefore, select option 4 over option 1 as the correct answer. **Review: carbidopa and levodopa.**
Level of Cognitive Ability: Analyzing
Client Needs: Physiological Integrity
Integrated Process: Nursing Process/Data Collection
Content Area: Pharmacology: Neurological Medications
Priority Concepts: Clinical Judgment, Mobility
Reference(s): Hodgson, Kizior (2015), pp. 192–193.

615. 1

Rationale: Phenytoin (Dilantin) is an anticonvulsant. Gingival hyperplasia, bleeding, swelling, and tenderness of the gums can occur with the use of this medication. The client needs to be taught good oral hygiene, gum massage, and the need for regular dentist visits. The client should not skip medication doses because this could precipitate a seizure. Capsules should not be chewed or broken, and they must be swallowed. The client needs to be instructed to report a sore throat, fever, glandular swelling, or any skin reaction because this indicates hematological toxicity.
Test-Taking Strategy: Focus on the subject, an understanding of the instructions. Eliminate option 3 because the client needs to be encouraged to take medications on time. Also, eliminate option 4 because the client needs to report these symptoms to the health care provider. From the remaining options, recalling that capsules should not be broken will direct you to option 1. **Review:** client instructions for **phenytoin (Dilantin).**
Level of Cognitive Ability: Evaluating
Client Needs: Physiological Integrity
Integrated Process: Nursing Process/Evaluation
Content Area: Pharmacology: Neurological Medications
Priority Concepts: Client Education, Intracranial Regulation
Reference(s): Hodgson, Kizior (2015), p. 960.

616. 2

Rationale: The therapeutic serum drug level range for phenytoin (Dilantin) is 10 to 20 mcg/mL. Therefore, options 1, 3, and 4 are incorrect.
Test-Taking Strategy: Knowledge regarding the subject, the therapeutic serum range of phenytoin, is required to answer the question. A helpful hint may be to remember that the theophylline therapeutic range and the acetaminophen (Tylenol) therapeutic range are the same as the phenytoin (Dilantin) therapeutic range. Remembering this may assist you when answering questions related to any of these three medications. **Review:** therapeutic **phenytoin level.**
Level of Cognitive Ability: Understanding
Client Needs: Physiological Integrity
Integrated Process: Nursing Process/Data Collection
Content Area: Pharmacology: Neurological Medications
Priority Concepts: Clinical Judgment, Intracranial Regulation
Reference(s): Hodgson, Kizior (2015), p. 960.

617. 1

Rationale: Ibuprofen is a nonsteroidal anti-inflammatory drug (NSAID). NSAIDs should be given with milk or food to prevent gastrointestinal irritation. Options 2, 3, and 4 are incorrect.
Test-Taking Strategy: Note that options 2, 3, and 4 are comparable or alike. Each of these options indicates administering the medication without food. Remember, NSAIDs can cause gastric irritation. **Review: nonsteroidal anti-inflammatory medications.**
Level of Cognitive Ability: Applying
Client Needs: Physiological Integrity
Integrated Process: Teaching and Learning
Content Area: Pharmacology: Neurological Medications
Priority Concepts: Client Education, Inflammation
Reference(s): Hodgson, Kizior (2015), p. 595.

618. 3

Rationale: Phenytoin (Dilantin) enhances the rate of estrogen metabolism, which can decrease the effectiveness of some birth control pills. Options 1, 2, are 4 are not accurate.
Test-Taking Strategy: Recall knowledge of the subject, medication interactions between phenytoin and birth control pills. Option 4 is not an appropriate statement because it would cause anxiety in the client. A client should not be instructed to stop anticonvulsant medication. Pregnancy does not need to be "avoided." **Review: phenytoin (Dilantin).**
Level of Cognitive Ability: Applying
Client Needs: Health Promotion and Maintenance
Integrated Process: Nursing Process/Implementation
Content Area: Pharmacology: Neurological Medications
Priority Concepts: Client Education, Reproduction
Reference(s): Lehne (2013), pp. 248–249.

619. 3

Rationale: Adverse effects of carbamazepine (Tegretol) appear as blood dyscrasias, including aplastic anemia, agranulocytosis, thrombocytopenia, leukopenia, cardiovascular disturbances, thrombophlebitis, dysrhythmias, and dermatological effects. Options 1, 2, and 4 identify normal laboratory values.
Test-Taking Strategy: Focus on the subject, the medication and normal laboratory values, to answer this question. If you are familiar with normal laboratory values, you will note that the only option that indicates an abnormal value is option 3. **Review:** adverse effects of **carbamazepine (Tegretol).**
Level of Cognitive Ability: Understanding
Client Needs: Physiological Integrity
Integrated Process: Nursing Process/Data Collection
Content Area: Pharmacology: Neurological Medications
Priority Concepts: Cellular Regulation, Pain
Reference(s): Lehne (2013), pp. 236, 249.

620. 3

Rationale: The antidote for cholinergic crisis is atropine sulfate. Acetylcysteine is the antidote for acetaminophen (Tylenol). Vitamin K is the antidote for warfarin (Coumadin) and protamine sulfate is the antidote for heparin.
Test-Taking Strategy: Knowledge regarding the subject, antidotes for various medications, is needed to answer this question. Remember that atropine sulfate is the antidote for cholinergic crisis. **Review: antidote for pyridostigmine (Mestinon).**
Level of Cognitive Ability: Applying
Client Needs: Physiological Integrity
Integrated Process: Nursing Process/Implementation
Content Area: Pharmacology: Neurological Medications
Priority Concepts: Clinical Judgment, Cellular Regulation
Reference(s): Hodgson, Kizior (2015), pp. 1020–1021.

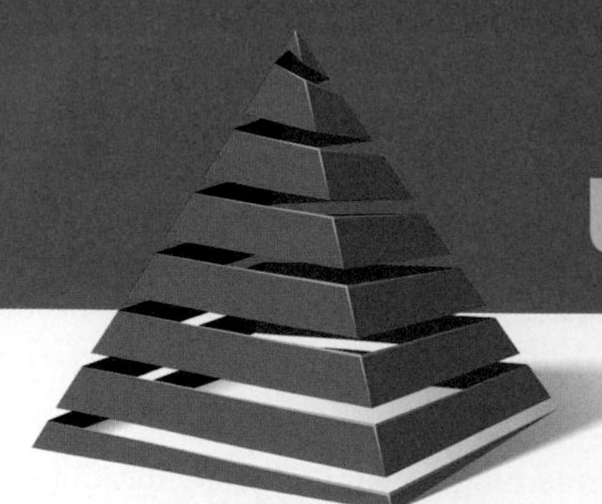

UNIT XVII

The Adult Client with a Musculoskeletal Disorder

PYRAMID TERMS

cast Stiff dressing or casting, made of plaster of Paris or synthetic material, to stabilize a part or parts of the body until healing occurs.

compartment syndrome Condition in which pressure increases in a confined anatomical space that leads to decreased blood flow, ischemia, and dysfunction of these tissues; initial ischemia with pain, pallor, paresthesia, muscle weakness, and loss of pulses may progress to necrosis and permanent muscle cellular dysfunction.

external fixation Stabilization of a fracture by the use of an external frame, with multiple pins applied through the bone.

fat embolism Sudden dislodgement of a fat globule that is freed into the circulation, where it can lodge in a blood vessel and obstruct blood flow to tissue that is distal to the obstruction.

internal fixation Stabilization of a fracture that involves the application of screws, plates, pins, or nails to hold the fragments in alignment.

reduction Correction or realignment of a bone fracture or joint dislocation.

traction Exertion of a pulling force to a fractured bone or dislocated joint to establish and maintain correct alignment for healing and to decrease muscle spasms and pain.

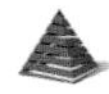

Pyramid to Success

The Pyramid to Success focuses on the emergency care for a client who sustains a fracture or other musculoskeletal injury, monitoring for complications related to fractures, and interventions if complications occur. Nursing care related to casts and traction is emphasized. Skill related to instructing the client on the use of an assistive device such as a cane, walker, or crutches is a Pyramid point. Pyramid points also include postoperative care following hip surgery or amputation, as well as care of the client with rheumatoid arthritis or osteoporosis. Focus on the points related to the psychosocial effects as a result of the musculoskeletal disorder, such as unexpected body-image changes, and the appropriate and available support services needed for the client.

Client Needs

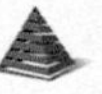

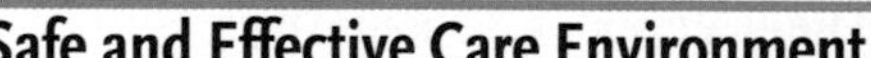

Safe and Effective Care Environment

Assisting with physical therapy and occupational therapy referrals
Ensuring that informed consent for diagnostic treatments and surgical procedures has been obtained
Establishing priorities
Handling hazardous and infectious materials safely
Maintaining asepsis related to wounds
Maintaining confidentiality regarding the disorder and plan of care
Maintaining standard and other precautions
Preventing accidents and injuries
Providing a dietary consultation
Upholding client rights

Health Promotion and Maintenance

Discussing expected body-image changes
Performing data collection techniques related to the musculoskeletal system
Promoting health related to diet and activity
Reinforcing home care instructions regarding care related to the musculoskeletal disorder
Reinforcing the importance of prescribed therapy
Teaching related to preventing diseases that occur as a result of the aging process

Psychosocial Integrity

Considering cultural, religious, and spiritual influences
Determining the client's ability to cope with feelings of isolation and loss of independence
Discussing situational role changes as a result of the musculoskeletal disorder

Identifying available support systems and use of community resources
Identifying unexpected body-image changes as a result of injury or disease
Identifying sensory and perceptual alterations
Mobilizing coping mechanisms

Physiological Integrity

Identifying complications of a fracture
Identifying complications related to procedures or injuries
Providing care related to casts and traction
Promoting normal elimination patterns
Promoting self-care measures
Providing emergency care for a fracture or other injury
Providing measures to promote comfort
Reinforcing measures about the use of assistive devices for mobility such as canes, walkers, and crutches
Reinforcing teaching about prescribed pharmacological therapy

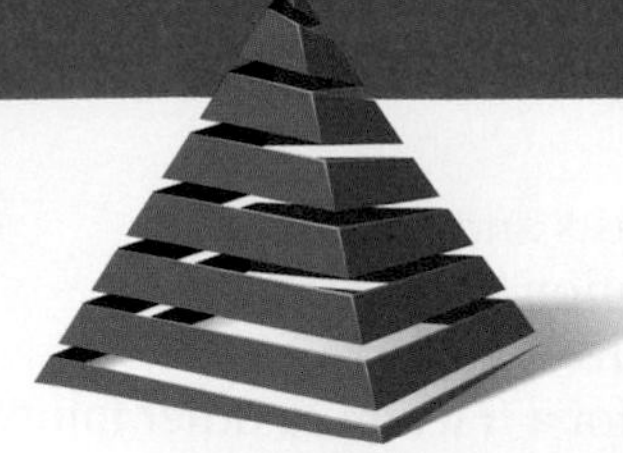

CHAPTER 59

Musculoskeletal System

CRITICAL THINKING What Should You Do?

The nurse employed in an industrial plant is called to an accident site in the plant in which an employee amputated his index finger on a saw. What should the nurse do?
Answer located on p. 855.

I. Anatomy and Physiology

A. Skeleton
1. Axial portion
a. Cranium
b. Vertebrae
c. Ribs
2. Appendicular portion
a. Limbs
b. Shoulders
c. Hips

B. Types of bones
1. Types include long, short, flat, and irregular
2. Spongy bone
a. Is located in the ends of long bones and the center of flat and irregular bones
b. Can withstand forces applied in many directions
3. Dense (compact) bone
a. Covers spongy bone
b. Forms a cylinder around a central marrow cavity
c. Better able to withstand longitudinal forces than horizontal forces
4. Characteristics of the bones
a. Support and protect structures of the body
b. Provide attachments for muscles, tendons, and ligaments
c. Contain tissue in the central cavities, which aids in the formation of blood cells
d. Assist in regulating calcium and phosphate concentrations
5. Bone growth
a. The length of bone growth results from the ossification of the epiphyseal cartilage at the ends of bones, and bone growth stops between the ages of 18 and 25 years.
b. The width of bone growth results from the activity of osteoblasts and occurs throughout life but does slow down with aging.

⚠ As aging occurs, bone resorption accelerates, decreasing bone mass and predisposing the client to injury.

C. Types of joints (Table 59-1)
1. Characteristics of the joints
a. Allow the movement between bones
b. Formed where two bones join
c. Surfaces are covered with cartilage
d. Enclosed in a capsule (synovial joints)
e. Contain a cavity filled with synovial fluid (synovial joints)
f. Ligaments hold the bone and joint in the correct position.
g. Articulation is the meeting point of two or more bones.
2. Synovial fluid
a. Found in the joint capsule
b. Formed by the synovial membrane, which lines the joint capsule
c. Lubricates the cartilage
d. Provides a cushion against shocks

D. Muscles
1. Characteristics of muscles
a. Made up of bundles of muscle fibers
b. Provide the force to move bones
c. Assist in maintaining posture
d. Assist with heat production

TABLE 59-1 Types of Joints

Type	Description
Amphiarthrosis	Cartilaginous joints Slightly movable joints
Diarthrosis	Synovial joints Ball-and-socket joints Permit free movement
Synarthrosis	Fibrous or fixed joints No movement associated with these joints

2. The process of contraction and relaxation
   a. Muscle contraction and relaxation require large amounts of adenosine triphosphate.
   b. Contraction also requires calcium, which functions as a catalyst.
   c. Acetylcholine released by the motor end plate of the motor neuron initiates an action potential.
   d. Acetylcholine is then destroyed by acetylcholinesterase.
   e. Calcium is required to contract muscle fibers and acts as a catalyst for the enzyme needed for the sliding-together action of actin and myosin.
   f. Following contraction, adenosine triphosphate transports calcium out to allow actin and myosin to separate and to allow the muscle to relax.
3. Skeletal muscles
   a. Skeletal muscles are attached to two bones and cross at least one joint.
   b. The point of origin is the point of attachment that does not move.
   c. The point of insertion is the point of attachment that moves when the muscle contracts.
   d. Skeletal muscles act in groups.
   e. Prime movers contract to produce movement.
   f. Antagonists relax.
   g. Synergists contract to stabilize body movement.
   h. Nerves activate and control the muscles.

E. Bone healing
1. Description: Bone union or healing is the process that occurs after the integrity of a bone is interrupted.
2. Stages (Fig. 59-1)

BOX 59-1 Risk Factors Associated with Musculoskeletal Disorders

Autoimmune disorders
Calcium deficiency
Falls
Hyperuricemia
Infection
Medications
Metabolic disorders
Neoplastic disorders
Obesity
Postmenopausal states
Trauma and injury

II. Risk Factors Associated with Musculoskeletal Disorders (Box 59-1)

III. Diagnostic Tests

A. Radiographs (x-rays)
1. Description: Radiography is a commonly used procedure to diagnose disorders of the musculoskeletal system.
2. Interventions 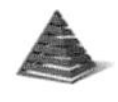
   a. Handle injured areas carefully and support extremities above and below the joint.
   b. Administer analgesics as prescribed before the procedure, particularly if the client is in pain.
   c. Remove any radiopaque objects, such as jewelry.
   d. Ask the client if she is pregnant; may be contraindicated in pregnancy.

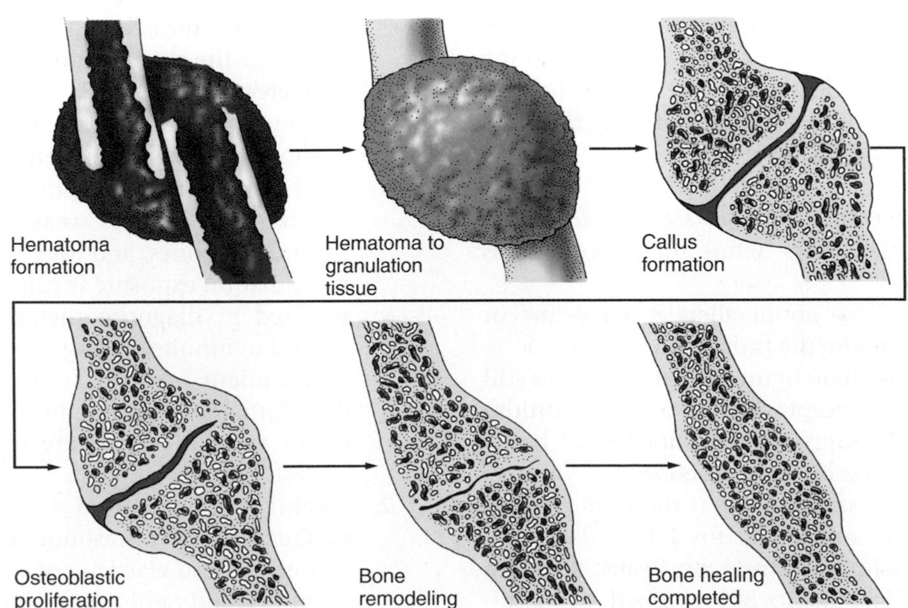

FIGURE 59-1 The stages of bone healing. (From Ignatavicius D, Workman ML: *Medical-surgical nursing: Patient-centered collaborative care*, ed 7, Philadelphia, 2013, Saunders.)

e. Shield client's testes, ovaries, or pregnant abdomen.

f. Reinforce instructions to lie still during a radiograph.

g. Inform the client that exposure to radiation is minimal and not dangerous.

h. The nurse must wear a lead apron if staying in the room with the client.

B. Arthrocentesis

1. Description: Arthrocentesis is used to diagnose joint inflammation and infection.

a. Arthrocentesis involves aspirating synovial fluid, blood, or pus via a needle inserted into a joint cavity.

b. Medication, such as corticosteroids, may be instilled into the joint if necessary to alleviate inflammation.

2. Interventions

a. Apply an elastic compression bandage postprocedure as prescribed.

b. Use ice to decrease pain and swelling.

c. Pain may worsen after aspirating fluid from the joint; analgesics may be prescribed.

d. Pain can continue up to 2 days after administration of corticosteroids into a joint.

e. Reinforce instructions to rest the joint for 8 to 24 hours postprocedure as prescribed.

f. Reinforce instructions to notify the health care provider (HCP) if a fever, increased redness, or swelling of the joint occurs.

C. Arthrography

1. Description: Arthrography is used in unexplained joint pain or inflammation to diagnose trauma to the joint capsule or ligaments.

a. Arthrography is a radiographic examination of the soft tissues of the joint structures.

b. A local anesthetic is used for the procedure.

c. A contrast medium or air is injected into the joint cavity, and the joint is moved through range of motion as a series of x-ray films are taken.

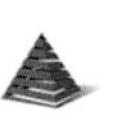

2. Interventions

a. Reinforce instructions to fast from food and fluids for 8 hours before the procedure, as prescribed.

b. Ask the client about allergies to iodine or shellfish before the procedure.

c. Inform the client of the need to remain as still as possible, except when asked to reposition.

d. Minimize the use of the joint for 12 hours after the procedure as prescribed.

e. Reinforce instructions that the joint may be edematous and tender for 1 to 2 days after the procedure and may be treated with ice packs and analgesics as prescribed.

f. Reinforce instructions to notify the HCP if edema and tenderness last longer than 2 days.

g. If knee arthrography was performed, an elastic compression wrap over the knee may be prescribed for 3 to 4 days and ice applied to decrease pain and swelling.

h. If air was used for injection, crepitus may be felt in the joint for up to 2 days.

D. Arthroscopy

1. Description: Arthroscopy is used to diagnose acute and chronic disorders of the joint.

a. Arthroscopy provides an endoscopic examination of various joints.

b. Articular cartilage abnormalities can be assessed, loose bodies can be removed, and the cartilage can be trimmed.

c. A biopsy may be performed during the procedure.

2. Interventions

a. Reinforce instructions to fast for 8 to 12 hours before the procedure.

b. Administer pain medication as prescribed postprocedure.

c. Monitor the neurovascular status of the affected extremity.

d. An elastic compression bandage should be worn for 2 to 4 days as prescribed postprocedure.

e. Reinforce instructions that walking without weight bearing is usually permitted after sensation returns but to limit activity for 1 to 4 days as prescribed postprocedure.

f. Reinforce instructions to elevate the extremity as often as possible for 2 days following the procedure and to place ice on the site to minimize swelling.

g. Reinforce instructions regarding the use of crutches, which may be used for 5 to 7 days postprocedure for walking.

h. Advise the client to notify the HCP if fever or increased knee pain occurs or if edema continues for more than 3 days postprocedure.

E. Bone mineral density measurements

1. Dual energy x-ray absorptiometry

a. Measures the bone mass of the spine, wrist and hip bones, and total body.

b. Radiation exposure is minimal.

c. Used to diagnose metabolic bone disease and to monitor changes in bone density with treatment

d. Inform the client that the procedure is painless.

e. All metallic objects are removed before the test.

2. Quantitative ultrasound

a. Quantitative ultrasound evaluates strength, density, and elasticity of various bones using ultrasound rather than radiation.

b. Inform the client that the procedure is painless.

F. Bone scan

1. Description: A bone scan is used to identify, evaluate, and stage bone cancer before and after treatment; it is also used to detect fractures.
   - **a.** Radioisotope is injected intravenously and will collect in areas that indicate abnormal bone metabolism and some fractures, if they exist.
   - **b.** The isotope is excreted in the urine and feces within 48 hours and is not harmful to others.
2. Interventions
   - **a.** Food and fluid may be withheld before the procedure.
   - **b.** Remove all jewelry and metal objects.
   - **c.** Following the injection of the radioisotope, the client must drink 32 oz of water (if not contraindicated) to promote renal filtering of the excess isotope.
   - **d.** From 1 to 3 hours after the injection, have the client void to clear excess isotope from the bladder before the scanning procedure is completed.
   - **e.** Inform the client of the need to lie supine during the procedure and that the procedure is not painful.
   - **f.** Monitor the injection site for redness and swelling.
   - **g.** Encourage oral fluid intake after the procedure.

No special precautions are required after a bone scan because a minimal amount of radioactivity exists in the radioisotope used for the procedure.

G. Bone or muscle biopsy

1. Description: A biopsy may be performed during surgery or through aspiration or punch or needle biopsy.
2. Interventions
   - **a.** Monitor for bleeding, swelling, hematoma, or severe pain.
   - **b.** Elevate the site for 24 hours following the procedure to reduce edema.
   - **c.** Apply ice packs as prescribed following the procedure to prevent the development of a hematoma and to decrease site discomfort.
   - **d.** Monitor for signs of infection following the procedure.
   - **e.** Inform the client that mild to moderate discomfort is normal following the procedure.

H. Electromyography (EMG)

1. Description: An EMG is used to evaluate muscle weakness.
   - **a.** Electromyography measures electrical potential associated with skeletal muscle contractions.
   - **b.** Needles are inserted into the muscle, and recordings of muscular electrical activity are traced on recording paper through an oscilloscope.
2. Interventions
   - **a.** Reinforce instructions that the needle insertion is uncomfortable.
   - **b.** Reinforce instructions not to take any stimulants or sedatives for 24 hours before the procedure.
   - **c.** Inform the client that slight bruising may occur at the needle insertion sites.
   - **d.** Mild analgesics can be used for the pain.

IV. Injuries

A. Strains

1. Strains are an excessive stretching of a muscle or tendon.
2. Management involves cold and heat applications, exercise with activity limitations, anti-inflammatory medications, and muscle relaxants.
3. Surgical repair may be required for a severe strain (ruptured muscle or tendon).

B. Sprains

1. Sprains are an excessive stretching of a ligament, usually caused by a twisting motion, such as in a fall or step on an uneven surface.
2. Sprains are characterized by pain and swelling.
3. Management involves RICE (rest, ice, a compression bandage, and elevation) to reduce swelling and provide joint support. RICE is considered a first-aid treatment rather than a cure for soft tissue injuries.
4. Casting may be required for moderate sprains to allow the tear to heal.
5. Surgery may be necessary for severe ligament damage.

C. Rotator cuff injuries

1. Musculotendinous or rotator cuff of the shoulder sustains a tear, usually as a result of trauma.
2. Injury is characterized by shoulder pain and the inability to maintain abduction of the arm at the shoulder (drop arm test).
3. Management involves nonsteroidal anti-inflammatory drugs (NSAIDs), physical therapy, sling support, and ice/heat applications. 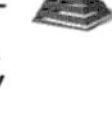
4. Surgery may be required if medical management is unsuccessful or for those who have a complete tear.

V. Fractures

A. Description: A fracture is a break in the continuity of the bone caused by trauma, twisting as a result of muscle spasm or indirect loss of leverage, or bone decalcification and disease that result in osteopenia.

B. Types of fractures (Box 59-2)

C. Data collection: Fracture of an extremity 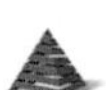

BOX 59-2 Types of Fractures

Closed or simple: Skin over the fractured area remains intact.
Comminuted: The bone is splintered or crushed, creating numerous fragments.
Complete: The bone is separated completely by a break into two parts.
Compression: A fractured bone is compressed by other bone.
Depressed: Bone fragments are driven inward.
Greenstick: One side of the bone is broken and the other is bent; these fractures occur most commonly in children.
Impacted: A part of the fractured bone is driven into another bone.
Incomplete: Fracture line does not extend through the full transverse width of the bone.
Oblique: The fracture line runs at an angle across the axis of the bone.
Open or compound: The bone is exposed to air through a break in the skin, and soft tissue injury and infection are common.
Pathological: The fracture results from weakening of the bone structure by pathological processes such as neoplasia; also called spontaneous fracture.
Spiral: The break partially encircles bone.
Transverse: The bone is fractured straight across.

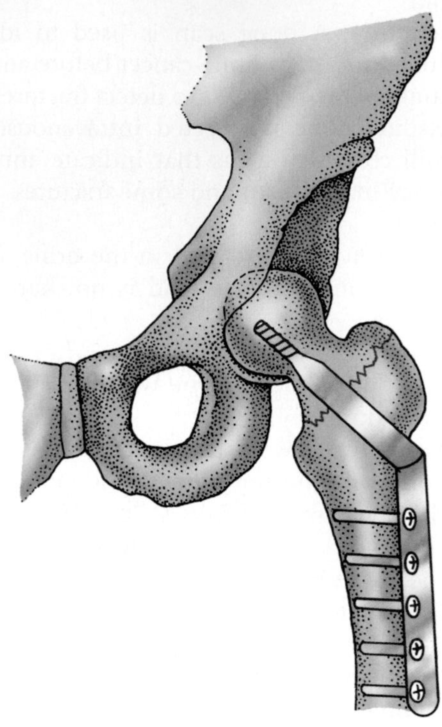

FIGURE 59-2 A compression hip screw used for open reduction with internal fixation. (From Ignatavicius D, Workman ML: *Medical-surgical nursing: Patient-centered collaborative care*, ed 7, Philadelphia, 2013, Saunders.)

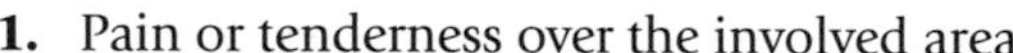

1. Pain or tenderness over the involved area
2. Decrease or loss of muscular strength or function
3. Obvious deformity of affected area
4. Crepitation, erythema, edema, or bruising
5. Muscle spasm and neurovascular impairment

D. Initial care of a fracture of an extremity
1. Immobilize affected extremity with **cast** or splint.
2. Check the neurovascular status of the extremity.
3. Interventions for a fracture include reduction, fixation, traction, and casting.

If a compound (open) fracture exists, splint the extremity and cover the wound with a sterile dressing.

E. **Reduction** restores the bone to proper alignment.
1. Closed reduction is a nonsurgical intervention that is performed by manual manipulation.
   a. Closed reduction may be performed under local or general anesthesia.
   b. A cast may be applied following reduction.
2. Open reduction involves a surgical intervention.
   a. Fracture may be treated with internal fixation devices.
   b. The client may be placed in traction or a cast following the procedure.

F. Fixation
1. **Internal fixation** follows an open reduction (Fig. 59-2).
   a. Internal fixation involves the application of screws, plates, pins, or intramedullary rods to hold the fragments in alignment.
   b. Internal fixation may involve the removal of damaged bone and replacement with a prosthesis.
   c. Internal fixation provides immediate bone strength.
2. **External fixation** is the use of an external frame to stabilize a fracture by attaching skeletal pins through bone fragments to a rigid external support.
   a. External fixation provides more freedom of movement than with traction.
   b. Monitor pin stability and provide pin care to decrease infection risks.
   c. Risk of infection exists with both fixation methods.
   d. External fixation is commonly used when massive tissue trauma is present.

G. **Traction** (Fig. 59-3)
1. Description
   a. Traction is the exertion of a pulling force applied in two directions to reduce and immobilize a fracture.
   b. Traction provides proper bone alignment and reduces muscle spasms.
2. Interventions 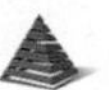
   a. Maintain proper body alignment.

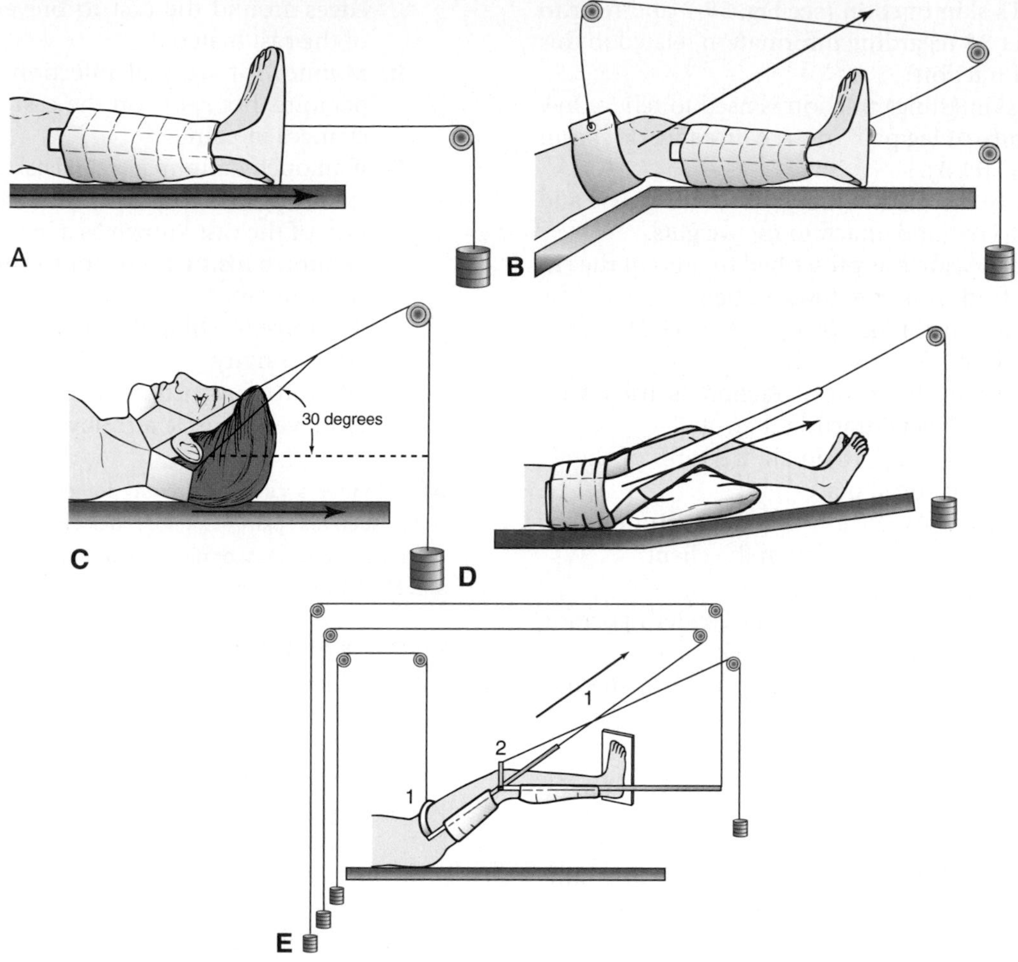

FIGURE 59-3 Types of traction. **A,** Buck's traction. **B,** Russell's traction. **C,** Head halter traction. **D,** Pelvic sling traction. **E,** Balanced suspension traction. (From Lewis S, Heitkemper M, Dirksen S: *Medical-surgical nursing: Assessment and management of clinical problems*, ed 7, St. Louis, 2007, Mosby.)

b. Ensure that the weights hang freely and do not touch the floor.
c. Do not remove or lift the weights without a HCP's prescription.
d. Ensure that pulleys are not obstructed and that ropes in the pulleys move freely.
e. Place knots in the ropes to prevent slipping.
f. Check the ropes for fraying.

H. Skeletal traction (see Fig. 59-3)
1. Description: Traction is applied mechanically to the bone with pins, wires, or tongs.
2. Interventions
a. Monitor color, motion, and sensation of the affected extremity.
b. Monitor the insertion sites for redness, swelling, drainage, or increased pain.
c. Provide insertion site care as prescribed.
3. Cervical tongs and a halo fixation device (refer to Chapter 57 regarding care of the client with these types of devices)

I. Skin traction
1. Description: Skin traction is applied by using elastic bandages or adhesive, foam boot, or sling.
2. Cervical skin traction relieves muscle spasms and compression in the upper extremities and neck (see Fig. 59-3).
a. Cervical skin traction uses a head halter and a chin pad to attach the traction.
b. Use powder to protect the ears from friction rub.
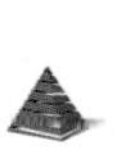
c. Position the client with the head of the bed elevated 30 to 40 degrees, and attach the weights to a pulley system over the head of the bed.
3. Buck's (extension) skin traction is used to alleviate muscle spasms and immobilize a lower limb by maintaining a straight pull on the limb with the use of weights (see Fig. 59-3).
a. A boot appliance is applied to attach to the traction.

b. Weight is attached to a pulley; allow the weights to hang freely over the edge of bed.
c. Not more than 8 to 10 lb of weight should be applied.
d. Elevate the foot of the bed to provide the traction.

4. Russell's skin traction (see Fig. 59-3 and refer to Chapter 38 regarding information related to this type of traction)
5. Pelvic skin (sling) traction is used to relieve low back, hip, or leg pain or to reduce muscle spasm (see Fig. 59-3).
   a. Apply the traction snugly over the pelvis and iliac crest and attach to the weights.
   b. Use measures as prescribed to prevent the client from slipping down in bed.

J. Balanced suspension traction (see Fig. 59-3)
1. Description
   a. Balanced suspension traction is used with skin or skeletal traction.
   b. It is used to approximate fractures of the femur, tibia, or fibula.
   c. Balanced suspension traction is produced by a counterforce other than the client.
2. Interventions
   a. Position the client in a low Fowler's position on either the side or the back.
   b. Maintain a 20-degree angle from the thigh to the bed.
   c. Protect the skin from breakdown.
   d. Provide pin care if pins are used with the skeletal traction.
   e. Clean the pin sites with sterile normal saline and hydrogen peroxide or povidone-iodine (Betadine) as prescribed or per agency policy.

K. Dunlop's traction
1. Description: Horizontal traction is used to align fractures of the humerus; vertical traction maintains the forearm in proper alignment.
2. Interventions: Nursing care is similar to that for Buck's skin traction.

L. Casts
1. Description: Plaster or fiberglass casts are used to immobilize bones and joints into correct alignment after a fracture or injury.
2. Interventions
   a. Keep the cast and extremity elevated.
   b. Allow a wet cast 24 to 72 hours to dry (synthetic casts dry in 20 minutes).
   c. Handle a wet cast with the palms of the hands until dry.
   d. Turn the extremity every 1 to 2 hours, unless contraindicated to allow air circulation and promote drying of the cast.
   e. Cool setting on a hair dryer can be used to dry a plaster cast. (Heat cannot be used on a plaster cast because the cast heats up and burns the skin.)
   f. Prepare for bivalving or cutting the cast if circulatory impairment occurs.
   g. Petal the cast or apply moleskin to the edges to protect the client's skin; maintain smooth edges around the cast to prevent crumbling of the cast material.
   h. Monitor for signs of infection such as temperature, hot spots on the cast, foul odor, or changes in pain.
   i. If an open draining area exists on the affected extremity, the HCP will make a cutout portion of the cast known as a *window.*
   j. Reinforce instructions not to stick objects inside the cast.
   k. Reinforce teaching the client to keep the cast clean and dry.
   l. Reinforce instructions on isometric exercises to prevent muscle atrophy.

Monitor a casted extremity for circulatory impairment such as pain, swelling, discoloration, tingling, numbness, coolness, or diminished pulse. Notify the RN and HCP immediately if circulatory compromise occurs.

VI. Complications of Fractures

A. Fat embolism
1. Description: A fat embolism originates in the bone marrow and occurs after a fracture when a fat globule is released into the bloodstream.
   a. Clients with long bone fractures are at the greatest risk for the development of fat embolism.
   b. Fat embolism can occur within the first 48 to 72 hours following the injury or when surgical manipulation occurs following surgery.
2. Data collection: Findings often suggest pulmonary embolism.
   a. Restlessness, hypoxemia, or mental status changes
   b. Tachycardia and hypotension
   c. Dyspnea and tachypnea
   d. Petechial rash over the upper chest and neck; these may fade quickly.
3. Interventions (see Priority Nursing Actions)

B. Compartment syndrome
1. Description
   a. Tough fascia surrounds muscle groups, forming compartments from which arteries, veins, and nerves enter and exit opposite ends.
   b. Compartment syndrome occurs when pressure increases within one or more compartments, leading to decreased blood flow, tissue ischemia, and neurovascular impairment.
   c. Within 4 to 6 hours after the onset of compartment syndrome, neurovascular damage is irreversible if not treated.

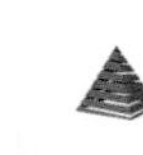

2. Data collection
   a. Unrelieved or increased pain in the limb
   b. Tissue that is distal to the involved area becomes pale, dusky, or edematous.

PRIORITY NURSING ACTIONS!

Actions to Take If the Client Develops a Fat Embolism

1. Notify the RN and HCP.
2. Administer oxygen.
3. Assist to monitor prescribed intravenous fluids.
4. Monitor vital signs and respiratory status.
5. Prepare to assist the RN and HCP with intubation and mechanical ventilation if necessary.
6. Document the event, actions taken, and the client's response.

A fat embolism originates in the bone marrow and occurs after a fracture when a fat globule is released into the bloodstream. Fat embolism can occur within the first 48 to 72 hours after the injury, and clients with long bone fractures are at the greatest risk for the development of a fat embolism. Findings are similar to those noted with pulmonary embolism and include restlessness, hypoxemia, mental status changes, dyspnea, tachypnea, tachycardia, and hypotension. Additionally, a petechial rash may present over the upper chest and neck. The RN and HCP are notified immediately while initiating emergency care. The client is maintained on bed rest and is repositioned only as necessary, and gently. Oxygen is administered, and IV hydration is administered to prevent hypovolemic shock. Vital signs and respiratory status are monitored closely, and the client is prepared for intubation and mechanical ventilation if necessary. Corticosteroids may also be prescribed for the client. The nurse then documents the event, actions taken, and the client's response.

Reference(s): deWit, D. & Kumagai, C. (2013). *Medical-surgical nursing: Concepts & practice.* (2nd ed., p. 741). St. Louis: Saunders.

c. Pain with passive movement and joint dysfunction
d. Loss of sensation (paresthesia)
e. Pulselessness (a late sign)

3. Interventions
   a. Notify the RN and HCP immediately and prepare to assist the RN.
   b. If severe, assist the HCP with fasciotomy to relieve pressure and restore tissue perfusion.
   c. Loosen tight dressings or bivalve restrictive cast as prescribed.

C. Infection and osteomyelitis
1. Description: Infection and osteomyelitis (inflammatory response in bone tissue) can be caused by the introduction of organisms into bones initially leading to localized bone infection.
2. Data collection
   a. Tachycardia and fever (usually above 101 °F)
   b. Erythema and pain in the area surrounding the infection
   c. Leukocytosis and elevated erythrocyte sedimentation rate (ESR)
3. Interventions
   a. Notify the RN and HCP immediately, and prepare to assist the RN.
   b. Initiation of aggressive, long-term intravenous antibiotic therapy is done.
   c. Hyperbaric oxygen therapy may be prescribed to promote client healing.
   d. Surgery may be performed for resistant osteomyelitis with sequestrectomy and/or bone grafts.

D. Avascular necrosis
1. Description: Occurs when a fracture interrupts the blood supply to a section of bone, leading to bone death

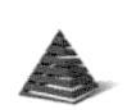

2. Data collection
   a. Pain
   b. Decreased sensation

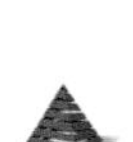

3. Interventions
   a. Notify the RN and HCP if pain or numbness occurs.
   b. Prepare the client for removal of necrotic tissue because it serves as a focus for infection.

E. Pulmonary embolism (see Priority Nursing Actions in Chapter 49)

VII. Crutch Walking

A. Description

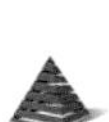
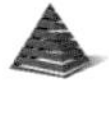

1. An accurate measurement of the client for crutches is important because an incorrect measurement could damage the brachial plexus.
2. The distance between the axillae and the arm pieces on the crutches should be two to three fingerwidths in the axilla space.
3. The elbows should be slightly flexed, 20 to 30 degrees, when the client is walking.
4. When ambulating with the client, stand on the affected side.
5. Reinforce instructions to never rest the axilla on the axillary bars.
6. Reinforce instructions to look up and outward when ambulating and to place the crutches 6 to 10 inches diagonally in front of the foot.
7. Reinforce instructions to stop ambulation if numbness or tingling in the hands or arms occurs.

B. Crutch gaits (Table 59-2)

C. Assisting the client with crutches to sit and stand.
1. Place the unaffected leg against the front of the chair.
2. Move the crutches to the affected side, and grasp the arm of the chair with the hand on the unaffected side.

TABLE 59-2 Crutch Gaits

Type of Gait	Use	Procedure
Two-point gait	Used with partial weight-bearing limitations and with bilateral lower extremity prostheses	The crutch on the affected side and the unaffected foot are advanced at the same time.
Three-point gait	Used for partial weight bearing or no weight bearing on the affected leg; requires that the client have strength and balance	Both crutches and the foot of the affected extremity are advanced together, followed by the foot of the unaffected extremity.
Four-point gait	Used if weight bearing is allowed and one foot can be placed in front of the other	The right crutch is advanced, then the left foot, then the left crutch, then the right foot.
Swing-to gait	Used when there is adequate muscle power and balance in the arms and legs	Both crutches are advanced together, then both legs are lifted and placed down on a spot behind the crutches; the feet and crutches form a tripod.
Swing-through gait	Used when there is adequate muscle power and balance in the arms and legs	Both crutches are advanced together, then both legs are lifted through and beyond the crutches and placed down again at a point in front of the crutches.

Adapted from Linton AD: *Introduction to medical-surgical nursing,* ed 4, St. Louis, 2007, Saunders.

3. Flex the knee of the unaffected leg to lower oneself into the chair while placing the affected leg straight out in front.
4. Reverse the steps to move from a sitting to a standing position.

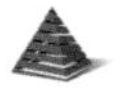

D. Going up and down stairs
1. Up the stairs
   a. The client moves the unaffected leg up first.
   b. The client moves the affected leg and the crutches up.
2. Down the stairs
   a. The client moves the crutches and the affected leg down.
   b. The client moves the unaffected leg down.

VIII. Canes and Walkers

A. Description: Canes and walkers are made of a lightweight material with a rubber tip at the bottom.

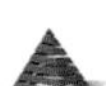

B. Interventions
1. Stand at the affected side of the client when ambulating.
2. The handle should be at the level of the client's greater trochanter.
3. The client's elbow should be flexed at a 15- to 30-degree angle.
4. Reinforce instructions to hold the cane 4 to 6 inches to the side of the foot.
5. Reinforce instructions to hold the cane in the hand on the unaffected side so that the cane and weaker leg can work together with each step.
6. Reinforce instructions to move the cane at the same time as the affected leg.
7. Reinforce instructions to inspect the rubber tips regularly for worn places.

C. Hemicanes or quadripod canes
1. Hemicanes or quadripod canes are used for clients who have the use of only one upper extremity.
2. Hemicanes provide more security than a quadripod cane; however, both types provide more security than a single-tipped cane.
3. Position the cane at the client's unaffected side, with the straight, nonangled side adjacent to the body.
4. Position the cane 6 inches from client's side, with the handgrips level with the greater trochanter.

D. Walker
1. Stand adjacent to the client on the affected side.
2. Reinforce instructions to put all four points of the walker flat on the floor before putting weight on the handpieces.
3. Reinforce instructions to move the walker forward and to walk into it.

⚠ Safety is the priority concern when the client uses an assistive device such as a cane, walker, or crutches. Be sure that the client demonstrates correct use of the device.

IX. Fractured Hip

A. Types
1. Intracapsular (femoral head is broken within the joint capsule)
   a. Femoral head and neck receive decreased blood supply and heal slowly.
   b. Skin traction is applied preoperatively to reduce fracture, immobilize bone, and help with muscle spasms.
   c. Treatment includes a total hip replacement or open reduction internal fixation (ORIF) with femoral head replacement.
   d. To prevent hip displacement postoperatively, avoid extreme hip flexion, and check the surgeon's prescriptions regarding positioning.

2. Extracapsular (fracture is outside the joint capsule)
   a. Fracture can occur at the greater trochanter or can be an intertrochanteric fracture.
   b. Trochanteric fracture is outside the joint.
   c. Preoperative treatment includes balanced suspension traction or skin traction to relieve muscle spasms and reduce pain.
   d. Surgical treatment includes ORIF with nail plate, screws, pins, or wires.

B. Postoperative interventions
1. Monitor for signs of delirium and institute safety measures.
2. Maintain leg and hip in proper alignment and prevent internal or external rotation; crossing over the midline with the operative leg needs to be avoided to prevent dislocation; avoid extreme hip flexion.
3. Follow the HCP's prescriptions regarding turning and repositioning; usually, turning to the unaffected side is allowed.
4. Elevate the head of the bed 30 to 45 degrees for meals only, unless otherwise prescribed.
5. Assist the client to ambulate as prescribed by the HCP.
6. Weight bearing is usually avoided on the affected leg as prescribed; instruct the client on the use of a walker to avoid weight bearing.
7. Weight bearing is often restricted after an ORIF and may not be restricted after total hip arthroplasty (THA); always refer to the HCP's prescriptions.
8. Keep the operative leg extended, supported, and elevated when getting the client out of bed.
9. Avoid hip flexion greater than 90 degrees and avoid low chairs when out of bed.
10. Monitor for wound infection or hemorrhage.
11. Perform neurovascular assessment of affected extremity: check color, pulses, capillary refill, movement, and sensation.
12. Maintain the compression of the wound drain to facilitate wound drainage if present.
13. Monitor and record drainage amount, which decreases consistently about 80 mL every 8 hours until 48 hours postoperatively.
14. Postoperative blood salvage may be done to collect, filter, and reinfuse salvaged blood into the client.
15. Use antiembolism stockings or sequential compression stockings and encourage the client to flex and extend the feet to reduce the risk of deep vein thrombosis (DVT).
16. Reinforce instructions to avoid crossing the legs and activities that require bending over.
17. Physical therapy will be instituted postoperatively with progressive ambulation as prescribed by the HCP.

Always check the HCP's postoperative prescriptions regarding positioning and activity restrictions following hip surgery. Restrictions may vary, depending on the type of surgery, surgical approach (anterior or posterior), and HCP preference.

X. Total Knee Replacement

A. Description: Total knee replacement is the implantation of a device to substitute for the femoral condyles and the tibial joint surfaces.

B. Postoperative interventions
1. Monitor surgical incision for drainage and infection.
2. Begin continuous passive motion 24 to 48 hours postoperatively if prescribed to exercise the knee and provide moderate flexion and extension.
3. Administer analgesics before continuous passive motion to decrease pain.
4. Prepare the client for out-of-bed activities as prescribed; have the client avoid leg dangling.
5. Avoid weight bearing, and instruct the client in the use of the prescribed assistive device, such as a walker or crutches.
6. Postoperative blood salvage to collect, filter, and reinfuse salvaged blood into the client may be prescribed.

XI. Joint Dislocation and Subluxation

A. Dislocation: Injury of the ligaments surrounding a joint that leads to displacement or separation of the articular surfaces of the joint

B. Subluxation: Incomplete displacement of joint surfaces when forces disrupt the soft tissue that surrounds the joints

C. Data collection
1. Asymmetry of the contour of affected body parts
2. Pain, tenderness, dysfunction, and swelling
3. Complications include neurovascular compromise, avascular necrosis, and open joint injuries.
4. X-rays are completed to determine joint shifting.

D. Interventions
1. Focus of treatment includes pain relief, joint support, and joint protection.
2. Immediate treatment is done to reduce the dislocation and realign the dislocated joint.
3. Open or closed reduction is done with a postprocedural joint immobilization.
4. Intravenous conscious sedation or local or general anesthesia is used during joint manipulation.
5. Initial activity restriction is followed by gentle range-of-motion activities and a gradual return of activities to normal levels while supporting the affected joint.

6. A weakened joint is prone to recurrent dislocation and may require extended activity restriction.

XII. Herniation: Intervertebral Disk

A. Description: The nucleus of the disk protrudes into the annulus, causing nerve compression.

B. Cervical disk herniation occurs at C5-C6 and C6-C7 interspaces.
   1. Cervical disk herniation causes pain radiation to shoulders, arms, hands, scapula, and pectoral muscles.
   2. Motor and sensory deficits can include paresthesia, numbness, and weakness of the upper extremities.
   3. Interventions
      a. Conservative management is used unless the client develops signs of neurological deterioration.
      b. Bed rest is prescribed to decrease pressure, inflammation, and pain.
      c. Immobilize the cervical area with a cervical collar, traction, or brace, as prescribed.
      d. Heat is used to reduce muscle spasms; ice is used to reduce inflammation and swelling.
      e. Maintain the head and spine in alignment.
      f. Reinforce instructions in the use of analgesics, sedatives, anti-inflammatory agents, and corticosteroids as prescribed.
      g. Prepare the client for a corticosteroid injection into the epidural space if prescribed.
      h. Assist and instruct client in the use of a cervical collar or cervical traction as prescribed.
   4. A cervical collar is used for cervical disk herniation.
      a. A cervical collar limits neck movement and holds the head in a neutral or slightly flexed position.
      b. The cervical collar may be worn intermittently or 24 hours a day.
      c. Inspect skin under the collar for irritation.
      d. When prescribed for use and after pain decreases, an exercise plan is designed to strengthen the muscles.
   5. Client education related to cervical disk conditions
      a. Avoid flexing, extending, and rotating the neck.
      b. Avoid the prone position, and maintain the neck, spine, and hips in neutral position while sleeping.
      c. Minimize long periods of sitting.
      d. Reinforce instructions regarding medications such as analgesics, sedatives, anti-inflammatory agents, and corticosteroids.

C. Lumbar disk herniation most often occurs at L4-L5 or L5-S1 interspaces.
   1. Herniation produces muscle weakness, sensory deficits, and diminished tendon reflexes.
   2. The client experiences pain and muscle spasms in the lower back, with radiation of the pain into one hip and down the leg (sciatica).
   3. Pain is relieved by bed rest and aggravated by movement, lifting, straining, and coughing.
   4. Interventions
      a. Conservative management is indicated unless neurological deterioration or bowel and bladder dysfunction occurs.
      b. Apply moist heat to decrease muscle spasms, and apply ice to decrease inflammation, as prescribed.
      c. Reinforce instructions to sleep on the side, with the knees and hips flexed, and place a pillow between the legs.
      d. Apply pelvic traction as prescribed to relieve muscle spasms and decrease pain.
      e. Begin progressive ambulation as inflammation, edema, and pain subside.

   5. Client education related to lumbar disk conditions
      a. Instruct in the use of prescribed medications such as analgesics, muscle relaxants, anti-inflammatory agents, or corticosteroids.
      b. Instruct about application techniques for corsets or braces to maintain immobilization and proper spine alignment.
      c. Instruct on correct posture while sitting, standing, walking, and working.
      d. Instruct on the correct technique to use when lifting objects such as bending knees, maintaining a straight back, and avoiding lifting objects above the elbow.
      e. Instruct in a weight-control program, as prescribed.
      f. Instruct in an exercise program to strengthen back and abdominal muscles, as prescribed.

D. Disk surgery is used when spinal cord compression is suspected or client symptoms do not respond to conservative treatment; minimally invasive procedures may be an option for the client.
   1. Preoperative interventions
      a. Provide routine preoperative instructions related to postoperative care.
      b. Reinforce instructions about logrolling and range-of-motion exercises.

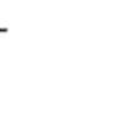

   2. Postoperative interventions: Cervical disk
      a. Monitor for respiratory difficulty from inflammation or hematoma.
      b. Encourage coughing, deep breathing, and early ambulation, as prescribed.
      c. Monitor for hoarseness and inability to cough effectively, because this may indicate laryngeal nerve damage.
      d. Use throat sprays or lozenges for sore throat, avoiding anesthetic lozenges that may numb the throat and increase choking risks.

e. Monitor the surgical wound for infection, swelling, redness, drainage, or pain
f. Provide a soft diet if the client complains of dysphagia.
g. Monitor for sudden return of radicular pain, which may indicate cervical spine instability.

3. Postoperative interventions: Lumbar disk
   a. Monitor for wound hemorrhage.
   b. Monitor lower extremities for sensation, movement, color, temperature, and paresthesia.
   c. Monitor for urinary retention, paralytic ileus, and constipation, which can result from decreased movement, opioid administration, or spinal cord compression.
   d. Prevent constipation by encouraging a high-fiber diet, increased fluid intake, and stool softeners, as prescribed.
   e. Administer opioids and sedatives as prescribed to relieve pain and anxiety.
   f. Assist and instruct the client to apply a prescribed back brace or corset while wearing cotton underwear to prevent skin irritation.
4. Postoperative lumbar disk positioning concerns
   a. In the immediate postoperative period, the client may be expected to lie supine or have other activity restrictions, depending on specific surgical intervention.
   b. Reinforce instructions to avoid spinal flexion or twisting and that the spine should be kept aligned.
   c. Reinforce instructions to minimize sitting, which may place a strain on the surgical site.
   d. When the client is lying supine, place a pillow under the neck and slightly flex the knees.
   e. Avoid extreme hip flexion when lying on the side.

Following disk surgery, instruct the client in correct logrolling techniques for turning and repositioning and for getting out of bed.

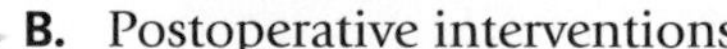

XIII. Amputation of a Lower Extremity

A. Description
1. Amputation (Fig. 59-4) is the surgical removal of a limb or part of the limb.
2. Complications include hemorrhage, infection, phantom limb pain, neuroma, and flexion contractures.

B. Postoperative interventions
1. Monitor for signs of complications.
2. Mark bleeding and drainage on the dressing if they occur.
3. Evaluate for phantom limb sensation and pain; explain sensation and pain to the client, and medicate the client as prescribed.
4. To prevent hip flexion contractures, do not elevate the residual limb on a pillow.

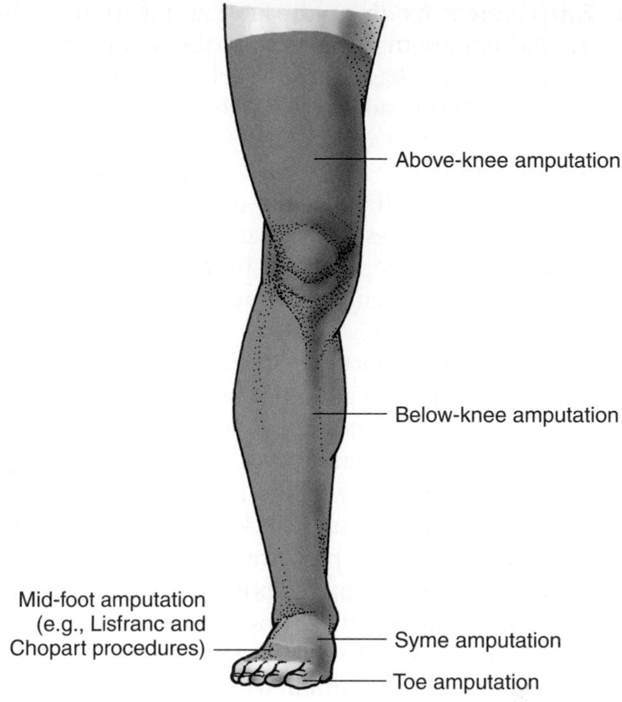

FIGURE 59-4 Common levels of lower-extremity amputation. (From Ignatavicius D, Workman ML: *Medical-surgical nursing: Patient-centered collaborative care*, ed 7, Philadelphia, 2013, Saunders.)

5. First 24 hours: Elevate the foot of the bed to reduce edema, and then keep the bed flat to prevent hip flexion contractures, if prescribed by the HCP.
6. After 24 to 48 hours postoperatively, position the client prone to stretch the muscles and prevent hip flexion contractures, if prescribed.
7. Maintain surgical application of dressing, elastic compression wrap, or elastic stump (residual limb) shrinker, as prescribed, to reduce swelling, minimize pain, and mold the residual limb in preparation for prosthesis.
8. As prescribed, wash the residual limb with mild soap and water and dry completely.
9. Massage the skin toward the suture line to mobilize scar and prevent its adherence to underlying bone.
10. Prepare for the prosthesis and reinforce instructions about progressive resistive techniques by gently pushing the residual limb against pillows and progressing to firmer surfaces.
11. Encourage verbalization regarding loss of the body part, and assist the client to identify coping mechanisms to deal with the loss.

C. Interventions for below-the-knee amputation
1. Prevent edema.
2. Do not allow the residual limb to hang over the edge of the bed.
3. Discourage long periods of sitting to lessen complications of knee flexion.

D. Interventions for above-the-knee amputation
1. Prevent internal or external rotation of the limb.
2. Place a sandbag, rolled towel, or trochanter roll along the outside of the thigh to prevent external rotation.

E. Rehabilitation
1. Instruct the client in the use of a mobility aid such as crutches or a walker.
2. Prepare the residual limb for a prosthesis.
3. Prepare the client for fitting of the residual limb for a prosthesis.
4. Reinforce instructions in exercises to maintain range of motion and upper body strengthening.
5. Provide psychosocial support to the client.

F. Traumatic amputation: Emergency care
1. Obtain emergency medical assistance (call 911).
2. Stay with the victim, check the amputation site, and apply direct pressure with gauze or cloth. Do not remove applied pressure dressing to prevent dislodging of a formed clot.
3. Elevate the extremity above heart level.
4. If finger(s) were amputated, place in a watertight sealed plastic bag and place the bag in ice water (not directly on ice) and transport to the emergency department with the victim.

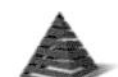

XIV. Rheumatoid Arthritis

A. Description
1. Rheumatoid arthritis is a chronic systemic inflammatory disease (immune complex–disorder); the cause may be related to a combination of environmental and genetic factors.
2. Rheumatoid arthritis leads to destruction of connective tissue and synovial membrane within the joints.
3. Rheumatoid arthritis weakens the joint, leading to dislocation and permanent deformity of the joint.
4. Formation of pannus occurs at the junction of synovial tissue and articular cartilage and projects into the joint cavity, causing necrosis.
5. Exacerbations of disease manifestations occur during periods of physical or emotional stress and fatigue.
6. Vasculitis can impede blood flow, leading to organ or organ system malfunction and failure because of tissue ischemia.

B. Data collection
1. Inflammation, tenderness, and stiffness of the joints

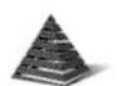

2. Moderate to severe pain with morning stiffness lasting longer than 30 minutes
3. Joint deformities, muscle atrophy, and decreased range of motion in affected joints
4. Spongy, soft feeling in the joints
5. Low-grade temperature, fatigue, and weakness
6. Anorexia, weight loss, and anemia
7. Elevated sedimentation rate and positive rheumatoid factor
8. Radiographic study showing joint deterioration
9. Synovial tissue biopsy reveals inflammation

C. Rheumatoid factor
1. A blood test used to assist in diagnosing rheumatoid arthritis
2. Values
   a. Nonreactive: 0 to 39 international units (IU)/mL
   b. Weakly reactive: 40 to 79 IU/mL
   c. Reactive: greater than 80 IU/mL

D. Medications: Combination of pharmacological therapies includes nonsteroidal anti-inflammatory drugs (NSAIDs), disease-modifying antirheumatic drugs (DMARDs), and glucocorticoids.

E. Physical mobility
1. Preserve joint function.
2. Provide range-of-motion exercises to maintain joint motion and muscle strengthening.
3. Balance rest and activity.
4. Splints may be used during acute inflammation to prevent deformity.
5. Prevent flexion contractures.
6. Apply heat or cold therapy to joints as prescribed.
7. Apply paraffin baths and massage as prescribed.
8. Encourage consistency with exercise program.
9. Use joint-protecting devices.
10. Avoid weight bearing on inflamed joints.

F. Self-care (Box 59-3)
1. Assess the need for assistive devices such as raised toilet seats, self-rising chairs, wheelchairs, and scooters to facilitate mobility.
2. Work with the RN and an occupational therapist or HCP to obtain assistive or adaptive devices.
3. Instruct the client in alternative strategies for providing activities of daily living.

G. Fatigue
1. Identify factors that may contribute to fatigue.
2. Monitor for signs of anemia, and administer iron, folic acid, and vitamins as prescribed.

BOX 59-3 Client Education for Rheumatoid Arthritis and Degenerative Joint Disease

Assist the client to identify and correct safety hazards in the home.
Instruct the client on the correct use of assistive or adaptive devices.
Instruct the client in energy conservation measures.
Review the prescribed exercise program.
Instruct the client to sit in a chair with a high, straight back.
Instruct the client to use only a small pillow when lying down.
Instruct the client on measures to protect the joints.
Instruct the client regarding prescribed medications.
Stress the importance of follow-up visits with the HCP.

3. Monitor for medication-related blood loss by testing the stool for occult blood.
4. Reinforce instructions in measures to conserve energy, such as pacing activities and obtaining assistance when possible.

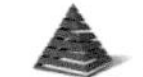
H. Disturbed body image
1. Determine the client's reaction to the body change.
2. Encourage the client to verbalize feelings.
3. Assist the client with self-care activities and grooming.
4. Encourage the client to wear street clothes.

I. Surgical interventions: Minimally invasive procedures may be prescribed.
1. Synovectomy: Surgical removal of the synovia to help maintain joint function
2. Arthrodesis: Bony fusion of a joint to regain some mobility
3. Joint replacement (arthroplasty): Surgical replacement of diseased joints with artificial joints; performed to restore motion to a joint and function to the muscles, ligaments, and other soft tissue structures that control a joint

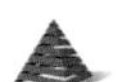

XV. Osteoarthritis (Degenerative Joint Disease)

A. Description
1. Osteoarthritis is marked by progressive deterioration of the articular cartilage.
2. It causes the formation of bony buildup and the loss of articular cartilage in peripheral and axial joints.
3. Osteoarthritis affects the weight-bearing joints and joints that receive the greatest stress, such as the hips, knees, and lower vertebral column and hands.
4. The cause of primary osteoarthritis is not known. Risk factors include trauma, aging, obesity, genetic changes, and smoking.

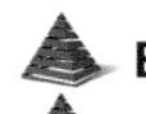
B. Data collection
1. Client experiences joint pain that diminishes after rest and intensifies after activity, noted early in the disease process.
2. As disease progresses, pain occurs with slight motion or even at rest.
3. Symptoms are aggravated by temperature change and climate humidity.
4. Presence of Heberden's nodes or Bouchard's nodes (hands)
5. Joint swelling (may be minimal), crepitus, and limited range of motion
6. Difficulty getting up after prolonged sitting
7. Skeletal muscle disuse atrophy
8. Inability to perform activities of daily living
9. Compression of the spine as manifested by radiating pain, stiffness, and muscle spasms in one or both extremities

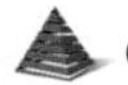
C. Pain
1. Administer medications as prescribed such as acetaminophen (Tylenol) or topical applications; if acetaminophen or topical agents do not relieve pain, then NSAIDs may be prescribed. Muscle relaxants may also be prescribed for muscle spasms, especially those occurring in the back.
2. Prepare the client for corticosteroid injections into joints as prescribed.
3. Position the joints in function position and avoid flexion of knees and hips.
4. Immobilize the affected joint with a splint or brace until inflammation subsides.
5. Avoid large pillows under the head or knees.
6. Provide a bed or foot cradle to keep linen off the feet.
7. Reinforce instructions on the importance of moist heat, hot packs or compresses, and paraffin dips as prescribed.
8. Apply cold applications as prescribed when the joint is acutely inflamed.
9. Encourage adequate rest.

D. Nutrition
1. Encourage a well-balanced diet.
2. Maintain weight within normal range to decrease stress on the joints.

E. Physical mobility
1. Reinforce instructions to balance activity with rest while participating in an exercise program that limits stressing affected joints.
2. Reinforce instructions that exercises should be active rather than passive and to stop exercise if pain occurs.
3. Reinforce instructions to limit exercise when joint inflammation is severe.

F. Surgical management: Minimally invasive procedures may be prescribed.
1. Osteotomy: The bone is resected to correct joint deformity, promote realignment, and reduce joint stress.
2. Total joint replacement or arthroplasty
   a. Total joint replacement is performed when all measures of pain relief have failed.
   b. Hips and knees are replaced most commonly.
   c. Total joint replacement is contraindicated in the presence of infection, advanced osteoporosis, or severe joint inflammation.

XVI. Osteoporosis

A. Description
1. Osteoporosis is a metabolic disease characterized by bone demineralization, with loss of calcium and phosphorus salts, leading to fragile bones and the subsequent risk for fractures.
2. Bone resorption accelerates as bone formation slows.
3. Osteoporosis occurs most commonly in the wrist, hip, and vertebral column.
4. Osteoporosis can occur postmenopausally or as a result of a metabolic disorder or calcium deficiency.

5. The client may be asymptomatic until the bones become fragile and a minor injury or movement causes a pathological fracture.
6. Primary osteoporosis
   a. Most often occurs in postmenopausal women; occurs in men with low testosterone levels
   b. Risk factors include decreased calcium intake, deficient estrogen, and sedentary lifestyle.
7. Secondary osteoporosis
   a. Causes include prolonged therapy with corticosteroids, thyroid-reducing medications, aluminum-containing antacids, or anticonvulsants
   b. Associated with immobility, alcoholism, malnutrition, or malabsorption
8. Risk factors (Box 59-4)

B. Data collection
1. Possibly asymptomatic
2. Back pain can occur after lifting, bending, or stooping.
3. Back pain that increases with palpation
4. Pelvic or hip pain, especially with weight bearing
5. Problems with balance
6. Decline in height from vertebral compression
7. Kyphosis of the dorsal spine, also known as "dowager's hump"
8. Degeneration of lower thorax and lumbar vertebrae on radiographic studies

⚠ The client with osteoporosis is at risk for pathological fractures.

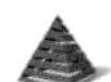

C. Interventions
1. Determine risk for injury, and institute measures to prevent injury in the client's personal environment.
   a. Assist the client to identify and correct hazards in his or her environment.
   b. Position household items and furniture for an unobstructed walkway.
   c. Use side rails to prevent falls.
   d. Reinforce instructions in the use of assistive devices such as a cane or walker.
   e. Encourage use of a firm mattress.
2. Provide personal care to the client to reduce injuries.
   a. Move the client gently when turning and repositioning.
   b. Assist with ambulation if the client is unsteady.
   c. Provide gentle range-of-motion exercises.
   d. Apply a back brace as prescribed during an acute phase to immobilize the spine and provide spinal column support.
3. Provide client instructions to promote optimal level of health and function.
   a. Reinforce instructions in the use of good body mechanics.
   b. Reinforce instructions in exercises to strengthen abdominal and back muscles to improve posture and provide support for the spine.
   c. Reinforce instructions to avoid activities that can cause vertebral compression.
   d. Reinforce instructions to eat a diet high in protein, calcium, vitamins C and D, and iron (see Chapter 12 for foods high in these vitamins and minerals).
   e. Reinforce instructions to avoid alcohol and coffee.
   f. Reinforce instructions to maintain an adequate fluid intake to prevent renal calculi.
4. Administer medication as prescribed to promote bone strength and decrease pain.

BOX 59-4 Risk Factors for Osteoporosis

Cigarette smoking
Early menopause
Excessive use of alcohol
Family history
Female gender
Increasing age
Insufficient intake of calcium
Sedentary lifestyle
Thin, small frame
White (European descent) or Asian race

XVII. Gout

A. Description
1. Gout is a systemic disease in which urate crystals deposit in joints and other body tissues.
2. Gout results from abnormal amounts of uric acid in the body.
3. Primary gout results from a disorder of purine metabolism.
4. Secondary gout involves excessive uric acid in the blood that is caused by another disease.

B. Phases
1. Asymptomatic: Client has no symptoms, but serum uric acid is elevated.
2. Acute: Client has excruciating pain and inflammation of one or more small joints, especially the great toe.
3. Intermittent: Client has intermittent periods without symptoms between acute attacks.
4. Chronic: Results from repeated episodes of acute gout
   a. Chronic gout results in deposits of urate crystals under the skin.
   b. Chronic gout results in deposits of urate crystals within major organs such as kidneys, leading to organ dysfunction.

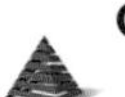

C. Data collection

1. Swelling and inflammation of the joints, leading to excruciating pain
2. Tophi: Hard, irregular-shaped nodules in the skin containing chalky deposits of sodium urate
3. Low-grade fever, malaise, and headache
4. Pruritus from urate crystals in the skin
5. Presence of renal stones from elevated uric acid levels

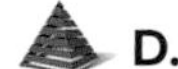

D. Interventions

1. Provide a low-purine diet as prescribed; foods such as organ meats, wines, and aged cheese should be avoided.
2. Encourage a high fluid intake of 2000 mL/day (unless contraindicated) to prevent stone formation.
3. Encourage a weight-reduction diet if required.
4. Instruct the client to avoid alcohol and starvation diets because they may precipitate a gout attack.
5. Increase urinary pH (above 6) by eating alkaline ash foods (see Chapter 53).
6. Provide bed rest during the acute attacks with affected extremity elevated.
7. Monitor joint range-of-motion ability and appearance of joints.
8. Position the joint in mild flexion during an acute attack.
9. Protect the affected joint from excessive movement or direct contact with sheets or blankets.
10. Provide heat or cold for local treatments to the affected joint as prescribed.
11. Administer medications such as analgesics, anti-inflammatory medications, and uricosuric agents, as prescribed.

CRITICAL THINKING What Should You Do?

Answer: In a traumatic amputation, the nurse should call 911 to transport the victim to the hospital. While awaiting emergency medical assistance, the nurse should immediately check the amputation site and apply direct pressure with dry gauze. This pressure dressing is not removed to prevent dislodgment of a formed clot. The extremity is elevated above heart level. The amputated finger is placed in a watertight sealed plastic bag, and the bag is placed in ice water (not directly on ice). The nurse stays with the victim until transport to the emergency department.

Reference(s): deWit, D. & Kumagai, C. (2013). *Medical-surgical nursing: Concepts & practice.* (2nd ed., p. 758). St. Louis: Saunders.

Ignatavicius, D., & Workman, M. (2013). *Medical-surgical nursing: Patient-centered collaborative care.* (7th ed., p. 1165). St. Louis: Saunders.

PRACTICE QUESTIONS

621. The nurse is one of several people who witness a vehicle hit a pedestrian at a fairly low speed on a small street. The individual is dazed and tries to get up, and the leg appears fractured. The nurse should plan to perform which action?

1. Try to manually reduce the fracture.
2. Assist the person to get up and walk to the sidewalk.
3. Leave the person for a few moments to call an ambulance.
4. Stay with the person and encourage the person to remain still.

622. The nurse witnesses a client sustain a fall and suspects that the client's leg may be fractured. Which action is the **priority**?

1. Take a set of vital signs.
2. Call the radiology department.
3. Immobilize the leg before moving the client.
4. Reassure the client that everything will be fine.

623. A client with a hip fracture asks the nurse why Buck's extension traction is being applied before surgery. The nurse's response is based on the understanding that Buck's extension traction has which **primary** function?

1. Allows bony healing to begin before surgery
2. Provides rigid immobilization of the fracture site
3. Lengthens the fractured leg to prevent severing of blood vessels
4. Provides comfort by reducing muscle spasms and provides fracture immobilization

624. The nurse is evaluating the pin sites of a client in skeletal traction. The nurse would be least concerned with which finding?

1. Inflammation
2. Serous drainage
3. Pain at a pin site
4. Purulent drainage

625. The nurse is caring for the client who has had skeletal traction applied to the left leg. The client is complaining of severe left leg pain. Which action should the nurse take **first**?

1. Provide pin care.
2. Call the health care provider (HCP).
3. Check the client's alignment in bed.
4. Medicate the client with an analgesic.

626. The nurse has provided instructions regarding specific leg exercises for the client immobilized in right skeletal lower leg traction. The nurse determines that the client **needs further teaching** if the nurse observes the client doing which activity?

1. Pulling up on the trapeze
2. Flexing and extending the feet
3. Doing quadriceps-setting and gluteal-setting exercises
4. Performing active range of motion (ROM) to the right ankle and knee

627. The nurse is checking the casted extremity of a client. The nurse should check for which sign indicative of infection?

1. Dependent edema
2. Diminished distal pulse
3. Presence of a "hot spot" on the cast
4. Coolness and pallor of the extremity

628. A client has sustained a closed fracture and has just had a cast applied to the affected arm. The client is complaining of intense pain. The nurse has elevated the limb, applied an ice bag, and administered an analgesic, which was ineffective in relieving the pain. The nurse interprets that this pain may be caused by which condition?

1. Infection under the cast
2. The anxiety of the client
3. Impaired tissue perfusion
4. The newness of the fracture

629. The nurse is assigned to care for a client with multiple traumas who is admitted to the hospital. The client has a leg fracture, and a plaster cast has been applied. In positioning the casted leg, the nurse should perform which intervention?

1. Keep the leg in a level position.
2. Elevate the leg for 3 hours, and put it flat for 1 hour.
3. Keep the leg level for 3 hours, and elevate it for 1 hour.
4. Elevate the leg on pillows continuously for 24 to 48 hours.

630. A client is complaining of skin irritation from the edges of a cast applied the previous day. The nurse should plan for which intervention?

1. Massaging the skin at the rim of the cast
2. Petaling the cast edges with adhesive tape
3. Using a rough file to smooth the cast edges
4. Applying lotion to the skin at the rim of the cast

❖ **631.** The nurse is preparing a list of cast care instructions for a client who just had a plaster cast applied to his right forearm. Which instructions should the nurse include on the list? **Select all that apply.**

- ❑ **1.** Keep the cast and extremity elevated.
- ❑ **2.** The cast needs to be kept clean and dry.
- ❑ **3.** Allow the wet cast 24 to 72 hours to dry.
- ❑ **4.** Expect tingling and numbness in the extremity.
- ❑ **5.** Use a hair dryer set on a warm to hot setting to dry the cast.
- ❑ **6.** Use a soft padded object that will fit under the cast to scratch the skin under the cast.

632. The nurse is planning to reinforce instructions to the client about how to stand on crutches. In the instructions, the nurse should plan to tell the client to place the crutches in which position?

1. 3 inches to the front and side of the client's toes
2. 8 inches to the front and side of the client's toes
3. 15 inches to the front and side of the client's toes
4. 20 inches to the front and side of the client's toes

633. The nurse is evaluating the client's use of a cane for left-sided weakness. The nurse should intervene and correct the client if the nurse observed that the client performed which action?

1. Holds the cane on the right side
2. Moves the cane when the right leg is moved
3. Leans on the cane when the right leg swings through
4. Keeps the cane 6 inches out to the side of the right foot

634. The nurse is caring for a client with fresh application of a plaster leg cast. The nurse should plan to prevent the development of compartment syndrome by which action?

1. Elevating the limb and applying ice to the affected leg
2. Elevating the limb and covering the limb with bath blankets
3. Keeping the leg horizontal and applying ice to the affected leg
4. Placing the leg in a slightly dependent position and applying ice

635. A client is being discharged home after application of a plaster leg cast. The nurse determines that the client understands proper care of the cast if the client makes which statement?

1. "I need to avoid getting the cast wet."
2. "I will use my fingertips to lift and move the leg."
3. "I need to cover the casted leg with warm blankets."
4. "I can use a padded coat hanger end to scratch under the cast."

ANSWERS

621. 4

Rationale: With a suspected fracture, the client is not moved unless it is dangerous to remain in that spot. The nurse should remain with the client and have someone else call for emergency help. A fracture is not reduced at the scene. Before moving the client, the site of the fracture is immobilized to prevent further injury.

Test-Taking Strategy: Focus on the subject, the action to take if a fracture is suspected. Eliminate options 1 and 2 first, because these actions are comparable or alike and could result in further injury to the client. From the remaining options, the most prudent action would be for the nurse to remain with the client and have someone else call for emergency assistance. **Review:** immediate care of the client with a **fracture**.

Level of Cognitive Ability: Applying
Client Needs: Physiological Integrity
Integrated Process: Nursing Process/Implementation
Content Area: Adult Health: Musculoskeletal
Priority Concepts: Mobility, Safety
Reference(s): Lewis et al (2014), p. 1518.

622. 3

Rationale: When a fracture is suspected, it is imperative that the area is splinted before the client is moved. Emergency help should be called if the client is not hospitalized; a health care provider is called for the hospitalized client. The nurse should remain with the client and provide realistic reassurance. The nurse does not prescribe radiology tests.

Test-Taking Strategy: Note the strategic word, *priority.* Eliminate option 2 because the nurse does not prescribe x-rays. Reassuring the client is eliminated next, because the nurse does not tell a client that "everything will be fine." From the remaining options, focus on the data in the question. Immobilizing the limb is imperative for the client's safety, which makes it a better choice than taking vital signs. **Review:** care of the client when a **fracture** is suspected.

Level of Cognitive Ability: Applying
Client Needs: Physiological Integrity
Integrated Process: Nursing Process/Implementation
Content Area: Adult Health: Musculoskeletal
Priority Concepts: Clinical Judgment, Mobility
Reference(s): deWit, Kumagai (2013), pp. 737–738; Lewis et al (2014), p. 1518.

623. 4

Rationale: Buck's extension traction is a type of skin traction often applied after hip fracture, before the fracture is reduced in surgery. It reduces muscle spasms and helps immobilize the fracture. It does not lengthen the leg for the purpose of preventing blood vessel severance. It also does not allow for bony healing to begin.

Test-Taking Strategy: Note the strategic word, *primary,* and focus on the subject, the function of traction. Recalling the purpose of traction will assist in eliminating options 1 and 3. From the remaining options, eliminate the option with the words *rigid immobilization.* **Review: Buck's traction.**

Level of Cognitive Ability: Applying
Client Needs: Physiological Integrity
Integrated Process: Nursing Process/Implementation
Content Area: Adult Health: Musculoskeletal
Priority Concepts: Pain, Safety
Reference(s): deWit, Kumagai (2013), p. 740.

624. 2

Rationale: A small amount of serous drainage is expected at pin insertion sites. Signs of infection such as inflammation, purulent drainage, and pain at the pin site are not expected findings and should be reported.

Test-Taking Strategy: Focus on the subject, the finding that the nurse would be least concerned with. Inflammation and purulent drainage indicate infection and are eliminated first; these options are comparable or alike. To select between the other options, look at them carefully. The complaint of pain is at "a pin site" only. It gives no indication that the pain is related to the fracture or muscle spasm. Because serous drainage is an expected finding, you would select this over the complaint of pain. **Review:** care of the client in **skeletal traction.**

Level of Cognitive Ability: Analyzing
Client Needs: Physiological Integrity
Integrated Process: Nursing Process/Data Collection
Content Area: Adult Health: Musculoskeletal
Priority Concepts: Clinical Judgment, Tissue Integrity
Reference(s): deWit, Kumagai (2013), p. 741.

625. 3

Rationale: A client who complains of severe pain may need realignment or may have had traction weights prescribed that are too heavy. The nurse realigns the client and, if ineffective, calls the HCP. Severe leg pain, once traction has been established, indicates a problem. Medicating the client should be done after trying to determine and treat the cause. Providing pin care is unrelated to the problem as described.

Test-Taking Strategy: Note the strategic word, *first.* Use the steps of the nursing process. The option describing checking the client's alignment is the only option that addresses data collection. **Review: skeletal traction.**

Level of Cognitive Ability: Applying
Client Needs: Physiological Integrity
Integrated Process: Nursing Process/Implementation
Content Area: Adult Health: Musculoskeletal
Priority Concepts: Clinical Judgment, Pain
Reference(s): deWit, Kumagai (2013), p. 744.

626. 4

Rationale: Exercise is indicated within therapeutic limits for the client in skeletal traction to maintain muscle strength and range of motion (ROM). The client may pull up on the trapeze, perform active ROM with uninvolved joints, and do isometric muscle-setting exercises (e.g., quadriceps- and gluteal-setting exercises). The client may also flex and extend his or her feet. Performing active ROM to the affected leg can be harmful.

Test-Taking Strategy: Note the strategic words, *needs further teaching.* This indicates a negative event query and the need to select the incorrect client action. Options 1 and 3 are most easily identified as correct actions and are therefore eliminated as possible answers. To select between the remaining options, imagine the lines of pull on the fracture site with the movements described. Although flexing and extending the feet do not disrupt the line of pull from the traction, performing

active ROM to the affected knee and ankle does. **Review:** care of the client in traction.
Level of Cognitive Ability: Evaluating
Client Needs: Physiological Integrity
Integrated Process: Teaching and Learning
Content Area: Adult Health: Musculoskeletal
Priority Concepts: Client Education, Tissue Integrity
Reference(s): deWit, Kumagai (2013), pp. 724–725.

627. 3
Rationale: Signs and symptoms of infection under a casted area include odor or purulent drainage from the cast or the presence of "hot spots," which are areas of the cast that are warmer than others. The health care provider should be notified if any of these occur. Signs of impaired circulation in the distal limb include coolness and pallor of the skin, diminished arterial pulse, and edema.
Test-Taking Strategy: Note the subject, a sign of infection. Begin to answer this question by thinking of what you would expect to find with infection: redness, swelling, heat, and purulent drainage. With these in mind, the options of diminished distal pulses and coolness of the extremity can be eliminated. *Dependent edema* is not necessarily indicative of infection; swelling would be continuous. The "hot spot" on the cast could signify infection underneath that area. **Review:** the complications of a cast.
Level of Cognitive Ability: Applying
Client Needs: Physiological Integrity
Integrated Process: Nursing Process/Data Collection
Content Area: Adult Health: Musculoskeletal
Priority Concepts: Infection, Tissue Integrity
Reference(s): Lewis et al (2014), p. 1518.

628. 3
Rationale: Most pain associated with fractures can be minimized with rest, elevation, application of cold, and administration of analgesics. Pain that is not relieved from these measures should be reported to the RN and health care provider because it may be the result of impaired tissue perfusion, tissue breakdown, or necrosis. Because this is a new closed fracture and cast, infection would not have had time to set in.
Test-Taking Strategy: Focus on the subject, interpretation of the cause of the client's intense pain. The options of anxiety and newness of the fracture can be eliminated first, based on the description in the question. Because the fracture and cast are so new, it is extremely unlikely that infection could have set in. The most likely option is impaired tissue perfusion, because pain from ischemia is not relieved by comfort measures and analgesics. **Review:** complications of a cast.
Level of Cognitive Ability: Analyzing
Client Needs: Physiological Integrity
Integrated Process: Nursing Process/Data Collection
Content Area: Adult Health: Musculoskeletal
Priority Concepts: Pain, Tissue Integrity
Reference(s): deWit, Kumagai (2013), pp. 741–742.

629. 4
Rationale: A casted extremity is elevated continuously for the first 24 to 48 hours to minimize swelling and to promote venous drainage. Therefore, the other options are incorrect.
Test-Taking Strategy: Focus on the subject, intervention used when positioning a casted leg. Recall that edema sets in after fracture and can be aggravated by casting. For this reason, options 1 and 3 are comparable or alike in keeping the leg level. These are the least helpful and can be eliminated first. There is no useful purpose for the timing in the option for elevating and then leaving the leg flat. **Review:** care of the client with a cast.
Level of Cognitive Ability: Applying
Client Needs: Physiological Integrity
Integrated Process: Nursing Process/Implementation
Content Area: Adult Health: Musculoskeletal
Priority Concepts: Inflammation, Mobility
Reference(s): deWit, Kumagai (2013), pp. 744–745.

630. 2
Rationale: The edges of the cast can be petaled with tape to minimize skin irritation. If a client has a cast applied and returns home, the client can be taught to do the same. Massaging and applying lotion will not alleviate the skin irritation from the cast edges. Filing the edges will cause cast material to fall into the cast and could lead to skin irritation under the cast.
Test-Taking Strategy: Focus on the subject, skin irritation. Options 1 and 4 are comparable or alike, and neither helps to get rid of the cause of the irritation, so they are eliminated first. Imagine the use of a "rough file"; it would create plaster chips and dust, which could go underneath the cast. **Review:** care of the client with a cast.
Level of Cognitive Ability: Applying
Client Needs: Physiological Integrity
Integrated Process: Nursing Process/Planning
Content Area: Adult Health: Musculoskeletal
Priority Concepts: Mobility, Tissue Integrity
Reference(s): deWit, Kumagai (2013), p. 739.

❖**631.** 1, 2, 3
Rationale: A plaster cast takes 24 to 72 hours to dry (synthetic casts dry in 20 minutes). The cast and extremity may be elevated to reduce edema. A wet cast is handled with the palms of the hands until it is dry, and the extremity is turned (unless contraindicated) so that all sides of the wet cast will dry. A cool setting on the hair dryer can be used to dry a plaster cast. (Heat cannot be used on a plaster cast because the cast heats up and burns the skin.) The cast needs to be kept clean and dry, and the client is instructed not to stick anything under the cast because of the risk of breaking skin integrity. The client is instructed to monitor the extremity for circulatory impairment such as pain, swelling, discoloration, tingling, numbness, coolness, or diminished pulse. The health care provider is notified immediately if circulatory impairment occurs.
Test-Taking Strategy: Focus on the subject, a plaster cast. Recalling that edema occurs following a fracture and recalling the complications associated with a cast will assist you in answering the question. **Review:** **cast care instructions.**
Level of Cognitive Ability: Analyzing
Client Needs: Physiological Integrity
Integrated Process: Teaching and Learning
Content Area: Adult Health: Musculoskeletal
Priority Concepts: Client Education, Tissue Integrity
Reference(s): deWit, Kumagai (2013), p. 739.

632. 2

Rationale: The classic tripod position is taught to the client before giving instructions on gait. The crutches are placed anywhere from 6 to 10 inches in front and to the side of the client, depending on the client's body size. This provides a wide enough base of support to the client and improves balance.
Test-Taking Strategy: Focus on the subject, the safe use of crutches. Three inches and 20 inches seem excessively short and long, respectively; therefore, these options can be eliminated first. Of the remaining options, 8 inches seems more in keeping with the normal length of a stride than 15 inches. Review: crutch walking.
Level of Cognitive Ability: Applying
Client Needs: Safe and Effective Care Environment
Integrated Process: Teaching and Learning
Content Area: Adult Health: Musculoskeletal
Priority Concepts: Client Education, Mobility
Reference(s): deWit, Kumagai (2013), pp. 730–731.

633. 2

Rationale: The cane is held on the stronger side to minimize stress on the affected extremity and provide a wide base of support. The cane is held 6 inches lateral to the fifth great toe. The cane is moved forward with the affected leg. The client leans on the cane for added support, while the stronger side swings through.
Test-Taking Strategy: Note the word, *intervene.* Therefore, the subject of the question is the incorrect client action. Knowing that the cane is held on the stronger side helps you eliminate options 1 and 4 first. To select from the remaining options, recall that the client moves the cane with the weaker leg and leans on it for support when the stronger leg swings through. Review: cane walking.
Level of Cognitive Ability: Applying
Client Needs: Safe and Effective Care Environment
Integrated Process: Nursing Process/Implementation
Content Area: Adult Health: Musculoskeletal
Priority Concepts: Client Education, Mobility
Reference(s): deWit, Kumagai (2013), p. 731.

634. 1

Rationale: Compartment syndrome is prevented by controlling edema. This is achieved most optimally with elevation and application of ice. Therefore, the other options are incorrect.
Test-Taking Strategy: Focus on the subject, compartment syndrome. Recalling that edema is controlled or prevented with limb elevation helps you eliminate options 3 and 4 first. From the remaining options, think about the effects of ice versus bath blankets. Ice will further control edema, but bath blankets will produce heat and prevent air circulation needed for the cast to dry. **Review: compartment syndrome.**
Level of Cognitive Ability: Applying
Client Needs: Physiological Integrity
Integrated Process: Nursing Process/Planning
Content Area: Adult Health: Musculoskeletal
Priority Concepts: Clinical Judgment, Perfusion
Reference(s): deWit, Kumagai (2013), pp. 741–742, 745.

635. 1

Rationale: A plaster cast must remain dry to keep its strength. The cast should be handled using the palms of the hands, not the fingertips, until fully dry. Air should circulate freely around the cast to help it dry; the cast also gives off heat as it dries. The client should never scratch under the cast; a cool hair dryer may be used to eliminate itching.
Test-Taking Strategy: Focus on the subject, proper cast care. Knowing that a wet cast can be dented with the fingertips, causing pressure underneath, helps you eliminate option 2 first. Knowing that the cast needs to dry helps you eliminate option 3 next. The option of using a coat hanger is dangerous to skin integrity and is also eliminated. Plaster casts, once they have dried after application, should not become wet. **Review:** home care instructions for a client with a cast.
Level of Cognitive Ability: Evaluating
Client Needs: Physiological Integrity
Integrated Process: Nursing Process/Evaluation
Content Area: Adult Health: Musculoskeletal
Priority Concepts: Client Education, Tissue Integrity
Reference(s): deWit, Kumagai (2013), p. 739.

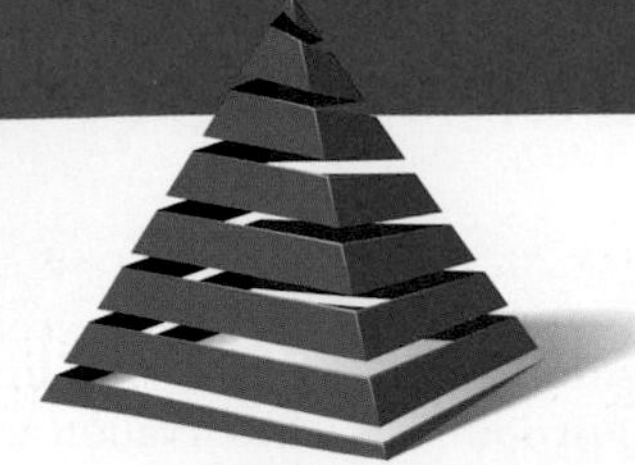

CHAPTER 60

Musculoskeletal Medications

CRITICAL THINKING What Should You Do?

Cyclobenzaprine (Flexeril) is prescribed for a client experiencing muscle spasms. The nurse reviews the client's record and notes that the client is currently taking phenelzine (Nardil). What should the nurse do?
Answer located on p. 864.

I. Skeletal Muscle Relaxants

A. Description
   1. Skeletal muscle relaxants (Box 60-1) act directly on the neuromuscular junction or act indirectly on the central nervous system (CNS).
   2. Centrally acting muscle relaxants depress neuron activity in the spinal cord or brain.
   3. Peripherally acting muscle relaxants act directly on the skeletal muscles, interfering with calcium release from muscle tubules and thus preventing the fibers from contracting.
   4. Skeletal muscle relaxants are used to prevent or relieve muscle spasms and treat spasticity associated with spinal cord disease or lesions, acute painful musculoskeletal conditions, and chronic debilitating disorders such as multiple sclerosis, brain attacks (stroke), or cerebral palsy.

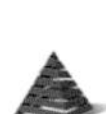

   5. Skeletal muscle relaxants are contraindicated in clients with severe liver, renal, or heart disease; these medications are often metabolized in the liver or excreted from the kidney.

BOX 60-1 Skeletal Muscle Relaxants

Baclofen
Carisoprodol (Soma)
Chlorzoxazone (Paraflex, Parafon Forte, Remular-S)
Cyclobenzaprine (Flexeril, Amrix)
Dantrolene (Dantrium)
Diazepam (Valium)
Metaxalone (Skelaxin)
Methocarbamol (Robaxin)
Orphenadrine (Norflex)
Tizanidine (Zanaflex)

   6. Skeletal muscle relaxants should not be taken with CNS depressants, such as barbiturates, opioids, alcohol, sedatives, hypnotics, or tricyclic antidepressants, unless specifically prescribed.

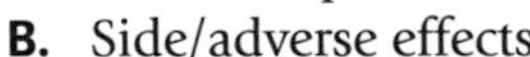

B. Side/adverse effects
   1. Dizziness and hypotension
   2. Drowsiness and muscle weakness
   3. Dry mouth
   4. Gastrointestinal upset
   5. Photosensitivity
   6. Liver toxicity

C. Interventions
   1. Obtain a medical history.
   2. Monitor vital signs.
   3. Monitor for CNS side/adverse effects.
   4. Determine risk for injury.
   5. Monitor involved joints and muscles for pain and mobility.
   6. Monitor renal function studies.
   7. Reinforce instructions to the client to take the medication with food to decrease gastrointestinal upset.
   8. Reinforce instructions to the client to report side/adverse effects.
   9. Reinforce instructions to the client to avoid alcohol and CNS depressants.
   10. Reinforce instructions to the client to avoid activities requiring alertness such as driving or operating equipment.

Monitor liver function tests when a client is taking a skeletal muscle relaxant because hepatotoxicity can occur.

D. Nursing considerations
   1. Baclofen
      a. Baclofen causes CNS effects such as drowsiness, dizziness, weakness, and fatigue, and nausea, constipation, and urinary retention.
      b. Administered with caution in the client with renal or hepatic dysfunction or a seizure disorder.
      c. Baclofen can be administered by the health care provider through intrathecal infusion using an implantable pump or by direct intrathecal administration over 1 minute.

d. The client with an implantable pump is instructed to maintain medication refill appointments to prevent the pump from emptying and experiencing sudden withdrawal symptoms (which could be life threatening).

2. Carisoprodol (Soma)
   a. The client is advised to take the medication with food to prevent gastrointestinal upset.
   b. Reinforce instructions to the client to report any rash or hypersensitivity to the health care provider (HCP).
3. Chlorzoxazone (Paraflex, Parafon Forte, Remular-S)
   a. Monitor the client for hypersensitivity reactions such as urticaria, redness or itching, and possibly angioedema.
   b. Chlorzoxazone may cause malaise and may cause the urine to turn orange or red.
   c. Chlorzoxazone can cause hepatitis and hepatic necrosis.
4. Cyclobenzaprine (Flexeril, Amrix)
   a. Cyclobenzaprine is contraindicated in clients who have received monoamine oxidase inhibitors (MAOIs) within 14 days of initiation of cyclobenzaprine therapy and in clients with cardiac disorders.
   b. Cyclobenzaprine has significant anticholinergic (atropine-like) effects and should be used with caution in clients with a history of urinary retention, angle-closure glaucoma, or increased intraocular pressure.
   c. Cyclobenzaprine should be used only for short-term therapy (2 to 3 weeks).
5. Dantrolene (Dantrium)
   a. Dantrolene acts directly on skeletal muscles to relieve spasticity.
   b. Liver damage is the most serious adverse effect.
   c. Liver function values should be monitored before the initiation of treatment and during treatment.
   d. Dantrolene can cause gastrointestinal bleeding, urinary frequency, impotence, photosensitivity, rash, and muscle weakness.
   e. Reinforce instructions to the client to wear protective clothing when in the sun.
   f. Reinforce instructions to the client to notify the HCP if rash, bloody or tarry stools, or yellow discoloration of the skin or eyes occurs.
6. Diazepam (Valium)
   a. Acts in the CNS to suppress spasticity; does not affect skeletal muscle directly
   b. Sedation is a common side effect.
7. Methocarbamol (Robaxin)
   a. The parenteral form is contraindicated in clients with renal impairment.
   b. The parenteral form can cause hypotension, bradycardia, anaphylaxis, and seizures, especially when the medication is given too rapidly. 
   c. Monitor site for extravasation, which can result in thrombophlebitis and tissue sloughing.
   d. Methocarbamol may cause the urine to turn brown, black, or green.
   e. The client is informed to notify the HCP if blurred vision, nasal congestion, urticaria, or rash occurs.
8. Tizanidine (Zanaflex) and metaxalone (Skelaxin): Can cause liver damage
9. Orphenadrine (Norflex) has significant anticholinergic (atropine-like) effects and should be used with caution in clients with a history of urinary retention, angle-closure glaucoma, or increased intraocular pressure.

Safety is a primary concern when the client is taking a skeletal muscle relaxant because these medications cause drowsiness.

II. Antigout Medications

A. Description
   1. Antigout medications allopurinol (Zyloprim), colchicine (Colcrys), probenecid, sulfinpyrazone reduce uric acid production and increase uric acid excretion (uricosuric) to prevent or relieve gout or to manage hyperuricemia.
   2. Nonsteroidal anti-inflammatory drugs (NSAIDs) are used for their anti-inflammatory effects and to relieve pain during an acute gouty attack (see Chapter 58 for information on NSAIDs).
   3. Glucocorticoids may be prescribed to reduce inflammation during an acute gouty attack (see Chapter 46 for information on glucocorticoids).
   4. Antigout medications should be used cautiously in clients with gastrointestinal, renal, cardiac, or hepatic disease. 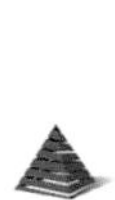
B. Side/adverse effects
   1. Headaches
   2. Nausea, vomiting, and diarrhea
   3. Blood dyscrasias, such as bone marrow suppression 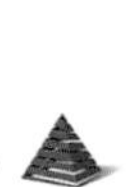
   4. Flushed skin and rash
   5. Uric acid kidney stones 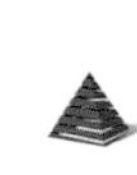
   6. Sore gums
   7. Metallic taste
C. Interventions
   1. Monitor serum uric acid levels.
   2. Monitor intake and output.
   3. Maintain a fluid intake of at least 2000 to 3000 mL/day to avoid kidney stones. 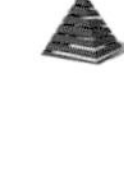 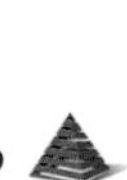
   4. Monitor complete blood cell count and renal and liver function.

5. Reinforce instructions to the client to avoid alcohol and caffeine because these products can increase uric acid levels.
6. The client is encouraged to comply with therapy to prevent elevated uric acid levels, which can trigger a gout attack.
7. Reinforce instructions to the client to avoid foods high in purine as prescribed, such as wine, alcohol, organ meats, sardines, salmon, scallops, and gravy.
8. Reinforce instructions to the client to take the medication with food to decrease gastric irritation.
9. Reinforce instructions to the client to report side/adverse effects to the HCP.
10. Reinforce instructions to the client not to take aspirin with these medications because this could trigger a gout attack.

D. Nursing considerations
1. Allopurinol (Zyloprim)
   a. Can increase the effect of warfarin (Coumadin) and oral hypoglycemic agents
   b. Reinforce instructions to the client not to take large doses of vitamin C while taking allopurinol, because kidney stones may occur.
   c. Hypersensitivity syndrome (rare) can occur, characterized by rash, fever, eosinophilia, and dysfunction of the liver and kidneys (medication is stopped and the HCP is notified).
   d. The client is advised to minimize exposure to sunlight and have an annual eye examination because visual changes can occur from prolonged use of allopurinol.
2. Colchicine (Colcrys)
   a. Used with caution in older clients, debilitated clients, and clients with cardiac, renal, and/or gastrointestinal disease
   b. If gastrointestinal symptoms occur (nausea, vomiting, diarrhea, and abdominal pain), the medication is stopped and the HCP is notified.
3. Probenecid
   a. Mild gastrointestinal effects can occur and can be reduced by taking the medication with food.
   b. Aspirin and other salicylates interfere with the uricosuric action of the medication.
4. Sulfinpyrazone
   a. Contraindicated in clients with active ulcer disease; used with caution in clients with a history of ulcer disease
   b. Salicylates counteract the uricosuric action of the medication.
   c. Inhibits hepatic metabolism of tolbutamide (Orinase), causing hypoglycemia, and of warfarin, causing bleeding tendencies

⚠ The concurrent use of antigout medications and aspirin causes elevated uric acid levels; the client should be instructed to take acetaminophen (Tylenol) if prescribed rather than aspirin.

III. Antiarthritic Medications (Box 60-2)

A. Description (Fig. 60-1)
1. Rheumatoid arthritis occurs as inflammation progresses into the synovia, cartilage, and bone; if this inflammation is not controlled, it will lead to joint destruction, thus affecting client mobility and comfort.
2. The focus of treatment is early diagnosis and aggressive treatment in order to preserve joint function.
3. Medication therapy includes NSAIDs, glucocorticoids, and disease-modifying antirheumatic drugs (DMARDs).
4. Gold salts: Use of gold salts has decreased, but their purpose is to reduce the progression of joint damage caused by arthritic processes. Gold toxicity, which includes pruritus, rash, metallic taste, stomatitis, and diarrhea, can occur; if toxicity occurs, dimercaprol (British antilewisite [BAL] in oil) may be prescribed to enhance gold excretion.

B. DMARDs
1. Description
   a. DMARDs are effective antirheumatic medications that are used to slow the degenerative effects of the disorder.
   b. DMARDs are usually prescribed secondary to NSAIDs but are often the first choice in the treatment of severe arthritis.
   c. Some medications are contraindicated during pregnancy.
2. Common side/adverse effects of DMARDs include injection site inflammation and pain, ecchymosis and edema, bone marrow suppression and infection, fatigue, headache, nausea, vomiting, flu-like symptoms, and allergic response. 

BOX 60-2 Antiarthritic Medications

Adalimumab (Humira)
Anakinra (Kineret)
Auranofin (Ridaura)
Aurothioglucose (Solganal)
Azathioprine (Imuran)
Cyclosporine (Neoral)
Etanercept
Gold sodium thiomalate (Aurolate, Myochrysine)
Infliximab (Remicade)
Leflunomide (Arava)
Methotrexate (Rheumatrex, Trexall)
Penicillamine (Cuprimine)
Sulfasalazine (Azulfidine)

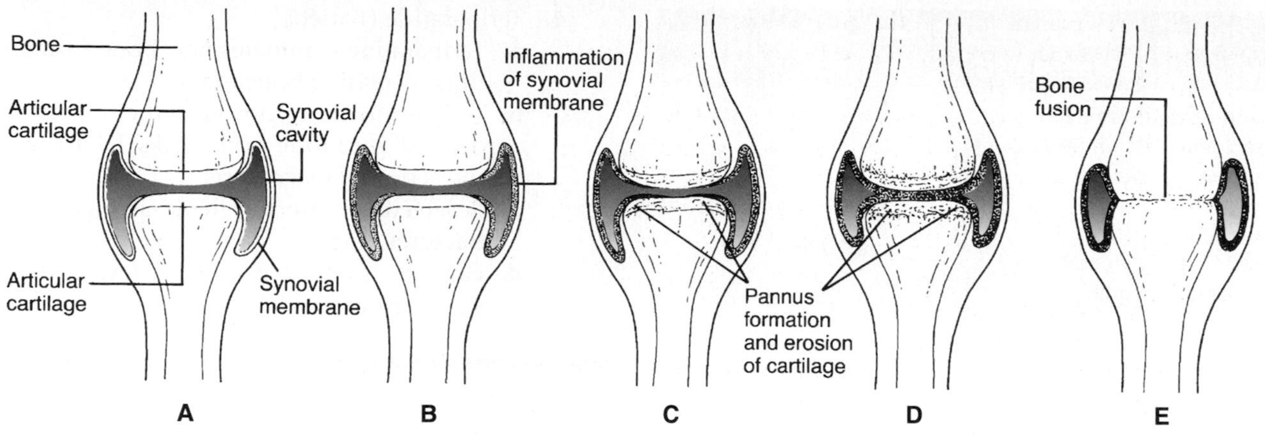

FIGURE 60-1 Progressive joint degeneration in rheumatoid arthritis. **A,** Healthy joint. **B,** Inflammation of synovial membrane. **C,** Onset of pannus formation and cartilage erosion. **D,** Pannus formation progresses and cartilage deteriorates further. **E,** Complete destruction of joint cavity together with fusion of articulating bones. (From Lehne R: *Pharmacology for nursing care*, ed 7, St. Louis, 2010, Saunders.)

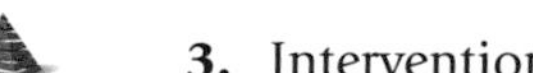

3. Interventions
   a. The client is instructed to monitor for signs of infection and report signs to the HCP.
   b. Monitor the injection site for signs of irritation, pain, inflammation, and swelling.
   c. Reinforce instructions to the client to consult with the HCP before receiving live vaccines and to avoid exposure to infections.
   d. The client is informed about the importance of laboratory tests for neutrophil counts, white blood cell counts, and platelet counts before initiation of treatment and during treatment.

4. Anakinra (Kineret): Injection site reactions are common (pruritus, erythema, rash, pain).

5. Adalimumab (Humira)
   a. Injection site reactions are common.
   b. Has been associated with neurological injury (numbness, tingling, dizziness, disturbed vision, weakness in the legs)

6. Auranofin (Ridaura): Oral gold preparation (not commonly used)

7. Gold sodium thiomalate (Aurolate, Myochrysine), aurothioglucose (Solganal): Intramuscular gold preparations (not commonly used)

8. Cyclosporine (Neoral): Immunosuppressive actions; can cause nephrotoxicity

9. Etanercept
   a. Injection site reactions are common.
   b. Poses a risk for heart failure; has been associated with central nervous system demyelinating disorders and hematological disorders

10. Hydroxychloroquine sulfate (Plaquenil): Associated with retinal damage; the client is informed to contact the HCP if visual disturbances occur.

11. Leflunomide (Arava): Side/adverse effects include diarrhea, respiratory infection, reversible alopecia, rash, and nausea; is hepatotoxic.

12. Methotrexate (Rheumatrex, Trexall): Can cause hepatic fibrosis, bone marrow suppression, gastrointestinal ulceration, and pneumonitis

13. Penicillamine (Cuprimine): Can cause bone marrow suppression and autoimmune disorders

14. Infliximab (Remicade): Can cause infusion reactions (fever, chills, pruritus, urticaria, chest pain); is hepatotoxic

15. Sulfasalazine (Azulfidine): Can cause gastrointestinal and dermatological reactions, bone marrow suppression, hepatitis

C. NSAIDs may be prescribed for their anti-inflammatory and analgesic effects. (See Chapter 58 for information on NSAIDs.)

D. Glucocorticoids may be prescribed for their anti-inflammatory effects. (See Chapter 46 for information on glucocorticoids.)

IV. Medications to Prevent and Treat Osteoporosis

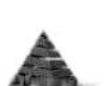

A. Description
   1. Osteoporosis is characterized by low bone mass and increased bone fragility.
   2. Calcium and vitamin D supplementation can reduce the risk of osteoporosis; calcium maximizes bone growth early in life and maintains bone integrity later in life, and vitamin D ensures calcium absorption. (See Chapter 46 for information on calcium and vitamin D supplements.)
   3. Treatment is aimed at reducing the occurrence of fractures by maintaining or increasing bone strength.
   4. Medications that decrease bone resorption (antiresorptive) and medications that promote bone formation are used (Box 60-3).

BOX 60-3 Medications to Prevent or Treat Osteoporosis

Alendronate (Fosamax)
Calcitonin, salmon (Miacalcin)
Calcium and vitamin D
Ibandronate
Raloxifene (Evista)
Risedronate (Actonel)
Teriparatide (Fortéo)

5. Antiresorptive medications include raloxifene (Evista), calcitonin, and bisphosphonates.
6. Teriparatide (Fortéo) promotes bone growth.

B. Interventions

1. Salmon calcitonin (Miacalcin)
   a. Calcitonin is secreted by the thyroid gland and inhibits osteoclastic bone resorption.
   b. Reinforce instructions to the client on how to administer the intranasal or subcutaneous form, depending on the route prescribed.
   c. Intranasal route: Examine the nares for irritation; alternate nostrils for doses.
   d. When calcitonin is taken, it is important to monitor for hypocalcemia.
2. Bisphosphonates (see Box 60-3)
   a. Bisphosphonates inhibit osteoclast-mediated bone resorption, thereby increasing total bone mass.
   b. Bisphosphonates include alendronate (Fosamax), risedronate (Actonel), and ibandronate (Boniva).
   c. Contraindicated for clients with esophageal disorders that can impede swallowing and for clients who cannot sit or stand for at least 30 minutes (60 minutes with ibandronate).
   d. Adverse effects include esophagitis, muscle pain, and ocular problems; the client is instructed to contact the HCP if adverse effects occur.

Because of the risk of esophagitis, bisphosphonates must be administered in the morning before eating or drinking with a full glass of water; the client must then remain sitting or standing for at least 30 minutes (60 minutes with ibandronate).

3. Raloxifene (Evista)
   a. Antiresorptive medication (nonbisphosphonate)
   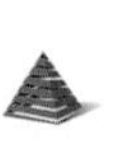
   b. Contraindicated in clients who have a history of venous thrombotic events
   c. Needs to be discontinued 72 hours before prolonged immobilization periods (such as with periods of extended bed rest)
   d. Reinforce instructions to the client to avoid extended periods of restricted activity (such as when traveling).
4. Teriparatide (Fortéo)
   a. Teriparatide stimulates new bone formation, thus increasing bone mass.
   b. Teriparatide is a portion of the human parathyroid hormone and works by increasing the action of osteoblasts.
   c. Reserved for use in clients at high risk for fractures
   d. Has been associated with the development of bone cancer 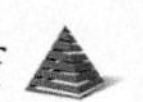

CRITICAL THINKING What Should You Do?

Answer: Cyclobenzaprine is a muscle relaxant and is contraindicated in clients who have received monoamine oxidase inhibitors (MAOIs) within 14 days of initiation of cyclobenzaprine therapy and in clients with cardiac disorders. Phenelzine (Nardil) is a MAOI medication. The nurse should inform the registered nurse and contact the health care provider and question the cyclobenzaprine prescription before the initiation of therapy.

Reference(s): Hodgson, B., & Kizior, R. (2015). *Saunders nursing drug handbook 2015.* (pp. 295–297) St. Louis: Saunders.

PRACTICE QUESTIONS

636. The client has been on treatment for rheumatoid arthritis for 3 weeks. During the administration of etanercept, it is **most important** for the nurse to collect which data?

1. The injection site for itching and edema
2. The white blood cell counts and platelet counts
3. A metallic taste in the mouth, with a loss of appetite
4. Whether the client is experiencing fatigue and joint pain

637. Alendronate (Fosamax) is prescribed for a client with osteoporosis and the nurse is providing instructions on administration of the medication. Which instruction should the nurse reinforce?

1. Take the medication at bedtime.
2. Take the medication in the morning with breakfast.
3. Lie down for 30 minutes after taking the medication.
4. Take the medication with a full glass of water after rising in the morning.

638. The nurse is monitoring a client receiving baclofen for side effects related to the medication. Which should indicate that the client is experiencing a side effect?

1. Polyuria
2. Diarrhea

3. Drowsiness
4. Muscular excitability

❖ **639.** In monitoring a client's response to disease-modifying antirheumatic drugs (DMARDs), which findings should the nurse interpret as acceptable responses? **Select all that apply.**
- ☐ 1. Symptom control during periods of emotional stress
- ☐ 2. Normal white blood cell, platelet, and neutrophil counts
- ☐ 3. Radiological findings that show nonprogression of joint degeneration
- ☐ 4. An increased range of motion in the affected joints 3 months into therapy
- ☐ 5. Inflammation and irritation at the injection site 3 days after injection is given
- ☐ 6. A low-grade temperature upon rising in the morning that remains throughout the day

640. A client with acute muscle spasms has been taking baclofen. The client calls the clinic nurse because of continuous feelings of weakness and fatigue and asks the nurse about discontinuing the medication. The nurse should make which appropriate response to the client?
1. "You should never stop the medication."
2. "It is best that you taper the dose if you intend to stop the medication."
3. "It is okay to stop the medication if you think that you can tolerate the muscle spasms."
4. "Weakness and fatigue commonly occur and will diminish with continued medication use."

641. The nurse is reviewing the laboratory studies on a client receiving dantrolene sodium (Dantrium). Which laboratory test(s) would identify an adverse effect associated with the administration of this medication?
1. Creatinine
2. Liver function tests
3. Blood urea nitrogen
4. Hematological function tests

642. The nurse is reviewing the record of a client who has been prescribed baclofen. Which disorder should alert the nurse to contact the health care provider?
1. Seizure disorders
2. Hyperthyroidism
3. Diabetes mellitus
4. Coronary artery disease

643. Cyclobenzaprine (Flexeril) is prescribed for a client to treat muscle spasms, and the nurse is reviewing the client's record. Which disorder would indicate a need to contact the health care provider regarding the administration of this medication?
1. Glaucoma
2. Emphysema
3. Hyperthyroidism
4. Diabetes mellitus

644. Dantrolene sodium (Dantrium) is prescribed for a client experiencing flexor spasms, and the client asks the nurse about the action of the medication. The nurse responds knowing that which is the therapeutic action of this medication?
1. Depresses spinal reflexes
2. Acts directly on the skeletal muscle to relieve spasticity
3. Acts within the spinal cord to suppress hyperactive reflexes
4. Acts on the central nervous system (CNS) to suppress spasms

645. The nurse is reinforcing discharge instructions to a client receiving baclofen. Which should the nurse include in the instructions?
1. Restrict fluid intake.
2. Avoid the use of alcohol.
3. Stop the medication if diarrhea occurs.
4. Notify the health care provider if fatigue occurs.

ANSWERS

636. 2

Rationale: Infection and suppression can occur as a result of etanercept. Laboratory studies are performed before and during medication treatment. The appearance of abnormal white blood cell counts and abnormal platelet counts can alert the nurse to a potentially life-threatening infection or potential bleeding. Injection site itching and edema are common occurrences following administration. A metallic taste and loss of appetite are not associated with this medication. Fatigue and joint pain occur with rheumatoid arthritis.

Test-Taking Strategy: Note the strategic words, *most important.* Option 3 can be eliminated because this is not associated with this medication. In early treatment, residual fatigue and joint pain may still be apparent. Option 2 monitors for a hematological disorder, which could indicate a reason for discontinuing this medication and should be reported. **Review:** etanercept.

Level of Cognitive Ability: Analyzing
Client Needs: Physiological Integrity
Integrated Process: Nursing Process/Data Collection
Content Area: Pharmacology: Musculoskeletal Medications
Priority Concepts: Infection, Inflammation

Reference(s): Hodgson, Kizior (2015), pp. 455–456; Lewis et al (2014), p. 1573.

637. 4

Rationale: Precautions need to be taken with the administration of alendronate to prevent gastrointestinal side/adverse effects (especially esophageal irritation) and to increase absorption of the medication. The medication needs to be taken with a full glass of water after rising in the morning. The client should not eat or drink anything for 30 minutes following administration and should not lie down after taking the medication.

Test-Taking Strategy: Focus on the subject, the administration of alendronate. Recalling that this medication can cause esophageal irritation will direct you to the correct option. Review: client teaching points for alendronate.

Level of Cognitive Ability: Applying

Client Needs: Physiological Integrity

Integrated Process: Teaching and Learning

Content Area: Pharmacology: Musculoskeletal Medications

Priority Concepts: Client Education, Safety

Reference(s): Hodgson, Kizior (2015), pp. 33–35.

638. 3

Rationale: Baclofen is a central nervous system (CNS) depressant and frequently causes drowsiness, dizziness, weakness, and fatigue. It can also cause nausea, constipation, and urinary retention. Clients should be warned about the possible reactions. Options 1, 2, and 4 are not side effects.

Test-Taking Strategy: Focus on the subject, side effect of baclofen. Recalling that baclofen is a CNS depressant used to treat muscle spasticity will direct you to the correct option. Review: side effects of baclofen.

Level of Cognitive Ability: Analyzing

Client Needs: Physiological Integrity

Integrated Process: Nursing Process/Data Collection

Content Area: Pharmacology: Musculoskeletal Medications

Priority Concepts: Clinical Judgment, Safety

Reference(s): Hodgson, Kizior (2015), pp. 116–117.

❖ **639. 1, 2, 3, 4**

Rationale: Because emotional stress frequently exacerbates the symptoms of rheumatoid arthritis, the absence of symptoms is a positive finding. DMARDs are given to slow progression of joint degeneration. In addition, the improvement in the range of motion after 3 months of therapy with normal blood work is a positive finding. Temperature elevation and inflammation and irritation at the medication injection site could indicate signs of infection.

Test-Taking Strategy: Focus on the subject, acceptable responses to therapy. Recalling that signs of an infection can indicate an unexpected finding will assist in eliminating options 5 and 6. **Review:** the expected effects of **disease-modifying antirheumatic drugs.**

Level of Cognitive Ability: Analyzing

Client Needs: Physiological Integrity

Integrated Process: Nursing Process/Data Collection

Content Area: Pharmacology: Musculoskeletal Medications

Priority Concepts: Mobility, Stress

Reference(s): Lehne (2013), pp. 928–929; Lilley et al (2014), pp. 767–769.

640. 4

Rationale: The client should be instructed that symptoms such as drowsiness, weakness, and fatigue are more intense in the early phase of therapy and diminish with continued medication use. The client should be instructed never to withdraw or stop the medication abruptly because abrupt withdrawal can cause visual hallucinations, paranoid ideation, and seizures. It is best for the nurse to inform the client that these symptoms will subside and encourage the client to continue the use of the medication.

Test-Taking Strategy: Focus on the subject, the effects of baclofen. Eliminate option 1 first because it is a rather extreme nursing response and uses the closed-ended word, *never.* Next, use general medication guidelines and eliminate options 2 and 3 because these responses do not represent the scope of nursing practice or nursing actions. **Review:** client teaching for **baclofen.**

Level of Cognitive Ability: Applying

Client Needs: Physiological Integrity

Integrated Process: Nursing Process/Implementation

Content Area: Pharmacology: Musculoskeletal Medications

Priority Concepts: Client Education, Mobility

Reference(s): Hodgson, Kizior (2015), p. 117.

641. 2

Rationale: Dose-related liver damage is the most serious adverse effect of dantrolene. To reduce the risk of liver damage, liver function tests should be performed before treatment and periodically throughout the treatment course. It is administered in the lowest effective dosage for the shortest time necessary. Options 1 and 3 are tests that assess kidney function.

Test-Taking Strategy: Focus on the subject, adverse effects of dantrolene. Eliminate options 1 and 3 because they are comparable or alike and assess kidney function. From the remaining options, it is necessary to recall that this medication affects liver function. **Review:** adverse effects of **dantrolene.**

Level of Cognitive Ability: Analyzing

Client Needs: Physiological Integrity

Integrated Process: Nursing Process/Data Collection

Content Area: Pharmacology: Musculoskeletal Medications

Priority Concepts: Cellular Regulation, Safety

Reference(s): Hodgson, Kizior (2015), p. 314.

642. 1

Rationale: Clients with seizure disorders may have a lowered seizure threshold when baclofen is administered. Concurrent therapy may require an increase in the anticonvulsive medication. The disorders in options 2, 3, and 4 are not a concern when the client is taking baclofen.

Test-Taking Strategy: Focus on the subject, contraindications of baclofen. Knowledge regarding the contraindications and the cautions associated with the administration of baclofen is required to answer this question. Remember, a lowered seizure threshold can occur when baclofen is administered. **Review:** contraindications and cautions of **baclofen.**

Level of Cognitive Ability: Analyzing

Client Needs: Safe and Effective Care Environment

Integrated Process: Nursing Process/Data Collection

Content Area: Pharmacology: Musculoskeletal Medications

Priority Concepts: Clinical Judgment, Safety

Reference(s): Hodgson, Kizior (2015), pp. 116–117.

643. 1

Rationale: Because this medication has anticholinergic effects, it should be used with caution in clients with a history of urinary retention, angle-closure glaucoma, and increased intraocular pressure. Cyclobenzaprine hydrochloride should be used only for short-term 2- to 3-week therapy. The disorders in options 2, 3, and 4 are not a concern when the client is taking cyclobenzaprine.

Test-Taking Strategy: Focus on the subject, contraindications of cyclobenzaprine. Recalling that this medication has anticholinergic effects will assist in directing you to the correct option. Review: contraindications with cyclobenzaprine (Flexeril).

Level of Cognitive Ability: Analyzing

Client Needs: Safe and Effective Care Environment

Integrated Process: Nursing Process/Data Collection

Content Area: Pharmacology: Musculoskeletal Medications

Priority Concepts: Clinical Judgment, Safety

Reference(s): Hodgson, Kizior (2015), pp. 294–296.

644. 2

Rationale: Dantrolene acts directly on skeletal muscle to relieve muscle spasticity. The primary action is the suppression of calcium release from the sarcoplasmic reticulum. This in turn decreases the ability of the skeletal muscle to contract. Options 1, 3, and 4 are not actions of the medication.

Test-Taking Strategy: Options 1, 3, and 4 are all comparable or alike in that they address central nervous system suppression and the depression of reflexes. Therefore, eliminate these options. Review: the action of dantrolene.

Level of Cognitive Ability: Applying

Client Needs: Physiological Integrity

Integrated Process: Nursing Process/Implementation

Content Area: Pharmacology: Musculoskeletal Medications

Priority Concepts: Client Education, Mobility

Reference(s): Hodgson, Kizior (2015), pp. 312–313.

645. 2

Rationale: Baclofen is a central nervous system (CNS) depressant. The client should be cautioned against the use of alcohol and other CNS depressants because baclofen potentiates the depressant activity of these agents. It is not necessary to restrict fluids, but the client should be warned that urinary retention can occur. Constipation rather than diarrhea is an adverse effect of baclofen. Fatigue is related to a CNS effect that is most intense during the early phase of therapy and diminishes with continued medication use. It is not necessary that the client notify the health care provider if fatigue occurs.

Test-Taking Strategy: Focus on the subject, discharge instructions with baclofen. Recalling that baclofen is a CNS depressant will direct you to the correct option. If you were unsure of the correct option, use general principles related to medication administration. Alcohol should be avoided with the use of medications. Review: discharge instructions/client teaching with baclofen.

Level of Cognitive Ability: Applying

Client Needs: Physiological Integrity

Integrated Process: Teaching and Learning

Content Area: Pharmacology: Musculoskeletal Medications

Priority Concepts: Client Education, Safety

Reference(s): Hodgson, Kizior (2015), p. 117.

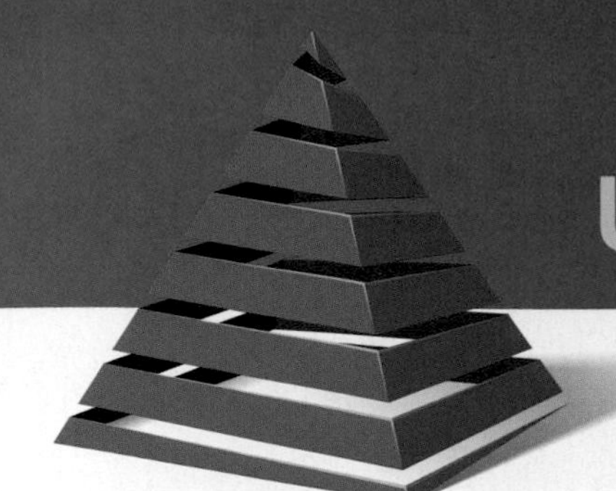

UNIT XVIII

The Adult Client with an Immune Disorder

PYRAMID TERMS

acquired immunity Immunity received passively from the mother's antibodies, animal serum, or production of antibodies in response to a disease; immunization produces active acquired immunity.

allergy An abnormal, individual response to certain substances that normally do not trigger such an exaggerated reaction.

cellular response A delayed response against slowly developing bacterial infections; also called delayed hypersensitivity.

humoral response An immediate response that provides protection against acute, rapidly developing bacterial and viral infections.

immunodeficiency The absence or inadequate production of immune bodies.

innate immunity Immunity present at birth and that is the first-line defense against pathogens; also known as natural immunity.

Kaposi's sarcoma Skin lesions that occur in individuals with a compromised immune system.

Lyme disease An infection acquired from a tick bite; ticks live in wooded areas and survive by attaching to a host.

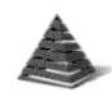

Pyramid to Success

Pyramid points focus on the effects of and complications associated with an immune deficiency. Specific focus relates to the nursing care related to the disorder, the impact of the treatment or disorder, and client adaptation. Acquired immunodeficiency syndrome is a Pyramid focus, along with protecting the client from infection and preventing the transmission of infection to other individuals. Psychosocial issues relate to social isolation and the body-image disturbances that can occur as a result of the immune disorder.

Client Needs

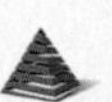

Safe and Effective Care Environment

Acting as an advocate related to the client's decisions
Addressing advance directives
Consulting with the RN and other members of the health care team
Ensuring that informed consent has been obtained for treatments and procedures
Establishing priorities
Handling hazardous and infectious materials safely
Implementing standard and other precautions
Maintaining asepsis
Maintaining confidentiality regarding diagnosis
Preventing infection
Upholding client rights

Health Promotion and Maintenance

Assisting with implementing health screening measures
Ensuring that the client receives recommended immunizations
Monitoring for expected body-image changes
Performing data collection techniques related to the immune system
Preventing disease related to infection
Respecting client lifestyle choices

Psychosocial Integrity

Assisting in mobilizing appropriate support and resource systems
Assisting the client and family to cope
Assisting the client to adapt and problem solve during illness or stressful events
Considering religious, spiritual, and cultural preferences

Discussing grief and loss related to death and the dying process
Promoting a positive environment to maintain optimal quality of life

Physiological Integrity

Managing medical emergencies
Managing pain
Monitoring for the expected and unexpected responses to treatments
Promoting nutrition
Protecting the client from infection
Providing basic care and comfort
Reviewing diagnostic test and laboratory test results

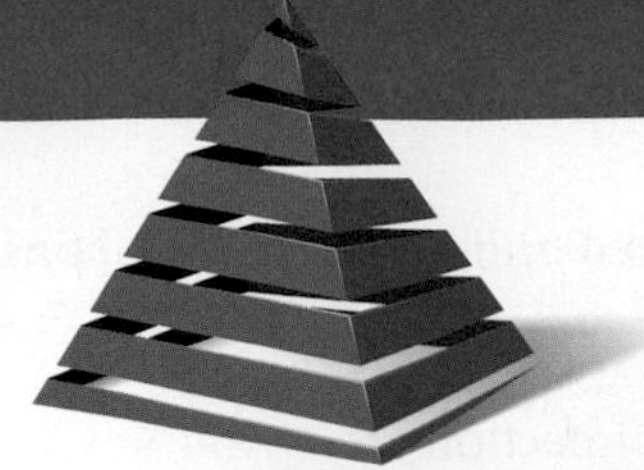

CHAPTER 61

Immune Disorders

CRITICAL THINKING What Should You Do?

The nurse notes that a client with scleroderma (systemic sclerosis) is having difficulty swallowing. What should the nurse do?

Answer located on p. 878.

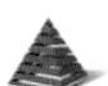

I. Functions of the Immune System

A. The immune system provides protection against invasion from microorganisms from outside the body.

B. The immune system protects the body from internal threats and maintains the internal environment by removing dead or damaged cells.

II. Immune Response

A. T lymphocytes and B lymphocytes

1. Lymphocytes are produced in the bone marrow and migrate to lymphoid tissue, where they remain dormant until they need to form sensitized lymphocytes for cellular immunity or antibodies for humoral immunity.
2. Some B lymphocytes lie dormant until a specific antigen enters the body, at which time they greatly increase in number and are available for defense.
3. Types of T lymphocytes include helper/inducer, suppressor, and cytotoxic/cytolytic.
4. T and B lymphocytes are necessary for a normal immune response.

B. Humoral response

1. Humoral response is immediate.
2. This type of response provides protection against acute, rapidly developing bacterial and viral infections.

C. Cellular response

1. Cellular response is delayed and is called *delayed hypersensitivity.*
2. This type of response is active against slowly developing bacterial infections and is involved in autoimmune response, some allergic reactions, and rejection of foreign cells.

III. Immunity

A. Innate immunity

1. Also called native or natural immunity
2. Present at birth and includes biochemical, physical, and mechanical barriers of defense as well as the inflammatory response

B. Acquired immunity

1. Acquired or adaptive immunity is received passively from the mother's antibodies, animal serum, or from the production of antibodies in response to a disease.
2. Immunization produces active acquired immunity.

IV. Immunizations (Refer to Chapter 39)

V. Laboratory Studies

A. Antinuclear antibody (ANA) titer

1. ANA titer is a blood test used in the differential diagnosis of rheumatic diseases and to detect antinucleoprotein factors and patterns associated with certain autoimmune diseases.
2. The test is positive at a titer of 1:20 or 1:40, depending on the laboratory.
3. A positive result does not necessarily confirm a disease.
4. The ANA titer is positive in most individuals diagnosed with systemic lupus erythematosus (SLE); it may also be positive in individuals with systemic sclerosis (scleroderma) or rheumatoid arthritis.
5. An ANA titer result can be false positive in some individuals.

B. Anti–double-stranded DNA (dsDNA) antibody test

1. The anti-dsDNA antibody test is a blood test done specifically to identify or differentiate DNA antibodies found in SLE.
2. The test supports a diagnosis, monitors disease activity and response to therapy, and establishes a prognosis for SLE.
3. Values
   a. Negative: Less than 70 units by enzyme-linked immunosorbent assay (ELISA)
   b. Borderline: 70 to 200 units
   c. Positive: Greater than 200 units

C. Refer to Chapter 11 for testing related to acquired immunodeficiency syndrome (AIDS).

D. Skin testing
 1. Description
  a. The administration of an allergen to the surface of the skin or into the dermis
  b. Administered by patch, scratch, or intradermal techniques
 2. Interventions: preprocedure
  a. Discontinue systemic corticosteroids or antihistamine therapy 5 days before the test, as prescribed.
  b. Ensure informed consent has been obtained.
 3. Interventions: Postprocedure
  a. Record the site, date, and time of the test.
  b. Record the date and the time for follow-up site reading.
  c. Have client remain in waiting room or office for at least 30 minutes after the injection to monitor for adverse effects.
  d. Inspect the site for erythema, papules, vesicles, edema, and wheal (Fig. 61-1).
  e. Measure flare along with the wheal, and document size and other findings.
  f. Provide the client with a list of potential allergens, if identified.

Have resuscitation equipment available if skin testing is performed because the allergen may induce an anaphylactic reaction.

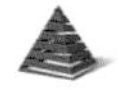

VI. Hypersensitivity and Allergy

A. Description
 1. An **allergy** is an abnormal, individual response to certain substances that normally do not trigger such an exaggerated reaction.
 2. In some types of allergies, a reaction occurs on a second and subsequent contact with the allergen.
 3. Skin testing may be done to determine the allergen.
 4. Types of hypersensitivity reactions (Table 61-1)

B. Data collection
 1. History of exposure to allergens
 2. Itching, tearing, and burning of eyes and skin
 3. Rashes
 4. Nose twitching and nasal stuffiness

C. Interventions
 1. Identification of the specific allergen
 2. Management of the symptoms with antihistamines, anti-inflammatory agents, or corticosteroids
 3. Ointments, creams, wet compresses, and soothing baths for local reactions
 4. Desensitization programs may be recommended.

Test Results	Interpretation
	Negative—Wheal less than 0.5 cm in diameter
	Positive—Wheal 0.5 cm in diameter (1+)
	Positive—Wheal 1.0 cm in diameter (2+)
	Positive—Wheal 1.5 cm in diameter (3+)
	Positive—Wheal 2.0 cm in diameter (4+)

FIGURE 61-1 Interpretation of intradermal allergy test results based on size of wheal after 15 to 30 minutes. (From Monahan F, Sands J, Neighbors M, Marek J, Green C: *Phipps' medical-surgical nursing: Health and illness perspectives*, ed 8, St. Louis, 2007, Mosby.)

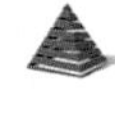

VII. Anaphylaxis

A. Description
 1. Anaphylaxis is a serious and immediate hypersensitivity reaction with the release of histamine from the damaged cells.
 2. Anaphylaxis can be systemic or cutaneous (localized).

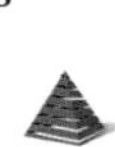

B. Data collection (Fig. 61-2)

C. Interventions (see Priority Nursing Actions)

VIII. Latex Allergy

A. Description
 1. Latex allergy is a hypersensitivity to latex.
 2. The source of the allergic reaction is thought to be the proteins in the natural rubber latex or the various chemicals used in the manufacturing process of latex gloves.
 3. Symptoms of the allergy can range from mild contact dermatitis to moderately severe symptoms of rhinitis, conjunctivitis, urticaria, and bronchospasm to severe life-threatening anaphylaxis.

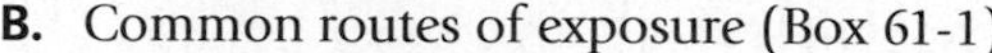

B. Common routes of exposure (Box 61-1)
 1. Cutaneous: Natural latex gloves and latex balloons
 2. Percutaneous and parenteral: IV lines and catheters; hemodialysis equipment
 3. Mucosal: Use of latex condoms, catheters, airways, and nipples
 4. Aerosol: Aerosolization of powder from latex gloves can occur when gloves are dispensed from the box or when gloves are removed from the hands.

TABLE 61-1 Types of Hypersensitivity Reactions

Type	Causative Component	Pathological Process	Reaction
I: Immediate, anaphylactic	IgE	Mast cell degranulation ↓ Histamine and leukotriene release	Anaphylaxis Atopic diseases Skin reactions
II: Cytolytic, cytotoxic	IgG IgM Complement	Complement fixation ↓ Cell lysis	ABO incompatibility Drug-induced hemolytic anemia
III: Immune complex	Antigen-antibody complexes	Deposition in vessels and tissue walls ↓ Inflammation	Arthus reaction Serum sickness Systemic lupus erythematosus Acute glomerulonephritis
IV: Cell-mediated, delayed	Sensitized T cells	Lymphokine release	Tuberculosis Contact dermatitis Transplant rejection

Ig, Immunoglobulin.

From Black J, Hawks J: *Medical-surgical nursing: Clinical management for positive outcomes,* ed 8, St. Louis, 2009, Saunders.

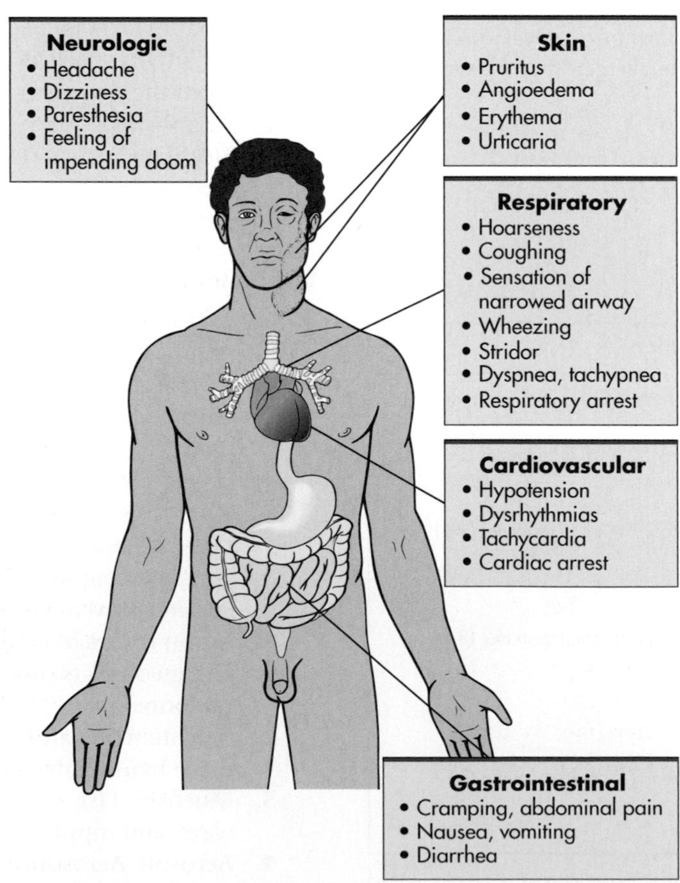

FIGURE 61-2 Clinical manifestations of a systemic anaphylactic reaction. (From Lewis S, Dirksen S, Heitkemper M, Bucher L, Camera I: *Medical-surgical nursing: Assessment and management of clinical problems,* ed 8, St. Louis, 2011, Mosby.)

PRIORITY NURSING ACTIONS!

Actions to Take If a Client Develops Anaphylaxis

1. Quickly check respiratory status and maintain a patent airway.
2. Call the RN, who will contact the health care provider (HCP) or Rapid Response Team.
3. Administer oxygen.
4. Assist the RN to prepare to start an intravenous (IV) line and infuse normal saline.
5. Prepare to administer diphenhydramine (Benadryl) and epinephrine (Adrenalin).
6. Document the event, actions taken, and the client's response.

If the client experiences an anaphylactic reaction, the immediate action would be to check the respiratory status quickly and maintain a patent airway. The nurse stays with the client and calls out for the RN, who will contact the HCP and/or Rapid Response Team. In the meantime, the nurse stays with the client and monitors the client's vital signs and for signs of shock. An IV device is inserted if one is not already in place, and normal saline is infused. The nurse then prepares to assist in the administration of diphenhydramine and epinephrine and other medications as prescribed. The head of the bed is elevated if the client's blood pressure is normal. The client's feet and legs may be raised if the blood pressure is low. The nurse documents the event, the actions taken, and the client's response.

Reference(s): deWit, D. & Kumagai, C. (2013). *Medical-surgical nursing: Concepts & practice.* (2nd ed., pp. 243, 1036–1037). St. Louis: Saunders.

Ignatavicius, D., & Workman, M. (2013). *Medical-surgical nursing: Patient-centered collaborative care.* (7th ed., p. 390). St. Louis: Saunders.

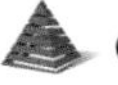

C. At-risk individuals
1. Health care workers
2. Individuals who work in the rubber industry
3. Individuals having multiple surgeries
4. Individuals with spina bifida
5. Individuals who wear gloves frequently such as food handlers, hairdressers, and auto mechanics
6. Individuals allergic to kiwis, bananas, pineapples, tropical fruits, grapes, avocados, potatoes, hazelnuts, and water chestnuts

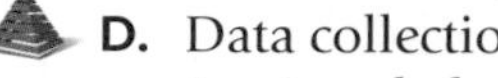

D. Data collection
1. Anaphylaxis or type I hypersensitivity is a response to natural rubber latex (Fig. 61-3; also see Fig. 61-2).
2. A delayed type IV hypersensitivity can occur within 6 to 48 hours. Symptoms of contact dermatitis include pruritus, edema, erythema, vesicles, papules, and crusting and thickening of the skin.

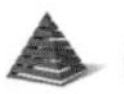

E. Interventions (Box 61-2)

BOX 61-1 Products That May Contain Natural Rubber Latex

Ace bandages (brown)
Adhesive or elastic bandages
Ambu Bag
Balloons
Blood pressure cuff (tubing and bladder)
Catheter leg bag straps
Catheters
Condoms
Diaphragms
Elastic pressure stockings
Electrocardiogram pads
Feminine hygiene pads
Gloves
Intravenous catheters, tubing, and rubber injection ports
Nasogastric tubes
Pads for crutches
Prepackaged enema kits
Rubber stoppers on medication vials
Stethoscopes
Syringes

Note: Health care agencies use as many nonlatex products as possible and have nonlatex supplies available for clients with a latex allergy.

IX. Immunodeficiency

A. Description
1. Immunodeficiency is the absence or inadequate production of immune bodies.
2. The disorder can be congenital (primary) or acquired (secondary).
3. Treatment depends on the inadequacy of immune bodies and its primary cause.

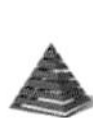

B. Data collection
1. Factors that decrease immune function
2. Frequent infections
3. Nutritional status
4. Medication history, such as use of corticosteroids for long periods
5. History of alcohol or drug abuse

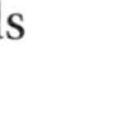

C. Interventions
1. Protect the client from infection.
2. Promote a balanced diet with adequate nutrition.
3. Use strict aseptic technique for all procedures.
4. Provide psychosocial care regarding lifestyle changes and role changes.
5. Reinforce instructions to the client in measures to prevent infection and to wear a Medic-Alert bracelet.

The priority concern for a client with immunodeficiency is infection.

X. Autoimmune Disease

A. Description

Adult—Immune

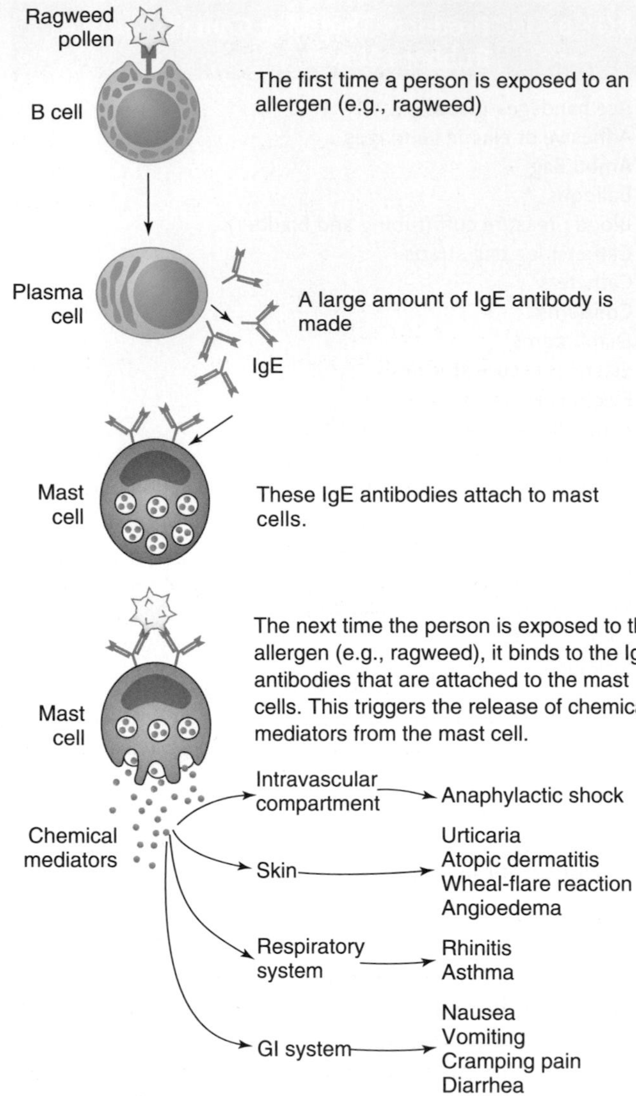
Ragweed pollen
B cell
The first time a person is exposed to an allergen (e.g., ragweed)
Plasma cell
A large amount of IgE antibody is made
IgE
Mast cell
These IgE antibodies attach to mast cells.
Mast cell
The next time the person is exposed to the allergen (e.g., ragweed), it binds to the IgE antibodies that are attached to the mast cells. This triggers the release of chemical mediators from the mast cell.
Chemical mediators
Intravascular compartment
Anaphylactic shock
Skin
Urticaria
Atopic dermatitis
Wheal-flare reaction
Angioedema
Respiratory system
Rhinitis
Asthma
GI system
Nausea
Vomiting
Cramping pain
Diarrhea

FIGURE 61-3 Steps in a type I allergic reaction. (From Lewis S, Dirksen S, Heitkemper M, Bucher L, Camera I: *Medical-surgical nursing: Assessment and management of clinical problems*, ed 8, St. Louis, 2011, Mosby.)

BOX 61-2 Interventions for the Client with a Latex Allergy

Ask the client about a known allergy to latex during the initial data collection procedures.
Identify risk factors to a latex allergy in the client.
Use nonlatex gloves and all latex-safe supplies.
Keep a latex-safe supply cart near the client's room.
Apply a cloth barrier to the client's arm under a blood pressure cuff.
Use latex-free syringes, medication containers (glass ampules), and latex-safe intravenous equipment.
Reinforce instructions to the client to wear a Medic-Alert bracelet.
Reinforce instructions to the client about the importance of informing health care providers and local and paramedic ambulance companies about the allergy.

1. The body is unable to recognize its own cells as a part of itself.
2. Autoimmune disease can affect collagenous tissue.

B. Systemic lupus erythematosus (SLE)
1. Description
   a. A chronic progressive systemic inflammatory disease that can cause major organs and systems to fail
   b. Connective tissue and fibrin deposits collect in blood vessels on collagen fibers and on organs.
   c. The deposits lead to necrosis and inflammation in blood vessels, lymph nodes, gastrointestinal tract, and pleura.
   d. No cure for the disease is known, but remissions are frequently experienced by clients who manage their care well.
2. Causes
   a. The cause of SLE is unknown, but it is thought to result from a defect in the immunological mechanisms and to have a genetic origin.
   b. Precipitating factors include medications, stress, genetic factors, sunlight or ultraviolet light, and pregnancy.
   c. Discoid lupus erythematosus is possible with some medications but totally disappears after the medication is stopped; the only manifestation is the skin rash that occurs in lupus.
3. Data collection 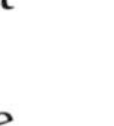
   a. Identify precipitating factors.
   b. Erythema of the face (malar rash; also called a butterfly rash)
   c. Dry, scaly, raised rash on the face or upper body
   d. Fever
   e. Weakness, malaise, and fatigue
   f. Anorexia
   g. Weight loss
   h. Photosensitivity
   i. Joint pain
   j. Erythema of the palms
   k. Anemia
   l. Positive antinuclear antibody (ANA) test and lupus erythematosus (LE) preparation
   m. Elevated sedimentation rate and C-reactive protein
4. Interventions 
   a. Monitor skin integrity and provide frequent oral care.
   b. Instruct the client to clean the skin with a mild soap, avoiding harsh and perfumed substances.
   c. Assist with the use of ointments and creams for the rash as prescribed.
   d. Identify factors contributing to fatigue.

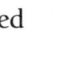

e. Administer iron, folic acid, or vitamin supplements as prescribed if anemia occurs.
f. Provide a high-vitamin and high-iron diet.
g. Provide a high-protein diet if there is no evidence of kidney disease.
h. Reinforce instructions in measures to conserve energy, such as pacing activities and balancing rest with exercise.
i. Administer topical or systemic corticosteroids, salicylates, and nonsteroidal anti-inflammatory drugs as prescribed for pain and inflammation.
j. Administer medications to decrease the inflammatory response, as prescribed.
k. Monitor intake and output, as well as daily weight for signs of fluid overload if corticosteroids are used.
l. Reinforce instructions to the client to avoid exposure to sunlight and ultraviolet light.
m. Monitor for proteinuria and red blood cell casts in the urine.
n. Monitor for bruising, bleeding, and injury.
o. Assist with plasmapheresis as prescribed to remove autoantibodies and immune complexes from the blood before organ damage occurs.
p. Monitor for signs of organ involvement such as pleuritis, nephritis, pericarditis, coronary artery disease, hypertension, neuritis, anemia, and peritonitis.
q. Note that lupus nephritis occurs early in the disease process.
r. Provide supportive therapy as major organs become affected.
s. Provide emotional support and encourage the client to verbalize feelings.
t. Provide information regarding support groups and encourage the use of community resources.

For the client with SLE, monitor the blood urea nitrogen and creatinine levels frequently for signs of renal impairment.

C. Scleroderma (systemic sclerosis)
1. Description
a. Scleroderma is a chronic connective tissue disease similar to SLE that is characterized by inflammation, fibrosis, and sclerosis.
b. This disorder affects the connective tissue throughout the body.
c. It causes fibrotic changes involving the skin, synovial membranes, esophagus, heart, lungs, kidneys, and gastrointestinal tract.

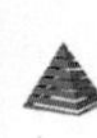

d. Treatment is directed toward forcing the disease into remission and slowing its progress.

2. Data collection
a. Pain
b. Stiffness and muscle weakness
c. Pitting edema of the hands and fingers that progresses to the rest of the body
d. Taut and shiny skin that is free from wrinkles
e. Skin tissue is tight, hard, and thick, and it loses its elasticity and adheres to underlying structures.
f. Dysphagia
g. Decreased range of motion
h. Joint contractures
i. Inability to perform activities of daily living
3. Interventions
a. Encourage activity as tolerated.
b. Maintain a constant room temperature.
c. Provide small, frequent meals, while eliminating foods that stimulate gastric secretions, such as spicy foods, caffeine, and alcohol.
d. Monitor for esophageal involvement; if present, advise the client to sit up for 1 to 2 hours after meals.
e. Provide supportive therapy as the major organs become affected.
f. Administer corticosteroids as prescribed for inflammation.
g. Provide emotional support and encourage the use of resources as necessary.

D. Polyarteritis nodosa
1. Description
a. Polyarteritis nodosa is a collagen disease and a form of systemic vasculitis that causes inflammation of the arteries in visceral organs, brain, and skin.
b. Treatment is similar to the treatment for SLE.
c. The cause is unknown, and prognosis is poor.
d. Renal disorders and cardiac involvement are the most frequent causes of death.
2. Data collection
a. Malaise, weakness, low-grade fever
b. Severe abdominal pain
c. Bloody diarrhea
d. Weight loss
e. Elevated sedimentation rate
3. Interventions
a. Provide supportive care as required.
b. Assist to administer corticosteroids and analgesics to control pain and inflammation.
c. Provide emotional support and encourage the client to verbalize feelings.
d. Initiate support services for the client.

E. Pemphigus
1. Description
a. Pemphigus is a rare autoimmune disease that occurs predominantly between middle and old age.
b. The cause is unknown, and the disorder is potentially fatal.

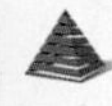
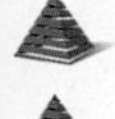
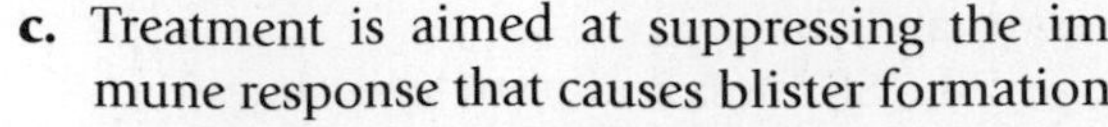

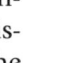

c. Treatment is aimed at suppressing the immune response that causes blister formation.

2. Data collection
   a. Fragile, partial-thickness lesions bleed, weep, and form crusts when bullae are disrupted
   b. Debilitation, malaise, pain, and dysphagia
   c. Nikolsky's sign: Separation of the epidermis caused by rubbing the skin
   d. Leukocytosis, eosinophilia, foul-smelling discharge from skin
3. Interventions
   a. Provide supportive care.
   b. Soothe oral lesions as prescribed, and assist with soothing baths as prescribed for relief of symptoms.
   c. Topical or systemic antibiotics may be prescribed for secondary infections.
   d. Corticosteroids and cytotoxic agents may be prescribed to bring about remission.

XI. Goodpasture's Syndrome

A. Description
   1. Goodpasture's syndrome is an autoimmune disorder; autoantibodies are made against the glomerular basement membrane and alveolar basement membrane.
   2. Goodpasture's syndrome is most common in males and young adults who smoke, and the exact cause is unknown.
   3. The lungs and the kidneys are affected primarily, and the disorder is usually not diagnosed until significant pulmonary or renal involvement occurs.

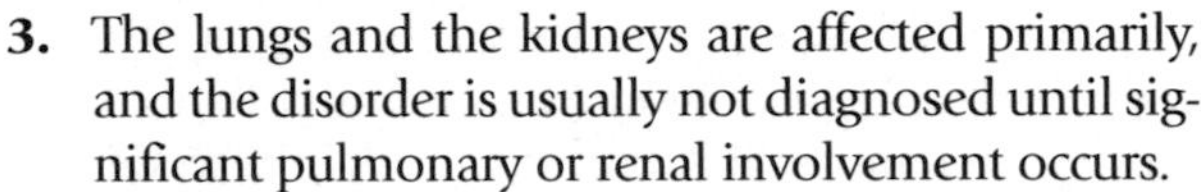

B. Data collection
   1. Clinical manifestations indicating pulmonary and renal involvement
   2. Shortness of breath
   3. Hemoptysis
   4. Decreased urine output
   5. Edema and weight gain
   6. Hypertension and tachycardia

C. Interventions
   1. Focus on suppressing the autoimmune response with medications such as corticosteroids and on plasmapheresis (filtration of the plasma to remove some proteins) to remove the autoantibodies.
   2. Provide supportive therapy for pulmonary and renal involvement.

XII. Lyme Disease

A. Description
   1. **Lyme disease** is an infection caused by the spirochete *Borrelia burgdorferi*, acquired from a tick bite (ticks live in wooded areas and survive by attaching to a host).
   2. Infection with the spirochete stimulates inflammatory cytokines and autoimmune mechanisms.

B. Data collection (Box 61-3)

BOX 61-3 Data Collection and Stages of Lyme Disease

First Stage

Symptoms can occur several days to months following the bite.
A small red pimple develops that spreads into a ring-shaped rash.
Rash may be large or small or may not occur at all.
Flu-like symptoms occur, such as headaches, stiff neck, muscle aches, and fatigue.

Second Stage

This stage occurs several weeks following the bite.
Joint pain occurs.
Neurological complications occur.
Cardiac complications occur.

Third Stage

Large joints become involved.
Arthritis progresses.

The typical ring-shaped rash of Lyme disease does not occur in all clients. Many clients never develop a rash. Additionally, if a rash does occur, it can occur anywhere on the body, not only at the site of the bite.

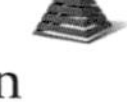

C. Interventions
   1. Gently remove the tick with tweezers, wash skin with antiseptic, and dispose of the tick by flushing it down the toilet; the tick may also be disposed of by placing it in a sealed jar so that the HCP can inspect it and determine its type.
   2. Obtain a blood test 4 to 6 weeks after a bite to detect the presence of the disease (testing before this time is not reliable).
   3. Reinforce instructions to the client in the administration of antibiotics; these are initiated immediately (even before the blood testing results are known).
   4. Instruct the client to avoid areas that contain ticks, such as wooded grassy areas, especially in the summer months.
   5. Instruct the client to wear long-sleeved tops, long pants, closed shoes, and hats while outside.
   6. Instruct the client to spray the body with tick repellent containing DEET before going outside.
   7. Instruct the client to examine the body when returning inside for the presence of ticks.

XIII. Immunodeficiency Syndromes

A. Acquired immunodeficiency syndrome (AIDS)
   1. AIDS is a viral disease caused by human immunodeficiency virus (HIV) that destroys T-cells, thereby increasing susceptibility to infection and malignancy (Fig. 61-4).

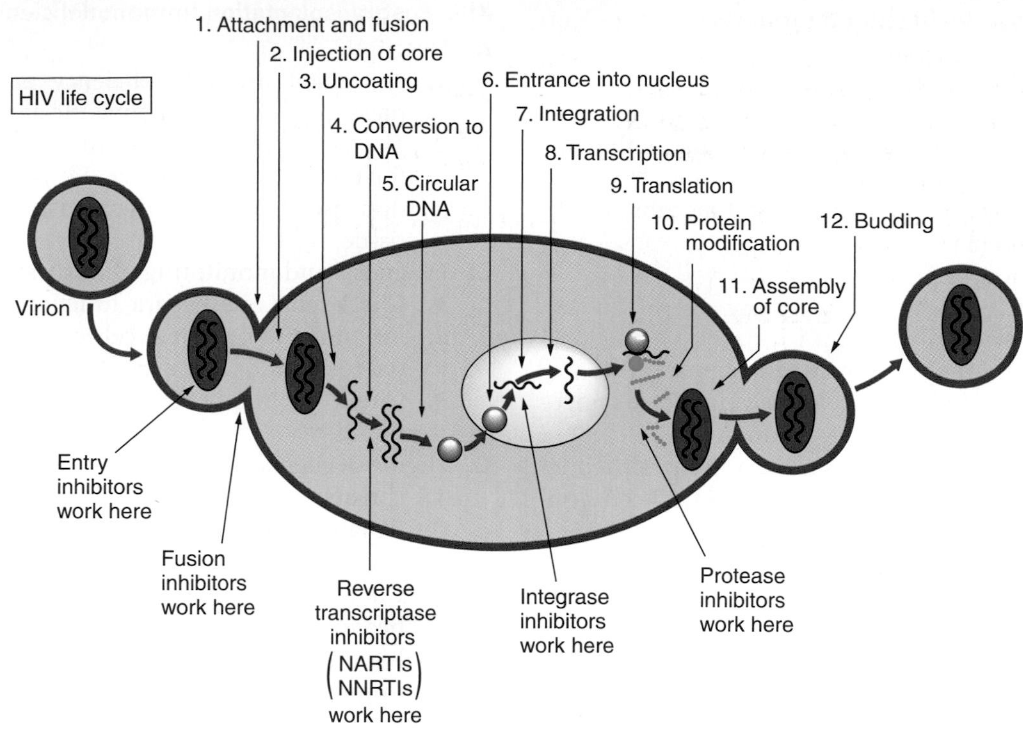

FIGURE 61-4 The life cycle of HIV. (From Ignatavicius D, Workman ML: *Medical-surgical nursing: Patient-centered collaborative care*, ed 7, Philadelphia, 2013, Saunders.)

2. The syndrome is manifested clinically by opportunistic infection and unusual neoplasms.
3. AIDS is considered a chronic illness.
4. The disease has a long incubation period, sometimes up to 10 years or more.
5. Manifestations may not appear until late in the infection.

B. Diagnosis and monitoring the client with AIDS
1. Refer to Chapter 11 for diagnostic tests.
2. Refer to Box 61-4 for tests used to evaluate the progression of HIV infection.

C. High-risk groups
1. Heterosexual or homosexual contact with high-risk individuals
2. Intravenous drug abusers, especially in those who share needles

BOX 61-4 Tests Used to Evaluate Progression of Human Immunodeficiency Virus (HIV) Infection

Complete Blood Cell Count
White blood cell (WBC) count normal to decreased
Lymphopenia (<30% of the normal number of WBCs)
Thrombocytopenia (decreased platelet count)

Lymphocyte Screen
Reduced $CD4^+/CD8^+$ T-cell ratio
$CD4^+$ (helper) lymphocytes decreased
$CD8^+$ lymphocytes increased

Quantitative Immunoglobin
Immunoglobulin G (IgG) increased
IgA frequently increased

Chemistry Panel
Lactate dehydrogenase increased (all fractions)
Serum albumin decreased
Total protein increased
Cholesterol decreased
AST and ALT elevated

Anergy Panel
Nonreactive (anergic) or poorly reactive to infectious agents or environmental materials (e.g., pokeweed, phytohemagglutinin mitogens and antigens, mumps, *Candida*)

Hepatitis B Surface Antigen
To detect the presence of hepatitis B

Blood Cultures
To detect septicemia

Chest Radiograph
To detect *Pneumocystis jiroveci* infection or tuberculosis

ALT, Alanine aminotransferase; *AST*, aspartate aminotransferase; immunoglobulin; *WBC*, white blood cell.

From Copstead L, Banasik J: *Pathophysiology*, ed 4, St. Louis, 2010, Saunders.

3. Persons receiving blood products
4. Health care workers
5. Babies born to infected mothers

D. Data collection
1. Malaise, fever, anorexia, weight loss, influenza-like symptoms
2. Lymphadenopathy of at least 3 months
3. Leukopenia
4. Diarrhea
5. Fatigue
6. Night sweats
7. Presence of opportunistic infections
8. Protozoal infections (*Pneumocystis jiroveci* pneumonia, a major source of mortality)
9. Neoplasms (Kaposi's sarcoma: purplish/red lesions of internal organs and skin), B-cell non-Hodgkin's lymphoma, cervical cancer)
10. Fungal infections (candidiasis, histoplasmosis)
11. Viral infections (cytomegalovirus, herpes simplex)
12. Bacterial infections

E. Interventions
1. Provide respiratory support.
2. Administer oxygen and respiratory treatments as prescribed.
3. Provide psychosocial support as needed.
4. Maintain fluid and electrolyte balance.
5. Monitor for signs of infection.
6. Prevent the spread of infection.
7. Initiate standard and other precautions as necessary.
8. Provide comfort as necessary.
9. Provide meticulous skin care.
10. Provide adequate nutritional support as prescribed.
11. Refer to Chapters 26 and 39 for additional information on AIDS.

F. **Kaposi's sarcoma**
1. Description: Skin lesions that occur primarily in individuals with a compromised immune system
2. Data collection
   a. Kaposi's sarcoma is a slow-growing tumor that appears as a raised, oblong, purplish/reddish-brown lesion; may be tender or nontender.
   b. Organ involvement includes the lymph nodes, airways, or lungs, or any part of the gastrointestinal tract from the mouth to anus.
3. Interventions
   a. Maintain standard and other precautions as necessary.
   b. Provide protective isolation if the immune system is depressed.
   c. Prepare the client for radiation therapy or chemotherapy, as prescribed.
   d. Immunotherapy may be prescribed to stabilize the immune system.

XIV. Posttransplantation Immunodeficiency

A. Description
1. Secondary immunodeficiency is immunosuppression caused by therapeutic agents.
2. The client must take immunosuppression agents for the rest of his or her life posttransplant to decrease rejection of the transplanted organ or tissue.

B. Diagnosis and monitoring of posttransplant clients
1. Check renal and hepatic function.
2. Monitor the complete cell count with differential to monitor for signs of infection.
3. Check all body secretions periodically for blood.

C. High-risk clients
1. Clients with a history of malignancy or premalignancy have an increased susceptibility to malignancy if immunosuppressed.
2. Clients with recent infection or exposure to tuberculosis, herpes zoster, or chickenpox have a high risk for severe generalized disease when on immunosuppressive agents.

D. Data collection
1. Monitor for signs of opportunistic infections.
2. Monitor nutritional status.
3. Monitor for signs of rejection (signs will depend on the organ or tissue transplant).

E. Interventions
1. Strict aseptic technique is necessary.
2. Reinforce teaching regarding asepsis and the signs of infection and rejection.
3. Provide psychosocial support as needed.
4. Reinforce client teaching about immunosuppressants.

CRITICAL THINKING What Should You Do?

Answer: Major organ damage can occur with diffuse scleroderma, with esophageal involvement being one complication. The nurse should continuously monitor the client's ability to swallow. If esophageal involvement is suspected, the nurse should collaborate with the RN and health care provider about scheduling a swallowing study. The nurse should also assist with collaboratation with the nutritionist about dietary changes, such as the need for small, frequent meals and minimizing the intake of foods and liquids that stimulate gastric secretion (spicy foods, caffeine, alcohol). The client should also sit up for 1 to 2 hours after meals.

Reference(s): Ignatavicius, D., & Workman, M. (2013). *Medical-surgical nursing: Patient-centered collaborative care.* (7th ed., pp. 347–348). St. Louis: Saunders.

PRACTICE QUESTIONS

646. Which individual is **least** at risk for the development of Kaposi's sarcoma?
1. A kidney transplant client
2. A male with a history of same-sex partners
3. A client receiving antineoplastic medications
4. An individual working in an environment where exposure to asbestos exists

647. The nurse prepares to give a bath and change the bed linens on a client with cutaneous Kaposi's sarcoma lesions. The lesions are open and draining a scant amount of serous fluid. Which should the nurse incorporate in the plan during the bathing of this client?
1. Wearing gloves
2. Wearing a gown and gloves
3. Wearing a gown, gloves, and a mask
4. Wearing a gown and gloves to change the bed linens and gloves only for the bath

648. A client is suspected of having systemic lupus erythematous. The nurse monitors the client, knowing that which is one of the initial characteristic signs/symptoms of systemic lupus erythematous?
1. Weight gain
2. Subnormal temperature
3. Elevated red blood cell count
4. Rash on the face across the nose and on the cheeks

649. A client with pemphigus is being seen in the clinic regularly. The nurse plans care based on which description of this condition?
1. The presence of tiny red vesicles
2. An autoimmune disease that causes blistering in the epidermis
3. The presence of skin vesicles found along the nerve caused by a virus
4. The presence of red, raised papules and large plaques covered by silvery scales

❖ **650.** Which interventions would apply in the care of a client at high risk for an allergic response to a latex allergy? **Select all that apply.**
- ❑ 1. Use nonlatex gloves.
- ❑ 2. Use medications from glass ampules.
- ❑ 3. Place the client in a private room only.
- ❑ 4. Do not puncture rubber stoppers with needles.
- ❑ 5. Keep a latex-safe supply cart available in the client's area.
- ❑ 6. Use a blood pressure cuff from an electronic device only to measure the blood pressure.

651. The nurse is assisting in planning care for a client with a diagnosis of immune deficiency. The nurse should incorporate which as a **priority** in the plan of care?
1. Protecting the client from infection
2. Providing emotional support to decrease fear
3. Encouraging discussion about lifestyle changes
4. Identifying factors that decreased the immune function

652. A client calls the office of his primary care health care provider and tells the nurse that he was just stung by a bumblebee while gardening. The client is afraid of a severe reaction because his neighbor experienced such a reaction just 1 week ago. Which is the appropriate nursing action?
1. Advise the client to soak the site in hydrogen peroxide.
2. Ask the client if he ever sustained a bee sting in the past.
3. Tell the client to call an ambulance for transport to the emergency room.
4. Tell the client not to worry about the sting unless difficulty with breathing occurs.

653. The nurse is assisting in administering immunizations at a health care clinic. The nurse understands that immunization provides which?
1. Protection from all diseases
2. Innate immunity from disease
3. Natural immunity from disease
4. Acquired immunity from disease

654. The nurse is assigned to care for a client with systemic lupus erythematosus (SLE). The nurse plans care considering which factor regarding this diagnosis?
1. A local rash occurs as a result of allergy.
2. It is a disease caused by overexposure to sunlight.
3. A continuous release of histamine in the body causes the disease.
4. It is an inflammatory disease of collagen contained in connective tissue.

655. The camp nurse prepares to instruct a group of children about Lyme disease. Which information should the nurse include in the instructions?
1. Lyme disease is caused by a tick carried by deer.
2. Lyme disease is caused by contamination from cat feces.
3. Lyme disease can be contagious by skin contact with an infected individual.
4. Lyme disease can be caused by the inhalation of spores from bird droppings.

656. The client is diagnosed with stage I of Lyme disease. The nurse should check the client for which characteristic of this stage?
1. Arthralgias
2. Flu-like symptoms
3. Enlarged and inflamed joints
4. Signs of neurological disorders

657. A female client arrives at the health care clinic and tells the nurse that she was just bitten by a tick and would like to be tested for Lyme disease. The client tells the nurse that she removed the tick and flushed it down the toilet. Which nursing action is appropriate?
1. Refer the client for a blood test immediately.
2. Inform the client that there is not a test available for Lyme disease.
3. Tell the client that testing is not necessary unless arthralgia develops.
4. Instruct the client to return in 4 to 6 weeks to be tested, because testing before this time is not reliable.

658. The nurse, a Cub Scout leader, is preparing a group of Cub Scouts for an overnight camping trip and instructs them about the methods to prevent Lyme disease. Which statement by one of the Cub Scouts indicates a **need for further teaching**?
1. "I need to bring a hat to wear during the trip."
2. "I should wear long-sleeved tops and long pants."
3. "I should not use insect repellent because it will attract the ticks."
4. "I need to wear closed shoes and socks that can be pulled up over my pants."

659. The client with acquired immunodeficiency syndrome is diagnosed with cutaneous Kaposi's sarcoma. Based on this diagnosis, the nurse understands that this has been confirmed by which?
1. Swelling in the genital area
2. Swelling in the lower extremities
3. Punch biopsy of the cutaneous lesions
4. Appearance of reddish-blue lesions on the skin

660. The client is brought to the emergency department and is experiencing an anaphylactic reaction from eating shellfish. The nurse should implement which **immediate** action?
1. Maintaining a patent airway
2. Administering a corticosteroid
3. Administering epinephrine (Adrenalin)
4. Instructing the client on the importance of obtaining a Medic-Alert bracelet

ANSWERS

646. 4

Rationale: Kaposi's sarcoma is a vascular malignancy that presents as a skin disorder and is a common acquired immunodeficiency syndrome indicator. It is seen frequently in men with a history of same-sex partners. Although the cause of Kaposi's sarcoma is not known, it is considered to be the result of an alteration or failure in the immune system. The renal transplant client and the client receiving antineoplastic medications are at risk for immunosuppression. Exposure to asbestos is not related to the development of Kaposi's sarcoma.

Test-Taking Strategy: Note the strategic word, *least.* Option 2 can be eliminated easily. Note that options 1 and 3 are comparable or alike; these clients are at risk for immunosuppression. Review: the risk factors associated with **Kaposi's sarcoma**.

Level of Cognitive Ability: Analyzing
Client Needs: Physiological Integrity
Integrated Process: Nursing Process/Data Collection
Content Area: Adult Health: Immune
Priority Concepts: Clinical Judgment, Immunity
References(s): deWit, Kumagai (2013), p. 225.

647. 2

Rationale: Gowns and gloves are required if the nurse anticipates contact with soiled items, such as wound drainage, or while caring for a client who is incontinent with diarrhea or a client who has an ileostomy or colostomy. Masks are not required unless droplet or airborne precautions are necessary. Regardless of the amount of wound drainage, a gown and gloves must be worn.

Test-Taking Strategy: Focus on the subject, preventing disease transmission. Think about the method of transmission of infection when answering a question of this type. Read the question, noting that the tasks presented in this case are bathing and changing bed linens. Eliminate option 3 because the method of transmission is not respiratory. Eliminate options 1 and 4 because neither provides adequate protection based on the method of transmission. Review: **standard and transmission-based precautions**.

Level of Cognitive Ability: Applying
Client Needs: Safe and Effective Care Environment
Integrated Process: Nursing Process/Planning
Content Area: Adult Health: Immune
Priority Concepts: Immunity, Infection
Reference(s): deWit, Kumagai (2013), pp. 109–110.

648. 4

Rationale: Skin lesions or a rash on the face across the bridge of the nose and on the cheeks is an initial characteristic sign of systemic lupus erythematosus (SLE). Fever and weight loss may also occur. Anemia is most likely to occur later in SLE.

Test-Taking Strategy: Focus on the subject, the characteristics of SLE. Recalling the characteristic butterfly rash associated with SLE will direct you to the correct option. **Review:** signs/symptoms of **systemic lupus erythematosus.**

Level of Cognitive Ability: Understanding
Client Needs: Physiological Integrity
Integrated Process: Nursing Process/Data Collection
Content Area: Adult Health: Immune
Priority Concepts: Immunity, Infection
Reference(s): deWit, Kumagai (2013), pp. 245–247.

649. 2
Rationale: Pemphigus is an autoimmune disease that causes blistering in the epidermis. The client has large flaccid blisters (bullae). Because the blisters are in the epidermis, they have a thin covering of skin and break easily, leaving large denuded areas of skin. On initial examination, clients may have crusting areas instead of intact blisters. Option 1 describes eczema, option 3 describes herpes zoster, and option 4 describes psoriasis.
Test-Taking Strategy: Focus on the **subject**, signs/symptoms of pemphigus. Recalling that pemphigus vulgaris is an autoimmune disorder will direct you to the correct option. **Review:** the signs/symptoms of **pemphigus.**
Level of Cognitive Ability: Understanding
Client Needs: Physiological Integrity
Integrated Process: Nursing Process/Planning
Content Area: Adult Health: Immune
Priority Concepts: Immunity, Tissue Integrity
Reference(s): Cooper, Gosnell (2015), pp. 1283–1284; Mosby (2013), p. 1356.

❖ **650. 1, 2, 4, 5**
Rationale: If a client is allergic to latex and is at high risk for an allergic response, the nurse would use nonlatex gloves and latex-safe supplies and would keep a latex-safe supply cart available in the client's area. Any supplies or materials that contain latex would be avoided. These include blood pressure cuffs and medication bottles with rubber stoppers that require puncture with a needle. It is not necessary to place the client in a private room.
Test-Taking Strategy: Focus on the **subject**, the client at high risk for an allergic response to a latex allergy. Recalling that items that contain rubber are likely to contain latex will direct you to the correct interventions. Also noting the **closed-ended word**, *only*, in options 3 and 6 will assist in eliminating these options. **Review:** care of the client with a latex allergy.
Level of Cognitive Ability: Analyzing
Client Needs: Safe and Effective Care Environment
Integrated Process: Nursing Process/Implementation
Content Area: Adult Health: Immune
Priority Concepts: Immunity, Safety
Reference(s): deWit, Kumagai (2013), p. 65.

651. 1
Rationale: The client with immune deficiency has inadequate or absent immune bodies and is at risk for infection. The priority nursing intervention would be to protect the client from infection. Options 2, 3, and 4 may be components of care but are not the priority.
Test-Taking Strategy: Use **Maslow's hierarchy of needs theory** and focus on the **strategic word**, *priority*. Remember that physiological needs are the priority. This will direct you to the correct option. **Review:** the care of a client with **immune deficiency.**
Level of Cognitive Ability: Applying
Client Needs: Physiological Integrity
Integrated Process: Nursing Process/Planning
Content Area: Adult Health: Immune
Priority Concepts: Immunity, Infection
Reference(s): deWit, Kumagai (2013), pp. 234–235.

652. 2
Rationale: In some types of allergies, a reaction occurs only on second and subsequent contacts with the allergen. Therefore, the appropriate action would be to ask the client if he ever received a bee sting in the past. Option 1 is not appropriate advice. Option 3 is unnecessary. The client should not be told "not to worry."
Test-Taking Strategy: Use the **steps of the nursing process.** Option 2 is the only option that addresses data collection. **Review: allergic reactions.**
Level of Cognitive Ability: Applying
Client Needs: Physiological Integrity
Integrated Process: Nursing Process/Implementation
Content Area: Adult Health: Immune
Priority Concepts: Immunity, Safety
References(s): deWit, Kumagai (2013), p. 238.

653. 4
Rationale: Acquired immunity can occur by receiving an immunization that causes antibodies to a specific pathogen to form. Natural (innate) immunity is present at birth. No immunization protects the client from all diseases.
Test-Taking Strategy: Eliminate option 1 first because of the **closed-ended word**, *all*. Next eliminate options 2 and 3 because they are **comparable or alike** and the same type of immunity. **Review: natural and acquired immunity.**
Level of Cognitive Ability: Understanding
Client Needs: Health Promotion and Maintenance
Integrated Process: Nursing Process/Implementation
Content Area: Adult Health: Immune
Priority Concepts: Clinical Judgment, Immunity
Reference(s): deWit, Kumagai (2013), pp. 204–205.

654. 4
Rationale: SLE is an inflammatory disease of collagen contained in connective tissue. Options 1, 2, and 3 are not associated with this disease.
Test-Taking Strategy: Focus on the **subject**, the characteristics of SLE. Eliminate option 1 because SLE is a systemic disorder, not a local one. Next, eliminate option 3 because of its similarity to option 1. From the remaining options, select option 4 because of its systemic characteristic. **Review: systemic lupus erythematosus.**
Level of Cognitive Ability: Understanding
Client Needs: Physiological Integrity
Integrated Process: Nursing Process/Planning
Content Area: Adult Health: Immune
Priority Concepts: Immunity, Inflammation
Reference(s): deWit, Kumagai (2013), pp. 245–246.

655. 1
Rationale: Lyme disease is a multisystem infection that results from a bite by a tick carried by several species of deer. Persons bitten by *Ixodes* ticks can be infected with the spirochete *Borrelia burgdorferi*. Lyme disease cannot be transmitted from one person to another. Toxoplasmosis is caused from the ingestion of cysts from contaminated cat feces. Histoplasmosis is caused by the inhalation of spores from bat or bird droppings.
Test-Taking Strategy: Focus on the **subject**, the characteristics and transmission of Lyme disease. Recalling that this disease is

caused by a bite will assist in eliminating the incorrect options. **Review:** cause of **Lyme disease.**
Level of Cognitive Ability: Applying
Client Needs: Health Promotion and Maintenance
Integrated Process: Teaching and Learning
Content Area: Adult Health: Immune
Priority Concepts: Client Education, Infection
Reference(s): deWit, Kumagai (2013), p. 745.

656. 2
Rationale: The hallmark of stage I is the development of a skin rash within 2 to 30 days of infection, generally at the site of the tick bite. The rash develops into a concentric ring, giving it a bull's-eye appearance. The lesion enlarges up to 50 to 60 cm, and smaller lesions develop farther away from the original tick bite. In stage I, most infected persons develop flu-like symptoms that last 7 to 10 days; these symptoms may reoccur later. Arthralgias and joint enlargements are most likely to occur in stage III. Neurological deficits occur in stage II.
Test-Taking Strategy: Eliminate options 1 and 3 first because they are **comparable or alike**. Next, note that the question asks for the characteristics of stage I. From the remaining two options, select the least serious one because the subject of the question relates to stage I. Expect neurological disorders to occur with progression of the disease. **Review:** stages of **Lyme disease.**
Level of Cognitive Ability: Understanding
Client Needs: Physiological Integrity
Integrated Process: Nursing Process/Data Collection
Content Area: Adult Health: Immune
Priority Concepts: Infection, Immunity
Reference(s): Ignatavicius, Workman (2013), pp. 352–353.

657. 4
Rationale: A blood test is available to detect Lyme disease; however, the test is not reliable if performed before 4 to 6 weeks following the tick bite. Antibody formation takes place in the following manner: immunoglobulin M is detected 3 to 4 weeks after Lyme disease onset, peaks at 6 to 8 weeks, and then gradually disappears; immunoglobulin G is detected 2 to 3 months after infection and may remain elevated for years. Options 1, 2, and 3 are incorrect.
Test-Taking Strategy: Focus on the **subject**, the instruction for the client who was bitten by a tick. Eliminate option 1 first. The word *immediately* should indicate that this is potentially an incorrect option. A blood test is available; therefore, eliminate option 2. Eliminate option 3 because treatment should begin before the arthralgia develops. **Review:** the method of diagnosing **Lyme disease.**
Level of Cognitive Ability: Applying
Client Needs: Physiological Integrity
Integrated Process: Nursing Process/Implementation
Content Area: Adult Health: Immune
Priority Concepts: Clinical Judgment, Infection
Reference(s): Ignatavicius, Workman (2013), pp. 352–353.

658. 3
Rationale: In the prevention of Lyme disease, individuals need to be instructed to use an insect repellent on the skin and clothes when in an area where ticks are likely to be found. Long-sleeved tops and long pants, closed shoes, and a hat or cap should be worn. If possible, one should avoid heavily wooded areas or areas with thick underbrush. Socks can be pulled up and over the pant legs to prevent ticks from entering under clothing.
Test-Taking Strategy: The **strategic words**, *need for further teaching*, indicate a **negative event query** and ask you to select an option that is an incorrect statement. Note that option 3 uses the words *should not*. Reading carefully will assist in directing you to this option. **Review:** measures to prevent contact with **ticks.**
Level of Cognitive Ability: Evaluating
Client Needs: Safe and Effective Care Environment
Integrated Process: Teaching and Learning
Content Area: Adult Health: Immune
Priority Concepts: Client Education, Infection
Reference(s): Lewis et al (2014), p. 1579.

659. 3
Rationale: Kaposi's sarcoma lesions begin as red, dark blue, or purple macules on the lower legs that change into plaques. These large plaques ulcerate or open and drain. The lesions spread by metastasis through the upper body and then to the face and oral mucosa. They can move to the lymphatic system, lungs, and gastrointestinal tract. Late disease results in swelling and pain in the lower extremities, penis, scrotum, or face. Diagnosis is made by punch biopsy of cutaneous lesions and biopsy of pulmonary and gastrointestinal lesions.
Test-Taking Strategy: Focus on the **subject**, diagnosing Kaposi's sarcoma. Eliminate options 1 and 2 first because these symptoms occur late in the development of Kaposi's sarcoma. From the remaining options, note the word *confirmed*. This word will assist in directing you to the option that will confirm the diagnosis: the biopsy of the lesions. **Review:** diagnostic measures for **Kaposi's sarcoma.**
Level of Cognitive Ability: Analyzing
Client Needs: Physiological Integrity
Integrated Process: Nursing Process/Data Collection
Content Area: Adult Health: Immune
Priority Concepts: Immunity, Infection
Reference(s): Ignatavicius, Workman (2013), p. 367.

660. 1
Rationale: If the client experiences an anaphylactic reaction, the immediate action would be to maintain a patent airway. The client then would receive epinephrine. Corticosteroids may also be prescribed. The client will need to be instructed about obtaining and wearing a Medic-Alert bracelet, but this is not the immediate action.
Test-Taking Strategy: Note the **strategic word**, *immediate*. Use the **ABCs—airway, breathing, and circulation**—to answer the question. Airway is always the priority. **Review:** care of the client experiencing an **anaphylactic reaction.**
Level of Cognitive Ability: Applying
Client Needs: Physiological Integrity
Integrated Process: Nursing Process/Implementation
Content Area: Critical Care: Emergency Situations
Priority Concepts: Gas Exchange, Immunity
Reference(s): deWit, Kumagai (2013), pp. 243, 1036–1037.

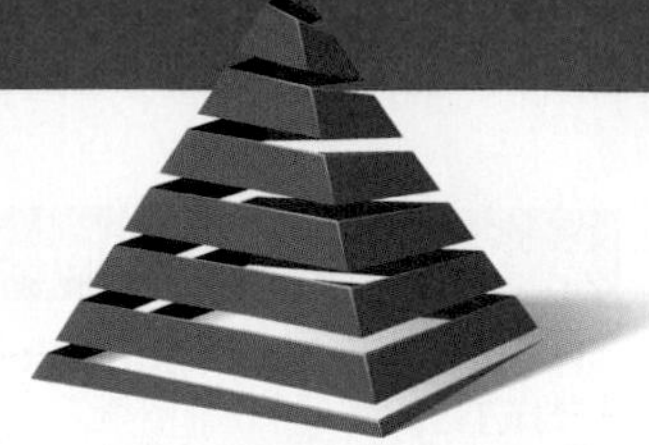

CHAPTER 62

Immunological Medications

Adult—Immune

CRITICAL THINKING What Should You Do?

A hospitalized client who is receiving ceftriaxone (Rocephin) to treat an infection develops severe diarrhea. What should the nurse do?

Answer located on p. 889.

I. Human Immunodeficiency Virus (HIV) and Acquired Immunodeficiency Syndrome (AIDS)

A. Medications include nucleoside-nucleotide reverse transcriptase inhibitors, nonnucleoside reverse transcriptase inhibitors, protease inhibitors, and fusion inhibitors (Box 62-1 and Fig. 62-1).

B. Nucleoside-nucleotide reverse transcriptase inhibitors and nonnucleoside reverse transcriptase inhibitors work by inhibiting the activity of reverse transcriptase.

C. Protease inhibitors work by interfering with the activity of the enzyme protease.

D. Fusion inhibitors work by inhibiting the binding of human **immunodeficiency** virus to cells.

E. Standard treatment consists of using three or four medications in regimens known as highly active antiretroviral therapy (HAART); this therapy is not curative but can delay or reverse loss of immune function, preserve health, and prolong life.

F. Other medications include those that are used to treat complications or opportunistic infections that develop (see Box 62-1).

G. Nucleoside-nucleotide reverse transcriptase inhibitors (NRTIs)
   1. Abacavir (Ziagen): Can cause nausea; monitor for hypersensitivity reaction, including fever, nausea, vomiting, diarrhea, lethargy, malaise, sore throat, shortness of breath, cough, and rash
   2. Abacavir/Lamivudine (Epzicom): In addition to the effects that can occur from abacavir and lamivudine, hypersensitivity reactions, lactic acidosis, and severe hepatomegaly can occur.
   3. Didanosine (Videx): Can cause nausea, diarrhea, peripheral neuropathy, hepatotoxicity, and pancreatitis
   4. Emtricitabine (Emtriva): Can cause headache, diarrhea, nausea, rash, hyperpigmentation of the palms and soles, lactic acidosis, and severe hepatomegaly
   5. Emtricitabine/Tenofovir (Truvada): In addition to the effects that can occur from emtricitabine and tenofovir, lactic acidosis and severe hepatomegaly can occur.
   6. Lamivudine (Epivir): Causes nausea and nasal congestion
   7. Lamivudine/Zidovudine (Combivir): Can cause anemia and neutropenia and lactic acidosis with hepatomegaly
   8. Lamivudine/Zidovudine/Abacavir (Trizivir): In addition to the effects that can occur from lamivudine, zidovudine, and abacavir, hypersensitivity reactions, anemia, neutropenia, lactic acidosis, and severe hepatomegaly can occur.
   9. Stavudine (d4t, Zerit): Can cause peripheral neuropathy and pancreatitis
   10. Tenofovir (Viread): Can cause nausea and vomiting
   11. Zalcitabine (ddC, Hivid): Can cause oral ulcers, peripheral neuropathy, hepatotoxicity, and pancreatitis
   12. Zidovudine (Retrovir): Can cause nausea, vomiting, anemia, leukopenia, myopathy, fatigue, and headache

H. Nonnucleoside reverse transcriptase inhibitors (NNRTIs)
   1. Delavirdine (Rescriptor): Can cause rash, liver function changes, and pruritus
   2. Efavirenz (Sustiva): Can cause rash, dizziness, confusion, difficulty concentrating, dreams, and encephalopathy
   3. Etravirine (Intelence): Can cause rash, gastrointestinal disturbances, headache, hypertension, and peripheral neuropathy
   4. Nevirapine (Viramune): Can cause rash, Stevens-Johnson syndrome, hepatitis, and increased transaminase levels

I. Protease inhibitors (PIs)
   1. Amprenavir/Vitamin E (Agenerase)

BOX 62-1 Medications for HIV and AIDS

Nucleoside-Nucleotide Reverse Transcriptase Inhibitors (NRTIs)
Abacavir (Ziagen)
Abacavir/Lamivudine (Epzicom)
Didanosine (Videx)
Emtricitabine (Emtriva)
Emtricitabine/Tenofovir (Truvada)
Emtricitabine/Tenofovir/Efavirenz (Atripla)
Lamivudine (Epivir)
Lamivudine/Zidovudine (Combivir)
Lamivudine/Zidovudine/Abacavir (Trizivir)
Stavudine (d4t, Zerit)
Tenofovir (Viread)
Zidovudine (Retrovir, azidothymidine, AZT, ZDV)

Nonnucleoside Reverse Transcriptase Inhibitors (NNRTIs)
Delavirdine (Rescriptor)
Efavirenz (Sustiva)
Etravirine (Intelence)
Nevirapine (Viramune)

Protease Inhibitors (PIs)
Amprenavir/Vitamin E (Agenerase)
Atazanavir (Reyataz)
Danunavir (Prezista)
Fosamprenavir (Lexiva)
Indinavir (Crixivan)
Lopinavir/Ritonavir (Kaletra)
Nelfinavir (Viracept)
Ritonavir (Norvir)
Saquinavir (Invirase)
Tipranavir (Aptivus)

Integrase Inhibitor
Raltegravir (Isentress)

Fusion Inhibitor
Enfuvirtide (Fuzeon)

CCR5 Antagonist
Maraviroc (Selzentry)

Anti-inflammatory Medication
Sulfasalazine (Azulfidine)

Anti-infective Medications
Atovaquone (Mepron)
Metronidazole (Flagyl)
Pentamidine isethionate (Pentam 300)
Sulfamethoxazole/Trimethoprim (Bactrim)

Antifungal Medications
Amphotericin B
Fluconazole (Diflucan)
Ketoconazole (Nizoral)

Antiviral Medications
Acyclovir (Zovirax)
Foscarnet
Ganciclovir

a. Can cause nausea, vomiting, headache, altered taste sensations, perioral paresthesia, rashes, and increased results of liver function studies
b. Oral solution contains an alcohol that can interact with metronidazole (Flagyl); can cause feelings of inebriation

2. Atazanavir (Reyataz): Can cause nausea, headache, infection, vomiting, diarrhea, drowsiness, insomnia, fever, hyperglycemia, hyperlipidemia, and increased bleeding in clients with hemophilia
3. Fosamprenavir (Lexiva): Similar to amprenavir; can cause nausea, vomiting, headache, altered taste sensations, perioral paresthesia, rashes, and increased results of liver function studies
4. Indinavir (Crixivan): Can cause nausea, diarrhea, hyperbilirubinemia, nephritis, and kidney stones
5. Lopinavir/ritonavir combination (Kaletra): Can cause nausea, diarrhea, altered taste sensations, circumoral paresthesia, and hepatitis
6. Nelfinavir (Viracept): Can cause nausea, flatulence, and diarrhea
7. Ritonavir (Norvir): Can cause nausea, vomiting, diarrhea, altered taste sensations, circumoral paresthesia, hepatitis, and increased triglyceride levels
8. Saquinavir (Invirase): Can cause nausea, diarrhea, photosensitivity, and headache
9. Tipranavir (Aptivus): Hepatotoxicity (liver damage); can also cause nausea, vomiting, diarrhea, headache, and fatigue

J. Integrase inhibitor: Raltegravor (Isentress)
1. Stops HIV replication and is used in combination with other antiretroviral medications
2. Common side/adverse effects include nausea, diarrhea, fatigue, headache, and itching.

K. Chemokine receptor 5 (CCR5) antagonist: Maraviroc (Selzentry)
1. Binds with CCR5 and blocks viral entry
2. Most common side/adverse effects are cough, dizziness, pyrexia, rash, abdominal pain, musculoskeletal symptoms, and upper respiratory tract infections; liver injury and cardiovascular events have occurred in some clients.

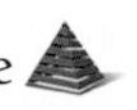

L. Fusion inhibitor: Enfuvirtide (Fuzeon) can cause skin irritation at injection site, fatigue, nausea, insomnia, and peripheral neuropathy.

M. Anti-infective medications: Used to treat opportunistic infections such as *Pneumocystis jiroveci* pneumonia; *Toxoplasma* encephalitis is treated with sulfamethoxazole-trimethoprim (Bactrim; see Box 62-1).

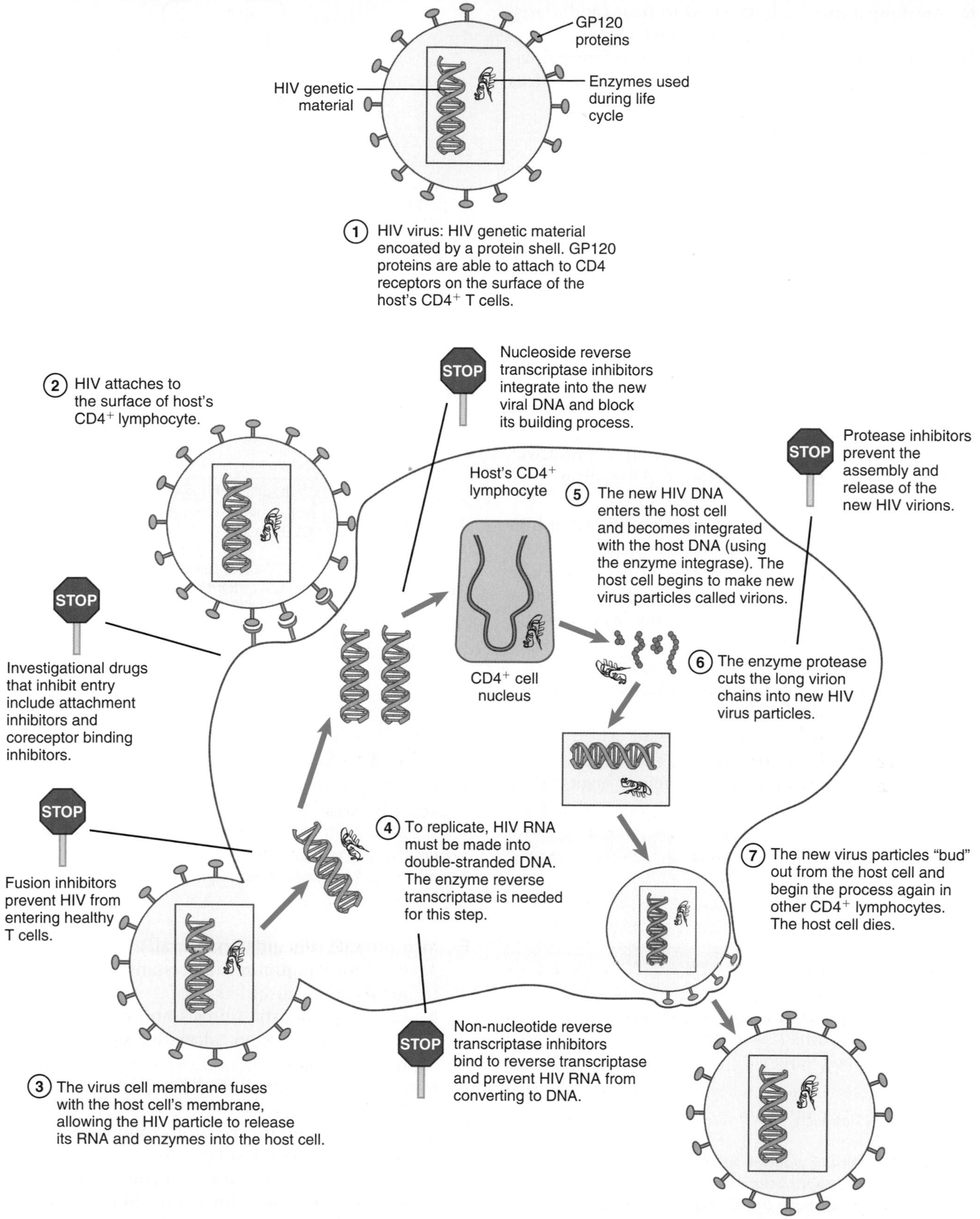

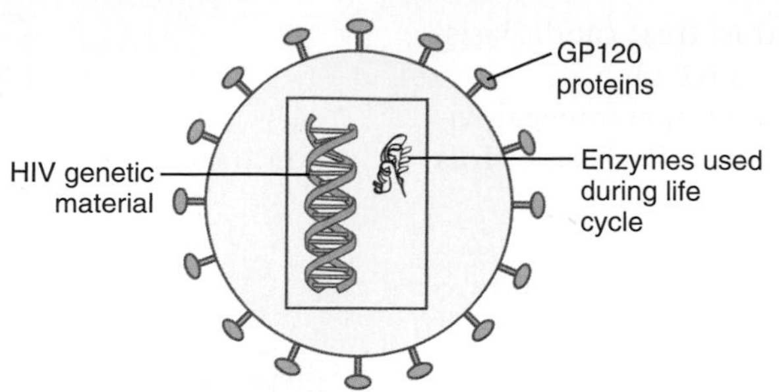

GP120 proteins
HIV genetic material
Enzymes used during life cycle
1 HIV virus: HIV genetic material encoated by a protein shell. GP120 proteins are able to attach to CD4 receptors on the surface of the host's CD4+ T cells.
2 HIV attaches to the surface of host's CD4+ lymphocyte.
STOP
Nucleoside reverse transcriptase inhibitors integrate into the new viral DNA and block its building process.
STOP
Protease inhibitors prevent the assembly and release of the new HIV virions.
Host's CD4+ lymphocyte
5 The new HIV DNA enters the host cell and becomes integrated with the host DNA (using the enzyme integrase). The host cell begins to make new virus particles called virions.
STOP
Investigational drugs that inhibit entry include attachment inhibitors and coreceptor binding inhibitors.
CD4+ cell nucleus
6 The enzyme protease cuts the long virion chains into new HIV virus particles.
STOP
Fusion inhibitors prevent HIV from entering healthy T cells.
4 To replicate, HIV RNA must be made into double-stranded DNA. The enzyme reverse transcriptase is needed for this step.
7 The new virus particles "bud" out from the host cell and begin the process again in other CD4+ lymphocytes. The host cell dies.
STOP
Non-nucleotide reverse transcriptase inhibitors bind to reverse transcriptase and prevent HIV RNA from converting to DNA.
3 The virus cell membrane fuses with the host cell's membrane, allowing the HIV particle to release its RNA and enzymes into the host cell.

FIGURE 62-1 Steps in the life cycle of the human immunodeficiency virus (HIV), with correlation to medications. (From Black J, Hawks J: *Medical-surgical nursing: Clinical management for positive outcomes*, ed 8, St. Louis, 2009, Saunders.)

Adult—Immune

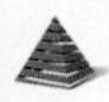

N. Antifungal medications: Used to treat candidiasis, cryptococcal meningitis (see Box 62-1)

O. Antiviral medications: Used to treat cytomegalovirus retinitis, herpes simplex, varicella-zoster virus (see Box 62-1)

The client with HIV or AIDS is at high risk for the development of opportunistic infections.

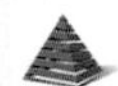

II. Immunosuppressants (Box 62-2 and Fig. 62-2)

A. Description: Immunosuppressants are used for transplant clients to prevent organ or tissue rejection and to treat autoimmune disorders such as systemic lupus erythematosus.

B. Cyclosporine (Sandimmune)
1. Used for prevention of rejection following allogeneic organ transplantation
2. Usually administered with a glucocorticoid and another immunosuppressant
3. Most common adverse effects are nephrotoxicity, infection, hypertension, and hirsutism.

C. Tacrolimus (Prograf)
1. Used for prevention of rejection following liver or kidney transplantation
2. Adverse effects include nephrotoxicity, neurotoxicity, gastrointestinal effects, hypertension, hyperkalemia, hyperglycemia, hirsutism, and gum hyperplasia.

D. Azathioprine (Imuran)
1. Generally used with renal transplant clients
2. Can cause neutropenia and thrombocytopenia

E. Cyclophosphamide (Neosar)
1. Used for its immunosuppressant action to treat autoimmune disorders
2. Can cause neutropenia and hemorrhagic cystitis

Box 62-2 Immunosuppressants

Calcineurin Inhibitors
Cyclosporine (Sandimmune)
Tacrolimus (Prograf)

Cytotoxic Medications
Azathioprine (Imuran)
Cyclophosphamide Methotrexate (Rheumatrex, Trexall)
Mycophenolate mofetil (CellCept)
Mycophenolic acid (Myfortic)

Antibodies
Basiliximab (Simulect)
Daclizumab
Lymphocyte immune globulin, an tithymocyte globulin (equine)
Muromonab-CD3 (Orthoclone OKT3)
$Rh_o(D)$ immune globulin (RhoGAM)

Other
Sirolimus (Rapamune)

Glucocorticoids
See Chapter 46.

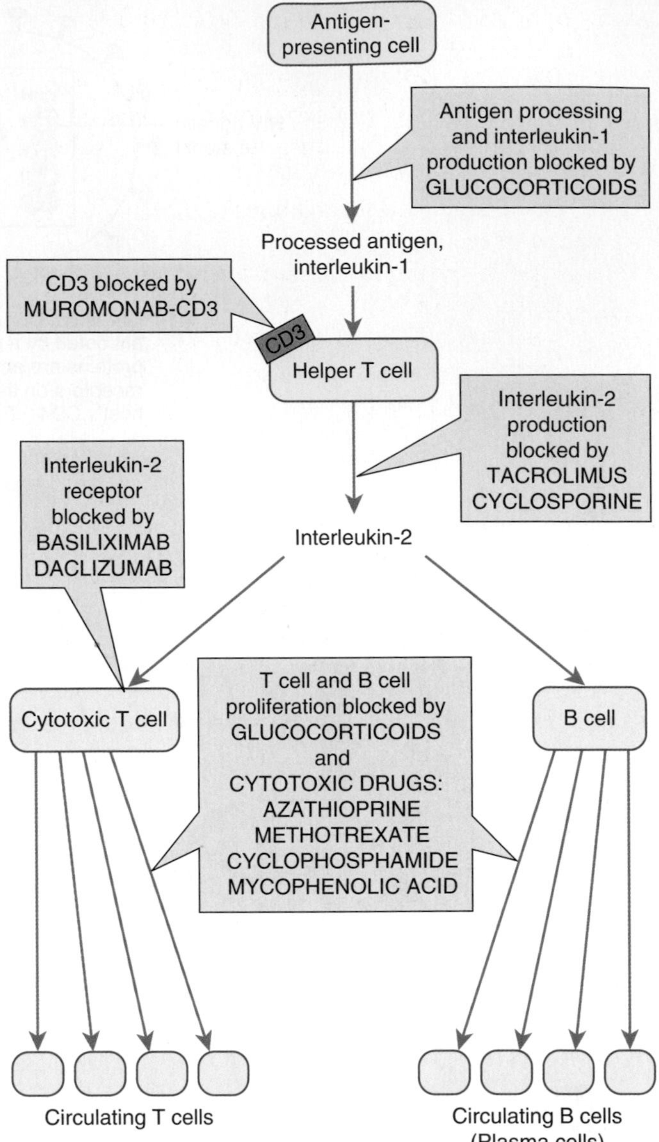

FIGURE 62-2 Sites of action of immunosuppressant drugs. (From Lehne R: *Pharmacology for nursing care*, ed 7, Philadelphia, 2010, Saunders.)

F. Methotrexate (Rheumatrex, Trexall)
1. Used for its immunosuppressant action to treat autoimmune disorders
2. Can cause hepatic fibrosis and cirrhosis, bone marrow suppression, ulcerative stomatitis, and renal damage

G. Mycophenolate mofetil (CellCept) and mycophenlic acid (Myfortic)
1. Used to prevent rejection following kidney, heart, and liver transplantation
2. Can cause diarrhea, vomiting, neutropenia, sepsis; increased risk of infection and malignancies, especially lymphomas

H. Basiliximab (Simulect); daclizumab (Zenapax)
1. Used to prevent rejection following kidney transplantation
2. Can cause severe acute hypersensitivity reactions including anaphylaxis

I. Lymphocyte immune globulin, antithymocyte globulin (equine)
 1. Used to prevent rejection following kidney, heart, liver, and bone marrow transplantation
 2. Side/adverse effects include fever, chills, leukopenia, and skin reactions.
 3. Can cause anaphylactoid reactions
J. Sirolimus (Rapamune)
 1. Used to prevent renal transplant rejection
 2. Increases the risk of infection; raises cholesterol and triglyceride levels; can cause renal injury
 3. Other side/adverse effects include rash, acne, anemia, thrombocytopenia, joint pain, diarrhea, and hypokalemia.

⚠ Monitor the client taking an immunosuppressant closely for signs of infection.

III. Immunizations (See Chapter 39)

IV. Antibiotics (Box 62-3)

A. Inhibit the growth of bacteria
B. Include medication classifications of aminoglycosides, cephalosporins, fluoroquinolones, macrolides,

BOX 62-3 Antibiotics

Aminoglycosides
Amikacin (Amikin)
Gentamicin
Kanamycin (Kantrex)
Neomycin (Neo-Fradin)
Streptomycin
Tobramycin

Antimycobacterials
Antituberculosis agents (see Chapter 50)
Leprostatics: Clofazimine

Antifungal Medications
Amphotericin B
Fluconazole (Diflucan)
Ketoconazole

Antiviral Medications
Acyclovir (Zovirax)
Foscarnet
Ganciclovir (Cytovene)

Cephalosporins
Cefaclor (Ceclor)
Cefazolin (Ancef, Kefzol)
Cefdinir (Omnicef)
Cefditoren (Spectracef)
Cefopodoxime (Vantin)
Cefotaxime (Claforan)
Cefotetan (Cefotan)
Cefoxitin (Mefoxin)
Cefprozil (Cefzil)
Ceftazidime (Ceptaz, Fortaz, Tazicef)
Ceftibuten (Cedax)
Ceftizoxime (Cefizox)
Ceftriaxone (Rocephin)
Cefuroxime (Ceftin)
Cephalexin (Keflex)
Loracarbef

Fluoroquinolones
Ciprofloxacin (Cipro)
Gatifloxacin
Gemifloxacin (Factive)
Levofloxacin (Levaquin)
Moxifloxacin (Avelox)
Norfloxacin (Noroxin)
Ofloxacin (Floxin)
Trovafloxacin (Trovan)

Lincosamides
Clindamycin (Cleocin)
Lincomycin (Lincocin)

Macrolides
Azithromycin (Zithromax)
Clarithromycin (Biaxin)
Dirithromycin
Erythromycin

Monobactam
Aztreonam (Azactam)

Penicillins
Amoxicillin (Amoxil)
Ampicillin (Principen)
Carbenicillin
Penicillin G (Bicillin L-A, Permapen, Pfizerpen, Wycillin)
Penicillin V (Veetids)
Piperacillin
Ticarcillin

Penicillinase-Resistant Penicillins
Dicloxacillin
Nafcillin
Oxacillin

Sulfonamides
Sulfadiazine
Sulfamethoxazole
Sulfasalizine
Sulfisoxazole
Trimethoprim/sulfamethoxazole (TMP-SMZ; Bactrim, Septra)

Tetracyclines
Demeclocycline (Declomycin)
Doxycycline (Vibramycin)
Minocycline (Minocin)
Oxytetracycline
Tetracycline (Sumycin)

lincosamides, monobactams, penicillins and penicillinase-resistant penicillins, sulfonamides, tetracyclines, antimycobacterials, antifungals (see Box 62-3)

C. Adverse effects (Table 62-1)

D. Nursing considerations

1. Check for allergies.
2. Monitor appropriate laboratory values before therapy as appropriate and during therapy to assess for adverse effects.
3. Monitor for adverse effects and report to the health care provider if any occur.
4. The appropriate method of administration is determined and instructions are provided to the client.
5. Monitor intake and output.
6. Encourage fluid intake (unless contraindicated).
7. Initiate safety precautions because of possible central nervous system effects.

TABLE 62-1 Antibiotics and their Adverse Effects

Classification	Adverse Effects
Aminoglycosides	Ototoxicity Confusion, disorientation Renal toxicity Gastrointestinal irritation Palpitations, blood pressure changes Hypersensitivity reactions
Cephalosporins	Gastrointestinal disturbances Pseudomembranous colitis Headache, dizziness, lethargy, paresthesias Nephrotoxicity Superinfections
Fluoroquinolones	Headache, dizziness, insomnia, depression Gastrointestinal effects Bone marrow depression Fever, rash, photosensitivity
Macrolides	Gastrointestinal effects Pseudomembranous colitis Confusion Superinfections Hypersensitivity reactions
Lincosamides	Gastrointestinal effects Pseudomembranous colitis Bone marrow depression
Monobactams	Gastrointestinal effects Hepatotoxicity Allergic reactions
Penicillins and penicillinase-resistant penicillins	Gastrointestinal effects, including sore mouth and furry tongue Superinfections Hypersensitivity reactions, including anaphylaxis
Sulfonamides	Gastrointestinal effects Hepatotoxicity Nephrotoxicity Bone marrow depression Dermatological effects, including hypersensitivity and photosensitivity Headache, dizziness, vertigo, ataxia, depression, seizures
Tetracyclines	Gastrointestinal effects Hepatotoxicity Teeth (staining) and bone damage Superinfections Dermatological reactions, including rash and photosensitivity Hypersensitivity reactions
Antimycobacterials, leprostatics	Gastrointestinal effects Neuritis, dizziness, headache, malaise, drowsiness, hallucinations
Antifungals	Gastrointestinal effects Headache, rash, anemia, hepatotoxicity, hearing loss, peripheral neuritis

8. Reinforce teaching the client about the medication and how to take the medication; the importance of completing the full prescribed course is emphasized.

CRITICAL THINKING What Should You Do?

Answer: Ceftriaxone (Rocephin) is a cephalosporin. Some adverse effects include gastrointestinal disturbances, pseudomembranous colitis, and superinfections. If the client develops severe diarrhea, the nurse should notify the RN and contact the health care provider immediately because of the potential development of an adverse effect. In some situations, antibiotic-associated gastrointestinal disturbances such as diarrhea may require contact precautions.

Reference(s): Hodgson, B., & Kizior, R. (2015). *Saunders nursing drug handbook 2015.* (pp. 228–229). St. Louis: Saunders.

PRACTICE QUESTIONS

❖ **661.** A client with human immunodeficiency virus is taking nevirapine (Viramune). The nurse should monitor for which side/adverse effects of the medication? **Select all that apply.**

- ☐ **1.** Rash
- ☐ **2.** Hepatotoxicity
- ☐ **3.** Hyperglycemia
- ☐ **4.** Peripheral neuropathy
- ☐ **5.** Reduced bone mineral density

662. The client with acquired immunodeficiency syndrome has begun therapy with zidovudine (Retrovir). The nurse should carefully monitor which laboratory result during treatment with this medication?

1. Blood culture
2. Blood glucose level
3. Blood urea nitrogen
4. Complete blood count

663. The nurse is reviewing the results of serum laboratory studies drawn on a client with acquired immunodeficiency syndrome who is receiving didanosine (Videx). The nurse interprets that the client may have the medication discontinued by the health care provider if which significantly elevated result is noted?

1. Serum protein
2. Blood glucose
3. Serum amylase
4. Serum creatinine

664. The nurse is caring for a postrenal transplant client taking cyclosporine (Sandimmune). The nurse notes an increase in one of the client's vital signs, and the client is complaining of a headache. Which is the vital sign that is **most likely** increased?

1. Pulse
2. Respirations
3. Blood pressure
4. Temperature

665. Amikacin (Amikin) is prescribed for a client with a bacterial infection. The client should be instructed to contact the health care provider (HCP) immediately if which occurs?

1. Nausea
2. Lethargy
3. Hearing loss
4. Muscle aches

666. The nurse is assigned to care for a client with cytomegalovirus retinitis and acquired immunodeficiency syndrome who is receiving foscarnet. The nurse should check the latest result of which laboratory study while the client is taking this medication?

1. $CD4^+$ cell count
2. Serum albumin
3. Serum creatinine
4. Lymphocyte count

667. The client with acquired immunodeficiency syndrome and *Pneumocystis jiroveci* infection has been receiving pentamidine isethionate (Pentam 300). The client develops a temperature of 101° F. The nurse should do further monitoring of the client, knowing that this sign would **most likely** indicate which?

1. The dose of the medication is too low.
2. The client is experiencing toxic effects of the medication.
3. The client has developed inadequacy of thermoregulation.
4. This is the result of another infection caused by the leukopenic effects of the medication.

668. Saquinavir (Invirase) is prescribed for the client who is human immunodeficiency virus seropositive. The nurse reinforces medication instructions and should provide the client with which health care measure?

1. Avoid sun exposure.
2. Eat low-calorie foods.
3. Eat foods that are low in fat.
4. Take the medication on an empty stomach.

❖ **669.** Ketoconazole is prescribed for a client with a diagnosis of candidiasis. Which interventions should the nurse include in the plan of care regarding this medication? **Select all that apply.**

- ❑ **1.** Restrict fluid intake.
- ❑ **2.** Instruct the client to avoid alcohol.
- ❑ **3.** Monitor hepatic and liver function studies.
- ❑ **4.** Administer the medication with an antacid.
- ❑ **5.** Instruct the client to avoid exposure to the sun.
- ❑ **6.** Administer the medication on an empty stomach.

670. The client who is human immunodeficiency virus seropositive has been taking stavudine (d4t, Zerit). Which should the nurse monitor closely while the client is taking this medication?

1. Gait
2. Appetite
3. Level of consciousness
4. Hemoglobin and hematocrit blood levels

ANSWERS

❖ **661. 1, 2**
Rationale: Nevirapine (Viramune) is a nonnucleoside reverse transcriptase inhibitor that is used to treat HIV infection. It is used in combination with other antiretroviral medications to treat HIV. Adverse effects include rash, Stevens-Johnson syndrome, hepatitis, and increased transaminase levels. Hyperglycemia, peripheral neuropathy, and reduced bone density are not side/adverse effects of this medication.
Test-Taking Strategy: Focus on the **subject**, side/adverse effects of neviparine (Viramune). Hyperglycemia, peripheral neuropathy, and reduced bone mineral density are not common side/adverse effects of commonly prescribed medications. Remember that rash, Stevens-Johnson syndrome, hepatitis, and increased transaminase levels are side/adverse effects of nevirapine. **Review:** side/adverse effects of **neviparine (Viramune)**.
Level of Cognitive Ability: Analyzing
Client Needs: Physiological Integrity
Integrated Process: Nursing Process/Data Collection
Content Area: Pharmacology: Immune Medications
Priority Concepts: Cellular Regulation, Infection
Reference(s): Hodgson, Kizior (2015), pp. 842–843.

662. 4
Rationale: A common side/adverse effect of therapy with zidovudine is leukopenia and anemia. The nurse monitors the complete blood count results for these changes. Options 1, 2, and 3 are unrelated to the use of this medication.
Test-Taking Strategy: Focus on the **subject**, zidovudine. Recalling that zidovudine causes leukopenia and anemia will direct you to the correct option. **Review:** side/adverse effects of **zidovudine**.
Level of Cognitive Ability: Analyzing
Client Needs: Physiological Integrity
Integrated Process: Nursing Process/Data Collection
Content Area: Pharmacology: Immune Medications
Priority Concepts: Cellular Regulation, Infection
Reference(s): Lehne (2013), pp. 1211–1212.

663. *Answer:* 3
Rationale: Didanosine (Videx) can cause pancreatitis. A serum amylase level that is increased 1.5 to 2 times normal may signify pancreatitis in the client with acquired immunodeficiency syndrome and is potentially fatal. The medication may have to be discontinued. The medication is also hepatotoxic and can result in liver failure.
Test-Taking Strategy: Focus on the **subject**, adverse effects of didanosine. Recalling that this medication can cause damage to the pancreas and is hepatotoxic will direct you to the correct option. **Review:** adverse effects of **didanosine**.
Level of Cognitive Ability: Analyzing
Client Needs: Physiological Integrity
Integrated Process: Nursing Process/Data Collection
Content Area: Pharmacology: Immune Medications
Priority Concepts: Cellular Regulation, Infection
Reference(s): Hodgson, Kizior (2015), pp. 359–360.

664. 3
Rationale: Hypertension can occur in a client taking cyclosporine (Sandimmune), and because this client is also complaining of a headache, the blood pressure is the vital sign to be monitoring most closely. Other adverse effects include infection, nephrotoxicity, and hirsutism. Options 1, 2, and 4 are unrelated to the use of this medication.
Test-Taking Strategy: Note the **strategic words**, *most likely.* Focus on the **subject**, cyclosporine, and note the data in the question. Recall that this medication can cause hypertension, which can be manifested by a headache. **Review:** the adverse effects of **cyclosporine**.
Level of Cognitive Ability: Analyzing
Client Needs: Physiological Integrity
Integrated Process: Nursing Process/Data Collection
Content Area: Pharmacology: Immune Medications
Priority Concepts: Immunity, Infection
Reference(s): Hodgson, Kizior (2015), pp. 301–302.

665. 3
Rationale: Amikacin (Amikin) is an aminoglycoside. Adverse effects of aminoglycosides include ototoxicity (hearing problems), confusion, disorientation, gastrointestinal irritation, palpitations, blood pressure changes, nephrotoxicity, and hypersensitivity. The nurse instructs the client to report hearing loss to the HCP immediately. Lethargy and muscle aches are not associated with the use of this medication. It is not necessary to contact the HCP immediately if nausea occurs. If nausea persists or results in vomiting, the HCP should be notified.
Test-Taking Strategy: Focus on the **subject**, contacting the HCP for an adverse effect of amikacin. Nausea, lethargy, and muscle aches do not usually require immediate contact of the HCP. Recalling that this medication is an aminoglycoside (most aminoglycoside medication names end in the letters *-cin*) and that aminogylcosides are ototoxic will direct you to the correct option. **Review:** the adverse effects of **aminoglycosides**.
Level of Cognitive Ability: Applying
Client Needs: Physiological Integrity
Integrated Process: Teaching and Learning

Content Area: Pharmacology: Immune Medications
Priority Concepts: Infection, Sensory Perception
Reference(s): Hodgson, Kizior (2015), p. 54.

666. 3
Rationale: Foscarnet is toxic to the kidneys. Serum creatinine is monitored before therapy, two to three times per week during induction therapy and at least weekly during maintenance therapy. Foscarnet may also cause decreased levels of calcium, magnesium, phosphorus, and potassium. Thus these levels are also measured with the same frequency.
Test-Taking Strategy: Focus on the **subject**, monitoring laboratory results for a client taking foscarnet. $CD4^+$ counts, serum albumin, and lymphocyte counts are not monitored frequently during use of most medications. Recalling that this medication is nephrotoxic will direct you to the correct option. **Review:** adverse effects of **foscarnet**.
Level of Cognitive Ability: Analyzing
Client Needs: Physiological Integrity
Integrated Process: Nursing Process/Data Collection
Content Area: Pharmacology: Immune Medications
Priority Concepts: Clinical Judgment, Infection
Reference(s): Hodgson, Kizior (2015), p. 523.

667. 4
Rationale: Frequent side/adverse effects of this medication include leukopenia, thrombocytopenia, and anemia. The client should be monitored routinely for signs and symptoms of infection. Options 1, 2, and 3 are inaccurate interpretations.
Test-Taking Strategy: Note the **strategic words**, *most likely*. Focus on the **subject**, the client develops a temperature of 101° F while taking Pentam 300. Note the relationship between these words and the correct option. Also note that low medication dose, toxic effects, and inadequacy of thermoregulation are not common side/adverse effects of commonly used medications. **Review:** side effects of **pentamidine**.
Level of Cognitive Ability: Analyzing
Client Needs: Physiological Integrity
Integrated Process: Nursing Process/Data Collection
Content Area: Pharmacology: Immune Medications
Priority Concepts: Infection, Thermoregulation
Reference(s): Lehne (2013), p. 1249.

668. 1
Rationale: Saquinavir (Invirase) is an antiretroviral (protease inhibitor) used with other antiretroviral medications to manage human immunodeficiency virus infection. Saquinavir is administered with meals and is best absorbed if the client consumes high-calorie, high-fat meals. Saquinavir can cause photosensitivity, and the nurse should instruct the client to avoid sun exposure.
Test-Taking Strategy: Focus on the **subject**, instructions to the client taking saquinavir. Options 2 and 3 can be eliminated first, knowing that these dietary measures would not likely be prescribed for this client. From the remaining options, you must know that this medication can cause photosensitivity. **Review:** medication instructions with **saquinavir**.
Level of Cognitive Ability: Applying
Client Needs: Physiological Integrity
Integrated Process: Teaching and Learning
Content Area: Pharmacology: Immune Medications
Priority Concepts: Client Education, Infection
Reference(s): Hodgson, Kizior (2015), p. 1088.

❖669. 2, 3, 5
Rationale: Ketoconazole is an antifungal medication. It is administered with food (not on an empty stomach), and antacids are avoided for 2 hours after taking the medication to ensure absorption. The medication is hepatotoxic, and the nurse monitors liver function studies. The client is instructed to avoid exposure to the sun because the medication increases photosensitivity. The client is also instructed to avoid alcohol. There is no reason for the client to restrict fluid intake. In fact, this could be harmful to the client.
Test-Taking Strategy: Focus on the **subject**, interventions when administering ketoconazole. Use general medication guidelines to assist in selecting the correct interventions. Also remember that this medication is administered with food and that it is hepatotoxic. **Review:** nursing interventions with **ketoconazole**.
Level of Cognitive Ability: Analyzing
Client Needs: Physiological Integrity
Integrated Process: Nursing Process/Implementation
Content Area: Pharmacology: Immune Medications
Priority Concepts: Clinical Judgment, Infection
Reference(s): Hodgson, Kizior (2015), p. 658; Lehne (2013), p. 1141.

670. 1
Rationale: Stavudine (d4t, Zerit) is an antiretroviral used to manage human immunodeficiency virus infection in clients who do not respond to or who cannot tolerate conventional therapy. The medication can cause peripheral neuropathy, and the nurse should monitor the client's gait closely and ask the client about paresthesia. Options 2, 3, and 4 are unrelated to the use of this medication.
Test-Taking Strategy: Focus on the **subject**, side/adverse effects of stavudine. Recalling that this medication causes peripheral neuropathy will direct you to the correct option. **Review:** side/adverse effects of **stavudine**.
Level of Cognitive Ability: Analyzing
Client Needs: Physiological Integrity
Integrated Process: Nursing Process/Data Collection
Content Area: Pharmacology: Immune Medications
Priority Concepts: Infection, Sensory Perception
Reference(s): Hodgson, Kizior (2015), pp. 1127–1129; Lehne (2013), pp. 1211–1212.

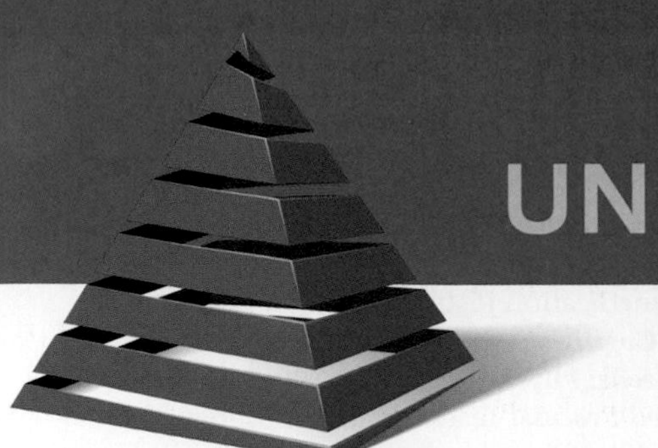

UNIT XIX

The Adult Client with a Mental Health Disorder

PYRAMID TERMS

abuse When directed toward another, includes acts of misuse, deceit, or exploitation; the wrong or improper use or action toward another individual that results in injury, damage, maltreatment, or corruption.

addiction State of dependence or compulsive use. In relation to drug dependence, addiction incorporates the concepts of loss of control with respect to the use of a drug, taking the drug despite related problems and complications, and a tendency to relapse.

coping mechanisms Method used to decrease anxiety.

crisis A temporary state of disequilibrium in which an individual's usual coping mechanisms or problem-solving methods fail. It can result in personality growth or personality disorganization.

defense mechanisms Coping mechanism used in an effort to protect the individual from feelings of anxiety. As anxiety increases and becomes overwhelming, the individual copes by using defense mechanisms to protect the ego and decrease anxiety.

milieu The physical and social environment in which an individual lives. Milieu therapy focuses on positive physical and social environmental manipulation to produce positive change.

restraints (security devices) Physical restraints include any manual method or mechanical device, material, or equipment that inhibits free movement. Chemical restraints include the administration of medications for the specific purpose of inhibiting a specific behavior or movement.

seclusion Placing a client alone in a specially designed room for protection and close supervision. It is the last measure in a process to maximize safety to the client and others.

suicide The ultimate act of self-destruction in which an individual purposefully ends his or her own life.

suicide attempt Any willful, self-inflicted, or life-threatening attempt by an individual that has not led to death.

Pyramid to Success

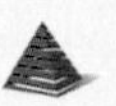

The Pyramid to Success focuses on the therapeutic nurse-client relationship, client rights, hospital admission procedures, ethical and legal issues related to the care of the client with a mental health disorder, and grief and loss. Pyramid points focus on the use of restraints, seclusion, and electroconvulsive therapy (ECT). Focus on care of the client with a substance-related or addictive disorder. Additional focus areas include anxiety disorders, depressive disorders, suicide, abuse and violence, rape crisis interventions, trauma- and stress-related disorders, obsessive-compulsive disorders, schizophrenia, and bipolar disorders. Pyramid points address the use of medications prescribed for the client with a mental health disorder.

Client Needs

Safe and Effective Care Environment

Ensuring client advocacy
Ensuring that informed consent related to treatments, such as restraints, seclusion, and electroconvulsive therapy (ECT), has been obtained
Implementing legal responsibilities related to reporting incidences of violence and abuse
Maintaining confidentiality
Providing safety to client and others
Upholding client rights
Using restraints (security devices) and seclusion appropriately and safely

Health Promotion and Maintenance

Identifying community resources for the client
Identifying individual lifestyle choices

Performing psychosocial data collection techniques
Providing health promotion programs related to substance-related or addictive disorders

Psychosocial Integrity

Addressing grief and loss issues
Caring for the client who has experienced trauma, such as sexual abuse
Considering religious, cultural, and spiritual influences on health
Developing a therapeutic nurse-client relationship
Identifying coping mechanisms
Identifying support systems
Implementing behavioral interventions as appropriate
Monitoring for abuse/neglect situations
Monitoring for domestic violence
Monitoring for substance-related or addictive disorders
Providing a therapeutic milieu
Reinforcing teaching about stress management techniques

Physiological Integrity

Administering medications as prescribed
Assessing for abusive and self-destructive behavior
Monitoring elimination patterns
Monitoring for alterations in body systems related to addictions
Monitoring for expected and untoward effects of medications
Monitoring for potential complications related to medications and electroconvulsive therapy
Monitoring laboratory values related to medication therapy
Monitoring rest and sleep patterns
Providing adequate nutrition
Providing personal hygiene measures

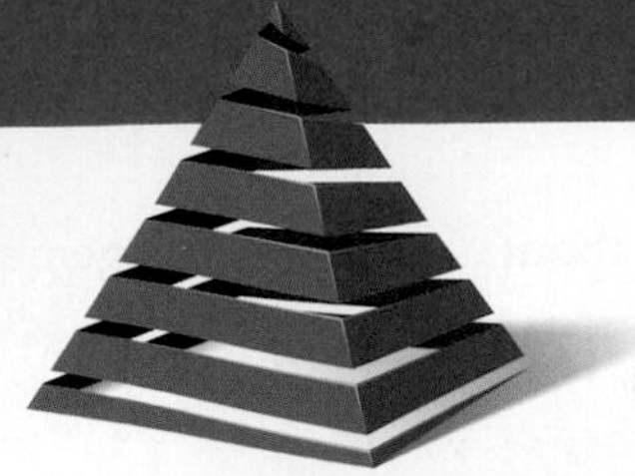

CHAPTER 63

Foundations of Psychiatric Mental Health Nursing

CRITICAL THINKING What Should You Do?

A client needs assistance in using coping mechanisms to decrease anxiety. What should the nurse do?
Answer located on p. 901.

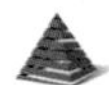

I. The Nurse–Client Relationship

A. Principles
1. Genuineness, respect, and empathic understanding are characteristics important to the development of a therapeutic nurse-client relationship.
2. The client should be cared for in a holistic manner.
3. The nurse considers the client's cultural beliefs and values in assessing the client's response to the nurse-client relationship and his or her adaptation to stressors.
4. Appropriate limits and boundaries define and facilitate a therapeutic nurse-client relationship.
5. Honest and open communication is an important cornerstone for the development of trust—an underpinning of the therapeutic nurse-client relationship.
6. The nurse uses therapeutic communication techniques to encourage the client to express thoughts and feelings as they address identified problem areas.
7. The nurse respects the client's confidentiality and limits discussion of the client to members of the treatment team.
8. The goal of the nurse-client relationship is to assist the client to develop problem-solving and coping mechanisms.

⚠ The nurse needs to consider the religious and spiritual practices of the client and whether these practices may give the client hope, comfort, and support while healing.

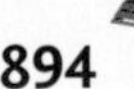

B. Phases of a therapeutic nurse-client relationship
1. Preinteraction phase
   a. The preinteraction phase begins before the nurse's first contact with the client.
   b. The nurse's task in the preinteraction phase is to focus on his or her own preconceived ideas, stereotypes, biases, and values that may impinge on the nurse-client relationship.
2. Orientation or introductory phase
   a. Acceptance, trust, and boundaries are established.
   b. Expectations and the time frame of the relationship are identified (establishing a contract).
   c. Client-centered goals are defined.
   d. Termination and separation of the relationship are discussed in anticipation of the time-limited nature of the relationship.
3. Working phase
   a. Exploring, focusing on, and evaluating the client's concerns and problems occurs; an attitude of acceptance and active listening assists the client to express thoughts and feelings.
   b. Encouraging independence in the client facilitates recovery and leads to readiness for termination.
4. Termination or separation phase
   a. Prepare the client for termination and separation on initial contact.
   b. Evaluate progress and achievement of goals.
   c. Identify responses related to termination and separation, such as anger, distancing from the relationship, a return of symptoms, and dependency.
   d. Encourage the client to express feelings about termination.
   e. Identify the client's strengths and anticipated needs for follow-up care.
   f. Refer the client to community resources and/or other support systems.

C. Family as an extension of the client
1. Family members should be viewed as collaborators in the management of a client's mental health needs (maintain confidentiality as necessary).

2. Competence and caring focused toward family members enhance the nurse's ability to identify client and family needs and to select and implement effective interventions directed toward promoting adaptive functioning.
3. Nurses have a professional obligation to be aware of and sensitive to the cultural and ethnic factors that affect the structure and resulting needs of the client and his or her family.
4. Educating family members regarding the client's illness, identification of symptoms, and effective management of maladaptive behaviors play a vital role in the client's quality of life.

D. Impact of culture, ethnicity, and spirituality on client care

1. Cultural competency allows the nurse to recognize the uniqueness of each client and the impact that culture, values, and spiritual beliefs have on an individual's mental health as well as the treatment required for existing mental illness.
2. A client's culture, ethnicity, value, and spiritual belief systems can impact all aspects of mental health care, including medication therapies, and can act as either protective or risk factors when dealing with the development and/or treatment of psychiatric disorders.
3. Nurses must be aware of the impact their own culture, values, and beliefs have on the care they provide and to avoid biases.
4. The treatment plan must be agreed upon by both client and nurse and take into consideration the needs of the client whenever possible.

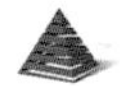

II. Therapeutic Communication Process

A. Principles

1. Communication includes verbal and nonverbal expression (Fig. 63-1).
2. Successful communication includes appropriateness, efficiency, flexibility, and feedback.
3. Anxiety in the nurse or client impedes communication.
4. Communication needs to be goal directed within a professional framework.

B. Therapeutic and nontherapeutic communication techniques (Box 63-1)

III. Mental Health

A. Mental health is a lifelong process of successful adaptation to a changing internal and external environment.

B. The mentally healthy individual is *in contact with reality,* is able to relate to people and situations in their environment, and can resolve conflicts within a problem-solving framework.

C. The mentally healthy individual has psychobiological resilience.

IV. Psychiatric/Mental Health Illness

A. Description

1. Psychiatric illness is the loss of ability to respond to the environment in ways that are in harmony with oneself or the expectations of society.
2. It is characterized by thought or behavior patterns that impair functioning and cause distress.

B. Personality characteristics

1. Self-concept is distorted.
2. Perception of strengths and weaknesses is unrealistic.
3. Thoughts and perceptions may not be reality-based.
4. The ability to find meaning and purpose in life may be impaired.
5. Life direction and productivity may be disturbed.
6. Meeting one's own needs may be problematic.
7. Excessive reliance or preoccupation on the thoughts, opinions, and actions of self or others may be present.

C. Adaptations to stress

1. The individual's sense of self-control may be affected.
2. Perception of the environment may be distorted.
3. Coping mechanisms may not exist or may be ineffective.

D. Interpersonal relationships

1. Interpersonal relationships may be minimally existent or may be negatively affected.
2. The ability to enjoy sustained intimacy in relationships is impaired.

V. Coping and Defense Mechanisms

A. Coping mechanisms

1. Coping involves any effort to decrease anxiety.
2. Coping mechanisms can be constructive or destructive, task or problem oriented in relation to direct problem solving, cognitively oriented in an attempt to neutralize the meaning of the problem, or defense or emotion oriented, thus regulating the response to protect oneself.

B. Defense mechanisms

1. As anxiety increases, the individual copes by using defense mechanisms.
2. A defense mechanism is a coping mechanism used in an effort to protect the individual from feelings of anxiety; as anxiety increases and becomes overwhelming, the individual copes by using defense mechanisms to protect the ego and decrease anxiety (Box 63-2).

Coping mechanisms and defense mechanisms are used by the client to decrease anxiety.

C. Interventions

1. Assist the client to identify the source of anxiety and to explore methods to reduce anxiety.
2. Assess the client's use of defense mechanisms.

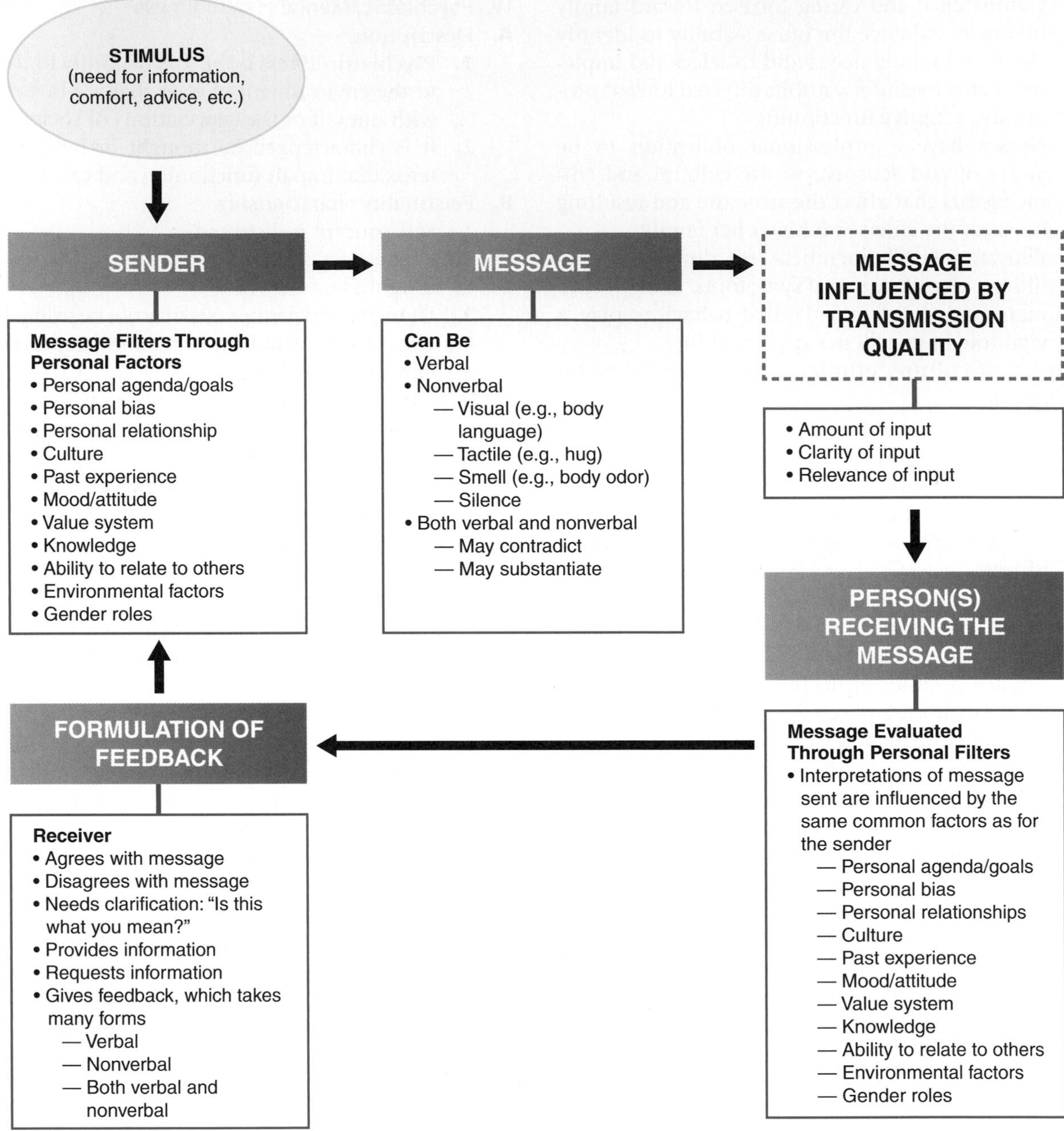

FIGURE 63-1 Operational definition of communication. (From Varcarolis E, Carson V, Shoemaker N: *Foundations of psychiatric mental health nursing*, ed 6, St. Louis, 2010, Saunders.)

3. Facilitate the appropriate use of defense mechanisms.
4. Determine whether the defense mechanisms used by the client are effective for him or her or create additional distress.
5. Avoid criticizing the client's behavior and use of defense mechanisms.

VI. *Diagnostic and Statistical Manual of Mental Health Disorders*

A. The *Diagnostic and Statistical Manual of Mental Health Disorders*, from the American Psychiatric Association, provides guidelines for health care personnel for identifying and categorizing mental illness.

B. The manual is a system used in clinical, research, and educational settings, in which diagnostic criteria are included for each mental health disorder.

C. The manual addresses culturally diverse populations and illness that may be associated with a particular culture.

D. The guidelines in the manual assist the health care team to plan and evaluate the treatment plan.

E. Dual diagnosis: Refers to the client who has both a mental health disorder and a substance-related disorder; also known as comorbidity or co-occurring disorders.

F. See American Psychiatric Association for updates: http://www.dsm5.org/Pages/Default.aspx

BOX 63-1 Therapeutic and Nontherapeutic Communication Techniques

Therapeutic Techniques

Clarifying and validating
Encouraging formulation of a plan of action
Focusing and refocusing
Giving information and presenting reality
Listening
Maintaining neutral responses
Maintaining silence
Providing acknowledgment and feedback
Providing nonverbal encouragement
Reflecting
Restating
Sharing perceptions
Summarizing
Using broad openings and open-ended questions

Nontherapeutic Techniques

Asking the client, "Why?"
Being defensive or challenging the client
Changing the subject
Giving advice or approval or disapproval
Making stereotypical comments
Making value judgments
Placing the client's feelings on hold
Providing false reassurance

VII. Types of Mental Health Admissions and Discharges

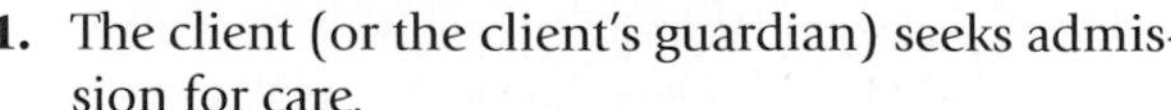

A. Voluntary admission
  1. The client (or the client's guardian) seeks admission for care.
  2. The voluntary client is free to sign out of the hospital with health care provider (HCP) notification and prescription.
  3. Detaining a voluntary client against his or her will is termed *false imprisonment.*
  4. Civil rights are retained fully by the client (Box 63-3).

B. Right to confidentiality

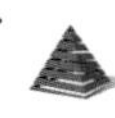

  1. A client has a right to confidentiality regarding his or her medical information. The Health Insurance Portability and Accountability Act (HIPAA) of 1996 ensures client confidentiality with regard to release and electronic transmission of data.
  2. Information sometimes must be released in life-threatening situations without the client's consent.
  3. In the event of a specific threat against an identified individual, the health care professional has a legal obligation to warn intended victim(s) of a client's threats of harm.

⚠ Except in an emergency situation, client information can be released only with the client's informed consent, which specifies the information that can be released and the time frame for which the release is valid.

BOX 63-2 Types of Defense Mechanisms

Compensation: Putting forth extra effort to achieve in areas where one has a real or imagined deficiency
Conversion: The expression of emotional conflicts through physical symptoms
Denial: Disowning consciously intolerable thoughts and impulses
Displacement: Feelings about one person are directed to another who is less threatening, thereby satisfying an impulse with a substitute object
Dissociation: The blocking off of an anxiety-provoking event or period of time from the conscious mind
Fantasy: Gratification by imaginary achievements and wishful thinking
Fixation: Never advancing to the next level of emotional development and organization; the persistence in later life of interests and behavior patterns appropriate to an earlier age
Identification: The unconscious attempt to change oneself to resemble an admired person
Insulation: Withdrawing into passivity and becoming inaccessible to avoid further threatening situations
Intellectualization: Excessive reasoning to avoid feelings; the thinking is disconnected from feelings, and situations are dealt with at a cognitive level
Introjection: A type of identification in which the individual incorporates the traits or values of another into himself or herself
Isolation: Response in which a person blocks feelings associated with an unpleasant experience
Projection: Transferring one's internal feelings, thoughts, and unacceptable ideas and traits to someone else
Rationalization: An attempt to make unacceptable feelings and behaviors acceptable by justifying the behavior
Reaction formation: Developing conscious attitudes and behaviors and acting out behaviors opposite to what one really feels
Regression: Returning to an earlier developmental stage to express an impulse to deal with anxiety
Repression: An unconscious process in which the client blocks undesirable and unacceptable thoughts from conscious expression
Sublimation: Replacement of an unacceptable need, attitude, or emotion with one more socially acceptable
Substitution: The replacement of a valued unacceptable object with an object that is more acceptable to the ego
Suppression: The conscious, deliberate forgetting of unacceptable or painful thoughts, ideas, and feelings
Symbolization: The conscious use of an idea or object to represent another actual event or object; many times the meaning is not clear because the symbol may be representative of something unconscious
Undoing: Engaging in behavior that is considered to be opposite of a previous unacceptable behavior, thought, or feeling

BOX 63-3 Client Rights

Right to accessible health care
Right to coordination and continuity of health care
Right to courteous and individualized health care
Right to information about the qualifications, names, and titles of personnel delivering care
Right to refuse observation by those not directly involved in care
Right to privacy and confidentiality
Right to informed consent
Right to treatment and to refuse treatment
Right to treatment in the least restrictive setting
Right not to be subjected to unnecessary restraints
Right to habeas corpus; may request a hearing at any time to be released from the hospital
Right to information about diagnosis, prognosis, and treatment
Right to information on the charges of service
Right to communicate with people outside the hospital through written correspondence, telephone, and personal visits
Right to keep clothing and personal effects
Right to be employed
Right to religious freedom
Right to execute wills
Right to retain licenses, privileges, or permits established by the law, such as a driver's or professional license

From Stuart G: *Principles and practice of psychiatric nursing*, ed 9, St. Louis, 2009, Mosby.

C. Involuntary admission
  1. Involuntary admission may be necessary when a person is mentally ill, is a danger to self or others, or is in need of psychiatric treatment or physical care.
  2. Involuntary admission occurs when a client is admitted or detained involuntarily for mental health treatment because of actual or imminent danger to self or others.
  3. The client who is admitted involuntarily retains his or her right for informed consent.
  4. The client retains the right to refuse treatments, including medications, unless a separate and specific treatment order is obtained from the court.
  5. The client loses the right to refuse treatment when the client poses an immediate danger to self or others, requiring immediate action by the health care team.
  6. An order from a judge is required for involuntary admissions, except in the case of an emergency, which allows time to obtain the necessary order from a judge. In the case of all involuntary admissions, legal counsel must be provided for the client.
  7. A court hearing is held by a judge within a specified time for clients admitted involuntarily. The specific time period varies by state.
  8. In most states, the client can institute a court hearing to seek an expedient judicial discharge (a writ of habeas corpus).
  9. At the court hearing, a determination is made as to whether the client may be released from the hospital or detained for further treatment and evaluation or committed to a mental health facility for an undetermined time period.
  10. The client has the right to treatment in the least restrictive treatment environment. If treatment objectives can be achieved, for example, by court-ordered treatment to an outpatient facility as opposed to an inpatient facility, the client has the right to be treated in the outpatient setting.
  11. The client is considered legally competent unless he or she has been declared incompetent through a legal hearing separate from the involuntary commitment hearing.
  12. In the course of providing nursing care and carrying out medical prescriptions, if the nurse believes that a client lacks competency to make informed decisions, action should be initiated to determine if a legal guardian needs to be appointed by the court.

D. Release from the hospital
  1. Description
     a. A client may be released voluntarily, against medical advice, or with conditions (conditional release).
     b. The client who sought voluntary admission has the right to be released upon request. 
  2. Voluntary release
     a. In the absence of an act of self-harm or danger to others, a voluntary client should never be detained.
     b. If a voluntary client wishes to be discharged from treatment but is considered potentially dangerous to self or others, the health care provider (HCP) can prescribe the client to be detained while legal proceedings for involuntary status are sought.
     c. Some states provide for conditional release of involuntarily hospitalized clients. This enables the treating HCP to prescribe continued treatment on an outpatient basis as opposed to discharging the client to follow up on his or her own initiative.
     d. Conditional release usually involves outpatient treatment for a specified period to determine the client's compliance with medication protocol, ability to meet basic needs, and ability to reintegrate into the community.
     e. An involuntary client who is released conditionally may be reinstitutionalized while the commitment is still in effect without recommencement of formal admission procedures.

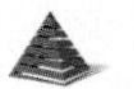

3. Discharge planning and follow-up care
   a. Discharge (unconditional release) is the termination of the client-institution relationship.
   b. This unconditional release may be prescribed by the psychiatrist, court, or administration for involuntarily admitted clients and may be requested by voluntary clients at any time.
   c. In most states, the client can institute a court hearing to seek an expedient judicial discharge (writ of habeas corpus).
   d. Discharge planning and follow-up care are important for the continued well-being of the client with a mental health disorder.
   e. After-care case managers are used to facilitate the client's adaptation back into the community and provide early referral if the treatment plan is not successful.

VIII. Milieu Therapy

A. Description
   1. The **milieu** refers to the physical and social environment in which an individual is receiving treatment.
   2. Milieu therapy uses a safe environment to meet the individual client's treatment needs.
   3. Safety is the number one priority in managing the milieu.
   4. Milieu therapy is staffed by persons educated to provide support, understanding, and individual attention. All encounters with the client have the goal of being "therapeutic."
   5. All members of the treatment team contribute to the planning and functioning of the milieu. The team generally includes the registered nurse, social worker, exercise therapist, recreational therapist, psychologist, psychiatrist, occupational therapist, clinical nurse specialist, or nurse practitioner.
   6. All treatment team members are viewed as significant and valuable to the client's successful treatment outcomes.

B. Focus of milieu therapy
   1. To use the physical and social environment to effect a positive change directed toward accomplishing the client's treatment goals
   2. To use community meetings, activity groups, social skills groups, and physical exercise programs to accomplish treatment goals
   3. To have one-to-one relationships with staff to examine client behaviors, feelings, and interactions within the context of the therapeutic group activities

The focus of milieu therapy is to empower the client through involvement in setting his or her own goals and to develop purposeful relationships with the staff to assist in meeting these goals.

IX. Interpersonal Psychotherapy

A. Description
   1. A treatment modality that uses a therapeutic relationship to modify the client's feelings, attitudes, and behaviors
   2. Therapeutic communication forms the foundation of the therapist–client relationship.

B. Focus of interpersonal psychotherapy.
   1. To establish a contract, clarify roles, and work within an agreed-upon time frame toward meeting the client's goals
   2. Focusing on the therapist-client relationship is used as a way for clients to examine other relationships in his or her life.

C. Levels of psychotherapy
   1. Supportive therapy
      a. Allows the client to express feelings, explore alternatives, and make decisions in a safe, caring environment
      b. The therapist reinforces the client's existing coping mechanisms.
   2. Re-educative therapy
      a. Involves learning new ways of perceiving and behaving
      b. The client enters into a contract that specifies desired changes of behavior.
      c. May include short-term psychotherapy, reality therapy, cognitive restructuring, behavior modification, and the development of coping skills
   3. Reconstructive therapy
      a. Emotional and cognitive restructuring of self takes place.
      b. Positive outcomes include a greater understanding of self and others, more emotional freedom, and the development of potential abilities.

X. Behavior Therapy

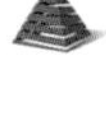

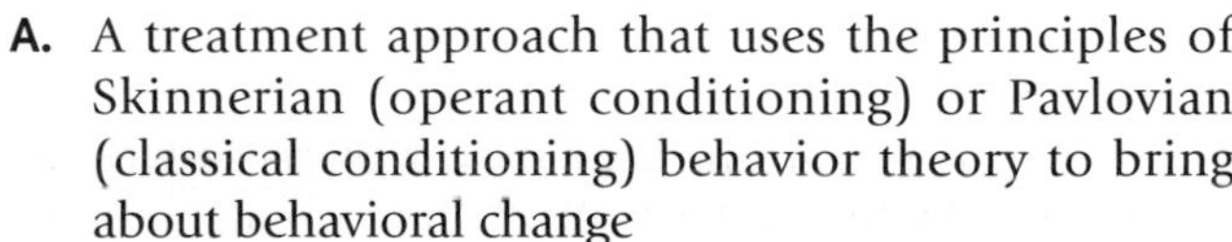

A. A treatment approach that uses the principles of Skinnerian (operant conditioning) or Pavlovian (classical conditioning) behavior theory to bring about behavioral change

B. The belief is that most behaviors are learned.

C. Operant conditioning refers to the manipulation of selected reinforcers to elicit and strengthen desired behavioral responses. The reinforcer refers to the consequence of the behavior, which is defined as anything that increases the occurrence of a behavior (Fig. 63-2).

D. In classical conditioning (respondent conditioning), the individual responds to a stimulus but is basically a passive agent (see Fig. 63-2).

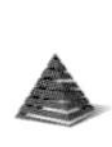

E. Desensitization is a form of behavior therapy by which exposure to increasing increments of a feared stimulus paired with increasing levels of relaxation helps to reduce the intensity of fear to a more tolerable level.

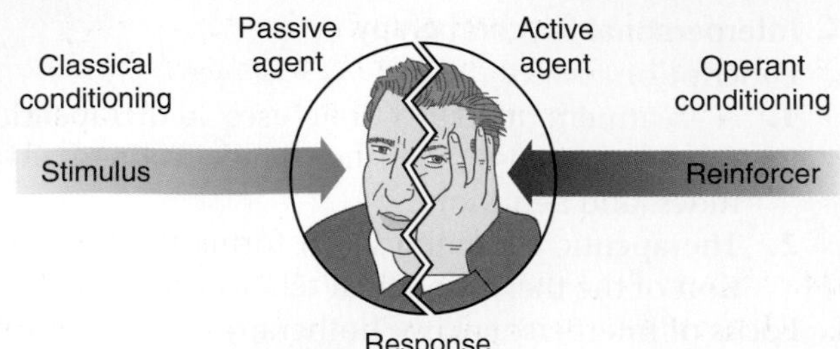

FIGURE 63-2 Respondent versus operant conditioning. (From Varcarolis E, Carson V, Shoemaker N: *Foundations of psychiatric mental health nursing*, ed 6, St. Louis, 2010, Saunders.)

F. Aversion therapy is a form of behavior therapy by which negative reinforcement is used to change behavior; for example, a stimulus *attractive* to the client is paired with an *unpleasant* event in hopes of endowing the stimulus with negative properties, thereby dissuading the behavior.

G. Modeling is behavioral therapy in which the therapist acts as a role model for specific identified behaviors so that the client learns through imitation.

XI. Cognitive Therapy

A. An active, directive, time-limited, structured approach used to treat a variety of disorders, including anxiety or depressive disorders

B. Based on the principle that how an individual feels and behaves is determined by how they think about the world and his or her place in it. The individual's cognitions are based on the attitudes or assumptions developed from previous experiences.

C. Therapeutic techniques are designed to identify, reality test, and correct distorted conceptualizations and the dysfunctional beliefs underlying these cognitions.

D. The therapist helps the individual to change the way he or she thinks, thereby reducing symptoms.

XII. Group Development and Group Therapy

A. Description: Group therapy involves a therapist and ideally five to eight members working on his or her individual goals within the context of a group, which presumably increases the opportunity for feedback and support.

B. Stages of group development
  1. Initial stage
     a. During this stage, group development involves superficial rather than open and trusting communication.
     b. Members become acquainted with one another and search for similarities among themselves.
     c. Members may be unclear about the purpose or goals of the group.
     d. Group norms, roles, and responsibilities are established.
  2. Working stage
     a. During this stage, the real work of the group is accomplished.
     b. Members are familiar with one another, the group leader, and the group roles, and they feel free to address and attempt to solve their problem.
     c. Both conflict and cooperation surface during the group's work as the members learn to work with one another.
  3. Termination stage
     a. Begins with the initial meeting.
     b. Members' feelings are explored regarding their accomplishments and the impending termination of the group.
     c. The termination stage provides an opportunity for members to learn to deal more realistically and comfortably with this normal part of human experience.

C. Self-help or support groups (Box 63-4)

Support groups are based on the premise that individuals who have experienced a problem are able to help others who have a similar problem.

XIII. Family Therapy

A. Family therapy is a specific intervention mode based on the premise that the member who has the presenting symptoms will signal the presence of problems in the entire family. This premise also assumes that a change in one member will bring about changes in other members.

B. The therapist works to assist family members to identify and express their thoughts and feelings; define family roles and rules; try new, more productive styles of relating; and restore strength to the family.

BOX 63-4 Examples of Self-Help or Support Groups

Adult Children of Alcoholics
Al-Anon
Alcoholics Anonymous
Bereavement groups
Cancer support groups
Co-dependents Anonymous
Gamblers Anonymous
Groups to help deal with unexpected body image changes, such as mastectomy or colostomy
Groups to help deal with caring for family members
Mental illness support groups
Narcotics Anonymous
Overeaters Anonymous
Parents without Partners
Recovery groups, such as for those who have experienced trauma
Smoking cessation groups

CRITICAL THINKING What Should You Do?

Answer: A coping mechanism involves any effort to decrease anxiety and can be constructive or destructive, task oriented, or defense oriented. The nurse should first help the client to identify the source of anxiety. Next, the nurse should explore with the client various methods to reduce anxiety, such as relaxation methods. A defense mechanism is a coping mechanism used in an effort to protect the individual from feelings of anxiety; as anxiety increases and becomes overwhelming, the individual copes by using defense mechanisms to protect the ego and decrease anxiety. The client may use a defense mechanism to protect self from anxiety. If so, the nurse should facilitate appropriate and constructive use of the defense mechanism and determine whether the defense mechanism used by the client is effective for him or her or creates additional distress. The nurse should never criticize the client's behavior or the use of defense mechanisms.

Reference(s): deWit, D. & Kumagai, C. (2013). *Medical-surgical nursing: Concepts & practice.* (2nd ed., pp. 1046, 1050). St. Louis: Saunders.

PRACTICE QUESTIONS

671. The nurse is assigned to care for a client experiencing disturbed thought processes. The nurse is told that the client believes that the food is being poisoned. Which communication technique should the nurse plan to use to encourage the client to eat?

1. Open-ended questions and silence
2. Focusing on self-disclosure regarding food preferences
3. Stating the reasons that the client may not want to eat
4. Offering opinions about the necessity of adequate nutrition

672. The nurse is assigned to care for a client admitted to the hospital after sustaining an injury from a house fire. The client attempted to save a neighbor involved in the fire, but despite the client's efforts, the neighbor died. Which action should the nurse take to enable the client to work through the meaning of the crisis?

1. Identifying the client's ability to function
2. Identifying the client's potential for self-harm
3. Inquiring about the client's feelings that may affect coping
4. Inquiring about the client's perception of the cause of the neighbor's death

673. The nurse is assisting with the data collection on a client admitted to the psychiatric unit. After review of the data obtained, the nurse should identify which as a **priority** concern?

1. The client's report of not eating or sleeping
2. The presence of bruises on the client's body
3. The client's report of self-destructive thoughts
4. The family member is disapproving of the treatment

674. Laboratory work is prescribed for a client who has been experiencing delusions. When the laboratory technician approaches the client to obtain a specimen of the client's blood, the client begins to shout, "You're all vampires. Let me out of here!" The nurse present at the time should respond by stating which?

1. "The technician will leave and come back later for your blood."
2. "What makes you think that the technician wants to hurt you?"
3. "Are you fearful and think that others may want to hurt you?"
4. "The technician is not going to hurt you but is going to help."

675. An intoxicated client is brought to the emergency department by local police. The client is told that the health care provider (HCP) will be in to see the client in about 30 minutes. The client becomes very loud and offensive and wants to be seen by the HCP immediately. The nurse assisting to care for the client should plan for which appropriate nursing intervention?

1. Watch the behavior escalate before intervening.
2. Attempt to talk with the client to de-escalate the behavior.
3. Offer to take the client to an examination room until he or she can be treated.
4. Inform the client that he or she will be asked to leave if the behavior continues.

676. A client is admitted to a psychiatric unit for treatment of a psychotic disorder. The client is at the locked exit door and is shouting, "Let me out! There's nothing wrong with me! I don't belong here!" The nurse identifies this behavior as which?

1. Denial
2. Projection
3. Regression
4. Rationalization

677. A client says to the nurse, "I'm going to die, and I wish my family would stop hoping for a 'cure'! I get so angry when they carry on like this! After all, I'm the one who's dying." Which therapeutic response should the nurse make to the client?

1. "Have you shared your feelings with your family?"
2. "I think we should talk more about your anger with your family."

3. "You're feeling angry that your family continues to hope for you to be 'cured'?"
4. "Well, it sounds like you're being pretty pessimistic. After all, years ago people died of pneumonia."

678. The nurse in a psychiatric unit is assigned to care for a client admitted to the unit 2 days ago. On review of the client's record, the nurse notes that the admission was a voluntary admission. Based on this type of admission, the nurse should expect which?
1. The client will be angry and will refuse care.
2. The client will participate in the treatment plan.
3. The client will be very resistant to treatment measures.
4. The client's family will be very resistant to treatment measures.

679. The nurse enters a client's room, and the client immediately demands to be released from the hospital. On review of the client's record, the nurse notes that the client was admitted 2 days ago for treatment of an anxiety disorder and that the admission was a voluntary admission. The nurse reports the findings to the registered nurse (RN) and expects that the RN will take which action?
1. Call the client's family.
2. Contact the health care provider (HCP).
3. Persuade the client to stay a few more days.
4. Tell the client that discharge is not possible at this time.

680. A client is admitted to the psychiatric nursing unit. When collecting data from the client, the nurse notes that the client was admitted on an involuntary status. Based on this type of admission, the nurse expects which?
1. The client presents a harm to self.
2. The client requested the admission.
3. The client consented to the admission.
4. The client provided written application to the facility for admission.

681. Following a group therapy session, a client approaches the nurse and verbalizes a need for seclusion because of uncontrollable feelings. The nurse reports the findings to the registered nurse (RN) and expects that the RN will take which action?
1. Call the client's family.
2. Place the client in seclusion immediately.
3. Inform the client that seclusion has not been prescribed.
4. Get a written prescription from the health care provider (HCP) and obtain an informed consent.

682. The nurse is providing care to a client admitted to the hospital with a diagnosis of anxiety disorder. The nurse is talking with the client, and the client says, "I have a secret that I want to tell you. You won't tell anyone about it, will you?" Which is the appropriate nursing response?
1. "No, I won't tell anyone."
2. "I cannot promise to keep a secret."
3. "If you tell me the secret, I will tell it to your doctor."
4. "If you tell me the secret, I will need to document it in your record."

❖**683.** The nurse in the mental health unit reviews the therapeutic and nontherapeutic communication techniques with a nursing student. Which are therapeutic communication techniques? **Select all that apply.**
- ☐ 1. Restating
- ☐ 2. Listening
- ☐ 3. Asking the client, "Why?"
- ☐ 4. Maintaining neutral responses
- ☐ 5. Giving advice or approval or disapproval
- ☐ 6. Providing acknowledgment and feedback

684. The nurse is preparing a client for the termination phase of the nurse-client relationship. Which task should the nurse appropriately plan for this phase?
1. Plan short-term goals.
2. Identify expected outcomes.
3. Assist in making appropriate referrals.
4. Assist in developing realistic solutions.

685. The psychiatric nurse is greeted by a neighbor in a local grocery store. The neighbor says to the nurse, "How is Carol doing? She is my best friend and is seen at your clinic every week." Which is the appropriate nursing response?
1. "I cannot discuss any client situation with you."
2. "I'm not supposed to discuss this, but since you are my neighbor, I can tell you that she is doing great!"
3. "You may want to know about Carol, so you need to ask her yourself so you can get the story firsthand."
4. "I'm not supposed to discuss this, but since you are my neighbor, I can tell you that she really has some problems!"

ANSWERS

671. 1

Rationale: Open-ended questions and silence are strategies used to encourage clients to discuss their problem. Options 3 and 4 do not encourage the client to express feelings. The nurse should not offer opinions and should not state the reasons but should encourage the client to identify the reasons for the behavior. Option 2 is not a client-centered intervention.

Test-Taking Strategy: Focus on the **subject**, communication techniques. Eliminate options 3 and 4 first because they do not support client expression of feelings. Eliminate option 2 next because it is not a client-centered intervention. Focusing on the client's feelings will direct you to option 1. **Review:** **therapeutic communication techniques**.

Level of Cognitive Ability: Applying

Client Needs: Psychosocial Integrity

Integrated Process: Caring

Content Area: Mental Health

Priority Concepts: Communication, Psychosis

Reference(s): Varcarolis (2013), pp. 120–123.

672. 3

Rationale: The client must first deal with feelings and negative responses before the client is able to work through the meaning of the crisis. Option 3 pertains directly to the client's feelings. Options 1, 2, and 4 do not directly address the client's feelings.

Test-Taking Strategy: Focus on the **subject**, adjustment to a crisis. Focusing on the feelings of the client will direct you to the correct option. **Review:** the nurse's actions in a **crisis** situation.

Level of Cognitive Ability: Applying

Client Needs: Psychosocial Integrity

Integrated Process: Nursing Process/Implementation

Content Area: Mental Health

Priority Concepts: Cognition, Coping

Reference(s): Stuart (2013), pp. 180, 190.

673. 3

Rationale: The client's thoughts are extremely important when verbalized. Self-destructive thoughts are the highest priority. Options 1, 2, and 4 will all affect the treatment of the client but are not of greatest importance at this time.

Test-Taking Strategy: The client is the focus of the question; therefore, eliminate option 4. Focus on the **strategic word**, *priority*, and use prioritizing skills. Remember, if the client verbalizes self-destructive thoughts, it is a priority concern. **Review:** data-collection techniques related to the client experiencing self-destructive thoughts.

Level of Cognitive Ability: Analyzing

Client Needs: Psychosocial Integrity

Integrated Process: Nursing Process/Data Collection

Content Area: Mental Health

Priority Concepts: Interpersonal Violence, Safety

Reference(s): Varcarolis (2013), pp. 448–449.

674. 3

Rationale: Option 3 is the only option that recognizes the client's need. This response helps the client focus on the emotion underlying the delusion but does not argue with it. If the nurse attempts to change the client's mind, the delusion may, in fact, be even more strongly held. Options 1, 2, and 4 do not focus on the client's feelings.

Test-Taking Strategy: Use **therapeutic communication techniques** and knowledge regarding the **subject**, the dynamics of delusions and how delusions meet the client's underlying needs. This will direct you to option 3. In addition, option 3 focuses on the client's feelings. **Review: therapeutic communication techniques.**

Level of Cognitive Ability: Applying

Client Needs: Psychosocial Integrity

Integrated Process: Communication and Documentation

Content Area: Mental Health

Priority Concepts: Communication, Psychosis

Reference(s): Varcarolis (2013), pp. 120–122, 321.

675. 3

Rationale: Safety of the client, other clients, and staff is of prime concern. Option 3 is in effect an isolation technique that allows for separation from others and provides a less stimulating environment where the client can maintain dignity. When dealing with an impaired individual, trying to talk may be out of the question. Waiting to intervene could cause the client to become even more agitated and a threat to others. Option 4 would only further aggravate an already agitated individual.

Test-Taking Strategy: Focus on the **subject** of the question, dealing with a loud and offensive client. Noting that the client is intoxicated will assist in directing you to option 3. Option 3 most directly addresses the situation and the behavior and feelings of the client. **Review:** nursing interventions for a client who is experiencing **agitation**.

Level of Cognitive Ability: Applying

Client Needs: Psychosocial Integrity

Integrated Process: Nursing Process/Planning

Content Area: Mental Health

Priority Concepts: Addiction, Clinical Judgment

Reference(s): Varcarolis (2013), pp. 467–468.

676. 1

Rationale: Denial is refusal to admit to a painful reality and is treated as if it does not exist. In projection, a person unconsciously rejects emotionally unacceptable features and attributes them to other people, objects, or situations. In regression, the client returns to an earlier, more comforting, although less mature, way of behaving. Rationalization is justifying the unacceptable attributes about oneself.

Test-Taking Strategy: Focus on the **subject**, the use of a defense mechanism. Note the words, *"There's nothing wrong with me!"* Select the option that recognizes the client's attempt to avoid looking at the reality of the situation. **Review: defense mechanisms.**

Level of Cognitive Ability: Understanding

Client Needs: Psychosocial Integrity

Integrated Process: Nursing Process/Data Collection

Content Area: Mental Health

Priority Concepts: Cognition, Psychosis

Reference(s): Varcarolis (2013), pp. 172–173.

677. 3

Rationale: Reflection is the therapeutic communication technique that redirects the client's feelings back to validate what

the client is saying. In option 2, the nurse attempts to use focusing, but the attempt to discuss central issues is premature. In option 4, the nurse makes a judgment and is nontherapeutic in the one-on-one relationship. In option 1, the nurse is attempting to assess the client's ability to openly discuss feelings with family members. Although this may be appropriate, the timing is somewhat premature and closes off facilitation of the client's feelings.
Test-Taking Strategy: Use **therapeutic communication techniques**. Note that option 3 uses the therapeutic technique of reflection and focuses on the client's feelings. Options 1, 2, and 4 are nontherapeutic at this time. **Review: therapeutic communication techniques.**
Level of Cognitive Ability: Applying
Client Needs: Psychosocial Integrity
Integrated Process: Communication and Documentation
Content Area: Mental Health
Priority Concepts: Cognition, Coping
Reference(s): Varcarolis (2013), pp. 122–124.

678. 2
Rationale: Generally, voluntary admission is sought by the client or client's guardian. If the client seeks voluntary admission, the most likely expectation is that the client will participate in the treatment program. Options 1 and 3 are not likely for a client seeking voluntary admission. Option 4 is not centered on the individual client.
Test-Taking Strategy: Note the **subject**, voluntary admission. This will direct you to option 2. In addition, note that options 1, 3, and 4 are **comparable or alike**. **Review:** the various types of **hospital admissions.**
Level of Cognitive Ability: Understanding
Client Needs: Psychosocial Integrity
Integrated Process: Nursing Process/Planning
Content Area: Mental Health
Priority Concepts: Adherence, Clinical Judgment
Reference(s): Varcarolis (2013), p. 81.

679. 2
Rationale: Generally, voluntary admission is sought by the client or client's guardian. Voluntary clients have the right to demand and obtain release. The best nursing action is to contact the HCP. Option 1 violates client confidentiality. Option 3 is not therapeutic or appropriate. Option 4 does not apply to a voluntary admission status.
Test-Taking Strategy: Focus on the **subject**, voluntary admission. Noting the type of hospital admission will assist in eliminating option 4. It is inappropriate to "persuade" a client to stay in the hospital. Option 1 should be eliminated simply based on the issues of client rights and confidentiality. **Review:** the various types of **hospital admission and discharge.**
Level of Cognitive Ability: Applying
Client Needs: Safe and Effective Care Environment
Integrated Process: Nursing Process/Implementation
Content Area: Mental Health
Priority Concepts: Anxiety, Clinical Judgment
Reference(s): Varcarolis (2013), p. 81.

680. 1
Rationale: Involuntary admission is made without the client's consent. Involuntary admission is necessary when a person is a danger to self or others or is in need of psychiatric treatment or physical care. Options 2, 3, and 4 describe the process of voluntary admission.
Test-Taking Strategy: Note the **subject**, involuntary status. This should direct you to the correct option. Also, note that options 2, 3, and 4 are **comparable or alike**. **Review:** process of **involuntary admission.**
Level of Cognitive Ability: Understanding
Client Needs: Psychosocial Integrity
Integrated Process: Nursing Process/Planning
Content Area: Mental Health
Priority Concepts: Interpersonal Violence, Safety
Reference(s): Varcarolis (2013), pp. 81–82.

681. 4
Rationale: A client may request to be secluded or restrained. Federal laws require the consent of the client unless an emergency situation exists in which an immediate risk to the client or others can be documented. The use of seclusion and restraint is permitted only on the written prescription of the health care provider (HCP), which must be reviewed and renewed every 24 hours, depending on state law requirements. It must also specify the type of restraint to be used.
Test-Taking Strategy: Focus on the **subject**, procedures for seclusion. There is no reason to call the family at this time; therefore, eliminate option 1. Knowing that a HCP's written prescription is necessary in this situation will assist in eliminating option 2. Option 3 is not the best choice because this information, if given to a client experiencing uncontrollable feelings, may cause escalation of the feelings. **Review:** the procedures for **seclusion.**
Level of Cognitive Ability: Applying
Client Needs: Safe and Effective Care Environment
Integrated Process: Nursing Process/Implementation
Content Area: Mental Health
Priority Concepts: Health Care Law, Interpersonal Violence
Reference(s): Varcarolis (2013), pp. 84–85.

682. 2
Rationale: The nurse should never promise to keep a secret. Secrets are appropriate in a social relationship but not in a therapeutic one. The nurse needs to be honest with the client and tell the client that a promise cannot be made to keep the secret.
Test-Taking Strategy: Use **therapeutic communication techniques** and think about safety. Option 1 can be eliminated because it is inappropriate. Also, options 3 and 4 are not only inappropriate but are threatening to an extent and may even block further communication. **Review:** the principles related to a **therapeutic nurse-client relationship.**
Level of Cognitive Ability: Applying
Client Needs: Psychosocial Integrity
Integrated Process: Communication and Documentation
Content Area: Mental Health
Priority Concepts: Clinical Judgment, Safety
Reference(s): Varcarolis (2013), p. 142.

❖**683. 1, 2, 4, 6**
Rationale: Some of the therapeutic communication techniques include listening, maintaining silence, maintaining neutral responses, using broad openings and open-ended questions, focusing and refocusing, restating, clarifying and

validating, sharing perceptions, reflecting, providing acknowledgment and feedback, giving information and presenting reality, encouraging formulation of a plan of action, providing nonverbal encouragement, and summarizing. Asking why, giving advice, and approving or disapproving are nontherapeutic.
Test-Taking Strategy: Use therapeutic communication techniques. This will assist you in selecting the correct answers. **Review: therapeutic and nontherapeutic techniques.**
Level of Cognitive Ability: Applying
Client Needs: Psychosocial Integrity
Integrated Process: Nursing Process/Implementation
Content Area: Mental Health
Priority Concepts: Caregiving, Communication
Reference(s): Varcarolis (2013), pp. 120, 123, 127–129.

684. 3
Rationale: Tasks of the termination phase include evaluating client performance, evaluating achievement of expected outcomes, evaluating future needs, making appropriate referrals, and dealing with the common behaviors associated with termination. Options 1, 2, and 4 identify the tasks of the working phase of the relationship.
Test-Taking Strategy: Focus on the subject, the tasks of the termination phase. Thinking about the definition of *termination* should direct you to the correct option. **Review: phases of the nurse-client relationship.**
Level of Cognitive Ability: Applying
Client Needs: Psychosocial Integrity
Integrated Process: Nursing Process/Planning
Content Area: Mental Health
Priority Concepts: Communication, Professionalism
Reference(s): Varcarolis (2013), pp. 144–145.

685. 1
Rationale: The nurse is required to maintain confidentiality regarding clients and their care. Confidentiality is basic to the therapeutic relationship and is a client's right. Option 3 is correct in a sense, but it is a rather blunt statement. Both options 2 and 4 identify statements that do not maintain client confidentiality.
Test-Taking Strategy: Focus on the subject of the question, maintaining confidentiality. This should assist in eliminating options 2 and 4. From the remaining options, select option 1 over option 3 because it is most direct and correct. Option 3 is a rather blunt and somewhat rude statement. **Review: confidentiality issues.**
Level of Cognitive Ability: Applying
Client Needs: Safe and Effective Care Environment
Integrated Process: Communication and Documentation
Content Area: Mental Health
Priority Concepts: Ethics, Professionalism
Reference(s): Varcarolis (2013), pp. 85, 144.

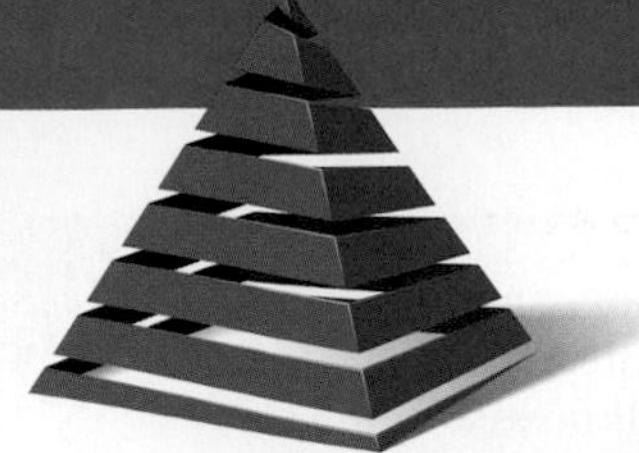

CHAPTER 64

Mental Health Disorders

CRITICAL THINKING What Should You Do?

A client is experiencing visual hallucinations. What should the nurse do?

Answer located on p. 920.

I. Anxiety

A. Description
1. Anxiety is a normal response to stress.
2. A subjective experience that includes feelings of apprehension, uneasiness, uncertainty, or dread
3. Occurs as a result of threats that may be misperceived or misinterpreted or as a result of a threat to identity or self-esteem
4. May result when values are threatened or preceding new experiences

B. Types of anxiety
1. Normal: A healthy type of anxiety
2. Acute: Precipitated by imminent loss or change that threatens one's sense of security
3. Chronic: Anxiety that persists as a characteristic response to daily activities

C. Levels of anxiety
1. Mild
   a. Associated with the tension of everyday life
   b. The individual is alert.
   c. The perceptual field is increased.
   d. Mild anxiety can be motivating, produce growth, enhance creativity, and increase learning.
2. Moderate
   a. The focus is on immediate concerns.
   b. Moderate anxiety narrows the perceptual field.
   c. Selective inattentiveness occurs.
   d. Learning and problem solving still occur.
3. Severe
   a. Severe anxiety is a feeling that something bad is about to happen.
   b. A significant narrowing in the perceptual field occurs.
   c. Focus is on minute or scattered details.
   d. All behavior is directed at relieving the anxiety.
   e. Learning and problem solving are not possible.
   f. The individual needs direction to focus.
4. Panic
   a. Panic is associated with dread and terror and a sense of impending doom.
   b. The personality is disorganized.
   c. The individual is unable to communicate or function effectively.
   d. Increased motor activity occurs.
   e. Loss of rational thoughts with distorted perception occurs.
   f. Inability to concentrate occurs.
   g. If prolonged, panic can lead to exhaustion and death.

D. Interventions: General nursing measures (see Priority Nursing Actions)
1. Recognize the anxiety.
2. Establish trust.
3. Protect the client.
4. Do not criticize **coping mechanisms**.
5. Do not force the client into situations that provoke anxiety.
6. Modify the environment by setting limits or limiting interaction with others.
7. Provide creative outlets.
8. Provide activities that limit the amount of time for destructive behavior.
9. Promote relaxation techniques such as breathing exercises or guided imagery.
10. Monitor vital signs and administer antianxiety medications as prescribed.

⚠ The immediate nursing action for a client with anxiety is to decrease stimuli in the environment and provide a calm and quiet environment.

E. Interventions: Mild to moderate levels
1. Help the client identify the anxiety.
2. Encourage the client to talk about feelings and concerns.
3. Help the client identify thoughts and feelings that occurred before the onset of anxiety.
4. Encourage problem solving.
5. Encourage gross motor exercise.

PRIORITY NURSING ACTIONS!

Actions to Take for a Client Experiencing Anxiety

1. Provide a calm environment, decrease environmental stimuli, and stay with the client.
2. Ask the client to identify what and how he or she feels.
3. Encourage the client to describe and discuss his or her feelings.
4. Help the client to identify the causes of the feelings if he or she is having difficulty doing so.
5. Listen to the client for expressions of helplessness and hopelessness.
6. Document the event, significant information, actions taken and follow-up actions, and the client's response.

If a client experiences anxiety, immediate actions are to provide a calm environment, decrease environmental stimuli, and stay with the client. Excess stimulation would escalate the anxiety. Next, asking the client to identify what and how he or she feels and helping the client to identify the causes of the feelings help to increase his or her awareness of the connection between behaviors and feelings. This awareness helps to decrease the anxiety. While listening to the client, the nurse observes for expressions of helplessness and hopelessness that could indicate self-harm intentions. The nurse provides follow-up care as needed based on observations and assessments. Finally, the nurse documents the event, significant information, actions taken and follow-up actions, and the client's response.

Reference(s): deWit, D. & Kumagai, C. (2013). *Medical-surgical nursing: Concepts & practice.* (2nd ed., p. 1046). St. Louis: Saunders.

F. Interventions: Severe to panic levels
- **1.** Reduce the anxiety quickly.
- **2.** Use a calm manner.
- **3.** Always remain with the client.
- **4.** Provide clear, simple statements.
- **5.** Use a low-pitched voice.
- **6.** Attend to the physical needs of the client.
- **7.** Provide gross motor activity.
- **8.** Administer antianxiety medications as prescribed.

II. Generalized Anxiety Disorder

A. Description
- **1.** Generalized anxiety disorder is an unrealistic anxiety about everyday worries that persists over time and is not associated with another psychiatric or medical disorder.
- **2.** Physical symptoms occur.

B. Data collection
- **1.** Restlessness and inability to relax
- **2.** Episodes of trembling and shakiness
- **3.** Chronic muscular tension
- **4.** Dizziness
- **5.** Inability to concentrate
- **6.** Chronic fatigue and sleep problems
- **7.** Inability to recognize the connection between the anxiety and physical symptoms
- **8.** Client is focused on the physical discomfort.

C. Panic disorder
- **1.** Description
  - **a.** Panic disorder produces a sudden onset of feelings of intense apprehension and dread.
  - **b.** The cause usually cannot be identified.
  - **c.** Severe, recurrent, intermittent anxiety attacks lasting 5 to 30 minutes occur.
- **2.** Data collection
  - **a.** Choking sensation
  - **b.** Labored breathing
  - **c.** Pounding heart
  - **d.** Chest pain
  - **e.** Dizziness
  - **f.** Nausea
  - **g.** Blurred vision
  - **h.** Numbness or tingling of the extremities
  - **i.** A sense of unreality and helplessness
  - **j.** A fear of being trapped
  - **k.** A fear of dying
- **3.** Interventions
  - **a.** Remain with the client.
  - **b.** Attend to the physical symptoms.
  - **c.** Assist the client to identify the thoughts that aroused the anxiety and identify the basis for these thoughts.
  - **d.** Assist the client to change the unrealistic thoughts to more realistic thoughts.
  - **e.** Use cognitive restructuring to replace distorted thinking.
  - **f.** Administer antianxiety medications if prescribed.

III. Posttraumatic Stress Disorder

A. Description: After experiencing a psychologically traumatic event, the individual is prone to reexperience the event and have recurrent and intrusive dreams or flashbacks.

B. Stressors
- **1.** Natural disaster
- **2.** Terrorist attack
- **3.** Combat experiences
- **4.** Accidents
- **5.** Rape
- **6.** Crime or violence
- **7.** Sexual, physical, or emotional **abuse**
- **8.** Re-experiencing the event as flashbacks

C. Data collection
- **1.** Emotional numbness
- **2.** Detachment

3. Depression
4. Anxiety
5. Sleep disturbances and nightmares
6. Flashbacks of the event
7. Hypervigilance
8. Guilt about surviving the event
9. Poor concentration and avoidance of activities that trigger the memory of the event

D. Interventions (Box 64-1)

IV. Phobias

A. Description
1. An irrational fear of an object or situation that persists, although the person may recognize it as unreasonable
2. Associated with panic level anxiety if the object, situation, or activity cannot be avoided
3. **Defense mechanisms** commonly used include repression and displacement.

B. Types (Box 64-2)

C. Interventions

BOX 64-1 Interventions for Posttraumatic Stress Disorder

Be nonjudgmental and supportive.
Assure the client that his or her feelings and behaviors are normal reactions.
Assist the client to recognize the association between his or her feelings and behaviors and the trauma experience.
Encourage the client to express his or her feelings. Provide individual therapy that addresses loss of control or anger issues.
Assist the client to develop adaptive coping mechanisms and use relaxation techniques.
Encourage the use of support groups.
Facilitate a progressive review of the trauma experience.
Encourage the client to establish and re-establish relationships.
Inform the client that hypnotherapy or systematic desensitization may be used as a form of treatment.

BOX 64-2 Types of Phobias

Acrophobia: Fear of heights
Agoraphobia: Fear of open spaces
Astraphobia: Fear of electrical storms
Claustrophobia: Fear of closed spaces
Hematophobia: Fear of blood
Hydrophobia: Fear of water
Monophobia: Fear of being alone
Mysophobia: Fear of dirt or germs
Nyctophobia: Fear of darkness
Pyrophobia: Fear of fires
Social phobia: Fear of situations in which one might be embarrassed or criticized and the fear of making a fool of oneself
Xenophobia: Fear of strangers
Zoophobia: Fear of animals

1. Identify the basis of the anxiety.
2. Allow the client to verbalize feelings about the anxiety-producing object or situation. Frequently talking about the feared object is the first step in the desensitization process.
3. Teach relaxation techniques such as breathing exercises, muscle relaxation exercises, and visualization of pleasant situations.
4. Promote desensitization by gradually introducing the individual to the feared object or situation in small doses.

⚠ Always stay with the client experiencing anxiety to promote safety and security. Never force the client to have contact with the phobic object or situation.

V. Obsessive-Compulsive Disorder

A. Obsessive-compulsive disorder includes disorders such as hoarding disorder and excoriation (skin-picking) disorder.

B. Obsessions: Preoccupation with persistent intrusive thoughts and ideas

C. Compulsion
1. A compulsion is the performance of rituals or repetitive behaviors designed to prevent some event, divert unacceptable thoughts, and decrease anxiety.
2. Obsessions and compulsions often occur together and can disrupt normal daily activities.
3. Anxiety occurs when one resists obsessions or compulsions and from being powerless to resist the thoughts or rituals.
4. Obsessive thoughts can involve issues of violence, aggression, sexual behavior, orderliness, or religion and can uncontrollably interrupt conscious thoughts and the ability to function.

D. Compulsive behavior patterns (behaviors or rituals)
1. Compulsive behavior patterns decrease the anxiety.
2. The patterns are associated with the obsessive thoughts.
3. The patterns neutralize the thought.
4. During stressful times, the ritualistic behavior increases.
5. Defense mechanisms include repression, displacement, and undoing.

E. Interventions (Box 64-3)

VI. Somatic Symptom Disorders

A. Description
1. Somatic symptom disorders are characterized by persistent worry or complaints regarding physical illness without supporting physical findings.
2. The client focuses on the physical signs and symptoms and is unable to control the signs and symptoms.
3. The physical signs and symptoms increase with psychosocial stressors.

BOX 64-3 Interventions for Obsessive-Compulsive Disorder

Ensure that basic needs (food, rest, grooming) are met.
Identify the situations that precipitate the compulsive behavior; encourage the client to verbalize concerns and feelings.
Be empathetic toward the client, and be aware of his or her need to perform the compulsive behavior.
Do not interrupt the compulsive behaviors unless they jeopardize the safety of the client or others (provide for client safety related to the behavior).
Allow time for the client to perform the compulsive behavior, but set limits on behaviors that may interfere with the client's physical well-being to protect the client from physical harm.
Implement a schedule for the client that distracts from the behaviors (structure simple activities, games, or tasks for the client).
Establish a written contract that will assist the client to decrease the frequency of compulsive behaviors gradually.
Recognize and reinforce positive nonritualistic behaviors.

4. The anxiety is redirected into a somatic concern.
5. The client may unconsciously use somatization for secondary gains such as increased attention and decreased responsibilities.

B. Conversion disorder
1. Description
    a. A physical symptom or a deficit suggesting loss or altered body function related to psychological conflict or a neurological disorder.
    b. Conversion disorder is an expression of a psychological conflict or need.
    c. The most common conversion symptoms are blindness, deafness, paralysis, and the inability to talk.
    d. Conversion disorder has no organic cause.
    e. Symptoms are beyond the conscious control of the client and are directly related to conflict.
    f. The development of physical symptoms reduces anxiety.
2. Data collection
    a. "La belle indifference": Unconcerned with symptoms
    b. Physical limitation or disability
    c. Feelings of guilt, anxiety, or frustration
    d. Low self-esteem and feelings of inadequacy
    e. Unexpressed anger or conflict
    f. Secondary gain

C. Interventions
1. Obtain a history and check for physical problems.
2. Explore with the client the needs being met by the physical symptoms.
3. Assist the client to identify alternative ways of meeting needs.
4. Assist the client to relate feelings and conflicts to the physical symptoms.
5. Convey understanding that the physical symptoms are real to the client.
6. Assure the client that physical illness has been ruled out.
7. Explore the source of anxiety and stimulate verbalization of anxiety.
8. Encourage the use of relaxation techniques as the anxiety increases.
9. Use a pain assessment scale if the client complains of pain, and implement pain-reduction measures as required.
10. Report and assess any new physical complaint.
11. Encourage diversional activities.
12. Provide positive feedback.
13. Assist the client in recognizing his or her own feelings and emotions.
14. Administer antianxiety medications if prescribed.

⚠ For a client with a somatic symptom disorder, allow a specific time period for the client to discuss physical complaints because the client will feel less threatened if this behavior is limited rather than stopped completely. However, avoid responding with positive reinforcement about the physical complaints.

VII. Dissociative Disorder

A. Description
1. Dissociative disorder is a disruption in integrative functions of memory, consciousness, or identity.
2. Dissociative disorder is associated with exposure to an extremely traumatic event.

B. Dissociative identity disorder (multiple personality)
1. Description
    a. Two or more fully developed distinct and unique personalities exist within the person.
    b. The host is the primary personality, and the other personalities are referred to as *alters*.
    c. Alter personalities may take full control of the client, one at a time, and may or may not be aware of one another.
    d. The alters may be aware of the host, but the host is not usually aware of the alter(s).
2. Data collection
    a. The client may have an inability to recall important information (unrelated to ordinary forgetfulness).
    b. Transition from one personality to the other is related to stress or a traumatic event and is sudden.
    c. Dissociation is used as a method of distancing and defending one's self from anxiety and traumatizing experiences.

C. Dissociative amnesia
1. Description
    a. The inability to remember important personal information because it provokes anxiety.

b. Memory impairment may range from partial to almost complete.
c. The client may assume a new identity in a new environment, may drift from place to place, develop few relationships, then return home unable to remember the amnesia.
2. Data collection
a. Localized: The client blocks out all memories about a specified period.
b. Selective: The client recalls some but not all memories about a specified period.
c. Generalized: The client has a loss of all memory about past life.

D. Depersonalization/derealization disorder
1. Description: An altered self-perception in which one's own reality is temporarily lost or changed
2. Data collection
a. Feelings of detachment
b. Intact reality testing

E. Interventions
1. Develop a trusting relationship with the client.
2. Encourage verbal expression of painful experiences, anxieties, and concerns.
3. Explore methods of coping.
4. Identify sources of conflict.
5. Focus on the client's strengths and skills.
6. Orient the client.
7. Provide nondemanding, simple routines.
8. Allow the client to progress at his or her own pace.
9. Implement stress-reduction techniques.
10. Plan for individual, group, and/or family psychotherapy to integrate dissociated aspects of personality or memory and expand self-awareness.

VIII. Mood Disorders

A. Bipolar disorder
1. Description (Box 64-4)
a. Bipolar disorder is characterized by episodes of mania and depression with periods of normal mood and activity in between.
b. The medication of choice has traditionally been lithium carbonate, which can be toxic and therefore requires the regular monitoring of serum lithium levels.
c. Other medications such as divalproex (Valproate), olanzapine (Zyprexa), and carbamazepine (Tegretol) may also be prescribed to reduce the symptoms of acute bipolar manic episodes.
2. Interventions for mania (Box 64-5)
a. Remove hazardous objects from the environment (this should be done for all clients).
b. Monitor the client closely for fatigue.
c. Monitor the client's sleep patterns; use comfort measures to promote sleep.
d. Provide frequent rest periods.
e. Provide a private room if possible.

BOX 64-4 Data Collection: Bipolar Disorder

Mania

Becomes angry quickly
Delusional self-confidence
Distracted by environmental stimuli
Extroverted personality
Flight of ideas
Grandiose and persecutory delusions
High and unstable affect
Inability to eat or sleep because of involvement in more important things
Inability to sleep yet still active
Inappropriate affect
Inappropriate dress
Initiation of activity
Pressured speech
Restlessness
Sexually promiscuous
Significant decrease in appetite
Unlimited energy
Urgent motor activity

Depression

Increased or decreased appetite
Decrease in activities of daily living
Decreased emotion and physical activity
Easily fatigued
Inability to make decisions
Poor concentration
Internalizing hostility
Introverted personality
Social isolation and withdrawn from groups
Lack of energy
Lack of initiative
Lack of self-confidence and low self-esteem
Lack of sexual interest
Psychomotor retardation
Suicidal thinking

f. Encourage the client to ventilate feelings.
g. Use calm, slow interactions.
h. Help the client focus on one topic during the conversation.
i. Ignore or distract the client from grandiose thinking; present reality to the client.
j. Do not argue with the client.
k. Limit group activities and assess the client's tolerance level; solitary activities may be necessary.
l. Provide high-calorie finger foods and fluids.
m. Supervise the client's choice of clothing.
n. Reduce environmental stimuli.
o. Set limits on inappropriate behaviors.
p. Provide physical activities and outlets for tension.
q. Avoid competitive games.
r. Provide gross motor activities such as walking.
s. Provide structured activities or one-to-one activities with the nurse.

BOX 64-5 Dealing with Inappropriate Behaviors Associated with Bipolar Disorder

Aggressive Behavior

Assist the client in identifying feelings of frustration and aggression.
Encourage the client to talk out instead of acting out feelings of frustration.
Assist the client in identifying precipitating events or situations that lead to aggressive behavior.
Describe the consequences of the behavior on self and others.
Assist in identifying previous coping mechanisms.
Assist the client in problem-solving techniques to cope with frustration or aggression.

De-escalation Techniques

Maintain safety for the client, other clients, and self.
Maintain a large personal space and use a nonaggressive posture.
Use a calm approach and communicate with a calm, clear tone of voice (be assertive, not aggressive).
Determine what the client considers to be his or her need.
Avoid verbal struggles.
Provide the client with clear options that deal with the client's behavior.
Assist the client with problem solving and decision making regarding the options.

Manipulative Behavior

Set clear, consistent, realistic, and enforceable limits, and communicate expected behaviors.
Be clear about the consequences associated with exceeding set limits, and follow through with the consequences in a nonpunitive manner if necessary.
Discuss the client's behavior in a nonjudgmental and nonthreatening manner.
Avoid power struggles with the client (avoid arguing with the client).
Assist the client in developing means of setting limits on personal behavior.

t. Provide simple and direct explanations for routine procedures.
u. Supervise the administration of medication.
3. Depression (See Section IX.)

IX. Depression

A. Description
1. Depression affects feelings, thoughts, and behaviors.
2. It can occur after a loss, including loss of self-esteem, the end of a significant relationship, the death of a loved one, or a traumatic event.
3. The loss is followed by grief and mourning; if this process does not resolve, depression results.
4. Depression may be mild, moderate, or severe.
5. Treatment includes counseling, antidepressant medication, and electroconvulsive therapy (ECT).
6. See Box 64-4 for general data collection findings.

B. Mild depression
1. Mild depression is triggered by an external event and follows the normal grief reaction.
2. Mild depression lasts less than 2 weeks.
3. Feeling sad
4. Feeling let down or disappointed
5. Mild alterations in sleep patterns
6. Feeling less alert
7. Irritability
8. Disinterested in spending time with others
9. Increased or decreased appetite
10. Increased use of alcohol or drugs

C. Moderate depression
1. Moderate depression persists over time.
2. The person experiences a sense of change and often seeks help.
3. Despondent and gloomy
4. Dejected
5. Low self-esteem
6. Helplessness and powerlessness
7. May experience intense anxiety and anger
8. Diurnal variation: The person may feel better at a certain time of the day
9. Slow thought processes and difficulty in concentrating
10. Rumination: Persistent thinking about and discussion of a particular subject
11. Negative thinking and suicidal thoughts (see Chapter 66)
12. Sleep disturbances
13. Social withdrawal
14. Anorexia, weight loss, and fatigue
15. Somatic complaints
16. Menstrual changes
17. Increased use of alcohol or drugs

D. Severe depression
1. Intense and pervasive
2. Despair and hopelessness
3. Guilt and worthlessness
4. Flat affect
5. May show agitation and pace about
6. Poor posture and unkempt appearance
7. Decreased speech
8. Self-destructive thoughts; however, the person may lack energy to act on the thought.
9. Social withdrawal
10. Poor concentration and overwhelmed by simple tasks
11. Severe psychomotor retardation
12. Anorexia and considerable weight loss
13. Constipation and urinary retention
14. Lack of sexual interest
15. Terminal insomnia
16. Diurnal variation: The person may feel better at a certain time of the day
17. Delusions and hallucinations

E. Interventions (Box 64-6)

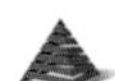

BOX 64-6 Interventions for Depressed Clients

Assess for suicidal ideation.
Provide safety from suicidal actions (be certain that there are no harmful objects in the environment).
Assist with activities of daily living.
Use gentle encouragement to participate in activities of daily living and unit therapies.
Do not push decision making or making complex choices. Make decisions that the client is not ready to make.
Monitor sleep patterns.
Monitor nutritional intake and weight.
Provide achievable activities in which the client can achieve success (focus on strengths).
Remind the client of times when he or she felt better and was successful.
Spend time with the client to convey the client's value.
Respond to anger therapeutically.

⚠ For a client at risk for self-harm, ask the client directly, "Have you thought of hurting yourself?"

X. Electroconvulsive Therapy (ECT)

A. Description
1. ECT is an effective treatment for depression (not a cure); a small amount of electrical current is delivered through electrodes attached to the temples that cause a brief seizure within the brain; outward movement is usually a slight movement of hands, feet, or a toe because premedication is given to relax the muscles. In addition, a short-acting anesthetic is given.
2. The usual course is 6 to 12 treatments given every 2 to 5 days; maintenance ECT once a month may help decrease the relapse rate for a client with recurrent depression.
3. ECT is not always effective in clients with dysthymic depression, depression and personality disorders, drug dependence, or depression secondary to situational or social difficulties.
4. At-risk clients include clients with recent myocardial infarction, brain attack (stroke), or intracranial mass lesions.

B. Uses (Box 64-7)

BOX 64-7 Electroconvulsive Therapy (ECT): Indications for Use

Antidepressant medications have no effect.
There is a need for a rapid, definitive response, such as when a client is suicidal or homicidal.
The client is in extreme agitation or stupor.
The risks of other treatments outweigh the risk of ECT.
The client has a history of poor medication response, a history of good ECT response, or both.
The client prefers ECT as a treatment.

1. Clients with severe depressive and bipolar depressive disorders, especially when psychotic symptoms are present.
2. Clients who have depression with marked psychomotor retardation and stupor
3. Manic clients whose conditions are resistant to lithium and antipsychotic medications and clients who are rapid cyclers (a client with a bipolar disorder who has many episodes of mood swings close together)
4. Clients with schizophrenia (especially catatonia), clients with schizoaffective syndromes, and psychotic clients

C. Preprocedure
1. Explain the procedure to the client.
2. Encourage the client to discuss feelings, including myths regarding ECT.
3. Teach the client and family what to expect.
4. Informed consent must be obtained when voluntary clients are being treated.
5. For involuntary clients, when informed consent cannot be obtained, permission may be obtained from the next of kin, although in some states the permission for ECT must be obtained from the court.
6. Maintain NPO status after midnight or at least 4 hours before treatment as prescribed.
7. Baseline vital signs are taken.
8. The client is requested to void.
9. Hairpins, contact lenses, and dentures are removed.
10. Administer preprocedure medication as prescribed.

D. During the procedure
1. Place a blood pressure cuff on one of the client's arms.
2. As the intravenous line is inserted, electroencephalographic and electrocardiographic electrodes are attached.
3. A pulse oximeter is placed on the client's finger.
4. Blood pressure is monitored throughout the treatment.
5. Medications administered may include a short-acting anesthetic and a muscle relaxant.
6. Throughout the procedure, 100% oxygen by mask via positive pressure is administered.
7. An airway is placed to prevent biting the tongue.
8. An electrical stimulus is administered; a brief seizure occurs.

E. Postprocedure
1. The client is transported to a recovery room with the blood pressure cuff and oximeter in place, where oxygen, suction, and other emergency equipment are available.
2. When the client is awake, talk to the client and take vital signs.
3. The client may be confused; provide frequent orientation (brief, distinct, and simple) and reassurance.

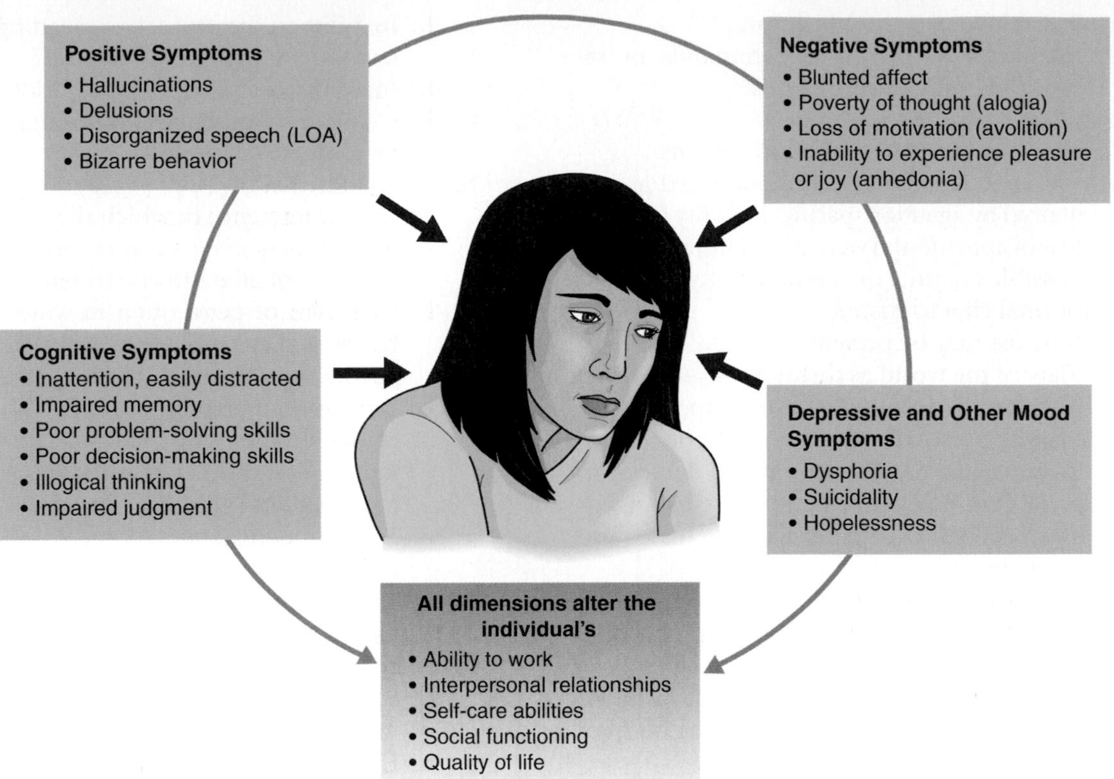

Positive Symptoms
• Hallucinations
• Delusions
• Disorganized speech (LOA)
• Bizarre behavior
Negative Symptoms
• Blunted affect
• Poverty of thought (alogia)
• Loss of motivation (avolition)
• Inability to experience pleasure or joy (anhedonia)
Cognitive Symptoms
• Inattention, easily distracted
• Impaired memory
• Poor problem-solving skills
• Poor decision-making skills
• Illogical thinking
• Impaired judgment
Depressive and Other Mood Symptoms
• Dysphoria
• Suicidality
• Hopelessness
All dimensions alter the individual's
• Ability to work
• Interpersonal relationships
• Self-care abilities
• Social functioning
• Quality of life

FIGURE 64-1 Treatment-relevant dimensions of schizophrenia. (From Varcarolis E, Carson V, Shoemaker N: *Foundations of psychiatric mental health nursing*, ed 6, St. Louis, 2010, Saunders.)

4. The client returns to the nursing unit when at least a 90% oxygen saturation level is maintained, vital signs are stable, and mental status is satisfactory.
5. Check for a gag reflex before giving the client fluids, food, or medication.

F. Potential side effects
1. Include confusion, disorientation, and short-term memory loss.
2. The client may be confused and disoriented on awakening.
3. Other side effects include headache, hypotension, muscle soreness, nausea, tachycardia.
4. Memory deficits may occur, but memory usually recovers completely, although some clients have memory loss lasting 6 months.

⚠ Monitor both a depressed client as well as a client who has recently been prescribed an antidepressant medication closely for signs of suicidal ideation. If the client presents with increased energy, monitor closely because it could mean that the client now has the energy to perform the suicide act.

XI. Schizophrenia

A. Description
1. Schizophrenia is a group of mental disorders characterized by psychotic features (hallucinations and delusions), disordered thought processes, and disrupted interpersonal relationships.
2. Disturbances in affect, mood, behavior, and thought processes occur.

B. Data collection (Fig. 64-1)
1. Physical characteristics
   a. Unkempt appearance
   b. Body image distortions
   c. May be preoccupied with somatic complaints
   d. May neglect hygiene, eating, sleeping, and elimination
2. Motor activity (Box 64-8)
   a. Catatonic posturing: Holding bizarre postures for long periods
   b. Catatonic excitement: Moving excitedly with no environmental stimuli present

BOX 64-8 Abnormal Motor Behaviors

Description

Abnormal motor behavior or activity displayed by the mentally ill client and occurring as a result of a psychiatric disorder

Types of Abnormal Motor Behaviors

Echolalia

Repeating the speech of another person

Echopraxia

Repeating the movements of another person

Waxy Flexibility

Having one's arms or legs placed in a certain position and holding that same position for hours

c. Possible total immobilization
d. Inability to respond to commands or responding only to commands
e. Waxy flexibility
f. Repetitive or stereotyped movements
g. Motor activity that may be increased as evidenced by agitation, pacing, inability to sleep, loss of appetite and weight, and impulsiveness
h. Possible inability to initiate activity (anergia)

3. Emotional characteristics
   a. Mistrust may be present.
   b. View of the world as threatening and unsafe
   c. Affect may be blunted, flat, or inappropriate.
   d. May display feelings of ambivalence, helplessness, anxiety, anger, guilt, or depression in response to hallucinations, delusions, or as a result of the grief related to losses imposed by this illness.
4. Compulsive rituals: Performed as an attempt to solve conflicting feelings by constant, repetitive activity
5. Overcompliance: Attempt to deny responsibility for any action by doing only what another instructs exactly
6. Affective disturbances
   a. Flat or incongruent affect or inappropriate affect
   b. Altered thought processes
7. Abnormal thought processes (Box 64-9)
   a. Impaired reality testing
   b. Fragmentation of thoughts
   c. Thought blocking
   d. Loose associations
   e. Echolalia
   f. Distorted perception of the environment
   g. Neologisms
   h. Magical thinking
   i. Inability to conceptualize meaning in words or thoughts
   j. Inability to organize facts logically
   k. Delusions associated with thought processes or content
8. Types of delusions (Box 64-10)
   a. Loss of reference in which the client believes that certain events, situations, or interactions are related directly to self
   b. Delusions of persecution in which the client believes that he or she is being harassed, threatened, or persecuted by some powerful force
   c. Delusions of grandeur in which the client attaches special significance to self in relation to others or the universe and has an exaggerated sense of self that has no basis in reality
   d. Somatic delusions in which the client believes that his or her body is changing or responding in an unusual way, which has no basis in reality
9. Perceptual distortions
   a. Illusions that may be brief experiences with a misinterpretation or misperception of reality
   b. Hallucinations (five senses) such as perceiving objects, sensations, or images with no basis in reality (Box 64-11)
10. Language and communication disturbances (Box 64-12)
   a. Related to disorders in thought process
   b. Inability to organize language
   c. Difficulty communicating clearly
   d. Inappropriate responses to a situation
   e. A single word or phrase that may represent the whole meaning of the conversation such that the client may feel that he or she has communicated adequately
   f. Development of a private language

BOX 64-9 Abnormal Thought Processes

Description

Abnormal thought processes displayed by the mentally ill client and occurring as a result of a psychiatric disorder

Circumstantiality

Before getting to the point or answering a question, the individual gets caught up in countless details and explanations

Confabulation

Filling a memory gap with detailed fantasy believed by the teller. The purpose of confabulation is to maintain self-esteem. This is seen in organic conditions such as Korsakoff's psychosis.

Flight of Ideas

A constant flow of speech in which the individual jumps from one topic to another in rapid succession. A connection between topics exists, although it is sometimes difficult to identify. This is seen in manic states.

Looseness of Association

Haphazard, illogical, and confused thinking and interrupted connections in thought. This is seen mostly in schizophrenic disorders.

Neologisms

Words that an individual makes up that only have meaning for the individual. This is often part of a delusional system.

Thought Blocking

A sudden cessation of a thought in the middle of a sentence; the client is unable to continue the train of thought. Often sudden new thoughts come up unrelated to the topic.

Word Salad

A mixture of words and phrases that have no meaning

BOX 64-10 Delusions

Description

A false belief held to be true even when there is evidence to the contrary

Types

Grandeur

The false belief that one is a powerful and important person

Jealousy

The false belief that one's partner or mate is being unfaithful.

Persecution

The thought that one is being singled out for harm by others

Interventions

Ask the client to describe the delusion.

Be open and honest in interactions to reduce suspiciousness.

Focus the conversation on reality-based topics rather than the delusion.

Encourage the client to express feelings and focus on the feelings that the delusions generate.

If the client obsesses on the delusion, set firm limits on the amount of time for talking about the delusion.

Do not dispute with the client or try to convince him or her that the delusions are false.

Validate if part of the delusion is real.

C. Interventions (Box 64-13)

D. Interventions: Active hallucinations

1. Monitor for hallucination cues and assess content of hallucinations.
2. Intervene with one-on-one contact.
3. Decrease stimuli or move the client to another area.
4. Avoid conveying to the client that others are also experiencing the hallucination.
5. Respond verbally to anything real that the client talks about.
6. Avoid touching the client.
7. Encourage the client to express feelings.
8. During a hallucination, attempt to engage the client's attention through a concrete activity.
9. Accept and do not joke about or judge the client's behavior.
10. Provide easy activities and a structured environment with routine activities of daily living.
11. Monitor for signs of increasing fear, anxiety, or agitation.
12. Decrease stimuli as needed.
13. Administer medications as prescribed.

BOX 64-12 Language and Communication Disturbances

Clang association: Repetition of words or phrases that are similar in sound but in no other way

Echolalia: Repetition of words or phrases heard from another person

Mutism: Absence of verbal speech

Neologism: A new word devised that has special meaning only to the client

Pressured speech: Speaking as if the words are being forced out quickly

Verbigeration: Purposeless repetition of words or phrases

Word salad: Form of speech in which words or phrases are connected meaninglessly

⚠ For a client with hallucinations, safety is the first priority. Ensure that the client does not have an auditory command telling him or her to harm self or others.

E. Interventions: Delusions

1. Interact based on reality.
2. Encourage the client to express feelings.
3. Do not dispute the client or try to convince the client that delusions are false.
4. Initially, initiate activities on a one-on-one basis.

BOX 64-11 Hallucinations

Description

A sense (occurs with one of the five senses) perception for which no external stimuli exist. This can have an organic or functional cause.

Types

Auditory

Hearing voices when none are present

Gustatory

Experiencing taste in the absence of stimuli

Olfactory

Smelling smells that do not exist

Tactile

Feeling touch sensations in the absence of stimuli

Visual

Seeing things that are not there

Command

"Voices" that direct a person to take action that is often harmful

Interventions

Ask the client directly about the hallucination.

Avoid reacting to the hallucination as if it were real.

Decrease stimuli or move the client to another area.

Do not negate the client's experience.

Focus on reality-based topics.

Attempt to engage the client's attention through a concrete activity.

Respond verbally to anything real that the client talks about.

Avoid touching the client.

Monitor for signs of increasing anxiety or agitation, which may indicate that the hallucinations are increasing.

BOX 64-13 Interventions for Schizophrenia

Assess the client's physical needs.
Set limits on the client's behaviors when it interferes with others and becomes disruptive.
Maintain a safe environment.
Initiate one-on-one interaction and progress to small groups as tolerated.
Spend time with the client even if he or she is unable to respond.
Monitor for altered thought processes.
Maintain ego boundaries and avoid touching the client.
Limit the time of interaction with the client.
Avoid an overly warm approach. A neutral approach is less threatening.
Do not make promises to the client that cannot be kept.
Establish daily routines.
Assist the client to improve grooming and accept responsibility for personal care.
Sit with the client in silence if necessary.
Provide brief and frequent contact with the client.
Tell the client when you are leaving.
Tell the client when you do not understand.
Do not "go along" with the client's delusions or hallucinations.
Provide simple, concrete activities, such as puzzles or word games.
Reorient the client as necessary.
Help the client establish what is real and unreal.
Stay with the client if he or she is frightened.
Speak to the client in a simple, direct, and concise manner.
Reassure the client that the environment is safe.
Remove the client from group situations if the client's behavior is too bizarre, disturbing, or dangerous to others.
Set realistic goals.
Initially, do not offer choices to the client, and gradually assist him or her in making decisions.
Use canned or packaged food, especially with the paranoid schizophrenic client.
Provide a radio or CD player at night for insomnia.
Explain to the client everything that is being done.
Set limits on the client's behavior if he or she cannot.
Decrease excessive stimuli in the environment.
Monitor for suicide risk.
Assist the client to use alternative means to express feelings through music or art therapy or writing.

5. Alter hospital routines as necessary, such as using canned or packaged food or food from home.
6. Recognize accomplishments and provide positive feedback for successes.

XII. Paranoid Disorders

A. Description
1. Paranoid disorder is a concrete, pervasive delusional system characterized by persecutory and grandiose beliefs.
2. The client demonstrates suspicion and mistrust of others.
3. The client is often viewed by others as hostile, stubborn, and defensive.

B. Behaviors
1. Suspicious and mistrustful
2. Emotionally distant
3. Distortion of reality
4. Poor insight and poor judgments
5. Hypervigilant
6. Low self-esteem
7. Highly sensitive, difficulty in admitting own error, and taking pride in being correct
8. Hypercritical and intolerant of others
9. Hostile, aggressive, and quarrelsome
10. Evasive
11. Exhibits concrete thinking

C. Delusions
1. Delusions serve a purpose in establishing identity and self-esteem.
2. Client may have grandiose and persecutory delusions.
3. Process of delusion includes denial, projection, and rationalization.
4. As trust in others increases, the need for delusions decreases.

D. Types of paranoid disorders
1. Paranoid personality disorder
   a. Suspicious
   b. Nonpsychotic
   c. No hallucinations or delusions
   d. No symptoms of schizophrenia
2. Paranoid-induced state
   a. Abrupt onset in response to stress and subsides when stress decreases
   b. No hallucinations but experiences paranoid delusions
   c. May be sensitive and suspicious before the development of delusions
   d. No symptoms of schizophrenia
3. Paranoia
   a. Exhibits an organized delusional system
   b. No hallucinations
   c. Reserved and sensitive before onset
   d. Psychotic state
   e. No symptoms of schizophrenia
4. Paranoid schizophrenia
   a. Before onset, the client becomes cold, withdrawn, distrustful, resentful, argumentative, sarcastic, and defiant.
   b. Bizarre, numerous, and changeable delusions occur.
   c. Delusions become less logical as the client becomes more disorganized.

BOX 64-14 Interventions for Paranoid Disorders

Assess for suicide risk.
Diminish suspicious behavior.
Avoid direct eye contact.
Establish a trusting relationship.
Promote increased self-esteem.
Remain calm, nonthreatening, and nonjudgmental.
Provide continuity of care.
Respond honestly to the client.
Follow through on commitments made to the client.
Acknowledge the client's feelings, but tell him or her that you do not share his or her interpretation of an event.
Provide a daily schedule of activities.
Assist the client to identify diversionary activities.
Gradually introduce the client to groups.
Refocus conversation to reality-based topics.
Use role playing to help the client identify thoughts and feelings.
Provide positive reinforcement for successes.
Do not argue with delusions.
Use concrete, specific words.
Do not be secretive with the client.
Do not whisper in the client's presence.
Assure the client that he or she will be safe.
Involve the client in noncompetitive tasks.
Provide the client opportunity to complete small tasks.
Monitor eating, drinking, sleeping, and elimination patterns.
Limit physical contact.
Monitor for agitation and decrease stimuli as needed.

- **d.** Persecutory hallucinations occur.
- **e.** Psychotic state ensues.
- **f.** All symptoms of schizophrenia are present.

E. Interventions (Box 64-14)

⚠ Do not whisper or laugh in front of a client with a paranoid disorder because the client will think that you are talking about or laughing at him or her. This increases the paranoia.

XIII. Personality Disorders

A. Description
1. Personality disorders include various inflexible maladaptive behavior patterns or traits that may impair functioning and relationships.
2. The individual usually remains in touch with reality and typically has a lack of insight into his or her behavior.
3. Stress exacerbates manifestations of the personality disorder.
4. In severe cases the personality disorder may deteriorate to a psychotic state.

B. Characteristics
1. Poor impulse control
   - **a.** Acting out to manage internal pain
   - **b.** Forms of acting out include physical and verbal attacks, such as yelling and swearing, and self-injurious behaviors such as cutting own skin, banging the head, punching self, manipulation, substance abuse, promiscuous sexual behaviors, and **suicide attempts**.
   - **c.** Client may be preoccupied with self, religion, or sex.
2. Mood characteristics
   - **a.** May experience abandonment and depression
   - **b.** Moods may include rage, guilt, fear, and emptiness.
3. Impaired judgment
   - **a.** Difficulty with problem solving
   - **b.** Inability to perceive the consequences of behavior
4. Impaired reality testing: Distortion of reality and often projection of own feelings onto others
5. Impaired object relations: Rigid and inflexible, with difficulty in intimate relationships
6. Impaired self-perception: Distorted self-perception and experience of self-hate or self-idealization
7. Impaired thought processes
   - **a.** Concrete or diffuse thinking
   - **b.** Difficulty concentrating
   - **c.** Impaired memory
8. Impaired stimulus barrier
   - **a.** Inability to regulate incoming sensory stimuli
   - **b.** Increased excitability
   - **c.** Excessive response to noise and light
   - **d.** Poor attention span
   - **e.** Agitated
   - **f.** Insomnia

C. Cluster A personality disorders include the odd/eccentric types: schizoid, schizotypal, and paranoid.
1. Schizoid personality disorder is characterized by an inability to form warm, close social relationships.
   - **a.** Social detachment and lack of close relationships
   - **b.** Interest in solitary activities
   - **c.** Aloof and indifferent
   - **d.** Restricted expression of emotions
   - **e.** Lack of interest in others
2. Schizotypal personality disorder is characterized by the display of abnormal or highly unusual thoughts, perceptions, speech, and behavior patterns.
   - **a.** Suspicious
   - **b.** Paranoia
   - **c.** Magical thinking
   - **d.** Odd thinking and speech
   - **e.** Relationship deficits
3. Paranoid personality disorder is characterized by suspiciousness and mistrust of others.
   - **a.** May be argumentative
   - **b.** May be hostile, aloof
   - **c.** May be rigid, critical, and controlling of others
   - **d.** May have thoughts of grandiosity

D. Cluster B personality disorders include the overemotional, erratic types: histrionic, narcissistic, borderline, and antisocial.
  1. Histrionic personality disorder is characterized by overly dramatic and intensely expressive behavior.
    a. Lively and dramatic and enjoys being the center of attention
    b. Has poor and shallow interpersonal relations
    c. May be sexually seductive or provocative
    d. Dramatizes their life and may appear theatrical
    e. Overly concerned with appearance
    f. Easily bored
  2. Narcissistic personality disorder is characterized by an increased sense of self-importance, preoccupation with fantasies and a sense of unlimited success.
    a. Need for admiration and inflation of accomplishments
    b. Overestimation of abilities and underestimation of contributions of others
    c. Lack of empathy and sensitivity to the needs of others
  3. Antisocial personality disorder is comprised of a pattern of irresponsible and antisocial behavior, selfishness, an inability to maintain lasting relationships, poor sexual adjustment, a failure to accept social norms, and a tendency toward irritability and aggressiveness.
    a. Perceives the world as hostile
    b. Superficial charm and hostility
    c. No shame or guilt
    d. Self-centered
    e. Unreliable
    f. Easily bored
    g. Poor work history
    h. Inability to tolerate frustration
    i. Views others as objects to be manipulated
    j. Poor judgment
    k. Impulsive
  4. Borderline personality disorder is characterized by instability in interpersonal relationships, unstable mood and self-image, and impulsive and unpredictable behavior.
    a. Unclear identity
    b. Unstable and intense
    c. Extreme shifts in mood
    d. Easily angered
    e. Easily bored
    f. Argumentative
    g. Depression
    h. Self-destructive behavior
    i. Manipulation
    j. Inability to tolerate anxiety
    k. Chronic feelings of emptiness and fear of being alone
    l. Splitting (sees others as all good or all bad; creates conflict between individuals by playing one person against another)

E. Cluster C Personality Disorders include the anxious, fearful types of personality disorders: obsessive-compulsive personality, avoidant, and dependent.
  1. Obsessive-compulsive personality disorder is characterized by difficulty expressing warm and tender emotions, perfectionism, stubbornness, the need to control others, and a devotion to work.
    a. Overly conscientious
    b. Inflexible and preoccupied with details and rules
    c. Extreme devotion to work to the exclusion of leisure activities and friendships
    d. Miserly and stubborn
    e. Hoarding behavior
    f. Engages in rituals
  2. Avoidant personality disorder is characterized by social withdrawal and extreme sensitivity to potential rejection
    a. Feelings of inadequacy
    b. Hypersensitive to reactions of others and poor reaction to criticism
    c. Social isolation
    d. Lack of support system
  3. Dependent personality disorder is characterized by intense lack of self-confidence and low self-esteem, and lack of ability to function independently, such that the individual passively allows others to make decisions and assume responsibility for major areas in the person's life. The dependent client has great difficulty making decisions.

F. General interventions for the client with a personality disorder
  1. Maintain safety against self-destructive behaviors.
  2. Allow the client to make choices and be as independent as possible.
  3. Encourage the client to discuss feelings rather than act them out.
  4. Provide consistency in response to the client's acting-out behaviors.
  5. Discuss expectations and responsibilities with the client.
  6. Discuss the consequences that follow certain behaviors.
  7. Inform the client that harm to self, others, and property is unacceptable.
  8. Identify splitting behavior.
  9. Assist the client to deal directly with anger.
  10. Develop a written safety and/or behavioral contract with the client.
  11. Encourage the client to keep a journal recording daily feelings.
  12. Encourage the client to participate in group activities, and praise nonmanipulative behavior.

13. Set and maintain limits to decrease manipulative behavior.
14. Remove the client from group situations in which attention-seeking behaviors occur.
15. Provide realistic praise for positive behaviors in social situations.

XIV. Cognitive Impairment Disorders

A. Autism: Refer to Chapter 37.
B. Attention deficit hyperactivity disorder: Refer to Chapter 37.
C. Dementia and Alzheimer's disease
  1. Dementia
    a. Dementia is a syndrome with progressive deterioration in intellectual functioning; secondary to structural or functional changes.
    b. Long- and short-term memory loss occurs with impairment in judgment, abstract thinking, problem-solving ability, and behavior.
    c. Dementia results in a self-care deficit.
    d. The most common type of dementia is Alzheimer's disease.
  2. Alzheimer's disease (Box 64-15)
    a. Alzheimer's disease is an irreversible form of senile dementia from nerve cell deterioration.
    b. Individuals with Alzheimer's disease experience cognitive deterioration and progressive loss of ability to carry out activities of daily living.
    c. The client experiences a steady decline in physical and mental functioning and usually requires long-term care facility placement in the final stages of the illness.
  3. Interventions
    a. Identify and reinforce retained skills.
    b. Provide continuity of care.
    c. Orient the client to the environment.
    d. Furnish the environment with familiar possessions.
    e. Acknowledge the client's feelings.
    f. Help the client and family members manage memory deficits and behavior changes.
    g. Encourage the family members to express feelings about caregiving.
    h. Provide the caregiver support, and identify the resources and support groups available.

BOX 64-15 Alzheimer's Disease

Agnosia: Failure to recognize or identify objects despite intact sensory function
Amnesia: Loss of memory caused by brain degeneration
Aphasia: Language disturbance in understanding and expressing the spoken word
Apraxia: Inability to perform motor activities despite intact motor function

    i. Monitor activities of daily living.
    j. Remind the client how to perform self-care activities.
    k. Help the client maintain independence.
    l. Provide the client with consistent routines.
    m. Provide exercise such as walking with an escort.
    n. Avoid activities that tax the memory.
    o. Allow the client plenty of time to complete a task.
    p. Use constant encouragement in a simple step-by-step approach.
    q. Provide activities that distract and occupy time, such as listening to music, coloring, and watching television.
    r. Provide the client with mental stimulation with simple games or activities.
  4. Wandering
    a. Provide a safe environment.
    b. Prevent unsafe wandering.
    c. Provide close supervision.
    d. Close and secure doors.
    e. Use identification bracelets and electronic surveillance.

⚠ Providing a safe environment is a priority in the care of a client with Alzheimer's disease.

  5. Communication
    a. Adapt to the communication level of the client.
    b. Use a firm volume and a low-pitched voice to communicate.
    c. Stand directly in front of the client and maintain eye contact.
    d. Call the client by name and identify self. Wait for a response.
    e. Use a calm and reassuring voice.
    f. Use pantomime gestures if the client is unable to understand spoken words.
    g. Speak slowly and clearly, using short words and simple sentences.
    h. Ask only one question at a time and give one direction at a time.
    i. Repeat questions if necessary but do not rephrase.
  6. Impaired judgment
    a. Remove throw rugs, toxic substances, and dangerous electrical appliances from the environment.
    b. Reduce hot water heater temperature.
  7. Altered thought processes
    a. Call the client by name.
    b. Orient the client frequently.
    c. Use familiar objects in the room.
    d. Place a calendar and clock in a visible place.
    e. Maintain familiar routines.
    f. Allow the client to reminisce.

g. Make tasks simple.
h. Allow time for the client to complete a task.
i. Provide positive reinforcement for positive behaviors.

8. Altered sleep patterns
   a. Allow the client to wander in a safe place until he or she becomes tired.
   b. Prevent shadows in the room by using indirect light.
   c. Avoid the use of hypnotics because they cause confusion and aggravate the sundown effect.
9. Agitation
   a. Assess the precipitant of the agitation.
   b. Reassure the client.
   c. Remove items that can be hazardous during the time of agitation.
   d. Approach the client slowly and calmly from the front, and then speak, gesture, and move slowly.
   e. Remove client to a less stressful environment; decrease excess stimuli.
   f. Use touch gently.
   g. Do not argue with or force the client.

XV. Psychosexual Alterations

A. Sexuality
   1. One's sense of being a sexual individual
   2. Includes how one looks, behaves, and relates to others
B. Sexual expression (Box 64-16)
C. Alterations in sexual behavior
   1. Gender dysphoria: Feeling that one's gender is inappropriate and desiring to acquire sexual characteristics of the opposite gender
   2. Exhibitionism: Sexual urges and fantasies and exposure of genitals to strangers to bring sexual gratification and/or arousal
   3. Fetishism: Using nonliving objects for sexual gratification
   4. Pedophilia: Desiring sexual activity with a child under age 13
   5. Sexual masochism: Sexual gratification that involves receiving pain
   6. Sexual sadism: Sexual gratification that involves inflicting pain
   7. Voyeurism: Sexual gratification through observing others disrobing or engaging in sexual activity
   8. Zoophilia: Intense sexual arousal or desire for sexual contact with animals
   9. Frotteurism: Intense sexual arousal or desire when rubbing against a nonconsenting person
D. Interventions
   1. Assess sexual history, history of trauma or abuse, and precipitating event for the sexual disorder.
   2. Encourage the client to explore personal beliefs.
   3. Provide a nonjudgmental attitude.
   4. Provide supportive psychotherapy.

BOX 64-16 Sexual Expression

Bisexuality: Sexual attraction to and activity with both genders
Heterosexuality: Male-female sexual relationships
Homosexuality: Sexual attraction to a member of the same gender
Gender dysphoria (Transvestism): Obsession with wearing clothing of the opposite gender

CRITICAL THINKING What Should You Do?

Answer: If a client is actively hallucinating, the nurse should intervene with one-on-one contact. The nurse should ask the client directly about the hallucination and avoid reacting to the hallucination as if it were real. The nurse should decrease stimuli or move the client to another area and avoid indicating to the client that others also are experiencing the hallucination. The nurse should encourage the client to express feelings, focus on reality-based topics, and respond verbally to anything real that the client talks about. The nurse also avoids touching the client. During a hallucination, the nurse also should attempt to engage the client's attention through a concrete activity and monitor for signs of increasing anxiety or agitation, which may indicate that the hallucinations are increasing.

Reference(s): deWit, D. & Kumagai, C. (2013). *Medical-surgical nursing: Concepts & practice.* (2nd ed., pp. 1104, 1110–1112). St. Louis: Saunders.

PRACTICE QUESTIONS

686. A client with delirium becomes agitated and confused at night. The **best initial** intervention by the nurse is which?
1. Move the client next to the nurse's station.
2. Use a night light and turn off the television.
3. Keep the television and a soft light on during the night.
4. Play soft music during the night and maintain a well-lit room.

687. The nurse is collecting data on a client who is actively hallucinating. Which nursing statement should be therapeutic at this time?
1. "I know you feel 'they are out to get you,' but it's not true."
2. "I can hear the voice, and she wants you to come to dinner."

3. "Sometimes people hear things or voices others can't hear."
4. "I talked to the voices you're hearing and they won't hurt you now."

688. The nurse is caring for a client with a diagnosis of depression. The nurse monitors for signs of constipation and urinary retention, knowing that these problems are likely caused by which?
1. Poor dietary choices
2. Lack of exercise and poor diet
3. Inadequate dietary intake and dehydration
4. Psychomotor retardation and side effects of medication

689. A client is admitted to the in-patient unit and is being considered for electroconvulsive therapy (ECT). The client appears calm, but the family is hypervigilant and anxious. The client's mother begins to cry and states, "My child's brain will be destroyed. How can the doctor do this?" The nurse should make which therapeutic response?
1. "It sounds as though you need to speak to the psychiatrist."
2. "Perhaps you'd like to see the ECT room and speak to the staff."
3. "Your child has decided to have this treatment. You should be supportive of the decision."
4. "It sounds as though you have some concerns about the ECT procedure. Why don't we sit down together and discuss any concerns you may have?"

❖ **690.** Which nursing interventions are appropriate for a hospitalized client with mania who is exhibiting manipulative behavior? **Select all that apply.**
- ☐ 1. Communicate expected behaviors to the client.
- ☐ 2. Ensure that the client knows that he or she is not in charge of the nursing unit.
- ☐ 3. Assist the client in developing means of setting limits on personal behavior.
- ☐ 4. Follow through about the consequences of behavior in a nonpunitive manner.
- ☐ 5. Enforce rules and inform the client that he or she will not be allowed to attend therapy groups.
- ☐ 6. Be clear with the client regarding the consequences of exceeding limits set regarding behavior.

691. The nurse is preparing for the hospital discharge of a client with a history of command hallucinations to harm self or others. The nurse instructs the client about interventions for hallucinations and anxiety and determines that the client understands the interventions when the client states which?
1. "My medications won't make me anxious."
2. "I'll go to a support group and talk so that I won't hurt anyone."
3. "I won't get anxious or hear things if I get enough sleep and eat well."
4. "I can call my therapist when I'm hallucinating so I can talk about my feelings and plans and not hurt anyone."

692. The nurse observes that a client is psychotic, pacing, and agitated and is making aggressive gestures. The client's speech pattern is rapid, and the client's affect is belligerent. Based on these observations, the nurse's **immediate priority** of care is which?
1. Provide safety for the client and other clients on the unit.
2. Provide the clients on the unit with a sense of comfort and safety.
3. Assist the staff in caring for the client in a controlled environment.
4. Offer the client a less-stimulating area to calm down and gain control.

693. The nurse is caring for a client diagnosed with catatonic stupor. The client is lying on the bed, with the body pulled into a fetal position. The appropriate nursing intervention is which?
1. Ask direct questions to encourage talking.
2. Leave the client alone and intermittently check on him.
3. Sit beside the client in silence and verbalize occasional open-ended questions.
4. Take the client into the dayroom with other clients so they can help watch him.

694. A mother of a teenage client with an anxiety disorder is concerned about her daughter's progress on discharge. She states that her daughter "stashes food, eats all the wrong things that make her hyperactive," and "hangs out with the wrong crowd." In helping the mother prepare for her daughter's discharge, the nurse should suggest which?
1. The mother should restrict the daughter's socializing time with her friends.
2. The mother should restrict the amount of chocolate and caffeine products in the home.
3. The mother should keep her daughter out of school until she can adjust to the school environment.
4. The mother should consider taking time from work to help her daughter readjust to the home environment.

695. A client is unwilling to go out of the house for fear of "doing something crazy in public." Because of this fear, the client remains homebound except when accompanied outside by the spouse. The nurse determines that the client has which?

1. Agoraphobia
2. Hematophobia
3. Claustrophobia
4. Hypochondriasis

696. A client has reported that crying spells have been a major problem over the past several weeks and that the doctor said depression is probably the reason. The nurse observes that the client is sitting slumped in the chair, and the clothes that the client is wearing do not fit well. The nurse interprets that further data collection should focus on which?

1. Weight loss
2. Sleep patterns
3. Medication compliance
4. Onset of the crying spells

697. A client was admitted to a medical unit with acute blindness. Many tests are performed, and there seems to be no organic reason why this client cannot see. The nurse later learns that the client became blind after witnessing a hit-and-run car crash in which a family of three was killed. The nurse suspects that the client may be experiencing which?

1. Psychosis
2. Repression
3. Conversion disorder
4. Dissociative disorder

698. A manic client announces to everyone in the dayroom that a stripper is coming to perform that evening. When the psychiatric nurse's aide firmly states that the client's behavior is not appropriate, the manic client becomes verbally abusive and threatens physical violence to the nurse's aide. Based on the analysis of this situation, the nurse determines that the appropriate action should be which?

1. Escort the manic client to his or her room.
2. Orient the client to time, person, and place.
3. Tell the client that the behavior is not appropriate.
4. Tell the client that smoking privileges are revoked for 24 hours.

699. The nurse notes documentation in a client's record that the client is experiencing delusions of persecution. The nurse understands that these types of delusions are characteristic of which?

1. The false belief that one is a very powerful person
2. The false belief that one is a very important person
3. The false belief that one's partner is being unfaithful
4. The false belief that one is being singled out for harm by others

700. A client who is diagnosed with pedophilia and recently has been paroled as a sex offender says, "I'm in treatment and I have served my time. Now this group has posters all over the neighborhood with my photograph and details of my crime." Which is an appropriate response by the nurse?

1. "When children are hurt the way you hurt them, people want you isolated."
2. "You're lucky it doesn't escalate into something pretty scary after your crime."
3. "You understand that people fear for their children, but you're feeling unfairly treated?"
4. "You seem angry, but you have committed serious crimes against several children, so your neighbors are frightened."

ANSWERS

686. 2

Rationale: It is important to provide a consistent daily routine and a low-stimulation environment when the client is agitated and confused. Noise levels including a radio and television may add to the confusion and disorientation. Moving the client next to the nurses' station is not the initial intervention.
Test-Taking Strategy: Note the strategic words, *best* and *initial*, in the question. Eliminate options 3 and 4 first because they are comparable or alike. From the remaining options, recalling that a low-stimulation environment is best will direct you to option 2. **Review:** measures related to the client with **agitation and confusion.**
Level of Cognitive Ability: Applying
Client Needs: Psychosocial Integrity
Integrated Process: Nursing Process/Implementation
Content Area: Mental Health
Priority Concept: Clinical Judgment, Thought Process
Reference(s): Varcarolis (2013), pp. 340–341.

687. 3

Rationale: It is important for the nurse to reinforce reality with the client. Options 1, 2, and 4 do not reinforce reality but reinforce the hallucination that the voices are real.
Test-Taking Strategy: Focus on the subject, hallucinations, and note that options 1, 2, and 4 all indicate reinforcement to the client that the voices are real. Option 3 is the only statement that indicates reality. **Review:** nursing interventions related to the client who is **hallucinating.**
Level of Cognitive Ability: Applying
Client Needs: Psychosocial Integrity
Integrated Process: Communication and Documentation
Content Area: Mental Health

Priority Concept: Cognition, Psychosis
Reference(s): Varcarolis (2013), p. 320.

688. 4
Rationale: In this situation, urinary retention is most likely caused by medications. Option 4 is the only option that addresses both constipation and urinary retention. Constipation can be related to inadequate food intake, lack of exercise, and poor diet.
Test-Taking Strategy: Focus on the data in the question. Options 1, 2, and 3 are all **comparable or alike** and address diet. Option 4 addresses both concerns of constipation and urinary retention. **Review:** the interventions for a client with **depression** and the effects of medications prescribed for this disorder.
Level of Cognitive Ability: Analyzing
Client Needs: Physiological Integrity
Integrated Process: Nursing Process/Data Collection
Content Area: Mental Health
Priority Concept: Elimination, Mood and Affect
Reference(s): Varcarolis (2013), p. 262.

689. 4
Rationale: The nurse needs to encourage the family and client to verbalize their fears and concerns. Option 4 is the only option that encourages verbalization. Options 1, 2, and 3 avoid dealing with the client or family concerns.
Test-Taking Strategy: Focus on the **subject**, therapeutic response. Use therapeutic communication techniques and focus on the client's and family's feelings and concerns. This will direct you to the correct option. **Review: therapeutic communication techniques.**
Level of Cognitive Ability: Applying
Client Needs: Psychosocial Integrity
Integrated Process: Nursing Process/Implementation
Content Area: Mental Health
Priority Concept: Anxiety, Communication
Reference(s): deWit, Kumagai (2013), p. 1057.

❖ **690. 1, 3, 4, 6**
Rationale: Interventions for dealing with the client exhibiting manipulative behavior include setting clear, consistent, and enforceable limits on manipulative behaviors; being clear with the client regarding the consequences of exceeding limits set; following through with the consequences in a nonpunitive manner; and assisting the client in developing means of setting limits on personal behaviors. Enforcing rules and informing the client that he or she will not be allowed to attend therapy groups are violations of a client's rights. Ensuring that the client knows that he or she is not in charge of the nursing unit is inappropriate; power struggles need to be avoided.
Test-Taking Strategy: Focus on the **subject**, manipulative behavior. Recalling clients' rights and that power struggles need to be avoided will assist in selecting the correct interventions. Review: care to the client with **manipulative behavior**.
Level of Cognitive Ability: Applying
Client Needs: Psychosocial Integrity
Integrated Process: Nursing Process/Implementation
Content Area: Mental Health
Priority Concept: Cognition, Psychosis
Reference(s): deWit, Kumagai (2013), p. 1113.

691. 4
Rationale: There may be an increased risk for impulsive and/or aggressive behavior if a client is receiving command hallucinations to harm self or others. Talking about the auditory hallucinations can interfere with the subvocal muscular activity associated with a hallucination. Option 4 is a specific agreement to seek help and evidences self-responsible commitment and control over his or her own behavior.
Test-Taking Strategy: Focus on the **subject**, hallucinations to harm self or others. Note the relationship between the word, *hallucinations,* in the question and the correct option. **Review:** care of the client with **command hallucinations**.
Level of Cognitive Ability: Evaluating
Client Needs: Psychosocial Integrity
Integrated Process: Nursing Process/Evaluation
Content Area: Mental Health
Priority Concept: Interpersonal Violence, Psychosis
Reference(s): deWit, Kumagai (2013), pp. 1108–1109.

692. 1
Rationale: Safety of the client and other clients is the priority. Option 1 is the only option that addresses the client and other clients' safety needs. Option 4 addresses the client's needs. Option 2 addresses other clients' needs. Option 3 is not client centered.
Test-Taking Strategy: Note the **strategic words**, *immediate priority*, and focus on the **subject**, safety. Option 1 is the **umbrella option** and addresses the safety of all. **Review:** care of the **psychotic client**.
Level of Cognitive Ability: Applying
Client Needs: Safe and Effective Care Environment
Integrated Process: Nursing Process/Implementation
Content Area: Mental Health
Priority Concept: Psychosis, Safety
Reference(s): Varcarolis (2013), pp. 340–341.

693. 3
Rationale: Clients with catatonic stupor may be immobile and mute and may require consistent, repeated approaches. The nurse facilitates communication with the client by sitting in silence, asking open-ended questions, and pausing to provide opportunities for the client to respond. The nurse would not leave the client alone. Fortunately, with pharmacotherapy and improved individual management, severe catatonic symptoms rarely occur. Option 4 relies on other clients to care for this one, which is an inappropriate expectation. Asking direct questions of this client is not therapeutic. Option 3 is the best action because it provides for client supervision and communication as appropriate.
Test-Taking Strategy: Focus on the **subject**, catatonic stupor. Eliminate option 2 because the nurse would not leave the client alone. Eliminate option 4 next because this action relies on other clients to care for this one. Eliminate option 1 because asking direct questions of this client is not therapeutic. **Review:** care of the client with **catatonic stupor**.
Level of Cognitive Ability: Applying
Client Needs: Psychosocial Integrity
Integrated Process: Nursing Process/Implementation
Content Area: Mental Health

Priority Concept: Communication, Mobility
Reference(s): deWit, Kumagai (2013), p. 1105; Varcarolis (2013), p. 314.

694. 2
Rationale: Clients with anxiety disorder should abstain from or limit their intake of caffeine, chocolate, and alcohol. These products have the potential of increasing anxiety. Options 1 and 3 are unreasonable and are an unhealthy approach. It may not be realistic for a family member to take time away from work.
Test-Taking Strategy: Options 1, 3, and 4 are **comparable or alike** and are concerned with monitoring or curtailing the client's physical activities. Option 2 addresses preparation of the client's environment and focuses on the concern or subject expressed in the question. **Review:** discharge planning for the client with an **anxiety disorder**.
Level of Cognitive Ability: Applying
Client Needs: Psychosocial Integrity
Integrated Process: Teaching and Learning
Content Area: Mental Health
Priority Concept: Anxiety, Nutrition
Reference(s): Varcarolis (2013), p. 159.

695. 1
Rationale: Agoraphobia is a fear of being alone in open or public places where escape might be difficult. Agoraphobia includes experiencing fear or a sense of helplessness or embarrassment if a phobic attack occurs. Avoidance of such situations usually results in the reduction of social and professional interactions. Hematophobia is the fear of blood. Claustrophobia is a fear of closed-in places. Clients with somatic symptom disorder focus their anxiety on physical complaints and are preoccupied with their health.
Test-Taking Strategy: Focus on the **subject** in the question, unwilling to go out of the house. Recalling the specific types of phobias and associated client behaviors will direct you to the correct option. **Review:** **phobia types** and associated client behaviors.
Level of Cognitive Ability: Understanding
Client Needs: Psychosocial Integrity
Integrated Process: Nursing Process/Data Collection
Content Area: Mental Health
Priority Concept: Coping, Psychosis
Reference(s): Varcarolis (2013), p. 176.

696. 1
Rationale: All the options are possible issues to address; however, the weight loss is the first item that needs further data collection because ill-fitting clothing could indicate a problem with nutrition. The client has already told the nurse that the crying spells have been a problem. Medication or sleep patterns are not mentioned or addressed in the question.
Test-Taking Strategy: Use **Maslow's Hierarchy of Needs Theory** to answer the question. Focusing on the data in the question will assist in eliminating the incorrect options. **Review:** the priorities of care for a client with **depression**.
Level of Cognitive Ability: Analyzing
Client Needs: Physiological Integrity
Integrated Process: Nursing Process/Data Collection
Content Area: Mental Health
Priority Concept: Mood and Affect, Nutrition
Reference(s): deWit, Kumagai (2013), p. 1058.

697. 3
Rationale: A conversion disorder is the alteration or loss of a physical function that cannot be explained by any known pathophysiological mechanism. It is thought to be an expression of a psychological need or conflict. In this situation, the client witnessed an accident that was so psychologically painful that the client became blind. A dissociative disorder is a disturbance or alteration in the normally integrative functions of identity, memory, or consciousness. Psychosis is a state in which a person's mental capacity to recognize reality, communicate, and relate to others is impaired, thus interfering with the person's capacity to deal with life's demands. Repression is a coping mechanism in which unacceptable feelings are kept out of awareness.
Test-Taking Strategy: Focus on the **subject**, blindness with no organic reason. Noting that the client evidences no organic reason to account for the blindness will direct you to the correct option. **Review:** **conversion disorders** and **defense mechanisms**.
Level of Cognitive Ability: Understanding
Client Needs: Psychosocial Integrity
Integrated Process: Nursing Process/Data Collection
Content Area: Mental Health
Priority Concept: Coping, Psychosis
Reference(s): Varcarolis (2013), pp. 196, 201.

698. 1
Rationale: The client is at risk for injury to self and others and therefore should be escorted out of the dayroom. Option 4 may increase the agitation that already exists in this client. Orientation will not halt the behavior. Telling the client that the behavior is not appropriate has already been attempted by the psychiatric nurse's aide.
Test-Taking Strategy: Focus on the **subject**, therapeutic interventions for the manic client. Options 2, 3, and 4 will not de-escalate the client's agitation. **Review:** appropriate interventions in dealing with a **manic client**.
Level of Cognitive Ability: Applying
Client Needs: Psychosocial Integrity
Integrated Process: Nursing Process/Implementation
Content Area: Mental Health
Priority Concept: Interpersonal Violence, Psychosis
Reference(s): deWit, Kumagai (2013), pp. 1053–1054.

699. 4
Rationale: A delusion is a false belief held to be true even when there is evidence to the contrary. A delusion of persecution is the thought that one is being singled out for harm by others. A delusion of grandeur is the false belief that he or she is a very powerful and important person. A delusion of jealousy is the false belief that one's partner is being unfaithful.
Test-Taking Strategy: Eliminate options 1 and 2 first because they are **comparable or alike**. From the remaining options, note the relationship between the word, *persecution*, in the question and the description in option 4. **Review:** description of the types of **delusions**.
Level of Cognitive Ability: Understanding
Client Needs: Psychosocial Integrity
Integrated Process: Nursing Process/Data Collection
Content Area: Mental Health
Priority Concept: Cognition, Psychosis
Reference(s): Varcarolis (2013), pp. 309–310.

700. 3

Rationale: Focusing and verbalizing the implied concern is the therapeutic response because it assists the client to clarify thinking and to re-examine what the client is really saying. Option 3 is the only option that reflects the use of this therapeutic communication technique. Option 1 is insensitive and anxiety-provoking. Option 4 does not facilitate the client's expression of feelings. Option 2 gives advice and does not facilitate the client's expression of feelings.

Test-Taking Strategy: Use **therapeutic communication techniques** to answer the question. Remembering to focus on the client's feelings and concerns will direct you to the correct option. **Review: therapeutic communication techniques.**

Level of Cognitive Ability: Applying

Client Needs: Psychosocial Integrity

Integrated Process: Communication and Documentation

Content Area: Mental Health

Priority Concept: Communication, Interpersonal Violence

Reference(s): Varcarolis (2013), pp. 527, 529.

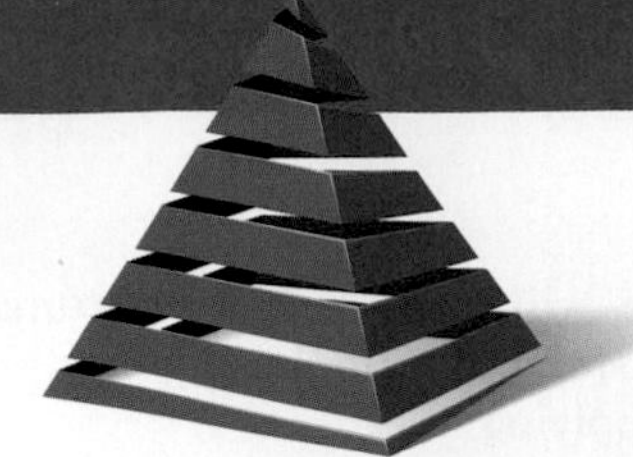

CHAPTER 65

Addictions

CRITICAL THINKING What Should You Do?

The nurse notes that a client is experiencing signs of alcohol withdrawal delirium. What should the nurse do?
Answer located on p. 933.

I. Eating Disorders

A. Description: Eating disorders are characterized by uncertain self-identification and grossly disturbed eating habits (Fig. 65-1).

B. Binge eating disorder

1. Binge eating is consuming a large amount of food in a short period of time, without purging.
2. Food consumption is out of the individual's control and occurs in a stereotyped fashion.
3. The client may be repulsed by eating, and the eating relieves tension but does not produce pleasure.
4. The client is aware that eating patterns are abnormal and feels depressed after eating.
5. The client eats secretly during a binge and consumes high-calorie and easily digestible foods.
6. The client repeatedly tries to diet but without success.
7. The client feels helpless and hopeless about weight.
8. When experiencing guilt, anger, depression, boredom, loneliness, inadequacy, or ambivalence, the client responds by eating.

C. Anorexia nervosa

1. Description
   - **a.** The onset often is associated with a stressful life event.
   - **b.** The client intensely fears obesity.
   - **c.** Body image is distorted, and the client has a disturbed self-concept.
   - **d.** The client is preoccupied with foods that prevent weight gain and has a phobia against foods that produce weight gain.
   - **e.** The eating disorder can be life threatening.
   - **f.** Death can occur from starvation, **suicide**, cardiomyopathies, or electrolyte imbalance.

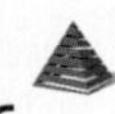

2. Data collection
   - **a.** Refusal to eat and appetite loss
   - **b.** Appetite denial
   - **c.** Feelings of lack of control
   - **d.** Self-induced vomiting and self-administered enemas
   - **e.** Compulsive exercising
   - **f.** Overachiever and perfectionist
   - **g.** Decreased temperature, pulse, and blood pressure
   - **h.** Weight loss
   - **i.** Gastrointestinal disturbances
   - **j.** Constipation
   - **k.** Electrolyte imbalances
   - **l.** Scaly, dry skin
   - **m.** Presence of lanugo on extremities
   - **n.** Sleep disturbances
   - **o.** Hormone deficiencies
   - **p.** Amenorrhea for at least three consecutive menstrual periods
   - **q.** Teeth and gum deterioration
   - **r.** Cyanosis and numbness of extremities
   - **s.** Esophageal varices from vomiting
   - **t.** Bone degeneration

⚠ The client with an eating disorder experiences an altered body image.

D. Bulimia nervosa

1. Description
   - **a.** The client indulges in eating binges, followed by purging behaviors.
   - **b.** Most clients remain within a normal weight range (due to purging) but feel that their lives are dominated by the eating-related conflict.
2. Data collection
   - **a.** Preoccupied with body shape and weight
   - **b.** Consumption of high-calorie foods in secret; guilt about secretive eating
   - **c.** Binge-purge syndrome
   - **d.** Attempts to lose weight through diets, vomiting, enemas, cathartics, and amphetamines or diuretics

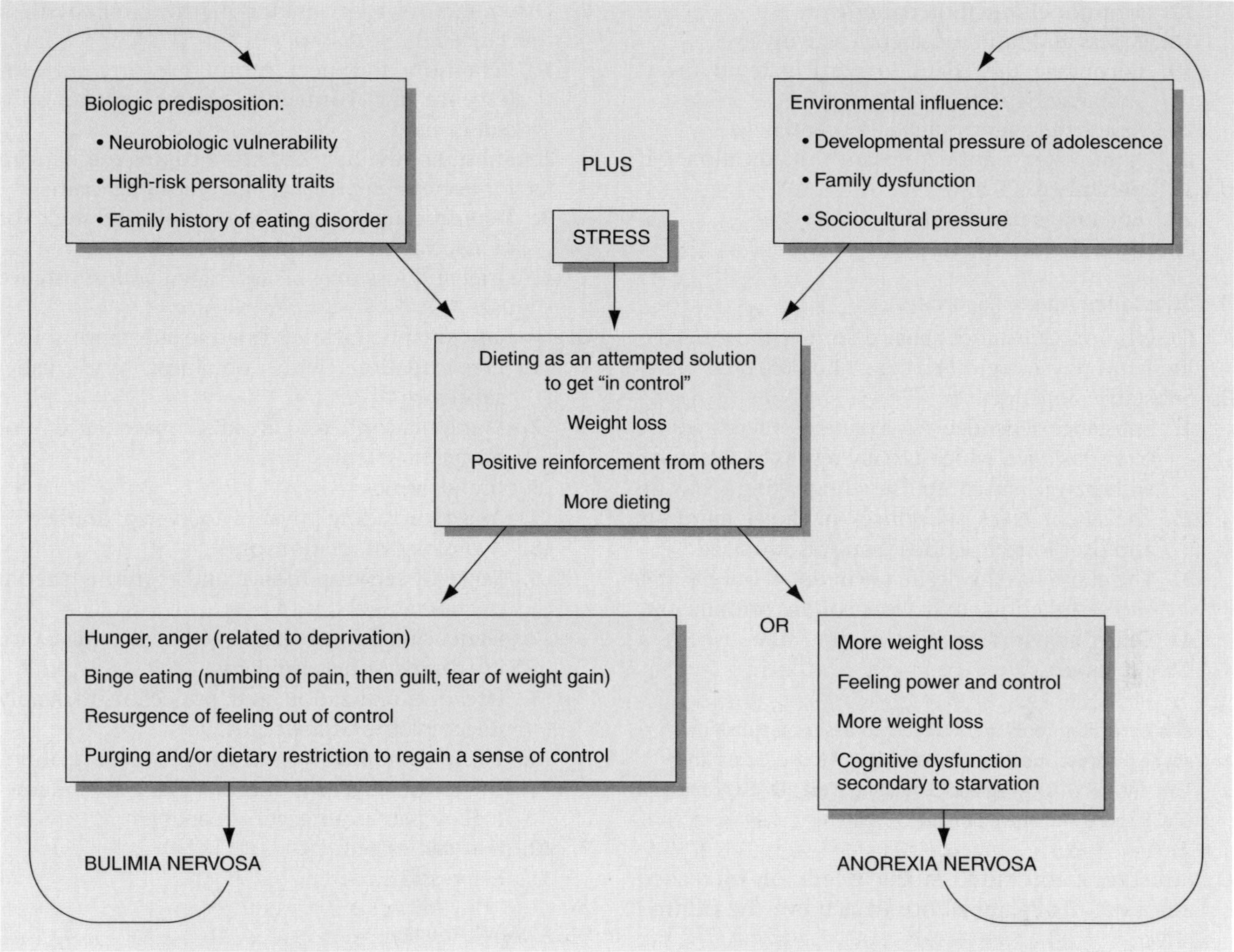

FIGURE 65-1 Cycle of eating disorders. (From Fortinash K, Holoday-Worret P: *Psychiatric mental health nursing*, ed 4, St. Louis, 2008, Mosby.)

- **e.** Has need for control yet experiences feelings of powerlessness or loss of control
- **f.** Low self-esteem
- **g.** Poor interpersonal relationships
- **h.** Decreased or absent interest in sex
- **i.** Mood swings
- **j.** Electrolyte imbalances
- **k.** Loss of tooth enamel and dental decay
- **l.** Stomach ulcers and rectal bleeding
- **m.** Esophageal varices from vomiting
- **n.** Cardiac disease and hypertension

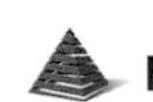 **E.** Interventions: Clients with an eating disorder

1. Assess the client's nutritional status and the severity of any medical problems.
2. Establish a one-to-one therapeutic relationship with the client. The nurse must establish trust and recognize any client reluctance to establish a relationship.
3. Set goals with the client concerning the nutritional plan for the day.
4. Assist the client to identify precipitants to the eating disorder.
5. Encourage the client to express feelings about the eating behavior and about how he or she feels about his/her body.
6. Be accepting and nonjudgmental.
7. Work with the client on exploring self-concept and establishing identity.
8. Implement behavior modification techniques.
9. Supervise the client during mealtimes and for a specified period after meals.
10. Set a time limit for each meal.
11. Provide a pleasant, relaxed environment for eating.
12. Monitor for signs of physical complications related to the eating disorder.
13. Record intake and output.
14. Weigh the client daily at the same time, using the same scale, after the client voids.
15. When weighing the client, ensure that the client is wearing the same clothing as when the previous weight was taken.
16. Monitor and restore fluid and electrolyte balance.

17. Monitor elimination patterns.
18. Assess and limit the client's activity level.
19. Encourage the client to participate in diversional activities.
20. Assess the client's suicidal potential.
21. Administer antidepressant medication if prescribed.
22. Encourage psychotherapy.
23. Refer the client to support groups.

II. Substance Abuse Disorders

A. Description: Substance **abuse** disorders cause behavioral and physiological changes (Box 65-1).

B. Substance dependence
1. Substance dependence is a pattern of repeated use of a substance, which usually results in tolerance, withdrawal, and compulsive drug-taking behavior.
2. The client takes substances in larger amounts and over longer periods than was intended.
3. The client has the desire to cut down but has unsuccessful efforts to decrease or discontinue use.
4. Daily activities revolve around the use of a substance.

Screening tools are available to assess a substance abuse disorder, including the Michigan Alcohol Screening Test (MAST), Drug Abuse Screening Test (DAST), and CAGE screening questionnaire.

C. Substance tolerance is the need for increased amounts of the substance to achieve the desired effect.

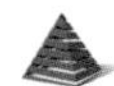

D. Substance abuse
1. The client recurrently uses substances.
2. The client experiences recurrent, significant harmful consequences related to the use of substances.
3. The client experiences a strong craving, desire, or urge to use the substance.

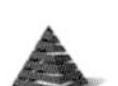

E. Substance withdrawal
1. Physiological and substance-specific cognitive symptoms occur.
2. Substance withdrawal occurs when an individual experiences a decrease in blood levels of a substance to which they are physiologically dependent.

BOX 65-1 CAGE Screening Test

C: Have you ever felt the need to *cut down* on your drinking/drug use?
A: Have you ever been *annoyed* at criticism of your drinking/drug use?
G: Have you ever felt *guilty* about something you have done when you have been drinking or taking drugs?
E: Have you ever had an *eye opener:* drinking or taking drugs first thing in the morning to get going or to avoid withdrawal symptoms?

F. Other factors to consider in the client with a substance-related disorder
1. Rebellion and peer group pressure in adolescence may contribute to the onset of substance use.
2. Substance use may become a coping mechanism for decreasing physical and emotional pain.
3. Depression may precede or occur as a result of or in association with substance use.
4. Grief and loss may be associated with substance use.

G. Dysfunctional behaviors related to substance abuse
1. Preoccupation with obtaining and using substance
2. Manipulation to avoid consequences of behavior
3. Impulsiveness
4. Anger, including physical and verbal abuse
5. Avoidance of relationships
6. Sense of self-importance and requiring special treatment
7. Denial; blaming everything but the substance use for his or her problems
8. Uses rationalization and projection to justify unacceptable behaviors
9. Likely to be involved in codependent relationships whereby a significant other also unknowingly serves as a significant enabler
10. Low self-esteem
11. Depression

III. Alcohol Abuse

A. Description
1. Alcohol is a central nervous system (CNS) depressant affecting all body tissues.
2. Physical dependence is a biological need for alcohol to avoid physical withdrawal symptoms, whereas psychological dependence refers to craving for the subjective effect of alcohol.

B. Risk factors
1. Biological predisposition. Genetic and familial predisposition may be a risk factor.
2. Depressed and highly anxious characteristics
3. Low self-esteem
4. Poor self-control
5. History of rebelliousness, poor school performance, or delinquency
6. Poor parental relationships

C. Data collection
1. Slurred speech
2. Uncoordinated movements
3. Unsteady gait
4. Restlessness
5. Belligerence
6. Confusion
7. Sneaking drinks, drinking in the morning, and experiencing blackouts

8. Binge drinking
9. Arguments about drinking
10. Missing work
11. Increased tolerance to alcohol
12. Intoxication, with blood alcohol levels of 0.1% (100 mg alcohol per deciliter of blood) or higher

⚠ Part of data collection should include the type of alcohol, how much consumed, for how many years, and date and time of the last drink.

D. Psychological symptoms
1. Depression
2. Hostility
3. Suspiciousness
4. Rationalization
5. Irritability
6. Isolation
7. Decrease in inhibitions
8. Decrease in self-esteem
9. Denial that a problem exists

E. Complications associated with chronic alcohol use
1. Vitamin deficiencies
   a. Vitamin B deficiency causing peripheral neuropathies
   b. Thiamine deficiency causing Korsakoff's syndrome (a form of amnesia)
2. Alcohol-induced persistent amnesic disorder causing severe memory problems
3. Wernicke's encephalopathy (degenerative condition of the brain) causing confusion, ataxia, and abnormal eye movements
4. Hepatitis; cirrhosis of the liver
5. Esophagitis and gastritis
6. Pancreatitis
7. Anemias
8. Immune system dysfunctions
9. Brain damage
10. Peripheral neuropathy
11. Cardiac disorders

IV. Alcohol Withdrawal

A. Description
1. Early signs develop within a few hours after cessation of alcohol intake.
2. These signs peak after 24 to 48 hours and then rapidly disappear, unless the withdrawal progresses to alcohol withdrawal delirium.
3. At the onset of withdrawal (Box 65-2), follow agency protocol using specified withdrawal assessment scales as indicated by unit or agency policy.
4. Chlordiazepoxide (Librium) is a commonly prescribed medication for acute alcohol withdrawal and is usually given orally unless a more immediate onset is required. Any benzodiazepine will decrease the withdrawal symptoms because of cross tolerance (see Chapter 67 for a list of benzodiazepines).
5. An intramuscular injection of vitamin B_1 (thiamine) followed by several days of oral administration may be prescribed to prevent Wernicke-Korsakoff's syndrome.

B. Withdrawal (see Box 65-2)

C. Withdrawal delirium: The state of delirium usually peaks 48 to 72 hours after cessation or reduction of intake (although can occur later) and lasts 2 to 3 days (Box 65-3).

⚠ Withdrawal delirium is a medical emergency. Death can occur from myocardial infarction, fat emboli, peripheral vascular collapse, electrolyte imbalance, aspiration pneumonia, or suicide.

D. Interventions
1. Provide care in a nonjudgmental manner.
2. Check the client frequently.
3. Monitor vital signs and neurological signs (as often as every 15 minutes) and provide one-to-one supervision.

BOX 65-2 Early Manifestations of Alcohol Withdrawal

Anorexia (nausea and vomiting may occur)
Anxiety
Being easily startled
Hyperalertness
Hypertension
Insomnia
Irritability
Jerky movements
Possibly experiences hallucinations, illusions, or vivid nightmares
Possibly reports a feeling of "shaking inside"
Seizures (usually appear 7 to 48 hours after cessation of alcohol)
Tachycardia
Tremors

BOX 65-3 Manifestations of Alcohol Withdrawal Delirium

Agitation
Anorexia
Anxiety
Delirium
Diaphoresis
Disorientation with fluctuating levels of consciousness
Fever (temperature of 100° to 103°F)
Hallucinations and delusions
Insomnia
Tachycardia and hypertension

4. Provide a quiet, nonstimulating environment. Encourage family members (one at a time) to stay with the client to minimize anxiety.
5. Orient the client frequently.
6. Explain all treatments and procedures in a quiet and simple manner.
7. Initiate seizure precautions.
8. Assist to administer sedating or anticonvulsant medication as prescribed.
9. Provide small, frequent, high-carbohydrate foods (administer antiemetic before meals as needed).
10. Monitor intake and output.
11. Assist to administer vitamins (multivitamin, vitamin B complex [including thiamine], and vitamin C).
12. Assist the client with activities of daily living and assist with ambulation if stable.
13. Allow the client to express fears.

E. Disulfiram (Antabuse) therapy
1. Description
   a. Disulfiram is an alcohol deterrent used for alcoholic dependence.
   b. The medication sensitizes the client to alcohol, so a disulfiram-alcohol reaction occurs if alcohol is ingested.
   c. The client must abstain from alcohol for at least 12 hours before the initial dose is administered.
   d. Adverse effects usually begin within minutes to a half hour after consuming alcohol and may last ½ to 2 hours.
   e. Alcohol consumption is avoided for up to 14 days after disulfiram therapy has been discontinued because it places the client at risk for a disulfiram-alcohol reaction.
2. Adverse reactions
   a. Facial flushing
   b. Sweating
   c. Throbbing headache
   d. Neck pain
   e. Nausea and vomiting
   f. Hypotension
   g. Tachycardia
   h. Respiratory distress
3. Client education
   a. Inform the client about the effects of the medication.
   b. Ensure that the client agrees to abstain from alcohol and any substances that contain alcohol.
   c. Inform the client that the effects of the medication may occur for several days after discontinuance.
   d. Other medications that may be used to assist with cravings include acamprosate calcium (Campral), naltrexone (ReVia), and nalmefene (Revex).

F. Dealing with the client who abuses alcohol (Boxes 65-4 and 65-5)

⚠ Inform the client who is on disulfiram (Antabuse) therapy to avoid the use of substances that contain alcohol, such as cough medicines, rubbing compounds, vinegar, mouthwashes, and aftershave lotions. The client needs to read the labels of all products.

V. Drug Dependency

A. Central nervous system (CNS) depressants
1. CNS depressants can include alcohol, benzodiazepines, and barbiturates, and they act as a depressant, sedative, and/or hypnotic.
2. Intoxication (Box 65-6)
3. Overdose can produce cardiovascular or respiratory depression, coma, shock, convulsions, and death.
4. Overdose: If the client is awake, vomiting is induced and activated charcoal is administered. If the client is comatose, airway establishment and maintenance and gastric lavage with activated charcoal are the priorities. Seizure precautions are indicated.
5. Flumazenil (Romazicon) intravenously may be used in benzodiazepine overdose to reverse the effects.

BOX 65-4 Dealing with the Client Who Abuses Alcohol

Direct the client's focus to the substance abuse problem.
Identify with the client those situations that precipitate angry feelings.
Set limits on manipulative behavior and verbal and physical abuse.
Hold the client firmly to reasonable limits, consistently reinforcing rules, with equitable consequences for breaking rules.
Hold the client accountable for all behaviors.
Assist the client to explore strengths and weaknesses.
Encourage focusing on strengths if the client is losing control.
Encourage the client to participate in group therapy and support groups.

BOX 65-5 Therapies for Substance Abuse Clients and Their Families

Behavior therapy, aversion conditioning with disulfiram (Antabuse) or another medication
Hospitalization
Psychotherapy (individual, group, family)
Support groups such as Alcoholics Anonymous; Narcotics Anonymous; Pills Anonymous; Al-Anon, Al-a-Teen, or Narc-Anon (for family members and friends of alcoholics or addicts); and Adult Children of Alcoholics
Transitional living programs (halfway houses)

BOX 65-6 Intoxication: Central Nervous System Depressants

Drowsiness
Hypotension
Impairment of memory, attention, judgment, and social or occupational functioning
Incoordination and unsteady gait
Irritability
Slurred speech

6. Withdrawal effects include nausea, vomiting, tachycardia, diaphoresis, irritability, tremors, insomnia, and seizures. Withdrawal must be treated with a carefully titrated similar drug (abrupt withdrawal can lead to death).
7. Withdrawal from CNS depressants such as barbiturates is generally treated with a barbiturate such as phenobarbital or a long-acting benzodiazepine.

B. CNS stimulants
1. CNS stimulants can include amphetamines, cocaine, and crack.
2. Intoxication (Box 65-7)
3. Overdose can produce respiratory distress, ataxia, hyperpyrexia, seizures, coma, brain attack (stroke), myocardial infarction, and death.
4. Overdose is treated with antipsychotics and management of associated effects.
5. Withdrawal effects include fatigue, depression, agitation, apathy, anxiety, insomnia, disorientation, lethargy, and craving.
6. Withdrawal is treated with antidepressants, a dopamine agonist, or bromocriptine (Parlodel). Withdrawal is primarily supportive, particularly when dealing with the severe depression and suicidal ideation that accompanies stimulant withdrawal.

C. Opioids
1. Opioids can include opium, heroin, meperidine (Demerol), morphine sulfate, codeine sulfate, methadone (Dolophine), hydromorphone (Dilaudid), and fentanyl (Sublimaze).
2. Intoxication (Box 65-8)
3. Overdose can produce respiratory depression, coma, shock, seizures, and death.
4. Overdose is treated with an opioid antagonist such as naloxone (Narcan).
5. Withdrawal effects include yawning, insomnia, irritability, rhinorrhea, diaphoresis, cramps, nausea and vomiting, muscle aches, chills, fever, lacrimation, and diarrhea.
6. Withdrawal may be treated by methadone detoxification or tapering dosage with other opioids.
7. Clonidine (Catapres) as an α-adrenergic blocker assists in reducing the severity of sympathetic nervous system–generated withdrawal discomfort.
8. Specific symptom management measures may also be used (e.g., bismuth subsalicylate [Kaopectate] for diarrhea, acetaminophen [Tylenol] for muscle aches).

D. Hallucinogens
1. Hallucinogens can include lysergic acid diethylamide (LSD), mescaline (peyote), psilocybin (mushrooms), or phencyclidine (PCP).
2. Intoxication (Box 65-9)
3. Overdose effects of LSD, peyote, and psilocybin include psychosis, brain damage, and death. Effects of PCP include psychosis, hypertensive **crisis**, hyperthermia, seizures, and respiratory arrest.

BOX 65-7 Intoxication: Central Nervous System Stimulants

Dilated pupils
Euphoria
Hypertension
Impaired judgment and social or occupational functioning
Insomnia
Nausea and vomiting
Paranoia, delusions, or hallucinations
Potential for violence
Tachycardia

BOX 65-8 Intoxication: Opioids

Constricted pupils
Decreased respirations
Drowsiness
Euphoria
Hypotension
Impaired memory, attention, and judgment
Psychomotor retardation
Slurred speech

BOX 65-9 Intoxication: Hallucinogens

Agitation and belligerence
Anxiety and depression
Bizarre, regressive, or violent behavior
Blank stare
Diaphoresis
Dilated pupils
Elevated vital signs including blood pressure
Hallucinations
Impaired judgment and social and occupational functioning
Incoordination
Muscular rigidity and chronic jerking
Paranoia
Seizures
Tachycardia
Tremors

4. Treatment (LSD, peyote, psilocybin) involves low environmental stimuli (speak slowly, clearly, and in a low voice) and medications to treat anxiety.
5. Treatment (PCP) involves possible gastric lavage (if alert), acidifying urine to assist in excreting drug, and interventions to treat behavioral disturbances, hyperthermia, hypertension, and respiratory distress.
6. Withdrawal is primarily supportive and may include medications to target particular problem behaviors, such as agitation.

E. Inhalants
1. Inhalants can include gases or liquids such as butane, paint thinner, paint and wax removers, airplane glue, nail polish remover, and nitrous oxide.
2. Intoxication (Box 65-10)
3. Overdose can cause damage to the nervous system and death.
4. Withdrawal management is mainly supportive, including treating affected body systems.

F. Marijuana (*Cannabis sativa*)
1. Marijuana generally is smoked but can be ingested.
2. Marijuana causes euphoria, detachment, relaxation, talkativeness, slowed perception of time, anxiety, or paranoia.
3. Long-term dependence can result in lethargy, difficulty concentrating, memory loss, and possibly chronic respiratory disorders.
4. Withdrawal management is mainly supportive.

G. Other recreational and club drugs
1. There are many recreational and club drugs, all of which have serious adverse and life-threatening effects. Some include ecstasy (methylenedioxymethamphetamine) GHB (gamma-hydroxybutyrate), methamphetamine (crank, meth, and other slang names), and ketamine.
2. Effects include euphoria, increased energy, increased self-confidence, and increased sociability.
3. Adverse effects include hyperthermia, rhabdomyolysis, renal failure, hepatotoxicity, depression, panic attacks, psychosis, cardiovascular collapse, and death.
4. Programs for addiction also address nicotine withdrawal and the pharmacologic and psychotherapeutic interventions for this problem, such as nicotine patches, nicotine inhalers, and bupropion (Zyban) for the reduction of withdrawal and cravings.
5. The use of anabolic steroids has been noted in the media to be the cause of adverse events, including death.

H. Interventions: Withdrawal
1. Initiate seizure precautions.
2. Hydrate the client.
3. Monitor vital signs every hour.
4. Monitor intake and output.
5. Orient client frequently.
6. Maintain minimal stimuli.
7. Approach the client in an accepting and nonjudgmental manner.
8. Direct the client's focus to the substance abuse problem.
9. Assist the client with identifying situations that precipitate angry feelings.
10. Assist the client to deal with emotions.
11. Limit the client's blame-placing or rationalizing to explain the substance abuse problem.
12. Assist the client to use assertive techniques rather than manipulation to meet needs.
13. Set limits on manipulative behavior and verbal and physical abuse.
14. Maintain firm and reasonable limits, consistently reinforcing rules, with reasonable consequences for breaking rules.
15. Hold the client accountable for all behaviors.
16. Assist the client to explore strengths and weaknesses.
17. Encourage focusing on strengths if the client is losing control.
18. Encourage the client to participate in unit activities.
19. Encourage the client to participate in group therapy and support groups.
20. Box 65-11 delineates nursing care for clients.

BOX 65-10 Intoxication: Inhalants

Enhancement of sexual pleasure
Euphoria
Excitation followed by drowsiness, light-headedness, disinhibition, and agitation
Giggling and laughter

BOX 65-11 Withdrawal: Nursing Care

Obtain information regarding the drug type and amount consumed.
Check vital signs.
Remove unnecessary objects from the environment.
Provide one-to-one supervision if necessary.
Provide a quiet, calm environment with minimal stimuli.
Maintain client orientation.
Ensure the client's safety by implementing seizure precautions.
Use restraints, if necessary and prescribed, to prevent the client from harming self and others.
Provide for physical needs.
Provide food and fluids as tolerated.
Assist to administer medications as prescribed to decrease withdrawal symptoms.
Collect blood and urine samples for drug screening.

I. Dual diagnoses
   1. Sometimes the use of alcohol and drugs masks underlying psychiatric pathology.
   2. Psychiatric pathology may also be precipitated by substance use and abuse.
   3. When psychiatric disorders and substance abuse are both present, it is often referred to as dual diagnosis.
   4. Separating out psychiatric diagnosis and substance dependence can only be done over time after a sustained period of abstinence.

⚠ Pyramid Alert: Gambling disorder is an addictive disorder and a type of impulse-control disorder. Compulsive gamblers cannot control the impulse to gamble, even when they know their gambling is hurting themselves or others. Gambling is all the compulsive gambler can think about and all he or she wants to do, no matter the consequences.

J. **Addiction** and abuse in health care professionals: Suspicious signs
   1. Frequently reporting that drugs have been wasted without being witnessed by another nurse
   2. Administering maximum dosages of controlled substances when other nurses do not
   3. A variance in usual pain relief in the absence of a change in dosage or frequency in their clients
   4. Work patterns include the following: always volunteering to carry opioid (narcotic) drug cabinet or drawer keys; choosing shifts in which less supervision is present; or choosing work areas in which the use of controlled substances is high, such as critical care units, operating rooms, anesthesia units, and trauma units.
   5. Nurses have a professional and ethical obligation to report impaired co-workers.
   6. The majority of impaired nurses are able to return to work through the State Board of Nursing assistance and monitoring programs. Such programs usually require strict adherence to clearly stated rules and regular reports and drug screens.

K. Codependency issues
   1. Codependency refers to the presence of coexisting behaviors present in a significant other, which serves to enable the addict or alcoholic to continue the irresponsible patterns of use without experiencing consequences.
   2. Examples of codependency include paying bills the addict or alcoholic is responsible for, bailing the addict or alcoholic out of jail, or helping the addict or alcoholic to call in sick.
   3. It is important to address codependency issues with the family to maximize the chance for recovery of both the client with the addiction and the person with codependent behaviors.

CRITICAL THINKING What Should You Do?

Answer: The nurse should immediately contact the health care provider if signs of alcohol withdrawal delirium occur, and the nurse should follow agency protocol using specified assessment scales. One-to-one supervision needs to be provided to ensure safety. The nurse should provide care in a nonjudgmental manner and monitor vital signs and neurological signs (every 15 minutes). The environment should be quiet and nonstimulating, and a family member should be encouraged to stay with the client to minimize anxiety. The nurse should orient the client frequently, explain all treatments and procedures in a quiet and simple manner, initiate seizure precautions, and administer sedating or anticonvulsant medication as prescribed. In addition, the nurse should provide small, frequent, high-carbohydrate foods (administer antiemetic before meals as needed).

Reference(s): deWit, D. & Kumagai, C. (2013). *Medical-surgical nursing: Concepts & practice.* (2nd ed., pp. 1068–1069, 1071). St. Louis: Saunders.

PRACTICE QUESTIONS

701. The nurse is caring for a female client who was recently admitted to the hospital for anorexia nervosa. The nurse enters the client's room and notes that the client is doing vigorous push-ups. Which nursing action is appropriate?
1. Interrupt the client and weigh her immediately.
2. Interrupt the client and offer to take her for a walk.
3. Allow the client to complete her exercise program.
4. Tell the client that she is not allowed to exercise vigorously.

❖**702.** Which are appropriate interventions for caring for the client in alcohol withdrawal? **Select all that apply.**
- ❑ 1. Monitor vital signs.
- ❑ 2. Maintain an NPO status.
- ❑ 3. Provide a safe environment.
- ❑ 4. Address hallucinations therapeutically.
- ❑ 5. Provide stimulation in the environment.
- ❑ 6. Provide reality orientation as appropriate.

703. The nursing student is developing a plan of care for the hospitalized client with bulimia nervosa. The nursing instructor intervenes if the student documents which incorrect intervention in the plan?
1. Monitor intake and output.
2. Monitor electrolyte levels.
3. Observe for excessive exercise.
4. Monitor for the use of laxatives and diuretics.

704. The nurse is monitoring a client who abuses alcohol for signs of alcohol withdrawal delirium. The nurse should monitor for which?
1. Hypotension, ataxia, vomiting
2. Stupor, agitation, muscular rigidity
3. Hypotension, bradycardia, agitation
4. Hypertension, disorientation, hallucinations

705. The spouse of a client admitted to the hospital for alcohol withdrawal says to the nurse, "I should get out of this bad situation." The **most** helpful response by the nurse should be which?
1. "Why don't you tell your husband about this?"
2. "This is not the best time to make that decision."
3. "What do you find difficult about this situation?"
4. "I agree with you. You should get out of this situation."

706. The nurse is caring for a client who is suspected of being dependent on drugs. Which question should be appropriate for the nurse to ask when collecting data from the client regarding drug abuse?
1. "Why did you get started on these drugs?"
2. "How much do you use and what effect does it have on you?"
3. "How long did you think you could take these drugs without someone finding out?"
4. The nurse does not ask any questions because of fear that the client is in denial and will throw the nurse out of the room.

707. A client who has been drinking alcohol on a regular basis admits to having "a problem" and is asking for assistance with the problem. The nurse should encourage the client to attend which community group?
1. Al-Anon
2. Fresh Start
3. Families Anonymous
4. Alcoholics Anonymous

708. A client with a diagnosis of anorexia nervosa, who is in a state of starvation, is in a two-bed hospital room. A newly admitted client will be assigned to this client's room. Which client should be an appropriate choice as this client's roommate?
1. A client with pneumonia
2. A client receiving diagnostic tests
3. A client who thrives on managing others
4. A client who could benefit from the client's assistance at mealtimes

709. The nurse is assigned to care for a client at risk for alcohol withdrawal. The nurse monitors the client, knowing that the **early** signs of withdrawal will usually develop within which time after cessation or reduction of alcohol intake?
1. In 7 days
2. In 14 days
3. In 21 days
4. Within a few hours

710. The nurse determines that the wife of an alcoholic client is benefiting from attending an Al-Anon group when the nurse hears the wife say which?
1. "I no longer feel that I deserve the beatings my husband inflicts on me."
2. "My attendance at the meetings has helped me to see that I provoke my husband's violence."
3. "I enjoy attending the meetings because they get me out of the house and away from my husband."
4. "I can tolerate my husband's destructive behaviors now that I know they are common in alcoholics."

711. A female client with anorexia nervosa is a member of a support group. The client has verbalized that she would like to buy some new clothes, but her finances are limited. Group members have brought some used clothes for the client to replace her old clothes. The client believes that the new clothes were much too tight, so she has reduced her calorie intake to 800 calories daily. The nurse identifies this behavior as which?
1. Normal
2. Regression
3. Indicative of the client's ambivalence
4. Evidence of the client's altered and distorted body image

712. A hospitalized client with a history of alcohol abuse tells the nurse, "I am leaving now. I have to go. I don't want any more treatment. I have things that I have to do right away." The client has not been discharged. In fact, the client is scheduled for an important diagnostic test to be performed in 1 hour. After the nurse discusses the client's concerns with the client, the client dresses and begins to walk out of the hospital room. The appropriate nursing action is which?
1. Call the nursing supervisor.
2. Call security to block all exit areas.
3. Restrain the client until the health care provider (HCP) can be reached.
4. Tell the client that she cannot return to this hospital again if she leaves now.

713. The nursing student is asked to identify the characteristics of bulimia nervosa. Which response by the student indicates a **need to further research** the disorder?
1. Dental erosion
2. Electrolyte imbalances
3. Enlarged parotid glands
4. Body weight well below ideal range

714. The nurse is caring for a client who has a history of opioid abuse and is monitoring the client for signs of withdrawal. Which manifestations are specifically associated with withdrawal from opioids?

1. Dilated pupils, tachycardia, and diaphoresis
2. Yawning, irritability, diaphoresis, cramps, and diarrhea
3. Tachycardia, hypertension, sweating, and marked tremors
4. Depressed feelings, high drug craving, fatigue, and agitation

715. The nurse is caring for a client with anorexia nervosa. The nurse is monitoring the behavior of the client and understands that the client with anorexia nervosa manages anxiety by which action?

1. Engaging in immoral acts
2. Always reinforcing self-approval
3. Observing rigid rules and regulations
4. Having the need to always make the right decision

ANSWERS

701. 2

Rationale: Clients with anorexia nervosa are frequently preoccupied with vigorous exercise and push themselves beyond normal limits to work off caloric intake. The nurse must provide for appropriate exercise as well as place limits on vigorous activities. Options 1, 3, and 4 are inappropriate nursing actions.

Test-Taking Strategy: Focus on the subject, anorexia nervosa. Recalling that the nurse needs to set firm limits with clients who have this disorder will direct you to option 2. **Review:** interventions for the client with anorexia nervosa.

Level of Cognitive Ability: Applying
Client Needs: Physiological Integrity
Integrated Process: Nursing Process/Implementation
Content Area: Mental Health
Priority Concepts: Nutrition, Safety
Reference(s): Varcarolis (2013), pp. 236–237.

❖ **702. 1, 3, 4, 6**

Rationale: When the client is experiencing withdrawal from alcohol, the priority for care is to prevent the client from harming himself or herself or others. The nurse would provide a low-stimulation environment to maintain the client in as calm a state as possible. The nurse would monitor the vital signs closely and report abnormal findings. The nurse would frequently reorient the client to reality and would address hallucinations therapeutically. Adequate nutritional and fluid intake must be maintained.

Test-Taking Strategy: Use therapeutic communication techniques to assist in selecting the correct interventions. Also, recalling the characteristics associated with alcohol withdrawal will assist in answering correctly. **Review:** interventions for alcohol withdrawal.

Level of Cognitive Ability: Applying
Client Needs: Psychosocial Integrity
Integrated Process: Nursing Process/Implementation
Content Area: Mental Health
Priority Concepts: Addiction, Safety
Reference(s): Stuart (2013), p. 454.

703. 3

Rationale: Excessive exercise is a characteristic of anorexia nervosa, not bulimia nervosa. Frequent vomiting, in addition to laxative and diuretic abuse, may lead to dehydration and electrolyte imbalance. Monitoring for both dehydration and electrolyte imbalance is an important nursing action. Option 3 is the only option that is not associated with care of the client with bulimia.

Test-Taking Strategy: Note the word, *incorrect,* in the question. This word indicates the need to select the incorrect intervention. Options 1, 2, and 4 are comparable or alike and directly or indirectly infer concern about fluid and electrolyte balance. Option 3 is different from the other options. **Review:** the characteristics associated with **bulimia nervosa.**

Level of Cognitive Ability: Analyzing
Client Needs: Physiological Integrity
Integrated Process: Nursing Process/Planning
Content Area: Mental Health
Priority Concepts: Fluid and Electrolyte Balance, Nutrition
Reference(s): Stuart (2013), p. 490.

704. 4

Rationale: The symptoms associated with alcohol withdrawal delirium typically are anxiety, insomnia, anorexia, hypertension, disorientation, visual or tactile hallucinations, agitation, fever, and delusions.

Test-Taking Strategy: Focus on the subject, signs of alcohol withdrawal. Review each option carefully to ensure that all the symptoms are contained in the correct option. Eliminate options 1 and 3 first, knowing that hypertension rather than hypotension occurs. From the remaining options, recalling that the client who is stuporous is not likely to exhibit agitation will direct you to option 4. **Review:** symptoms associated with alcohol withdrawal.

Level of Cognitive Ability: Analyzing
Client Needs: Physiological Integrity
Integrated Process: Nursing Process/Data Collection
Content Area: Mental Health
Priority Concepts: Addiction, Psychosis
Reference(s): deWit, Kumagai (2013), p. 1068.

705. 3

Rationale: The most helpful response is the one that encourages the client to problem solve. Giving advice implies that the nurse knows what is best and can also foster dependency. The nurse should not agree with the client, nor should the nurse request that the client provide explanations.

Test-Taking Strategy: Note the strategic word, *most.* Use therapeutic communication techniques. Eliminate option 1 because of the word *why,* which should be avoided

in communication. Eliminate option 2 because this option places the client's feelings on hold. Eliminate option 4 because the nurse is agreeing with the client. Option 3 is the only option that addresses the client's feelings. **Review: therapeutic communication techniques.**
Level of Cognitive Ability: Applying
Client Needs: Psychosocial Integrity
Integrated Process: Communication and Documentation
Content Area: Mental Health
Priority Concepts: Addiction, Communication
Reference(s): deWit, Kumagai (2013), pp. 1076–1077; Varcarolis (2013), pp. 120–123, 382.

706. 2
Rationale: Whenever the nurse collects data from a client who is dependent on drugs, it is best for the nurse to attempt to elicit information by being nonjudgmental and direct. Option 1 is incorrect because it is judgmental, off focus, and reflects the nurse's bias. Option 3 is incorrect because it is judgmental, insensitive, and aggressive, which is nontherapeutic. Option 4 is incorrect because it indicates passivity on the nurse's part and uses rationalization to avoid the therapeutic nursing intervention.
Test-Taking Strategy: Use **therapeutic communication techniques** to answer the question. Option 2 is the statement that is nonjudgmental and direct. **Review:** data collection of a client who is a **drug abuser.**
Level of Cognitive Ability: Applying
Client Needs: Psychosocial Integrity
Integrated Process: Nursing Process/Data Collection
Content Area: Mental Health
Priority Concepts: Addiction, Communication
Reference(s): deWit, Kumagai (2013), pp. 1076–1077; Varcarolis (2013), pp. 120–123, 382.

707. 4
Rationale: Alcoholics Anonymous is a major self-help organization for the treatment of alcoholism. Option 1 is a group for families of alcoholics. Option 3 is for parents of children who abuse substances. Option 2 is for nicotine addicts.
Test-Taking Strategy: Focus on the **subject**, self-help groups for an alcoholic. If you are unfamiliar with these support groups, note the relation between *drinking* in the question and *Alcoholics* in the correct option. **Review:** purposes of specific **support groups.**
Level of Cognitive Ability: Applying
Client Needs: Safe and Effective Care Environment
Integrated Process: Nursing Process/Implementation
Content Area: Mental Health
Priority Concepts: Addiction, Communication
Reference(s): Varcarolis (2013), p. 391.

708. 2
Rationale: The client receiving diagnostic tests is an appropriate roommate. The client with anorexia is most likely experiencing hematological complications, such as leukopenia. Having a roommate with pneumonia would place the client with anorexia nervosa at risk for infection. The client with anorexia nervosa should not be put in a situation in which he or she can focus on the nutritional needs of others or be managed by others, because this may contribute to sublimation and suppression of his or her own hunger.
Test-Taking Strategy: Note the **subject**, a state of starvation. Recalling the characteristics and complications associated with anorexia nervosa will direct you to the correct option. **Review:** care of the client with **anorexia nervosa.**
Level of Cognitive Ability: Analyzing
Client Needs: Safe and Effective Care Environment
Integrated Process: Nursing Process/Planning
Content Area: Mental Health
Priority Concepts: Infection, Nutrition
Reference(s): Stuart (2013), p. 481.

709. 4
Rationale: Early signs of alcohol withdrawal develop within a few hours after cessation or reduction of alcohol and peak after 24 to 48 hours.
Test-Taking Strategy: Note the **strategic word**, *early*. This will assist in directing you to the correct option. **Review:** the signs/symptoms associated with **alcohol withdrawal.**
Level of Cognitive Ability: Understanding
Client Needs: Physiological Integrity
Integrated Process: Nursing Process/Data Collection
Content Area: Mental Health
Priority Concepts: Addiction, Clinical Judgment
Reference(s): deWit, Kumagai (2013), p. 1068.

710. 1
Rationale: Al-Anon support groups are a protected, supportive opportunity for spouses and significant others to learn what to expect and to obtain suggestions about successful behavioral changes. Option 1 is the healthiest response because it exemplifies an understanding that the alcoholic partner is responsible for his behavior and cannot be allowed to blame family members for loss of control. The nonalcoholic partner should not feel responsible when the spouse loses control (option 2). Option 4 indicates that the wife remains codependent. Option 3 indicates that the group is being seen as an escape, not a place to work on issues.
Test-Taking Strategy: Focus on the **subject** of the question, benefiting from attending an Al-Anon group. This will direct you to the correct option. **Review:** the purpose of **Al-Anon.**
Level of Cognitive Ability: Evaluating
Client Needs: Psychosocial Integrity
Integrated Process: Nursing Process/Evaluation
Content Area: Mental Health
Priority Concepts: Addiction, Interpersonal Violence
Reference(s): deWit, Kumagai (2013), p. 1078.

711. 4
Rationale: Altered or distorted body image is a concern with clients with anorexia nervosa. Although the client may struggle with ambivalence and present with regressed behavior, the client's coping pattern relates to the basic issue of distorted body image. The client's behavior is not normal.
Test-Taking Strategy: Focus on the information provided in the question to determine that the **subject** relates to a distorted body image. This will direct you to the correct option. **Review:** characteristics associated with the client with **anorexia nervosa.**
Level of Cognitive Ability: Understanding
Client Needs: Psychosocial Integrity
Integrated Process: Nursing Process/Data Collection

Content Area: Mental Health
Priority Concepts: Coping, Nutrition
Reference(s): Stuart (2013), p. 494.

712. 1
Rationale: The nurse can be charged with false imprisonment if a client is made to wrongfully believe that he or she cannot leave the hospital. Notifying the nurse supervisor is the correct option. Most health care facilities have documents that the client is asked to sign that relate to the client's responsibilities when he or she leaves against medical advice (AMA). The client should be asked to sign this document before leaving. The nurse should request that the client wait to speak to the HCP before leaving, but if the client refuses to do so, the nurse cannot hold the client against his or her will. Restraining the client and calling security to block exits constitutes false imprisonment. Any client has a right to health care (option 4) and cannot be told otherwise.
Test-Taking Strategy: Keeping the concept of false imprisonment in mind, eliminate options 2 and 3 because they are **comparable or alike**. Eliminate option 4, knowing that any client has a right to health care. **Review:** points related to false **imprisonment.**
Level of Cognitive Ability: Applying
Client Needs: Safe and Effective Care Environment
Integrated Process: Nursing Process/Implementation
Content Area: Mental Health
Priority Concepts: Addiction, Health Care Law
Reference(s): Varcarolis (2013), pp. 87–88.

713. 4
Rationale: Clients with bulimia nervosa may not initially appear to be physically or emotionally ill. They are often at or slightly below ideal body weight. On further inspection, the client demonstrates enlargement of the parotid glands with dental erosion and caries if he or she has been inducing vomiting. Electrolyte imbalances are present.
Test-Taking Strategy: Focus on the **subject**, bulimia nervosa. Note the **strategic words**, *need to further research*. These words indicate a **negative event query** and the need to select the incorrect characteristic of bulimia nervosa. Focusing on the client's diagnosis will direct you to option 4. Option 4 is a characteristic sign of anorexia nervosa, not bulimia nervosa. **Review:** characteristics of **anorexia nervosa**.
Level of Cognitive Ability: Evaluating
Client Needs: Physiological Integrity
Integrated Process: Teaching and Learning
Content Area: Mental Health
Priority Concepts: Fluid and Electrolyte Balance, Nutrition
Reference(s): Varcarolis (2013), pp. 240–241.

714. 2
Rationale: Opioids are central nervous system (CNS) depressants. Withdrawal effects include yawning, insomnia, irritability, rhinorrhea, diaphoresis, cramps, nausea and vomiting, muscle aches, chills, fever, lacrimation, and diarrhea. Withdrawal is treated by methadone tapering or medication detoxification. Option 2 identifies the clinical manifestations associated with withdrawal from opioids. Option 3 describes withdrawal from alcohol. Option 1 describes intoxication from hallucinogens. Option 4 describes withdrawal from cocaine.
Test-Taking Strategy: Focus on the **subject** of the question, the clinical manifestations associated with withdrawal from opioids. Recalling that opioids are CNS depressants will direct you to option 2. **Review:** the manifestations associated with **opioid withdrawal.**
Level of Cognitive Ability: Analyzing
Client Needs: Physiological Integrity
Integrated Process: Nursing Process/Data Collection
Content Area: Mental Health
Priority Concepts: Clinical Judgment, Addiction
Reference(s): deWit, Kumagai (2013), p. 1073.

715. 3
Rationale: Clients with anorexia nervosa have the desire to please others. Their need to be correct or perfect interferes with rational decision-making processes. These clients are moralistic. Rules and rituals help the clients manage their anxiety. Options 1, 2, and 4 are incorrect.
Test-Taking Strategy: Focus on the **subject**, managing anxiety. Eliminate options 2 and 4 because of the closed-ended word, *always*. Eliminate option 1 because it is not characteristic of the client with anorexia. **Review:** characteristics associated with **anorexia nervosa.**
Level of Cognitive Ability: Understanding
Client Needs: Psychosocial Integrity
Integrated Process: Nursing Process/Data Collection
Content Area: Mental Health
Priority Concepts: Cognition, Nutrition
Reference(s): Stuart (2013), p. 483.

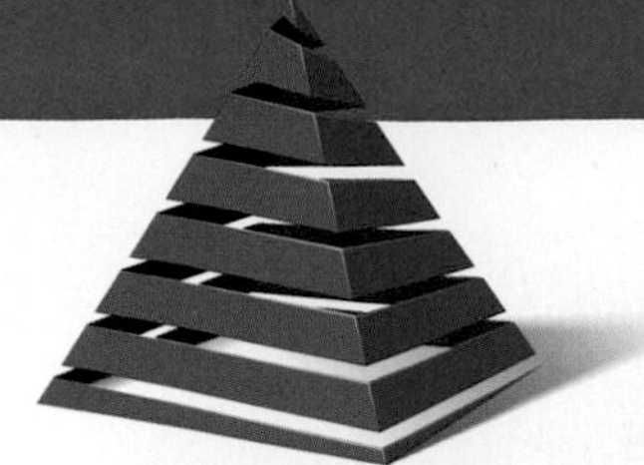

CHAPTER 66

Crisis Theory and Intervention

CRITICAL THINKING What Should You Do?

A female victim of rape has just arrived at the emergency department. What should the nurse do?
Answer located on p. 946.

I. Crisis Intervention

A. Description
   1. **Crisis** is a temporary state of severe emotional disorganization caused by failure of **coping mechanisms** and lack of support.
   2. Decision making and problem solving are inadequate.
   3. Treatment is aimed at assisting the client and the family through the stressful situation.

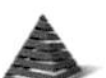

B. Phases of a crisis
   1. Phase 1: External precipitating event
   2. Phase 2
      a. Perception of the threat
      b. Increase in anxiety
      c. Client may cope or resolve the crisis.
   3. Phase 3
      a. Failure of coping
      b. Increasing disorganization
      c. Emergence of physical symptoms
      d. Relationship problems
   4. Phase 4
      a. Mobilization of internal and external resources
      b. Goal is to return the individual to at least a precrisis level of functioning.

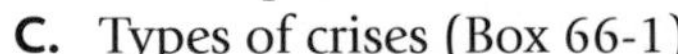

C. Types of crises (Box 66-1)

D. Crisis intervention
   1. Treatment is immediate, supportive, and directly responsive to the immediate crisis.
   2. Interventions are goal directed.
   3. Feelings of the client are acknowledged.
   4. Intervention provides opportunities for expression and validation of feelings.
   5. Connections are made between the meaning of the event and the crisis.
   6. Client explores alternative coping mechanisms and tries out new behaviors.

II. Grief

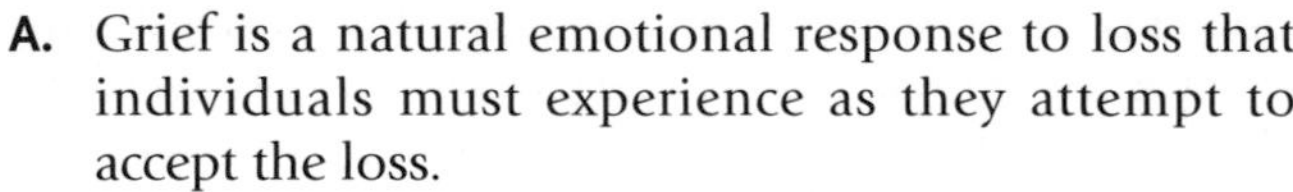

A. Grief is a natural emotional response to loss that individuals must experience as they attempt to accept the loss.

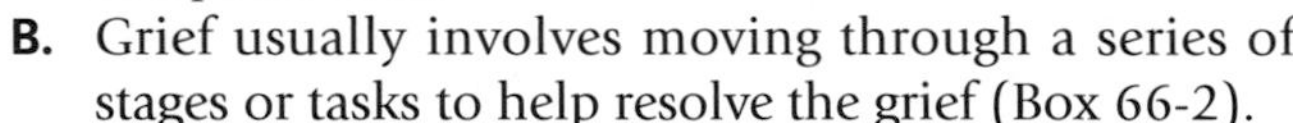

B. Grief usually involves moving through a series of stages or tasks to help resolve the grief (Box 66-2).

C. Feelings associated with grief can include anger, frustration, loneliness, sadness, guilt, regret, or peace.

D. Healing can occur when the pain of the loss has lessened and the survivor has adapted to life without the deceased. The survivor will continue to experience memories of the deceased.

E. Types of grief
   1. Normal grief: Physical, emotional, cognitive, or behavioral reactions can occur. The process of resolution can take months to years.
   2. Anticipatory grief occurs before the loss and is associated with an acute, chronic, or terminal illness.
   3. Disenfranchised grief occurs when a loss is experienced and cannot be acknowledged openly. (Societal norms do not define the loss as a loss within its traditional definition.)
   4. Dysfunctional grief occurs with prolonged emotional instability and a lack of progression to successful coping with the loss.
   5. Children's grief is based on their developmental level (Box 66-3).

III. Loss

A. Loss is the absence of something desired or previously thought to be available.

B. Actual loss can be identified by others and can arise in response to or in anticipation of a situation.

C. Perceived loss is experienced by one person and cannot be verified by others.

D. Anticipatory loss is experienced before the loss occurs.

E. Mourning
   1. The outward and social expression of loss
   2. May be dictated by cultural and religious beliefs

F. Bereavement
   1. Includes the inner feelings and the outward reactions of the survivor
   2. Includes grief and mourning

BOX 66-1 Types of Crises

Maturational Crisis

Relates to developmental stages and associated role changes; examples include marriage, birth of a child, and retirement.

Situational Crisis

Arises from an external source, is often unanticipated, and is associated with a life event that upsets an individual or a group's psychological equilibrium; examples include loss of a job or a change in job, a change in financial status, death of a loved one, divorce, abortion, and severe physical or mental illness.

Adventitious Crisis

Relates to a crisis of disaster or an event that is not a part of everyday life and is unplanned and accidental. This type of crisis may result from a natural disaster such as a flood, earthquake, hurricane, fire, or tornado; a national disaster such as war, riots, or acts of terrorism; or a crime of violence such as rape, assault, murder, spousal or child abuse.

BOX 66-2 The Grief Response

Stage 1: Shock and Disbelief

The survivor may have feelings of numbness, difficulties with decision making, emotional outbursts, denial, and isolation.

Stage 2: Experiencing the Loss

The survivor may feel angry at the loved one who died or may feel guilt about the death.

Bargaining and/or depression may also occur in this stage.

Stage 3: Reintegration

The survivor begins to reorganize his or her life and accepts the reality of the loss.

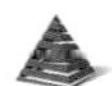 IV. Nurse's Role: Grief and Loss (Box 66-4)

A. Allow ongoing opportunities for fully informed choices.

B. Facilitate the grief process. Assess grief and assist the survivor to feel the loss and complete the tasks of the grief process.

C. Grief affects survivors physically, psychologically, socially, and spiritually; therefore, a multidisciplinary team approach including a bereavement specialist facilitates the grief process.

⚠ The nurse's role in the grief and loss process includes communicating with the client, family members, and significant other. The nurse must consider the survivor's culture, religion, family structure, individual life experiences, coping skills, and support systems.

BOX 66-3 Children's Grief

Birth to 1 Year

The infant has no concept of death.

The infant reacts to the loss of mother or caregiver.

1 to 2 Years

The child may see death as reversible.

The grief response occurs only to the death of the significant person in the child's life.

The child may scream, withdraw, or become disinterested in the environment.

2 to 5 Years

The child may see death as reversible.

The child has a sense of loss and is concerned about who will provide care.

Regression or aggressive behavior may occur.

5 to 9 Years

The child begins to see death as permanent.

The child may feel responsible for the occurrence.

The child has difficulty concentrating.

Preadolescent Through Adolescence

The adolescent sees death as permanent.

The adolescent experiences a strong emotional reaction.

The adolescent may regress.

BOX 66-4 Communication during Grief and Loss

Determine how much the client and family want to know.

Determine whether there is a spokesperson for the family.

Be aware of cultural and religious beliefs and how they may affect the communication process. Consider personal space issues, eye contact, and touch.

Obtain an interpreter if necessary.

Allow opportunity for informed choices.

Assist with the decision-making process if asked. Use problem solving to assist in decision making, and avoid interjecting personal views or opinions.

Encourage expression of feelings, concerns, and fears.

Be honest and truthful, and let the client and family know that you will not abandon them.

Ask the client and family about their expectations and needs.

Be a sensitive listener. Sit in silence if necessary and appropriate.

Extend touch and hold the client's or family member's hand if appropriate.

Encourage reminiscing.

If you do not know what to do in a particular situation, seek assistance.

If you do not know what to say to a client or family who is talking about death, listen attentively and use therapeutic communication techniques such as open-ended questions or reflection.

Acknowledge your own feelings. Let the client and family know that the topic of conversation is a difficult one and that you do not know what to say.

Realize that it is acceptable to cry with the client and family during the grief process.

Mental Health

V. Suicidal Behavior

A. Description
   1. Suicidal clients characteristically have feelings of worthlessness, guilt, and hopelessness that are so overwhelming that they feel unable to go on with life and feel unfit to live.
   2. The nurse caring for a depressed client always considers the possibility of suicide.

B. High-risk groups
   1. Those with a history of previous **suicide attempts**
   2. Family history of suicide attempts
   3. Adolescents
   4. Older clients
   5. Disabled or terminally ill adults
   6. Clients with personality disorders
   7. Clients with organic brain syndrome or dementia
   8. Depressed or psychotic clients
   9. Substance abusers

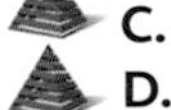
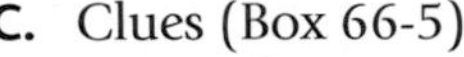

C. Clues (Box 66-5)

D. Data collection (Box 66-6)

E. Interventions
   1. Initiate suicide precautions.
   2. Do not leave the client alone.
   3. Provide a nonjudgmental, caring attitude.
   4. Develop a contract (per psychiatrist prescription and agency procedures) that is written, dated, and signed and that indicates alternative behavior at times of suicidal thoughts.
   5. Encourage the client to talk about feelings and identify positive aspects about self.
   6. Encourage active participation in own care.
   7. Keep the client active by assigning achievable tasks.
   8. Check that visitors do not leave harmful objects in the client's room.
   9. Identify support systems.
   10. Do not allow the client to leave the unit unless accompanied by a staff member.
   11. Continue to assess the client's suicide potential.

⚠ Provide one-to-one supervision at all times for the client at risk for suicide.

BOX 66-5 Suicidal Clues

Giving away personal, special, and prized possessions
Canceling social engagements
Making out or changing a will
Taking out or changing insurance policies
Positive or negative changes in behavior
Poor appetite
Sleeping difficulties
Feelings of hopelessness
Difficulty in concentrating
Loss of interest in activities
Client statements that indicate intent to attempt suicide
Sudden calmness or improvement in a depressed client
Client questions about poisons, guns, or other lethal objects

BOX 66-6 Suicidal Client: Data Collection

The Plan

Does the client have a plan?
What is the plan, how lethal is the plan, and how likely is death to occur?
Does the client have the means to carry out the plan?

Client History of Attempts

What suicide attempts occurred in the past, and what were the outcomes (i.e., physiological injuries)?
Was the client accidentally rescued?
Have the past attempts and methods been the same, or have methods increased in lethality?

Psychosocial

Is the client alone or alienated from others?
Is hostility or depression present?
Do hallucinations exist?
Is substance abuse present?
Has the client had any recent losses or physical illness?
Has the client had any environmental or lifestyle changes?

VI. Abusive Behaviors

A. Anger
   1. A feeling of annoyance that may be displaced onto an object or person
   2. Used to avoid anxiety and gives a feeling of power in situations in which the person feels out of control

B. Aggression can be harmful and destructive when not controlled.

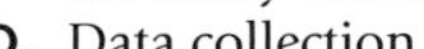
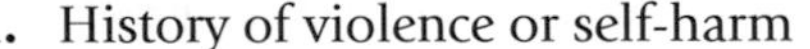
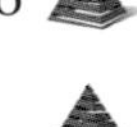
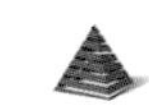

C. Violence is the physical force that is threatening to the safety of self and others.

D. Data collection
   1. History of violence or self-harm
   2. Poor impulse control and low tolerance of frustration
   3. Defiance and argumentativeness
   4. Raising of voice
   5. Making verbal threats
   6. Pacing and agitation
   7. Muscle rigidity
   8. Flushed face
   9. Glaring at others

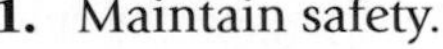

E. Interventions
   1. Maintain safety.
   2. Use a calm approach and communicate with a calm, clear tone of voice. (Be assertive but not aggressive, and avoid verbal struggles.)
   3. Maintain a large personal space, and use a nonaggressive posture.
   4. Listen actively and acknowledge the client's anger.
   5. Determine what the client considers to be his or her need.

6. Provide the client with clear options that deal with the client's behavior, set limits on behavior, and make the client aware of the consequences of anger and violence.
7. Discuss the use of restraints or seclusion if the client is unable to control angry behavior that may lead to violence.
8. Assist the client with problem solving and decision making regarding the options.

F. Restraints (security devices) and seclusion
1. Description
   a. Physical **restraints**: Any manual method or mechanical device, material, or equipment that inhibits free movement
   b. **Seclusion**: A process in which a client is placed alone in a specially designed room for protection and close supervision
   c. Chemical restraints: Medications given for a specific purpose of inhibiting a specific behavior or movement and that have an impact on the client's ability to relate to the environment
2. Use of restraints and seclusion

Restraints require a written prescription by the health care provider, which must be reviewed and renewed every 24 hours. The prescription must specify the type of restraint or seclusion and the criteria for release. (Agency policy and procedures must be followed.)

   a. Restraints and seclusion should never be used as punishment or for the convenience of the health care staff.
   b. Restraints and seclusion are used when behavior is physically harmful to the client or others and when alternative or less restrictive measures are insufficient in protecting the client or others from harm.
   c. The nurse must document the behavior leading to the use of restraints or seclusion.
   d. Restraints and seclusion are used when the client anticipates that a controlled environment would be helpful and requests seclusion.
   e. In an emergency, the qualified nurse may place a client in restraints or seclusion and obtain a written or verbal prescription as soon as possible thereafter.
   f. Within 1 hour of the initiation of restraints or seclusion, the psychiatrist must make a face-to-face assessment and evaluation of the client and must continuously re-evaluate the need for continued restraint or seclusion.
   g. While in restraints or seclusion, the client must be protected from all sources of harm by having one-to-one supervision with a staff member within an arm's length of the client.
   h. The client in restraints or seclusion needs constant one-to-one supervision. Physical, safety, and comfort needs must be assessed every 15 to 30 minutes, and these observations are also documented (such as food, fluids, bathroom needs, range-of-motion exercise, and ambulation).

VII. Bullying

A. Bullying is the **abuse** of power by an individual on another through repeated aggressive acts.
B. It most often occurs in children and in high school or college environments but can also occur in the workplace or other environments.
C. The bully feels power from sources such as physical strength, maturity, a higher status within a peer group, from knowing the victim's weaknesses, or from support of others.
D. Bullying can occur in the form of physical harm, relational aggression, isolation and exclusion, and verbal harm such as slander, rumors, or threats; it is both intentionally cruel and unprovoked.
E. Cyberbullying is also a form of bullying and occurs in the form of Internet messages on social media networks, text messages, e-mails, photos being posted, and rumors.
F. The bullied person is repeatedly experiencing negative actions from the bully(s).
G. These bully acts can lead to depression, low self-esteem, humiliation, isolation, and social withdrawal in the victim; it could result in suicide and murder.
H. The nurse's responsibility is to observe for signs of bullying and to educate teachers, school administrators, and parents about bullying behaviors and signs that it may be occurring.

VIII. Family Violence

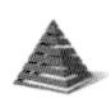

A. Description (Fig. 66-1)
1. The violence begins with threats or verbal or physical minor assaults (tension building), and the victim attempts to comply with the requests of the abuser.
2. The abuser loses control and becomes destructive and harmful (acute battering), while the victim attempts to protect himself or herself.
3. After the battering, the abuser then becomes loving and attempts to make peace (calmness and a diffusion of tension).
4. The abuser justifies that violence is normal and the victim is responsible for the **abuse**.
5. Outsiders are usually not aware of what is happening in the family.
6. Family members are isolated socially and lack autonomy and trust among one another. Caring and intimacy in the family are absent.

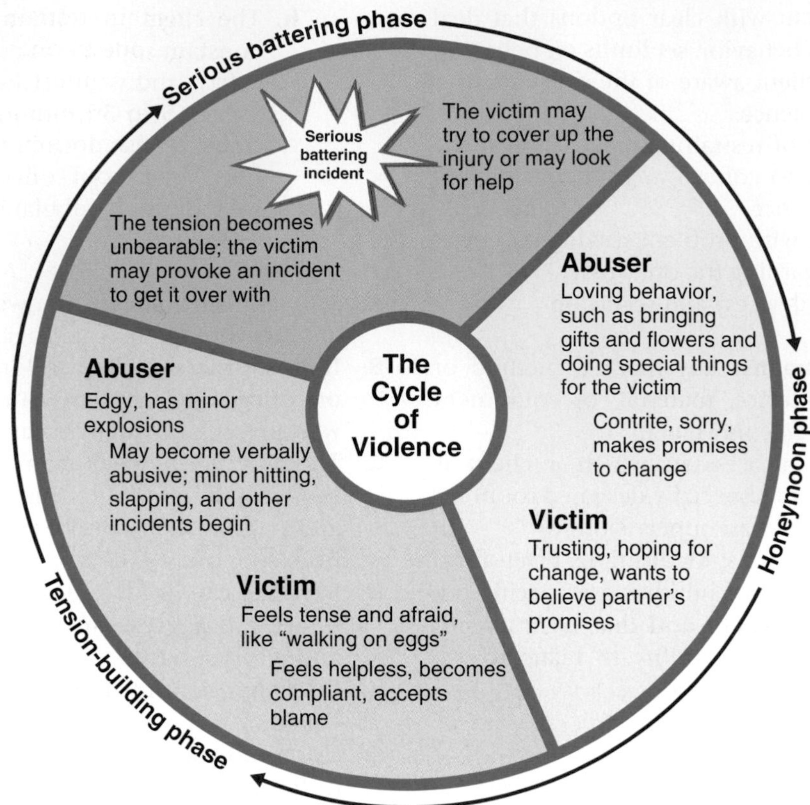

FIGURE 66-1 The cycle of violence. (Redrawn from YWCA of Annapolis and Anne Arundel County, 1517 Ritchie Highway, Arnold, MD 21012.)

7. Family members expect other members of the family to meet their needs, but none are able to do so.
8. The abuser threatens to abandon the family.

B. Types of violence (Box 66-7)

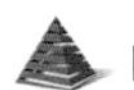 C. The vulnerable person
1. The vulnerable person is the one in the family unit against whom violence is perpetrated.
2. Those most vulnerable are children and older adults.
3. The perpetrator of violence and the person targeted by the violence can be male or female.
4. Battering is a crime.

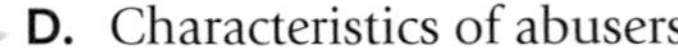 D. Characteristics of abusers
1. Impaired self-esteem
2. Strong dependency needs
3. Narcissistic and suspicious
4. History of abuse during childhood
5. Perceive victims as their property and believe that they are entitled to abuse them

E. Characteristics of victims
1. Victims feel trapped, dependent, helpless, and powerless.
2. Victims of abuse may become depressed as they are trapped in the abuser's power and control cycle (see Fig. 66-1).
3. As victims' self-esteem becomes diminished with chronic abuse, they may blame themselves for the violence and be unable to see a way out of the situation.

BOX 66-7 Types of Violence

Physical violence: Infliction of physical pain or bodily harm
Sexual violence: Any form of sexual contact without consent
Emotional violence: Infliction of mental anguish
Physical neglect: Failure to provide health care to prevent or treat physical or emotional illnesses
Developmental neglect: Failure to provide physical and cognitive stimulation needed to prevent developmental deficits
Educational neglect: Depriving a child of education
Economic exploitation: Illegal or improper exploitation of money, funds, or other resources for one's personal gain

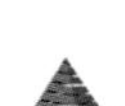
F. Interventions
1. Report suspected or actual cases of child abuse or abuse to the older adult to appropriate authorities. (Follow state and agency guidelines.)
2. Check for evidence of physical injuries.
3. Ensure privacy and confidentiality during data collection, and provide a nonjudgmental and empathetic approach to foster trust. Reassure the victim that he or she has not done anything wrong. (See Box 66-8 for examples of data collection questions.)
4. Assist the victim to develop self-protective abilities and other problem-solving abilities.

BOX 66-8 Data Collection Questions for Violence and Abuse

"Has anyone ever touched you in a way that made you uncomfortable?"
"Is anyone hurting you now?"
"How do you and your partner deal with anger (or disagreement)?"
"Has your partner ever hit you?"
"Have you ever been threatened by ______?"
"Does your partner prevent you from seeing family or friends?"
"Does your partner ever use the children to manipulate you?"
"Did (or does) anyone in your family deal with anger by hitting?"
"Whom do you play with most often? Is there anyone you do not like playing with? Are there games you don't like playing?"

5. Even if the victim is not ready to leave the situation, encourage the victim to develop a specific safety plan (a fast escape if the violence resumes) and the best place to obtain help (hotlines, safe houses, and shelters). An abused person is usually reluctant to call the police.
6. Assess the suicidal potential of the victim.
7. Assess the potential for homicide.
8. Check for the use of drugs and alcohol.
9. Determine family coping patterns and support systems.
10. Provide support and assistance in coping with contacting the legal system.
11. Assist in resolving family dysfunction with prescribed therapies.
12. Encourage individual therapy as prescribed for the victim that promotes coping with the trauma and prevents further psychological conflict.
13. Individual therapy that focuses on preventing violent behavior and repairing relationships is encouraged for abusers.
14. Encourage as prescribed, psychotherapy, counseling, group therapy, and support groups to assist family members to develop coping strategies.
15. Assist the family to access community and personal resources.
16. Maintain accurate and thorough medical health records.

IX. Child Abduction

A. Description

1. Child abduction is the kidnapping of a child (or infant) by an older person.
2. Occurrences
   a. A stranger may kidnap a child for criminal or mischievous purposes.
   b. A stranger may kidnap a child (or infant) to bring up him or her as that person's own child.
   c. A parent removes or retains a child from the other parent's care (often in the course of or after divorce proceedings).
3. Because of the increased independence that occurs in the preschool-age child, parents are less able to provide the constant protection they once did when the child reaches this age; interventions (including teaching the child) that ensure protection are necessary.

B. Interventions

1. Instruct the parents to teach a child basic guidelines about personal safety that include the following:
   a. Do not go anywhere alone.
   b. Always tell an adult where he or she is going and when he or she will return.
   c. Say *no* if he or she feels uncomfortable with a situation.
   d. Do not talk with strangers or get into their cars.
   e. Do not help anyone look for a lost dog or cat and do not accept candy from a stranger.
   f. If lost in a store, do not wander around looking for the parent; go at once to a clerk or guard.
2. Children need to learn their full name, address, and parent's name.
3. Watch for posttraumatic stress disorder in any child who has experienced an abduction.

X. Child Abuse

A. Description

1. Abuse is the nonaccidental physical injury or the nonaccidental act of omission of care by a parent or person responsible for a child; abuse comprises neglect and physical, sexual, and emotional maltreatment.
2. Neglect can be in the form of physical or emotional neglect and involves the deprivation of basic needs, supervision, medical care, or education and failure to meet a child's needs for attention and affection.
3. Sexual abuse can involve incest, molestation, exhibitionism, pornography, prostitution, or pedophilia; findings associated with sexual abuse may not be easily apparent in a child.
4. Shaken baby syndrome is caused by the violent shaking of an infant and results in intracranial (usually subdural hemorrhage) trauma; this can lead to cerebral edema and death.

B. Data Collection (Box 66-9)

C. Interventions

1. Support the child during a thorough physical assessment.

BOX 66-9 Child Neglect and Abuse: Data Collection Findings

Neglect
- Inadequate weight gain
- Poor hygiene
- Consistent hunger
- Inconsistent school attendance
- Constant fatigue
- Reports of lack of child supervision
- Delinquency

Physical Abuse
- Unexplained bruises, burns, or fractures
- Bald spots on the scalp
- Apprehensive child
- Extreme aggressiveness or withdrawal
- Fear of parents
- Lack of crying (older infant, toddler, or young preschool child) when approached by a stranger
- Spinal fractures without history of trauma from a sports injury

Emotional Abuse
- Speech disorders
- Habit disorders such as sucking, biting, and rocking
- Psychoneurotic reactions
- Learning disorders
- Suicide attempts

Sexual Abuse
- Difficulty walking or sitting
- Torn, stained, or bloody underclothing
- Pain, swelling, or itching of genitals
- Bruises, bleeding, or lacerations in genital or anal area
- Unwillingness to change clothes or unwillingness to participate in gym activities
- Poor peer relations

Shaken Baby Syndrome
- External signs of trauma are usually absent
- Ophthalmoscopic examination reveals retinal hemorrhages
- Full bulging fontanels and head circumference greater than expected

2. Check for injuries.
3. If shaken baby syndrome is suspected, monitor the infant for a decrease in level of consciousness, which can indicate increased intracranial pressure (ICP).
4. Report a case of suspected abuse; nurses are legally required to report all cases of suspected child abuse to the appropriate local or state agency.
5. Place the child in an environment that is safe, preventing further injury.
6. Document information related to the suspected abuse in an objective manner.
7. Assist to assess parents' strengths and weaknesses, normal coping mechanisms, and presence or absence of support systems.
8. Assist the family in identifying stressors, support systems, and resources.
9. Refer the family to appropriate support groups.

⚠ Nurses are legally required to report all cases of suspected child abuse to the appropriate local or state agency.

XI. Latchkey Children

A. Description
1. Children who do not have adult supervision before or after school hours; they are left to care for themselves during these times
2. Occurs when children are members of a single-parent family or both parents work and need to leave the home before children are brought to school
3. This situation induces a stress-provoking environment for the children and places the children at risk for an unsafe situation, injury, and delinquent behavior.

B. Interventions
1. Identify the latchkey child.
2. Encourage the parent to teach the child about self-care and self-help skills.
3. Assist the parent to identify possible alternatives rather that leaving the children alone
4. Inform the parent about available community resources such as after-school programs for children

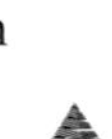

XII. Abuse of the Older Adult

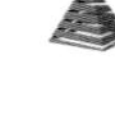

A. Description
1. Abuse of an older adult involves physical, emotional, or sexual abuse; neglect; and economic exploitation.
2. Older adults at most risk include individuals who are dependent because of illness, immobility, or altered mental status.
3. Factors that contribute to abuse and neglect include long-standing family violence, caregiver stress, and the older adult's increasing dependence on others.
4. Victims may attempt to dismiss injuries as accidental, and abusers may prevent victims from receiving proper medical care to avoid discovery.
5. Victims often are isolated socially by their abusers.

B. Data Collection
1. Physical abuse
   a. Sprains, dislocations, or fractures
   b. Abrasions, bruises, or lacerations
   c. Pressure sores
   d. Puncture wounds
   e. Burns
   f. Skin tears

2. Sexual abuse
   a. Torn or stained underclothing
   b. Discomfort or bleeding in the genital area
   c. Difficulty in walking or sitting
   d. Unexplained genital infections or disease
3. Emotional abuse
   a. Confusion
   b. Fearful and agitated
   c. Changes in appetite and weight
   d. Withdrawn and loss of interest in self and social activities
4. Neglect
   a. Disheveled appearance
   b. Dressed inadequately or inappropriately
   c. Dehydration and malnutrition
   d. Lacking physical needs, such as glasses, hearing aids, and dentures
5. Signs of medication overdose
6. Economic exploitation
   a. Inability to pay bills and fearful when discussing finances
   b. Confused, inaccurate, or no knowledge of finances

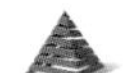 C. Interventions
1. Check for physical injuries and treat physical injuries.
2. Report cases of suspected abuse to appropriate authorities (follow state and agency guidelines).
3. Separate the older adult from the abusive environment, if possible, and contact adult protective services for assistance in placement while the abuse is being investigated.
4. Explore alternative living arrangements that are least restrictive and disruptive to the victim.
5. The older adult who has been abused may need assistance for financial or legal matters.
6. Provide referrals to emergency community resources.
7. When working with caregivers, determine the need for respite care or counseling if needed to deal with caregiver stress (see Priority Nursing Actions).

PRIORITY NURSING ACTIONS!

Actions to Take When an Older Client Is Physically Abused

1. Assess and treat the wounds.
2. Remove the victim from immediate danger.
3. Adhere to mandatory abuse reporting laws.
4. Notify the caseworker of the family situation.
5. Document the occurrence, findings, actions taken, and the victim's response.

When a victim is abused, the priority is to assess and treat any physical injuries. The nurse stays with the victim and provides comfort and support. After physical injuries are treated, the nurse ensures that the client is safe and is removed from the threatening environment. The nurse assists the registered nurse in making appropriate contacts. Elder abuse needs to be reported, so the nurse would adhere to the mandatory abuse reporting laws of the state. The nurse also contacts the caseworker of the family situation so that the incident is reported and follow-up with the family can occur. If there is no caseworker, the nurse contacts social services or the appropriate service to initiate this process. Finally, the nurse documents the occurrence, findings, actions taken, and the victim's response.

Reference(s): deWit, D. & Kumagai, C. (2013). *Medical-surgical nursing: Concepts & practice.* (2nd ed., p. 1042). St. Louis: Saunders.

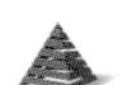

XIII. Rape and Sexual Assault

A. Description
1. Rape (sexual assault) is engaging another person in a sexual act and/or sexual intercourse through the use of force and without the consent of the sexual partner.
2. The victim is not required by law to report the rape or assault.
3. Often, the victim is blamed by others and receives no support from significant others.
4. Acquaintance rapes involve someone known to the victim.
5. Statutory rape is the act of sexual intercourse with a person under the age of legal consent, even if the minor consents.
6. Marital rape
   a. The belief that marriage bestows rights to sex whenever wanted and without consent of the partner contributes to the occurrence of marital rape.
   b. Victims of marital rape describe being forced to perform acts they did not wish to perform and being physically abused during sex.

B. Data collection
1. Female client
   a. Obtain the date of the last menstrual period.
   b. Determine the form of birth control used and the last act of intercourse before rape.
   c. Determine the duration of intercourse, orifices violated, and whether penile penetration occurred.
   d. Determine the use of a condom by the perpetrator.
2. Shame, embarrassment, and humiliation
3. Anger and revenge
4. Fear of telling others for fear of not being believed

C. It is important to note that males may be sexually abused both as children and as adults and are the usual targeted victim of pedophiles. Males may have more difficulty with disclosing their abuse.

D. Rape trauma syndrome
1. Sleep disturbances and nightmares
2. Loss of appetite
3. Fears, anxiety, phobias, and suspicion

4. Decrease in activities and motivation
5. Disruptions in relationships with partner, family, and friends
6. Self-blame, guilt, and shame
7. Lowered self-esteem and feelings of worthlessness
8. Somatic complaints

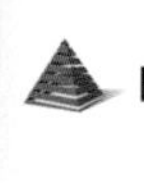

E. Interventions
1. Perform data collection in a quiet, private area.
2. Stay with the victim.
3. Assess the victim's stress level before performing treatments and procedures.
4. Victim should not shower, bathe, douche (female), or change clothing until an examination is performed.
5. Ensure that written consent is obtained for the examination, photographs, laboratory tests, release of information, and laboratory samples.
6. Assist with the female pelvic examination, and obtain specimens to detect semen (the pelvic examination may trigger a flashback of the attack). A shower and fresh clothing should be made available to the client after the examination.
7. Preserve any evidence.
8. Treat physical injuries and provide client safety.
9. Document all events in the care of the victim.
10. Reinforce to the victim that surviving the assault is most important. If the victim survived the rape, he or she did exactly what was necessary to stay alive.
11. Refer the victim to crisis intervention and support groups.

CRITICAL THINKING What Should You Do?

Answer: The nurse should first take the victim to a quiet and private room and assess the victim's stress level before performing treatments and procedures. The nurse needs to stay with the victim. The victim should not shower, bathe, douche (female), or change clothing until an examination is performed. The nurse should obtain consent for an examination, photographs, laboratory tests, release of information, and laboratory samples. The nurse should assist with the female pelvic examination (the pelvic examination may trigger a flashback of the attack). A shower and fresh clothing should be made available to the client after the examination. Any evidence needs to be preserved, and physical injuries need to be treated. The nurse should provide for client safety, document all events in the care of the victim, and reinforce to the victim that surviving the assault is most important; if the victim survived the rape, he or she did exactly what was necessary to stay alive. When appropriate, the nurse should refer the victim to crisis intervention and support groups.

Reference(s): Varcarolis, E. (2013). *Essentials of Psychiatric Mental Health Nursing: A communication approach to evidence-based care.* (2nd ed., pp. 426–427). St. Louis: Saunders.

PRACTICE QUESTIONS

716. The nurse is caring for an older adult client who has recently lost her husband. The client says, "No one cares about me anymore. All the people I loved are dead." Which response by the nurse is therapeutic?
1. "Right! Why not just 'pack it in'?"
2. "That seems rather unlikely to me."
3. "I don't believe that, and neither do you."
4. "You must be feeling all alone at this point."

717. The nurse is planning care for a client who is being hospitalized because the client has been displaying violent behavior and is at risk for potential harm to others. The nurse should avoid which intervention in the plan of care?
1. Facing the client when providing care
2. Ensuring that a security officer is within the immediate area
3. Keeping the door to the client's room open when with the client
4. Assigning the client to a room at the end of the hall to prevent disturbing the other clients

718. Which behaviors observed by the nurse might lead to the suspicion that a depressed adolescent client could be suicidal?
1. The client gives away a DVD and a cherished autographed picture of the performer.
2. The client runs out of the therapy group swearing at the group leader and then runs to her room.
3. The client gets angry with her roommate when the roommate borrows her clothes without asking.
4. The client becomes angry while speaking on her cell phone and slams the phone down on her bed.

719. A client is admitted to the psychiatric unit after a serious suicidal attempt by hanging. The nurse's **most important** aspect of care is to maintain client safety and do which?
1. Request that a peer remain with the client at all times.
2. Remove the client's clothing and place the client in a hospital gown.
3. Assign a staff member to the client who will remain with him or her at all times.
4. Admit the client to a seclusion room where all potentially dangerous articles are removed.

720. The police arrive at the emergency room with a client who has seriously lacerated both wrists. The **initial** nursing action is which?
1. Administer an antianxiety agent.
2. Examine and treat the wound sites.
3. Secure and record a detailed history.
4. Encourage and assist the client to vent feelings.

721. The nurse is caring for a client with severe depression. Which activity is appropriate for this client?
1. A puzzle
2. Drawing
3. Checkers
4. Paint by number

722. A client experiencing a severe major depressive episode is unable to address activities of daily living. The appropriate nursing intervention is which?
1. Feed, bathe, and dress the client as needed until the client can perform these activities independently.
2. Offer the client choices and consequences to the failure to comply with the expectation of maintaining activities of daily living.
3. Structure the client's day so that adequate time can be devoted to the client's assuming responsibility for the activities of daily living.
4. Have the client's peers confront the client about how the noncompliance in addressing activities of daily living affects the milieu.

❖ **723.** The nurse is preparing to care for a dying client, and several family members are at the client's bedside. Which therapeutic techniques should the nurse use when communicating with the family? **Select all that apply.**
- ❑ 1. Discourage reminiscing.
- ❑ 2. Make the decisions for the family.
- ❑ 3. Encourage expression of feelings, concerns, and fears.
- ❑ 4. Explain everything that is happening to all family members.
- ❑ 5. Extend touch, and hold the client's or family member's hand if appropriate.
- ❑ 6. Be honest and truthful, and let the client and family know that you will not abandon them.

724. The nurse is assisting in planning care for a client being admitted to the nursing unit who has attempted suicide. Which **priority** nursing intervention should the nurse include in the plan of care?
1. One-to-one suicide precautions
2. Suicide precautions, with 30-minute checks
3. Checking the whereabouts of the client every 15 minutes
4. Asking that the client report suicidal thoughts immediately

725. The nurse is reviewing the health care record of a client admitted to the psychiatric unit. The nurse notes that the admission nurse has documented that the client is experiencing anxiety as a result of a situational crisis. The nurse should determine that this type of crisis could be caused by which?
1. Witnessing a murder
2. The death of a loved one
3. A fire that destroyed the client's home
4. A recent rape episode experienced by the client

726. The nurse is gathering data from a client in crisis. When determining the client's perception of the precipitating event that led to the crisis, the **most appropriate** question to ask is which?
1. "With whom do you live?"
2. "Who is available to help you?"
3. "What leads you to seek help now?"
4. "What do you usually do to feel better?"

727. The nurse is assisting in developing a plan of care for the client in a crisis state. When developing the plan, the nurse should consider which?
1. A crisis state indicates that the individual is suffering from a mental illness.
2. A crisis state indicates that the individual is suffering from an emotional illness.
3. Presenting symptoms in a crisis situation are similar for all individuals experiencing a crisis.
4. A client's response to a crisis is individualized, and what constitutes a crisis for one person may not constitute a crisis for another person.

728. The nurse observes that a client with a potential for violence is agitated, pacing up and down in the hallway, and making aggressive and belligerent gestures at other clients. Which statement is appropriate to make to this client?
1. "You need to stop that behavior now!"
2. "You will need to be placed in seclusion!"
3. "What is causing you to become agitated?"
4. "You will need to be restrained if you do not change your behavior."

729. During a conversation with a depressed client on a psychiatric unit, the client says to the nurse, "My family would be better off without me." The nurse should make which therapeutic response to the client?
1. "Have you talked to your family about this?"
2. "Everyone feels this way when they are depressed."
3. "You will feel better once your medication begins to work."
4. "You sound very upset. Are you thinking of hurting yourself?"

730. An older client is a victim of elder abuse, and the client's family has been attending weekly counseling sessions. Which statement by the abusive family member indicates the client has learned positive coping skills?

1. "I will be more careful to make sure that my father's needs are met."
2. "Now that my father is moving into my home, I will need to change my ways."
3. "I feel better able to care for my father now that I know where to obtain assistance."
4. "I am so sorry and embarrassed that the abusive event occurred. It won't happen again."

ANSWERS

716. 4

Rationale: The client is experiencing loss and is feeling hopeless. The therapeutic response by the nurse is the one that attempts to translate words into feelings. In option 1, the nurse uses sarcasm, which gives advice and is nontherapeutic as a nursing response. In option 2, the nurse is voicing doubt, which is often used when a client verbalizes delusional ideas. In option 3, the nurse is disagreeing with the client, which implies that the nurse has passed judgment on the client's ideas or opinions.
Test-Taking Strategy: Use **therapeutic communication techniques**. Option 4 is the only option that focuses on the client's feelings. **Review: therapeutic communication techniques.**
Level of Cognitive Ability: Applying
Client Needs: Psychosocial Integrity
Integrated Process: Communication and Documentation
Content Area: Mental Health
Priority Concepts: Communication, Coping
Reference(s): Varcarolis (2013), pp. 120–123, 489.

717. 4

Rationale: The client should be placed in a room near the nurses' station and not at the end of a long, relatively unprotected corridor. The nurse should not isolate himself or herself with a potentially violent client. The door to the client's room should be kept open, and the nurse should never turn away from the client. A security officer or male aide should be within immediate call in case the possibility of violence is suspected.
Test-Taking Strategy: Focus on the **subject**, the intervention to avoid. This indicates the need to select the incorrect intervention. Keeping in mind that safety is the subject will direct you to the correct option. **Review:** guidelines for caring for the **violent client**.
Level of Cognitive Ability: Applying
Client Needs: Safe and Effective Care Environment
Integrated Process: Nursing Process/Planning
Content Area: Mental Health
Priority Concepts: Interpersonal Violence, Safety
Reference(s): Varcarolis (2013), p. 469.

718. 1

Rationale: A depressed, suicidal client often gives away that which is of value as a way of saying "good-bye" and wanting to be remembered. Options 2, 3, and 4 identify acting-out behaviors.
Test-Taking Strategy: Options 2, 3, and 4 are **comparable or alike** in that they deal with anger and "acting-out behaviors," which are often typical of some adolescents. Option 1 is different in nature and could indicate that the client may be saying good-bye. **Review:** clues that indicate **suicide**.
Level of Cognitive Ability: Analyzing
Client Needs: Psychosocial Integrity
Integrated Process: Nursing Process/Data Collection
Content Area: Mental Health
Priority Concepts: Coping, Mood and Affect
Reference(s): Varcarolis (2013), p. 452.

719. 3

Rationale: Hanging is a serious suicide attempt. The plan of care must reflect action that will promote the client's safety. Constant observation status (one-on-one) with a staff member who is never less than an arm's length away is the safest intervention.
Test-Taking Strategy: Note the **strategic words**, *most important*. Also focus on the **subject**, suicide. Eliminate option 4 because seclusion should not be the initial intervention. Eliminate option 1 next because the responsibility to safeguard a client is not the peer's responsibility. Eliminate option 2 because removing one's clothing will not maximize all possible safety strategies. **Review:** nursing interventions for the client at **risk for suicide**.
Level of Cognitive Ability: Applying
Client Needs: Safe and Effective Care Environment
Integrated Process: Nursing Process/Implementation
Content Area: Mental Health
Priority Concepts: Mood and Affect, Safety
Reference(s): Varcarolis (2013), pp. 452–453.

720. 2

Rationale: The initial nursing action is to examine and treat the self-inflicted injuries. Injuries from lacerated wrists can lead to a life-threatening situation. Other interventions may follow after the client has been treated medically.
Test-Taking Strategy: Note the **strategic word**, *initial*. Use **Maslow's Hierarchy of Needs Theory** to prioritize. Physiological needs come first. Option 2 addresses the physiological need. **Review:** care of the client who has **attempted suicide**.
Level of Cognitive Ability: Applying
Client Needs: Physiological Integrity
Integrated Process: Nursing Process/Implementation
Content Area: Mental Health
Priority Concepts: Interpersonal Violence, Mood and Affect
Reference(s): Varcarolis (2013), p. 452.

721. 2

Rationale: Concentration and memory are poor in a client with severe depression. When a client has a diagnosis of severe

depression, the nurse needs to provide activities that require little concentration. Activities that have no right or wrong choices or decisions minimize opportunities for the client to put down himself or herself. The nurse can also process the client's feelings by sitting with the client and talking or encouraging the client to write in a journal.
Test-Taking Strategy: Note that options 1, 3, and 4 are comparable or alike in that they all require concentration. It is important to remember that clients with depression have difficulty concentrating and need activities that require little concentration. **Review:** care of the client with severe depression.
Level of Cognitive Ability: Applying
Client Needs: Psychosocial Integrity
Integrated Process: Nursing Process/Implementation
Content Area: Mental Health
Priority Concepts: Coping, Mood and Affect
Reference(s): Stuart (2013), pp. 315, 373.

722. 1
Rationale: The client with depression may not have the energy or interest to complete activities of daily living. Often, severely depressed clients are unable to perform even the simplest activities of daily living. The nurse assumes this role and completes these tasks with the client. Options 2 and 3 are incorrect because the client lacks the energy and motivation to perform these tasks independently. Option 4 will increase the client's feelings of poor self-esteem and unworthiness.
Test-Taking Strategy: Note the subject, severe major depressive episode. Eliminate options 2 and 3 because the client lacks the energy and motivation to do these independently. In addition, option 2 may lead to increased feelings of worthlessness as the client fails to meet expectations. Option 4 will increase the client's feelings of poor self-esteem and unworthiness. **Review:** care of the client with **severe depression**.
Level of Cognitive Ability: Applying
Client Needs: Physiological Integrity
Integrated Process: Nursing Process/Implementation
Content Area: Mental Health
Priority Concepts: Caregiving, Mood and Affect
Reference(s): Varcarolis (2013), p. 262.

❖ 723. 3, 5, 6
Rationale: The nurse must determine whether there is a spokesperson for the family and how much the client and family want to know. The nurse needs to allow the family and client the opportunity for informed choices and assist with the decision-making process if asked. The nurse should encourage expression of feelings, concerns, and fears, as well as reminiscing. The nurse needs to be honest and truthful and let the client and family know that they will not be abandoned. It is important to extend touch and hold the client's or family member's hand if appropriate.
Test-Taking Strategy: Recalling therapeutic communication techniques and client and family rights will assist you in answering this question. **Review: therapeutic communication** and care to the **dying client**.
Level of Cognitive Ability: Applying
Client Needs: Psychosocial Integrity
Integrated Process: Caring
Content Area: Developmental Stages: End of Life Care
Priority Concepts: Communication, Coping
Reference(s): Varcarolis (2013), pp. 491–492.

724. 1
Rationale: One-to-one suicide precautions are required for the client who has attempted suicide. Options 2 and 3 are not appropriate, considering the situation. Option 4 may be an appropriate nursing intervention, but the priority is stated in option 1. The best option is constant supervision so that the nurse may intervene as needed if the client attempts to cause harm to him or herself.
Test-Taking Strategy: Note the strategic word, *priority.* Recalling that one-to-one suicide precautions are the priority in caring for a suicidal client will direct you to the correct option. **Review:** interventions for the **suicidal client**.
Level of Cognitive Ability: Applying
Client Needs: Safe and Effective Care Environment
Integrated Process: Nursing Process/Implementation
Content Area: Mental Health
Priority Concepts: Communication, Mood and Affect
Reference(s): deWit, Kumagai (2013), p. 1060.

725. 2
Rationale: A situational crisis is associated with a life event. External situations that could precipitate a situational crisis include loss or change of a job, the death of a loved one, abortion, change in financial status, divorce, and severe illness. Options 1, 3, and 4 identify adventitious crises. An adventitious crisis relates to a crisis, disaster, or event that is not a part of everyday life, is unplanned, and is accidental.
Test-Taking Strategy: Focus on the subject, situational crisis. This will assist in eliminating options 1, 3, and 4 because they are comparable or alike. **Review: types of crisis.**
Level of Cognitive Ability: Understanding
Client Needs: Psychosocial Integrity
Integrated Process: Nursing Process/Data Collection
Content Area: Mental Health
Priority Concepts: Anxiety, Coping
Reference(s): Varcarolis (2013), p. 400.

726. 3
Rationale: The nurse's initial task when gathering data from a client in crisis is to assess the individual or family and the problem. The more clearly the problem can be defined, the better the chance a solution can be found. Option 3 will assist in determining data related to the precipitating event that led to the crisis. Options 1 and 2 identify situational supports. Option 4 identifies personal coping skills.
Test-Taking Strategy: Note the strategic words, *most appropriate* and focus on the subject, precipitating event. Eliminate options 1 and 2 because these data will determine support systems. Eliminate option 4 because this question would be asked when determining coping skills. **Review:** data collection methods for a client in **crisis**.
Level of Cognitive Ability: Applying
Client Needs: Psychosocial Integrity
Integrated Process: Nursing Process/Data Collection
Content Area: Mental Health
Priority Concepts: Communication, Coping
Reference(s): Varcarolis (2013), pp. 402–403.

727. 4

Rationale: Although each crisis response can be described in similar terms as far as presenting symptoms are concerned, what constitutes a crisis for one person may not constitute a crisis for another person because each is a unique individual. Being in a crisis state does not mean that the client is suffering from an emotional or mental illness.

Test-Taking Strategy: Eliminate option 3 because of the closed-ended word, *all*. Next, eliminate options 1 and 2 because a crisis does not indicate "illness." **Review:** characteristics of a **crisis state**.

Level of Cognitive Ability: Understanding

Client Needs: Psychosocial Integrity

Integrated Process: Nursing Process/Data Collection

Content Area: Mental Health

Priority Concepts: Communication, Coping

Reference(s): Varcarolis (2013), p. 399.

728. 3

Rationale: The best statement is to ask the client what is causing the agitation. This will assist the client to become aware of the behavior and will assist the nurse in planning appropriate interventions for the client. Option 1 is demanding behavior, which could cause increased agitation in the client. Options 2 and 4 are threats to the client and are inappropriate.

Test-Taking Strategy: Focus on the subject, an aggressive client. Eliminate option 1 because of the demand that it places on the client. Eliminate options 2 and 4 because they indicate threats to the client. **Review:** appropriate nursing interventions for the **agitated client**.

Level of Cognitive Ability: Applying

Client Needs: Psychosocial Integrity

Integrated Process: Communication and Documentation

Content Area: Mental Health

Priority Concepts: Communication, Interpersonal Violence

Reference(s): Varcarolis (2013), pp. 120–123.

729. 4

Rationale: Clients who are depressed may be at risk for suicide. It is critical for the nurse to assess suicidal ideation and plan. The client should be directly asked if a plan for self-harm exists. Options 1, 2, and 3 are not therapeutic responses.

Test-Taking Strategy: Use therapeutic communication techniques. Option 4 is the only option that deals directly with the client's feelings. Additionally, clients at risk for suicide need to be directly assessed regarding the potential for self-harm. **Review:** data collection techniques for the **depressed client**.

Level of Cognitive Ability: Applying

Client Needs: Psychosocial Integrity

Integrated Process: Nursing Process/Data Collection

Content Area: Mental Health

Priority Concepts: Communication, Mood and Affect

Reference(s): Varcarolis (2013), p. 451.

730. 3

Rationale: Elder abuse sometimes occurs with family members who are being expected to care for their aging parents. This can cause family members to become overextended, frustrated, or financially depleted. Knowing where in the community to turn for assistance in caring for aging family members can bring much-needed relief. Taking advantage of these alternatives is a positive alternative coping strategy, which many families use.

Test-Taking Strategy: Focus on the subject, a coping strategy. Only option 3 identifies a means of coping with the subjects. The other options are statements of good faith or promises, which may or may not be kept in the future. Option 3 outlines a definitive plan for how to handle the pressure associated with the father's care. **Review:** effective **coping strategies**.

Level of Cognitive Ability: Evaluating

Client Needs: Psychosocial Integrity

Integrated Process: Nursing Process/Evaluation

Content Area: Mental Health

Priority Concepts: Coping, Interpersonal Violence

Reference(s): Varcarolis (2013), p. 428.

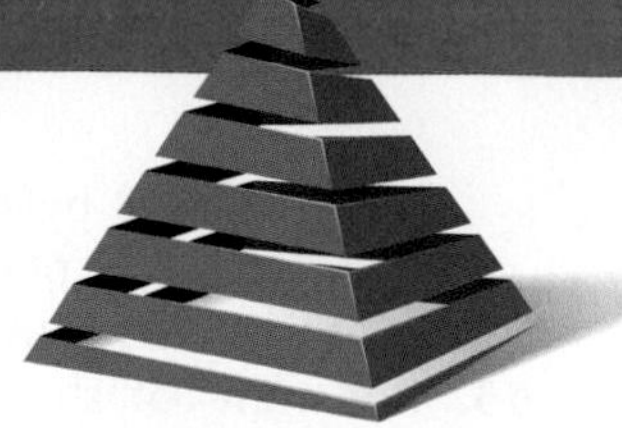

CHAPTER 67

Psychiatric Medications

CRITICAL THINKING What Should You Do?

A client has been taking alprazolam (Xanax) on a long-term basis for the treatment of anxiety. The health care provider has informed the nurse that the medication will be discontinued and the client needs instructions about tapering off of the medication. What should the nurse do?

Answer located on p. 960.

I. Selective Serotonin Reuptake Inhibitors (SSRIs) (Box 67-1)

A. Description
   1. Inhibit serotonin uptake and elicit an antidepressant response.
   2. The potential for medication interactions is high, and complete medication assessments must be obtained and evaluated. The nurse should inquire about the use of herbal therapies, especially St. John's wort.

B. Side/adverse effects
   1. Nausea, vomiting, cramping, and diarrhea

BOX 67-1 Reuptake Inhibitors

Selective Serotonin Reuptake Inhibitors
Citalopram (Celexa)
Escitalopram (Lexapro)
Fluoxetine (Prozac)
Fluvoxamine (Luvox)
Paroxetine hydrochloride (Paxil, Pexeva)
Sertraline hydrochloride (Zoloft)
Vilazodone hydrochloride (Viibryd)

Serotonin-Norepinephrine Reuptake Inhibitors
Venlafaxine (Effexor)
Duloxetine (Cymbalta)
Desvenlafaxine (Pristiq)

Atypical Antidepressants
Bupropion hydrochloride (Wellbutrin, Budeprion)
Mirtazapine (Remeron)
Nefazodone
Trazodone (Oleptro)

   2. Dry mouth
   3. Central nervous system (CNS) stimulation, including akathisia (restlessness, agitation) 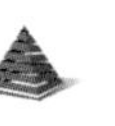
   4. Increased sweating
   5. Photosensitivity
   6. Insomnia, somnolence (sleepy, drowsy), apathy
   7. Nervousness
   8. Headache, dizziness
   9. Weight loss or gain
   10. Decreased libido
   11. Tremors
   12. Seizure activity

C. Interventions
   1. Monitor the vital signs, because SSRIs can potentially lower or elevate blood pressure.
   2. Monitor weight.
   3. Initiate safety precautions, particularly if dizziness occurs.
   4. Administered with a snack or meal to reduce the risk of dizziness and light-headedness.
   5. The client is instructed to avoid alcohol.
   6. Monitor the suicidal client, especially during improved mood and increased energy levels.
   7. The client taking fluoxetine (Prozac) and bupropion (Wellbutrin) is instructed to take the medication early in the day to prevent interference with sleep.
   8. For the client on long-term therapy, monitor liver and renal function test results. Altered values may occur requiring dosage adjustments.
   9. Monitor white blood cell and neutrophil counts. The medication may be discontinued if levels fall below normal.
   10. If priapism (painful, prolonged penile erection) occurs, the medication is withheld and the health care provider (HCP) is notified.
   11. The client is informed about the possibility of decreased libido.
   12. Reinforce instructions to the client to change positions slowly to avoid a hypotensive effect.
   13. Caution the client about photosensitivity and to take measures to prevent exposure to sunlight.
   14. Educate about the potential for discontinuation syndrome if medication is stopped abruptly rather than tapered. The syndrome is

characterized by gastrointestinal (GI) distress, behavioral or perceptual oddities, movement problems, and sleep disturbances.

15. Be aware of the potential for serotonin syndrome characterized by elevated temperature, muscle rigidity, and elevated creatine phosphokinase (CPK) levels. This risk is greatly increased when SSRIs are given with monoamine oxidase inhibitors (MAOIs). Thus this medication combination needs to be avoided.
16. Reinforce instructions to the client that over-the-counter (OTC) cold medicines can increase the likelihood of serotonin syndrome.
17. In pregnancy, consultation with an obstetrician is recommended regarding taking these medications.
18. Monitor the medication response in children, adolescents, and the older client closely because the response may be different from in an adult client.
19. Psychotherapy is encouraged.

II. Tricyclic Antidepressants (Box 67-2)

A. Description
  1. Block the reuptake of norepinephrine (and serotonin) at the presynaptic junction. It is used to treat depression.
  2. May reduce seizure threshold
  3. May reduce effectiveness of antihypertensive agents
  4. Concurrent use with alcohol or antihistamines can cause CNS depression.
  5. Concurrent use with MAOIs can cause hypertensive **crisis**.
  6. Cardiac toxicity can occur, and all clients should undergo electrocardiographic evaluation before treatment and periodically thereafter.
  7. Overdose is life-threatening, necessitating immediate treatment (see Priority Nursing Actions).
  8. The tricyclic antidepressant clomipramine (Anafranil) may be used to treat obsessive-compulsive disorder.

B. Side/adverse effects
  1. Anticholinergic effects: Dry mouth, difficulty voiding, dilated pupils and blurred vision, decreased gastrointestinal motility, constipation

BOX 67-2 Tricyclic Antidepressants

Amoxapine
Amitriptyline (Elavil)
Clomipramine (Anafranil)
Desipramine (Norpramin)
Doxepin (Sinequan)
Imipramine (Tofranil)
Nortriptyline
Protriptyline (Vivactil)
Trimipramine (Surmontil)

PRIORITY NURSING ACTIONS!

Actions to Take for a Tricyclic Antidepressant Overdose

1. Check airway and maintain a patent airway.
2. Administer oxygen.
3. Check vital signs.
4. Assist to obtain an electrocardiogram (ECG).
5. Prepare to assist with gastric lavage with activated charcoal.
6. Prepare to assist with the administration of physostigmine (a cholinesterase inhibitor) and antidysrhythmic medications.
7. Document the event, actions taken, and the client's response.

A tricyclic antidepressant overdose can be life-threatening. Signs and symptoms include dysrhythmias, including tachycardia, intraventricular blocks, complete atrioventricular block, ventricular fibrillation; hypothermia; flushing; dry mouth; dilation of the pupils; confusion, agitation, and hallucinations; and seizures, followed by coma. The immediate action is to check the airway and institute measures such as oxygen to maintain a patent airway. Vital signs are checked and monitored, and an ECG is obtained to check for dysrhythmias. Gastric lavage with activated charcoal is done to prevent further medication absorption. Physostigmine (a cholinesterase inhibitor) is given to counteract anticholinergic effects, and antidysthythmics are administered as needed. The nurse assists the registered nurse and documents the event, the actions taken, and the client's response.

Reference(s): deWit, D. & Kumagai, C. (2013). *Medical-surgical nursing: Concepts & practice.* (2nd ed., p. 1022). St. Louis: Saunders.
Lehne, R. (2013). *Pharmacology for nursing care* (8th ed., pp. 377–378). St. Louis: Saunders.

  2. Photosensitivity
  3. Cardiovascular disturbances such as tachycardia, dysrhythmias; orthostatic hypotension
  4. Sedation
  5. Seizures (with bupropion)
  6. Weight gain
  7. Anxiety, restlessness, irritability
  8. Decreased or increased libido with ejaculatory and erection disturbances

C. Interventions 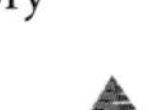
  1. Monitor the suicidal client, especially during improved mood and increased energy levels.
  2. The client is instructed to change positions slowly to avoid a hypotensive effect.
  3. Monitor pattern of daily bowel activity.
  4. Monitor for urinary retention.
  5. For the client on long-term therapy, monitor liver and renal function test results.
  6. Administer with food or milk if gastrointestinal distress occurs.

7. Administer the entire daily oral dose at one time, preferably at bedtime because of the sedative effect.
8. The client is instructed to avoid alcohol and nonprescription medications to prevent adverse medication interactions.
9. The client is instructed to avoid driving and other activities requiring alertness until the response is known. Sedation is expected in early therapy and may subside with time.
10. When the medication is discontinued by the health care provider, it should be tapered gradually.
11. The potential for medication interactions with OTC cold medication exists.
12. The client is cautioned about photosensitivity and to take measures to prevent exposure to sunlight.
13. Good oral hygiene and the use of hard candies and mouth rinses to relieve dry mouth are encouraged.
14. Psychotherapy is encouraged.

The client is informed that antidepressant medication may take several weeks to produce the desired effect. (The client response may not occur until 2 to 4 weeks after the first dose.)

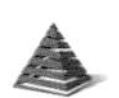

III. Monoamine Oxidase Inhibitors (MAOIs) (Box 67-3)

A. Description
1. Inhibit the enzyme monoamine oxidase, which is present in the brain, blood platelets, liver, spleen, and kidneys.
2. Monoamine oxidase metabolizes amines, norepinephrine, and serotonin, so the concentration of these amines increases with MAOI.
3. Clients who have depression and have not responded to other antidepressant therapies, including electroconvulsive therapy, may be given MAOIs.
4. Concurrent use with amphetamines, antidepressants, dopamine, epinephrine, guanethidine, levodopa, methyldopa, nasal decongestants, norepinephrine, reserpine, tyramine-containing foods, or vasoconstrictors may cause hypertensive crisis.
5. Concurrent use with opioid analgesics may cause hypertension, hypotension, coma, or seizures.

B. Side/adverse effects
1. Orthostatic hypotension
2. Restlessness
3. Insomnia
4. Dizziness
5. Weakness, lethargy
6. Gastrointestinal upset
7. Dry mouth
8. Weight gain
9. Peripheral edema
10. Anticholinergic effects
11. CNS stimulation (anxiety, agitation, mania)
12. Delay in ejaculation

C. Hypertensive crisis
1. Hypertension
2. Occipital headache radiating frontally
3. Neck stiffness and soreness
4. Nausea and vomiting
5. Sweating
6. Fever and chills
7. Clammy skin
8. Dilated pupils
9. Palpitations, tachycardia, or bradycardia
10. Constricting chest pain
11. Antidote for hypertensive crisis: Phentolamine by intravenous injection

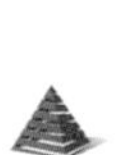

D. Interventions
1. Monitor blood pressure frequently for hypertension.
2. Monitor for signs of hypertensive crisis.
3. If palpitations or frequent headaches occur, the medication is withheld and the HCP is notified.
4. Administered with food if gastrointestinal distress occurs.
5. The client is instructed that the medication effect may be noted during the first week of therapy, but maximum benefit may take up to 3 weeks.
6. The client is instructed to report headache, neck stiffness, or neck soreness immediately.
7. The client is instructed to change positions slowly to prevent orthostatic hypotension.
8. The client is instructed to avoid caffeine or OTC preparations such as weight-reducing pills or medications for hay fever and colds.
9. Monitor for client compliance with medication administration.
10. The client is instructed to carry a Medic-Alert card indicating that an MAOI medication is being taken.
11. Administering the medication in the evening is avoided because insomnia may result.
12. When the medication is discontinued by the HCP, it should be discontinued gradually.
13. Reinforce instructions to the client to avoid foods that require bacteria or molds for their preparation or preservation and those that contain tyramine (Fig. 67-1 and Box 67-4).

The client is taught about the foods that contain tyramine. Consuming tyramine-containing foods when taking an MAOI can cause hypertensive crisis.

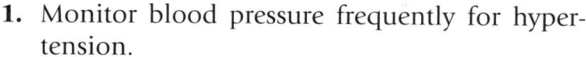

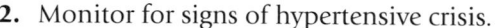

BOX 67-3 Monoamine Oxidase Inhibitors

Phenelzine sulfate (Nardil)
Tranylcypromine (Parnate)
Isocarboxazid (Marplan)
Selegiline (Emsam)

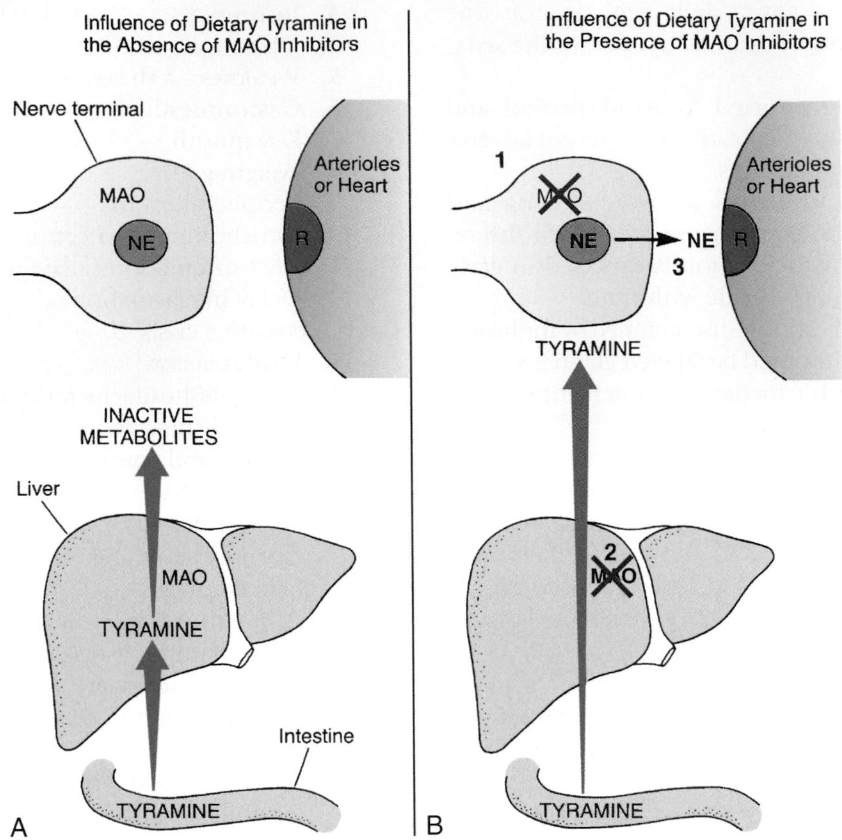

FIGURE 67-1 Interaction between dietary tyramine and monoamine oxidase inhibitors (MAOIs). **A,** In the absence of MAOIs, dietary tyramine is absorbed from the intestine, transported to the liver, and then immediately activated by MAO. No tyramine reaches the general circulation. **B,** Three events occur in the presence of MAOIs: (1) inhibition of neuronal MAO raises levels of norepinephrine (NE) in sympathetic nerve terminals; (2) inhibition of hepatic MAO allows dietary tyramine to pass through the liver and enter systemic circulation intact; and (3) on reaching peripheral sympathetic nerve terminals, tyramine promotes the release of accumulated NE stores, thereby causing massive vasoconstriction and excessive stimulation of the heart. *MAO,* Monoamine oxidase; *R,* receptor for NE. (From Lehne R: *Pharmacology for nursing care*, ed 7, Philadelphia, 2010, Saunders.)

BOX 67-4 Foods to Avoid That Contain Tyramine

Avocados
Bananas
Beef or chicken liver
Brewer's yeast
Broad beans
Caffeine, such as in coffee, tea, or chocolate
Cheese, especially aged, except cottage cheese
Eggplant
Figs
Meat extracts and tenderizers
Overripe fruit
Papaya
Pickled herring
Raisins
Red wine, beer, sherry
Sausage, bologna, pepperoni, salami
Sour cream
Soy sauce
Yogurt

Note: These foods need to be avoided in the client taking an MAOI. Even a small amount of tyramine can increase the blood pressure and the force and/or rate of heart contractions.

IV. Mood Stabilizers (Box 67-5)

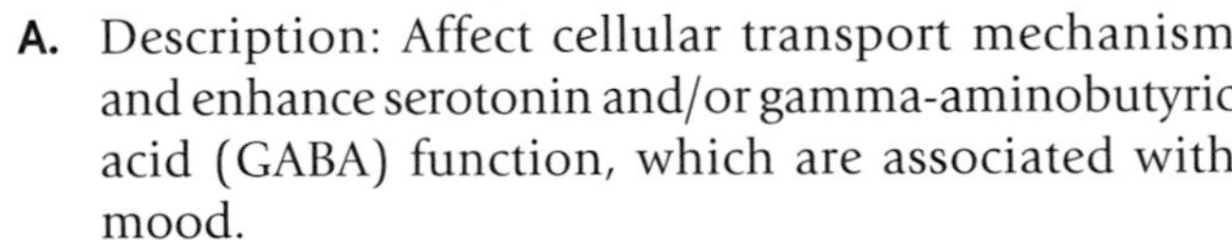

A. Description: Affect cellular transport mechanism and enhance serotonin and/or gamma-aminobutyric acid (GABA) function, which are associated with mood.

B. Lithium

1. Concurrent use with diuretics, fluoxetine (Prozac), methyldopa, or nonsteroidal anti-inflammatory drugs (NSAIDs) increases lithium reabsorption by the kidney or inhibits lithium excretion, either of which increases the risk of lithium toxicity.
2. Acetazolamide (Diamox), theophylline, phenothiazines, or sodium bicarbonate may increase renal excretion of lithium, reducing its effectiveness.
3. The therapeutic dose is only slightly less than the amount producing toxicity.
4. The therapeutic drug serum level of lithium is 0.6 to 1.2 mEq/L. The actual dose at which the therapeutic effect is achieved and the levels at which toxicity appears are highly variable among individuals. 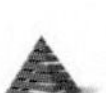

BOX 67-5 Mood Stabilizers

Lithium Preparations
Lithium carbonate
Lithium citrate

Other Mood Stabilizers
Aripiprazole (Abilify)
Carbamazepine (Tegretol)
Gabapentin (Neurontin)
Lamotrigine (Lamictal)
Olanzapine (Zyprexa)
Olanzapine/fluoxetine (Symbyax)
Oxcarbazepine (Trileptal)
Quetiapine (Seroquel)
Risperidone (Risperdal)
Valproate sodium (Depacon, Depakene, Depakote)
Ziprasidone (Geodon)

5. The causes of an increase in the lithium level include decreased sodium intake; fluid and electrolyte loss associated with severe sweating, dehydration, diarrhea, or diuretic therapy; and illness or overdose.
6. Serum lithium levels should be checked frequently after initiation of therapy and then every 1 to 2 months or whenever any behavioral change suggests an altered serum level.
7. Blood samples to check serum lithium levels should be drawn in the morning, 12 hours after the last dose was taken.
8. Lithium is classified as pregnancy category D; it crosses the placental barrier freely and has been associated with fetal toxicity.

C. Side/adverse effects
1. Polyuria
2. Polydipsia
3. Anorexia, nausea
4. Dry mouth
5. Mild thirst
6. Weight gain
7. Abdominal bloating
8. Soft stools or diarrhea
9. Fine hand tremors
10. Inability to concentrate
11. Muscle weakness
12. Lethargy, fatigue
13. Headache
14. Hair loss
15. Hypothyroidism

D. Interventions
1. Monitor the suicidal client, especially during improved mood and increased energy levels.
2. The medication is administered with food to minimize gastrointestinal irritation.
3. Reinforce instructions to the client to avoid excessive amounts of coffee, tea, or cola, which have a diuretic effect.
4. Diuretics are not administered while the client is taking lithium.
5. Reinforce instructions to the client to avoid alcohol.
6. Reinforce instructions to the client to avoid OTC medications.
7. Reinforce instructions to the client that he or she may take a missed dose within 2 hours of the scheduled time. Otherwise, the client should skip the missed dose and take the next dose at the scheduled time.
8. Reinforce instructions to the client not to adjust or stop the medication without consulting the HCP because lithium should be tapered and not discontinued abruptly.
9. Reinforce instructions to the client in the signs and symptoms of lithium toxicity.
10. Reinforce instructions to the client to notify the HCP if polyuria, prolonged vomiting, diarrhea, or fever occurs.
11. Reinforce instructions to the client that the therapeutic response to the medication will be noted in 1 to 3 weeks.
12. Monitor the electrocardiogram (ECG), renal function tests, and thyroid tests (ensure that these tests are performed before the start of therapy).
13. Monitor weight.

The client taking lithium (Lithobid) is instructed to maintain a fluid intake of six to eight glasses of water a day and an adequate salt intake to prevent lithium toxicity.

E. Lithium toxicity 
1. Description
   a. Occurs when ingested lithium cannot be detoxified and excreted by the kidneys
   b. Symptoms of toxicity begin to appear when the serum lithium level is 1.5 to 2 mEq/L.
2. Mild toxicity
   a. Serum lithium level is 1.5 mEq/L.
   b. Apathy
   c. Lethargy
   d. Diminished concentration
   e. Mild ataxia
   f. Coarse hand tremors
   g. Slight muscle weakness
3. Moderate toxicity
   a. Serum lithium level between 1.5 to 2.5 mEq/L
   b. Nausea, vomiting
   c. Severe diarrhea
   d. Mild to moderate ataxia and incoordination
   e. Slurred speech
   f. Tinnitus
   g. Blurred vision
   h. Muscle twitching
   i. Irregular tremor

4. Severe toxicity
   a. Serum lithium level is higher than 2.5 mEq/L.
   b. Nystagmus
   c. Muscle fasciculations
   d. Deep tendon hyperreflexia
   e. Visual or tactile hallucinations
   f. Oliguria or anuria
   g. Impaired level of consciousness
   h. Tonic-clonic seizures or coma, leading to death
5. Interventions for lithium toxicity
   a. Lithium is withheld and the HCP is notified.
   b. Monitor vital signs and level of consciousness.
   c. Monitor cardiac status.
   d. Prepare to obtain samples to monitor lithium, electrolyte, blood urea nitrogen, and creatinine levels and perform a complete blood cell count.
   e. Monitor for suicidal tendencies and institute **suicide** precautions.

V. Antianxiety or Anxiolytic Medications

A. Description
1. Antianxiety medications depress the CNS, thereby increasing the effects of GABA, which produces relaxation and may depress the limbic system.
2. Benzodiazepines have anxiety-reducing (anxiolytic), sedative-hypnotic, muscle-relaxing, and anticonvulsant actions (Box 67-6).
3. Benzodiazepines are contraindicated in clients with acute narrow-angle glaucoma and should be used cautiously in children and older clients.
4. Benzodiazepines interact with other CNS medications, producing an additive effect.
5. Abrupt withdrawal of benzodiazepines can be potentially life-threatening, and withdrawal should occur only under medical supervision.

B. Side/adverse effects
1. Daytime sedation
2. Ataxia
3. Dizziness
4. Headaches
5. Blurred or double vision
6. Hypotension
7. Tremor
8. Amnesia
9. Slurred speech
10. Urinary incontinence
11. Constipation
12. Paradoxical CNS excitement
13. Lethargy
14. Behavioral change

C. Acute toxicity
1. Somnolence
2. Confusion
3. Diminished reflexes and coma
4. Flumazenil (Romazicon) is a benzodiazepine antagonist that will reverse benzodiazepine intoxication in 5 minutes (it is administered intravenously).
5. The client being treated for an overdose of a benzodiazepine may experience agitation, restlessness, discomfort, and anxiety.

D. Interventions
1. Monitor for motor responses such as agitation, trembling, and tension.
2. Monitor for autonomic responses such as cold, clammy hands and sweating.
3. Monitor for paradoxical CNS excitement during early therapy, particularly in older and debilitated individuals.
4. Monitor for visual disturbances because the medications can worsen glaucoma.
5. Monitor liver and renal function test results and complete blood cell counts.
6. Reduce the medication dose as prescribed for the older adult client and for the client with impaired liver function.
7. Initiate safety precautions, because the older adult client is at risk for falling when taking the medication for sleep or anxiety.
8. Assist with ambulation if drowsiness or lightheadedness occurs.
9. Inform the client that drowsiness usually disappears during continued therapy.
10. Inform the client to avoid tasks that require alertness until the response to the medication is established.
11. Inform the client to avoid alcohol.
12. Reinforce instructions to not take other medications without consulting the HCP.
13. Reinforce instructions not to stop the medication abruptly (can result in seizure activity).

E. Withdrawal
1. To lessen withdrawal symptoms, the dosage of a benzodiazepine should be tapered gradually over 2 to 6 weeks.

BOX 67-6 Benzodiazepines

Alprazolam (Xanax, Niravam)
Chlordiazepoxide (Librium)
Clonazepam (Klonopin)
Clorazepate (Tranxene)
Diazepam (Valium)
Lorazepam (Ativan)
Midazolam Oxazepam (Serax)
Temazepam (Restoril)
Triazolam (Halcion)

Nonbenzodiazepine Anxiolytics

Buspirone (BuSpar)

2. Abrupt or too-rapid withdrawal results in the following:
   a. Restlessness
   b. Irritability
   c. Insomnia
   d. Hand tremors
   e. Abdominal or muscle cramps
   f. Sweating
   g. Vomiting
   h. Seizures

VI. Barbiturates and Sedative-Hypnotics (Box 67-7)

A. Description
   1. These medications depress the reticular activating system by promoting the inhibitory synaptic action of the neurotransmitter GABA.
   2. These medications are used for short-term treatment of insomnia or for sedation to relieve anxiety, tension, and apprehension.

B. Side/adverse effects
   1. Dizziness and drowsiness
   2. Confusion
   3. Irritability
   4. Allergic reactions
   5. Agranulocytosis
   6. Thrombocytopenic purpura
   7. Megaloblastic anemia

C. Overdose
   1. Tachycardia
   2. Hypotension
   3. Cold and clammy skin
   4. Dilated pupils
   5. Weak and rapid pulse
   6. Signs of shock
   7. Depressed respirations
   8. Absent reflexes
   9. Coma and death may result from respiratory and cardiovascular collapse.

D. Withdrawal
   1. Severe withdrawal symptoms begin within 24 hours after the medication is discontinued in an individual with severe medication dependence.
   2. Gradual withdrawal is used to detoxify a dependent client.
   3. Anxiety
   4. Insomnia
   5. Nightmares
   6. Daytime agitation
   7. Tremors
   8. Delirium
   9. Seizures
   10. Behavioral changes

E. Interventions
   1. Lower doses are administered as prescribed for the older client.
   2. Medications should be used with caution in the client who has suicidal tendencies or has a history of drug **addiction**.
   3. Maintain safety by supervising ambulation and using side rails at night.
   4. Reinforce instructions to take the medication as directed.
   5. Reinforce instructions to avoid driving or operating hazardous equipment if drowsiness, dizziness, or unsteadiness occurs.
   6. The client needs to avoid alcohol.
   7. For insomnia, the client should take the medication 30 minutes before bedtime; avoid taking with a large amount of food to help absorption.
   8. Inform the client that a hangover effect may occur in the morning.
   9. The client should not discontinue the medication abruptly.
   10. Inform the client taking chloral hydrate to take the medication with food and a full glass of water, fruit juice, or ginger ale to prevent gastric irritation.

BOX 67-7 Barbiturates and Sedative-Hypnotics

Barbiturates

Amobarbital (Amytal)
Butabarbital (Butisol)
Pentobarbital (Nembutal)
Phenobarbital (Luminal)
Secobarbital (Seconal)

Sedative-Hypnotics

Chloral hydrate (Somnote)
Eszopiclone (Lunesta)
Meprobamate (Trancot)
Ramelteon (Rozerem)
Zaleplon (Sonata)
Zolpidem (Ambien)

VII. Antipsychotic Medications (Box 67-8)

A. Description
   1. Improve the thought processes and the behavior of the client with psychotic symptoms, especially the client with schizophrenia
   2. Affect dopamine receptors in the brain, thereby reducing the psychotic symptoms
   3. Typical antipsychotics are more effective for positive symptoms of schizophrenia such as hallucinations, aggression, and delusions. Typical antipsychotic medications also block the chemoreceptor trigger zone and vomiting center in the brain, producing an antiemetic effect.
   4. Atypical antipsychotics are more effective for the negative symptoms of schizophrenia, such as avolition, apathy, and alogia.
   5. The effects of antipsychotic medications will be potentiated when given with other medications acting on the CNS.

BOX 67-8 Antipsychotic Medications

Typical Antipsychotics
Chlorpromazine
Fluphenazine decanoate (Prolixin Decanoate)
Haloperidol
Loxapine (Loxitane)
Molindone hydrochloride
Perphenazine pimozide (Orap)
Thiothixene (Navane)
Trifluoperazine

Atypical Antipsychotics
Aripiprazole (Abilify)
Clozapine (Clozaril)
Olanzapine (Zyprexa)
Palperidone (Invega)
Quetiapine (Seroquel)
Risperidone (Risperdal)
Ziprasidone (Geodon)

B. Side/adverse effects (Box 67-9)

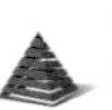
C. Extrapyramidal syndrome
1. Parkinsonism
   a. Tremors
   b. Mask-like facies
   c. Dysphagia, drooling
   d. Rigidity, shuffling gait
2. Dystonia
   a. Facial grimacing
   b. Abnormal or involuntary eye movements
3. Akathisia
   a. Restlessness
   b. Constant moving about
4. Tardive dyskinesia
   a. Protrusion of the tongue
   b. Chewing motions
   c. Involuntary movements of the body and extremities

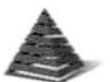
D. Interventions
1. Monitor vital signs.
2. Monitor for symptoms of neuroleptic malignant syndrome (refer to Section VIII).
3. Monitor urine output.
4. Monitor serum glucose level.
5. Administer the medication with food or milk to decrease gastric irritation.
6. For oral use, the liquid form might be preferred because some clients hide tablets to avoid taking them.
7. Note that the absorption rate is faster with the liquid form of oral medication.
8. Skin contact with the liquid concentrate is avoided to prevent contact dermatitis.
9. Protect the liquid concentrate from light.
10. Dilute the liquid concentrate with fruit juice.

BOX 67-9 Side/Adverse Effects of Antipsychotic Medications

Anticholinergic Effects
Dry mouth
Increased heart rate
Urinary retention
Constipation
Hypotension

Extrapyramidal Side/Adverse Effects

Parkinsonism
Tremors
Mask-like facies
Rigidity
Shuffling gait
Dysphagia
Drooling

Dystonias
Abnormal or involuntary eye movements, including oculogyric crisis
Facial grimacing
Twisting of the torso or other muscle groups

Akathisia
Restlessness
Constant moving about

Tardive Dyskinesia
Protrusion of the tongue
Chewing motion
Involuntary movements of the body and extremities

Other Side/Adverse Effects
Drowsiness
Blood dyscrasias
Pruritus
Photosensitivity
Elevated blood glucose level
Increased weight
Impaired body temperature regulation
Gynecomastia
Lactation

11. The client is informed that a full therapeutic effect of the medication may not be evident for 3 to 6 weeks after initiation of therapy. However, an observable therapeutic response may be apparent after 7 to 10 days.
12. The client is informed that some medications may cause a harmless change in urine color to pinkish to red-brown.
13. Reinforce instructions to use sunscreen, hats, and protective clothing when outdoors.
14. Inform the client to avoid alcohol or other CNS depressants.
15. Reinforce instructions to change positions slowly to avoid orthostatic hypotension.
16. Reinforce instructions to report signs of agranulocytosis, including sore throat, fever, and malaise.

17. Reinforce instructions to report signs of liver dysfunction, including jaundice, malaise, fever, and right upper abdominal pain.
18. When antipsychotics are discontinued, the medication dosage is reduced gradually to avoid sudden recurrence of psychotic symptoms.

⚠ Monitor for extrapyramidal side/adverse effects in the client taking an antipsychotic medication.

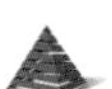

VIII. Neuroleptic Malignant Syndrome

A. Description
1. A potentially fatal syndrome that may occur at any time during therapy with neuroleptic (antipsychotic) medications
2. Although rare, neuroleptic malignant syndrome more commonly occurs at the initiation of therapy, after the client has changed from one medication to another, after a dosage increase, or when a combination of medications is used.

B. Data collection
1. Dyspnea or tachypnea
2. Tachycardia or irregular pulse rate
3. Fever
4. High or low blood pressure
5. Increased sweating
6. Loss of bladder control
7. Skeletal muscle rigidity
8. Pale skin
9. Excessive weakness or fatigue
10. Altered level of consciousness
11. Seizures
12. Severe extrapyramidal side/adverse effects
13. Difficulty swallowing
14. Excessive salivation
15. Oculogyric crisis
16. Dyskinesia
17. Elevated white blood cell count, liver function results, and creatinine phosphokinase level

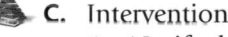

C. Interventions
1. Notify the registered nurse, who will then notify the HCP.
2. Monitor the vital signs.
3. Initiate safety and seizure precautions.
4. Prepare to discontinue the medication.
5. Monitor the level of consciousness.
6. Administer antipyretics as prescribed.
7. Use a cooling blanket to lower the body temperature.
8. Monitor electrolyte levels and assist to administer fluids intravenously as prescribed.

IX. Medications to Treat Attention-Deficit/Hyperactivity Disorder (Box 67-10)

A. Attention-deficit/hyperactivity disorder (ADHD) is categorized as a neurodevelopmental disorder (brain development correlates with this disorder).

BOX 67-10 Medications to Treat Attention-Deficit/Hyperactivity Disorder

Amphetamine
Atomoxetine (Strattera)
Dexmethylphenidate (Focalin)
Dextroamphetamine
Dextroamphetamine and amphetamine (Adderall XR, Adderall)
Lisdexamfetamine (Desoxyn)
Methamphetamine (Desoxyn)
Methylphenidate (Ritalin, Concerta, Metadate CD, Methylin)

B. It is characterized by inattentive or hyperactive-impulsive symptoms; onset criterion is that symptoms were present prior to age 12.

C. Children with ADHD may require medication to reduce hyperactive behavior and lengthen attention span.

D. CNS stimulants are effective in controlling this disorder; these medications, which increase agitation and activity in adults, have a calming effect on children with ADHD and increase alertness and sensitivity to stimuli.

E. Side/adverse effects
1. Tachycardia
2. Anorexia and weight loss
3. Elevated blood pressure
4. Dizziness
5. Agitation

F. Interventions
1. Monitor for CNS side/adverse effects.
2. Obtain a baseline ECG.
3. Monitor the blood pressure.
4. The child and parents are instructed that OTC medications need to be avoided.
5. The child and parents are instructed that the last dose of the day should be taken at least 6 hours before bedtime (14 hours for extended-released forms) to prevent insomnia.
6. Monitor height and weight (particularly in children).
7. Reinforce that several weeks of therapy may be necessary before the therapeutic effect is noted.
8. Reinforce instructions to the child and parents that a drug-free period may be prescribed to allow growth of the child if the medication has caused growth retardation.

X. Medications to Treat Alzheimer's Disease (Box 67-11)

A. Acetylcholinesterase inhibitors may be used to treat Alzheimer's disease to improve cognitive functions in the early stages.

B. Donepezil (Aricept)
1. An inhibitor of acetylcholinesterase used to treat mild to moderate dementia of Alzheimer's disease
2. Side/adverse effects include nausea and diarrhea.
3. Donepezil can slow the heart rate through its vagotonic effect. 

BOX 67-11 Medications to Treat Alzheimer's Disease

Donepezil (Aricept)
Galantamine (Razadyne)
Memantine (Namenda)
Rivastigmine (Exelon)

C. Galantamine (Razadyne)
1. An inhibitor of cholinesterase used to treat mild to moderate dementia of Alzheimer's disease
2. Side/adverse effects include nausea, vomiting, diarrhea, anorexia, and weight loss.
3. Can cause bronchoconstriction. Used with caution in clients with asthma and chronic obstructive pulmonary disease.

D. Memantine (Namenda)
1. An NMDA (*N*-methyl-D-aspartate) receptor antagonist is indicated for moderate to severe Alzheimer's disease.
2. Side/adverse effects include dizziness, headache, confusion, and constipation.
3. Should not be used in combination with other NMDA antagonists such as amantadine (Symmetrel) or ketamine (Ketalar). Such combinations produce undesirable additive effects.
4. Sodium bicarbonate and other medications that alkalinize the urine can decrease renal excretion of memantine. Accumulation to toxic levels can result.

E. Rivastigmine (Exelon)
1. Cholinesterase inhibitor used to treat mild to moderate dementia of Alzheimer's disease
2. Side/adverse effects include nausea, vomiting, diarrhea, abdominal pain, and anorexia.
3. Used with caution in clients with peptic ulcer disease, bradycardia, sick sinus syndrome, urinary obstruction, and lung disease because it enhances cholinergic transmission, thus intensifying symptoms of these disorders

CRITICAL THINKING What Should You Do?

Answer: Alprazolam is a benzodiazepine, and to prevent withdrawal or lessen withdrawal symptoms, the nurse should reinforce instructions to the client to taper the dose gradually over 2 to 6 weeks as specifically prescribed by the health care provider. The nurse should inform the client that abrupt or too rapid withdrawal can result in restlessness, irritability, insomnia, hand tremors, abdominal or muscle cramps, sweating, vomiting, and seizures. The nurse informs the client that if any of these manifestations occur during tapering, they should be reported immediately to the health care provider.

Reference(s): Hodgson, B., & Kizior, R. (2015). *Saunders nursing drug handbook 2015.* (pp. 42–44). St. Louis: Saunders.

PRACTICE QUESTIONS

731. The nurse is caring for a hospitalized client who has been taking clozapine (Clozaril) for the treatment of a schizophrenic disorder. Which laboratory study prescribed for the client should the nurse specifically review to monitor for an adverse effect associated with the use of this medication?
1. Platelet count
2. Cholesterol level
3. White blood cell count
4. Blood urea nitrogen level

732. Disulfiram (Antabuse) is prescribed for a client seen in the psychiatric health care clinic. The nurse is collecting data on the client and is reinforcing instructions regarding the use of this medication. Which is **most important** for the nurse to determine before administration of this medication?
1. A history of hyperthyroidism
2. A history of diabetes insipidus
3. When the last full meal was consumed
4. When the last alcoholic drink was consumed

733. The nurse is collecting data from a client, and the client's spouse reports that the client is taking donepezil hydrochloride (Aricept). Which disorder should the nurse suspect that this client may have based on the use of this medication?
1. Dementia
2. Schizophrenia
3. Seizure disorder
4. Obsessive-compulsive disorder

734. Fluoxetine (Prozac) is prescribed for the client, and the nurse reinforces instructions to the client regarding the administration of the medication. Which statement by the client indicates an understanding about administration of the medication?
1. "I should take the medication with my evening meal."
2. "I should take the medication at noon with an antacid."
3. "I should take the medication in the morning when I first arise."
4. "I should take the medication right before bedtime with a snack."

735. A client receiving a tricyclic antidepressant arrives at the mental health clinic. Which observation indicates that the client is correctly following the medication plan?
1. Reports not going to work for the past week
2. Complains of not being able to "do anything" anymore

3. Arrives at the clinic neat and appropriate in appearance
4. Reports sleeping 12 hours per night and 3 to 4 hours during the day

❖ **736.** A hospitalized client is started on phenelzine sulfate (Nardil) for the treatment of depression. The nurse reinforces instructions to the client and tells the client to avoid consuming which foods while taking this medication? **Select all that apply.**

- ❑ 1. Figs
- ❑ 2. Yogurt
- ❑ 3. Crackers
- ❑ 4. Aged cheese
- ❑ 5. Tossed salad
- ❑ 6. Oatmeal cookies

737. A client taking buspirone (BuSpar) for 1 month returns to the clinic for a follow-up visit. Which should indicate medication effectiveness?

1. No rapid heartbeats or anxiety
2. No paranoid thought processes
3. No thought broadcasting or delusions
4. No reports of alcohol withdrawal symptoms

738. A client taking lithium carbonate reports vomiting, abdominal pain, diarrhea, blurred vision, tinnitus, and tremors. The lithium level is checked as a part of the routine follow-up, and the level is 3.0 mEq/L. The nurse knows that this level is which?

1. Toxic
2. Normal
3. Slightly above normal
4. Excessively below normal

739. A client arrives at the health care clinic and tells the nurse that he has been doubling his daily dosage of bupropion hydrochloride (Wellbutrin) to help him get better faster. The nurse understands that the client is now at risk for which?

1. Insomnia
2. Weight gain
3. Seizure activity
4. Orthostatic hypotension

740. The nurse is performing a follow-up teaching session with a client discharged 1 month ago who is taking fluoxetine (Prozac). Which information should be important for the nurse to gather regarding the adverse effects related to the medication?

1. Cardiovascular symptoms
2. Gastrointestinal dysfunctions
3. Problems with mouth dryness
4. Problems with excessive sweating

Mental Health

ANSWERS

731. 3

Rationale: Hematological reactions can occur in the client taking clozapine and include agranulocytosis and mild leukopenia. The white blood cell count should be checked before initiating treatment and should be monitored closely during the use of this medication. The client should also be monitored for signs indicating agranulocytosis, which may include sore throat, malaise, and fever. Options 1, 2, and 4 are unrelated to this medication.

Test-Taking Strategy: Focus in the subject, an adverse effect of clozapine. Remember, clozapine can cause agranulocytosis and mild leukopenia. **Review:** adverse effects of clozapine.

Level of Cognitive Ability: Analyzing
Client Needs: Physiological Integrity
Integrated Process: Nursing Process/Data Collection
Content Area: Pharmacology: Psychiatric Medications
Priority Concepts: Cellular Regulation, Cognition
Reference(s): Hodgson, Kizior (2015), pp. 279–281.

732. 4

Rationale: Disulfiram is used as an adjunct treatment for selected clients with chronic alcoholism who want to remain in a state of enforced sobriety. Clients must abstain from alcohol intake for at least 12 hours before the initial dose of the medication is administered. The most important data are to determine when the last alcoholic drink was consumed. The medication is used with caution in clients with diabetes mellitus, hypothyroidism, epilepsy, cerebral damage, nephritis, and hepatic disease. It is contraindicated in severe heart disease, psychosis, or hypersensitivity related to the medication.

Test-Taking Strategy: Note the strategic words, *most important.* Recall that the medication is used as an adjunct treatment for selected clients with chronic alcoholism. This will assist in directing you to the correct option. **Review: disulfiram.**

Level of Cognitive Ability: Analyzing
Client Needs: Physiological Integrity
Integrated Process: Nursing Process/Data Collection
Content Area: Pharmacology: Psychiatric Medications
Priority Concepts: Addiction, Safety
Reference(s): Lehne (2013), pp. 446–447, 449; Varcarolis (2013), p. 373.

733. 1

Rationale: Donepezil hydrochloride is a cholinergic agent used in the treatment of mild to moderate dementia of the Alzheimer type. It enhances cholinergic functions by increasing the concentration of acetylcholine. It slows the progression of Alzheimer's disease. This medication is not used to treat the disorders in options 2, 3, and 4.

Test-Taking Strategy: Focus on the subject, the use of donepezil hydrochloride. Remember, this medication is used to treat mild to moderate dementia. **Review: donepezil.**

Level of Cognitive Ability: Analyzing
Client Needs: Physiological Integrity

Integrated Process: Nursing Process/Data Collection
Content Area: Pharmacology: Psychiatric Medications
Priority Concepts: Caregiving, Cognition
Reference(s): Hodgson, Kizior (2015), pp. 387–388.

734. 3
Rationale: Fluoxetine is a selective serotonin reuptake inhibitor. It is administered in the early morning without consideration to meals. Options 1, 2, and 4 are incorrect.
Test-Taking Strategy: Focus on the subject, the administration of fluoxetine. Use medication guidelines to eliminate option 2. Next, eliminate options 1 and 4 because they are comparable or alike and indicate taking the medication with food. Review: **fluoxetine client-teaching points.**
Level of Cognitive Ability: Evaluating
Client Needs: Physiological Integrity
Integrated Process: Nursing Process/Evaluation
Content Area: Pharmacology: Psychiatric Medications
Priority Concepts: Client Education, Mood and Affect
Reference(s): Lehne (2013), p. 376.

735. 3
Rationale: Depressed individuals will sleep for long periods, are not able to go to work, and feel as if they cannot "do anything." Once they have had some therapeutic effect from their medication, they will report resolution of many of these complaints, as well as demonstrate an improvement in their appearance.
Test-Taking Strategy: Focus on the subject, the effects of tricyclic antidepressants. Observations identified in options 1, 2, and 4 are all symptoms of depression. The improvement in appearance indicates a therapeutic response to the medication, thus indicating compliance with the medication regimen. **Review:** the expected effects of **tricyclic antidepressants.**
Level of Cognitive Ability: Evaluating
Client Needs: Physiological Integrity
Integrated Process: Nursing Process/Evaluation
Content Area: Pharmacology: Psychiatric Medications
Priority Concepts: Cognition, Mood and Affect
Reference(s): Lehne (2013), p. 366.

❖ **736. 1, 2, 4**
Rationale: Phenelzine sulfate (Nardil) is a monoamine oxidase inhibitor. The client should avoid consuming foods that are high in tyramine. Eating these foods could trigger a potentially fatal hypertensive crisis. Some foods to avoid include yogurt, aged cheeses, smoked or processed meats, red wines, and fruits such as avocados, raisins, and figs.
Test-Taking Strategy: Focus on the subject, foods to avoid when taking a monoamine oxidase inhibitor. Recall that phenelzine sulfate is a monoamine oxidase inhibitor and foods high in tyramine must be avoided. Next, from the food items listed in the question, identify the food that contains tyramine. **Review:** the food items to avoid with **monoamine oxidase inhibitors.**
Level of Cognitive Ability: Applying
Client Needs: Physiological Integrity
Integrated Process: Nursing Process/Implementation
Content Area: Pharmacology: Psychiatric Medications
Priority Concepts: Client Education, Safety
Reference(s): Hodgson, Kizior (2015), p. 952.

737. 1
Rationale: Buspirone hydrochloride is not recommended for the treatment of drug or alcohol withdrawal, paranoid thought disorders, or schizophrenia (thought broadcasting or delusions). Buspirone hydrochloride is most often indicated for the treatment of anxiety and aggression.
Test-Taking Strategy: Focus on the subject, the use of buspirone hydrochloride. Recalling that this medication is an antianxiety medication will direct you to the correct option. Review: **buspirone.**
Level of Cognitive Ability: Evaluating
Client Needs: Physiological Integrity
Integrated Process: Nursing Process/Evaluation
Content Area: Pharmacology: Psychiatric Medications
Priority Concepts: Anxiety, Mood and Affect
Reference(s): Hodgson, Kizior (2015), pp. 167–168.

738. 1
Rationale: The therapeutic serum level of lithium is 0.6 to 1.2 mEq/L. A level of 3 mEq/L indicates toxicity.
Test-Taking Strategy: Focus on the subject, the therapeutic serum level of lithium. Remember the therapeutic level is 0.6 to1.2 mEq/L. **Review: serum lithium levels.**
Level of Cognitive Ability: Understanding
Client Needs: Physiological Integrity
Integrated Process: Nursing Process/Data Collection
Content Area: Pharmacology: Psychiatric Medications
Priority Concepts: Cellular Regulation, Safety
Reference(s): Hodgson, Kizior (2015), p. 711.

739. 3
Rationale: Bupropion is an atypical antidepressant and does not cause significant orthostatic blood pressure changes. Seizure activity is common in dosages greater than 450 mg daily. Bupropion frequently causes a drop in body weight. Insomnia is a side effect, but seizure activity causes a greater client risk.
Test-Taking Strategy: Focus on the subject, the effects of doubling a dose of bupropion. Recalling that seizure activity can occur with higher-than-recommended doses will direct you to option 3. **Review: bupropion.**
Level of Cognitive Ability: Analyzing
Client Needs: Physiological Integrity
Integrated Process: Nursing Process/Data Collection
Content Area: Pharmacology: Psychiatric Medications
Priority Concepts: Clinical Judgment, Intracranial Regulation
Reference(s): Hodgson, Kizior (2015), p. 167.

740. 2
Rationale: The most common adverse effects related to fluoxetine include central nervous system (CNS) and gastrointestinal (GI) system dysfunction. This medication affects the GI system by causing nausea and vomiting, cramping, and diarrhea. Options 1, 3, and 4 are not adverse effects of this medication.
Test-Taking Strategy: Focus on the subject, adverse effects related to fluoxetine. It is necessary to recall that this medication causes CNS and GI system dysfunction. **Review: fluoxetine.**
Level of Cognitive Ability: Analyzing
Client Needs: Physiological Integrity
Integrated Process: Nursing Process/Data Collection
Content Area: Pharmacology: Psychiatric Medications
Priority Concepts: Clinical Judgment, Mood and Affect
Reference(s): Hodgson, Kizior (2015), p. 506.

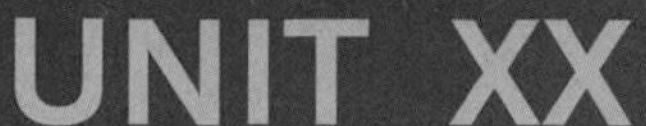
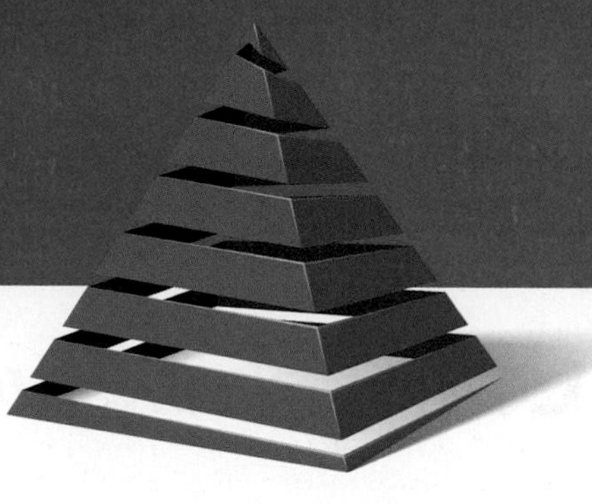

Comprehensive Test

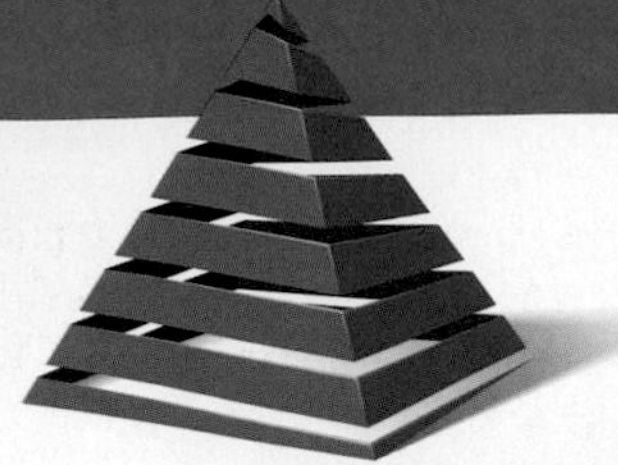

Comprehensive Test

741. The nurse reinforces home care instructions to the parents of a child hospitalized with pertussis. The child is in the convalescent stage and is being prepared for discharge. Which statement by the parents indicates a **need for further teaching**?
1. "We need to encourage adequate fluid intake."
2. "Coughing spells may be triggered by dust or smoke."
3. "We need to maintain respiratory precautions and a quiet environment for at least 2 weeks."
4. "Good hand-washing techniques need to be instituted to prevent spreading the disease to others."

❖ **742.** A client enters the emergency department confused, twitching, and having seizures. His family states he recently was placed on corticosteroids for arthritis and was feeling better and exercising daily. Upon assessment, he has flushed skin, dry mucous membranes, an elevated temperature, and poor skin turgor. His serum sodium level is 172 mEq/L. Which interventions would the health care provider likely prescribe? **Select all that apply.**
- ❑ 1. Monitor the vital signs.
- ❑ 2. Monitor intake and output.
- ❑ 3. Increase water intake orally.
- ❑ 4. Monitor the electrolyte levels.
- ❑ 5. Provide a sodium-reduced diet.
- ❑ 6. Administer sodium replacements.

743. The nurse is monitoring a client receiving glipizide (Glucotrol). Which outcome indicates an ineffective response from the medication?
1. A decrease in polyuria
2. A decrease in polyphagia
3. A fasting plasma glucose of 100 mg/dL
4. A glycosylated hemoglobin level of 12%

744. The nurse is reinforcing discharge instructions to a client receiving sulfisoxazole. Which should be included in the plan of care for instructions?
1. Maintain a high fluid intake.
2. Discontinue the medication when feeling better.
3. If the urine turns dark brown, call the health care provider immediately.
4. Decrease the dosage when symptoms are improving to prevent an allergic response.

745. Before administering an intermittent tube feeding through a nasogastric tube, the nurse checks for gastric residual volume. Which is the **best** rationale for checking gastric residual volume before administering the tube feeding?
1. Observe the digestion of formula.
2. Check fluid and electrolyte status.
3. Evaluate absorption of the last feeding.
4. Confirm proper nasogastric tube placement.

746. A postoperative client requests medication for flatulence (gas pains). Which medication from the following PRN list should the nurse administer to this client?
1. Ondansetron (Zofran)
2. Simethicone (Mylicon)
3. Acetaminophen (Tylenol)
4. Magnesium hydroxide (milk of magnesia, MOM)

747. A client is admitted to the hospital with a diagnosis of major depression. During the admission interview, the nurse determines that a major concern is the client's altered nutrition related to poor nutritional intake. Which nursing intervention related to altered nutrition should be the **initial** choice?
1. Weigh the client three times per week, before breakfast.
2. Explain to the client the importance of a good nutritional intake.
3. Report the nutritional concern to the psychiatrist and obtain a nutritional consult as soon as possible.
4. Offer the client several small, frequent meals daily, and schedule brief nursing interactions with the client during these times.

748. A client received 20 units of NPH insulin subcutaneously at 8:00 AM. The nurse should check the client for a potential hypoglycemic reaction at which time?

1. 5:00 PM
2. 10:00 AM
3. 11:00 AM
4. 11:00 PM

749. The nurse assists in developing a plan of care for a client with hyperparathyroidism receiving calcitonin-human (Cibacalcin). Which outcome has the **highest priority** regarding this medication?

1. Relief of pain
2. Absence of side effects
3. Reaching normal serum calcium levels
4. Verbalization of appropriate medication knowledge

750. The nursing instructor asks a nursing student about the cause of hemophilia. The student correctly responds by telling the instructor which fact about hemophilia?

1. Hemophilia is a Y-linked hereditary disorder.
2. A splenectomy resolves the bleeding disorders.
3. Hemophilia A results from deficiency of factor VIII.
4. A bone marrow transplant is the treatment of choice.

751. A 4-year-old child is admitted to the hospital with suspected acute lymphocytic leukemia (ALL). The nurse understands that which diagnostic study should confirm this diagnosis?

1. A platelet count
2. A lumbar puncture
3. Bone marrow biopsy
4. White blood cell (WBC) count

752. A child with leukemia is experiencing nausea related to medication therapy. The nurse, concerned about the child's nutritional status, should offer which during an episode of nausea?

1. Low-calorie foods
2. Cool, clear liquids
3. Low-protein foods
4. The child's favorite foods

753. To ensure a safe environment for a child admitted to the hospital for a craniotomy to remove a brain tumor, the nurse should include which in the plan of care?

1. Initiating seizure precautions
2. Using a wheelchair for out-of-bed activities
3. Assisting the child with ambulation at all times
4. Avoiding contact with other children on the nursing unit

❖ **754.** The nurse is preparing to suction an adult client through the client's tracheostomy tube. Which interventions should the nurse perform for this procedure? **Select all that apply.**

- ☐ 1. Apply suction for up to 10 to 15 seconds.
- ☐ 2. Hyperoxygenate the client before suctioning.
- ☐ 3. Set the wall suction unit pressure at 160 mm Hg.
- ☐ 4. Apply suction while gently inserting the catheter.
- ☐ 5. Apply intermittent suction while rotating and withdrawing the catheter.
- ☐ 6. Advance the catheter until resistance is met and then pull the catheter back 1 cm.

755. The nurse is assisting in caring for a client who has a placenta previa. The nurse understands that a cervical examination should not be performed on the client primarily because it could do which?

1. Cause hemorrhage
2. Initiate premature labor
3. Rupture the fetal membranes
4. Increase the chance of infection

756. A mother is breastfeeding her newborn. The mother complains to the nurse that she is experiencing severe nipple soreness. The nurse should provide which suggestion to the client?

1. Avoid rotating breastfeeding positions so that the nipple will toughen.
2. Stop nursing during the period of nipple soreness to allow the nipples to heal.
3. Nurse the newborn infant less frequently and substitute a bottle feeding until the nipples become less sore.
4. Position the newborn infant with the ear, shoulder, and hip in straight alignment and with the baby's stomach against the mother's.

757. On data collection, which behavior should the nurse expect a client diagnosed with agoraphobia to describe?

1. A fear of leaving the house
2. A fear of riding in elevators
3. A fear of speaking in public
4. A fear of uncleanliness and the need to bathe every hour

758. The nurse checks the food on a tray delivered for an Orthodox Jewish client and notes that the client has received a cheeseburger and potato fries with whole milk as a beverage. Which action should the nurse take?

1. Deliver the food tray to the client.
2. Replace the whole milk with lactose-free milk.
3. Call the dietary department and ask for a different meal.
4. Ask the dietary department to replace the beef with pork.

759. A client is brought to the emergency department by the ambulance team after collapse at home. Cardiopulmonary resuscitation is attempted but is unsuccessful. The wife of the client tells the nurse that the client is an organ donor and that his eyes are to be donated. Which action should the nurse take **next**?
1. Place dry, sterile dressings over the eyes of the deceased.
2. Call the National Donor Association to confirm that the client is a donor.
3. Close the eyes, elevate the head of the bed, and place a small ice pack on the eyes.
4. Ask the wife to obtain the legal documents regarding organ donation from the lawyer.

760. The nurse prepares to administer a prescribed dose of scopolamine (Transderm-Scop). The nurse should monitor for which side effect of this medication?
1. Dry mouth
2. Diaphoresis
3. Excessive urination
4. Pupillary constriction

761. The nurse is caring for a newborn diagnosed with Down syndrome. The parents are asking questions about the disorder. The nurse should provide which information when discussing Down syndrome?
1. The condition is characterized by above-average intellectual functioning with deficits in adaptive behavior.
2. The condition is characterized by average intellectual functioning and the absence of deficits in adaptive behavior.
3. The condition is characterized by subaverage intellectual functioning with the absence of deficits in adaptive behavior.
4. The condition is congenital and results in moderate to severe retardation and has been linked to an extra chromosome 21 (group G).

762. A client with a diagnosis of major depression becomes more anxious, reports sleeping poorly, and seems to display increased anger. The nurse should make which interpretation about the client's behavior?
1. The client is at increased risk for suicide.
2. The client is dealing with pertinent issues.
3. The client may need some time off the unit.
4. The client is responding normally to hospitalization.

763. Which electrocardiogram changes would the nurse note on the cardiac monitor with a client whose potassium (K^+) level is 2.7 mEq/L?
1. U waves
2. Flat P waves
3. Elevated T waves
4. Prolonged PR interval

764. An adult client with hepatic encephalopathy has a serum ammonia level of 120 mcg/dL and receives treatment with lactulose (Chronulac) syrup. The nurse determines that the client has the **best** response if the level changes to which after medication administration?
1. 2 mcg/dL
2. 5 mcg/dL
3. 70 mcg/dL
4. 100 mcg/dL

765. The nurse assists in developing a plan of care for the child with meningitis. Which would be the **priority** client problem for a child with a meningitis diagnosis?
1. Pain
2. Inadequate knowledge
3. Neurological dysfunction
4. Difficult family coping processes

766. The nurse is caring for a postoperative client who has been NPO and the health care provider has prescribed a clear liquid diet. In planning to initiate this diet, which **priority** item should the nurse place at the client's bedside?
1. A straw
2. Code cart
3. Blood pressure cuff
4. Suction equipment

767. The nurse reinforces client instructions about ethambutol (Myambutol). The nurse determines that the client understands the instructions if the client indicates to report which occurrence?
1. Impaired sense of hearing
2. Distressing gastrointestinal side effects
3. Orange-red discoloration of body secretions
4. Difficulty discriminating the color red from green

768. The nurse is caring for an older client with a diagnosis of myasthenia gravis and has reinforced self-care instructions. Which statement by the client indicates a **need for further teaching**?
1. "I rest each afternoon after my walk."
2. "I cough and deep breathe many times during the day."
3. "If I get abdominal cramps and diarrhea, I should call my doctor."
4. "I can change the time of my medication on the mornings that I feel strong."

❖769. The nurse should implement which in the care of a child who is having a seizure? **Select all that apply.**

- ❑ 1. Time the seizure.
- ❑ 2. Restrain the child.
- ❑ 3. Stay with the child.
- ❑ 4. Insert an oral airway.
- ❑ 5. Place the child in a supine position.
- ❑ 6. Loosen clothing around the child's neck.

❖770. The nurse is preparing to administer 35 mg of a prescribed intramuscular (IM) dose of medication to a client. The medication label reads 50 mg/mL. How many milliliters should the nurse administer to the client? **Fill in the blank.**

Answer: ______________ mL

❖771. The nurse is calculating a client's 24-hour fluid intake. The client consumed coffee (8 oz), water (8 oz), and orange juice (6 oz) for breakfast; soup (4 oz) and iced tea (8 oz) for lunch; and milk (10 oz), tea (8 oz), and water (8 oz) for dinner. The client also consumed 24 oz of water during the day. How many milliliters of fluid did the client consume in the 24-hour period? **Fill in the blank.**

Answer: ______________ mL

772. A client with diabetes mellitus who has been controlled with daily insulin has been placed on atenolol (Tenormin) for the control of angina pectoris. Because of the effects of atenolol, the nurse determines that which is the **most** reliable indicator of hypoglycemia?

1. Sweating
2. Tachycardia
3. Nervousness
4. Low blood glucose level

❖773. The nurse is asked to regulate the flow rate of an intravenous (IV) solution being administered to a client. The IV bag contains 50 mL of solution and the solution is to be administered over 30 minutes. The administration set has a drop factor of 10 drops (gtts)/mL. The nurse should regulate the roller clamp on the infusion set to deliver how many drops per minute? **Fill in the blank. Round answer to the nearest whole number.**

Answer: __________ gtts/minute

774. Which data would indicate a potential complication associated with age-related changes in the musculoskeletal system?

1. Decrease in height
2. Overall sclerotic lesions
3. Diminished lean body mass
4. Changes in structural bone tissue

775. The nurse reinforces home care instructions to the mother of a child recovering from Reye's syndrome. Which statement by the mother indicates a **need for further teaching**?

1. "I need to check for jaundiced skin and eyes every day."
2. "I need to have my child nap during the day to provide rest."
3. "I need to decrease the stimuli at home to prevent intracranial pressure."
4. "I need to give frequent, small, nutritious meals if my child starts to vomit."

❖776. A health care provider prescribes potassium chloride (KCl) elixir, 20 mEq orally daily. The medication label states potassium chloride (KCl), 30 mEq/15 mL. How many milliliters should the nurse prepare to administer the dose? **Fill in the blank.**

Answer: ______________ mL

777. The nurse reinforces medication instructions to a client with peptic ulcer disease. Which statement by the client indicates the **best** understanding of the medication therapy?

1. "Antacids will coat my stomach."
2. "Omeprazole (Prilosec) will coat the ulcer and help it heal."
3. "Sucralfate (Carafate) will change the fluid in my stomach."
4. "The nizatidine (Axid) will cause me to produce less stomach acid."

778. In planning activities for the depressed client, especially during the early stages of hospitalization, which is **best**?

1. Plan nothing until the client asks to participate in the milieu.
2. Encourage the client to participate in a structured daily program of activities.
3. Give the client a menu of daily activities and insist that the client participate in all activities offered.
4. Provide an activity that is quiet and solitary in nature to avoid increased fatigue, such as drawing or reading a book.

779. The nurse is assisting in preparing a plan of care for a 4-year-old child hospitalized with nephrotic syndrome. Which intervention is **most appropriate** for this child?

1. Provide a high-salt diet.
2. Provide a high-protein diet.
3. Discourage visitors at mealtimes.
4. Encourage the child to eat in the playroom.

780. The nursing instructor asks a student to describe the pathophysiology that occurs in Cushing's disease. Which statement by the student indicates an accurate understanding of this disorder?
1. "Cushing's disease is characterized by an oversecretion of insulin."
2. "Cushing's disease is characterized by an oversecretion of glucocorticoid hormones."
3. "Cushing's disease is characterized by an undersecretion of corticotropic hormones."
4. "Cushing's disease is characterized by an undersecretion of glucocorticoid hormones."

781. The nursing instructor asks the nursing student about the physiology related to the cessation of ovulation that occurs during pregnancy. Which response by the student indicates an understanding of this physiological process?
1. "Ovulation ceases during pregnancy because the circulating levels of estrogen and progesterone are high."
2. "Ovulation ceases during pregnancy because the circulating levels of estrogen and progesterone are low."
3. "The low levels of estrogen and progesterone increase the release of follicle-stimulating hormone and luteinizing hormone."
4. "The high levels of estrogen and progesterone promote the release of follicle-stimulating hormone and luteinizing hormone."

782. The nurse is assisting in collecting data on a child with seizures. The nurse is interviewing the child's parents to establish their adjustment to caring for their child with a chronic illness. Which statement by the parents indicates a **need for further teaching**?
1. "Our child sleeps in our bedroom at night."
2. "We worry about injuries when our child has a seizure."
3. "Our child is involved in a swim program with neighbors and friends."
4. "Our babysitter just completed first-aid and child resuscitation training."

783. A client is taking lansoprazole (Prevacid) for the chronic management of Zollinger-Ellison syndrome. If prescribed, which medication would be appropriate for the client if needed for a headache?
1. Naprosyn (Aleve)
2. Ibuprofen (Advil)
3. Acetaminophen (Tylenol)
4. Acetylsalicylic acid (aspirin)

784. A depressed client verbalizes feelings of low self-esteem and self-worth typified by statements such as "I'm such a failure. I can't do anything right!" Which action should the nurse take?
1. Tell the client that this is not true and that we all have a purpose in life.
2. Remain with the client and sit in silence until the client verbalizes feelings.
3. Identify recent behaviors or accomplishments that demonstrate skill or ability.
4. Reassure the client that you know how the client is feeling and that things will get better.

785. The nurse is assigned to care for an infant with cryptorchidism. The nurse anticipates that diagnostic studies will be prescribed to evaluate which?
1. DNA synthesis
2. Babinski reflex
3. Kidney function
4. Chromosomal analysis

786. The nurse is caring for a client with a diagnosis of pemphigus vulgaris. The nurse understands that which is a characteristic of this condition?
1. Dry skin
2. Hard skin
3. Leathery skin
4. Blistering skin

787. A client asks the nurse about the causes of acne. The nurse should respond by making which statement to the client?
1. "It is caused by oily skin."
2. "The exact cause of acne is not known."
3. "It is caused as a result of exposure to heat and humidity."
4. "Acne is caused by eating chocolate, nuts, and fatty foods."

❖ **788.** The nurse notes the appearance of skin breakdown on a client's hand at the site of an intravenous catheter that had medication infusing. The nurse determines that which adverse effect occurred? **Refer to figure.**
1. Phlebitis
2. Infiltration

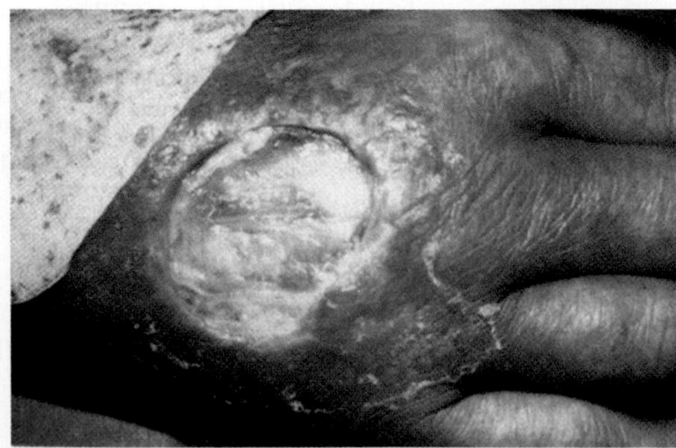

(Figure from Lewis S, Dirksen S, Heitkemper M, Bucher L, Camera I: *Medical-surgical nursing: Assessment and management of clinical problems*, ed 8, St. Louis, 2011, Mosby.)

3. Thrombosis
4. Extravasation

789. The nurse is reviewing the health record of a pregnant client at 16 weeks' gestation. The nurse should expect to note documentation that the fundus of the uterus is located at which area?
1. At the umbilicus
2. Just above the symphysis pubis
3. At the level of the xiphoid process
4. Midway between the symphysis pubis and the umbilicus

790. The nurse is assigned to care for a child with a compound (open) fracture of the arm that occurred as a result of a fall. The nurse plans care knowing that this type of fracture involves which specific characteristic?
1. The entire bone fractured straight across
2. A greater risk of infection than a simple fracture
3. The bone being fractured but not producing a break in the skin
4. One side of the bone being broken and the other side being bent

791. The nursing student is asked to discuss the topic of clubfoot at a clinical conference. The student plans to tell the group which fact about clubfoot?
1. It is a congenital anomaly.
2. It always occurs bilaterally.
3. It affects girls more often than boys.
4. It is a rare deformity of the skeletal system.

792. A client with type 1 diabetes mellitus is to begin an exercise program, and the nurse is reinforcing instructions to the client regarding the program. Which should the nurse include in the instructions?
1. Try to exercise before mealtime.
2. Administer insulin after exercising.
3. Take a blood glucose test before exercising.
4. Exercise should be performed during peak times of insulin.

793. The nurse is caring for an older client who is terminally ill. Which signs indicate to the nurse that death may be imminent?
1. Rubor and warm skin
2. Eupnea and normal body temperature
3. Irregular, noisy breathing and cold, clammy skin
4. Presence of swallowing reflex and active bowel sounds

794. The nurse has reinforced instructions to a client with tuberculosis about proper handling and disposal of respiratory secretions. The nurse determines that the client understands the instructions if the client verbalizes to take which measure?
1. Discard used tissues in a plastic bag.
2. Wash hands at least four times a day.
3. Brush teeth and rinse the mouth once a day.
4. Turn the head to the side if coughing or sneezing.

795. A client who has been taking isoniazid for 1½ months complains to the nurse about numbness, paresthesia, and tingling in the extremities. The nurse interprets that the client is experiencing which adverse effect?
1. Hypercalcemia
2. Peripheral neuritis
3. Small blood vessel spasm
4. Impaired peripheral circulation

796. The nurse is preparing a 2-year-old child with suspected nephrotic syndrome for a renal biopsy to confirm the diagnosis. The mother asks the nurse, "Will my child ever look thin again?" The nurse should respond by giving which statement?
1. "Do you feel guilty about your child's weight gain?"
2. "In most cases, medication and diet will control fluid retention."
3. "Wearing loose-fitting clothing should help conceal the extra weight."
4. "When children are little, it's expected that they'll look a little chubby."

❖ **797.** The nurse is caring for a client hospitalized with acute exacerbation of chronic obstructive pulmonary disease (COPD). Which should the nurse expect to note in this client? **Select all that apply.**
- ❑ **1.** Hypocapnia
- ❑ **2.** Dyspnea on exertion
- ❑ **3.** Presence of a productive cough
- ❑ **4.** Difficulty breathing while talking
- ❑ **5.** Increased oxygen saturation with exercise
- ❑ **6.** A shortened expiratory phase of respiration

❖ **798.** The nurse is preparing to administer an enema to an adult client. Which interventions should the nurse plan to perform for this procedure? **Select all that apply.**
- ❑ **1.** Apply disposable gloves.
- ❑ **2.** Place the client in the right Sims' position.
- ❑ **3.** Lubricate the enema tube and insert it approximately 4 inches.
- ❑ **4.** Clamp the tubing if the client expresses discomfort during the procedure.
- ❑ **5.** Hang the container containing the enema solution 24 inches above the client's anus.
- ❑ **6.** Ensure that the temperature of the solution is between 100°F (37.8°C) and 105°F (40.5°C).

❖ **799.** The nurse is assigned to care for an adult client who had a stroke and is aphasic. Which interventions should the nurse use for communicating with the client? **Select all that apply.**
- ❑ 1. Face the client when talking.
- ❑ 2. Speak slowly and maintain eye contact.
- ❑ 3. Use gestures when talking to enhance words.
- ❑ 4. Avoid the use of body language when talking to the client.
- ❑ 5. Give the client directions using short phrases and simple terms.
- ❑ 6. Phrase what was said differently the second time, if there is a need to repeat it.

800. The nurse observes that a client with a nasogastric tube connected to continuous gastric suction is mouth breathing, has dry mucous membranes, and has a foul breath odor. In planning care, which nursing intervention would be **best** to maintain the integrity of this client's oral mucosa?
1. Offer small sips of water frequently.
2. Encourage the client to suck on sour, hard candy.
3. Use lemon glycerin swabs to provide oral hygiene.
4. Use diluted mouthwash and water to rinse the mouth after brushing teeth.

801. A client is admitted to the hospital with possible rheumatic endocarditis. The nurse should check for a history of which type of infection?
1. Viral infection
2. Yeast infection
3. Streptococcal infection
4. Staphylococcal infection

802. A client who is taking hydrochlorothiazide (HydroDIURIL, HCTZ) has been started on triamterene (Dyrenium) as well. The client asks the nurse why both medications are required. Which response is the **most** accurate to give to the client?
1. Both are weak potassium-excreting diuretics.
2. The combination of these medications prevents renal toxicity.
3. Hydrochlorothiazide is an expensive medication, so using a combination of diuretics is cost-effective.
4. Triamterene is a potassium-retaining diuretic, whereas hydrochlorothiazide is a potassium-excreting diuretic.

803. A client who has begun taking fosinopril (Monopril) is very distressed, telling the nurse that he cannot taste food normally since beginning the medication 2 weeks ago. Which suggestion would provide the **best** support for the client?
1. Tell the client not to take the medication with food.
2. Suggest that the client taper the dose until taste returns to normal.
3. Inform the client that impaired taste is expected and generally disappears in 2 to 3 months.
4. Tell the client that a request will be made to the health care provider (HCP) to change the prescription.

804. The nurse is planning to administer amlodipine (Norvasc) to a client. The nurse should plan to check which before giving the medication?
1. Respiratory rate
2. Blood pressure and heart rate
3. Heart rate and respiratory rate
4. Level of consciousness and blood pressure

805. A client had an aortic valve replacement 2 days ago. This morning, the client tells the nurse, "I don't feel any better than I did before surgery." Which response by the nurse is **most appropriate**?
1. "You will feel better in a week or two."
2. "It's only the second day post-op. Cheer up."
3. "This is a normal frustration. It'll get better."
4. "You are concerned that you don't feel any better after surgery?"

❖ **806.** The nurse is preparing a list of home care instructions regarding stoma and laryngectomy care to a client. Which instructions should be included in the list? **Select all that apply.**
- ❑ 1. Restrict fluid intake.
- ❑ 2. Obtain a Medic-Alert bracelet.
- ❑ 3. Keep the humidity in the home low.
- ❑ 4. Prevent debris from entering the stoma.
- ❑ 5. Avoid exposure to people with infections.
- ❑ 6. Avoid swimming and use care when showering.

807. The nurse administers an injection to a client with a diagnosis of acquired immunodeficiency syndrome (AIDS). After administering the medication, the nurse should dispose of the used needle by which method?
1. Asking the client to recap the needle
2. Placing the needle and syringe in a puncture-resistant container
3. Recapping the needle before placing it in a puncture-resistant container
4. Laying the needle and syringe on the bedside table and carefully recapping the needle

808. The nurse is assisting in identifying clients in the community at risk for latex allergy. Which client population is **most** at risk for developing this type of allergy?
1. Children in day care centers
2. Individuals with spina bifida
3. Individuals with cardiac disease
4. Individuals living in a group home

809. A client has just had a cast removed and the underlying skin is yellow-brown and crusted. The nurse determines that **further skin care instructions are required** if the client makes which statement?
1. "I will soak the skin and then wash it gently."
2. "I need to scrub the skin vigorously with soap and water."
3. "I need to apply an emollient lotion to enhance softening."
4. "I need to use a sunscreen on the skin if it will be directly exposed to the sun."

810. A client has had skeletal traction applied to the right leg and has an overhead trapeze available for use. The nurse should monitor which as a high-risk area for pressure and breakdown?
1. Scapulae
2. Left heel
3. Right heel
4. Back of the head

811. A client has been placed in Buck's extension traction. Which technique provided by the nurse will provide countertraction?
1. Using a footboard
2. Providing an overhead trapeze
3. Slightly elevating the foot of the bed
4. Slightly elevating the head of the bed

❖ **812.** The nurse should expect to note which interventions in the plan of care for a client with hypothyroidism? **Select all that apply.**
- ❑ 1. Provide a cool environment for the client.
- ❑ 2. Instruct the client to consume a high-fat diet.
- ❑ 3. Instruct the client about thyroid replacement therapy.
- ❑ 4. Encourage the client to consume fluids and high-fiber foods in the diet.
- ❑ 5. Inform the client that iodine preparations will be prescribed to treat the disorder.
- ❑ 6. Instruct the client to contact the health care provider if episodes of chest pain occur.

813. The nurse is admitting a client with Guillain-Barré syndrome to the nursing unit. The client has an ascending paralysis to the level of the waist. Knowing the complications of the disorder, the nurse should bring which items into the client's room?
1. Nebulizer and pulse oximeter
2. Blood pressure cuff and flashlight
3. Flashlight and incentive spirometer
4. Electrocardiographic monitoring electrodes and intubation tray

814. A client with chronic kidney disease is receiving ferrous sulfate (Feosol). The nurse should monitor the client for which common side effect associated with this medication?
1. Diarrhea
2. Weakness
3. Headache
4. Constipation

815. The nurse is attempting to communicate with a hearing-impaired client. Which strategy by the nurse would be least helpful when talking to this client?
1. Reducing any background noise
2. Smiling continuously during conversation
3. Facing the client so that there is light on the nurse's face
4. Avoiding showing frustration through facial expression

816. The nurse is preparing to administer digoxin (Lanoxin), 0.125 mg orally, to a client with heart failure. Which vital sign is **most important** for the nurse to check before administering the medication?
1. Heart rate
2. Temperature
3. Respirations
4. Blood pressure

❖ **817.** A postoperative client has a prescription to receive an intravenous (IV) infusion of 1000 mL normal saline solution over a period of 10 hours. The drop (gtt) factor for the IV infusion set is 15 gtts/mL. The nurse sets the flow rate at how many drops per minute? **Fill in the blank.**

Answer: ________________ gtts/minute

❖ **818.** The nurse is preparing to set up a sterile field using the principles of aseptic technique to perform a dressing change. Which should the nurse include in the preparations? **Select all that apply.**
- ❑ 1. Use a dry table that is below waist level.
- ❑ 2. Open the distal flap of a sterile package first.
- ❑ 3. Prepare the sterile field just before the planned procedure.
- ❑ 4. Don clean gloves before touching items on the sterile field.
- ❑ 5. Place the sterile field 1 foot behind the working area and out of view of the client.
- ❑ 6. Avoid placing items within 1 inch of any area surrounding the outer edge of the sterile field.

819. The nurse is performing nasotracheal suctioning of a client. The nurse interprets that the client is adequately tolerating the procedure if which observation is made?
1. Skin color becomes cyanotic.
2. Secretions are becoming bloody.

3. Coughing occurs with suctioning.
4. Heart rate decreases from 78 to 54 beats/minute.

820. The nurse inspects the oral cavity of a client with cancer and notes white patches on the mucous membranes. The nurse interprets this occurrence as which?

1. Common
2. Suggests that the client is anemic
3. Characteristic of a thrush infection
4. Indicative that oral hygiene needs to be improved

821. The nurse is monitoring the laboratory results of a client preparing to receive chemotherapy. The nurse determines that the white blood cell count (WBC) is normal if which result is present?

1. 2000 cells/mm^3
2. 3000 cells/mm^3
3. 5000 cells/mm^3
4. 15,000 cells/mm^3

822. The nurse reinforces instructions to the client about breast self-examination (BSE). The nurse instructs the client to lie down and examine the left breast. Which is the correct area for placing a pillow when examining the left breast?

1. Under the left shoulder
2. Under the right scapula
3. Under the right shoulder
4. Under the small of the back

823. A client suspected of having an abdominal tumor is scheduled for a computed tomography (CT) scan with dye injection. The nurse should tell the client which about the test?

1. The test may be painful.
2. Fluids will be restricted after the test.
3. The test takes approximately 2 to 3 hours.
4. The dye injected may cause a warm, flushing sensation.

824. The nurse is caring for a client dying of ovarian cancer. During care, the client states, "If I can just live long enough to attend my daughter's graduation, I'll be ready to die." Which phase of coping is this client experiencing?

1. Anger
2. Denial
3. Bargaining
4. Depression

❖ **825.** The nurse is caring for a client who has been prescribed furosemide (Lasix) and is monitoring for adverse effects associated with this medication. Which should the nurse recognize as potential adverse effects? **Select all that apply.**

- ❑ 1. Nausea
- ❑ 2. Tinnitus
- ❑ 3. Hypotension
- ❑ 4. Hypokalemia
- ❑ 5. Photosensitivity
- ❑ 6. Increased urinary frequency

ANSWERS

741. 3

Rationale: Pertussis is transmitted by direct contact or respiratory droplets from coughing. The communicable period occurs primarily during the catarrhal stage. Respiratory precautions are not required during the convalescent phase. Options 1, 2, and 4 are components of home care instructions.

Test-Taking Strategy: Note the strategic words, *need for further teaching*. These words indicate a negative event query and the need to select the incorrect statement. Options 1 and 4 can be easily eliminated because they are general interventions associated with convalescence. Knowing that coughing spells are associated with pertussis will assist in directing you to the correct option from the remaining options. In addition, a 2-week period of respiratory precautions is not required. **Review:** home care instructions for the child with **pertussis.**

Level of Cognitive Ability: Evaluating

Client Needs: Safe and Effective Care Environment

Integrated Process: Nursing Process/Evaluation

Content Area: Child Health: Infectious and Communicable Diseases

Priority Concepts: Gas Exchange, Infection

Reference(s): Hockenberry, Wilson (2013), pp. 428, 653–654.

❖ **742. 1, 2, 3, 4, 5**

Rationale: Hypernatremia is described as having a serum sodium level that exceeds 145 mEq/L. Signs and symptoms would include dry mucous membranes, loss of skin turgor, thirst, flushed skin, elevated temperature, oliguria, muscle twitching, fatigue, confusion, and seizures. Interventions include monitoring fluid balance, monitoring vital signs, reducing dietary intake of sodium, monitoring electrolyte levels, and increasing oral intake of water. Sodium replacement therapy would not be prescribed for a client with hypernatremia.

Test-Taking Strategy: Focus on the subject, a sodium level of 172 mEq/L. Knowledge that this level is elevated and knowledge of the treatment for hyperkalemia will direct you to the correct options. **Review: hypernatremia.**

Level of Cognitive Ability: Analyzing

Client Needs: Physiological Integrity

Integrated Process: Nursing Process/Planning

Content Area: Fundamental Skills: Fluids & Electrolytes

Priority Concepts: Clinical Judgment, Fluid and Electrolyte Balance

Reference(s): deWit, Kumagai (2013), pp. 41–42.

743. 4

Rationale: Glipizide (Glucotrol) is an oral hypoglycemic agent administered to decrease the serum glucose level and the signs and symptoms of hyperglycemia. Therefore, a decrease in both polyuria and polyphagia would indicate a therapeutic response. Laboratory values are also used to monitor a client's response to treatment. A fasting blood glucose level of 100 mg/dL is within normal limits. However, glycosylated hemoglobin of 12% indicates poor glycemic control.

Test-Taking Strategy: Focus on the subject, an ineffective response to the medication. Recalling that glipizide is an oral hypoglycemic agent tells you to look for an option that would indicate hyperglycemia (lack of response to the medication). Options 1 and 2 are **comparable or alike options** and are eliminated first. Next, eliminate option 3 because it is a normal blood glucose level. **Review: glipizide (Glucotrol).**

Level of Cognitive Ability: Evaluating

Client Needs: Physiological Integrity

Integrated Process: Nursing Process/Evaluation

Content Area: Pharmacology: Endocrine Medications

Priority Concepts: Adherence, Glucose Regulation

Reference(s): deWit, Kumagai (2013), pp. 827, 862.

744. 1

Rationale: Each dose of sulfisoxazole should be administered with a full glass of water, and the client should maintain a high fluid intake. The medication is more soluble in alkaline urine. The client should not be instructed to taper or discontinue the dose. Some forms of sulfisoxazole cause the urine to turn dark brown or red. This does not indicate the need to notify the health care provider.

Test-Taking Strategy: Focus on the subject, instructions for a client taking a sulfonamide. General principles related to medication administration will assist in eliminating options 2 and 4. Options 2 and 4 are also **comparable or alike** options. Next, it is necessary to know that the client should maintain a high fluid intake. **Review: sulfisoxazole.**

Level of Cognitive Ability: Applying

Client Needs: Physiological Integrity

Integrated Process: Teaching and Learning

Content Area: Pharmacology: Renal and Urinary Medications

Priority Concepts: Client Education, Elimination

Reference(s): deWit, Kumagai (2013), p. 786.

745. 3

Rationale: All the stomach contents are aspirated and measured before administering a tube feeding. This procedure measures the gastric residual volume. The gastric residual volume is checked to confirm whether undigested formula from a previous feeding remains and thereby evaluates the absorption of the last feeding. It is important to check the gastric residual before administration of a tube feeding. A full stomach could result in overdistention, thus predisposing the client to regurgitation and possible aspiration. If residual feeding is obtained, the health care provider's prescription and agency policy are checked to determine the course of action (hold or reduce the volume of the intermittent tube feeding).

Test-Taking Strategy: Note the **strategic word**, *best*. Next, note the subject, the purpose of checking residual volume. Think about the complications associated with tube feedings and the risk of aspiration with an overdistended stomach. **Review:** the purpose for checking **gastric residual** volume.

Level of Cognitive Ability: Applying

Client Needs: Physiological Integrity

Integrated Process: Nursing Process/Data Collection

Content Area: Adult Health: Gastrointestinal

Priority Concepts: Clinical Judgment, Nutrition

Reference(s): Cooper, Gosnell (2015), pp. 676, 680.

746. 2

Rationale: Simethicone is an antiflatulent used in the relief of pain caused by excessive gas in the gastrointestinal tract. Ondansetron is used to treat postoperative nausea and vomiting. Acetaminophen is a nonopioid analgesic. Magnesium hydroxide is an antacid and laxative.

Test-Taking Strategy: Note the subject, a medication to treat flatulence (gas pains). Recalling the classifications of the medications in the options will direct you to the correct option. Review: **simethicone (Mylicon).**

Level of Cognitive Ability: Applying

Client Needs: Physiological Integrity

Integrated Process: Nursing Process/Implementation

Content Area: Pharmacology: Gastrointestinal Medications

Priority Concepts: Clinical Judgment, Pain

Reference(s): Hodgson, Kizior (2015), pp. 1104–1105.

747. 4

Rationale: Change in appetite is one of the major symptoms of depression. Offering the client several small, frequent meals and the nurse's presence at that time to support, encourage, or perhaps even feed the client is the most appropriate intervention. A client with depression experiences poor concentration and will not understand the importance of an adequate nutritional intake. Weighing the client does not address how to increase nutritional intake. Reporting the nutritional problems to the psychiatrist is correct to some degree, but it does not address how one might increase food intake.

Test-Taking Strategy: Note the **strategic word**, *initial*, and focus on the subject, the poor nutritional intake. The correct option is the only option that addresses the altered nutrition concretely and designs a method in which the client will feasibly increase the nutritional intake. **Review:** nutritional concerns with **depression**.

Level of Cognitive Ability: Applying

Client Needs: Physiological Integrity

Integrated Process: Nursing Process/Implementation

Content Area: Mental Health

Priority Concepts: Mood and Affect, Nutrition

Reference(s): deWit, Kumagai (2013), p. 1058.

748. 1

Rationale: NPH is intermediate-acting insulin. Its onset of action is 1 to 2½ hours, it peaks in 4 to 12 hours, and its duration of action is 24 hours. Hypoglycemic reactions most likely occur during peak time.

Test-Taking Strategy: Focus on the subject, NPH insulin. Recalling that peak action is between 4 and 12 hours will direct you to the correct option. **Review:** the characteristics of **NPH insulin**.

Level of Cognitive Ability: Applying

Client Needs: Physiological Integrity

Integrated Process: Nursing Process/Implementation

Content Area: Pharmacology: Endocrine Medications

Priority Concepts: Clinical Judgment, Glucose Regulation
Reference(s): Lehne (2013), p. 712.

749. 3
Rationale: Hypercalcemia can occur in clients with hyperparathyroidism, and calcitonin is used to lower plasma calcium levels. The highest-priority outcome in this client situation would be a reduction in serum calcium level. Option 1 is unrelated to this medication. Although options 2 and 4 are expected outcomes, they are not the highest priority for administering this medication.
Test-Taking Strategy: Note the **strategic words**, *highest priority*. Focus on the **subject**, a client with hyperparathyroidism who is receiving calcitonin-human (Cibacalcin). Also note the relation between the name of the medication and the word *calcium* in the correct option. **Review: calcitonin-human (Cibacalcin).**
Level of Cognitive Ability: Evaluating
Client Needs: Physiological Integrity
Integrated Process: Nursing Process/Planning
Content Area: Pharmacology: Endocrine Medications
Priority Concepts: Clinical Judgment, Fluid and Electrolyte Balance
Reference(s): deWit, Kumagai (2013), p. 825; Hodgson, Kizior (2015), pp. 176–177.

750. 3
Rationale: The term *hemophilia* refers to a group of bleeding disorders. The identification of the specific factor deficiencies allows for definitive treatment with replacement agents. Hemophilia A results from a deficiency of factor VIII. Hemophilia B (Christmas disease) is a deficiency of factor IX. Hemophilia is inherited in a recessive manner via a genetic defect on the X chromosome, not the Y chromosome. Neither a bone marrow transplant nor a splenectomy is used to treat this disorder.
Test-Taking Strategy: Focus on the **subject**, the definition of hemophilia. Knowledge regarding hemophilia and its related causes and treatment is needed to answer the question. Remember, hemophilia A results from a deficiency of factor VIII. **Review: hemophilia.**
Level of Cognitive Ability: Understanding
Client Needs: Physiological Integrity
Integrated Process: Teaching and Learning
Content Area: Child Health: Hematological
Priority Concepts: Clotting, Perfusion
Reference(s): McKinney et al (2013), p. 1252.

751. 3
Rationale: The confirmatory test for leukemia is microscopic examination of bone marrow obtained by bone marrow aspirate and biopsy. The WBC count may be high or low in leukemia. A lumbar puncture may be done to look for blast cells in the spinal fluid that are indicative of central nervous system disease. An altered platelet count occurs as a result of chemotherapy.
Test-Taking Strategy: Note the **subject**, diagnosing leukemia. Thinking about the pathophysiology of leukemia and recalling that the bone marrow is affected will direct you to the correct option. **Review:** diagnostic studies related to **leukemia.**
Level of Cognitive Ability: Understanding
Client Needs: Physiological Integrity
Integrated Process: Nursing Process/Data Collection
Content Area: Child Health: Oncological
Priority Concepts: Cellular Regulation, Clinical Judgment
Reference(s): McKinney et al (2013), p. 1274.

752. 2
Rationale: When the child is nauseated, it is best to offer frequent intake of cool, clear liquids in small amounts because small portions are usually better tolerated. Cool, clear fluids are also soothing and better tolerated when a client is nauseated. It is best not to offer favorite foods when the child is nauseated because foods eaten during times of nausea will be associated with being sick. It is best to offer small, frequent meals of high-protein and high-calorie content once the nausea has been controlled with medication or has subsided.
Test-Taking Strategy: The **subject** of the question relates to nutritional status in a child with nausea. You should easily be able to eliminate options 1 and 3 because of the word *low* in these options. For the remaining options, remember that it is best not to offer favorite foods when the child is nauseated because of their association with being sick. **Review:** interventions to relieve **nausea.**
Level of Cognitive Ability: Applying
Client Needs: Physiological Integrity
Integrated Process: Nursing Process/Implementation
Content Area: Fundamental Skills: Nutrition
Priority Concepts: Cellular Regulation, Nutrition
Reference(s): Hockenberry, Wilson (2013), pp. 781–782.

753. 1
Rationale: Safety of the child is the nursing priority. Seizure precautions should be implemented for any child with a brain tumor, both preoperatively and postoperatively. A thorough neurological assessment should be performed on the child, and the child's safety should be assessed before allowing the child to get out of bed without help. Assessment of the child's gait should be assessed daily. However, options 2 and 3 are not required unless functional deficits exist. Isolating the child, option 4, is not necessary.
Test-Taking Strategy: Note the **subject**, care for a child with a brain tumor. Eliminate options 2 and 3 first because they are **comparable or alike**. In addition, note the **closed-ended word**, *all*, in option 3. Eliminate option 4 because it is unnecessary. **Review:** care of the child with a **brain tumor.**
Level of Cognitive Ability: Analyzing
Client Needs: Safe and Effective Care Environment
Integrated Process: Nursing Process/Planning
Content Area: Child Health: Neurological
Priority Concepts: Intracranial Regulation, Safety
Reference(s): Hockenberry, Wilson (2013), pp. 965–966; McKinney et al (2013), pp. 1282–1283.

❖ **754. 1, 2, 5, 6**
Rationale: Intermittent suction is applied while rotating the catheter for 10 to 15 seconds. The nurse should hyperoxygenate the client with a resuscitator bag/Ambu-bag connected to an oxygen source before suctioning because suction depletes the client's oxygen supply (option 2). The catheter should be inserted gently until resistance is met or the client coughs, then pulled back 1 cm or ½ inch. Intermittent suction is applied

while rotating and withdrawing the catheter. Option 3 is incorrect because wall suction should be set to 80 to 120 mm Hg. Pressure set at a higher level can cause trauma to respiratory tract tissues. Strict asepsis needs to be maintained, and the nurse would wear sterile gloves to perform this procedure. Suction is never applied when inserting the catheter because it will deplete oxygen and can traumatize tissues.
Test-Taking Strategy: Focus on the subject, suctioning procedure through a tracheostomy tube. The priority issues to think about when answering this question include maintaining oxygenation, maintaining asepsis, and preventing tissue trauma. **Review: suctioning procedure.**
Level of Cognitive Ability: Analyzing
Client Needs: Physiological Integrity
Integrated Process: Nursing Process/Implementation
Content Area: Adult Health: Respiratory
Priority Concepts: Gas Exchange, Tissue Integrity
Reference(s): Cooper, Gosnell (2015), pp. 653–654; deWit, Kumagai (2013), p. 272.

755. 1
Rationale: Because the placenta is implanted low in the uterus, cervical examination could cause the disruption of the placenta and initiate profound hemorrhage. The other options are also correct, but the profound hemorrhage is of the greatest concern in this case.
Test-Taking Strategy: Focus on the subject, reason to not perform a cervical examination on a client with placenta previa. Think about the pathophysiology associated with placenta previa. Recall that bleeding is a primary concern. **Review: placenta previa.**
Level of Cognitive Ability: Applying
Client Needs: Physiological Integrity
Integrated Process: Nursing Process/Implementation
Content Area: Maternity: Antepartum
Priority Concepts: Reproduction, Safety
Reference(s): McKinney et al (2013), pp. 583–584.

756. 4
Rationale: Severe nipple soreness most often occurs as a result of poor positioning, incorrect latch-on, improper suck, or monilial infection. Comfort measures for nipple soreness include positioning the newborn with the ear, shoulder, and hip in straight alignment and with the baby's stomach against the mother's. Options 1, 2, and 3 do not identify measures that will alleviate the nipple soreness.
Test-Taking Strategy: Focus on the subject, correct positioning for breastfeeding. Eliminate options 2 and 3 because they are comparable or alike. To select between the remaining options, visualize each and note the word *toughen* in the incorrect option. **Review: breastfeeding.**
Level of Cognitive Ability: Applying
Client Needs: Health Promotion and Maintenance
Integrated Process: Teaching and Learning
Content Area: Maternity: Postpartum
Priority Concepts: Client Education, Nutrition
Reference(s): McKinney et al (2013), pp. 535, 542–543.

757. 1
Rationale: Agoraphobia is a fear of open spaces (i.e., leaving the house); panic attacks may occur when doing so. Option 2 describes a fear of closed spaces (claustrophobia). Option 3 describes a fear of public speaking (social phobia). Option 4 describes an obsessive-compulsive behavior.
Test-Taking Strategy: Focus on the subject, agoraphobia. It is necessary to recall the definition of agoraphobia to direct you to the correct option. **Review: phobias.**
Level of Cognitive Ability: Understanding
Client Needs: Psychosocial Integrity
Integrated Process: Nursing Process/Data Collection
Content Area: Mental Health
Priority Concepts: Anxiety, Mood and Affect
Reference(s): Varcarolis (2013), p. 176.

758. 3
Rationale: In the Orthodox Jewish tradition, members avoid meat from carnivores, pork products, and certain fish. The nurse should not deliver the food tray to the client and should ask the dietary department to deliver a different meal. Meat and dairy are served separately, thus the dairy–meat combination is not acceptable, making option 2 incorrect. Option 4 is incorrect because pork and pork products are also not allowed in the diet.
Test-Taking Strategy: Focus on the subject, nutrition in the Orthodox Jewish tradition. Recall that the dairy-meat combination is not acceptable in the Orthodox Jewish tradition. **Review:** the dietary rules of the **Orthodox Jewish** population.
Level of Cognitive Ability: Applying
Client Needs: Psychosocial Integrity
Integrated Process: Nursing Process/Implementation
Content Area: Fundamental Skills: Cultural Awareness
Priority Concepts: Culture, Nutrition
Reference(s): Giger (2013), pp. 516–517, 522.

759. 3
Rationale: When a corneal donor dies, antibiotic eyedrops may be prescribed and instilled. The eyes are closed and a small ice pack is placed on the closed eyes. The head of the bed is raised to 30 degrees to prevent edema. Within 2 to 4 hours, the eyes are enucleated. The cornea is usually transplanted within 24 to 48 hours. Option 1 is incorrect because dry dressings are not applied. Some organ donation protocols indicate using normal saline-moistened gauze. Option 2 is not an immediate action. In addition, the client should have a signed donor card, living will, or an organ donor–identified driver's license stating his or her wishes. Additional legal documentation should not be required. Agency procedures regarding donor care should be followed.
Test-Taking Strategy: Note the strategic word, *next.* Also note that the subject relates to preservation of the corneas and donation of the eyes. This should assist in eliminating options 2 and 4. From the remaining options, think about the effects of gravity and edema formation and recalling that the head of the bed should be elevated will direct you to the correct option. **Review: organ donation.**
Level of Cognitive Ability: Applying
Client Needs: Safe and Effective Care Environment
Integrated Process: Nursing Process/Implementation
Content Area: Leadership/Management: Ethical/Legal
Priority Concepts: Clinical Judgment, Ethics
Reference(s): Ignatavicius, Workman (2013), p. 1059.

760. 1
Rationale: Scopolamine is an anticholinergic medication that causes the frequent side effects of dry mouth, urinary retention, decreased sweating, and dilation of the pupils. The other options describe the opposite effects of cholinergic-blocking agents and therefore are incorrect.
Test-Taking Strategy: Focus on the subject, the side effects of an anticholinergic. It is necessary to know the effects of these medications to answer correctly. **Review:** the side effects associated with **anticholinergics.**
Level of Cognitive Ability: Applying
Client Needs: Physiological Integrity
Integrated Process: Nursing Process/Data Collection
Content Area: Fundamental Skills: Safety
Priority Concepts: Clinical Judgment, Safety
Reference(s): Hodgson, Kizior (2015), pp. 1091–1092.

761. 4
Rationale: Down syndrome is a form of mental retardation. It is a congenital condition that results in moderate to severe mental retardation. The syndrome has been linked to an extra group G chromosome, chromosome 21 (trisomy 21). Options 1, 2, and 3 are incorrect descriptions.
Test-Taking Strategy: Focus on the subject, Down syndrome. It is necessary to know that this condition is associated with an extra chromosome. **Review:** the characteristics of **Down syndrome.**
Level of Cognitive Ability: Understanding
Client Needs: Physiological Integrity
Integrated Process: Nursing Process/Implementation
Content Area: Child Health: Neurological
Priority Concepts: Client Education, Intracranial Regulation
Reference(s): Hockenberry, Wilson (2013), p. 576.

762. 1
Rationale: The behaviors identified in the question may be manifested by the client who is contemplating suicide. In clients who are depressed, anger may be self-directed in the form of suicide. Many of these symptoms are those of the depressed client; however, with this client, these behaviors have increased. Hospitalization may actually lessen these symptoms in the depressed client because a feeling of hope or relief may occur once treatment begins. Dealing with pertinent issues may be traumatic, but this is not the best interpretation of the behavior. Time off the unit for this client could put the client at risk for injury.
Test-Taking Strategy: Focus on the subject, a client with major depression. Noting the client's diagnosis and the words *becomes more anxious* will direct you to the correct option. **Review: suicide.**
Level of Cognitive Ability: Analyzing
Client Needs: Psychosocial Integrity
Integrated Process: Nursing Process/Data Collection
Content Area: Mental Health
Priority Concepts: Anxiety, Mood and Affect
Reference(s): Varcarolis (2013), p. 255.

763. 1
Rationale: A serum potassium level less than 3.5 mEq/L is indicative of hypokalemia. Potassium deficit is the most common electrolyte imbalance and is potentially life-threatening. Cardiac changes with hypokalemia may include peaked P waves, flattened T waves, depressed ST segment, and the presence of U waves.
Test-Taking Strategy: Focus on the subject, a potassium level of 2.7 mEq/L, and that this represents hypokalemia. It is necessary to recall the cardiac changes for a client with hypokalemia. Options 2, 3, and 4 are all characteristic cardiac changes noted with hyperkalemia. **Review: hypokalemia.**
Level of Cognitive Ability: Analyzing
Client Needs: Physiological Integrity
Integrated Process: Nursing Process/Data Collection
Content Area: Fundamental Skills: Fluids & Electrolytes
Priority Concepts: Fluid and Electrolyte Balance, Perfusion
Reference(s): Cooper, Gosnell (2015), pp. 543–544; deWit, Kumagai (2013), pp. 42, 44.

764. 3
Rationale: The normal serum ammonia level is 10 to 80 mcg/dL. In the client with hepatic encephalopathy, the serum level is not likely to drop below normal. The most optimal yet realistic change from the options provided would be to 70 mcg/dL, which falls in the normal range. A level of 100 mcg/dL represents an insufficient effect of the medication. Lactulose is administered for its hyperosmotic laxative effect, thus removing ammonia from the colon. The client should also be monitored for hypokalemia resulting from the severe purging lactulose causes.
Test-Taking Strategy: Note the strategic word, *best.* Familiarity with the subject, the normal serum ammonia level, is needed to answer this question. It is also necessary to understand the association between hepatic encephalopathy and this laboratory value. Recalling that the normal level is 10 to 80 mcg/dL will direct you to the correct option. **Review: serum ammonia levels.**
Level of Cognitive Ability: Analyzing
Client Needs: Physiological Integrity
Integrated Process: Nursing Process/Data Collection
Content Area: Pharmacology: Gastrointestinal Medications
Priority Concepts: Cellular Regulation, Fluid and Electrolyte Balance
Reference(s): deWit, Kumagai (2013), pp. 630, 696.

765. 3
Rationale: Neurological dysfunction is the priority client care concern for the child with meningitis. Pain related to meningeal irritation may also be a concern, but it is not the priority. There are no data in the question to indicate that there are psychosocial issues.
Test-Taking Strategy: Note the strategic word, *priority.* Use Maslow's Hierarchy of Needs theory to assist in eliminating options 2 and 4 because they are psychosocial problems. Next, focus on the child's diagnosis to direct you to the correct option. **Review: meningitis.**
Level of Cognitive Ability: Analyzing
Client Needs: Physiological Integrity
Integrated Process: Nursing Process/Planning
Content Area: Child Health: Neurological
Priority Concepts: Clinical Judgment, Intracranial Regulation
Reference(s): Hockenberry, Wilson (2013), p. 952; McKinney et al (2013), p. 1440.

766. 4

Rationale: In a postoperative client, a concern related to initiating a diet is aspiration. Initiating postoperative oral fluids may lead to distention and vomiting. Suction equipment must be available. A blood pressure cuff may be necessary but is not the priority from the options provided. A code cart is unnecessary. A straw may help the client sip fluids but is not necessary.

Test-Taking Strategy: Note the strategic word, *priority.* Use the ABCs—airway, breathing, and circulation—to answer this question. The correct option will maintain airway clearance. Review: care to the **postoperative client**.

Level of Cognitive Ability: Applying

Client Needs: Safe and Effective Care Environment

Integrated Process: Nursing Process/Planning

Content Area: Fundamental Skills: Perioperative Care

Priority Concepts: Gas Exchange, Nutrition

Reference(s): Perry, Potter, Ostendorf (2014), pp. 766–767.

767. 4

Rationale: Ethambutol causes optic neuritis, which decreases visual acuity and the ability to discriminate between the colors red and green. This poses a potential safety hazard when driving a motor vehicle. The client is taught to report this symptom immediately. The client is also taught to take the medication with food if gastrointestinal upset occurs. Impaired hearing results from antitubercular therapy with streptomycin. Orange-red discoloration of secretions occurs with rifampin (Rifadin).

Test-Taking Strategy: Focus on the subject, adverse effects of ethambutol. Option 2 is the least likely symptom to report; rather, it should be managed by taking the medication with food. Thus, this option can be eliminated first. From the remaining options, it is necessary to know that ethambutol may cause optic neuritis and difficulty with red-green discrimination. **Review: ethambutol**.

Level of Cognitive Ability: Evaluating

Client Needs: Physiological Integrity

Integrated Process: Nursing Process/Evaluation

Content Area: Pharmacology: Respiratory Medications

Priority Concepts: Safety, Sensory Perception

Reference(s): Hodgson, Kizior (2015), pp. 456–458.

768. 4

Rationale: The client with myasthenia gravis should be taught that timing of anticholinesterase medication is critical. It is important to instruct the client to administer the medication on time to maintain a chemical balance at the neuromuscular junction. If not given on time, the client may become too weak to swallow. Options 1, 2, and 3 include the necessary information that the client needs to understand to maintain health with this neurological degenerative disease.

Test-Taking Strategy: Note the strategic words, *need for further teaching.* These words indicate a negative event query and the need to select the incorrect client statement. Basic principles related to medication administration will direct you to the correct option. Remember, clients should not adjust dosage and medication times. **Review: myasthenia gravis**.

Level of Cognitive Ability: Evaluating

Client Needs: Physiological Integrity

Integrated Process: Teaching and Learning

Content Area: Pharmacology: Neurological Medications

Priority Concepts: Client Education, Safety

Reference(s): deWit, Kumagai (2013), p. 564; Ignatavicius, Workman (2013), p. 996.

❖ **769. 1, 3, 6**

Rationale: During a seizure, the child is placed on his or her side in a lateral position. Positioning on the side will prevent aspiration because saliva will drain out of the corner of the child's mouth. The child is not restrained because this could cause injury to the child. The nurse would loosen clothing around the child's neck and ensure a patent airway. Nothing is placed into the child's mouth during a seizure because this action may cause injury to the child's mouth, gums, or teeth. The nurse would stay with the child to reduce the risk of injury and allow for observation and timing of the seizure.

Test-Taking Strategy: Focus on the subject, interventions during a seizure. Recalling that airway patency and safety are the priorities will assist in determining the appropriate interventions. **Review:** care for the child experiencing a **seizure**.

Level of Cognitive Ability: Analyzing

Client Needs: Physiological Integrity

Integrated Process: Nursing Process/Implementation

Content Area: Child Health: Neurological

Priority Concepts: Intracranial Regulation, Safety

Reference(s): Hockenberry, Wilson (2013), p. 965.

❖ **770. 0.7 mL**

Rationale: Use the medication calculation formula and note the prescribed (35 mg) and available doses (50 mg/mL).

Formula:

$$\frac{Desired}{Available} \times Volume = mL\ per\ dose$$

$$\frac{35\text{ mg}}{50\text{ mg}} \times 1\text{ mL} = 0.7\text{ mL}$$

Test-Taking Strategy: The subject of the question is medication dosage calculation. Follow the formula for the calculation of the correct dose, noting the prescribed dose and the available dose. Note that the prescribed dose is a smaller amount than the dose available. This indicates that the amount to be given will be less than 1 mL. Once you have done the calculation, use a calculator to verify the answer. **Review: medication calculations**.

Level of Cognitive Ability: Applying

Client Needs: Physiological Integrity

Integrated Process: Nursing Process/Implementation

Content Area: Fundamental Skills: Medication/IV Calculations

Priority Concepts: Clinical Judgment, Safety

Reference(s): Cooper, Gosnell (2015), pp. 559, 567.

❖ **771. 2520 mL**

Rationale: The client consumed a total of 84 oz of fluid. Because 1 oz is equal to 30 mL, multiply 84 oz by 30 mL/oz. This yields 2520 mL.

Test-Taking Strategy: The subject of the question is dosage fluid intake calculation. First, count the total milliliters that the client consumed in a 24-hour period. Next, multiply the total milliliters by 30, recalling that 1 oz equals 30 mL. Use a calculator to verify the amount. **Review:** the procedure for calculating intake and changing **ounces to milliliters**.

Level of Cognitive Ability: Applying
Client Needs: Physiological Integrity
Integrated Process: Nursing Process/Data Collection
Content Area: Fundamental Skills: Fluids & Electrolytes
Priority Concepts: Fluid and Electrolyte Balance, Nutrition
Reference(s): Potter et al (2013), pp. 573–574.

772. 4
Rationale: β-Adrenergic blocking agents, such as atenolol, inhibit the appearance of signs and symptoms of acute hypoglycemia, which would include nervousness, increased heart rate, and sweating. Therefore, the client receiving this medication should adhere to the therapeutic regimen and monitor blood glucose levels carefully. Option 4 is the most reliable indicator of hypoglycemia.
Test-Taking Strategy: Note the strategic word, *most,* in the question. This indicates that more than one option could be partially or completely correct. Each option is, in fact, an indicator of hypoglycemia. Recalling the masking effects of β-adrenergic blocking agents helps you to choose the blood glucose level as the most reliable indicator. **Review: atenolol.**
Level of Cognitive Ability: Analyzing
Client Needs: Physiological Integrity
Integrated Process: Nursing Process/Data Collection
Content Area: Pharmacology: Cardiovascular Medications
Priority Concepts: Clinical Judgment, Glucose Regulation
Reference(s): Hodgson, Kizior (2015), pp. 93–94.

❖ **773. 17 gtt/minute**
Rationale: Use the IV flow rate formula.
Formula:

$$\frac{(\textit{Total volume} \times \textit{drop factor})}{\textit{Time (in minutes)}} = \textit{drops per minute}$$

$$\frac{50\text{ mL} \times 10\text{ gtt/mL}}{30\text{ minutes}} = 16.66, \text{ or } 17\text{ gtt/minute}$$

Test-Taking Strategy: The subject of the question is an IV flow rate calculation. To calculate the answer to this question correctly, you must be familiar with the standard formula for calculating IV flow rates. Use the formula and check your answer with a calculator. Remember to round to the nearest whole number. **Review: calculating IV rates.**
Level of Cognitive Ability: Applying
Client Needs: Physiological Integrity
Integrated Process: Nursing Process/Implementation
Content Area: Fundamental Skills: Medication/IV Calculations
Priority Concepts: Clinical Judgment, Safety
Reference(s): Cooper, Gosnell (2015), pp. 607–608.

774. 2
Rationale: Sclerotic lesions occur as bone resorption increases and results in replacement of original bone with fibrous material. This condition occurs in Paget's disease, an age-related disorder. Options 1, 3, and 4 identify normal age-related changes in the musculoskeletal system.
Test-Taking Strategy: Focus on the subject, age related changes in the musculoskeletal system. Note the words, *potential complication.* Recalling the normal age-related musculoskeletal findings will assist in directing you to the correct option. **Review:** normal findings in the **musculoskeletal system** in the **aging process.**
Level of Cognitive Ability: Understanding
Client Needs: Physiological Integrity
Integrated Process: Nursing Process/Data Collection
Content Area: Developmental Stages: Early Adulthood to Later Adulthood
Priority Concepts: Development, Tissue Integrity
Reference(s): Cooper, Gosnell (2015), pp. 729, 1087.

775. 4
Rationale: The vomiting that occurs in Reye's syndrome is caused by cerebral edema and is a symptom of increased intracranial pressure. Small, frequent meals will not affect the amount of vomiting, and the health care provider is notified if vomiting occurs. Options 1, 2, and 3 are all correct statements. Decreasing stimuli and providing rest decrease stress on the brain tissue. Checking for jaundice will assist in identifying the presence of liver complications, which are characteristic of Reye's syndrome.
Test-Taking Strategy: Note the strategic words, *need for further teaching.* These words indicate a negative event query and the need to select the incorrect client statement. Recalling the causes of vomiting with Reye's syndrome will direct you to the correct option. **Review: Reye's syndrome.**
Level of Cognitive Ability: Evaluating
Client Needs: Physiological Integrity
Integrated Process: Teaching and Learning
Content Area: Child Health: Neurological
Priority Concepts: Client Education, Intracranial Regulation
Reference(s): Hockenberry, Wilson (2013), p. 956; McKinney et al (2013), pp. 1004–1005, 1444.

❖ **776. 10**
Rationale: Follow the formula for dosage calculation.
Formula:

$$\frac{\textit{Desired}}{\textit{Available}} \times \textit{Volume} = \textit{mL per dose}$$

$$\frac{20\text{ mEq}}{30\text{ mEq}} \times 15\text{ mL} = 10\text{ mL}$$

Test-Taking Strategy: The subject of the question is a medication dosage calculation. Follow the formula for the calculation of the correct dose, and focus on the key information, 30 mEq/15 mL. Verify the answer with a calculator. **Review: medication calculations.**
Level of Cognitive Ability: Applying
Client Needs: Physiological Integrity
Integrated Process: Nursing Process/Implementation
Content Area: Fundamental Skills: Medication/IV Calculations
Priority Concepts: Clinical Judgment, Safety
Reference(s): Cooper, Gosnell (2015), pp. 559, 567.

777. 4
Rationale: Nizatidine, a histamine H_2-receptor blocker, is frequently used in the management of peptic ulcer disease. Histamine H_2-receptor blockers decrease the secretion of gastric acid (HCL). Antacids are used as adjunct therapy and neutralize acid in the stomach. Omeprazole is a proton pump inhibitor. Sucralfate (Carafate) promotes healing by covering the ulcer, thus protecting it from erosion caused by gastric acids.
Test-Taking Strategy: Note the strategic word, *best.* Also, focus on the subject, the pathophysiology associated with peptic

ulcer disease. Next, recalling the actions of the medications in the options will direct you to the correct one. **Review:** medications used to treat **peptic ulcer disease.**
Level of Cognitive Ability: Evaluating
Client Needs: Physiological Integrity
Integrated Process: Nursing Process/Evaluation
Content Area: Pharmacology: Gastrointestinal Medications
Priority Concepts: Client Education, Tissue Integrity
Reference(s): Hodgson, Kizior (2015), pp. 862–863.

778. 2
Rationale: A depressed person suffers with depressed mood and is often withdrawn. Also, the person experiences difficulty concentrating, loss of interest or pleasure, low energy, fatigue, and feelings of worthlessness and poor self-esteem. The plan of care needs to provide successful experiences in a stimulating yet structured environment rather than a quiet and solitary one.
Test-Taking Strategy: Note the **strategic word**, *best.* Also, focus on the **subject**, activities for the client with depression. Options 1 and 4 are eliminated first because they are too restrictive and offer little or no structure and stimulation. Option 3 is eliminated next because of the word *insist* and the **closed-ended word** *all* in this option. **Review:** care of the client with **depression.**
Level of Cognitive Ability: Applying
Client Needs: Psychosocial Integrity
Integrated Process: Nursing Process/Planning
Content Area: Mental Health
Priority Concepts: Mood and Affect, Safety
Reference(s): Stuart (2013), pp. 315, 373.

779. 4
Rationale: Mealtimes should center on pleasurable socialization. The child should be encouraged to eat meals with other children on the unit. A diet that is normal in protein with a sodium restriction is normally prescribed for a child with nephrotic syndrome. Parents or other family members should be encouraged to be present at mealtimes with a hospitalized child.
Test-Taking Strategy: The **subject** of the question is interventions for the child with nephrotic syndrome. Also note the **strategic words**, *most appropriate.* Eliminate options 1 and 2 first. A diet that is normal in protein with a sodium restriction is normally prescribed. Option 3 diminishes the importance of socialization at mealtime. **Review:** care to the child with **nephrotic syndrome.**
Level of Cognitive Ability: Applying
Client Needs: Physiological Integrity
Integrated Process: Nursing Process/Planning
Content Area: Child Health: Renal and Urinary
Priority Concepts: Fluid and Electrolyte Balance, Nutrition
Reference(s): Hockenberry, Wilson (2013), p. 914; McKinney et al (2013), p. 1132.

780. 2
Rationale: Cushing's syndrome is characterized by an oversecretion of glucocorticoid hormones. Addison's disease is characterized by the failure of the adrenal cortex to produce and secrete adrenocortical hormones. Options 1 and 4 are inaccurate regarding Cushing's syndrome.
Test-Taking Strategy: The **subject** of the question is the definition of Cushing's syndrome. Option 1 can be eliminated first because Cushing's syndrome is not associated with insulin. Remembering that in Cushing's ("u" as in "up") syndrome there is an oversecretion and in Addison's ("d" as in "down") there is an undersecretion will direct you to the correct option. **Review: Cushing's syndrome.**
Level of Cognitive Ability: Understanding
Client Needs: Physiological Integrity
Integrated Process: Teaching and Learning
Content Area: Adult Health: Endocrine
Priority Concepts: Cellular Regulation, Client Education
Reference(s): Cooper, Gosnell (2015), pp. 1746–1747.

781. 1
Rationale: Ovulation ceases during pregnancy because the circulating levels of estrogen and progesterone are high, thus inhibiting the release of follicle-stimulating hormone and luteinizing hormone, which are necessary for ovulation. Options 2, 3, and 4 are incorrect.
Test-Taking Strategy: Focus on the **subject**, the hormonal changes that occur during the menstrual cycle and during pregnancy. Remember, ovulation ceases during pregnancy because the circulating levels of estrogen and progesterone are high. **Review: hormonal changes in pregnancy.**
Level of Cognitive Ability: Understanding
Client Needs: Physiological Integrity
Integrated Process: Teaching and Learning
Content Area: Adult Health: Reproductive
Priority Concepts: Development, Reproduction
Reference(s): McKinney et al (2013), pp. 215, 751–752.

782. 1
Rationale: Parents are especially concerned about seizures that might go undetected at night. The nurse should suggest a baby monitor. Reassurance by the nurse should ensure parental confidence and decrease parental overprotection. Option 2 is a common concern. Options 3 and 4 demonstrate the parents' ability to choose respite care and activities appropriately. The parents need to be reminded that as the child grows, they cannot always observe their child, but their knowledge of seizure activity and care is appropriate to minimize complications.
Test-Taking Strategy: Note the **strategic words**, *need for further teaching.* These words indicate a **negative event query** and the need to select the incorrect client statement. The correct option identifies a need to provide the parents with an alternative method to monitor for night seizures. **Review:** parent teaching regarding **seizures.**
Level of Cognitive Ability: Evaluating
Client Needs: Psychosocial Integrity
Integrated Process: Teaching and Learning
Content Area: Child Health: Neurological
Priority Concepts: Family Dynamics, Intracranial Regulation
Reference(s): Hockenberry, Wilson (2013), p. 964.

783. 3
Rationale: Zollinger-Ellison syndrome is a hypersecretory condition of the stomach. The client should avoid taking medications that are irritating to the stomach lining. Irritants would include aspirin and nonsteroidal anti-inflammatory drugs (NSAIDs) such as naprosen and ibuprofen. Acetaminophen

would likely be prescribed for headache for this client because it would not be irritating to the stomach.

Test-Taking Strategy: Remember that comparable or alike options are not likely to be correct. With this in mind, eliminate options 1 and 2 first because they are NSAIDs. Choose acetaminophen over aspirin because it is least irritating to the stomach. **Review:** medication use in **Zollinger-Ellison syndrome**.

Level of Cognitive Ability: Applying
Client Needs: Physiological Integrity
Integrated Process: Nursing Process/Implementation
Content Area: Pharmacology: Gastrointestinal
Priority Concepts: Pain, Safety
Reference(s): Hodgson, Kizior (2015), pp. 672–674; Lewis et al (2014), p. 944.

784. 3

Rationale: Feelings of low self-esteem and worthlessness are common symptoms of the depressed client. An effective plan of care is to provide successful experiences for the client that are challenging but will not be met with failure to enhance the client's personal self-esteem. Reminders of the client's past accomplishments or personal successes are ways to interrupt the client's negative self-talk and distorted cognitive view of himself or herself. Options 1 and 4 offer false reassurances. Option 2 is not a therapeutic intervention with a depressed client.

Test-Taking Strategy: Use therapeutic communication techniques. Eliminate options 1 and 4 because the nurse is offering an opinion and false reassurance. Eliminate option 2 because, in this situation, silence can be interpreted as agreeing with the client's feelings. **Review:** care of the client with **depression**.

Level of Cognitive Ability: Applying
Client Needs: Psychosocial Integrity
Integrated Process: Nursing Process/Implementation
Content Area: Mental Health
Priority Concepts: Communication, Mood and Affect
Reference(s): Varcarolis (2013), pp. 255, 257.

785. 3

Rationale: Cryptorchidism may be the result of hormone deficiency, intrinsic abnormality of a testis, or a structural problem. Diagnostic tests would assess kidney function because the kidneys and testes arise from the same germ tissue. Babinski's reflex tests neurological function and is unrelated to this diagnosis. DNA synthesis and a chromosomal analysis are also unrelated to this diagnosis.

Test-Taking Strategy: The subject is diagnostic studies with cryptorchidism. Cryptorchidism, undescended or hidden testicles, relates to the genitourinary system. Option 2 relates to neurological function. Options 1 and 4 relate to the structure of cells. Option 3 is the only option that relates to the genitourinary system. **Review: cryptorchidism or undescended testes.**

Level of Cognitive Ability: Evaluating
Client Needs: Physiological Integrity
Integrated Process: Nursing Process/Data Collection
Content Area: Child Health: Renal and Urinary
Priority Concepts: Cellular Regulation, Clinical Judgment
Reference(s): McKinney et al (2013), p. 1126.

786. 4

Rationale: Pemphigus vulgaris is a rare, chronic, blistering disease caused by an autoimmune disorder that occurs most often during middle and old age. The lesions occur on normal-appearing skin or mucous membrane surfaces as fragile, flaccid bullae. Breaking the bullae leaves partial-thickness wounds that bleed, weep, and eventually form crusts. The skin is not dry, hard, or leathery.

Test-Taking Strategy: Knowledge of the subject, pemphigus vulgaris, is needed to answer the question. Eliminate options 2 and 3 first because they are comparable or alike. Next, it is necessary to know that this condition results in blistering. Review: the characteristics of **pemphigus vulgaris**.

Level of Cognitive Ability: Understanding
Client Needs: Physiological Integrity
Integrated Process: Nursing Process/Data Collection
Content Area: Adult Health: Integumentary
Priority Concepts: Immunity, Tissue Integrity
Reference(s): Lewis et al (2014), pp. 209, 217.

787. 2

Rationale: The exact cause of acne is unknown. Exacerbations that coincide with the menstrual cycle result from hormonal activity. Oily skin alone is not the cause of acne. Heat, humidity, and excessive perspiration also play a role in exacerbation of acne. There is no evidence that consumption of foods such as chocolate, nuts, or fatty foods affects acne.

Test-Taking Strategy: Focus on the subject, the causes of acne. Specific knowledge about this condition is needed to answer correctly. Options 1, 3, and 4 are not causes of acne. Remember that the exact cause is unknown. **Review: acne** and its causes.

Level of Cognitive Ability: Applying
Client Needs: Physiological Integrity
Integrated Process: Nursing Process/Implementation
Content Area: Adult Health: Integumentary
Priority Concepts: Cellular Regulation, Tissue Integrity
Reference(s): deWit, Kumagai (2013), pp. 967–968.

❖ **788. 4**

Rationale: Extravasation refers to the tissue injury that occurs from leakage of medication into surrounding skin and subcutaneous tissue; it can also cause tissue necrosis. Phlebitis is an inflammation of the vein that can occur from mechanical or chemical (medication) trauma or from a local infection. Phlebitis can cause the development of a clot (thrombophlebitis). Infiltration is seepage of the intravenous fluid out of the vein and into the surrounding interstitial spaces. It is a form of tissue injury, but the injury is not to the extent that occurs with extravasation.

Test-Taking Strategy: Focus on the subject, the characteristics of the tissue injury noted in the figure. Eliminate options 1 and 3 first because they are comparable or alike and relate to vein injury. Next, noting that the injury in the figure illustrates an open wound will direct you to the correct option. **Review:** the characteristics of **extravasation**.

Level of Cognitive Ability: Analyzing
Client Needs: Physiological Integrity
Integrated Process: Nursing Process/Data Collection
Content Area: Critical Care: Medications and Intravenous Therapy
Priority Concepts: Clinical Judgment, Tissue Integrity
Reference(s): deWit, Kumagai (2013), p. 54.

789. 4

Rationale: At 12 weeks' gestation, the uterus extends out of the maternal pelvis and can be palpated above the symphysis pubis. At 16 weeks, the fundus reaches midway between the symphysis pubis and the umbilicus. At 20 weeks, the fundus is located at the umbilicus. By 36 weeks, the fundus reaches its highest level at the xiphoid process.

Test-Taking Strategy: Focus on the subject, uterine growth at 16 weeks' gestation. Think about the growth of the fetus to assist in answering. **Review: uterine growth pattern.**

Level of Cognitive Ability: Understanding

Client Needs: Physiological Integrity

Integrated Process: Nursing Process/Data Collection

Content Area: Maternity: Antepartum

Priority Concepts: Development, Reproduction

Reference(s): McKinney et al (2013), p. 223.

790. 2

Rationale: In a compound (open) fracture, a wound in the skin leads to the broken bone, and there is an added danger of infection. Option 1 describes a transverse fracture. Option 3 describes a closed or simple fracture. Option 4 describes a greenstick fracture.

Test-Taking Strategy: Focus on the subject, an open fracture. Visualize this type of fracture. An open wound provides the entry to bacteria. **Review:** various types of **fractures.**

Level of Cognitive Ability: Applying

Client Needs: Physiological Integrity

Integrated Process: Nursing Process/Planning

Content Area: Child Health: Musculoskeletal

Priority Concepts: Infection, Tissue Integrity

Reference(s): Hockenberry, Wilson (2013), p. 1057.

791. 1

Rationale: Clubfoot, one of the most common deformities of the skeletal system, is a congenital anomaly characterized by a foot that has been twisted inward or outward. The condition generally affects both feet, and boys are affected twice as often as girls.

Test-Taking Strategy: Eliminate option 2 because of the closed-ended word, *always,* and option 4 because of the word *rare.* From the remaining options, it is necessary to know that this disorder is a congenital anomaly. **Review:** congenital **clubfoot.**

Level of Cognitive Ability: Understanding

Client Needs: Physiological Integrity

Integrated Process: Nursing Process/Planning

Content Area: Child Health: Musculoskeletal

Priority Concepts: Development, Mobility

Reference(s): Hockenberry, Wilson (2013), pp. 1071–1072.

792. 3

Rationale: A blood glucose test performed before exercising provides information to the client regarding the need to eat a snack first. Exercising during the peak times of insulin effect or before mealtime places the client at risk for hypoglycemia. Insulin should be administered as prescribed.

Test-Taking Strategy: The subject of the question relates to the occurrence of a hypoglycemic reaction. Keep this subject in mind and think about the effects of insulin and exercise on the blood glucose level. **Review: insulin, exercise, and the blood glucose level.**

Level of Cognitive Ability: Applying

Client Needs: Health Promotion and Maintenance

Integrated Process: Teaching and Learning

Content Area: Adult Health: Endocrine

Priority Concepts: Glucose Regulation, Safety

Reference(s): Cooper, Gosnell (2015), pp 517, 1755–1756.

793. 3

Rationale: The clinical signs of impending or approaching death include inability to swallow; pitting edema; decreased gastrointestinal and urinary tract activity; bowel and bladder incontinence; loss of motion, sensation, and reflexes; cold or clammy skin; cyanosis; lowered blood pressure; noisy or irregular respiration; and Cheyne-Stokes respirations.

Test-Taking Strategy: The subject of the question is the signs of impending death. Eliminate options 2 and 4 because these identify normal findings. Eliminate option 1 because warm skin is a normal finding. **Review: the signs of impending death.**

Level of Cognitive Ability: Understanding

Client Needs: Physiological Integrity

Integrated Process: Nursing Process/Data Collection

Content Area: Developmental Stages: End-of-Life Care

Priority Concepts: Caregiving, Gas Exchange

Reference(s): Cooper, Gosnell (2015), p. 757.

794. 1

Rationale: Used tissues are discarded in a plastic bag, so contaminated respiratory secretions can be contained. The client with tuberculosis should wash hands carefully after each contact with respiratory secretions. Oral care should be performed more than once a day. The client should be instructed to cover the mouth and nose when laughing, sneezing, or coughing and to wear a mask when in contact with others until drug therapy suppresses the infection.

Test-Taking Strategy: Note that the question specifically relates to the subject of handling and disposal of secretions. The only options that address this topic directly are options 1 and 4. Because turning the head to the side for coughing and sneezing does not specifically address the handling of secretions, eliminate option 4. Disposal of tissues in a plastic bag is correct. **Review:** home care instructions related to **tuberculosis.**

Level of Cognitive Ability: Evaluating

Client Needs: Safe and Effective Care Environment

Integrated Process: Nursing Process/Evaluation

Content Area: Fundamental Skills: Infection Control

Priority Concepts: Infection, Safety

Reference(s): deWit, Kumagai (2013), p. 301.

795. 2

Rationale: An adverse effect of isoniazid is peripheral neuritis. This is manifested by numbness, tingling, and paresthesias in the extremities. This adverse effect can be minimized with pyridoxine (vitamin B_6) intake.

Test-Taking Strategy: Focus on the subject, the adverse effects of isoniazid. Options 3 and 4 would not cause the symptoms presented in the question but instead would be manifested by pallor and coolness. Thus options 3 and 4 can be eliminated first. From the remaining options, it is necessary to know either that peripheral neuritis is an adverse effect of the medication or that the client's symptoms do not correlate with hypercalcemia. **Review:** adverse effects of **isoniazid.**

Level of Cognitive Ability: Analyzing
Client Needs: Physiological Integrity
Integrated Process: Nursing Process/Data Collection
Content Area: Adult Health: Respiratory Medications
Priority Concepts: Clinical Judgment, Safety
Reference(s): deWit, Kumagai (2013), p. 300.

796. 2
Rationale: It is important to give the mother information that addresses the issue that is the parent's concern. Most children experience remission with treatment. Options 1 and 3 are nontherapeutic and may add to the mother's guilt. Option 4 does not acknowledge the concern and is a stereotypical response.
Test-Taking Strategy: Use **therapeutic communication techniques**, and focus on the mother's concern. Options 1, 3, and 4 do not address the mother's concern and are inappropriate and nontherapeutic responses. Remember to always address the client's feelings and concerns. **Review: nephrotic syndrome and therapeutic communication techniques.**
Level of Cognitive Ability: Applying
Client Needs: Physiological Integrity
Integrated Process: Communication and Documentation
Content Area: Child Health: Renal and Urinary
Priority Concepts: Communication, Fluid and Electrolyte Balance
Reference(s): Hockenberry, Wilson (2013), p. 915; McKinney et al (2013), pp. 30–31.

❖ **797. 2, 3, 4**
Rationale: Clinical manifestations of COPD include hypoxemia, hypercapnia, dyspnea on exertion and at rest, oxygen desaturation with exercise, use of accessory muscles of respiration, and a prolonged expiratory phase of respiration. The client may also exhibit difficulty breathing while talking, and may have to take breaths between every one or two words. Some clients with COPD, especially those with a history of smoking, often have a productive cough especially on arising in the morning. The chest x-ray will reveal a hyperinflated chest and a flattened diaphragm if the disease is advanced.
Test-Taking Strategy: Think about the **subject**, the manifestations noted in chronic obstructive pulmonary disease (COPD). Think about the pathophysiology associated with COPD. Eliminate option 5 because oxygen desaturation rather than saturation would occur. Next, eliminate option 6 because, in the client with COPD, a prolonged expiratory phase of respiration would be noted. From the remaining options, reading carefully will assist in eliminating option 1 because hypercapnia would occur. **Review:** signs/symptoms associated with **chronic obstructive pulmonary disease.**
Level of Cognitive Ability: Analyzing
Client Needs: Physiological Integrity
Integrated Process: Nursing Process/Data Collection
Content Area: Adult Health: Respiratory
Priority Concepts: Gas Exchange, Perfusion
Reference(s): Cooper, Gosnell (2015), pp. 1657–1658, 1660; deWit, Kumagai (2013), pp. 303–304.

❖ **798. 1, 3, 4, 6**
Rationale: The administration of an enema is a clean procedure, and standard precautions must be used. The nurse applies disposable gloves when administering an enema to prevent the transfer of microorganisms. To administer an enema, the nurse places the client in the left Sims' position because the enema solution will flow downward by gravity along the natural curve of the sigmoid colon and rectum, improving retention of the enema solution. The tube is lubricated for easy insertion and is inserted approximately 3 to 4 inches in an adult. If the client complains of cramping or discomfort during the procedure, the nurse clamps the tubing until the discomfort subsides. The container containing the enema solution is hung about 12 to 18 inches above the client's anus. A flow of solution that is too forceful can damage the bowel. The temperature of the solution should be between 100°F (37.8°C) and 105°F (40.5°C). Solution that is too hot will burn the client, and solution that is too cool will cause cramping.
Test-Taking Strategy: Focus on the **subject**, procedure for administering an enema. Thinking about the anatomy of the bowel and the precautions that need to be taken to prevent trauma to rectal tissue will assist in identifying the correct interventions. **Review:** the procedure for administering an enema.
Level of Cognitive Ability: Applying
Client Needs: Physiological Integrity
Integrated Process: Nursing Process/Implementation
Content Area: Fundamental Skills: Elimination
Priority Concepts: Elimination, Safety
Reference(s): Cooper, Gosnell (2015), pp. 686–688.

❖ **799. 1, 2, 3, 5**
Rationale: A client who is aphasic has difficulty expressing or understanding language. The nurse should face the client when talking, establish and maintain eye contact, and speak slowly and distinctly. The nurse should use gestures and pantomime when talking to enhance words and use body language to enhance the message. The nurse should give the client directions using short phrases and simple terms, and phrase questions so that they can be answered with a yes or no. If there is a need to repeat something, the nurse should use the same words a second time.
Test-Taking Strategy: Aphasia is the **subject** of the question. Recall that a client who is aphasic has difficulty expressing or understanding language. Using the principles related to communicating to a hearing-impaired client will assist in identifying the correct interventions for the client with aphasia. **Review:** the guidelines for communicating with a client who is aphasic.
Level of Cognitive Ability: Applying
Client Needs: Physiological Integrity
Integrated Process: Communication and Documentation
Content Area: Adult Health: Neurological
Priority Concepts: Communication, Intracranial Regulation
Reference(s): Cooper, Gosnell (2015), pp. 75, 1100.

800. 4
Rationale: After the nasogastric tube is in place, mouth care is extremely important. With one naris occluded, the client tends to mouth breathe, drying the mucous membranes. Frequent oral hygiene may be required to prevent or care for dry, irritated mucous membranes. Frequent, small sips of water would be contraindicated when the client is on gastric suction. The hard candy would increase the salivation but would not be useful in cleaning the oral cavity. Lemon glycerin swabs have a drying or irritating effect on the mucous membranes.

Test-Taking Strategy: Note the strategic word, *best,* and focus on the subject, maintaining the integrity of the oral mucosa. Recalling that a client on gastric suction will be NPO and swallowing water or other liquids would be prohibited will assist in eliminating options 1 and 2. From the remaining options, eliminate option 3 because lemon glycerin swabs are drying to the mucosa. **Review:** care of the client with a **nasogastric tube**.
Level of Cognitive Ability: Applying
Client Needs: Physiological Integrity
Integrated Process: Nursing Process/Implementation
Content Area: Adult Health: Gastrointestinal
Priority Concepts: Clinical Judgment, Tissue Integrity
Reference(s): Cooper, Gosnell (2015), p. 678.

801. 3
Rationale: Rheumatic endocarditis, also called rheumatic carditis, is a major indicator of rheumatic fever, which is a complication of infection with group A β-hemolytic streptococcal infections. It is frequently triggered by streptococcal pharyngitis. Options 1, 2, and 4 are incorrect.
Test-Taking Strategy: Focus on the subject, the type of infection associated with rheumatic endocarditis. Think about the pathophysiology associated with this disorder. Remember that streptococcal infections can result in rheumatic heart disease. **Review:** the causes of **endocarditis**.
Level of Cognitive Ability: Applying
Client Needs: Physiological Integrity
Integrated Process: Nursing Process/Data Collection
Content Area: Adult Health: Cardiovascular
Priority Concepts: Infection, Inflammation
Reference(s): Lewis et al (2014), p. 819.

802. 4
Rationale: Potassium-retaining diuretics include amiloride (Midamor), spironolactone (Aldactone), and triamterene (Dyrenium). They are weak diuretics that are used in combination with potassium-excreting diuretics. This combination is useful when medication and dietary supplement of potassium is not appropriate. The use of two different diuretics does not prevent renal toxicity. Hydrochlorothiazide is an effective and inexpensive generic form of the thiazide classification of diuretics.
Test-Taking Strategy: Note the strategic word, *most.* Focus on the medications in the question and their classifications. Hydrochlorothiazide is a potassium-excreting diuretic, and triamterene is a potassium-retaining diuretic; thus option 1 can be eliminated. Toxicity from these medications is the result of fluid and electrolyte imbalances, so option 2 can be eliminated. Hydrochlorothiazide is a common and inexpensive diuretic, so option 3 can be eliminated. **Review: diuretics.**
Level of Cognitive Ability: Applying
Client Needs: Physiological Integrity
Integrated Process: Nursing Process/Implementation
Content Area: Pharmacology: Cardiovascular Medications
Priority Concepts: Clinical Judgment, Fluid and Electrolyte Balance
Reference(s): Lehne (2013), pp. 486–487.

803. 3
Rationale: ACE inhibitors, such as fosinopril, cause temporary impairment of taste (dysgeusia). The nurse can tell the client that this effect usually disappears in 2 to 3 months, even with continued therapy, and provide nutritional counseling if appropriate to avoid weight loss. Options 1, 2, and 4 are inappropriate actions. Taking this medication with or without food does not affect absorption and action. The dosage should never be tapered without HCP approval, and the medication should never be stopped abruptly.
Test-Taking Strategy: Note the strategic word, *best,* and use general medication administration guidelines to answer correctly. Eliminate option 2 first because it is an inappropriate nursing action. The nurse does not advise the client to make dosage changes for any prescribed medication. Taking the medication with or without food is not going to change the taste of the food, so option 1 can be eliminated next. **Review:** the effects of ACE **inhibitors**.
Level of Cognitive Ability: Applying
Client Needs: Physiological Integrity
Integrated Process: Nursing Process/Implementation
Content Area: Pharmacology: Cardiovascular Medications
Priority Concepts: Adherence, Sensory Perception
Reference(s): Cooper, Gosnell (2015), p. 1568; Lehne (2013), pp. 512–513.

804. 2
Rationale: Amlodipine is a calcium channel blocker. This medication decreases the rate and force of cardiac contraction. Before administering a calcium channel blocking agent, the nurse should check the blood pressure and heart rate, which could both decrease in response to the action of this medication. This action will help to prevent or identify early problems related to decreased cardiac contractility, heart rate, and conduction.
Test-Taking Strategy: Focus on the subject, the action to take before administering amlodipine. Recall that this medication is a calcium channel blocker. This group of medications decreases the rate and force of cardiac contraction. This in turn lowers the pulse rate and blood pressure. Option 1 can be eliminated first because it is unrelated to the medication. With options 3 and 4, note that only half of the option is correct. When answering questions with two items per option, both of the items must be correct for that option to be correct. **Review: amlodipine.**
Level of Cognitive Ability: Applying
Client Needs: Physiological Integrity
Integrated Process: Nursing Process/Data Collection
Content Area: Pharmacology: Cardiovascular Medications
Priority Concepts: Clinical Judgment, Perfusion
Reference(s): Hodgson, Kizior (2015), pp. 59–60.

805. 4
Rationale: Paraphrasing is restating the client's message in the nurse's own words. Paraphrasing may be in the form of a question. Option 4 uses the therapeutic communication technique of paraphrasing. The client is frustrated and is searching for understanding. Options 1, 2, and 3 are inappropriate communication techniques. Option 1 belittles the client's concerns. Options 2 and 3 offer false reassurance by the nurse.
Test-Taking Strategy: Note the strategic words, *most appropriate.* Use therapeutic communication techniques to answer the question. Option 4 focuses on the client's feelings. **Review: therapeutic communication techniques.**

Level of Cognitive Ability: Applying
Client Needs: Psychosocial Integrity
Integrated Process: Communication and Documentation
Content Area: Fundamental Skills: Perioperative Care
Priority Concepts: Communication, Coping
Reference(s): Cooper, Gosnell (2015), pp. 62–68; deWit, Kumagai (2013), p. 446.

❖ 806. 2, 4, 5, 6
Rationale: The nurse should teach the client how to care for the stoma, depending on the type of laryngectomy performed. Most interventions focus on protection of the stoma and the prevention of infection. Interventions include avoiding swimming and using caution when showering, avoiding exposure to people with infections, preventing debris from entering the stoma, and obtaining a Medic-Alert bracelet. Additional interventions include wearing a stoma guard or high-collar clothing to cover the stoma, increasing the humidity in the home, and increasing fluid intake to 3000 mL/day to keep the secretions thin.
Test-Taking Strategy: Focus on the subject, protecting a laryngectomy stoma. Think about the complications that can occur with this type of stoma and the interventions that protect the stoma and prevent infection. This will assist in identifying the client instructions for home care. **Review:** home care instructions for a **laryngectomy stoma.**
Level of Cognitive Ability: Analyzing
Client Needs: Physiological Integrity
Integrated Process: Teaching and Learning
Content Area: Fundamental Skills: Safety
Priority Concepts: Infection, Tissue Integrity
Reference(s): Lewis et al (2014), p. 517.

807. 2
Rationale: The correct procedure for needle disposal is to discard uncapped needles and sharps in a hard-walled, puncture-resistant, leak-proof container immediately after use. Discarding the uncapped needle and attached syringe in a designated sharps container prevents injury to the client and health care personnel. Recapping needles increases the risk of needle-stick injury. Options 1, 3, and 4 are unsafe actions.
Test-Taking Strategy: Focus on the subject, safe disposal of needles. Note that options 1, 3, and 4 are comparable or alike in that they all address recapping the needle. **Review:** principles of **safe disposal of needles.**
Level of Cognitive Ability: Applying
Client Needs: Safe and Effective Care Environment
Integrated Process: Nursing Process/Implementation
Content Area: Fundamental Skills: Safety
Priority Concepts: Infection, Safety
Reference(s): deWit, Kumagai (2013), p. 230.

808. 2
Rationale: Individuals at risk for developing a latex allergy include health care workers; individuals who work with manufacturing latex products; individuals with spina bifida; individuals who wear gloves frequently such as food handlers, hairdressers, and auto mechanics; and individuals allergic to kiwis, bananas, pineapples, passion fruit, avocados, and chestnuts.
Test-Taking Strategy: Note the strategic word, *most.* Focus on the subject, a latex allergy. Recalling the cause and the source of the allergic reaction will easily direct you to the correct option. **Review:** the cause of this type of **latex allergy** and the individuals at risk.
Level of Cognitive Ability: Analyzing
Client Needs: Health Promotion and Maintenance
Integrated Process: Nursing Process/Data Collection
Content Area: Adult Health: Immune
Priority Concepts: Clinical Judgment, Immunity
Reference(s): Perry, Potter, Ostendorf (2014), p. 191.

809. 2
Rationale: The skin under a casted area may be discolored and crusted with dead skin layers. The client should gently soak and wash the skin for the first few days. The skin should be patted dry, and a lubricating lotion should be applied. Clients often want to scrub the dead skin away, which irritates the skin. The client should avoid direct exposure of the skin to the sunlight.
Test-Taking Strategy: Note the strategic words, *further skin care instructions are required.* These words indicate a negative event query and the need to select the incorrect option. Option 3 is obviously helpful and therefore cannot be the answer to the question as stated. Option 4 is a safe measure and is eliminated next. Because vigorous scrubbing is more likely to be irritating than providing a gentle wash, option 2 is the likely choice as the answer to the question. **Review:** skin care measures after **cast removal.**
Level of Cognitive Ability: Evaluating
Client Needs: Physiological Integrity
Integrated Process: Teaching and Learning
Content Area: Adult Health: Musculoskeletal
Priority Concepts: Client Education, Tissue Integrity
Reference(s): deWit, Kumagai (2013), p. 745.

810. 2
Rationale: Common areas that are under pressure and are at risk for breakdown include the elbows (if they are used for repositioning instead of a trapeze) and the heel of the good leg (which is used as a brace when pushing up in bed). Other pressure points caused by the traction include the ischial tuberosity, popliteal space, and Achilles tendon.
Test-Taking Strategy: Focus in the subject, high-risk area for skin breakdown. Thus you should compare each of the options in terms of their relative risk and choose the one that is highest. The right heel is eliminated first because it is off the bed in the traction setup. The overhead trapeze would diminish the likelihood that the scapulae and back of the head would be immobiled. This leaves the left heel as the answer. This makes sense, given that the client would use the unaffected heel to push into the mattress during repositioning. With repeated use, this could cause the left heel to become reddened and break down. **Review:** the complications of **skeletal traction.**
Level of Cognitive Ability: Applying
Client Needs: Physiological Integrity
Integrated Process: Nursing Process/Data Collection
Content Area: Adult Health: Musculoskeletal
Priority Concepts: Mobility, Tissue Integrity
Reference(s): deWit, Kumagai (2013), p. 744.

811. 3
Rationale: The part of the bed under an area in traction is usually elevated to aid in countertraction. For the client in Buck's

extension traction (which is applied to a leg), the foot of the bed is elevated. Option 1 places undue pressure on the client's unaffected foot. Option 2 is not used for the purpose of countertraction. Buck's extension traction is applied to the leg, so you can eliminate option 4.
Test-Taking Strategy: The subject of the question is traction and countertraction. To answer this question correctly, you need to understand the principles of traction and countertraction and be familiar with Buck's extension traction. Option 2 is not used for the purpose of countertraction and is eliminated first. Knowing that Buck's extension traction is applied to the leg helps you eliminate option 4. Of the two remaining options, option 1 places undue pressure on the client's unaffected foot. Furthermore, a footboard is not used for the purpose of providing countertraction. Option 3 provides a force that opposes the traction force effectively without harming the client. **Review:** care of the client in **Buck's extension traction**.
Level of Cognitive Ability: Applying
Client Needs: Physiological Integrity
Integrated Process: Nursing Process/Implementation
Content Area: Adult Health: Musculoskeletal
Priority Concepts: Mobility, Safety
Reference(s): deWit, Kumagai (2013), p. 744.

❖ 812. 3, 4, 6
Rationale: The clinical manifestations of hypothyroidism are the result of decreased metabolism from low levels of thyroid hormone. Interventions are aimed at replacement of the hormones and providing measures to support the signs and symptoms related to a decreased metabolism. The nurse encourages the client to consume a well-balanced diet that is low in fat for weight reduction and high in fluids and high-fiber foods to prevent constipation. The client often has cold intolerance and requires a warm environment. The client would notify the health care provider if chest pain occurs because it could be an indication of overreplacement of thyroid hormone. Iodine preparations are used to treat hyperthyroidism. These medications decrease blood flow through the thyroid gland and reduce the production and release of thyroid hormone.
Test-Taking Strategy: Focus on the subject, client teaching points for hypothyroidism. Recalling that the client has a decreased metabolic rate in this disorder will assist in determining the appropriate interventions. **Review:** interventions for the client with **hypothyroidism** and **hyperthyroidism**.
Level of Cognitive Ability: Analyzing
Client Needs: Physiological Integrity
Integrated Process: Nursing Process/Implementation
Content Area: Adult Health: Endocrine
Priority Concepts: Caregiving, Thermoregulation
Reference(s): Cooper, Gosnell (2015), p. 1737; deWit, Kumagai (2013), p. 844.

813. 4
Rationale: The client with Guillain-Barré syndrome is at risk for respiratory failure because of ascending paralysis. An intubation tray should be available for use. Another complication of this syndrome is cardiac dysrhythmia, which necessitates the use of ECG monitoring. Because the client is immobilized, the nurse should routinely assess for deep vein thrombosis and pulmonary embolism.
Test-Taking Strategy: Use the ABCs—airway, breathing, and circulation. With an ascending paralysis, the client is at risk for involvement of respiratory muscles and subsequent respiratory failure. This knowledge makes you look for an option that coincides with this line of thought. The correct option is the only one that includes an intubation tray, which would be needed if the client's status deteriorated to needing intubation and mechanical ventilation. It also addresses cardiac monitoring. **Review:** care of the client with **Guillain-Barré syndrome**.
Level of Cognitive Ability: Applying
Client Needs: Physiological Integrity
Integrated Process: Nursing Process/Implementation
Content Area: Adult Health: Neurological
Priority Concepts: Gas Exchange, Safety
Reference(s): deWit, Kumagai (2013), pp. 560–561.

814. 4
Rationale: Feosol is an iron supplement used to treat anemia. Constipation is a frequent and uncomfortable side effect associated with the administration of oral iron supplements. Stool softeners are often prescribed to prevent constipation. Options 1, 2, and 3 are not associated with this medication.
Test-Taking Strategy: Focus on the subject, a side effect of ferrous sulfate. Think about the classification of this medication. Recalling that oral iron can cause constipation will direct you to the correct option. **Review:** the side effects of **ferrous sulfate**.
Level of Cognitive Ability: Applying
Client Needs: Physiological Integrity
Integrated Process: Nursing Process/Data Collection
Content Area: Pharmacology: Hematological Medications
Priority Concepts: Cellular Regulation, Elimination
Reference(s): Hodgson, Kizior (2015), pp. 486–488.

815. 2
Rationale: Hearing-impaired clients rely on visual cues to help them comprehend the conversation of others. Smiling continuously is the least helpful strategy, because the smile distorts the appearance of the mouth if the client is trying to read lips. When beginning the conversation, it helps to reduce background noise such as turning off or lowering the volume of the television. Facing the client and standing so there is light on the nurse's face are helpful strategies, because it assists the client to lip-read. Taking care not to show frustration or annoyance with the client's impairment is also helpful to preserve the client's self-esteem.
Test-Taking Strategy: Focus on the subject, the least-helpful strategy for communicating with the hearing-impaired client. Noting the words, *smiling continuously,* in option 2 will direct you to this option. **Review: communication strategies.**
Level of Cognitive Ability: Applying
Client Needs: Psychosocial Integrity
Integrated Process: Communication and Documentation
Content Area: Adult Health: Ear
Priority Concepts: Communication, Sensory Perception
Reference(s): deWit, Kumagai (2013), p. 587.

816. 1
Rationale: Digoxin is a cardiac glycoside that is used to treat heart failure and acts by increasing the force of myocardial contraction. Because bradycardia may be a clinical sign of toxicity, the nurse counts the apical heart rate for 1 full minute before administering the medication. If the pulse rate is less

than 60 beats/minute in an adult client, the nurse would withhold the medication and report the pulse rate to the registered nurse, who would then contact the health care provider.
Test-Taking Strategy: Note the strategic words, *most important*, and focus on the subject, the parameter to measure before administering digoxin. Recalling that this medication is a cardiac glycoside and the action and nursing interventions related to administering this medication will assist in answering this question. Remember that bradycardia is a sign of toxicity. Review: nursing interventions related to the administration of digoxin.
Level of Cognitive Ability: Applying
Client Needs: Physiological Integrity
Integrated Process: Nursing Process/Implementation
Content Area: Pharmacology: Cardiovascular Medications
Priority Concepts: Clinical Judgment, Perfusion
Reference(s): Hodgson, Kizior (2015), p. 363.

❖ 817. 25 gtt/min
Rationale: Use the formula for calculating IV flow rates.
Formula:

$$\frac{\textit{Total volume to infuse} \times \textit{gtt factor}}{\textit{Time in minutes}} = \textit{gtt/minute}$$

$$\frac{1000\ \text{mL} \times 15\ \text{gtt/mL}}{600\ \text{minutes}} = 25\ \text{gtt/min}$$

Test-Taking Strategy: Focus on the subject, calculating an IV flow rate. Use the IV flow rate formula, and remember to change hours to minutes. Once you have done the calculation, recheck your work using a calculator and make sure that the answer makes sense. Review: **IV flow rates**.
Level of Cognitive Ability: Applying
Client Needs: Physiological Integrity
Integrated Process: Nursing Process/Implementation
Content Area: Fundamental Skills: Medication/IV Calculations
Priority Concepts: Clinical Judgment, Safety
Reference(s): Cooper, Gosnell (2015), pp. 607–608.

❖ 818. 2, 3, 6
Rationale: Sterile packages are opened away from the nurse's body, and the distal flap of a sterile package is opened first. This prevents contaminating the pack by reaching over the exposed sterile contents after the other flaps are opened (option 2). To avoid contamination, the sterile field should be prepared just before the planned procedure, and supplies should be used immediately (option 3). The outer 1-inch border of the sterile field must be considered unsterile, and sterile items are not placed within this 1-inch area (option 6). A dry table that is at waist level is used to set up a sterile field. Moisture will contaminate the sterile field, and anything below waist level is considered contaminated, according to the principles of surgical asepsis. The sterile field must be kept in sight at all times, and the nurse should not turn away from it. If this happens, the nurse cannot be sure that it is still sterile. Sterile gloves, not clean gloves, are used. An unsterile item touching a sterile item contaminates the sterile item.
Test-Taking Strategy: Focus on the subject, the principles of aseptic technique. Thinking about these principles and visualizing each intervention will assist in identifying those that are appropriate. Review: principles of **aseptic technique**.
Level of Cognitive Ability: Applying
Client Needs: Safe and Effective Care Environment
Integrated Process: Nursing Process/Implementation
Content Area: Fundamental Skills: Infection Control
Priority Concepts: Infection, Safety
Reference(s): Cooper, Gosnell (2015), pp. 116–117, 121.

819. 3
Rationale: Coughing is a normal response to suctioning for the client with an intact cough reflex, and it is not an indication that the client is not tolerating the procedure. The client should be encouraged to cough to help with removal of secretions from the lungs. The nurse should monitor for the adverse effects of suctioning, which include cyanosis (pulse oximetry falls below 90% or 5% from baseline), excessively rapid or slow heart rate (a 20 beat/minute change), or the sudden development of bloody secretions. If they occur, the nurse stops suctioning, administers oxygen as appropriate, and reports these signs to the health care provider immediately.
Test-Taking Strategy: Note the subject, adequately tolerating nasotracheal suctioning. Cyanosis and bradycardia are abnormal findings and are eliminated first. From the remaining options, the use of the word *becoming* in association with bloody secretions tells you that this has not been an ongoing occurrence, making this an incorrect option. Because the cough reflex is normally present and suction triggers coughing, option 3 is preferable. Review: **nasotracheal suctioning**.
Level of Cognitive Ability: Evaluating
Client Needs: Physiological Integrity
Integrated Process: Nursing Process/Evaluation
Content Area: Adult Health: Respiratory
Priority Concepts: Clinical Judgment, Gas Exchange
Reference(s): Cooper, Gosnell (2015), pp. 660–661.

820. 3
Rationale: Candidiasis is a fungal infection caused by *Candida albicans*. When it occurs in the mouth, it is called thrush and appears as white plaques. Although it can occur in an immunocompromised client, it is not considered to be common. Options 2 and 4 are not accurate regarding this infection.
Test-Taking Strategy: Focus on the subject, white patches on the mucous membranes. Options 1 and 4 can be eliminated first because this is not a common manifestation and is unrelated to the need for improved oral hygiene. Recalling that the anemic client is more likely to exhibit pallor will assist in eliminating option 2 and will direct you to the correct option. Review: manifestations associated with **thrush**.
Level of Cognitive Ability: Analyzing
Client Needs: Physiological Integrity
Integrated Process: Nursing Process/Data Collection
Content Area: Adult Health: Integumentary
Priority Concepts: Cellular Regulation, Infection
Reference(s): Cooper, Gosnell (2015), pp. 1988–1989.

821. 3
Rationale: The normal WBC count ranges from 4500 to 11,000 cells/mm^3. Options 1 and 2 identify values lower than normal. Option 4 identifies a value higher than normal.
Test-Taking Strategy: Focus on the subject, a normal white blood cell count. Recalling that the normal white blood cell

count ranges from 4500 to 11,000 cells/mm^3 will direct you to the correct option. **Review: the normal white blood cell count.**
Level of Cognitive Ability: Understanding
Client Needs: Physiological Integrity
Integrated Process: Nursing Process/Data Collection
Content Area: Fundamental Skills: Laboratory Values
Priority Concepts: Cellular Regulation, Clinical Judgment
Reference(s): deWit, Kumagai (2013), p. 207.

822. 1
Rationale: The nurse would instruct the client to lie down and place a towel or pillow under the shoulder on the side of the breast to be examined. If the left breast is to be examined, the pillow would be placed under the left shoulder. Options 2 and 4 are incorrect.
Test-Taking Strategy: The **subject** of the question is the correct procedure for breast self-examination. Visualize this procedure. Remember, to examine the left breast, the pillow is placed under the left shoulder; to examine the right breast, the pillow is placed under the right shoulder. **Review: breast self-examination.**
Level of Cognitive Ability: Applying
Client Needs: Health Promotion and Maintenance
Integrated Process: Teaching and Learning
Content Area: Adult Health: Oncology
Priority Concepts: Client Education, Health Promotion
Reference(s): deWit, Kumagai (2013), pp. 892–893.

823. 4
Rationale: The CT scan causes no pain and takes about 15 to 60 minutes to perform. The dye may cause a warm flushing sensation when injected. Fluids are encouraged following the procedure. If an iodine dye is used, the client should be asked about allergies to seafood or iodine.
Test-Taking Strategy: Focus on the **subject**, client information about a CT scan. Note that the question indicates that the client will be receiving a dye injection. Next, note the relationship between these words and option 4. **Review: computed tomography (CT) scan.**
Level of Cognitive Ability: Applying
Client Needs: Physiological Integrity
Integrated Process: Nursing Process/Implementation
Content Area: Fundamental Skills: Diagnostic Tests
Priority Concepts: Cellular Regulation, Client Education
Reference(s): Pagana, Pagana (2013), pp. 282–283.

824. 3
Rationale: Denial, bargaining, anger, depression, and acceptance are recognized stages that a person experiences when facing a life-threatening illness. The client's statement is indicative of bargaining. Denial is expressed as shock and disbelief and may be the first response to hearing bad news. Depression may be manifested by hopelessness, weeping openly, or remaining quiet or withdrawn. Anger may also be a first response to upsetting news, and the predominant theme is "Why me?" or the blaming of others.
Test-Taking Strategy: Focus on the **subject**, a phase of coping. Note the client's statement and focus on the words, *"If I can just live long enough."* This should direct you to the correct option. **Review: coping and grief.**
Level of Cognitive Ability: Analyzing
Client Needs: Psychosocial Integrity
Integrated Process: Nursing Process/Data Collection
Content Area: Adult Health: Oncology
Priority Concepts: Communication, Coping
Reference(s): Potter et al (2013), p. 333.

❖ **825. 2, 3, 4**
Rationale: Furosemide is a loop diuretic; therefore, an expected effect is increased urinary frequency. Nausea is a frequent side effect, not an adverse effect. Photosensitivity is an occasional side effect. Adverse effects include tinnitus (ototoxicity), hypotension, and hypokalemia and occur as a result of sudden volume depletion.
Test-Taking Strategy: Focus on the **subject**, adverse effects of furosemide. Recalling that this medication is a loop diuretic and thinking about the expected and unexpected effects of the medication will assist in answering correctly. **Review:** the side and adverse effects of **furosemide.**
Level of Cognitive Ability: Analyzing
Client Needs: Physiological Integrity
Integrated Process: Nursing Process/Data Collection
Content Area: Pharmacology: Cardiovascular Medications
Priority Concepts: Clinical Judgment, Fluid and Electrolyte Balance
Reference(s): Hodgson, Kizior (2015), pp. 530–532.

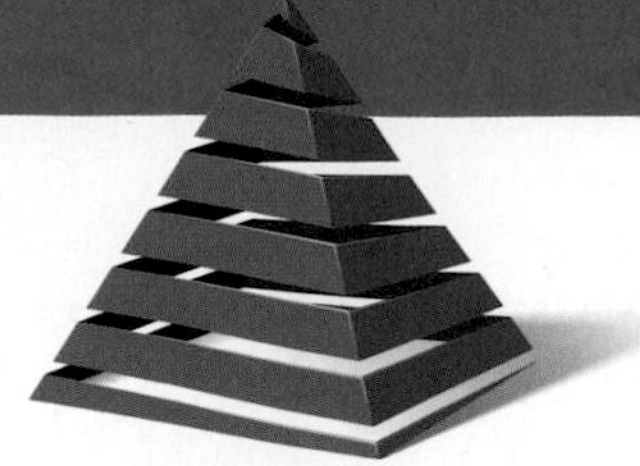

References

American Hospital Association: *The patient care partnership: understanding expectations, rights and responsibilities*. Available at http://www.aha.org/content/00-10/pcp_english_030730.pdf.

Berg RA, et al: American Heart Association guidelines for cardiopulmonary resuscitation and emergency cardiovascular care, *Circulation* 122:S685–S705, 2010. Available online at, http://circ.ahajournals.org/cgi/reprint/122/18_suppl_3/S685.

Bryant R, Nix D: *Acute & chronic wounds: current management concepts*, ed 4, St. Louis, 2012, Mosby.

CDC: *Guidelines for the prevention of intravascular catheter-related infections*. www.cdc.gov/hicpac/pdf/guidelines/bsi-guidelines-2011.pdf.

Chernecky C, Berger B: *Laboratory tests and diagnostic procedures*, ed 6, St. Louis, 2013, Saunders.

Cooper K, Gosnell K: *Foundations and adult health nursing*, ed 7, St. Louis, 2015, Elsevier.

deWit D, Kumagai C: *Medical-surgical nursing: concepts & practice*, ed 2, St. Louis, 2013, Saunders.

Dolan B, Holt L: *Accident & emergency theory into practice*, ed 3, St. Louis, 2013, Elsevier.

Gahart B, Nazareno A: *2015 Intravenous medications*, ed 31, St. Louis, 2015, Mosby.

Giger J: *Transcultural nursing assessment & intervention*, ed 6, St. Louis, 2013, Mosby.

Hammond B, Zimmermann P: *Sheehy's manual of emergency care*, ed 7, St. Louis, 2013, Elsevier.

Hockenberry M, Wilson D: *Wong's essentials of pediatric nursing*, ed 9, St. Louis, 2013, Mosby.

Hockenberry M, Wilson D: *Wong's nursing care of infants and children*, ed 10, St. Louis, 2015, Mosby.

Hodgson B, Kizior R: *Saunders nursing drug handbook 2014*, St. Louis, 2014, Saunders.

Hodgson B, Kizior R: *Saunders nursing drug handbook 2015*, St. Louis, 2015, Saunders.

Huber D: *Leadership and nursing care management*, ed 5, St. Louis, 2014, Saunders.

Ignatavicius D, Workman M: *Medical-surgical nursing: patient-centered collaborative care*, ed 7, St. Louis, 2013, Saunders.

Jarvis C: *Physical examination and health assessment*, ed 6, St. Louis, 2012, Saunders.

Kee J, Hayes E, McCuistion L: *Pharmacology: a nursing process approach*, ed 7, St. Louis, 2012, Saunders.

Lehne R: *Pharmacology for nursing care*, ed 8, St. Louis, 2013, Saunders.

Leifer G: *Introduction to maternity and pediatric nursing*, ed 7, St. Louis, 2015, Elsevier.

Lewis S, Dirksen S, Heitkemper M, Bucher L: *Medical-surgical nursing: assessment and management of clinical problems*, ed 9, St. Louis, 2014, Mosby.

Lilley L, Rainforth Collins S, Harrington S, Snyder J: *Pharmacology and the nursing process*, ed 7, St. Louis, 2014, Mosby.

Linton A: *Introduction to medical-surgical nursing*, ed 5, St. Louis, 2012, Saunders.

Lowdermilk D, Perry S, Cashion K, Alden K: *Maternity & women's health care*, ed 10, St. Louis, 2012, Mosby.

McKinney E, James S, Murray S, Nelson K, Ashwill J: *Maternal-child nursing*, ed 4, St. Louis, 2013, Elsevier.

Mosby's dictionary of medicine nursing & health professions, ed 9, St. Louis, 2013, Elsevier.

Nix S: *Williams' basic nutrition and diet therapy*, ed 14, St. Louis, 2013, Mosby.

Pagana K, Pagana T: *Mosby's diagnostic and laboratory tests reference*, ed 11, St. Louis, 2013, Mosby.

Perry A, Potter P, Elkin M: *Nursing interventions & clinical skills*, ed 5, St. Louis, 2012, Mosby.

Perry A, Potter P, Ostendorf W: *Clinical nursing skills & techniques*, ed 8, St. Louis, 2014, Mosby.

Potter P, Perry AG, Stockert PA, Hall AM: *Fundamentals of nursing*, ed 8, St. Louis, 2013, Mosby.

Skidmore-Roth L: *Mosby's nursing drug reference*, ed 27, St. Louis, 2014, Mosby.

Stuart G: *Principles & practice of psychiatric nursing*, ed 10, St. Louis, 2013, Mosby.

Swearingen P: *All-in-one care planning resource: medical-surgical, pediatric, maternity, & psychiatric nursing care plans*, ed 3, St. Louis, 2012, Mosby.

U.S. Department of Health and Human Services Office for Civil Rights: *Health information privacy*. Available at http://www.hhs.gov/ocr/privacy/.

Varcarolis E: *Essentials of psychiatric mental health nursing: a communication approach to evidence-based care*, ed 2, St. Louis, 2013, Saunders.

Zerwekh J, Zerwekh A: *Nursing today: transition and trends*, p ed 8, St. Louis, 2015, Elsevier.

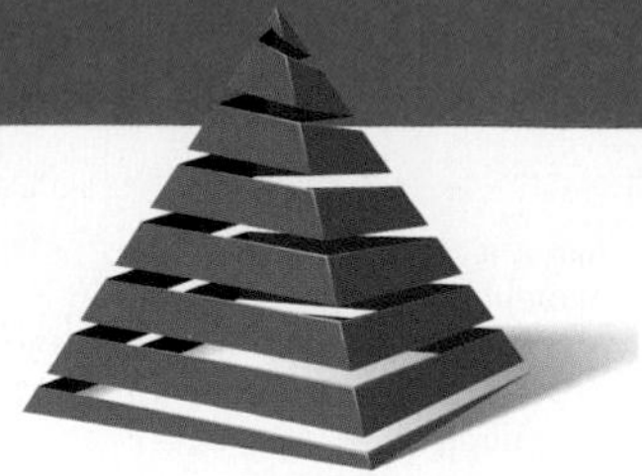

Index

Note: Page numbers followed by *f* indicate figures, *t* indicate tables, and *b* indicate boxes.

C

D

E

F

H

M

P

Q

R

S

U

V

W

X

Y

Z